M000101194

Mayo Clinic Cardiology

Concise Textbook

THIRD EDITION

Mayo Clinic Cardiology

Concise Textbook

THIRD EDITION

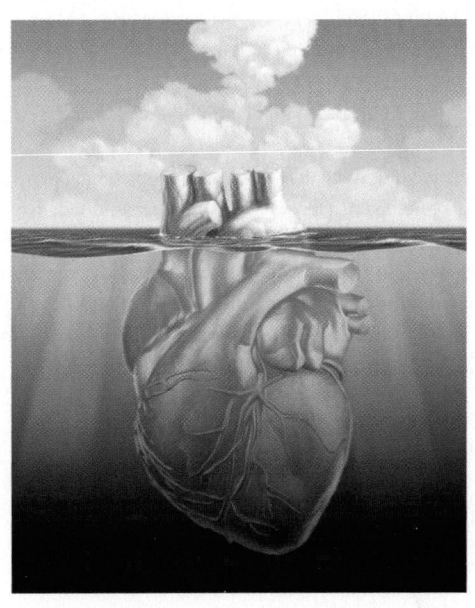

Editors

Joseph G. Murphy, MD
Margaret A. Lloyd, MD

Associate Editors

Gregory W. Barsness, MD
Arshad Jahangir, MD
Garvan C. Kane, MD
Lyle J. Olson, MD

MAYO CLINIC SCIENTIFIC PRESS
AND INFORMA HEALTHCARE USA, INC.

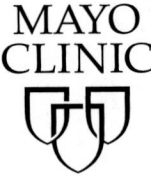

ISBN 0-8493-9057-5

For order inquiries, contact Taylor & Francis Group, 6000 Broken Sound Parkway NW, Suite #300, Boca Raton, FL 33487.

www.taylorandfrancis.com

Catalog record is available from the Library of Congress.

Care has been taken to confirm the accuracy of the information presented and to describe generally accepted practices. However, the authors, editors, and publisher are not responsible for errors or omissions or for any consequences from application of the information in this book and make no warranty, express or implied, with respect to the contents of the publication. This book should not be relied on apart from the advice of a qualified health care provider.

The authors, editors, and publisher have exerted efforts to ensure that drug selection and dosage set forth in this text are in accordance with current recommendations and practice at the time of publication. However, in view of ongoing research, changes in government regulations, and the constant flow of information relating to drug therapy and drug reactions, the reader is urged to check the package insert for each drug for any change in indications and dosage and for added warnings and precautions. This is particularly important when the recommended agent is a new or infrequently employed drug.

Some drugs and medical devices presented in this publication have Food and Drug Administration (FDA) clearance for limited use in restricted research settings. It is the responsibility of the health care providers to ascertain the FDA status of each drug or device planned for use in their clinical practice.

Printed in Canada
10 9 8 7 6 5 4 3

DEDICATION

This book is dedicated to my parents, my wife Marian,
without whose support and encouragement this textbook would not have been possible,
and my children Owen, Sinéad, and Aidan, as well as Tornados, Spartans, Pink Panthers, and Tommies everywhere.

Joseph G. Murphy, MD

For my parents, who taught me to love books. Booksellers everywhere, thank you as well.

Margaret A. Lloyd, MD

FOREWORD

It is a distinct honor and pleasure to write this foreword for the third edition of *Mayo Clinic Cardiology: Concise Textbook*.

I have had the pleasure of working on the staff of Mayo Clinic's Division of Cardiovascular Diseases for the past 25 years. Although the diagnosis and treatment of cardiovascular diseases and the day-to-day practice of medicine have changed greatly during that time, the Mayo Clinic tradition of clinical excellence in cardiovascular disease has not. The unique strength of the Division is its breadth of clinical expertise across the areas of acute coronary care, electrophysiology, intervention, adult congenital heart disease, valvular heart disease, vascular disease, heart failure, and others. This expertise covers both common conditions in the practice of cardiovascular disease and those that are very uncommon, even in major tertiary referral centers. The breadth of that expertise is reflected in the range of topics covered in this book. The common conditions include ST-segment elevation myocardial infarction, for which Mayo Clinic conducted one of the first clinical trials comparing thrombolytic therapy with acute angioplasty, and chronic mitral insufficiency, to which Mayo Clinic investigators have made multiple major contributions to both diagnosis and the timing and benefit of mitral valve repair. The uncommon conditions include adult congenital heart disease, hypertrophic cardiomyopathy, and pericardial disease, on which the size of our practice has permitted a few of my colleagues to focus their expertise.

This book began as an outgrowth of the syllabus for the Mayo Cardiovascular Review Course for Cardiology Boards and Recertification. This highly successful course attracts an annual attendance of more than 700, including cardiology fellows preparing for their initial boards, practicing cardiologists preparing for recertification, and experienced clinicians who simply want to ensure that they are up-to-date on the latest cardiovascular science and care. Readers from any one of these broad categories will find this book very useful.

Both the education of cardiology fellows and the practice of cardiovascular medicine are increasingly subject to time constraints. Our fellows complain that 3 or 4 years is simply inadequate to master the rapidly expanding scope of cardiovascular science and practice. Practicing physicians find that their working day grows ever longer, leaving less time for continuing medical education. The strength of this book is its concise presentation of the existing state of cardiovascular practice, as emphasized by its subtitle.

There is a growing crisis in the health care system, focused on rapid increases in health care costs and evidence of suboptimal quality. The practice of cardiovascular medicine will be under increasing pressure to shift from the more-care-is-better paradigm that dominated in the past to a focus on improving quality and efficiency. The *Dartmouth Atlas of Health Care* identified the Medicare referral region centered on Rochester, Minnesota, as a "high-quality, low-cost" region. The principles underlying that efficiency are evident throughout this text. It is hoped that it will assist the reader in his or her personal quest to improve the quality of cardiovascular care in clinical practice.

Raymond J. Gibbons, MD
Consultant, Division of Cardiovascular Diseases
Mayo Clinic
Arthur M. & Gladys D. Gray Professor of Medicine
Mayo Clinic College of Medicine
Rochester, Minnesota

PREFACE

The cover art of the "iceberg" heart is meant to symbolize the significant extent of occult cardiovascular disease in our society and the ruthless "icy" nature of cardiovascular death that curses the sea of humanity.

It has been a great honor to oversee the publication of this, the third, edition of *Mayo Clinic Cardiology: Concise Textbook* (formerly titled *Mayo Clinic Cardiology Review*). Large textbooks are never the work of one or two individuals but rather the product of a team of dedicated professionals, as has been the case for this book. This textbook from a single institution was written by a diverse faculty of more than 100 cardiologists from more than 17 countries.

This textbook is primarily a teaching and learning textbook of cardiology rather than a reference textbook. In response to welcome feedback from readers of our two previous textbook editions, we have maintained a relatively large typeface to make the textbook easily readable and have avoided the temptation to reduce the font size to increase content. Newer electronic search modalities have made textbook references less timely and we have deleted most chapter references and all multiple-choice questions to save space.

This textbook is designed to present the field of cardiology in a reader-friendly format that can be read in about 12 months. Many small cardiology textbooks are bare-bones compilations of facts that do not explain the fundamental concepts of cardiovascular disease, and many large cardiology textbooks are voluminous and describe cardiology in great detail. *Mayo Clinic Cardiology: Concise Textbook* is designed to be a bridge between these approaches. We sought to present a solid framework of ideas with sufficient depth to make the matter interesting yet concise, aimed specifically toward fellows in training or practicing clinicians wanting to update their knowledge. The book contains 1,400 figures, 483 of which are color photographs to supplement the text. Teaching points and clinical pearls have been added to make the textbook come alive and challenge the reader.

The concept for this textbook originated from the first syllabus for the Mayo Cardiovascular Review Course, a function the textbook continues to fulfill. The impetus to produce this textbook owes much to the encouragement of Rick Nishimura, MD, and Steve Ommen, MD, the directors of the Mayo Cardiovascular Review Course now in its 11th year.

This third edition is a complete revision of all previous chapters of the textbook and has been expanded at the suggestion of cardiology fellows to now include 40 new chapters, including newer aspects of electrophysiology, interventional cardiology, noninvasive imaging, and randomized clinical trials.

The text is intended primarily for cardiology fellows studying for cardiology board certification and practicing cardiologists studying for board recertification. It will also be useful for physicians studying for examinations of the Royal Colleges of Physicians, anesthesiologists, critical care physicians, internists and general physicians with a special interest in cardiology, and coronary care and critical care nurses.

We thank all our colleagues in the Mayo Clinic Division of Cardiovascular Diseases at Rochester, Arizona, and Jacksonville who generously contributed to this work. We also thank William D. Edwards, MD, for permission to use slides from the Mayo Clinic cardiology pathologic image database. LeAnn Stee and Randall J. Fritz, DVM, at Mayo Clinic, contributed enormously through their editorial guidance. Sandy Beberman at Informa Healthcare patiently guided this project through countless tribulations. We thank both Mayo Clinic and the Informa Healthcare production teams: at Mayo—Roberta Schwartz (production editor), Sharon Wadleigh (scientific publications specialist), Jane Craig and Virginia Dunt (editorial assistants), Kenna Atherton and John Hedlund (proofreaders), Karen Barrie (art director), Jonathan Goebel (graphic designer) and Charlene Wibben (Continuing Medical Education); at Informa Healthcare—Suzanne Lassandro (project editor), and Rick Beardsley (production and manufacturing). We specifically acknowledge colleagues from outside North America who contributed many ideas to this book and who translated previous editions of the book into several foreign languages. We have included a short SI conversion table for common laboratory values to aid their reading of the book.

We would appreciate comments from our readers about how we might improve this textbook or, specifically, about any errors that you find.

Joseph G. Murphy, MD
Consultant, Division of Cardiovascular
 Diseases, and Chair, Section of Scientific Publications,
 Mayo Clinic
Professor of Medicine
 Mayo Clinic College of Medicine
Rochester, Minnesota
murphy.joseph@mayo.edu

Margaret A. Lloyd, MD
Consultant, Division of Cardiovascular Diseases,
 Mayo Clinic
Assistant Professor of Medicine
 Mayo Clinic College of Medicine
Rochester, Minnesota

SI Units and Alternative Scientific Names

SI Units

Cholesterol (Total Cholesterol, LDL Cholesterol, HDL Cholesterol)

200 mg/dL = 5.2 mmol/L
160 mg/dL = 4.2 mmol/L
130 mg/dL = 3.4 mmol/L
100 mg/dL = 2.6 mmol/L
70 mg/dL = 1.8 mmol/L
40 mg/dL = 1.0 mmol/L

Triglycerides

100 mg/dL = 1.1 mmol/L
200 mg/dL = 2.2 mmol/L

Glucose

100 mg/dL = 5.5 mmol/L
200 mg/dL = 11.0 mmol/L

Creatinine

1 mg/dL = 88.4 μmol/L
2 mg/dL = 177 μmol/L
3 mg/dL = 265 μmol/L

Alternative Scientific Names

Epinephrine = adrenaline
Norepinephrine = noradrenaline
Isoproterenol = isoprenaline

CONTRIBUTORS

Michael J. Ackerman, MD, PhD
Consultant, Divisions of Cardiovascular Diseases and Pediatric Cardiology and Department of Molecular Pharmacology and Experimental Therapeutics*
Associate Professor of Medicine, Pediatrics, and Pharmacology[†]

Thomas G. Allison, PhD
Consultant, Division of Cardiovascular Diseases*
Associate Professor of Medicine[†]

Naser M. Ammash, MD
Consultant, Division of Cardiovascular Diseases*
Associate Professor of Medicine[†]

Nandan S. Anavekar, MB, BCh
Chief Medical Resident and Instructor in Medicine[†]

Christopher P. Appleton, MD
Consultant, Division of Cardiovascular Diseases[‡]
Professor of Medicine[†]

Samuel J. Asirvatham, MD
Consultant, Division of Cardiovascular Diseases*
Associate Professor of Medicine[†]

John W. Askew III, MD
Fellow in Nuclear Cardiology[†]

Luciano Babuin, MD
Research Collaborator, Mayo School of Graduate Medical Education[†]

Gregory W. Barsness, MD
Consultant, Division of Cardiovascular Diseases*
Assistant Professor of Medicine[†]

Malcolm R. Bell, MD
Consultant, Division of Cardiovascular Diseases*
Professor of Medicine[†]

Patricia J. M. Best, MD
Senior Associate Consultant, Division of Cardiovascular Diseases*
Assistant Professor of Medicine[†]

Joseph L. Blackshear, MD
Consultant, Division of Cardiovascular Diseases[§]
Professor of Medicine[†]

David J. Bradley, MD, PhD
Consultant, Division of Cardiovascular Diseases*
Assistant Professor of Medicine[†]

Peter A. Brady, MD
Consultant, Division of Cardiovascular Diseases*
Assistant Professor of Medicine[†]

Jerome F. Breen, MD
Consultant, Department of Radiology*
Assistant Professor of Radiology[†]

John F. Bresnahan, MD
Consultant, Division of Cardiovascular Diseases*
Associate Professor of Medicine[†]

Frank V. Brozovich, MD, PhD
Senior Associate Consultant, Division of Cardiovascular Diseases and Department of Physiology and Biomedical Engineering*
Professor of Medicine and of Physiology[†]

T. Jared Bunch, MD
Fellow in Cardiovascular Diseases and Assistant Professor of Medicine[†]

John C. Burnett, Jr, MD
Consultant, Division of Cardiovascular Diseases*
Professor of Medicine and of Physiology[†]

Mark J. Callahan, MD
Consultant, Division of Cardiovascular Diseases*
Assistant Professor of Medicine[†]

Yong-Mei Cha, MD
Consultant, Division of Cardiovascular Diseases*
Assistant Professor of Medicine[†]

Krishnaswamy Chandrasekaran, MD
Consultant, Division of Cardiovascular Diseases*
Professor of Medicine[†]

Panithaya Chareonthaitawee, MD
Consultant, Division of Cardiovascular Diseases*
Assistant Professor of Medicine[†]

Frank C. Chen, MD
Fellow in Cardiovascular Diseases[†]

Horng H. Chen, MD
Consultant, Division of Cardiovascular Diseases*
Associate Professor of Medicine[†]

Stuart D. Christenson, MD
Senior Associate Consultant, Division of Cardiovascular Diseases*
Assistant Professor of Medicine[†]

Alfredo L. Clavell, MD
Consultant, Division of Cardiovascular Diseases*
Assistant Professor of Medicine[†]

Heidi M. Connolly, MD
Consultant, Division of Cardiovascular Diseases*
Professor of Medicine[†]

*Mayo Clinic, Rochester, Minnesota.
[†]Mayo Clinic College of Medicine, Rochester, Minnesota.
[‡]Mayo Clinic, Scottsdale, Arizona.
[§]Mayo Clinic, Jacksonville, Florida.

Leslie T. Cooper, Jr, MD
 Consultant, Division of Cardiovascular Diseases*
 Associate Professor of Medicine†
Richard C. Daly, MD
 Consultant, Division of Cardiovascular Surgery*
 Associate Professor of Surgery†
Brooks S. Edwards, MD
 Consultant, Division of Cardiovascular Diseases*
 Professor of Medicine†
Robert P. Frantz, MD
 Consultant, Division of Cardiovascular Diseases*
 Assistant Professor of Medicine†
Paul A. Friedman, MD
 Consultant, Division of Cardiovascular Diseases*
 Professor of Medicine†
Robert L. Frye, MD
 Consultant, Division of Cardiovascular Diseases*
 Professor of Medicine†
Apoor S. Gami, MD
 Fellow in Cardiovascular Diseases and
 Assistant Professor of Medicine†
Gerald T. Gau, MD
 Consultant, Division of Cardiovascular Diseases*
 Professor of Medicine†
Thomas C. Gerber, MD, PhD
 Consultant, Division of Cardiovascular Diseases and
 Department of Radiology§
 Associate Professor of Medicine and of Radiology†
Bernard J. Gersh, MB, ChB, DPhil
 Consultant, Division of Cardiovascular Diseases*
 Professor of Medicine†
Jason M. Golbin, DO
 Fellow in Thoracic Diseases and Critical Care Medicine†
Martha A. Grogan, MD
 Consultant, Division of Cardiovascular Diseases*
 Assistant Professor of Medicine†
Richard J. Gumina, MD
 Senior Associate Consultant, Division of Cardiovascular Diseases*
Stephen C. Hammill, MD
 Consultant, Division of Cardiovascular Diseases*
 Professor of Medicine†
David L. Hayes, MD
 Chair, Division of Cardiovascular Diseases*
 Professor of Medicine†

Sharonne N. Hayes, MD
 Consultant, Division of Cardiovascular Diseases*
 Associate Professor of Medicine†
Anthony A. Hilliard, MD
 Fellow in Cardiovascular Diseases†
Michael J. Hogan, MD, MBA
 Consultant, Division of Regional and International Medicine‡
 Assistant Professor of Medicine†
David R. Holmes, Jr, MD
 Consultant, Division of Cardiovascular Diseases*
 Professor of Medicine†
Allan S. Jaffe, MD
 Consultant, Division of Cardiovascular Diseases*
 Professor of Medicine†
Arshad Jahangir, MD
 Consultant, Division of Cardiovascular Diseases*
 Associate Professor of Medicine†
Traci L. Jurrens, MD
 Fellow in Cardiovascular Diseases†
Ravi Kanagala, MD
 Senior Associate Consultant, Division of Cardiovascular Diseases*
 Assistant Professor of Medicine†
Garvan C. Kane, MD
 Fellow in Cardiovascular Diseases and Instructor in Medicine†
Birgit Kantor, MD, PhD
 Senior Associate Consultant, Division of Cardiovascular Diseases*
 Assistant Professor of Medicine†
Tomas Kara, MD, PhD
 Research Fellow in Hypertension and Assistant Professor of Medicine†
Bijoy K. Khandheria, MD
 Chair, Division of Cardiovascular Diseases‡
 Professor of Medicine†
Stephen L. Kopecky, MD
 Consultant, Division of Cardiovascular Diseases*
 Professor of Medicine†
Iftikhar J. Kullo, MD
 Consultant, Division of Cardiovascular Diseases*
 Associate Professor of Medicine†
Sudhir S. Kushwaha, MD
 Consultant, Division of Cardiovascular Diseases*
 Associate Professor of Medicine†
André C. Lapeyre III, MD
 Consultant, Division of Cardiovascular Diseases*
 Assistant Professor of Medicine†
Hon-Chi Lee, MD, PhD
 Consultant, Division of Cardiovascular Diseases*
 Professor of Medicine†

*Mayo Clinic, Rochester, Minnesota.
†Mayo Clinic College of Medicine, Rochester, Minnesota.
‡Mayo Clinic, Scottsdale, Arizona.
§Mayo Clinic, Jacksonville, Florida.

Amir Lerman, MD
    Consultant, Division of Cardiovascular Diseases*
    Professor of Medicine†
Margaret A. Lloyd, MD
    Consultant, Division of Cardiovascular Diseases*
    Assistant Professor of Medicine†
Francisco Lopez-Jimenez, MD, MS
    Consultant, Division of Cardiovascular Diseases*
    Assistant Professor of Medicine†
Verghese Mathew, MD
    Consultant, Division of Cardiovascular Diseases*
    Associate Professor of Medicine†
Robert D. McBane, MD
    Consultant, Division of Cardiovascular Diseases*
    Associate Professor of Medicine†
Marian T. McEvoy, MD
    Consultant, Division of Dermatology*
    Associate Professor of Dermatology†
Michael D. McGoon, MD
    Consultant, Division of Cardiovascular Diseases*
    Professor of Medicine†
Shaji C. Menon, MD
    Fellow in Pediatric Cardiology†
Fletcher A. Miller, Jr, MD
    Consultant, Division of Cardiovascular Diseases*
    Professor of Medicine†
Todd D. Miller, MD
    Consultant, Division of Cardiovascular Diseases*
    Professor of Medicine†
Wayne L. Miller, MD, PhD
    Consultant, Division of Cardiovascular Diseases*
    Associate Professor of Medicine†
Andrew G. Moore, MD
    Consultant, Division of Cardiovascular Diseases*
    Instructor in Medicine†
Thomas M. Munger, MD
    Consultant, Division of Cardiovascular Diseases*
    Assistant Professor of Medicine†
Joseph G. Murphy, MD
    Consultant, Division of Cardiovascular Diseases*
    Professor of Medicine†
Ajay Nehra, MD
    Consultant, Department of Urology*
    Professor of Urology†

Rick A. Nishimura, MD
    Consultant, Division of Cardiovascular Diseases*
    Professor of Medicine†
Jae K. Oh, MD
    Consultant, Division of Cardiovascular Diseases*
    Professor of Medicine†
Lyle J. Olson, MD
    Consultant, Division of Cardiovascular Diseases*
    Professor of Medicine†
Steve Ommen, MD
    Consultant, Division of Cardiovascular Diseases*
    Associate Professor of Medicine†
Oyere K. Onuma, BS
    Research Trainee, Division of Cardiovascular Diseases*
Thomas A. Orszulak, MD
    Consultant, Division of Cardiovascular Surgery*
    Professor of Surgery†
Michael J. Osborn, MD
    Consultant, Division of Cardiovascular Diseases*
    Associate Professor of Medicine†
Narith N. Ou, PharmD
    Pharmacist*
Lance J. Oyen, PharmD
    Pharmacist*
    Assistant Professor of Pharmacy†
Douglas L. Packer, MD
    Consultant, Division of Cardiovascular Diseases*
    Professor of Medicine†
John G. Park, MD
    Consultant, Division of Pulmonary and Critical Care Medicine*
    Assistant Professor of Medicine†
Robin Patel, MD
    Consultant, Division of Infectious Diseases*
    Associate Professor of Microbiology and Professor of Medicine†
Patricia A. Pellikka, MD
    Consultant, Division of Cardiovascular Diseases*
    Professor of Medicine†
Sabrina D. Phillips, MD
    Senior Associate Consultant, Division of Cardiovascular Diseases*
    Assistant Professor of Medicine†
Co-burn J. Porter, MD
    Consultant, Division of Pediatric Cardiology*
    Professor of Pediatrics†
Udaya B. S. Prakash, MD
    Consultant, Division of Pulmonary and Critical Care Medicine*
    Professor of Medicine,†

*Mayo Clinic, Rochester, Minnesota.
†Mayo Clinic College of Medicine, Rochester, Minnesota.
‡Mayo Clinic, Scottsdale, Arizona.
§Mayo Clinic, Jacksonville, Florida.

Abhiram Prasad, MD
  Consultant, Division of Cardiovascular Diseases*
  Assistant Professor of Medicine†
Sarinya Puwanant, MD
  Research Fellow in Cardiovascular Diseases†
Robert F. Rea, MD
  Consultant, Division of Cardiovascular Diseases*
  Associate Professor of Medicine†
Margaret M. Redfield, MD
  Consultant, Division of Cardiovascular Diseases*
  Professor of Medicine†
Guy S. Reeder, MD
  Consultant, Division of Cardiovascular Diseases*
  Professor of Medicine†
Charanjit S. Rihal, MD
  Consultant, Division of Cardiovascular Diseases*
  Professor of Medicine†
Richard J. Rodeheffer, MD
  Consultant, Division of Cardiovascular Diseases*
  Professor of Medicine†
Brian P. Shapiro, MD
  Fellow in Cardiovascular Diseases†
Win-Kuang Shen, MD
  Consultant, Division of Cardiovascular Diseases*
  Professor of Medicine†
Raymond C. Shields, MD
  Consultant, Division of Cardiovascular Diseases*
  Instructor in Medicine†
Clarence Shub, MD
  Consultant, Division of Cardiovascular Diseases*
  Professor of Medicine†
Justo Sierra Johnson, MD, MS
  Research Fellow in Cardiovascular Diseases†
Robert D. Simari, MD
  Consultant, Division of Cardiovascular Diseases*
  Professor of Medicine†
Lawrence J. Sinak, MD
  Consultant, Division of Cardiovascular Diseases*
  Assistant Professor of Medicine†
Virend K. Somers, MD, PhD
  Consultant, Division of Cardiovascular Diseases*
  Professor of Medicine†
Peter C. Spittell, MD
  Consultant, Division of Cardiovascular Diseases*
  Assistant Professor of Medicine†

James M. Steckelberg, MD
  Chair, Division of Infectious Diseases*
  Professor of Medicine†
Thoralf M. Sundt III, MD
  Consultant, Division of Cardiovascular Surgery*
  Professor of Surgery†
Imran S. Syed, MD
  Fellow in Cardiovascular Diseases†
Deepak R. Talreja, MD
  Fellow in Cardiovascular Diseases and Instructor in Medicine†
Zelalem Temesgen, MD
  Consultant, Division of Infectious Diseases*
  Associate Professor of Medicine†
Andre Terzic, MD
  Consultant, Department of Molecular Pharmacology*
  Professor of Medicine and of Pharmacology†
Randal J. Thomas, MD, MS
  Consultant, Division of Cardiovascular Diseases*
  Assistant Professor of Medicine†
Henry H. Ting, MD
  Consultant, Division of Cardiovascular Diseases*
  Assistant Professor of Medicine†
Cindy W. Tom, MD
  Research Fellow in Cardiovascular Diseases†
Laurence C. Torsher, MD
  Consultant, Division of Anesthesia*
  Assistant Professor of Anesthesiology†
Teresa S. M. Tsang, MD
  Consultant, Division of Cardiovascular Diseases*
  Professor of Medicine†
Eric M. Walser, MD
  Senior Associate Consultant, Department of Radiology§
  Professor of Radiology†
Carole A. Warnes, MD
  Consultant, Division of Cardiovascular Diseases*
  Professor of Medicine†
Paul W. Wennberg, MD
  Consultant, Division of Cardiovascular Diseases*
  Assistant Professor of Medicine†
Robert Wolk, MD, PhD
  Research Collaborator in Cardiovascular Diseases*
R. Scott Wright, MD
  Consultant, Division of Cardiovascular Diseases*
  Professor of Medicine†
Waldemar E. Wysokinski, MD
  Consultant, Division of Cardiovascular Diseases*
  Assistant Professor of Medicine†
Leonid V. Zingman, MD
  Research Associate, Division of Cardiovascular Diseases*
  Assistant Professor of Medicine and Instructor in Pharmacology†

*Mayo Clinic, Rochester, Minnesota.
†Mayo Clinic College of Medicine, Rochester, Minnesota.
‡Mayo Clinic, Scottsdale, Arizona.
§Mayo Clinic, Jacksonville, Florida.

TABLE OF CONTENTS

SECTION I

Fundamentals of
Cardiovascular Disease

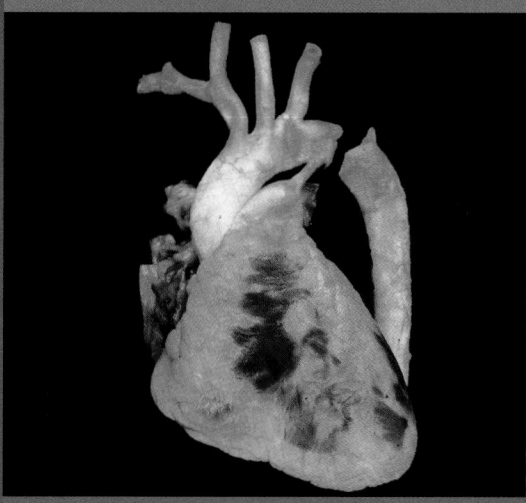

Transected Aorta: Motor Vehicle Accident

1

CARDIOVASCULAR EXAMINATION

Clarence Shub, MD

GENERAL APPEARANCE

The physical examination, including the general appearance of the patient, is an extremely important component of cardiology examinations. Almost every question has physical examination findings that provide critical clues to the answer in the stem of the question. Important clues to a cardiac diagnosis can be obtained from inspection of the patient (Table 1).

BLOOD PRESSURE

Blood pressure should always be determined in both arms and in the legs if there is any suspicion of coarctation of the aorta. A difference in systolic blood pressure between both arms of more than 10 mm Hg is abnormal (Table 2).

ABNORMALITIES ON PALPATION OF THE PRECORDIUM

The patient should be examined in both the supine and the left lateral decubitus position. Examining the apical impulse by the posterior approach with the patient in the sitting position may at times be the best method to appreciate subtle abnormalities of precordial motion. The normal apical impulse occurs during early systole with an outward motion imparted to the chest wall. During mid and late systole, the left ventricle (LV) is diminishing in volume and the apical impulse moves away from the chest wall. Thus, outward precordial apical motion occurring in late systole is abnormal. Remember that *point of maximal impulse* is not synonymous with *apical impulse*.

Palpation of the Apex

Constrictive pericarditis or tricuspid regurgitation produces a subtle systolic precordial retraction.

The apical impulse of LV enlargement is usually widened or diffuse (>3 cm in diameter), can be palpated in two interspaces, and is displaced leftward. A subtle presystolic ventricular rapid filling wave (A wave)—frequently associated with LV hypertrophy—may be better visualized than palpated by observing the motion of the stethoscope applied lightly on the chest wall, with appropriate timing during simultaneous auscultation. Likewise, a palpable A wave can be detected in this manner. The apical impulse of LV hypertrophy without dilatation is sustained and localized but should not be displaced.

Causes of a palpable A wave (presystolic impulse) include the following:
1. Aortic stenosis
2. Hypertrophic obstructive cardiomyopathy
3. Systemic hypertension

Table 1.   Clinical Clues to Specific Cardiac Abnormalities Detectable From the General Examination

Condition	Appearance	Associated cardiac abnormalities
Marfan syndrome	Tall	Aortic root dilatation
	Long extremities	Mitral valve prolapse
Acromegaly	Large stature	Cardiac hypertrophy
	Coarse facial features	
	"Spade" hands	
Turner syndrome	Web neck	Aortic coarctation
	Hypertelorism	Pulmonary stenosis
	Short stature	
Pickwickian syndrome	Severe obesity	Pulmonary hypertension
	Somnolence	
Friedreich ataxia	Lurching gait	Hypertrophic cardiomyopathy
	Hammertoe	
	Pes cavus	
Duchenne type muscular dystrophy	Pseudohypertrophy of calves	Cardiomyopathy
Ankylosing spondylitis	Straight back syndrome	Aortic regurgitation
	Stiff ("poker") spine	Heart block (rare)
Jaundice	Yellow skin or sclera	Right-sided congestive heart failure
		Prosthetic valve dysfunction (hemolysis)
Sickle cell anemia	Cutaneous ulcers	Pulmonary hypertension
	Painful "crises"	Secondary cardiomyopathy
Lentigines (LEOPARD syndrome*)	Brown skin macules that do not increase with sunlight	Hypertrophic obstructive cardio-myopathy
		Pulmonary stenosis
Hereditary hemorrhagic telangiectasia (Osler-Weber-Rendu disease)	Small capillary hemangiomas on face or mouth, with or without cyanosis	Pulmonary arteriovenous fistula
Pheochromocytoma	Pale, diaphoretic skin	Catecholamine-induced secondary dilated cardiomyopathy
	Neurofibromatosis—café-au-lait spots	
Lupus	Butterfly rash on face	Verrucous endocarditis
	Raynaud phenomenon—hands	Myocarditis
	Livedo reticularis	Pericarditis
Sarcoidosis	Cutaneous nodules	Secondary cardiomyopathy
	Erythema nodosum	Heart block
Tuberous sclerosis	Angiofibromas (face; adenoma sebaceum)	Rhabdomyoma
Myxedema	Coarse, dry skin	Pericardial effusion
	Thinning of lateral eyebrows	Left ventricular dysfunction
	Hoarseness of voice	
Right-to-left intracardiac shunt	Cyanosis and clubbing of distal extremities	Any of the lesions that cause Eisenmenger syndrome
	Differential cyanosis and clubbing	Reversed shunt through patent duc-tus arteriosus

Table 1. (continued)

Condition	Appearance	Associated cardiac abnormalities
Holt-Oram syndrome	Rudimentary or absent thumb	Atrial septal defect
Down syndrome	Mental retardation	Endocardial cushion defect
	Simian crease of palm	
	Characteristic facies	
Scleroderma	Tight, shiny skin of fingers with contraction	Pulmonary hypertension
		Myocardial, pericardial, or endocardial disease
	Characteristic taut mouth and facies	
Rheumatoid arthritis	Typical hand deformity	Myocardial, pericardial, or endocardial disease (often subclinical)
	Subcutaneous nodules	
Thoracic bony abnormality	Pectus excavatum	Pseudocardiomegaly
	Straight back syndrome	Mitral valve prolapse
Carcinoid syndrome	Reddish cyanosis of face	Right-sided cardiac valve stenosis or regurgitation
	Periodic flushing	

*LEOPARD syndrome: *l*entigines, *e*lectrocardiographic changes, *o*cular hypertelorism, *p*ulmonary stenosis, *a*bnormal genitalia, *r*etardation of growth, *d*eafness.

- The apical impulse of LV hypertrophy without dilatation is sustained and localized. It should not be displaced but may be accompanied by a palpable presystolic outward movement, the A wave.
- Outward precordial apical motion occurring in late systole is abnormal.
- Multiple abnormal outward precordial movements may occur: presystolic, systolic, or late systolic rebound and an A wave in late diastole.

Palpation of the Lower Sternal Area
Precordial motion in the lower sternal area usually reflects right ventricular (RV) motion. RV hypertrophy due to systolic overload (such as in pulmonary stenosis) causes a sustained outward lift. Diastolic overload (such as in atrial septal defect [ASD]) causes a vigorous nonsustained motion. In severe mitral regurgitation, the left atrium expands in systole but is limited in its posterior motion by the spine. The RV may then be pushed forward, and the parasternal region is "lifted" indirectly.

Significant *overlap* of sites of maximal pulsation occurs in LV and RV overload states. For example, in RV overload, the abnormal impulse can overlap with

the LV in the apical sternal region (between the apex and the left lower sternal border). An LV apical aneurysm may produce a delayed outward motion and cause a "rocking" motion.

Palpation of the Left Upper Sternal Area
Abnormal pulsations at the left upper sternal border (pulmonic area) can be due to a dilated pulmonary artery (e.g., poststenotic dilatation in pulmonary valve stenosis, idiopathic dilatation of the pulmonary artery, or increased pulmonary flow related to ASD or pul-

Table 2. Causes of Blood Pressure Discrepancy Between Arms or Between Arms and Legs

Arterial occlusion or stenosis of any cause
Dissecting aortic aneurysm
Coarctation of the aorta
Patent ductus arteriosus
Supravalvular aortic stenosis
Thoracic outlet syndrome

monary hypertension). Pulsations of increased blood flow are dynamic and quick, whereas pulsations due to pressure overload cause a sustained impulse.

■ If the apical impulse is not palpable and the patient is hemodynamically unstable, consider cardiac tamponade as the first diagnosis.

Palpation of the Right Upper Sternal Area
Abnormal pulsations at the right upper sternal border (aortic area) should suggest an aortic aneurysm. An enlarged left lobe of the liver associated with severe tricuspid regurgitation may be appreciated in the epigastrium, and the epigastric site may be the location of the maximal cardiac impulse in patients with emphysema or an enlarged RV.

■ RV hypertrophy due to systolic overload causes a sustained outward lift. Diastolic overload (as in ASD) causes a vigorous nonsustained motion.
■ In severe mitral regurgitation, the left atrium expands in systole but is limited in its posterior motion by the spine. The RV may then be pushed forward, and the parasternal region is "lifted" indirectly.
■ Significant *overlap* of sites of maximal pulsation occurs in LV and RV overload states.
■ Pulsations of increased blood flow are dynamic and quick, whereas pulsations due to pressure overload cause a sustained impulse.

JUGULAR VEINS

Abnormal waveforms in the jugular veins reflect abnormal hemodynamics of the right side of the heart. In the presence of normal sinus rhythm, there are two positive or outward moving waves (*a* and *v*) and two visible negative or inward moving waves (*x* and *y*) (Fig. 1). The *x* descent is sometimes referred to as the *systolic collapse*. Ordinarily, the *c* wave is not readily visible. The *a* wave can be identified by simultaneous auscultation of the heart and inspection of the jugular veins. The *a* wave occurs at about the time of the first heart sound (S_1). The *x* descent follows. The *v* wave, a slower, more undulating wave, occurs near the second heart sound (S_2). The *y* descent follows. The *a* wave is normally larger than the *v* wave, and the *x* descent is more marked than the *y* descent (Tables 3 and 4).

Normal jugular venous pressure decreases with inspiration and increases with expiration. Veins that fill at inspiration (Kussmaul sign), however, are a clue to constrictive pericarditis, pulmonary embolism, or RV infarction (Table 5).

■ Jugular veins that fill at inspiration (Kussmaul sign) are a clue to constrictive pericarditis, pulmonary embolism, or RV infarction.

"Hepatojugular" (Abdominojugular) Reflux Sign
The neck veins distend with steady (>10 seconds) upper abdominal compression while the patient continues to breathe normally without straining. Straining may cause a false-positive "hepatojugular" reflux sign. The neck veins may collapse or remain distended. Jugular venous pressure that remains increased and then falls abruptly (≥4 cm H_2O) indicates an abnormal response. It may occur in LV failure with secondary pulmonary hypertension. In patients with chronic congestive heart failure, a positive hepatojugular reflux sign (with or without increased jugular venous pressure), a third heart sound (S_3), and radiographic pulmonary vascular redistribution are independent predictors of increased pulmonary capillary wedge pressure. The

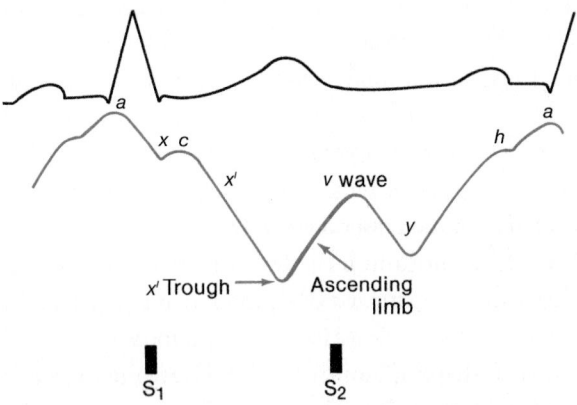

Fig. 1. Normal jugular venous pulse. The jugular *v* wave is built up during systole, and its height reflects the rate of filling and the elasticity of the right atrium. Between the bottom of the *y* descent (*y* trough) and the beginning of the *a* wave is the period of relatively slow filling of the "atrioventricle" or diastasis period. The wave built up during diastasis is the *h* wave. The *h* wave height also reflects the stiffness of the right atrium. S_1, first heart sound; S_2, second heart sound.

Table 3.   Timing of Jugular Venous Pulse Waves

a wave—precedes the carotid arterial pulse and is simultaneous with S_4, just before S_1
x descent—between S_1 and S_2
v wave—just after S_2
y descent—after the *v* wave in early diastole

abdominojugular maneuver can also be useful for eliciting venous pulsations if they are difficult to visualize.

- A positive "hepatojugular" (abdominojugular) reflux sign may be found in LV failure with secondary pulmonary hypertension.
- If the jugular veins are engorged but not pulsatile, consider superior vena caval obstruction.

ARTERIAL PULSE

Abnormalities of the Carotid Pulse

Hyperdynamic Carotid Pulse
A vigorous, hyperdynamic carotid pulse is consistent with aortic regurgitation. It may also occur in other states of high cardiac output or be caused by the wide pulse pressure associated with atherosclerosis, especially in the elderly.

Dicrotic and Bisferiens Pulses
A dicrotic carotid pulse occurs in myocardial failure, especially in association with hypotension, decreased cardiac output, and increased peripheral resistance. *Dicrotic* and *bisferious* are the Greek and Latin terms, respectively, for *twice beating*, but in cardiology they are not equivalent. The second impulse occurs in early diastole with the dicrotic pulse and in late systole with the bisferiens pulse. The bisferiens pulse usually occurs in combined aortic regurgitation and aortic stenosis, but occasionally it occurs in pure aortic regurgitation.

Aortic Stenosis
Pulsus parvus (soft or weak) classically occurs in aortic stenosis but can also result from severe stenosis of any cardiac valve or can occur with low cardiac output of

Table 4.   Abnormal Jugular Venous Pulse Waves

Increased *a* wave
  1. Tricuspid stenosis
  2. Decreased right ventricular compliance due to right ventricular hypertrophy in severe pulmonary hypertension
        Pulmonary stenosis
        Pulmonary vascular disease
  3. Severe left ventricular hypertrophy due to pressure by the hypertrophied septum on right ventricular filling (Bernheim effect)
        Hypertrophic obstructive cardiomyopathy
Rapid *x* descent
    Cardiac tamponade
Increased *v* wave
    Tricuspid regurgitation
    Atrial septal defect
Rapid *y* descent (Friedreich sign)
    Constrictive pericarditis

any cause. Severe aortic stenosis also produces a slowly increasing delayed pulse (pulsus tardus). Because of the effects of aging on the carotid arteries, the typical findings of pulsus parvus and pulsus tardus may be less apparent or absent in the elderly, even with severe degrees of aortic stenosis.

Hypertrophic Obstructive Cardiomyopathy
In hypertrophic obstructive cardiomyopathy, the ventricular obstruction begins in mid systole, increases as

Table 5.   Differentiation of Internal Jugular Vein Pulse and Carotid Pulse

Jugular vein pulse	Carotid pulse
Double peak when in sinus rhythm	Single peak
Obliterated by gentle pressure	Unaffected by gentle pressure
Changes with position and inspiration	Unaffected by position or inspiration

contraction proceeds, and decreases in late systole. The initial carotid impulse is brisk. The pulse may be bifid as well (Table 6).

Inequality of the carotid pulses can be due to carotid atherosclerosis, especially in elderly patients. In a young patient, consider supravalvular aortic stenosis. (The right side then should have the stronger pulse.) Aortic dissection and thoracic outlet syndrome may also produce inequality of arterial pulses. A pulsating cervical mass, usually on the right, may be caused by atherosclerotic "buckling" of the right common carotid artery and give the false impression of a carotid aneurysm.

Transmitted Murmurs

Transmitted murmurs of aortic origin, most often due to aortic stenosis (less often due to coarctation, patent ductus arteriosus, pulmonary stenosis, and ventricular septal defect), decrease in intensity as the stethoscope ascends the neck, whereas a carotid bruit is usually louder higher in the neck and decreases in intensity as the stethoscope is inched proximally toward the chest. Both conditions may coexist, especially in elderly patients. An abrupt change in the acoustic characteristics (pitch) of the bruit as the stethoscope is inched upward may be a clue to the presence of combined lesions.

Pulsus Paradoxus

Paradoxical pulse is an exaggeration of the normal (≤10 mm) inspiratory decline in arterial pressure. It occurs classically in cardiac tamponade but occasionally with other restrictive cardiac abnormalities, severe conges-tive heart failure, pulmonary embolism, or chronic obstructive pulmonary disease (Table 7).

Pulsus Alternans

Pulsus alternans (alternation of stronger and weaker beats) rarely occurs in healthy subjects and then is transient after a premature ventricular contraction. It usually is associated with severe myocardial failure and is frequently accompanied by an S3, both of which impart an ominous prognosis. Pulsus alternans may be affected by alterations in venous return and may disappear as congestive heart failure progresses. Electrical alternans (alternating variation in the height of the QRS complex) is unrelated to pulsus alternans (Table 8).

- A dicrotic carotid pulse occurs in myocardial failure, often in association with hypotension, decreased cardiac output, and increased peripheral resistance.
- Pulsus parvus (soft or weak) classically occurs in aortic stenosis but can also result from severe stenosis of any cardiac valve or can occur with severely low cardiac output of any cause.
- Because of the effects of aging on the carotid arteries, the typical findings of pulsus parvus and

---

Table 6.   Causes of a Double-Impulse Carotid Arterial Pulse

Dicrotic pulse (systolic + diastolic impulse)
   Cardiomyopathy
   Left ventricular failure
Bisferiens pulse (two systolic impulses)
   Aortic regurgitation
   Combined aortic valve stenosis and regurgitation (dominant regurgitation)
Bifid pulse (two systolic impulses with intervening pulse collapse)
   Hypertrophic cardiomyopathy

Table 7.   Causes of Pulsus Paradoxus

Constrictive pericarditis
Pericardial tamponade
Severe emphysema
Severe asthma
Severe heart failure
Pulmonary embolism
Morbid obesity

Table 8.   Pulsus and Electrical Alternans

Pulsus alternans
   Severe heart failure
Electrical alternans
   Pericardial tamponade
   Large pericardial effusions

pulsus tardus may be less apparent or absent in the elderly, even with severe degrees of aortic stenosis.

- Inequality of the carotid pulses can be due to carotid atherosclerosis, especially in elderly patients. In a young patient, consider supravalvular aortic stenosis. (The right side then should have the stronger pulse.)
- Transmitted murmurs of aortic origin, most often due to aortic stenosis (less often due to coarctation, patent ductus arteriosus, pulmonary stenosis, or ventricular septal defect), decrease in intensity as the stethoscope ascends the neck, whereas a carotid bruit is usually louder higher in the neck and decreases in intensity as the stethoscope is inched proximally toward the chest.
- Paradoxical pulse occurs classically in cardiac tamponade but occasionally with other restrictive cardiac abnormalities, severe congestive heart failure, pulmonary embolism, or chronic obstructive pulmonary disease.
- Pulsus alternans usually is associated with severe myocardial failure and is frequently accompanied by an S_3, both of which impart an ominous prognosis.

Abnormalities of the Femoral Pulse

In hypertension, simultaneous palpation of radial and femoral pulses may reveal a delay or relative weakening of the femoral pulses, suggesting aortic coarctation. The finding of a femoral (or carotid) bruit in an adult suggests diffuse atherosclerosis. Fibromuscular dysplasia is less common and occurs in younger patients.

HEART SOUNDS

First Heart Sound

Only the mitral (M_1) and tricuspid (T_1) components of S_1 are normally audible. M_1 occurs before T_1 and is the loudest component. Wide splitting of S_1 occurs with right bundle branch block and Ebstein anomaly.

Factors Influencing the Intensity of S_1

PR Interval

The PR interval varies inversely with the loudness of S_1—with a long PR interval, the S_1 is soft; conversely, with a short PR interval, the S_1 is loud.

Mitral Valve Disease

Mitral stenosis produces a loud S_1 if the valve is pliable. When the valve becomes calcified and immobile, the intensity of S_1 decreases. The S_1 may also be soft in severe aortic regurgitation (related to early closure of the mitral valve) caused by LV filling from the aorta.

The Rate of Increase of Systolic Pressure Within the LV

A loud S_1 can be produced by hypercontractile states, such as fever, exercise, thyrotoxicosis, and pheochromocytoma. Conversely, a soft S_1 can occur in LV failure.

If S_1 seems louder at the lower left sternal border than at the apex (implying a loud T_1), suspect ASD or tricuspid stenosis. Atrial fibrillation produces a variable S_1 intensity. (The intensity is inversely related to the previous RR cycle length; a longer cycle length produces a softer S_1.) A variable S_1 intensity during a wide complex, regular tachycardia suggests atrioventricular dissociation and ventricular tachycardia. The marked delay of T_1 in Ebstein anomaly is related to the late billowing effect of the deformed (sail-like) anterior leaflet of the tricuspid valve as it closes in systole. Table 9 lists causes of an abnormal S_1.

- If S_1 seems to be louder at the base than at the apex, suspect an ejection sound masquerading as S_1. If the S_1 is louder at the lower left sternal border than at the apex (implying a loud T_1), suspect ASD or tricuspid stenosis.

Table 9.   Abnormalities of S_1 and Their Causes

Loud S_1
Short PR interval
Mitral stenosis
Left atrial myxoma
Hypercontractile states
Soft S_1
Long PR interval
Depressed left ventricular function
Early closure of mitral valve in acute severe aortic incompetence
Ruptured mitral valve leaflet or chordae
Left bundle branch block

- A variable S$_1$ intensity during a wide complex, regular tachycardia suggests atrioventricular dissociation and ventricular tachycardia.
- The marked delay of T$_1$ in Ebstein anomaly is related to the late billowing effect of the deformed (sail-like) anterior leaflet of the tricuspid valve as it closes in systole.

Systolic Ejection Clicks (or Sounds)

The ejection click (sound) follows S$_1$ closely and can be confused with a widely split S$_1$ or, occasionally, with an early nonejection click. Clicks can originate from the left or right side of the heart.

The three possible mechanisms for production of the clicks are as follows:

1. Intrinsic abnormality of the aortic or pulmonary valve, such as congenital bicuspid aortic valve
2. Pulsatile distention of a dilated great artery, as occurs in increased flow states such as truncus arteriosus (aortic click) or ASD (pulmonary click) or in idiopathic dilatation of the pulmonary artery
3. Increased pressure in the great vessel, such as in aortic or pulmonary hypertension

Because an aortic click is not usually heard with uncomplicated coarctation, its presence should suggest associated bicuspid aortic valve. In the latter condition, the click diminishes in intensity, becomes "buried" in the systolic murmur, and ultimately disappears as the valve becomes heavily calcified and immobile later in the course of the disease. Although a click implies cusp mobility, its presence does not necessarily exclude severe stenosis. A click would be expected to be absent in subvalvular stenosis. The timing of the pulmonary click in relationship to S$_1$ (reflecting the isovolumic contraction period of the RV) is associated with hemodynamic severity in valvular pulmonary stenosis. With higher systolic gradient and lower pulmonary artery systolic pressure, the isovolumic contraction period shortens and thus the earlier the click occurs in relationship to S$_1$. A pulmonary click can occur in idiopathic dilatation of the pulmonary artery, and this condition may be a masquerader of ASD, especially in young adults. The pulmonary click due to valvular pulmonary stenosis is the only right-sided heart sound that *decreases* with inspiration. Most other right-sided auscultatory events either increase in intensity with inspiration (most commonly) or show minimal change. The pulmonary click is best heard along the upper left sternal border, but if it is loud enough or if the RV is markedly dilated, it may be heard throughout the precordium. The aortic click radiates to the aortic area and the apex and does not change with respiration. The causes of ejection clicks are listed in Table 10.

- The presence, absence, or loudness of the ejection click does not correlate with the degree of valvular stenosis.
- An aortic click is not heard with uncomplicated coarctation; its presence should suggest associated bicuspid aortic valve.
- A click is absent in subvalvular or supravalvular aortic stenosis or hypertrophic obstructive cardiomyopathy.
- A pulmonary click can occur in idiopathic dilatation of the pulmonary artery, a condition that may mimic ASD, especially in young adults.
- The pulmonary click is best heard along the upper left sternal border. The aortic click radiates to the aortic area and the apex and does not change with respiration.

Mid-to-Late Nonejection Clicks (Systolic Clicks)

Nonejection clicks are most commonly due to mitral valve prolapse. Rarely, nonejection clicks can be caused by papillary muscle dysfunction, rheumatic mitral valve disease, or hypertrophic obstructive cardiomyopathy.

Table 10. Causes of Ejection Clicks

Aortic click
    Congenital valvular aortic stenosis
    Congenital bicuspid aortic valve
    Truncus arteriosus
    Aortic incompetence
    Aortic root dilatation or aneurysm
Pulmonary click
    Pulmonary valve stenosis
    Atrial septal defect
    Chronic pulmonary hypertension
    Tetralogy of Fallot with pulmonary valve stenosis (absent if there is only infundibular stenosis)
    Idiopathic dilated pulmonary artery

Other rare causes of nonejection clicks (that can masquerade as mitral prolapse) include ventricular or atrial septal aneurysms, ventricular free wall aneurysms, and ventricular and atrial mobile tumors, such as myxoma. A nonejection click not due to mitral valve prolapse does not have the typical responses to bedside maneuvers found with mitral valve prolapse, as outlined below.

Mitral Valve Prolapse
Maneuvers that decrease LV volume, such as standing or the Valsalva maneuver, move the click earlier in the cardiac cycle. Conversely, maneuvers that increase LV volume, such as assuming the supine position and elevating the legs, move the click later in the cardiac cycle. With a decrease in LV volume, a systolic murmur, if present, would become longer. Interventions that increase systemic blood pressure make the murmur louder.

- Miscellaneous causes of nonejection clicks (that can masquerade as mitral prolapse) include ventricular or atrial septal aneurysms, ventricular free wall aneurysms, and ventricular and atrial mobile tumors, such as myxoma.
- Maneuvers that decrease LV volume, such as standing or the Valsalva maneuver, move the click earlier in the cardiac cycle. Conversely, maneuvers that increase LV volume, such as assuming the supine position and elevating the legs, move the click later in the cardiac cycle.

Second Heart Sound
S_2 is often best heard along the upper and middle left sternal border. Splitting of S_2 (Fig. 2) is best heard during normal breathing with the subject in the sitting position.

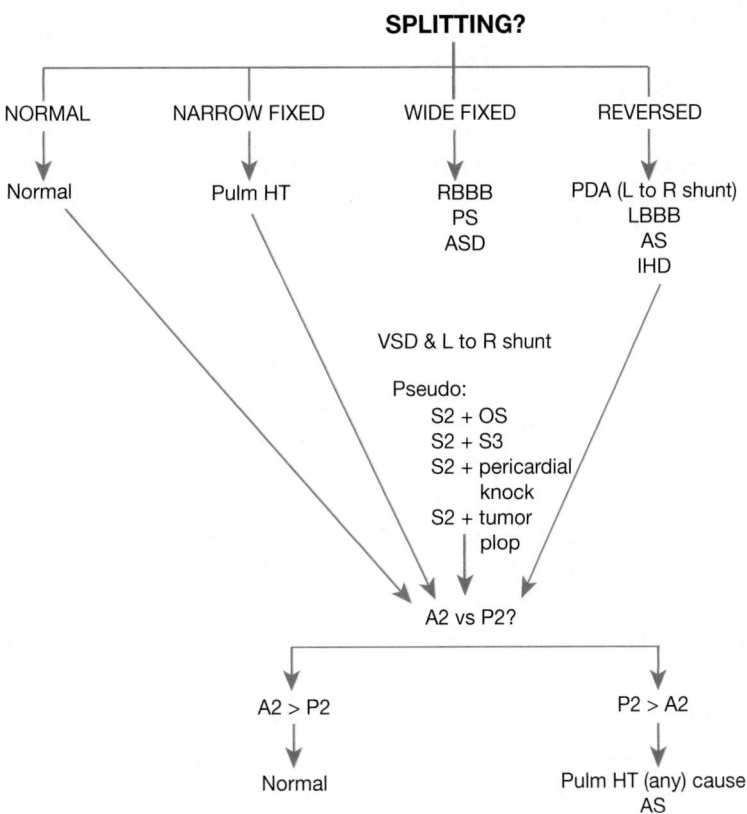

Fig. 2. Branching logic tree for second heart sound (S_2) splitting. A2, aortic closure sound; AS, aortic stenosis; ASD, atrial septal defect; HT, hypertension; IHD, ischemic heart disease; LBBB, left bundle branch block; L to R, left-to-right; OS, opening snap; P2, pulmonic closure sound; PDA, patent ductus arteriosus; PS, pulmonary stenosis; Pulm HT, pulmonary hypertension; RBBB, right bundle branch block; S3, third heart sound; VSD, ventricular septal defect.

Determinants of S2 include the following:

1. Ventricular activation (bundle branch block delays closure of the ventricle's respective semilunar valve)
2. Ejection time
3. Valve gradient (increased gradient with low pressure in the great vessel delays closure)
4. Elastic recoil of the great artery (decreased elastic recoil delays closure, such as in idiopathic dilatation of the pulmonary artery)

Splitting of S2

Wide but physiologic splitting of S2 (Fig. 3) may be due to the following:

1. Delayed electrical activation of the RV, such as in right bundle branch block or premature ventricular contraction originating in the LV (which conducts with a right bundle branch block pattern)
2. Delay of RV contraction, such as in increased RV stroke volume and RV failure
3. Pulmonary stenosis (prolonged ejection time)

In ASD, there is only minimal respiratory variation in S2 splitting. This is referred to as *fixed splitting*. Fixed splitting should be verified with the patient in the sitting or standing position because healthy subjects occasionally appear to have fixed splitting in the supine position. When the degree of splitting is unusually wide, especially when the pulmonary component of the second heart sound (P2) is diminished, suspect concomitant pulmonary stenosis. Indeed, this condition is the cause of the most widely split S2 that can be recorded.

Wide, fixed splitting, although considered typical of ASD, occurs in only 70% of patients with ASD. However, persistent expiratory splitting is audible in most. Normal respiratory variation of the S2 occurs in up to 8% of patients with ASD. With Eisenmenger physiology, the left-to-right shunting decreases and the degree of splitting narrows. A pulmonary systolic ejection murmur (increased flow) is common in patients with ASD, and with a significant left-to-right shunt, a diastolic tricuspid flow murmur can be heard as well. As with aortic stenosis, as pulmonary stenosis increases in severity, P2 decreases in intensity, and ultimately S2 becomes single.

The wide splitting of S2 in mitral regurgitation and ventricular septal defect is related to early aortic valve closure (in ventricular septal defect, P2 is delayed

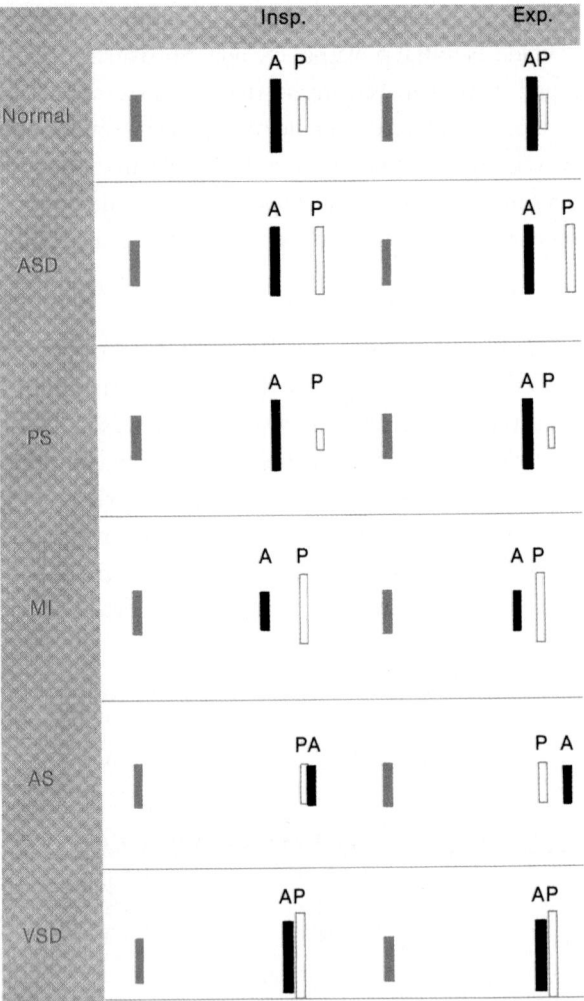

Fig. 3. Diagrammatic representation of normal and abnormal patterns in the respiratory variation of the second heart sound. The heights of the bars are proportional to the sound intensity. A, aortic component; AS, aortic stenosis; ASD, atrial septal defect; Exp., expiration; Insp., inspiration; MI, mitral incompetence; P, pulmonary component; PS, pulmonary stenosis; VSD, ventricular septal defect.

as well), which, in turn, is due to decreased LV ejection time, but the loud pansystolic regurgitant murmur often obscures the wide splitting of S2 so that the S2 *appears* to be single.

Partial anomalous pulmonary venous connection may occur alone or in combination with ASD (most often of the sinus venosus type). Wide splitting of S2 occurs in both conditions, but it usually shows normal respiratory variation in isolated partial anomalous pulmonary venous connection.

Pulmonary hypertension may cause wide splitting of S_2, although the intensity of P_2 is usually increased and widely transmitted throughout the precordium.

■ Fixed splitting should be verified with the patient in the sitting or standing position because healthy subjects occasionally appear to have fixed splitting in the supine position.

■ Wide, fixed splitting, although considered typical of ASD, occurs in only 70% of patients with ASD.

■ Wide splitting of S_2 occurs in both partial anomalous pulmonary venous connection and ASD, but it usually shows normal respiratory variation in isolated partial anomalous pulmonary venous connection.

■ Pulmonary hypertension may cause wide splitting of S_2, although the intensity of P_2 is usually increased and widely transmitted throughout the precordium.

Paradoxical (Reversed) Splitting of S_2
Paradoxical splitting of S_2 is usually caused by conditions that delay aortic closure. Examples include the following:

1. Electrical delay of LV contraction, such as left bundle branch block (most commonly)
2. Mechanical delay of LV ejection, such as aortic stenosis and hypertrophic obstructive cardiomyopathy
3. Severe LV systolic failure of any cause
4. Patent ductus arteriosus, aortic regurgitation, and systemic hypertension are other rare causes of paradoxic splitting

Paradoxical splitting of S_2 (that is, with normal QRS duration) may be an important bedside clue to significant LV dysfunction. In severe aortic stenosis, the paradoxical splitting is only rarely recognized because the late systolic ejection murmur obscures S_2. However, when paradoxical splitting of S_2 is found in association with aortic stenosis, usually in young adults (assuming left bundle branch block is absent), severe aortic obstruction is suggested. Similarly, paradoxical splitting in hypertrophic obstructive cardiomyopathy implies a significant resting LV outflow tract gradient. Transient paradoxical splitting of S_2 can occur with myocardial ischemia, such as during an episode of angina, either alone or in combination with an apical systolic murmur of mitral regurgitation (papillary muscle dysfunction) or prominent fourth heart sound (S_4).

■ When paradoxical splitting of S_2 is found in association with aortic stenosis, usually in young adults (assuming left bundle branch block is absent), severe aortic obstruction is suggested. Similarly, paradoxical splitting in hypertrophic obstructive cardiomyopathy implies a significant resting LV outflow tract gradient.

■ Transient paradoxical splitting of S_2 can occur with myocardial ischemia, such as during an episode of angina, either alone or in combination with an apical systolic murmur of mitral regurgitation (papillary muscle dysfunction) or a prominent S_4.

Intensity of S_2

Loud S_2
Ordinarily, the intensity of the aortic component of the second heart sound (A_2) exceeds that of the P_2. In adults, a P_2 that is louder than A_2, especially if P_2 is transmitted to the apex, implies either pulmonary hypertension or marked RV dilatation, such that the RV now occupies the apical zone. The latter may occur in ASD (approximately 50% of patients). Hearing two components of the S_2 at the apex is abnormal in adults, because ordinarily only A_2 is heard at the apex. Thus, when both components of S_2 are heard at the apex in adults, suspect ASD or pulmonary hypertension.

Soft S_2
Decreased intensity of A_2 or P_2, which may cause a single S_2, reflects stiffening and decreased mobility of the aortic or pulmonary valve (aortic stenosis or pulmonary stenosis, respectively). A single S_2 may also be heard in older patients and the following cases:

1. With only one functioning semilunar valve, such as in persistent truncus arteriosus, pulmonary atresia, or tetralogy of Fallot
2. When one component of S_2 is enveloped in a long systolic murmur, such as in ventricular septal defect
3. With abnormal relationships of great vessels, such as in transposition of the great arteries

■ When both components of S_2 are heard at the apex in adults, implying an increased pulmonary component of S_2, suspect ASD or pulmonary hypertension.

Opening Snap

A high-pitched snapping sound related to mitral or tricuspid valve opening, when present, is abnormal and is referred to as an opening snap (OS). This may arise from either a doming stenotic mitral valve or tricuspid valve, more commonly the former. The intensity of an OS correlates with valve mobility. Rarely, an OS occurs in the absence of atrioventricular valve stenosis in conditions associated with increased flow through the valve, such as significant mitral regurgitation.

In mitral stenosis, the presence of an OS, often accompanied by a loud S_1, implies a pliable mitral valve. The OS is often well transmitted to the left sternal border and even to the aortic area. In mitral stenosis, the absence of an OS implies the following:

1. Severe valvular immobility and calcification (note that an OS can still be heard in some of these cases)
2. Mitral regurgitation is the predominant lesion

■ Significant mitral stenosis may be present in the absence of an OS if the mitral valve leaflets are fixed and immobile.

S2-OS Interval

The S_2–mitral OS interval reflects the isovolumic relaxation period of the LV. With increased severity of mitral stenosis and greater increase in left atrial pressures, the S_2-OS interval becomes shorter and may be confused with a split S_2. The S_2-OS interval should not vary with respiration. The S_2-OS interval widens on standing, whereas the split S_2 either does not change or narrows. Mild mitral stenosis is associated with an S_2-OS interval of more than 90 ms, and severe mitral stenosis with an interval of less than 70 ms. However, the S_2-OS interval is an unreliable predictor of the severity of mitral stenosis. Other factors that increase left atrial pressures, such as mitral regurgitation or LV failure, can also affect this interval. When the S_2-OS interval is more than 110 to 120 ms, the OS may be confused with an LV S_3. In comparison, the LV S_3 is usually low-pitched and is localized to the apex.

A tricuspid valve OS caused by tricuspid stenosis can be recognized by its location along the left sternal border and its increase with inspiration. In normal sinus rhythm, a prominent A wave can be seen in the jugular venous pulse, along with slowing of the Y descent.

An LV S_3, which implies that rapid LV filling can occur, is rare in pure mitral stenosis. Also, an RV S_3 can occur in mitral stenosis with severe secondary pulmonary hypertension and RV failure. An RV S_3 is found along the left sternal border and increases with inspiration. A tumor "plop" due to an atrial myxoma has the same early diastolic timing as an OS and can be confused with it.

■ In mitral stenosis, the presence of an OS, often accompanied by a loud S_1, implies a pliable mitral valve that is not heavily calcified. (In such cases, the patient may be a candidate for mitral commissurotomy or balloon valvuloplasty rather than mitral valve replacement.)

■ In general, mild mitral stenosis is associated with an S_2-OS interval >90 ms, and severe mitral stenosis with an interval <70 ms.

■ A tumor "plop" due to atrial myxoma has the same early diastolic timing as an OS and can be confused with it.

Third Heart Sound

The exact mechanism of S_3 production remains controversial, but its timing relates to the peak of rapid ventricular filling with rapid flow deceleration. Factors related to S_3 intensity include the following:

1. Volume and velocity of blood flow across the atrioventricular valve
2. Ventricular relaxation and compliance

Although a physiologic S_3 can be heard in young healthy subjects, it should not be audible after age 40. An RV S_3 may be augmented with inspiration. The physiologic S_3 may disappear in the standing position; the pathologic S_3 persists. An S_3 in a patient with mitral regurgitation implies severe regurgitation or a failing LV or both. The presence of a diastolic flow rumble ("relative" mitral stenosis) after the S_3 suggests severe mitral regurgitation. An S_3 is less common in conditions that cause thick, poorly compliant ventricles, for example, LV hypertrophy that occurs with pressure overload states (such as aortic stenosis or hypertension), until late in the disease. An S_3 may occur in hypertrophic obstructive cardiomyopathy with normal systolic function.

The pericardial knock of constrictive pericarditis is similar to an S_3 and is associated with sudden arrest of ventricular expansion in early diastole. The pericardial knock is of higher frequency than S_3, occurs slightly earlier in diastole, may vary with respiration, and is more widely transmitted. The causes of S_3 are listed in Table 11.

- An S_3 in a patient with mitral regurgitation implies severe regurgitation or a failing LV or both.
- An S_3 is less common in conditions that cause thick, poorly compliant ventricles, for example, LV hypertrophy that occurs with pressure overload states.
- The pericardial knock is of higher frequency than S_3, occurs slightly earlier in diastole, may vary with respiration, and is more widely transmitted.

Fourth Heart Sound

The S_4 is thought to originate within the ventricular cavity and results from a forceful atrial contraction into a ventricle having limited distensibility, such as in hypertrophy or fibrosis. It is not heard in healthy young persons or in atrial fibrillation.

Common pathologic states in which an S_4 is often present include the following:

1. Aortic stenosis
2. Hypertension
3. Hypertrophic obstructive cardiomyopathy
4. Pulmonary stenosis
5. Ischemic heart disease

As the S_4 becomes closer to S_1, the intensity of the latter increases. Sitting or standing may attenuate the S_4. A loud S_4 can be heard in acute mitral regurgitation (e.g., with ruptured chordae tendineae) or regurgitation of recent onset (the left atrium has not yet significantly dilated). With chronic mitral regurgitation due to rheumatic disease, the left atrium dilates, becomes more distensible, and generates a less forceful contraction. Under these circumstances, an S_4 is usually absent. An S_4 can still be heard in patients with LV hypertrophy or ischemic heart disease, despite enlargement of the left atrium.

Although an S_4 can be heard in otherwise healthy elderly patients, a palpable S_4 (*a* wave) should not be present unless the LV is abnormal. An S_4 can originate from the RV. A right-sided S_4 is increased in intensity with inspiration, is often associated with large jugular venous *a* waves, and is best heard along the left sternal border rather than at the apex (this is the usual site of an LV S_4).

Table 11. Causes of S_3

Physiologic in young adults and children
Severe left ventricular dysfunction of any cause
Left ventricular dilatation without failure due to
Mitral regurgitation
Ventricular septal defect
Patent ductus arteriosus
Right ventricular S_3 in right ventricular failure and severe tricuspid regurgitation
Pericardial knock in constrictive pericarditis
S_3 is augmented in intensity with an increase in venous return due to
Leg elevation
Exercise
Release phase of Valsalva maneuver
S_3 is augmented in intensity with increased systemic peripheral resistance due to sustained handgrip

In patients with aortic stenosis who are younger than 40 years, the presence of an S_4 usually indicates significant obstruction. Similarly, the presence of right-sided S_4, in association with pulmonary stenosis, indicates severe pulmonary valve obstruction. An S_4 is present in most patients with hypertrophic obstructive cardiomyopathy and in patients with acute myocardial infarction and is often heard in patients with systemic hypertension.

- A loud S_4 can be heard in acute mitral regurgitation (e.g., with ruptured chordae tendineae) and can be a clue that the regurgitation is of recent onset.
- Although an S_4 can be heard in otherwise healthy elderly patients, a palpable S_4 (*a* wave) should not be present unless the LV is abnormal.
- An S_4 is present in most patients with hypertrophic obstructive cardiomyopathy and in patients with acute myocardial infarction and is often heard in patients with systemic hypertension.

CARDIAC MURMURS

Systolic Murmurs

Systolic murmurs (Fig. 4) may be divided into two categories:

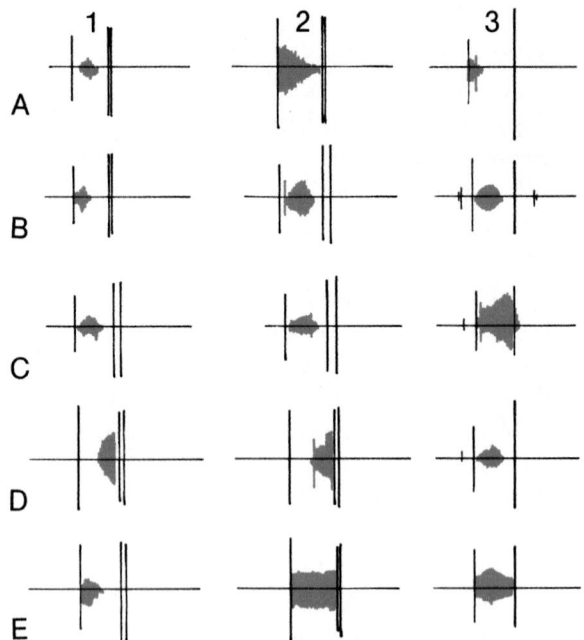

1. Ejection types, such as aortic or pulmonary stenosis
2. Pansystolic or regurgitant types, such as mitral regurgitation, tricuspid regurgitation, or ventricular septal defect

Most, but not all, systolic murmurs fit into this simple classification scheme. Factors that differentiate the various causes of LV outflow tract obstruction are shown in Table 12. The effects of various maneuvers on murmurs and S_2 are shown in Figure 5.

Aortic and Pulmonary Stenosis

Stenosis of the aortic or pulmonary valves causes a delay in the peak intensity of the systolic murmur related to prolongation of ejection. The magnitude of the delay is proportional to the severity of obstruction. The intensity (loudness) of an ejection systolic murmur may not reflect the severity of obstruction. Thus, for example, a patient with mild aortic stenosis or a normal mechanical aortic prosthesis and increased cardiac output may have a loud murmur (grade 3 or 4). Conversely, a patient with severe aortic stenosis and low cardiac output may have only a grade 1 or 2 murmur. However, the timing of peak intensity may still be delayed. For valvular pulmonary stenosis, early timing of the ejection click, a widely split S_2, and delayed peak intensity of systolic murmur suggest severe stenosis.

Fig. 4. Sketches of various murmurs and heart sounds.
A1, Short, midsystolic murmur with normal aortic (A_2) and pulmonic (P_2) components of the second heart sound (S_2)—findings consistent with an innocent murmur.
A2, Holosystolic murmur that decreases in the latter part of systole—a configuration observed in acute mitral regurgitation.
A3, An ejection sound and a short early systolic murmur, plus accentuated, closely split S_2—consistent with pulmonary hypertension, as with an Eisenmenger ventricular septal defect.
B1, Early to midsystolic murmur with vibratory component—typical of an innocent murmur.
B2, An ejection sound followed by a diamond-shaped murmur and wide splitting of S_2 that may be present with atrial septal defect or mild pulmonic stenosis; an ejection sound is more likely with valvular pulmonic stenosis.
B3, Crescendo-decrescendo systolic murmur, not holosystolic; the third heart sound (S_3) and fourth heart sound (S_4) are present—findings consistent with mitral systolic murmur heard in congestive cardiomyopathy or coronary artery disease with papillary muscle dysfunction and cardiac decompensation.
C1, Longer, somewhat vibratory crescendo-decrescendo systolic murmur with wide splitting of S_2. If S_2 becomes fused with expiration, atrial septal defect is less likely; if the remainder of the cardiovascular evaluation is normal, this finding is consistent with an innocent murmur.
C2, Midsystsolic murmur and wide splitting of S_2 that was "fixed"—findings typical of atrial septal defect.
C3, Prolonged diamond-shaped systolic murmur masking A_2 with delayed P_2, S_4, and ejection sound—findings typical of valvular pulmonic stenosis of moderate severity.
D1, Late apical systolic murmur of prolapsing mitral valve leaflet.
D2, Systolic click—late apical systolic murmur of prolapsing mitral leaflet syndrome.
D3, S_4 and midsystolic murmur consistent with mitral systolic murmur of cardiomyopathy or ischemic heart disease.
E1, Early crescendo-decrescendo systolic murmur ending in midsystole consistent with innocent murmur and small ventricular septal defect.
E2 and E3, Holosystolic murmur consistent with mitral or tricuspid regurgitation, and ventricular septal defect.

Table 12. Factors That Differentiate the Various Causes of Left Ventricular Outflow Tract Obstruction

Feature	Valvular	Supravalvular	Discrete subvalvular	HOCM
Valve calcification	Common after age 40 y	Absent	Absent	Absent
Dilated ascending aorta	Common	Rare	Rare	Rare
PP after VPB	Increased	Increased	Increased	Decreased
Valsalva effect on SM	Decreased	Decreased	Decreased	Increased
Murmur of AR	Common	Rare	Sometimes	Absent
Fourth heart sound (S₄)	If severe	Uncommon	Uncommon	Common
Paradoxical splitting	Sometimes*	Absent	Absent	Common*
Ejection click	Most (unless valve calcified)	Absent	Absent	Uncommon or absent
Maximal thrill & murmur	2nd RIS	1st RIS	2nd RIS	4th LIS
Carotid pulse	Normal to anacrotic* (parvus et tardus)	Unequal	Normal to anacrotic	Brisk, jerky; systolic rebound

AR, aortic regurgitation; HOCM, hypertrophic obstructive cardiomyopathy; LIS, left intercostal space; PP, pulse pressure; RIS, right intercostal space; SM, systolic murmur; VPB, ventricular premature beat.

Hypertrophic Obstructive Cardiomyopathy

Patients with hypertrophic obstructive cardiomyopathy can have three different types and locations of systolic murmurs:

1. Mid to lower left sternal border (LV outflow tract obstruction)
2. Apex (associated mitral regurgitation)
3. Upper left sternal border (RV outflow tract obstruction)—uncommon (a bedside clue is a prominent jugular venous *a* wave).

Frequently, the louder systolic murmur at the mid left sternal border, which can be widely transmitted, may merge with or mask the others.

Aortic Stenosis Versus Aortic Sclerosis

A frequent clinical problem is the differentiation of aortic stenosis from benign aortic sclerosis. With aortic sclerosis, there should be no other clinical, electrocardiographic, or radiographic evidence of heart disease. The systolic murmur is generally of grade 1 or 2 intensity and peaks early. The carotid upstroke should be normal. A normal S₂ (that is, A₂ preserved) supports a benign process, but remember that S₂ can appear single in healthy elderly subjects. The systolic murmur of aortic stenosis, in contrast, is delayed (peaking late in systole) and is usually louder, and the carotid pulse is weakened and delayed (parvus et tardus) (remember the exception of the elderly, who may have normal carotid pulses despite having significant aortic stenosis). The apical impulse in aortic stenosis is frequently abnormal also (see the "Abnormalities on Palpation of the Precordium" section above).

Supravalvular Aortic Stenosis

The systolic murmur of supravalvular aortic stenosis is maximal in the first or second right intercostal space, and a carotid pulse inequality may be present (see the "Abnormalities of the Carotid Pulse" section above). Patients are usually young. (The differential diagnosis of LV outflow tract obstruction is shown in Table 12.)

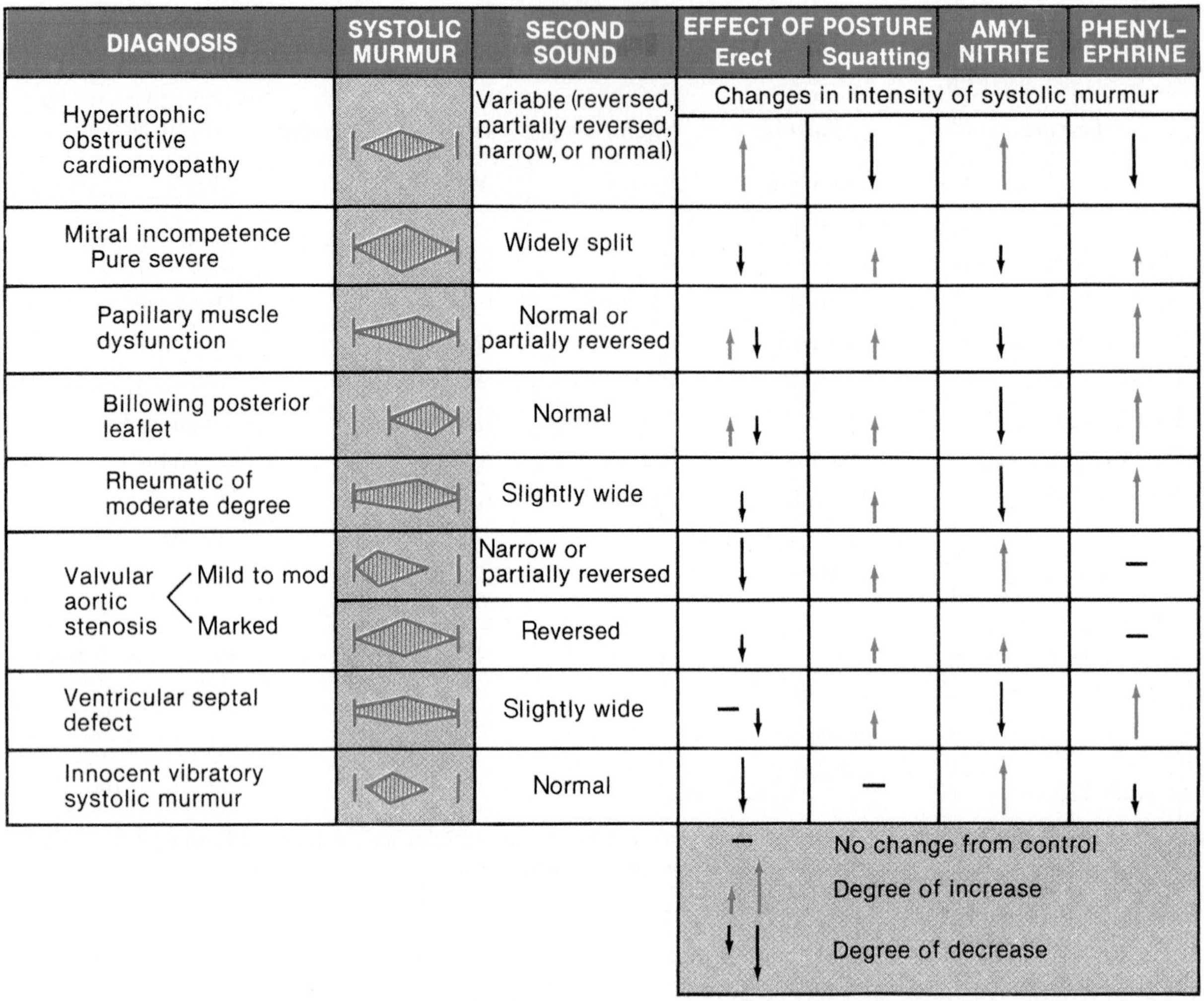

DIAGNOSIS	SYSTOLIC MURMUR	SECOND SOUND	EFFECT OF POSTURE Erect	EFFECT OF POSTURE Squatting	AMYL NITRITE	PHENYL-EPHRINE
			Changes in intensity of systolic murmur			
Hypertrophic obstructive cardiomyopathy	◁▷	Variable (reversed, partially reversed, narrow, or normal)	↑	↓	↑	↓
Mitral incompetence Pure severe	◁▷	Widely split	↓	↑	↓	↑
Papillary muscle dysfunction	◁▷	Normal or partially reversed	↑ ↓	↑	↓	↑
Billowing posterior leaflet	▷	Normal	↑ ↓	↑	↓	↑
Rheumatic of moderate degree	▭	Slightly wide	↓	↑	↓	↑
Valvular aortic stenosis — Mild to mod	◁▷	Narrow or partially reversed	↓	↑	↑	—
Valvular aortic stenosis — Marked	◁▷	Reversed	↓	↑	↑	—
Ventricular septal defect	▭	Slightly wide	— ↓	↑	↓	↑
Innocent vibratory systolic murmur	◁▷	Normal	↓	—	↑	↓

Legend:
— No change from control
↑ Degree of increase
↓ Degree of decrease

Fig. 5. Diagrammatic representation of the character of the systolic murmur and of the second heart sound in 5 conditions. The effects of posture, amyl nitrite inhalation, and phenylephrine injection on the intensity of the murmur are shown. mod, moderate.

Mitral Regurgitation

Although mitral regurgitation is usually pansystolic, the timing can be late systolic (in this case, suspect mitral prolapse, papillary muscle dysfunction, and, less commonly, rheumatic disease). The systolic murmur of mitral regurgitation can also be early systolic in timing; this can be heard in cases of acute, severe mitral regurgitation with markedly increased left atrial pressures, reducing the late systolic LV–left atrial gradient. In such cases, the patients are usually hemodynamically unstable and have evidence of significant pulmonary congestion. The systolic murmur of severe chronic mitral regurgitation is usually loud (grade 3-4 or louder). The systolic murmur of severe acute mitral regurgitation can be variable, especially in the presence of low cardiac output states or shock (such as acute myocardial infarction with LV dysfunction and papillary muscle dysfunction). Under these circumstances, the systolic murmur may be unimpressive or even absent. The systolic murmur of *posterior mitral leaflet syndrome* can be well transmitted to the aortic area and be confused with aortic stenosis. Except in the elderly, palpation of the carotid pulse helps differentiate these two conditions. In about 15% of cases, pure aortic stenosis can cause a localized apical systolic murmur. Auscultation during inhalation of amyl nitrite can help differentiate this murmur from mitral regurgitation (Tables 13 and 14). The systolic murmur of *anterior mitral leaflet syndrome* is transmitted posteriorly and can be heard along the thoracic spine and even at the base of the skull.

Table 13. Effect of Selected Physiologic Changes and Physical or Pharmacologic Maneuvers on Common Cardiac Murmurs

Feature	Effect on murmur		
	Augmented	Little or no change	Decreased
Amyl nitrite	HOCM		MR
	AS, PS		VSD ⎤ SM
	Innocent SM		
	MS		AR
	TS		Austin Flint ⎤ DM
Handgrip	AR	AS, TR	HOCM
	MR	PR	
	VSD	TS	
	MS*		
Long cardiac cycle length	AS	MR	
(e.g., atrial fibrillation	PS	AR	
or with premature	HOCM		
ventricular contraction)			
Valsalva maneuver	HOCM		AS
	MV prolapse†		PS
Posture			
Standing	HOCM		AS
	MV prolapse†		PS
Squatting	AR, MR, VSD		HOCM
			MV prolapse‡

AR, aortic regurgitation; AS, aortic stenosis; DM, diastolic murmur; HOCM, hypertrophic obstructive cardiomyopathy; MR, mitral regurgitation; MS, mitral stenosis; MV, mitral valve; PR, pulmonary regurgitation; PS, pulmonary stenosis; SM, systolic murmur; TR, tricuspid regurgitation; TS, tricuspid stenosis; VSD, ventricular septal defect.
*Related to increased cardiac output.
†Duration of systolic murmur increased (earlier onset); variable augmentation effect.
‡Duration of systolic murmur decreased (later onset); variable intensity effect.

Tricuspid Regurgitation
The systolic murmur of tricuspid regurgitation is usually best heard at the lower left sternal border or over the xiphisternum, but it may also be heard to the right of the sternum, over the apicosternal area, or over the apex (if the RV is sufficiently dilated and occupies the position usually taken by the LV). The systolic murmur of significant tricuspid regurgitation may be subtle or even inaudible clinically, but large *v* waves can be seen in the jugular venous pulse. Inspiration may accentuate the murmur of tricuspid regurgitation, but not consistently so, and the absence of inspiratory augmentation does not exclude tricuspid regurgitation (with severe tricuspid regurgitation, the *x* descent becomes obliterated).

Ventricular Septal Defect
Depending on the size of the defect and the pressure gradient between the LV and the RV, the systolic murmur of ventricular septal defect is typically pansystolic and associated with a thrill along the left sternal border, but the murmur can be variable in contour and the thrill absent. The murmur parallels the pressure difference between the two ventricles (in turn related to pulmonary and systemic vascular resistances). With significant pulmonary hypertension, the murmur duration shortens

Table 14. Effect of Amyl Nitrite and Vasopressors on Various Murmurs

Diagnosis	Amyl nitrite	Phenylephrine
	Systolic murmurs	
Mitral insufficiency	Decrease	Increase
Ventricular septal defect	Decrease	Increase
Patent ductus arteriosus	Decrease	Increase
Tetralogy of Fallot	Decrease	Increase
Atrial septal defect	Increase	Increase or no change
Idiopathic hypertrophic subaortic stenosis	Increase	Decrease
Aortic stenosis (valvular)	Increase	No change
Pulmonary stenosis (valvular and muscular)	Increase	No change
Tricuspid insufficiency	Increase	No change
Systolic ejection murmur (innocent)	Increase	Decrease
	Diastolic murmurs	
Aortic insufficiency	Decrease	Increase
Austin Flint murmur	Decrease	Increase
Mitral stenosis	Increase	Decrease
Pulmonary insufficiency	Increase	No change
Pulmonary insufficiency due to Eisenmenger syndrome	Decrease	Increase
Tricuspid stenosis	Increase	No change

and may resemble an early systolic ejection-type murmur. If the maximal intensity of the systolic murmur is in the first and second left intercostal spaces with radiation to the left clavicle, suspect supracristal ventricular septal defect or patent ductus arteriosus. The systolic murmur of multiple ventricular septal defects is indistinguishable from that of single defects. The same is true for LV–right atrial shunts. The loud pansystolic murmur of ventricular septal defect may mask associated defects, such as patent ductus arteriosus. A wide pulse pressure suggests the latter or associated aortic regurgitation. The combination of ventricular septal defect and aortic regurgitation may suggest patent ductus arteriosus, but the systolic murmur in patent ductus arteriosus peaks at S_2 and it does not in the combination of ventricular septal defect and aortic regurgitation. A systolic murmur in the posterior thorax may be caused by the following:

1. Coarctation
2. Aortic dissection
3. Anterior mitral leaflet syndrome (with posteriorly directed jet of mitral regurgitation)
4. Peripheral pulmonary artery stenosis
5. Pulmonary arteriovenous fistula

- Stenosis of a semilunar valve causes a delay in the peak intensity of the systolic murmur related to prolongation of ejection. The magnitude of the delay is proportional to the severity of obstruction.
- For valvular pulmonary stenosis, early timing of the ejection click, a widely split S_2, and delayed peak intensity of systolic murmur suggest severe stenosis.
- The systolic murmur of supravalvular aortic stenosis is maximal in the first or second right intercostal space, and a carotid pulse inequality may be present.
- Although mitral regurgitation is usually pansystolic, the timing can be late systolic (in this case, suspect mitral prolapse, papillary muscle dysfunction, and, less commonly, rheumatic disease).
- Mitral regurgitation that is early systolic in timing can be heard in acute, severe cases with markedly increased left atrial pressures, reducing the late systolic LV–left atrial gradient.
- The systolic murmur of posterior mitral leaflet syndrome can be transmitted to the aortic area and be confused with aortic stenosis.
- The systolic murmur of anterior mitral leaflet syndrome is transmitted posteriorly and can be heard

along the thoracic spine and even at the base of the skull.

- Inspiration may accentuate the murmur of tricuspid regurgitation, but not consistently so, and the absence of inspiratory augmentation does not exclude tricuspid regurgitation.
- The systolic murmur of ventricular septal defect is typically pansystolic and associated with a thrill along the left sternal border, but the murmur can be variable in contour.
- If the maximal intensity of a systolic murmur is in the first and second left intercostal spaces with radiation to the left clavicle, suspect supracristal ventricular septal defect or patent ductus arteriosus.
- A loud pansystolic murmur of ventricular septal defect may mask associated defects, such as patent ductus arteriosus. A wide pulse pressure suggests the latter or associated aortic regurgitation.
- The combination of ventricular septal defect and aortic regurgitation may suggest patent ductus arteriosus, but the murmur in the latter peaks at S_2, and it does not in the combination of ventricular septal defect and aortic regurgitation.

Innocent Systolic Murmurs

Innocent systolic murmurs are generally related to increased blood flow or turbulence across a semilunar valve, especially the aortic valve. These murmurs are common at all ages. In young patients, they are apt to be heard over the pulmonary area. Innocent systolic murmurs usually are soft (≤grade 2), are short (never pansystolic), and have no associated abnormal clinical findings (e.g., S_2 is normal and there are no clicks). In older patients, they generally emanate from a sclerotic aortic valve or dilated aortic root. Such murmurs can be heard at the aortic area, left sternal border, or apex. If heard at the apex, they may be confused with the murmur of mitral regurgitation. In younger patients, an innocent systolic murmur may originate from the RV outflow tract or pulmonary artery. Remember that a patent ductus arteriosus or ventricular septal defect also can masquerade as an innocent murmur.

An innocent systolic murmur heard at the lower left sternal border should be differentiated from the systolic murmur of ventricular septal defect, tricuspid regurgitation, infundibular pulmonary stenosis, or hypertrophic obstructive cardiomyopathy. When uncertain about the cause of a systolic murmur, a Valsalva maneuver should be performed (Table 13). The findings that suggest that a systolic murmur is pathologic are listed in Table 15.

- Innocent systolic murmurs usually are soft (≤grade 2 or less), are short, and have no associated abnormal clinical findings.
- In younger patients, an innocent systolic murmur often originates from the RV outflow tract or pulmonary artery.
- Remember that a patent ductus arteriosus or ventricular septal defect can masquerade as an innocent murmur.

Diastolic Murmurs

In general, the loudness of a diastolic murmur correlates with the severity of the underlying abnormality.

Aortic Regurgitation

The murmur of mild aortic regurgitation (AR) may be difficult to hear and may be clinically "silent." This murmur is best heard with the patient in the sitting position, leaning forward, in held expiration. Consider AR when there is a wide arterial pulse pressure, especially in young or middle-aged patients (older patients may have generalized atherosclerosis causing wide pulse pressure). The murmur of AR is typically early diastolic (immediately after S_2) and decrescendo in timing. In the presence of mitral stenosis, an early diastolic murmur may be caused by AR or pulmonary

Table 15. Findings That Suggest That a Systolic Murmur Is Pathologic

Loud (≥grade 3)
Long duration
Associated with ejection or nonejection click
Loud S_1, A_2, or P_2
Presence of an opening snap
Presence of left or right ventricular hypertrophy or heave
Fixed or expiratory splitting of S_2

A_2, aortic component of S_2; P_2, pulmonary component of S_2; S_1, first heart sound; S_2, second heart sound.

regurgitation (Graham Steell murmur) but more often by AR. Severe AR, especially if acute, may be associated with markedly increased LV end-diastolic pressures. These pressures will decrease the gradient between the aorta and the LV in diastole, and the murmur will taper rapidly. Thus, a short, early diastolic murmur does not exclude significant acute AR, especially if the patient has evidence of acute heart failure. A patient with severe AR due to infective endocarditis may present in this way. In mild AR, the LV end-diastolic pressure remains normal, the gradient persists throughout most of diastole, and the murmur may persist longer into diastole. With severe, chronic AR, there is often a wide pulse pressure (with hyperdynamic pulses), a systolic ejection murmur that usually peaks early (related to increased aortic flow), reduced diastolic blood pressure, and LV enlargement by palpation.

Remember that the anatomical location of the aortic valve is not under the second right intercostal space (the "aortic area") but is situated lower in the thorax under the mid sternum, although the "jet" of aortic stenosis is often best heard in the aortic area. The murmur of AR is often best heard along the left sternal border. It can be primarily transmitted down the right sternal border. If so, one should suspect diseases of the aortic root, such as aortic aneurysm or dissection. The combination of hypertension, chest pain, and right sternal border transmission of the AR murmur should suggest proximal aortic dissection. When the AR is of valvular origin, the murmur can be heard at the aortic area, but it is also transmitted along the left sternal border and to the apex.

- Consider AR when there is a wide arterial pulse pressure, especially in young or middle-aged patients.
- In the presence of mitral stenosis, an associated early diastolic murmur may be due to AR or pulmonary regurgitation (Graham Steell murmur) but more often to AR.
- A short, early diastolic murmur does not exclude significant acute AR, especially if the patient has evidence of acute heart failure.
- The murmur of AR, although often heard at the left sternal border, can be primarily transmitted down the right sternal border. If so, one should suspect diseases of the aortic root, such as aortic aneurysm or dissection.

- The combination of hypertension, chest pain, and right sternal border transmission of the AR murmur should suggest proximal aortic dissection.

Austin Flint Murmur

An Austin Flint murmur is related to mitral inflow turbulence caused by the AR jet and implies a significant AR leak. Because this may produce an apical diastolic rumble that is mid-diastolic in timing with presystolic accentuation, it may be confused with mitral stenosis. The presence of radiographic left atrial enlargement or atrial fibrillation favors mitral stenosis rather than isolated AR. Administration of amyl nitrite can help differentiate these murmurs (Table 14): the Austin Flint murmur decreases (as the LV afterload decreases), whereas the mitral stenosis murmur increases (as do all valvular stenotic murmurs in response to amyl nitrite). Also, there should be no OS or other features of mitral valve disease. Obviously, a patient with rheumatic heart disease can have both AR and mitral stenosis. When AR has a "honking" or "cooing" quality, consider a perforated, everted, or ruptured aortic cusp, such as with infective endocarditis.

- With administration of amyl nitrite, the Austin Flint murmur decreases (as the LV afterload decreases), whereas the murmur of mitral stenosis increases (as do all valvular stenotic murmurs in response to amyl nitrite).
- When AR has a "honking" or "cooing" quality, consider a perforated, everted, or ruptured aortic cusp, such as with infective endocarditis.

Pulmonary Regurgitation

Although pulmonary regurgitation may sound similar to the murmur of AR, it is usually localized to the pulmonary area and, like most right-sided events, gets louder with inspiration. The murmur characteristics depend on the cause. The murmur of pulmonary regurgitation due to pulmonary hypertension begins in early diastole (immediately after P2) and is long and high-pitched. In comparison, the murmur of pulmonary regurgitation due to organic pulmonary valve disease is lower pitched, harsher, and rumbling, beginning slightly later in diastole and often ending in mid diastole. Pulmonary regurgitation, especially when mild or even moderate, is frequently inaudible. In the presence of mitral stenosis, an early diastolic murmur heard at the left sternal border is more likely to be AR than pulmonary regurgitation.

■ The murmur of pulmonary regurgitation due to pulmonary hypertension begins in early diastole and is long and high-pitched. In comparison, the murmur of pulmonary regurgitation due to organic pulmonary valve disease is lower pitched, harsher, and rumbling, begins slightly later in diastole, and often ends in mid diastole.

Mitral Stenosis

The diastolic murmur of mitral stenosis is very localized (to the apex), is low-pitched, and begins at the time of mitral valve opening. The presence of a loud S_1 or an OS should prompt a careful search for this easily overlooked diastolic murmur. With the patient in the left lateral decubitus position, the stethoscope may have to be inched around the apical region to find the highly localized, subtle, flow rumble of mitral stenosis. If the murmur is not audible, exercise (such as sit-ups) may augment mitral flow and bring out the murmur. Other provocative maneuvers that increase flow across the mitral valve, such as administration of amyl nitrite, also augment the murmur of mitral stenosis (Table 13). The duration of the diastolic murmur is related to the severity of mitral stenosis, persisting as long as there is a significant pressure gradient across the mitral valve. Therefore, a pandiastolic murmur implies severe mitral stenosis. The murmur may crescendo in late diastole (presystolic accentuation), even in atrial fibrillation, suggesting that atrial contraction is not required for this phenomenon.

Rarely in mitral stenosis, the diastolic murmur is not heard ("silent" mitral stenosis). The usual reasons for silent mitral stenosis are as follows:
1. Improper auscultation (most commonly)
2. Very mild mitral stenosis
3. A decrease in flow rates across the mitral valve, such as in severe congestive heart failure or concomitant aortic or tricuspid stenosis
4. Abnormal chest wall configuration limiting auscultation, such as in obesity or severe chronic obstructive pulmonary disease, in which case all sounds should be indistinct or distant

Consider mitral stenosis and focus the cardiac examination accordingly with new onset of atrial fibrillation or when atrial fibrillation is found in association with any of the following clinical scenarios:
1. Stroke or other systemic or peripheral embolus (an atrial myxoma may also present in this way)
2. "Unexplained" pulmonary hypertension
3. "Unexplained" congestive heart failure
4. "Unexplained" recurrent pleural effusions

■ The duration of the diastolic murmur is related to the severity of mitral stenosis, persisting as long as there is a significant pressure gradient across the mitral valve.
■ Even in the apparent absence of a murmur, important auscultatory clues to the presence of mitral stenosis include a loud S_1 and an OS.
■ Consider mitral stenosis when atrial fibrillation is found in association with any of the following clinical scenarios: 1) stroke or other systemic or peripheral embolus, 2) "unexplained" pulmonary hypertension, 3) "unexplained" congestive heart failure, and 4) "unexplained" recurrent pleural effusions.

Tricuspid Stenosis

The bedside differentiation of tricuspid and mitral stenosis includes the following:
1. Response to inspiration—murmur of tricuspid stenosis increases
2. Location—the diastolic murmur of tricuspid stenosis is best heard at the left sternal border, whereas the murmur of mitral stenosis is localized to the apex. The associated OS, if present, augments with inspiration
3. Frequency—tricuspid stenosis is higher in frequency and begins earlier in diastole than mitral stenosis (these differences may be difficult to appreciate at the bedside)
4. Large jugular venous *a* wave with a slow *y* descent—suggestive of tricuspid stenosis (other causes of large *a* waves, including pulmonary stenosis and pulmonary hypertension, should not interfere with RV filling and therefore are not associated with a slow *y* descent)

Rarely, there may be a diastolic thrill palpable along the lower left sternal border and hepatic (presystolic) pulsation. Other causes of RV inflow obstruction, such as thrombus or extrinsic RV compression, can masquerade as tricuspid stenosis.

Note that tricuspid stenosis usually occurs in patients with rheumatic heart disease (although there are other, rarer causes, such as carcinoid). In patients with rheumatic heart disease, especially females, concomitant mitral valve disease is almost always present. The clinical finding of left-sided valve lesions often overshadow the tricuspid involvement, and the murmur of tricuspid stenosis may be mistaken for aortic or pulmonary regurgitation.

■ A large jugular venous *a* wave with a slow *y* descent should suggest tricuspid stenosis.

■ The clinical finding of left-sided valve lesions often overshadows the tricuspid involvement, and the murmur of tricuspid stenosis may be mistaken for aortic or pulmonary regurgitation.

Mid-Diastolic Flow Murmurs

Almost any condition that increases flow across atrioventricular valves (such as mitral regurgitation, patent ductus arteriosus, intracardiac shunts, or complete heart block) can also cause a short mid-diastolic flow rumble (functional diastolic murmur) in the absence of organic atrioventricular valve stenosis. (Actually, the rumble begins in early rather than mid diastole, but it is delayed in comparison with the early diastolic murmur of semilunar valve regurgitation.) The murmur may begin after a prominent S_3 and does not show presystolic accentuation.

■ Almost any condition that increases flow across atrioventricular valves (such as mitral regurgitation, patent ductus arteriosus, intracardiac shunts, or complete heart block) can also cause a short mid-diastolic flow rumble (functional diastolic murmur) in the absence of organic atrioventricular valve stenosis.

Continuous Murmurs

Continuous murmurs should be differentiated from to-and-fro murmurs (such as occur in combined aortic stenosis and AR). In AR, the systolic component decreases before S_2, whereas the continuous murmur of patent ductus arteriosus, for example, typically peaks at S_2. Murmurs caused by coronary arteriovenous fistula, venous hum, and ruptured sinus of Valsalva aneurysm peak later in diastole. Murmurs due to dilated bronchial

vessels, such as in pulmonary atresia, can be heard anywhere in the chest, axillae, or back. When a continuous murmur is loudest in the posterior thorax, consider the following:

1. Coarctation
2. Pulmonary arteriovenous fistula
3. Peripheral pulmonary stenosis

■ Continuous murmurs should be differentiated from to-and-fro murmurs (such as occur in combined aortic stenosis and AR). In AR, the systolic component decreases before S_2, whereas the continuous murmur of patent ductus arteriosus typically peaks at S_2.

Bedside Physiologic Maneuvers to Differentiate Different Types of Murmurs

Several bedside physiologic maneuvers can be used to distinguish types of murmurs (Table 13).

Valsalva Maneuver

The Valsalva maneuver is useful for differentiating right-sided from left-sided murmurs. During the active strain phase, with decreased venous return, most murmurs decrease in intensity. There are two important exceptions to this rule:

1. The murmur of hypertrophic obstructive cardiomyopathy typically gets louder.
2. The murmur of mitral valve prolapse may get longer (and possibly louder).

After the release of the Valsalva maneuver, with a sudden increase in venous return, right-sided murmurs return immediately (within one or two cardiac cycles), whereas left-sided murmurs gradually return after several cardiac cycles. Thus, differentiation between aortic and pulmonary stenosis and between aortic and pulmonary regurgitation is possible.

Respiration

The effect of normal respiration is also useful for distinguishing right-sided and left-sided murmurs. In general, right-sided murmurs are augmented with inspiration (frequent exceptions occur with tricuspid regurgitation). In cases of severe RV failure, the RV may be unable to augment its output with inspiration, and pulmonary or tricuspid murmurs may fail to become louder with inspiration.

RR Cycle Length

Varying RR cycle length (such as in atrial fibrillation or with frequent premature ventricular contractions) affects murmurs in specific ways that can be of diagnostic value at the bedside. In general, systolic ejection murmurs (such as with aortic or pulmonary stenosis) increase after a long cycle length, whereas regurgitant murmurs (such as with mitral or tricuspid regurgitation) do not. The systolic murmur of hypertrophic obstructive cardiomyopathy is augmented with the increased contractility of a post–premature ventricular contraction beat, but the peripheral arterial pulse volume decreases because LV outflow tract obstruction worsens.

Handgrip

Isometric exercise (such as handgrip), by increasing systemic blood pressure (afterload), augments the murmurs of mitral and aortic regurgitation or ventricular septal defect but does not significantly alter the murmur of aortic stenosis and tends to decrease the murmur of hypertrophic obstructive cardiomyopathy.

Squatting

Prompt squatting causes a rapid transient increase in venous return and a sustained increase in peripheral resistance. The latter may augment the murmurs of mitral and aortic regurgitation. Because LV volume and peripheral resistance increase, the murmur of hypertrophic obstructive cardiomyopathy becomes softer. Then, after the upright position is assumed, with decreased LV volume and peripheral resistance, the murmur of hypertrophic obstructive cardiomyopathy becomes louder.

Amyl Nitrite

Administration of amyl nitrite is simple, inexpensive, and, in most patients, safe (exceptions are in acute myocardial infarction or critical carotid artery stenosis, in which even transient hypotension should be avoided if possible). Amyl nitrite causes acute systemic vasodilation, resulting in a transient (30-45 seconds) decline in systemic blood pressure, followed by reflex tachycardia and an increase in venous return and cardiac output. All stenotic murmurs, including those with hypertrophic obstructive cardiomyopathy,

become louder. The murmur of mitral regurgitation usually decreases because of the decrease in LV afterload (during the vasodilation phase). The diastolic murmur of AR diminishes, whereas the murmur of mitral stenosis becomes louder because of the increased flow across the mitral valve, especially during the tachycardia phase. The systolic murmur of mitral prolapse may become longer (as LV volume decreases initially) but not necessarily louder, because LV pressures also are decreased. The major usefulness of amyl nitrite is to differentiate within the following pairs (Tables 13 and 14):

1. A small ventricular septal defect (murmur decreases) and pulmonary stenosis (murmur increases)
2. Aortic stenosis (increase) and mitral regurgitation (decrease)
3. AR (decrease) and mitral stenosis (increase)
4. AR (decrease) and pulmonary regurgitation (increase)
5. Mitral regurgitation (decrease) and tricuspid regurgitation (increase)

- After release of the Valsalva maneuver, with a sudden increase in venous return, right-sided murmurs return immediately (within one or two cardiac cycles), whereas left-sided murmurs gradually return after several cardiac cycles.
- Systolic ejection murmurs (such as with aortic or pulmonary stenosis) increase after a long cycle length, whereas regurgitant murmurs (such as with mitral or tricuspid regurgitation) do not.
- Amyl nitrite causes all stenotic murmurs, including those with hypertrophic obstructive cardiomyopathy, to become louder.

Miscellaneous

The mammary soufflé can be continuous and can mimic patent ductus arteriosus. It can be obliterated by pressure with the examining finger next to the stethoscope. Innocent venous hums are loudest in the neck but can be transmitted to the precordium and be mistaken for patent ductus arteriosus or atrioventricular fistula. The venous hum is loudest in the sitting or standing position. Motion of the neck or jugular vein compression affects the intensity of the murmur.

- The innocent venous hum is loudest in the neck but can be transmitted to the precordium and be mistaken for patent ductus arteriosus or atrioventricular fistula.

- The venous hum is of variable quality, is loudest in the sitting or standing position, and decreases in the supine position.

Applied Anatomy of the Heart and Great Vessels

Joseph G. Murphy, MD

R. Scott Wright, MD

Mediastinum

The mediastinum contains the heart, great vessels, distal portion of the trachea, right and left bronchi, esophagus, thymus, autonomic nerves (cardiac and splanchnic, left recurrent laryngeal, and bilateral vagal and phrenic), various small arteries (such as bronchial and esophageal) and veins (such as bronchial, azygos, and hemiazygos), lymph nodes, cardiopulmonary lymphatics, and thoracic duct.

Enlargement of a cardiac chamber or great vessel may displace or compress an adjacent noncardiac structure. An enlarged left atrium may displace the left bronchus superiorly and the esophagus rightward. An aberrant retroesophageal right subclavian artery indents the esophagus posteriorly and may cause dysphagia. Mediastinal neoplasms can compress the atria, superior vena cava, or pulmonary veins.

Pericardium

The pericardium surrounds the heart and consists of fibrous and serous portions. The fibrous pericardium forms a tough outer sac, which envelops the heart and attaches to the great vessels. The ascending aorta, pulmonary artery, terminal 2 to 4 cm of superior vena cava, and short lengths of the pulmonary veins and inferior vena cava are intrapericardial.

The fibrous pericardium is inelastic and limits the diastolic distention of the heart during exercise. Cardiac enlargement or *chronic* pericardial effusions, if they develop slowly, will stretch the fibrous pericardium. The fibrous pericardium cannot stretch *acutely*, and the rapid accumulation of as little as 200 mL of fluid may produce fatal cardiac tamponade. Hemopericardium results from perforation of either the heart or the intrapericardial great vessels.

The serous pericardium is a delicate mesothelial layer that lines the inner aspect of the fibrous pericardium (parietal pericardium) and the outer surface of the heart and intrapericardial great vessels (visceral pericardium). The visceral pericardium, or epicardium, contains the coronary arteries and veins, autonomic nerves, lymphatic channels, and variable amounts of adipose tissue.

In obese subjects, excessive epicardial fat may encase the heart, but because pericardial fat is liquid at body temperature, cardiac motion is generally unhindered.

Modified from Edwards WD. Applied anatomy of the heart. In: Giuliani ER, Gersh BJ, McGoon MD, et al, editors. Mayo Clinic practice of cardiology. 3rd ed. St Louis: Mosby; 1996. p. 422-89. By permission of Mayo Foundation.

Between the great arteries (aorta and pulmonary artery) and the atria is a tunnel-like transverse sinus. Posteriorly, the pericardial reflection forms an inverted U-shaped cul-de-sac known as the oblique sinus.

A sequential saphenous vein bypass graft to the left coronary system may be positioned posteriorly through the transverse sinus. A persistent left superior vena cava occupies the expected site of the ligament of Marshall, along the junction between the appendage and body of the left atrium.

Between the parietal and visceral layers of the serous pericardium is the pericardial cavity, which normally contains 10 to 20 mL of serous fluid that allows the tissue surfaces to glide over each other with minimal friction.

Thick and roughened surfaces associated with fibrinous pericarditis lead to an auscultatory friction rub, and organization of such an exudate may result in fibrous adhesions between the epicardium and the parietal pericardium. Focal adhesions are usually unimportant, but occasionally they may allow the accumulation of loculated fluid or, rarely, tamponade of an individual cardiac chamber, usually the right ventricle. After cardiac surgery, the opened pericardial cavity may become sealed again if the parietal pericardium adheres to the sternum; in this setting, the raw pericardial surfaces, which are lined by fibrovascular granulation tissue, may ooze enough blood to cause cardiac tamponade.

Densely fibrotic adhesions, with or without calcification, can hinder cardiac motion and may restrict cardiac filling. The pericardium is thickened in subjects with chronic constriction but may be of normal thickness in persons with constriction that develops relatively rapidly. In the setting of constrictive pericarditis, surgical excision of only the anterior pericardium (between the phrenic nerves) is often inadequate, because the remaining pericardium surrounds enough of the heart to maintain constriction.

Most postoperative pericardial adhesions are usually functionally unimportant, but they may obscure the location of the coronary arteries at subsequent cardiac operation.

■ The fibrous pericardium cannot stretch acutely, and the rapid accumulation of as little as 200 mL of fluid may produce fatal cardiac tamponade.

■ A sequential saphenous vein bypass graft to the left circumflex coronary artery may be positioned posteriorly through the transverse sinus.

GREAT VEINS

Bilaterally, the subclavian and internal jugular veins merge to form bilateral innominate (or brachiocephalic) veins. The latter then join to form the superior vena cava (or superior caval vein) (Fig. 1).

Superior Vena Cava

The right internal jugular vein, right innominate vein, and superior vena cava afford a relatively straight intravascular route to the right atrium and tricuspid orifice. This route may be used for passage of a stiff

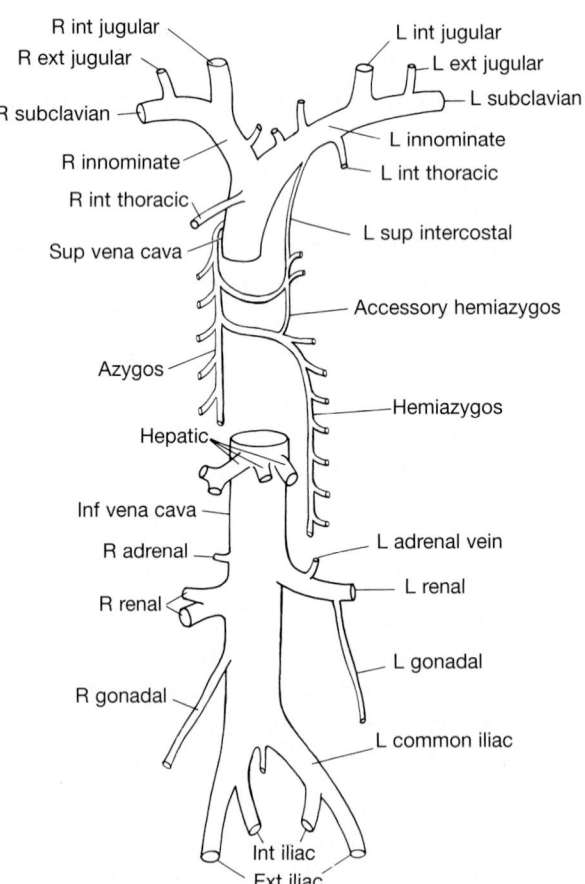

Fig. 1. Systemic veins, excluding the portal circulation. (See Appendix at end of chapter for abbreviations.)

endomyocardial bioptome across the tricuspid valve and into the right ventricular apex to obtain a cardiac biopsy specimen. Similarly, both temporary and permanent transvenous pacemaker leads are inserted via either the subclavian or the internal jugular vein and are threaded into the right ventricular apex.

Catheters and pacemakers within the innominate veins and superior vena cava become partially coated with thrombus and may be associated with thrombotic venous obstruction, pulmonary thromboembolism, or secondary infection. Mediastinal neoplasms, fibrosis, and aortic aneurysms may compress the thin-walled veins and result in the superior vena cava syndrome.

Inferior Vena Cava

The inferior vena cava receives systemic venous drainage from the legs and retroperitoneal viscera and, at the level of the liver, from the intra-abdominal systemic venous drainage (portal circulation) via the hepatic veins.

The inferior vena cava, which is retroperitoneal, may become trapped and compressed between the vertebral column posteriorly and either an adjacent retroperitoneal structure (e.g., an abdominal aortic aneurysm) or an intraperitoneal structure (e.g., a neoplasm) and thereby produce the inferior vena cava syndrome.

Venous thrombi in the lower extremities may extend into the inferior vena cava or may become dislodged and embolize to the right heart and pulmonary circulation. Renal cell carcinomas may extend intravascularly within the renal veins and inferior vena cava and may even form tethered intracavitary right-sided cardiac masses. Hepatocellular carcinomas often involve the hepatic veins and occasionally may enter the suprahepatic inferior vena cava or right atrium.

The superior and inferior pulmonary veins from each lung enter the left atrium. The proximal 1 to 3 cm of the pulmonary veins contain cardiac muscle within the media and may thereby function like sphincters during atrial systole as well as when significant mitral valve disease exists.

The thin-walled and low-pressure pulmonary veins may be compressed extrinsically by mediastinal neoplasms or fibrosis. Pulmonary vein stenosis is a rare complication of electrophysiology radiofrequency ablation.

Congenital Anomalies of the Venous System

Congenital anomalies of the systemic veins include a persistent left superior vena cava (with or without a left innominate vein) joining the coronary sinus or, rarely, the left atrium; an unroofed or absent coronary sinus; a large right sinus venosus valve (so-called cor triatriatum dexter); azygos continuity of the inferior vena cava; and bilateral subrenal inferior venae cavae.

Anomalous Venous Connection

In total anomalous pulmonary venous connection, the confluence of pulmonary veins does not join the left atrium but rather maintains connection to derivatives of the cardinal or umbilicovitelline veins, such as the left innominate vein, coronary sinus, or ductus venosus. An interatrial communication must also be present.

In partial anomalous pulmonary venous connection, only some veins (usually from the right lung) lack left atrial connections. Connection of the right pulmonary veins to the right atrium commonly accompanies sinus venosus atrial septal defects, whereas connection of these veins to the suprahepatic inferior vena cava is usually part of the scimitar syndrome.

Cor Triatriatum

Cor triatriatum (sinistrum) results when the junction between the common pulmonary vein and the left atrium is stenotic. A fenestrated membranous or muscular shelf subdivides the left atrium into a posterosuperior chamber, which receives the pulmonary veins, and an anteroinferior chamber, which contains the atrial appendage and mitral orifice.

- Mediastinal neoplasms, fibrosis, and aortic aneurysms may compress the thin-walled veins and result in the superior vena cava syndrome.
- The inferior vena cava may become trapped and compressed between the vertebral column posteriorly and either an adjacent retroperitoneal structure or an intraperitoneal structure and thereby produce the inferior vena cava syndrome.
- The thin-walled, low-pressure pulmonary veins may be compressed extrinsically by mediastinal neoplasms or fibrosis.
- Connection of one (usually the upper) or both right pulmonary veins to the right atrium commonly accompanies sinus venosus atrial septal defects.

Cardiac Chambers

Right Atrium

The right atrium and the superior vena cava form the right lateral border of the frontal chest radiographic cardiac silhouette. The right atrium receives the systemic venous return from the superior and inferior venae cavae and receives most of the coronary venous return via the coronary sinus and numerous small thebesian veins. The ostium of the inferior vena cava is bordered anteriorly by a crescentic eustachian valve, which may be large and fenestrated and form a so-called Chiari network. The coronary sinus ostium is partly shielded by a fenestrated thebesian valve. The right atrium free wall has a smooth-walled posterior portion, which receives the caval and coronary sinus blood flow, and a muscular anterolateral portion, which contains ridge-like pectinate muscles and a large pyramid-shaped appendage. Separating the two regions is a prominent C-shaped muscle bundle, the crista terminalis (or terminal crest). The right atrial appendage abuts the right aortic sinus and overlies the proximal right coronary artery.

The thickness of the right atrial free wall varies considerably. The atrial wall between the pectinate muscles is paper-thin and can be perforated by a stiff catheter.

With atrial enlargement and blood flow stasis, mural thrombi may form within the recesses between the pectinate muscles, particularly in the atrial appendage. Indwelling cardiac catheters or pacemaker wires tend to injure the endocardium at the cavoatrial junction and are often associated with shallow linear mural thrombi. An atrial pacing lead can be inserted into the muscle bundles within the appendage.

Atrial Septum

The atrial septum has interatrial and atrioventricular components (Fig. 2). The interatrial portion contains the fossa ovalis (or oval fossa), which includes an arch-shaped outer muscular rim (the limbus or limb) and a central fibrous membrane (the valve). The foramen ovale (or oval foramen, which is patent throughout fetal life) represents a potential interatrial shunt, which courses between the anterosuperior limbic rim and the valve of the fossa ovalis and then through the natural valvular perforation (ostium secundum or second ostium) into the left atrium. In approximately two-

thirds of subjects, the foramen ovale closes anatomically during the first year of life as the valve of the fossa ovalis becomes permanently sealed to the limbus. In the remaining third, this flap-valve closes functionally only when left atrial pressure exceeds right atrial pressure; this constitutes a so-called valvular-competent (or probe-patent) patent foramen ovale (Fig. 3). If right atrial pressure exceeds left atrial pressure, as in right heart failure or during the Valsalva maneuver, right-to-left shunting will occur.

Through a patent foramen ovale, systemic venous emboli may enter the systemic arterial circulation. Such paradoxical emboli may be thrombotic (e.g., from the legs) or nonthrombotic (e.g., air emboli).

Pronounced atrial dilatation may so stretch the atrial septum that the limbus no longer covers the ostium secundum in the valve of the fossa ovalis. As a result, interatrial shunting may occur across the valvular-incompetent patent foramen ovale. In some subjects, aneurysms of the valve of the fossa ovalis may develop and may undulate during the cardiac cycle. Atrial dilatation stimulates the release of natriuretic peptide.

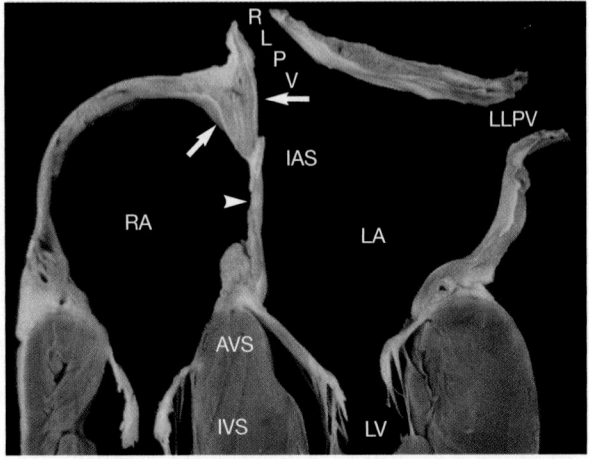

Fig. 2. Atrial anatomy with tricuspid and mitral valves in profile. The atrioventricular septum is anterior to the interatrial septum and posterior to the interventricular septum; note also the infolded nature of the limbus (*arrows*) and the relative thinness of the valve of the fossa ovalis (*arrowhead*). The origin of the normal tricuspid valve is below that of the mitral valve, allowing the possibility of a right atrial–to–left ventricular shunt. (Four-chamber view from 15-year-old boy.) (See Appendix at end of chapter for abbreviations.)

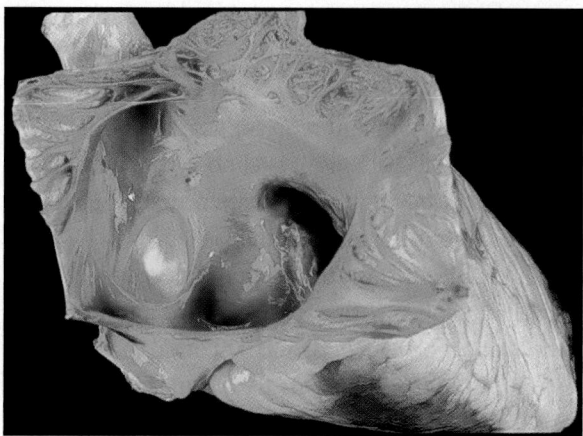

Fig. 3. Thin wall of foramen ovale (transilluminated).

The atrioventricular component of the atrial septum, which separates the right atrium from the left ventricle, is primarily muscular but also has a small fibrous component (the atrioventricular portion of the membranous septum) (Fig. 2).

Triangle of Koch

The atrioventricular septum corresponds to the triangle of Koch, an important anatomical landmark that contains the atrioventricular node (Fig. 4); it is bound by the septal tricuspid anulus, the coronary sinus ostium, and the tendon of Todaro.

Tendon of Todaro

The tendon of Todaro is a subendocardial fibrous cord that extends from the eustachian-thebesian valvular commissure to the anteroseptal tricuspid commissure (at the membranous septum); it very roughly corresponds to the level of the mitral anulus.

The thickness of the atrial septum varies considerably. The valve of the fossa ovalis is a paper-thin translucent membrane at birth but becomes more fibrotic with time and may achieve a thickness of 1 to 2 mm. The limbus of the fossa ovalis ranges from 4 to 8 mm in thickness; however, lipomatous hypertrophy may produce a bulging mass more than three times this thickness. The muscular atrioventricular septum forms the summit of the ventricular septum and may range from 5 to 10 mm in thickness; this may be greatly increased in the setting of hypertrophic cardiomyopathy or concentric left ventricular hypertrophy. The membranous septum generally is less than 1 mm thick.

Left Atrium

The left atrium, a posterior midline chamber, receives pulmonary venous blood and expels it across the mitral orifice and into the left ventricle. The esophagus and descending thoracic aorta abut the left atrial wall. Thus, the left atrium, atrial septum, and mitral valve are particularly well visualized with transesophageal echocardiography. The body of the left atrium does not contribute to the frontal cardiac silhouette; however, the left atrial appendage, when enlarged, may form the portion of the left cardiac border between the left ventricle and the pulmonary trunk. Normally the appendage, shaped like a windsock, abuts the pulmonary artery and overlies the bifurcation of the left main coronary artery.

With chronic obstruction to left atrial emptying (e.g., rheumatic mitral stenosis), the dilated left atrium may shift the atrial septum rightward and in severe cases may actually form the right cardiac border on chest x-ray films. Moreover, the esophagus can be shifted rightward, and the left bronchus may be elevated. Mural thrombi often develop within the atrial appendage or, less commonly, the atrial body, and in severe cases can virtually fill the chamber except for small channels leading from the pulmonary veins to the mitral orifice. In contrast to left atrial mural thrombi, which tend to involve the free wall, most myxomas arise from the left side of the atrial septum.

Comparison of Atria

The right atrial free wall contains a crista terminalis and pectinate muscles, whereas the left atrial free wall

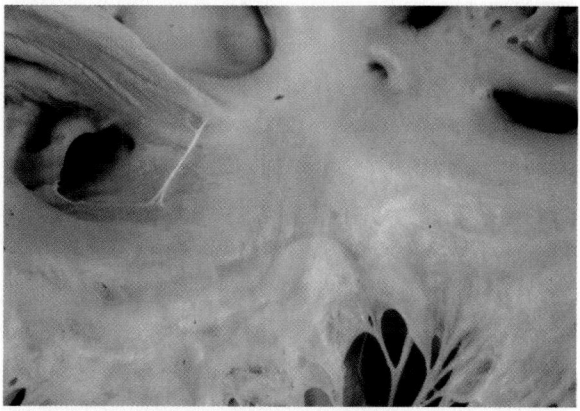

Fig. 4. Position of atrioventricular node (triangle of Koch).

has neither. The right atrial appendage is large and pyramidal, in contrast to the windsock-like left atrial appendage. Finally, the atrial septum is characterized by the fossa ovalis on the right side and by the ostium secundum on the left (Fig. 5).

Owing to hemodynamic streaming within the right atrium during intrauterine life, superior vena caval blood is directed toward the tricuspid orifice, and inferior vena caval blood, carrying well-oxygenated placental blood, is directed by the eustachian valve toward the foramen ovale. As a result, the most-well-oxygenated blood in the fetal circulation is directed, via the left heart, to the coronary arteries, the upper extremities, and the brain. Even postnatally, the superior vena cava maintains its orientation toward the tricuspid anulus, and the inferior vena cava maintains its orientation toward the atrial septum (Fig. 6).

Consequently, an endomyocardial biopsy specimen of the right ventricular apex is much more easily obtained via a superior vena caval approach than via an inferior vena caval approach. In contrast, the passage of a catheter from the right atrium into the left atrium via the foramen ovale is much more easily performed via an inferior vena caval approach. In subjects in whom the foramen ovale is anatomically sealed, the valve of the fossa ovalis may be intentionally perforated (transseptal approach); however, this membrane becomes thicker and more fibrotic with age.

Atrial Septal Defect
A secundum atrial septal defect involves the fossa ovalis region of the interatrial septum. It is the most common form of atrial septal defect and often is an isolated anomaly.

A primum atrial septal defect involves the atrioventricular septum and represents a malformation of the endocardial cushions; it is almost invariably associated with mitral and tricuspid abnormalities, particularly a cleft in the anterior mitral leaflet.

A sinus venosus atrial septal defect involves the posterior aspect of the atrial septum and is usually associated with an anomalous right atrial connection of the right pulmonary veins. A coronary sinus atrial septal defect is usually associated with an absent (unroofed) coronary sinus and connection of the left superior vena cava to the left atrium.

- Most myxomas arise from the left side of the atrial septum.
- A secundum atrial septal defect involves the fossa ovalis region of the interatrial septum.
- A coronary sinus atrial septal defect is usually associated with an absent coronary sinus and connection of the left superior vena cava to the left atrium.

Right Ventricle
The right ventricle does not contribute to the borders of the frontal cardiac silhouette radiographically. It is crescent-shaped in short-axis and triangular-shaped when viewed in long-axis (Fig. 7).

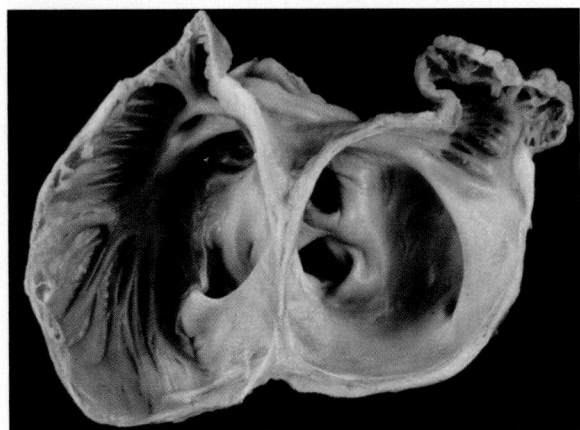

Fig. 5. Normal atria.

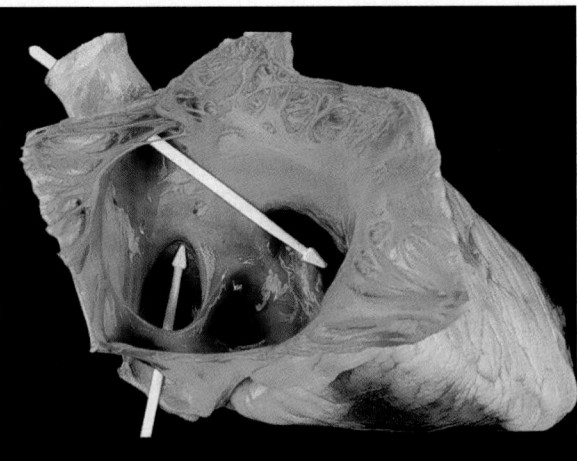

Fig. 6. Right atrial hemodynamic streaming. Superior vena caval blood is directed toward the tricuspid orifice, and inferior vena caval blood is directed toward the fossa ovalis. (Opened right atrium from 31-year-old man.)

Conditions, such as pulmonary hypertension, that impose a pressure overload on the right ventricle cause straightening of the ventricular septum such that both ventricles attain a "D" shape on cross-section. In extreme cases, such as Ebstein anomaly or total anomalous pulmonary venous connection, leftward bowing of the ventricular septum may result not only in a circular right ventricle and crescentic left ventricle but also in possible obstruction of the left ventricular outflow tract.

The right ventricular chamber consists of three regions—inlet, trabecular, and outlet. The inlet region receives the tricuspid valve and its cordal and papillary muscle attachments. A complex meshwork of muscle bundles characterizes the anteroapical trabecular region. In contrast, the outlet region is smoother-walled and is also known as the infundibulum, conus, or right ventricular outflow tract. Along the outflow tract, an arch of muscle separates the tricuspid and pulmonary valves. The arch consists of a parietal band, outlet septum, and septal band, known collectively as the crista supraventricularis (supraventricular crest).

During right ventricular endomyocardial biopsy, the bioptome is directed septally, not only to avoid injury to the cardiac conduction system and tricuspid apparatus but also to prevent possible perforation of the relatively thin free wall. Tissue is more often procured from the meshwork of apical trabeculations than from the septal surface per se. When permanent transvenous pacemaker electrodes are inserted into the right ventricle, the apical trabeculations trap the tined tip and thereby prevent dislodgment.

During vigorous cardiopulmonary resuscitation in which ribs are fractured, the jagged bones may be forced through the parietal pericardium anteriorly and may lacerate an epicardial coronary artery or may perforate the right atrial or right or left ventricular free wall. Furthermore, if the force of closed chest cardiac massage during cardiopulmonary resuscitation is at the midsternum rather than the xiphoid area, the right ventricular outflow tract may be compressed; the resultant high right ventricular pressure may cause apical rupture.

Left Ventricle

The left ventricle forms the left border of the frontal cardiac silhouette radiographically. It is circular in short-axis views and is approximated in three dimensions by a truncated ellipsoid.

Pressure Overload

Conditions such as aortic stenosis and chronic hypertension, which impose a pressure overload on the left ventricle, induce concentric left ventricular hypertrophy without appreciable dilatation. Although the short-axis chamber diameter does not increase significantly, the wall thickness generally increases 25% to 75%, and the heart may double or triple in weight.

Volume Overload

Disorders that impose a volume overload on the left ventricle, such as chronic aortic or mitral regurgitation or dilated cardiomyopathy, are attended not only by hypertrophy but also by chamber dilatation. They thereby produce a globoid heart with increased base-apex and short-axis dimensions. Although the heart weight may double or triple, the left ventricular wall thickness generally remains within the normal range because of the thinning effect of dilatation. Accordingly, when the left ventricle is dilated, wall thickness cannot be used as a reliable indicator of hypertrophy. The term *volume hypertrophy* is favored in this situation. Hypertrophy, with or without chamber dilatation, decreases myocardial compliance and impairs diastolic filling.

Like the right ventricle, the left ventricle can be divided into inlet, apical, and outlet regions. The inlet receives the mitral valve apparatus, the apex contains fine trabeculations, and the outlet is angled away from

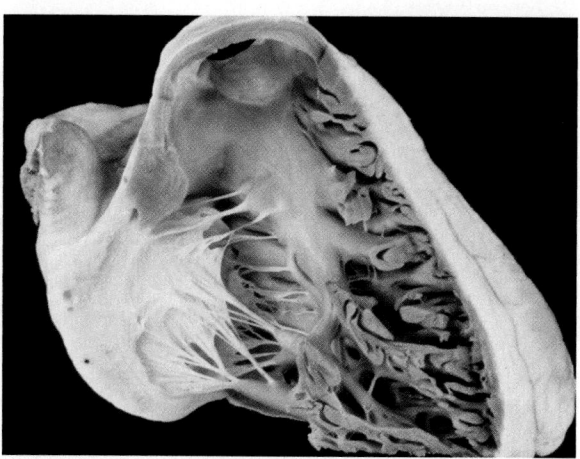

Fig. 7. Right ventricle, showing marked trabeculation and tricuspid valve.

the remainder of the chamber. Inflow and outflow tracts are separated by the anterior mitral leaflet, which forms an intracavitary curtain between the two.

The anterior mitral leaflet is also in direct contact, at its anulus, with the left and posterior aortic valve cusps. For comparison, the membranous septum (Fig. 8) abuts the right and posterior aortic cusps, and the outlet septum lies beneath the right and left aortic cusps.

For practical purposes, the base-apex length of the left ventricle is divided into thirds—basal (corresponding to the mitral leaflets and tendinous cords), midventricular (corresponding to the mitral papillary muscles), and apical levels. Each level is then further divided into segments, thus forming the basis for regional analysis of the left ventricle (e.g., the evaluation of regional wall motion abnormalities) (Fig. 9 and Table 1).

Hypertrophic cardiomyopathy is characterized by asymmetric (nonconcentric) left ventricular hypertrophy that disproportionately involves the septum. Cardiac amyloid may mimic hypertrophic cardiomyopathy.

In the normal elderly heart, left ventricular geometry is altered (the septum is more sigmoid in shape) and in concert with mild fibrosis and calcification of the aortic and mitral valves may contribute to the low-grade systolic ejection murmurs that are so common in the elderly. With advancing age, the aortic anulus dilates appreciably and tilts rightward and less posteriorly, thereby altering the shape and direction of the left ventricular outflow tract, which may simulate

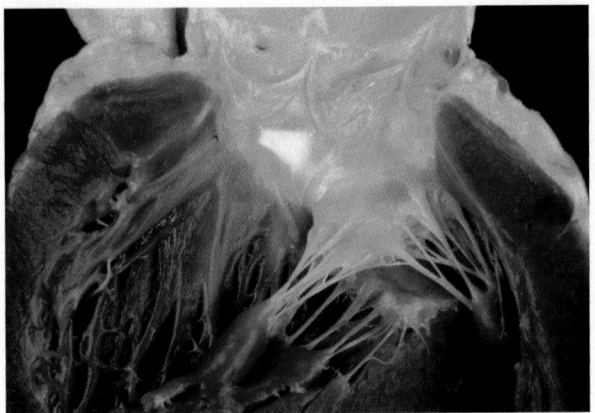

Fig. 8. Left ventricle with thin-walled membranous septum transilluminated.

hypertrophic cardiomyopathy.

Left ventricular trabeculae carneae are small, and permanent apical entrapment of a tined transvenous pacemaker electrode is difficult to achieve and may necessitate the placement of epicardial electrodes (e.g., in patients with corrected transposition of the great

Table 1.   Percentage of Regional Left Ventricular (LV) Mass

Level	% LV volume per segment	No. of segments	Total, %
Basal	7.2	6	43
Middle	6.0	6	36
Apical	5.3	4	21

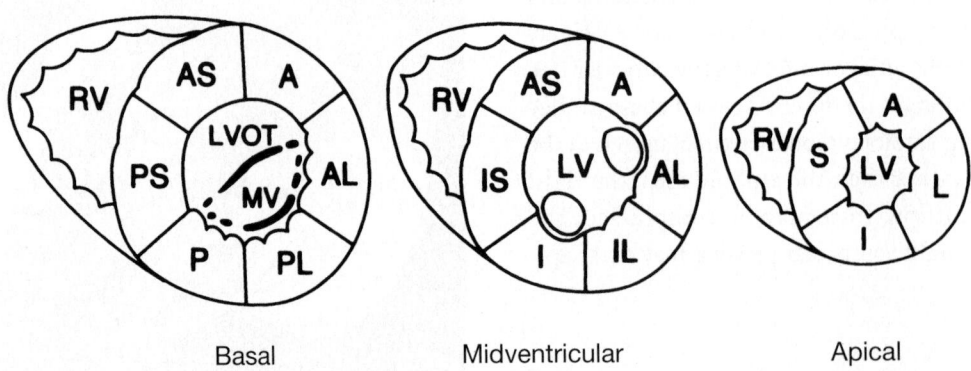

Basal   Midventricular   Apical

Fig. 9. Regional analysis of the left ventricle. Short-axis views show the recommended 16-segment system. (See Appendix at end of chapter for abbreviations.)

arteries or with complete transposition of the great arteries and a previous Mustard or Senning operation).

When left ventricular endomyocardial biopsy is performed, care must be taken not to injure the mitral apparatus or left bundle branch and not to perforate the apex (Fig. 10).

In some persons, apical or anteroseptal trabeculae carneae may form a prominent spongy meshwork that may be misinterpreted as apical mural thrombus on imaging studies.

Comparison of Ventricles

Normally, left ventricular wall thickness is three to four times that of the right ventricle. In short-axis, the left ventricle is circular and the right is crescentic. Whereas the tricuspid and pulmonary valves are separated from one another, the mitral and aortic valves are in direct continuity. The right ventricular apex is much more heavily trabeculated than the left.

By two-dimensional echocardiography, ventricular morphology is best inferred from the morphology of the atrioventricular valves, particularly by differences in their anular levels at the cardiac crux.

Ventricular Septal Defect

The most common ventricular septal defect, either isolated or associated with other cardiac anomalies, is the membranous (perimembranous) type, which involves the membranous septum. An infundibular (also called outlet, supracristal, or subarterial) ventricular septal defect is commonly encountered in tetralogy of Fallot

and truncus arteriosus. A malalignment ventricular septal defect occurs when one of the great arteries overrides the septum and attains biventricular origin, or both great arteries arise from one ventricle. Muscular defects involve the muscular septum and can be solitary or multiple (so-called Swiss cheese septum). A defect of the atrioventricular septum is considered to be an atrioventricular canal defect, and straddling of an atrioventricular valve most commonly occurs across a defect of this type.

Tetralogy of Fallot

Within the spectrum of cyanotic congenital heart disease is a group of anomalies that share in common a maldevelopment of the conotruncal septum. Tetralogy of Fallot, the most common anomaly in this group, results from displacement of the infundibular septum and is characterized by a large malalignment ventricular septal defect, an overriding aorta, and variable degrees of infundibular and valvular pulmonary stenosis. When the pulmonary valve is atretic, pulmonary blood flow may come from the ductus arteriosus or systemic collateral arteries.

Transposition of the Great Arteries

Complete transposition of the great arteries is associated with abnormal conotruncal septation and parallel rather than intertwined great arteries, such that the aorta arises from the right ventricle and the pulmonary artery emanates from the left ventricle; a ventricular septal defect is present in about one-third of cases.

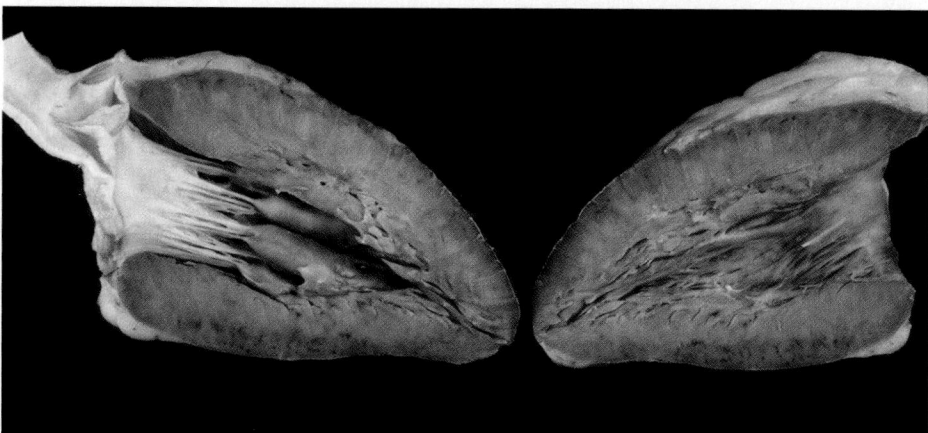

Fig. 10. Left ventricle (free wall and septum) with mitral valve and papillary muscles on free wall.

Truncus Arteriosus

Truncus arteriosus implies absent conotruncal septation and is characterized by a single arterial trunk from which the aorta, pulmonary arteries, and coronary arteries arise; the ventricular septal defect is of the membranous or infundibular type.

Double-Outlet Right Ventricle

Double-outlet right ventricle is characterized by the origin of both great arteries from the right ventricle, a malalignment ventricular septal defect, and infundibular septal displacement that differs from the type observed in tetralogy of Fallot.

Myocyte Response to Injury

Myocardial cells are by volume one-half contractile elements and one-third mitochondria. They are exquisitely sensitive to oxygen deprivation, and ischemia represents the most common form of myocardial injury. Other injurious agents include viruses, chemicals, and excessive cardiac workload (volume or pressure).

The heart has only a limited response to stress or injury. Adaptive responses include hypertrophy and dilatation, whereas sublethal cellular injury is characterized by various degenerative changes. Necrosis is the histologic hallmark of lethal cellular injury, and it elicits an inflammatory response with subsequent healing by scar formation.

Hypertrophy of cardiac muscle cells is accompanied by degenerative changes, an increase in interstitial collagen, and a decrease in ventricular compliance. In dilated hearts, hypertrophied myocytes are also stretched, but with relatively normal diameters. In dilated hearts, the best histologic indicators of hypertrophy are nuclear alterations.

Acute myocardial ischemia is characterized by intense sarcoplasmic staining with eosin dyes, prominent sarcoplasmic contraction bands, and, occasionally, stretched and wavy myocardial cells. When ischemic cells are irreversibly injured, the changes of coagulative necrosis appear. Nuclei fade away (karyolysis) or fragment (karyorrhexis), and the sarcoplasm develops a glassy homogeneous appearance, although in many cases the cross-striations remain intact for several days. Necrotic myocardium elicits an inflammatory infiltrate of neutrophils and macrophages, which serves histologically to differentiate acute infarction from acute ischemia. Because myocardial cells have a very limited ability to replicate, healing is by organization, with scar formation.

CARDIAC VALVES

Atrioventricular Valves

The right (tricuspid) and left (mitral) atrioventricular valves have five components, three of which form the valvular apparatus (anulus, leaflets and commissures) and two of which form the tensor apparatus (chordae tendineae and papillary muscles).

Valve Anulus

The anulus of each atrioventricular valve is saddle-shaped. As part of the fibrous cardiac skeleton at the base of the heart, each anulus electrically insulates atrium from ventricle. Since the tricuspid anulus is an incomplete fibrous ring, loose connective tissue maintains insulation at the points of fibrous discontinuity. The mitral anulus, in contrast, constitutes a continuous ring of fibrous tissue.

Valve Leaflet

The valve leaflets are delicate fibrous tissue flaps that close the anatomical valvular orifice during ventricular systole (Fig. 11). The leading edge of each leaflet is its free edge, and its serrated appearance results from direct cordal insertions into this border. The closing edge, in contrast, represents a slightly thickened nodular ridge several millimeters above the free edge. When the valve closes, apposing leaflets contact one another along their closing edges, and interdigitation of these nodular ridges ensures a competent seal. Each leaflet comprises two major layers—namely, the fibrosa, which forms the strong structural backbone of the valve, and the spongiosa, which acts as a shock absorber along the atrial surface, particularly at the closing edge (rough zone), where one leaflet coapts with an adjacent leaflet.

Chordae Tendineae

The chordae tendineae are strong, fibrous tendinous cords that act as guidewires to anchor and support the leaflets. They restrict excessive valvular excursion during ventricular systole and thereby prevent valvular

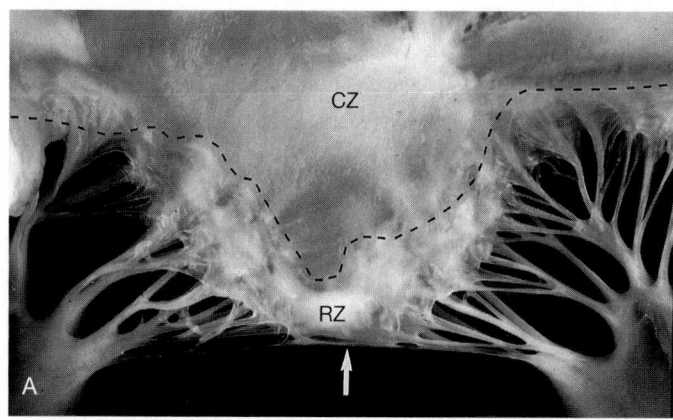
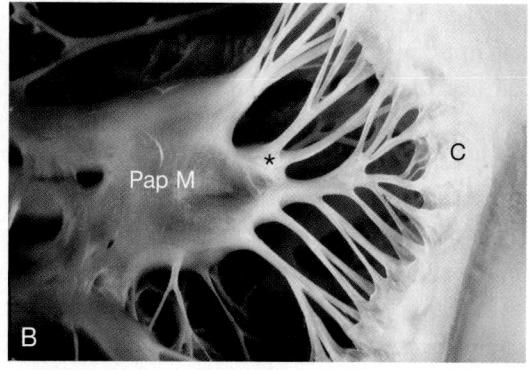

Fig. 11. Components of an atrioventricular valve (from the mitral valve of an 8-year-old girl). *A*, Each leaflet has a large clear zone (CZ) and a smaller rough zone (RZ) between its free edge (*arrow*) and closing edge (*dashed line*). *B*, Each commissure (C) separates two leaflets and overlies a papillary muscle (Pap M); a fan-like commissural tendinous cord (*) connects the tip of the papillary muscle to the commissure.

prolapse into the atria. Most tendinous cords branch one or more times, so that generally more than 100 cords insert into the free edge of each atrioventricular valve. By virtue of these numerous cordal insertions, the force of systolic ventricular blood is evenly distributed throughout the undersurface of each leaflet.

Papillary Muscles

The papillary muscles, which may have multiple heads, are conical mounds of ventricular muscle that receive the majority of the tendinous cords (Fig. 12). Because of their position directly beneath a commissure, each papillary muscle receives cords from two adjacent leaflets. As a result, papillary muscle contraction tends to pull the two leaflets toward each other and thereby facilitates valve closure.

In the elderly, mild mitral anular dilatation may occur, with or without atrial dilatation. Leaflets become thicker, with increasing nodularity of the rough zone and with mild hooding deformity of the entire leaflet. Contributing to the latter is a decrease in ventricular base-apex length, which makes the thickened cords appear relatively longer than necessary, thus simulating mitral valve prolapse.

Tricuspid Valve

The plane of the tricuspid anulus faces toward the right ventricular apex. Along the free wall, the anulus inserts into the atrioventricular junction, whereas along

the septum, it separates the atrioventricular and interventricular portions of the septum.

In living subjects, the tricuspid annular circumference varies with the cardiac cycle: it is maximum during ventricular diastole (about 11 cm^2) and decreases by about 30% during ventricular systole. The reduction in area is due to contraction of the underlying basal right ventricular myocardium, since the incomplete tricuspid anulus cannot adequately constrict by itself.

The three tricuspid leaflets are not always well separated from one another. The septal (medial) leaflet lies parallel to the ventricular septum, and the posterior (inferior) leaflet lies parallel to the diaphragmatic

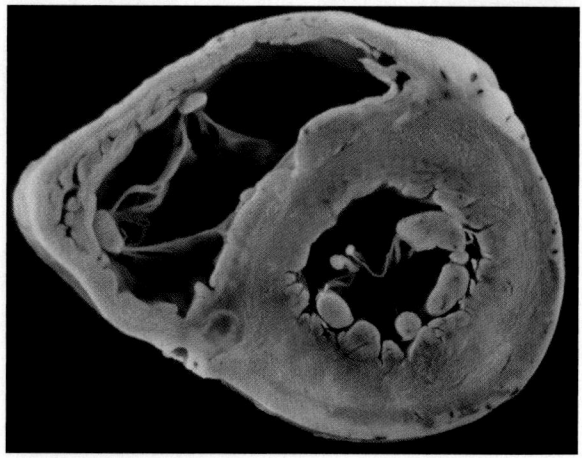

Fig. 12. Mitral valve papillary muscles (short-axis).

aspect of the right ventricular free wall. In contrast, the anterior (anterosuperior) tricuspid leaflet forms a large sail-like intracavitary curtain that partially separates the inflow tract from the outflow tract.

Because of differences in leaflet size and cordal length, the excursion of the posterior and septal leaflets is less than that of the anterior leaflet. In the setting of anular dilatation, leaflet excursion is inadequate to effect central coaptation, and valvular incompetence results. Because the tricuspid anulus is incomplete, and because the basal right ventricular myocardium forms a subjacent muscular ring, dilatation of the right ventricle commonly produces anular dilatation and tricuspid regurgitation. Right atrial dilatation alone, as in constrictive pericarditis, usually does not cause significant tricuspid insufficiency.

Valvular incompetence also may be observed in conditions that limit leaflet and cordal excursion, such as rheumatic disease (fibrosis and scar retraction), carcinoid endocardial plaques (thickening and retraction), and eosinophilic endomyocardial diseases (thrombotic adherence to the underlying myocardium). In normal hearts, mild degrees of tricuspid regurgitation commonly exist.

Tricuspid stenosis involves commissural and cordal fusion and may occur in rheumatic or carcinoid heart disease.

Mitral Valve

Mitral Anulus

The plane of the mitral anulus faces toward the left ventricular apex (Fig. 13). The orifice changes shape during the cardiac cycle, from elliptical during ventricular systole to more circular during diastole. In living subjects, the normal mitral anular circumference is maximal during ventricular diastole (about 7 cm^2) and decreases 10% to 15% during systole.

Mitral anular calcification almost invariably involves only the posterior mitral leaflet and forms a C-shaped ring of anular and subanular calcium which may impede basal ventricular contraction and thereby produce mitral regurgitation. Similarly, inadequate basal ventricular contraction may contribute to valvular incompetence in the setting of pronounced left ventricular dilatation; however, because only part of the mitral anulus is in direct contact with the basal ventricular myocardium, dilatation of the ventricle rarely increases anular circumference more than 25%.

Secondary left atrial dilatation may contribute to the progression of preexisting mitral incompetence by displacing the posterior leaflet and its anulus and thereby hindering the excursion of this taut leaflet (Fig. 14).

Mitral Leaflets

The mitral leaflets form a continuous funnel-shaped veil with two prominent indentations, the anterolateral and posteromedial commissures. Although the two commissures do not extend entirely to the anulus, they effectively separate the two leaflets. In contrast to the

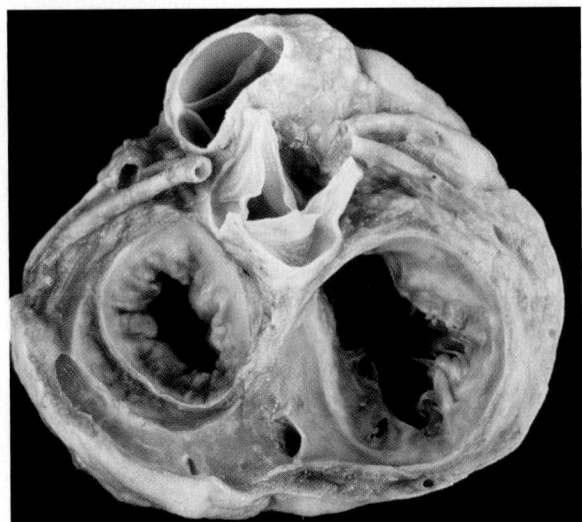

Fig. 13. Four valves at base of heart.

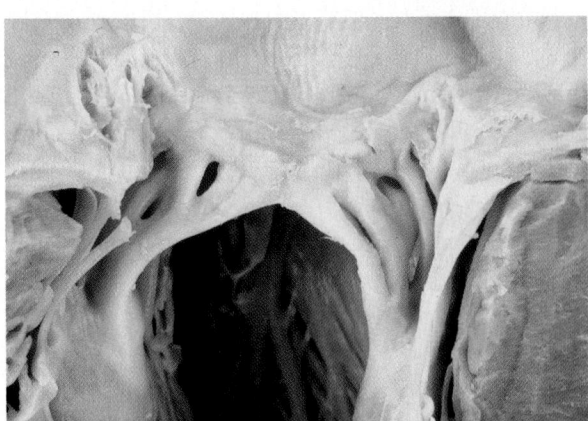

Fig. 14. Valve fibrosis in rheumatic mitral stenosis.

three other cardiac valves, which each comprise three leaflets or cusps, the mitral valve has only two leaflets. At midleaflet level, the mitral orifice is elliptical or football-shaped, and its long axis aligns with the two commissures and their papillary muscles.

Although the anterior leaflet occupies only about 35% of the anular circumference, its leaflet area is almost identical to the area of the posterior leaflet, about 5 cm². The total mitral leaflet surface area is 10 cm², nearly twice that necessary to close the systolic anular orifice, 5.2 cm². However, some folding of leaflet tissue is needed to ensure a competent seal, and the normal leaflets are not as redundant as they might appear (Fig. 15 and 16).

The myxomatous (or floppy) mitral valve is characterized by anular dilatation, stretched tendinous cords, and redundant hooded folds of leaflet tissue, which are prone to prolapse, incomplete coaptation, cordal rupture, and mitral regurgitation. In contrast, rheumatic mitral insufficiency results from scar retraction of leaflets and cords. In the setting of infective endocarditis, virulent organisms may perforate the leaflet tissue and produce acute mitral regurgitation. In hypertrophic cardiomyopathy, the anterior mitral leaflet contacts the ventricular septum during systole and contributes both to left ventricular outflow tract obstruction and to mitral incompetence.

In chronic aortic insufficiency, the regurgitant stream may strike the anterior mitral leaflet and produce not only a fibrotic jet lesion but also the leaflet flutter and premature valve closure that are so characteristic echocardiographically.

Papillary Muscles

A fan-shaped cord emanates from the tip of each of the two papillary muscles and inserts into its overlying commissure and into both adjacent leaflets (Fig. 11 *B*). Similarly, a smaller commissural cord inserts into each minor commissure between their posterior scallops. Two particularly prominent cords insert along each half of the ventricular surface of the anterior mitral leaflet, and these so-called strut cords offer additional support for this mid-cavitary leaflet that also forms part of the wall of the left ventricular outflow tract. Cordal length is generally 1 to 2 cm.

Rheumatic mitral stenosis is characterized by cordal and commissural fusions, which obliterate the secondary intercordal orifices and narrow the primary valve orifice. Cordal rupture may occur in a myxomatous (floppy) valve, an infected valve, or, rarely, an apparently normal valve and lead to acute mitral regurgitation.

The mitral papillary muscles occupy the middle third of the left ventricular base-apex length. Two prominent muscles originate from the anterolateral and posteromedial (inferomedial) free wall, beneath their respective mitral commissures. Trabeculations not only anchor the papillary muscles but also may form a muscle bridge between the two papillary groups and thereby contribute to valve closure.

The anterolateral muscle is a single structure with a midline groove in 70% to 85% of cases, whereas the posteromedial muscle is multiple or is bifid or trifid in 60% to 70%. The anterolateral muscle is generally larger and extends closer to the anulus than the postero-

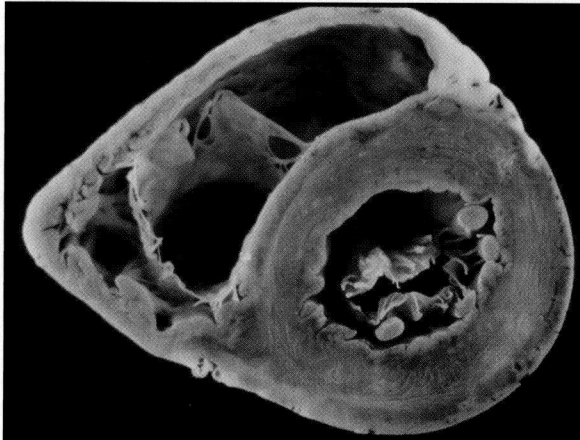

Fig. 15. Mitral valve leaflets and cords (short-axis).

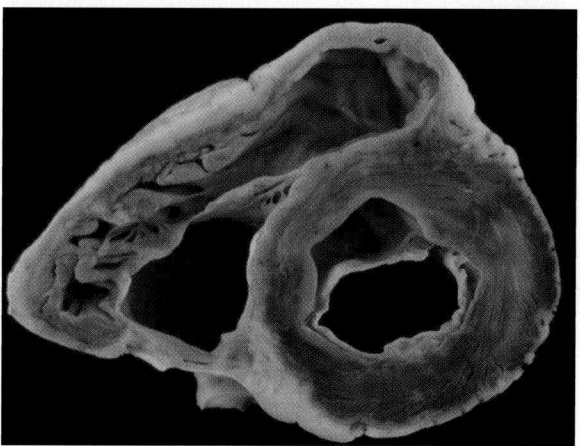

Fig. 16. Mitral valve leaflets and anulus (short-axis).

medial muscle. Occasionally, an accessory papillary muscle is interposed between the two major muscles along the free wall. No papillary muscles or tendinous cords originate from the septum and terminate on the mitral leaflets. However, in about 50% of subjects, one or more cord-like structures, known as left ventricular false tendons, or pseudotendons, arise from a papillary muscle and insert either onto the septal surface or onto the opposite papillary muscle.

Chronic postinfarction mitral regurgitation is associated with papillary muscle atrophy and scarring, thinning and scarring of the subjacent left ventricular free wall, and left ventricular dilatation. Acute postinfarction mitral regurgitation may be associated with rupture of a papillary muscle (almost invariably the posteromedial) and can involve the entire muscle or only one of its multiple heads.

Competent function of the mitral valve requires the harmonious interaction of all valvular components, including the left atrium and left ventricle.

- Right atrial dilatation alone usually does not cause significant tricuspid insufficiency.
- In normal hearts, mild degrees of tricuspid regurgitation commonly exist.
- Secondary left atrial dilatation may contribute to the progression of preexisting mitral incompetence.
- In hypertrophic cardiomyopathy, the anterior mitral leaflet may contact the ventricular septum during systole and contribute both to left ventricular outflow tract obstruction and to mitral incompetence.
- Chronic postinfarction mitral incompetence is associated with papillary muscle atrophy and scarring.

Semilunar Valves

The right (pulmonary) and left (aortic) semilunar valves, in contrast to the atrioventricular valves, have no tensor apparatus and, therefore, are structurally simpler valves (Fig. 17). They consist of anulus, cusps, and commissures. Behind each cusp is an outpouching of the arterial root, known as a sinus (of Valsalva). There are three aortic sinuses and three pulmonary sinuses, which impart a cloverleaf shape to the arterial roots.

The anuli of the semilunar valves are part of the fibrous cardiac skeleton. They are nonplanar structures, shaped like a triradiate crown.

The cusps are half-moon–shaped (semilunar),

pocket-like flaps of delicate fibrous tissue which close the valvular orifice during ventricular diastole. The leading edge of each cusp is its free edge. The closing edge, in contrast, represents a slightly thickened ridge that lies a few millimeters below the free edge, along the ventricular surface of the cusp. At the center of each cusp, the closing edge meets the free edge and forms a small fibrous mound, the nodule of Arantius. When the valve closes, apposing cusps contact one another along the surfaces between their free and closing edges (i.e., the lunular areas), forming a competent seal.

Like the atrioventricular valves, the semilunar valves contain two major layers histologically. The fibrosa forms the structural backbone of the valve and is continuous with the anulus, whereas the spongiosa acts more like a shock absorber along the ventricular surface, especially at the closing edge. Cusps contain little elastic tissue and, accordingly, have no appreciable elastic recoil. The opening and closing of the semilunar valves is a passive process that entails cusp excursion and anulocuspid hinge-like motion.

In the elderly, degenerative changes in the aortic valve may result in low-grade systolic ejection murmurs. The closing edges become thickened and, along the nodules of Arantius, may form whisker-like projections called Lambl's excrescences. Lunular fenestrations also tend to develop with increasing age.

Disease processes that tend to increase cusp rigidity, such as fibrosis or calcification, or that lead to commissural fusion, such as rheumatic valvulitis, tend to

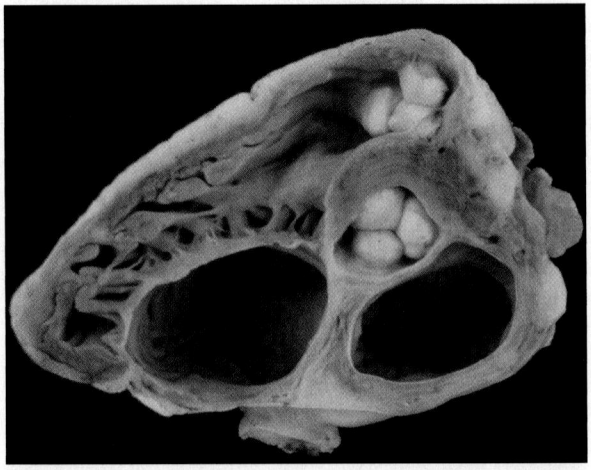

Fig. 17. Aortic valve and pulmonary valve (from below).

narrow the effective valvular orifice and, as a consequence, produce stenosis. In contrast, processes that straighten the cuspid line between commissures and thereby hold the commissures open, such as arterial root dilatation or rheumatic cuspid scar retraction, tend to produce regurgitation.

Pulmonary Valve

The plane of the pulmonary anulus faces toward the left mid-scapula, with an area of about 3.5 cm2 (Fig. 18). The cusps are usually similar in size, although minor variations are commonly observed.

Pulmonary incompetence occurs in conditions that produce dilatation of the pulmonary artery and anulus, such as pulmonary hypertension or heart failure. Combined pulmonary stenosis and incompetence are features of carcinoid heart disease, in which the anulus becomes constricted and stenotic and in which the cusps are also retracted and insufficient. Pure pulmonary stenosis is almost always congenital in origin.

Aortic Valve

The plane of the aortic valve faces the right shoulder. In the living subject, the normal aortic anular area averages about 3 cm2 (Fig. 19).

Unoperated symptomatic aortic stenosis has a worse prognosis than many malignancies. The vast majority of stenotic aortic valves are calcified. Most commonly, the valve represents either degenerative (senile) calcification or a calcified congenitally bicuspid

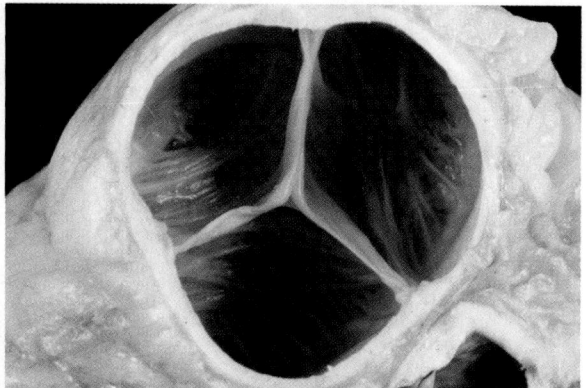

Fig. 18. Pulmonary valve.

valve (Fig. 20). Only rarely are heavily calcified valves the site of active infective endocarditis.

Aortic root dilatation stretches open the commissures and thereby produces aortic insufficiency in either a tricuspid or a bicuspid aortic valve. Acute aortic regurgitation may be produced by infective aortic endocarditis with cuspid perforation or by acute aortic dissection with commissural prolapse. Chronic aortic regurgitation with coexistent aortic stenosis is most commonly associated with postrheumatic cuspid retraction, which yields a fixed triangular orifice.

Among cases of infective endocarditis, perhaps none present so varied a clinical spectrum as those associated with aortic anular abscesses. The possible clinical presentations depend to a great extent on the particular cusp(s) involved. Subvalvular extension may

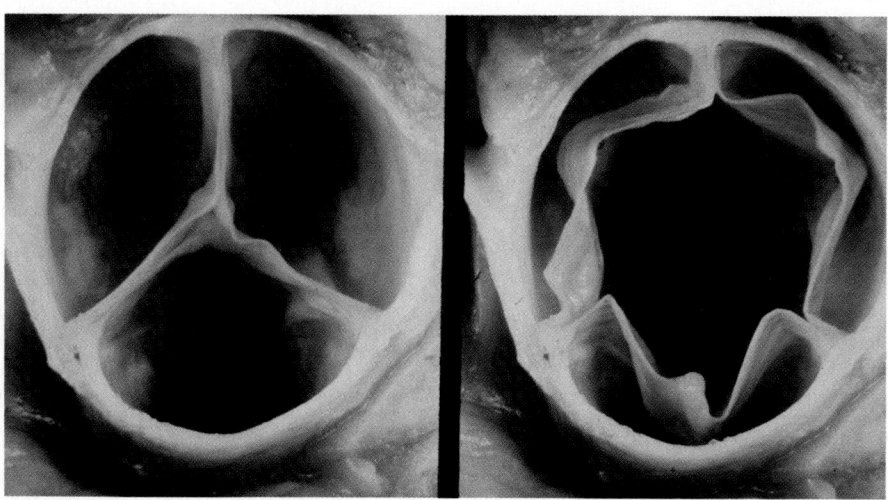

Fig. 19. Normal aortic valve, closed (*left*) and opened (*right*).

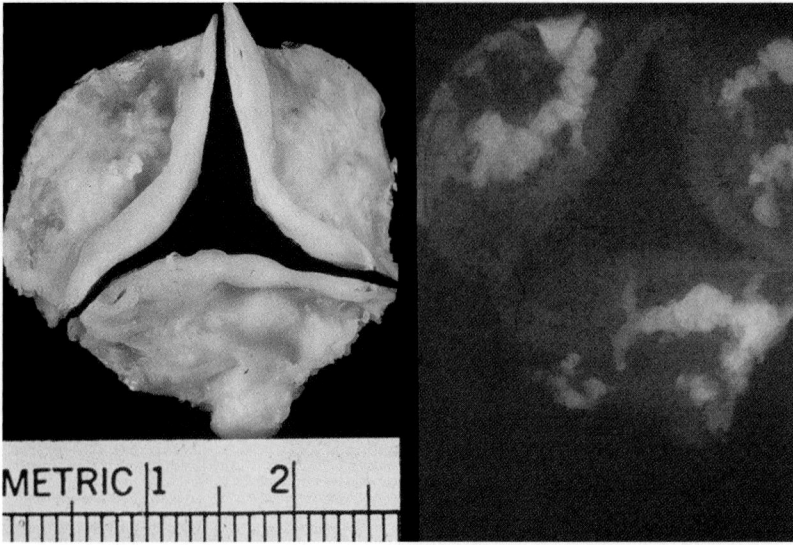

Fig. 20. Calcification of aortic valve in degenerative aortic stenosis. *Left*, Gross specimen. *Right*, Matched radiograph of valve shows calcium deposition.

involve the anterior mitral leaflet, left bundle branch, or ventricular septal myocardium; involvement of the ventricular septal myocardium may produce a large abscess cavity or result in rupture into a ventricular chamber with the formation of either an aorto–right ventricular or an aorto–left ventricular fistula. An aortic anular abscess may expand laterally and enter the pericardial cavity and thereby produce purulent pericarditis or fatal hemopericardium, or it may expand into adjacent cardiac chambers or vessels and produce various fistulas (aorto–right atrial, aorto–left atrial, or aortopulmonary).

Fibrous Cardiac Skeleton

At the base of the heart, the fibrous cardiac skeleton encircles the four cardiac valves. It comprises not only the four valvular anuli but also their intervalvular collagenous attachments (the right and left fibrous trigones, the intervalvular fibrosa, and the conus ligament) and the membranous septum and tendon of Todaro. This fibrous scaffold is firmly anchored to the ventricles but is rather loosely attached to the atria. Thus, the cardiac skeleton not only electrically insulates the atria from the ventricles but also supports the cardiac valves and provides a firm foundation against which the ventricles may contract.

Because of the intervalvular attachments of the fibrous cardiac skeleton, disease or surgery on one valve can affect the size, shape, position, or relative angula-

tion of its neighboring valves and also can affect the adjacent coronary arteries or cardiac conduction system. Tricuspid annuloplasty or replacement may be complicated by injury to the right coronary artery or atrioventricular conduction tissues, whereas mitral valve replacement may be attended by trauma to the circumflex coronary artery, coronary sinus, or aortic valve. At aortic valve replacement, the anterior mitral leaflet, left bundle branch, or coronary ostia may be injured inadvertently.

Most congenital anomalies of the pulmonary valve are associated with stenosis. Isolated pulmonary stenosis is almost always due to a dome-shaped acommissural valve, with congenital fusion of all three commissures. However, forms of pulmonary stenosis associated with other cardiac malformations, such as tetralogy of Fallot, usually result from a bicuspid or unicommissural valve (often with a hypoplastic anulus) or from a dysplastic valve with three thickened cusps.

Congenitally bicuspid aortic valves affect 1% to 2% of the general population and constitute the most common form of congenital heart disease. Although they usually are neither stenotic nor insufficient at birth, most bicuspid valves become stenotic during adulthood as the cusps calcify, and some become insufficient as a result of infective endocarditis or aortic root dilatation. In contrast, the congenitally unicommissural aortic valve is usually stenotic at birth and becomes progressively more obstructive as calcification develops in adulthood. Aortic atresia is associated with the hypoplastic left heart syndrome and is usually fatal during the first week of life. All congenital anomalies of the aortic valve are much more common in males than in females.

In truncus arteriosus, the truncal valve most commonly comprises three cusps and resembles a normal aortic valve. However, it may be quadricuspid, bicuspid, or, rarely, pentacuspid and may contain one or more raphes; such nontricuspid valves are often incompetent, particularly if the truncal root is dilated.

- Disease processes that tend to increase cusp rigidity tend to narrow the effective valvular orifice and produce stenosis.
- Processes that straighten the cuspid line between commissures tend to produce regurgitation.
- Pulmonary incompetence occurs in conditions that produce dilatation of the pulmonary trunk and anulus, such as pulmonary hypertension or heart failure.
- Pure pulmonary stenosis is almost always congenital in origin.
- An aortic anular abscess may expand laterally and enter the pericardial cavity.
- Congenitally bicuspid aortic valves affect 1%-2% of the general population.

GREAT ARTERIES

Pulmonary Arteries
The pulmonary artery arises anteriorly and to the left of the ascending aorta and is directed toward the left shoulder. In adults, it is slightly greater in diameter than the ascending aorta, although its wall thickness is roughly half that of the aorta. At the bifurcation, the right pulmonary artery travels horizontally beneath the aortic arch and behind the superior vena cava, and the left pulmonary artery courses over the left main bronchus (Fig. 21). The main and left pulmonary arteries contribute to the left border of the frontal cardiac silhouette radiographically.

In pulmonary hypertension, especially in children with pliable tracheobronchial cartilage, the tense and dilated pulmonary arteries can compress the left bronchus and the left upper and right middle lobar

bronchi and thereby contribute to recurrent bronchopneumonia in those lobes. Furthermore, the dilated pulmonary artery may displace the aortic arch rightward and secondarily produce tracheal indentation and, occasionally, hoarseness as a result of compression of the left recurrent laryngeal nerve.

Aorta
The aorta arises at the level of the aortic valve anulus and terminates at the aortic bifurcation, approximately at the level of the umbilicus and the fourth lumbar vertebra. The aorta has four major divisions: ascending aorta, aortic arch, descending thoracic aorta, and abdominal aorta (Fig. 22).

The ascending aorta lies almost entirely within the pericardial sac and includes sinus and tubular portions, which are demarcated by the aortic sinotubular junction. The aortic valve leaflets are related to the three sinuses, and the right and left coronary arteries arise from the right and left aortic sinuses, respectively. The ascending aorta lies posterior and to the right of the pulmonary artery.

With age or with the development of atherosclerosis, the aortic sinotubular junction can become heavily calcified, particularly above the right cusp, and may produce coronary ostial stenosis. Among the causes of aortic root dilatation, perhaps aging, mucoid medial

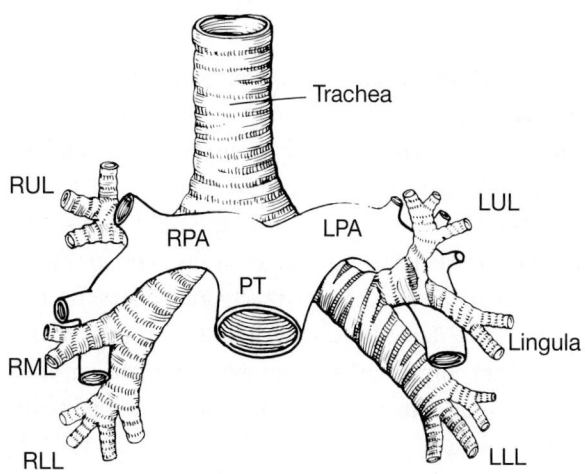

Fig. 21. Pulmonary arteries and bronchi. The right and left pulmonary arteries do not exhibit mirror-image symmetry. (See Appendix at end of chapter for abbreviations.)

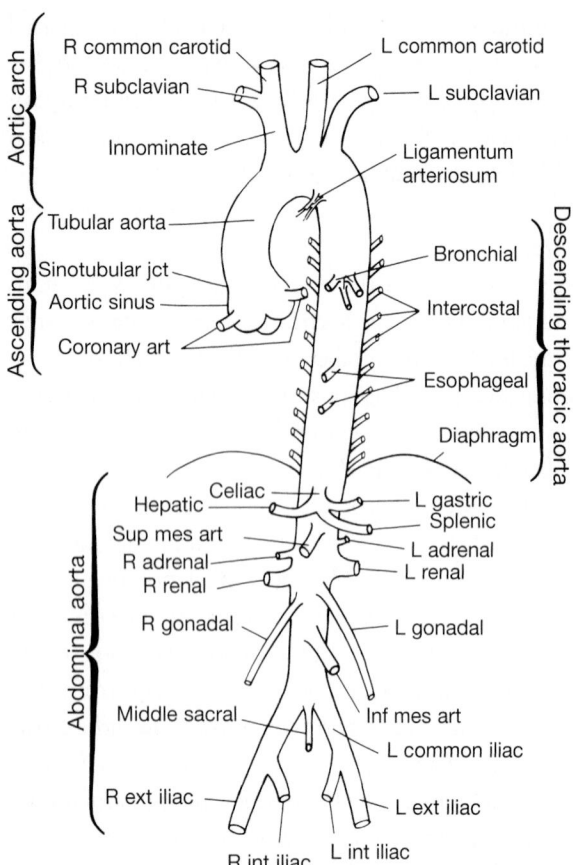

Fig. 22. Systemic arteries. The aorta may be divided into ascending, arch, descending thoracic, and abdominal regions. (See Appendix at end of chapter for abbreviations.)

degeneration (so-called cystic medial necrosis), and chronic hypertension are the most common and may produce an ascending aortic aneurysm, aortic valvular regurgitation, or acute aortic dissection.

The aortic arch travels over the right pulmonary artery and the left bronchus. From its superior aspect emanate the innominate (or brachiocephalic), left common carotid, and left subclavian arteries, in that order. In 11% of subjects, the innominate and left common carotid arteries form a common ostium, and in 5%, the left vertebral artery arises directly from the aortic arch, between the left common carotid and left subclavian arteries. The ligamentum arteriosum represents the obstructed fibrotic or fibrocalcific remnant of the fetal ductus arteriosus (ductal artery), which joins the proximal left pulmonary artery to the undersurface of the

aortic arch. The aortic arch contributes to the left superior border of the frontal cardiac silhouette and forms the radiographic aortic knob.

Aortic Dissection

When aortic dissections do not involve the ascending aorta (type III or type B), the intimal tear is commonly near the ligamentum arteriosum or the ostium of the left subclavian artery. By virtue of severe torsional and shear stresses placed on the heart and great vessels during nonpenetrating decelerative chest trauma, as can occur in motor vehicle accidents, the aorta may be transected at the junction between the aortic arch and the descending thoracic aorta. When the tear is incomplete, a posttraumatic pseudoaneurysm can develop with time. Aneurysms of the aortic arch may be associated with hypertension, atherosclerosis, or aortitis, or they may be idiopathic.

Descending Thoracic Aorta

The descending thoracic aorta abuts the left anterior surface of the vertebral column and lies adjacent to the esophagus and the left atrium. Its posterolateral branches are the bilateral intercostal arteries, and its anterior branches include the bronchial, esophageal, mediastinal, pericardial, and superior phrenic arteries. The bronchial arteries, most commonly two left and one right, nourish the bronchial walls and the pulmonary arterial and venous walls. Uncommonly, bronchial arteries may arise from intercostal or subclavian arteries or, rarely, from a coronary artery. The bronchial veins drain not only into the azygos and hemiazygos veins but also into the pulmonary veins.

If the bronchial circulation is adequate, pulmonary emboli usually do not cause pulmonary infarction. In several forms of pulmonary hypertension, the bronchial arteries become quite enlarged and tortuous.

Aneurysms of the descending thoracic aorta may be associated with aortic dissection, aortitis, atherosclerosis, hypertension, or trauma. They may or may not extend below the diaphragm.

Abdominal Aorta

The abdominal aorta travels along the left anterior surface of the vertebral column and lies adjacent to the inferior vena cava. The major lateral (retroperitoneal) branches include the renal, adrenal, right and left lumbar, and inferior phrenic arteries. The gonadal arteries arise somewhat more anteriorly but remain retroperitoneal. The intraperitoneal branches arise anteriorly and include the celiac artery (with its left gastric, splenic, and hepatic branches) and the superior and inferior mesenteric arteries. The distal aortic branches include the right and left common iliac arteries and a small middle sacral artery.

Atherosclerotic abdominal aortic aneurysms are most commonly infrarenal. They tend to bulge anteriorly and thereby stretch and compress the gonadal and inferior mesenteric arteries. Such aneurysms are generally filled with laminated thrombus and so their residual lumens often appear normal or even narrowed rather than dilated. Rupture of an atherosclerotic abdominal aortic aneurysm may be associated with extensive retroperitoneal hemorrhage, with or without intraperitoneal hemorrhage.

Aortopulmonary Window

An aortopulmonary septal defect represents a large opening between the ascending aorta and the pulmonary trunk and hemodynamically resembles a patent ductus arteriosus. Rarely, one pulmonary artery originates from the ascending aorta or ductus arteriosus, while the other arises normally from the pulmonary trunk. Congenital stenosis of the pulmonary arteries is usually associated with maternal rubella during the first trimester. In pulmonary atresia with ventricular septal defect, the pulmonary arteries may be derived from the right or left ductus arteriosus and from bronchial or other systemic collateral arteries (analogous to total anomalous pulmonary venous connection).

Aortic Arch Congenital Abnormalities

Various anomalies result from faulty development of the aortic arches. A right aortic arch results from persistence of the right fourth aortic arch and disappearance of its left counterpart; it most commonly accompanies tetralogy of Fallot, pulmonary atresia with ventricular septal defect, and truncus arteriosus. A double aortic arch results from persistence of both fourth aortic arches. An aberrant retroesophageal right subclavian artery is a relatively common anomaly, which may cause dysphagia; it probably results from persistence of the right dorsal aorta and resorption of the right fourth aortic arch.

Ductus Arteriosus

The patent ductus arteriosus may be isolated or may accompany other cardiac malformations. A left ductus arteriosus joins the proximal left pulmonary artery to the aortic arch, whereas a right ductus arteriosus joins the proximal right pulmonary artery to the right subclavian artery; in cases of right aortic arch with mirror-image brachiocephalic branching, the opposite pertains.

Coarctation of the Aorta

Coarctation of the aorta represents an obstructive infolded ridge just distal to the left subclavian artery and opposite the ductus arteriosus; it is associated with a congenitally bicuspid aortic valve in at least half of the cases.

- Acute aortic dissection is commonly associated with an intimal tear above the right aortic cusp and with eventual rupture into the pericardial sac.
- When aortic dissections do not involve the ascending aorta (type III or type B), the intimal tear is commonly near the ligamentum arteriosum or the ostium of the left subclavian artery.

CORONARY CIRCULATION

Right Coronary Artery

The right coronary artery arises nearly perpendicularly from the right aortic sinus (Fig. 23). In 50% of subjects, one or more conus arteries also originate from the right aortic sinus, anterior to the right coronary ostium. Rarely, the descending septal artery or the sinus nodal artery originates directly from the aorta.

The left coronary artery arises from the left aortic sinus and tends to arise at an acute angle and to travel parallel to the aortic sinus wall. When the left main artery is exceptionally short, its ostium may assume a double-barrel appearance.

Among the various causes of coronary ostial stenosis, perhaps the most common is degenerative calcification of the aortic sinotubular junction, which often affects the right aortic sinus. Stenosis of the right coronary ostium occurs six to eight times more often than that of the left. Aortitis associated with syphilis or ankylosing spondylitis also may be complicated by

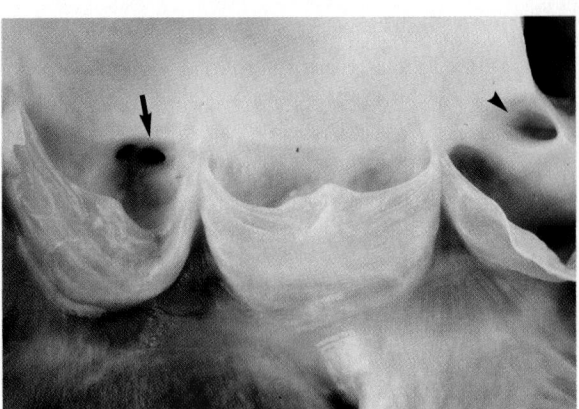

Fig. 23. Coronary ostia. The conus artery and right coronary artery (*arrow*) arise separately from the right cusp in this specimen. The *arrowhead* points to the left coronary ostium.

coronary ostial obstruction. Iatrogenic ostial injury may complicate coronary arteriography, intraoperative coronary perfusion, or aortic valve replacement.

The right coronary artery travels within the right atrioventricular sulcus (or groove) (Fig. 24). In 50% of subjects, the first anterior branch is the conus artery, which nourishes the right ventricular outflow tract; in the remainder, this artery arises independently from the right aortic sinus. The descending septal artery, which arises from the proximal right coronary artery or, rarely, from the conus artery or right aortic sinus, supplies the infundibular septum and, in some individuals, the distal atrioventricular (His) bundle. Along the acute cardiac margin, from base to apex, courses a prominent acute marginal branch, and between this vessel and the conus artery, several smaller marginal branches arise and travel parallel to the acute margin; these vessels nourish the lateral two-thirds of the anterior right ventricular free wall.

Beyond the acute margin, along the inferior surface of the heart, the length of the right coronary artery varies inversely with that of the circumflex coronary artery. However, in 90% of human hearts, the right coronary artery gives rise not only to the posterior descending artery, which travels in the inferior interventricular sulcus, but also to branches that supply the inferior left ventricular free wall. Accordingly, these arteries nourish the inferior third of the ventricular septum (the inlet septum), including the right bundle branch and the posterior portion of the left bundle branch, and the inferior left ventricular free wall, including the posteromedial mitral papillary muscle.

Left Main Coronary Artery

The left main coronary artery travels between the pulmonary artery and the left atrium and is covered in part by the left atrial appendage. In two-thirds of subjects, it bifurcates into left anterior descending and circumflex branches, and in the remaining one-third, it trifurcates into the aforementioned branches and an intermediate artery (ramus intermedius), which follows a course similar to that of either the first diagonal or first marginal branch.

Left Anterior Descending Coronary Artery

The left anterior descending coronary artery travels within the anterior interventricular sulcus (or groove) and, after wrapping around the apex, may ascend a variable distance along the inferior interventricular sulcus. Septal perforating branches nourish not only the anterosuperior two-thirds and entire apical one-third of the ventricular septum but also the atrioventricular (His) bundle and the right and anterior left bundle branches (Fig. 25). The proximal septal perforators anastomose with the descending septal artery. Epicardial branches, called diagonals, nourish the anterior left ventricular free wall and the medial third of the anterior right ventricular free wall. Myocardial bridges may be demonstrated angiographically in 12% of subjects and almost invariably involve the anterior descending artery; they produce critical systolic luminal narrowing in only 1% to 2% of hearts and probably have a benign prognosis in most cases (Fig. 26).

Circumflex Coronary Artery

The circumflex coronary artery travels within the left atrioventricular sulcus (or groove) and often terminates just beyond the obtuse marginal branch. The circumflex artery nourishes the lateral left ventricular free wall; however, in the 10% of subjects in whom the circumflex artery gives rise to the posterior descending branch, it also supplies the inferior left ventricular free wall and the inferior third of the ventricular septum. The circumflex and anterior descending arteries nourish the anterolateral mitral papillary muscles, and the circumflex and right coronary arteries supply the posteromedial mitral papillary muscles.

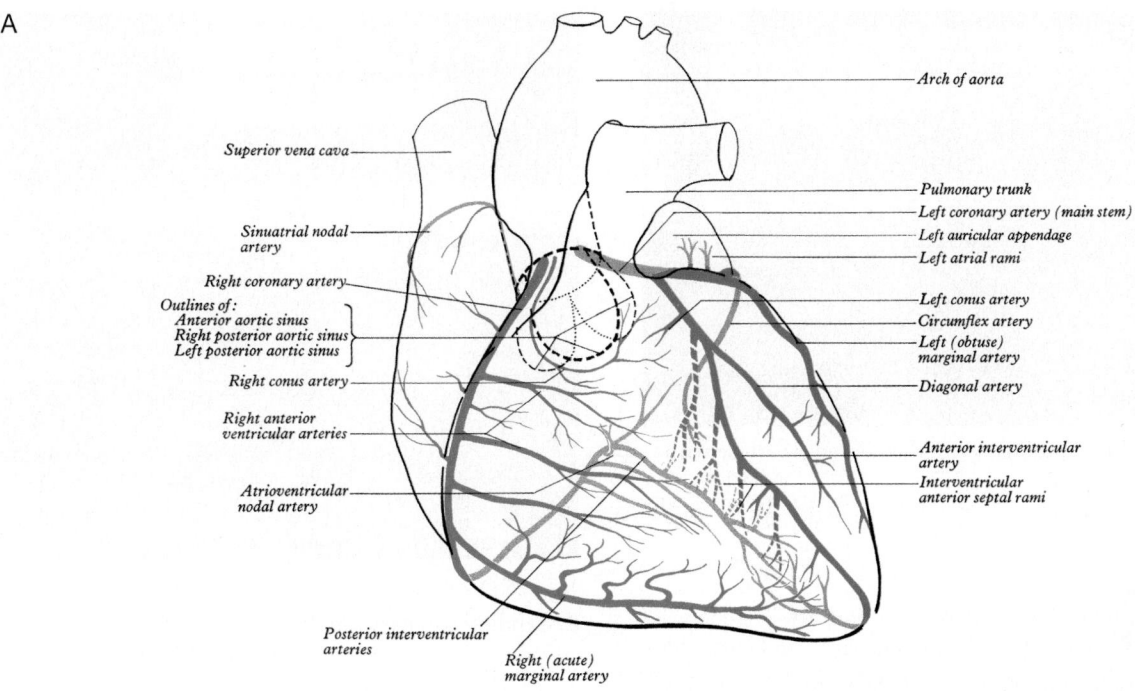

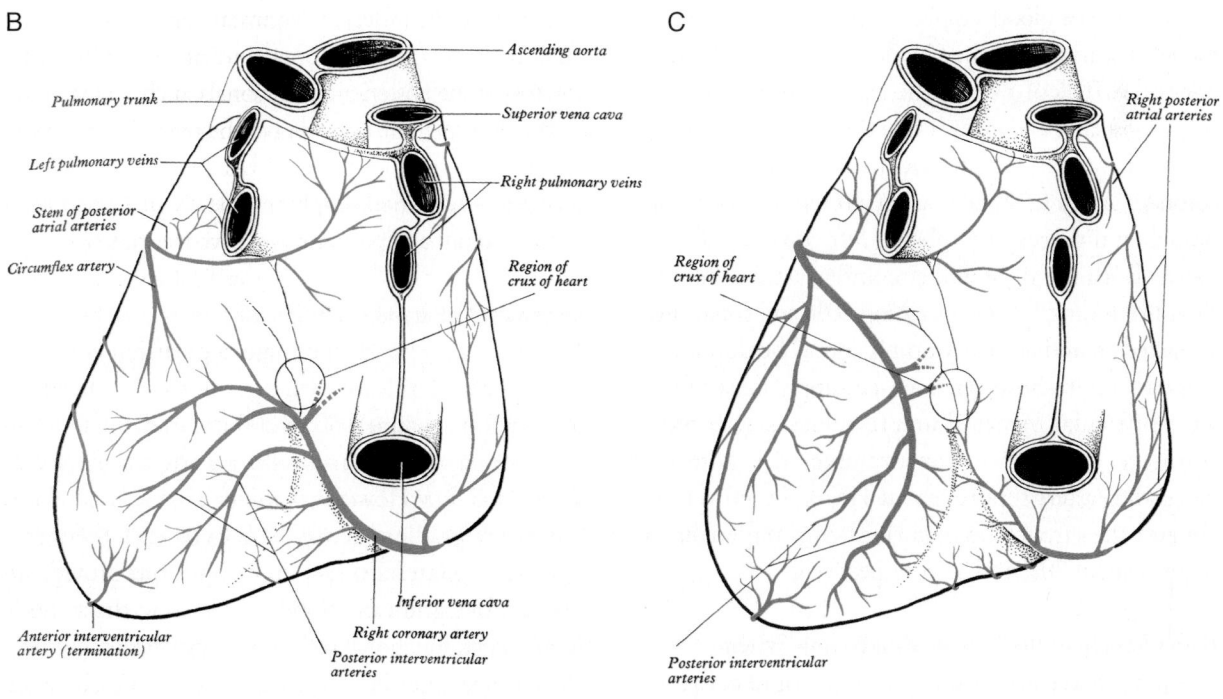

Fig. 24. Coronary arterial system. *A*, Anterior view. *B* and *C*, Posteroinferior views showing right dominance (*B*) and left dominance (*C*).

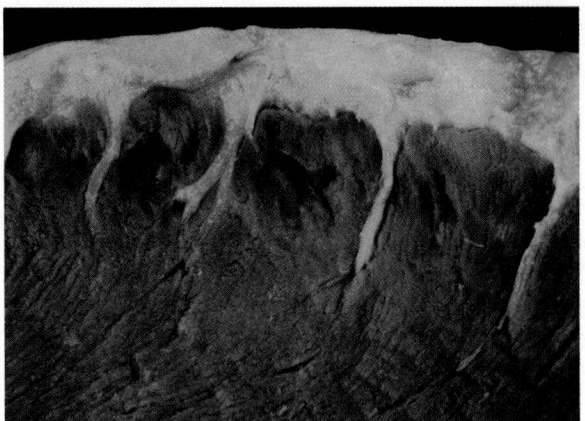

Fig. 25. Left anterior descending coronary artery with septal perforators.

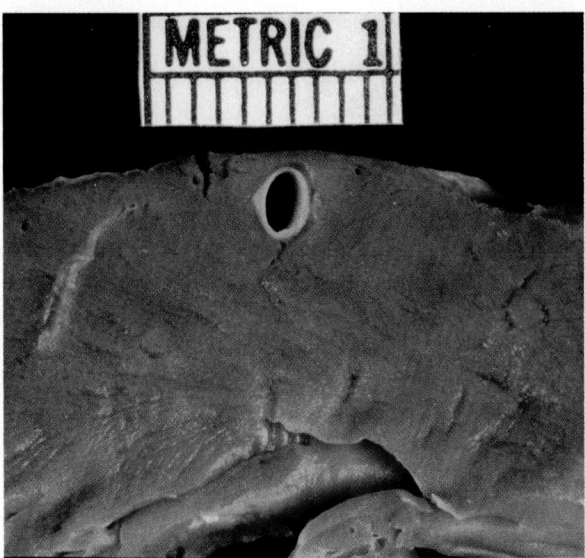

Fig. 26. Myocardial bridge over the left anterior descending coronary artery.

The four major epicardial coronary arteries occupy only two planes of the heart. The right and circumflex arteries delineate the plane of the atrioventricular sulcus (cardiac base), and the left main artery and anterior and posterior descending arteries delineate the plane of the ventricular septum.

The origin of the posterior descending artery determines the blood supply to the inferior portion of the left ventricle and thereby defines coronary dominance. In 70% of hearts, the right coronary artery crosses the crux and gives rise to this branch, establishing right coronary dominance. In 10%, the circumflex coronary artery terminates as the posterior descending branch and thereby establishes left coronary dominance. Both the right and circumflex arteries supply the cardiac crux in the remaining 20% and constitute so-called shared coronary dominance. The dominant coronary artery, however, does *not* supply most of the left ventricular myocardium. In subjects with right coronary dominance, for example, the anterior descending artery supplies about 45% of the left ventricle and the circumflex and right coronary arteries nourish about 20% and 35%, respectively.

Blood Supply of the Cardiac Conduction System

The sinus nodal artery arises from the right coronary artery in 60% of subjects and from the circumflex artery in 40%, but its artery of origin does not depend on patterns of coronary arterial dominance. The atrioventricular nodal artery originates from the dominant artery and, accordingly, arises from the right coronary in 90%

and the circumflex in 10%. The atrioventricular nodal artery and the first septal perforator of the anterior descending artery offer dual blood supply to the atrioventricular (His) bundle. Other septal perforating branches of the anterior descending artery supply the anterior aspect of the left bundle branch, and septal perforators of the posterior descending branch, an extension of the dominant artery, supply the posteroinferior portion of the left bundle branch. The right bundle branch receives a dual blood supply from the septal perforators of the anterior and posterior descending arteries.

Coronary Collateral Circulation

In the human heart, the major epicardial coronary arteries communicate with one another by means of anastomotic channels 50 to 200 μm in diameter (Fig. 27). Normally, these small collateral arteries afford very little blood flow. However, if arterial obstruction induces a pressure gradient across such a channel, then with time the collateral vessel may dilate and provide an avenue for significant blood flow beyond the stenotic lesion. Such functional collaterals may develop between the terminal branches of two coronary arteries, between the side branches of two arteries, between branches of the same artery, or within the same branch (via the vasa vasorum). They are most numerous in the ventricular septum (between septal perforators of anterior and posterior descending arteries), in the ventricular apex

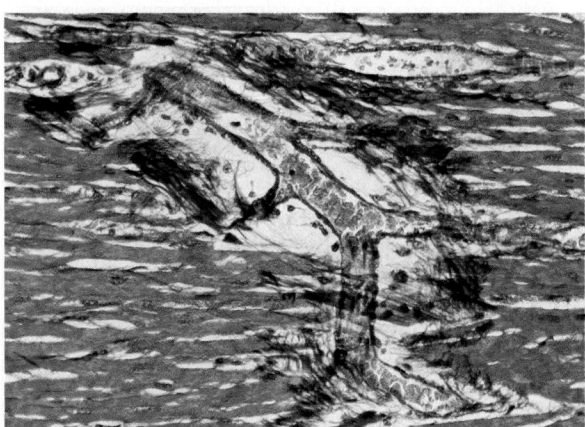

Fig. 27. Myocardial arteriole.

(between anterior descending septal perforators), in the anterior right ventricular free wall (between anterior descending and right or conus arteries), in the anterolateral left ventricular free wall (between anterior descending diagonals and circumflex marginals), at the cardiac crux (between the right and circumflex arteries), and along the atria (Kugel anastomotic artery between right and circumflex arteries). Smaller subendocardial anastomoses also exist (Fig. 28).

The most common sites for high-grade atherosclerotic lesions are the proximal one-half of the anterior descending and circumflex arteries and the origin and entire length of the right coronary artery. The distribution and severity of atherosclerotic plaques do not differ significantly among patients with angina pectoris, acute myocardial infarction, end-stage ischemic heart disease, or sudden death.

Congenital malformations of the coronary arteries include anomalous ostial origin, anomalous arterial branching patterns, and anomalous arterial anastomoses.

Coronary Veins

The venous circulation of the heart comprises a coronary sinus system, an anterior cardiac venous system, and the thebesian venous system (Fig. 29). Small thebesian veins drain directly into a cardiac chamber, particularly the right atrium or right ventricle; the ostia of these veins are easily recognized along the relatively smooth atrial walls but are difficult to identify in the trabeculated ventricles.

During cardiac electrophysiologic studies among patients with Wolff-Parkinson-White syndrome and left-sided bypass tracts, a catheter electrode may be positioned within the coronary sinus and great cardiac vein, adjacent to the mitral anulus, to localize the aberrant conduction pathways.

Cardiac Lymphatics

Myocardial lymphatics drain toward the epicardial surface, where they are joined by lymphatic channels from the conduction system, atria, and valves. Larger epicardial lymphatics then travel in a retrograde manner with the coronary arteries back to the aortic root, where a confluence of right and left cardiac lymphatics drains into a pretracheal lymph node and eventually empties into the right lymphatic duct.

The coronary veins and cardiac lymphatics work in concert to remove excess fluid from the myocardial interstitium and pericardial sac. Accordingly, obstruction of either system or of both systems may result in myocardial edema and pericardial effusion.

CARDIAC CONDUCTION SYSTEM

Sinus Node

The sinus node is the primary pacemaker of the heart. It is an epicardial structure that measures approximately 15×5×2 mm and is located in the sulcus terminalis (intercavarum) near the superior cavoatrial junction

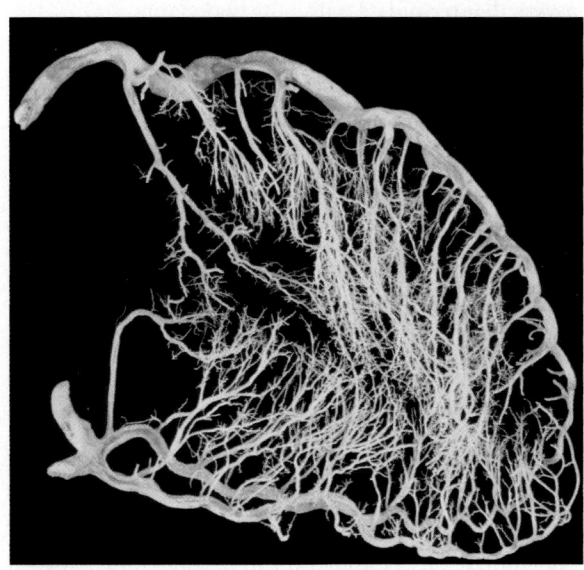

Fig. 28. Septal perforators (coronary cast).

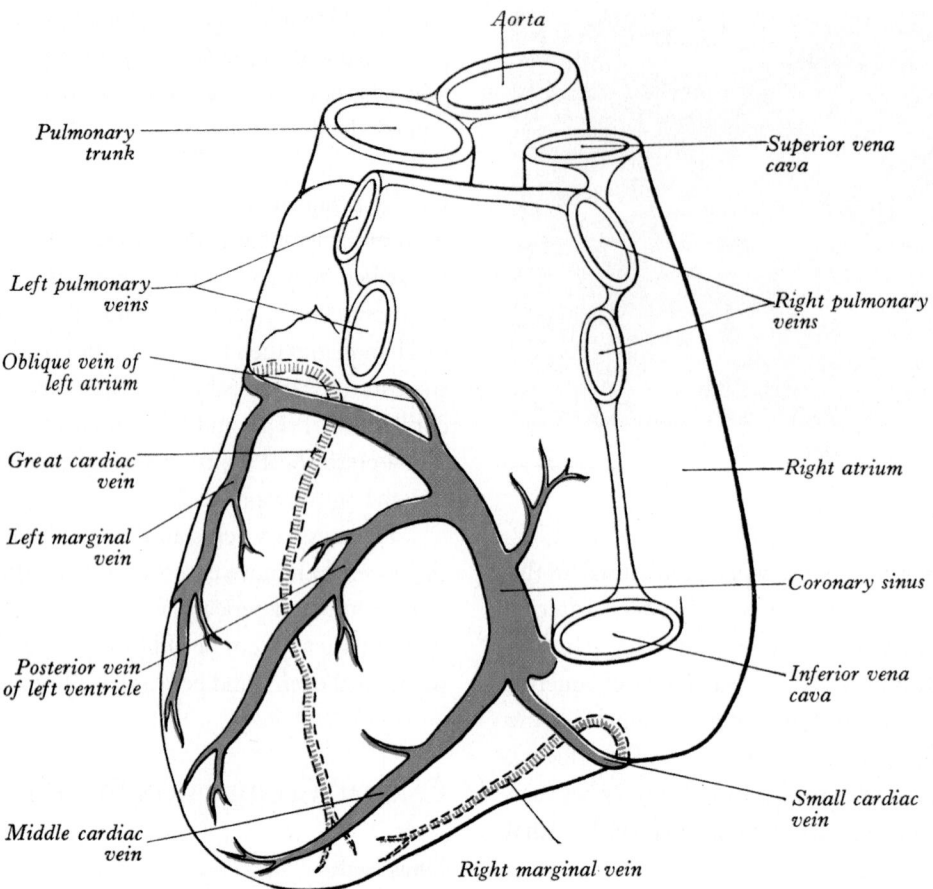

Fig. 29. Coronary veins from posterior aspect of heart.

(Fig. 30). Through its center passes a relatively large sinus nodal artery. Sinus nodal function is greatly influenced by numerous sympathetic and parasympathetic nerves that terminate within its boundaries.

Histologically, the sinus node consists of specialized cardiac muscle cells embedded within a prominent collagenous stroma. Its myocardial cells are smaller than ventricular muscle cells and contain only scant contractile elements. Ultrastructurally, the sinus node comprises transitional cells and variable numbers of P cells centrally and atrial myocardial cells peripherally. The P cells are thought to be the source of normal cardiac impulse formation.

Because the sinus node occupies an epicardial position, its function may be affected by pericarditis or metastatic neoplasms. In the setting of cardiac amyloidosis, extensive fibrosis or amyloid deposition may involve the sinus node. Although the sinus node is rarely infarcted, its function can be altered by adjacent atrial infarction.

Internodal Tracts

There are no morphologically distinct conduction pathways between the sinus and the atrioventricular nodes by light microscopy, but electrophysiologic studies support the concept of three functional preferential conduction pathways. In ultrastructural studies, some investigators have observed specialized cardiac muscle cells in these internodal tracts.

Lipomatous hypertrophy of the atrial septum may interfere with internodal conduction and induce various atrial arrhythmias. Because the functional preferential pathways travel only in the limbus and not in the valve of the fossa ovalis, internodal conduction disturbances do not occur with intentional septal perforation at cardiac catheterization (transseptal approach), with the Rashkind balloon atrial septostomy, or with the Blalock-Hanlon partial (posterior) atrial septectomy. With the Mustard operation for complete transposition of the great arteries, in which the entire atrial septum is resected and in which the surgical atriotomy

A

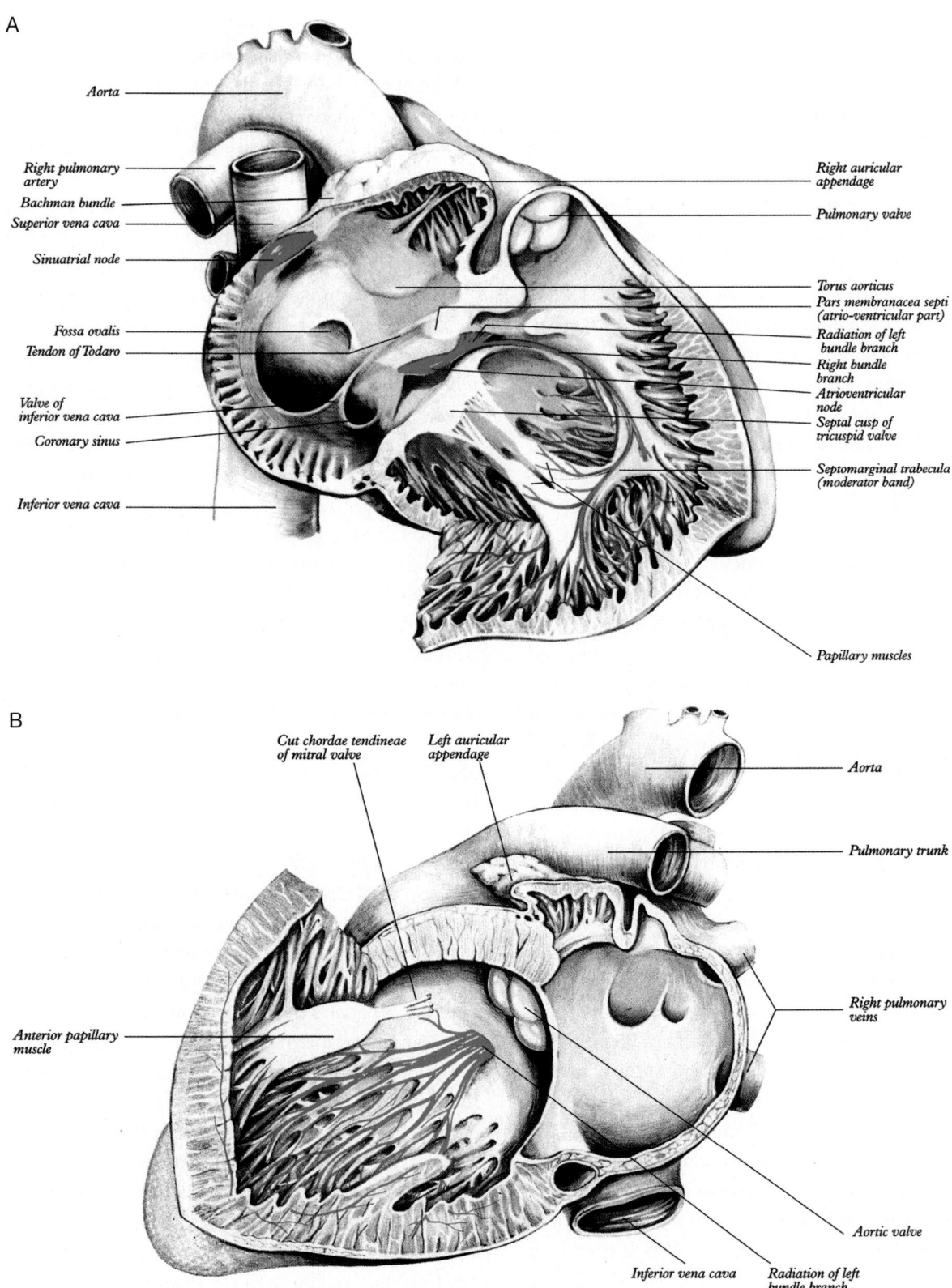

Aorta

Right pulmonary artery
Bachman bundle
Superior vena cava

Sinuatrial node

Fossa ovalis
Tendon of Todaro

Valve of inferior vena cava
Coronary sinus

Inferior vena cava

Right auricular appendage

Pulmonary valve

Torus aorticus
Pars membranacea septi (atrio-ventricular part)
Radiation of left bundle branch
Right bundle branch
Atrioventricular node
Septal cusp of tricuspid valve

Septomarginal trabecula (moderator band)

Papillary muscles

B

Cut chordae tendineae of mitral valve

Left auricular appendage

Aorta

Pulmonary trunk

Right pulmonary veins

Anterior papillary muscle

Aortic valve

Inferior vena cava
Radiation of left bundle branch

Fig. 30. Cardiac conduction system. *A*, Right heart. The sinus (sinuatrial) and atrioventricular nodes are both right atrial structures. *B*, Left heart. The left bundle branch forms a broad sheet that does not divide into distinct anterior and posterior fascicles.

may disrupt the crista terminalis, severe disturbances of internodal conduction may result.

Atrioventricular Node

The atrioventricular node is a subendocardial right atrial structure that measures approximately 6×4×1.5 mm. It is located within the triangle of Koch (bordered by the tendon of Todaro, septal tricuspid anulus, and coronary sinus ostium) and abuts the right fibrous trigone (central fibrous body). The atrioventricular nodal artery courses near the node but not necessarily through it. Sympathetic and parasympathetic nerves enter the atrioventricular node and greatly influence its function.

Like the sinus node, the atrioventricular node histologically consists of a complex interwoven pattern of small specialized cardiac muscle cells within a fibrous stroma. With advanced age, the atrioventricular node acquires progressively more fibrous tissue, although not as extensively as the sinus node.

The so-called mesothelioma of the atrioventricular node is a small and rare primary neoplasm which, by virtue of its position, produces various arrhythmias and may cause sudden death. Metastatic neoplasms may rarely infiltrate the atrioventricular node but do not necessarily alter its function. Sarcoid granulomas tend to involve the basal ventricular myocardium and may destroy the atrioventricular conduction system. Because of its subendocardial position, the atrioventricular node may be ablated nonsurgically at the time of electrophysiologic study.

Atrioventricular Bundle

The atrioventricular (His) bundle arises from the distal portion of the atrioventricular node and courses through the central fibrous body to the summit of the muscular ventricular septum, adjacent to the membranous septum. It affords the only normal physiologic avenue for electrical conduction between ventricles. By virtue of its position within the central fibrous body (right fibrous trigone), the atrioventricular bundle is closely related to the annuli of the aortic, mitral, and tricuspid valves. The atrioventricular bundle has a dual blood supply—from the atrioventricular nodal artery and the first septal perforating branch of the anterior descending artery. In some subjects, a septal branch of the proximal right coronary artery also nourishes the atrioventricular bundle.

The atrioventricular bundle is made up of numerous parallel bundles of specialized cardiac muscle cells, which are separated by delicate fibrous septa. The entire atrioventricular bundle is insulated by a collagenous sheath. With increasing age, the fibrous septa become thicker, and the functional elements may be partially replaced by adipose tissue. Ultrastructurally, the atrioventricular bundle contains Purkinje cells and ventricular myocardial cells in parallel arrangement.

In some subjects, alternate conduction pathways exist between the atria and the ventricles, either within the existing atrioventricular conduction system or elsewhere along the fibrous cardiac skeleton, and may produce various arrhythmias. Atrionodal bypass tracts (of James) connect the atria to the distal atrioventricular node, and atriofascicular tracts (of Brechenmacher) connect the atria to the atrioventricular bundle. Nodoventricular and fasciculoventricular bypass fibers (of Mahaim) connect the atrioventricular node and atrioventricular bundle, respectively, to the underlying ventricular septal summit. These bypass fibers are quite commonly observed histologically and are apparently nonfunctional in most persons, although they may produce ventricular preexcitation in some instances.

Ventricular preexcitation is usually associated with aberrant atrioventricular bypass tracts that bridge the tricuspid or mitral annuli. These tracts often travel within the adipose tissue of the atrioventricular sulcus rather than through a defect in the valvular annuli. Such bypass tracts can be single or multiple and may be identified by electrophysiologic mapping.

Acquired complete heart block may involve the atrioventricular node and bundle or both bundle branches. That occurring with acute myocardial infarction is usually transient and more commonly complicates inferoseptal than anteroseptal infarction. Usually the atrioventricular node and atrioventricular bundle are edematous, or the bundle branches are focally infarcted. Acute heart block also can complicate aortic infective endocarditis. Chronic heart block may be associated with ischemic heart disease or with fibrocalcific disorders of the aortic or mitral valves, but it is most commonly due to idiopathic fibrosis of the atrioventricular bundle and bilateral bundle branches. Heart block may also complicate aortic or mitral valve replacement.

Congenital complete heart block presents as persistent bradycardia in utero and can represent an isolated anomaly or may accompany other cardiac malformations. It results from interruption of atrioventricular conduction pathways, either at the junction between atrial muscle and the atrioventricular node or at the junction between the atrioventricular node and the atrioventricular bundle. The different embryologic origins of these three regions account for the specific sites of disrupted conduction tissue.

Bundle Branches

As an extension of the atrioventricular bundle, the right bundle branch forms a cordlike structure, approximately 50 mm in length and 1 mm in diameter, which courses along the septal and moderator bands to the level of the anterior tricuspid papillary muscle. The left bundle branch forms a broad fenestrated sheet of conduction fibers which spreads along the septal subendocardium of the left ventricle and separates incompletely and variably into two or three indistinct fascicles. The fascicles travel toward the left ventricular apex and both mitral papillary muscle groups. The bundle branches are nourished by septal perforators arising from the anterior and posterior descending coronary arteries. Histologically, the bundle branches consist of parallel tracts of specialized cardiac muscle cells which are insulated by a delicate fibrous sheath. Ultrastructurally, Purkinje cells and ventricular myocardial cells form the bundle branches.

Right bundle branch block may be idiopathic or be associated with ischemic heart disease, chronic systemic hypertension, or pulmonary hypertension. Right ventriculotomy usually produces the electrocardiographic features of right bundle branch block, even though the bundle may not have been transected.

Chronic left bundle branch block may be associated with fibrocalcific degeneration of the ventricular septal summit as a result of chronic ischemia, left ventricular hypertension, calcification of the aortic or mitral valves, or any form of cardiomyopathy.

- The sinus node comprises transitional cells and variable numbers of P cells centrally and atrial myocardial cells peripherally.
- With the Mustard operation for complete transposition of the great arteries, in which the entire atrial septum is resected, severe disturbances of internodal conduction may result.

- The atrioventricular bundle has a dual blood supply—from the atrioventricular nodal artery and the first septal perforating branch of the anterior descending artery.
- Acute heart block may complicate aortic infective endocarditis.

Cardiac Innervation

Because the embryonic heart tube first forms in the future neck region, its autonomic innervation also arises from this level. From the cervical ganglia originate three pairs of cervical sympathetic cardiac nerves, which intermingle as they join the cardiac plexus, between the great arteries and the tracheal bifurcation. Several thoracic sympathetic cardiac nerves arise from the upper thoracic ganglia and also join the cardiac plexus. From the parasympathetic vagus nerves emanate the superior and inferior cervical vagal cardiac nerves and the thoracic vagal cardiac nerves, which likewise interweave within the cardiac plexus. The various sympathetic and parasympathetic nerves then descend from this plexus onto the heart and thereby innervate the coronary arteries, cardiac conduction system, and myocardium. Furthermore, afferent nerves concerned with pain and various reflexes ascend from the heart toward the cardiac plexus.

The transplanted human heart is completely denervated and responds only to circulating (humoral) substances and not to autonomic impulses. Similarly, afferent pathways are also lost, including pain tracts and various reflexes. Consequently, if chronic cardiac transplant rejection produces diffuse coronary arterial obstruction, subsequent myocardial ischemia and infarction will be asymptomatic.

The asplenia syndrome is characterized by bilateral right-sided symmetry and is generally associated with right atrial isomerism, right pulmonary isomerism, abdominal situs ambiguus, and, in some instances, bilateral sinus nodes. In contrast, the sinus node may be congenitally absent or malpositioned in cases of polysplenia with left atrial isomerism.

- The transplanted heart is completely denervated and responds only to circulating (humoral) substances and not to autonomic impulses.
- Congenital complete heart block may present as persistent bradycardia in utero.

APPENDIX

Abbreviations Used in Figures

A	Anterior	LUL	Left upper lobe
Art	Artery	LV	Left ventricle
AL	Anterolateral	LVOT	Left ventricular outflow tract
AS	Anteroseptal	Mes	Mesenteric
AVS	Atrioventricular septum	MV	Mitral valve
Ext	External	P	Posterior
I	Inferior	PL	Posterolateral
IAS	Interatrial septum	PS	Posteroseptal
IL	Inferolateral	PT	Pulmonary trunk
Inf	Inferior	R	Right
Int	Internal	RA	Right atrium
IS	Inferoseptal	RLL	Right lower lobe
IVS	Interventricular septum	RLPV	Right lower pulmonary vein
Jct	Junction	RML	Right middle lobe
L	Left	RPA	Right pulmonary artery
LA	Left atrium	RUL	Right upper lobe
LLL	Left lower lobe	RV	Right ventricle
LLPV	Left lower pulmonary vein	S	Septal
LPA	Left pulmonary artery	Sup	Superior

3

EVIDENCE-BASED MEDICINE AND STATISTICS IN CARDIOLOGY

Apoor S. Gami, MD

Charanjit S. Rihal, MD

EVIDENCE-BASED MEDICINE

Evidence-based medicine is the conscientious and explicit use of the current best evidence from systematic research to guide medical decision making in the care of individual patients. Its practice takes into consideration three elements: clinical setting, scientific evidence, and physician-patient factors.

Clinical Setting

The clinical setting includes specific information about the patient (history, physical examination, imaging, and laboratory studies) and where the medical decision occurs. The latter includes culture, societal values, characteristics of the practice site, and constraints due to time, reimbursement, and the availability of technology (i.e., primary angioplasty may be better than thrombolysis *if* access to a referral center is possible within a reasonable time).

Scientific Evidence

Any observation about the relationship between events is considered evidence; however, a hierarchy of evidence exists. A randomized controlled trial (RCT) with a sample size of one provides definite evidence about the effects of treatment in an *individual patient*. Among studies of *populations*, the best evidence comes from meta-analyses of methodologically sound RCTs that have consistent results. The next best evidence is from single RCTs, which are better than meta-analyses of observational studies and single observational studies. At the bottom of the hierarchy are unsystematic observations of clinical phenomena.

The results of one RCT (the Heart and Estrogen Replacement Study, published in 1998) reversed decades of thought on the cardiovascular effects of female hormone therapy that had been based on an abundance of misinterpreted or biased observational data. Judicious use of the evidence requires exhaustive searches for all relevant evidence and careful appraisal of its validity, results, and applicability.

Patient-Physician Factors

Evidence alone cannot direct management of an individual patient. Physician expertise and patient preferences are crucial in making the final medical decision, which is influenced by the prior experiences, expectations, ethics, and cultural beliefs of both parties.

STATISTICS IN CARDIOLOGY

Statistics is the analysis of numerical data to infer proportions in a population from those in a representative sample and to measure the probability that observed results are chance findings. In cardiology examinations, an understanding of the basic principles of biostatistics and their use in medical decision making is tested with statistical questions about 1) the probability of disease or therapeutic outcomes and 2) the evaluation of diagnostic test results.

DISEASE AND THERAPEUTIC OUTCOMES

Prevalence and Incidence

The *prevalence* of a disease is the proportion of people in a population who have the disease at a given time. The *incidence* of a disease in a population is the proportion of people at risk of the disease who develop the disease during a specific period.

Consider the following example: In a county of 100,000 people, 2,000 have atrial fibrillation. Ten years later in the county, 300 people had died (of whom 25 had atrial fibrillation), 250 people had been born (none had atrial fibrillation), and 500 other people had atrial fibrillation. The baseline prevalence of atrial fibrillation in the population was 2% (2,000/100,000), the incidence of atrial fibrillation in the baseline population during those 10 years was 0.5% (500/100,000), and the prevalence of atrial fibrillation at the end of the 10 years was 2.5% (2,475/99,950). Note that incidence must be used in the context of a specific time period.

Measures of Effect

Measures of effect are summarized in Table 1 and defined as follows:

- *Event rate* is the number of people who have an event during follow-up divided by the number of people at baseline who were at risk of having the event. Event rates are usually described for experimental and control groups in RCTs and observational studies.
- *Relative risk*, which is synonymous with *risk ratio* (both are abbreviated as *RR*), is the event rate in the experimental group divided by the event rate in the control group.
- *Odds ratio* (OR) is a measure of the strength of association between a condition or exposure and a disease or outcome. The odds of an event is the probability of it occurring divided by the probability of it not occurring. The OR is the odds of an event

Table 1.   Summary of Measures of Effect

$$RR = \frac{EER}{CER}$$

$$ARR = CER - EER$$

$$ARI = EER - CER$$

$$RRR = 1 - \frac{EER}{CER}$$

$$NNT = \frac{1}{ARR}$$

$$NNH = \frac{1}{ARI}$$

CER, control event rate; EER, experimental event rate. (See text for other abbreviations.)

in one group (i.e., an exposure group) divided by the odds of the event in another group (i.e., a control group). It is the measure of effect used in cross-sectional and case-control studies.

- *Absolute risk reduction* (ARR) is the event rate in the control group minus the event rate in the experimental group—but only if the difference is a positive number. If it is a negative number, its absolute value is the *absolute risk increase* (ARI).
- *Relative risk reduction* (RRR) is the ARR divided by the event rate in the control group. It can also be calculated as 1 minus the RR. If the event rate in the experimental group is larger than the event rate in the control group, the *relative risk increase* (RRI) is calculated as the ARI divided by the event rate in the control group, or the absolute value of 1 minus the RR. The RRR is often the statistic used in pharmaceutical promotional material because it shows the largest numerical effect. When the event rate in the control group is small, a large RRR may reflect a small ARR that does not have clinical importance.
- *Number needed to treat* (NNT) better conceptualizes the risk relationships described above. NNT is the number of patients who need to receive an intervention to prevent one unfavorable outcome. This is calculated by rounding the reciprocal of the ARR to

the next higher integer. NNT must always be accompanied by duration of treatment or follow-up.

■ *Number needed to harm* (NNH) is a concept similar to NNT, but it is the number of patients who need to receive an intervention for one patient to have an unfavorable outcome. This is calculated by rounding the reciprocal of the ARI to the next higher integer. Like NNT, it must be accompanied by a duration of treatment or follow-up.

Null Hypothesis

The *null hypothesis* of a study states that any observed difference (usually in treatment effects) between groups is due to chance alone and that no true difference exists between groups. When the probability that the study result is due to chance is less than a specific value (α level), the null hypothesis is rejected and the difference between groups is considered statistically significant.

α Level

The *α level* is the threshold value for statistical significance of a test for differences between groups. The α level is the probability that a statistical test erroneously supports the conclusion that a chance observed difference between groups is real (a *type I error*). The α level is determined by the researcher, typically at 0.05 or 0.01. It is important to correctly interpret the *P* value in the results of a study: If *P* is less than 0.05, there is less than a 5% chance that the observed difference between groups is due to chance.

β Level

The *β level* is the probability that a statistical test erroneously supports the conclusion that a real observed difference between groups is due to chance (a *type II error*). The β level is determined by the researcher, typically at 0.2 or 0.1. The *power* of a statistical test is the ability to detect a given difference between groups if one exists, and it is calculated as 1 minus β. A β of 0.2 gives a statistical power of 0.8 (i.e., an 80% chance of observing a real difference).

Confidence Intervals

A *confidence interval* (CI) is a range of values in which the true value for the total population (from which the study sample was selected) is likely to exist. A 95% CI means that the true value will be outside the CI 5% of

the time. A CI that spans the *line of no difference* (0 for ARR and RRR; 1 for RR and OR) represents a result that is *not* statistically significant. In this case, comparing the clinical significance of the lower and upper limits of the CI might help identify a beneficial or harmful trend that could be confirmed in larger trials. The CI is narrower (and the results more precise) as the sample size increases. It is important to correctly interpret the CI in the results of a study: A 95% CI is a range of values that 95% of the time will contain the real value for the phenomenon being observed in the source population.

An example of how the different measures of effect are calculated and how these statistical concepts are interpreted is shown below with the published data of the SHOCK (Should We Emergently Revascularize Occluded Coronaries for Cardiogenic Shock) Trial (N Engl J Med 1999;341:625-34). This was a multicenter RCT of 302 patients with cardiogenic shock complicating acute myocardial infarction. Patients were randomly assigned to emergency revascularization (experimental group, *n*=152) or initial medical stabilization (control group, *n*=150). The primary end point was 30-day mortality. At 30 days, 71 patients had died in the revascularization group and 84 patients had died in the medical group. Thus the event rate in the revascularization group was 47% (71/152), and the event rate in the medical therapy group was 56% (84/150). The RR of death at 30 days for patients in the revascularization group compared with the medical therapy group was 84% (0.47/0.56). The ARR of death at 30 days for patients in the revascularization group was 9.0% (0.56–0.47). The RRR of death at 30 days for patients in the revascularization group was 16% (1–0.84 or 0.09/0.56). The NNT to prevent one death at 30 days by performing emergent revascularization instead of using medical stabilization was 12 (1/0.09 = 11.1). The *P* value for the ARR was 0.11, which means that there was an 11% chance that the observed difference was due to chance and not a real difference between the groups. Thus, with a predetermined α level of 0.05, the null hypothesis was not rejected and the primary study result was not statistically significant. The 95% CI for the RR was 0.67 to 1.04, which means that 95% of the times that this protocol is reproduced in the same population, the real RR will be between 0.67 and 1.04. Since the CI spans the line of no difference (i.e., 1), the result is not statistically significant.

DIAGNOSTIC TESTS

Medical decision making requires the appropriate understanding and application of diagnostic test results, which include historical information, physical examination findings, and laboratory evaluations. The performance of a diagnostic test is assessed by comparing the results of the diagnostic test with the results of a criterion standard in a study population. Several terms are useful for describing the features of a diagnostic test (Table 2).

Sensitivity and Specificity

The *sensitivity* of a test is the proportion of patients with the disease who have a positive test. Sensitivity is calculated as the number of true positives (a) divided by the total number of patients with the disease (i.e., true positives [a] + false negatives [b]). If the test has a high sensitivity and the result is negative, the disease is ruled out. A mnemonic for this concept is *SnNout* (which refers to the phrase "*Se*nsitive test when *N*egative rules *out* disease").

The *specificity* of a test is the proportion of patients without the disease who have a negative test. Specificity is calculated as the number of true negatives (d) divided by the total number of patients without the disease (i.e., true negatives [d] + false positives [c]). If the test has a high specificity and the result is positive, the disease is ruled in. A mnemonic for this concept is *SpPin* (which refers to the phrase "*Sp*ecific test when *P*ositive rules *in* disease").

The sensitivity and specificity of a test depend on the inherent quality of the test and the characteristics of the specific population in which it is tested. They might be most helpful when the values are high and can be used to rule in or rule out disease; however, they are not usually practical to the clinician since they do not help revise the probability of disease in an individual patient.

Predictive Values

The positive predictive value (PPV) and negative predictive value (NPV) of a test provide the answer to the specific question a clinician might ask: What is the probability that the test result (positive or negative) for this patient is true? It is important to note that the predictive values are affected by the prevalence of disease in the population in which the test is applied.

Table 2. A 2×2 Table and Derivation of Diagnostic Test Features

		Criterion standard	
		+	−
Diagnostic test	+	a	c
	−	b	d

$$\text{Sensitivity} = \frac{a}{a+b}$$

$$\text{Specificity} = \frac{d}{c+d}$$

$$\text{PPV} = \frac{a}{a+c}$$

$$\text{NPV} = \frac{d}{b+d}$$

$$+\text{LR} = \frac{a/(a+b)}{c/(c+d)} = \frac{\text{Sensitivity}}{1-\text{Specificity}}$$

$$-\text{LR} = \frac{b/(a+b)}{d/(c+d)} = \frac{1-\text{Sensitivity}}{\text{Specificity}}$$

See text for abbreviations.

The PPV of a test is the probability that a patient with a positive test result actually has the disease. This is calculated as the number of true positives (a) divided by the total number of positives (true positives [a] + false positives [c]).

The NPV of a test is the probability that a patient with a negative test result actually does not have the disease. This is calculated as the number of true negatives (d) divided by the total number of negatives (true negatives [d] + false negatives [b]).

Likelihood Ratios

The positive likelihood ratio (+LR) and negative likelihood ratio (−LR) of a test are extremely useful measures because they facilitate probabilistic medical decision making (i.e., the use of Bayes theorem). They can be used to combine the results of multiple and serial diagnostic tests, and they can be used directly to calculate posttest probability of disease. Also, they are less affected by the prevalence of disease in a patient population.

The +LR is calculated as the probability of having a positive test in the presence of disease (a/a+b) divided by the probability of having a positive test in the absence of disease (c/c+d). This is equivalent to the sensitivity divided by (1 minus the specificity).

The –LR is calculated as the probability of having a negative test in the presence of disease (b/a+b) divided by the probability of having a negative test in the absence of disease (d/c+d). This is equivalent to (1 minus the sensitivity) divided by the specificity.

The posttest probability of disease can be obtained in two ways. The first is by use of a nomogram (Fig. 1). The second is by converting the pretest probability to odds, multiplying by the LR (or multiple LRs for serial tests), and then converting the posttest odds to probability, as follows:

$$\text{Probability} = \frac{\text{Odds}}{\text{Odds}+1}$$

$$\text{Odds} = \frac{\text{Probability}}{1-\text{Probability}}$$

Pretest odds × LR = Posttest odds

The following formula simplifies the above conversions and directly relates pretest probability to posttest probability without converting to odds:

$$\text{Posttest probability} = \frac{\text{Pretest probability} \times \text{LR}}{1 + \text{Pretest probability} \times (\text{LR}-1)}$$

Use the +LR if a test is positive, and use the –LR if a test is negative. An LR greater than 1 increases the probability of disease, and an LR less than 1 decreases the probability of disease. When the pretest probability of disease is intermediate, an LR greater than 10 essentially rules in the disease, whereas an LR less than 0.1 essentially rules out the disease.

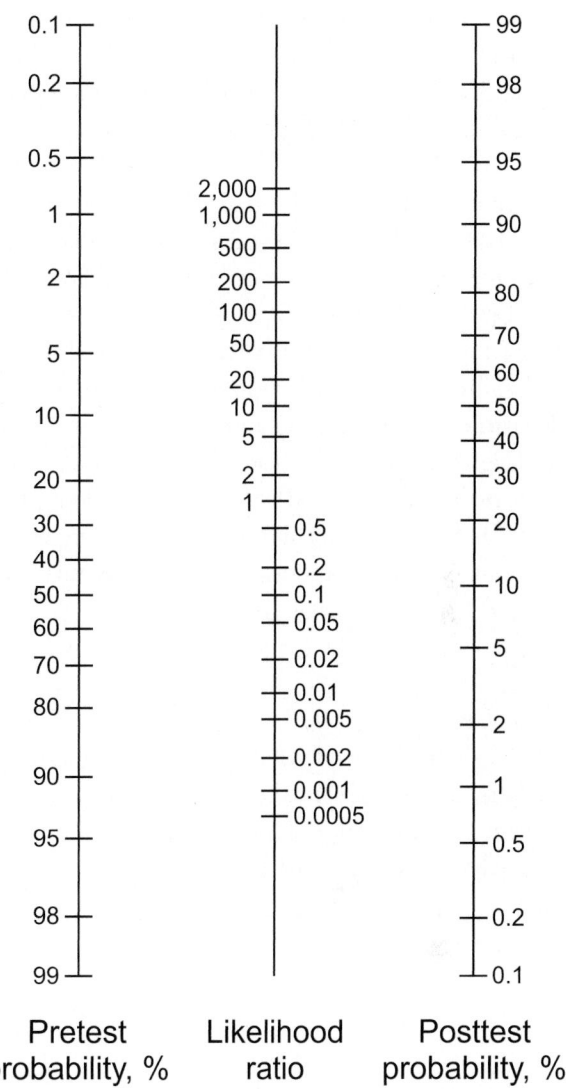

Fig. 1. Likelihood ratio nomogram for converting pretest probability to posttest probability.

An example of how to evaluate diagnostic tests is shown below with the published data of the Breathing Not Properly Multicenter Study (Circulation 2002;106:416-22). This was a prospective study of 1,538 patients presenting to emergency departments with a chief complaint of dyspnea. The accuracy of using a brain natriuretic peptide (BNP) concentration greater than 100 pg/mL (a threshold derived from a receiver operating characteristic curve in the same population) as a diagnostic test for heart failure was compared with the criterion standard, which was consensus of 2 independent cardiologists who reviewed the entire medical record and classified the cause of dyspnea as either heart failure or noncardiac. The cardiologists' review identified 722 patients with heart failure, of whom 650 had a BNP level greater than 100 pg/mL. Another 220 patients also had a BNP level greater than 100 pg/mL. From these data, one can derive the sensitivity, specificity, predictive values, and LRs for a BNP level greater than 100 pg/mL for the diagnosis of HF. After first trying this yourself, review Table 3. Thus, for a patient with dyspnea in the emergency department, with a history and physical examination findings that yield a pretest probability of 25% for acute heart failure, a BNP level less than 100 pg/mL provides a posttest probability of 4%, by using either the nomogram or the posttest probability formula: $0.25 \times 0.14/[1 + 0.25 \times (0.14 - 1)]$.

RESOURCE

The Evidence-Based Medicine Working Group. Users' guides to the medical literature: essentials of evidence-based clinical practice. Guyatt G, Rennie D, editors. Chicago: AMA Press; 2002.

Table 3.   Evaluation of Brain Natriuretic Peptide (BNP) Concentration as a Diagnostic Test for Heart Failure

		Criterion standard (cardiologists' review)	
		+	−
Diagnostic test	+	a=650	c=220
BNP>100 pg/mL	−	b	d

a+b=722   a+b+c+d=1,538

Values for b and d are calculated by use of simple algebra. The following are derived using the formulas in Table 2:

Sensitivity = 650/722 = 90%
Specificity = 596/816 = 73%
PPV = 650/870 = 75%
NPV = 596/668 = 89%
+LR = 0.9/0.27 = 3.3
−LR = 0.1/0.73 = 0.14

See text for abbreviations.

4

Noncardiac Surgery in Patients With Heart Disease

Traci L. Jurrens, MD

Clarence Shub, MD

The American College of Cardiology and the American Heart Association (ACC/AHA) have published guidelines for the perioperative evaluation and management of patients with heart disease who are to have noncardiac operations. The guidelines recommend a conservative approach. Expensive testing, invasive strategies, and revascularization are rarely, if ever, warranted just to "get the patient through an operation." Rather, the indications for extensive perioperative testing or revascularization are generally similar to those in a nonoperative setting.

■ Testing or revascularization is *not* indicated just to "get the patient through an operation."

EFFECT OF CORONARY ARTERY DISEASE
The risk of a perioperative myocardial infarction in patients without clinical evidence of heart disease is approximately 0.15%. In patients with clinical heart disease, the risk of a perioperative myocardial infarction can be stratified according to the *cardiovascular profile of the patient* (major, intermediate, minor, or no clinical predictors of increased risk) and according to the *cardiac stress of the operation* (high, medium, or low stress or risk).

■ Patients without clinical evidence of heart disease are at low risk (about 0.15%) of perioperative myocardial infarction.

The mortality rate in association with perioperative myocardial infarction is significantly higher than that with an infarct unrelated to an operation. Previously, the risk of perioperative myocardial infarction was less well recognized and the antemortem diagnosis was more difficult. Increased awareness of the problem, better patient selection, improved anesthetic and operative techniques, improved perioperative monitoring and management, and improved diagnostic techniques (including the newer biomarkers such as serum troponin) have all contributed to a significant reduction in mortality from perioperative myocardial infarction.

The risk of perioperative reinfarction is increased in the first 6 months after an index myocardial infarction. This risk decreases with increasing time between the index infarction and the planned operation. After percutaneous revascularization, patients have a high-risk period of 6 weeks and then an intermediate-risk period of 3 to 6 months. Ideally, noncardiac surgery is delayed at least 3 months. Sometimes clinical circumstances may warrant proceeding with surgery sooner than recommended (e.g., rapidly spreading tumors,

61

impending aortic aneurysm rupture, major fractures, and infections requiring drainage).

According to the ACC/AHA guidelines, an elective surgical procedure can be performed before 6 months has elapsed as long as the patient undergoes postinfarction risk stratification. Absence of postinfarction ischemia, a negative postinfarction stress test, and complete myocardial revascularization after infarction suggest a reduced risk of reinfarction with an elective operation. The ACC/AHA guidelines do suggest that it is prudent to wait at least 4 to 6 weeks after infarction before proceeding with an elective operation.

- Risk of perioperative reinfarction varies inversely with the time between the index infarction and the operation.
- Patients with a negative postinfarction stress test or complete postinfarction myocardial revascularization can proceed with an elective operation at 4 to 6 weeks after infarction.

The risk of perioperative reinfarction is *not* significantly different between patients who have had a Q-wave infarction and those who have had a non–Q-wave infarction.

- Recent Q-wave and non–Q-wave myocardial infarctions are associated with the same risk of perioperative reinfarction.

PREOPERATIVE CARDIAC RISK INDEXES

Risk factors in patients undergoing noncardiac operations include 1) type of operation (intrathoracic and intra-abdominal procedures have a higher risk than limb operations); 2) presence and severity of coronary artery disease, especially if unstable (heart failure or unstable angina); 3) status of left ventricular function (ejection fraction); 4) age of patient; 5) severe valvular heart disease, especially aortic stenosis; 6) serious cardiac arrhythmias; 7) associated medical conditions (e.g., chronic obstructive pulmonary disease, hypoxemia, diabetes mellitus, and renal insufficiency); and 8) overall functional status.

Clinical risk stratification tools can identify patients at high risk of perioperative ischemic events and guide appropriate perioperative medical strategies. The Revised Cardiac Risk Index identifies six independent predictors of major cardiac complications: high-risk surgery, history of ischemic heart disease, history of congestive heart failure, history of cerebrovascular disease, preoperative treatment with insulin, and preoperative creatinine level greater than 2.0 mg/dL (Table 1). One can easily calculate the risk of major cardiac complications by using the number of predictors (Table 2).

Perioperative risks can be stratified further into major, intermediate, and low (minor) risks (Table 3). Active conditions are more important than dormant ones, and the degree of abnormality is also important. The presence of major risk predictors warrants further evaluation and (usually) treatment that may delay or cancel the elective operation. The urgency of a noncardiac operation may dictate patient management. Thus, a patient with a recent myocardial infarction and an acute abdominal crisis generally requires laparotomy without delay. The presence of intermediate predictors of increased perioperative risk warrants careful clinical assessment and, when appropriate, use of additional cardiac testing. Minor predictors have relatively less clinical importance.

Table 1. Predictors in the Revised Cardiac Risk Index

1. High-risk surgery
2. History of ischemic heart disease
3. History of congestive heart failure
4. History of cerebrovascular disease
5. Preoperative treatment with insulin
6. Preoperative creatinine >2.0 mg/dL

Table 2. Rates of Major Cardiac Complications in the Revised Cardiac Risk Index

No. of predictors	Cardiac risk, %
0	0.4
1	0.9
2	7
≥3	11

Risk stratification based on the type of operation planned is also important (Table 4). *High-risk operations* include 1) major intrathoracic procedures, 2) abdominal (intraperitoneal) operations, 3) aortic surgi-

cal procedures (e.g., aortic aneurysmectomy), and 4) peripheral vascular operations.

High-risk operations have been associated with a higher incidence of postoperative congestive heart failure and a threefold greater incidence of myocardial infarction in comparison with other general surgical procedures. A major operation is often associated with large extravascular and intravascular fluid shifts or blood loss and postoperative hypoxemia. The magnitude and anticipated duration of the procedure are also important. Patients undergoing peripheral vascular operations are at high risk, primarily because of the increased incidence of associated coronary artery disease. Emergency major operations, especially in the elderly, are also considered high risk.

Intermediate-risk operations include 1) carotid endarterectomy, 2) head and neck procedures, 3) orthopedic and prostate operations, and 4) less extensive intraperitoneal and intrathoracic procedures.

Low-risk operations include 1) ophthalmologic procedures, 2) endoscopic surgery, 3) breast surgery, and 4) uncomplicated herniorrhaphy.

- High-risk operations include major intrathoracic, abdominal (intraperitoneal), and aortic surgical procedures (e.g., aortic aneurysmectomy).
- Patients undergoing peripheral vascular operations are also at high risk, primarily because of the increased incidence of associated coronary artery disease.

NONVASCULAR VERSUS VASCULAR SURGERY

Overall, perioperative cardiac event rates recently have decreased markedly, especially for patients undergoing *nonvascular* operations, partly because of improved patient selection, anesthetic techniques, and perioperative management. Most studies have focused on patients having *vascular* procedures, because they are at higher risk.

Routine coronary angiography performed before a vascular operation has demonstrated that more than one-half of patients with clinically suspected coronary artery disease have severe multivessel or inoperable coronary artery disease. Even patients with peripheral vascular disease and no previous history of heart disease may have severe coronary artery disease, especially those with diabetes mellitus.

Table 3.   Clinical Predictors of Increased Perioperative Cardiovascular Risk (Myocardial Infarction, Congestive Heart Failure, and Death)

Major risk
   Unstable coronary syndromes
      Recent myocardial infarction* with evidence of important ischemic risk by clinical symptoms or noninvasive study
      Unstable or severe† angina (Canadian class III or IV)
   Decompensated congestive heart failure
   Significant arrhythmias
      High-grade atrioventricular block
      Symptomatic ventricular arrhythmias in the presence of underlying heart disease
      Supraventricular arrhythmias with uncontrolled ventricular rate
   Severe valvular disease
Intermediate risk
   Mild angina pectoris (Canadian class I or II)
   Prior myocardial infarction by history of pathologic Q waves
   Compensated or prior congestive heart failure
   Diabetes mellitus
Minor risk
   Advanced age
   Abnormal ECG (left ventricular hypertrophy, left bundle branch block, ST-T abnormalities)
   Rhythm other than sinus (e.g., atrial fibrillation)
   Low functional capacity (e.g., inability to climb 1 flight of stairs with a bag of groceries)
   History of stroke
   Uncontrolled systemic hypertension

ECG, electrocardiogram.
*The American College of Cardiology National Database Library defines *recent myocardial infarction* as myocardial infarction occurring >7 days but ≤30 days previously.
†May include "stable" angina in patients who are unusually sedentary.

■ Even patients with peripheral vascular disease and no previous history of heart disease may have severe coronary artery disease, especially those with diabetes mellitus.

VALVULAR HEART DISEASE

In patients with valvular heart disease, the risk of a noncardiac operation depends on 1) the type, anatomical location, and severity of the valve lesion; 2) left ventricular systolic function; and 3) New York Heart Association (NYHA) functional class.

Patients with severe, symptomatic aortic stenosis have the greatest risk and, ideally, should undergo a corrective aortic valve operation or, in selected cases, balloon valvuloplasty before having a noncardiac operation. However, aortic balloon valvuloplasty has inherent risks, including serious vascular access complications, especially in the elderly. A selected, small group of Mayo Clinic patients who had severe aortic stenosis and who were not candidates for (or who refused) an aortic valve operation or valvuloplasty had noncardiac operations with a low risk of having major complications; nonetheless, most patients with aortic stenosis should be considered high risk and aortic valve replacement is generally warranted. Patients with severe mitral stenosis are at increased risk of perioperative congestive heart failure, especially if tachycardia occurs. Patients with milder degrees of aortic or mitral stenosis have a lower risk.

Generally, patients with aortic or mitral regurgitation, especially if they have only mild symptoms, seem to be at lower risk than those with stenotic lesions. Patients with advanced symptoms (NYHA class III or IV) of congestive heart failure and those with severe valvular regurgitation and left ventricular systolic dysfunction are at greater risk (regardless of the mechanism) and should undergo further evaluation and treatment before having a noncardiac operation, especially if it includes a high-risk surgical procedure (Table 4).

■ Patients with severe, symptomatic aortic stenosis have the greatest risk and, ideally, should undergo a corrective aortic valve operation before having a noncardiac operation.
■ Patients with severe mitral stenosis are at increased risk of perioperative congestive heart failure, especial-

Table 4.   Cardiac Risk* Stratification for Noncardiac Surgical Procedures

High (reported cardiac risk often >5%)
  Emergency major operations, particularly in the elderly
  Aortic and other major vascular
  Peripheral vascular
  Anticipated prolonged surgical procedures associated with large fluid shifts or blood loss
Intermediate (reported cardiac risk generally <5%)
  Carotid endarterectomy
  Head and neck
  Intraperitoneal and intrathoracic
  Orthopedic
  Prostate
Low† (reported cardiac risk generally <1%)
  Endoscopic procedures
  Superficial procedures
  Cataract
  Breast

*Combined incidence of cardiac death and nonfatal myocardial infarction.
†Does not generally require further preoperative cardiac testing.

ly if tachycardia occurs.
■ Patients with advanced symptoms (NYHA class III or IV) of congestive heart failure and those with severe valvular regurgitation and left ventricular systolic dysfunction are at greater risk (regardless of the mechanism) and should undergo further evaluation and treatment before having a noncardiac operation, especially if it includes a high-risk surgical procedure.

HYPERTROPHIC OBSTRUCTIVE CARDIOMYOPATHY

In general, patients with hypertrophic obstructive cardiomyopathy tolerate noncardiac operations reasonably well. However, some of them are at increased risk. In general, these patients require closer perioperative monitoring. Hemodynamic changes associated with an anesthetic-related decrease in peripheral resistance, hypovolemia, or adrenergic stimulation may increase the left ventricular outflow tract gradient and lead to hemodynamic deterioration.

■ In patients with hypertrophic obstructive cardiomyopathy, hemodynamic changes associated with an anesthetic-related decrease in peripheral resistance, hypovolemia, or adrenergic stimulation may increase the left ventricular outflow tract gradient and lead to hemodynamic deterioration.

PREOPERATIVE CARDIOVASCULAR FUNCTIONAL ASSESSMENT

The ability of a patient to exercise is an important indicator of how well he or she will tolerate a noncardiac operation. If a patient is able to exercise moderately (4-5 metabolic equivalents [METs]) without symptoms, the risk is relatively low. Preoperative exercise stress testing is an important objective means of functional assessment before a noncardiac operation (Table 5) and is especially important when the functional status of the patient is unclear.

Postoperative cardiac risk is increased in patients with abnormal findings on a preoperative exercise stress test and in those who are unable to exercise to a moderate workload (e.g., 4-5 METs). In one study of patients undergoing symptom-limited exercise radionuclide angiography before a peripheral vascular operation, perioperative cardiac events occurred only in those unable to exercise at a relatively low workload of 400 kg-m/min (4.5 METs for a 70-kg patient). Activities such as digging in the garden and walking at a brisk pace (3.5-4 mph) are associated with energy costs of about 5 METs. Climbing a flight of stairs, scrubbing floors, and playing golf generally exceed 4 METs. Participating in strenuous sports (swimming or tennis) exceeds 10 METs (Table 6).

■ If a patient is able to exercise moderately (4-5 METs) without symptoms, the perioperative risk is relatively low.
■ In general, postoperative cardiac events occur more frequently in patients with abnormal findings on a preoperative exercise stress test and in those who are unable to exercise to a moderate workload (e.g., 4-5 METs).
■ Activities such as digging in the garden and walking

Table 5. Prognostic Gradient of Ischemic Responses During an ECG-Monitored Exercise Test

Patients with suspected or proven CAD
High risk
   Ischemia induced by low-level exercise* (<4 METs or heart rate <100 bpm [<70% age predicted]), manifested by 1 or more of the following:
      Horizontal or downsloping ST depression >0.1 mV
      ST-segment elevation >0.1 mV in non-infarct lead
      ≥5 abnormal leads
      Persistent ischemic response >3 min after exertion
      Typical angina
Intermediate risk
   Ischemia induced by moderate-level exercise (4-6 METs or heart rate 100-130 bpm [70%-85% age predicted]), manifested by 1 or more of the following:
      Horizontal or downsloping ST depression >0.1 mV
      Typical angina
      Persistent ischemic response >1-3 min after exertion
      3 or 4 abnormal leads
Low risk
   No ischemia or ischemia induced at high-level exercise (>7 METs or heart rate >130 bpm [<85% age predicted]), manifested by
      Horizontal or downsloping ST depression >0.1 mV
      Typical angina
      1 or 2 abnormal leads
Inadequate test
   Inability to reach adequate target workload or heart rate response for age without an ischemic response. For patients undergoing a noncardiac operation, ability to exercise to at least the intermediate-risk level without ischemia should be considered a low risk for perioperative ischemic events

bpm, beats per minute; CAD, coronary artery disease; ECG, electrocardiographically; MET, metabolic equivalent.

*Workload and heart rate estimates for risk severity require adjustment for patient age. Maximal target heart rates for 40- and 80-year-old subjects taking no cardioactive medication are 180 and 140 bpm, respectively.

at a brisk pace (3.5-4 mph) are associated with energy costs of about 5 METs. Climbing a flight of stairs, scrubbing floors, and playing golf generally exceed 4 METs.

PREOPERATIVE FUNCTIONAL ASSESSMENT OF PATIENTS UNABLE TO EXERCISE

In patients unable to exercise adequately, pharmacologic stress testing (intravenous dipyridamole [or adenosine] thallium [or sestamibi] imaging or dobutamine stress echocardiography) has been used as an alternative means of stress testing, and each type of pharmacologic stress testing demonstrates similar patterns of risk prediction. The stress testing data are most valuable if the test results are negative (i.e., they have a high *negative* predictive value). Patients with normal scans are at low risk. The opposite is not true, however: positive stress tests have a low *positive* predictive value for perioperative events. The incorporation of clinical factors improves the specificity and predictive value of a positive scan. For example, patients with a thallium redistribution defect in patients with one or more *clinical* risk factors has been associated with a higher incidence of perioperative cardiac complications than in patients with a reversible thallium defect but without such clinical risk factors. Severe ischemia has greater predictive value than mild ischemia. In addition to thallium redistribution, ischemic electrocardiographic changes during the test are predictive of perioperative events. Dobutamine stress testing allows identification of the heart rate when ischemia first appears and calculation of the ischemic threshold, based on the expected age-related heart rate response. Ischemic thresholds less than 70% have been shown to increase perioperative risk.

CLINICAL APPROACH TO PREOPERATIVE ASSESSMENT AND MANAGEMENT

Generally, the perioperative risk for nonvascular non–high-risk operations is low, limiting the predictive value of stress testing. Standard clinical evaluation should suffice in most of these low-risk patients.

Functionally active patients without major- or intermediate-risk factors for whom there is no clinical suspicion of coronary artery disease do not need to undergo *routine* stress testing before a noncardiac operation, especially for a low-risk procedure. Patients with chronic stable angina who are active and able to perform activities of daily living (4-5 METs) probably can tolerate most types of low- or intermittent-risk noncardiac operations. This group of patients routinely would not require preoperative stress testing.

For optimal use of resources, the ACC/AHA guidelines recommend that if a patient has had coronary revascularization within the past 5 years and if the clinical status has remained stable without recurrent symptoms or signs of ischemia, additional cardiac testing generally is not needed. For patients with ischemic heart disease who have not had coronary revascularization but who have undergone coronary evaluation in the past 2 years (assuming adequate testing and a

Table 6. Estimated Requirements for Various Activities

1 MET	Can you take care of yourself?
	Eat, dress, or use the toilet?
	Walk indoors around the house?
	Walk a block or two on level ground at 2-3 mph or 3.2-4.8 km/h?
	Do light work around the house such as dusting or washing dishes?
4 METs	Climb a flight of stairs or walk up a hill?
	Walk on level ground at 4 mph or 6.4 km/h?
	Run a short distance?
	Do heavy work around the house like scrubbing floors or lifting or moving heavy furniture?
	Participate in moderate recreational activities such as golf, bowling, dancing, doubles tennis, or throwing a baseball or football?
>10 METs	Participate in strenuous sports such as swimming, singles tennis, football, basketball, or skiing?

MET, metabolic equivalent.

favorable outcome of testing), it usually is unnecessary to repeat testing unless there has been an acceleration of angina or new symptoms of ischemia have appeared during the interim.

For patients at intermediate clinical risk, consideration of both the functional capacity and the level of operation-specific risk is necessary. Further noninvasive testing should be considered for patients with poor functional capacity or moderate functional capacity before a high-risk procedure is performed. Patients about to undergo a high-risk operation, especially if they have serious clinical risk factors, should be considered for preoperative stress testing. In selected patients with known coronary artery disease and significant (class III or IV) symptomatic limitation or accelerating angina, preoperative coronary angiography is often indicated, as it would be even if a noncardiac operation were not being contemplated.

The CASS (Coronary Artery Surgery Study) registry showed that coronary revascularization before a noncardiac operation can decrease perioperative cardiac mortality to approximately 1% or less, compared with 2.4% for patients with similar coronary artery disease treated medically. There are no randomized trials showing benefit of coronary revascularization before noncardiac surgery. The potential risks (morbidity and mortality) of coronary artery bypass grafting itself, especially in patients older than 70 years, must also be considered before a noncardiac operation is performed.

A recent Veterans Administration study demonstrated that perioperative outcomes are as good with perioperative medical treatment as with revascularization (percutaneous coronary intervention [PCI] or coronary artery bypass graft [CABG]) in carefully screened patients undergoing vascular surgery. This study excluded patients with left main coronary artery disease, severe systolic dysfunction, unstable angina, and severe aortic stenosis.

A multicenter study of percutaneous transluminal coronary angioplasty (PTCA) has demonstrated an overall mortality of 1% (2.8% in the presence of triple-vessel disease), a 4.3% incidence of nonfatal myocardial infarction, and a need for emergency CABG in 3.4% of patients. Coronary stenting (which is increasingly used during PCI) affects the timing of surgery. The strategy of performing coronary angiography and PTCA before a noncardiac operation to reduce the risk of a noncar-

diac procedure depends on individual circumstances and has not proved beneficial in controlled clinical trials. Prolonged antiplatelet therapy using clopidogrel after coronary stenting mandates delaying noncardiac surgery. The frequency of perioperative cardiac events in a patient who has had PTCA is highest immediately after the operative procedure and decreases thereafter with a second increase in cardiac events 90 days after PTCA because of neointimal hyperplasia. Although brief clopidogrel treatment can be used with bare metal stents (vs. drug-eluting stents), there is an increased risk of perioperative cardiac complications in the first 6 weeks after stenting procedures. The risk of converting a stable but flow-limiting coronary lesion into a less stable, nonflow-limiting lesion as a result of PCI should be taken into account. Stent thrombosis is most common in the first 2 weeks after stent placement but can occur later as well. The rate of stent thrombosis diminishes after endothelialization of the stent occurs (4-8 weeks).

In patients who require noncardiac surgery after placement of bare metal stents, noncardiac surgery should be delayed at least 6 weeks after stent placement, at which time stents are generally endothelialized and antiplatelet therapy can be safely discontinued. There are no studies currently available on drug-eluting stents, but if they are used, delaying surgery for at least 6 months should be considered. The potential risk of stent thrombosis due to prematurely stopping clopidogrel has to be considered in the overall perioperative risk assessment.

In most ambulatory patients who are active enough to perform adequate stress testing, the exercise electrocardiographic treadmill test is usually preferred because it provides an estimate of both functional capacity and ischemic response. In patients with an abnormal resting electrocardiogram (e.g., left ventricular hypertrophy, left bundle branch block, digitalis effect, and nonspecific ST-T abnormalities), a cardiac imaging exercise test such as exercise echocardiography or myocardial perfusion imaging should be considered. The choice of the specific test depends on various factors, especially local expertise with a specific technique.

Interventional procedures rarely are needed just to lower the risk of a noncardiac operation, unless the intervention is thought to be indicated anyway (i.e., if the patient were not undergoing a noncardiac operation). Thus, the strategy of performing coronary revascularization just to avoid perioperative cardiac complications should be reserved for only a small subset of very high-risk patients.

According to the ACC/AHA guidelines, class I indications for preoperative coronary angiography for patients with suspected or proven coronary artery disease include the following (Table 7):

1. High-risk results of noninvasive testing
2. Severe (class III or IV) angina unresponsive to medical therapy
3. Unstable angina
4. Nondiagnostic or equivocal noninvasive test results in a high-risk patient, for example, multiple clinical risk factors in a patient undergoing a high-risk operation (see above)

Coronary angiography generally is not indicated in low-risk patients or in those who are asymptomatic after coronary revascularization and have good exercise capacity.

- Generally, the perioperative risk for nonvascular non–high-risk operations is low, limiting the predictive value of cardiac stress testing. Standard clinical evaluation should suffice in most of these low-risk patients.
- Patients with chronic stable angina who are active and able to perform activities of daily living (4-5 METs) probably can tolerate the stress of most types of noncardiac operations.
- If a patient has undergone coronary revascularization within the past 5 years and if the clinical status has remained stable without recurrent symptoms or signs of ischemia, additional cardiac testing generally is not needed.
- For patients with ischemic heart disease who have not had coronary revascularization but who have undergone coronary evaluation in the past 2 years (assuming adequate testing and a favorable outcome of testing), it usually is unnecessary to repeat testing unless there has been an acceleration of angina or new symptoms of ischemia have appeared during the interim.
- In selected patients with known coronary artery disease and significant (class III or IV) symptomatic limitation or accelerating angina, preoperative coronary angiography is often indicated, as it would be even if a noncardiac operation were not being contemplated.

Table 7.   Recommendations for Coronary Angiography in Perioperative Evaluation

Class I: Patients with suspected or known CAD
   Evidence for high risk of adverse outcome based on noninvasive test results
   Angina unresponsive to adequate medical therapy
   Unstable angina, particularly when facing intermediate-risk or high-risk noncardiac surgery
   Equivocal noninvasive test results in patients at high clinical risk undergoing high-risk surgery

Class IIa
   Multiple markers of intermediate clinical risk and planned vascular surgery (noninvasive testing should be considered first)
   Moderate to large region of ischemia on noninvasive testing but without high-risk features and without lower LVEF
   Nondiagnostic noninvasive test results in patients of intermediate clinical risk undergoing high-risk noncardiac surgery
   Urgent noncardiac surgery while convalescing from acute MI

Class IIb
   Perioperative MI
   Medically stabilized class III or IV angina and planned low-risk or minor surgery

Class III
   Low-risk noncardiac surgery with known CAD and no high-risk results on noninvasive testing
   Asymptomatic after coronary revascularization with excellent exercise capacity (≥7 METs)
   Mild stable angina with good left ventricular function and no high-risk noninvasive test results
   Noncandidate for coronary revascularization owing to concomitant medical illness, severe left ventricular dysfunction (e.g., LVEF <0.20), or refusal
   Candidate for liver, lung, or renal transplant who is more than 40 years old as part of evaluation for transplantation, unless noninvasive testing reveals high risk

CAD, coronary artery disease; LVEF, left ventricular ejection fraction; MET, metabolic equivalent; MI, myocardial infarction.

■ The strategy of performing coronary angiography and "preventive" PTCA or coronary stenting preoperatively to reduce the risk of noncardiac surgery has not been proved in controlled clinical trials.

■ In carefully screened patients with stable coronary artery disease scheduled for vascular surgery, perioperative medical treatment is an acceptable option.

■ After placement of bare metal stents, patients should preferably wait 6 weeks before undergoing noncardiac surgery.

PREOPERATIVE HEMODYNAMIC ASSESSMENT AND INTRAOPERATIVE HEMODYNAMIC MONITORING

If overt congestive heart failure is present, medical therapy should be optimized preoperatively, but dehydration and hypotension from overly aggressive diuretic and vasodilator therapy must be avoided. In patients with overt congestive heart failure, preoperative or intraoperative monitoring with Swan-Ganz catheters may be useful in selected cases, especially with high-risk procedures, so that intravenous fluid and drug therapy can be guided optimally. Monitoring should be continued into the postoperative period, when major extravascular fluid mobilization could precipitate pulmonary edema in patients with severe valvular heart disease or left ventricular dysfunction. The risks of invasive hemodynamic monitoring must be balanced against the potential benefits. Many patients can be managed adequately on a clinical basis without the need for invasive hemodynamic monitoring. Randomized trials have not proved a major benefit from invasive hemodynamic monitoring for decreasing perioperative cardiac morbidity. Preoperative serum brain natriuretic peptide (BNP) determinations may be useful as a predictor of perioperative outcome in selected patients.

■ If overt congestive heart failure is present, medical therapy should be optimized preoperatively.

■ In patients with overt congestive heart failure, preoperative or intraoperative monitoring with Swan-Ganz catheters may be useful, especially with high-risk procedures, so that intravenous fluid and drug therapy can be guided optimally.

■ Randomized trials have not proved a major benefit from invasive hemodynamic monitoring for decreasing perioperative cardiac morbidity.

PREOPERATIVE MEDICATIONS AND MANAGEMENT

Patients should continue to take their cardiovascular medications up to the time of the operation and should resume taking them as soon after the operation as possible. There appears to be benefit for use of β-blockers in high-risk patients; however, further information is needed about their use in low- and intermediate-risk patients. Treatment with β-blockers, which reduce postoperative ischemia and improve perioperative outcomes, should remain uninterrupted as long as possible, especially in patients with coronary artery disease. Postoperative sinus tachycardia should be prevented in these patients, especially if ischemia developed on preoperative stress testing. In selected patients, treatment with β-blockers, and other cardiac medications if needed, can be continued until the morning of the operation. Patients taking β-blockers who have an operation may experience involuntary "drug withdrawal" if the medication is not administered early in the postoperative period. This problem has been prevented in recent years by temporary intravenous administration of β-blockers, such as esmolol, until the patient can resume taking medications orally. Low-risk patients may not benefit from initiation of preoperative β-blocker therapy: the potential adverse side effects (e.g., hypotension or bradycardia) may outweigh the cardioprotective effects. Although calcium channel blockers and anesthetics have additive vasodilator and negative inotropic effects, most patients who take these agents can be anesthetized safely. Calcium channel blockers, especially diltiazem, have been shown to reduce perioperative ischemia, supraventricular tachycardia, and major cardiac events.

There is preliminary evidence that the use of statin therapy preoperatively may decrease perioperative cardiac events, and in small randomized trials clonidine has also been shown to reduce perioperative ischemia and death.

Although mild or moderate hypertension usually does not warrant delaying the operation, severe hypertension (i.e., systolic pressure >180 mm Hg and diastolic pressure >110 mm Hg) should be controlled before the operation is performed. Patients with hypertension whose blood pressure is controlled with medication usually tolerate anesthesia better than those with poorly controlled blood pressure. The decision to delay the operation to achieve improved blood pressure control should take into account the urgency of the operation. Significant perioperative hypertension occurs in approximately 25% of patients with hypertension, appears unrelated to preoperative control, and occurs frequently in patients undergoing abdominal aortic aneurysm repair and other peripheral vascular procedures, including carotid endarterectomy. If oral intake of antihypertensive medications must be interrupted, parenteral therapy may be needed perioperatively. Various antihypertensive medications can be used, including intravenous β-blockers, vasodilators, calcium channel blockers, and angiotensin-converting enzyme inhibitors. For patients taking clonidine orally, it may be helpful to switch to a long-acting clonidine cutaneous patch preoperatively to avoid "rebound hypertension" perioperatively. Preoperative myocardial ischemia occurs in up to 35% of elderly patients before hip fracture surgery. Early preoperative administration of epidural analgesia may lessen overall perioperative risks. Appropriate analgesia is especially important in this elderly group.

- Treatment with β-blockers should remain uninterrupted as long as possible, especially in patients with coronary artery disease. Routine use of β-blockers should be used in high-risk patients undergoing surgery.
- Although calcium channel blockers and anesthetics have additive vasodilator and negative inotropic effects, most patients who take these agents can be anesthetized safely.
- Although mild or moderate hypertension usually does not warrant delaying the operation, severe hypertension should be controlled before the operation is performed.

ARRHYTHMIAS AND CONDUCTION DISTURBANCES

Rapid postoperative atrial arrhythmias affect almost 1 million patients annually. In contrast, bradyarrhythmias or ventricular arrhythmias severe enough to require treatment affect less than 1% of patients undergoing noncardiac surgery. Clinical evaluation should seek to uncover any underlying heart or pulmonary disease, drug toxicity, and electrolyte or metabolic abnormality that might be causing arrhythmias or conduction disturbances. Symptomatic or hemodynamically significant arrhythmias should be treated before the patient undergoes a noncardiac operation; the indications for treatment are similar to those in the nonoperative setting. It is important to correct even mild degrees of preoperative hypokalemia in patients taking digitalis. The respiratory alkalosis that usually occurs during general anesthesia may cause a decrease in extracellular potassium concentration and provoke arrhythmias. Asymptomatic conduction system disease such as bundle branch block, bifascicular block, or even trifascicular block does not predict high-grade or complete heart block during a noncardiac operation and does not by itself mandate prophylactic temporary pacing. Atrial tachyarrhythmia is a common complication after thoracic surgery and is associated with longer hospital stay. Calcium channel blockers and β-blockers reduce the risk of atrial tachyarrhythmias.

- Symptomatic or hemodynamically significant arrhythmias should be treated before the patient undergoes a noncardiac operation.
- It is important to correct even mild degrees of preoperative hypokalemia in patients taking digitalis.
- Asymptomatic conduction system disease such as bundle branch block, bifascicular block, or even trifascicular block does not predict high-grade or complete heart block during a noncardiac operation and does not by itself mandate prophylactic temporary pacing.

APPROACH TO PATIENTS REQUIRING LONG-TERM ORAL ANTICOAGULATION

The issue of discontinuation of oral anticoagulation in the perioperative setting requires balancing the thromboembolic potential of the patient's cardiovascular disease with the hemorrhagic risk of the operation. For most cardiovascular situations, including patients with bioprosthetic valves, the acute thromboembolic potential is low. The thromboembolic potential is high for patients with mechanical prosthetic valves, especially those in the tricuspid or mitral position, and for patients with recent embolic episodes from, for example, cardiomyopathies, atrial fibrillation, ventricular aneurysms, or acute infarctions. Unfortunately, there are no large randomized trials studying the risk of thromboembolism versus the risk of hemorrhage in various conditions and types of operation.

Several small studies have suggested that patients with low or moderate risk can have an international normalized ratio (INR) less than 2.0 for 5 to 7 days with relative safety. A reasonable approach to these patients would be to discontinue the use of warfarin several days in advance of the operation, which should be performed as soon as the INR is 1.5 or less. Oral anticoagulation is resumed as soon as possible postoperatively, and heparin is reserved for patients whose INR is less than 2.0 for 5 days or more. In patients at high risk of thromboembolic complications (Table 8), intravenous heparin coverage can be instituted until 6 hours before the operation and then resumed as soon as possible postoperatively. The use of heparin can be discontinued after the use of warfarin has been resumed and the INR is in the therapeutic range.

Recent studies have shown that standardized periprocedural use of subcutaneous low-molecular-weight heparin (LMWH) is associated with a low risk of thromboembolic and major bleeding complications. LMWH is an alternative to unfractionated heparin for bridging therapy. The use of LMWH is appealing because it can be given in an outpatient setting. In patients who have mechanical valves and require interruption of warfarin therapy for emergency noncardiac surgery, fresh frozen plasma is preferred over high-dose vitamin K.

Five days of subtherapeutic INR for patients with low to moderate thromboembolic risk is probably reasonable.

- Perioperative heparin coverage should be used in patients with a high thromboembolic risk.
- Perioperative use of subcutaneous LMWH is being used as an alternative to standard anticoagulation with unfractionated heparin.

Examination Strategy

For the purposes of cardiology examinations, the most important information to remember about evaluating

Table 8.   High-Risk Factors for Thromboembolism

Older generation thrombogenic valves (Björk-Shiley)
Mechanical mitral valve replacement
Mechanical aortic valve replacement with *any* risk factor or multiples of the following risk factors in the absence of a prosthetic heart valve:
1. Atrial fibrillation
2. Left ventricular dysfunction
3. Previous thromboembolism
4. Hypercoagulable condition

patients with heart disease before noncardiac operations includes the following:

1. The clinical indicators of high, intermediate, and low risk for a cardiac event in the perioperative period
2. The surgical procedures associated with high, intermediate, and low risk for precipitating perioperative myocardial infarction and cardiac complications
3. Patients with peripheral vascular disease are at high risk of a perioperative cardiac event, and most of these patients should have some type of stress test before an elective vascular operation
4. The indications for preoperative testing and revascularization are similar to those in the nonoperative setting and are not based on getting the patient through the planned operation

Not all patients with peripheral vascular disease need preoperative stress tests (e.g., patients who had complete coronary revascularization <5 years earlier and who remain moderately active and asymptomatic). Patients can generally have a favorable operative outcome even in the presence of significant cardiac disease, and so the indications for preoperative testing and revascularization are similar to those in the nonoperative setting and are based on a patient's long-term cardiac requirements.

5

ESSENTIAL MOLECULAR BIOLOGY OF CARDIOVASCULAR DISEASES

Cindy W. Tom, MD

Robert D. Simari, MD

BASICS OF MOLECULAR BIOLOGY

Deoxyribonucleic acid (DNA), the fundamental genetic material of life, specifies the amino acid sequence of the large number of proteins that make up cells. *Nucleotides* are the building blocks of DNA. DNA consists of nucleotide chains, and each nucleotide consists of a nitrogenous base (purine or pyrimidine), a pentose sugar (2-deoxyribose in DNA and ribose in ribonucleic acid [RNA]), and a phosphate group. The four bases in DNA are adenine (A), guanine (G), cytosine (C), and thymine (T); uridine (U) replaces thymine in RNA (Fig. 1). The nucleotide sequence determines the amino acids encoded. It is the sequence-specific pairing of these nucleotides that is the basis for inheritance of the genetic code. A binds to T, and G binds to C: it is from this pairing that the double helical structure of DNA is derived, with its unique ability to reproduce very accurately over many generations (each chain acting as a unique template to which complementary base pairs bind). The genetic information in DNA is transferred to RNA through a process called *transcription* and from RNA to peptides (proteins) through *translation*.

- Pyrimidines (A and G) bind only to purines (C, T, and U).
- A binds to T.
- G binds to C.
- DNA is double-stranded.
- Messenger RNA (mRNA) is single-stranded.

- DNA $\xrightarrow{\text{transcription}}$ RNA $\xrightarrow{\text{translation}}$ Protein.

Gene Structure

A *gene* is a collection of adjacent nucleotides that specify the amino acids of a unique polypeptide. A *chromosome* is a microscopically visible long thread of DNA that contains many genes. The human genome has 23 pairs of chromosomes (44 autosomal and 2 sex chromosomes) containing about 3 billion base pairs of DNA and approximately 20,000 to 30,000 genes. The primary structure of DNA is determined by its base pair composition (Fig. 2). The tertiary structure is *not* determined by its base pair sequence. Rather, double-stranded DNA in chromosomes forms a double helical structure that undergoes subsequent supercoiling to pack the DNA into the nucleus in such a way as to avoid torsion and uncontrolled double strand breakage. Later, for replication and transcription, a protein can introduce negative supercoiling so that strand separation is favored and the base pairs are exposed.

The human genome contains 3.2 gigabases. More than 50% of chromosomal DNA is long, repeated

73

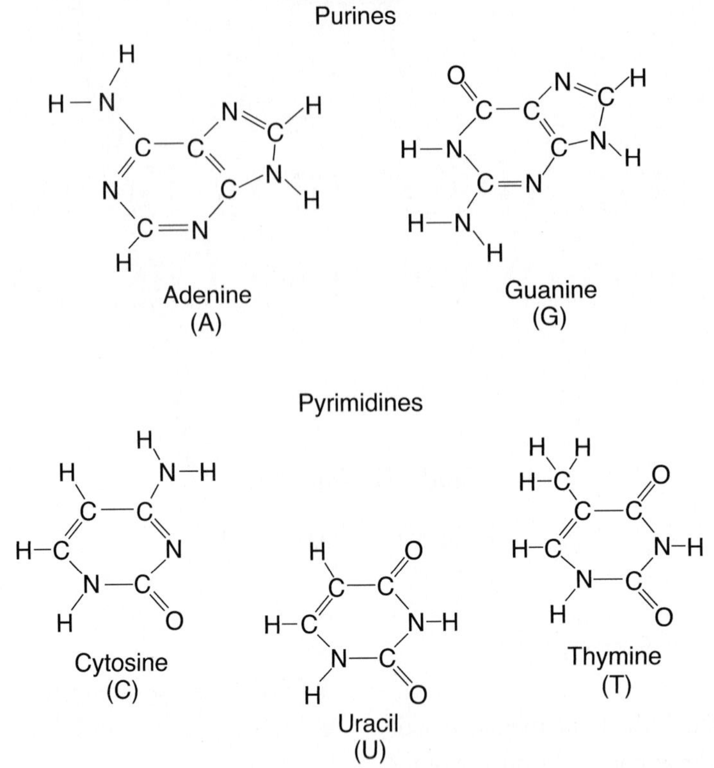

Purines

Adenine
(A)

Guanine
(G)

Pyrimidines

Cytosine
(C)

Uracil
(U)

Thymine
(T)

Fig. 1. Chemical structure of purines and pyrimidines.

elements. Only 25% of the genome is transcribed, and 1% encodes for protein.

A gene is an ordered unit of DNA that contains important structural elements necessary for creating a functional product (whether it be protein or an RNA molecule). The "average" gene encodes for 400 amino acids. Genes are divided into exons and introns.

Introns are DNA sequences whose RNA products are nonfunctional and are removed from mRNA. Each intron contains specific identifying base pair sequences at its boundaries. In contrast, *exons* are DNA sequences whose fully functional RNA products exit the nucleus and enter the cytoplasm, where they are translated into specific proteins (Fig. 3).

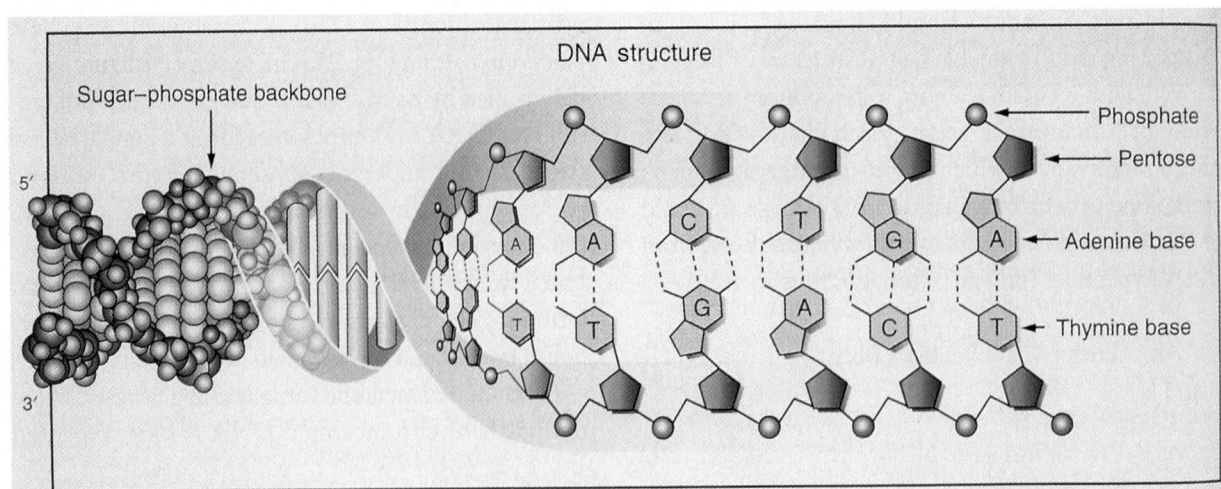

Fig. 2. The structure of DNA. C, cytosine; G, guanine.

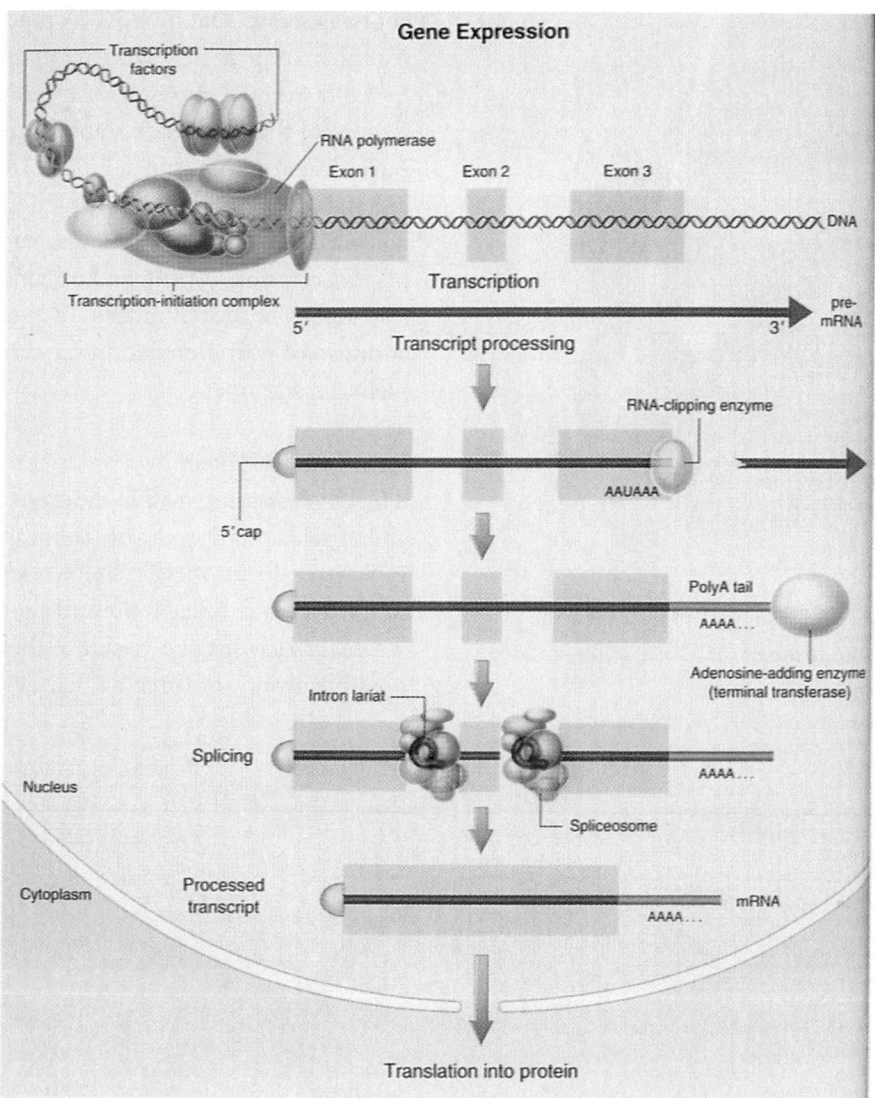

Fig. 3. Gene expression.

All chromosomes are organized with two arms attached to a centromere. The centromere is the point where a chromosome is attached to a spindle during cell division. The short arm is designated *p* and the long arm *q*, so that mutations and genes can be referred to by the chromosome number followed by the arm, the band, and the subband where the gene of interest lies (e.g., *7q31* is on the long arm of chromosome 7, band 3, subband 1). A chromosome consists of both nucleic acids and proteins. DNA is complexed with proteins, called *histones* (Fig. 4), into nucleoprotein fibers, called *chromatin*. It is chromatin that gives DNA its beadlike appearance.

Every nucleic acid chain has an orientation that refers to the orientation of its sugar phosphate backbone. The end that terminates with the 5' carbon is the *5' end*, and the end that terminates with the 3' carbon is the *3' end*. Because double-stranded DNA helices contain identical copies, it is standard to refer to DNA in the 5' to 3' direction. DNA and RNA chains form in the 5' to 3' direction, and proteins are formed in the same direction, which is from the amino to the carboxy terminus of the polypeptide chain.

Genes contain DNA sequences that are involved in the control of production of mRNA (transcription) and protein (translation). *Promoters* are upstream regu-

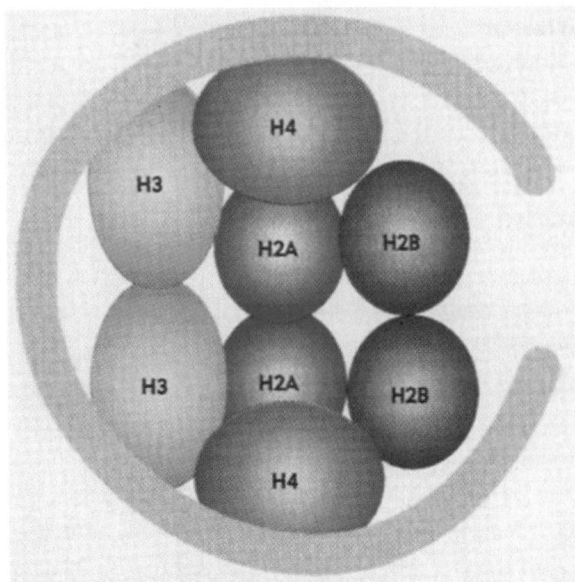

Fig. 4. Diagram of nucleosome demonstrating the relationship between histones 2A, 2B, 3, and 4 and associated DNA.

latory elements that bind RNA polymerases and the complex of proteins that regulate transcription. *Enhancers* and *suppressors* are bidirectional DNA sequences that modulate transcription of DNA and can be found within or at a distance from a gene. These enhancer and suppressor sequences bind proteins known as *transcription factors* that regulate the process of transcription. At the end of genes are sequences responsible for the termination of transcription and the addition of polyadenylation sequences required for mRNA transport.

From Gene to Protein

The DNA sequence within the exons of a gene and the amino acids that it codes are colinear (Fig. 5). That is, DNA encodes for specific amino acids in a linear fashion, with three bases representing one amino acid. There is a lack of a one-to-one relationship between all possible groups of three nucleic acids (codons) and

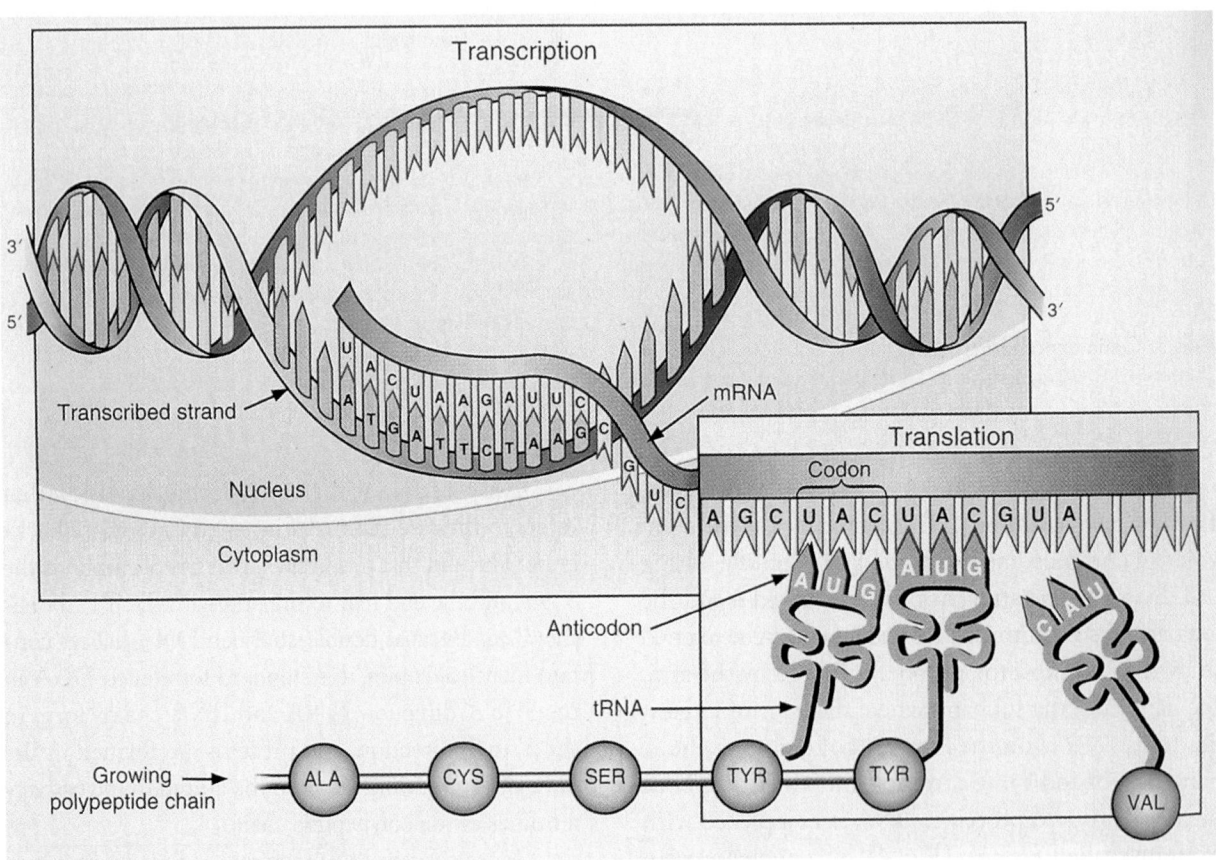

Fig. 5. Transcription and translation. A, adenine; ALA, alanine; C, cytosine; CYS, cysteine; G, guanine; SER, serine; T, thymine; TYR, tyrosine; U, uridine; VAL, valine.

amino acids. Thus, the genetic code is a degenerate code with 64 possible codons specifying only 20 amino acids. Each amino acid has one to six specifying codons.

Transcription, the formation of RNA from DNA, is a complex process that involves many known and unknown proteins in a highly regulated fashion (Fig. 5). Transcription in eukaryotic cells is in three forms, using different RNA polymerases. Transcription that results in mRNA (which makes up only 3%-5% of the total RNA within a cell) is dependent on RNA polymerase II. The RNA polymerases are made up of several subunits and bind DNA sequences (promoters) through separate DNA binding proteins known as *transcription factors*. The RNA strand produced by the polymerase is formed upon a single-strand DNA template. This resulting mRNA is complementary to the template DNA.

- A *codon* is three successive nucleotides of mRNA that code for a single amino acid.
- *Stop* (UAA, UGA, and UAG) and *Start* (AUG) codons signal the start and termination of protein RNA translation.
- AUG (start codon) codes for methionine.

The primary mRNA (pre-mRNA) transcript must undergo several processing steps before protein translation can occur in the cytoplasm. The ends of the initial transcript must be modified with methyl capping of the 5' terminal end and polyadenylation of the 3' terminal end. The removal of introns by splicing in the nucleus results in a mature mRNA that is transported to the cytoplasm for translation. Complementary DNA (cDNA) is a product of reverse transcribing mRNA and, as such, does not contain introns.

Translation is the complex interaction between three types of RNA: mRNA acts as a template, ribosomal RNA (rRNA) forms the ribosomes, and transfer RNA (tRNA) acts as a carrier of the amino acids to be incorporated into the polypeptide. mRNA contains the genetic code in the form of codons that identify the sequence of amino acids to be added to the growing polypeptide chain. The resulting protein is then released and can have either an intracellular or extracellular role.

Regulation of Gene Expression

Genes are expressed in a regulated manner throughout an organism. It is this gene regulation that ultimately underlies the variability among cells, tissues, and organisms. Gene expression may be regulated at several levels. Transcriptional regulation modulates the production of mRNA. Translational and posttranslational regulation can modulate the production and activity of proteins that are expressed.

Regulation of transcription can be direct or indirect. An example of indirect regulation is the effect of modifying histones by enzymes capable of acetylation or deacetylation of histones that affect the formation of nucleosomes and, thus, the accessibility of RNA polymerases to DNA. A more direct form of regulation is through transcription factors. Transcription factors are specific proteins capable of binding specific DNA sequences and modulating the rate of transcription (Fig. 6). Several groups of transcription factors have been identified and are classified by similarities in their protein structure. Zinc finger, helix-loop-helix, and leucine zippers are separate groups of transcription factors known to regulate gene expression.

Translational and posttranslational regulation vary in importance with the proteins studied. Some proteins (clotting factors) are made in a precursor form and activated by other proteins (posttranslational regulation). Other gene products are regulated either solely or partially at the transcriptional level.

TOOLS OF THE CARDIOVASCULAR MOLECULAR BIOLOGIST

When heated, DNA can be *denatured*, that is, separated into two complementary strands. With cooling, these strands can be reannealed. Complementary sequences of DNA from other sources, such as short oligonucleotides, can bind in a species-specific manner to single-stranded DNA templates. This binding is referred to as *hybridization*.

DNA Techniques

To facilitate handling of short segments of DNA, fragments are often inserted into *plasmids*, which are circular double-stranded DNA structures (Fig. 7). Plasmids have their origin in bacteria and are often associated with the transfer of antibiotic resistance. Plasmids can

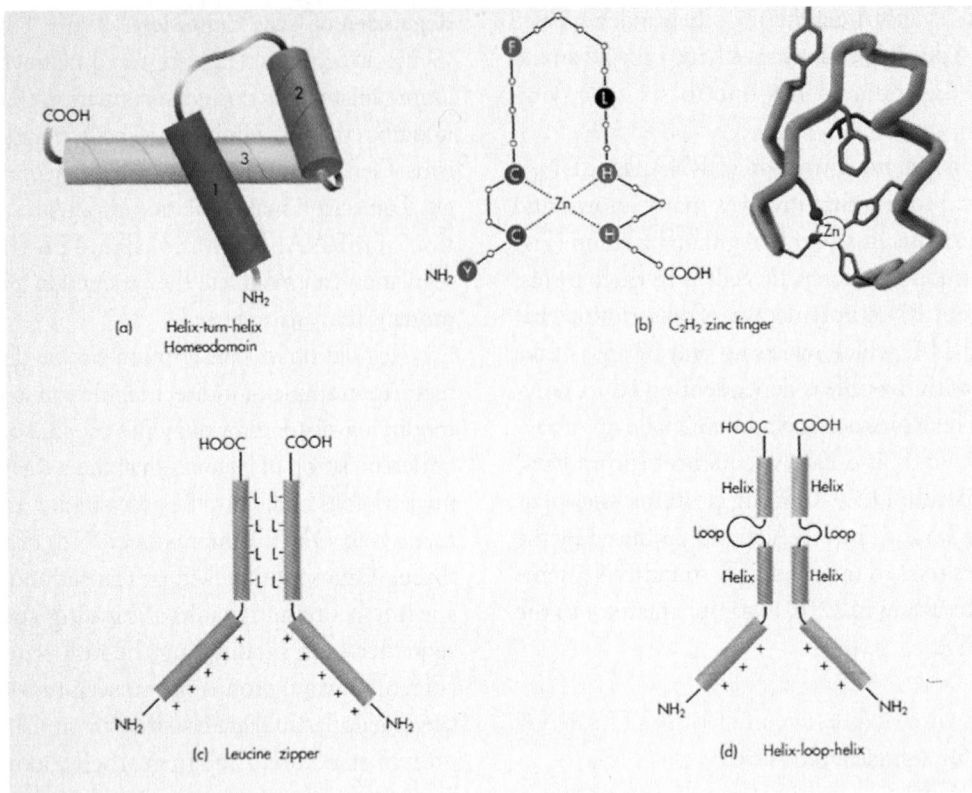

Fig. 6. Representative types of transcription factors.

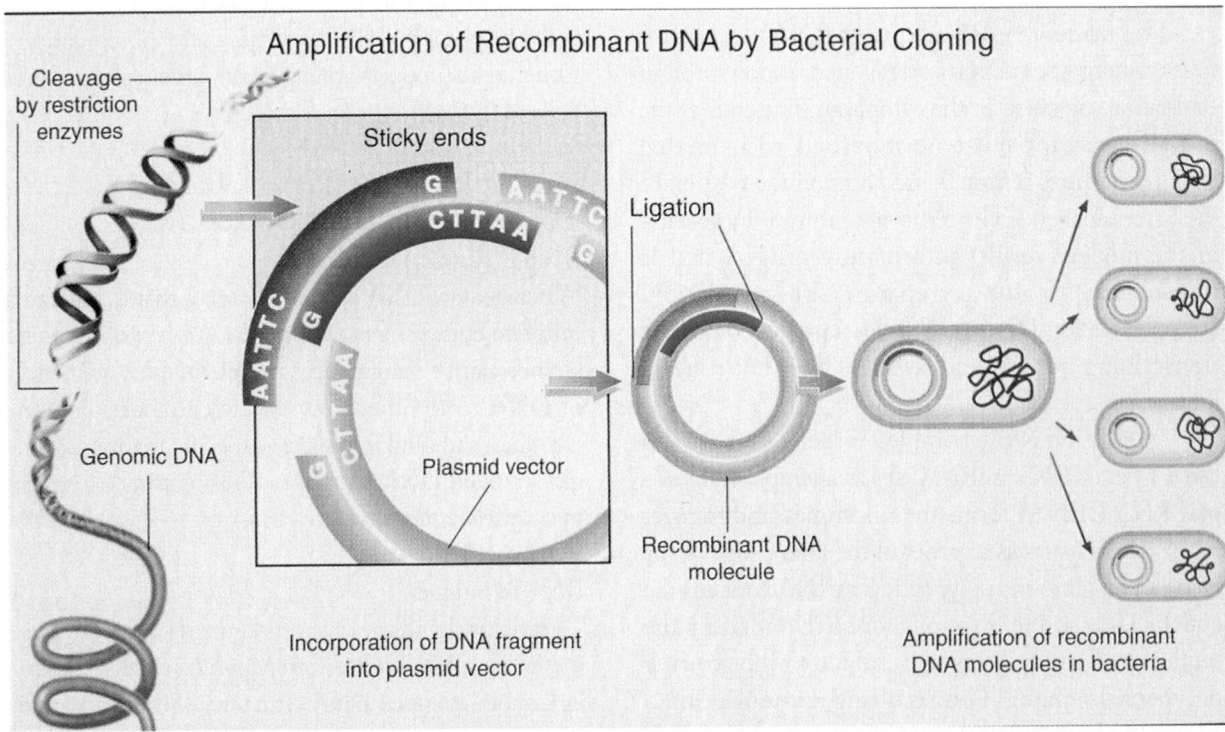

Fig. 7. Amplification of DNA by bacterial cloning. A, adenine; C, cytosine; G, guanine; T, thymine.

be used to carry DNA fragments for manipulation and to express genes in vitro or in vivo.

Manipulating DNA Fragments

Portions of DNA, whether genomic or cellular, can be cut, ligated, and extended using a set of powerful enzymes. *Restriction endonucleases* are bacterial proteins that are capable of cutting DNA at specific DNA sequences (Fig. 8). Restriction endonucleases cut within DNA sequences and leave either a 3' or a 5' overlap or blunt ends. Exonucleases are capable of cutting DNA ends that are free in order to tailor recombination events.

Enzymes called *DNA polymerases* can be used to extend DNA fragments. Ligases are capable of joining either blunt or complementary (sticky) ends of DNA, creating a recombinant DNA molecule. This process is often referred to as *cloning*.

Analyzing DNA Fragments

The base pair sequence of a fragment of DNA can be

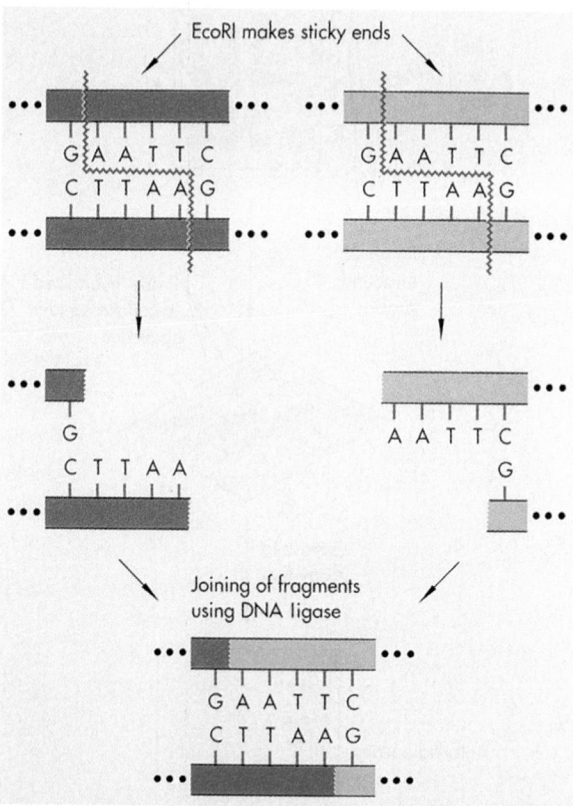

Fig. 8. Restriction endonucleases. A, adenine; C, cytosine; G, guanine; T, thymine.

determined at a gross level or at an exact level. The use of restriction digests can be very helpful in determining the relative composition of a DNA sequence. Because restriction endonucleases identify specific DNA sequences and the distance between adjacent cuts can be determined with agarose gel electrophoresis, non-detailed maps of DNA fragments can be made.

Sequencing

Sequencing is a powerful tool that enables molecular biologists to create a detailed map containing each base within a portion of DNA. The two classic techniques for sequencing DNA are the Sanger method and the Maxam-Gilbert method. The Sanger method sequences a template DNA using four labeled dideoxynucleotides and a primer (short oligonucleotide complementary to one end). With the use of DNA polymerase, the dideoxynucleotides, when incorporated, terminate the chain. By altering the composition of the dideoxynucleotides, the resulting chains can be identified and, thus, the sequence determined. The Maxam-Gilbert method depends on a series of chemicals that destroy certain bases or combinations of bases. When a portion of radiolabeled DNA is subjected to these reactions and the products are isolated and electrophoresed, the sequences can be inferred.

Southern Blotting

Hybridization of a radiolabeled probe (oligonucleotide) to a template DNA can be used to identify specific DNA fragments (Fig. 9). Hybridization to immobilized DNA was first performed by E. M. Southern and is referred to as *Southern blotting*. First, a radiolabeled probe is created that is complementary to the target to be identified. Second, the DNA to be analyzed is cut with restriction endonucleases and the resulting fragments are electrophoresed. Third, the DNA is transferred from the agarose to a nylon membrane and fixed to it. Fourth, the probe is hybridized to the membrane. Finally, after washes to remove nonspecific binding, the membrane is exposed to x-ray film. The label exposes the film, identifying specific hybridization to a DNA fragment.

- Southern blotting is used to analyze DNA.
- Northern blotting is used to analyze RNA.
- Western blotting is used to analyze proteins.

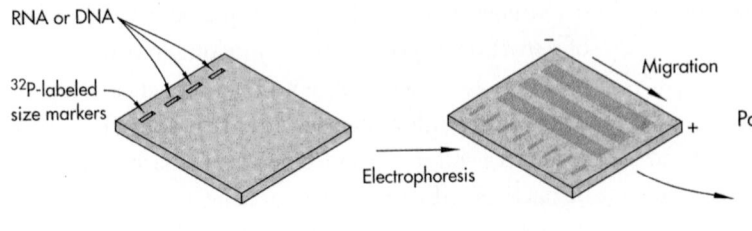

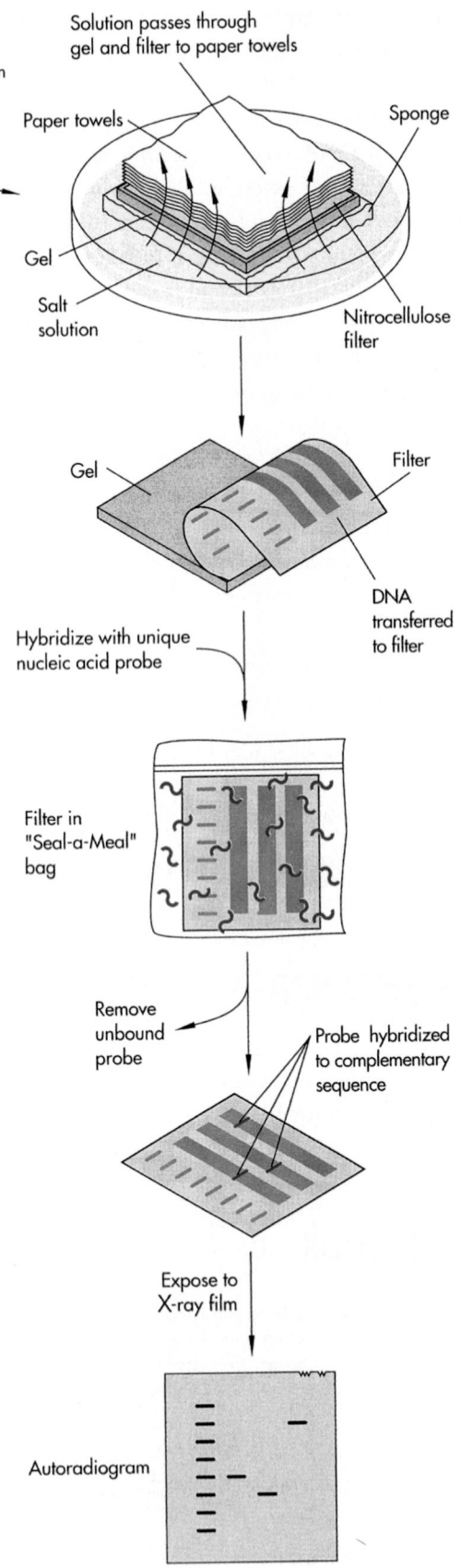

Fig. 9. Analyzing DNA and RNA by gel electrophoresis and blotting.

Polymerase Chain Reaction

The polymerase chain reaction (PCR) takes advantage of the heat stability of the DNA polymerase from *Thermus aquaticus* (Taq) (Fig. 10). The goal of PCR is to amplify a target DNA fragment. The procedure mixes the DNA sample being used as a template, free nucleotides, and the Taq polymerase at 94°C. After DNA denaturation (separation into complementary strands), the temperature is decreased to 55°C, allowing the target sequence to polymerize. This results in an exact copy of the target sequence. Repeating this process 30 to 40 times can generate up to 2^{40} copies of the target DNA. PCR is a powerful tool for amplifying minute portions of DNA for analysis.

Because they can amplify minute quantities of DNA, sensitive PCR tests have been developed for various diseases that can be tested by extracting DNA from a small blood sample. Current tests for Chagas disease involve PCR methods for the detection of parasitic DNA in collected blood samples. These tests are superior to xenodiagnosis or hemoculture in some selected patients in highly endemic areas. PCR is also being developed for the detection of pathogens in valve tissue samples from patients with infectious endocarditis that is negative on blood culture.

■ PCR is used to amplify small amounts of DNA.

RNA Techniques

Unlike DNA, which is stable for relatively long periods even at room temperature, RNA is an unstable molecule that is susceptible to degradation from ubiquitous ribonucleases. Thus, great care is required to obtain and analyze RNA from cells or tissue. In addition, mRNA representing the genes that are expressed in any cell makes up only a minority of the total RNA within a cell.

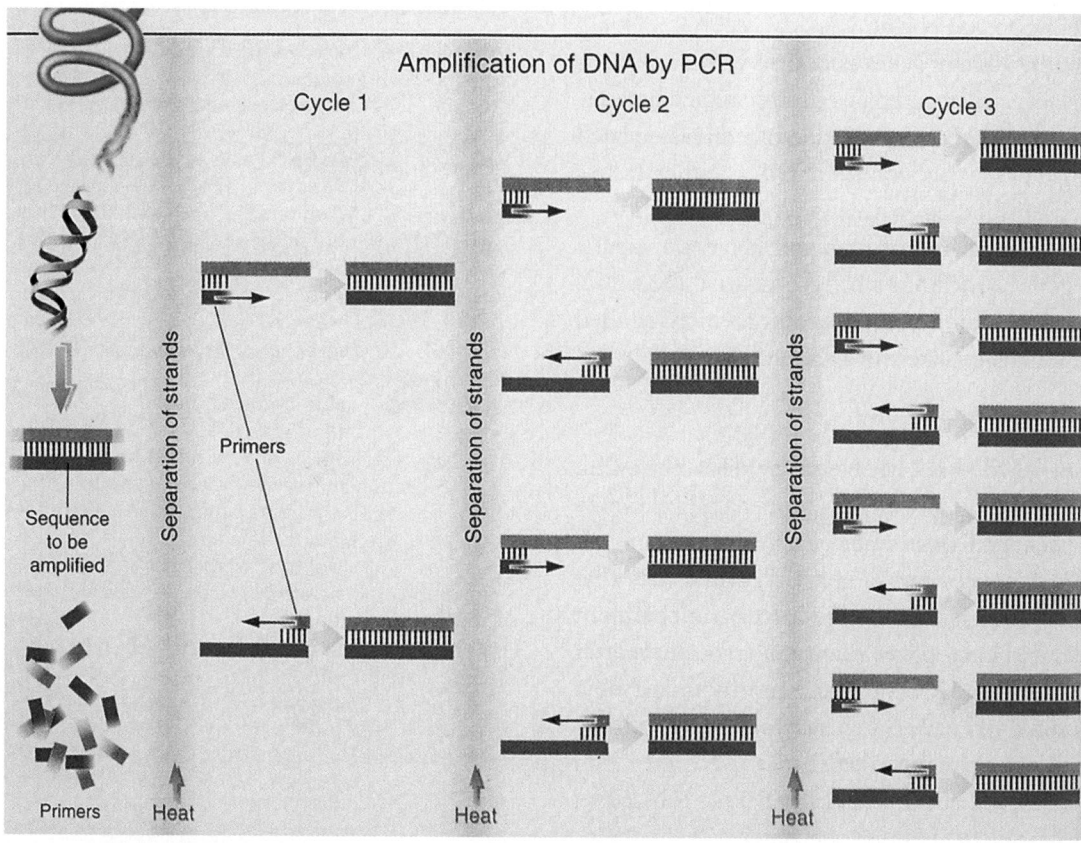

Fig. 10. Amplification of DNA by the polymerase chain reaction (PCR).

Northern Blotting

As with DNA, RNA can be electrophoresed and transferred to membranes and hybridized with labeled probes (Fig. 9). These probes can be either DNA or RNA. This process is called *Northern blotting*. It provides a means for identifying and quantifying the amount of an RNA species in a sample.

Reverse Transcriptase-Polymerase Chain Reaction

Amplification of mRNA can be performed using reverse transcriptase-PCR (RT-PCR). RT-PCR requires that mRNA undergo reverse transcription to cDNA before the initial amplification steps. This can be performed with a retroviral reverse transcriptase enzyme.

Analysis of DNA-Protein Interactions

As mentioned above, much of the important gene regulation is based on the interactions between proteins and DNA. Techniques have been developed to analyze proteins that bind in a sequence-specific manner to DNA. A popular technique to assess this protein-DNA interaction is the electrophoretic mobility shift assay (EMSA). EMSA is based on the fact that the electrophoretic migration of DNA fragments bound to protein is slower than that of unbound DNA. Thus, nuclear protein extracts are isolated and exposed to short fragments of radiolabeled double-stranded DNA in a binding buffer. The resulting mixture is electrophoresed and exposed to x-ray film. Unbound DNA runs faster, whereas DNA bound to protein is delayed ("shifted"). The bound protein can be identified further by adding to the mixture antibodies specific for the proteins, resulting in further electrophoretic delay ("supershift").

Western Blotting

Western blotting is used to sequence proteins by gel electrophoresis, using antibody probes analogous to Southern blotting for DNA analysis.

MOLECULAR GENETICS

The identification of genes associated with disease has been the focus of an enormous effort in biomedical science. Classically, the identification of a disease-related protein led to the development of probes, either nucleic acids or antibodies, with which to screen DNA libraries. The screening of a genomic library can identify the gene associated with the disease (Fig. 11). However, the number of diseases for which detailed biochemical defects are known is few.

Gene Mapping

Without detailed knowledge of the disease protein, positional cloning techniques (gene mapping) can be used to identify disease-related genes. Gene mapping is based on Mendel's laws of genetics, which state that genes sort independently. Thus, truly independent genes should have a 50% chance of association after meiotic sorting. Genes that are tightly linked on a chromosome will have less chance to cross over during meiosis, creating an increased chance of cosegregation (linkage) (Fig. 12 and 13). Linkage analysis is based on the statistical chances that the genes will sort independently. For instance, genes in disparate locations will sort independently, whereas two genes in proximity are less likely to sort independently.

An increasing number of chromosomal markers are available for linkage analysis. Pedigree analysis of families is needed to determine the patterns of coinheritance and the potential linkage with known markers. A likelihood ratio is determined for the coinheritance. For instance, if the likelihood for cosegregation is 1,000:1, the log of the odds (LOD) score is 3 (log 1,000=3). An LOD score of 3 is the lower limit for statistically significant linkage (95% probability of linkage). After a linkage has been determined, the chromosomal region can be analyzed further to isolate the gene of interest.

- LOD score is the statistical chance that the disease gene is located near the marker gene.
- An LOD score of 3 corresponds to a probability of linkage of 95% and is the lower limit for significance.

In certain situations, reasonable guesses can be made from the knowledge of a disease which would

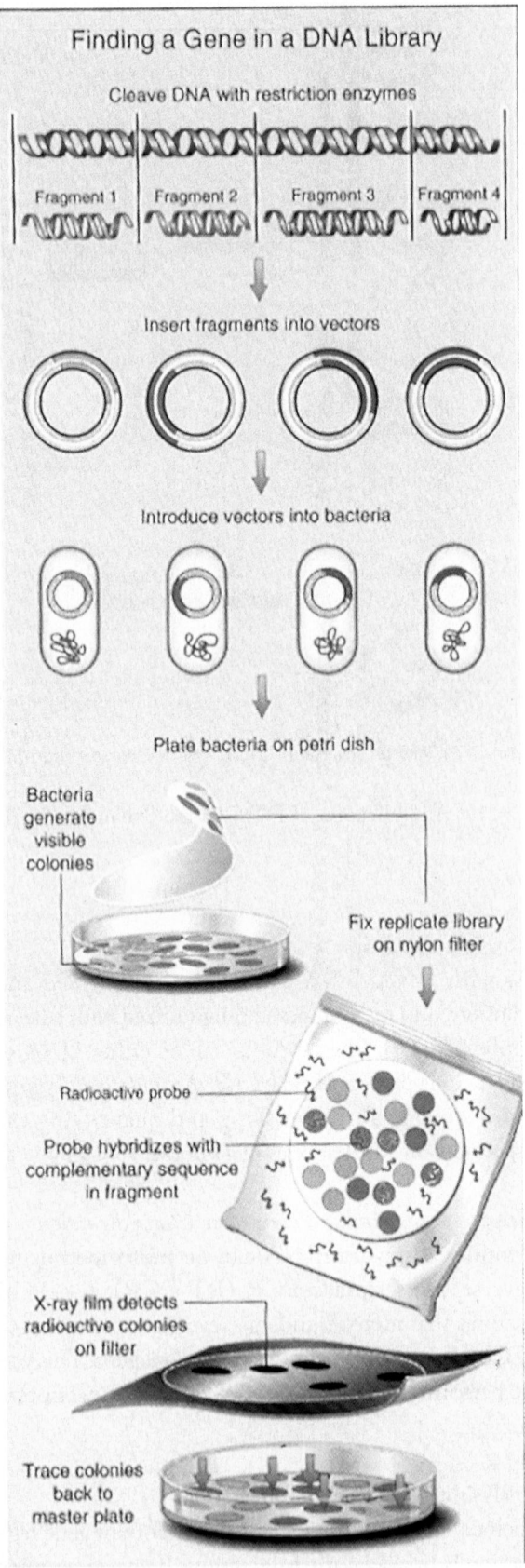

Fig. 11. Identifying a gene in a DNA library.

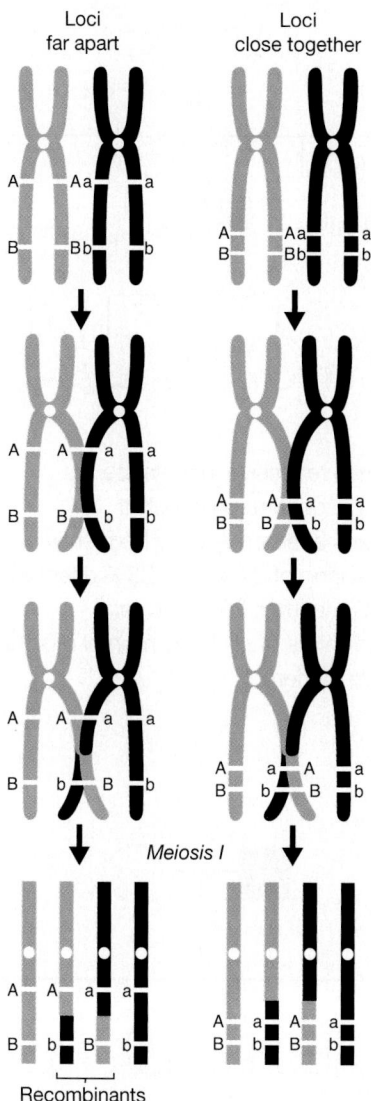

Fig. 12. Segregation of chromosomes depicting differences between close and distant loci.

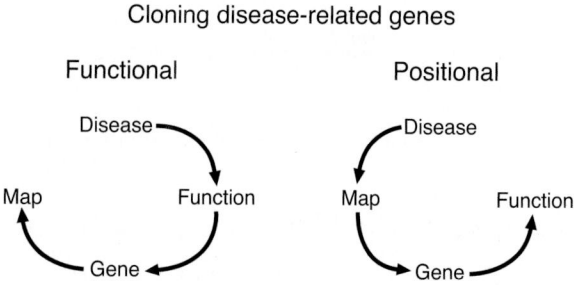

Fig. 13. Functional and positional cloning of disease-related genes.

allow for a list of potential genes that might be responsible for the disease (*candidate genes*). This candidate approach is improved if linkage data are available to narrow the search to a limited list of reasonable candidates. Some of the genes associated with hypertrophic cardiomyopathy have been identified with the candidate gene approach.

Genetic diseases can be associated with single-gene or multigene abnormalities. Single-gene defects provide a model for understanding the mendelian inheritance of disease (Fig. 14). Autosomally related disorders are associated with abnormalities of the autosomes (non–sex chromosomes). These disorders can be dominant or recessive. *Autosomal dominant* (AD) disorders require only one copy (of the two) of the mutant gene to cause the disease. In dominant disorders, a child has a 50% chance of inheriting the gene and, thus, the disease. Healthy siblings do not possess the mutation, but every patient has an affected parent. Males and females are affected equally. Penetrance and late or variable expression of the disorder may affect the course of the disease. *Autosomal recessive* (AR) disorders require two mutant copies of the gene. A single copy of the mutant gene results in the person being a carrier. The offspring of two carriers have a 1-in-4 chance of having the disease and a 1-in-2 risk of being a carrier. All of the offspring of affected individuals are carriers.

X-linked disorders result from mutant genes on the X chromosome. Because males have one X chromosome, these disorders act like dominant mutations. In females, they usually act like recessive mutations. Women act as carriers, and transmission of disease is only from females to sons. Transmission of carrier status can come from females to daughters or from males who give their diseased X chromosome exclusively to their daughters. Mutations in the mitochondrial genome are passed from mother to son. Multigenic disorders result from the interaction of multiple genes, and their inheritance pattern is difficult—if not impossible—to discern.

■ Know the mendelian patterns of inheritance and the risk of transmission for common cardiovascular disorders such as hypertrophic cardiomyopathy, familial hyperlipidemia, and long QT syndrome.

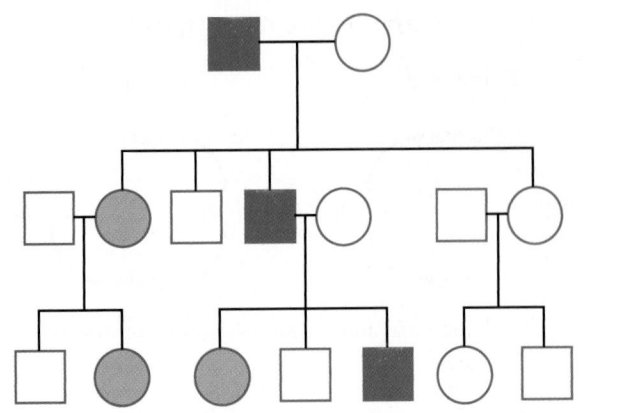

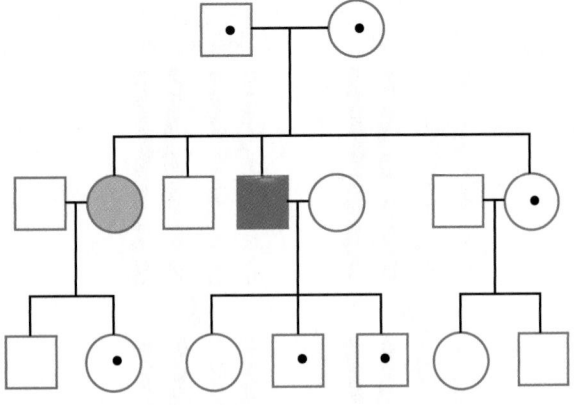

A—Autosomal dominant inheritance
  Multiple generations affected
  Sexes affected equally frequently
  In familial cases, only one parent
    need be affected
  Male-to-male transmission occurs
  Offspring of affected parent have a 50%
    chance of being affected

B—Autosomal recessive inheritance
  Single generation affected
  Sexes affected equally frequently
  Offspring of 2 carriers: 25% affected,
    50% carrier, 25% normal
  Two-thirds of clinically normal offspring
    are carriers

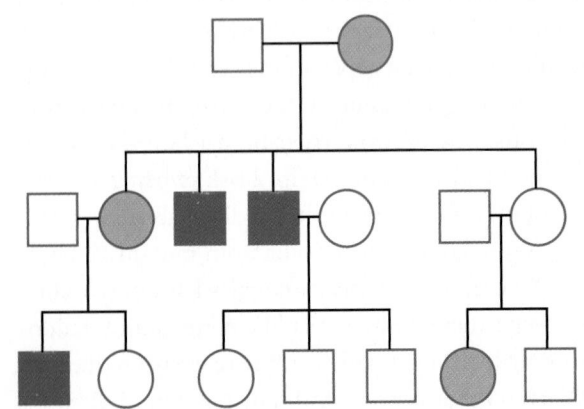

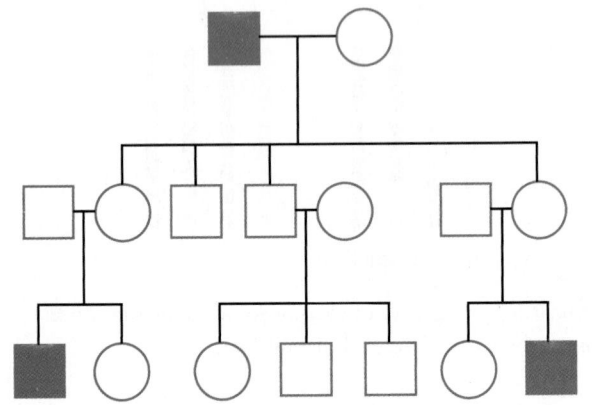

C—Mitochondrial inheritance
  Sexes equally frequently and severely
    affected
  Transmission only through women;
    offspring of affected men are
    unaffected
  All offspring of affected women may be
    affected

D—X-linked inheritance
  No male-to-male transmission
  All daughters of affected males are
    carriers
  Sons of carrier mother have 50% chance
    of being affected; daughters have 50%
    chance of being carriers

Fig. 14. *A-D*, Mendelian inheritance patterns.

MOLECULAR BASIS OF CARDIOVASCULAR DISEASES

Variation in genetic sequences may be responsible for differences between individuals or be associated with disease. *Polymorphisms* are differences in DNA sequence which are frequently found in populations. Many polymorphisms are thought to have arisen after selective pressure for alleles conferred adaptive advantages in different habitats. A classic example of gene polymorphism among individuals is the variability in hepatic metabolism of medications by cytochrome P-450. Research into gene polymorphisms that are responsible for aspirin resistance, sensitivity of adrenergic receptors to β-blockers, and lipid homeostasis has contributed to an understanding of optimal medical therapy.

Mutations are changes in the DNA sequence associated with disease. Mutations can arise from 1) point mutations, where single nucleotide substitutions cause a single amino acid change (designated by the amino acid intended, a number designating where the mutation happened, and the new amino acid product); 2) deletion; or 3) insertion of extra DNA. Millions of single nucleotide polymorphisms (SNPs) exist in the human genome, and thousands of mutations have been identified for human disease.

Of the many types of diseases that affect the cardiovascular system, an increasing number have been identified as resulting from single-gene (monogenic) or polygenic mutations. The cardiac diseases about which the genetic basis is known include hypertrophic cardiomyopathy (HCM) and the long QT syndrome.

Myocardial Diseases

Hypertrophic Cardiomyopathy

HCM has been recognized as a familial disorder for more than 30 years. It is characterized by great clinical heterogeneity, with architectural disorganization at every level from molecule to ventricle. It has great genetic heterogeneity and the pattern of inheritance for HCM is AD (Fig. 15). More than 200 mutations in 10 known genes are associated with HCM. HCM is a disease of sarcomeric proteins, and the genetic variability (defects both within and among genes) and variable penetrance may account for the clinical spectrum of disease.

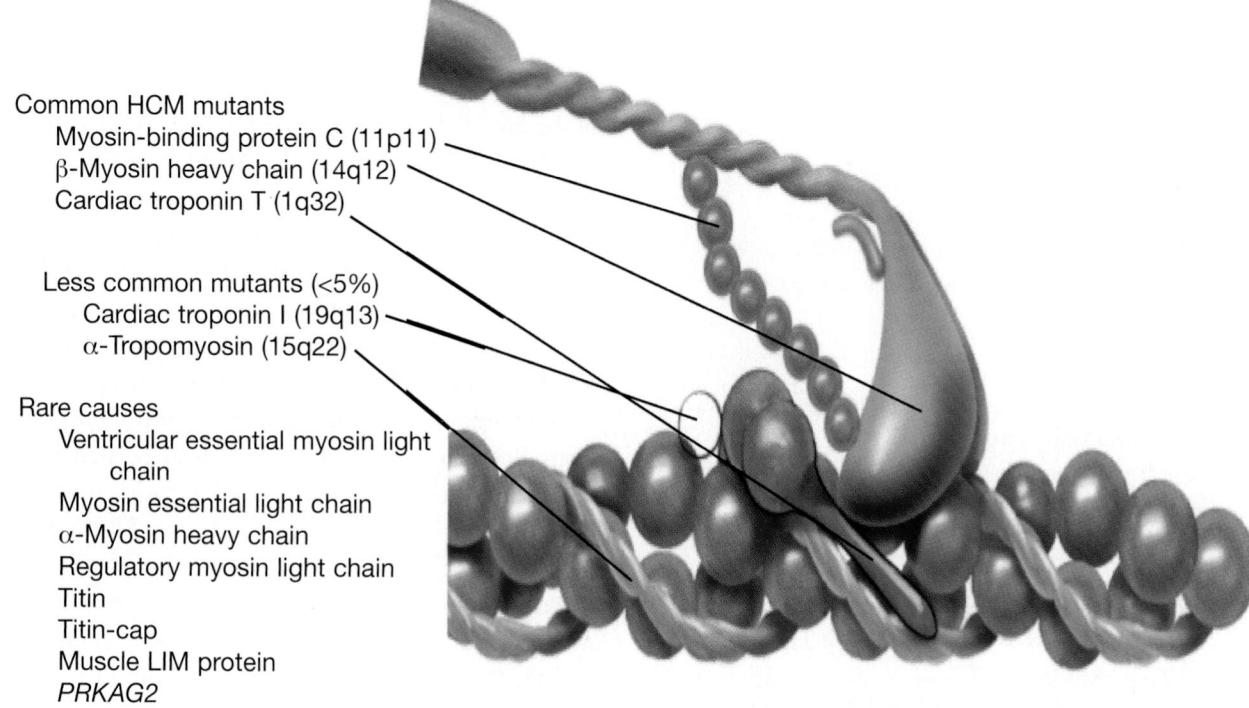

Common HCM mutants
    Myosin-binding protein C (11p11)
    β-Myosin heavy chain (14q12)
    Cardiac troponin T (1q32)

    Less common mutants (<5%)
        Cardiac troponin I (19q13)
        α-Tropomyosin (15q22)

Rare causes
    Ventricular essential myosin light
        chain
    Myosin essential light chain
    α-Myosin heavy chain
    Regulatory myosin light chain
    Titin
    Titin-cap
    Muscle LIM protein
    PRKAG2

Fig. 15. Commonly mutated proteins in hypertrophic cardiomyopathy (HCM).

HCM originally was associated with mutations for β-myosin heavy chain (β-MHC) (chromosome 14q11-12; 15%-25% of patients); α-tropomyosin (chromosome 15q22; <5% of patients); and cardiac troponin T (chromosome 1q32; 5%-15% of patients). Recent studies have suggested that one of the more common causes of HCM is mutations for cardiac myosin-binding protein C (chromosome 11p11.2; 15%-25% of patients), which is important embryologically for generating myofibril, as well as for sarcomere function.

Other mutations (Table 1) associated with HCM have been found in essential myosin light chain (chromosome 3), the regulatory myosin light chain (chromosome 12), and cardiac troponin I (chromosome 19).

Mutations in the gene *PRKAG2* (encoding a subunit of an adenosine monophosphate-activated protein kinase on chromosome 7q36) have been linked to familial cardiac hypertrophy with the Wolff-Parkinson-White syndrome. Overactivity of the protein kinase leads to excess glycogen, resulting in large vacuoles within the myocytes. Structurally, the myofibrils are not in disarray as they are in classic HCM, leading researchers to classify this as a form of myocardial metabolic storage disease. Another protein that is similarly associated with severe, early cardiac hypertrophy with ventricular preexcitation is lysosome-associated membrane protein-2 (LAMP-2), which is associated with a form of glycogen storage disease.

Table 1. Mutations in Genes for Cardiac Sarcomeric Proteins Causally Linked to Hypertrophic Cardiomyopathy (HCM)

Sarcomeric protein	Chromosome
β-Myosin heavy chain	14
Cardiac troponin T	1
Cardiac troponin I	19
Regulatory myosin light chains	3
	12
HCM with Wolff-Parkinson-White syndrome	7
α-Tropomyosin	15
Cardiac myosin-binding protein C	11

The spectrum of genetic defects associated with HCM has led to the correlation between genotype and phenotype. Clinical studies of β-MHC and cardiac troponin T demonstrated that certain troponin T mutations may result in a significant risk of sudden death in spite of minimal hypertrophy. The Arg^{403}Gln mutation in β-MHC leads to a malignant course similar to that of troponin T defects and more severe than the relatively benign variant of β-MHC, Val^{606}Met, with attenuated myocardial energetics and increased beat-to-beat QT variability. The development of clinical techniques to screen for these defects in families will allow early detection, limit the need for repeated screening, and provide for better prognosis.

- HCM is associated with mutations in 10 genes on at least 8 different chromosomes.
- Arg^{719}Trp, Arg^{403}Gln, and Arg^{453}Cys mutations in β-MHC are associated with a high risk of sudden death.
- The Leu^{908}Val mutation in β-MHC is associated with a low risk of sudden death.
- The Ser^{179}Phe mutation in troponin T is associated with early sudden cardiac death and severe HCM, whereas the Phe^{110}Ile troponin T mutation is relatively benign.

Dilated Cardiomyopathy

Dilated cardiomyopathy (DCM) is a primary disorder of the myocardium characterized by increased left ventricular size, decreased ejection fraction, and, in later stages, symptoms of congestive heart failure. In up to 20% to 30% of cases, DCM may have a genetic cause. Some forms of DCM are related to systemic diseases such as muscular dystrophy, whereas others appear as distinct clinical entities (Table 2). Understanding of the genetic basis in both types of disease is increasing.

Duchenne muscular dystrophy and its milder form, Becker muscular dystrophy, are associated with defects in the dystrophin gene (*Xp21*); cardiac involvement is common and is manifested as DCM and heart failure. This is an X-linked disorder. The defective dystrophin gene results in altered expression of dystrophin in cardiac and skeletal muscles. In X-linked DCM, the defect in dystrophin is limited to the myocardium and may be associated with specific mutations within the gene. Other forms of muscular dystrophy associated with DCM include limb-girdle muscular dystrophy (inherited in an autosomal recessive pattern and associated with defects in the dystrophin-associated glycoprotein complex) and congenital muscular dystrophy (an AD disorder associated with defects in laminin).

Genetic defects in DCM not associated with muscular dystrophy have been identified recently. Two unrelated families with DCM have been shown to have mutations in cardiac actin. Unlike HCM, which is associated with deficits in proteins associated with force generation, it has been hypothesized that defects in actin may be associated with deficits in force transmission. Familial DCM is predominantly AD in transmission and frequently asymptomatic; it is found on screening of family members of an affected person. About 10% of asymptomatic family members have a normal ejection fraction with an enlarged left ventricular volume.

Mitochondria contain a small amount of DNA that codes for 13 genes involved in mitochondrial metabolism. The Kearns-Sayre syndrome is an example of a mitochondrial cardiomyopathy due to a mitochondrial DNA deletion with maternal inheritance (all children of affected mothers will have the mutation).

Congenital Heart Disease

Two common examples of the known molecular basis for congenital heart disease are Marfan syndrome and supravalvular aortic stenosis. Marfan syndrome is an AD inherited disease with high penetrance, characterized by skeletal, cardiovascular, and ocular abnormalities. The incidence of Marfan syndrome is about 1/10,000 births. Premature deaths are due to progressive aortic dilatation with associated aortic insufficiency and aortic dissection. Genetic linkage analysis led to the identification of fibrillin as the abnormal protein responsible for this disease. Thirty mutations have been found in the fibrillin gene on chromosome 15 associated with Marfan syndrome.

Linkage analysis has determined that alterations in the elastin gene on chromosome 7 are responsible for supravalvular aortic stenosis. Like Marfan syndrome, this disorder is inherited in an AD fashion with high penetrance. Supravalvular aortic stenosis in combination with mental retardation, connective tissue abnormalities, and hypercalcemia is called *Williams syndrome*.

Several other single-gene defects are associated with congenital heart disease, including familial atrial septal defects, Holt-Oram syndrome on chromosome 12, and the atrioventricular canal defects associated with Down syndrome. In general, the genetic abnormalities associated with congenital heart disease may result in several clinical presentations.

Arrhythmias

An increasing understanding of the molecular biology of myocardial ion channels has led to a better understanding of the genetic basis of life-threatening arrhythmias in certain patients. The best described model for this is the long QT syndrome. This syndrome, known previously as *Romano-Ward* or *Jervell and Lange-Nielsen syndrome*, is a group of related disorders of arrhythmias (torsades de pointes) associated with prolongation of the QT interval. The long QT syndrome is now recognized as having a distinct genetic basis (Table 3). More than 35 mutations in four cardiac ion channels are associated with this syndrome.

Arrhythmogenic right ventricular dysplasia (ARVD) is a form of right ventricular cardiomyopathy inherited in an AD manner. It is associated with fatty infiltration and fibrosis of the right ventricle, and it may cause sudden death. Like HCM, the molecular basis of the ARVD phenotype can be recapitulated by several different genotype mutations linked to chromosomes 1, 2, 6, 10, 12, and 14.

The Romano-Ward syndrome is a cluster of disorders inherited in an AD pattern associated with at least six genotypes, including mutations in the I_{Ks} channel, the *HERG* (human ether-a-go-go related gene) I_{Kr} channel, and the *SCNA5* I_{Na} channel and mutations in unidentified genes for three additional variants. The Jervell and Lange-Nielsen syndrome is an AR disorder associated with sensorineural hearing loss and mutations in the voltage-gated potassium channel gene (*KVLQT1*) and its subunit *minK*. These genotypes have some associated phenotypic changes on electrocardiography. For example, isolated prolongation of the ST segment is associated with mutations in the *SCNA5* I_{Na} channel, whereas a double-humped T wave is associated with the *HERG* genotype. In the future as genotype-phenotype relationships are developed, a therapeutic goal will be to prevent sudden death in high-risk patients.

Table 2. Cardiomyopathy Mutants

Disease	Phenotype	Mutation	Inheritance	Chromosome	Mechanism
Kearns-Sayre syndrome	DCM, heart block, short stature, ataxia, cognitive impairment, ptosis, weakness, deafness	Mitochondrial DNA	mt	mt	Deletions in mitochondrial DNA result in impaired electron transport chain & mitochondrial function
Duchenne muscular dystrophy	DCM, conduction abnormalities, distal muscle weakness, Gowers sign, lordosis, mental retardation	Dystrophin	XR	Xp21	Loss of stabilizing glycoprotein complex on muscle fiber's plasma membrane → muscle fiber degradation
Fabry disease	Late-onset LVH, CAD, conduction defects, aortic root dilatation, skin lesion, valvulopathy, neuropathy, TIA/CVA, proteinuria, and renal disease	α-Galactosidase A	XR	Xq22	Abnormal lysosomal deposits
Cardiac hypertrophy with Wolff-Parkinson-White syndrome	HCM, ventricular pre-excitation, palpitations, chest pain (myalgia in 15%)	*PRKAG2* (subunit of AMP-activated protein kinase)	AD	7q36	Overactive AMP activity → excess glycogen granules, large cardiomyocytes
Marfan syndrome	Dilatation of aorta & sinuses of Valsalva, aortic root dilatation/ dissection, scoliosis, arachnodactyly, ectopia lentis, dural ectasia	Fibrillin 1	AD	15q21	Suspected altered calcium binding to growth-factor–like domain in protein needed for fibrillogenesis in connective tissues
Williams syndrome	Supravalvular aortic stenosis, pulmonary artery stenosis, microcephaly, micrognathia/ "elfin facies," mental retardation, hypercalcemia, renal artery stenosis, hypertension	Elastin	AD*	7q11	Unclear; thought to be due to gene deletion of the transcription factor involved
ARVD	Arrhythmia, SCD	Desmoplakin	AD	6p24	Mutant has disruption & loss of desmosome function & tight gap junctions

Table 2   (continued)

Disease	Phenotype	Mutation	Inher-itance	Chromo-some	Mechanism
ARVD (cont'd)		Plakophilin 2	AD	12p11	→ when shear stress, get myo-cardial injury/in-flammation → fatty infiltration & cell death → fibrosis of the right ventricle
ARVD (Naxos disease)	ARVD with hyper-keratosis of palms/soles, woolly hair	Plakoglobin	AR	17q21	Deletion results in gap junction abnor-mality, loss of cell-cell adhesion → ? problems with myocyte integrity → fibrofatty infiltrate/ cell death

AD, autosomal dominant; AMP, adenosine monophosphate; AR, autosomal recessive; ARVD, arrhythmogenic right ventricu-lar dysplasia; CAD, coronary artery disease; CVA, cerebrovascular accident; DCM, dilated cardiomyopathy; HCM, hyper-trophic cardiomyopathy; LVH, left ventricular hypertrophy; mt, mitochondrial; SCD, sudden cardiac death; TIA, transient ischemic attack; XR, X-linked recessive.
*Sporadic new mutations.

The Brugada syndrome is a clinical complex asso-ciated with syncope and sudden death. It is associated with an electrocardiographic pattern of ST-segment elevation in leads V_1 through V_3. Brugada syndrome is also linked to mutations in the SCN5A subunit of the sodium channel. It is inherited in an AD pattern with incomplete penetrance.

- Patients with *SCN5A* genotype may benefit from sodium channel blocking agents.
- Patients with *HERG* may benefit from β-blockers.

The inheritance of arrhythmias is discussed fur-ther in the chapter on channelopathies.

Risk Factors for Atherosclerosis
Atherosclerosis is a complex disease associated with acquired and genetic factors. The genetic background is clearly polygenic and associated with a complex interplay with environmental factors. Of the known risk factors for atherosclerosis, two provide models for a genetic understanding: hyperlipidemia and hyper-homocysteinemia.

Hyperlipidemia
One of the most widely understood cardiovascular genetic disorders is associated with familial hypercho-lesterolemia (Table 4). Familial hypercholesterolemia is a relatively common cause of increased levels of low-density lipoprotein (LDL) and is associated with a defective LDL receptor gene on chromosome 19. Familial hypercholesterolemia is an AD disorder in which the heterozygotes are affected to an intermedi-ate degree. Homozygotes have LDL cholesterol levels of 650 to 1,000 mg/dL and are often affected by coro-nary atherosclerosis before the age of 10 years. The homozygote phenotype is notable for the presence of planar cutaneous xanthomas. The heterozygotes have

Table 3. Arrhythmia Mutants

Disease	Phenotype	Mutation	Inheritance	Chromosome	Mechanism
Long QT mutants					
LQT1 (most common, least severe)	Heightened sensitivity to arousal as triggers (noise, emotion, exercise) Homozygous mutants have an increased risk of arrhythmias, deafness	*LQT1 KVLQT1* (aka *KCNQ1*)	AD or AR	11p15	Mutated α subunit → channel assembles improperly → ↓ function of delayed rectifier K channel → (I_{Ks}) reduces repolarizing current and prolongs AP
LQT2 (common— 1/3 to 2/5 of cases)	Event triggers more likely auditory (ringing/alarm)	*HERG* (aka *KCNH2*)	AD	7q35-36	Reduced repolarizing current (I_{Kr}) from loss of function mutation of the fast delayed rectifier K channel (*HERG, MiRP*)
LQT3	Event triggers highest while resting/asleep	*SCN5A* (aka *NaV1.5*)	AD	3p21-24	Faster inactivation of mutant Na channels, possibly reopens during AP, getting prolonged Na^+ influx
LQT4	Sinus node dysfunction (sinus bradycardia, junctional escapes), AF, SCD with exertion or emotion	Ankyrin B	AD	4q25-27	Loss of function of adapter/coordination protein thought to coordinate Na ion pump, Na/Ca exchanger, and signaling receptors
LQT5					
Romano-Ward syndrome	Arrhythmia	*KCNQ1* or *KCNE1* mutant	AD	21q22	Mutant K channel β subunit *minK*
Jervell and Lange-Nielsen syndrome	Arrhythmia, deafness (also in double mutation of *KCNQ1* and *KCNE1*)	Homozygous *KCNQ1* or heterozygous *KCNQ1* & *KCNE1*	AR		
LQT6	Usually clinically silent, but VF possible from sensitivity to long QT with medications (sulfamethoxazole)	*MiRP1* (*minK*-related peptide 1 or *KCNE2*)	AD	21q22	Problems with mutant *MiRP1* causing decreased K current (I_{Kr}) with slow opening/fast closing of *HERG* channels

Table 3   (continued)

Disease	Phenotype	Mutation	Inheritance	Chromosome	Mechanism
LQT7 (Andersen-Tawil syndrome)	Spontaneous hypokalemic periodic paralysis in childhood, variable phenotype: short stature, low-set ears, mandible hypoplastic/micrognathia, broad nose	*KCNJ2* (inward rectifying K channel *Kir2.1*)	AD	17q23	Reduced function of inward rectifying K channels (Kir) prolongs terminal phase of AP If K is low, can get delayed afterpotentials
LQT8 (Timothy syndrome)	Long QT, variable abnormalities: syndactyly, autism, paroxysmal hypoglycemia, altered immune response, cardiac malformations	Missense mutation of *CACNA1c*	Sporadic	12p13	Gain of function: mutant *CaV1.2* L-type Ca channel → lose voltage-dependent inactivation → continuous Ca inward current, delayed myocyte repolarization
Catecholamine-induced polymorphic ventricular tachycardia (70% with 1 of the 2 genes)	Family history of juvenile sudden death, emotional/physical stress → VT/VF → syncope	*RyR2*	AD	14q42	Gain of function: missense → myocyte Ca overload
	Bedouin families with SCD, syncope/seizure at age 6-12 y	*CASQ2* (calsequetrin 2)	AR	1p13	Unclear; possibly a problem with Ca reservoir in SR of myocytes
Idiopathic (familial) VF	Sudden unexplained death syndrome, structurally normal heart, 26% recurrent VF over 11 mo	*SCN5A*	AD	3p21-24	Loss of function → ↓ number of functional Na channels, short AP, slow conduction velocity
Brugada syndrome (15%-30% of families)	Many carriers asymptomatic from incomplete penetrance	*SCN5A*	AD	3p21-24	Defective myocardial Na channels, ↓ I_{Na}, ↓ duration of AP

AD, autosomal dominant; AF, atrial fibrillation; aka, also known as; AP, action potential; AR, autosomal recessive; Ca, calcium; I_{Kr}, rapidly activating delayed rectifier potassium current; I_{Ks}, slowly activating component of the delayed rectifier potassium current; I_{Na}, late sodium current; K, potassium; Kir, inward rectifier potassium current; Na, sodium; SCD, sudden cardiac death; SR, sarcoplasmic reticulum; VF, ventricular fibrillation; VT, ventricular tachycardia.

Table 4. Genetic Causes of Hypercholesterolemia and Hyperhomocysteinemia

Disease	Phenotype	Mutation	Inheritance	Chromosome	Mechanism
Cholesterol mutants					
FH	Xanthomas, xanthelasma, aortic stenosis in 50% of homozygotes	*LDLR*	AD	19p13	LDL receptor dysfunction results in failure to take up cholesterol from plasma
Sitosterolemia	Tendon xanthomas, premature atherosclerosis	*ABCG5* or *ABCG8*	AR	2p21	ATP-binding cassette
Familial defective apo B-100	Similar to FH	Apo B-100 (ligand on LDL particle)	AD	2p24-23	Impaired binding of LDL to the LDL (apo B/E) receptor
Cerebrotendinous xanthomatosis	Ataxia, Achilles tendon xanthomata, premature atherosclerosis, cataracts	Mitochondrial 27-hydroxylase (*CYP27*)	AR	2q33	Bile acid synthesis blocked; ? cholestanol causing neurologic toxicity
Hyperhomocysteinemia					Prothrombotic in ACS
Most common form from T mutation	Homozygotes (TT): marfanoid appearance, premature CAD/cerebrovascular disease Heterozygotes (T): normal appearance, may have vascular disease	5,10-methylenetetrahydrofolate reductase (*MTHFR*)	AR	21q22	Enzymatic activity of *MTHER* reduced (T mutation) from Ala-to-Val substitution causing ↑ homocysteine, especially with low folate

ACS, acute coronary syndrome; AD, autosomal dominant; apo, apolipoprotein; AR, autosomal recessive; ATP, adenosine triphosphate; CAD, coronary artery disease; FH, familial hypercholesterolemia; LDL, low-density lipoprotein.

LDL levels that are twice normal, and they are at high risk of premature coronary artery disease. At least 150 different mutations of the LDL receptor gene are associated with familial hypercholesterolemia.

The genetic determinants for other abnormalities of lipoprotein metabolism are being studied. The clinical clues to a potential genetic cause for lipoprotein disorders include the presence of premature atherosclerosis in the patient or a first-degree relative, the presence of xanthomas, and extremely high levels of total cholesterol (>300 mg/dL) or triglycerides (>500 mg/dL).

Hyperhomocysteinemia

Hyperhomocysteinemia is associated with an increased risk of premature vascular disease. Both genetic and nutritional deficiencies can lead to hyperhomocysteinemia. Classic hyperhomocysteinemia-homocystinuria is caused by defects in the cystathione β-synthetase gene (chromosome 21q22) and is inherited in an AR pattern. Homozygotes have a marfanoid appearance and develop premature vascular disease. Heterozygotes, who appear healthy, may have an increased risk of vascular disease. Defects in the gene for 5,10-methylenetetrahydrofolate reductase are also associated with hyperhomocysteinemia and premature vascular disease. Treatment with folate and vitamins B_6 and B_{12} can decrease homocysteine levels in these patients. Fortification of flour has decreased the incidence of hyperhomocystinemia.

Potential Molecular-Based Therapies for Cardiovascular Disease

Genetically based treatments can be divided into two categories: those dependent on genetic technology for development and those that use genetic material as drugs.

Recombinant Approaches to Drug Development

Recombinant DNA technology has played an important part in the development of revolutionary drugs based on naturally occurring enzymes. Mammalian cells with recombinant DNA of a certain desired enzyme can be grown to secrete the recombinant forms of glycoproteins into culture medium. These proteins can then be purified into a powder form for sterile reconstitution and intravenous infusion. An important example of this is recombinant tissue plasminogen activator (r-tPA) (alteplase). The use of r-tPA as a fibrinolytic agent to treat myocardial infarction helped usher in a new age of rapid reperfusion therapy and has been shown in large international trials to decrease mortality. Nesiritide (Natrecor) is a recombinant form of brain natriuretic peptide (BNP) that has been approved by the Federal and Drug Administration for acutely decompensated heart failure to promote natriuresis; it is currently under further study. Similar to other synthesized peptides, nesiritide is designed for intravenous infusion (to avoid protein degradation by oral routes); after being reconstituted, these drugs must be used as a single dose and the remainder discarded.

Recombinant DNA technology can also be used to generate antibody fragments that can bind to and block certain molecular targets. Abciximab (ReoPro), which is made of the antigen-binding fragment (Fab fragment) of a chimeric antibody to the glycoprotein IIb/IIIa receptor on platelets, has proved useful in treating high-risk patients undergoing percutaneous transluminal coronary angioplasty (PTCA). Other monoclonal antibodies are also under clinical trial investigation for use as adjunctive therapy for acute myocardial infarction, including the anti–C5 complement antibody pexelizumab (many monoclonal antibody generic names have the suffix –*mab*).

Gene Therapies for Cardiovascular Disease

Gene transfer is the modulation of foreign or native gene expression by the introduction of new genetic material into a cell or organism. Gene therapy strategies for cardiovascular disease have been limited to somatic cells (non-germline cells). Genes are introduced into cells through the use of *vectors*, which can contain elements that are both viral and nonviral.

The initial demonstration of vascular gene transfer used plasmid DNA and retroviral vectors to deliver reporter genes to the vasculature. These studies were limited by the low efficiency of gene transfer because retroviral vectors are capable of infecting only dividing cells, which are rarely present in normal arteries.

The development of adenoviral vectors led to the ability to demonstrate potential therapeutic benefits from vascular gene transfer. Adenoviruses are DNA viruses capable of infecting dividing and nondividing cells. The ability to clone transgenes into replication-deficient adenoviral vectors has resulted in more efficient (yet transient) transgene expression in vascular tissue.

A prime target for gene transfer has been restenosis after PTCA. Restenosis occurs as a result of cellular proliferation, matrix production, thrombosis, and chronic renarrowing. Gene transfer approaches have targeted cellular proliferation as a means to limit restenosis. Gene transfer strategies aimed at killing proliferating cells include the use of the herpesvirus thymidine kinase gene (*tk*) and the prodrug ganciclovir. The *tk* gene product sensitizes infected cells to the killing effects of ganciclovir. Clinical trials using these strategies have been delayed by the lack of effective and safe intracoronary delivery catheters.

Another major target for cardiovascular gene transfer has been the development of strategies to create angiogenesis within ischemic tissue by delivering genes encoding for growth factors. Genes for vascular endothelial growth factor and members of the fibroblast growth factor family have been used for this purpose. Vascular endothelial growth factor and fibroblast growth factor are highly potent secreted peptides; as such, their genes can be delivered to relatively few cells within the vessel, resulting in locally increased concentrations of protein. This angiogenic strategy is currently being tested in clinical studies. A phase 3 study of adenoviral-mediated gene transfer of fibroblast growth factor 4 is underway in subjects with chronic stable angina.

6

MEDICAL ETHICS

John G. Park, MD

Medical ethics are the moral principles and practices that govern physician conduct in the treatment of patients. Ethical obligations typically exceed the minimal legal duties of the physician to patients. Medical ethics cannot be adequately learned from a textbook. The following outline of principles should be considered a guide only.

PRINCIPLES OF MEDICAL ETHICS

The three major principles are 1) autonomy, 2) beneficence and nonmaleficence, and 3) justice.

Autonomy

Autonomy involves respect for a patient's right to self-determination and implies *decisional capability*, that is, the ability to think about the available information and to draw conclusions. Clinical evidence of confusion, disorientation, and psychosis resulting from organic diseases, metabolic disturbances, and iatrogenic causes can adversely affect decision-making ability. In clinical practice, the lack of decisional capability should be proved and not presumed. Decisionally capable patients have the right to refuse medical therapy, even at the risk of death. If a previously decisionally capable patient had indicated, clearly and convincingly, whether life-sustaining therapy should be administered or withheld in the event of permanent unconsciousness, that wish should be respected, unless it was subsequently clearly rescinded. An updated advance directive may aid in maintaining a patient's autonomy, even when the patient no longer has decision-making capability.

- Autonomy involves respecting the patient's right to self-determination.
- Autonomy implies decisional capability (the right to refuse medical therapy, even at the risk of death).
- Lack of decisional capability should be proved and not presumed.

Substituted Judgment

Substituted judgment is the ability of family members or other duly appointed person(s) to make decisions about therapy on behalf of the patient on the basis of what they believe the patient, if decisionally capable, would have chosen.

Modified from Prakash UBS, editor. Mayo internal medicine board review 1996-97. Mayo Foundation for Medical Education and Research, 1996. Used with permission.

Surrogate Decision Maker

The surrogate represents the patient's interests and previously expressed wishes in the context of the medical issues. The surrogate is ideally designated by the patient before the critical illness. One type of surrogate is the durable power of attorney for health, in which a legally binding proxy directive authorizes a designated individual to speak on behalf of the patient. A second type of surrogate is the patient's family, physician, or the court. A third type is a moral surrogate (usually a family member) who best knows the patient and has the patient's interest at heart.

■ Ideally, a surrogate is designated by a patient before the critical illness.

Living Will

This is a type of advance directive or health-care declaration. This document commonly includes a declaration of durable power of attorney for health-care matters (proxy). The living will reflects a patient's autonomy and can aid greatly in medical decision making and may alleviate any confusion for a surrogate decision maker or for family members. Any decisionally capable person 18 years or older can have a living will.

■ A living will is a type of advance directive or health-care declaration.
■ The living will reflects a patient's autonomy.
■ Legal reliability may vary from state to state.

Disclosure

To make the principle of autonomy function, the physician must provide decisionally capable patients with adequate and truthful information on which to base medical decisions. Honesty on the part of the physician is an integral part of patient autonomy. This discussion, however, may be limited because of cultural or religious barriers or difficulty in accurately predicting death or survival. Such predictions are especially difficult with chronic diseases such as end-stage congestive heart failure or emphysema, whereas illnesses such as terminal cancer may have a slightly more predictable course. Severity-of-illness scoring systems hold promise in assisting physicians in quantifying the risk of mortality, thereby providing the patient more precise input to aid in decision making than has been available

in the past. Scoring systems such as Acute Physiology and Chronic Health Evaluations and Simplified Acute Physiology Scores continue to evolve; they have been validated for groups of patients with similar diseases but remain inadequate for predicting individual risk of mortality.

A serious issue is the availability of more than one acceptable form of therapy for a disease. In a patient with a cancer amenable to surgical resection, chemotherapy or radiation may provide a similar long-term outlook, albeit with different complications and side effects. However, a physician may be biased toward one of the three treatments. In this situation, it is the duty of the physician to set aside personal bias and provide detailed information on each treatment and its potential complications and to allow the well-informed patient to express personal preferences.

■ Physicians must provide decisionally capable patients with adequate and truthful information on which to base medical decisions.
■ Physicians must consider ethical issues and a patient's values and preferences.
■ Honesty is an integral part of autonomy.
■ Severity-of-illness scoring systems may assist in assessment of mortality risk, but current systems remain imprecise for predicting mortality for a given individual.

Informed Consent

Informed consent is voluntary acceptance of physician recommendations by decisionally competent patients or surrogates who have been furnished with ample truthful information regarding risks, benefits, and alternatives and who clearly indicate their comprehension of the information. Informed consent is especially important when performing new, innovative, nonstandard surgical procedures and research procedures, in an effort to maintain a patient's autonomy, and it is essential before initiation of any treatments or procedures. Informed consent from surrogates is necessary to perform an autopsy (except in specific instances such as coroners' cases, in which the decision is made by outside authorities) or to practice intubation, placement of intravascular lines, or other procedures on the newly dead. The amount of information needed by the patient to give informed consent is not that which the physician feels is adequate (professional practice standard) but that which the average prudent person would need to make a decision (reasonable person standard). In rare exceptions, the physician can treat a patient without truly informed consent (e.g., in an emotionally unstable patient who requires urgent treatment, informing the patient of the details may produce further problems). Many informed-consent forms in clinical use may not meet the reasonable person standard and therefore should be reviewed with caution.

- The amount of information needed by a patient is that which the average prudent person would need to make a decision (reasonable person standard).
- Many informed-consent forms may not meet reasonable person standard and need to be scrutinized carefully to uphold its moral and legal value.

Confidentiality

Patient confidentiality provides the patient the right to keep medical information solely within the realm of the physician-patient relationship. The physician is obliged to maintain the medical information in strict confidence. Exceptions to this include instances when data, if not released to appropriate agencies, have the potential to cause greater societal harm. Typical examples include positive results of the human immunodeficiency virus (HIV) test, a sputum culture that is positive for *Mycobacterium tuberculosis*, or a known or suspected criminal in hiding who is currently undergoing treatment. Patients who voluntarily request the HIV test should be informed by the physician that the result, if positive, will be automatically reported to the appropriate health agency. Confidentiality also may be breached when patients ask about the health information of deceased family members. Although genetic information is protected by law (Health Insurance Portability and Accountability Act regulation), health information about deceased family members may be disclosed for treatment purposes without prior authorization.

- Physicians are obliged to maintain medical information in strict confidence.
- Exceptions include instances when data, if not released to appropriate agencies, may cause greater societal harm (e.g., positive HIV test, positive sputum culture for *Mycobacterium tuberculosis*).

Group-Specific Beliefs

Certain religious practices preclude or compromise accepted medical practices. The principle of autonomy provides that adult patients who refuse life-saving measures (e.g., blood transfusion) should be allowed to maintain their religious practices after the physician ensures that the patient fully understands the ramification of the decision. However, in cases involving children, the courts have overruled the religious objections.

- Adult patients who refuse life-saving measures (e.g., blood transfusion) should be allowed to maintain their religious practices.

Beneficence and Nonmaleficence

Beneficence is acting to benefit patients by preserving life, restoring health, relieving suffering, and restoring or maintaining function. The physician (acting in good faith) is obligated to help patients attain their own interests and goals as determined by the patient, *not* the physician. Relief of suffering is essential for patients receiving palliative care, but the extent of such relief has limitations. For example, physician-assisted suicide remains controversial and illegal in most states.

- Beneficence involves preservation of life, restoration of health, relief of suffering, and restoration or maintenance of function.

The principle of nonmaleficence is based on "do no harm, prevent harm, and remove harm." This principle addresses unprofessional behavior; verbal, physical, and sexual abuse of patients; and uninformed and undisclosed experimentation on patients with drugs and procedures with the potential to cause harmful side effects. Breach of physician-patient confidentiality which results in harm to the patient is another example of maleficence. The caveat to this principle is that of "double effect." This caveat implies that unintentional hastening of death while primarily providing relief from pain and suffering is acceptable as long as the primary goal of such therapy is to provide such relief.

- Nonmaleficence is based on "do no harm, prevent harm, and remove harm."

Implied Consent

The principle of implied consent is invoked when true informed consent is not possible because the patient (or surrogate) is unable to express a decision regarding treatment, specifically in emergency situations in which physicians are compelled to provide medically necessary therapy without which harm would result. This clarifies that there is a duty to assist a person in urgent need of care. This principle has been legally accepted, and it provides the physician a legal defense against battery (although not negligence).

■ Implied consent is invoked when true informed consent is not possible.

Treatment of Minors

Minors, that is, persons aged 17 years or younger, in all states require parental permission for nonemergency cardiac treatment, with several exceptions. Emancipated minors can be treated without parental permission. This group includes married minors, minors in the armed services, students living away from home in college, and minors clearly living independent of their parents.

Incurable Disease and Death

The following guidelines are suggested in dealing with incurable disease and death. The patient and family (if the patient so desires) must be provided ample opportunity to talk with the physician and ask questions. An unhurried openness and willing-to-listen attitude on the part of the physician are critical for a positive outcome. Patients often find it easier to share their feelings about death with their physician, who is likely to be more objective and less emotional, than with family and friends. Nevertheless, the physician should not remain or appear completely detached from the patient's feelings and emotions. Even an attempt on the part of the physician to enter the inner feelings of the patient will have a soothing, if not therapeutic, effect.

■ The patient and family must be provided every opportunity to talk with the physician and ask questions.
■ An unhurried openness and willing-to-listen attitude on the part of the physician are critical for a positive outcome.

The physician should assume the responsibility to furnish or arrange for physical, emotional, and spiritual support. Adequate control of pain, maintenance of human dignity, and close contact with the family are crucial; numerous studies have suggested that these critical aspects of palliative care remain inadequate but are of utmost importance to the patient and family. The emotional and spiritual support available through local clergy (as appropriate, given the patient's personal beliefs) should not be underestimated. At no other time in life is the reality of human mortality so real as in the terminal phases of disease. It is always preferable to allay the anxiety of the dying patient through adequate emotional and spiritual support rather than by sedation. The physician should constantly remind herself or himself that despite all the medical technology that surrounds the patient, the patient must not be dehumanized.

■ Adequate pain control, maintenance of human dignity, and close contact with family are crucial.
■ Despite all the technology that surrounds the patient, human-to-human contact should be the most important aspect of treatment.
■ It is always preferable to allay anxiety by adequate emotional and spiritual support rather than by sedation.

Control of Pain

The principle of beneficence calls for relief of suffering. Adequate analgesia, particularly in patients with incurable disease, is the responsibility of the physician. If death ensues in a terminally ill patient because of respiratory depression from analgesia, the physician has not acted immorally (principle of double effect). Patients allowed to die after removal from ventilators are commonly treated in this fashion. Nevertheless, it is necessary to stress that the primary objective of analgesia is relief of pain and not the hastening of death, even in terminally ill patients.

■ Beneficence calls for relief of suffering.
■ Adequate analgesia, particularly in patients with incurable disease, is the responsibility of the physician.
■ A physician has not performed immorally if death in a terminally ill patient is the result of respiratory depression from analgesic therapy; euthanasia is not the goal.

Nonabandonment

Abandonment connotes leaving the patient (for whom the physician has provided—or agreed to provide—health care in the past) without care. This conduct is unacceptable and has been "universally condemned as a serious and punishable infraction of both the legal and ethical obligations that physicians owe patients." In contrast, nonabandonment denotes a requisite ethical obligation of physicians to provide optimal care once the patient and physician mutually agree to enter into a relationship. Noncompliance by the patient, in terms of taking medications or following a physician's instructions, is not grounds for abandonment. Such conflicts may be resolved by discussing termination of the physician-patient contract. Physicians should strive to respond to the needs of their patients over time, but they should not trespass their own values in the process.

Conflict of Interest

The principle of beneficence requires that the physician not engage in activities that are not in the patient's best interest. Some studies have suggested that physicians' prescribing practices are influenced by financial and other substantial rewards from pharmaceutical or medical equipment companies. If the physician does not ardently avoid areas of potential conflict of interest (because of the principle of beneficence), the result may be maleficence.

Conscientious Objection by the Physician

Physicians may refuse to perform a treatment or procedure that they judge immoral by their moral standards. Treatment should not be refused to patients whom a physician dislikes on moral grounds.

Justice

Every patient deserves and must be provided optimal care as warranted by the underlying medical condition. Allocation of medical resources fairly and according to medical need is the basis for this principle. The decision to provide optimal medical care should be based on the medical need of each patient and the perceived medical benefit to the patient. The patient's social status, ability to pay, or perceived social worth should not dictate the quality or quantity of medical care. The physician's clear-cut responsibility is to the patient's well-being (beneficence). Physicians should not make decisions about individual care of their patients based on larger societal needs. The bedside is not the place to make general policy decisions.

- Justice is allocation of medical resources fairly and according to a patient's medical need.
- Physicians should not make decisions about individual care of patients based on larger societal needs.

TRIAGE

Triage is a term applied to the decisions made in emergency situations about whom to select for treatment. The moral principle is to do the greatest good for the greatest number of patients. In this situation, preference for treatment is given to moderately and severely injured patients in whom emergency treatment can affect clinical outcome. In patients with minor injuries and those with a high probability of death even with advanced treatment, care is delayed.

MANAGED CARE

Health maintenance organizations are the most common model of managed care. They seek to provide their members with appropriate medical care at generally lower costs than fee-for-service practice models. Incentives for physicians to be cost-conscious and cost-effective are usually part of the practice plan.

Physicians owe a professional responsibility to the patient to investigate symptoms appropriately and to recommend the best therapeutic option even if this is the more expensive option. Never should financial issues be allowed to interfere with the provision of conscientious, high-quality care.

DO-NOT-RESUSCITATE ORDER

Do-not-resuscitate (DNR) orders affect administration of cardiopulmonary resuscitation (CPR) only; other therapeutic options should not be influenced by the DNR order. Every person whose medical history is unclear or unavailable should receive CPR in the event of cardiopulmonary arrest. CPR is not recommended when it merely prolongs life in a patient with terminal illness or when the fatal outcome is clinically evident.

Of paramount importance are the patient's knowledge of the extent of disease and the prognosis, the physician's estimate of the potential efficacy of CPR, and the wishes of the patient (or surrogate) regarding CPR as a therapeutic tool. The DNR order should be reviewed frequently because clinical circumstances may dictate other measures (e.g., a patient with dilated cardiomyopathy who had initially turned down heart transplantation and wanted to be considered a DNR candidate may change her or his mind and now opt for the transplantation). Physicians should discuss the appropriateness of CPR or DNR with patients at high risk for cardiopulmonary arrest and with the terminally ill. The discussion should optimally take place in the outpatient setting, during the initial period of hospitalization, and periodically during hospitalization, if appropriate. DNR orders (and rationale) should be entered into a patient's medical records. In some institutions, separate discussions can be held or decisions made regarding other therapeutic interventions such as intubations.

- DNR orders affect CPR only.
- Other therapeutic options should not be influenced by the DNR order.
- Every patient should be considered a candidate for CPR unless clear indications exist otherwise.
- CPR is not recommended when it merely prolongs life in a patient with a terminal illness, but ideally the decision to withhold CPR remains with the patient or surrogate in an effort to maintain patient autonomy.
- DNR orders should be reviewed frequently.
- DNR orders (and rationale) should be entered in a patient's medical records.

WITHHOLDING AND WITHDRAWING LIFE SUPPORT

This decision may be compatible with beneficence, nonmaleficence, and autonomy. The right of a decisionally capable person to refuse lifesaving hydration and nutrition was upheld by the U.S. Supreme Court, but a surrogate decision maker's right to refuse treatment for decisionally incapable persons can be restricted by states. Brain death is not a necessary requirement for withdrawing or withholding life support. The value of each medical therapy (risk:benefit ratio) should be

assessed for each patient. The American Medical Association has issued certain guidelines, and one of them states that a life-sustaining medical intervention can be limited without the consent of the patient or surrogate when the intervention is judged to be futile. Three states (California, Texas, and Virginia), for example, have permitted medical institutions to withhold futile treatments even against a patient's or surrogate's wishes. The extent to which these guidelines will be upheld by legal authorities is as yet unclear. When appropriate, the withholding or withdrawal of life support is best accomplished with input from more than one experienced clinician and institutional ethics authorities. Various institutions and organizations have published guidelines for withdrawing life support. The primary objective in such situations is to provide patient comfort (through analgesia or sedation) before and after withdrawal of support. It is emphasized, however, that if a patient had been paralyzed, reversal of paralysis is ensured before withdrawal of support.

- Withholding or withdrawing life support does not conflict with the principles of beneficence, nonmaleficence, and autonomy.
- Brain death is not a necessary requirement for withdrawing or withholding life support.

PERSISTENT VEGETATIVE STATE

A persistent vegetative state is a chronic state of unconsciousness (loss of self-awareness) lasting for more than a few months (criteria must be met at least 1 year after traumatic brain injury in young patients or at least 3 months after nontraumatic illnesses), characterized by the presence of wake and sleep cycles but without behavioral or cerebral metabolic evidence of cognitive function or of being able to respond in a perceptive manner to external events or stimuli. The body retains functions necessary to sustain vegetative survival, if provided nutritional and other supportive measures. The American Academy of Neurology has published practice guidelines that define persistent vegetative states. In such states, however, the patient may continue to exhibit variable cranial nerve and spinal reflexes such as moving, yawning, or mouth opening as long as these movements remain non-intentional or meaningful. Note that the U.S. Supreme Court has ruled that there is no distinction between artificial feeding and hydration versus mechanical ventilation.

- Persistent vegetative state is unconsciousness (loss of self-awareness) lasting for more than a few months.
- U.S. Supreme Court ruling states that there is no distinction between artificial feeding and hydration versus mechanical ventilation.

DEFINITION OF DEATH

Death is irreversible cessation of circulatory and respiratory function or irreversible cessation of all functions of the entire brain, including the brain stem. Clinical criteria (at times substantiated, but not necessary, by electroencephalographic testing or assessment of cerebral perfusion) permit the reliable diagnosis of cerebral death.

The family should be informed of the brain death but should not be asked to decide whether further medical therapy should be continued. One exception is when the patient had earlier directed the family to make certain decisions, such as organ donation, in case of brain death.

Once it is ascertained that the patient is brain dead and that no further therapy can be offered, the primary physician, preferably after consultation with another physician involved in the care of the patient, may withdraw supportive measures.

The imminent possibility of harvesting organs for transplantation should in no way affect any of the above-outlined decisions. When organ donation is possible after the determination of brain death, the family should be approached, preferably before cessation of cardiac function, regarding organ donation.

- Death is irreversible cessation of circulatory and respiratory function or irreversible cessation of all functions of entire brain, including brain stem.
- Electroencephalography is not necessary to establish death.

7

Restrictions on Drivers and Aircraft Pilots With Cardiac Disease

Stephen L. Kopecky, MD

This chapter is divided into three sections:

1. Restrictions for patients operating a private motor vehicle: These restrictions are from the National Highway Traffic Safety Administration (NHTSA), which is an agency of the US Department of Transportation. There are no clear-cut statutory rules for who can drive and who cannot. The recommendations are designed to aid the physician when performing a medical evaluation and making recommendations.

2. Restrictions for patients operating a commercial motor vehicle: Drivers of these vehicles must be certified as fit-to-drive by a medical practitioner, although there are no statutory rules to follow. The guidelines are recommendations.

3. Restrictions for patients operating an aircraft: The Federal Aviation Administration (FAA) requires all pilots to obtain an airman medical certificate and, although a cardiologist can evaluate a patient, the ultimate decision to grant a license to an individual pilot is made by the FAA.

Noncommercial License: Medical Conditions That May Impair Driving a Private Vehicle

This section contains a reference list of medical conditions that may impair driving skills and recommendations for each one (Table 1). These recommendations apply only to drivers of private motor vehicles and should not be applied to commercial drivers. The corresponding recommendations are based on scientific evidence whenever possible, but the use of these recommendations has not been proved to reduce crash risk. (Although scientific evidence links certain medical conditions and levels of functional impairment with crash risk, more research is needed to establish that driving restrictions based on these medical conditions and levels of functional impairment significantly reduce crash risk.) As such, these recommendations are provided to assist physicians in the decision-making process and are not intended to be formal practice guidelines nor substitutes for the physician's clinical judgment. These recommendations were adapted from

Table 1.   Driving Restrictions and Waiting Periods Before Resumption of Driving for Patients With Cardiovascular Disease

Condition	Restrictions and waiting periods*
Angina pectoris	
Stable	No additional restrictions; no waiting period
Unstable	Patients should not drive if they experience symptoms at rest or at the wheel
Angioplasty	Driving may usually resume 2-7 d after successful percutaneous coronary intervention if stable and asymptomatic
Myocardial infarction (acute)	
Uncomplicated	Waiting period of 2 wk before resuming driving
Complicated (e.g., arrhythmia, congestive heart failure, dizziness, recurrent myocardial infarction)	Waiting period of 1 mo *and* complete assessment by a cardiologist before resuming driving
Cardiac surgery involving median sternotomy	Driving may usually resume 4 wk after coronary artery bypass graft or valve replacement surgery and 8 wk after heart transplantation, depending on the resolution of cardiac symptoms and the patient's course of recovery
	In the absence of surgical and postsurgical complications, the main limitation to driving is the risk of sternal disruption after median sternotomy
	For patients undergoing a coronary artery graft operation using the minimally invasive surgery technique, the waiting period may be considerably shorter
Atrial fibrillation/flutter with bradycardia or rapid ventricular response	No further restrictions after heart rate and symptoms have been controlled
	Patients should not drive after an acute episode that causes dizziness or syncope until the condition is stabilized
High-grade AV/intraventricular block	For symptomatic block corrected without a pacemaker (e.g., by stopping the use of medications that caused the block), the patient may resume driving when asymptomatic for 4 wk and electrocardiographic documentation shows resolution of the block
Isolated block	No restriction
LBBB, bifascicular block, Mobitz type I AV block, first degree AV block, and bifascicular block	No restrictions if there are no associated signs of cerebral ischemia
Mobitz type II AV block, trifascicular block, acquired third degree AV block	Should not drive unless satisfactorily treated
Congenital third degree AV block	No restrictions if there are no associated signs of cerebral ischemia

Table 1 (continued)

Condition	Restrictions and waiting periods*
PSVT (including WPW syndrome), brief nonsustained paroxysmal VT, paroxysmal supraventricular tachycardia, paroxysmal atrial fibrillation/flutter	No restrictions if the patient is asymptomatic during documented episodes Patients with a history of symptomatic tachycardia may resume driving after they have been asymptomatic for 6 mo during antiarrhythmic therapy Patients who undergo radiofrequency ablation may resume driving after 6 mo if there is no recurrence of symptoms or sooner if no preexcitation or arrhythmias are induced at subsequent EP testing No restrictions with the following: 1. No associated signs of cerebral ischemia and no underlying heart disease 2. Ventricular preexcitation and no associated cerebral ischemia 3. Satisfactory control with resolved signs of cerebral ischemia 4. Satisfactory control with underlying heart disease
Sick sinus syndrome, sinus bradycardia, sinus exit block, sinus arrest	No restrictions if patient is asymptomatic Regular medical follow-up is recommended to monitor progression
Prolonged, nonsustained VT	No restrictions if the patient is asymptomatic during documented episodes Patients with symptomatic VT may resume driving after 3 mo if they are receiving antiarrhythmic therapy (with or without an ICD) guided by EP testing and if VT is noninducible at subsequent EP testing Patients may resume driving after 6 mo if they are receiving empirical antiarrhythmic therapy (with or without an ICD) without arrhythmic events or if they have an ICD without additional antiarrhythmic therapy
Sustained VT, ventricular fibrillation, cardiac arrest, ICDs	Patients may resume driving after 3 mo if they are receiving antiarrhythmic therapy (with or without an ICD) guided by EP testing and if VT is noninducible at subsequent EP testing Patients may resume driving after 6 mo without arrhythmic events if they are receiving empirical antiarrhythmic therapy (with or without an ICD) or if they have an ICD without additional antiarrhythmic therapy For long-distance or sustained high-speed travel, patients should be encouraged to have an adult companion drive Patients should avoid the use of cruise control
Cardiac arrest	After recovery, patients need a certificate from an appropriate specialist before they resume driving; the underlying cause should have been treated and the other relevant criteria in this table met
Pacemaker (insertion or revision)	The patient may resume driving after 1 wk if *all* the following are met: 1. The patient no longer experiences presyncope or syncope 2. The electrocardiogram shows normal sensing and capture 3. The pacemaker performs within the manufacturer's specifications
Hypertrophic cardiomyopathy	Patients who experience syncope or presyncope should not drive until they have been treated

Table 1 (continued)

Condition	Restrictions and waiting periods*
Congenital heart disease	Assessment should be based on the presence or absence of myocardial ischemia, left ventricular dysfunction, valvular lesions, or disturbances of cardiac rhythm and on the relevant guidelines in the sections of this table
Congestive heart failure	Physicians should reassess patients for driving fitness every 6 mo to 2 y as needed, depending on clinical course and control of symptoms Patients with functional class III (marked limitation of activity but no symptoms at rest; working capacity 2-4 METs) should be reassessed at least every 6 mo Patients have no restrictions if they meet the following criteria: 1. Functional class I (no functional limitations and able to achieve 7 METs without symptoms or objective evidence of cardiac dysfunction) 2. Functional class II (mild functional limitations and able to achieve 7 METs) 3. Functional class III (moderate limitations, working capacity <2 METs, and symptoms at rest) if no signs of cerebral ischemia (e.g., dizziness, palpitations, lightheadedness, and loss of consciousness) or dyspnea Patients should *not* drive if they are in functional class IV (severe impairment, working capacity <2 METs, and symptoms at rest)
Heart transplantation	Waiting period of 2 mo before resuming driving Waiting period may be shortened at the discretion of the specialist Annual reassessment recommended
Hypotension	Not a contraindication to driving unless it has caused episodes of loss of consciousness (syncope) or confusion caused by cerebral ischemia or hypoperfusion If cerebral ischemia or hypoperfusion has occurred, the patient should discontinue driving If treatment can prevent further attacks, the patient may resume driving
Hypertension	No driving restrictions for any type of hypertension other than uncontrolled malignant hypertension

Valvular heart disease
    Medically treated or
    untreated
	No restrictions if there is no associated cerebral ischemia
	Patients who experience syncope or presyncope should not drive until they have been treated, (*especially* if they have aortic stenosis)

Surgically treated (e.g., mechanical prostheses, mitral bioprostheses, or valvuloplasty with nonsinus rhythm	Waiting period of 6 wk No restrictions if no thromboembolic complications or symptoms of cerebral ischemia

AV, atrioventricular; EP, electrophysiologic; ICD, implantable cardioverter defibrillator; LBBB, left bundle branch block; MET, metabolic equivalent; PSVT, paroxysmal supraventricular tachycardia; VT, ventricular tachycardia; WPW, Wolff-Parkinson-White syndrome.

*The recommendations are general guidelines that all drivers with cardiovascular disease should satisfy. These are federal restrictions—private and commercial drivers may have additional restrictions imposed by individual states.

the June 2000 "Preliminary Guidelines for Physicians" published under the auspices of the NHTSA. The review and guidelines were developed by the Association for the Advancement of Automotive Medicine in cooperation with NHTSA.

In the inpatient setting, whenever appropriate, driving should be addressed before the patient is discharged. Even for patients whose symptoms clearly preclude driving, it should not be assumed that they are aware that they should not drive. The physician should counsel the patient about driving and discuss a future plan (e.g., resumption of driving after symptoms resolve, driver rehabilitation after symptoms stabilize, and permanent driving cessation).

Cardiac Conditions That May Cause a Sudden, Unpredictable Loss of Consciousness

The main consideration in determining medical fitness to drive for patients with cardiac conditions is the risk of presyncope or syncope due to a bradyarrhythmia or tachyarrhythmia. For the patient with a known arrhythmia, the physician should identify and treat the underlying cause of arrhythmia, if possible, and recommend temporary driving cessation until symptoms have been controlled.

CERTIFICATION OF COMMERCIAL DRIVERS

A *commercial motor vehicle* (CMV) is a motor vehicle used in commerce to transport passengers or property. Drivers of these vehicles must be certified as medically fit-to-drive by a medical practitioner. Although medical examiners are not required to have specific training or to demonstrate any special competence to medically certify CMV drivers, examiners are expected to exercise good medical judgment during the evaluation, and they could face litigation in the case of an undesirable outcome.

In September 2005, the US Department of Transportation issued preliminary guidelines for examiners to assess medical fitness-to-drive. This report, entitled "Medical Conditions and Driving: A Review of the Literature (1960-2000)," is a practical compendium that serves as a resource for physicians and caregivers, along with state department of motor vehicle personnel and others, and provides a comprehensive and integrative review of past and current research (to

the year 2000) on the effects of medical conditions on driving performance. Unlike regulations, which are codified and have a statutory basis, the fitness-to-drive recommendations in the report were established simply to guide the medical examiner in determining a driver's medical qualifications pursuant to Section 391.41 of the Federal Motor Carrier Safety Regulations. The Office of Motor Carrier Research and Standards routinely sends copies of these guidelines to medical examiners to assist them in making an evaluation. The medical examiner may accept the recommendations but is not required to accept them.

With regard to cardiovascular disease, the current federal regulations state that a person is physically qualified to drive a commercial motor vehicle if that person meets *either* of the following criteria:

1. Has no current clinical diagnosis of myocardial infarction, angina pectoris, coronary insufficiency, or thrombosis
2. Has no other cardiovascular disease of a variety known to be accompanied by syncope, dyspnea, collapse, or congestive heart failure

Because the CMV license does not provide the opportunity for the examiner to restrict work activity, the commercial driver must be able to perform very heavy work in order to be certified. For commercial drivers, an exercise treadmill test (ETT) requires exercising to a workload capacity of at least 6 metabolic equivalents (METs) (through stage 2 of a Bruce protocol), attaining a heart rate greater than 85% of the predicted maximum (unless the patient is receiving β-blocker therapy), having an increase in the systolic blood pressure of more than 20 mm Hg without angina, and having no significant ST-segment depression or elevation. Stress radionuclide or echocardiographic imaging should be performed for symptomatic individuals, individuals with an abnormal resting electrocardiogram, patients receiving digoxin, and drivers who do not meet the minimal requirements of the standard ETT.

An abnormal ETT result is defined as an inability to exceed 6 METs on a standard Bruce protocol or as the presence of ischemic symptoms or signs (e.g., characteristic anginal pain or 1-mm ST depression or elevation in two or more leads), inappropriate systolic blood pressure or heart rate responses (e.g., inability of the maximal heart rate to meet or exceed 85% of the age-predicted maximal heart rate), or ventricular dysrhythmia.

Ischemic electrocardiographic changes are defined as the presence of new 1-mm ST-segment elevation or depression or marked T wave abnormality.

Driving ability may be compromised with the following cardiovascular conditions if they are associated with cerebral ischemia (e.g., paroxysmal arrhythmias such as nonsustained paroxysmal ventricular tachycardia, paroxysmal supraventricular tachycardia, paroxysmal atrial fibrillation or flutter, and sinus node dysfunction):

1. Cardiac arrhythmias
2. Artificial cardiac pacemakers
3. Hypertrophic cardiomyopathy
4. Congestive heart failure
5. Valvular heart disease

Table 2 is a compendium of conditions with specific guidelines for medical approval or disapproval for CMV certification.

FAA MEDICAL CERTIFICATION

Heart disease is the number one cause of medical certificate denial for aircraft pilots of all classes. The FAA requires all pilots of fixed- or rotor-wing aircraft that exceed certain weight limitations to obtain an airman medical certificate. There are more than 5,000 designated private physicians (called aviation medical

Table 2. Compendium of Conditions and Guidelines for Medical Approval or Disapproval for Commercial Motor Vehicle (CMV) Certification

Condition	Guideline	Medical approval*†
Without known coronary artery disease	Asymptomatic, high-risk person (CHD risk-equivalent condition defined as presence of diabetes mellitus, peripheral vascular disease, or Framingham risk score predicting a 20% CHD event risk during the next 10 years)	Yes
	Asymptomatic high-risk person older than 45 y with multiple risk factors for CHD with abnormal ETT	No
Essential hypertension		
Stage 1 (systolic BP 140-159 mm Hg or diastolic BP 90-99 mm Hg)	May be certified to drive for 1 y; annual examination systolic BP ≤140/90 mm Hg (if <160/100 mm Hg, certification may be extended 1 time for 3 mo)	Yes
Stage 2 (BP 160-179/100-109 mm Hg)	May have a one-time certification for 3 mo; at recheck, if BP ≤140/90 mm Hg certification may be extended for 1 y from initial examination; annual BP ≤140/90 mm Hg	Yes
Stage 3 (BP >180/110 mm Hg)	This is immediately disqualifying	No
	If at recheck, BP ≤140/90 mm Hg and treatment is well tolerated, may be certified for 6 mo from initial examination; evaluate every 6 mo; BP ≤140/90 mm Hg	Yes
Angina pectoris	Should have biennial ETT at minimum	
	Rest angina or change in anginal pattern within 3 mo of examination; abnormal ETT; ischemic changes on resting ECG; intolerance to cardiovascular therapy	No

Table 2 (continued)

Condition	Guideline	Medical approval[*][†]
Myocardial infarction (MI)	Should have biennial ETT at minimum (if test is positive or inconclusive, imaging stress test may be indicated)	
	At least 2 mo after MI; approved by cardiologist; no angina; post-MI EF ≥40% (by echocardiogram or ventriculogram); tolerance to current cardiovascular medications	Yes
	Recurrent anginal symptoms; post-MI EF <40% (by echocardiogram or ventriculogram); abnormal ETT demonstrated before planned work return; ischemic changes on resting ECG; poor tolerance to current cardiovascular medications	No
Percutaneous coronary intervention (PCI)	At least 1 wk after procedure; asymptomatic; no injury to the vascular access site; approved by cardiologist; tolerance to medications	Yes
	Incomplete healing or complication at vascular access site; rest angina; ischemic ECG changes	No
	After uncomplicated, elective PCI to treat *stable angina*, a commercial driver may return to work as soon as 1 wk after the procedure	
	Criteria for continuing to work after PCI: 1. ETT 3-6 mo after PCI, then annual medical qualification examination 2. Commercial driver should have negative ETT at least every other year (criteria above) 3. Tolerance of all cardiovascular medications 4. Driver *should not* experience orthostatic symptoms, including symptomatic lightheadedness, a resting systolic BP <95 mm Hg, or a systolic BP decline >20 mm Hg upon standing	
Coronary artery bypass graft (CABG) surgery	Asymptomatic; ≥3 mo after CABG surgery; tolerance to medications without orthostatic symptoms; LVEF >40% on resting echocardiogram at the first qualifying examination after CABG surgery (a documented report of an echocardiogram performed in-hospital after CABG surgery is equally sufficient); approval by cardiologist	Yes
	Left ventricular dysfunction (EF <40%)	No
	After CABG surgery, a patient should have annual medical evaluation; after 5 y, an annual ETT (with imaging if indicated by standard criteria)	

Table 2 (continued)

Condition	Guideline	Medical approval*†
CABG surgery (continued)	Acceptable exercise capacity: the maximal heart rate achieved is >85% of the age-predicted maximum (unless the patient is receiving β-blockers), no ischemic signs or symptoms, a workload of at least 6 METs, appropriate systolic BP and heart rate responses, and no ventricular dysrhythmias	
	The examiner should have a low threshold for requiring stress imaging studies instead of a standard ETT	
Supraventricular tachycardias		
Atrial fibrillation/flutter	May be certified if asymptomatic and anticoagulated adequately for ≥1 mo; anticoagulation monitored by at least monthly INR; and rate/rhythm control deemed adequate	Yes
Multifocal atrial tachycardia	Symptomatic	No
AVNRT, WPW syndrome, atrial tachycardia, junctional tachycardia	Symptomatic	No
	WPW with atrial fibrillation	No
Ventricular arrhythmias	CHD and sustained VT with poor prognosis and high risk	No
	NSVT with LVEF ≥40% and symptoms of cerebral hypoperfusion	No
	Dilated cardiomyopathy with NSVT (LVEF ≤40%) *or* sustained VT (any LVEF) *or* syncope/near syncope (any LVEF)	No
	Long QT-interval syndrome, Brugada syndrome, or any cardiovascular diagnosis with symptomatic VT	No
	Any indication for PPM with symptoms (without PPM implantation)	No
	Neurocardiogenic syncope and hypersensitive carotid sinus with syncope	No
	If 3 mo after PPM implantation with documented correct function by pacemaker center and absence of symptom recurrence	Yes
Permanent pacemaker	More than 1 million people in the United States have pacemakers; when assessing the risk for sudden, unexpected incapacitation in a patient with a PPM, the underlying disease responsible for the PPM indication must be considered	

Table 2 (continued)

Condition	Guideline	Medical approval*†
Permanent pacemaker (continued)	If the patient has no symptoms 3 mo after implantation and correct function of the PPM has been documented	Yes
	If patients have neurocardiogenic syncope with both vasodepressor and negative chronotropic components and maintaining the heart rate can attenuate the vasodepressor aspect and if asymptomatic	Yes
Implantable cardioverter-defibrillator (ICD)	ICDs do not prevent arrhythmias; patients who have had a cardiac arrest and who have received ICD implantation	No
	Patients who have received an ICD for primary prevention (at risk of an arrest due to electrophysiologic testing or other evaluation), the risk of loss of consciousness is considerable	No
Hypertrophic cardiomyopathy		No
Idiopathic dilated cardiomyopathy and congestive heart failure	Symptomatic congestive heart failure	No
	Ventricular arrhythmias, LVEF ≤50%, and asymptomatic	No
	Ventricular arrhythmias, LVEF <40%, and asymptomatic	No
	No ventricular arrhythmias, LVEF 40%-50%, and asymptomatic	Yes
Restrictive cardiomyopathy		No
Mitral stenosis	Moderate and asymptomatic with annual evaluation and echocardiography	Yes
	Severe (mitral valve area ≤1.0 cm², New York Heart Association class II or higher, atrial fibrillation, pulmonary artery pressure ≥50% of systemic pressure, and inability to exercise for >6 METs on Bruce protocol (stage II)	No
Repair or replacement of any valve	≥4 wk after percutaneous balloon mitral valvotomy or ≥3 mo after surgical commissurotomy	Yes
Mitral regurgitation	Moderate and asymptomatic, with normal LV size and function and normal pulmonary artery pressure on annual echocardiogram	Yes
	Severe and asymptomatic with echocardiogram every 6-12 mo	Yes
	Severe and symptomatic with inability to achieve >6 METs on Bruce protocol, ruptured chordae or flail leaflet, atrial fibrillation, LV dysfunction (LVEF <60%), thromboembolism or pulmonary artery pressure >50% of systolic arterial pressure	No

Table 2 (continued)

Condition	Guideline	Medical approval*†
Aortic stenosis	Moderate (aortic valve area ≥1.0-1.5 cm²) and asymptomatic, with echocardiogram every 1-2 y	Yes
	Moderate with angina, heart failure, syncope, atrial fibrillation, LV dysfunction with EF <50%, or thromboembolism	No
	Severe (aortic valve area <1.0 cm²) (irrespective of symptoms or LV function)	No
Aortic regurgitation	Severe and asymptomatic, with normal LV function (EF ≥50%), mild LV dilatation (LVEDD <60 mm and LVESD <50 mm), and echocardiogram every 6-12 mo	Yes
	Severe and symptomatic; unable to complete Bruce protocol stage II, with LVEF <50%, and LVEDD >70 mm or LVESD >55 mm	No
Mechanical valves	Symptomatic, LV dysfunction (EF <40%), thromboembolic complication after the procedure, pulmonary hypertension >50% of systemic, and unable to maintain adequate anticoagulation (based on monthly INR checks)	No
Congenital heart disease	Patients with milder forms of congenital heart disease or in whom the condition has spontaneously resolved (e.g., spontaneous closure of a ventricular septal defect) or who have had surgical repair of a malformation	Yes
	A minimal waiting period of 3 mo after cardiac surgery is recommended for clinical and hemodynamic evaluation of results; evaluation by a cardiologist should be performed every 1-2 y, owing to the risk of subsequent cardiovascular complications	
	Bicuspid aortic valve with aortic transverse diameter >5.5 cm	No
	Marfan syndrome with any aortic root enlargement, more than moderate aortic valve regurgitation, more than mild mitral valve regurgitation related to mitral valve prolapse, or LV dysfunction (without associated valvular lesion) with EF <40%	No
	Atrial septal defect that is asymptomatic (i.e., no history of paradoxical embolus)	Yes

Table 2 (continued)

Condition	Guideline	Medical approval*†
Congenital heart disease (continued)	Atrial septal defect—ostium secundum with symptoms of dyspnea, palpitation, or paradoxical embolus; pulmonary artery pressure >50% systemic; right-to-left shunt; or pulmonary-to-systemic flow ratio >1.5:1	No
	Ventricular septal defect—small with symptoms of dyspnea, palpitations, or syncope; pulmonary artery pressure >50% systemic; right-to-left shunt; LV enlargement or reduced function; or pulmonary-systemic flow ratio >1.5:1	No
	Ventricular septal defect—moderate size (risk of sudden incapacitation from a paradoxical embolism or progressive pulmonary hypertension)	No
	Certification 3 mo after surgical closure if absence of the disqualifying criteria outlined above, QRS complex <120 ms on ECG, and no serious dysrhythmia on 24-h ambulatory ECG	Yes
	If the right ventricular conduction is >120 ms on ECG, the driver may still be certified if invasive His bundle studies show no infra-His block or other serious electrophysiologic disorders indicating a high risk of incapacitation, as determined by a cardiologist with expertise in cardiac electrophysiology	Yes
	Pulmonary hypertension that is >50% systemic from any cause	No

AVNRT, atrioventricular nodal reentrant tachycardia; BP, blood pressure; CHD, coronary heart disease; ECG, electrocardiogram; EF, ejection fraction; ETT, exercise treadmill test; INR, international normalized ratio; LV, left ventricular; LVEDD, left ventricular end-diastolic diameter; LVEF, left ventricular ejection fraction; LVESD, left ventricular end-systolic diameter; MET, metabolic equivalent; NSVT, nonsustained ventricular tachycardia; PPM, permanent pacemaker; VT, ventricular tachycardia; WPW, Wolff-Parkinson-White.

*For medical approval for a CMV license ("Yes"), all criteria must be present. For disapproval ("No"), only one criterion must be present.

†Restrictions are national. Individual states may impose additional restrictions on private and commercial drivers.

examiners [AMEs]) around the world who are designated to provide medical applications, give forensic examinations, and issue FAA medical certificates to qualified airmen. There are three standards of medical fitness (examinations for classes I, II, and III), each designed for the type of flying in which a pilot participates. The most stringent standards are required for a class I medical certificate: An examination is required for airline captains of scheduled air carriers and is valid for 6 calendar months. A class II medical certificate is required for cocaptains (first officers) and other professional pilots (e.g., agricultural spray pilots). A class III medical certificate is required for recreational pilots. The cardiovascular evaluation of a pilot with underlying cardiac conditions may be done by a cardiologist in conjunction with an AME, although ultimate certification involves review by the FAA at either the office of the applicable regional flight surgeon or the

Aeromedical Certification Division of the FAA in Oklahoma City, Oklahoma.

Of the 15 disqualifying medical conditions facing pilots, seven are related to cardiovascular disease:

1. Angina pectoris
2. Coronary heart disease that has been treated or, if untreated, has been symptomatic or clinically significant
3. Myocardial infarction
4. Cardiac valve replacement
5. Permanent cardiac pacemaker
6. Heart replacement
7. Disturbance of consciousness without satisfactory explanation of cause

Of these, only persistent angina pectoris, having more than one heart valve replaced (except for the Ross procedure), and heart transplantation are absolutely disqualifying.

If an implantable cardioverter-defibrillator (ICD) is implanted for cardiac arrest, for ventricular tachycardia or ventricular fibrillation, or for any of the standard criteria for ICD, the pilot is automatically disqualifed; however, all other indications (i.e., atrial fibrillation) are evaluated by the FAA on a case-by-case basis.

Using a waiver system outlined in Federal Aviation Regulation 67.401, the FAA may allow a pilot to fly if medical stability can be established. This is also known as *special issuance authorization.*

If the systolic blood pressure is greater than 155 mm Hg, or if the diastolic blood pressure is greater than 95 mm Hg, a pilot is grounded until the blood pressure is under control and the FAA is satisfied that no serious underlying cardiovascular disease is the cause.

For consideration of special issuance, the FAA usually asks three questions that the evaluating cardiologist must answer:

1. Is the coronary artery risk factor controlled (e.g., lipid levels, fasting blood glucose level, and exercise tolerance)?
2. Is there reversible ischemia?
3. Does the patient require any medications? Are there any side effects of the medications?

Pilots who have a myocardial infarction or undergo any invasive procedure such as stent insertion, valve replacement, or coronary artery bypass grafting require a mandatory 6-month stand-down time to establish condition stability before forensic testing may be performed for certification purposes. All pilots must undergo testing 6 months after a percutaneous coronary intervention; class I pilots must undergo coronary angiography to show patency, but class II and class III pilots may undergo noninvasive imaging to show absence of ischemia. Pilots who require insertion of a permanent pacemaker require 6 weeks of condition stability before forensic testing may ensue.

Heart valve replacement cases are considered by the Aeromedical Certification Division of the FAA on a case-by-case basis. The FAA is developing specialized centers of excellence for forensic examinations involving pilots with complex cardiovascular and other potentially disqualifying medical conditions (Mayo Clinic is one of those centers).

Currently, AMEs cannot approve certification of cardiovascular conditions that would be otherwise disqualifying without approval from the FAA directly. Therefore, they will typically defer the application (FAA form 8500-8) for authorization. Because the review process involves a decision from an external review panel of academic cardiologists, the pilot's certification decision may require up to 6 months for final approval.

SECTION II

Noninvasive Imaging

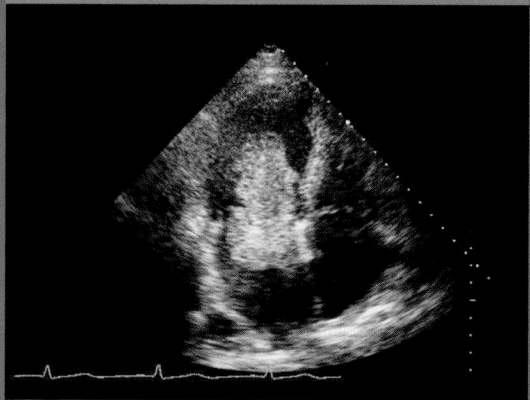

Cardiac Myxoma

PRINCIPLES OF ECHOCARDIOGRAPHY

Teresa S. M. Tsang, MD

This chapter summarizes the central role of echocardiography in both the initial diagnosis and the quantification of the nature and severity of specific cardiovascular diseases. It is important to appreciate the relative strengths, weaknesses, and incremental value of information obtained by different echocardiographic methods. The American College of Cardiology, the American Heart Association, and the American Society of Echocardiography jointly published practice guidelines in 2003 for the use of echocardiography. These guidelines make recommendations about appropriate and inappropriate uses of echocardiography.

The guidelines divide indications into the following categories: I, generally indicated; IIa, evidence is conflicting but in favor of usefulness; IIb, conflicting evidence with less well-established indications; and III, generally thought to be either not useful or contraindicated. The ensuing sections discuss some of the generally accepted indications and their technologic considerations; Table 1 lists important class III examples.

TRANSTHORACIC ECHOCARDIOGRAPHY

Anatomical and functional assessment of cardiac chambers, valves, myocardium, pericardium, and the aorta are important aspects of the echocardiographic examination.

M-MODE AND TWO-DIMENSIONAL ECHOCARDIOGRAPHY

M-mode imaging, which dates from the early days of echocardiography, is still a useful part of a complete ultrasonographic examination and can be acquired using two-dimensional (2D) guidance. The typical views obtained with the transducer placed at the left parasternal region, sweeping from the ventricular level to the mitral valve level to the aortic valve level, are shown in Figure 1.

Measurements of the left ventricular (LV) dimensions and wall thickness can be readily derived from M-mode recordings and are usually made according to the recommendations of the American Society of Echocardiography at end diastole (the onset of the QRS complex) and end systole (the point of maximal upward motion of the LV posterior wall endocardium). These measurements are made from leading edge to leading edge. LV ejection fraction can be readily calculated from measurements obtained by M-mode or 2D assessments (see "Assessment of Ventricular Function" section in this chapter).

2D imaging provides important structural and functional information on cardiac disease. The American Society of Echocardiography has recommended that cardiac imaging be performed in three orthogonal planes: long-axis (from the aortic root to the apex),

Table 1. ACC/AHA/ASE Guidelines for Clinical Applications of Echocardiography: Conditions for Which Echocardiography is Generally Not Recommended

1. Patients for whom the results of the study would have no effect on the diagnosis, clinical decision making, or management
2. Routine repetition of echocardiography in past users of anoretic drugs with prior normal studies or known trivial valvular abnormalities
3. Asymptomatic heart murmur thought to be functional by an experienced clinician
4. Routine reevaluation of asymptomatic, mild aortic stenosis in patients with stable physical signs and normal left ventricular systolic function
5. Routine reevaluation of asymptomatic, mild to moderate mitral stenosis in patients with stable signs
6. Routine reevaluation of asymptomatic, mild to moderate mitral or aortic regurgitation in patients with stable signs in the absence of chamber dilatation
7. Exclusion of mitral valve prolapse in patients without clinical symptoms or signs or family history
8. Routine repetition of echocardiography for patients with mitral valve prolapse who have no or mild regurgitation and no change of symptoms or signs
9. Routine reevaluation of patients who have uncomplicated endocarditis during antibiotic therapy when there are no changes in symptoms or signs
10. Transient fever without evidence of bacteremia
11. Routine reevaluation of valve replacement when there are no clinical symptoms or signs to suggest dysfunction or a failing prosthesis
12. Evaluation of chest pain when a clear-cut noncardiac cause is responsible
13. Assessment of prognosis more than 2 years after myocardial infarction
14. Patients who have been receiving long-term therapeutic anticoagulation and who do not have mitral valve disease or hypertrophic cardiomyopathy before cardioversion (unless there are other reasons for anticoagulation, e.g., prior embolus or thrombus known from previous transesophageal echocardiography)
15. Routine screening echocardiogram for participation in competitive sports if patients have a normal cardiovascular history, electrocardiogram, and physical examination
16. Suspected myocardial contusion in hemodynamically stable patients who have a normal electrocardiogram and no abnormal cardiothoracic physical findings or no mechanism of injury that suggests cardiovascular contusion

ACC, American College of Cardiology; AHA, American Heart Association; ASE, American Society of Echocardiography.

short-axis (perpendicular to the long axis), and four-chamber (traversing both ventricles and atria through the mitral and tricuspid valves). *Long-axis* and *short-axis* refer to axes of the heart not the body. The three planes can be visualized with four standard transducer positions: parasternal, apical, subcostal, and suprasternal. The views obtained are depicted in Figure 2.

DOPPLER ECHOCARDIOGRAPHY

Doppler echocardiography uses the Doppler effect, that is, the change in the frequency of sound waves as the sound source moves toward or away from the observer (Equation 1).

Equation 1. Frequency Shift (Δf)

$$\Delta f = \frac{2 f_t v \cos \theta}{c}$$

Δf = Doppler frequency shift

f_t = transmitted frequency

$\cos \theta$ = (angle theta) angle between the vector of the moving object and the interrogating beam

c = (constant), velocity of sound in tissue or water (1,560 m/s)

v = velocity of the moving object

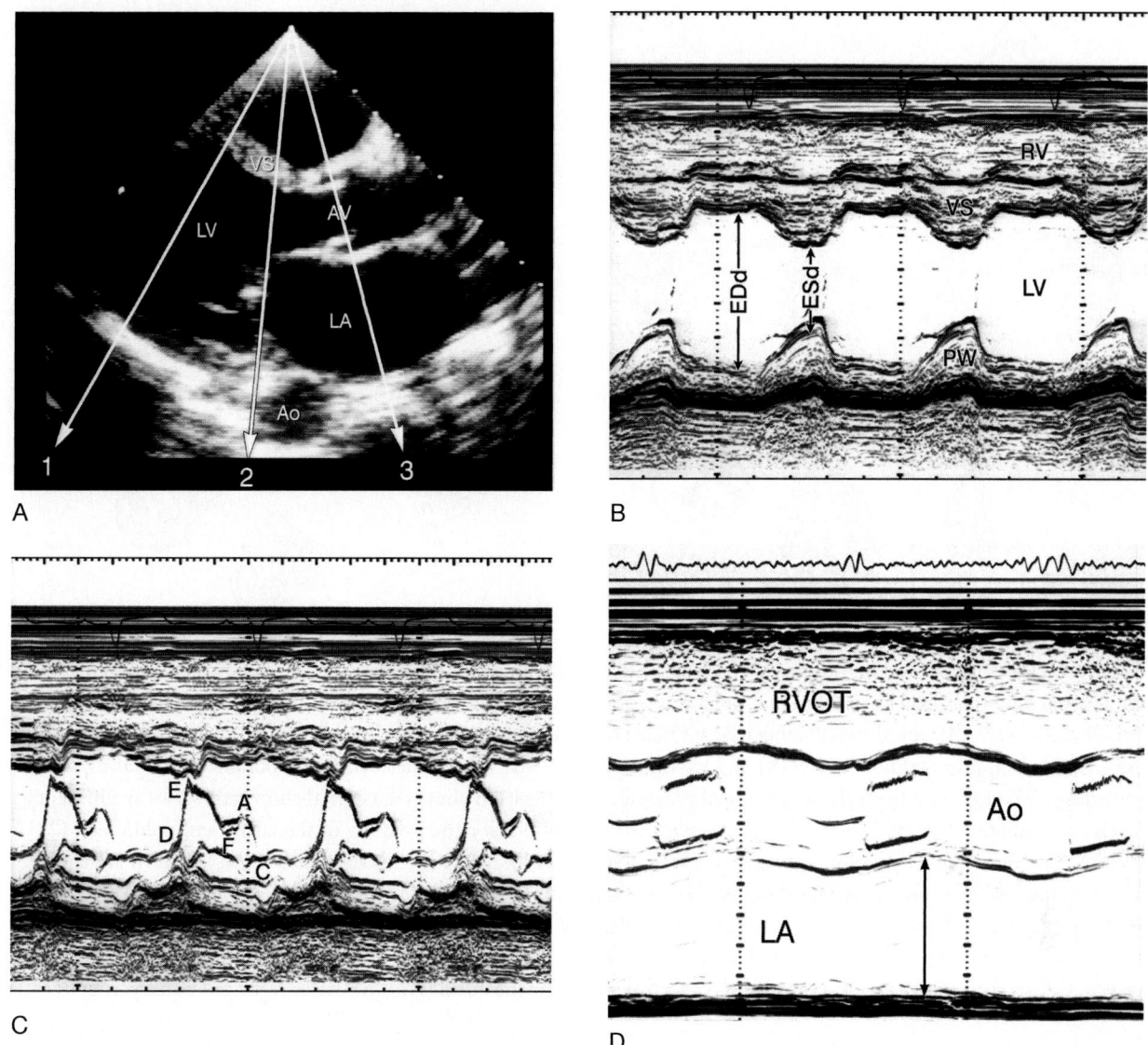

Fig. 1. *A,* An M-mode cursor is placed along different levels (1, ventricular level; 2, mitral valve level; 3, aortic valve level) of the heart, with parasternal long-axis two-dimensional echocardiographic guidance. *B-D,* Representative normal M-mode echocardiograms at the midventricular, mitral valve, and aortic valve levels, respectively. *Arrows* in *B* indicate end-diastolic (EDd) and end-systolic (ESd) dimensions of the left ventricle. *C,* The M-mode echocardiogram of the anterior mitral leaflet: A, peak of late opening with atrial systole; C, closure of the mitral valve; D, end systole before mitral valve opening; E, peak of early opening; F, mid-diastolic closure. The *double-headed arrow* in *D* indicates the dimension of the left atrium at end systole. Ao, aorta; AV, aortic valve; LA, left atrium; LV, left ventricle; PW, posterior wall; RVOT, right ventricular outflow tract; VS, ventricular septum.

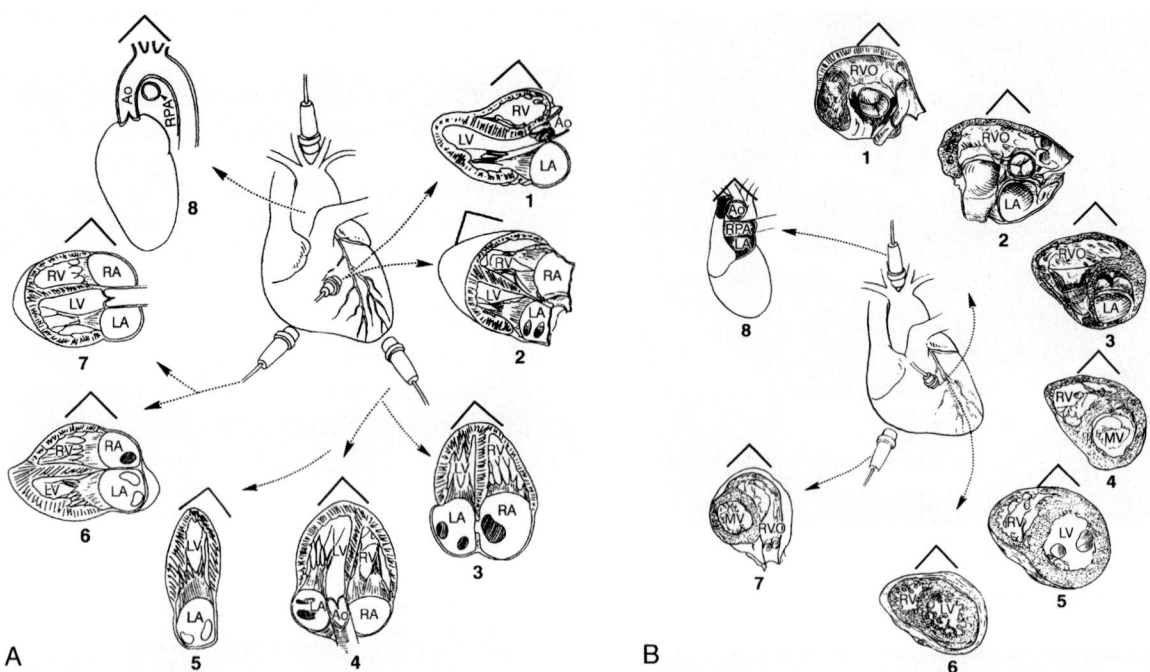

Fig. 2. *A,* Drawings of the longitudinal views from the four standard transthoracic transducer positions. Shown are the parasternal long-axis view (1), parasternal right ventricular (RV) inflow view (2), apical four-chamber view (3), apical five-chamber view (4), apical two-chamber view (5), subcostal four-chamber view (6), subcostal long-axis (five-chamber) view (7), and suprasternal notch view (8). *B,* Drawings of short-axis views. These views are obtained by rotating the transducer 90° clockwise from the longitudinal position. Drawings 1-6 show parasternal short-axis views at different levels by angulating the transducer from a superior medial position (for the imaging of the aortic and pulmonary valves) to an inferolateral position, tilting toward the apex (from level 1 to level 6 short-axis views). Shown are short-axis views of the right ventricular outflow (RVO) tract and pulmonary valve (1), aortic valve and left atrium (LA) (2), RVO tract (3), and short-axis views at the left ventricular (LV) basal (mitral valve [MV] level) (4), the LV midlevel (papillary muscle) (5), and the LV apical level (6). A good view to visualize the RVO tract is the subcostal short-axis view (7). Also shown is the suprasternal notch short-axis view of the aorta (Ao) (8). RPA, right pulmonary artery.

This Doppler frequency shift is detected and translated into a blood flow velocity (Equation 2) by the Doppler transducer and instrument.

Equation 2. Velocity (v), m/s

$$v = \frac{\Delta f \, c}{2 f_t \cos \theta}$$

(Definitions as in Equation 1)

The velocity of blood can be used to determine gradients, intracardiac pressures, volumetric flow, and valve areas.

Pulsed wave Doppler echocardiography and continuous wave Doppler echocardiography are the two most commonly used spectral Doppler modalities (Table 2). Pulsed wave Doppler echocardiography is "site specific," allowing the measurement of blood velocities at a particular region of interest. The disadvantage is aliasing of the signal when velocities reach one-half of the pulse repetition frequency, or the Nyquist limit (Fig. 3). This property limits the maximal velocity that can be measured with pulsed wave Doppler echocardiography.

Continuous wave Doppler echocardiography measures all velocities in the path of the ultrasound beam, is not site specific, and is not limited by aliasing. The disadvantage is that although very high velocities

Table 2. Appropriate Utilization of Doppler Modalities

Pulsed wave	Continuous wave
Flow volume	Valvular and other stenotic gradients
Diastolic filling variables	
Pulmonary/hepatic vein flow	Intracardiac pressure
	Mitral regurgitant velocities
Localizing site of flow disturbance	Pressure half-time measurements
	Intracavitary gradients

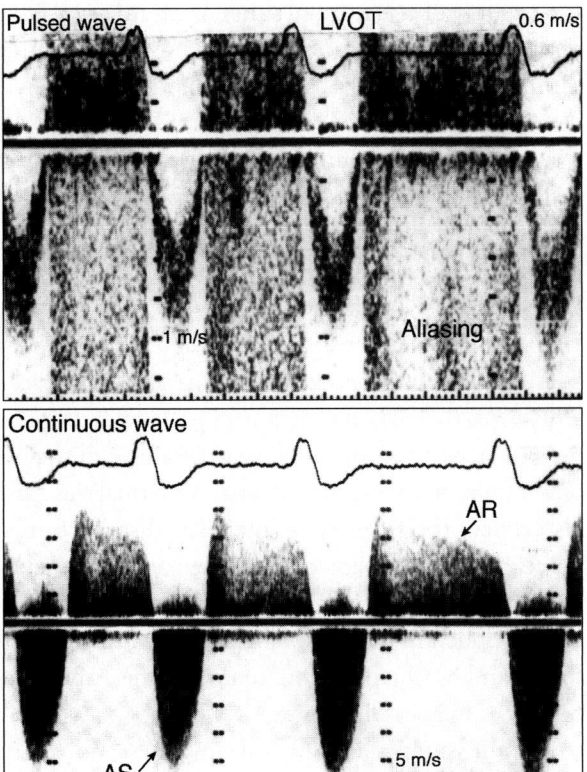

Fig. 3. Pulsed wave and continuous wave Doppler spectra from a patient with aortic stenosis (AS) and aortic regurgitation (AR). The pulsed wave sample volume is in the left ventricular outflow tract (LVOT) and demonstrates aliasing and "wrapping around" the baseline of the high-velocity AR signal. The continuous wave signal displays the entire AS and AR signals.

can be recorded, the specific anatomical site where the highest velocity is present cannot be accurately localized (but it can be inferred). Continuous wave Doppler echocardiography is typically used to measure high-velocity jets and gradients.

Color flow imaging is computer-enhanced pulsed wave Doppler echocardiography that displays the velocity and directional information of blood flow. Red depicts blood flow toward the transducer and blue, away from the transducer. Color flow imaging, like pulsed wave Doppler imaging, has a Nyquist limit and displays aliasing. Color flow imaging is used to detect, localize, and semiquantitate abnormal flow, such as that resulting from valvular regurgitation, shunts, or intracavitary obstruction.

Tissue Doppler imaging is now an integral part of routine electrocardiography and is most commonly used for assessment of mitral anular motion, which is part of a comprehensive diastolic function assessment (see "Diastolic Function Assessment" section). The velocity of the mitral anulus motion represents the velocity of changes in the LV long-axis dimensions. The diastolic velocity has been considered a measure of the intrinsic speed of myocardial relaxation. Early diastolic velocity is recorded at the septal or lateral mitral anulus using a pulse wave technique with a 1.5-mm sample volume. The ratio of peak early mitral diastolic LV filling velocity (E) to the mitral anulus velocity (e') by tissue Doppler imaging (i.e., E/e') provides an excellent assessment of LV diastolic filling pressures in sinus rhythm and in atrial fibrillation. Cutoff values differ among echocardiographic laboratories, depending on specificities and sensitivities chosen. In the laboratory at Mayo Clinic, E/e' is high if it is more than 15 and low or normal if it is less than 8. However, between 8 and 15, there is considerably variability in filling pressures.

CONTRAST ECHOCARDIOGRAPHY

Identification of intracardiac shunts is one of the most frequent indications for contrast echocardiography, and agitated saline solution remains the most commonly used contrast agent. Saline bubbles do not cross the pulmonary vascular bed, and this precludes opacification of left-sided chambers without an intracardiac shunt.

In recent years, stabilized solutions of microbubbles have been developed that can traverse the pulmonary capillary bed in high concentration after intravenous injection. These microbubble agents are capable of producing high-intensity signals not only within the LV but also within the myocardium following intravenous injection. Contrast agent facilitates the identification of the endomyocardial border and is most often used in stress echocardiography when visualization of the endocardium is essential for assessment of ischemia.

Second harmonic imaging enhances the ultrasonic backscatter from contrast microbubbles (which resonate in an ultrasonic field) while decreasing the returning signal from myocardium (which does not resonate).

ASSESSMENT OF CHAMBER SIZE AND WALL THICKNESS

The American Society of Echocardiography has recently published updated guidelines for cardiac chamber quantitation.

Left Ventricular Size

It is recommended that LV end-diastolic diameter (LVED$_D$), end-systolic diameter (LVES$_D$), and wall thicknesses be measured at the level of the LV minor axis, approximately at the mitral valve leaflet tips (Fig. 1 *A*). These linear measurements can be made directly from 2D images (Fig. 1 *A*) or by using 2D-targeted M-mode echocardiography (Fig. 1 *B*). It is not always possible to align the M-mode cursor perpendicularly to the long axis of the ventricle, a requirement that is critical for measurement of a true minor-axis dimension. As an alternative, chamber dimension and wall thicknesses can be acquired from the parasternal short-axis view using direct 2D measurements or targeted M-mode echocardiography, provided that the M-mode cursor can be positioned perpendicularly to the septum and LV posterior wall. As a general guideline, the upper limit of a normal LVED$_D$ is approximately 5.5 cm, but it varies according to body surface area. LV enlargement is an important finding, especially in patients with valvular regurgitant lesions, hypertension, cardiomyopathy, and LV remodeling after myocardial infarction. Thus, accurate measurement of LV diameter with serial echocardiographic monitoring is important for many clinical diagnoses. *LV size* is often interpreted as LV end-diastolic diameter.

Left Ventricular Wall Thickness

LV wall thickness is routinely measured in a standard echocardiographic study. LV septal wall thickness (SWT) and posterior wall thickness (PWT) are measured at end-diastole (d) from 2D or M-mode recordings routinely. The measurements of the septal and posterior walls are obtained at the same level of the ventricle as the LV diameter (Fig. 1 *B*). LV mass can then be calculated from the following formula:

$$LV\ mass = 0.8 \times [1.04\ (LVED_D + PWTd + SWTd)^3 - (LVED_D)^3 + 0.6\ g$$

Left Atrial Size

Traditionally, a single-dimension M-mode left atrial (LA) dimension has been used for assessment of LA size (Fig. 1 *D*). Recently, LA volume, indexed to body surface area, has been shown to be more accurate. The upper limit of the normal range is 28 mL/m^2. The biplane area-length method (Fig. 4) and biplane Simpson summation of discs method (Fig. 5) have been considered valid for assessment of LA volume. At Mayo Clinic, LA volume by the biplane area-length method is routinely assessed.

Right Ventricular Size, Right Atrial Size, and Right Ventricular Wall Thickness

Right ventricular and right atrial size assessment is qualitatively described in most clinical laboratories. This is particularly important in patients with pulmonary hypertension, pulmonary diseases, and tricuspid or pulmonary valvular lesions. Abnormalities may also reflect the severity of left heart disease. Some guidelines with respect to assessment and interpretation of the right ventricular and right atrial sizes have been included in the most recent "Recommendations for Chamber Quantitation" report by the American Society of Echocardiography.

Right ventricular free wall thickness, normally less than 0.5 cm, is measured using either M-mode or 2D imaging. Although right ventricular free wall thickness can be assessed from the apical and parasternal long-axis views, the subcostal view at the level of the tricuspid valve chordae tendineae, measured at the peak of the R wave, provides less variation and closely correlates with right ventricular peak systolic pressure.

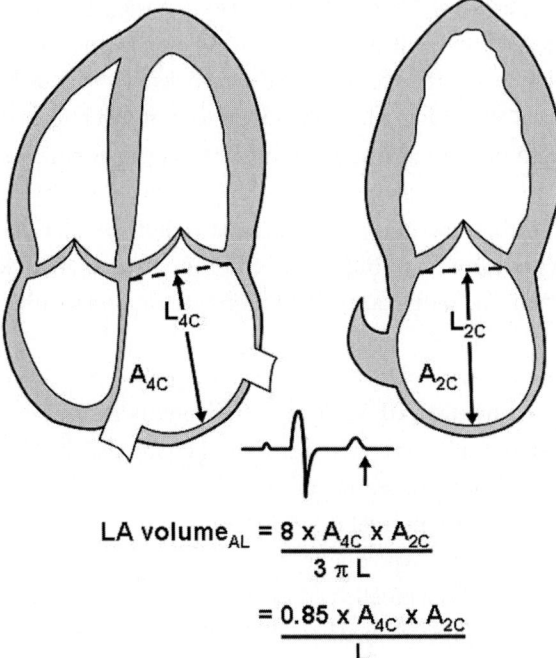

$$LA \; volume_{AL} = \frac{8 \times A_{4C} \times A_{2C}}{3 \pi L}$$

$$= \frac{0.85 \times A_{4C} \times A_{2C}}{L}$$

Fig. 4. The four-chamber (4C) and two-chamber (2C) lengths should be within 5 mm of each other; otherwise, foreshortening should be considered. In the formula, L is the average of the two lengths. (Note: the smaller of the two lengths has been used for L, which is acceptable if the difference between the two is no more than 5 mm). The *arrow* in the electrocardiographic tracing indicates the stage of the cardiac cycle represented by the drawings. A, area; AL, area-length; L, length; LA, left atrial.

ASSESSMENT OF VENTRICULAR FUNCTION (SYSTOLIC, DIASTOLIC, GLOBAL, AND REGIONAL)

Systolic Function Assessment

LV global systolic function can be evaluated with several echocardiographic techniques. These include 2D volumes derived from two- and four-chamber areas and length measurements (area-length method) and the modified Simpson method (or summation of discs). Formulae for calculating LV ejection fraction from 2D volumes (Equation 3) or 2D-directed M-mode (Equation 4), and fractional shortening (Equation 5) are shown below.

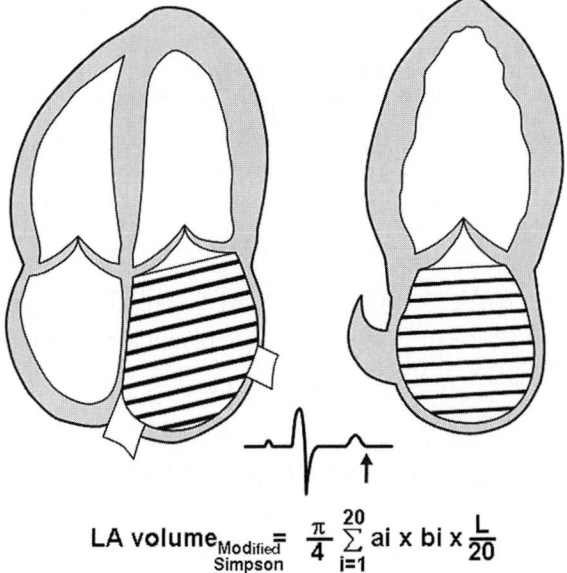

$$LA \; volume_{\substack{Modified \\ Simpson}} = \frac{\pi}{4} \sum_{i=1}^{20} ai \times bi \times \frac{L}{20}$$

Fig. 5. The length (L) is the dimension perpendicular to the discs, from the plane of the mitral anulus to the superior aspect of the left atrium (LA). The *arrow* in the electrocardiographic tracing indicates the stage of the cardiac cycle represented by the drawings. ai, area by integration along chord in four-chamber view; bi, area by integration along chord in two-chamber view.

Equation 3. Ejection Fraction (EF), %

$$EF = \frac{LVED_V - LVES_V}{LVED_V} \times 100$$

$LVED_V$ = LV end-*diastolic* volume
$LVES_V$ = LV end-*systolic* volume
(This formula can be applied to any contracting cavity; volumes are measured by the modified Simpson method with online software.)

Equation 4. Ejection Fraction (EF), %

$$EF = \frac{LVED_D^{\;2} - LVES_D^{\;2}}{LVED_D^{\;2}} \times 100$$

$LVED_D$ = LV end-*diastolic* diameter
$LVES_D$ = LV end-*systolic* diameter

Equation 5. Fractional Shortening (FS), %

$$FS = \frac{LVED_D - LVES_D}{LVED_D} \times 100$$

$LVED_D$ = LV end-*diastolic* diameter
$LVES_D$ = LV end-*systolic* diameter

Cardiac output can be derived from 2D volumes or from use of Doppler echocardiographic techniques (Equations 6-9).

Equation 6. Stroke Volume (SV), mL

$$SV = LVED_V - LVES_V$$
(Definitions as in Equation 3)

Equation 7. Stroke Volume (SV), mL

SV = area × TVI
Area = πr^2 (i.e., the cross-sectional area [cm2]
    through which velocity is recorded)

$$\pi r^2 = \pi \left(\frac{d}{2}\right)^2 = 0.785 d^2$$

d = diameter
r = radius
TVI = time-velocity integral = stroke distance (cm),
    which is the distance over which blood travels
    in one cardiac cycle (the cycle velocity [cm/s]
    divided by time [s])

Equation 8. Cardiac Output (CO), L/min

$$CO = \text{Stroke volume} \times \text{Heart rate}$$

Equation 9. Cardiac Index (CI), L/min per m2

$$CI = \frac{\text{Cardiac output}}{\text{Body surface area}}$$

Regional LV function is based on the 2D assessment of the contractility of 16 LV wall segments (six segments at the base and mid-ventricle and four at the apical level) (Fig. 6). A numerical score is given to each segment depending on contractility: 1, normal; 2, hypokinetic; 3, akinetic; 4, dyskinetic; and 5, aneurysm. A wall motion score index can then be derived (Equation 10). Studies have demonstrated adverse prognostic significance from high wall motion scores.

Equation 10. Wall Motion Score Index
Sum of wall scores ÷ Number of segments visualized
    Scoring of segmental contraction
        1 = normal
        2 = hypokinetic
        3 = akinetic
        4 = dyskinetic
        5 = aneurysm
    (Hyperdynamic walls are considered normal [i.e., score = 1].)

Diastolic Function Assessment

Mitral inflow assessment is fundamental to the evaluation of diastolic function. Mitral E (early filling phase) and A (atrial contraction) velocities, deceleration time, and isovolumic relaxation time (IVRT) are measured (Fig. 7). In general, three abnormal patterns are recognized: impaired relaxation (grade 1 diastolic dysfunction), pseudonormal filling (grade 2 diastolic dysfunction), and restrictive filling (grade 3 [reversible] and grade 4 [irreversible] diastolic dysfunction) (Fig. 8). At Mayo Clinic, abnormal relaxation with elevated filling pressures (grade 1A) is distinguished from that without elevated filling pressures (grade 1).

Mitral inflow patterns change depending on loading conditions. Therefore, other assessments are also necessary to provide a more comprehensive evaluation, especially to distinguish pseudonormal from normal. The Valsalva maneuver can be used to decrease preload and unmask the seemingly normal pattern of pseudonormal filling to reveal a pattern characteristic of relaxation abnormality. The pulmonary venous flow pattern, the tissue Doppler mitral anular velocity profile (Fig. 9), left atrial size, and color M-mode all contribute to the assessment of diastolic function and filling pressures,

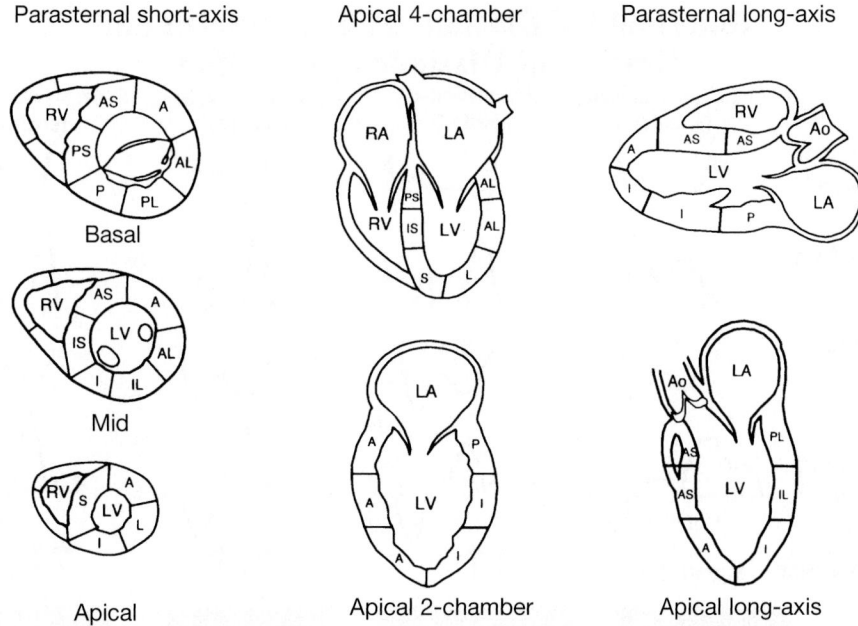

Parasternal short-axis   Apical 4-chamber   Parasternal long-axis

Basal

Mid

Apical   Apical 2-chamber   Apical long-axis

Fig. 6. Schema of the 16 left ventricular wall segments used to assess regional systolic function and wall motion score index. A, anterior; AL, anterolateral; Ao, aorta; AS, anteroseptal; I, inferior; IL, inferolateral; IS, inferoseptal; L, lateral; LA, left atrium; LV, left ventricle; P, posterior; PL, posterolateral; PS, posteroseptal; RA, right atrium; RV, right ventricle; S, septal.

allowing classification of diastolic function and LV filling pressures (Fig. 8). At Mayo Clinic, left atrial size is measured as left atrial volume.

HEMODYNAMIC ASSESSMENT

The following is a list of commonly used echocardiographic hemodynamic variables and their clinical usefulness:

1. Pressure gradients (maximal instantaneous and mean)—valvular stenosis, prosthetic valve, left and right ventricular outflow tract obstruction, and coarctation of aorta

2. Intracardiac pressures—right ventricular, pulmonary artery, and LV systolic and end-diastolic pressures

3. Volumetric flow—stroke volume, cardiac output, regurgitant volume and fraction, and, less commonly,

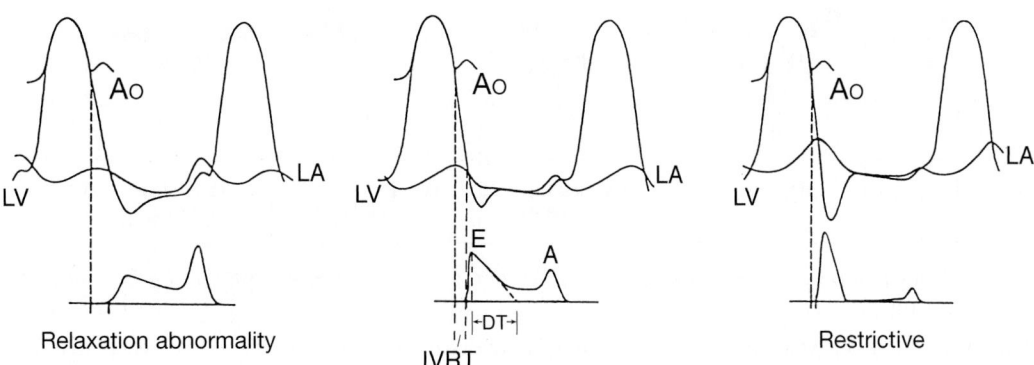

Relaxation abnormality   IVRT   Restrictive

Fig. 7. Schematic left ventricular (LV), aortic (Ao), and left atrial (LA) pressure tracings and corresponding mitral inflow Doppler spectrum. A, atrial contraction; DT, deceleration time; E, early filling phase; IVRT, isovolumic relaxation time.

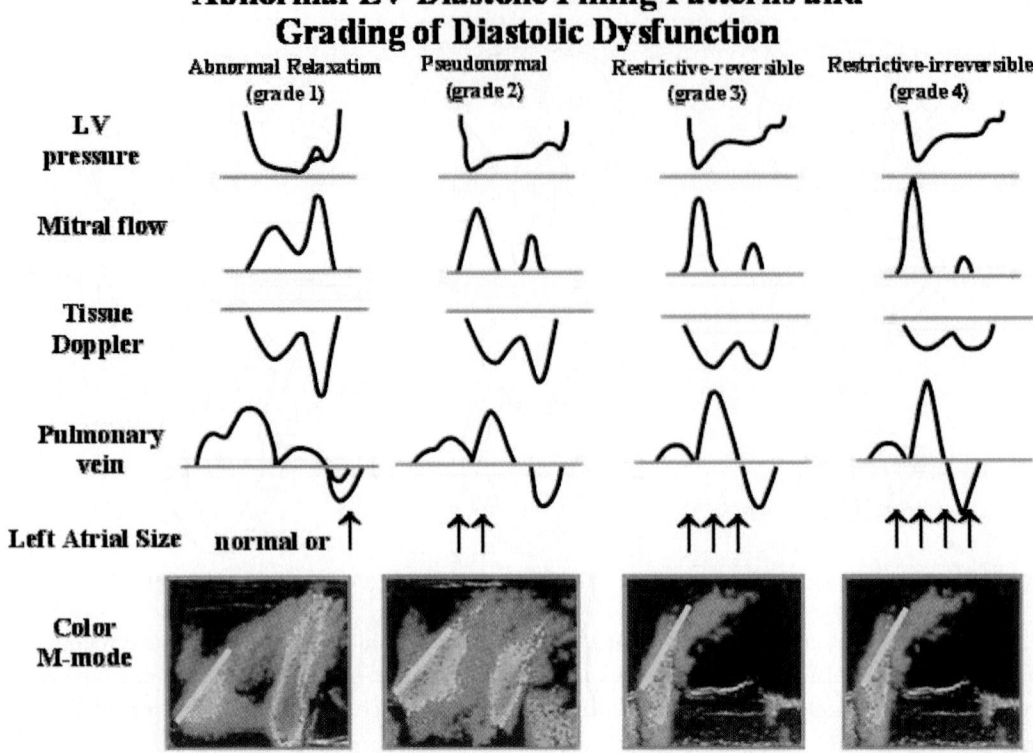

Fig. 8. Diastolic function assessment using mitral inflow, pulmonary venous flow, tissue Doppler imaging, left atrial size, and color M-mode. LV, left ventricular.

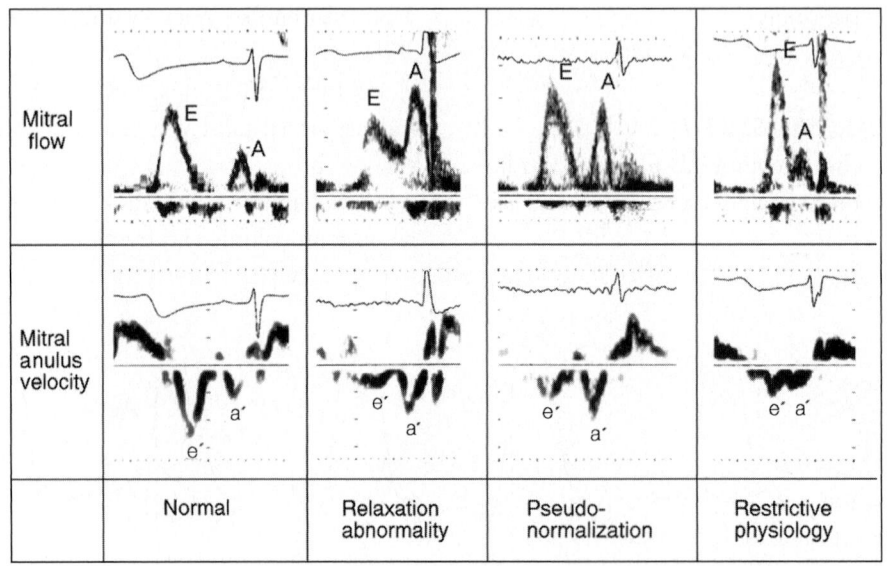

Fig. 9. Patterns of mitral inflow and mitral anulus velocity from normal to restrictive physiology. The mitral anulus velocity was obtained from the septal side of the mitral anulus with tissue Doppler imaging. Each calibration mark in the recording of mitral anulus velocity represents 5 cm/s. Early diastolic anulus velocity (e') is greater than late diastolic anulus velocity (a') in a normal pattern. In all other patterns, e' is not greater than a'. In relaxation abnormality, e' and a' parallel early (E) and late (A) velocities of mitral inflow. However, when filling pressure is increased (pseudonormalization and restrictive physiology), e' remains decreased (i.e., persistent underlying relaxation abnormality) while mitral inflow E velocity increases. Hence, E/e' may be useful in estimating left ventricular filling pressure.

shunt fraction (pulmonary stroke volume/systemic stroke volume [Qp/Qs])

4. Valve areas—continuity equation and pressure half-time

5. Diastolic filling variables

To make these measurements, it is essential to understand and use the modified Bernoulli equation (Equation 11 and Fig. 10), in which the decrease in pressure across a stenosis is equal to $4v^2$, and the concept of the time-velocity integral (TVI), or "stroke distance" (Fig. 11).

Equation 11. Gradient (ΔP), mm Hg

$$\Delta P = 4(v_2{}^2 - v_1{}^2)$$

or

$$\Delta P = 4v^2$$

P = pressure
v_2 = accelerated velocity across a stenosis
v_1 = velocity proximal to a stenosis
Note: Normally v_1 is much smaller than v_2 and can usually be omitted. Therefore, the equation can be simplified to $4v^2$
v = velocity across any vessel, chamber, or valve

When comparing Doppler-derived gradients with those measured invasively, it is important to remember that the maximal instantaneous gradient measured by Doppler is not equal to the peak-to-peak gradient measured at catheterization (Fig. 12). The maximal instantaneous gradient is always higher than the "non-physiologic" (i.e., nonsimultaneous) peak-to-peak gradient. Doppler- and catheter-derived mean pressure gradients are comparable.

By using the modified Bernoulli equation (Equation 11) and the measured Doppler velocity of a regurgitant or restrictive flow jet, the pressure difference between the two chambers can be calculated. If the pressure in one of the chambers can be measured accurately or estimated noninvasively, the pressure in the other chamber can be derived as shown in the following examples:

1. RV or PA systolic pressure = 4 (TR systolic velocity)^2 + RA pressure

2. PA diastolic pressure = 4 (PR end-diastolic velocity)^2 + RA pressure

3. LA pressure = systolic BP – 4 (MR systolic velocity)^2

4. RV systolic pressure = systolic BP – 4 (VSD velocity)^2

where BP = blood pressure, LA = left atrium, MR = mitral regurgitation, PA = pulmonary artery, PR = pulmonary regurgitation, RA = right atrium, RV = right ventricle, TR = tricuspid regurgitation, and VSD = ventricular septal defect.

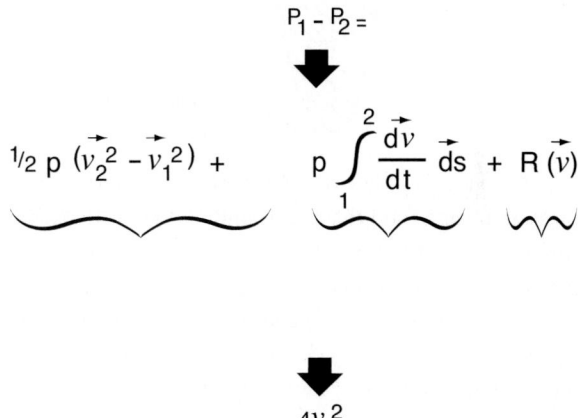

Fig. 10. Derivation of the modified Bernoulli equation, which measures the pressure difference ($P_1 - P_2$) across a restrictive orifice. In most clinical situations, the viscous friction and flow acceleration components are negligible and can be ignored. If the proximal velocity (v_1) is very small compared with the distal velocity (v_2), as in severe aortic stenosis, the proximal velocity term can be omitted, resulting in the simplified equation $\Delta P = 4v^2$.

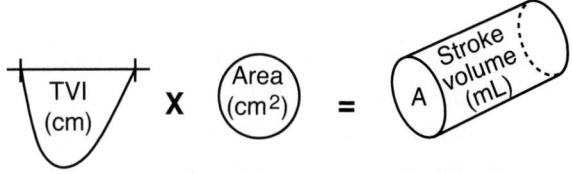

Fig. 11. The time-velocity integral (TVI) is the calculated area under the Doppler spectrum over time. It is also known as "stroke distance" because it represents the distance (cm) that blood travels with each stroke or beat. The stroke volume (mL) is the volume of the cylinder formed by the product of the cross-sectional area (cm^2) of the blood vessel or orifice and the distance (TVI) that the blood moves in a specified time period (i.e., systole or diastole).

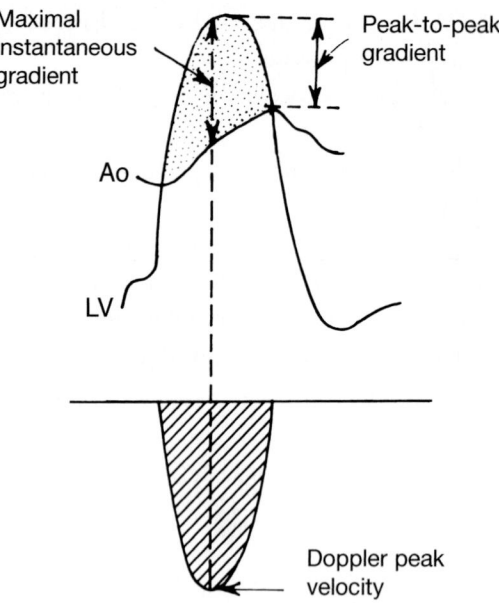

Fig. 12. Schema of left ventricular (LV) and aortic (Ao) pressure tracings and the corresponding Doppler velocity spectrum demonstrating the difference between peak-to-peak and maximal instantaneous gradients. The mean gradient (hatched area) is the area under the curve of the Doppler spectrum and is closely correlated with the mean gradient measured invasively (stippled area).

Right atrial pressure can be estimated by any one or a combination of techniques, including clinical estimate of central venous pressure, nomograms derived from Doppler catheter correlation studies, and echocardiographic estimates based on right atrial and inferior vena caval size and inferior vena caval reactivity to inspiratory effort. In practice, if the right atrium and inferior vena cava appear normal, 5 mm Hg is used for right atrial pressure estimates. If the inferior vena cava is mildly dilated or has blunted inspiratory collapse, 10 to 14 mm Hg is assumed. If the inferior vena cava is plethoric, has little or no inspiratory motion, or the clinical examination findings are consistent with marked increase of central venous pressure, 20 mm Hg or more is added to the pressure difference measured by Doppler echocardiography.

Regurgitant volume and fraction (Equations 12 and 13) and Qp/Qs (Equation 14) are obtained by comparing the flow through a nonregurgitant reference valve with flow through the affected valve or chamber.

Equation 12. Regurgitant Volume, mL

$$\text{Regurgitant volume} = SV_{valve} - SV_{systemic}$$

SV = stroke volume

$SV_{systemic}$ = systemic flow measured elsewhere in an unaffected area of the heart (area × TVI)

SV_{valve} = flow volume (area × TVI) across the regurgitant valve (forward plus regurgiant flow)

TVI = time-velocity integral

Equation 13. Regurgitant Fraction, %

$$\text{Regurgitant fraction} = \frac{SV_{valve} - SV_{systemic}}{SV_{valve}}$$

(Definitions as in Equation 12)

Equation 14. Pulmonary-to-Systemic Flow Ratio (Qp/Qs)

$$\frac{Qp}{Qs} = \frac{Area_{PV} \times TVI_{PV}}{Area_{LVOT} \times TVI_{LVOT}}$$

Qp = pulmonary stroke volume (usually measured at pulmonary valve anulus [PV])

Qs = systemic stroke volume (usually measured at left ventricular outflow tract [LVOT])

TVI = time-velocity integral

The continuity equation, which is based on the principle of conservation of mass ("what goes in must come out"), states that flow proximal and distal to an orifice must be equal in a closed system (Equation 15). Rearrangement of the continuity equation allows calculation of stenotic and regurgitant orifice areas by measuring three variables and solving for the fourth (Equation 16).

Equation 15. Continuity Equation

$Flow_{proximal} = Flow_{distal}$
$A_1 \times TVI_1 = A_2 \times TVI_2$

$A_1 \times TVI_1$ = proximal flow
$A_2 \times TVI_2$ = flow across valve

A_1 = reference area
A_2 = area of the stenotic valve (cm^2)
TVI = time-velocity integral

Equation 16. Valve Area, cm^2

(Rearrangement of continuity equation [Equation 15])

$$A_2 = A_1 \times \frac{TVI_1}{TVI_2}$$

A_1 = reference area
A_2 = area of the stenotic valve (cm^2)
TVI = time-velocity integral

Mitral valve area can be measured with the continuity equation (Equation 15) or the pressure half-time method (Equations 17 and 18).

Equation 17. Pressure Half-Time (PHT), ms

$$PHT = DT \times 0.29$$

PHT = time required for the peak gradient to decrease by one-half
DT = deceleration time (time [ms] from the maximal velocity to zero velocity)
0.29 = an algebraic constant that converts velocity to gradient

---

Equation 18. Mitral Valve Area (MVA) by Half-Time Measurement, cm^2

$$MVA = \frac{220}{PHT} \text{ or } \frac{759}{DT}$$

220 and 759 = empirical time constants equating to an MVA of approximately 1 cm^2

(Definitions as in Equation 17)

The proximal isovelocity surface area (PISA) method (Fig. 13) is used most frequently in the context of quantifying mitral and aortic regurgitation. This method represents a variation of the continuity equation and uses the property of flow convergence of fluid as it approaches a restrictive orifice. Blood forms multiple concentric "shells" or "hemispheres" of isovelocity. As the surface area decreases, the velocity increases. The velocity at a given distance from the orifice (v_r) can be measured by altering the aliasing velocity of the color flow Doppler signal. The flow rate through the orifice can be calculated (Equation 19). The effective regurgitant orifice (ERO), also referred to as regurgitant orifice area (ROA), and regurgitant volume can be calculated using the continuity equation and the peak velocity and TVI of the continuous-wave mitral regurgitant signal (Equations 20 and 21). Variations of the PISA technique also allow calculation of flow rate and volume and orifice area of stenotic mitral valves, atrial and ventricular septal defects, and aortic coarctation.

Equation 19. Proximal Isovelocity Surface Area (PISA) Flow Rate, mL/s

$$Flow = 2 \pi^2 \times v_r$$

Flow = instantaneous flow rate (mL/s)
r = radial distance of isovelocity shell from orifice (cm)
v_r = flow velocity radius r (cm/s)

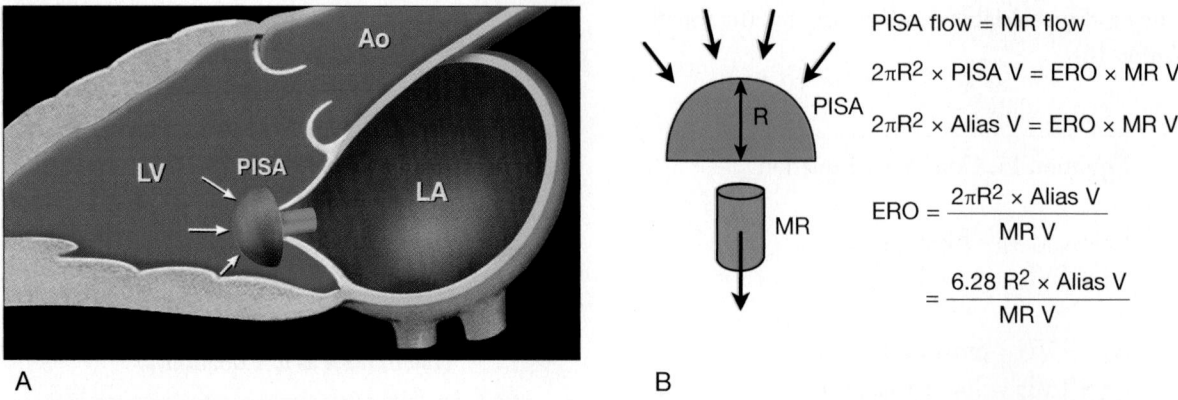

PISA flow = MR flow

$2\pi R^2 \times PISA\ V = ERO \times MR\ V$

$2\pi R^2 \times Alias\ V = ERO \times MR\ V$

$$ERO = \frac{2\pi R^2 \times Alias\ V}{MR\ V}$$

$$= \frac{6.28\ R^2 \times Alias\ V}{MR\ V}$$

A   B

Fig. 13. *A*, Diagram of proximal isovelocity surface area (PISA) (*arrows*) of mitral regurgitation. As blood flow converges toward the mitral regurgitant orifice, blood-flow velocity increases gradually and forms multiple isovelocity hemispheric shells. The flow rate calculated at the surface of the hemisphere is equal to the flow rate going through the mitral regurgitant orifice. Ao, aorta; LA, left atrium; LV, left ventricle. *B*, Calculation and derivation of effective regurgitant orifice (ERO) area of mitral regurgitation (MR) with the PISA method. R, PISA radius; V, velocity.

Equation 20. Effective Regurgitant Orifice (ERO) (cm2) for Quantifying Mitral Regurgitation

$$ERO = \frac{Flow\ (mL/s)}{v_{MR}\ (cm/s)}$$

v_{MR} = peak velocity of continuous-wave mitral regurgitant signal

---

Equation 21. Regurgitant Volume (mL) for Quantifying Mitral Regurgitation

Regurgitant volume = ERO (cm2) × TVI$_{MR}$ (cm)
ERO = effective regurgitant orifice
TVI$_{MR}$ = time-velocity integral of continuous-wave mitral regurgitant signal

---

For cardiology examinations, be able to identify the Doppler signals and assess the hemodynamic significance of the following conditions:

1. Aortic stenosis—transvalvular velocity, gradient, and aortic valve area by the continuity equation (Fig. 14)

2. Aortic regurgitation—pressure half-time and diastolic flow reversals in aorta (Fig. 15)

3. Mitral stenosis—transvalvular gradient, pressure half-time, and mitral valve area (Fig. 16)

4. Mitral regurgitation—regurgitant volume, fraction, and systolic flow reversals in pulmonary veins

5. Pulmonary artery pressure—tricuspid regurgitant velocity

6. Hypertrophic cardiomyopathy—left ventricular outflow tract gradient

7. Tricuspid regurgitation—systolic flow reversals in hepatic veins and marked dilated inferior vena cava and hepatic veins

Evaluation of Specific Disorders

Aortic Stenosis

1. M-mode/2D echocardiography—valve morphology (unicuspid, bicuspid, or tricuspid) and calcification.

2. Doppler echocardiography—peak aortic velocity, TVI, mean gradient (Fig. 14), and aortic valve area by the continuity equation (Equation 16).

Severe aortic stenosis is usually present if the peak aortic velocity is 4.5 m/s or greater, the mean pressure gradient is 50 mm Hg or greater, the valve area is less than 0.80 cm2, or the left ventricular outflow tract–aortic valve TVI ratio is 0.25 or less. A small calculated aortic valve area associated with a low gradient and a

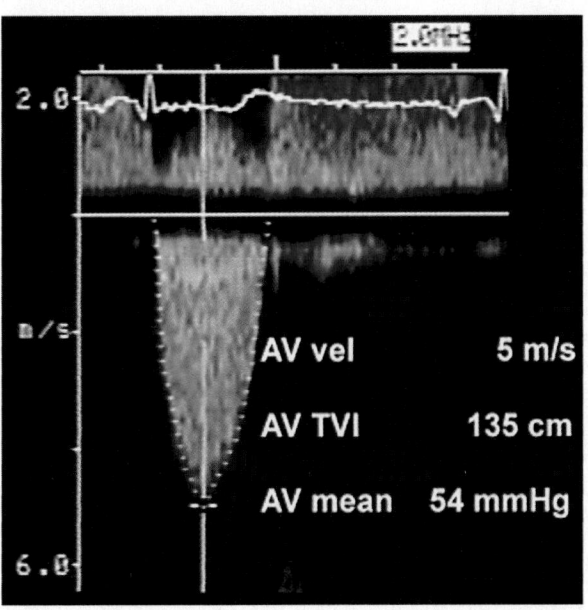

Fig. 14. Doppler signal obtained from the apical window in a patient with severe, symptomatic calcific aortic stenosis. LVOT vel = 1 m/s; LVOT TVI = 20 cm; LVOT diameter = 2.0 cm. By the continuity equation, the aortic valve area = 0.47 cm². AV vel = 5 m/s; AV TVI = 135 cm; mean gradient across the aortic valve = 54 mm Hg. AV, aortic valve; LVOT, left ventricular outflow tract; TVI, time-velocity integral; vel, velocity.

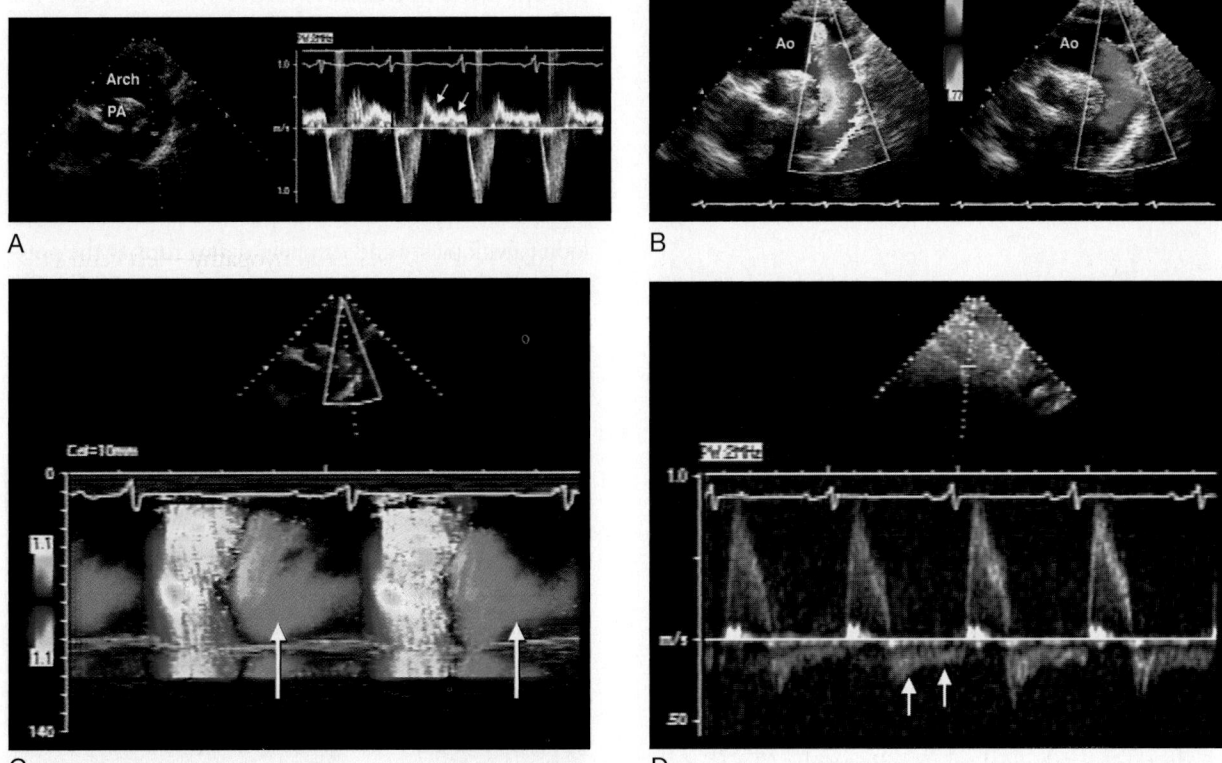

Fig. 15. *A,* Holodiastolic reversal flow (*arrows*) in the descending aorta indicates severe aortic regurgitation. Similar diastolic reversal can be seen in a descending thoracic aneurysm or shunt into the aorta during diastole (as in Blalock-Taussig shunt). The sample volume usually is located just distal to the takeoff of the left subclavian artery. PA, pulmonary artery. *B,* Two-dimensional color flow imaging of the descending thoracic aorta during diastole. The orange-red flow in the descending aorta during diastole indicates flow toward the transducer, that is, reversal flow due to severe aortic regurgitation. Ao, aorta. *C,* Color M-mode from the descending thoracic aorta shows holodiastolic reversal flow (*arrows*). *D,* Pulsed-wave Doppler recording of abdominal aorta showing diastolic flow reversal (*arrows*) in severe aortic regurgitation.

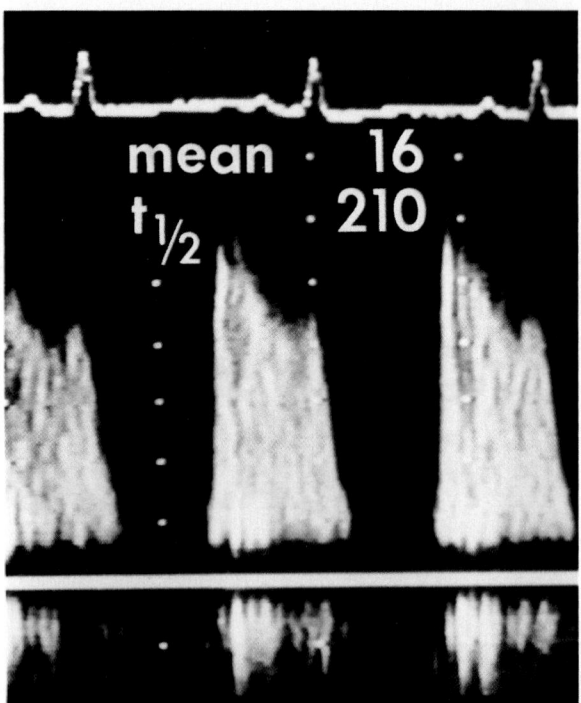

Fig. 16. Continuous wave Doppler signal from a patient with severe mitral stenosis. Mean gradient is 16 mm Hg. Pressure half-time ($t_{1/2}$) is 210 ms. Mitral valve area by pressure half-time method is 1.0 cm².

low cardiac output state requires careful evaluation to differentiate decreased LV systolic function due to truly severe aortic stenosis from milder aortic stenosis and the presence of unrelated myocardial dysfunction. Dobutamine echocardiography has been used to increase contractility and to increase cardiac output to differentiate anatomical from "relative" aortic stenosis.

The major pitfall in assessment of aortic stenosis is underestimation of the gradient and overestimation of the valve area when the highest velocity Doppler signal is not obtained because of technical or anatomical factors. When there is a discrepancy between clinical assessment and calculated valve area by transthoracic study, transesophageal echocardiography (TEE) may be required for more sensitive assessment of the valve morphology and degree of stenosis, and planimetry of the valve area can also be performed.

Mitral Stenosis

1. M-mode/2D echocardiography—valve morphology, doming or "hockey stick" (long-axis view)

(Fig. 17), "fish mouth" (short-axis view), leaflet and subvalvular thickening, calcification and mobility (Abascal echocardiographic score), commissural anatomy, and left atrial size.

2. Doppler echocardiography—mean gradient, mitral valve area by continuity equation, pressure half-time, and planimetry methods (Equations 16-18); pulmonary artery pressure; and degree of mitral regurgitation. All three methods of echocardiographic assessment of mitral valve area correlate well with invasive measures, but each has unique features that render it more or less accurate in a given patient (Table 3). Therefore, all three methods should be performed to achieve an integrated approach to the severity of mitral stenosis.

A high transvalvular gradient with normal pressure half-time may reflect severe mitral regurgitation rather than mitral stenosis. Severe mitral stenosis is usually present if the mitral valve area is 1.0 cm² or less, the mean resting pressure gradient is 10 mm Hg or greater, or the pressure half-time is 220 ms or longer. Exercise Doppler echocardiography can be very useful to assess stress-induced changes in gradient, mitral valve area, and pulmonary artery pressures.

TEE is essential before percutaneous mitral balloon valvuloplasty and can help define further the presence or absence of commissural fusion and calcification. The presence of heavy calcification at both commissures, significant subvalvular disease, and

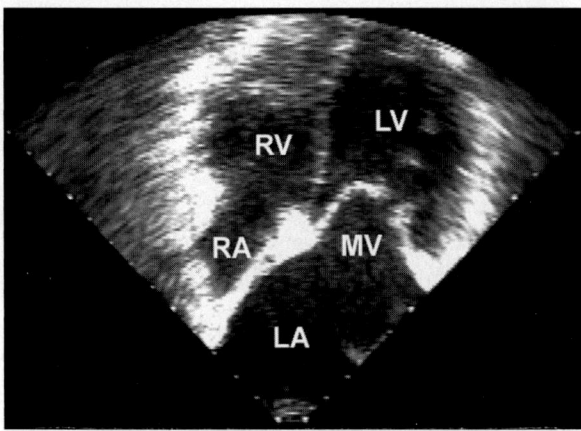

Fig. 17. Rheumatic mitral stenosis with left atrial (LA) enlargement and obvious doming of the anterior mitral leaflet. LV, left ventricle; MV, mitral valve; RA, right atrium; RV, right ventricle.

Table 3.   Limitations and Pitfalls in Assessing Mitral Valve Area

Two-dimensional (2D) planimetry
    Dependent on 2D image quality, gain-setting, and ability to visualize the minimal orifice area
    Less accurate when extensive calcification is present
    Difficult after commissurotomy because of irregular orifice
Doppler pressure half-time
    Tachycardia
    Nonlinear pressure decay
    Significant or acute aortic regurgitation increases the rate of increase in left ventricular pressure and shortens
        pressure half-time (mitral valve area overestimated)
    Immediately after percutaneous mitral valvuloplasty when hemodynamics are not stable (mitral valve area
        overestimated)
Continuity equation
    Cumbersome to perform, multiple measurements are subject to error
    Mitral valve area underestimated when significant mitral regurgitation is present

marked leaflet thickening and immobility predict suboptimal results for valvuloplasty. Left atrial thrombus must be excluded to avoid embolic complications.

Aortic Regurgitation

1. M-mode/2D echocardiography—valve morphology, LV size and function, premature mitral valve closure, diastolic opening of the aortic valve (severe aortic regurgitation), fluttering of the mitral valve, and etiology: Marfan syndrome, bicuspid aortic valve, endocarditis, and dissection.

2. Color flow imaging—ratio of jet width or area to LV outflow tract width or area (mild, <30%; severe, >60%).

3. Pulsed wave Doppler echocardiography—holodiastolic flow reversals in the descending or abdominal aorta are indicative of significant regurgitation.

4. Continuous wave Doppler echocardiography—pressure half-time (mild, ≥400 ms; severe, ≤250 ms). High LV end-diastolic pressure can shorten pressure half-time, causing overestimation of the severity of regurgitation.

5. Quantitative methods—Regurgitant fraction (mild <30%; severe >55%) or regurgitant volume ≥60 mL; effective regurgitant orifice (mild, <0.10 cm^2; severe, ≥0.30 cm^2); LV diastolic dimension in chronic aortic regurgitation (mild, <6.0 cm; severe, ≥7.5 cm).

An integrated approach using these quantitative and semiquantitative methods of evaluation should be used because all the above can be influenced by factors other than the degree of aortic regurgitation (Fig. 15).

A restrictive mitral inflow pattern may be seen in acute severe aortic regurgitation.

Mitral Regurgitation

1. M-mode/2D echocardiography—valve morphology, LV size and function, and cause: mitral valve prolapse, flail leaflet, mitral anular calcification, papillary muscle dysfunction or rupture, and endocarditis.

2. Color flow imaging—jet size and jet–left atrial area ratio. Color flow imaging jet size is influenced by instrument settings (pulse repetition frequency, depth, etc.), loading conditions, and jet direction. An eccentric jet, or one that "hugs" the left atrial wall, carries more regurgitant volume than a similarly sized "central" or "free" jet.

3. Pulsed wave Doppler echocardiography—systolic reversals in the pulmonary vein indicate severe mitral regurgitation.

4. Quantitative methods—regurgitant volume and fraction. The PISA method allows assessment of regurgitant volume and ERO area using the concept of the continuity equation and flow convergence.

5. TEE—useful in assessing mitral valve morphology and the cause of regurgitation, useful for visualizing the color flow jet and pulmonary veins, and useful intraoperatively before and after mitral valve repair or replacement.

Tricuspid Regurgitation

M-mode/2D echocardiography—valve morphology and right ventricular size and function to determine cause of tricuspid regurgitation (rheumatic valve, prolapse, Ebstein anomaly, carcinoid valve, right ventricular infarct, pulmonary hypertension, or tricuspid valve injury). Severe tricuspid regurgitation is suggested by a color flow regurgitant jet area of 30% or more of the right atrium, anular dilatation of 4 cm or more, increased tricuspid inflow velocity greater than 1.0 m/s, or systolic flow reversals in the hepatic veins.

Prosthetic Valves

The range of "normal" hemodynamic variables (gradient, effective orifice area, etc.) for a given prosthetic valve type and location is broad. There are published reference values for these variables that serve as guidelines. The best approach for assessing a patient is to perform a baseline transthoracic 2D and hemodynamic evaluation early postoperatively to establish the patient's own "normal values" for later comparison.

"Normal" regurgitation is present in virtually all prosthetic valves and has been well characterized in vitro and in vivo. This "physiologic" regurgitation is usually of low volume and velocity, appearing as a non-aliased jet, and should be differentiated from pathologic regurgitation. Normal prosthetic valves are inherently "stenotic," with higher transvalvular gradients than native valves.

Prosthetic valve dysfunction includes valvular and perivalvular regurgitation, pannus formation, obstruction, endocarditis, abscess, dehiscence, and thromboembolism. A complete transthoracic 2D evaluation may be limited by acoustical shadowing from the prosthesis. Doppler echocardiography usually can assess valve gradients and effective orifice areas accurately, detect and quantitate regurgitation, and provide ancillary information about pulmonary pressures and LV systolic and diastolic function.

Unexpectedly high transvalvular gradients or small effective orifice areas should be assessed further to exclude valve dysfunction. If available, comparison with a previous echocardiographic study is invaluable. If no change has occurred and the patient is clinically stable, it is likely that the hemodynamics are "normal" for that patient and valve or that a prosthesis-patient mismatch is present; that is, the valve is relatively undersized for the patient's body size and hemodynamics. High gradients may also occur in the presence of increased transvalvular flow, such as anemia or other high-output states, but effective orifice areas should remain relatively normal in these conditions. High velocities present in otherwise normal valves may be due to localized high-velocity jets and distal pressure recovery, which may lead to Doppler gradients that are higher than those measured by catheter. This has been observed most commonly in smaller Starr-Edwards and St. Jude prosthetic valves.

TEE is invaluable and often complementary for visualizing valve motion, ring abscess, thrombus, pannus, endocarditis, or the degree of regurgitation if a transthoracic study cannot address the clinical question or concern adequately, or if there are abnormalities detected from transthoracic examination but the cause remains uncertain.

Chest Pain/Acute Myocardial Infarction

Echocardiography is useful for the assessment of causes of chest pain (pericarditis, large pulmonary embolus, aortic dissection, etc.), global and regional LV systolic function, and region and extent of myocardial infarction and for the identification of patients who may benefit from revascularization. The absence of regional wall motion abnormalities during chest pain makes ischemia unlikely as a cause of the chest pain and so may be useful to aid in triaging patients presenting emergently. A restrictive pattern of LV diastolic filling or a high wall motion score index (or both) predicts a poor prognosis. Infarct-related complications may be readily assessed with echocardiography (Table 4).

Hypertrophic Cardiomyopathy

M-mode and 2D echocardiography are useful in establishing the diagnosis of hypertrophic cardiomyopathy, evaluating the severity of hypertrophy and its morphology (asymmetric, symmetric, apical, etc.), and assessing the presence and degree of LV outflow obstruction. Typical M-mode features of hypertrophic cardiomyopathy include mid-systolic aortic valve notching and systolic anterior motion of the mitral apparatus. Also, 2D echocardiography is useful for demonstrating presence or absence of systolic anterior motion and for assessing mitral valve morphology.

Pulsed wave Doppler and color flow imaging are

Table 4. Detection of Complications of
Myocardial Infarction by
Echocardiography

Right ventricular infarction
    Dilated right atrium and right ventricle with
        regional wall motion abnormalities
    Significant tricuspid regurgitation
    Inferior vena cava dilation or plethora
Pericardial effusion/tamponade
Mitral regurgitation
    Ischemic—papillary muscle dysfunction or
        anular dilatation
    Ruptured papillary muscle
Ventricular septal defect
    Color flow localization
    Right ventricular dilatation
    Elevated right ventricular pressure
    Inferior vena cava plethora
Left ventricular free wall rupture
    Pericardial effusion/tamponade
    Pericardial thrombus
    Extracardiac flow
Pseudoaneurysm (contained rupture)
    Narrow neck, thin-walled
Aneurysm
    Myocardial thinning, 90% located at apex
Left ventricular thrombus

useful in localizing the presence and site of LV outflow tract or mid-ventricular obstruction. The degree of obstruction (pressure gradient) is defined by a characteristic continuous wave Doppler late-peaking, dagger-shaped signal. The peak gradient is calculated using the modified Bernoulli equation ($4v^2$). Measurement of the gradient during the Valsalva maneuver, administration of amyl nitrite, or exercise can demonstrate the dynamic nature of the obstruction.

Diastolic abnormalities in hypertrophic cardiomyopathy are strongly associated with symptoms of dyspnea and exercise intolerance and should be carefully assessed. Isovolumic relaxation period flow is present occasionally and is due to asynchronous ventricular relaxation. Normally, there is little or no flow during the isovolumic relaxation period when both the mitral and the aortic valves are closed. It is important not to confuse this flow with the mitral E wave.

Infective Endocarditis

Echocardiography is the diagnostic procedure of choice for detecting valvular vegetations (Fig. 18). It has the additional benefit of being able to detect abscesses, valve perforation, rupture or aneurysm, fistula, dehiscence of a prosthetic valve, and hemodynamic consequences (shunt or regurgitation). The combination of transthoracic echocardiography and TEE has a sensitivity for vegetations in the range of 90% to 95% for native valves and 85% to 90% for prosthetic valves. Patients with suspected infective endocarditis should have a baseline transthoracic study and, in most cases, a transesophageal study. TEE is superior to transthoracic echocardiography in diagnosing valve ring abscess. Serial echocardiographic examinations may be helpful, especially in patients with congestive heart failure, fever, or persistently positive blood cultures.

The false-negative rate for detection of vegetations is low (<5%), but in patients with clinical features consistent with infective endocarditis and negative initial TEE findings, it may be reasonable to repeat the study in 1 to 2 weeks.

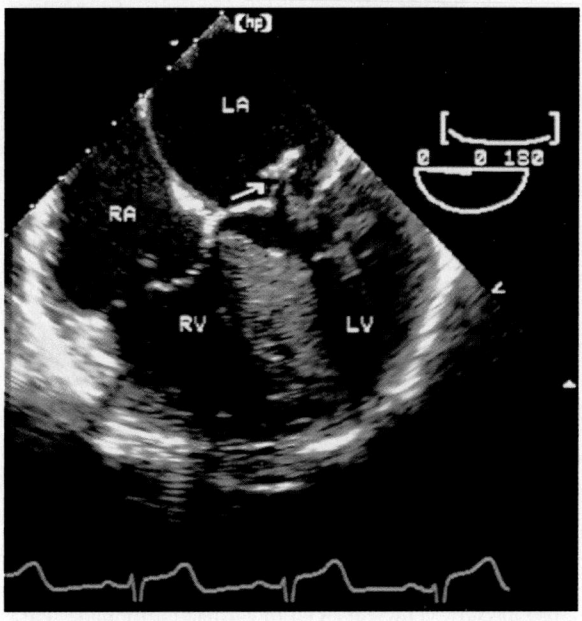

Fig. 18. Vegetation (*arrow*) on the mitral valve with flail in endocarditis. RA, right atrium; RV, right ventricle; LA, left atrium; LV, left ventricle.

Pericardial Disease

Effusion

Echocardiography is the diagnostic procedure of choice for detecting and evaluating pericardial effusion. An effusion is defined as "an echo-free space present throughout the cardiac cycle." Large effusions may be associated with a "swinging heart" (Fig. 19 *A*).

Tamponade

2D and M-mode features of tamponade are not sensitive but can be quite specific. These include diastolic collapse of the right atrium or right ventricle (Fig. 19 *B*) and inferior vena cava plethora with blunted inspiratory collapse. Doppler findings of cardiac tamponade are more sensitive and are based on ventricular interdependence due to the relatively fixed cardiac volume and reduced response of intrapericardial pressures to changes in intrathoracic pressures. With inspiration, LV filling is impaired, whereas right ventricular filling is favored. Doppler findings include an inspiratory increase in IVRT and decreased mitral E-wave velocity, with reciprocal changes in tricuspid valve inflow tracings. Pulmonary venous, hepatic venous, and LV outflow tract tracings show similar respiratory flow changes. Echocardiographically guided pericardiocentesis is the initial therapy of choice for most patients with tamponade (except for patients who have aortic dissection with tamponade). The use of an indwelling pigtail catheter for complete drainage until fluid return is less

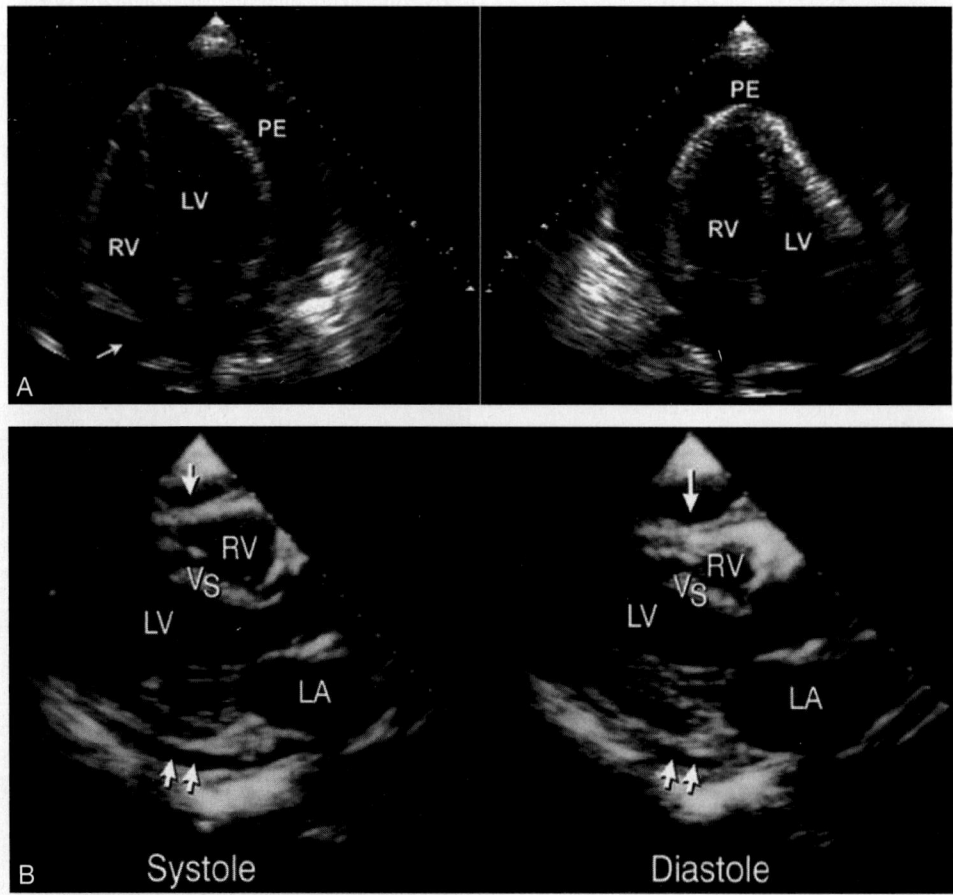

Fig. 19. *A*, "Swinging heart" in cardiac tamponade. With a large amount of fluid, the position of the heart changes dramatically during the cardiac cycle. *Left*, Diastole with right atrial inversion (*arrow*). *Right*, Systole. *B*, Diastolic collapse of right ventricle (RV) in cardiac tamponade. Parasternal long-axis view of tamponade during systole (*left*) and diastole (*right*). The RV collapses during diastole. The single *arrows* indicate anterior pericardial effusion; the *pairs of arrows* indicate posterior pericardial effusion compressing the RV free wall. LA, left atrium; LV, left ventricle; PE, pericardial effusion; V$_S$, ventricular septum.

than 25 mL over 24 hours is associated with a much lower likelihood of recurrence of pericardial effusion. The need for surgical management of pericardial effusion has become uncommon with the introduction of echocardiographically guided pericardiocentesis techniques and the adaptation of pigtail catheter drainage for decreasing recurrence of effusion. Sclerotherapy is no longer used at Mayo Clinic and is generally not recommended because of significant pain associated with instilling a sclerosing agent into the pericardial space.

Constrictive Pericarditis

2D and M-mode features of constrictive pericarditis include thickened or hyperechoic pericardium, abnormal "jerky" septal motion, respiratory variation in ventricular size, and a dilated inferior vena cava. Doppler features of constriction are similar to those of tamponade, with an inspiratory decrease in left-sided flow (Fig. 20). Expiratory hepatic vein diastolic flow reversals are

often prominent. There is an absence of significant inspiratory augmentation of systolic forward flow in the superior vena cava. Restrictive cardiomyopathy usually shows no significant respiratory changes in mitral inflow; therefore, Doppler echocardiography is useful in differentiating constriction from restriction. Tissue Doppler imaging is also helpful in distinguishing constriction from restriction. In constriction, mitral anulus septal early velocity, e', is well preserved, usually >0.08 m/s. In restriction, e' is usually of low velocity.

THE THORACIC AORTA

Although transthoracic echocardiography is usually useful for visualizing the aortic root and arch, most of the aorta cannot be evaluated satisfactorily. With TEE, the entire thoracic aorta can be seen in most patients. Dissection can be evaluated with TEE (Fig. 21) as well as with computed tomography, magnetic resonance

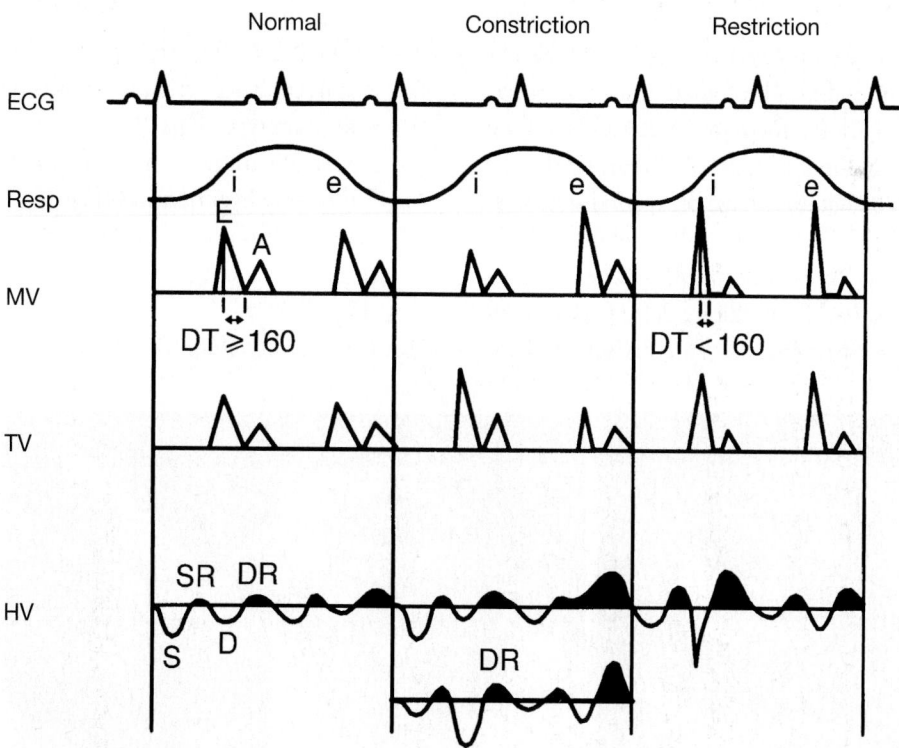

Fig. 20. Schema of Doppler velocities from mitral inflow (MV), tricuspid inflow (TV), and hepatic vein (HV). Electrocardiographic (ECG) and respirometer (Resp) recordings with inspiration (i) and expiration (e) are also represented. The relative changes from normal caused by restrictive or constrictive pericarditis are represented. Both restriction and constriction are characterized by short deceleration time (DT), but patients with constriction demonstrate reciprocal changes in filling of the left and right sides of the heart with respiration, whereas patients with restriction do not. A, atrial contraction; D, diastolic; DR, diastolic reversal; E, early filling phase; S, systolic; SR, systolic reversal.

imaging, or aortography. Because time is often critical in suspected acute dissection, TEE has the added advantages of 1) portability to bedside for any patient whose condition is unstable, 2) simultaneous assessment of cardiac function and associated conditions (aortic regurgitation and pericardial effusion), and 3) no need for contrast agents. Other thoracic aorta conditions that can be readily evaluated with TEE include aortic aneurysm, rupture, ulcer, debris, abscess, and coarctation.

SOURCE OF EMBOLUS

Cardiovascular sources of emboli may account for 20% to 40% of all strokes. Potential sources of emboli detectable with transthoracic echocardiography or TEE include intracardiac thrombus (Fig. 5) or mass, valvular vegetation, thoracic aortic debris, atrial septal aneurysm, and patent foramen ovale. In the absence of overt cardiac disease on the basis of history, physical examination, or electrocardiographic findings, the yield from a transthoracic echocardiogram for identification of a cardiac source of embolus is less than 1% and is not routinely recommended. The transthoracic examination, if performed, should focus on LV function and on excluding abnormalities such as valvular heart disease and tumors. Several studies have concluded that proceeding directly to TEE is a clinically useful and cost-effective strategy for evaluation of stroke. TEE is particularly well suited for excluding left atrial and left atrial appendage thrombi, spontaneous echocardio-graphic contrast, patent foramen ovale, and mobile lesions in the thoracic aorta. In recent years, echocardiographically guided percutaneous device closure of patent foramen ovale has been performed for the prevention of recurrent cerebrovascular events in selected patients (i.e., patients whose patent foramen ovale is thought to be a potential culprit for their cerebrovascular events), generally after thorough investigations that have eliminated other potential causes or sources of stroke.

SELECTED ABNORMALITIES THAT ARE DIAGNOSTIC BY TRANSTHORACIC OR TRANSESOPHAGEAL ECHOCARDIOGRAPHY

1. Left atrial myxoma (Fig. 22)
2. Left atrial thrombus (Fig. 23)
3. Patent foramen ovale (Fig. 24)
4. Hypertrophic obstructive cardiomyopathy (Fig. 25)
5. Ruptured mitral valve chordae tendineae with flail leaflet (Fig. 26)
6. Aortic dissection (Fig. 21)
7. Aortic debris (Fig. 27)
8. Atrial septal defect: sinus venosus type (Fig. 28) and secundum type (Fig. 29)
9. Rheumatic mitral stenosis (Fig. 17)
10. Pulmonary hypertension (Fig. 30)
11. Cardiac effusion and tamponade: "swinging heart" (Fig. 19 *A*) and right ventricular diastolic collapse (Fig. 19 *B*)
12. Endocarditis (Fig. 18)

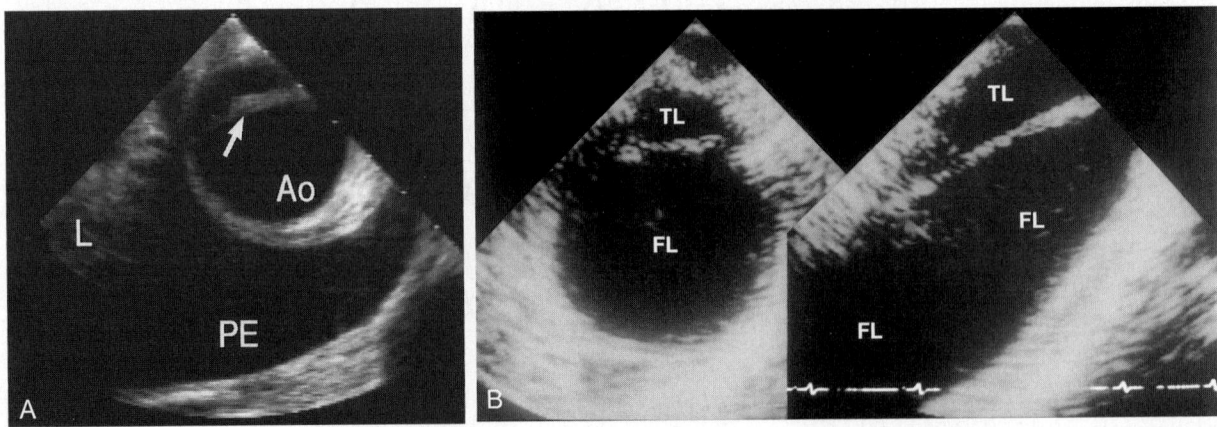

Fig. 21. *A,* Acute aortic dissection complicated by pleural effusion. Left pleural effusion within the posteromedial costophrenic angle highlights the dissected (*arrow*) descending thoracic aorta (Ao); a portion of the left lung (L) is also noted within the effusion. PE, pleural effusion. *B,* Transesophageal echocardiogram of the descending thoracic aorta with dissection present. TL, true lumen; FL, false lumen.

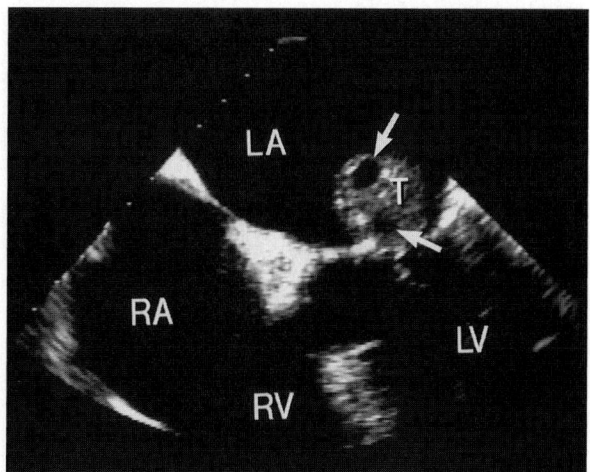

Fig. 22. Left atrial (LA) myxoma; transverse four-chamber transesophageal echocardiographic plane. Cystic echolucencies (*arrows*) are clearly seen within this myxoma (T); they were not evident on transthoracic examination. The myxoma appears to be attached to the mitral valve but was found to be attached to the mitral anulus on off-axis imaging. LV, left ventricle; RA, right atrium; RV, right ventricle.

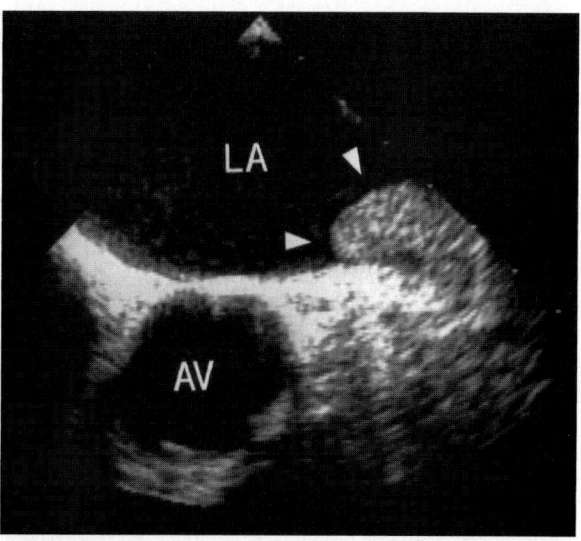

Fig. 23. Left atrial (LA) appendage thrombus; transverse transesophageal echocardiographic plane, basal short-axis view. A protruding thrombus (*arrowheads*) fills the appendage of the left atrium. This thrombus was slightly mobile on real-time evaluation. AV, aortic valve.

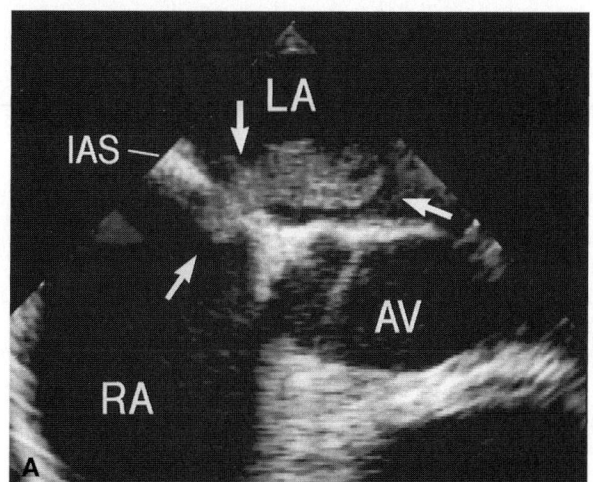

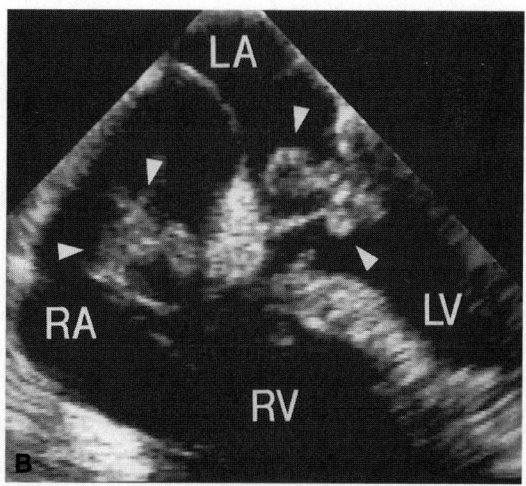

Fig. 24. Examples of transesophageal echocardiographic findings in patients with paradoxical embolism. In each case, a thrombus (*arrows* or *arrowheads*) is crossing through a patent foramen ovale. AV, aortic valve; IAS, interatrial septum. Other abbreviations as in Figure 22.

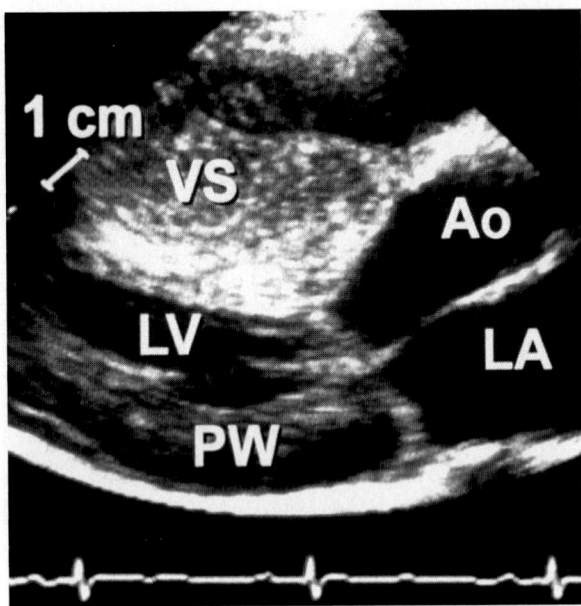

Fig. 25. Hypertrophic obstructive cardiomyopathy. Ao, aorta; LA, left atrium; LV, left ventricle; PW, posterior wall; VS, ventricular septum.

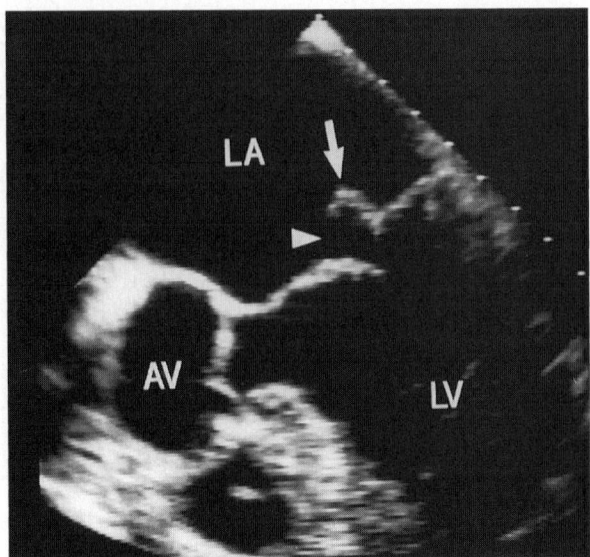

Fig. 26. Mitral valve prolapse with flail leaflet; left ventricular (LV) outflow view in the transverse plane. There is prolapse of the posterior mitral leaflet, with a flail leaflet segment (*arrow*) producing a large deficiency in coaptation (*arrowhead*) with the anterior leaflet. AV, aortic valve; LV, left ventricle.

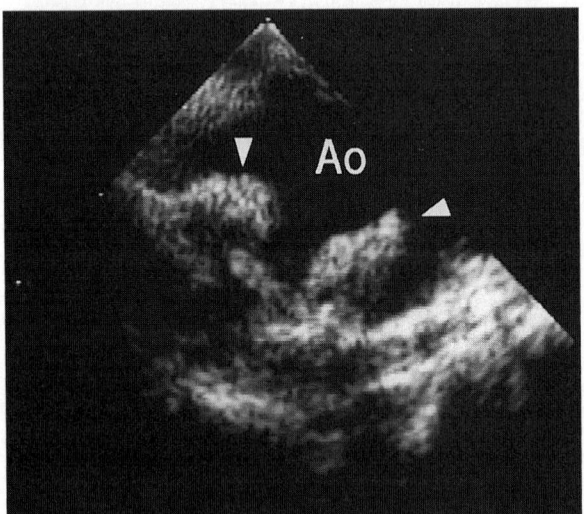

Fig. 27. Extensive atherosclerotic debris within the descending thoracic aorta; transverse transesophageal echocardiographic plane. A "shaggy" appearance of the lumen of the aorta (Ao) is produced by several partially mobile lesions (*arrowheads*) projecting far into the aortic lumen. This patient presented with diffuse atheroembolic cutaneous infarcts of the feet and "blue toe" syndrome.

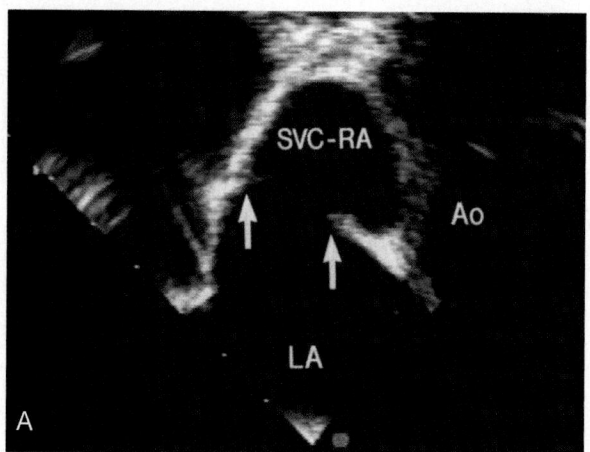 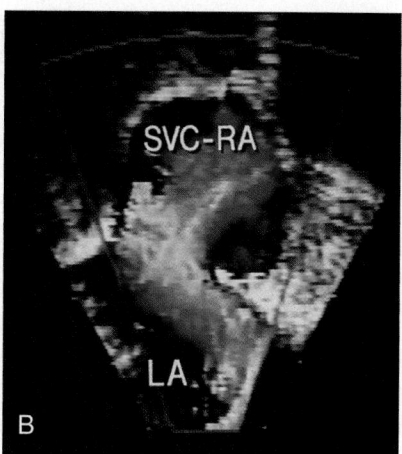

Fig. 28. Sinus venosus atrial septal defect. Short-axis scan (midesophageal transducer, horizontal plane, withdrawn to the high atrial level just below the superior vena cava at the caval-atrial junction [SVC-RA]). *A*, The transducer is posterior to the left atrium (LA). Note the typical sinus venosus atrial septal defect (*arrows*) between the LA and the SVC-RA. *B*, Color flow Doppler study (the color polarity has been reversed to better illustrate the atrial septal defect left-to-right shunt) (i.e., LA to SVC-RA). Ao, ascending aorta.

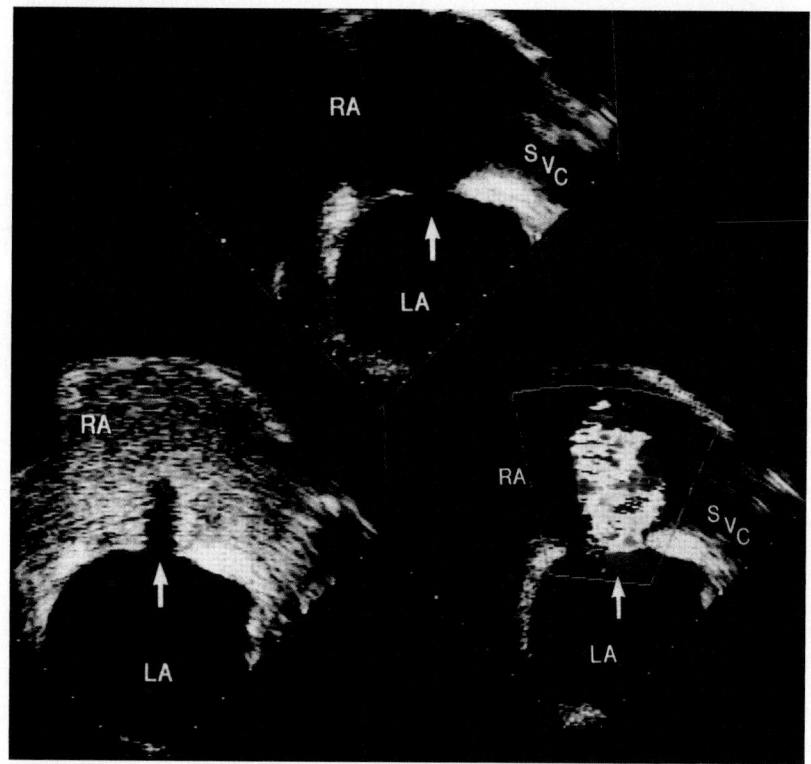

Fig. 29. Secundum atrial septal defect with contrast and color flow echocardiographic study. These are longitudinal scans of the atrial septum from midesophagus. *Top*, Long-axis view of the atrial septum with a 1-cm atrial septal defect (*arrow*). The transducer is within the esophagus posterior and adjacent to the left atrium (LA). Anteriorly, the right atrium (RA) and superior vena cava (SVC) are visualized. *Bottom left*, After an upper extremity venous injection, the RA is densely opacified. Left-to-right shunt (*arrow*) across the atrial septal defect appears as a negative contrast effect in the RA. *Bottom right*, Color flow Doppler study shows left-to-right shunt (*arrow*) across the same atrial septal defect.

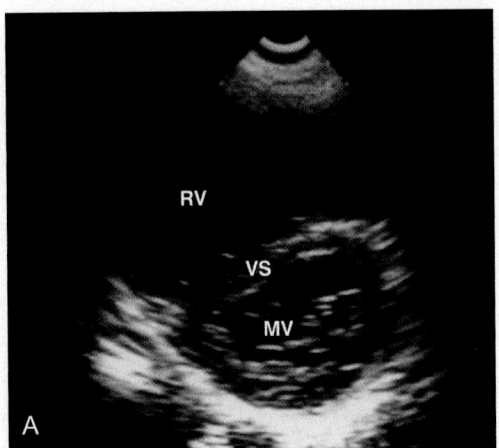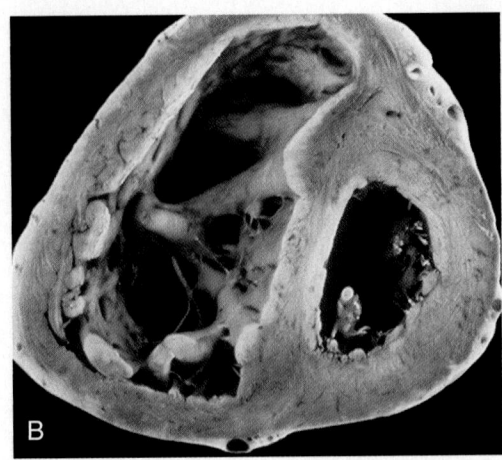

Fig 30. *A*, Parasternal short-axis view demonstrating the *D*-shaped left ventricular cavity and enlarged right ventricular (RV) cavity in pulmonary hypertension. Similar appearances are present in RV volume overload; however, flattening of the ventricular septum (VS) persists during the entire cardiac cycle in RV and pulmonary artery pressure overload, whereas it disappears during systole in RV volume overload. MV, mitral valve. *B*, Corresponding pathology specimen.

9

STRESS ECHOCARDIOGRAPHY

Patricia A. Pellikka, MD

Stress echocardiography, introduced in 1979, is used for detection of coronary artery disease. Subsequently, the technique has evolved into a widely used, versatile technique not only for diagnosis of ischemic heart disease but also for determination of prognosis. The rationale for stress echocardiography is that stress results in wall motion abnormalities in regions subtended by a stenosed coronary artery; these wall motion abnormalities can be detected with echocardiography.

METHODS

Various methods of stress have been combined with echocardiography. Treadmill exercise echocardiography is the most widely used form of exercise echocardiography. Images are obtained before and immediately after symptom-limited treadmill exercise. Attention is directed toward assessment of regional wall motion and evaluation of changes in ejection fraction and systolic volume. The standard views are parasternal long- and short-axis and apical four- and two-chamber views. Additional views, including apical long-axis and apical short-axis, also are obtained. Rest and stress images are compared side by side to appreciate subtle changes. Alternatively, the test may be performed with either supine or upright bicycle imaging. Bicycle imaging offers the advantage that images can be obtained during exercise. This is useful if Doppler data are obtained in addition to regional wall motion assessment.

For patients who are unable to perform physical exercise, pharmacologic stress testing with dobutamine or the vasodilators dipyridamole or adenosine can be used. Dobutamine is the most common pharmacologic stress agent used in combination with echocardiography. Dobutamine is predominantly a β_1-adrenergic stimulating agent. Its half-life in plasma is approximately 2 minutes, and therefore it must be administered with a continuous intravenous infusion. A typical protocol involves administration at a starting dosage of 5 µg/kg per minute, increasing at 3-minute intervals to 10, 20, 30, and 40 µg/kg per minute. End points are intolerable symptoms, uncontrolled hypertension, hypotension, or significant arrhythmias. The infusion is continued to achievement of 85% of the age-predicted maximal heart rate (220 – age). If this is not achieved with dobutamine infusion, atropine at a dose of 0.5 mg is administered intravenously and repeated at 1-minute intervals to a maximal total dose of 2 mg. Used in this way, atropine has been shown to increase the sensitivity of dobutamine stress echocardiography, especially in patients receiving β-blocker therapy. Dynamic intracavitary or left ventricular outflow tract obstruction can be detected with Doppler echocardiography in approximately 20% of patients undergoing dobutamine stress echocardiography.

Dipyridamole is a coronary vasodilator, the effects of which are mediated by increased interstitial levels of endogenous adenosine. Dipyridamole decreases coronary vascular resistance and increases coronary blood

143

flow but seems to have little effect on vascular resistance in ischemic areas where small vessels are already maximally dilated. Adenosine offers the advantages of greater coronary vasodilation and a shorter half-life (less than 10 seconds). Vasodilator stress echocardiography typically produces a mild to moderate increase in heart rate and a mild decrease in blood pressure. Contraindications include bronchospastic lung disease, severe obstructive lung disease, or current aminophylline use. The methylxanthine caffeine, another antagonist of adenosine, should not be ingested 12 hours before testing. Use of oral dipyridamole should be discontinued 24 hours before testing. Adenosine is contraindicated in patients with heart block.

A newer method for patients who are unable to exercise is transesophageal atrial pacing stress echocardiography. An 10F flexible catheter is inserted orally or nasally after a topical anesthetic is applied to the patient's posterior pharynx. Initial pacing occurs at 10 beats per minute more than the patient's baseline heart rate at the lowest current that provides stable atrial capture (usually 15 mA). At 2-minute stages, the paced heart rate is increased to levels of 85% and 100% of the age-predicted maximum. Wenckebach second-degree heart block may occur, necessitating atropine administration. The advantage of this protocol is very few side effects related to the method and rapid return to baseline conditions on discontinuation of atrial pacing.

In patients with a temporary or permanent pacemaker, a pacing stress echocardiogram can be obtained by temporarily reprogramming the pacemaker to a higher heart rate. Ergonovine or hyperventilation has been used in conjunction with stress echocardiography to detect coronary vasospastic disease. Ergonovine testing has the potential to produce severe or prolonged ischemia and should not be performed in patients with previous infarction or documented ischemia. This form of testing is most safely performed in the angiography laboratory, where nitrates can be infused locally and the coronary artery opened mechanically if complications occur.

Interpretation

During stress echocardiography, images obtained at rest are compared with those obtained during stress. With supine bicycle or dobutamine stress echocardiography, imaging is performed during gradual increases in stress. This approach permits recognition of the heart rate or level of stress at which ischemia first develops. The normal response to stress is the development of hyperdynamic wall motion, a decrease in end-systolic volume, and an increase in ejection fraction (Fig. 1). Regional wall motion is assessed in each left ventricular segment at rest and with stress. A 16-segment model of the left ventricle is most frequently used; a 17-segment model, which includes an additional segment at the left ventricular apex, has recently been proposed for echocardiographic perfusion imaging. The development of new or worsening regional wall motion abnormalities is considered a manifestation of ischemia (Fig. 2). Resting wall motion abnormalities that are unchanged with stress are considered to represent infarction. A biphasic response, that is, with a low level of exercise or pharmacologic stress, an improvement in contractility of regions that are hypokinetic or akinetic at rest followed by worsening with continued stress, is considered a marker of viability. This may be seen in segments subtended by severe coronary stenosis. Regional wall motion abnormalities correlate with coronary artery anatomical distribution of blood flow. A regional wall motion score is calculated at rest and at stress as a sum of the scores of the individual segments divided by the number of segments. A 5-point scoring system is most commonly used, in which 1 = normal, 2 = hypokinesis, 3 = akinesis, 4 = dyskinesis, and 5 = aneurysm. A decrease in the ejection fraction or an increase in end-systolic volume with stress is a marker of extensive ischemia.

Harmonic imaging is beneficial for improving image quality. Intravenous administration of contrast (sonicated microbubbles) is recommended if images are technically inadequate or if more than one segment cannot be adequately visualized at rest. With current state-of-the-art ultrasound equipment and use of contrast agent as needed, technically adequate transthoracic images can be expected in 97% of patients.

STRESS ECHOCARDIOGRAPHY FOR DETECTION OF CORONARY ARTERY DISEASE

Stress echocardiography is widely used for the detection of coronary artery disease and for assessment of its functional significance. Stress echocardiography has been shown to be a cost-effective method for assessment

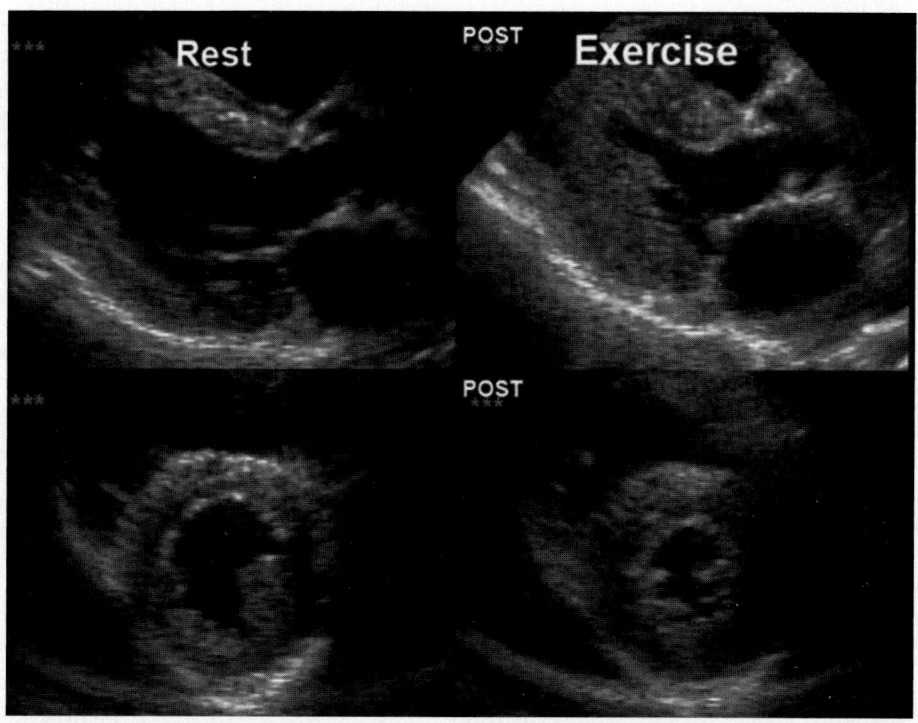

Fig. 1. Parasternal long- (top) and short- (bottom) axis images at rest (*left*) and immediately after (POST) exercise (*right*) show normal systolic contraction at rest and with stress. With exercise, ejection fraction markedly increases and all walls become hyperdynamic. Mild concentric left ventricular hypertrophy also is noted in this patient, who had a history of hypertension.

of patients with known or suspected coronary artery disease. Coronary artery disease may be manifested by either a resting wall motion abnormality or a stress-induced abnormality. The accuracy of stress echocardiography has been shown to be superior to that of exercise electrocardiography. The accuracy of stress echocardiography has been directly compared with that of radionuclide perfusion imaging in laboratories of similar proficiency. In this situation, the techniques performed similarly. Recent meta-analyses also have compared stress echocardiographic with radionuclide techniques and have found a higher specificity with stress echocardiography.

Advantages of stress echocardiography include its relatively lower cost than other imaging tests and its versatility, that is, cardiac structure and function, including wall thicknesses, chamber sizes, valves, the proximal aortic root, and presence of pericardial effusion, can be evaluated simultaneously. For the detection of coronary artery disease, the sensitivity has been reported to range from 72% to 97% depending on lesion severity and

extent of coronary artery disease. As with all forms of stress testing, the sensitivity for detection of single-vessel disease is lower than that of multivessel disease. Sensitivity is highest if coronary artery disease is defined as stenosis of 70% or more diameter narrowing and less when stenosis is defined as 50% or more diameter narrowing. However, specificity varies conversely. The apparent accuracy of stress echocardiography can be affected by referral bias in that only patients with positive test results are likely to be referred for angiography, a practice leading to an artificially higher sensitivity and lower specificity.

Although regional wall motion abnormalities are the hallmark of ischemic heart disease, they also may occur in cardiomyopathy and microvascular disease and may be precipitated by a hypertensive response to stress. False-negative studies can occur in patients with single-vessel disease or in those in whom a small regional myocardium is subtended by a stenosed vessel. False negative results also can occur if there is a delay in acquisition of images after peak exercise, if the patient

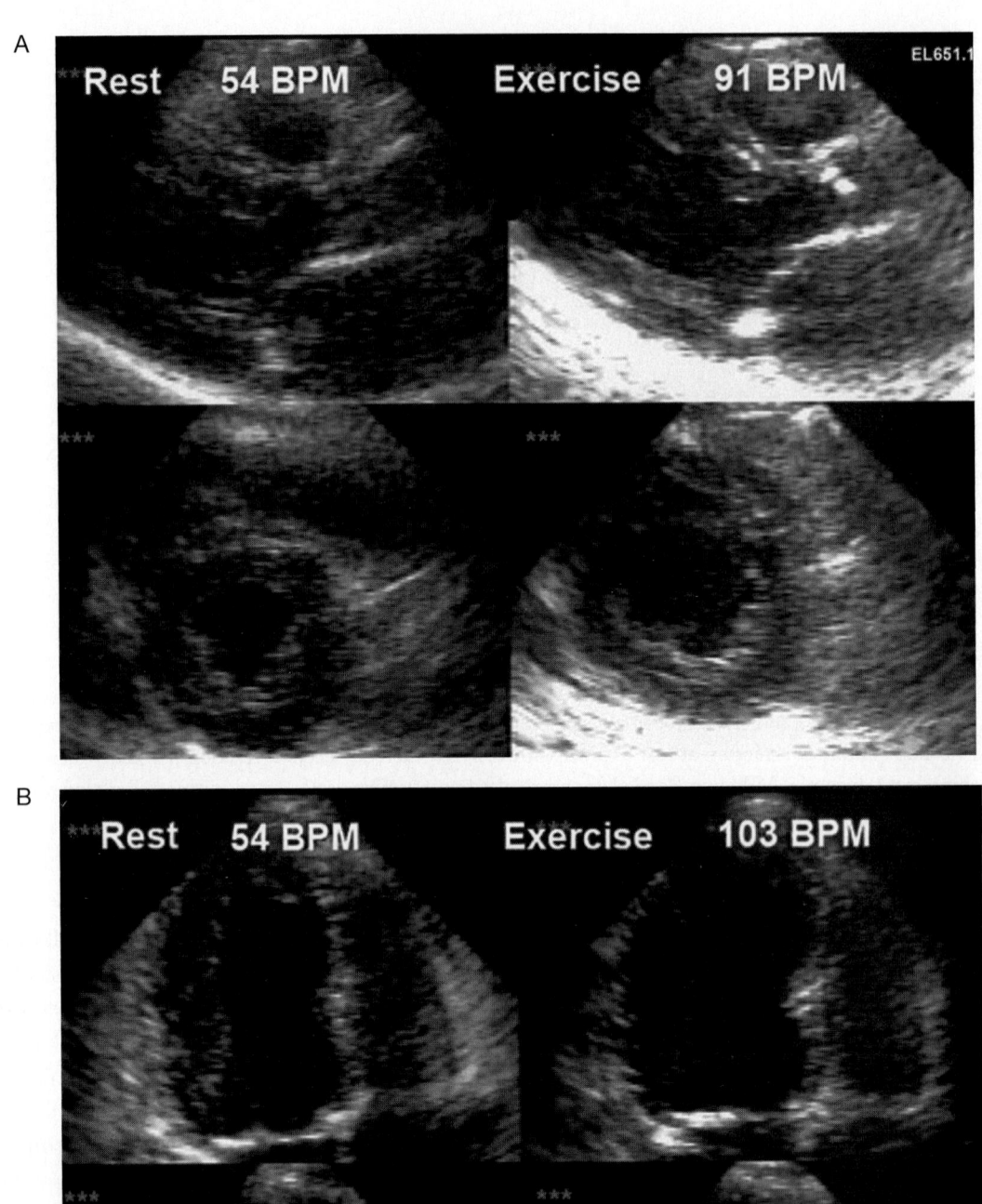

Fig. 2. Parasternal (*A*) and apical (*B*) images show the development of hypokinesis of the apex and anterior wall after the stress of exercise. In contrast to Figure 1, there has been an increase in systolic cavity size with exercise, which was accompanied by a decrease in ejection fraction. Aortic valve sclerosis also was noted. BPM, beats per minute.

performs a low level of exercise, or if the heart rate response to exercise or dobutamine stress is suboptimal.

PROGNOSTIC VALUE OF STRESS ECHOCARDIOGRAPHY

Numerous large studies from various centers have shown the prognostic value of stress echocardiography. It provides information incremental to that which can be gleaned by assessing clinical variables, exercise duration, electrocardiographic changes, and resting echocardiographic function to identify patients at risk of all-cause mortality and cardiac events, including cardiac death and myocardial infarction. This prognostic value has been found in various subgroups, including both men and women, the elderly, patients who have had coronary artery bypass grafting, patients who have had percutaneous intervention, and patients with diabetes mellitus. Not only the presence of ischemia but also the extent and severity of ischemia as shown by the percentage of abnormal segments at peak stress, the stress wall motion score index, a multivessel distribution of abnormalities, the change in wall motion score index with stress, the ejection fraction response to stress, and end-systolic volume response to stress are useful for identifying patients at highest risk. Risk indices combining clinical, exercise test, and stress echocardiographic variables have been developed and validated. In patients with a normal exercise echocardiogram, the prognosis is excellent, with an event rate including cardiac death, myocardial infarction, or coronary revascularization of less than 1% per year. Exercise echocardiography has been shown to be a cost-effective method for assessment of patients with known or suspected coronary artery disease.

Stress echocardiography has been used to predict risk in patients who have had a myocardial infarction. The presence of residual or remote ischemia manifested as a stress-induced wall motion abnormality or worsening of ventricular function with stress identifies patients with a worse prognosis. Stress testing may be done early after myocardial infarction, and dobutamine stress testing allows recognition of myocardial viability.

Cardiac risk assessment before noncardiac operation is a frequent application of stress echocardiography and is especially beneficial in patients with risk factors, cardiac symptoms, or known coronary artery disease. Stress echocardiography has been shown to provide incremental information beyond that which can be obtained from clinical variables, resting left ventricular function, or exercise electrocardiography. This advantage has been shown in patients undergoing both vascular and nonvascular operation. Pharmacologic stress echocardiography with dobutamine is used frequently because orthopedic, peripheral vascular, or other comorbid conditions may limit a patient's ability to exercise. With dobutamine stress echocardiography, the ischemic threshold, that is, the heart rate at which ischemia first develops, can be used to monitor the patient perioperatively. If ischemia is extensive or occurs at a low heart rate, preoperative coronary angiography and revascularization are indicated. Alternatively, if the ischemia begins at a higher heart rate, perioperative β-blocker therapy should suffice.

Stress echocardiography also has an important role for detection of myocardial viability. Systolic dysfunction may indicate hibernating or stunned myocardium. Augmentation of regional function in dysfunctional segments with a low dose of dobutamine and reworsening of function with high doses (Fig. 3) has been shown to be predictive of recovery of function after coronary revascularization. Stunned myocardium, that is, myocardium that is viable but dysfunctional after prolonged severe ischemia but for which blood flow has been restored also improves contractility during dobutamine administration. Myocardial thickness is also an indicator of viability. Segments that are less than 5 or 6 mm in thickness have a low likelihood of recovery of function after coronary revascularization. In patients with myocardial viability and ischemia who do not undergo revascularization, prognosis has been shown to be unfavorable.

STRESS ECHOCARDIOGRAPHY AND NONISCHEMIC HEART DISEASE

Stress echocardiography also may be used to assess valvular heart disease, hypertrophic cardiomyopathy and pulmonary hypertension and to recognize abnormalities of diastolic function which occur with stress. In most patients with valvular heart disease, resting echocardiography and Doppler assessment suffice. However, for patients in whom exertional symptoms do not correlate with resting echocardiographic findings, a stress test may be beneficial. In patients with mitral stenosis or regurgitation, changes in severity of

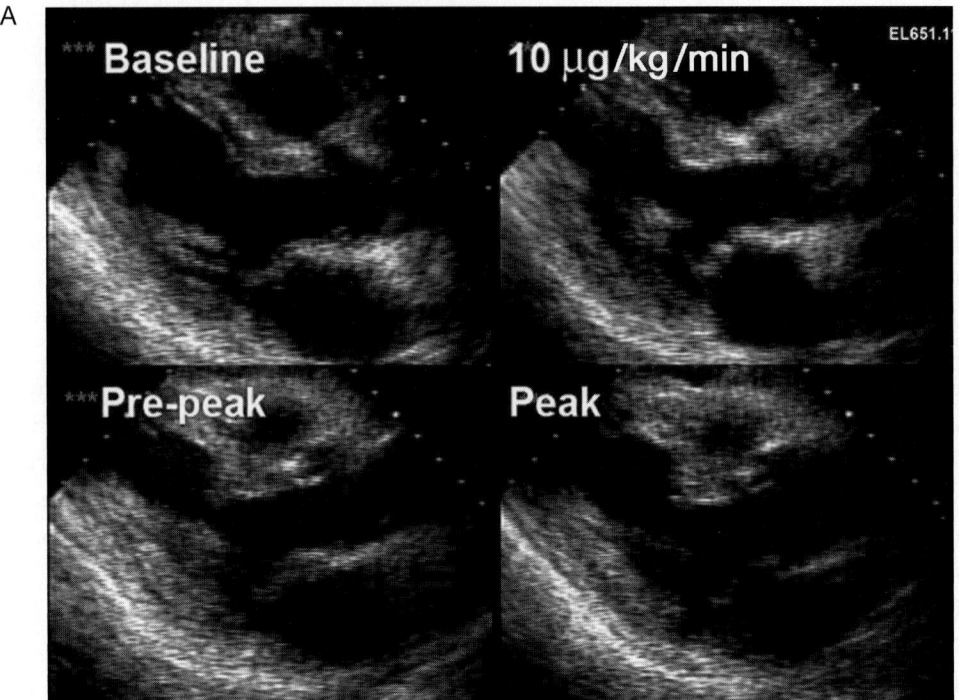

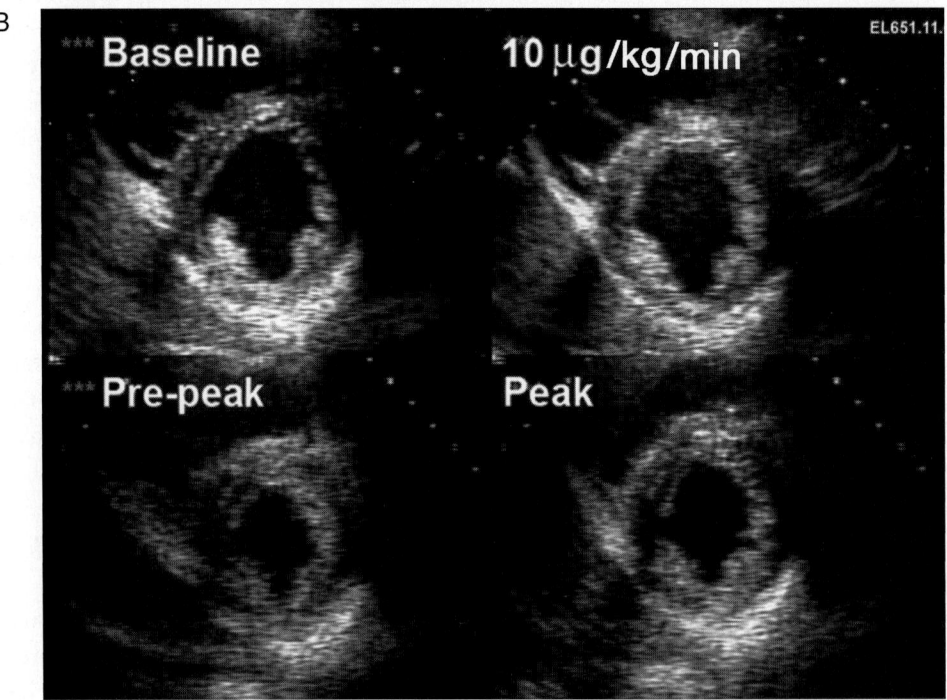

Fig. 3. Dobutamine stress echocardiographic parasternal images (*A*, long axis; *B*, short axis) in a patient with a recent anterior wall myocardial infarction show improvement of contraction of the distal anteroseptum, apex, and mid anterior wall with low-dose dobutamine. At peak dose, there is reworsening of systolic function, accompanied by an increase in end-systolic size. This biphasic response—with initial improvement of hypokinetic segments followed by worsening at higher doses of dobutamine—is characteristic of hibernating myocardium. The patient, who had received thrombolysis at the time of acute infarction, was found to have a residual high-grade stenosis of the left anterior descending coronary artery and underwent percutaneous coronary intervention.

regurgitation may occur with exercise. Alteratively, marked increases in the gradient across the mitral valve may occur with exercise in patients with mitral stenosis, contributing to exertional symptoms. Lung disease and mitral valve disease can be differentiated by assessing relative changes in the gradient across the mitral valve with relative changes in pulmonary artery pressure as assessed by tricuspid regurgitation velocity.

In patients with aortic stenosis and reduced left ventricular systolic function (low output, low-gradient aortic stenosis), low doses of dobutamine can be administered to augment the stroke volume; the Doppler-derived aortic valve area can then be recalculated under these different hemodynamic conditions. If the stenosis is significant, the Doppler-derived aortic valve area remains reduced despite augmentation of ventricular function. Furthermore, dobutamine administration can be used to identify cases in which no contractile reserve is present. Changes in pulmonary artery systolic pressure with exercise echocardiography may be useful for identifying patients limited by pulmonary hypertension. Changes in diastolic function, most commonly measured from the mitral inflow and mitral anulus tissue Doppler profiles and the ratio of the diastolic mitral inflow velocity (E) to mitral anulus velocity (e'), can identify patients with increases in filling pressure during exercise.

NEW DEVELOPMENTS

New technologies, including color kinesis, tissue Doppler, and strain and strain rate imaging, can be applied to assess segmental function and may provide quantitative assessment of left ventricular response to stress. Myocardial perfusion may be assessed with contrast echocardiography performed in conjunction with regional wall motion assessment. These techniques have been shown to be feasible with exercise, vasodilator, or dobutamine stress. Real-time three-dimensional imaging has become feasible and permits acquisition of stress echocardiographic data very quickly at or immediately after peak stress. These techniques all offer the potential to further improve the accuracy of stress echocardiography.

SUMMARY

Stress echocardiography is a well-validated, relatively inexpensive, and widely available means of detecting coronary artery disease and assessing prognosis. Newer techniques will permit increased accuracy and quantification of extent and severity of ischemia. The test is highly versatile and additionally has applications to evaluation of valvular heart disease, diastolic dysfunction, and exertional cardiac symptoms.

10

Transesophageal Echocardiography

Sarinya Puwanant, MD

Lawrence J. Sinak, MD

Krishnaswamy Chandrasekaran, MD

Multiplane transesophageal echocardiography (TEE) allows excellent visualization of all cardiac structures and great vessels. The common clinical indications for TEE are assessment of complications of myocardial infarction, detection of aortic dissection, diagnosis of infective endocarditis and its complications in native and prosthetic valves, determination of embolic source (left atrial appendage, ventricle, valves, aorta), visualization of cardiac tumors, evaluation of congenital heart diseases, and assessment of critically ill patients. TEE is also a valuable adjunctive imaging method during cardiovascular surgery and percutaneous cardiac interventions (Table 1).

Complications of Acute Myocardial Infarction

TEE is an excellent diagnostic imaging method in patients with acute myocardial infarction (Fig. 1) with heart failure, hemodynamic collapse, or hypoxia. TEE can identify the cause of ventricular septal rupture, acute mitral regurgitation from papillary muscle or chordal rupture, acute hypoxia from right-to-left shunt across a patent foramen ovale, and cardiogenic shock due to ventricular pump failure or right ventricular infarction.

Aortic Dissection

TEE is the diagnostic imaging method of choice when aortic dissection is suspected (Fig. 2). It has a sensitivity of 97% to 99% and a specificity of 98%. Mortality from aortic dissection increases at the rate of 1% to 2% per hour; thus, the most important role of TEE is the reliable, rapid diagnosis of aortic dissection. It can be performed within 15 minutes at the bedside. The diagnosis of aortic dissection is based on identification of an intimal flap, which creates a double lumen in the aorta. TEE can identify all major complications of aortic dissection, including pericardial effusion, tamponade, aortic regurgitation, and coronary artery dissection. Important information for surgical planning includes the finding of involvement of the ascending aorta (type A dissection), the entry site of the intimal tear, the extent of dissection, the morphologic features of the true and false lumen, aortic root integrity, and the presence of pericardial hematoma. TEE provides valuable information about the entire thoracic aorta; however, visualization of the distal part of the ascending aorta and aortic arch frequently is obscured by the air-filled left main bronchus.

Table 1. Summary of Clinical Applications of Transesophageal Echocardiography

Diseases of aorta
  Aortic dissection
    Anatomical diagnostic information
      Intimal flap and mobility
      Site of intimal tear
      True and false lumen
      Size of false lumen
      Location of major blood flow
    Management information
      Pericardial effusion and tamponade
      Coronary involvement: RWMA
      Expansion of false lumen
      Aortic regurgitation
        Aortic valve and root integrity
  Intramural hematoma
  Aortic ulcer
  Aortic rupture or transection
  Aortic atheromatous disease: assessment of extent, complexity, and thickness of plaques
  Aortoarteritis syndrome: assessment of aortic root in Marfan syndrome

Surgical planning
  Involvement of ascending aorta
  Entry site and extent of dissection
  Morphologic features of the true and false lumen
  Aortic root integrity
  Pericardial hematoma
  Expansion of false lumen

Infective endocarditis and its complications
  Diagnosis:
    Suspected endocarditis with poor TTE
    Persistent bacteremia with negative TTE
    Persistent bacteremia in a patient with prosthetic valve
    Bacteremia in patients with devices (pacemaker lead, AICD)
    Preoperatively for endocarditis

  TEE after TTE should be performed in patients with the following:
    Prosthetic valves
    Virulent organisms
    Clinical suspicion of development of perivalvular extension
    Congenital defects
    Persistent bacteremia and clinical deterioration

  Initial TEE should be performed in patients with the following:
    Staphylococcus aureus bacteremia with indwelling catheter, pacer lead, AICD lead
    Intermediate probability (Duke criteria)

  Serial TEE should be performed in patients with:
    An initial negative TEE but with high clinical suspicion of infective endocarditis
    Clinical deterioration or persistent bacteremia for assessment of disease progression

Assessment of prosthetic valves
  Mechanism of stenosis (thrombus, leaflet degeneration, pannus)
  Mechanism of regurgitation: prosthetic (malfunction of occluder or disk, leaflet degeneration) or
    periprosthetic (location and severity)
  Unexplained anemia (hemolytic RBC morphologic features)

Assessment of native valves
  Mitral valve morphologic features (balloon valvuloplasty, mechanism of regurgitation, mass lesions)
  Aortic valve morphology (poor TTE with enlarged aortic root, unusually high gradients with normal
    morphologic features—subaortic membrane, mass lesions)
  Tricuspid valve morphologic features (Ebstein anomaly, mechanism of regurgitation in patients with a device)

Table 1   (continued)

Assessment of native valves (continued)
  Suspected endocarditis with negative TTE or infection with organisms of low virulency

Determination of source of embolism
  LAA and aortic thrombus
  Spontaneous echo contrast
  Intracardiac mass (vegetation, tumor)
  Interatrial shunt

Congenital heart disease
  Atrial septal defects, Ebstein anomaly, coarctation of the aorta, etc.

Intraoperative TEE
  Mitral valve repair
    Preoperative data (mechanisms and pathology of valvular dysfunction)
    Postoperative data (residual regurgitation, LVOT obstruction from SAM)
  Valve replacement
    Postoperative valve function and paravalvular regurgitation, aortic valve integrity
  Myectomy in patients with hypertrophic cardiomyopathy
    Preoperative data (myectomy site, mitral apparatus and location of papillary muscle, mitral valve disease,
      SAM, subaortic membrane)
    Postoperative data (adequacy of myectomy, aortic valve integrity, aortic regurgitation, ventricular septal
      defect, SAM)
  Coronary artery bypass grafting (RWMA, ventricular function, position of tips of intra-aortic balloon pump)
  Detecting air in ventricular chambers and great vessels
  Surgery of the aorta (evaluation of aortic graft anastomosis)
  Heart or heart-lung transplantation (evaluation of anastomosis; LV and RV function)

Critically ill patients
  Unexplained hypotension (volume status, LV contractility, RV contractility, RWMA, pericardial effusion,
    pulmonary thromboembolism)
  Unexplained hypoxemia (right-to-left shunt across PFO, undetected ASD, shunt from arteriovenous
    malformation, pulmonary embolism)
  Sepsis (endocarditis, line infection)
  Evaluation of cardiac function in patients with brain death who are candidates for transplantation

Cardioversion
  Identification of thrombus in LA or LAA before cardioversion
  Assessment of LV function and LAA function in terms of predictor of successful restoration of sinus rhythm

Interventional cardiology
  Transseptal puncture
  Guiding the position of catheter during the following:
    Radiofrequency ablation
    Percutaneous valvular intervention
    Transcatheter closure of interatrial communication and VSD
    Novel transcatheter LAA occluder device
  Percutaneous stent graft of aorta
  Stent angioplasty of coarctation of aorta
  Endomyocardial biopsy
  Pacemaker lead extraction

AICD, automatic implantable cardioverter-defibrillator; ASD, atrial septal defect; LA, left atrium; LAA, left atrial appendage;
  LV, left ventricular; LVOT, left ventricular outflow tract; PFO, patent foramen ovale; RBC, red blood cell; RV, right ventric-
  ular; RWMA, regional wall motion abnormality; SAM, systolic anterior motion; TEE, transesophageal echocardiography;
  TTE, transthoracic echocardiography; VSD, ventricular septal defect.

A

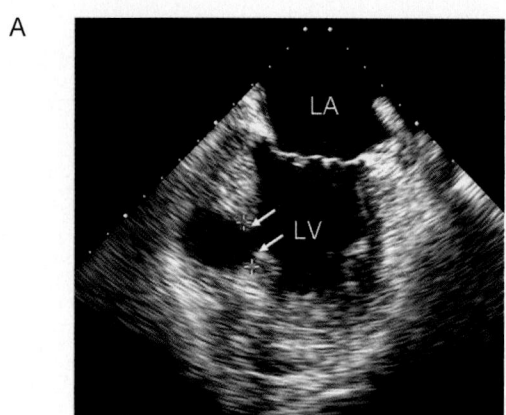

B

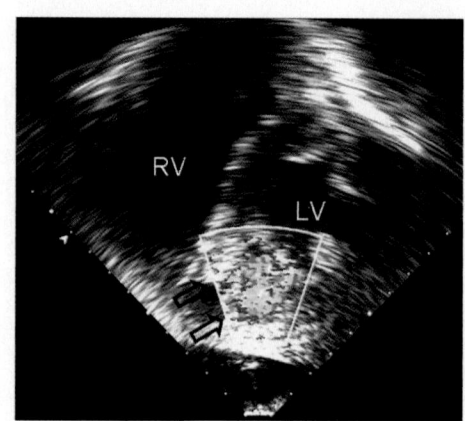

Fig. 1. Patient with inferior myocardial infarction and heart failure. *A*, Multiplane transesophageal echocardiogram, showing complex intramyocardial rupture (*arrows*) through posterior wall of left ventricle (LV) resulting in acquired ventricular septal defect. *B*, Transgastric short-axis view, showing disruption of posterior wall of LV (*open arrows*) that extends through posterior wall of right ventricle (RV) and septum with left-to-right shunt. LA, left atrium.

INFECTIVE ENDOCARDITIS AND ITS COMPLICATIONS

TEE aids in the diagnosis of infective endocarditis (Duke major criteria) and is useful for detecting complications of native valve and prosthetic valve endocarditis (Fig. 3). TEE is more sensitive than transthoracic echocardiography (TTE) for detecting vegetations, perivalvular abscess or fistula (Fig. 4), valve leaflet perforation (Fig. 5), bioprosthetic valve dehiscence, and paravalvular leakage, all suggestive echocardiographic signs of infective endocarditis. With use of high-resolution imaging, TEE is superior to TTE for detecting small vegetations (1-2 mm), prosthetic valve endocarditis, and pulmonary valve endocarditis, which can be missed by TTE. The anterior portion of an aortic prosthesis or of the aortic root is often better visualized with TTE than TEE. Recent data have shown that TEE improves the sensitivity of the Duke criteria to diagnose definite infective endocarditis and seems particularly useful for evaluation of patients with suspected prosthetic valve endocarditis. The specificity of TEE for the diagnosis of infective endocarditis is 85% to 98%. False-positive findings of vegetation may be caused by thrombus, suture materials, and pannus in patients with prosthetic valves. Although negative results of TEE have a negative predictive value of 98% to 100% in native valve endocarditis and of 90% in prosthetic valve endocarditis, serial TEE should be considered if clinical suspicion is high. A false-negative result of TEE can occur because of early infection when vegetation and abscess are not well formed,

unsatisfactory image quality due to prosthetic valve artifact, or a previously embolized vegetation.

Even when the results of TTE support the diagnosis of infective endocarditis, TEE is required for evaluation of the extent and complications of infective endocarditis,

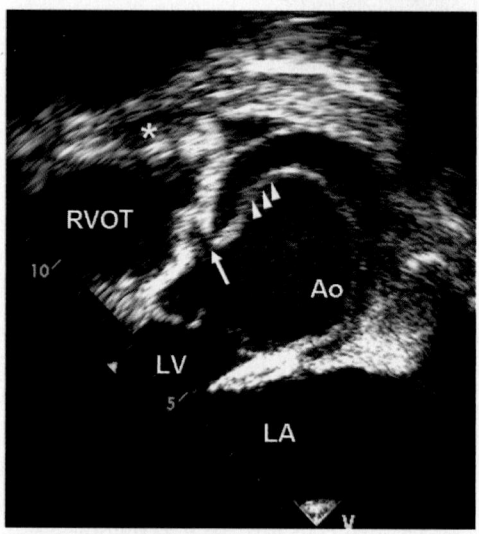

Fig. 2. Transesophageal echocardiogram obtained at bedside on an emergency basis for patient with shock and chest pain. Basal short-axis view at the 158° transducer position, showing type A aortic dissection with a mobile intimal flap separating true lumen from false lumen, and intimal flap (*arrowheads*) extending into ostium of right coronary artery (*arrow*). Small amount of pericardial effusion is also seen (*asterisk*). Ao, ascending aorta; LA, left atrium; LV, left ventricle; RVOT, right ventricular outflow tract.

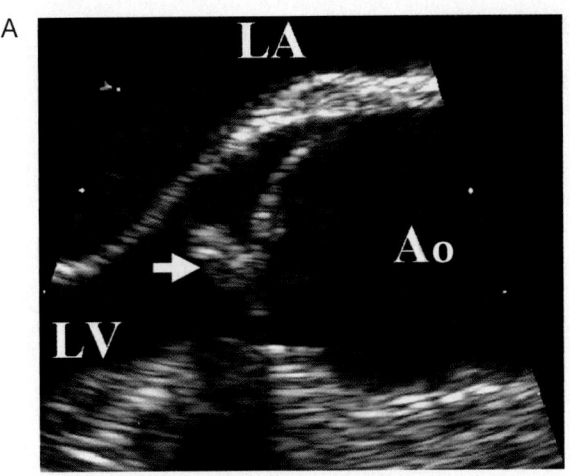

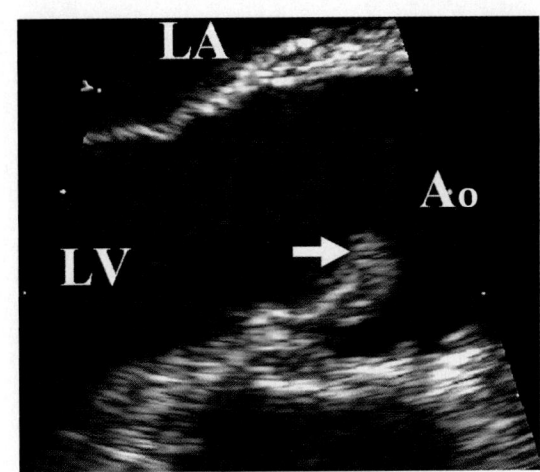

Fig. 3. Transesophageal echocardiograms, long-axis view, from patient with bicuspid aortic valve and persistent bacteremia. End-diastolic (*A*) and end-systolic (*B*) frames, showing oscillating vegetation on right coronary cusp of aortic valve (*arrow*). Ao, aorta; LA, left atrium; LV, left ventricle.

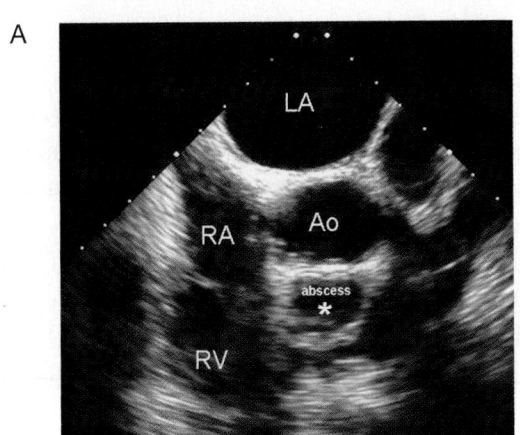

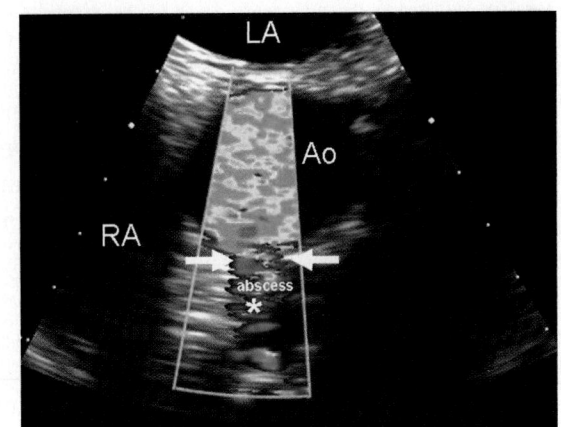

Fig. 4. *A*, Transesophageal echocardiogram, short-axis view, from patient with aortic prosthetic valve endocarditis, showing abscess cavity in base of anterior septum (*asterisk*). *B*, Color Doppler study, showing 4-mm communication (*arrows*) from anterior aortic root just below prosthetic valve into abscess cavity. Ao, aorta; LA, left atrium; RA, right atrium; RV, right ventricle.

particularly in patients with virulent organisms, clinical suspicion of perivalvular extension, specific congenital heart defects, prosthetic valves, aortic valve endocarditis, persistent bacteremia, and clinical hemodynamic deterioration. Recent studies support initial TEE as a useful and cost-effective diagnostic approach in patients with *Staphylococcus aureus* bacteremia or an intermediate clinical probability of infective endocarditis.

When TEE shows perivalvular abscess or fistula, mycotic aortic aneurysm, new valvular dehiscence, or paravalvular leakage, cardiac surgery should be considered (Fig. 6). Other indications for cardiac surgery are early prosthetic valve endocarditis (<2 months after surgery),

prosthetic valve endocarditis associated with heart failure, infective endocarditis not responsive to standard treatment, or infection with virulent organisms (*Staphylococcus aureus*) or difficult-to-eradicate organisms (fungi). Echocardiographic data that relate vegetation size and the need for surgery with the risk of subsequent embolization are controversial.

CRITICALLY ILL PATIENTS
Many critically ill patients are managed with mechanical ventilation with an endotracheal tube. This both hinders image quality on TTE and facilitates examina-

A

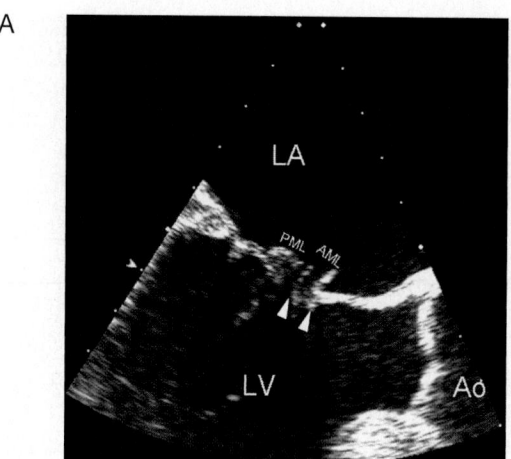

B

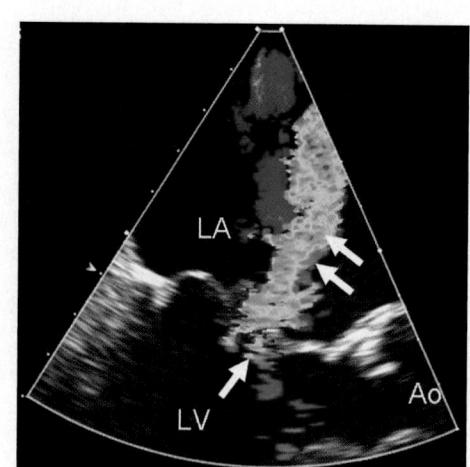

Fig. 5. *A*, Intraoperative transesophageal echocardiogram, long-axis view systolic frame, from patient undergoing mitral valve operation for regurgitation, showing prolapse of myxomatous mitral valve and perforated (*arrowheads*) mycotic aneurysm of anterior mitral leaflet from healed endocarditis. *B*, Color Doppler study, showing severe mitral valve regurgitation through perforation (*arrows*). Ao, aorta; AML, anterior mitral leaflet; LA, left atrium; LV, left ventricle; PML, posterior mitral leaflet.

tion with TEE. TEE is useful in critically ill patients with unexplained hypotension, hypoxemia, or systemic and pulmonary embolism (Fig. 7). In patients declared brain dead who are donor candidates for organ transplantation, TEE can determine the suitability of the donor organ for transplant.

CARDIOVERSION

The Assessment of Cardioversion Using Transesophageal Echocardiography (ACUTE) study found

that cardioversion in patients with atrial fibrillation can be safely performed when TEE shows an absence of left atrial or left atrial appendage thrombus (Fig. 8). This is also a more clinically effective alternative strategy to conventional anticoagulation therapy for several weeks before elective cardioversion. In addition to the safety consideration, TEE is helpful for identifying patients who are most likely to recover sinus rhythm. Left ventricular function and left atrial appendage anatomy and function assessed by two-dimensional and Doppler TEE have been reported to accurately

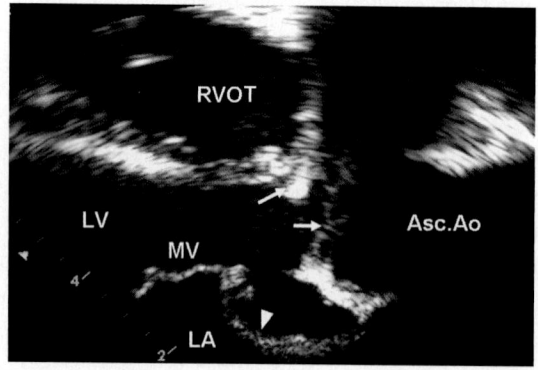

Fig. 6. Transesophageal echocardiogram, long-axis view, showing large mitral aortic intervalvular fibrosa pseudoaneurysm (*arrowhead*) below aortic valve prosthesis (*arrows*) in a patient who had aortic valve replacement for aortic valve endocarditis. Asc.Ao, ascending aorta; LA, left atrium; LV, left ventricle; MV, mitral valve; RVOT, right ventricular outflow tract.

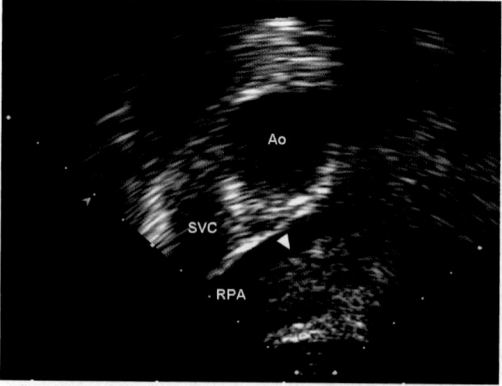

Fig. 7. Transesophageal echocardiogram, basal short-axis view, for critically ill patient with hypotension, showing large thrombus at bifurcation of main pulmonary artery and right pulmonary artery (*arrowhead*). Ao, aorta; RPA, right pulmonary artery; SVC, superior vena cava.

predict rhythm restoration and maintenance of sinus rhythm after cardioversion.

INTRAOPERATIVE TEE

Intraoperative TEE is now widely used before, during, and after cardiac surgery. It is particularly useful in mitral valve repair, for providing information to aid the surgical plan, including preoperative details of the mechanisms of regurgitation and valve abnormality (Fig. 9), and for providing postoperative details of residual regurgitation (Fig. 10) and systolic anterior motion. Additionally, after aortic or mitral valve replacement, intraoperative TEE can recognize prosthetic valve dysfunction and determine the significance of paravalvular regurgitation. It also has been recommended to help determine the extent and site of ventricular myectomy in patients with hypertrophic cardiomyopathy (Fig. 11). Furthermore, it is helpful for identifying mitral valve structural abnormalities associated with hypertrophic cardiomyopathy, which may require valve repair, and complications associated with postoperative myectomy, including aortic regurgitation and ventricular septal defect. In patients undergoing coronary artery bypass grafting, intraoperative TEE is helpful for defining chamber size and function (to help guide fluid and drug administraton) and for evaluating segmental regional wall motion abnormalities. In addition, intraoperative TEE is particularly useful for detecting air in the left ventricle and aorta immediately after cardiopulmonary bypass surgery, which if undetected can

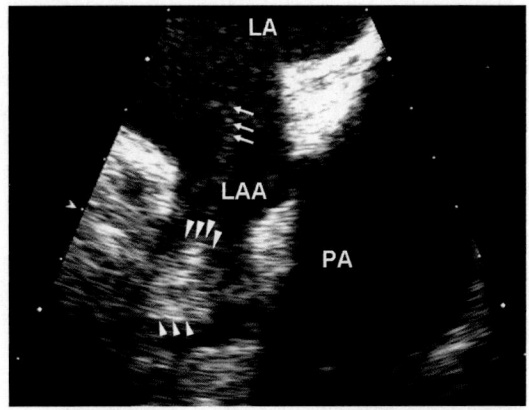

Fig. 8. Transesophageal echocardiogram obtained before cardioversion in patient with atrial fibrillation, showing large thrombus (*arrowheads*) in left atrial appendage (LAA) with spontaneous echo contrast (*arrows*). LA, left atrium; PA, pulmonary artery.

lead to myocardial ischemia due to coronary artery air embolization. Moreover, in high-risk patients undergoing coronary artery bypass grafting in which an intra-aortic balloon pump is used, intraoperative TEE is helpful for positioning the tip of the balloon pump in the aorta. It is also valuable in the assessment of anastomoses of great vessels in surgery of the aorta and heart-lung transplantation.

CARDIOVASCULAR INTERVENTIONS

TEE-guided cardiovascular intervention results in a

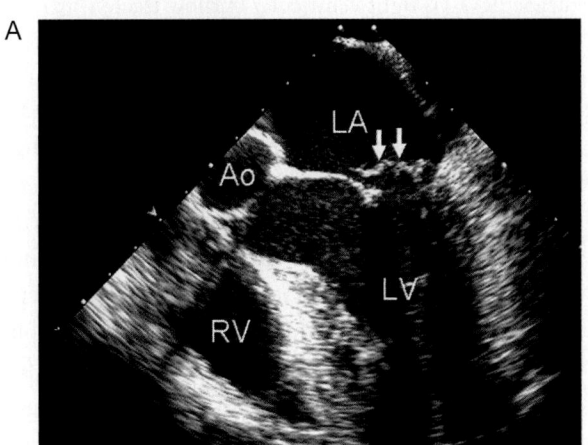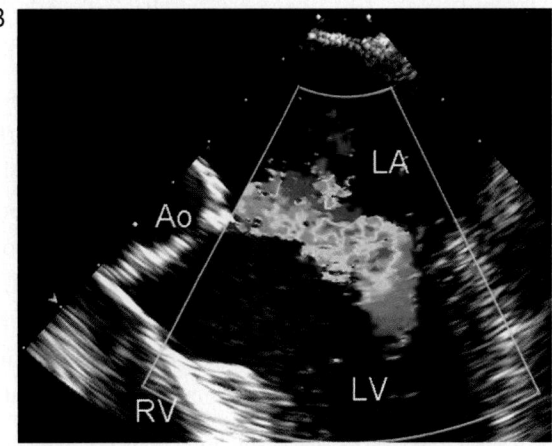

Fig. 9. *A*, Intraoperative transesophageal echocardiogram, showing mitral valve prolapse with flail (*arrows*) middle scallop of posterior leaflet. *B*, Color Doppler study, showing severe mitral valve regurgitation. Ao, aorta; LA, left atrium; LV, left ventricle; RV, right ventricle.

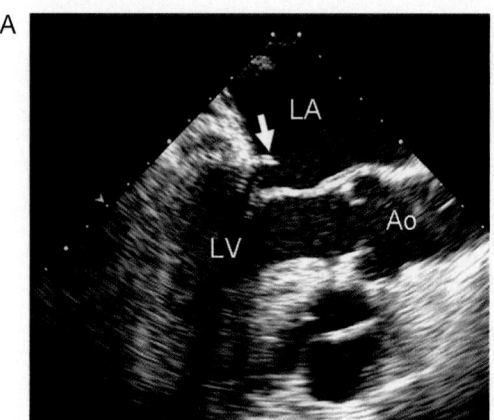

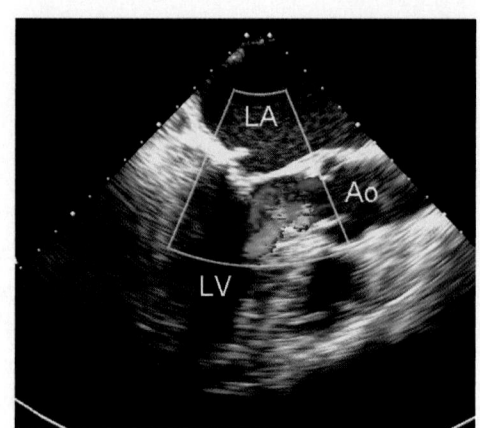

Fig. 10. *A*, Transesophageal echocardiogram, systolic frame, obtained after bypass for same patient described in Figure 5, showing repair of anterior mitral valve perforation and ring anuloplasty (*arrow*). *B*, Color Doppler study, showing no residual mitral valve regurgitation. Ao, aorta; LA, left atrium; LV, left ventricle.

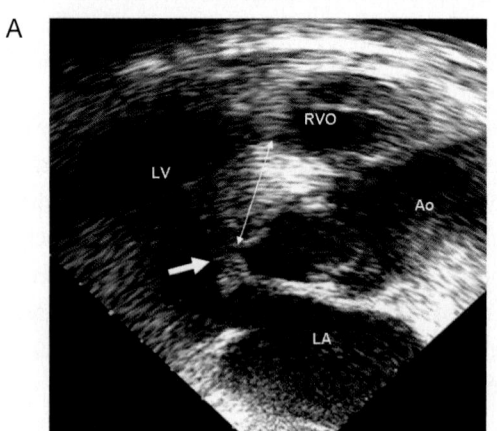

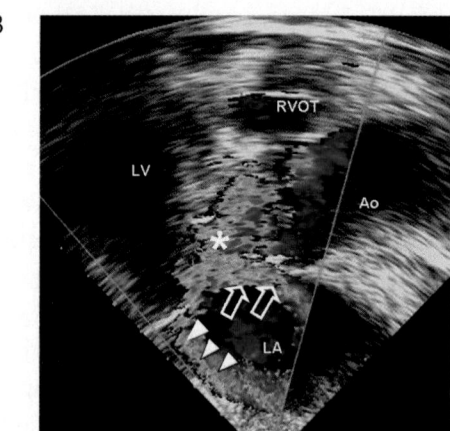

Fig. 11. *A*, Preoperataive transesophageal echocardiogram, long-axis systolic frame, in patient with hypertrophic cardiomyopathy, showing markedly increased thickness of basal septum (*double-headed arrow*) and systolic anterior motion of mitral valve (*arrow*). *B*, Color Doppler study, showing systolic flow turbulence in left ventricular outflow tract (*asterisk*) and eccentric mitral regurgitation, a predominant posterior-directed jet (*arrowheads*), and a less severe anterior jet (*open arrows*). Ao, aorta; LA, left atrium; LV, left ventricle; RVOT, right ventricular outflow tract.

substantial reduction of fluoroscopic X-ray exposure to patients and operator. TEE is useful for guiding the position of the catheter during radiofrequency ablation, transseptal puncture, balloon valvuloplasty, novel percutaneous valvular intervention, novel percutaneous left atrial appendage transcatheter occlusion (Fig. 12), and transcatheter device closure of interatrial communication and ventricular septal defect. Furthermore, TEE is helpful for guiding the placement of percutaneous stent graft of the aorta and stent angioplasty of coarctation of the aorta. Sporadically, TEE has been used as a guide during high-risk endomyocardial biopsy and pacemaker implantation.

DETERMINATION OF SOURCES OF EMBOLISM

Ischemic stroke is the leading cause of morbidity and mortality. TEE permits excellent visualization of potential thromboembolic sites: the left atrial appendage, the arch of the aorta, and the descending thoracic aorta. In addition, it can image the atrial septum for possible shunts, which have been implicated in paradoxical embolism. However, the yield of TEE for detecting the cause of embolism is high in younger individuals. Improved visualization by TEE allows easy recognition of potential sources of embolism, including small thrombi, cardiac tumors such as myxoma (Fig. 13), papillary fibroelastoma, vegetations, and interatrial

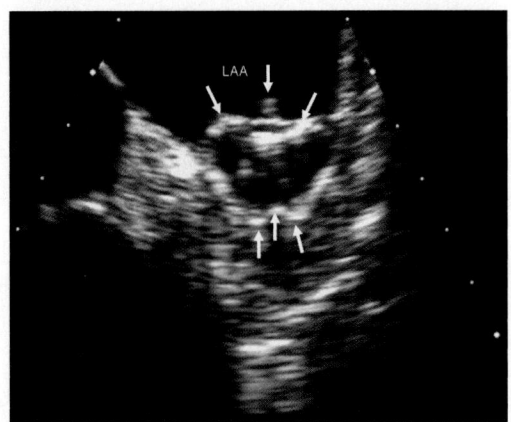

Fig. 12. Transesophageal echocardiogram, showing percutaneous left atrial appendage (LAA) occluder device (*arrows*).

are difficult to visualize by TTE because of ultrasonographic artifacts as well as masking. Prosthetic valve obstruction often results from thrombus in the mitral position and is commonly on the atrial side of the prosthesis; hence, TEE is essential to identify them. Prosthetic valve obstruction in the aortic position often results from panus, which may be difficult to separate from the housing unit by TTE, and TEE can define them more easily in most cases. TEE is essential to define the site and mechanism of regurgitation for both aortic and mitral prostheses (Fig. 15). Furthermore, in cases of suspected endocarditis, TEE is essential not only to confirm the diagnosis but also to identify high-risk patients, those with abscesses and fistulae.

septum abnormality, especially patent foramen ovale and atrial septal defect. Previous studies have demonstrated that a protruding, noncalcified aortic plaque ≥4 mm detected by TEE is a significant risk factor of ischemic stoke and peripheral embolism. With TEE, those atheroma as well as aortic plaque compositions can be easily detected and visualized (Fig. 14).

PROSTHETIC VALVE EVALUATION

Clinically suspected prosthetic valve malfunction commonly requires both TTE and TEE. TTE provides hemodynamic information indicating the dysfunction; however, delineating the mechanism of dysfunction often requires TEE. Although the ventricular aspect of the mitral and aortic prosthesis can be well visualized by TTE, the atrial and aortic aspects of the prosthesis

CONGENITAL HEART DISEASES

TEE is helpful in evaluation of complex congenital as well as simple congenital lesions, such as atrial septal defect (Fig. 16), the cleft of atrioventricular valves, and anomalies of the aorta associated with bicuspid aortic valve. In addition, it is essential in previously operated patients to identify the residual defects, right ventricular outflow tract or pulmonary obstruction, the patency of the conduits and baffles, the patency of the superior vena cava or inferior vena cava, especially in the post-Fontan procedure, and the function of an atrioventricular valve prosthesis in individuals who require atrioventricular valve replacement. Furthermore, in post-Fontan patients, right pulmonary vein compression can occur from an enlarged right atrium or atrial baffle bulging into the left atrium. In those patients, TEE is superior to TTE in the assessment of the pulmonary venous flow pattern.

A
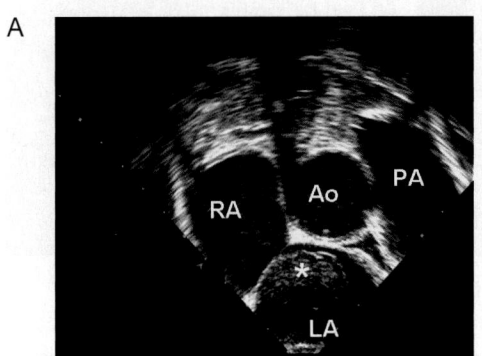

B
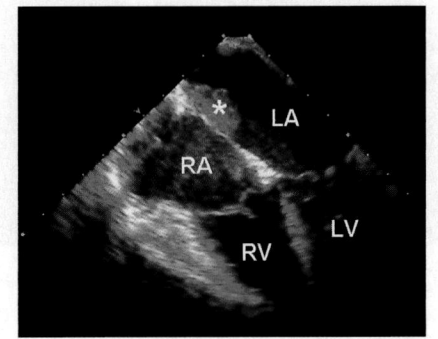

Fig. 13. Transesophageal echocardiograms, showing left atrial myxoma (*asterisk*) attached to interatrial septum in short-axis (*A*) and four-chamber (*B*) views. Ao, aorta; LA, left atrium; LV, left ventricle; PA, pulmonary artery; RA, right atrium; RV, right ventricle.

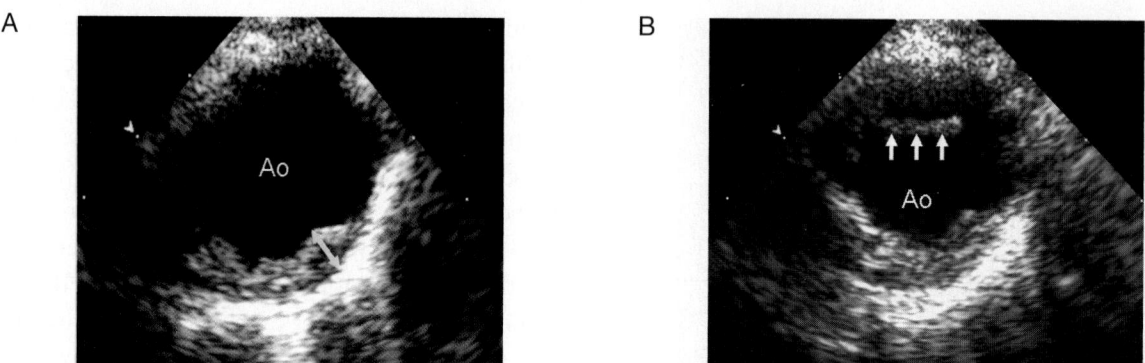

Fig. 14. Transesophageal echocardiography in a patient with a transient ischemic attack demonstrates a 5-mm-thick complex atherosclerosis (*double-head arrow*) of the proximal descending thoracic aorta (Ao) (*A*) and a highly mobile thrombus (*arrows*) just distal to the left subclavian artery origin (*B*).

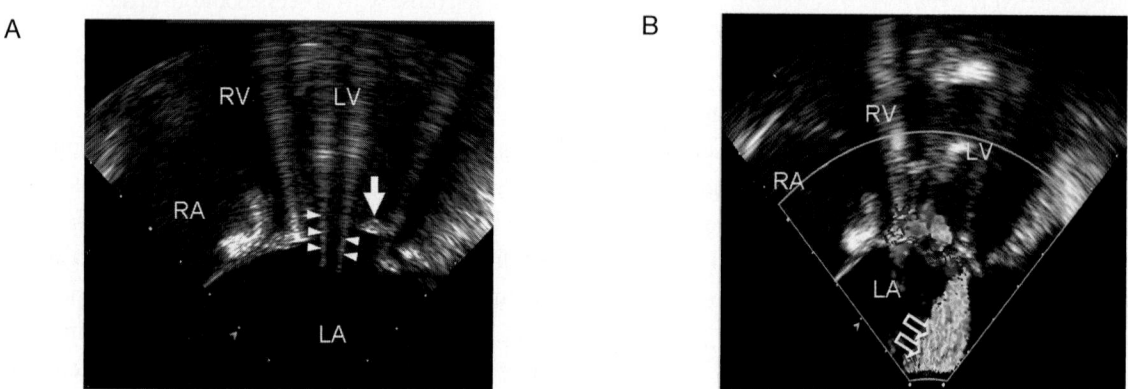

Fig. 15. *A,* Transesophageal echocardiographic diastolic frame in a patient with mitral valve replacement who had recurrent heart failure. A mobile thrombus (*arrow*) is on the ventricular surface of the prosthesis. *Arrowheads* indicate normal open position of both leaflets of St. Jude mechanical prosthesis. *B,* Color Doppler image demonstrates that the thrombus protrudes in and out, causing intermittent impaired closure of the lateral orifice of the mitral prosthetic valve, resulting in moderate to severe mitral prosthetic regurgitation (*open arrows*). LA, left atrium; LV, left ventricle; RA, right atrium; RV, right ventricle.

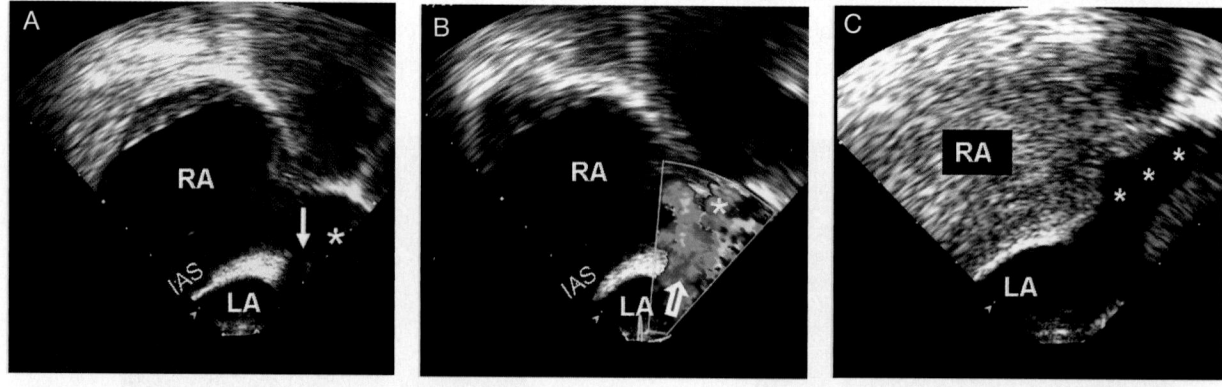

Fig. 16. *A,* Transesophageal echocardiography in a patient with a heart murmur demonstrates a sinus venosus atrial septal defect (ASD) (*arrow*) in the superior portion of the interatrial septum (IAS) near the orifice of the superior vena cava (SVC) (∗). *B,* Color Doppler shows a left-to-right shunt through the ASD and the flow from the pulmonary vein draining into the posterior aspect of the SVC (∗). *C,* Contrast echocardiography demonstrates a negative contrast created by the flow from the left atrium (LA) to the right atrium (RA) across the ASD and by the right upper pulmonary vein flow draining into the SVC (∗).

11

NUCLEAR IMAGING

John W. Askew III, MD

Todd D. Miller, MD

Nuclear cardiology imaging techniques are commonly used to evaluate myocardial perfusion at rest and with stress, to measure left ventricular function and volume, and to determine the presence or absence of myocardial viability.

RADIONUCLIDE IMAGING

Radiopharmaceuticals

Nuclear cardiology is based on the administration of a radiopharmaceutical consisting of a radionuclide (isotope) with or without a complexing agent (depending on the type of study) in order to image the cardiovascular system. A radionuclide is an unstable element that decays spontaneously and, as a result, emits energy in the form of radiation or charged particles. Radiation that is emitted from the decay of the nucleus of an atom is called gamma radiation. With some isotopes, the radiation is reabsorbed by the orbiting electrons and then re-emitted as x-rays. Gamma rays are high-energy electromagnetic radiation. By comparison, light is considered low-energy electromagnetic radiation. The energy of a gamma ray is described in units of electron volts, typically between 50,000 and 200,000 electron volts (abbreviated as 50-200 keV). Radiopharmaceuticals also may consist of a complexing agent (sestamibi or tetrofosmin) that helps

to facilitate stabilization, biodistribution, and delivery of the radionuclide to the intended target. If the emitted gamma rays from the administered radionuclide are not absorbed or scattered by soft tissue or bone and pass out of the body, they can be detected and used to create an image.

Radioisotopes

Two important radioisotopes (Table 1) used in nuclear cardiology are thallium 201 (^{201}Tl) and technetium 99m (^{99m}Tc).

^{201}Tl is a metallic element in group IIIA of the periodic table and is a cyclotron-generated, monovalent cation with properties similar to that of potassium. ^{201}Tl is rapidly extracted from the blood (extraction fraction close to 85%), enters the myocardium by using the Na-K-ATPase pump, and has an initial distribution proportional to that of myocardial blood flow and an equilibrium distribution proportional to that of potassium. ^{201}Tl displays the property of redistribution; after its initial extraction, there is a continuous exchange involving the myocyte and the extracellular space. The rate of "wash in" and "wash out" is largely due to coronary blood flow. The maximal percentage of myocardial uptake of the original dose is between 4% and 5%. ^{201}Tl decays to mercury 201 by electron capture. ^{201}Tl emits some gamma rays with energies of 135 and 167

Table 1. Isotope Characteristics

Characteristic	Isotope	
	Thallium 201	Technetium 99m sestamibi
Class	Element	Isonitrile
Charge	Cation	Cation
Production	Cyclotron generated	Molybdenum-99m generator
Half-life, h	73	6
Extraction fraction, %	85	65
Maximal myocardial uptake, % injected dose	3-5	1.2-1.5
Mechanism of myocardial uptake	Na-K-ATPase pump	Mitochondrial-derived gradient
Whole-body radiation dose, mrad/mCi	240	16
Gamma rays/x-rays (photopeak), keV	68-80, 135, 167	140
Myocardial redistribution	Yes	Minimal

keV; however, the principal (most abundant) radiation emissions are x-rays emitted in the range of 69 to 83 keV. The relatively low-energy 80-keV protons are more susceptible to scattering and attenuation. The long physical half-life (73 hours) limits the ability to administer higher doses of ^{201}Tl. The low x-ray energy and low administered dose can result in a reduction of image quality.

^{99m}Tc, a lipophilic monovalent cation, is formed through the decay of molybdenum-99 (^{99}Mo), which is available commercially from a ^{99}Mo generator. The "m" in ^{99m}Tc is present because it is metastable, eventually decaying to ^{99}Tc. Sodium pertechnetate (^{99m}TcO$_4$) is obtained by passing a sodium chloride solution through the ^{99}Mo generator to elute the ^{99m}Tc continuously being formed by the constant decay of ^{99}Mo (half-life, 66 hours). Because ^{99m}Tc is acquired by eluting a ^{99}Mo generator, an important quality control step that should be performed the first time the generator is eluted is to ensure that very little ^{99}Mo is eluted from the generator. Because of the long half-life of ^{99}Mo, too much ^{99}Mo results in an increased radiation dose to the patient. The permissible amount must be less than 0.15 µCi ^{99}Mo/mCi ^{99m}Tc. ^{99m}Tc has a lower myocardial extraction fraction (65%) than ^{201}Tl and is sequestered in the cardiac myocyte by the mitochondria. Uptake of both ^{99m}Tc sestamibi and tetrofosmin plateaus at a lower myocar-

dial blood flow rate than ^{201}Tl. In contrast to ^{201}Tl, ^{99m}Tc does not seem to be dependent on the Na-K-ATPase pump and undergoes minimal redistribution. The decay of ^{99m}Tc emits a higher-energy gamma ray with a photopeak of 140 keV. The shorter half-life (6 hours) and the higher-energy photon (140 keV) improve image resolution through the ability to administer higher doses and limit photon scatter and attenuation. The ability to use a higher energy gamma ray can limit the number of scattered photons, thereby accepting a greater percentage of valid counts, and consequently image quality is improved and gating is enhanced.

Instrumentation

In nuclear cardiology, the most commonly used device to detect photons is the gamma camera. The gamma camera consists of multiple components with the primary function of detecting photons and converting that energy into an electrical current. The primary components of the gamma camera are the collimator, the sodium iodide crystal, and the photomultiplier tubes. The collimator serves as a shield by allowing photons traveling at an approximate 90° angle to pass through; image resolution is thereby improved in the intended area of interest. Not all photons passing through the collimator result in an accurate image because photons from other areas may be scattered and ultimately pass through the collimator. In an effort to correct these events, an energy window is used to identify scattered photons, because they typically will have a lower-energy level and thus can be identified and excluded from analysis. Appropriate incoming photons strike the sodium iodide crystal and are converted to visible light. The light strikes the photomultiplier tube and is amplified and converted to a measurable electrical signal. With the aid of computer processing, the spatial image of interest is reconstructed. A separate detection system occasionally used in nuclear cardiology is the multicrystal camera, which contains several sodium iodide crystals with separate photomultiplier tubes. The multicrystal camera allows for high count sensitivity but low spatial resolution. The improved temporal resolution of the multicrystal camera enables its use for first-pass imaging (described later).

Numerous computer programs are available for display and analysis of the planar/projection images and the reconstructed tomographic slices. The standard planes (short axis, horizontal long axis, and vertical long axis) used for analysis of the reconstructed tomographic slices are shown in Figure 1. The reconstructed short-axis slices typically are divided into 16 segments and can be assigned to coronary artery perfusion territories (Fig. 2).

GATED SPECT

Electrocardiogram-gated single-photon emission computed tomography (SPECT) is an accurate and reproducible technique to measure left ventricular (LV) ejection fraction (EF) and volume. In addition to quantifying LV function and volume, gating permits the assessment of regional wall motion. Performing a gated SPECT study requires the typical equipment used in acquiring a standard SPECT image set with the addition of a three-lead electrocardiogram-gating device. Each cardiac cycle is identified using the RR interval. A gating rate is set (typically 8 frames for each RR interval). All of the counts acquired at each projection are placed into a designated bin (frame) that corresponds to the time the counts were acquired during the cardiac cycle. The pre-set RR interval can remain the same for the entire study (fixed acquisition mode) or

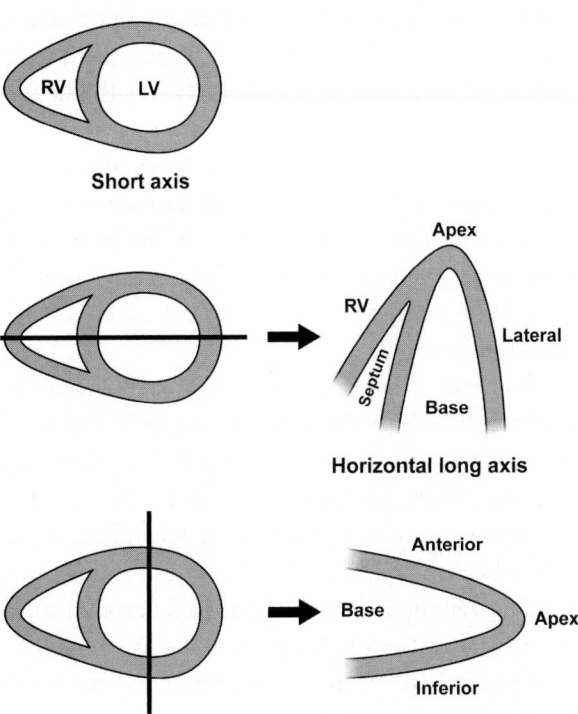

Fig. 1. Standard imaging planes used in nuclear cardiology: short axis, horizontal long axis, and vertical long axis. LV, left ventricle; RV, right ventricle.

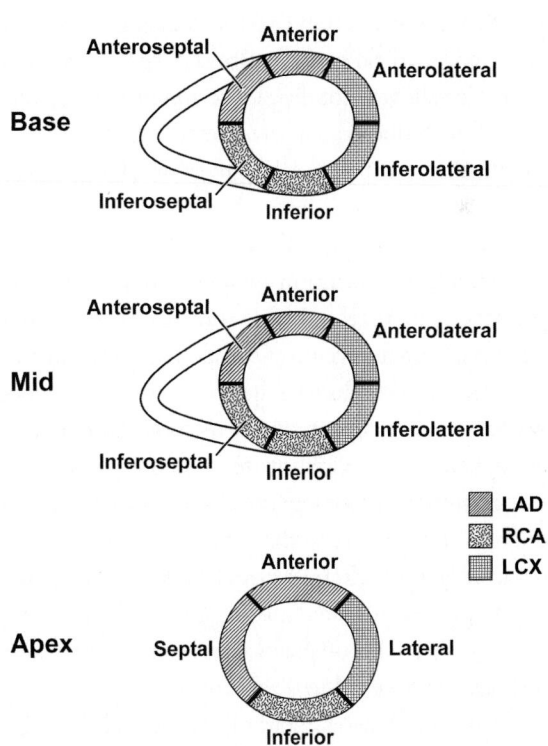

Fig. 2. Nomenclature and location of the 16 myocardial segments and assignment of coronary arterial perfusion territories on the short-axis model. LAD, left anterior descending coronary artery; LCX, left circumflex coronary artery; RCA, right coronary artery.

can be monitored and recalculated during each projection (variable acquisition mode). Because the heart rate may be dynamic, acceptance windows can be specified to reject cycle lengths that do not fall within a predetermined range of the expected RR interval. Use of acceptance windows allows for improved accuracy and reliability of the gated information and avoids potential perfusion image artifacts (flashing, blurring, and streaking) related to arrhythmias. In contrast to the count-based technique used to calculate EF by blood-pool imaging, gated SPECT is based on volume. Computer algorithms are applied to identify the endocardial borders. Volumes at end-diastole (EDV) and end-systole (ESV) are measured, and LVEF can then be calculated: LVEF (%) = (EDV − ESV)/EDV × 100. Limitations to quantifying LVEF can occur in patients with a small LV cavity, in that the ESV is underestimated because of obliteration of the LV cavity, with subsequent over-estimation of the LVEF.

MYOCARDIAL PERFUSION IMAGING

Stress SPECT is the standard for assessing myocardial perfusion in clinical practice. Stress SPECT has been extensively validated for diagnostic and prognostic purposes. The hallmark of myocardial ischemia is a reversible defect, which may be either partial or complete (Fig. 3). Severe fixed defects represent myocardial infarction (Fig. 4). Mild fixed defects can represent nontransmural infarction or attenuation artifacts. Assessment of regional wall motion on the gated images can help resolve this issue. SPECT imaging is a relative perfusion technique; because myocardial blood flow during stress is reduced in regions subtended by hemodynamically significant stenoses, the radioisotope tracer content in these regions also is reduced. Global reduction in flow due to three-vessel coronary artery disease (balanced ischemia) can result in normal perfusion images. Available data suggest that this occurs uncommonly in clinical practice and can be detected by other variables (see below).

Even though assessment of myocardial perfusion is the primary reason for performing SPECT studies, other important findings can be seen on the planar/rotating images. Cardiac size at rest and after stress can be qualitatively assessed. Transient ischemic dilatation refers to the apparent increase in LV size on the stress images compared with the rest images and can be measured qualitatively or quantitatively (Fig. 5). Transient ischemic dilatation implies extensive myocardial ischemia or severe (left main or multivessel) coronary artery disease. Severe stress-induced ischemia may result in prolonged wall motion abnormalities visible on the post-stress gated images. Isotope uptake in the right ventricle can occasionally be seen and allow for evaluation of right ventricular enlargement and hypertrophy (Fig. 6). Increased lung tracer uptake (lung-heart ratio >0.5) with ^{201}Tl is suggestive of increased LV filling pressures, LV dysfunction, or extent of ischemia (Fig. 7). Additional noncardiac findings can relate to areas of increased isotope uptake (thyroid disease, ectopic parathyroids, lymphomas, breast and lung malignancies) and, conversely, reduced isotope uptake (ascites, cysts, pleural and pericardial effusions).

Types

The most common forms of stress testing performed in conjunction with SPECT imaging include treadmill exercise or pharmacologic stress (adenosine, dipyridamole, or dobutamine). Pharmacologic stress tests are performed in patients unable to adequately exercise or in patients with selected electrocardiographic findings (left bundle branch block or paced ventricular rhythm). Adenosine increases myocardial blood flow through its interaction with adenosine receptors (primarily A_2) in the coronary bed. Activation of the A_2 receptor results in coronary vasodilatation. Dipyridamole exerts its vasodilatory actions by blocking the intracellular transport of adenosine, thus raising extracellular adenosine levels which in turn activate A_2 receptors, resulting in coronary vasodilatation.

Potential side effects of adenosine and dipyridamole include light-headedness, headache, flushing, nausea, chest discomfort, abdominal discomfort, and dyspnea. More serious side effects can include hypotension, profound bradycardia, second- or third-degree heart block, and bronchospasm (these effects usually resolve with decreasing the dose, discontinuation of the infusion, or administration of aminophylline). Changes on the electrocardiogram can occur with adenosine. ST-segment depression (≥1 mm) is suggestive of ischemia and may indicate severe (left main or three-vessel) coronary artery disease. In patients with contraindications to vasodilating agents, dobutamine

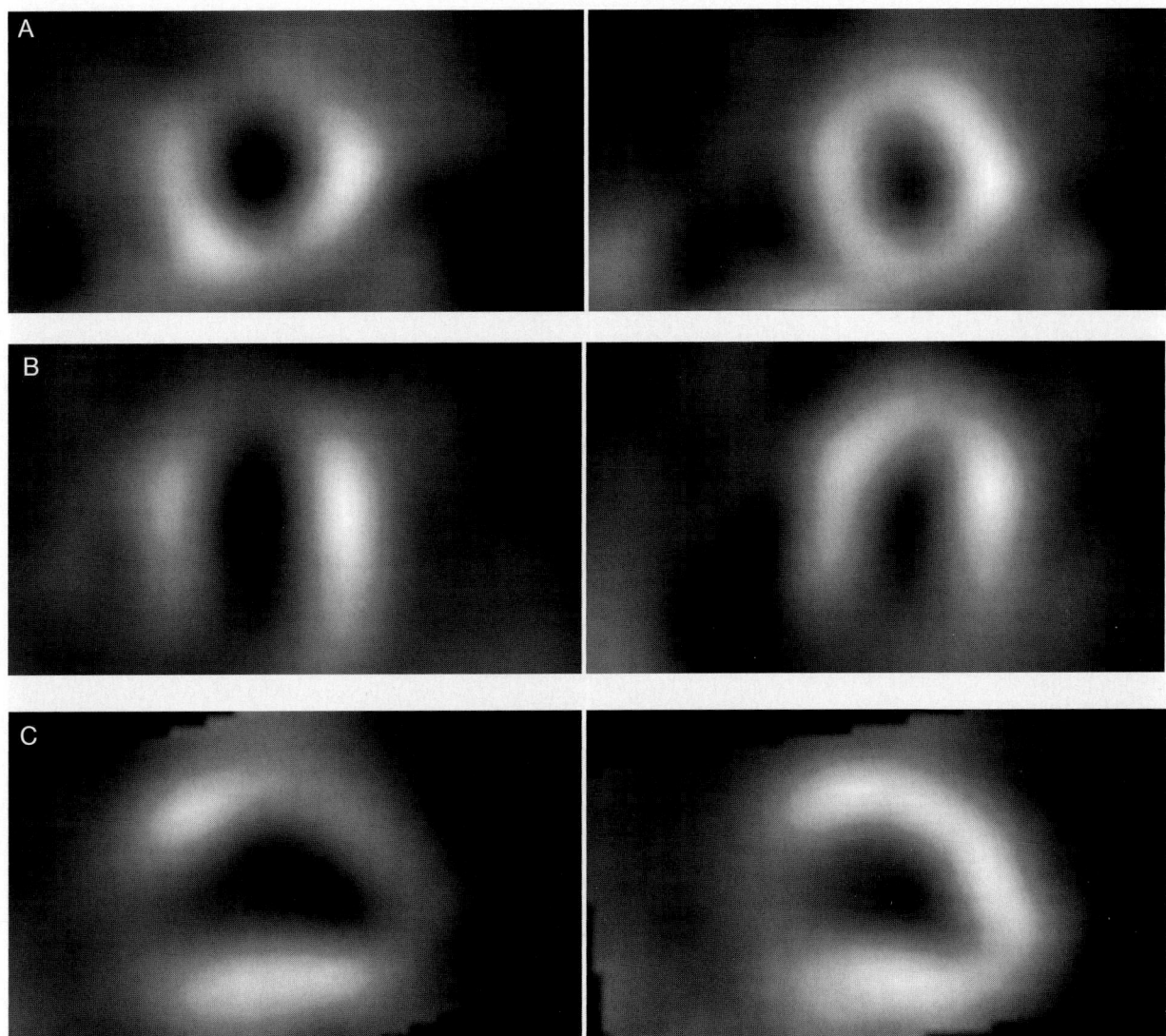

Fig. 3. Stress images (*left*) and rest images (*right*) show a large area of ischemia (involving the apex, septum, anterior, and anterolateral segments) on the short-axis (*A*), horizontal long-axis (*B*), and vertical long-axis (*C*) views.

can be used. Dobutamine is an inotropic agent that exerts its catecholamine effect of increasing heart rate and contractility through activation of cardiac adrenergic receptors. Potential side effects include chest pain, dyspnea, flushing, palpitations, and nausea.

Indications and relative contraindications for adenosine, dipyridamole, and dobutamine are listed in Table 2. Protocols for administering adenosine, dipyridamole, and dobutamine vary. Standard protocols include adenosine infusion of 140 μg/kg per minute for 6 minutes with radioisotope injection 3 minutes into the infusion, dipyridamole infusion of 0.56 mg/kg over 4 minutes with radioisotope injection 3 to 4 minutes

after infusion is complete, and stepwise titration of dobutamine up to 40 to 50 μg/kg per minute with the addition of atropine (to a total dose ≤2 mg) as needed to achieve 85% of the age-adjusted maximal heart rate.

Imaging Protocols

Various imaging protocols can be used, including same-day rest-stress or stress-rest imaging with a single isotope, a 2-day protocol with the same isotope, or a dual-isotope study in which the rest imaging is performed with one isotope and the stress imaging, with another (201Tl, 99mTc sestamibi). Acquisition protocols vary but typically consist of acquiring 60 to 64 projections

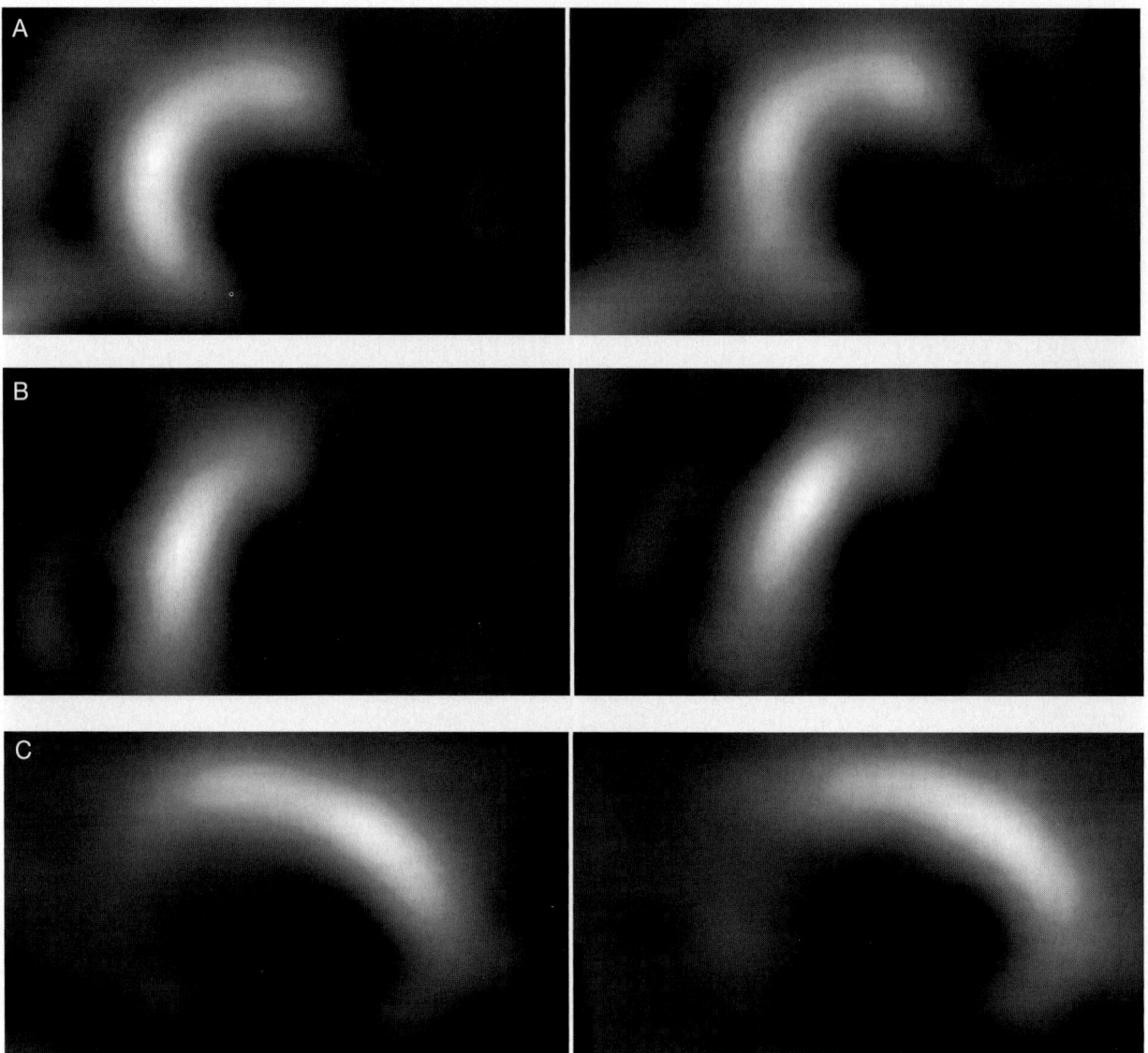

Fig. 4. Stress images (*left*) and rest images (*right*) show a large, dense infarction (involving the lateral and inferior walls) on the short-axis (*A*), horizontal long-axis (*B*), and vertical long-axis (*C*) views.

at 15 to 20 seconds per projection over a 180° arc (45° right anterior oblique to 45° left posterior oblique) with the patient in the supine position. Prone imaging is occasionally performed in addition to supine imaging because it can minimize diaphragmatic attenuation artifacts by increasing the separation of the inferior wall and the diaphragm.

The total acquisition time depends on the number and configuration of the detectors, the number of degrees between each projection, and the length of acquisition time at each projection. The total acquisition time to obtain either a rest or a stress image with

dual-head (90°) detectors with a 180° orbit and 60 projections at 20 seconds per projection can be under 12 minutes. Time from injection of the isotope to image acquisition varies according to the imaging protocol, the type of isotope (shorter times for ^{201}Tl), and the method of stress (shorter times with exercise). These times vary and are in an effort to minimize artifacts by allowing for activity in the liver to decrease yet avoiding the impact of subdiaphragmatic activity from isotope activity in the stomach and intestines.

Several types of artifacts can occur and may be related to the patient and the imaging equipment.

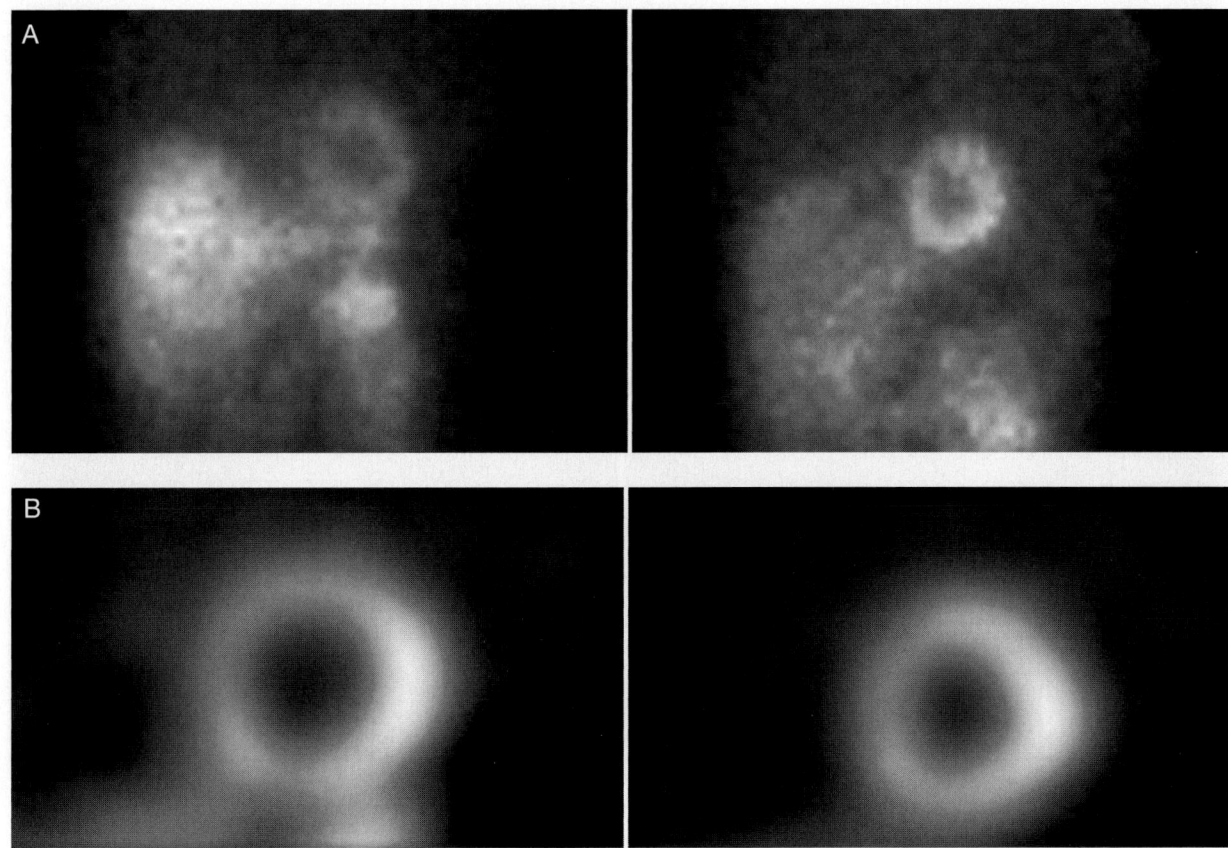

Fig. 5. Stress images (*left*) and rest images (*right*) show transient ischemic dilatation of the left ventricle on the planar projection (*A*) and short-axis (*B*) view. Coronary angiography showed multivessel coronary artery disease.

Patient-related artifacts include attenuation from soft tissue, breast, chest wall, diaphragm, and overlapping visceral activity. Patient movement can occur during the acquisition of images and may result in vertical or horizontal motion artifacts. A phenomenon referred to as "upward creep" has been described with exercise ^{201}Tl stress studies when the stress images are acquired soon after exercise. Immediately after exercise, diaphragmatic excursion is increased because of the depth of respiration; as the depth of respiration decreases, the position of the diaphragm rises in the chest with a resulting upward movement of the heart during the acquisition of images, giving rise to the diaphragmatic "creep" artifact. Septal artifacts can be seen with left bundle branch block or paced rhythms. The dyssynchronous septal motion due to left bundle branch block seen in many patients at rest is intensified with the heart rate acceleration that occurs with exercise. Studies suggest that septal blood flow may be altered. Substituting a pharmacologic

vasodilator stress agent (dipyridamole or adenosine) can reduce this problem by avoiding significant tachycardia and is generally recommended in patients with a left bundle branch block or paced rhythm.

Assessment of Left Ventricular Size and Function

Equilibrium radionuclide angiography, commonly known as multiple-gated blood pool imaging, is an imaging technique of the intravascular blood pool using an isotope. The accuracy and reproducibility of the technique as a noninvasive assessment of ventricular function have made it a valuable imaging tool for many years. 99mTc is the most commonly used radioisotope for equilibrium radionuclide angiography. If images that reflect the intravascular blood volume are to be obtained, the isotope (99mTc) must be linked to a carrier that will remain within the circulation and be uniformly

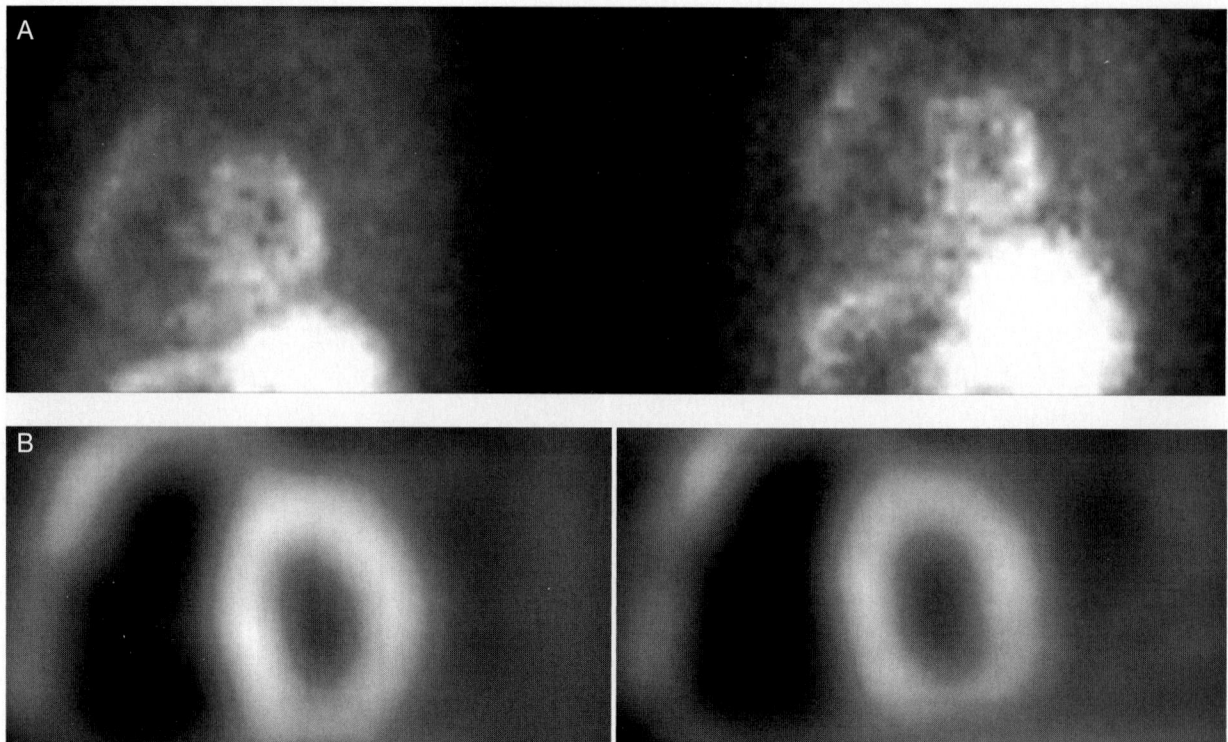

Fig. 6. Severe right ventricular enlargement and hypertrophy noted on the planar projection (*A*) and short-axis (*B*) image.

distributed. Currently, red blood cells are used as the carrier. Labeling the patient's red blood cells with ^{99m}Tc can be accomplished with either in vitro or in vivo techniques. Both techniques require the use of a reducing agent (stannous ions) that helps facilitate red blood cell binding to ^{99m}Tc by providing a lower oxidation state.

After labeling of the red blood cells, a gamma camera is used to acquire the images. An electrocardiographic monitoring device is used for R-wave triggering, which allows each cardiac cycle to be timed. Each cardiac cycle is divided into "frames" (usually between 16 and 32). The summation of data from the same frames of each cardiac cycle can be processed and displayed for review, providing images of the cardiac chambers acquired over multiple cardiac cycles. Typically more than 2 million counts are needed from the field of view for acceptable image resolution, accurate assessment of wall motion, and reproducible quantification calculations, requiring the sampling of many (>200) cardiac cycles. As with all gating techniques, a fairly regular heart rate is required. Orientation and separation of the

cardiac chambers are important for assessing wall motion and quantitating ventricular volumes and ejection fractions because all chambers will contain radiolabeled red blood cells.

Standard views of the left ventricle at rest include anterior, left anterior oblique (45°), and left lateral (Fig. 8).

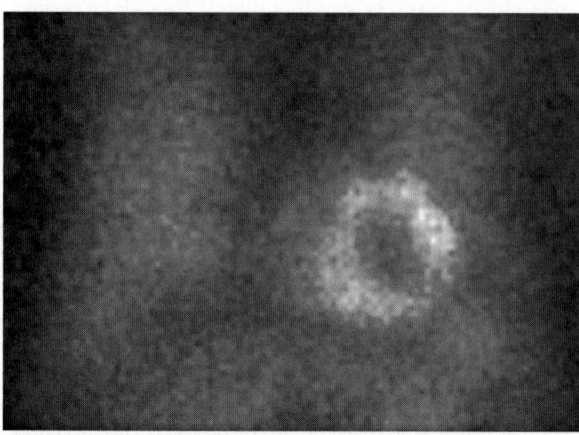

Fig. 7. Thallium planar projection image with increased pulmonary uptake (lung-heart ratio, 0.66).

Table 2. Indications for Choosing Adenosine, Dipyridamole, or Dobutamine

Indication	Adenosine	Dipyridamole	Dobutamine
Asthma	No*	No*	Yes
COPD	No*	No*	Yes
Patient taking dipyridamole	No	Yes	Yes
Patient taking theophylline	No†	No†	Yes
High-grade AV block	No	No	Yes
Caffeine use (<24 h)	No‡	No‡	Yes
Left bundle branch block	Yes	Yes	No

AV, atrioventricular; COPD, chronic obstructive pulmonary disease.
*May be tolerated if forced expiratory volume in 1 second is >40 L/s and bronchodilator change <31%.
†May use if theophylline use is discontinued ≥48 hours before the test.
‡May use; however, potential problem of false-negative results.

The left anterior oblique view results in optimal separation of the ventricular chambers. Stress equilibrium radionuclide angiography can be performed during cycle ergometry exercise with 3-minute stages. Usually, only one left anterior oblique view is used because of acquisition times at each exercise level (approximately 2 minutes) and the importance of measuring LVEF during exercise. Equilibrium radionuclide angiography can be used to assess ventricular volumes, LVEF, regional wall motion, right ventricular function, and diastolic variables (early diastolic filling, rate of peak filling, and time to peak filling). Because the measurements are count-based and do not require assumptions about cardiac (ventricular) geometry, the technique provides an accurate, reproducible, and operator-independent assessment of ventricular function.

First-pass radionuclide angiography, although technically different from equilibrium radionuclide angiography, is an alternative to quantifying ventricular function. Red blood cell labeling is not required because the radioisotope (commonly ^{99m}Tc) is directly administered as a bolus injection into the venous circulation and recorded during its first pass through the circulation. The radioisotope bolus is tracked from the superior vena cava through the right atrium, right ventricle, pulmonary circulation, left atrium, left ventricle, and ascending aorta with a multicrystal camera to enhance temporal resolution of the bolus as it passes through each region of interest. The most common

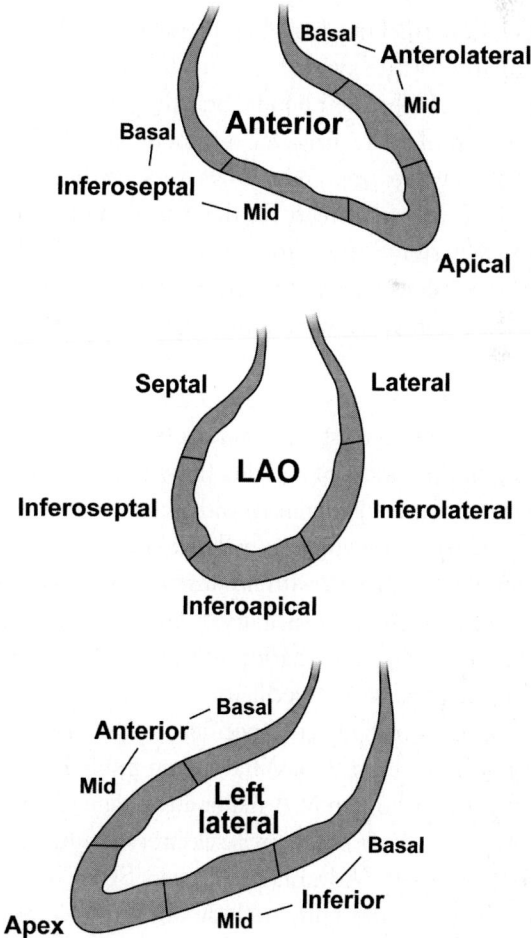

Fig. 8. Standard views (anterior, left anterior oblique [LAO], left lateral) and nomenclature of the left ventricle for equilibrium radionuclide angiography.

application of the first-pass technique is quantification of LVEF. Other applications include quantification of right ventricular EF, assessment of LV wall motion, quantification of ventricular volumes, and detection of right-to-left shunts.

CLINICAL APPLICATIONS

Chronic Coronary Artery Disease (Known or Suspected)

Diagnostic Assessment

Stress SPECT is most beneficial for diagnostic purposes in patients at intermediate risk for coronary artery disease (Bayes theorem) who are not candidates for standard exercise treadmill testing, because of, for example, inability to exercise or baseline electrocardiographic abnormalities, including preexcitation (Wolff-Parkinson-White syndrome), electronically paced ventricular rhythm, left bundle branch block, or more than 1 mm of resting ST-segment depression. Published values are 85% to 90% for sensitivity and 70% to 75% for specificity for the detection of angiographically significant coronary artery disease (Table 3). These values have not been corrected for referral bias, also known as verification bias. Referral bias describes the effect of primarily referring patients with abnormal test results to angiography to verify the results of the stress test. The number of patients in the angiographic cohort of patients (in whom sensitivity and specificity are determined) with positive test results (both true-positive and false-positive) greatly exceeds the number of patients with negative test results (both true-negative and false-negative). The net impact of referral bias is overestimation of test sensitivity and underestimation of test specificity.

Similar sensitivity and specificity values (also not corrected for referral bias) have been published for stress echocardiography. A major advantage of stress imaging procedures over exercise electrocardiography is higher sensitivity. Advantages of stress SPECT over stress echocardiography include obtaining quality images in a greater percentage of patients despite body habitus or other confounding factors (e.g., chronic obstructive pulmonary disease) and greater accuracy for detecting ischemia in the presence of resting wall

Table 3.   Sensitivity and Specificity* of Myocardial Perfusion SPECT for Detecting Coronary Artery Disease

Test	Sensitivity, %	Specificity, %
Exercise SPECT	87	73
Vasodilator SPECT	89	75

SPECT, single-photon emission computed tomography.
*Because of the impact of referral bias on specificity, the normalcy rate is occasionally used and refers to the frequency of normal test results in patients with a low likelihood of coronary artery disease (91% for stress SPECT).

motion abnormalities or dyssynchronous contraction patterns related to left bundle branch block or paced ventricular rhythm.

Prognostic Assessment

Stress SPECT has the largest published prognostic database of any noninvasive stress imaging technique. The prognostic value of stress SPECT imaging has been well validated in numerous studies. Many prognostic variables have been identified, most importantly, LVEF and perfusion. Patients with normal perfusion images, in general, are at very low risk and have an annual "hard" event rate (cardiac death or nonfatal myocardial infarction) of less than 1%. This statement may not apply to selected subsets of patients, including those with diabetes and those undergoing pharmacologic stress, especially if they have ischemic electrocardiographic changes with adenosine or dipyridamole. In patients with abnormal images, the risk of a cardiac event is proportional to the degree of abnormality. Both the size and the severity of the perfusion defect are prognostically important and have been incorporated into the calculation of summed scores. The summed stress score is a reflection of both infarcted and ischemic myocardium and has modestly greater prognostic value than the summed difference score (the extent and severity of ischemic myocardium).

The prognostic information obtained with stress SPECT adds incremental value over clinical and exercise variables. The prognostic value of stress SPECT has been shown in numerous patient subsets, including women, the elderly, patients with diabetes, and patients with an intermediate-risk treadmill test result. Stress SPECT has also been well validated for preoperative assessment of patients at intermediate clinical risk undergoing an intermediate risk or high-risk operation. The risk of a perioperative event is 15% to 20% in patients with ischemic images and 2% to 3% in patients with normal images.

Assessment After Revascularization

Stress SPECT has been validated for risk stratification in patients who previously have had coronary artery bypass grafting or percutaneous intervention. Guidelines recommend stress imaging over treadmill testing for assessment of patients who have had revascularization and experience a change in symptom status (class I indication). The frequency with which stress imaging should be performed in asymptomatic patients after revascularization is controversial. Guidelines currently suggest that testing should not be performed more often than every 3 years.

Acute Coronary Syndromes

Myocardial perfusion imaging plays an important role in assessing patients who present with symptoms ranging from atypical chest pain to acute myocardial infarction. Rest myocardial perfusion imaging is occasionally used to evaluate patients presenting to the emergency department with chest pain and nondiagnostic electro-cardiography who are suspected of having an acute coronary syndrome. The characteristic of minimal redistribution with ^{99m}Tc-labeled agents allows them to be injected while the patient is having chest pain and imaging is performed at a later time, after resolution of the chest pain. The sensitivity and negative predictive value of acute rest imaging are high; however, if perfusion defects are present, distinguishing between acute ischemia, acute infarct, or chronic infarct is not possible on the basis of rest images alone.

Stress SPECT imaging in patients with unstable angina or non–ST-segment elevation myocardial infarction also can be used for risk stratification in patients treated with an early conservative strategy or for assessment of the hemodynamic significance of a coronary stenosis after coronary angiography. Patients with an ST-segment elevation myocardial infarction are not candidates for acute imaging. In clinically

low- and intermediate-risk patients in the chronic phase of ST-segment elevation myocardial infarction (days 3-21) treated with an initial conservative approach, stress SPECT can be used for risk stratification and for identification of appropriate patients for coronary angiography. Useful information includes perfusion, LVEF, regional wall motion, and detection of viable myocardium. The presence of ischemia or a perfusion defect outside the infarct zone identifies patients at higher risk.

Myocardial Viability

The term *hibernation* refers to a chronic condition of contractile dysfunction in patients with coronary artery disease due to long-standing underperfusion in whom restoration of myocardial blood flow results in recovery of function. Hibernation is usually distinguished from *myocardial stunning*, which is a reduction in myocardial contractility resulting from transient reduction in blood flow. Viable myocardium typically has characteristics of preserved cell membrane integrity, preserved glucose metabolism, and inotropic reserve. These characteristics can be evaluated with nuclear (SPECT and positron emission tomography) techniques.

Rest ^{201}Tl viability protocols consist of immediate images and delayed images at 4 and 24 hours. Initial ^{201}Tl uptake on the immediate images is proportional to myocardial blood flow. Washout of ^{201}Tl occurs more rapidly in normally perfused myocardium and more slowly in areas that are poorly perfused. Over time, the ^{201}Tl concentration can redistribute and equalize between these areas, thereby showing viability on the delayed images (Fig. 9). Myocardial segments that have reduced or absent ^{201}Tl uptake at rest and no further uptake over time reflect areas of myocardial scar. Viability studies with ^{99m}Tc-sestamibi also can be performed, in which uptake is dependent on an intact cell membrane and functioning mitochondria. Studies with ^{99m}Tc-sestamibi may underestimate viability in areas with a critically severe stenosis because of its minimal redistribution. Efforts to improve the ability of ^{99m}Tc-sestamibi to correctly identify viable myocardium include performing a 4-hour redistribution image, quantification of the degree of ^{99m}Tc activity in a perfusion defect, use of gated wall motion in combination with radioisotope uptake, and obtaining a nitrate-enhanced image. Currently, the optimal

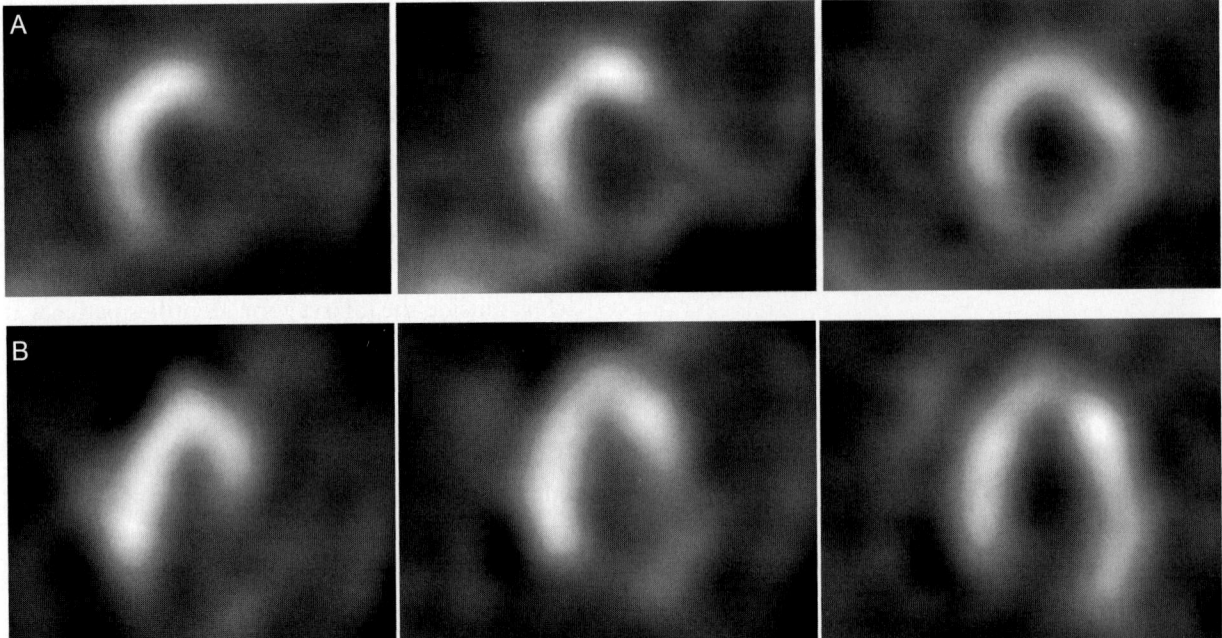

Fig. 9. Thallium viability study (images from left to right represent time 0, 4 hours, and 24 hours), showing viability of the lateral wall on the short-axis (*A*) and horizontal long-axis (*B*) views.

technique for assessing viability is the demonstration of preserved glucose metabolism using fluorine-18-labeled fluorodeoxyglucose on positron emission tomography.

Additional Applications

Although metabolic imaging is ideally assessed with positron emission tomography, imaging of iodine 123 (123I)-labeled fatty acids can be performed with SPECT to assess fatty acid metabolism for detection of myocardial ischemia. Radionuclide imaging has been used to visualize areas of myocardial infarct through the use of 99mTc-pyrophosphate or indium 111-labeled antibodies to cardiac myosin (hot-spot imaging). These agents localize to areas of infarct. Unfortunately, the images are often of poor quality, and these approaches are not being currently used. In addition to use in myocardial infarct imaging, antimyosin imaging has been used to assess myocarditis and rejection after

cardiac transplantation. Imaging in congestive heart failure is expanding to include the use of 123I-m-iodobenzylguanidine and carbon 11-hydroxy-ephedrine for evaluating cardiac innervation and the potential use of 99mTc-labeled annexin V for the non-invasive imaging of apoptosis. Further research is ongoing in radionuclide imaging of atherosclerotic lesions and vulnerable plaques.

LIMITATIONS

Nuclear cardiology is a valuable technique in clinical practice, but it does have limitations. Accurate nuclear cardiology imaging necessitates well-qualified and experienced personnel at all steps in the process, including image acquisition, processing, and interpretation. Nuclear imaging requires radiation exposure and is expensive. For these reasons, it should be applied in patients who have appropriate indications.

12

POSITRON EMISSION TOMOGRAPHY

Panithaya Chareonthaitawee, MD

PRINCIPLES OF POSITRON EMISSION TOMOGRAPHY

Cardiac positron emission tomography (PET), previously used primarily in research, is gaining wider acceptance as a valuable diagnostic tool. Several inherent characteristics of PET contribute to its high spatial, temporal, and contrast resolution; high diagnostic accuracy; and utility for quantifying physiologic processes in absolute terms. These characteristics include high-energy tracers, coincidence detection, and built-in attenuation correction.

PET tracers emit positrons, which collide with electrons of nearby atoms in annihilation reactions. Each reaction releases two high-energy (511 keV) photons that travel at 180° to each other. When a pair of radiation detectors is set up at opposite ends of the 180° line (in a coincidence circuit), the time difference from when one photon strikes one radiation detector to when the other photon strikes the other detector in the coincidence circuit is used to localize precisely the source of the annihilation event. Hundreds of such pairs of radiation detectors are arranged in a circular fashion around the PET gantry to detect millions of counts per second. This unique coincidence detection scheme for forming tomographic images is used for all PET tracers.

PET has built-in attenuation correction. When a radioactive tracer is administered to a subject, the photons traveling outward may be attenuated in the setting of large body habitus, dense tissue (e.g., breasts), or overlying diaphragm. This can lead to an apparent reduction in the observed amount of tracer uptake (Fig. 1, *top row*). An external radiation source on the PET scanner (either germanium-68 line sources or computed tomography [CT] in hybrid PET-CT systems) allows a transmission scan to be acquired for correction of the emission image (image after PET tracer administration) to yield a superior attenuation-corrected image (Fig. 1, *middle* and *bottom rows*).

Another unique feature of PET is the ability to radiolabel many naturally occurring compounds and to quantify specific physiologic processes in absolute terms through tracer kinetic modeling. Such measurements include global and regional myocardial blood flow (MBF), myocardial glucose utilization (MGU), oxidative metabolism, and cardiac neuronal function, among others.

CARDIAC PET RADIOPHARMACEUTICALS

The general principles of radiopharmaceuticals are discussed in Chapter 11 ("Nuclear Imaging"). While many single-photon emission CT (SPECT) tracers are generator-produced, the majority of PET tracers are produced by a cyclotron, a particle accelerator that

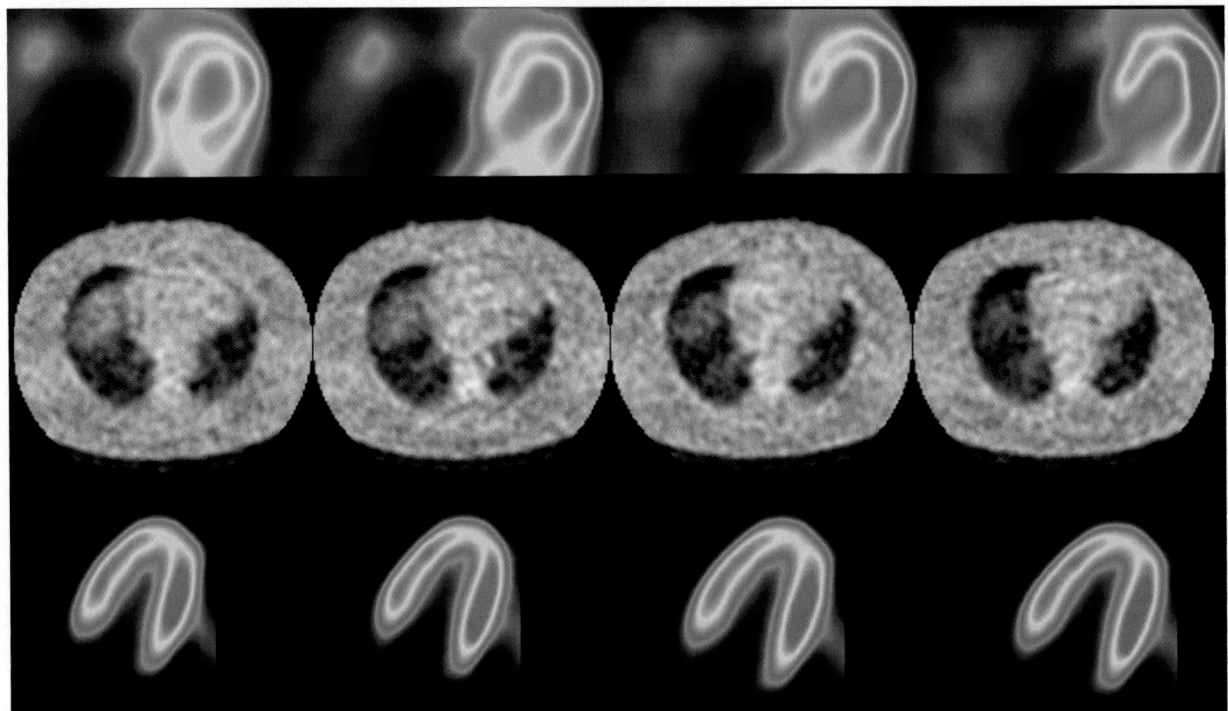

Fig. 1. *Top row*, Positron emission tomographic (PET) rubidium-82 (^{82}Rb) emission image without attenuation correction. *Middle row*, PET transmission image using germanium-68 line sources. *Bottom row*, Same PET ^{82}Rb image after attenuation correction demonstrates more homogeneous tracer uptake with overall improved image quality.

requires specialized facilities. The most commonly used PET tracers in clinical cardiology and their characteristics are listed in Table 1. In cardiology practice, there are two main categories of PET tracers: those predominantly measuring myocardial perfusion and those predominantly measuring myocardial metabolism.

PET Perfusion Tracers

The most commonly used PET perfusion tracers in clinical practice in the United States are nitrogen-13 (^{13}N)-ammonia and rubidium-82 (^{82}Rb)-chloride. Oxygen-15 (^{15}O)-water deserves mention because it has properties of an ideal perfusion tracer.

^{13}N must be produced by an in-house or a very nearby cyclotron because its physical half-life is only 9.8 minutes. ^{13}N-ammonia has a high first-pass extraction fraction of nearly 100%. Tissue retention of ^{13}N-ammonia is prolonged owing to metabolic trapping by the glutamine synthetase pathway. The net extraction fraction is approximately 80% with flows in the resting range, but it decreases with hyperemic flow values. The presence of ^{13}N-ammonia myocardial uptake is also a marker of myocardial viability. However, the absence of uptake may reflect poor perfusion, in which case additional viability studies are needed. Despite some dependence on myocardial metabolism and possible flow underestimation at very high flow rates, ^{13}N-ammonia provides the best quality perfusion images for visual analysis owing to the relatively long physical half-life, the relatively high extraction fraction, and the low background and low liver activity (Fig. 2). Absolute quantification of MBF in milliliters per minute per gram can also be performed with use of ^{13}N-ammonia dynamic imaging and well-validated tracer kinetic models. The duration of each ^{13}N-ammonia image acquisition is approximately 10 to 20 minutes, depending on the mode of acquisition (static or dynamic; two-dimensional or three-dimensional) and the PET scanner characteristics. Simultaneous gated acquisition for assessment of left ventricular (LV) volumes and systolic function is feasible and adds incremental value to perfusion data. ^{13}N-ammonia is approved by the Food and Drug Administration

Table 1.   Characteristics of the Most Commonly Used Positron Emission Tomographic Tracers in Cardiology

Feature	N-13 ammonia	Rubidium-82	O-15 water	[18]FDG
Production	Cyclotron	Generator (strontium 82)	Cyclotron	Cyclotron
Physical half-life	9.8 min	75 s	122 s	110 min
Positron range	0.4 mm	2.8 mm	1.1 mm	0.3 mm
Physiology	Extracted (first pass 100%; net 80% at rest)	Extracted (60% at rest)	Freely diffusible	Glucose analogue
Visual image quality	+++++	++++	+	+++++
Measures	Predominantly perfusion	Predominantly perfusion	Perfusion	Myocardial glucose metabolism (viability)
FDA approval	Yes	Yes	No	Yes
Medicare reimbursement	Yes	Yes	No	Yes

FDA, Food and Drug Administration; [18]FDG, fluorine-18–labeled fluorodeoxyglucose; N, nitrogen; O, oxygen.

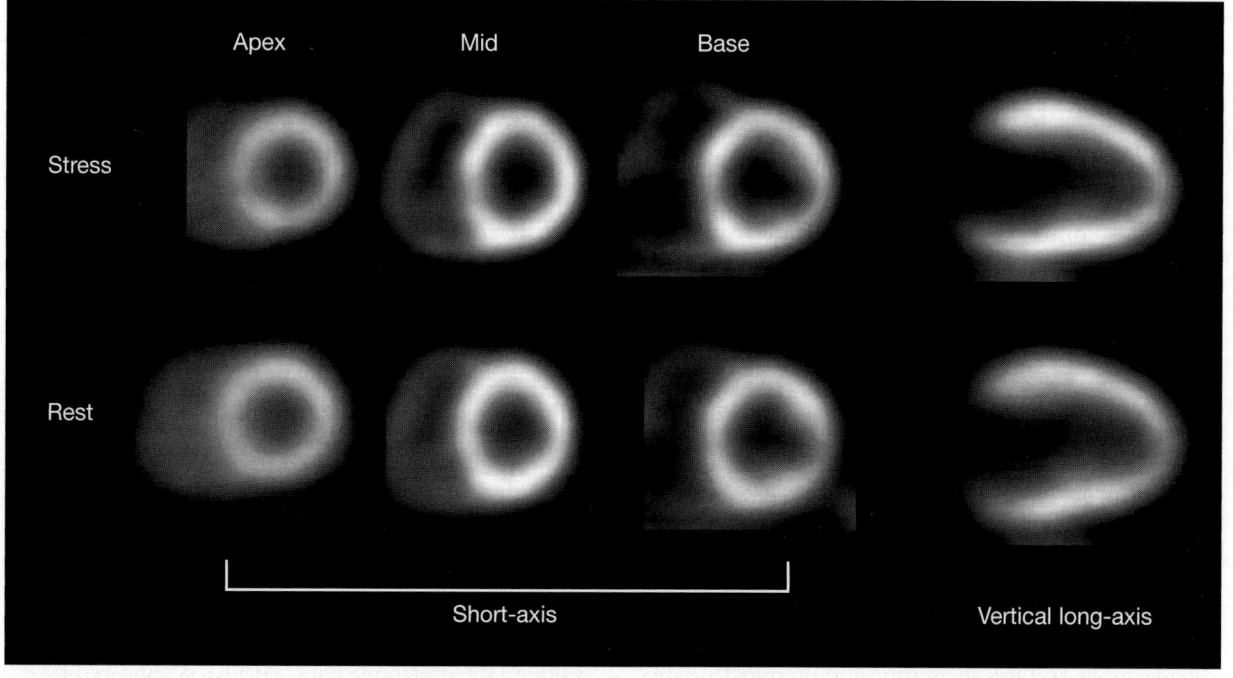

Fig. 2. Short-axis and vertical long-axis positron emission tomography nitrogen-13 ammonia rest and stress myocardial perfusion images. There is homogeneous tracer uptake, consistent with normal perfusion at rest and with stress.

(FDA) and is reimbursed by Medicare for the assessment of myocardial perfusion.

82Rb is produced from a commercially available strontium-82 generator, which has a physical half-life of 23 days and can elute the tracer every 10 minutes. The major advantage of 82Rb is the ability to obtain myocardial perfusion images without a cyclotron, which can add considerable capital and maintenance costs. However, the strontium-82 generator must be replaced every month, and this expense should be considered in the context of patient volumes. 82Rb has a physical half-life of 75 seconds. Its uptake in tissue is similar to that of potassium, and like thallium-201, it requires an active sodium-potassium–adenosine triphosphatase pump for intracellular transport. The first-pass extraction fraction is 50% to 60% for resting flow, decreasing to 25% to 30% with high flow, and is reduced in ischemic myocardium. In addition to its role as a perfusion tracer, 82Rb uptake is also a marker of viability since cell membrane disruption may cause its rapid loss from the myocardium. The short physical half-life of 82Rb and its higher energy (thus long positron tract) mildly impair the spatial resolution of the images (Fig. 3). Because of this very short physical half-life of 82Rb, a large dose of tracer must be administered. Absolute quantification of MBF with 82Rb is feasible but is not as well validated as for 13N-ammonia or 15O-water. The duration of each 82Rb image acquisition is approximately 5 to 10 minutes. Simultaneous gated acquisition is also possible (Fig. 4). 82Rb is approved by the FDA and is reimbursed by Medicare for the assessment of myocardial perfusion.

A less commonly used PET perfusion tracer is 15O-water. 15O is produced by a cyclotron and has a physical half-life of 122 seconds. Theoretically, 15O-water is an ideal perfusion tracer because it is freely diffusible and metabolically inert. Its tissue accumulation is almost exclusively a function of flow and it does not underestimate flow at high flow rates. However, its freely diffusible state and very short physical half-life result in poor image contrast resolution (Fig. 5). Visual analysis is generally not feasible and quantification of absolute MBF must be performed, which somewhat limits its use for clinical purposes owing to longer processing times and less diagnostic and prognostic data. 15O-water differs from 13N-ammonia and 82Rb in that gating is not possible with 15O-water and it is

neither approved by the FDA nor reimbursed by Medicare for the assessment of myocardial perfusion.

PET Metabolic Tracers

The most commonly used PET metabolic tracer in cardiology practice is fluorine-18–labeled fluorodeoxyglucose (18FDG). Fluorine 18 is produced by a cyclotron; however, because of its longer physical half-life of 110 minutes, it may be purchased from nearby locations, thus obviating the need for an on-site cyclotron. 18FDG is a glucose analogue and, like glucose, is transported intracellularly by the glucose transporters GLUT-1 and GLUT-4. 18FDG traces the initial transmembranous exchange of glucose from blood into tissue and its subsequent hexokinase-mediated phosphorylation into glucose-6-phosphate. Unlike phosphorylated glucose, FDG-6-phosphate is not a substrate for the glycolytic pathway, the pentose shunt, glycogenesis, or dephosphorylation, and it remains trapped within the myocytes. Under normal fasting conditions, the human heart primarily uses free fatty acids for its energy production. With resting or stress-induced ischemia, a switch from aerobic to anaerobic metabolism is in part responsible for increased MGU. Uptake of 18FDG is also dependent on myocardial substrate use, being low when plasma free fatty acid levels are high and high when plasma glucose and insulin levels are high. Adequate patient preparation is therefore crucial to obtain images of high diagnostic quality, with fasting conditions yielding more inadequate images than glucose-loading protocols. The hyperinsulinemic-euglycemic clamp technique provides controlled metabolic conditions with steady-state plasma insulin and glucose levels and yields high-quality 18FDG images but is time-consuming and difficult to implement. Acipimox, a nicotinic acid derivative, indirectly promotes myocardial glucose uptake but is not approved by the FDA for this purpose. For the assessment of myocardial viability, visual image analysis is generally preferred, but quantification of absolute MGU is also feasible if the hyperinsulinemic-euglycemic clamp is used. The duration of 18FDG acquisition varies from 20 to 60 minutes, depending on the mode of acquisition and scanner type. Electrocardiographic (ECG) gating provides incremental value to the metabolic data. 18FDG is approved by the FDA and reimbursed by Medicare for the assessment of myocardial viability.

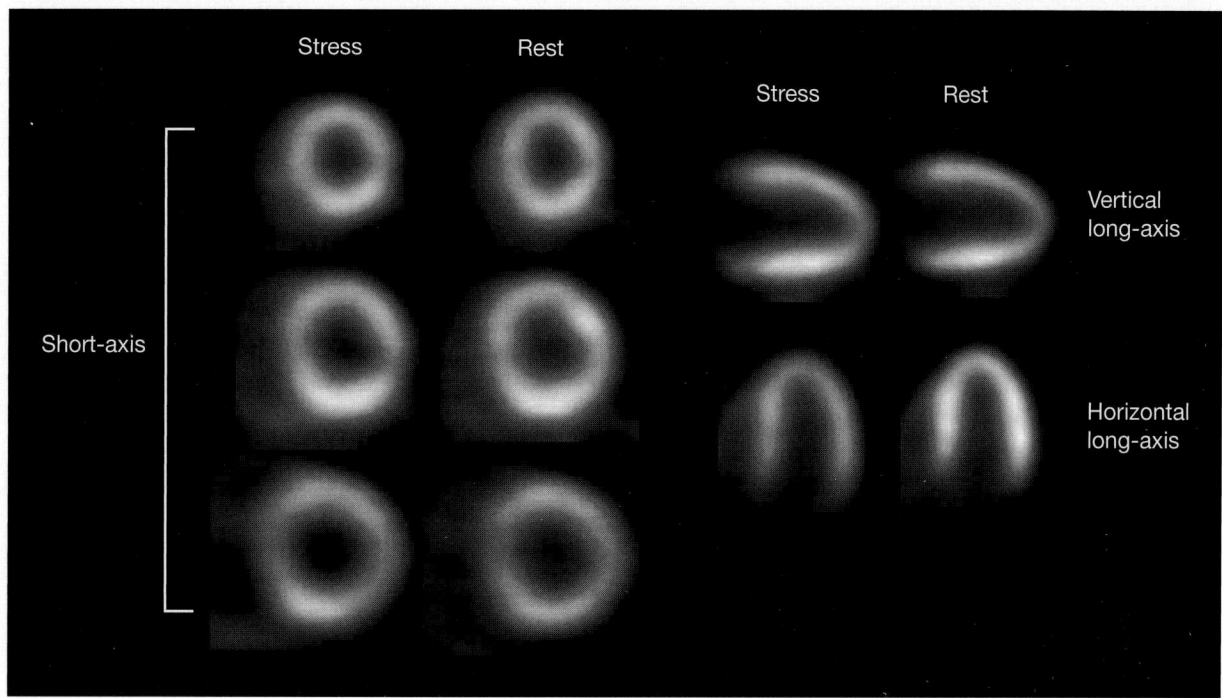

Fig. 3. Short-axis, horizontal long-axis, and vertical long-axis positron emission tomography rubidium-82 rest and stress myocardial perfusion images. There is homogeneous tracer uptake, consistent with normal perfusion at rest and with stress. In the short-axis images (2 columns on left), the 3 rows are apex (*top*), mid (*middle*), and base (*bottom*), and the 2 columns are images with stress (*left*) and at rest (*right*). In the long-axis images (2 columns on right), the 2 rows are vertical long-axis (*top*) and horizontal long-axis (*bottom*), and the 2 columns are images with stress (*left*) and at rest (*right*).

CLINICAL APPLICATIONS

The main clinical applications of cardiac PET are diagnosis of coronary artery disease (CAD) and identification of myocardial viability.

Diagnosis of CAD

A PET rest-stress myocardial perfusion study may be performed for indications similar to those for SPECT, including diagnosing CAD, assessing risk and prognosis, and guiding therapy. PET is particularly useful in technically challenging situations, such as when body habitus is large (e.g., obesity) or tissue is dense (e.g., breasts), when the hemodynamic significance of intermediate angiographic coronary stenosis is assessed, or when inconclusive results are present with other noninvasive imaging methods. PET rest-stress myocardial perfusion studies with approved PET perfusion tracers are reimbursed by Medicare for these appropriate indications.

The PET rest-stress protocol is similar to those of SPECT (see Chapter 11, "Nuclear Imaging"). Because PET perfusion tracers have short physical half-lives, they must be administered at rest and again with stress. Image acquisition must occur simultaneously with tracer administration to avoid the effects of radioactivity decay. Pharmacologic stress is therefore highly preferable, since treadmill exercise cannot be performed simultaneously with image acquisition and supine bicycle stress may introduce considerable upper body motion. Vasodilators such as adenosine or dipyridamole are generally used but may be replaced with dobutamine in patients with a contraindication to vasodilators (see Chapter 11, "Nuclear Imaging"). Treadmill exercise testing with ^{13}N-ammonia injection at peak stress followed immediately by image acquisition has been performed at a few institutions but requires considerable technical expertise. Examples of ^{13}N-ammonia and [82]Rb rest-stress protocols are shown in Figure 6.

For the diagnosis of CAD, visual analysis of PET

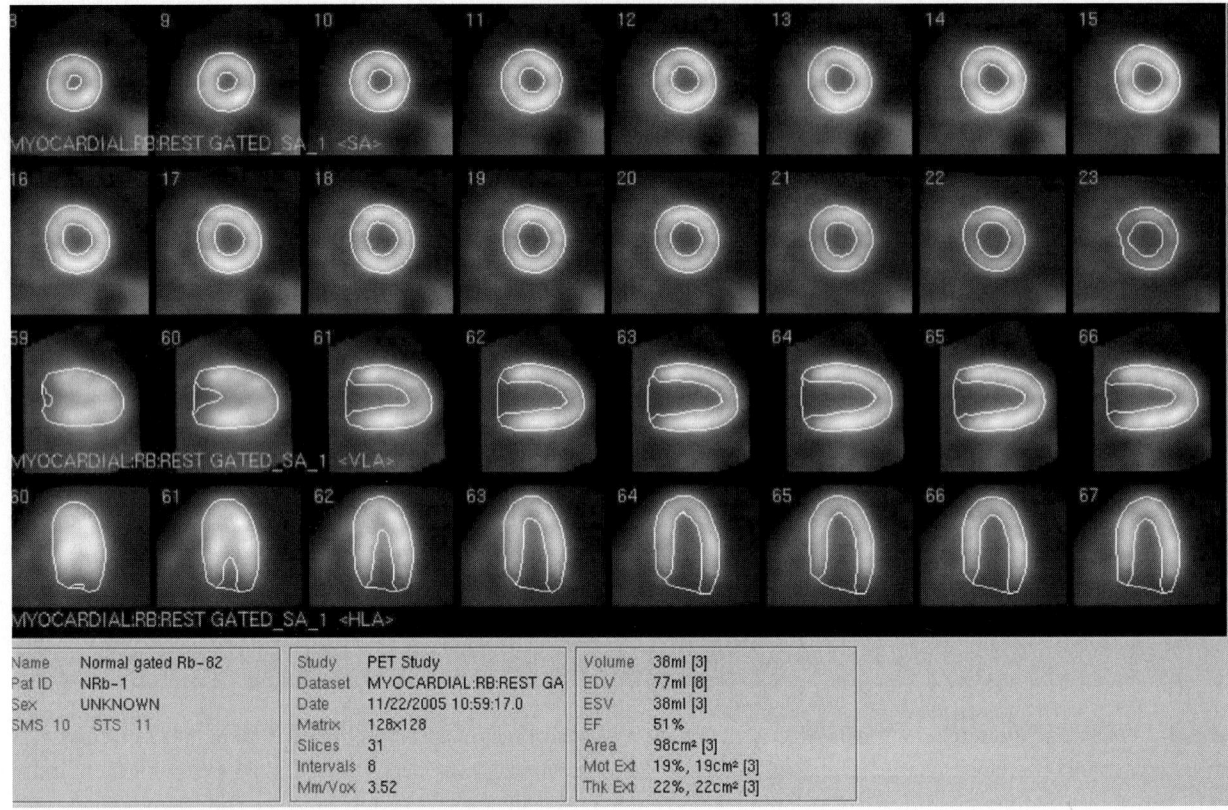

Name	Normal gated Rb-82	Study	PET Study	Volume	38ml [3]
Pat ID	NRb-1	Dataset	MYOCARDIAL:RB:REST GA	EDV	77ml [8]
Sex	UNKNOWN	Date	11/22/2005 10:59:17.0	ESV	38ml [3]
SMS 10 STS 11		Matrix	128x128	EF	51%
		Slices	31	Area	98cm² [3]
		Intervals	8	Mot Ext	19%, 19cm² [3]
		Mm/Vox	3.52	Thk Ext	22%, 22cm² [3]

Fig. 4. Sample computer display of rubidium-82 gated data.

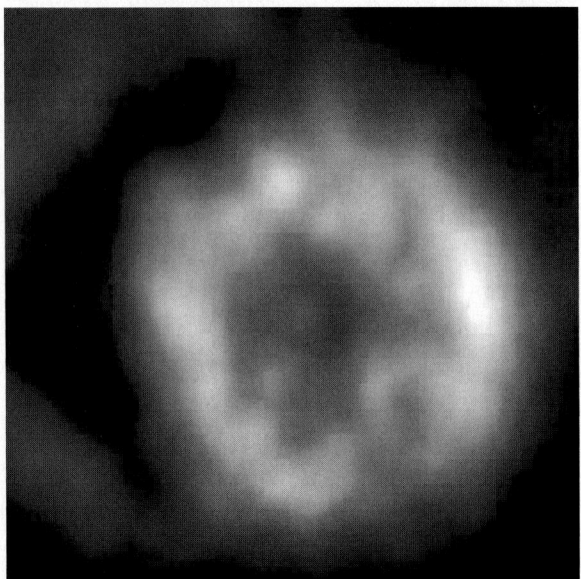

Fig. 5. Short-axis oxygen-15 water perfusion image illustrates poor contrast resolution.

perfusion images is similar to that of SPECT images. Cardiac size and global LV systolic function may be visually assessed but can also be correlated with software-generated ECG-gated LV volumes and LV ejection fraction. Visual assessment of regional LV systolic function can also be performed. Although transient ischemic dilatation (TID) (see Chapter 11, "Nuclear Imaging") has been noted with PET perfusion images and likely implies extensive myocardial ischemia or severe CAD (or both), quantitative measurements of PET TID and their prognostic significance have not been validated as extensively as for SPECT. With visual analysis, PET perfusion in each segment (usually a 16- or 17-segment model) is generally graded using a semiquantitative approach of side-by-side rest and stress images in multiple views (horizontal long-axis, vertical long-axis, and short-axis) to determine the extent, severity, and reversibility of the perfusion defect (Fig. 7). A polar map display or other software-generated quantitative perfusion defect may also be used. A report that incorporates the extent, severity, and reversibility of the perfusion abnormality, along with gated data, is

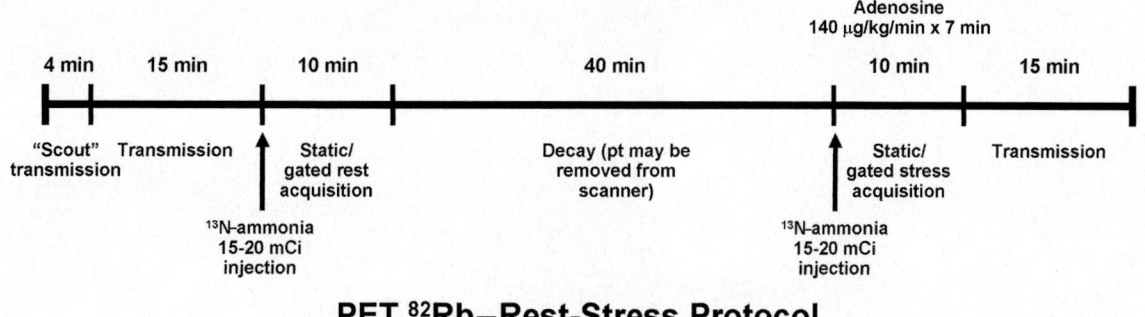

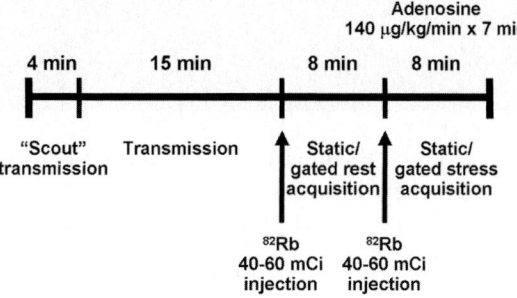

Fig. 6. Examples of positron emission tomographic (PET) nitrogen-13 (^{13}N)-ammonia and rubidium-82 (^{82}Rb)–rest-stress protocols. pt, patient.

most helpful clinically (Fig. 8).

The diagnostic performance of PET ^{13}N-ammonia or ^{82}Rb for detecting obstructive CAD was documented in seven studies published between 1986 and 1992. The mean sensitivity for detecting more than 50% angiographic stenosis was 89% (range, 83%-100%), and the mean specificity was 86% (range, 73%-100%). Two earlier studies performed a head-to-head comparison of the diagnostic accuracy of ^{82}Rb PET and ^{201}thallium SPECT in the same patient population. One study (202 patients) demonstrated a higher sensitivity with PET than with SPECT (93% vs. 76%) and no significant difference in specificity (80% vs. 78%). The second study (81 patients) showed a higher specificity with PET than with SPECT (83% vs. 53%) but no significant difference in sensitivity (84% vs. 86%). Overall diagnostic accuracy was higher with PET than with SPECT (89% vs. 78%) in the second study.

More recently, a study that used contemporary technology compared 112 PET studies with 112 SPECT studies in which patient populations were matched by sex, body mass index, and presence and extent of CAD. Diagnostic accuracy was reported to be higher in the PET studies for the following: 50% and 70% angiographic stenosis, men and women, obese and nonobese patients, and correct identification of multivessel CAD. Many confounding factors challenge the validity of these observational studies, particularly referral bias and the absence of clinical outcomes data.

The prognostic implications of PET rest-stress perfusion findings have been examined in few studies. One study of 685 patients reported the independent prognostic value of PET ^{82}Rb defect extent and severity in predicting cardiac death and total cardiac events and their incremental value to clinical and angiographic data.

In patients with known CAD, absolute coronary blood flow and flow reserve with PET ^{13}N-ammonia or ^{15}O-water are inversely and nonlinearly related to stenosis severity by quantitative angiography. Quantification of flow has the potential to define the functional

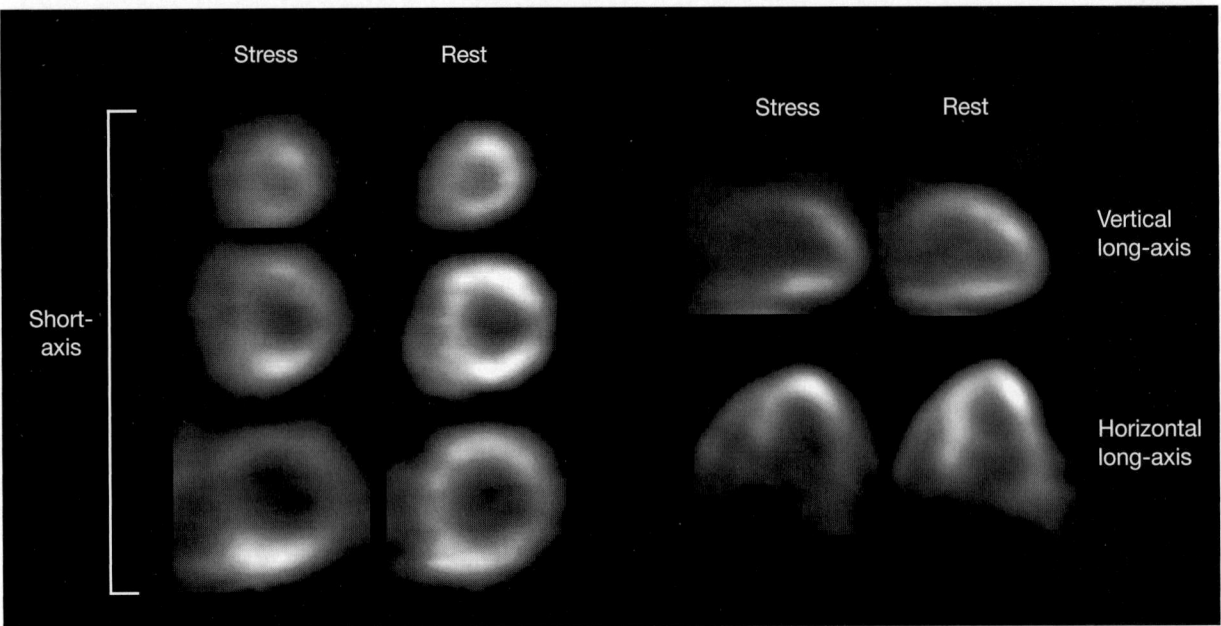

Fig. 7. Short-axis, horizontal long-axis, and vertical long-axis positron emission tomographic rubidium-82 rest and stress myocardial perfusion images. There is a very large, mainly reversible apical, anterior, septal, and lateral perfusion defect consistent with ischemia.

PET Myocardial Perfusion, Multiple Study, Rest & Stress

Isotope: Rubidium 82

Injected dose: rest 44.30 mCi/stress 44.60 mCi

Cardiac enlargement: Yes

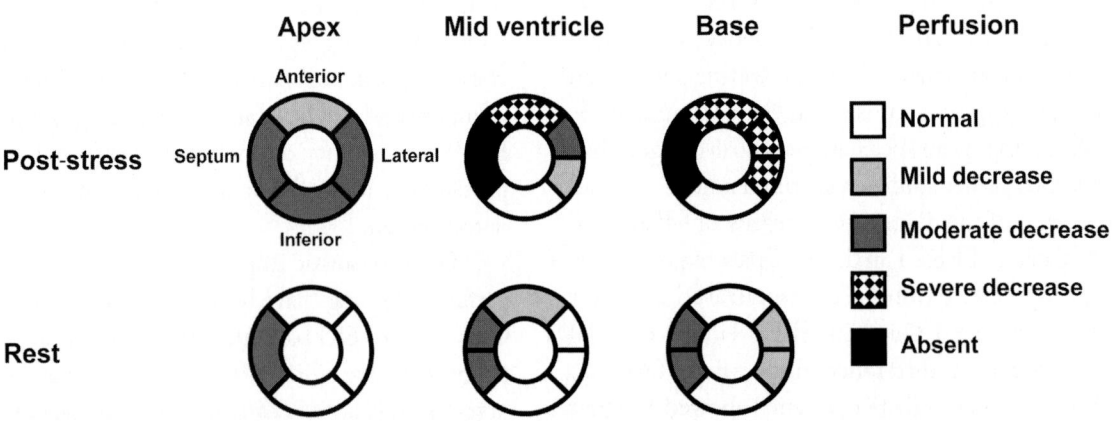

Comments: Very large, mainly reversible apical, anterior, septal, and lateral defect consistent with abnormal flow reserve with areas of partial viability. ECG changes in the presence of adenosine suggest ischemia and severe CAD. The rest gated PET LVEF was 32%. The post-stress gated PET LVEF was 25%; this decrease in LVEF is consistent with severe ischemia. There is also post-stress LV dilatation. Gated PET wall motion was moderately hypokinetic globally with preserved motion only in the inferior wall.

Fig. 8. Sample positron emission tomographic (PET) rest-stress report corresponding to the PET images in Figure 7. CAD, coronary artery disease; ECG, electrocardiographic; LV, left ventricular; LVEF, left ventricular ejection fraction.

importance of known epicardial coronary stenosis and, in the setting of "balanced ischemia," may help to uncover additional areas of at-risk myocardium that otherwise would not be identified with relative perfusion techniques. More studies are needed in these areas.

Identification of Myocardial Viability

In patients with CAD, the myocardium has short-term and long-term responses to ischemic processes, which may result in stunned or hibernating but viable myocardium (see Chapter 11, "Nuclear Imaging"). Accurate identification of this viable myocardium in specific subsets of patients with ischemic LV systolic dysfunction has crucial therapeutic and prognostic implications. Specifically, revascularization may improve LV systolic function, symptoms, and survival in patients with a substantial amount of hypocontractile but viable myocardium.

PET has traditionally been considered the criterion standard for viability assessment. In patients with moderate to severe ischemic cardiomyopathy or prior myocardial infarction (or both), PET is indicated for the determination of myocardial viability either as the initial diagnostic study or after inconclusive SPECT, particularly if the patient is a potential candidate for revascularization. PET viability studies are reimbursed by Medicare for these appropriate indications.

The most commonly used PET viability protocol consists of an assessment of resting regional myocardial perfusion, generally with ^{13}N-ammonia or ^{82}Rb, in conjunction with an assessment of resting regional MGU, with ^{18}FDG. Visual assessment of regional perfusion and regional glucose uptake can be performed using a semiquantitative approach of side-by-side perfusion and ^{18}FDG images in multiple views. With this approach, three distinct perfusion and metabolism patterns in dysfunctional myocardium have been described: 1) normal blood flow and normal ^{18}FDG uptake; 2) decreased blood flow with preserved or enhanced ^{18}FDG uptake (perfusion-metabolism mismatch) (Fig. 9); and 3) proportional decrease in perfusion and ^{18}FDG uptake (perfusion-metabolism match). A severe PET perfusion-metabolism match (Fig. 10) indicates scar tissue with a low likelihood of contractile recovery after revascularization. The PET perfusion-metabolism mismatch is considered the hallmark of hibernating myocardium and has a high

likelihood of contractile recovery after revascularization. Pattern 1 (i.e., normal blood flow and normal ^{18}FDG uptake) also represents viable tissue with potential benefit from revascularization on the basis of stress-induced ischemia or repetitive stunning, if the anatomical features are appropriate. There is uncertainty about the benefits of revascularization in patients with mild or moderate PET matched perfusion-metabolism defects. The reverse mismatch pattern (normal perfusion and reduced ^{18}FDG uptake) has been described in myocardial stunning and left bundle branch block or paced rhythm. Knowledge of regional contractile function is crucial to the interpretation of PET perfusion and ^{18}FDG images, and LV functional parameters by gated ^{18}FDG PET add incremental prognostic value. Other important information in the interpretation of PET perfusion and ^{18}FDG images includes the clinical history, the patient's metabolic status and preparation protocol, and the coronary anatomy, if available.

The current literature on the diagnostic accuracy of noninvasive viability techniques has many limitations, including the following: use of contractile recovery after revascularization as a surrogate for viability, observational and nonrandomized nature of studies, early contractile assessment and follow-up after revascularization, small sample size of studies, referral bias, varied protocols, limited follow-up, and lack of graft or vessel patency information at follow-up.

In a 2001 analysis of 20 studies and 598 patients with ^{18}FDG PET, the mean sensitivity for detecting regional contractile recovery after revascularization was 93% (range, 71%-100%) and mean specificity was 58% (range, 33%-91%). However, the studies with the lowest specificity did not use the combined perfusion-metabolism approach; instead, they used a quantitative ^{18}FDG PET approach with a threshold absolute MGU value. In comparative studies, PET showed evidence of viability in approximately 15% of patients with large, severe, fixed SPECT defects, and its diagnostic accuracy appears to be less affected by the severity of regional and global LV systolic dysfunction than the accuracy of other techniques that rely on the assessment of changes in contractile function.

The magnitude of improvement in global LV systolic function after revascularization is related to the amount of viable myocardium identified by PET

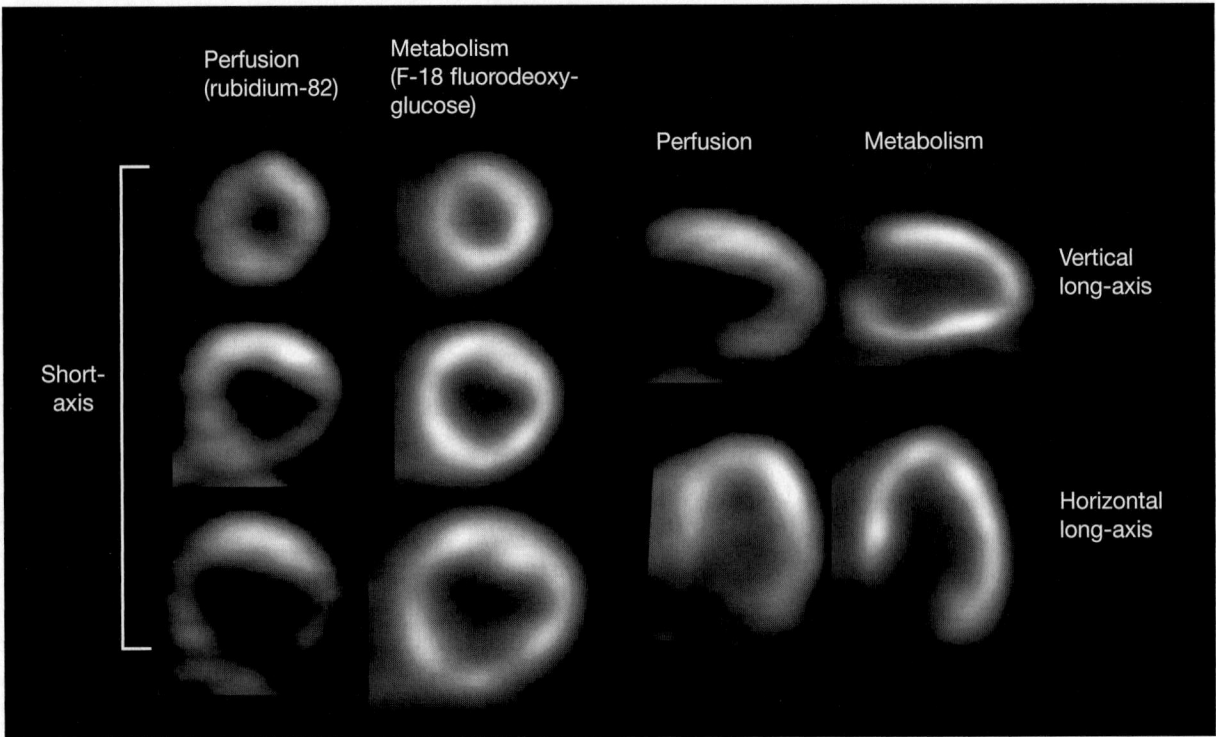

Fig. 9. Short-axis, horizontal long-axis, and vertical long-axis positron emission tomographic viability (rest rubidium-82 perfusion and rest fluorine-18–labeled fluorodeoxyglucose metabolism) images demonstrating a large perfusion-metabolism mismatch in the apical, septal, inferior, and lateral regions. This pattern, considered the hallmark of hibernating myocardium, indicates a high likelihood of functional recovery after revascularization.

before revascularization. This amount has ranged from 17% to 67% of the LV in various [18]FDG PET studies. It has been suggested that 25% of the LV is the minimal amount of dysfunctional but viable myocardium that is required before revascularization in order to observe an improvement in global LV systolic function after revascularization.

PET viability imaging is also used to predict prognosis and functional outcome for patients with ischemic cardiomyopathy. Medically treated patients with a significant amount of viable myocardium on PET imaging have the lowest survival rate. Survival is significantly improved with revascularization compared with medical therapy only if a significant amount of viable myocardium is present. Similarly, there is no difference in survival between medical therapy and revascularization in the absence of viable myocardium. In several small studies, improvement in symptoms and exercise capacity after revascularization was modestly related to the preoperative presence

and extent of dysfunctional but viable (on PET) myocardium.

FUTURE DIRECTIONS

Newer hybrid PET/multidetector CT technology provides the potential of combined assessments of coronary anatomy, atherosclerotic burden, and possible plaque characterization, along with the physiologic significance and cardiac anatomy and function in a single session. Several approaches to assess microvascular dysfunction with PET are also being developed. More studies are needed in these areas.

LIMITATIONS

PET lacks standardization in many areas, including patient preparation, particularly for viability studies, tracer administration, image acquisition, and data analysis and interpretation. Fewer data are available on the normal

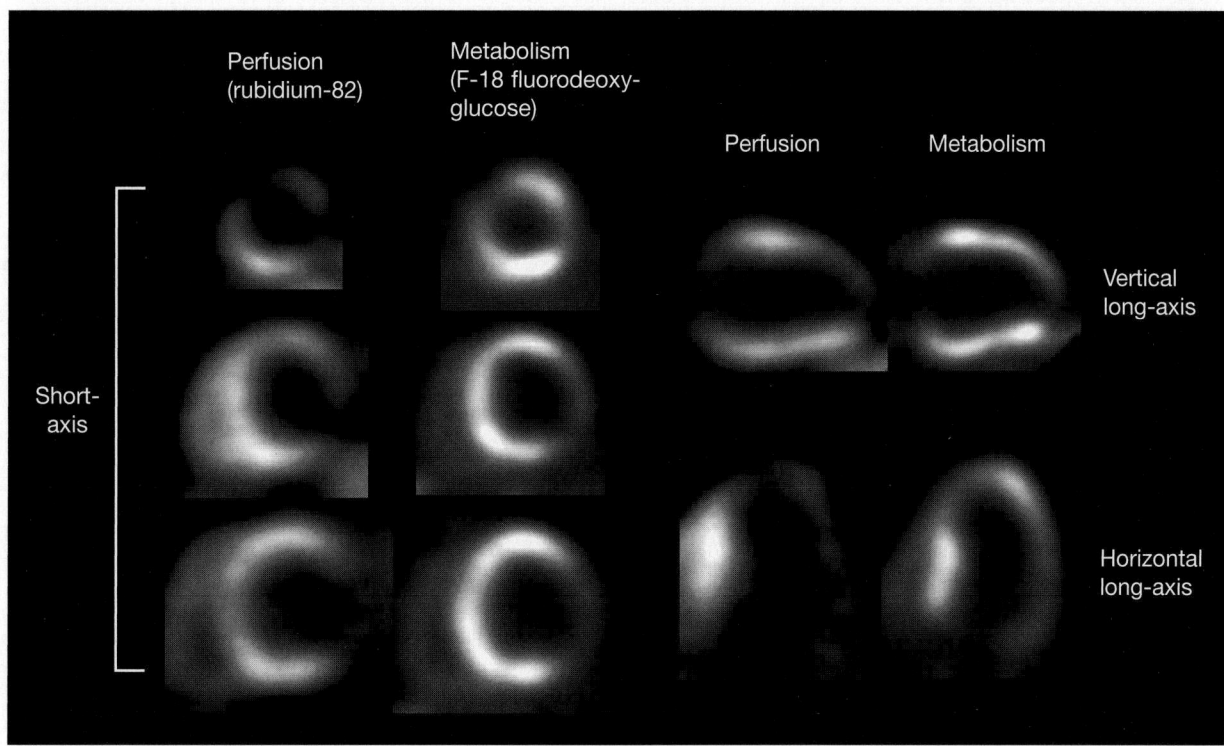

Fig. 10. Short-axis, horizontal long-axis, and vertical long-axis positron emission tomographic viability (rest rubidium-82 perfusion and rest fluorine-18–labeled fluorodeoxyglucose metabolism) images demonstrating a large, severe perfusion-metabolism match in the lateral wall, consistent with scar tissue that has a low likelihood of functional recovery after revascularization. On the same images, there is also evidence of a medium-sized apical and anterior perfusion-metabolism mismatch consistent with hibernating myocardium.

distribution of PET tracer uptake than on SPECT imaging. Limited commercial software is an issue, particularly for quantitative analysis. Coregistration between transmission and emission and between CT and PET images is still problematic. Exercise PET remains particularly challenging because of the short physical half-lives of PET perfusion tracers. Capital costs for equipment and an in-house cyclotron are substantial. More studies are needed on the diagnostic performance, cost-effectiveness, and prognostic significance of PET studies.

CARDIOVASCULAR COMPUTED TOMOGRAPHY AND MAGNETIC RESONANCE IMAGING

Thomas C. Gerber, MD, PhD

Eric M. Walser, MD

Image formation in clinical computed tomography (CT) relies on the mathematical conversion, by filtered back-projection, of projection data that have been obtained by measuring with detectors the attenuation of a fan-shaped x-ray beam from many angles around the patient. Image formation in clinical magnetic resonance imaging (MRI) relies on the alignment of hydrogen nuclei or protons along an external magnetic field. The alignment and angular momentum (spin) of these particles can be excited if radiofrequency pulses are applied at the so-called Lamor frequency. The relaxation of the particles toward their original alignment in the magnetic field produces an MRI signal that can measured by external receiver coils. Each excitation-relaxation sequence results in one line of data to be used for image reconstruction, typically by Fourier transformation.

With current technology, CT examinations are faster and easier to perform than MRI examinations and, therefore, are more widely offered. Current CT scanners acquire a complete three-dimensional dataset that can be reformatted in any arbitrary plane after the examination is complete. Most MR pulse sequences acquire multiple parallel slices or slab-shaped volumes that do, for example, not encompass the entire heart. Most MRI examinations consist of many image acquisitions, and experience is needed to obtain the desired views. As a means to avoid misregistration and motion artifacts, data acquisition or image reconstruction with both methods is performed relative to the electrocardiogram and often also to the respiratory cycle. However, such gating increases the time required to complete a scan.

Depending on the type of scanner used, the x-ray dose received from a cardiac CT examination can be higher than that received from selective, invasive coronary angiography and similar to that received from several hundred chest x-rays. Compared with CT, MRI can have higher temporal resolution but has lower spatial resolution. Gadolinium, the contrast agent used in MRI, is less nephrotoxic than the iodinated contrast media needed for many CT examinations. MRI cannot safely be performed in the presence of many metallic medical implants, including the growing number of patients with coronary artery disease who have received an implantable cardioverter-defibrillator. However, the presence of coronary artery stents is not a contraindication to performing MRI, even if placed more recently than 6 to 8 weeks previously. Device compatibility and MRI safety information is available on the Internet at http://www.mrisafety.com/ and from other sources, such as the U. S. Food and Drug Administration.

CARDIAC CT AND MRI

High temporal and spatial resolution are needed to obtain images of the beating heart and of the small-caliber, often tortuous coronary arteries which are detailed and free of motion artifact. Attaining high temporal and spatial resolution is difficult and can be mutually exclusive. Recent developments in CT scanner technology and the programming of MRI pulse sequences have made cardiac CT (CCT) and cardiac MR (CMR) widely available and frequently used.

Two types of CT scanners can be used for CCT imaging: multirow detector CT and electron beam CT. Multirow detector CT is much more widely available than electron beam CT, but much of the evidence base, particularly for coronary calcium scanning, has been developed with electron beam CT. Contemporary multirow detector CT scanners acquire at least 64 image slices simultaneously, and each gantry rotation lasts 330 milliseconds or less.

Most CMR examinations are performed on scanners with a field strength of 1.5 T, but initial experience with 3-T scanners has been reported. Spin echo sequences (black-blood technique) are used for anatomical imaging, and gradient echo sequences (bright-blood technique) are used for functional imaging.

With current technology, CCT and CMR have distinct areas of strength, and which method is to be used often depends on the clinical objective. To date, neither the American Heart Association nor the American College of Cardiology has guidelines for the use of CCT and CMR.

The field of view in CCT and CMR imaging is not limited to the heart. Frequent incidental findings on these examinations include patent foramen ovale (Fig. 1), atrial or ventricular thrombi (Fig. 2), and calcified lymph nodes and pulmonary nodules.

Cardiac CT

A frequent, appropriate noncoronary indication for CCT is pericardial disease, for example, to visualize pericardial thickness and calcifications (Fig. 3).

Coronary Artery Calcium Scanning

Coronary artery calcification is an active process that begins in the early stages of atherosclerosis and is regulated similar to the calcification of bone. Because calcium has high x-ray attenuation, it can be detected sensitively by CT. The quantity of coronary calcium, usually determined as Agatston score, volume score, or calcium mass, is roughly proportional to, but represents only approximately one-fifth of, the coronary plaque burden. Race and socioeconomic factors affect the prevalence of coronary artery calcification in ways not explained solely by differences in risk factor profiles.

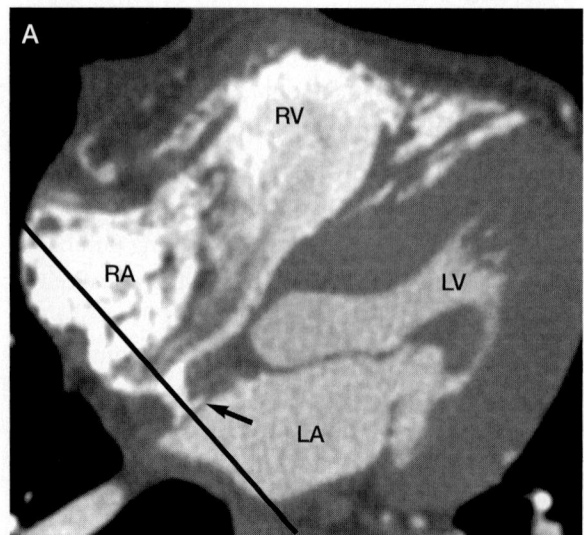 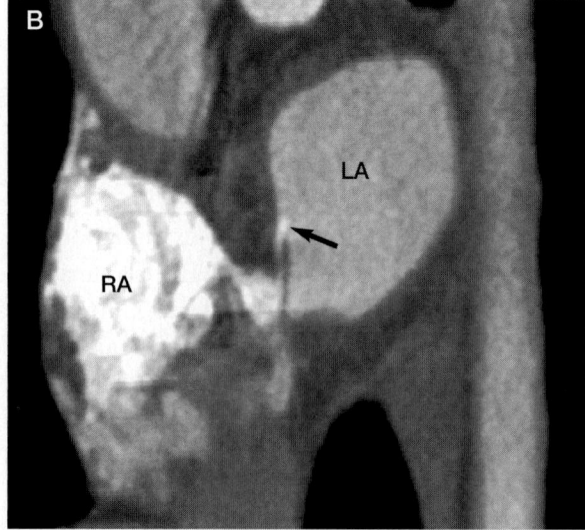

Fig. 1. Computed tomograms of patent foramen ovale (PFO). *A*, Horizontal long-axis view. The fossa ovalis membrane (*arrow*) is visible. Line indicates plane in which Figure 1 *B* is reformatted. *B*, A small amount of contrast (*arrow*) traverses through the PFO from the right atrium (RA) into the left atrium (LA). LV, left ventricle; RV, right ventricle.

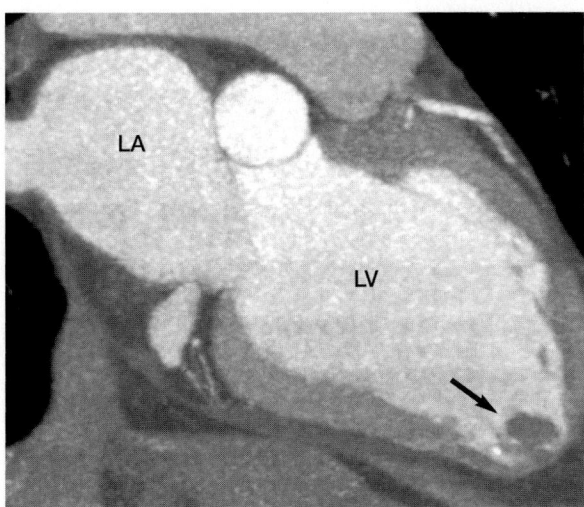

Fig. 2. Vertical long-axis view of thrombus (*arrow*) in left ventricular apex seen with computed tomography. LA, left atrium; LV, left ventricle.

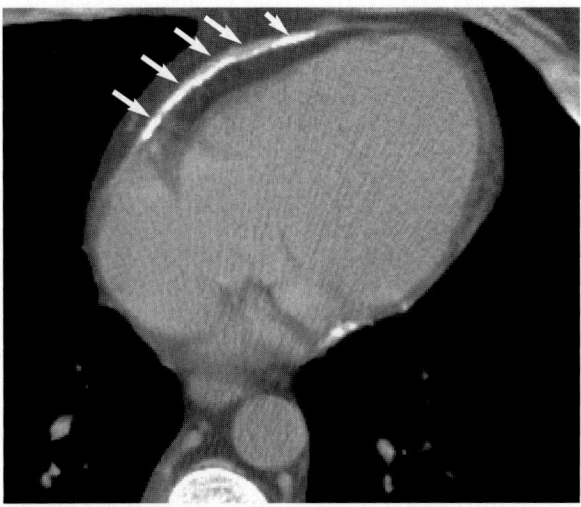

Fig. 3. Computed tomogram of thickened and calcified anterior pericardium (*arrows*) in a patient with catheter-proven constrictive pericarditis.

Because of the variable biologic process of vascular remodeling, not all plaque results in luminal narrowing. A high quantity of calcium may be present on CCT in the absence of coronary stenoses. In asymptomatic patients, a high coronary calcium score alone should not trigger a decision to perform coronary angiography. However, in patients symptomatic with chest pain, the presence of coronary calcification predicts the presence of coronary luminal diameter stenoses exceeding 50% of a reference segment with high sensitivity (~90%) but only moderate specificity (~50%). Diagnostic accuracy can be improved if the quantity, not just the presence, of coronary calcium is considered and if age- and sex-specific threshold values for the calcium score are used to predict the presence of coronary stenoses. The absence of coronary artery calcium predicts the absence of coronary artery stenoses with very high accuracy.

The exact relationship between coronary artery calcification and the presence of plaque likely to cause acute coronary syndromes is poorly understood. Various theories hold that calcification stabilizes plaque and makes it less likely to rupture, that spotty calcification of plaques creates interfaces between tissue with differing mechanical properties at which shear stress can mechanically induce plaque rupture, or that calcified plaques and plaques likely to rupture colocalize.

Despite these uncertainties, coronary calcium scanning with CT is increasingly used as a screening technique to predict future cardiac events.

Most of the studies examining the prognostic value of coronary calcium reported to date have important methodologic shortcomings, and well-designed population-based studies are currently ongoing. The current data suggest that the rates of adverse cardiac events are higher in patients with coronary calcification (Fig. 4 *A*) than in patients without (Fig. 4 *B*) and that the odds ratio and relative risk increase with increasing calcium scores (adjusted relative risk for death or myocardial infarction, between 2.1 and 17.0). Coronary calcification may allow refining risk prediction in patients with an intermediate risk of cardiovascular events based on the Framingham risk score, particularly if the calcium score is high (e.g., Agatston score >300). Currently, it is not clear whether absolute calcium scores or age- and sex-adjusted percentiles are the better predictor of cardiovascular risk. However, there is no evidence that the rate of progression of coronary calcification measured by serial CT can be attenuated by pharmacologic preventive therapy. Similarly, to date, no outcomes studies suggest that making the findings on coronary calcium scanning the basis of decisions for pharmacologic management of risk factors will improve the prognosis of patients with high coronary artery calcium scores.

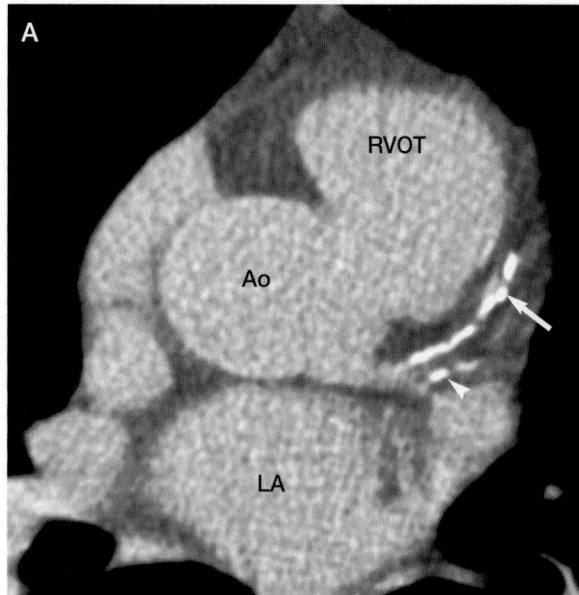 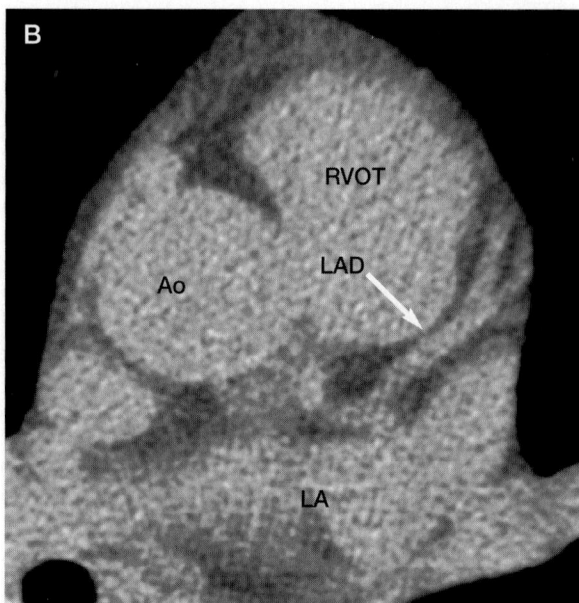

Fig. 4. Transaxial computed tomograms without contrast enhancement. *A*, Patient with calcification of left anterior descending artery (*arrow*) and intermediate branch (*arrowhead*). *B*, Patient without coronary artery calcifications. Ao, aorta; LA, left atrium; LAD, left anterior descending artery; RVOT, right ventricular outflow tract.

Coronary CT Angiography

CT angiography (CTA) can, under many circumstances, create detailed and appealing images of epicardiacal coronary artery branches with a diameter of approximately 1.5 mm or more (Fig. 5). The diagnostic accuracy of coronary CTA improves with every new generation of CT scanners. Numerous single-center studies at experienced institutions, each including limited numbers of patients, suggest that coronary CTA with contemporary 64-slice multidetector scanners can identify, with high sensitivity (88%-100%) and specificity (85%-97%), among patients referred for catheter-based, selective coronary angiography, those with at least one coronary luminal diameter stenosis exceeding 50% of a reference segment (Fig. 6). To date, no studies support the use of coronary CTA as a first-line approach to the diagnosis of coronary artery disease in place of stress testing. Similarly, no studies have examined the prognostic value of screening coronary CTA in asymptomatic patients at intermediate or high risk of cardiac events. In particular, the prognostic implications of detecting noncalcified plaque (Fig. 7) not large enough to cause high-grade luminal stenosis are not established, although some comparative studies with histopathologic results or intravascular ultrasono-

graphic findings suggest that such plaques can have features associated with an increased likelihood of vulnerability or rupture.

Coronary CTA can, with sensitivity and specificity of 95% or more, detect luminal diameter stenoses exceeding 50% of a reference segment in, or occlusion of, coronary artery bypass grafts (Fig. 8). Coronary CTA can also with greater ease than invasive, catheter-based coronary angiography determine whether the proximal course of coronary arteries with congenitally abnormal origin is between the pulmonary artery and the aorta (Fig. 9). It is important to unequivocally make this determination because such congenital coronary anomalies can be associated with sudden cardiac death. However, in younger patients, CMR imaging may be preferred to coronary CTA for this purpose to avoid radiation exposure.

The following might be considered appropriate indications for coronary CTA: clarifying the anatomy of suspected or known congenital anomalies of coronary artery origin, examining clinically important coronary artery bypass grafts that could not be engaged selectively during cardiac catheterization, patients with typical symptoms or abnormal results of stress testing who refuse cardiac catheterization or are at high risk for

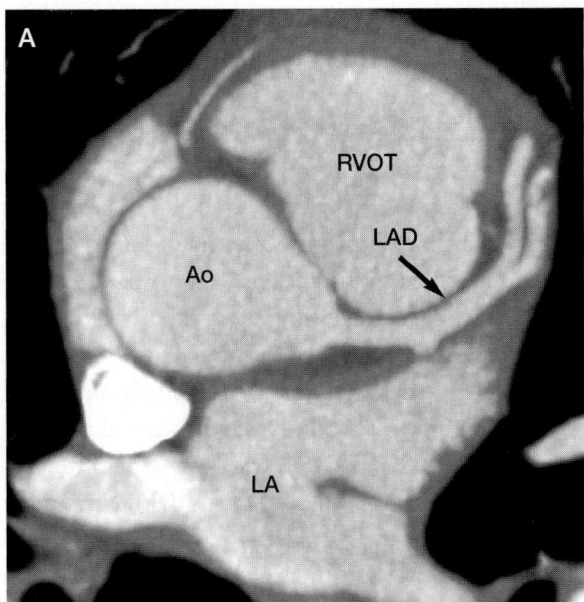
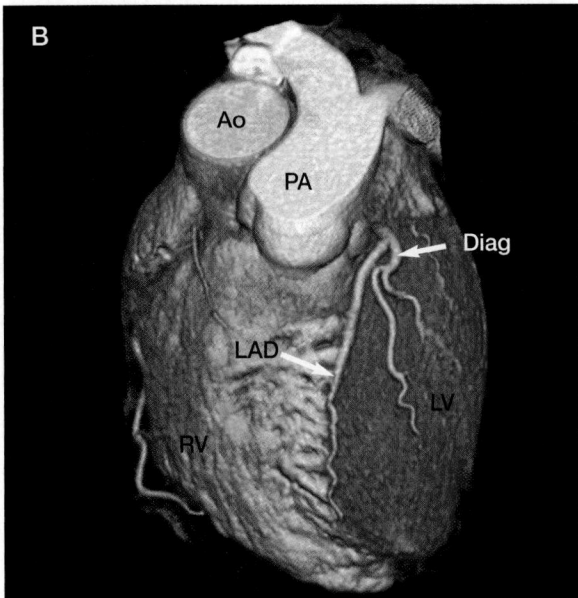

Fig. 5. Coronary computed tomographic angiograms obtained from a patient without coronary calcifications or coronary artery stenoses. *A*, Contrast-enhanced transaxial view. *B*, Volume rendering. Ao, aorta; Diag, diagonal branch; LA, left atrium; LAD, left anterior descending artery; PA, pulmonary artery; RV, right ventricle; RVOT, right ventricular outflow tract.

atheroembolic complications, and patients with atypical symptoms or nondiagnostic results of stress tests in whom coronary disease could not convincingly be established.

Coronary CTA with current technology should not be considered an alternative if invasive, selective coronary angiography seems indicated. In particular, the following scenarios are not acceptable indications

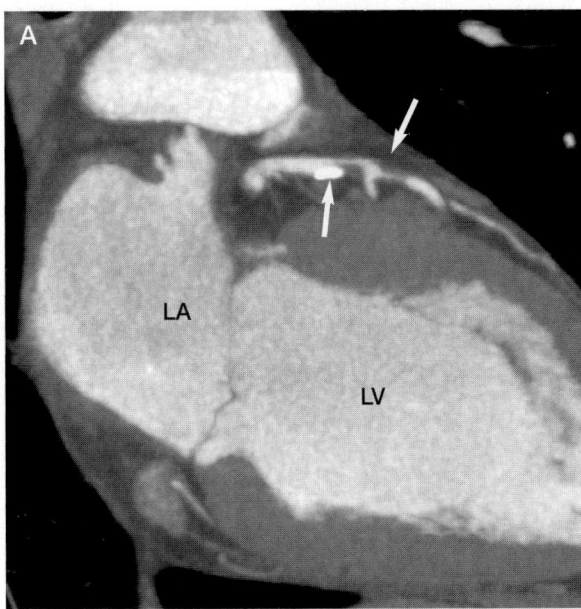
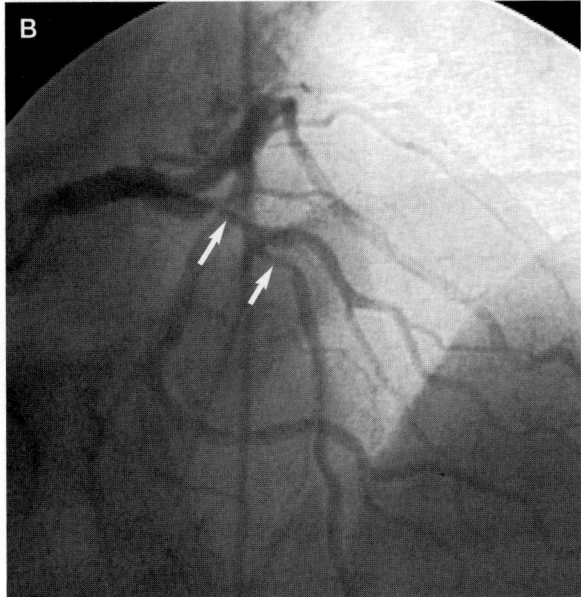

Fig. 6. Tandem high-grade coronary artery stenoses (*arrows*) in left anterior descending artery, proximal and distal to a diagonal branch. *A*, Coronary computed tomographic angiogram, reformatted in vertical long axis. *B*, Invasive selective coronary angiogram. LA, left atrium; LV, left ventricle.

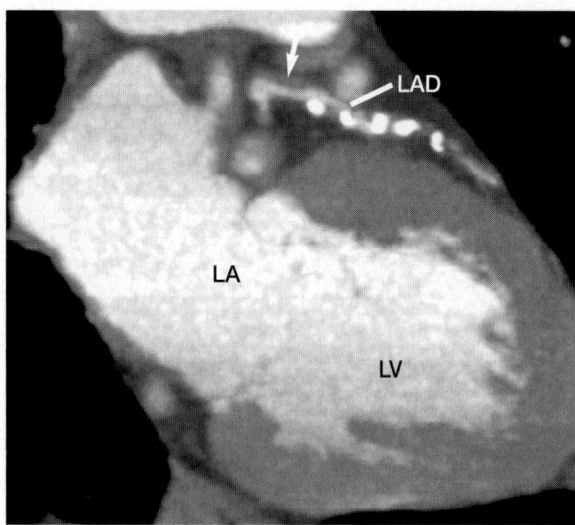

Fig. 7. Partially obstructive noncalcified plaque (*arrow*) in proximal segment of left anterior descending artery (LAD) seen in a computed tomographic vertical long-axis view. Diffuse calcification is distal to plaque. LA, left atrium; LV, left ventricle.

for coronary CTA: screening of asymptomatic patients with risk factors for coronary artery disease, establishing or ruling out progession of disease in patients with known coronary artery stenoses, possible in-stent restenosis (except stents in the left main coronary artery), and unequivocally abnormal results of stress testing (if patient is willing and able to undergo cardiac catheterization).

Cardiac MRI

CMR determines left and right ventricular volumes without geometric assumptions and provides accurate measurements of stroke volume, ejection fraction, and myocardial mass.

In patients with hypertrophic cardiomyopathy, the precise anatomical distribution of myocardial thickening can be well characterized with CMR (Fig. 10), and the systolic anterior motion of the mitral valve and the dynamic outflow tract obstruction can be visualized. In patients with valvular heart disease, gradient echo CMR can show the turbulent flow created by valvular stenosis and regurgitation. Aortic and mitral valve areas determined planimetrically from CMR images correlate well with data derived from echocardiographic assessment. Velocity-encoded CMR, a variant of gradient echo, allows quantitation of regurgitant volumes and calculation of regurgitation fractions or pressure gradients.

In patients with simple (Fig. 11) or complex (Fig. 12) congenital heart disease, CMR can determine with high resolution the connections between the heart chambers and the great vessels, the function of the

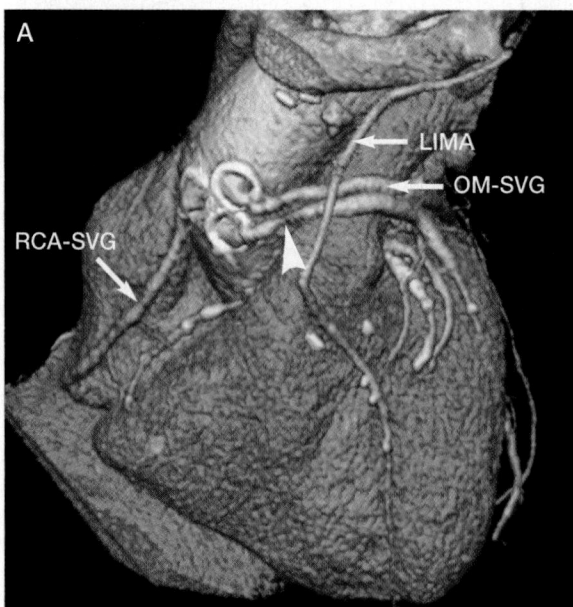

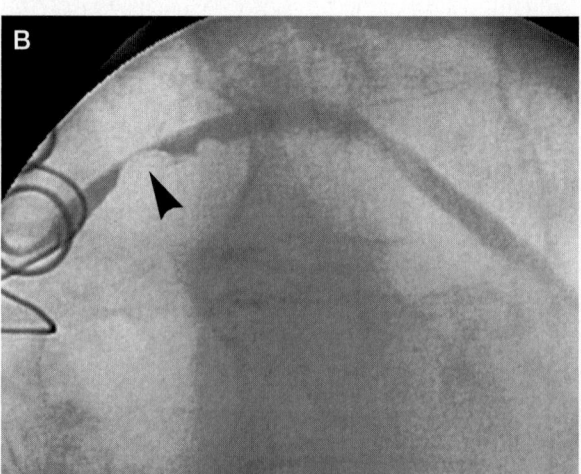

Fig. 8. High-grade stenosis (*arrowhead*) in proximal portion of saphenous vein graft to diagonal branch. *A*, Volume-rendered coronary computed tomographic angiogram. *B*, Invasive, selective coronary angiogram. LIMA, left internal mammary artery; OM-SVG, saphenous vein graft to obtuse marginal branch; RCA-SVG, saphenous vein graft to right coronary artery.

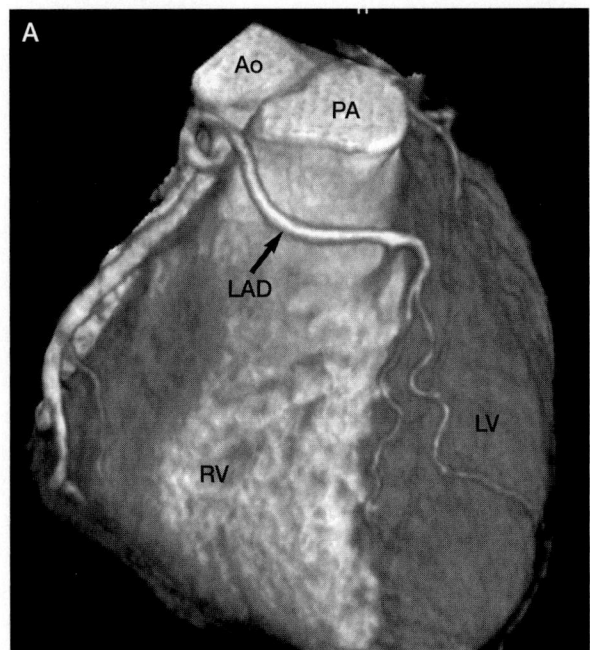

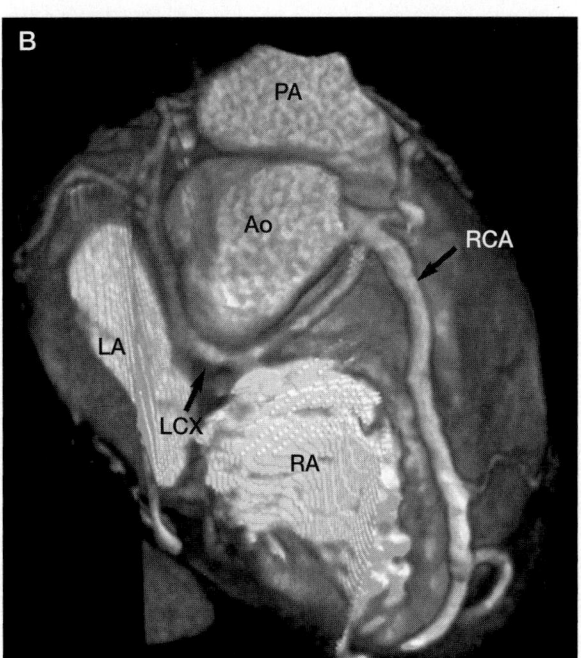

Fig. 9. Volume-rendered coronary computed tomographic angiograms of a single coronary artery arising from the right sinus of Valsalva. *A*, Anterior view. Left anterior descending artery (LAD) courses in front of the pulmonary artery (PA). *B*, Posterior view. Circumflex coronary artery (LCX) courses behind aorta (Ao). Parts of left atrium (LA) and right atrium (RA) have been removed by image processing. LV, left ventricle; RCA, right coronary artery; RV, right ventricle.

heart chambers, and the hemodynamic consequences (e.g., shunt volume) of the anomaly. Although CCT may image anatomy with greater spatial resolution, many imagers prefer CMR for the assessment of congenital cardiovascular disease to avoid repeated, substantial radiation exposure in the often young or very young patients.

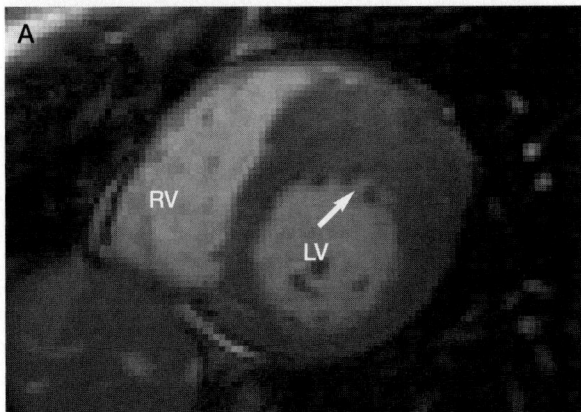

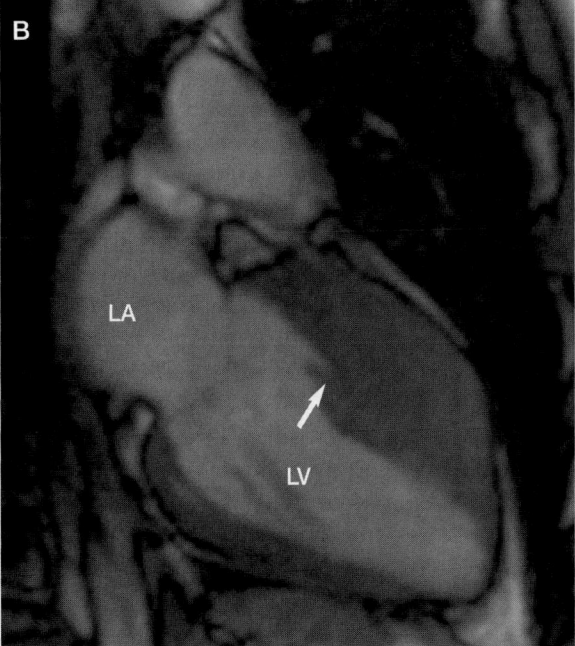

Fig. 10. Gradient echo cardiac magnetic resonance images of hypertrophic cardiomyopathy affecting anterior wall and anterior septum (*arrows*). *A*, Short-axis view at mid ventricular level. *B*, Vertical long-axis view. Maximal wall thickness was 26 mm; left ventricular outflow tract obstruction was not present. LA, left atrium; LV, left ventricle; RV, right ventricle.

Stress Imaging

Although coronary MR angiography is currently inferior to coronary CTA, CMR is useful for the assessment of coronary artery disease. Exercise CMR is logistically difficult. Among the pharmacologic approaches, adenosine stress CMR is more widely performed than dobutamine stress CMR, mostly because of higher patient acceptance, although dobutamine stress-induced regional wall motion abnormalities are the overall most accurate predictor (sensitivity, 90%; specificity, 80%) of hemodynamically significant coronary artery stenoses. Adenosine stress-induced regional wall motion abnormalities are highly specific (95%), whereas adenosine stress-induced myocardial perfusion abnormalities, currently the most widely used stress CMR approach, are very sensitive (90%) for the detection of hemodynamically significant coronary artery stenoses. Quantitative measurement of myocardial perfusion by MRI is possible but requires complex mathematical modeling. Therefore, assessment of myocardial perfusion is typically performed by visual assessment of myocardial first-pass enhancement by a bolus of gadolinium.

Delayed Myocardial Enhancement

A bolus of gadolinium washes in and out of normal myocardium quickly. Expanded extracellular space in the presence of myocyte necrosis can cause retention of gadolinium molecules, and delayed (15-20 minutes after gadolinium administration) myocardial enhancement (DME) on inversion-recovery prepared gradient echo images signifies myocardial damage.

Different patterns of DME can help distinguish between different causes of myocardial damage. DME as the result of myocardial infarction typically occurs in coronary perfusion territories and involves at least the subendocardium. The volume of DME correlates well with myocyte necrosis on triphenyltetrazolium chloride staining and can therefore be used to quantify infarct size. The transmural extent of DME is a measure of myocardial viability and predicts the likelihood of functional recovery after revascularization of hypokinetic or akinetic myocardial segments. For example, if more than 75% of myocardial thickness shows delayed enhancement, the likelihood of functional recovery is less than 2% (Fig. 13).

In contrast, myocyte damage due to idiopathic dilated cardiomyopathy, hypertrophic cardiomyopathy, myocarditis, sarcoidosis, Anderson-Fabry disease, or

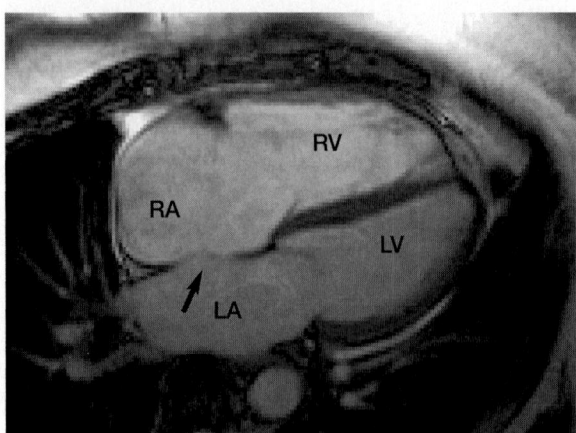

Fig. 11. Gradient echo cardiac magnetic resonance image of an atrial septal aneurysm *(arrow)* and an atrial septal defect of 5 mm with enlargement of right atrium (RA) and right ventricle (RV). Pulmonary/systemic blood flow ratio was 2.0. LA, left atrium; LV, left ventricle.

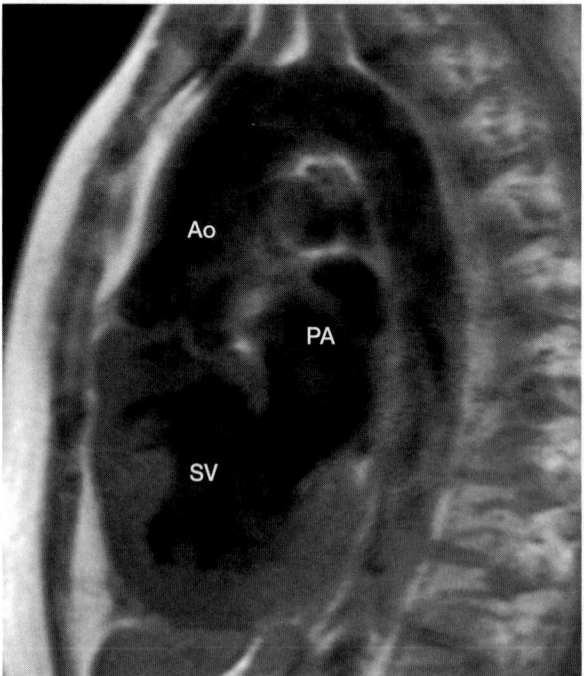

Fig. 12. Spin echo cardiac magnetic resonance image of repaired complex congenital heart disease with D-transposition of great arteries. Aorta (Ao) and pulmonary artery (PA) arise from a single ventricle (SV) with left ventricular morphologic features.

Chagas disease typically shows a midmyocardial or subepicardial pattern of DME. Amyloidosis can have a subendocardial pattern of DME similar to that of myocardial infarction, but the DME is patchy, does not follow coronary perfusion territories, and may involve the right ventricular myocardium (Fig. 14).

Vascular CT and MRI

Technical Issues

Recent technical developments in CT and MRI have facilitated vascular imaging because an entire scan can now be completed during the transit time of one intravenous bolus administration of contrast material. The newer, 64-slice CT scanners and the newer pulse sequences for MRI have essentially replaced diagnostic angiography for large and medium-sized vessels. Additionally, a single intravenous injection of contrast agent permits three-dimensional and multiplanar representation not only of the vessel lumen and wall in multiple projections but also of surrounding structures (Fig. 15), whereas during standard catheter-based angiography only intraluminal anatomy can be visualized.

CT Angiography Versus MR Angiography

Because MR angiography (MRA) requires no iodinated contrast material and allows imaging in multiple different planes of acquisition, it is the safest and most flexible imaging technique for evaluating large and medium-sized blood vessels. MRA is not as affected by severe vascular calcification as is CT. Heavily calcified arteries may still induce artifact by MRA, but luminal narrowings and irregularities are better seen with MRA in this situation. However, MR is very sensitive to the presence of metal, and clips or stents can severely distort MRA and lead to false diagnoses (Fig. 16).

CTA, especially when done with the newer and faster scanners, allows very high-resolution axial imaging. Complex vessel morphologic features, as seen in dissections, irregular aneurysms, and vascular tortuosity, are better delineated by CT because of artifacts that turbulent or multidirectional blood flow can cause on MRI. Indications for CTA overlap those for MRA, but there is bias for CTA in cases requiring a high degree of image detail (Fig. 17). Additionally, if the surrounding anatomy is important to evaluate, CTA provides better resolution of solid organs, particularly the lungs. Because of its high spatial resolution, CTA is also very well suited for the evaluation of aneurysms and dissecting hematomas, especially abdominal aortic aneurysms and intracerebral aneurysms. CT provides the best imaging results for planning vascular surgical or endovascular procedures. CT is particularly important for the increasing numbers of endovascular stent repairs of thoracic and abdominal aortic aneurysms and dissections. Planning these procedures requires very exact measurements of the vessel diameters, angulations, and

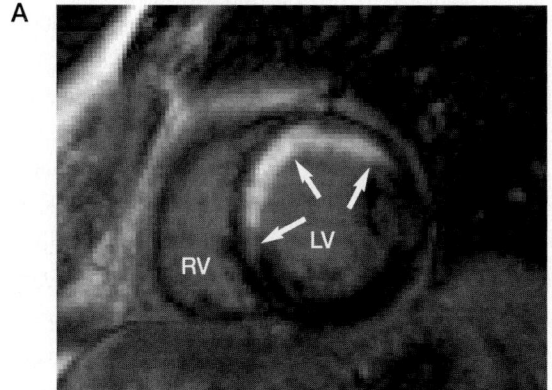
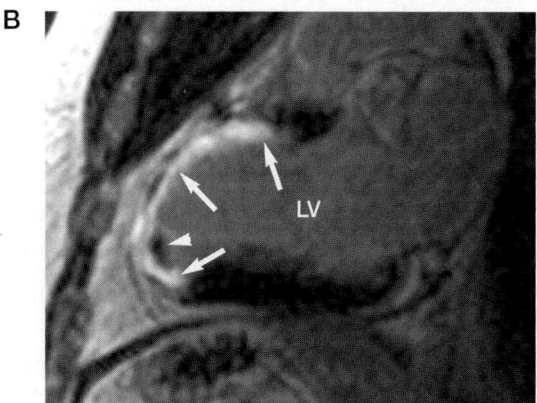

Fig. 13. Anterior myocardial infarction after failed placement of stent, complicated by vessel occlusion, in left anterior descending artery. More than 75% of thickness of anterior wall and anterior septum from base to apex show delayed myocardial enhancement (*arrows*). *A*, Short-axis view at mid ventricular level. *B*, Vertical long-axis view. *Arrowhead*, apical thrombus. LV, left ventricle; RV, right ventricle.

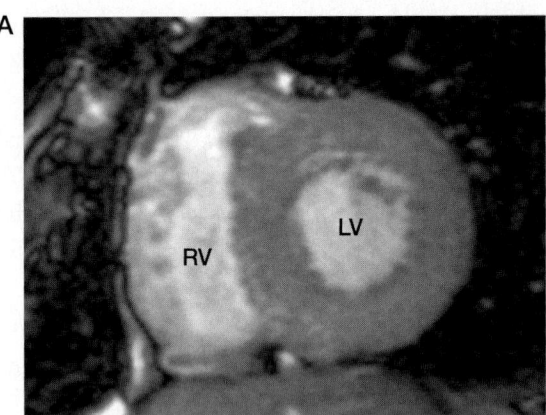
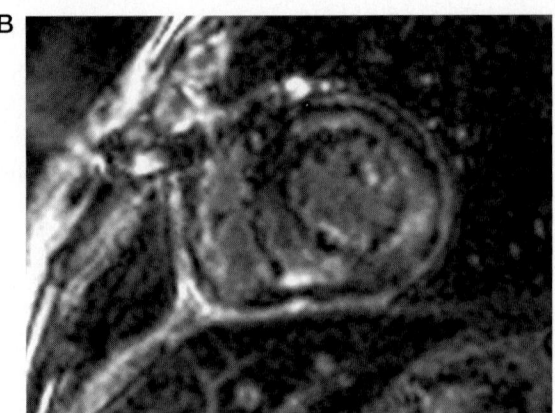

Fig. 14. Biopsy-proven cardiac amyloid. *A*, Gradient echo cardiac magnetic resonance short-axis view at mid ventricular level, showing symmetric left ventricular hypertrophy. LV, left ventricle; RV, right ventricle. *B*, Corresponding inversion recovery-prepared image, showing patchy, delayed myocardial enhancement that does not follow any coronary artery perfusion territory and includes right ventricle.

lengths in order to choose the appropriate device. In patients who already have vascular stents in place, better images are obtained with CT than MR because of the metallic artifact created in MR (Fig. 18 and 19). Other metallic structures such as clips or prostheses also tip the balance in favor of CTA rather than MRA, although CT images also may be degraded by streak artifact from large metallic objects such as hip prostheses.

Technique of CTA and MRA

MRA and CTA are tailored to the specific purpose of the examination. Standard principles of cross-sectional imaging to facilitate reformatting images in three dimensions include thin sections (2-5 mm) and rapid bolus administration of contrast material at 4 to 5 mL/s. Large-bore venous access is required to perform CTA or MRA (18 gauge at the least). Secondary multiplanar or three-dimensional reconstructions of vascular anatomy are now easily done with standard software; however, such image processing can introduce artifacts and errors of its own, and reformatted images should always be reviewed in conjunction with source images.

Because of the current limitations in resolution, MRA and CTA are not appropriate imaging methods for evaluating small vessels and diagnosing problems such as vasculitis or embolic disease to the hand or foot. CTA and particularly MRA tend to overestimate stenoses, a feature that makes them sensitive screening tools. False-positive findings occur most often in obese patients, uncooperative patients, or patients with tortuous

vessels, in whom reduced signal-to-noise ratio, motion, or turbulent flow, respectively, create image artifacts.

Specific Indications for MRA and CTA

Pulmonary Arteries

Pulmonary CTA has evolved into the primary imaging method of screening for pulmonary embolism, effectively replacing ventilation-perfusion imaging and catheter-based pulmonary angiography. Ventilation-perfusion scanning and pulmonary angiography cannot detect other abnormalities in the chest which can cause acute-onset dyspnea and chest pain. In patients allergic to iodinated contrast material or with decreased renal function, diagnostic multidetector pulmonary CTA can be performed with intravenous gadolinium, although gadolinium is less radiopaque than iodine-based contrast material. Pulmonary MRA is currently limited by lack of resolution.

Studies comparing older single-detector CT with pulmonary angiography show a sensitivity of 60% to 100% and specificity of 80% to 100% for the diagnosis of pulmonary embolus. Pulmonary artery CT is very sensitive for central pulmonary emboli, and the lower sensitivities and specificities were primarily due to very peripheral emboli in third- or higher-generation pulmonary artery branches (Fig. 20).

Multidetector CT scanners are now fast enough to image the entire chest and pulmonary circulation with 2-mm collimation in one breath hold, even in acutely

A

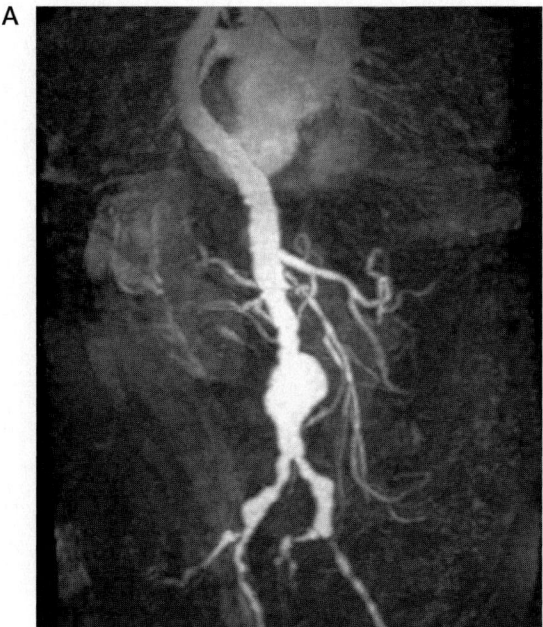

C

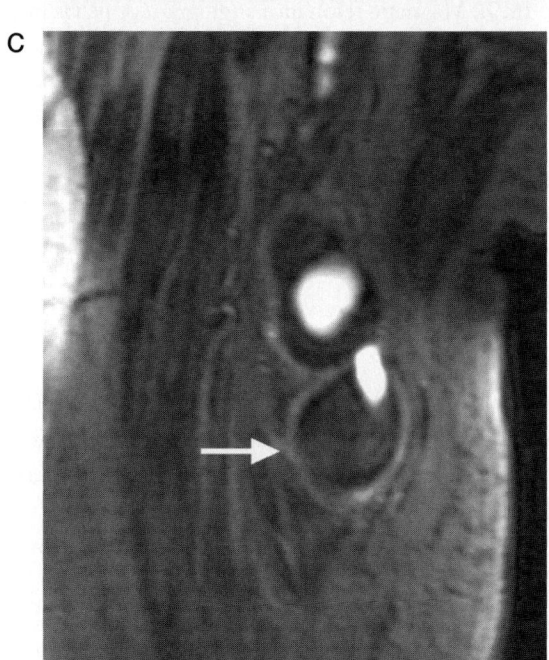

B

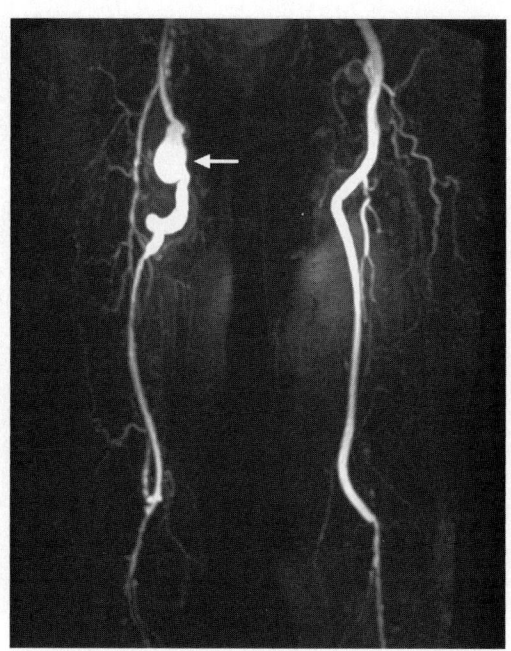

Fig. 15. Magnetic resonance angiograms of abdomen, pelvis, and lower extremities, showing abdominal aortic aneurysm (*A*) and aneurysmal degeneration of right femoral popliteal bypass graft (*arrow* in *B*). Coronal sources image, showing anatomical location of degenerated bypass and thrombus within aneurysm (*arrow* in *C*).

dyspneic patients (Fig. 21). Up to 30% of patients undergoing CT for suspected pulmonary embolus have some other cause for their symptoms which is readily apparent on the high-resolution CT scans. For example, spiral CT of the pulmonary arteries is able to detect even a small patent ductus arteriosus because of the unopacified jet of blood entering the pulmonary artery at the level of the aorticopulmonary window.

Aortic Arch Branches and Central Venous Structures
Vascular stenoses of the great vessels are also easily seen with CTA or MRA, similar to stenoses in other medium-sized to large vessels (Fig. 22). MR detects great artery stenoses with a sensitivity of 90% and a specificity of 96%. In brachiocephalic or subclavian arterial stenoses, delayed imaging helps to visualize the retrograde vertebral artery and distal subclavian artery in cases of subclavian steal. In the presence of great vessel stenoses, it is important to include the carotid bifurcations in the field of view, particularly if surgical subclavian carotid bypass grafting is an option (Fig. 23). Anomalies of the aortic arch, such as aberrant subclavian arteries and coarctation and bicuspid aortic valves, can be seen with both CTA and MRA (Fig. 24 and 25).

Aortic Arch and Thoracic Aorta
MRA and CTA are extremely accurate for the evaluation of aortic aneurysms and dissections. In the case of dissections, multidetector CT is preferred because of its

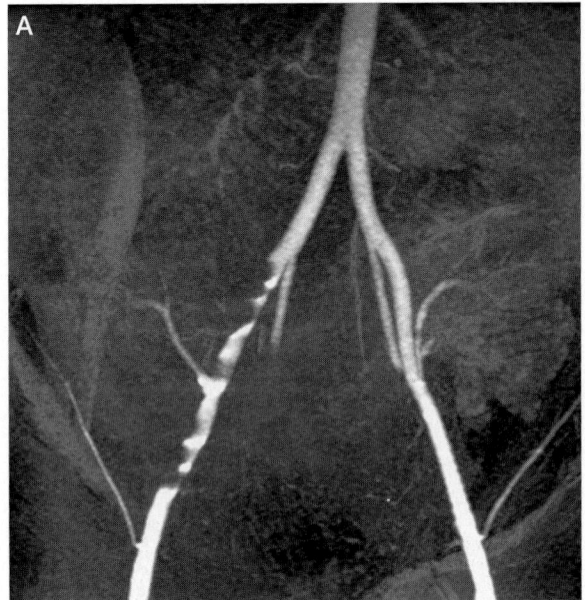

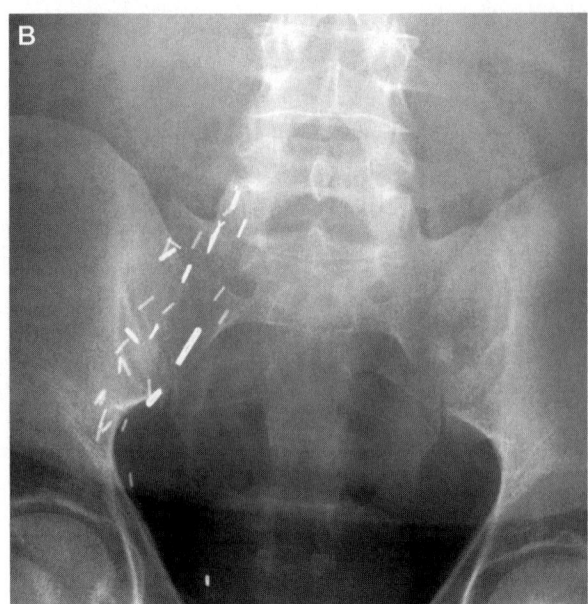

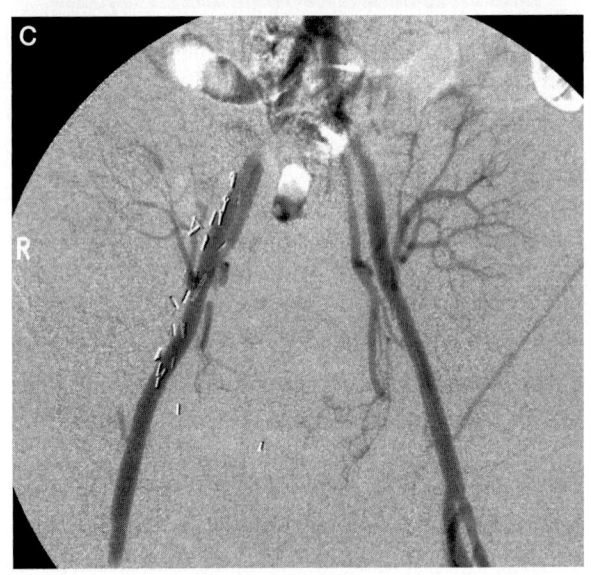

Fig. 16. *A*, Magnetic resonance angiogram of pelvis in a renal transplant recipient. Donor renal artery is normal, but there is unusual scalloping along the common and external iliac arteries. *B*, Plain radiograph, showing multiple metal clips along course of iliac vessels. *C*, Angiogram, showing no iliac arterial stenoses. The pseudostenoses were artifacts from metal clips during magnetic resonance angiography of pelvis.

improved resolution and ability to visualize small intimal flaps or ulcerations. Recent studies report 99% sensitivity and 100% specificity for multirow detector CT of acute dissections (Fig. 26). CT performed in the setting of back pain in hypertensive patients is positive for dissection in about 18% of patients. The rare false-negative examination usually occurs in patients with small penetrating atherosclerotic ulcers or minimal intramural hematomas that may escape detection by CTA.

Thoracic aneurysms can be similarly imaged with MRA or CTA, but some advantage is given to MRA because it does not require iodinated contrast and

radiation exposure. When a thoracic aneurysm is being followed, resolution requirements are reduced because only aortic diameter and branch vessel patency are evaluated (Fig. 27).

Abdominal Aorta

MRA and CTA of the abdominal aorta are used to evaluate abdominal aneurysms or dissections and to image the inflow arteries in patients with known peripheral vascular disease. In patients with aneurysms considered for stent-graft repair, CTA is preferred because of its improved resolution (Fig. 28). CTA shows the contraction of the aneurysm sac, indicating successful treatment, and monitors for endoleaks, which appear as contrast material filling the persistent or enlarging aneurysm sac. After a patient has undergone endovascular stenting, it is important for early and delayed scanning to be performed, because endoleaks around the stent graft may become visible only late

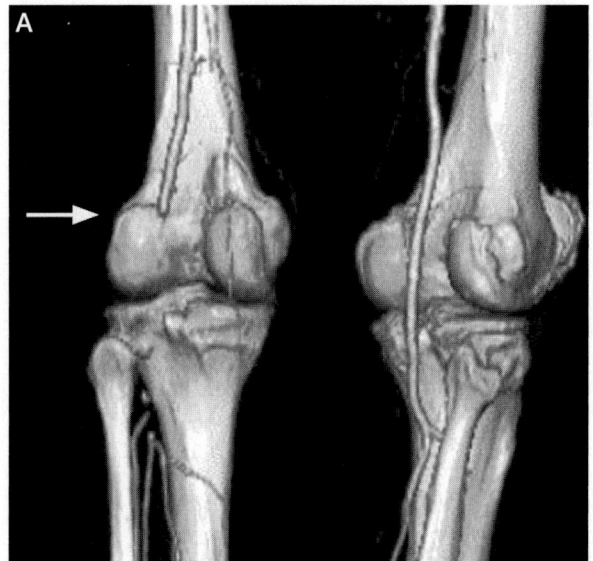
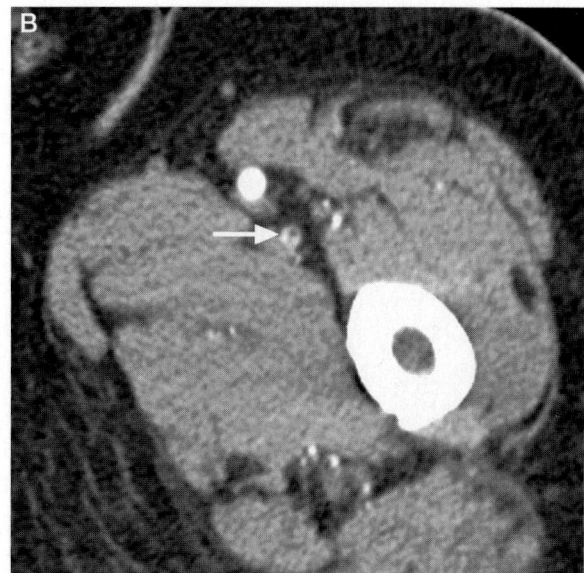

Fig. 17. *A*, Posterior volume-rendered computed tomographic angiogram of knees, showing left popliteal occlusion (*arrow*). *B*, Thin-section transverse image, showing tiny filling defect in left profunda femoral artery (*arrow*). These findings allowed the diagnosis of acute embolic disease to the lower extremities.

after contrast injection (Fig. 29). Branch vessel or iliac occlusions can complicate endovascular stent grafts and can be easily seen and characterized with CTA.

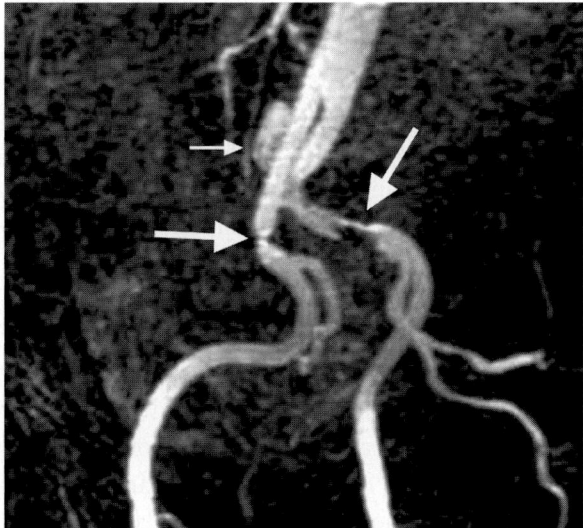

Fig. 18. Magnetic resonance angiogram, showing a patent aortic stent graft with small endoleak (*small arrow*). Metal-related artifact at proximal and iliac limbs of stent graft is due to metal stents in these locations (*large arrows*). Arteriography showed no stenoses at iliac segments.

Renal Artery Stenosis

It is generally agreed that screening patients for renal artery stenosis is best done with CTA or MRA. CTA and MRA tend to overestimate stenoses, and a small percentage of false-positive screening results, which are insignificant lesions by angiography, can be expected. MR and CT are equivalent for evaluating suspected renal artery stenosis, but MR generally is preferred because of the diminished renal function in many patients (Fig. 30-32). For renal artery stenosis, MRA for the detection of hemodynamically significant arterial stenosis has a sensitivity of 93% and a specificity of 99%. Similarly, CTA has a sensitivity of 92% and a specificity of 99%.

A second common application of MRA and CTA is evaluation of vascular anatomy in living renal donors or, more recently, liver donors before transplantation. Advantages of MRA and CTA over standard angiography in this setting include the ability to see renal parenchyma and the rest of the abdomen to screen for potential tumors, cysts, or stone disease before transplantation.

Mesenteric Ischemia

Similar to the situation for renal arteries, MRA and CTA have essentially replaced angiography for the

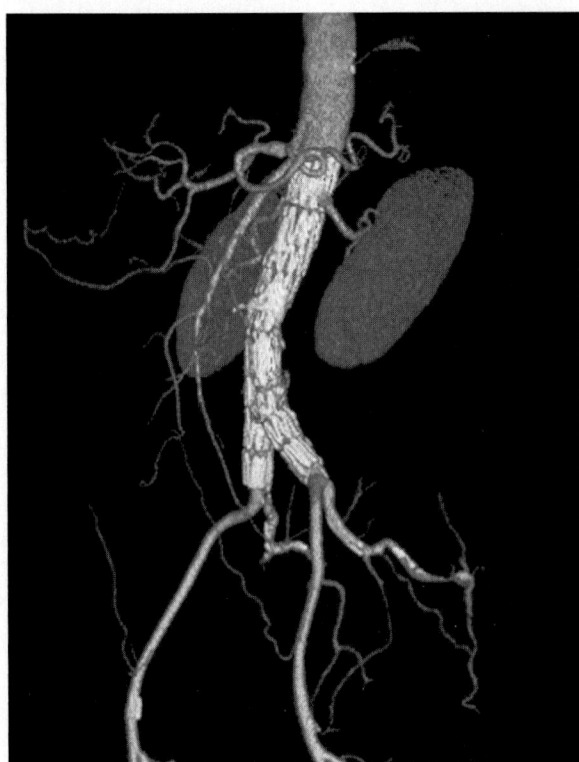

Fig. 19. Computed tomographic angiogram of aorta and iliac arteries obtained after stent grafting. This method has better precision and fewer artifacts than magnetic resonance angiography.

evaluation of patients with postprandial abdominal pain and weight loss. MR evaluation of the abdominal aorta in suspected mesenteric ischemia generally is performed in the sagittal plane rather than the axial plane because of the orientation of the mesenteric vessels along the long axis of the aorta compared with the lateral exit of the renal arteries off the aorta (Fig. 33). For detection of mesenteric artery stenosis, CT has a reported sensitivity of 100% and a specificity of 89%. Similarly, MRA has a reported sensitivity of 100% and a specificity of 95% for mesenteric arterial stenoses greater than 75%.

RESOURCES

Budoff MJ, Cohen MC, Garcia MJ, et al, American College of Cardiology Foundation; American Heart Association; American College of Physicians Task Force on Clinical Competence and Training; American Society of Echocardiography; American Society of Nuclear Cardiology; Society of Atherosclerosis Imaging; Society for Cardiovascular Angiography & Interventions. ACCF/AHA clinical competence statement on cardiac imaging with computed tomography and magnetic resonance: a report of the American College of Cardiology Foundation/ American Heart Association/American College of Physicians Task Force on Clinical Competence and Training. J Am Coll Cardiol. 2005;46:383-402.

Cerqueira MD, Weissman NJ, Dilsizian V, et al, American Heart Association Writing Group on Myocardial Segmentation and Registration for Cardiac Imaging. Standardized myocardial segmentation and nomenclature for tomographic imaging of the heart: a statement for healthcare professionals from the Cardiac Imaging Committee of the Council on Clinical Cardiology of the American Heart Association. Circulation. 2002;105:539-42.

Gibbons RJ, Abrams J, Chatterjee K, et al, American College of Cardiology; American Heart Association Task Force on Practice Guidelines. Committee on the Management of Patients With Chronic Stable Angina. ACC/AHA 2002 guideline update for the management of patients with chronic stable angina— summary article: a report of the American College of Cardiology/American Heart Association Task Force on Practice Guidelines (Committee on the Management of Patients With Chronic Stable Angina). Circulation. 2003;107:149-58.

Mieres JH, Shaw LJ, Arai A, et al, Cardiac Imaging Committee, Council on Clinical Cardiology, and the Cardiovascular Imaging and Intervention Committee, Council on Cardiovascular Radiology and Intervention, American Heart Association. Role of noninvasive testing in the clinical evaluation of women with suspected coronary artery disease: consensus statement from the Cardiac Imaging Committee, Council on Clinical Cardiology, and the Cardiovascular Imaging and Intervention Committee, Council on Cardiovascular Radiology and Intervention, American Heart Association. Circulation. 2005 Feb 8;111:682-96. Epub 2005 Feb 1.

O'Rourke RA, Brundage BH, Froelicher VF, et al, American College of Cardiology/American Heart Association Expert Consensus document on elec-

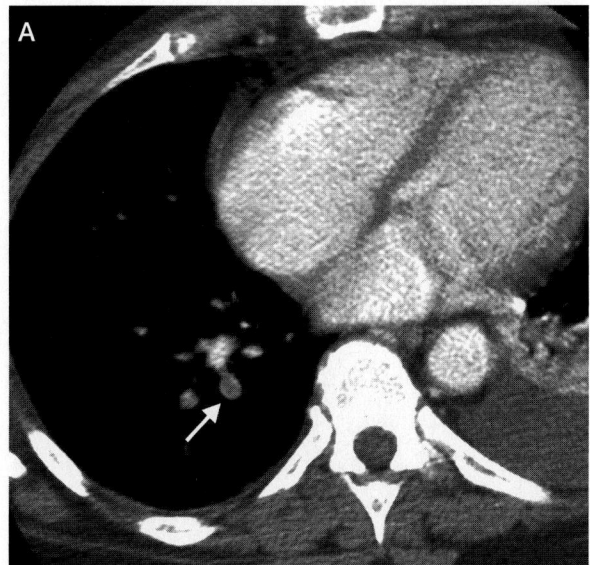 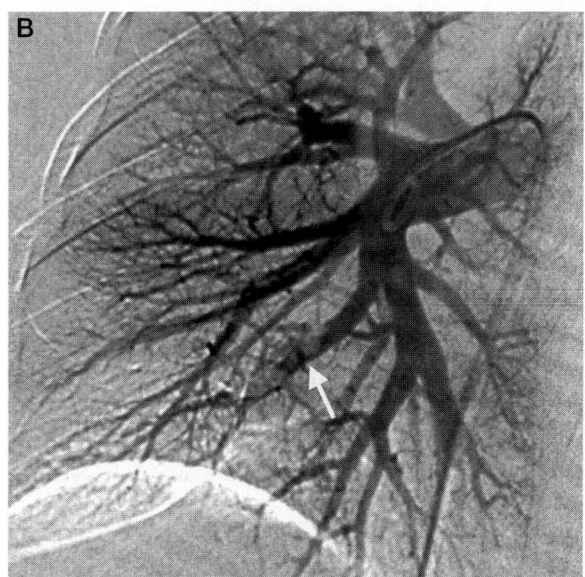

Fig. 20. *A,* Computed tomographic angiogram, showing small filling defect in a basilar segmental right pulmonary artery (*arrow*). *B,* Pulmonary angiogram confirmed defect (*arrow*). Pulmonary embolus in this third-generation branch is near the limit of resolution of computed tomographic angiography, although sensitivity continues to improve with newer generation scanners.

tron-beam computed tomography for the diagnosis and prognosis of coronary artery disease. Circulation. 2000;102:126-40.

Pennell DJ, Sechtem UP, Higgins CB, et al, Society for Cardiovascular Magnetic Resonance; Working Group on Cardiovascular Magnetic Resonance of the European Society of Cardiology. Clinical indications for cardiovascular magnetic resonance (CMR): consensus panel report. Eur Heart J. 2004;25:1940-65.

Weinreb JC, Larson PA, Woodard PK, et al, American College of Radiology. American College of Radiology clinical statement on noninvasive cardiac imaging. Radiology. 2005 Jun;235:723-7. Epub 2005 Apr 21.

Wexler L, Brundage B, Crouse J, et al, American Heart Association Writing Group. Coronary artery calcification: pathophysiology, epidemiology, imaging methods, and clinical implications; a statement for health professionals from the American Heart Association. Circulation. 1996;94:1175-92.

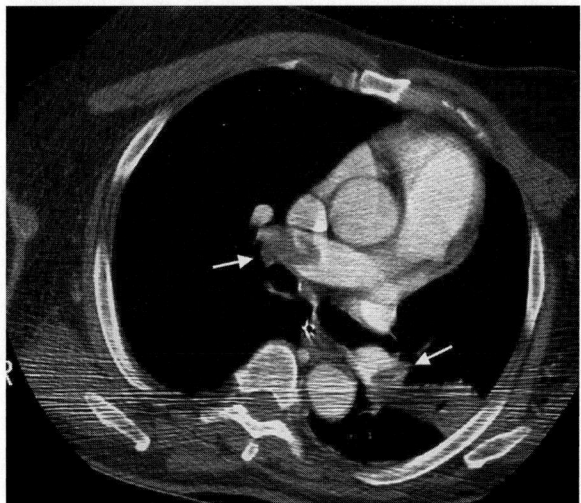

Fig. 21. Computed tomographic angiogram, showing large central pulmonary emboli on the left and right (*arrows*) in acutely dyspneic patient. Although the patient was severely ill and marginally stable, diagnostic images were obtained with minimal breath holding.

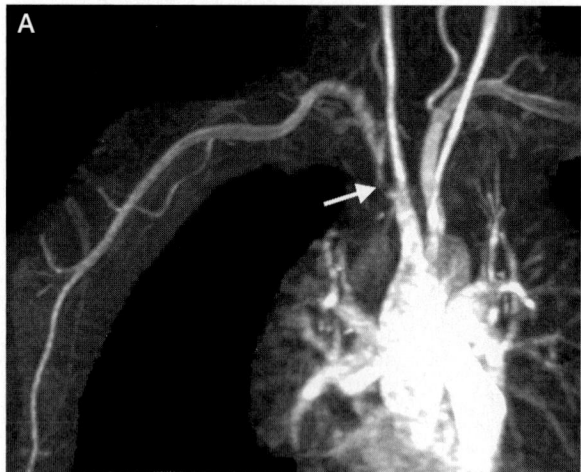

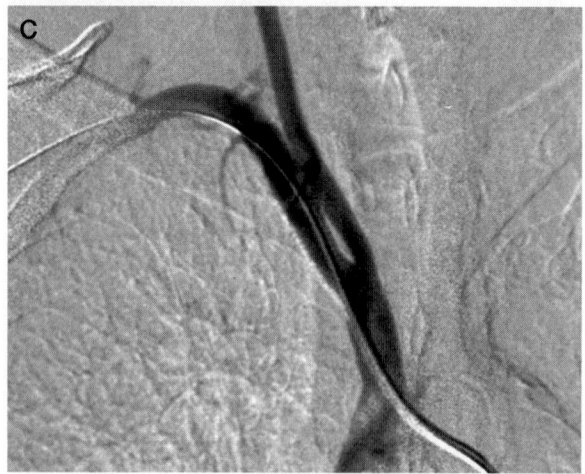

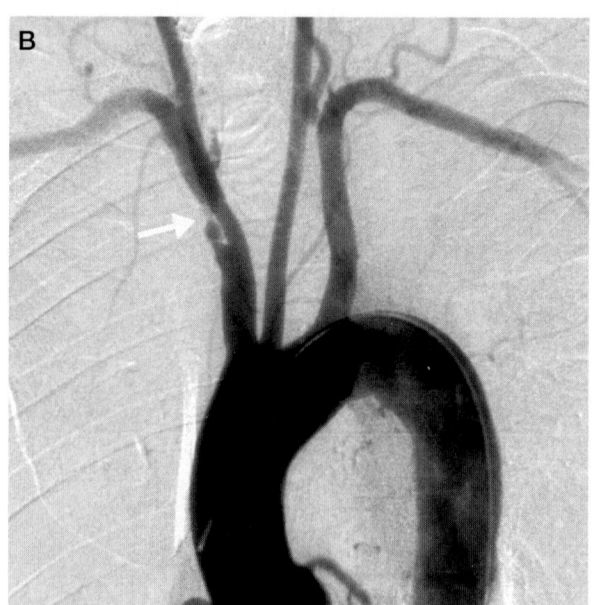

Fig. 22. *A*, Magnetic resonance angiogram, showing irregular severe stenosis in proximal right subclavian artery (*arrow*). *B* and *C*, Catheter angiograms confirmed the diagnosis and allowed successful angioplasty and stenting of this lesion.

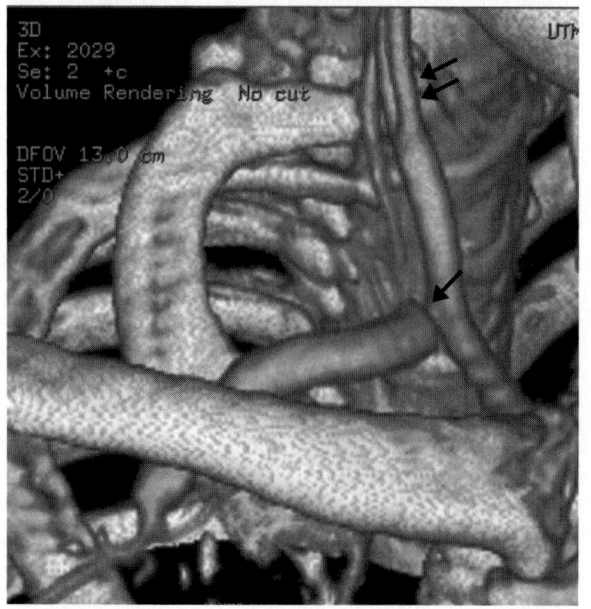

Fig. 23. Computed tomographic angiogram obtained from a patient who had carotid subclavian bypass for right subclavian artery occlusion. Patient had recurrent ischemic right arm pain, and computed tomographic angiogram showed intimal hyperplasia narrowing the proximal anastomosis (*arrow*). Notice inclusion of carotid bifurcation (*double arrows*). Significant internal carotid stenosis would alter surgical mangement of the dysfunctional bypass graft because carotid endarterectomy also might be required.

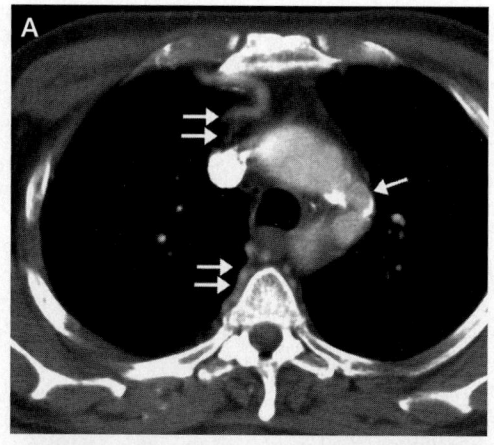

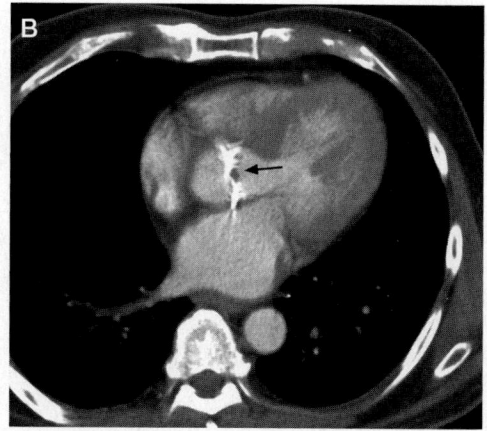

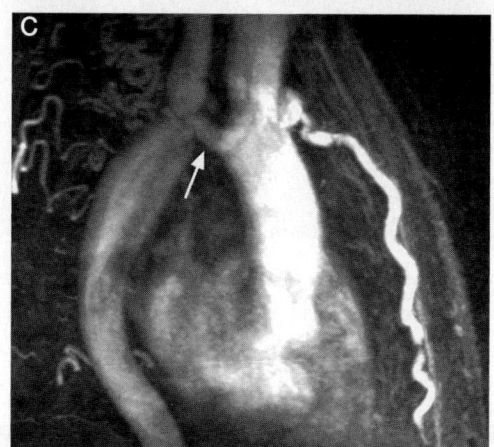

Fig. 24. Patient with coarctation of the aorta. *A* and *B*, Computed tomographic angiograms, showing calcific arch stenosis (*arrow* in *A*) and enlarged internal mammary artery and intercostal collaterals (*double arrows* in *A*). A bicuspid aortic valve is also apparent (*arrow* in *B*). *C*, Magnetic resonance angiogram, showing similar findings with coarctation visible in arch (*arrow*).

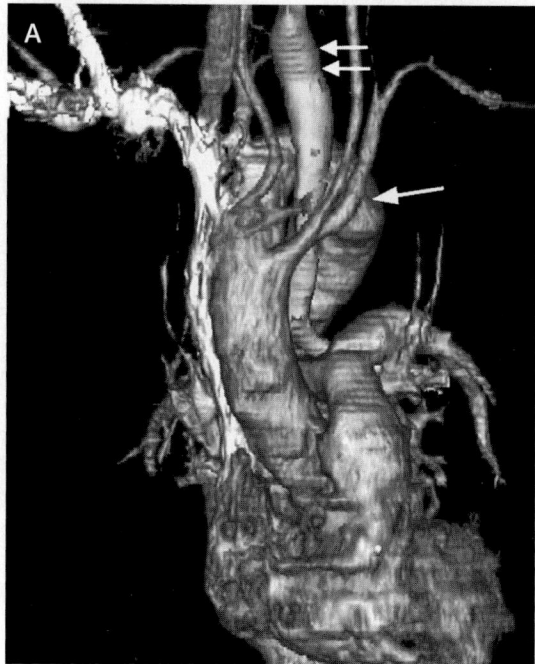

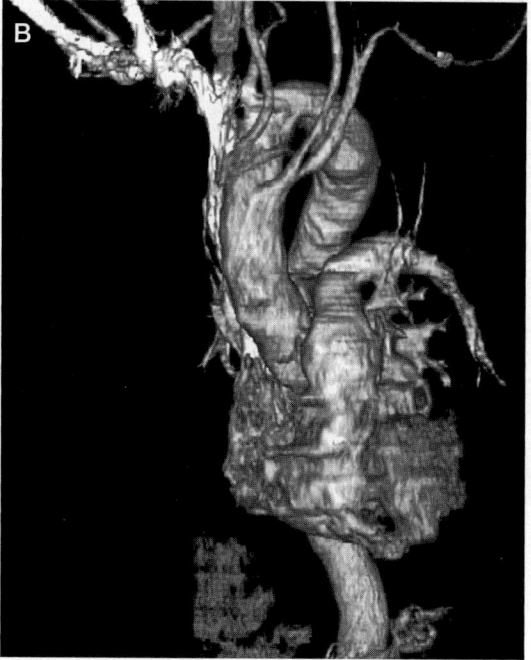

Fig. 25. *A* and *B*, Computed tomographic angiograms of right aortic arch with vascular ring formed by left subclavian artery and aortic diverticulum (*arrow* in *A*) surrounding trachea (*double arrow* in *A*). Left oblique view showing vascular structures forming the ring (*B*).

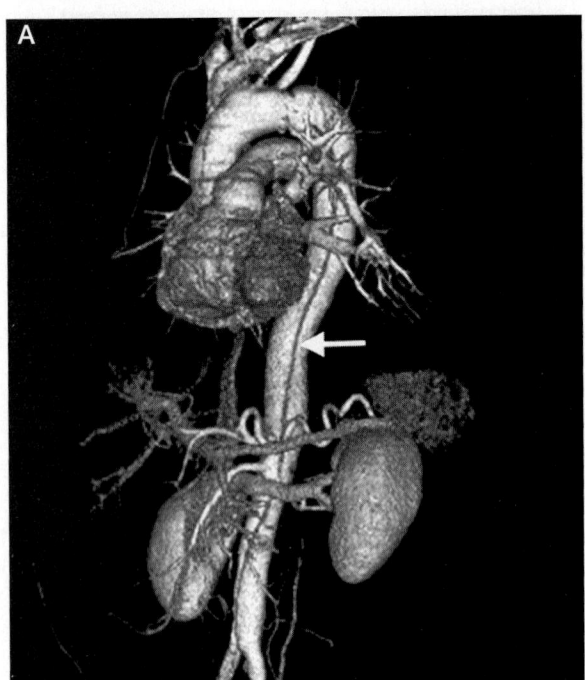
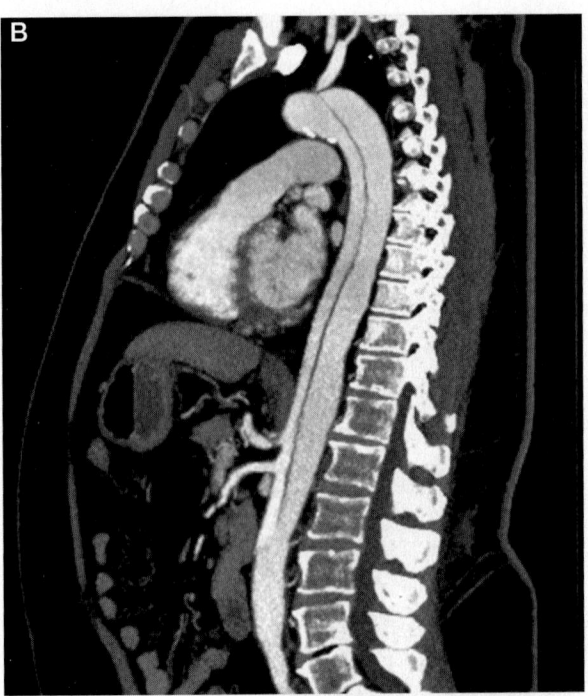

Fig. 26. Computed tomographic angiograms of type III aortic dissection. *A*, Volume-rendered image, showing thin dissection flap extending from left subclavian artery to distal aortic bifurcation (*arrow*). *B*, Sagittal reformatted image, showing intimal flap and mesenteric arteries.

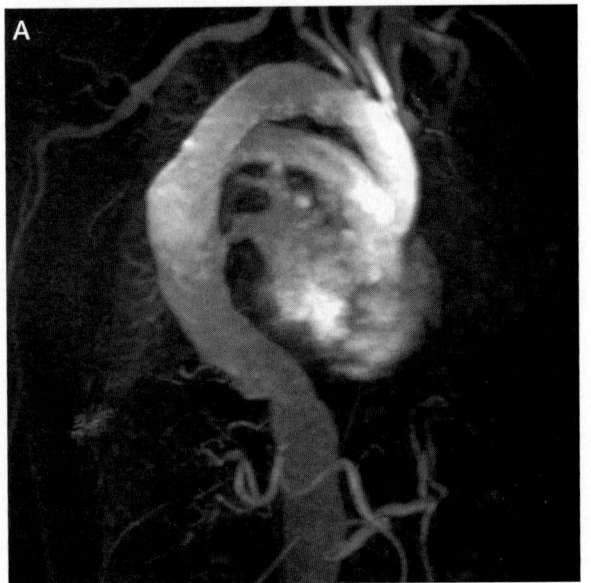
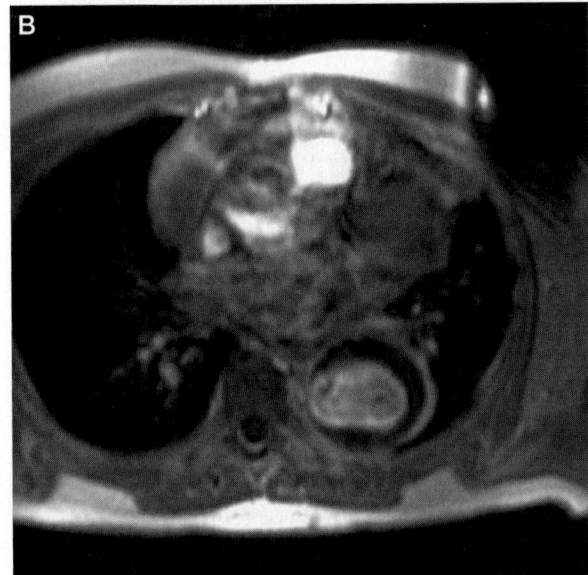

Fig. 27. *A* and *B*, Magnetic resonance angiograms of thoracoabdominal aneurysm. Transverse image (*B*) allows evaluation of luminal thrombus and aneurysm diameter.

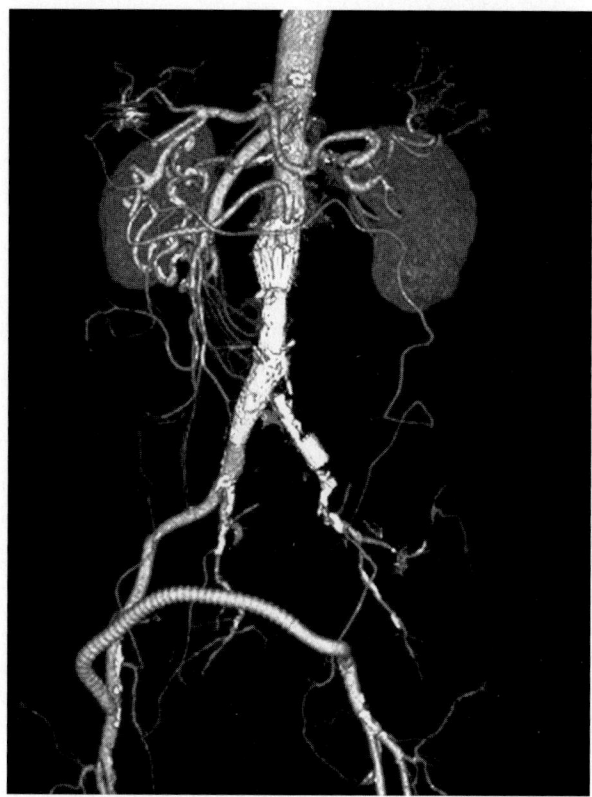

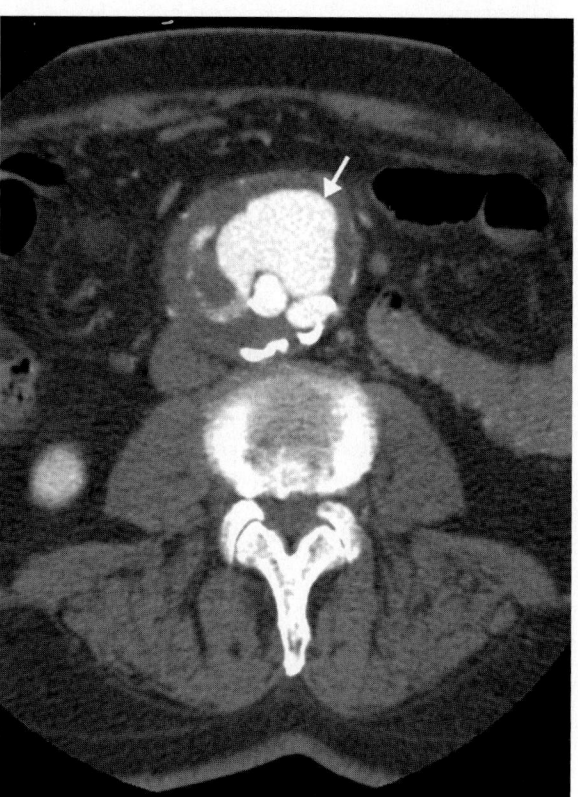

Fig. 28. Computed tomographic angiogram obtained from a patient after aorto–uni-iliac stent graft placement and left iliac artery occlusion with crossed femoral bypass for aortoiliac aneurysmal disease.

Fig. 29. Computed tomographic angiogram obtained after aortic stent graft repair of infrarenal aortic aneurysm. There is a large endoleak (*arrow*) with persistent enlargement and enhancement of aneurysm sac.

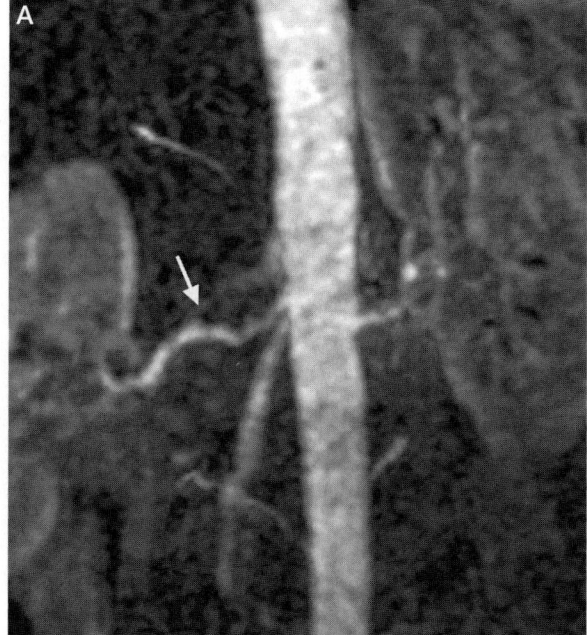

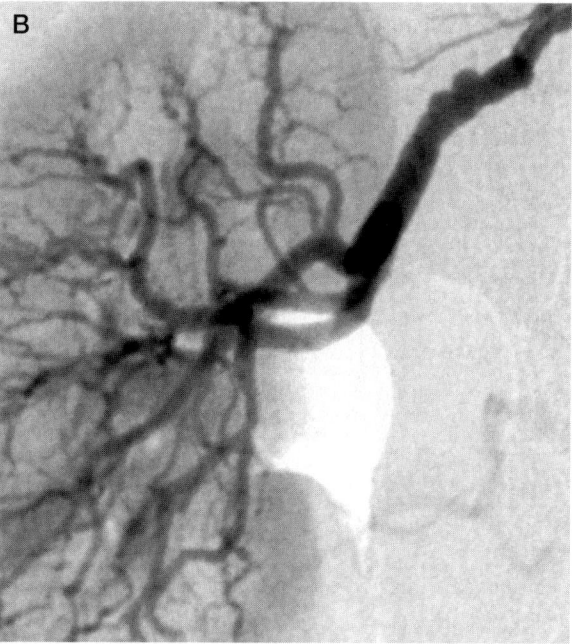

Fig. 30. *A*, Magnetic resonance angiogram of right renal artery, showing corrugation and possible stenosis of proximal renal artery (*arrow*). *B*, Angiogram showing fibromuscular dysplasia and stenosis, successfully treated with angioplasty.

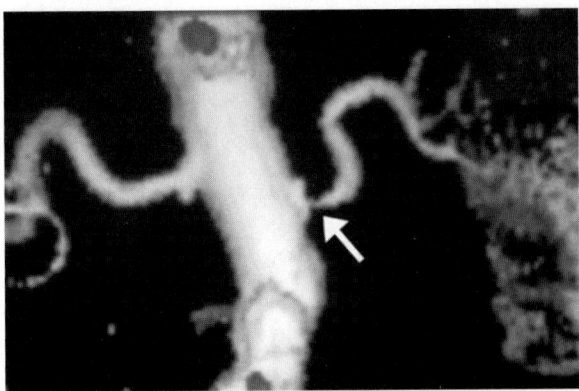

Fig. 31. Computed tomography angiogram of left renal artery ostial stenosis (*arrow*).

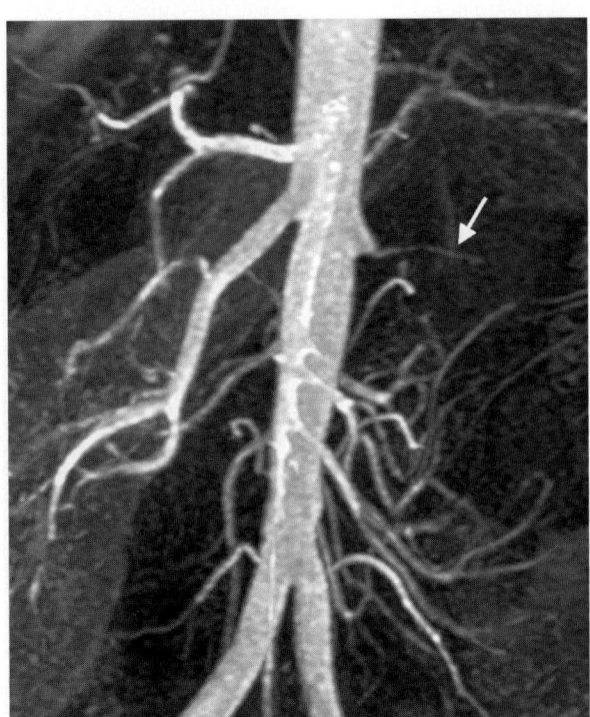

Fig. 32. Magnetic resonance angiogram of kidneys, showing compensatory hypertrophy of right kidney and severe, long-segment stenosis and distal occlusion of left renal artery (*arrow*). There was little function in the left kidney, and it was surgically resected.

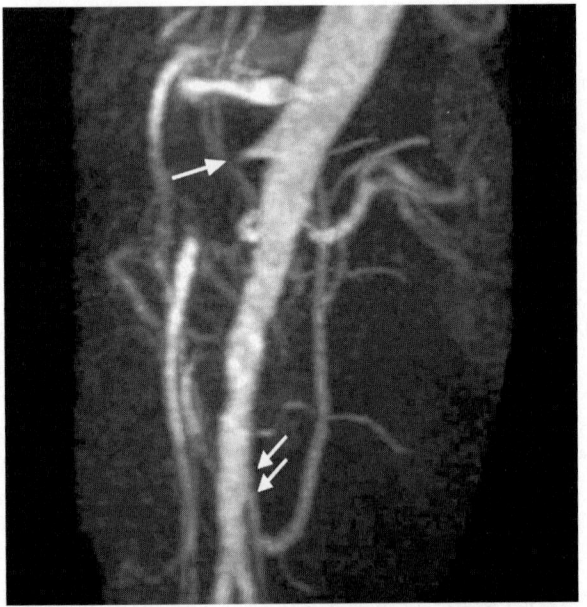

Fig. 33. Magnetic resonance angiogram, showing long-segment superior mesenteric artery occlusion (*arrow*) in a patient with weight loss and abdominal pain. Although the inferior mesenteric artery (*double arrows*) was patent, it was severely stenotic at its origin. Chronic mesenteric ischemia symptoms are generally not evident until two of the three mesenteric arteries are significantly stenosed or occluded.

CARDIAC RADIOGRAPHY

Jerome F. Breen, MD

Mark J. Callahan, MD

The conventional upright posteroanterior and lateral x-ray projections of the chest are obtained with high kilovoltage technique at maximal inspiration to permit short exposure times, which freeze cardiac motion. Interstitial markings are accentuated on a poor inspiratory effort radiograph. A tube-to-film distance of at least 6 feet minimizes distortion and magnification.

■ Chest radiographs that show cardiac abnormality are a very important part of the cardiology examinations.

■ Always take a systematic approach to interpreting chest radiographs. Always identify the border-forming structures of the heart on both the frontal and the lateral views. Use the pulmonary blood vessels to help explain all abnormal contours.

■ Always try to compare a chest radiograph with any available previous study.

■ Postoperatively, suspect new abnormalities on chest radiographs to be related to the surgical procedure.

■ If a computed tomogram or magnetic resonance image is shown on the cardiology boards, look carefully for pericardial or aortic disease.

CARDIAC SILHOUETTE AND CHAMBER SIZE

The image of the heart and great vessels on the chest radiograph is a two-dimensional display of dynamic

three-dimensional structures (Fig. 1-10). The cardiovascular silhouette varies not only with the abnormality but also with body habitus, age, respiratory depth, cardiac cycle, and position of the patient.

Posteroanterior Projection

The right mediastinal contour consists of a straight upper vertical border formed by the superior vena cava and a smooth convex lower cardiac contour formed by

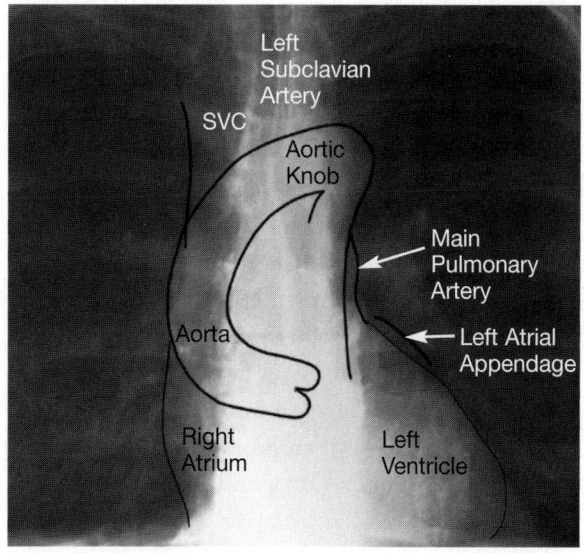

Fig. 1. Posteroanterior projection of the heart. SVC, superior vena cava.

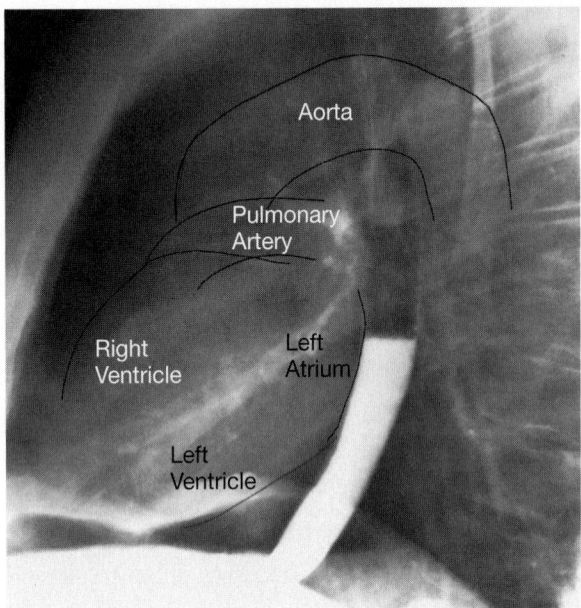

Fig. 2. Lateral projection of the heart.

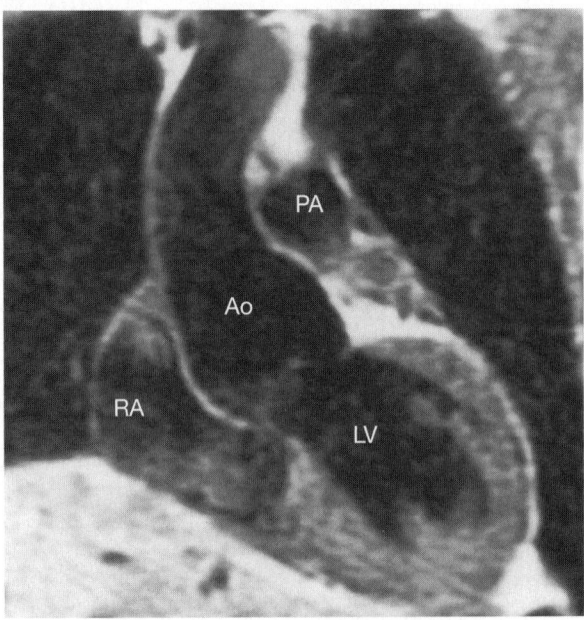

Fig. 3. Magnetic resonance imaging of the heart in the frontal plane. Ao, aorta; LV, left ventricle; PA, pulmonary artery; RA, right atrium.

the right atrium. Occasionally, a short segment of inferior vena cava is seen where the right atrium meets the diaphragm.

The normal left mediastinal contour is formed by a series of convexities: from superior to inferior, the aortic knob, the pulmonary trunk, and the left ventricle abutting the diaphragm. The left atrial appendage may be seen projecting between the pulmonary trunk and the left ventricle in the normal heart, primarily in young females. The shape of the pulmonary trunk segment varies with age and body habitus. Most frequently, this segment is only slightly convex; however, it can be prominent in women 20 to 40 years old and straight or even concave in older patients and still be within normal limits. Occasionally, the cardiophrenic junction of the cardiac silhouette is not formed by the left ventricle but by a fat pad. Less common is a border-forming fat pad in the right cardiophrenic angle, which should not be confused with a cardiac mass.

- The left atrial appendage may be seen projecting between the pulmonary trunk and left ventricle, especially in young females.
- The left cardiophrenic junction may be formed by a fat pad and give a false impression of cardiomegaly.

Lateral Projection

Routinely, the patient's left side is positioned against the film cassette to minimize distortion of the heart due to geometric magnification. Superiorly, the anterior border is formed by the ascending aorta posterior to the retrosternal air space; inferiorly, the right ventricle and right ventricular outflow tract abut the sternum and blend into the main pulmonary artery, which then courses posteriorly to its bifurcation. The posterior cardiac contour is formed by the left atrium superiorly beneath the carina and the left ventricle curving inferiorly to the diaphragm, where the straight vertical edge of the inferior vena cava is often apparent within the thorax as it enters the right atrium.

Heart Size on Chest Radiographs

The cardiothoracic ratio—the ratio of the transverse cardiac diameter to the maximal internal diameter of the thorax at the level of the diaphragm on an upright posteroanterior chest radiograph—corrects for body size and magnification produced by slight differences in radiographic techniques. In adults, a ratio more than 0.5 is considered to indicate cardiomegaly. In aortic regurgitation, the left ventricle is often enlarged downward rather than horizontally. A high diaphragm

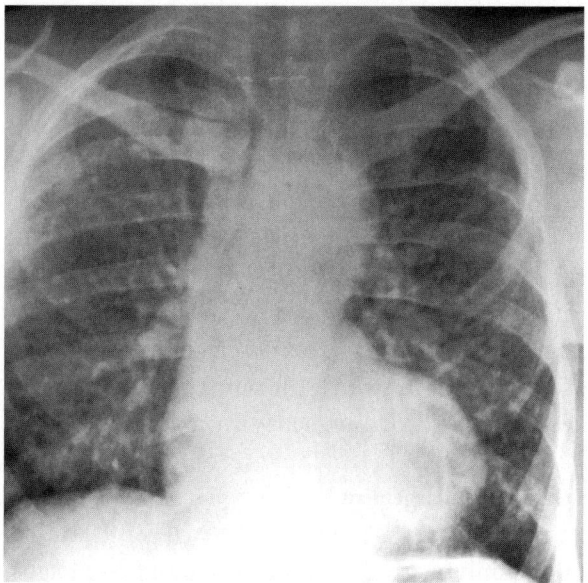

Fig. 4. Tetralogy of Fallot. Indentation in the region of the left pulmonary artery and elevation of the apex due to right ventricular hypertrophy give rise to a boot-shaped contour, typical for this condition.

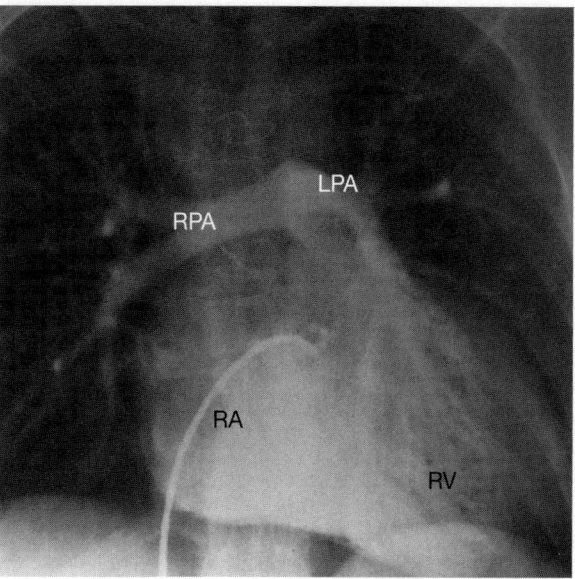

Fig. 5. Angiogram showing relative positions of right heart chambers on the posteroanterior projection. LPA, left pulmonary artery; RA, right atrium; RPA, right pulmonary artery; RV, right ventricle.

position, as seen with obesity or shallow inspiration, produces an erroneous ratio more than 0.5. Pectus excavatum and the absence of pericardium displace the heart posteriorly and rotate the apex laterally, resulting in a ratio more than 0.5 in the presence of a normal-sized heart. Large pericardial fat pads may give a falsely

increased cardiothoracic ratio. Because of these factors, relying on the cardiothoracic ratio alone to diagnose cardiomegaly can be misleading; however, it does serve as a baseline for future comparisons.

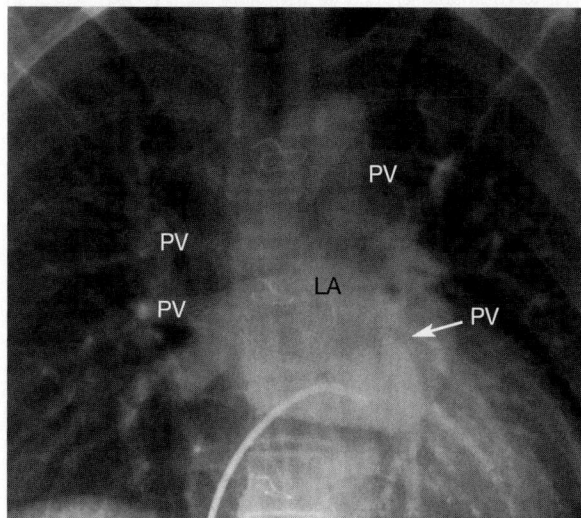

Fig. 6. Angiogram showing drainage of the pulmonary veins (PV) into the left atrium (LA).

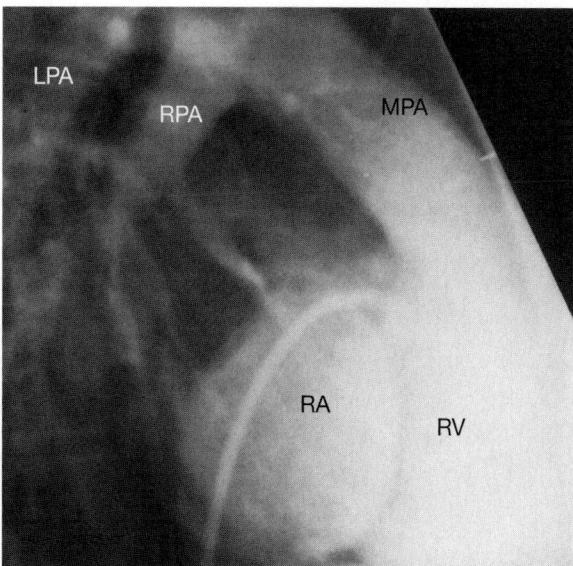

Fig. 7. Angiogram showing the relative positions of right heart chambers on lateral projection. LPA, left pulmonary artery; MPA, main pulmonary artery; RA, right atrium; RPA, right pulmonary artery; RV, right ventricle.

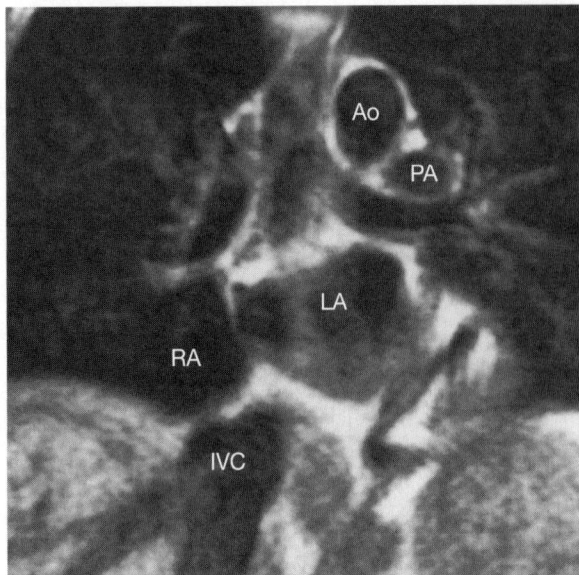

Fig. 8. Magnetic resonance image of heart showing the close anatomical relationship of right and left atria (RA and LA), aorta (Ao), and pulmonary artery (PA). IVC, inferior vena cava.

■ A cardiothoracic ratio >0.5 with a normal heart size occurs with absent pericardium, pectus excavatum, obesity, and poor inspiration.

Generalized Cardiac Enlargement

Global heart enlargement, with maintenance of an otherwise normal cardiac contour, usually is due to diffuse myocardial disease, abnormal volume or pressure overload as a consequence of valvular heart disease, hyperthyroidism, hypothyroidism, or anemia. Pericardial effusions also produce generalized enlargement of the cardiac silhouette (Fig. 11). Asymmetric enlargement with left ventricular prominence can be seen in the late stages of essential hypertension and other left-sided obstructive lesions with secondary left ventricular failure or in left-sided regurgitant valvular lesions (Fig. 12).

Left Atrial Enlargement

The left atrium sits just below the angle of the carina, in proximity with the left bronchus and esophagus; thus, enlargement is readily reflected by the displacement of these neighboring structures. Enlargement usually produces a double density behind the right atrial margin on a frontal projection as the left atrium bulges out from the mediastinum into the right lung. Occasionally, a double density is seen in the presence of a normal-sized left atrium in patients with a prominent right pulmonary venous confluence.

Additional signs of left atrial enlargement on the posteroanterior projection include upward and posterior displacement of the left main bronchus, resulting in

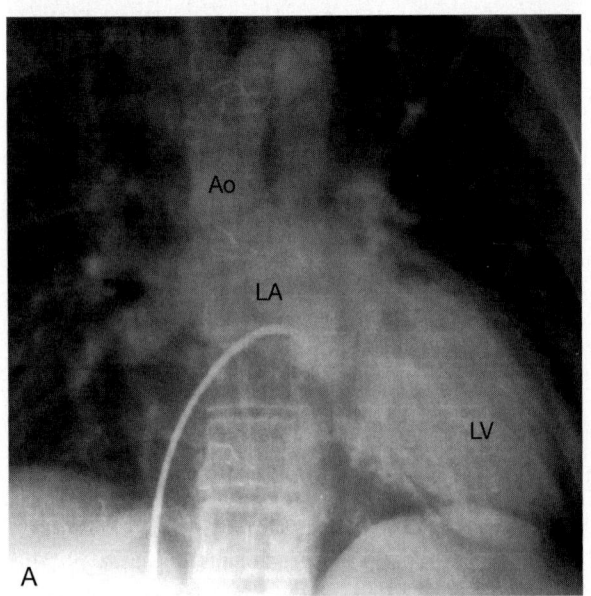
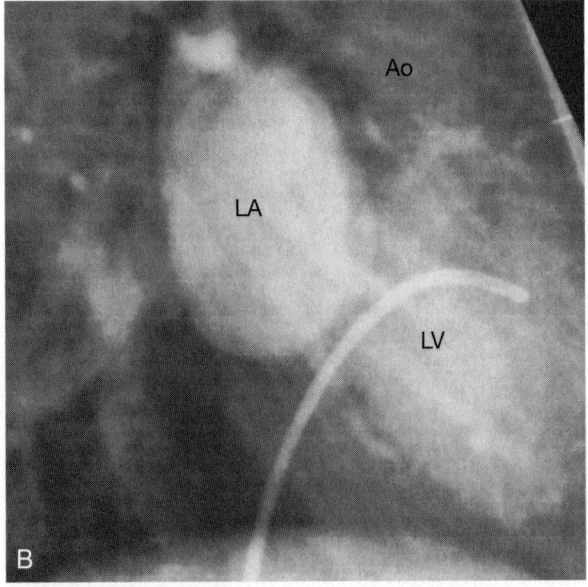

Fig. 9. Angiograms showing relative position of left heart chambers on frontal (*A*) and lateral (*B*) projections. Ao, aorta; LA, left atrium; LV, left ventricle.

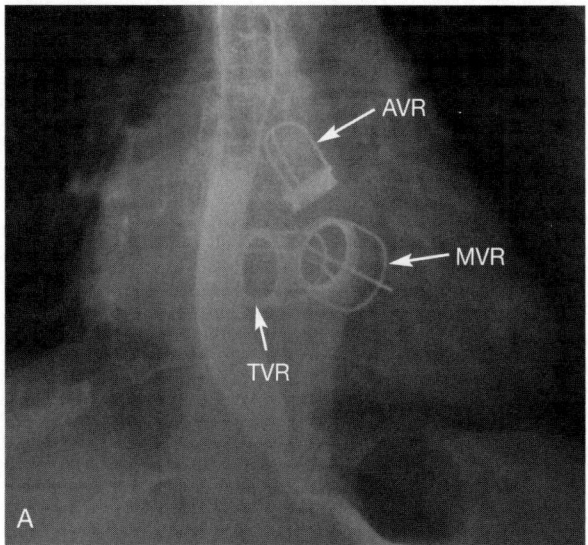

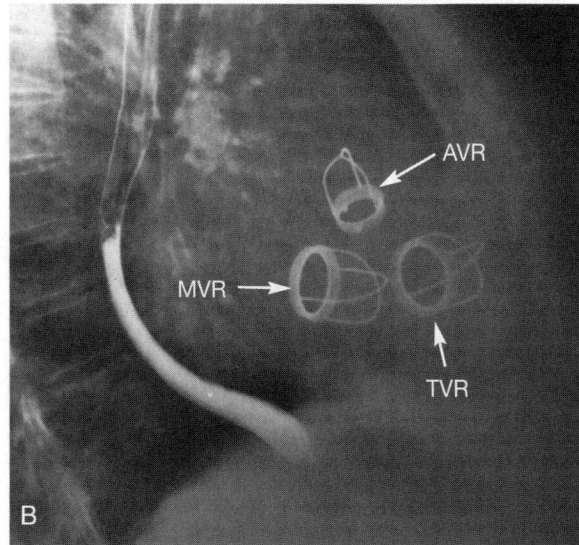

Fig. 10. Prosthetic Starr-Edwards valves seen on frontal (*A*) and lateral (*B*) projections. AVR, aortic valve prosthesis; MVR, mitral valve prosthesis; TVR, tricuspid valve prosthesis.

a less acute carinal angle. Enlargement of the left atrial appendage initially causes straightening and, subsequently, a convexity in the upper left cardiac contour. In the presence of a giant left atrium, the left atrium itself may project beyond the right atrium and form a portion of the right cardiac contour. On the lateral projection, left atrial enlargement can be recognized by posterior and upward displacement of the left main stem bronchus. The left atrium itself enlarges upward and posteriorly to form an increasing convex density.

■ Signs of left atrial enlargement are double density of right heart border and upward and posterior displacement of left main bronchus—widening of carinal angle.

Isolated left atrial enlargement most commonly is due to mitral valve stenosis caused by rheumatic heart disease (Fig. 13 and 14). Left atrial myxoma and cor triatriatum can also cause isolated left atrial enlargement.

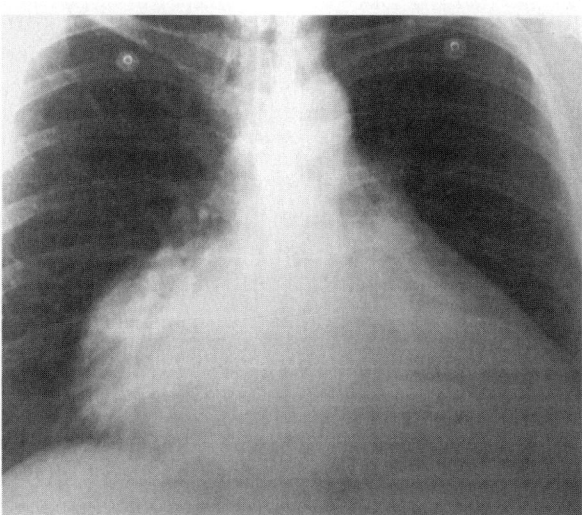

Fig. 11. Markedly enlarged cardiac silhouette primarily due to a large malignant pericardial effusion resulting from a sarcoma invading the heart chambers on the right.

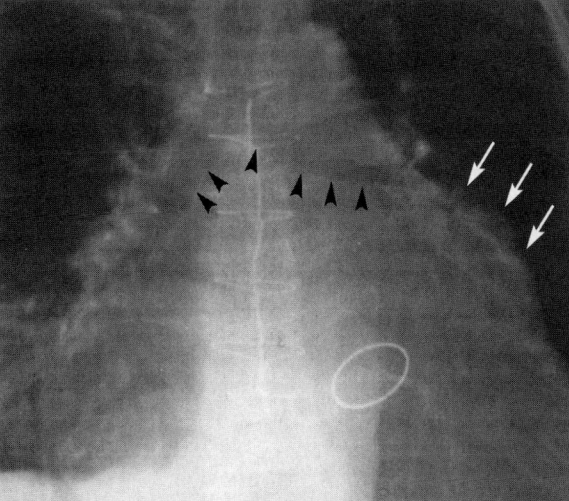

Fig. 12. Multichamber cardiac enlargement resulting from rheumatic heart disease. The left atrium is the most dilated chamber. Note prominence of the left atrial appendage (*arrows*) and marked splaying of the carina (*arrowheads*). A Hancock valve is in mitral position.

Isolated enlargement of the left atrial appendage or apparent enlargement due to a pericardial defect and focal herniation of the appendage may cause a localized bulge in the upper left cardiac contour without other signs of left atrial dilatation. Left atrial enlargement in combination with additional chamber involvement may be produced by various conditions, such as left ventricular failure, left-sided obstructive lesions, and certain shunts (e.g., ventricular septal defect, patent ductus arteriosus, and aortopulmonary window). However, left atrial enlargement does not occur with simple atrial septal defects. When left atrial enlargement is marked, it most often is due to rheumatic valvular disease.

- Isolated left atrial enlargement most commonly is due to mitral valve disease.
- Rarely, cor triatriatum or left atrial myxoma causes isolated left atrial enlargement.
- Left atrial enlargement does not occur with simple atrial septal defects.

Left Ventricular Enlargement

Left ventricular enlargement can be due to dilatation or hypertrophy or both. Considerable hypertrophy must be present to cause the cardiac shadow to enlarge appreciably. The classic appearance of left ventricular hypertrophy on the posteroanterior projection is rounding of the cardiac apex, with downward and lateral displacement without cardiac enlargement. Left ventricular dilatation causes an increase in the transverse diameter of the heart and cardiothoracic ratio, together with an apparent increase in the length of the left heart border. The cardiac apex may be displaced to the extent that it projects below the diaphragm. On the lateral projection, dilatation increases the posterior convexity of the left ventricular contour, which will project behind the edge of the vertical inferior vena cava. Obstruction to left ventricular emptying or increased afterload, as caused by systemic hypertension, aortic coarctation, or aortic valve stenosis, leads to hypertrophy initially, with rounding of the cardiac apex (Fig. 15). Left ventricular dilatation with cardiac failure may follow. Dilated cardiomyopathy, especially ischemic cardiomyopathy, primarily enlarges the left ventricle. Aortic valve regurgitation and mitral valve regurgitation enlarge the left ventricle and are associated with dilatation of the aorta and left atrium, respectively.

Left ventricular aneurysms, usually the result of a previous myocardial infarction, occasionally result in a localized bulge that projects beyond the normal ventricular contour or an angulation of the left ventricular contour (Fig. 16). A large apical aneurysm can appear similar to simple left ventricular chamber dilatation. Sometimes with true aneurysms of the left ventricle, the heart appears normal in size and contour. False

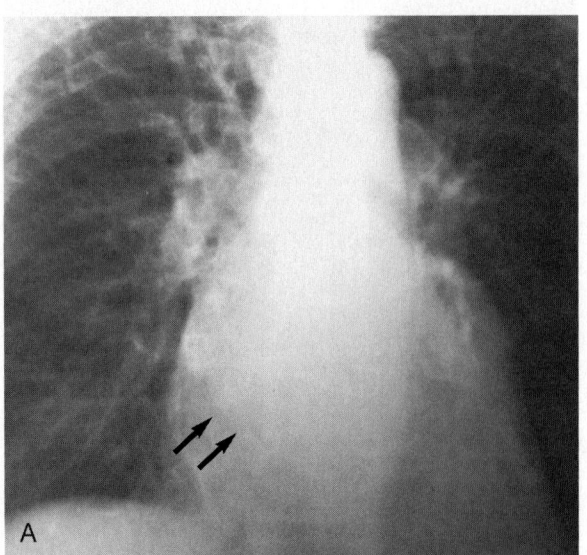
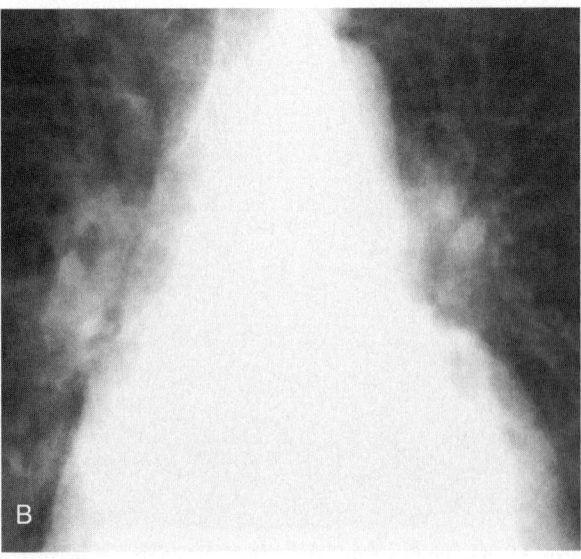

Fig. 13. Mitral stenosis resulting in left atrial enlargement, pulmonary venous hypertension, and right ventricular dilatation. Note double density projected over the right atrium (*arrows*) because of dilatation of left atrium.

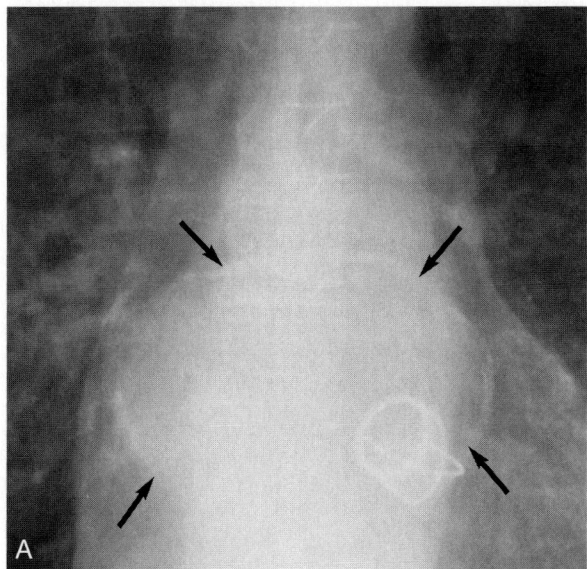 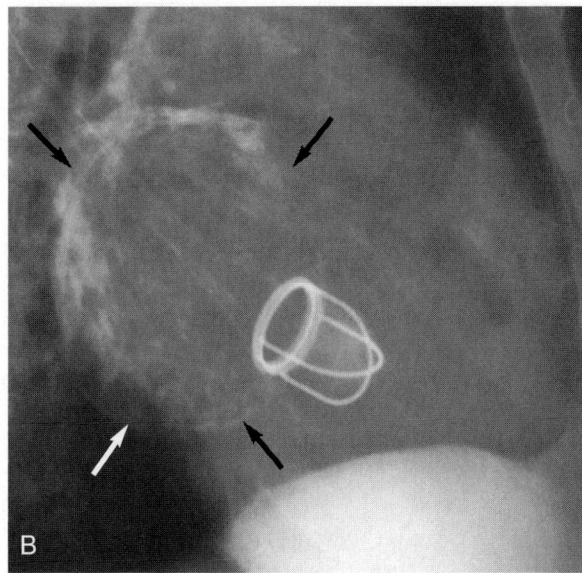

Fig. 14. *A*, Posteroanterior and, *B*, lateral projections showing mitral stenosis with left atrial enlargement (*arrows*) and calcification of atrial wall.

aneurysms often are paracardiac in location, posterior and inferior to the left ventricle. All cardiac chambers have been reported to be involved with aneurysm formation, although atrial aneurysms are extremely rare.

■ In the absence of heart failure, left ventricular hypertrophy must be massive before the heart shadow enlarges.

Right Atrial Enlargement

Isolated right atrial enlargement is detected best on a frontal radiograph. Enlargement is to the right and causes increased fullness and convexity of the right cardiac contour and angulation of the junction of the superior vena cava and right atrium. There may be associated dilatation of the superior and inferior venae cavae which causes widening of the right superior

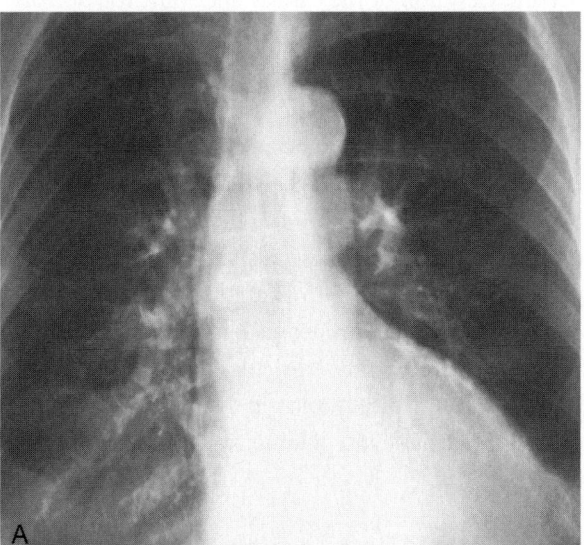 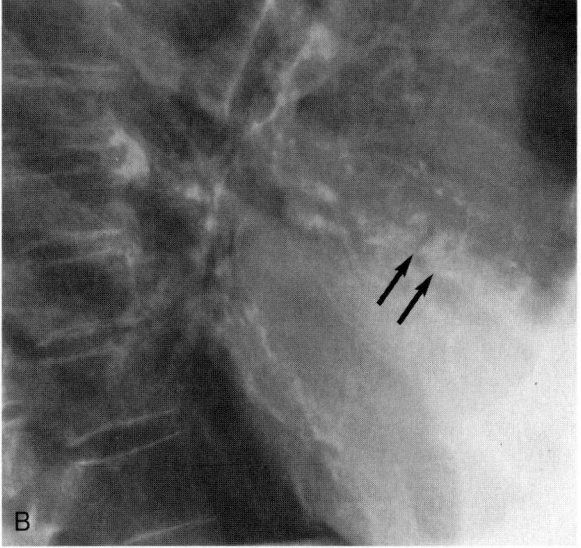

Fig. 15. *A*, Posteroanterior and, *B*, lateral projections of an enlarged left ventricle with dilatation of ascending aorta due to combined aortic insufficiency and aortic stenosis. The aortic valve is calcified (*arrows*) and pulmonary arteries are enlarged in this patient, who also has chronic obstructive pulmonary disease.

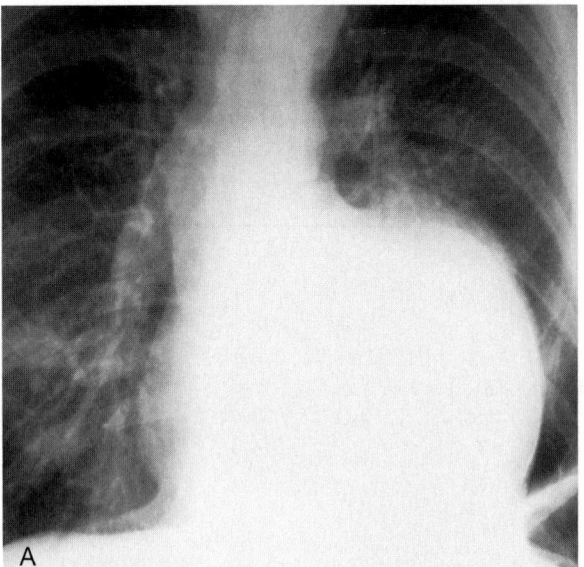
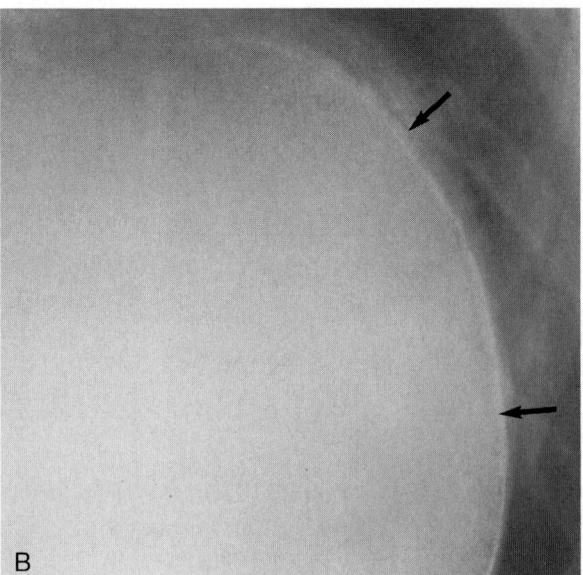

Fig. 16. *A*, Posteroanterior projection showing marked enlargement of left ventricle due to left ventricular aneurysm. *B*, Curvilinear calcification outlines aneurysm (*arrows*).

mediastinum and an additional border in the right cardiophrenic angle. On the lateral projection, right atrial dilatation is often difficult to appreciate. It causes a filling-in of the retrosternal clear space anteriorly and superiorly, with the cardiac silhouette extending behind the sternum more than one-third the way above the cardiophrenic angle, similar to that seen with right ventricular enlargement. There may be a double density that merges with the inferior vena caval shadow, which may be a slightly convex structure. Left atrial enlargement can be simulated by marked right atrial dilatation.

■ Right atrial enlargement fills in the retrosternal clear space on the lateral projection.

Isolated right atrial enlargement is uncommon and usually is due to tricuspid stenosis or right atrial tumor. Right atrial dilatation associated with other chamber enlargement, primarily right ventricular enlargement, occurs in several conditions, such as tricuspid regurgitation, pulmonary arterial hypertension, shunts to the right atrium, and cardiomyopathies (Fig. 17 and 18). Marked isolated right atrial enlargement resulting in a box-shaped heart occurs in Ebstein malformation of the tricuspid valve (Fig. 19). This configuration of the heart is the result of marked angulation at the superior vena caval-right atrial junction as the right atrium enlarges.

■ Ebstein anomaly causes a box-shaped heart.

Right Ventricular Enlargement

The right ventricle enlarges by broadening its triangular shape in the superior and leftward direction. With increasing right ventricular enlargement, the entire heart rotates to the left around its long axis and displaces the left ventricle posteriorly. This displacement causes increased convexity of the left upper heart border and elevation of the cardiac apex. The rotation also makes the pulmonary trunk appear relatively small. With marked dilatation, the right ventricle may form the left heart border on the posteroanterior projection.

On the lateral projection, the right ventricle extends cranially behind the sternum, with increased bulk anteriorly. Normally, the heart does not extend more than one-third of the distance from the cardiophrenic angle to the sternal angle or the level of the carina; however, normal extension can vary with body habitus. Isolated right ventricular enlargement is very unusual. More typically, there is associated prominence of the right atrium and pulmonary trunk.

PULMONARY VASCULATURE

Because the pulmonary vasculature reflects the physiologic effects of a cardiac lesion, it provides important clues to the diagnosis. Radiographic

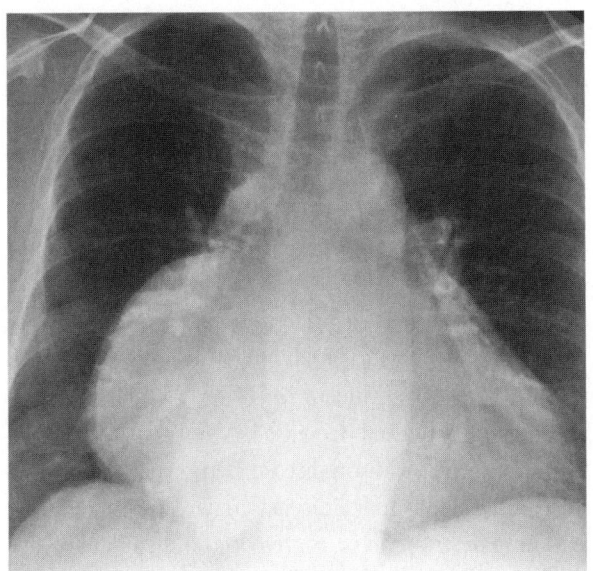

Fig. 17. Marked right atrial dilatation and right ventricular dilatation due to severe tricuspid regurgitation related to traumatic injury of tricuspid valve.

abnormalities are primarily the result of an increase in pulmonary blood flow or an obstruction to flow somewhere in the pulmonary circuit.

Normal Pulmonary Blood Flow

The pulmonary arteries and veins extend outward from each hilum in an orderly branching fashion, gradually tapering peripherally. The hilar density is composed of the proximal pulmonary arteries, and the left hilum normally projects more cranially than the right one because of the course of the left pulmonary artery over the left main bronchus. In the upper lobes, the veins and arteries are essentially parallel, the veins lying lateral to their corresponding arteries. The major arteries and veins in the lower lung fields cross each other, the veins taking a more horizontal course toward the left atrium. In the upright position, there is increased flow to the base of the lungs (largely due to the effects of gravity), which causes the lower-lobe vessels to increase in size. It may be difficult to identify the apical vessels clearly because pulmonary flow to the apices is negligible in the upright position. Therefore, position has a marked effect on flow distribution.

Increased Pulmonary Blood Flow

As pulmonary flow increases, the pulmonary vessels, both arteries and veins, become enlarged. These enlarged vessels become apparent when pulmonary flow is approximately twice normal. The overcirculation pattern may be symmetric or asymmetric. High-output states with increased circulating blood volume, such as anemia, pregnancy, thyrotoxicosis, overhydration, and fever, result in a symmetric increase in vascularity, as do various congenital defects characterized by left-to-right

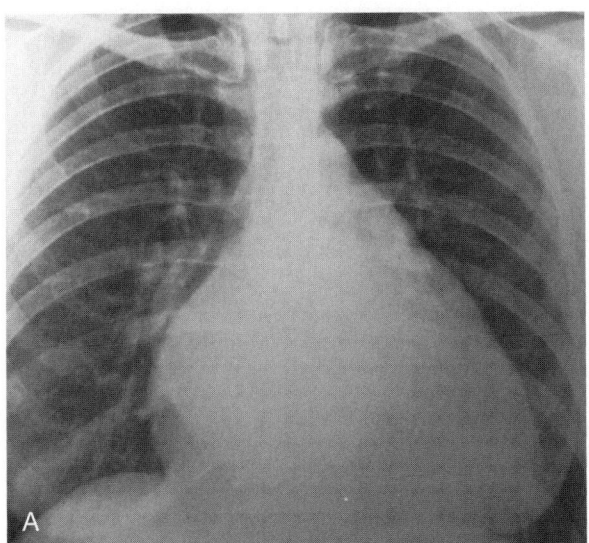
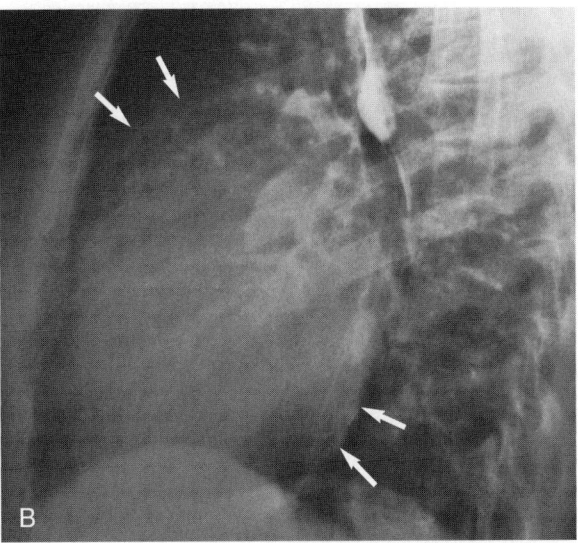

Fig. 18. *A*, Posteroanterior and, *B*, lateral projections showing combined mitral stenosis and mitral insufficiency resulting in left atrial enlargement, marked right ventricular enlargement, and slight left ventricular enlargement. Dilated ventricles (*arrows*) are appreciated best on lateral view.

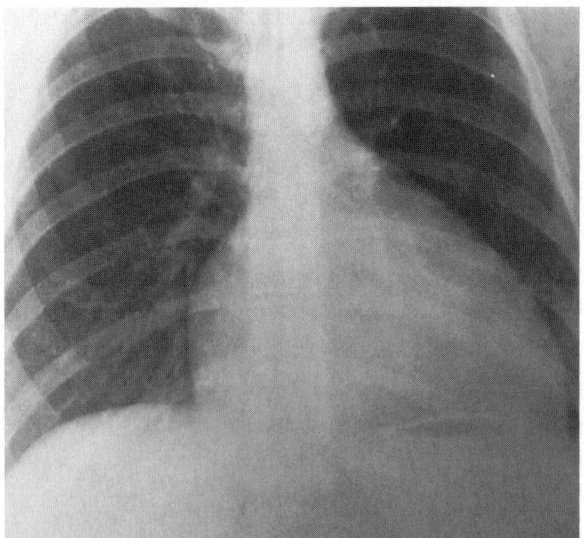

Fig. 19. Enlarged box-shaped heart with decreased pulmonary vascularity typical of Ebstein anomaly.

shunts (Fig. 20 and 21). An asymmetric increase in pulmonary flow may be congenital in origin (e.g., pulmonary arteriovenous malformation, anomalous origin of a pulmonary artery) but is more commonly the result of surgical intervention to create a systemic-to-pulmonary shunt to improve pulmonary blood flow in the presence of severe pulmonary stenosis or atresia (e.g., a Blalock-Taussig shunt).

Decreased Pulmonary Blood Flow

Essentially all the linear shadows in the normal lung fields are due to pulmonary vasculature. When flow and, therefore, vessel size are diminished, the lung fields appear abnormally radiolucent. Both symmetric and asymmetric patterns of abnormal vascularity can be observed. Generalized undercirculation can be due to an obstructive lesion in the right heart, as in tetralogy of Fallot, pulmonary atresia, right ventricular tumor, or tricuspid valve atresia. Small-caliber pulmonary vessels with relatively hyperlucent lungs and a small heart are evidence of a marked decrease in the circulating blood volume (e.g., in Addison disease, hemorrhage). Chronic obstructive pulmonary disease may result in generalized lung destruction or, more commonly, a patchy distribution of decreased vascularity. Segmental and asymmetric decreases in pulmonary vascularity are seen with pulmonary embolic disease (Westermark sign), segmental chronic obstructive pulmonary disease, partial pneumonectomy, and branch pulmonary artery stenoses (Fig. 22). Rarely, postinflammatory changes (e.g., granulomatous mediastinitis), extrinsic compression (e.g., aortic aneurysm), and congenital hypoplasia as seen in the scimitar syndrome result in areas of decreased pulmonary flow. Bronchial collateral circulation may become prominent, with a somewhat disordered pattern, when there is a decrease in pulmonary

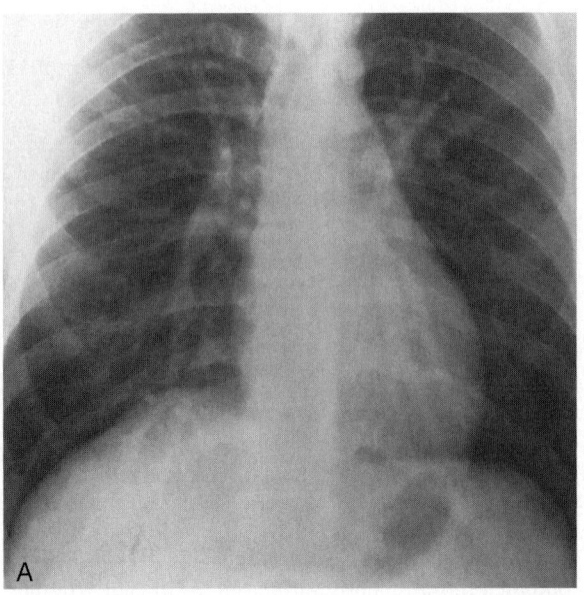

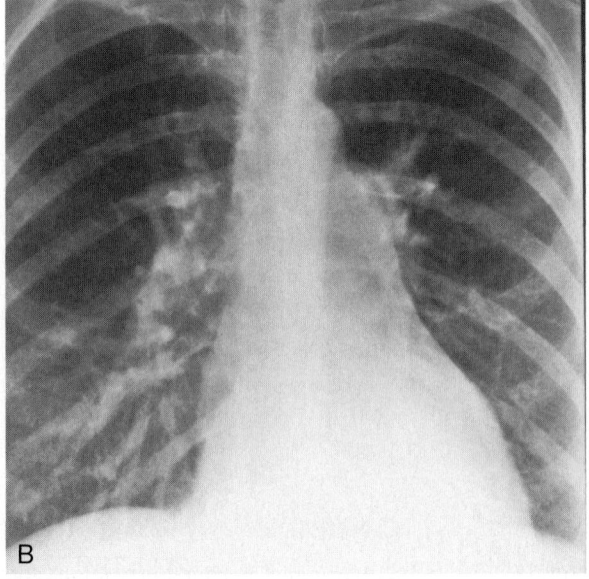

Fig. 20. Two examples of patients with atrial septal defects. *A*, Mild right ventricular dilatation in an asymptomatic patient. *B*, More prominent shunt vascularity and cardiac enlargement in a patient with very mild dyspnea on exertion.

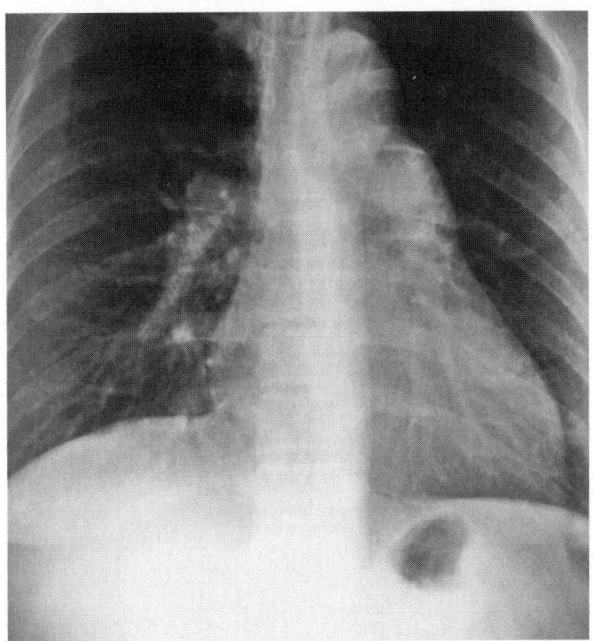

Fig. 21. Patent ductus arteriosus resulting in prominence of the aortic arch and shunt vascularity. There is mild left ventricular enlargement.

artery blood flow, and occasionally it gives the illusion that the overall vascularity is actually normal or even increased. Small hila in tetralogy of Fallot or pulmonary atresia and loss of the normal branching pattern of pulmonary vasculature should be evident on the chest radiograph.

■ If the lung hila are small, consider tetralogy of Fallot or pulmonary atresia.

Increased Resistance to Pulmonary Blood Flow

Pulmonary hypertension with redistribution of flow is the result of increased resistance in the pulmonary circuit. Recognition of the various redistribution patterns seen on chest radiographs often allows the level of the increased resistance and the possible underlying abnormality to be identified.

Pulmonary Venous Hypertension

Lesions acting beyond the pulmonary capillary level result in increase of the pulmonary venous pressure. Left ventricular dysfunction and mitral valve disease are the most common causes of pulmonary venous hypertension; other obstructive lesions at the left atrial level (e.g., atrial myxoma, cor triatriatum, thrombus) or pulmonary vein level (e.g., stenosis, veno-occlusive disease, or thrombosis) are relatively rare.

Initially, because of the increase in venous pressure, venous dilatation occurs throughout the lungs. However, the radiographic pattern typically seen is that of prominent upper lung vessels, both arteries and veins. This phenomenon is thought to be due to a localized segmental reflex initiated by the increase in pulmonary venous pressure above a critical level of about 10 to 15 mm Hg. An additional factor is the

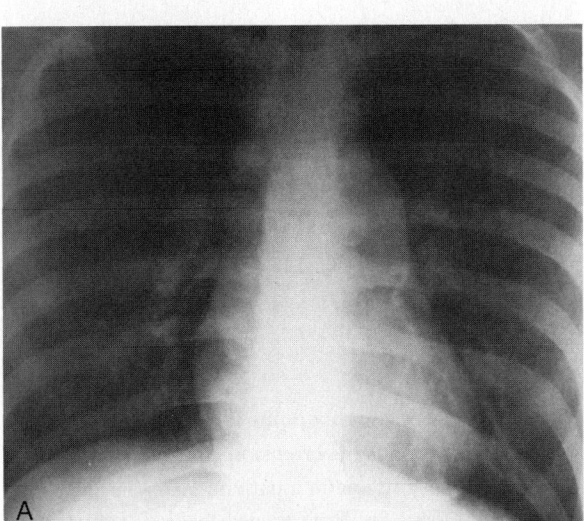

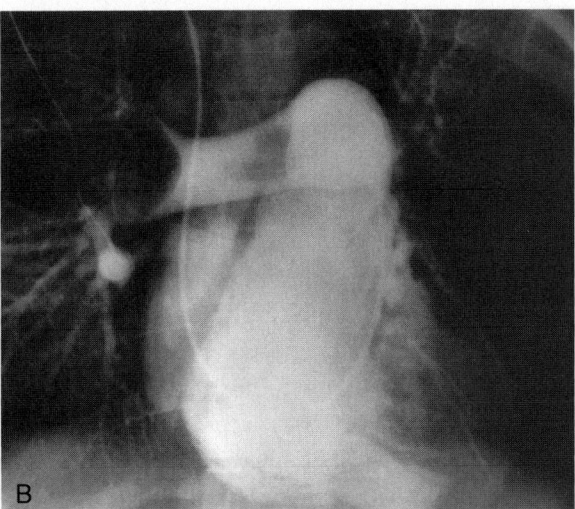

Fig. 22. *A*, Posteroanterior projection showing decreased vascular markings in both lungs, most marked in right upper lobe. *B*, Angiogram showing large bilateral emboli, resulting in little flow to right upper lobe and left lower lobe.

accumulation of fluid around compressible small vessels when plasma oncotic pressure is exceeded by pulmonary venous pressure. When a person is in the upright position, the pressure in the lower lung is greater because of hydrostatic forces; therefore, vasoconstriction of both arteries and veins occurs here first and increases resistance to flow, thereby reducing the circulatory volume through these vessels. To overcome the increased resistance and to maintain a gradient in the presence of increased pulmonary venous pressure, the pulmonary artery pressure must increase, resulting in increased flow to the apices. The diverted pulmonary flow increases the size and visibility of the upper-lobe vessels (Fig. 23). As pulmonary venous hypertension increases to the order of 25 mm Hg, there is increased transudation of plasma from the lower lung capillaries which results in interstitial edema. In addition to obscuring further the now smaller and crowded lower-lobe vessels, this transudation results in the radiographic appearance of septal lines (Kerley lines), which are due to fluid within the interlobular septa (Fig. 24). Still further increase in pulmonary venous pressure results in transudation of plasma into the alveoli, producing classic alveolar edema when the pressure exceeds 30 mm Hg.

Pulmonary Arterial Hypertension

Increased resistance at the pulmonary capillary or arteriolar level increases pulmonary artery pressure. The causes of pulmonary arterial hypertension include 1) obstructive processes (e.g., chronic pulmonary emboli, idiopathic or primary pulmonary arterial hypertension, pulmonary schistosomiasis), 2) obliterative processes (e.g., pulmonary fibrosis, chronic obstructive pulmonary disease), 3) constrictive processes (e.g., chronic hypoxia), and 4) increased flow as seen in large left-to-right shunts with development of Eisenmenger syndrome (Fig. 25 and 26). Radiographically, pulmonary arteries are dilated centrally, with an abrupt disparity in the caliber of the central and intrapulmonary arteries or "pruning" of the intrapulmonary branches. This uneven response is thought to be due to constriction of the muscular intrapulmonary branches in response to the increased intraluminal pressures, with dilatation of the more elastic central arteries.

■ The classic chest radiographic findings in pulmonary arterial hypertension are dilated distal proximal pulmonary arteries and "pruning" of intrapulmonary branches.

PERICARDIAL DISEASE

Normal pericardium is seldom identified on plain chest radiographs. It may be visible as a sharp line at the cardiac apex, outlined by epicardial and mediastinal fat.

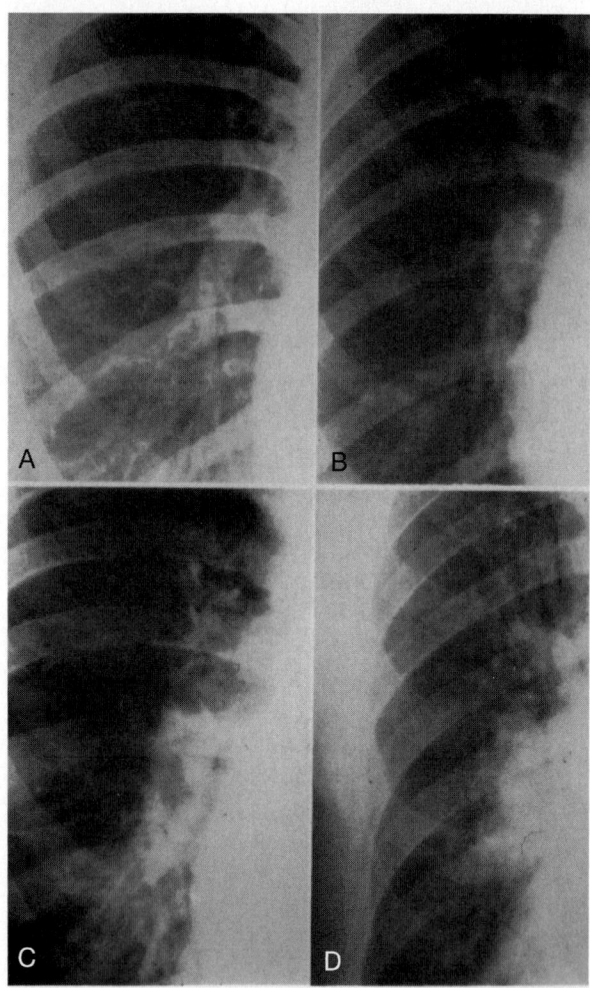

Fig. 23. *A-D*, Serial radiographs showing development of pulmonary venous hypertension continuing on to florid pulmonary edema in a patient with a large myocardial infarction. Note progressive redistribution of the prominence of the pulmonary vessels to the right upper lobe. The hilar vessels become much less distinct as the edema develops.

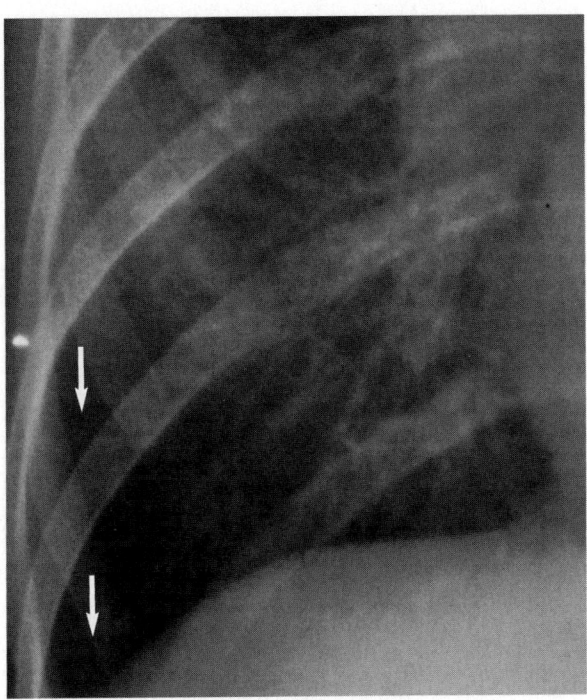

Fig. 24. Interstitial edema with appearance of Kerley lines (*arrows*) due to fluid within the interlobular septa.

Pericardial Effusion

A pericardial stripe wider than 2 mm that parallels the lower heart border, usually in the lateral projection and best identified in the sternophrenic angle, is diagnostic of a pericardial effusion. The only clue to a relatively small effusion may be a noticeable change in heart size compared with that on previous studies. The classic water-flask configuration of a large effusion may not be present, and the appearance of the cardiac silhouette may be identical to that in dilated cardiomyopathy with no significant distortion other than enlargement. A large heart with a prominent superior vena cava and azygos vein in combination with decreased pulmonary vasculature should raise the question of cardiac tamponade. Acutely, a relatively small effusion can cause tamponade with minimal enlargement of the cardiac shadow.

Pericardial Calcification

Constrictive pericarditis may occur as the result of pericarditis and pericardial effusion of any cause. Calcification of the pericardium is highly suggestive but not pathognomonic of constrictive pericarditis. In more

than 50% of patients with constrictive pericarditis, calcifications do not show on the plain chest radiograph. Calcifications are found frequently on the anterior and diaphragmatic surfaces, but they may be over any part of the heart. Linear or plaque-like calcifications, often best seen on the lateral view, are typically projected over the right ventricle or the atrioventricular groove (Fig. 27). The entire heart may appear encased in a shell. The calcification may be dense and thick.

■ In more than 50% of patients with constrictive pericarditis, pericardial calcification does not show on chest radiography.

Pericardial Defects

Congenital or surgical absence of the pericardium may result in changes in the cardiac contours. Congenital absence is more commonly left-sided and rarely right-sided. Partial defects may allow a portion of the heart (usually the left atrial appendage in congenital defects) to herniate outside the pericardial sac, with the herniated portion producing a bulge in the contour of the heart. "Complete" absence of the pericardium is actually a unilateral defect and nearly always left-sided. The heart appears shifted to the left without a shift in the trachea (Fig. 28). The left cardiac contour has an elongated appearance. The pulmonary artery often appears prominent and sharply defined. A somewhat similar appearance is seen on the frontal projection when the heart is rotated because of compression of the chest wall in patients with pectus excavatum deformity.

■ Partial or "complete" absence of the pericardium is usually left-sided.

CARDIAC MASSES

The role of plain chest radiographs in the identification of cardiac masses is often limited. Radiographic manifestations are dependent on tumor size, location, and type. With many intracavitary and intramural tumors of even moderate size, no changes are seen on plain radiographs unless hemodynamic alterations are produced, such as the mimicking of mitral stenosis by a left atrial myxoma. Left ventricular aneurysms, pericardial cysts, extracardiac mediastinal masses, loculated pericardial cysts, and loculated pericardial effusions are all

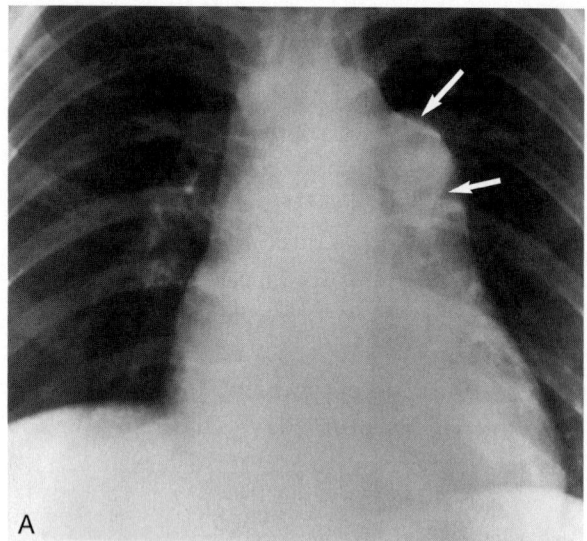

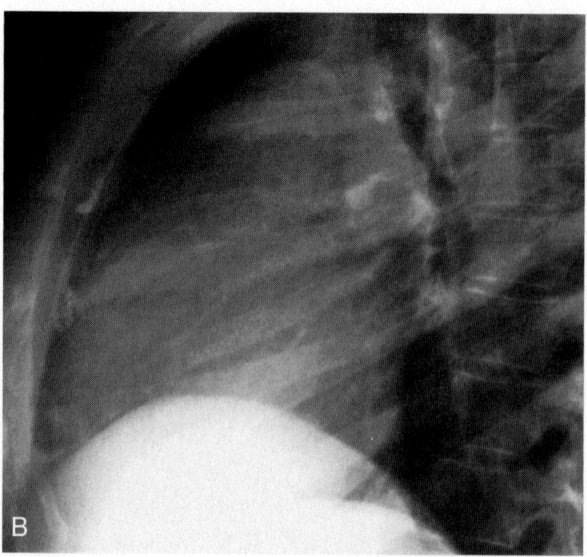

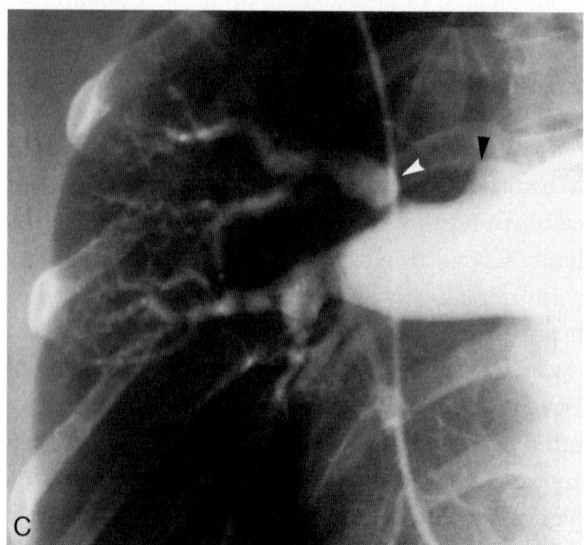

Fig. 25. Pulmonary hypertension due to chronic pulmonary emboli. Note the central pulmonary artery enlargement (*arrows*) (*A*) and right ventricular dilatation seen best in the lateral projection (*B*). The angiogram shows classic arterial occlusions and stenoses (*arrowheads*) (*C*).

causes of abnormal contours that can be indistinguishable from neoplasms (Fig. 29 and 30). The presence of calcification may help in the detection of a mass, but calcification patterns are not specific, and differentiation from calcification of thrombus or normal structures usually requires additional imaging methods.

AORTIC DISEASE

The aortic knob, representing the foreshortened transverse aortic arch, is the only border-forming portion of the normal thoracic aorta that is otherwise hidden within the mediastinum. The descending thoracic aorta parallels the thoracic spine on the left. With the development of atherosclerotic aortic disease,

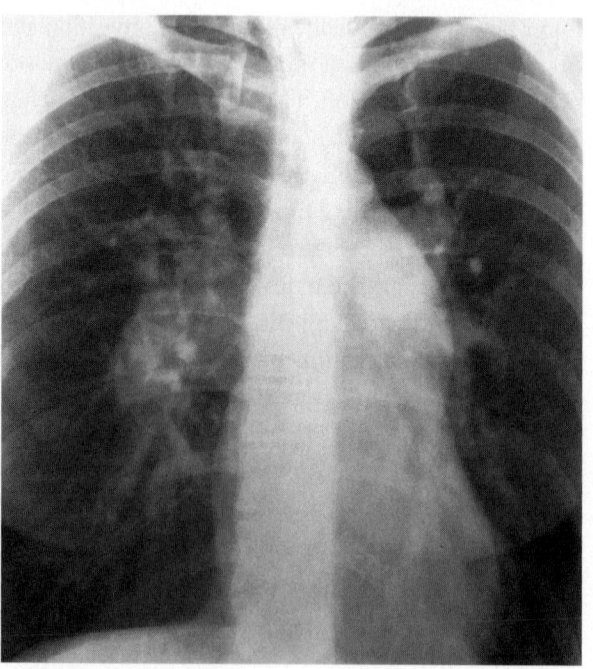

Fig. 26. Marked enlargement of the pulmonary arteries centrally due to Eisenmenger syndrome caused by longstanding atrial septal defect.

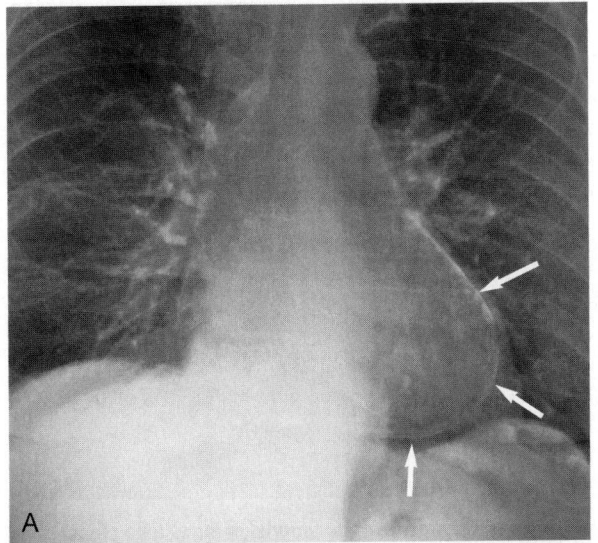

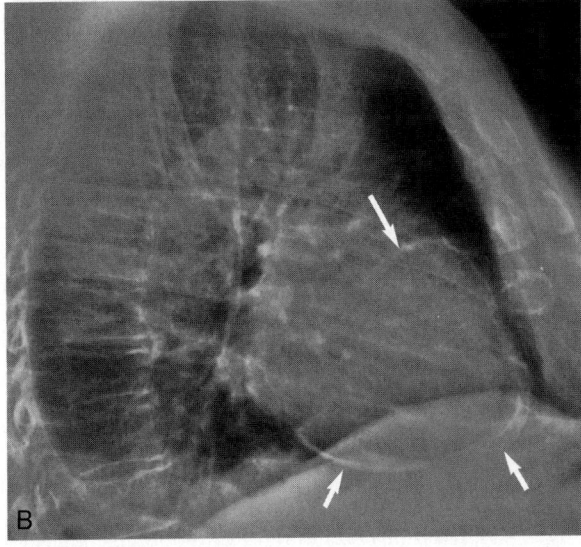

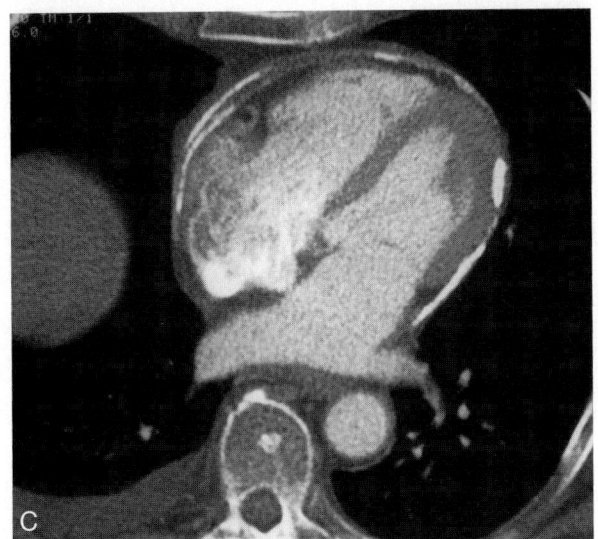

Fig. 27. *A* and *B*, Plain radiographs showing constrictive pericarditis with circumferential pericardial calcifications (*arrows*). Note the pulmonary venous hypertension and right pleural effusion. *C*, Computed tomographic image through the mid ventricles better shows the circumferential nature of the relatively coarse calcifications.

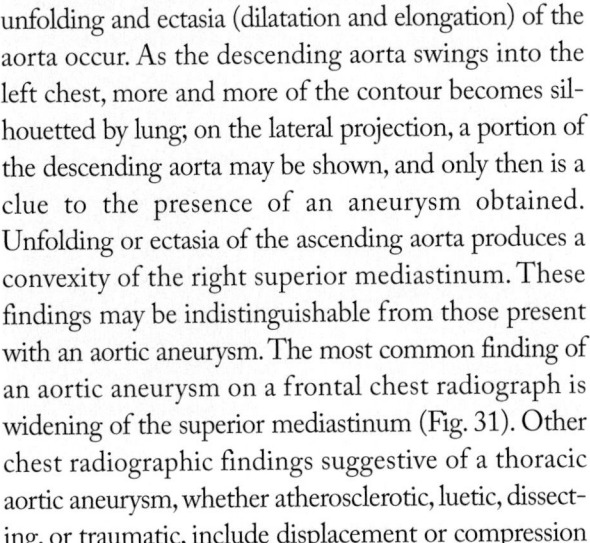

unfolding and ectasia (dilatation and elongation) of the aorta occur. As the descending aorta swings into the left chest, more and more of the contour becomes silhouetted by lung; on the lateral projection, a portion of the descending aorta may be shown, and only then is a clue to the presence of an aneurysm obtained. Unfolding or ectasia of the ascending aorta produces a convexity of the right superior mediastinum. These findings may be indistinguishable from those present with an aortic aneurysm. The most common finding of an aortic aneurysm on a frontal chest radiograph is widening of the superior mediastinum (Fig. 31). Other chest radiographic findings suggestive of a thoracic aortic aneurysm, whether atherosclerotic, luetic, dissecting, or traumatic, include displacement or compression

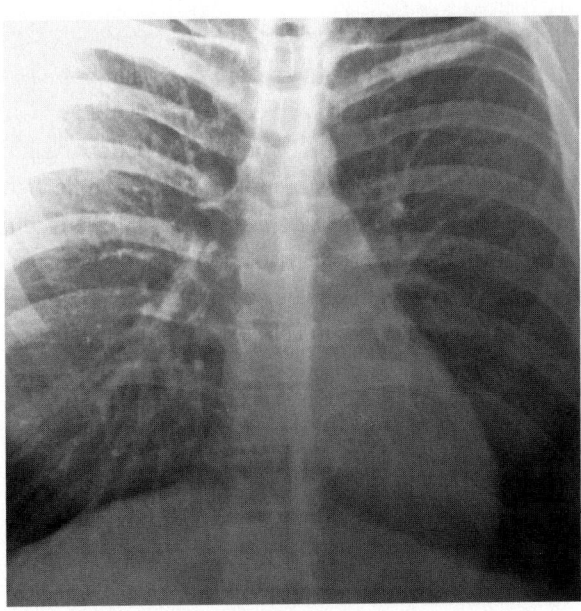

Fig. 28. Absence of pericardium resulting in displacement of cardiac apex to the left, mimicking an oblique projection.

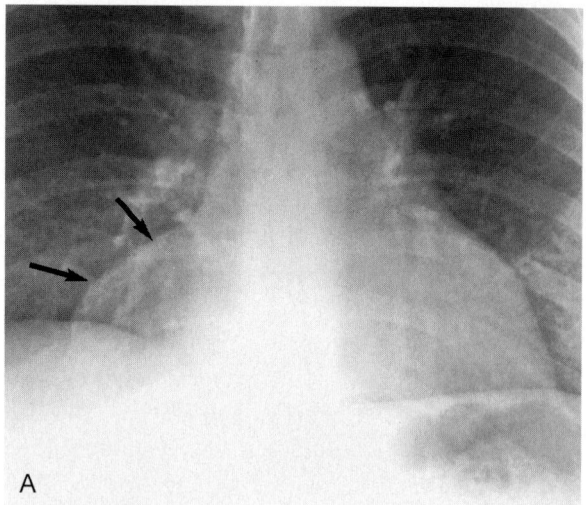
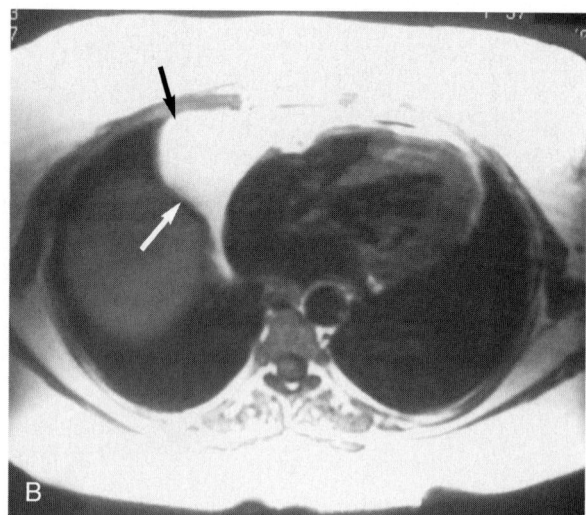

Fig. 29. *A*, Mass (*arrows*) in right cardiophrenic angle consistent with a prominent cardiac fat pad. *B*, High signal of adipose tissue (*arrows*) is shown with magnetic resonance imaging of this region.

(or both) of the trachea and esophagus either to the left and posteriorly by an aneurysm of the ascending aorta or to the right and anteriorly by an aneurysm of the descending aorta. Calcification in the aorta is a common finding in atherosclerotic aortic disease. Because

the aorta is largely hidden by the mediastinal silhouette, the cross-sectional methods, such as computed tomography and magnetic resonance imaging, provide greater detail in the evaluation and follow-up of aortic disease (Fig. 32-34).

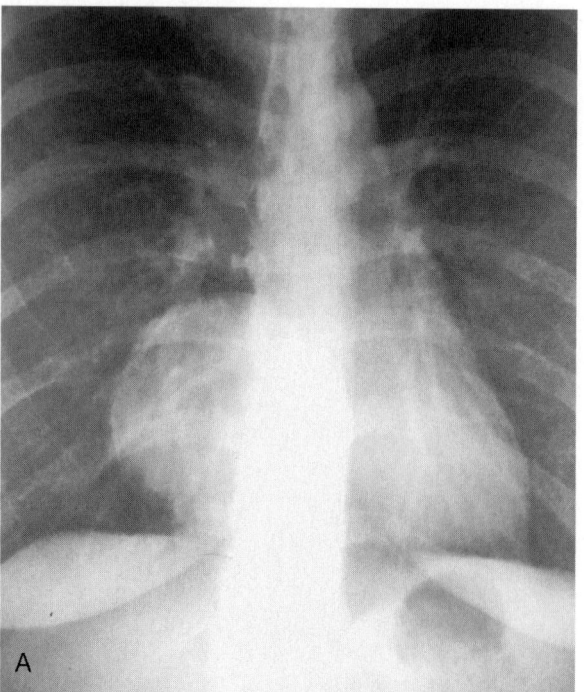
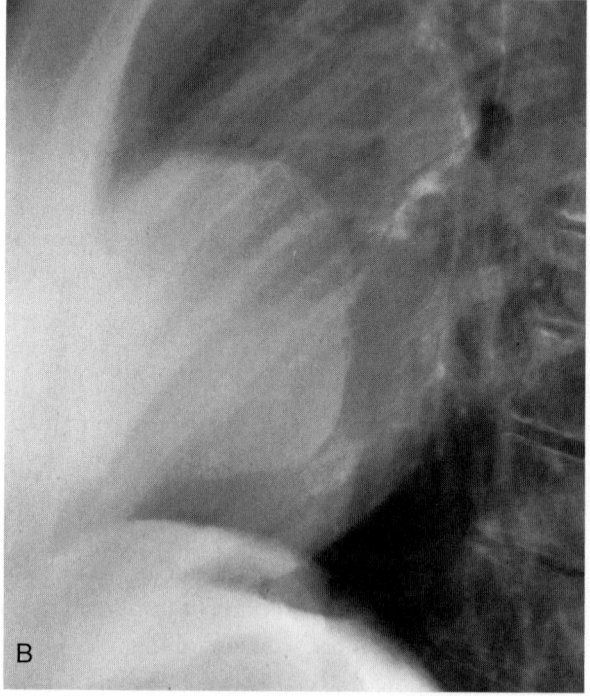

Fig. 30. *A*, Posteroanterior and, *B*, lateral projections showing a well-defined rounded mass projected adjacent to right atrium. Heart and pulmonary vasculature are otherwise normal. Appearance is typical of a pericardial cyst.

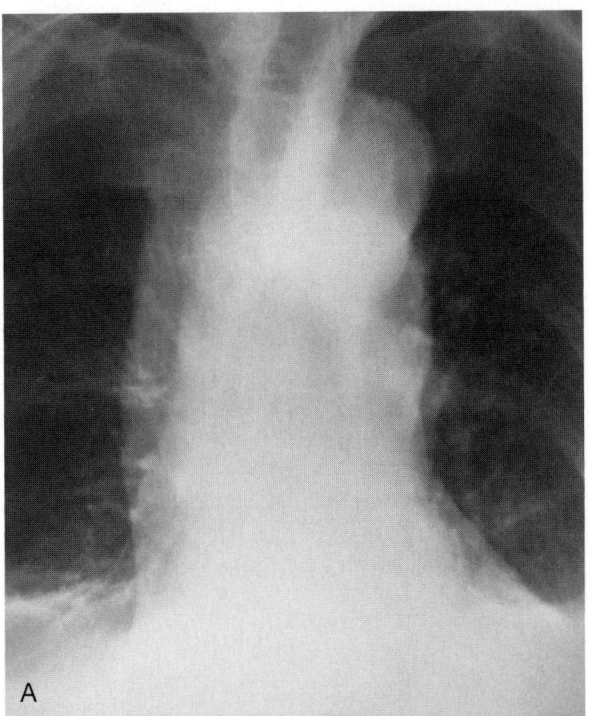

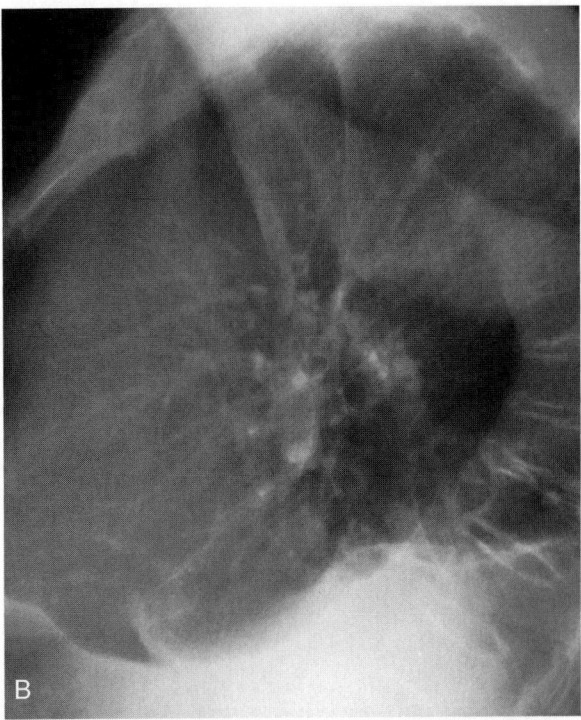

Fig. 31. *A*, Posteroanterior and, *B*, lateral projections showing marked enlargement of aortic knob and widening of mediastinum due to a large ascending aortic aneurysm. The size of the ascending aorta is appreciated better on the lateral view. The patient has significant aortic regurgitation with bilateral pleural effusions.

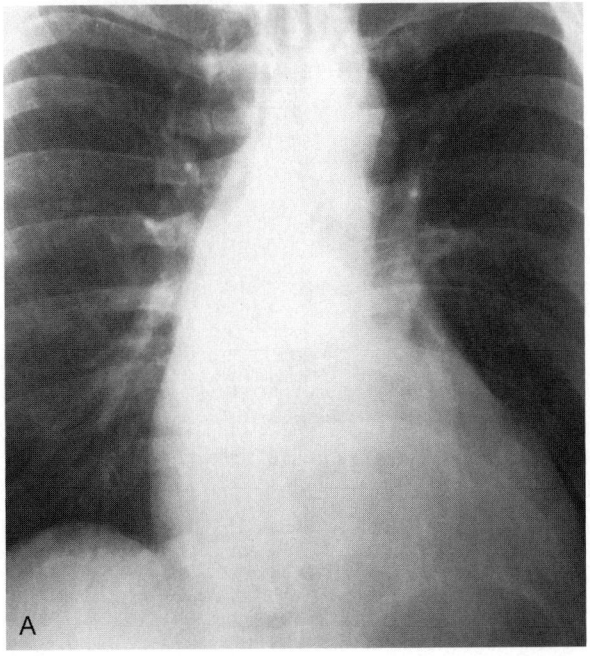

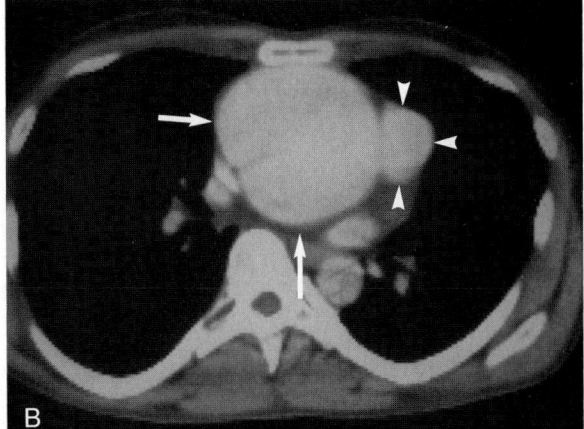

Fig. 32. *A*, Posteroanterior projection showing marked enlargement of ascending aorta caused by a dissecting aneurysm. *B*, This is appreciated better on a computed tomographic scan. Note discrepancy in size between the ascending aorta (*arrows*) and the main pulmonary artery (*arrowheads*).

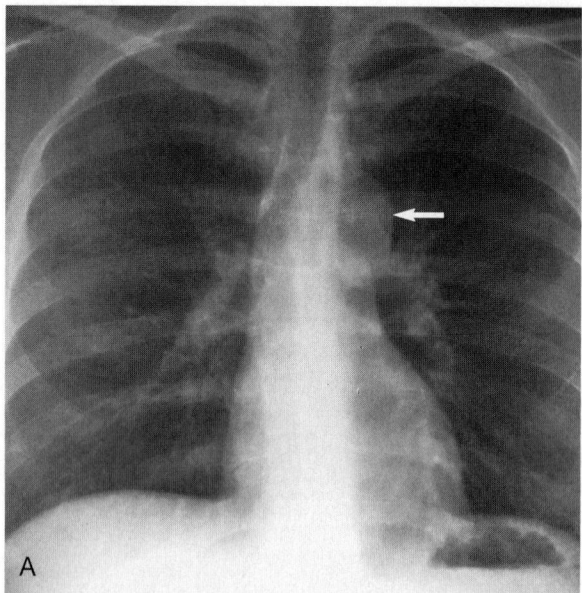

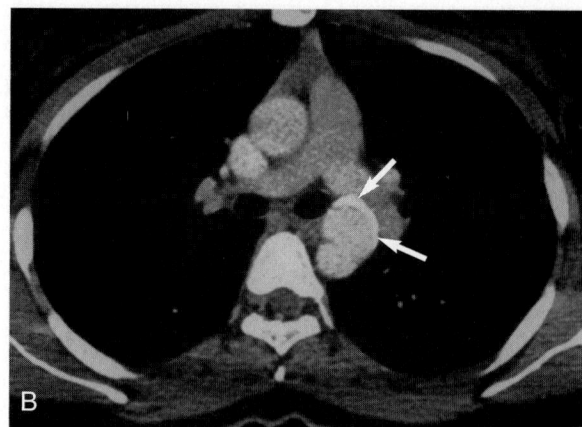

Fig. 33. *A*, Enlargement of aortic arch containing curvilinear calcification (*arrow*). *B*, Computed tomographic scan shows better the small pseudoaneurysm containing peripheral calcification (*arrows*), the result of remote trauma.

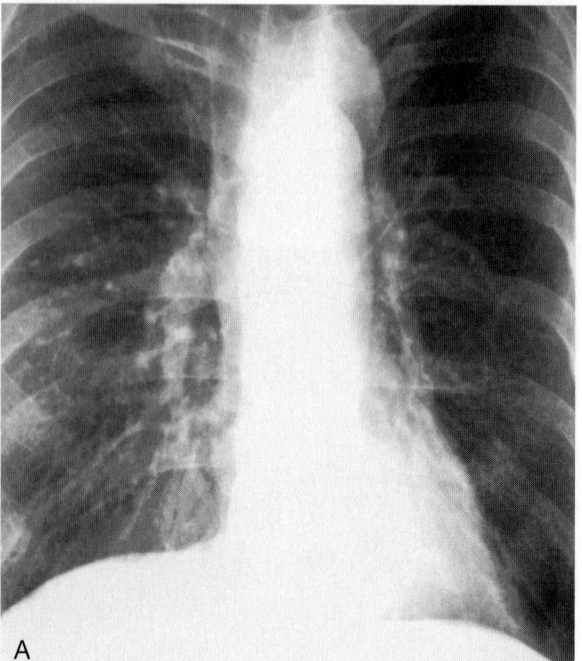

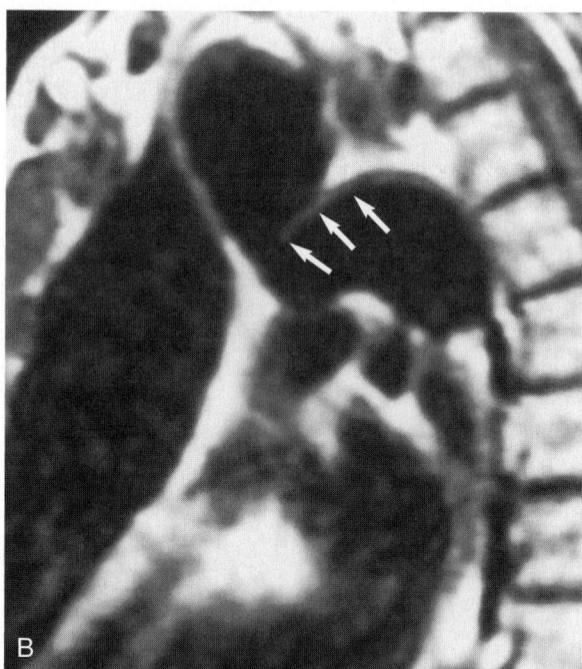

Fig. 34. *A*, Double contour to aortic arch typical of coarctation. *B*, Magnetic resonance image nicely shows the focal narrowing and resulting kinking (*arrows*) of proximal descending aorta.

15

ATLAS OF RADIOGRAPHS OF CONGENITAL HEART DEFECTS

Sabrina D. Phillips, MD

Joseph G. Murphy, MD

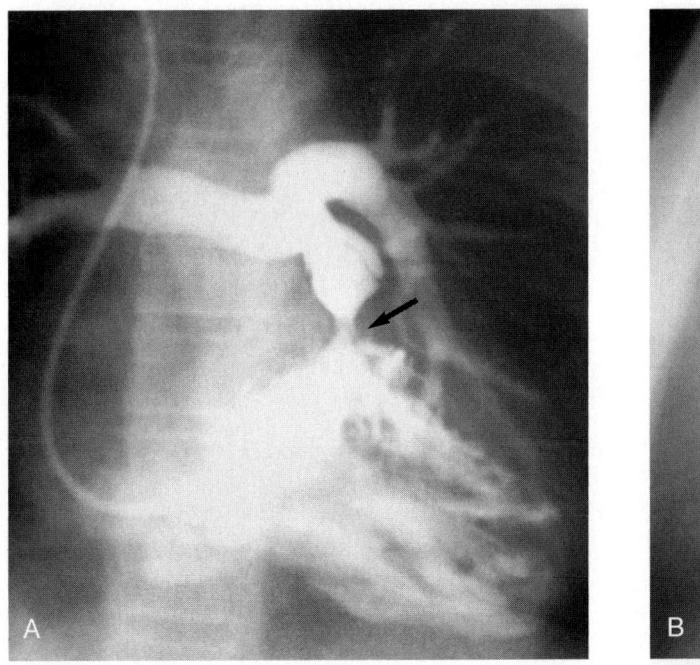 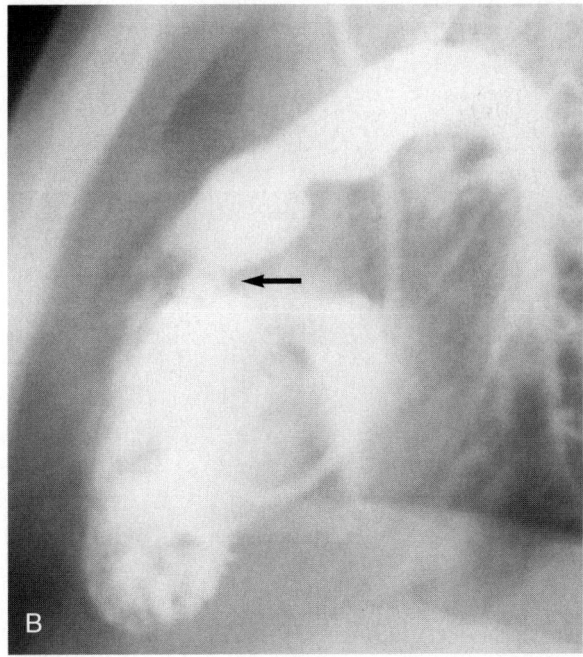

Fig. 1. Tetralogy of Fallot. Right ventriculograms show marked infundibular stenosis (*arrows*) in both frontal (*A*) and lateral (*B*) projections.

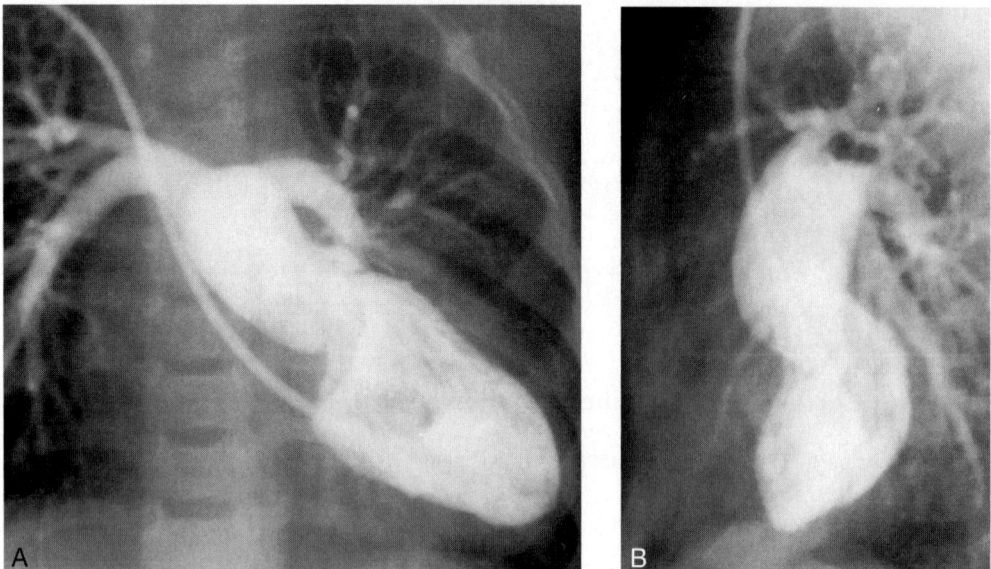

Fig. 2. D-Transposition with intact ventricular septum. Frontal (*A*) and lateral (*B*) views.

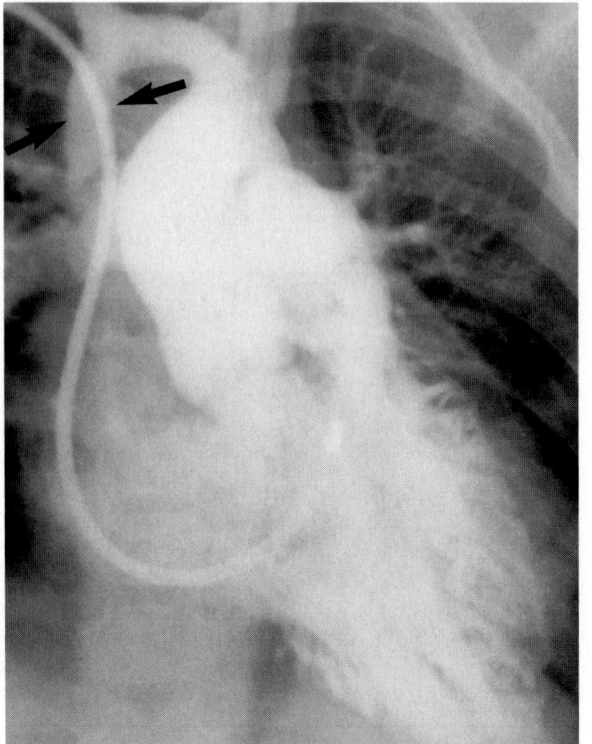

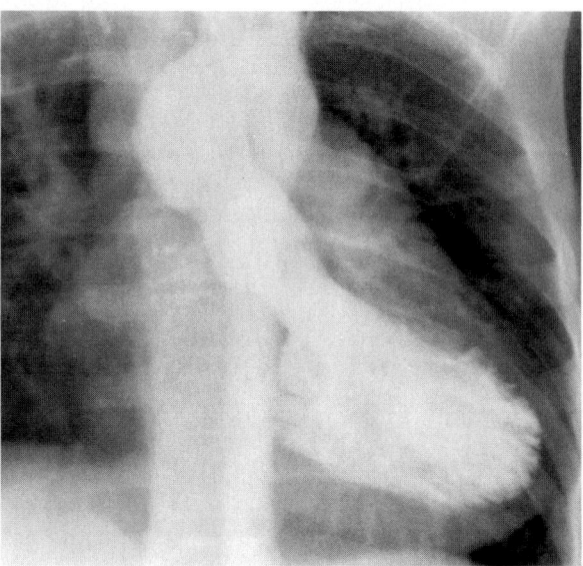

Fig. 4. Partial atrioventricular canal defect. Catheter in left ventricle.

Fig. 3. Tetralogy of Fallot with right subclavian artery-to-right pulmonary artery anastomosis (*arrows*) (right Blalock operation).

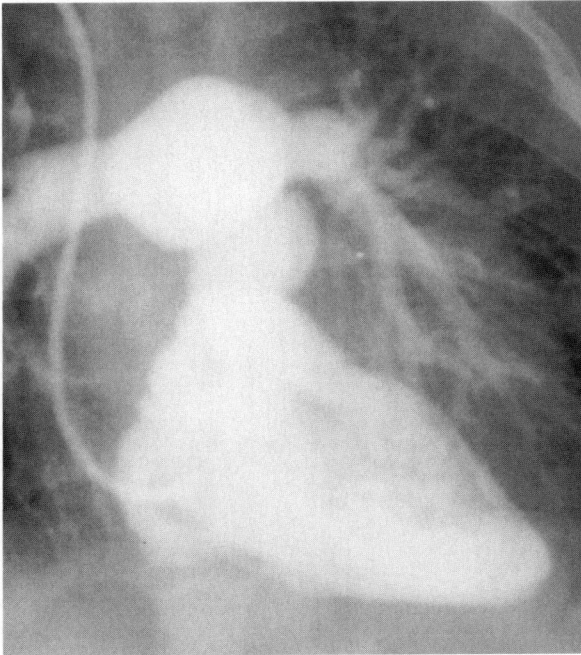

Fig. 5. Corrected transposition with intact ventricular septum.

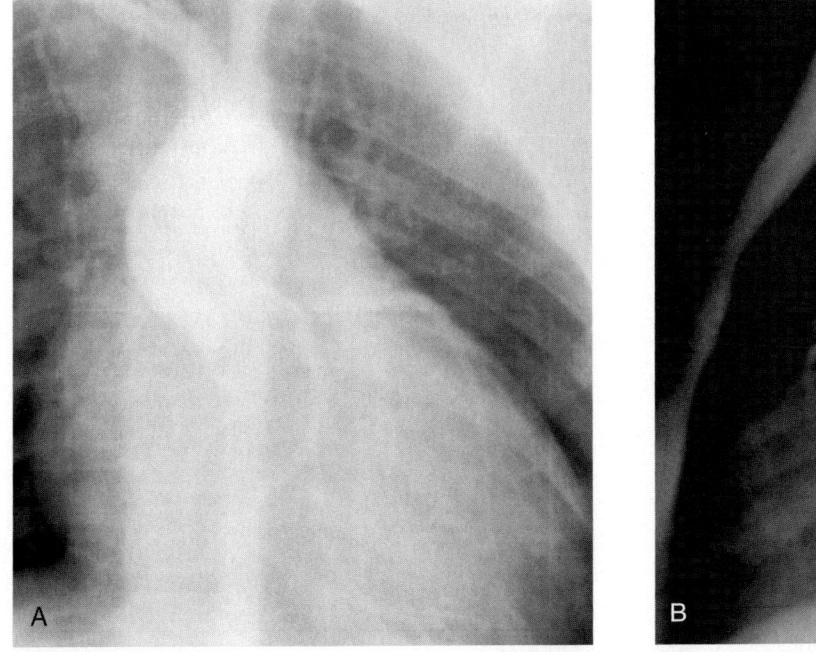

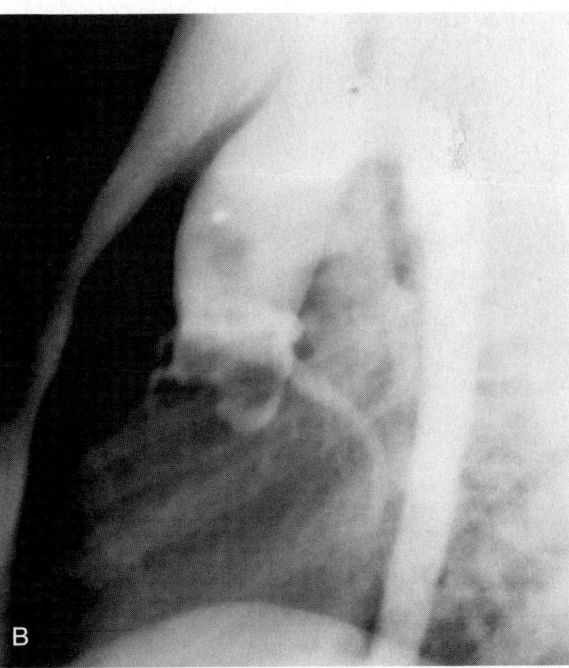

Fig. 6. Congenital aortic stenosis. *A*, Left anterior oblique projection. *B*, Right anterior oblique projection.

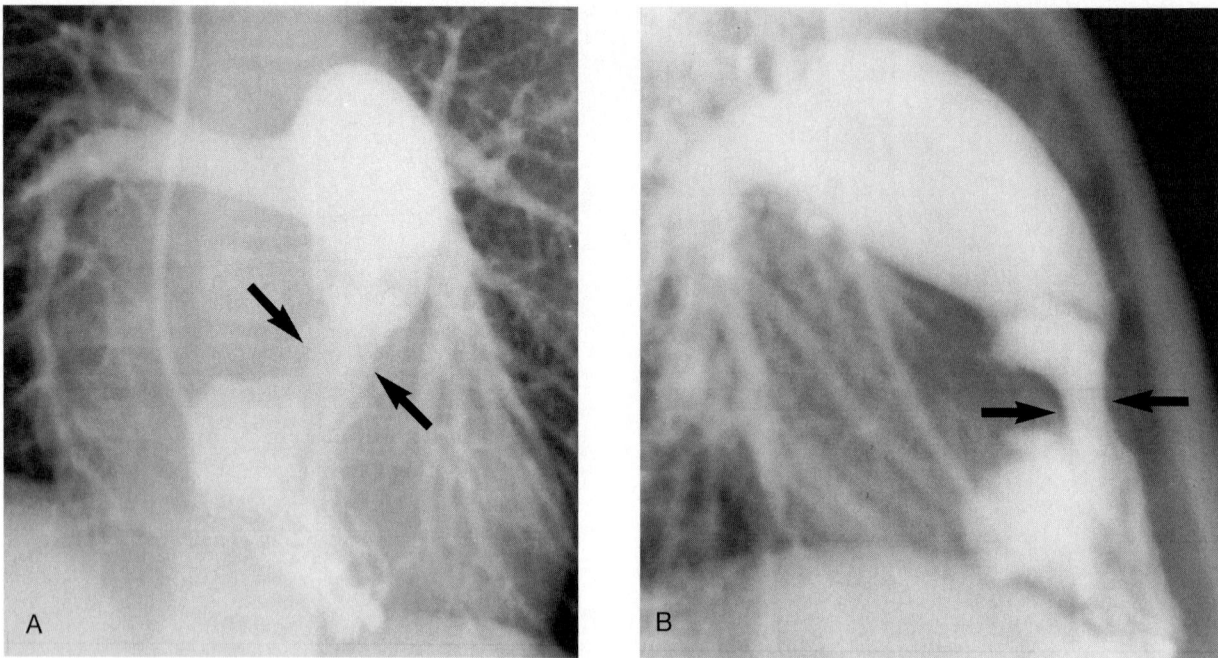

Fig. 7. Pulmonary stenosis (*arrows*). Right ventriculograms in frontal (*A*) and lateral (*B*) projections.

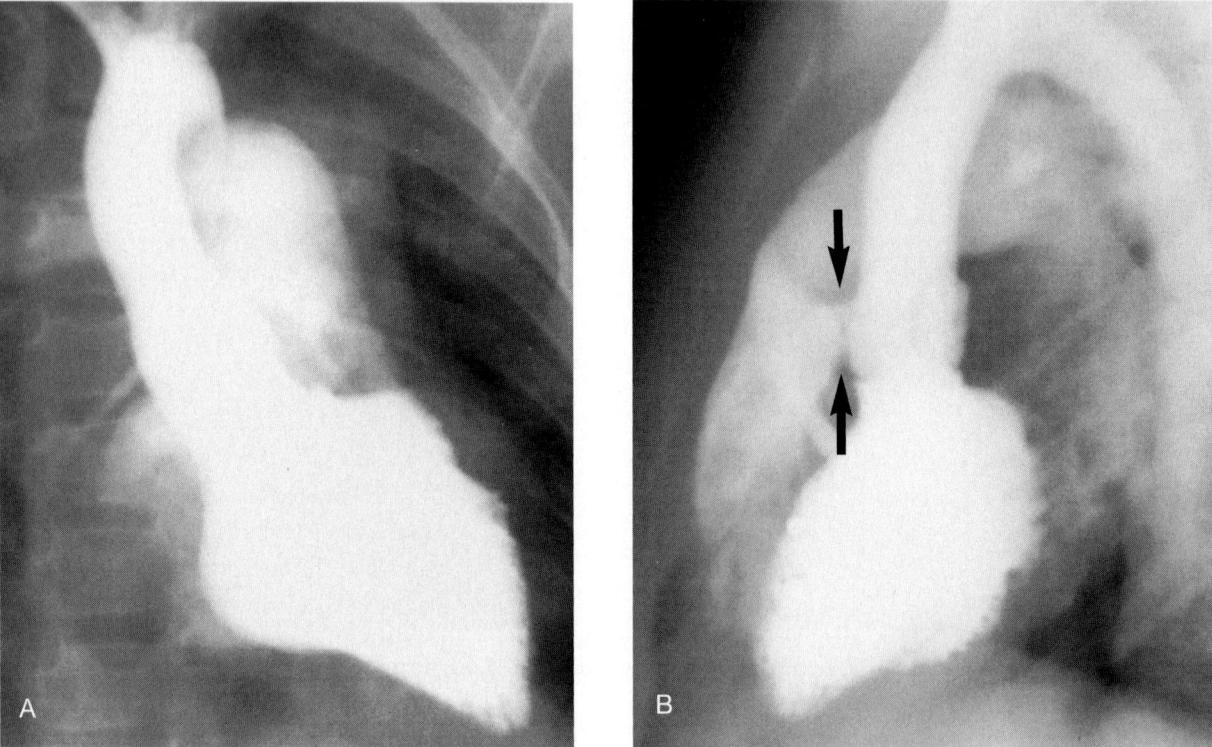

Fig. 8. Left ventriculograms, showing a small ventricular septal defect (*arrows* in *B*) in frontal (*A*) and lateral (*B*) projections.

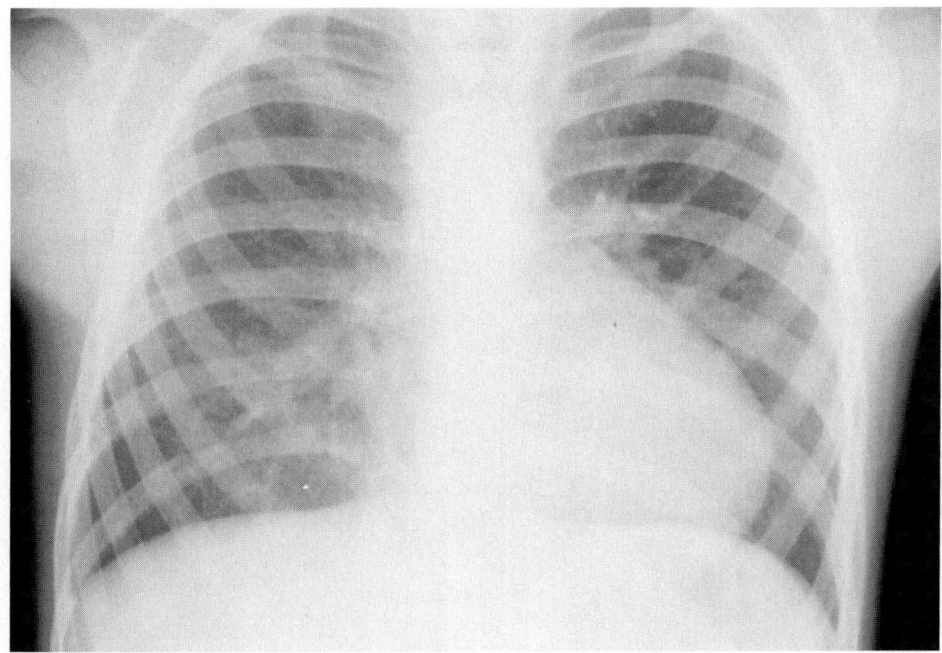

Fig. 9. Chest radiograph in tetralogy of Fallot.

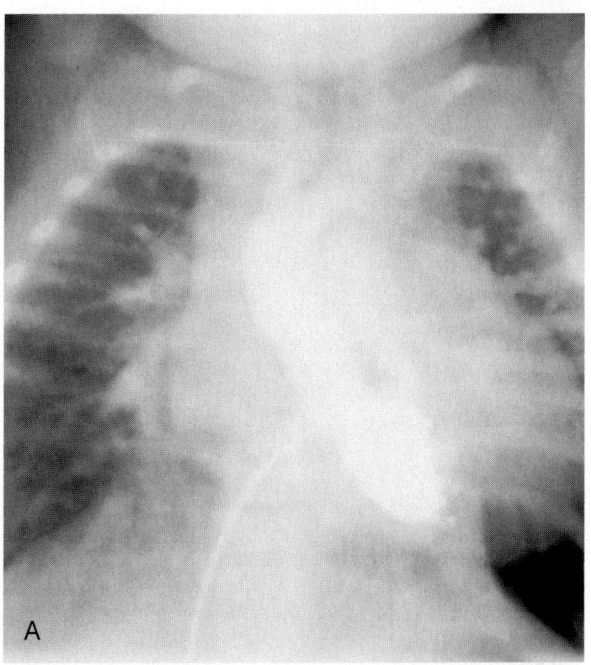

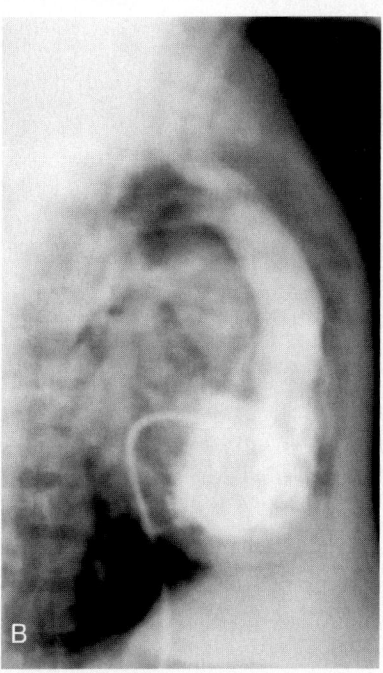

Fig. 10. Transposition of the great vessels with a ventricular septal defect. Frontal (*A*) and lateral (*B*) views.

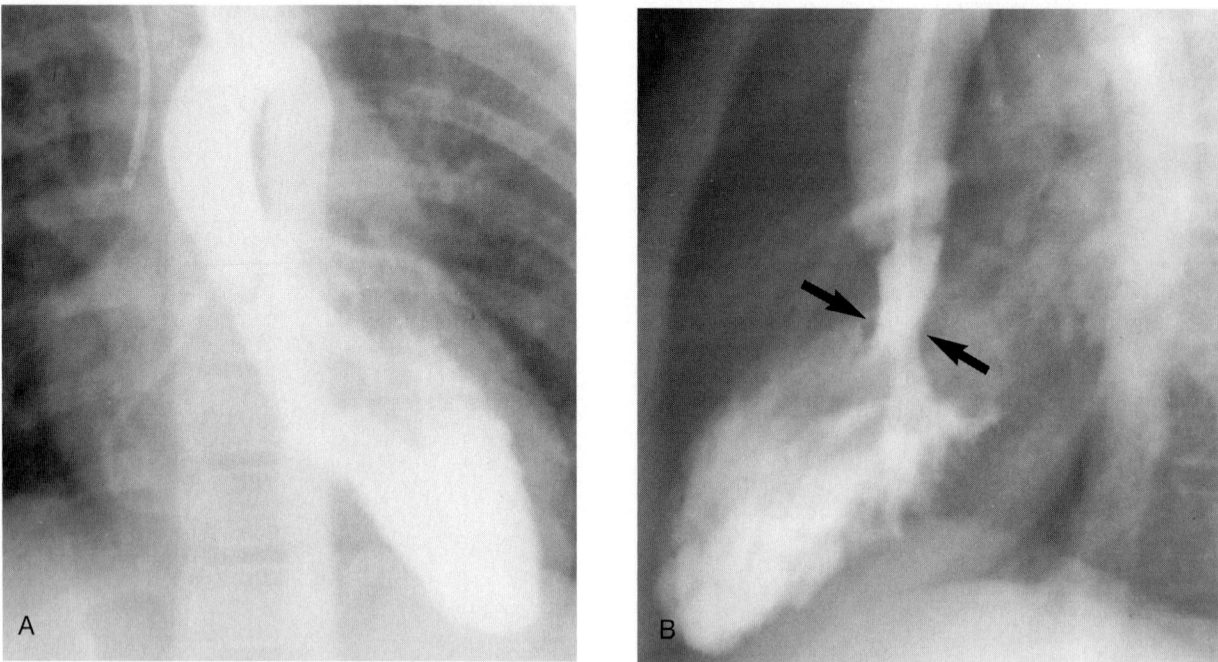

Fig. 11. Valvular and subvalvular aortic stenosis (*arrows* in *B*). Frontal (*A*) and lateral (*B*) views.

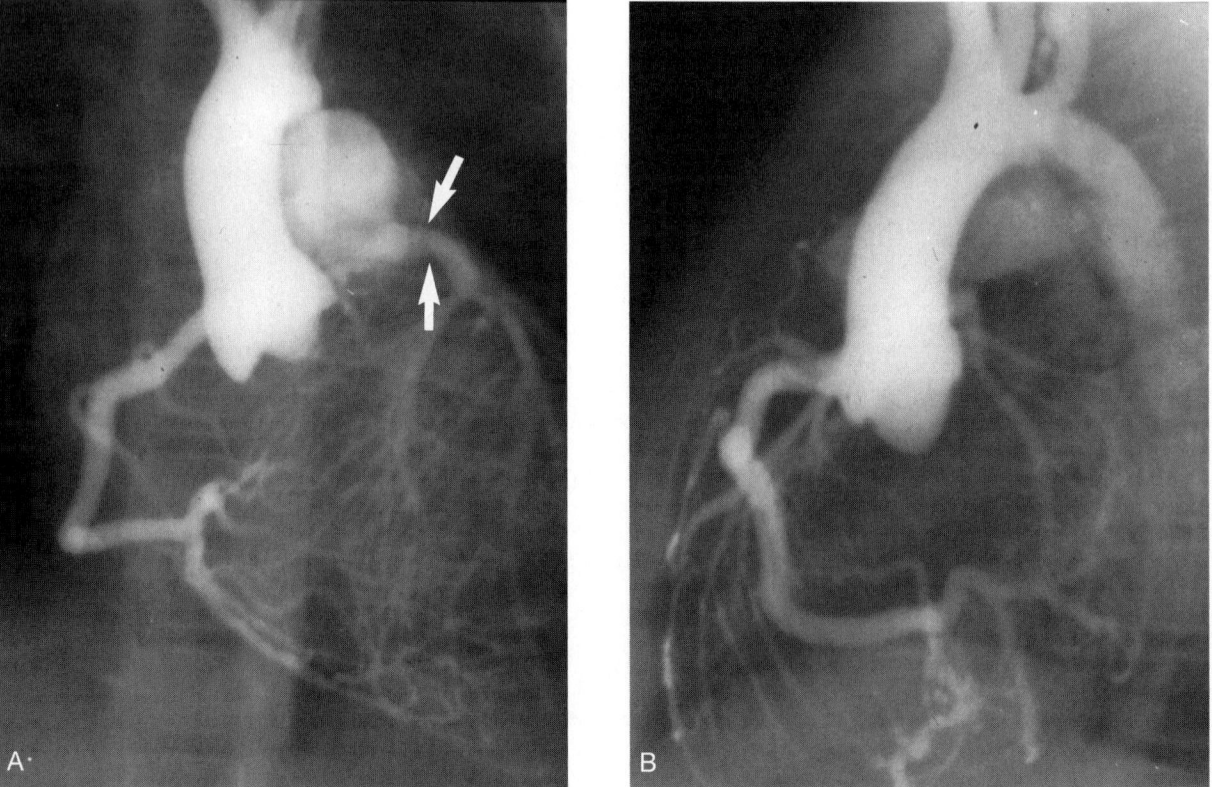

Fig. 12. Origin of the left coronary artery from the pulmonary artery (*arrows*). The right coronary artery arises normally from the right coronary sinus. *A*, Left anterior oblique projection. *B*, Right anterior oblique projection.

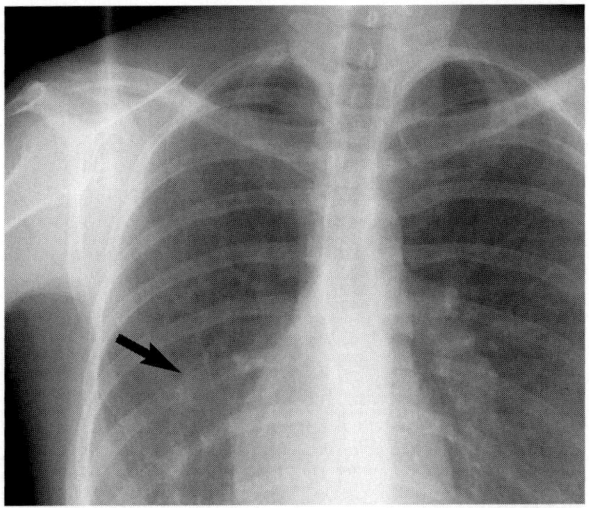

Fig. 13. Scimitar syndrome: partial anomalous pulmonary venous return of right pulmonary vein(s) to the inferior vena cava, below the diaphragm. This results in dextroposition of the heart, right lung hypoplasia with a small right hemithorax, and a curvilinear structure (*arrow*) in the right lung field (the scimitar), which represents the anomalous pulmonary vein(s).

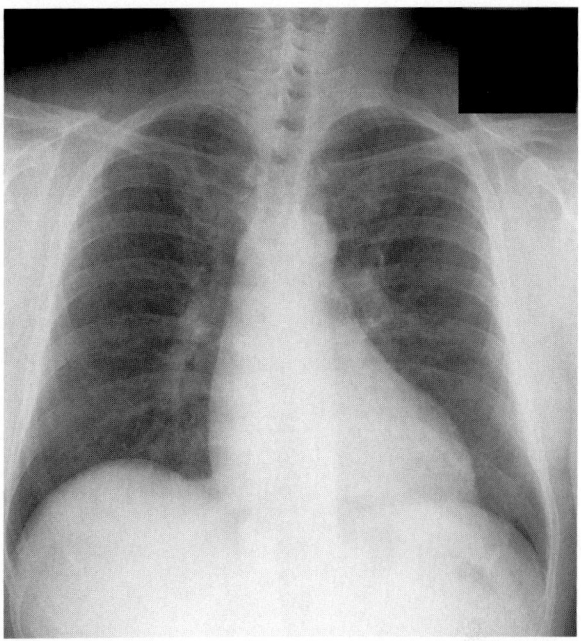

Fig. 14. Atrial septal defect. There is enlargement of the central pulmonary arteries with prominent vascularity throughout the lung fields. There is mild cardiac enlargement. This is consistent with pulmonary overcirculation from a significant left-to-right intracardiac shunt.

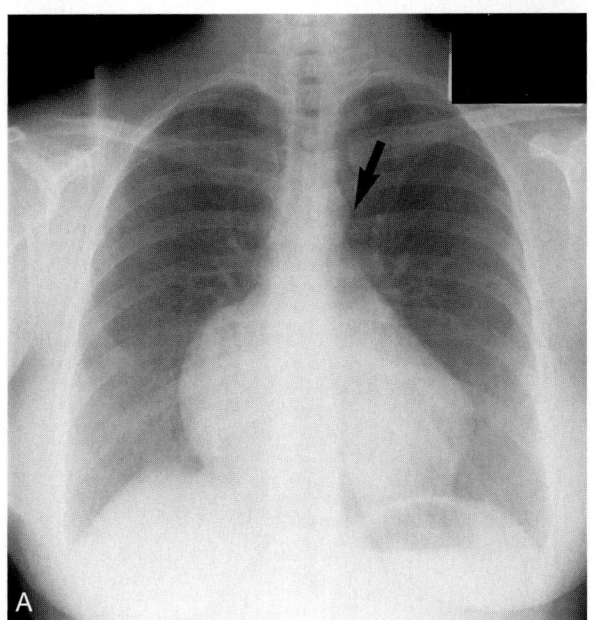

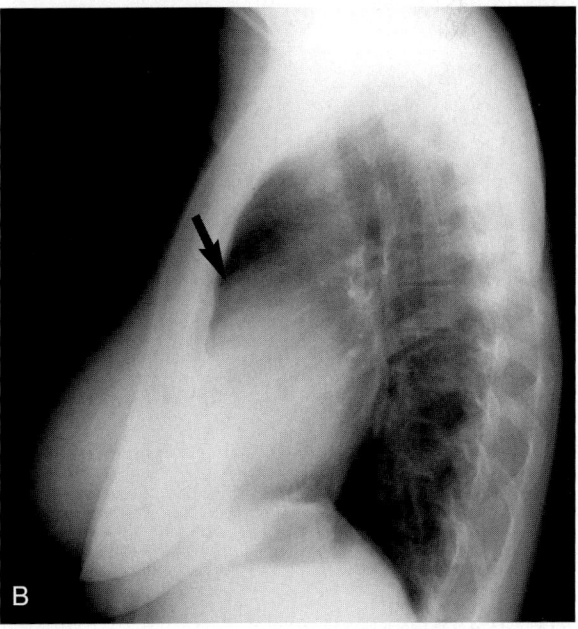

Fig. 15. Ebstein anomaly. *A*, Note cardiac enlargement with rounded contour of the cardiac silhouette, consistent with right chamber enlargement. Also note small aortic arch (*arrow*). *B*, Obliteration of the retrosternal space (*arrow*) in the lateral projection confirms right-sided chamber enlargement.

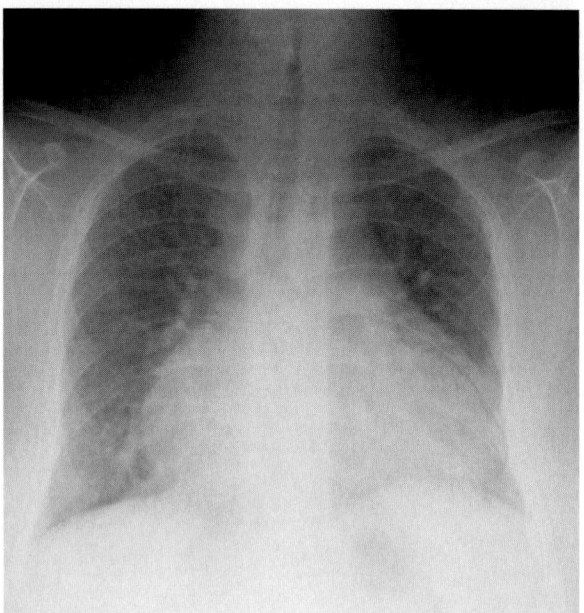

Fig. 16. Eisenmenger syndrome. Note marked cardiac enlargement with large central pulmonary arteries and "pruned" distal pulmonary arteries.

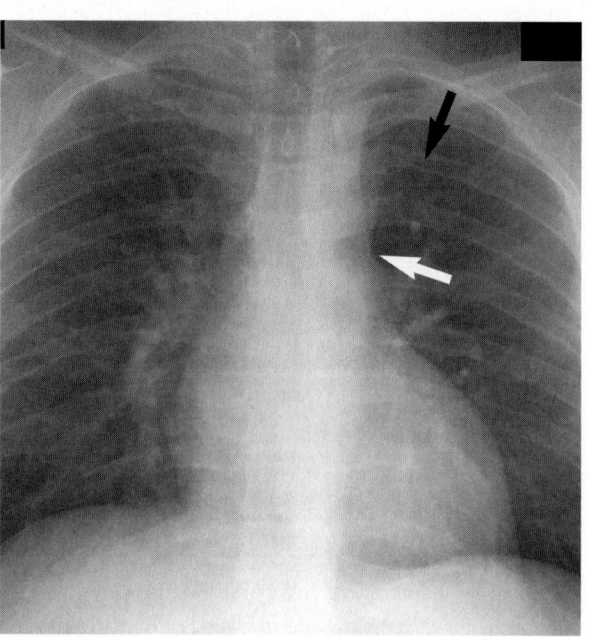

Fig. 17. Coarctation of the aorta. Note rib notching due to intercostal collaterals (*black arrow*). Contour of the descending aorta is abnormal, consistent with coarctation (*white arrow*).

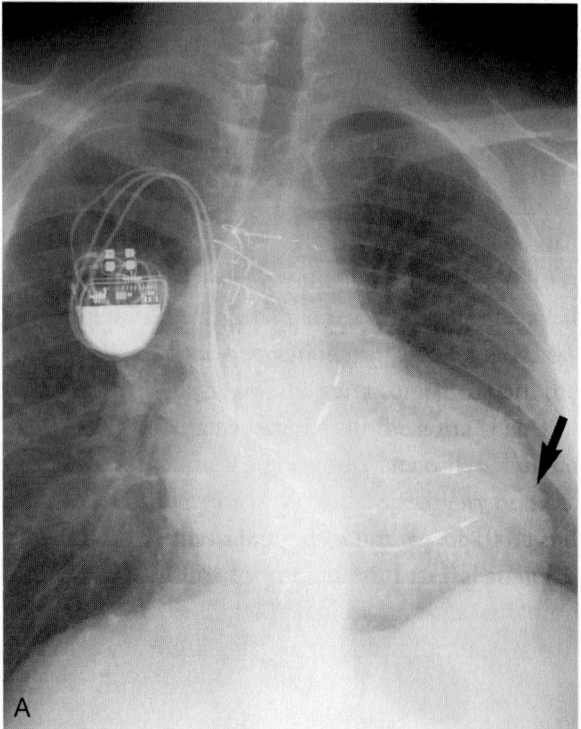

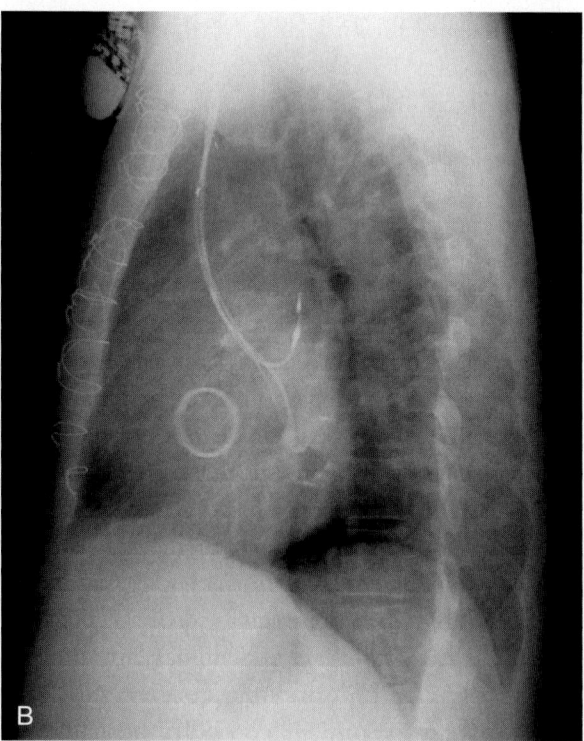

Fig. 18. *A*, D-Transposition of the great arteries after Mustard operation (atrial switch). Note rounded cardiac border (*arrow*), indicative of morphologic right ventricular enlargement. Right ventricle serves as systemic ventricle in this situation. *B*, Note that pacemaker is in posterior chamber of the heart, which is the morphologic left ventricle serving as the subpulmonic ventricle after a Mustard procedure.

16

CARDIOPULMONARY EXERCISE TESTING

Thomas G. Allison, PhD

HISTORY OF CARDIOPULMONARY EXERCISE TESTING

Cardiopulmonary exercise testing—also known as *metabolic testing* and $\dot{V}O_2max$ *testing*—is an important tool in a state-of-the-art, comprehensive cardiovascular program. Cardiopulmonary exercise testing was originally developed for testing the fitness of athletes such as long-distance runners and cross-country skiers; maximal oxygen consumption ($\dot{V}O_2max$) is the most important predictor of performance in endurance events.

Measurement of oxygen (O_2) consumption during various forms of physical works, an important early use of cardiopulmonary exercise testing, was initially cumbersome and labor intensive because expired air had to be collected in meteorologic balloons made of large canvas bags (Douglas bags). The balloons were then evacuated into large, calibrated tanks (Tissot tanks) to measure the volume of expired gas, and samples of mixed gas were manually analyzed for O_2 and carbon dioxide (CO_2) content by using instruments that measured the gas volume before and after O_2 or CO_2 were selectively removed by chemicals. Finally, the measurements were used to calculate $\dot{V}O_2max$ by use of specified equations and the Haldane conversion based on the nonmetabolic

properties of nitrogen. Fortunately, fully automated, accurate systems have been developed that enable breath-to-breath measurement of O_2 consumption without the need to collect large volumes of gas or to perform either analysis or calculations by hand. The automated systems are compact—especially when a laptop computer is used—and they calibrate in a few minutes and integrate with either a treadmill or a cycle ergometer and electrocardiographic (ECG) stress monitor. Relatively little additional technician time or patient inconvenience is needed to add cardiopulmonary measurements to the standard exercise test. The amount of additional time and cost of cardiopulmonary exercise testing compared with conventional treadmill testing with only ECG monitoring is relatively small.

Additional instrumentation for the cardiopulmonary exercise test includes 1) a small, light, and disposable mouthpiece or face mask through which the flow of expired gas and continuous O_2 and CO_2 concentrations are measured and 2) a forehead sensor to measure O_2 saturation transcutaneously. Numeric and graphic real-time displays of O_2 consumption and other cardiopulmonary exercise variables are provided, and final reports are available within 5 minutes of test completion.

Relationship of $\dot{V}O_2max$ to Cardiac Output

Mathematically, $\dot{V}O_2max$ is equal to the product of cardiac output and arteriovenous oxygen difference (AVO_2diff). In turn, cardiac output is a product of heart rate (HR) and stroke volume (Fig. 1). Stroke volume is the difference between end-diastolic and end-systolic volumes. End-diastolic volume is affected by compliance of the ventricle and by filling pressure (blood volume); end-systolic volume is related to inherent contractility, preload, and afterload. It is well known from the Starling principle that modest increases in preload and end-diastolic volume increase stroke volume, even in a heart weakened by severe ischemia or various myopathic preocesses, whereas larger increases distend the ventricle to a point at which contractility decreases and stroke volume is reduced.

AVO_2diff is affected by hemoglobin concentration, alveolar ventilation and O_2 tension, and pulmonary diffusing capacity (Fig. 2). O_2 content of mixed venous blood is determined by the mass of the working muscles and the amount of O_2 extracted, which is dependent on regional blood flow, capillary density, and oxidative enzyme levels in the active muscle mass.

In healthy individuals, several of these factors affecting $\dot{V}O_2max$ are in part determined by the following:

1. Genetics—particularly heart and lung size, muscle fiber type distribution (the relative mix of fast twitch glycolytic and slow twitch oxidative), and maximal heart rate.
2. Sex—an influence on $\dot{V}O_2max$ through effects on heart and lung size, skeletal muscle mass, and hemoglobin concentration.
3. Aging—a reduction in muscle mass, peak heart rate, and vital capacity of the lung.
4. Aerobic exercise training—a very important influence on $\dot{V}O_2max$; parts of the system affected by aerobic training include skeletal muscle mass and oxidative enzyme capacity, peripheral muscle capillary density, blood volume, and contractile properties of the heart.
5. Body weight—generally expressed as milliliters of O_2 per kilogram of body weight per minute; in particular, excess adipose tissue, which is relatively metabolically inactive, reduces $\dot{V}O_2max$.

These various influences on $\dot{V}O_2max$ produce a wide range of "normal values." Women have roughly 80% to 90% of the $\dot{V}O_2max$ of men at similar levels of training, whereas $\dot{V}O_2max$ declines by 5% to 10% per decade of age, depending on the level of physical activity. A value of 20 mL/kg per minute for $\dot{V}O_2max$ might be considered "normal" for a sedentary, overweight, 70-year-old woman, whereas healthy and lean elite male endurance athletes in their 20s may have levels of $\dot{V}O_2max$ that are 70 mL/kg per minute or higher. For predicting $\dot{V}O_2max$ during treadmill exercise in healthy adults, many laboratories use the following equations:

$$\text{For men, predicted } \dot{V}O_2max = (60 - 0.5 \times age) \text{ mL/kg per min}$$

$$\text{For women, predicted } \dot{V}O_2max = (48 - 0.4 \times age) \text{ mL/kg per minute}$$

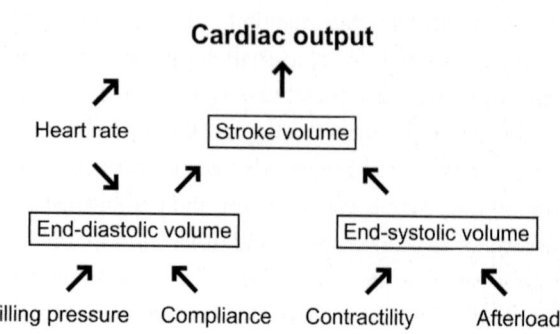

Fig. 1. Cardiac outout is a product of heart rate and stroke volume.

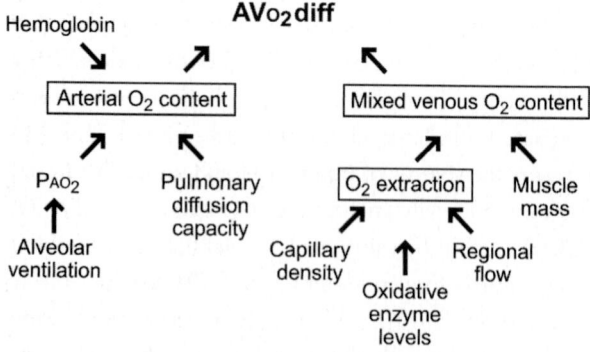

Fig. 2. The arteriovenous oxygen difference (AVO_2diff) is affected by hemoglobin concentration, alveolar ventilation and oxygen (O_2) tension, and pulmonary diffusing capacity.

ADVANTAGES OF CARDIOPULMONARY EXERCISE TESTING

The advantages of cardiopulmonary exercise testing over conventional exercise testing include the following:

1. An objective measure of fatigue is provided.
2. $\dot{V}O_2$max provides a better measure of functional capacity than treadmill time alone.
3. The reason(s) for a low $\dot{V}O_2$max can be identified: poor cardiac reserve, ventilation limitation or other pulmonary abnormalities, claudication, musculoskeletal problems, poor effort, or severe deconditioning.

During conventional exercise testing, the degree of effort or fatigue is estimated from subjective reports of the patient (ratings of perceived exertion [RPE]), the percentage of the predicted maximal heart rate to which the patient exercises, and of course, the opinion of the personnel monitoring the test. Unfortunately, RPE do not always accurately reflect the degree of cardiopulmonary effort or fatigue because they may be influenced by factors such as claudication or other causes of musculoskeletal pain, pulmonary abnormalities, and fearfulness or anxiety during the test. Maximal heart rate has a standard deviation of approximately 12 beats per minute and is affected both by drugs commonly used to treat cardiovascular disease (most notably β-blockers) and by physiologic effects of various disease states (e.g., autonomic impairment in diabetes). During cardiopulmonary exercise testing, the monitored objective measure of fatigue is the respiratory exchange ratio (RER), which is the ratio of CO_2 production ($\dot{V}CO_2$) to O_2 consumption ($\dot{V}O_2$). That is, RER = $\dot{V}CO_2/\dot{V}O_2$. RER values greater than 1.0 indicate the presence of some degree of anaerobic metabolism. Empirically, at least in healthy individuals, exercising to an RER greater than 1.15 is necessary to attain.

In the United States, most exercise testing is done on a motor-driven treadmill. In young, healthy individuals, there is a high correlation between treadmill performance time and $\dot{V}O_2$max, but the correlation is much weaker in older patients, especially those with cardiac disease. Patients with left ventricular dysfunction have impaired cardiac output and thus rely more heavily on anaerobic energy sources for treadmill work, so their $\dot{V}O_2$ is lower at any given workload. Excessive use of handrails for support also lowers $\dot{V}O_2$ at a given workload. Thus, $\dot{V}O_2$max—and cardiac reserve—are over-estimated from the performance time on the test. In contrast, gait abnormalities due to degenerative joint disease of the lower extremities, obesity, or lack of experience with walking on a motor-driven treadmill increase $\dot{V}O_2$ at a given workload, causing an underestimate of cardiac reserve for a given performance time. So, although the estimated metabolic equivalent (MET) level from a treadmill is a reasonable surrogate for $\dot{V}O_2$max, it is often an imperfect surrogate, especially in various cardiac disease states. Cycle ergometer tests show a more consistent relationship between $\dot{V}O_2$ and performance time, but patients generally do not achieve cardiac output levels that are as high as on treadmill tests, and most of the norms for functional capacity with which US cardiologists are familiar are based on treadmill time. Sometimes nonstandard ergometers (e.g., combined arm and leg cycle) or protocols are used for exercise testing in patients with particular orthopedic problems, and no standard prediction equations related to performance time are available. In these cases, measurement of $\dot{V}O_2$max is the only means of identifying functional capacity and cardiac reserve.

INTERPRETATION OF THE CARDIOPULMONARY EXERCISE TEST

A low $\dot{V}O_2$max may be a sign of poor cardiac reserve if the RER reaches an adequate level, but obese and severely deconditioned patients may have a low $\dot{V}O_2$max with normal cardiac function. Therefore, several other measures of cardiac performance are examined to determine whether the limitation is truly due to poor cardiac reserve. One is an early plateau in $\dot{V}O_2$ as plotted against time during graded exercise. Extending the measurement of $\dot{V}O_2$ during active recovery increases the sensitivity of the curve of $\dot{V}O_2$ versus time because a plateau or further increase in $\dot{V}O_2$ during active recovery has also been associated with poor cardiac reserve. Second, the curve of oxygen pulse plotted against exercise time for $\dot{V}O_2$ can be examined. Oxygen pulse ($\dot{V}O_2/HR$), mathematically equivalent to the product of stroke volume and arteriovenous O_2 difference, is even more sensitive to cardiac output impairment than $\dot{V}O_2$ itself. An early plateau or even a decrease in oxygen pulse is generally considered an indication of decreasing stroke volume with increasing work. Other indications of impaired cardiac output include the ventilatory equivalent for CO_2 (ratio of expired ventilation [$\dot{V}_E$] to CO_2 production = $\dot{V}_E/\dot{V}CO_2$) and the breathing reserve (BR) (BR = 1 − $\dot{V}_E$/MVV [maximal voluntary ventilation, measured by spirometry or estimated from age, sex, and height]). An elevated $\dot{V}_E/\dot{V}CO_2$ (defined in various ways, most simply by a value at peak exercise >40) or a large breathing reserve (>35% of the MVV) in the absence of clinically significant pulmonary disease is associated with clinically significant cardiac disease. Thus, with the additional information gained from cardiopulmonary exercise testing, the severity of a cardiac output limitation can be more fully defined than by looking only at treadmill performance along with HR and blood pressure responses.

Termination of the test at a low RER may indicate poor effort, musculoskeletal limitations, or ventilation limitation. Comparison of MVV, as measured during standard spirometry, with the maximal $\dot{V}_E$ during exercise should provide an indication of whether exercise was ventilation limited. Sorting out poor effort from musculoskeletal limitation would be based on the specific complaints identified by the patient during the test and the physical examination and medical history.

Sample Cardiopulmonary Tests

Examples of three actual exercise tests from clinical practice are given below. They illustrate important points in the use of exercise testing discussed in the previous section.

Test 1

A healthy, fit, 49-year-old man who underwent cardiopulmonary exercise testing (Fig. 3) had the following data: body mass index (BMI) 26.4 kg/m2, $\dot{V}O_2$max 56.5 mL/kg per minute (159% predicted), time 14.9 min, peak HR 193 beats per minute, RER 1.25, BR 6%, and $\dot{V}_E/\dot{V}CO_2$ 27.

Test 2

A healthy but unfit, 44-year-old man who underwent cardiopulmonary exercise testing (Fig. 4) data: BMI 32.2 kg/m2, $\dot{V}O_2$max 33.4 mL/kg per minute (88% predicted), time 10.6 min, peak HR 164 beats per minute, RER 1.13, BR 30%, and $\dot{V}E/\dot{V}CO_2$ 27. This patient is slightly younger than the patient in test 1 but

is considerably more overweight and less fit from a cardiovascular standpoint. The degree of effort is only near maximal (peak RER, 1.13).

Test 3

A 48-year-old man with chronic heart failure who underwent cardiopulmonary exercise testing (Fig. 5) had the following data: BMI 25.0 kg/m2, $\dot{V}O_2$max 15.3 mL/kg per minute (43% predicted), time 6.0 min, peak HR 114 beats per minute, RER 1.25, BR 61%, and $\dot{V}_E/\dot{V}CO_2$ 41. This test is markedly different from test 1 or test 2, not just in terms of poorer performance and lower $\dot{V}O_2$max (despite a maximal effort [RER, 1.25]).

Prognosis Based on $\dot{V}O_2$max

Perhaps the most widely recognized use of cardiopulmonary exercise testing in clinical cardiology is for the evaluation of patients with chronic heart failure. Several studies have established that $\dot{V}O_2$max is a strong predictor of survival in this patient group. As a result, $\dot{V}O_2$ max has been used in the risk stratification of heart failure patients for cardiac transplantation, and serial cardiopulmonary exercise testing is routinely performed to adjust risk level and time of transplantation as heart failure progresses (or stabilizes). Although criteria for cardiac transplantation have broadened in recent years, $\dot{V}O_2$max remains one of several critical factors used by insurance companies in determining the appropriateness (and hence reimbursement) of cardiac transplantation.

It has also been reported that $\dot{V}O_2$max can be used to predict long-term survival among cardiac rehabilitation patients who as a group are considerably healthier than heart failure patients and represent a much broader spectrum of cardiovascular disease (Fig. 6).

Other cardiac conditions for which patients might be referred for cardiopulmonary exercise testing include hypertrophic cardiomyopathy, valvular heart disease, congenital heart disease, and pulmonary hypertension. Cardiopulmonary exercise testing not only helps to determine cardiac reserve and establish prognosis in these patients but it also helps to determine the effects of various therapies such as drugs, pacing, and rehabilitation and will allow for periodic evaluation for the timing of surgical interventions.

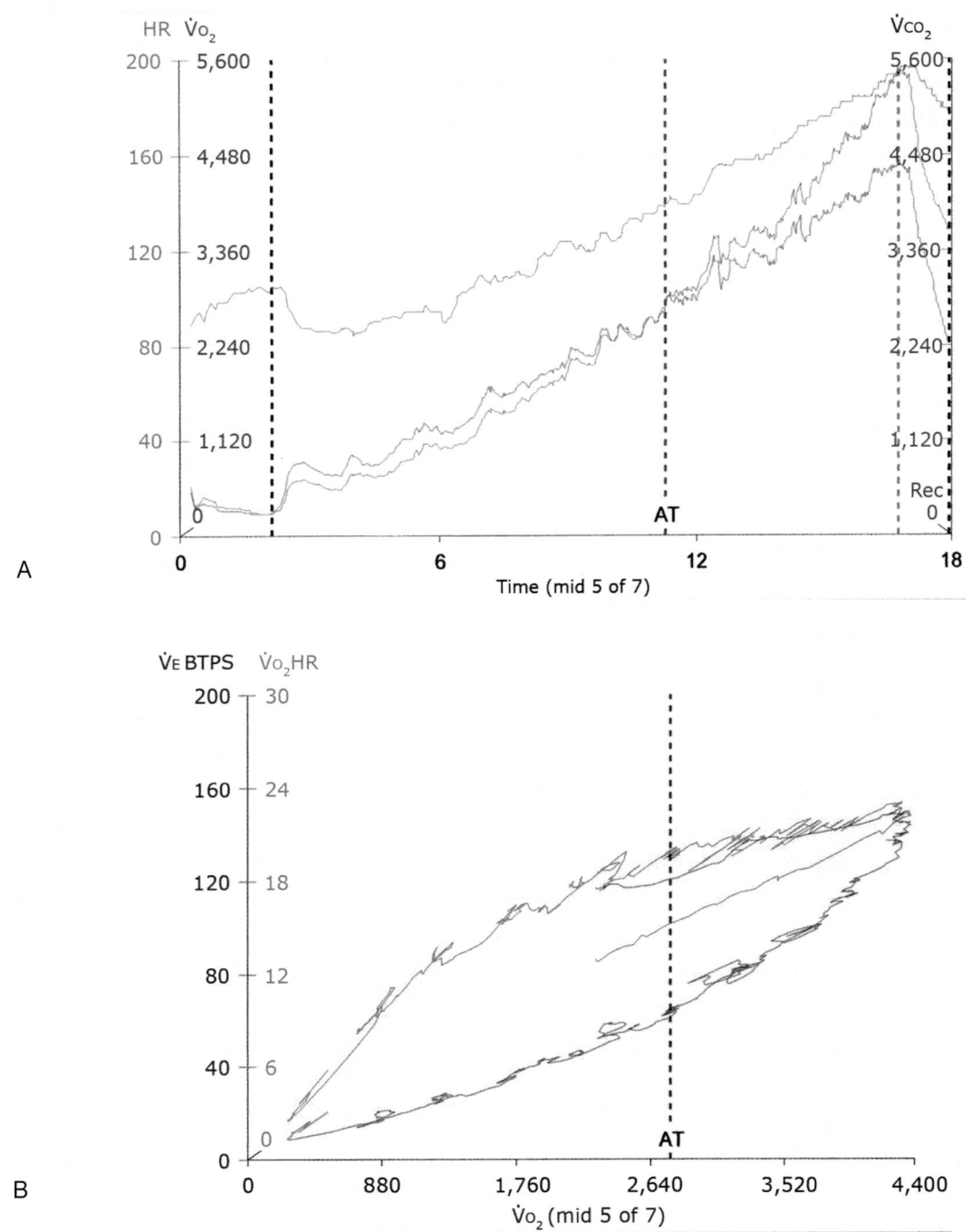

Fig. 3. Cardiopulmonary exercise test 1. *A*, Heart rate (HR) in beats per minute, oxygen consumption ($\dot{V}O_2$) (in milliliters/kilogram per minute), and carbon dioxide production ($\dot{V}CO_2$) (in milliliters/kilogram per minute) are plotted against time of exercise. Note that $\dot{V}O_2$ increases normally throughout exercise (to the right of the first black dashed line) and decreases rapidly in active recovery (to the right of the red dashed line). $\dot{V}CO_2$ increases to a higher level because of the contribution of anaerobic metabolism, indicating a maximal effort (peak RER, 1.25). AT, anaerobic threshold; Rec, recovery. *B*, In the second figure, oxygen pulse ($\dot{V}O_2$/HR) and expired ventilation ($\dot{V}_E$) in milliliters/ kilogram per minute are plotted against $\dot{V}O_2$. Oxygen pulse increases rapidly during exercise but then rises at a slower rate throughout the remainder of the test. Ventilation rises continuously in a curvilinear manner with a greater increase per unit of $\dot{V}O_2$ above the AT. The breathing reserve is small (6%), which is consistent with high cardiac output.

RANGES FOR $\dot{V}O_2MAX$

By the prediction equations given above, the average $\dot{V}O_2max$ for a 50-year-old, healthy but untrained man would be 35 mL/kg per minute compared with 28 mL/kg per minute for a 50-year-old woman similarly healthy but untrained. However, the range for $\dot{V}O_2max$ is quite broad with champion endurance athletes having values greater than 80 mL/kg per minute, whereas patients with severe heart failure may have levels less than 10 mL/kg per minute. As previously

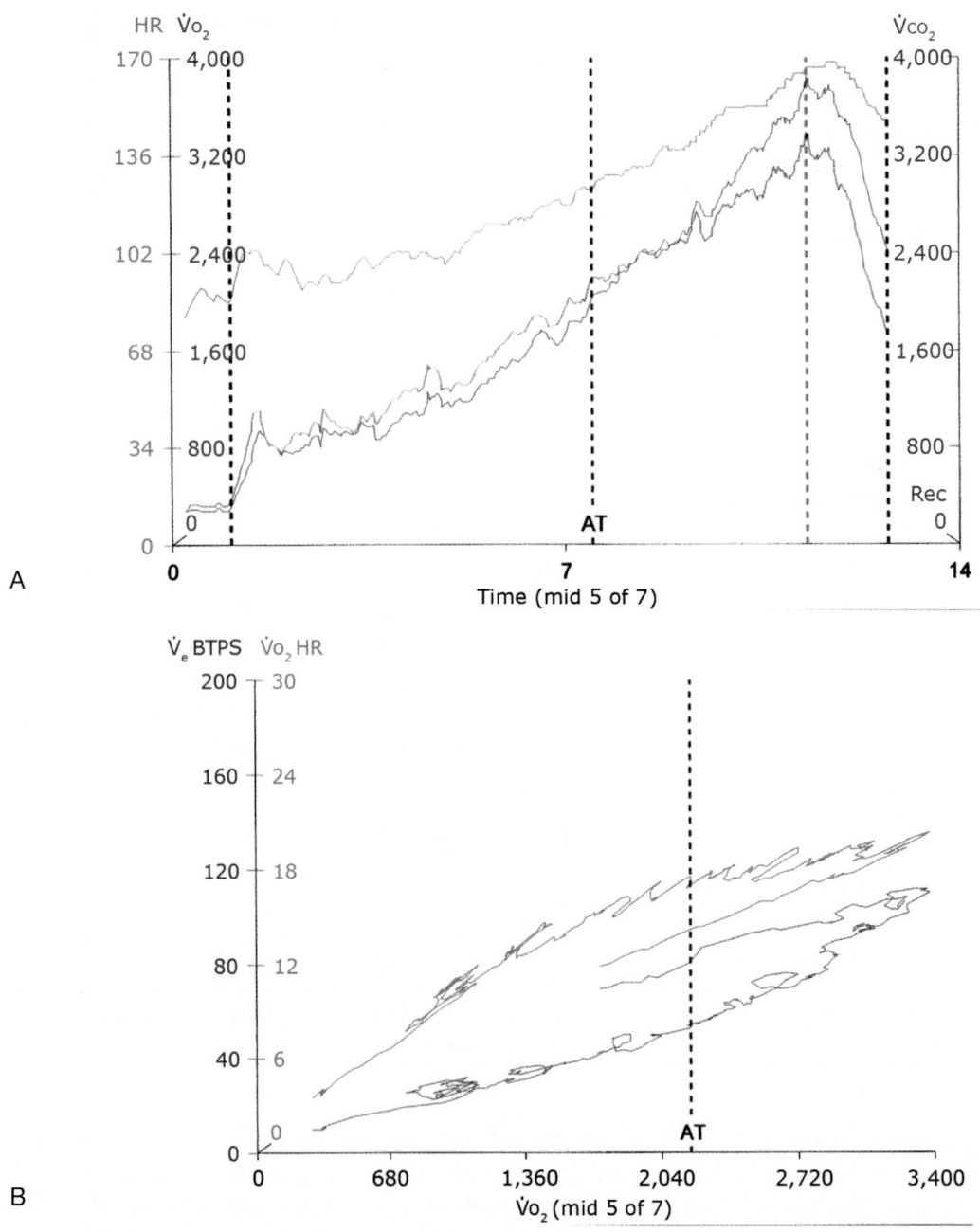

Fig. 4. Cardiopulmonary exercise test 2. Although $\dot{V}O_2max$ is much lower, the shapes of all curves are similar to those shown for the healthy, fit man in test 1. The breathing reserve is higher (30%), but still within the normal range. Breathing efficiency (expired ventilation/carbon dioxide production [$\dot{V}_E/\dot{V}CO_2$]) is similar to test 1. Thus, the conclusion is that this was a normal test result and that the patient's oxygen consumption ($\dot{V}O_2$) was limited by his weight, deconditioning, and to some extent a near-maximal effort. AT, anaerobic threshold; HR, heart rate; Rec, recovery.

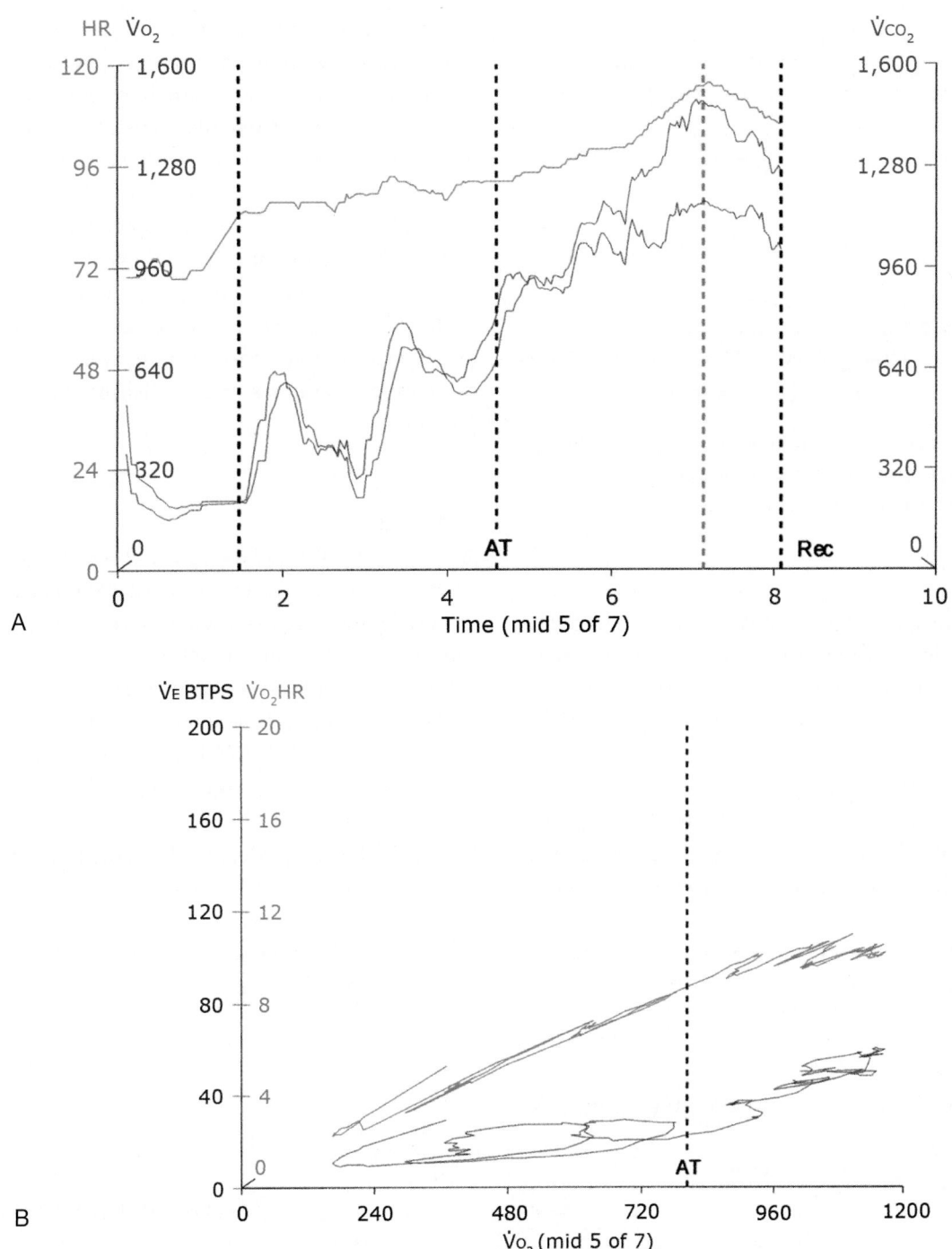

Fig. 5. Cardiopulmonary exercise test 3. Oxygen consumption ($\dot{V}O_2$) appears to plateau during late exercise and early recovery (Rec). Oxygen pulse ($\dot{V}O_2/HR$) increases initially but the plateaus during later exercise, suggesting a drop in stroke volume. The breathing reserve is quite large (61%), again suggesting limited cardiac output, and the elevated $\dot{V}_E/\dot{V}CO_2 = 41$ may indicate a secondary pulmonary vascular abnormality. All of the signs of impaired cardiac output described in the previous section are present in test 3: 1. low $\dot{V}O_2max$, 2. plateau in $\dot{V}O_2$ against time of exercise, 3. plateau in oxygen pulse, 4. large breathing reserve, and 5. elevated $\dot{V}_E/\dot{V}CO_2$. AT, anaerobic threshold; HR, heart rate; Rec, recovery.

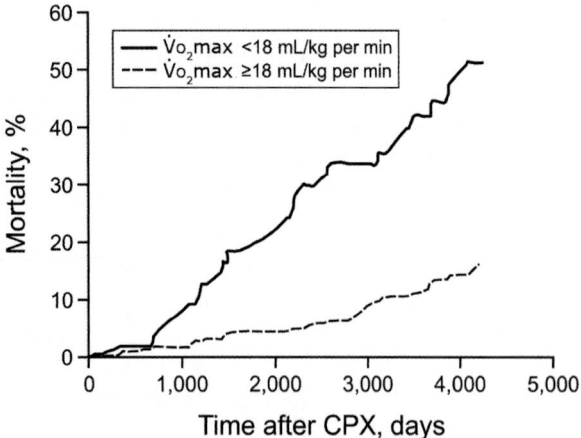

Fig. 6. Maximal oxygen consumption ($\dot{V}O_2$max) and survival among cardiac rehabilitation patients. CPX, cardiopulmonary exercise testing.

noted, many factors influence $\dot{V}O_2$max, including age, sex, BMI, level of physical activity, left ventricular function, and ability to achieve a normal maximal heart rate. Examples of values for $\dot{V}O_2$max that might be expected for various patients are given in Table 1.

The American Heart Association suggests that 18 mL/kg per minute is a critical value for $\dot{V}O_2$max: Patients with $\dot{V}O_2$max less than 18 mL/kg per minute have a high degree of disability and a poor long-term prognosis, and patients with $\dot{V}O_2$max between 18 and 22.5 mL/kg per minute are considered to have an intermediate risk.

In summary, cardiopulmonary exercise testing provides more accurate assessment of both $\dot{V}O_2$max and cardiac reserve than conventional treadmill testing in many cardiac disease states. Thus, the impact of the disease on functional capacity and long-term prognosis can be established more accurately.

Table 2 shows uses for cardiopulmonary exercise testing. Although conventional exercise testing is considered useful in many of these instances, cardiopulmonary exercise testing has the potential to provide additional information relevant to making the correct diagnosis or establishing an accurate prognosis.

RESOURCES

American Heart Association guidelines and policy statements on exercise testing [cited 2006 June 26]. Available from: http://www.americanheart.org/presenter.jhtml?identifier=3004540

American Thoracic Society/American College of Chest Physicians statement on cardiopulmonary exercise testing [cited 2006 June 26]. Available from: http://ajrccm.atsjournals.org/cgi/content/full/167/2/211

Milani RV, Lavie CJ, Mehra MR. Cardiopulmonary exercise testing: how do we differentiate the cause of dyspnea? Circulation. 2004 [cited 2006 June 27]; 110: e27-e31. Available from: http://circ.ahajournals.org/cgi/content/full/110/4/e27

Table 1.   Examples of VO2max for Various Patients

Patient			
Age, y	Sex	Condition	$\dot{V}O_2$max, mL/kg per minute
30	M	Lean, active	52
30	F	Competitive long-distance runner	60
40	M	Overweight, deconditioned	35
40	F	Class II heart failure	18
60	M	Asymptomatic CHD treated with β-blocker	25
60	F	Lean, active	28

CHD, coronary heart disease; VO_{2max}, maximal oxygen consumption.

Table 2. Uses for Cardiopulmonary Exercise
          Testing

Diagnosis	Uses for cardio-pulmonary exercise testing
Heart failure	Establish prognosis
	Pretransplantation evaluation
	Effect of therapy (e.g., biventricular pacing)
Valvular heart disease	Functional status
	Severity of impairment
Hypertrophic cardio-myopathy	Severity of cardiac output limitation
	Effect of therapy
Coronary artery disease	Establish prognosis
	Exercise prescription
Combined cardiac/pulmonary disease	Primary cause of dyspnea
Disability evaluation	Objective assessment of effort
	True functional capacity
Congenital heart disease	Functional capacity
	Cardiac versus non-cardiac limitations
Endurance athlete	Performance potential
	Evaluation of training
	Exercise prescription
Chronic fatigue	Objective assessment of effort
Exercise intolerance of unknown cause	True functional capacity
	Rule out cardiac limitation
Orthopedic condition	Accurate assessment of fitness despite gait abnormality or non-standard ergometry results

17

Stress Test Selection

Stuart D. Christenson, MD

Introduction

Cardiac stress testing is an integral part of clinical cardiology. The safe performance of high-quality stress testing with imaging techniques has led to an increase in the number of stress procedures in recent years. This has prompted the development of national guidelines and appropriateness criteria for cardiac stress testing and imaging techniques. Although the particular techniques of exercise electrocardiographic (ECG) stress testing, stress echocardiography, and myocardial perfusion imaging are discussed in more detail in other chapters of this text, this chapter focuses on the relative advantages and limitations of each technique to ensure that the appropriate test is performed on the appropriate patient.

Stress Testing for the Diagnosis of Coronary Artery Disease

Three basic questions need to be addressed when considering stress testing for the diagnosis of coronary artery disease (CAD):

1. What is the pretest probability of CAD?
2. Can the patient exercise?
3. Are there conditions precluding a diagnostic exercise ECG stress test?

Pretest Probability

An estimate of the pretest probability of having CAD can be determined for each patient on the basis of clinical history. Age, sex, and the characterization of chest pain are powerful predictors of CAD. Chest pain can be categorized into one of three groups:

1. Typical or definite angina
    a) Substernal chest discomfort with characteristic quality and duration
    b) Provoked by exertion or emotional stress
    c) Relieved with rest or nitroglycerin
2. Atypical or probable angina—chest discomfort with two of the above typical angina characteristics
3. Noncardiac chest pain—chest discomfort with one or none of the above typical angina characteristics

Additional clinical characteristics that have strengthened prediction models include diabetes mellitus, smoking, hypercholesterolemia, and resting ECG changes. With these models, patients can be classified as having a low (<10%), intermediate (10%-90%), or high probability (>90%) of having CAD. Current guidelines suggest that stress testing for the diagnosis of CAD be performed only in patients with an intermediate likelihood of having CAD. Patients with a low pretest probability of CAD are unlikely to benefit from further testing owing to a high rate of false-positive test results. Similarly, stress testing offers little additional diagnostic information for patients with high pretest probability, because the posttest probability of CAD remains high even after a negative test result. In clinical practice, stress testing is still performed at times in these high-probability patients to gather prognostic information that can be used to guide therapy beyond the initial detection of disease.

Standard Stress Test Techniques

Exercise is the stress test modality of choice in most patients capable of exercise. It is generally safe, widely available, and the least costly of available diagnostic stress options. However, exercise ECG testing alone is limited in certain patient groups. Patients who should be considered for stress testing with myocardial imaging techniques include those with any of the following:

1. More than 1-mm ST-segment depression on baseline ECG
2. Complete LBBB
3. Ventricular paced rhythms
4. Preexcitation syndromes
5. Left ventricular hypertrophy
6. Digoxin use
7. Inability to adequately exercise
8. Previous revascularization

   Stress echocardiography can be performed with either exercise or pharmacologic stress. Additional information obtained from echocardiographic images includes left ventricular size and function, global and regional wall motion and thickening, and further assessment of ischemic threshold. Myocardial contrast perfusion echocardiography may have a valuable role in the future but is not currently part of standard practice.

   Myocardial perfusion imaging typically uses the radionuclides thallium Tl 201– or technetium Tc 99m–labeled sestamibi or tetrofosmin, all of which appear to provide similar diagnostic accuracy in CAD. Imaging with single-photon emission computed tomography (SPECT) is now performed more commonly than planar techniques. Testing can be performed with either exercise or pharmacologic stress. Additional information obtained from perfusion imaging includes the severity and extent of perfusion deficits, left ventricular ejection fraction, and limited information

on global and regional wall motion. Positron emission tomography (PET) is also being used increasingly for myocardial perfusion imaging with improved accuracy in patients with indeterminate SPECT scans or soft tissue attenuation. However, cardiac PET imaging is not yet widely available and will not be considered further in this chapter. Stress radionuclide angiography is now performed infrequently and will not be discussed further.

   Computed tomographic (CT) and *magnetic resonance imaging* (MRI) techniques are also used to assess cardiovascular risk and prognosis. Although emerging data are beginning to validate the techniques, their role in the general management of patients with chest pain is still being determined.

Advantages and Limitations of Stress Test Modalities

Exercise ECG Testing

Standard treadmill assessment is widely available and can be performed with limited expense (Table 1). Its use has been well validated in several different populations. The sensitivity of exercise ECG testing (typically 45%-67%) is generally lower than that of other stress imaging techniques. The sensitivity appears to be higher in elderly patients and in those with multivessel disease. Exercise ECG testing maintains a relatively high specificity (72%-90%), but it is decreased in patients with resting ST-segment depression, left ventricular hypertrophy, LBBB, ventricular paced rhythms, or valvular heart disease and in those taking digoxin. In addition, there appears to be a higher false-positive rate in women, possibly reflecting the decreased prevalence of disease in women than in men of similar age. Finally, exercise ECG testing alone is not useful for localizing the distribution or extent of myocardial ischemia, which can greatly influence patient management decisions.

Exercise Stress Echocardiography

Stress echocardiography is widely available and can be performed at an intermediate cost (Table 1). Sensitivity (range, 70%-97%; overall average, 85%) and specificity (range, 72%-100%; overall average, 86%) are both greater with stress echocardiography than with exercise ECG testing alone. Echocardiography can provide pertinent information on the distribution and extent of CAD, chamber size, global and regional function, and valvular function. Imaging allows accurate detection of

CAD even in the presence of resting ECG abnormalities and digoxin use. Image interpretation can be more difficult when resting regional wall motion abnormalities exist, and interobserver variability remains a limitation. Finally, image quality can be reduced in certain patients because of body habitus or pulmonary disease.

Exercise Myocardial Perfusion Imaging
Perfusion imaging has been well validated for both the detection of CAD and the assessment of prognosis, with widely reproducible results (Table 1). In general, the sensitivity and specificity for detecting CAD with myocardial perfusion imaging are similar to those with stress echocardiography. Several meta-analyses have suggested that sensitivity is higher and specificity is lower with myocardial perfusion imaging than with stress echocardiography. Myocardial perfusion imaging can accurately localize the distribution and extent of ischemia as well as provide basic information on myocardial viability, global ventricular size and function, and regional wall motion in patients with regular rhythms.

Limitations of exercise myocardial perfusion imaging include additional equipment and personnel requirements, radionuclide administration with both rest and stress imaging, and an increased cost compared with other stress test modalities. Soft tissue attenuation and motion artifact may also limit image interpretation. Finally, patients who have LBBB or ventricular paced rhythms have an increased risk of false-positive results with exercise myocardial perfusion imaging.

Pharmacologic Stress Testing
The vasodilators adenosine and dipyridamole are the pharmacologic agents of choice when performing myocardial perfusion imaging in patients who cannot exercise. Despite frequent mild side effects (50% with dipyridamole and 80% with adenosine), both agents are safe and well tolerated. Side effects from dipyridamole can be attenuated with aminophylline, but this is ordinarily not needed with adenosine owing to its very short half-life. Both agents may cause severe bronchospasm in patients who have asthma or chronic obstructive pulmonary disease with reversible airway disease, so they should be used with *extreme* caution or

Table 1. Relative Benefit of Stress Test Modalities

Feature	Standard exercise ECG test	Stress echocardiography	Stress myocardial perfusion imaging
Sensitivity for CAD	Adequate	Very good	Very good*
Specificity for CAD	Good	Very good	Very good*
Accuracy with limited ability to exercise	Poor	Very good	Very good
Accuracy with baseline ST-segment abnormalities	Poor	Very good	Very good
Accuracy for ischemia with baseline wall motion abnormalities	Not applicable	Good	Very good
Ability to localize ischemia	Poor	Very good	Very good
Ability to assess viability	Poor	Good	Good
Ability to assess prognosis	Good	Very good†	Very good
Cost	Relatively inexpensive	Intermediate expense	Expensive

CAD, coronary artery disease; ECG, electrocardiographic.
*Several studies suggest that sensitivity is higher and specificity lower with myocardial perfusion imaging than with stress echocardiography.
†Data on prognosis are more limited with stress echocardiography than with the other modalities.

avoided altogether in these patients. Their use is also limited in patients with heart block, oral dipyridamole or theophylline use, and recent caffeine ingestion. Vasodilator stress with perfusion imaging has been well validated and can detect the presence of CAD with a high sensitivity and an acceptable specificity that are similar to those of exercise imaging. Pharmacologic stress perfusion imaging appears to produce fewer false-positive test results in patients with LBBB or ventricular paced rhythms than exercise perfusion imaging and should be strongly considered as the preferred stress modality in those patients.

Dobutamine is the stress agent of choice for pharmacologic stress echocardiography. By increasing heart rate, systolic blood pressure, and myocardial contractility, dobutamine increases myocardial oxygen demand and may provoke ischemia. Dobutamine is also relatively safe, and side effects may be terminated with discontinuation of the infusion or administration of a β-blocker. Patients with severe CAD, depressed left ventricular function, or recent myocardial injury have an increased risk of ventricular arrhythmias during dobutamine infusion. Dobutamine stress echocardiography has a much higher sensitivity for detection of CAD than vasodilator stress echocardiography (which is used infrequently in the United States), with an estimated sensitivity of 82% and specificity of 85%. In addition, dobutamine echocardiography can provide additional information on myocardial viability and ischemic threshold. Dobutamine stress can also be used during myocardial perfusion imaging with reasonable diagnostic accuracy, although its use should be restricted to patients with contraindications to adenosine or dipyridamole since it does not provoke as great an increase in coronary flow.

CHOICE OF APPROPRIATE STRESS TEST MODALITY

A recommended strategy for determining the appropriate stress test modality (Fig. 1) is based on the three questions noted previously.

1. What is the pretest probability of CAD? If a patient has a very low (<10%) or very high (>90%) pretest probability of CAD by clinical history, stress testing may not be an appropriate diagnostic strategy since the results would be unlikely to alter management decisions. If a patient has contraindications to stress testing or high-risk clinical findings, consider direct referral for coronary angiography.
2. Can the patient exercise? If a patient has an intermediate likelihood of CAD and no contraindications to stress testing, the patient's ability to exercise should be assessed. If the patient cannot exercise, consider a pharmacologic imaging study.
3. Are there conditions precluding a diagnostic exercise ECG stress test? These conditions include baseline ECG abnormalities, digoxin use, and history of prior revascularization. If none of these barriers are present, standard exercise ECG testing can be performed. Otherwise, consider exercise testing with imaging. Patients with LBBB or ventricular paced rhythms require special consideration because pharmacologic myocardial perfusion imaging may offer more diagnostic utility than exercise stress imaging.

With this strategy in mind, review the following three cases.

Case 1

Report of Case

A 45-year-old woman presents with substernal chest pain that can last for hours and is most prominent while lying supine at night. She has no cardiovascular risk factors and has a normal ECG.

Comment

This patient's age, sex, and noncardiac character of chest pain would place her at low pretest probability of CAD (approximately 2%). Her lack of other risk factors further supports a low pretest probability of CAD. She does not require any further cardiac stress testing. Even though stress testing is often performed clinically, the likelihood of false-positive results prompting further unnecessary testing may lead to unwarranted risk and expense.

Case 2

Report of Case

A 45-year-old woman presents with substernal chest pain that occurs at times of high anxiety and is relieved after several minutes of relaxation. She has a history of asthma and diabetes mellitus but denies other cardiovascular risk factors and has a normal ECG.

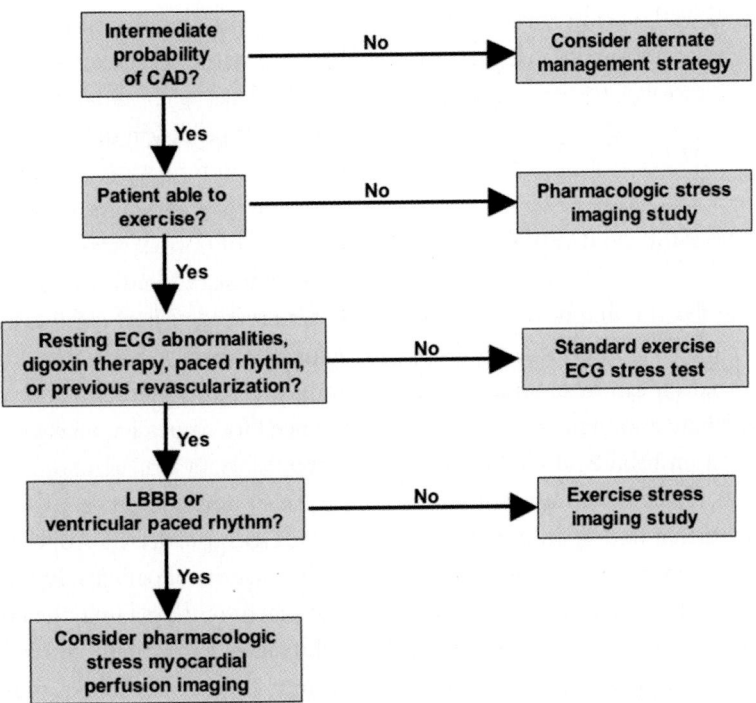

Fig. 1. Choice of stress test modality for the diagnosis of coronary artery disease (CAD). Most patients with either low or high probability of CAD do not require cardiac stress testing and should be considered for alternative management strategies such as noncardiac testing, medical therapy, or coronary angiography. *Pharmacologic stress testing* refers primarily to dobutamine echocardiography and adenosine or dipyridamole myocardial perfusion imaging. ECG, electrocardiographic; LBBB, left bundle branch block.

Comment

This patient's pretest probability is greater than that for the patient in case 1, primarily because of the more typical character of her chest pain, placing her at intermediate probability of CAD (approximately 40%-50%). Diabetes mellitus is another strong predictor of her intermediate risk. If she can exercise, a standard exercise ECG stress test should be performed since she has a normal baseline ECG and has not had prior revascularization. (Although this is still an area of controversy because of the risk of false-positive results in females with exercise ECG testing, some cardiologists would recommend that she have an exercise ECG stress test. If she is still at intermediate risk after a positive exercise ECG test, she could proceed to subsequent stress imaging.) If she cannot exercise, a pharmacologic stress test with dobutamine (typically stress echocardiography) should be performed. Note that she has asthma, and stress with adenosine or dipyridamole should be avoided owing to the risk of life-threatening bronchospasm.

Case 3

Report of Case

A 55-year-old man presents with substernal chest pain that occurs with activity and improves with ibuprofen but not necessarily rest. He is a current smoker but denies other cardiovascular risk factors, and his ECG demonstrates an LBBB.

Comment

Although sometimes difficult to assess, this patient's chest pain is most characteristic of atypical angina. Along with his age, sex, and smoking history, this would place him at intermediate probability of CAD (50%-70%). However, exercise ECG testing would be nondiagnostic for the presence of CAD because he has LBBB. Patients with these characteristics are typically referred for adenosine or dipyridamole stress myocardial perfusion imaging. Exercise perfusion imaging in patients with LBBB may lead to a false-positive test, and the baseline regional wall motion abnormalities from LBBB make stress echocardiography interpretation more difficult.

STRESS TESTING FOR RISK STRATIFICATION AND PROGNOSIS

Although stress testing for the diagnosis of CAD should be restricted to patients at intermediate risk of CAD, prognostic information can be obtained from patients at both intermediate and high risk of CAD. Patients with a low pretest probability of CAD have a low event rate regardless of stress testing results and therefore do not require further testing. In general, the same principles that determined appropriate stress testing for the diagnosis of CAD may also be applied to risk stratification. Exercise testing should be performed with patients who can do the requisite level of activity. The inability to perform an exercise test has by itself been shown to be a marker of poor prognosis. Several predictors of poor outcome have been identified, including poor exercise capacity (<5 metabolic equivalents), the degree (>2 mm) and duration (>5 min) of ST-segment depression, ST-segment elevation, and a low Duke treadmill score. Other predictors that continue to be validated include low peak systolic blood pressure (<130 mm Hg), blunted heart rate response to exercise, delayed heart rate recovery after exercise, and exercise-induced LBBB.

In patients with a normal resting ECG who are not taking digoxin, the modest incremental benefit of additional stress imaging for the prediction of subsequent events does not appear to justify the added cost. However, a stress imaging technique should be considered as the initial stress test in patients with ST-segment depression of more than 1 mm, LBBB, ventricular paced rhythms, or preexcitation. The extent and severity of exercise-induced left ventricular dysfunction that occurs with exercise echocardiography can add incremental prognostic value beyond the Duke treadmill score alone. Similarly, with dobutamine echocardiography, the number of territories with both resting and exercise-induced regional wall motion abnormalities is a predictor of mortality.

The prognostic value of myocardial perfusion imaging with either exercise or pharmacologic stress has also been well validated. The presence, extent, and severity of perfusion defects can provide independent prognostic information beyond exercise data. A normal perfusion scan predicts a low event rate comparable with that of normal stress echocardiography. A mildly abnormal scan identifies a group with low mortality but increased risk of cardiac events requiring more aggressive medical management. Moderate or severely abnormal scans predict a poor prognosis and suggest the need for aggressive management with angiography and possible revascularization.

In summary, exercise ECG testing can ultimately provide adequate detection of CAD and risk stratification in the majority of patients. In those who require further assessment with imaging, the choice of stress imaging technique requires careful consideration of the individual patient characteristics. In many cases, either stress echocardiography or myocardial perfusion imaging may be appropriate; the preferred test often depends on local expertise, available facilities, and considerations of cost-effectiveness.

RESOURCES

Brindis RG, Douglas PS, Hendel RC, et al. ACC/ASNC appropriateness criteria for single-photon emission computed tomography myocardial perfusion imaging (SPECT MPI): a report of the American College of Cardiology Foundation Quality Strategic Directions Committee Appropriateness Criteria Working Group and the American Society of Nuclear Cardiology. Available from: http://www.acc.org/clinical/pdfs/SPECTMPIACPub File.pdf.

Gibbons RJ, Antman EM, Alpert JS, et al. ACC/AHA 2002 guideline update for the management of patients with chronic stable angina. Available from: http://www.acc.org/clinical/guidelines/stable/update_index.htm.

Gibbons RJ, Balady GJ, Bricker JT, et al. ACC/AHA 2002 guideline update for exercise testing—full text. Available from: http://www.acc.org/clinical/guidelines/exercise/dirindex.htm.

SECTION III

Electrophysiology

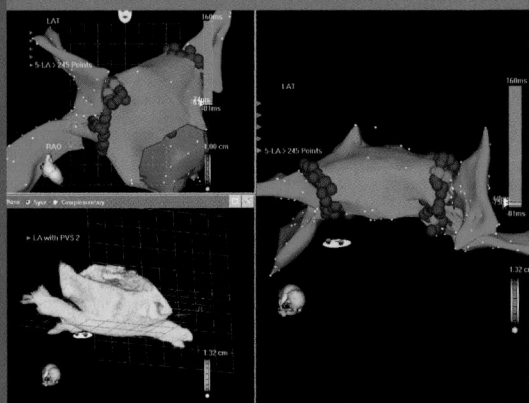

Voltage Map

ELECTROCARDIOGRAPHIC DIAGNOSES: CRITERIA AND DEFINITIONS OF ABNORMALITIES

Stephen C. Hammill, MD

This chapter is a diagnostic guide for all physicians who evaluate electrocardiograms (ECGs), and the criteria are of specific value to persons taking professional examinations in cardiology and internal medicine. The criteria are those used in clinical practice at Mayo Clinic, and thus they may differ in minor ways from those used on examinations. Check the specific diagnoses available on the answer sheet. These criteria are not endorsed by any professional examination body or organization.

EXAMINATION STRATEGY

When reviewing ECGs, be sure to evaluate the tracing systematically for abnormalities of the rate, rhythm, and axis and to examine the configuration, duration, and relationship of the P, QRS, and T waves. Most examination ECGs have one to three major findings. Cardiology examinations emphasize the correct identification of the major diagnoses on the tracing; points are subtracted for important oversights and misdiagnoses. The ancillary minor diagnoses are given minimal or neutral credit.

This chapter includes a score sheet similar to that used in cardiology examinations. Minor changes are made to the numbering of the examination answer

codes from year to year. In this chapter, letters are purposely used for codes to avoid confusion between the numbering scheme of examinations and the criteria in this chapter. Initially this chapter lists all the ECG diagnoses; in subsequent pages criteria for each diagnosis are defined on the score sheet.

Do not guess the ECG diagnoses on the examination, because wrong diagnoses receive negative credits. If the ECG looks normal, be aware that it may not be normal. Always double-check for subtle ECG changes, including the delta wave of Wolff-Parkinson-White syndrome, QT interval prolongation, the prominent U waves of hypokalemia, the tall R wave in lead V_1 associated with a posterior wall infarct, and PR-segment depression in acute pericarditis.

Systematic Evaluation of an ECG Tracing

1. Standardization and leads shown; review for reversed leads, right chest leads, and 1/2 voltage standardization in left ventricular hypertrophy
2. Heart rate: determine separately for QRS and P waves if the rhythm is other than sinus
3. Heart rhythm
4. Cardiac axis
5. Configuration and duration of P, QRS, and T waves
6. Relationship of P wave to QRS complex

7. Intervals: PR, QRS, and QT
8. ECG diagnosis
9. Suggested clinical diagnosis

ECG DIAGNOSES

1. General Features

   a. Normal ECG
   b. Borderline normal ECG or normal variant
   c. Incorrect electrode placement
   d. Artifact due to tremor

2. Atrial Rhythms

   a. Sinus rhythm
   b. Sinus arrhythmia
   c. Sinus bradycardia (<60 beats/min)
   d. Sinus tachycardia (>100 beats/min)
   e. Sinus pause or arrest
   f. Sinoatrial exit block
   g. Ectopic atrial rhythm
   h. Wandering atrial pacemaker
   i. Atrial premature complexes, normally conducted
   j. Atrial premature complexes, nonconducted
   k. Atrial premature complexes with aberrant intraventricular conduction
   l. Atrial tachycardia (regular, sustained, 1:1 conduction)
   m. Atrial tachycardia, repetitive (short paroxysms)
   n. Atrial tachycardia, multifocal (chaotic atrial tachycardia)
   o. Atrial tachycardia with atrioventricular (AV) block
   p. Supraventricular tachycardia, unspecified
   q. Supraventricular tachycardia, paroxysmal
   r. Atrial flutter
   s. Atrial fibrillation
   t. Retrograde atrial activation

3. AV Junctional Rhythms

   a. AV junctional premature complexes
   b. AV junctional escape complexes
   c. AV junctional rhythm, accelerated
   d. AV junctional rhythm

4. Ventricular Rhythms

   a. Ventricular premature complex(es), uniform, fixed coupling
   b. Ventricular premature complex(es), uniform, nonfixed coupling
   c. Ventricular premature complex(es), multiform
   d. Ventricular premature complexes, in pairs (2 consecutive)
   e. Ventricular parasystole
   f. Ventricular tachycardia (≥3 consecutive beats)
   g. Accelerated idioventricular rhythm
   h. Ventricular escape complexes or rhythm
   i. Ventricular fibrillation

5. Atrioventricular Interactions in Arrhythmias

   a. Fusion complexes
   b. Reciprocal (echo) complexes
   c. Ventricular capture complexes
   d. AV dissociation
   e. Ventriculophasic sinus arrhythmia

6. AV Conduction Abnormalities

   a. AV block, first degree
   b. AV block, second degree–Mobitz type I (Wenckebach)
   c. AV block, second degree–Mobitz type II
   d. AV block, 2:1
   e. AV block, third degree
   f. AV block, variable
   g. Short PR interval (with sinus rhythm and normal QRS duration)
   h. Wolff-Parkinson-White pattern

7. Intraventricular Conduction Disturbances

   a. Right bundle branch block (RBBB), incomplete
   b. RBBB, complete
   c. Left anterior fascicular block
   d. Left posterior fascicular block
   e. Left bundle branch block (LBBB), complete with ST-T waves suggestive of acute myocardial injury or infarction
   f. LBBB, complete

g. LBBB, intermittent

h. Intraventricular conduction disturbance, nonspecific type

i. Aberrant intraventricular conduction with supraventricular arrhythmia (specify rhythm)

8. P-Wave Abnormalities

    a. Right atrial abnormality

    b. Left atrial abnormality

    c. Nonspecific atrial abnormality

9. Abnormalities of QRS Voltage or Axis

    a. Low voltage, limb leads only

    b. Low voltage, limb and precordial leads

    c. Left-axis deviation (>−30°)

    d. Right-axis deviation (>+100°)

    e. Electrical alternans

10. Ventricular Hypertrophy

    a. Left ventricular hypertrophy by voltage only

    b. Left ventricular hypertrophy by both voltage and ST-T–segment abnormalities

    c. Right ventricular hypertrophy

    d. Combined ventricular hypertrophy

11. Transmural Myocardial Infarction

	Probably acute or recent	Probably old or age indeterminate
Anterolateral	**a.**	**g.**
Anterior	**b.**	**h.**
Anteroseptal	**c.**	**i.**
Lateral or high lateral	**d.**	**j.**
Inferior (diaphragmatic)	**e.**	**k.**
Posterior	**f.**	**l.**

    m. Probable ventricular aneurysm

12. ST-, T-, and U-Wave Abnormalities

    a. Normal variant, early repolarization

    b. Normal variant, juvenile T waves

c. Nonspecific ST- or T-wave abnormalities

d. ST-segment or T-wave abnormalities suggesting myocardial ischemia

e. ST-segment or T-wave abnormalities suggesting myocardial injury

f. ST-segment or T-wave abnormalities suggesting acute pericarditis

g. ST-segment or T-wave abnormalities due to intraventricular conduction disturbance or hypertrophy

h. Post-extrasystolic T-wave abnormality

i. Isolated J-point depression

j. Peaked T waves

k. Prolonged QT interval

l. Prominent U waves

13. Pacemaker Function and Rhythm

    a. Atrial or coronary sinus pacing

    b. Ventricular demand pacing

    c. AV sequential pacing

    d. Ventricular pacing, fixed rate (asynchronous)

    e. Dual-chamber, atrial-sensing pacemaker

    f. Pacemaker malfunction, not constantly capturing (atrium or ventricle)

    g. Pacemaker malfunction, not constantly sensing (atrium or ventricle)

    h. Pacemaker malfunction, not firing

    i. Pacemaker malfunction, slowing

14. Suggested or Probable Clinical Disorders

    a. Digitalis effect

    b. Digitalis toxicity

    c. Antiarrhythmic drug effect

    d. Antiarrhythmic drug toxicity

    e. Hyperkalemia

    f. Hypokalemia

    g. Hypercalcemia

    h. Hypocalcemia

    i. Atrial septal defect, secundum

    j. Atrial septal defect, primum

    k. Dextrocardia, mirror image

    l. Mitral valve disease

    m. Chronic lung disease

    n. Acute cor pulmonale, including pulmonary embolus

o. Pericardial effusion

p. Acute pericarditis

q. Hypertrophic cardiomyopathy

r. Coronary artery disease

s. Central nervous system disorder

t. Myxedema

u. Hypothermia

v. Sick sinus syndrome

w. Ebstein anomaly

CRITERIA FOR SCORE SHEET DIAGNOSIS

1. General Features

   a. Normal ECG

   - No abnormalities of the rhythm, rate, or axis
   - The configurations of the P wave, QRS complex, and T wave are within normal limits (Fig. 1)

   b. Borderline normal ECG or normal variant

   - Early repolarization (see item **12a**)
   - Juvenile T waves (see item **12b**)
   - S_1, S_2, and S_3
     A terminal negative deflection is present in

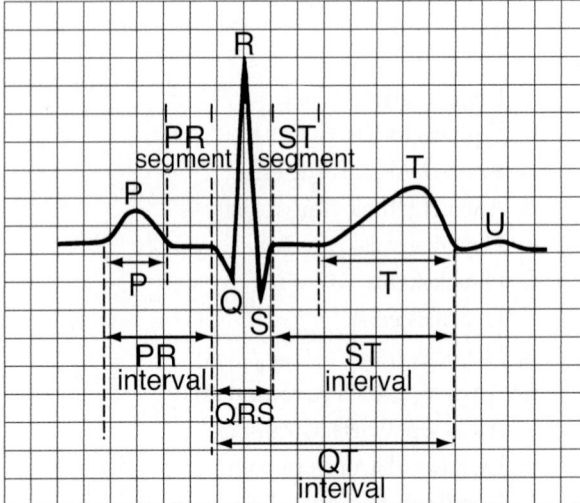

Fig. 1. Components of the scalar electrocardiogram with standard wave labeling (P, Q, R, S, T, U) and clinically useful interval and segment measurements.

the QRS complexes in the standard limb leads in up to 20% of healthy adults—it should be distinguished from abnormal left axis deviation

   - rSR′ or rSr′ in lead V_1 (2.4% of normals)
     - QRS duration <0.10 second and <7 mm in height
     - Amplitude of r′ smaller than amplitude of r or S

   c. Incorrect electrode placement—most commonly the following:

   - Reversal of right and left arm leads (Fig. 2). Resultant ECG mimics dextrocardia in limb leads with P, QRS, and T inversion in limb leads I and aVL. However, the precordial leads remain normal and thus rule out dextrocardia.
   - Reversal of chest V leads (Fig. 3). There is a sudden decrease in the R-wave amplitude with return in the next V lead.

   d. Artifact due to tremor

   - Parkinson tremor simulates atrial flutter with a rate of approximately 300/min (4-6/s) (Fig.4)
   - Physiologic tremor rate is 500/min (7-9/s)
   - Most prominent in limb leads

2. Atrial Rhythms

   a. Sinus rhythm

   - Rate 60-100/min
   - P axis normal (+15° to +75°)

   b. Sinus arrhythmia—requires the following:

   - P-wave morphology and axis normal
   - PP interval varies by >0.16 second or 10%

   c. Sinus bradycardia (<60 beats/min)—requires the following:

   - Rate < 60 beats/min
   - Normal P-wave axis

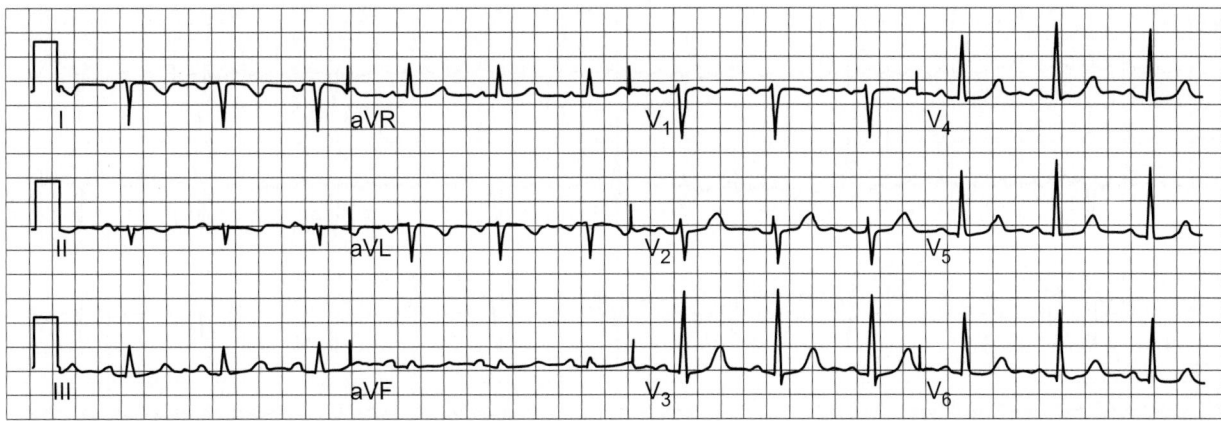

Fig. 2. Reversal of right and left arm leads.

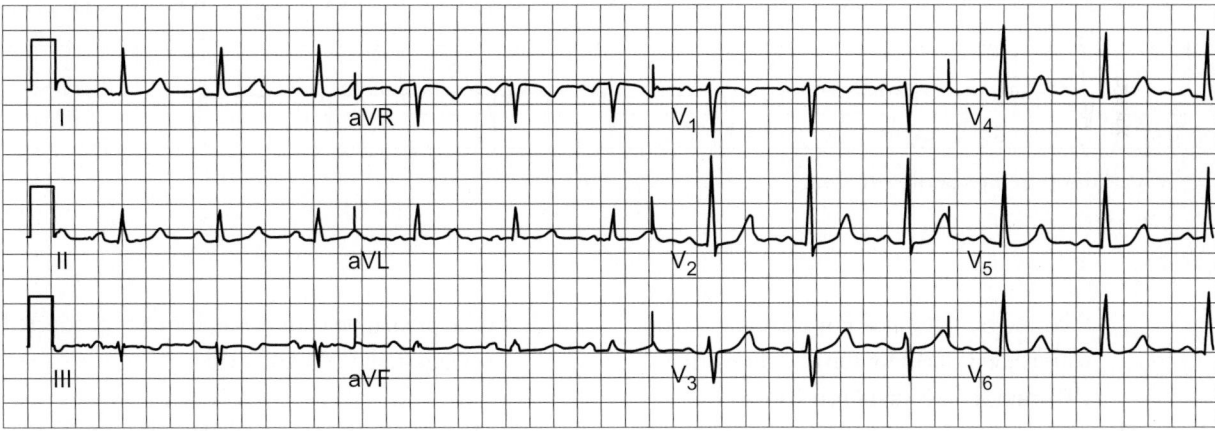

Fig. 3. Reversal of V_2 and V_3 leads in a 61-year-old woman.

Note: If rate <40/min, consider 2:1 sinoatrial exit block

d. Sinus tachycardia (>100 beats/min)—requires the following:

- Rate >100 beats/min
- Normal P-wave axis

Note: P amplitude often increases and PR interval shortens with increasing rate

e. Sinus pause or arrest—pause >2.0 seconds without a P wave

Note: The differential diagnosis includes the following:

- Sinus arrhythmia—phasic, gradual PP-interval change

- Sinoatrial exit block—pause is multiple (2 times, 3 times, etc.) of usual PP interval
- Nonconducted atrial premature complexes—look for P wave deforming the preceding T wave
- Sinus arrest

f. Sinoatrial exit block

- First- and third-degree not detectable on surface ECG
- Second-degree
  - Type I (Mobitz I)—Group beating with shortening of the PP interval, constant PR interval, and a PP pause that is less than twice the normal PP interval
  - Type II (Mobitz II)—Constant PP interval

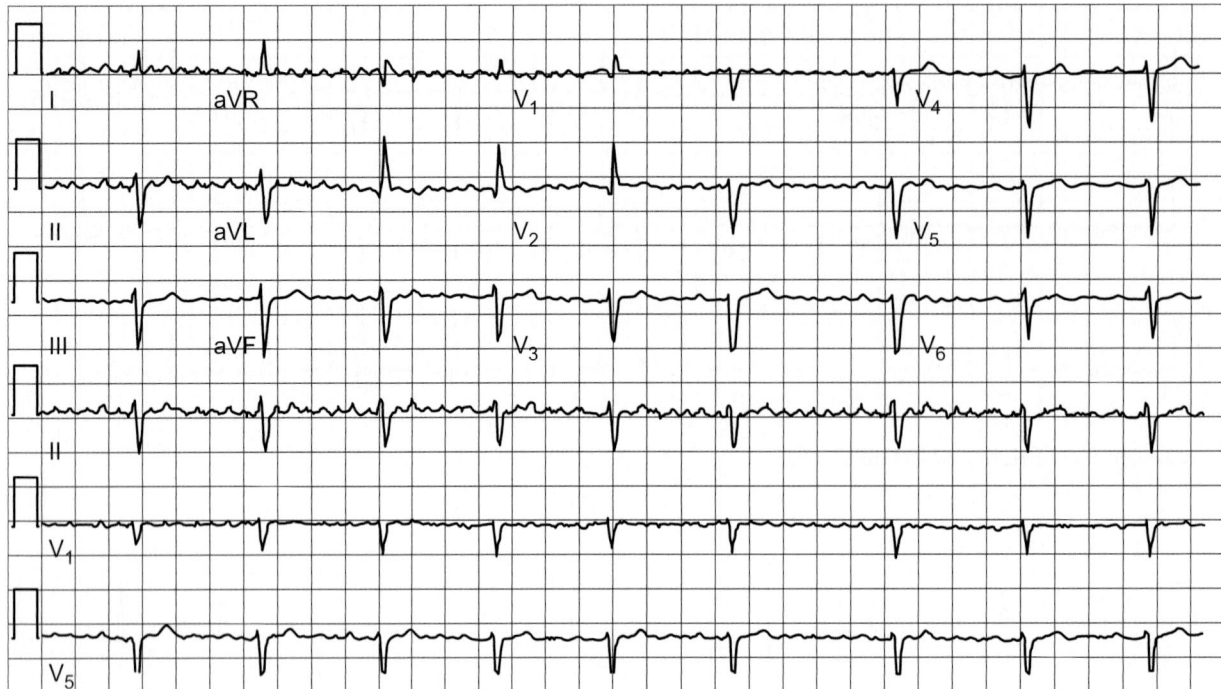

Fig. 4. Parkinson tremor causing artifact.

followed by a dropped P wave, the pause being a near multiple of the normal PP interval. Interval of pause may be slightly less than twice the normal PP interval but usually within 0.10 second

g. Ectopic atrial rhythm—requires all the following:

- P-wave axis or morphology different from sinus rhythm
- Rate <100 beats/min
- PR interval >0.11 second

Note: Low atrial focus may activate atrium retrogradely (P inverted in II, III, and aVF), but PR interval >0.11 second, distinguishing it from AV junctional rhythm

h. Wandering atrial pacemaker—requires the following:

- Rate <100 beats/min
- Varying P waves with ≥3 morphologic patterns

i. Atrial premature complexes, normally conducted —suggested by the following:

- Premature P wave in relation to normal sinus rhythm
- P wave usually abnormal in configuration
- PR interval may be normal, increased, or decreased
- Post-extrasystolic pause is noncompensatory unless sinoatrial entrance block is present and sinoatrial node is not reset, resulting in either an interpolated beat or a full compensatory pause
- QRS complex similar in morphology to the QRS complex present during sinus rhythm

j. Atrial premature complexes, nonconducted (Fig. 5 and 6)—suggested by the following:

- Premature P waves that are abnormal in morphology but not followed by QRS
- P waves that are often hidden in T wave (look for deformed T wave)
- The sinus node is usually reset, resulting in

RR interval pause

k. Atrial premature complexes with aberrant intra-ventricular conduction (Fig. 7)—suggested by the following:

- P wave that occurs very early
- RBBB pattern is most common, but LBBB or even variable QRS morphology may occur
Note: Also see item **7i**

l. Atrial tachycardia (regular, sustained, 1:1 conduction)—suggested by the following:

- Abnormal P waves that are different in morphology from sinus P waves
- Three or more beats in succession
- The atrial rate is generally 100-180 beats/min
- Regular rhythm (constant RR interval), except for a warm-up period in the automatic type
- A QRS complex follows each P wave—the QRS complex usually resembles the morphology present during sinus rhythm unless aberrantly conducted
- PR interval may be within normal limits or

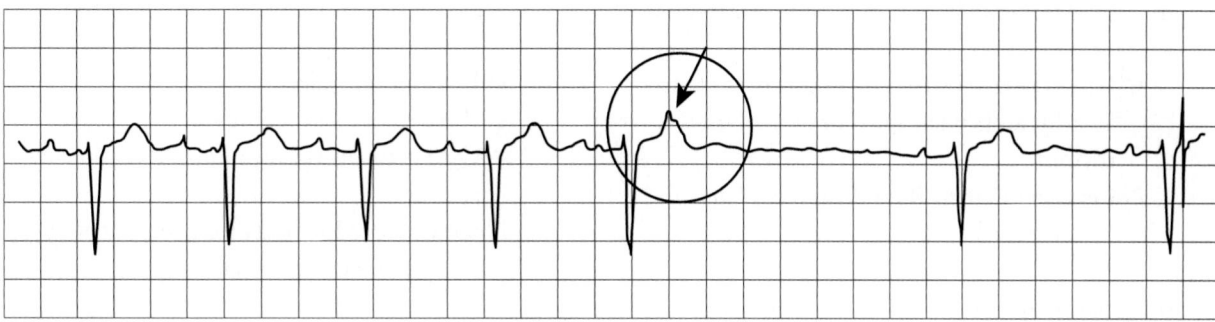

Fig. 5. Nonconducted atrial premature complex (*arrow*) causing a pause.

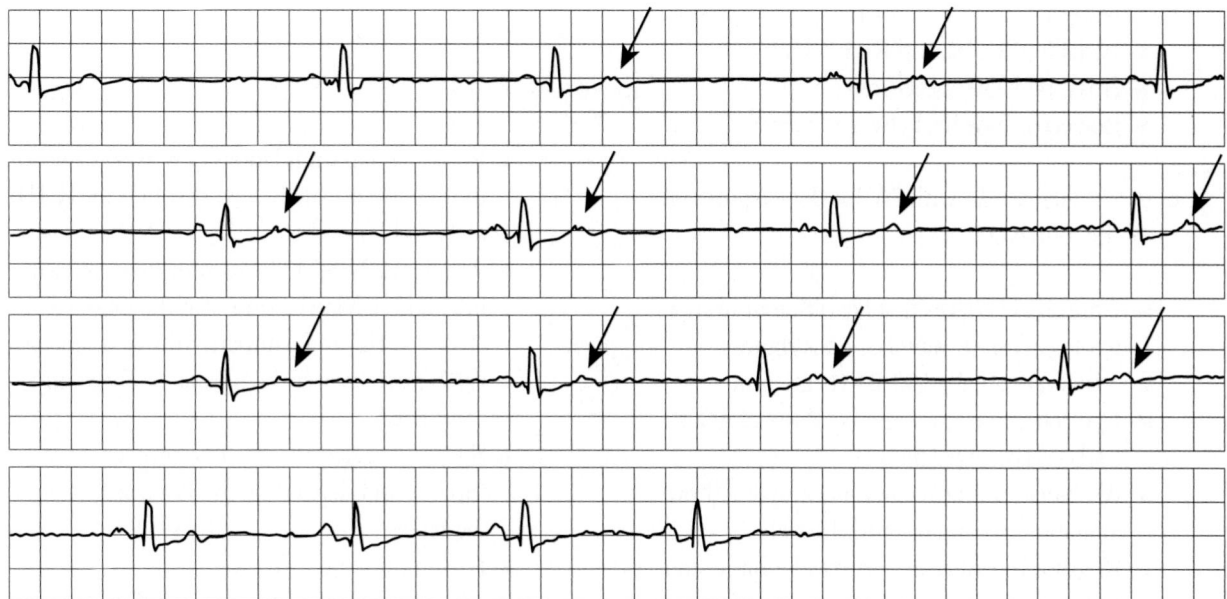

Fig. 6. Nonconducted atrial premature complexes (*arrows*) in bigeminy causing bradycardia. Strip is continuous.

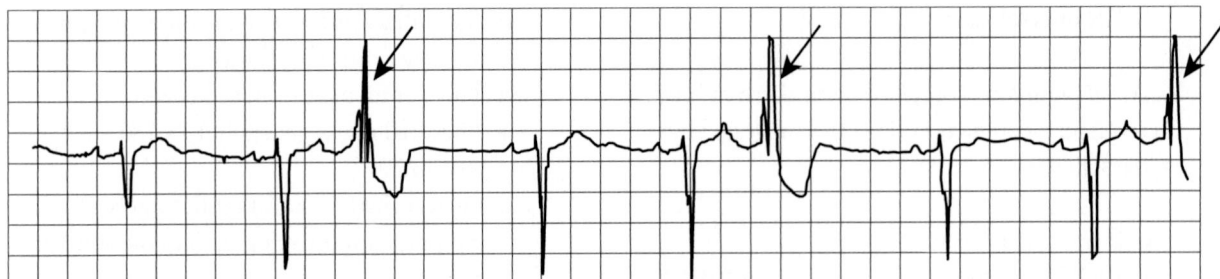

Fig. 7. Atrial premature complexes with aberrant intraventricular conduction (*arrows*).

prolonged
- Secondary ST- and T-wave changes may occur

m. Atrial tachycardia, repetitive (short paroxysms)

- Characterized by recurring short runs of atrial tachycardia interrupted by normal sinus rhythm
Note: Refer to item **2l** for definition of *atrial tachycardia*

n. Atrial tachycardia, multifocal (chaotic atrial tachycardia)—requires *all* of the following:

- P waves of at least 3 morphologic patterns
- Absence of 1 dominant atrial pacemaker (in contradistinction to normal sinus rhythm with multifocal atrial premature complexes)
- Variable PR, RR, and RP intervals
- Atrial rate >100 beats/min
- Isoelectric baseline between P waves

o. Atrial tachycardia with AV block—requires *all* of the following:

- Abnormal P waves that are different in morphology from P waves of sinus rhythm
- Atrial rate usually 150-240 beats/min
- Isoelectric intervals between P waves in all leads (unlike atrial flutter)
- AV block to a degree beyond simple PR prolongation (second or third degree)
- Rhythm is regular, but ventriculophasic sinus arrhythmia may occur (refer to item **5e** for definition)

Note: Most cases are due to digitalis toxicity (refer to item **14b**)

p. Supraventricular tachycardia, unspecified

- Rhythm is regular
- P wave not easily identified
- QRS complex usually narrow (occasionally aberrant)
Note: If rate is 150 beats/min, rule out atrial flutter with 2:1 block

q. Supraventricular tachycardia, paroxysmal

- Onset and termination sudden
- May have retrograde P wave (see item **2t**)
- Refer to item **2p** for definition of *supraventricular tachycardia*

r. Atrial flutter

- Rapid regular undulations (F waves), sawtooth pattern usually seen best in leads II, III, aVF, and V_1
- Atrial rate 240-340 beats/min. May be faster in children. May be slower in the presence of class 1A, 1C, and 3 antiarrhythmic drugs
- QRS complex may be normal or aberrantly conducted
- Rate and regularity of QRS complexes are variable and depend on the AV conduction sequence
- AV conduction
  - Complete block may occur with or without AV junctional tachycardia (usually digoxin

toxicity)
- May have varying degrees of block (2:1, 4:1, or more)

s. Atrial fibrillation

- P waves are absent. Atrial activity is represented by fibrillation (f) waves of varying amplitudes, duration, and morphology causing random oscillation of the baseline
- The ventricular rhythm, in the absence of third-degree AV block, is irregularly irregular
- Atrial activity is best seen in the right precordial and inferior leads
- Rate is usually 100-180 beats/min in the absence of drugs. If rate is <100 beats/min, conduction system disease is likely to be present. If rate is >200 beats/min with a QRS complex >0.12 second in duration, consider Wolff-Parkinson-White syndrome.
- Differential diagnosis:
  - Multifocal atrial tachycardia
  - Paroxysmal atrial tachycardia with block
  - Atrial flutter

t. Retrograde atrial activation

- Inverted P waves in leads II, III, and aVF
- Look for retrograde P waves after ventricular premature complexes and other ectopic junctional or ventricular beats

3. AV Junctional Rhythms

a. AV junctional premature complexes—require *all* of the following:

- Occur early in cycle, in contrast to escape beats
- P wave is inverted in leads II, III, and aVF and upright in leads I and aVL
- P wave may precede the QRS by ≤0.11 second or may be superimposed on or follow the QRS
- Ventricular complex may show aberration
- Coupling interval is usually constant
- Noncompensatory pause is usually seen
Note: Consider also item **2t**

b. AV junctional escape complexes

- There is decreased sinus impulse formation or conduction from the sinoatrial node, or high-degree AV block at or proximal to the bundle of His. Atrial mechanism may be sinus rhythm, paroxysmal atrial tachycardia, atrial flutter, or atrial fibrillation.
- May be seen with post-extrasystolic pause after atrial tachycardia, atrial flutter, or atrial fibrillation

c. AV junctional rhythm, accelerated—requires *all* of the following:

- Rate >60 beats/min
- Variable relationship between atrial and ventricular rates. If retrograde block is present, atria remain in sinus rhythm and AV dissociation will be present. If retrograde activation occurs, constant QRS-P interval will be present
- May be seen with atrial fibrillation or atrial flutter with complete heart block (consider digoxin toxicity)
- Exit block also occurs with digoxin toxicity
Note: Consider items **2t** and **14b**

d. AV junctional rhythm (rate ≤60 beats/min)

- RR interval of escape rhythm usually constant (<0.04-second variation)
- May have isorhythmic AV dissociation (consider item **5d**)
- P wave inverted in leads II, III, and aVF and upright in leads I and aVL (consider item **2t**)

4. Ventricular Rhythms

a. Ventricular premature complex(es), uniform, fixed coupling (Fig. 8)—*all* of the folowing are required:

- Premature in relation to normal cycles, not preceded by P wave (or shorter than expected PR interval or "collapsing PR")
- Coupling interval usually the same for each site or focus (variation usually <0.08 second)

- Abnormal QRS configuration that is almost always >0.12 second in duration
- Retrograde capture of atria may occur (consider item **2t**)
- Initial direction of QRS complex is often different from that observed during sinus rhythm
- Usually full compensatory pause is noted
- Compensatory pause requires an undisturbed sinus depolarization due to one of the following:
  - Ventriculoatrial block
  - Sinoatrial entrance block if atrial capture occurs
  - Sinoatrial node discharged before arrival of retrograde wavefront, and thus refractory

b. Ventricular premature complex(es), uniform, nonfixed coupling

- Ventricular premature complexes with variable temporal relationship to regular sinus beats

c. Ventricular premature complex(es), multiform
- Two or more morphologic patterns of ventricular premature complexes present

d. Ventricular premature complexes, in pairs (2 consecutive)

- Two consecutive ventricular premature complexes of not necessarily the same morphology
Note: Refer to item **4a** for criteria

e. Ventricular parasystole—an automatic ventricular focus with entrance block and all of the following:

- Rates usually 30-56 beats/min
- Varying relationship with the preceding sinus beats
- All interectopic intervals are a multiple of a constant shortest interval
- When fusion beats and lack of fixed coupling are noted, consider parasystole

f. Ventricular tachycardia (≥3 consecutive beats)—rapid succession of ≥3 beats of ventricular origin (Fig. 9 and 10)
- Abnormal and wide QRS complexes with secondary ST-T changes
Note: Ventricular tachycardia originating in the

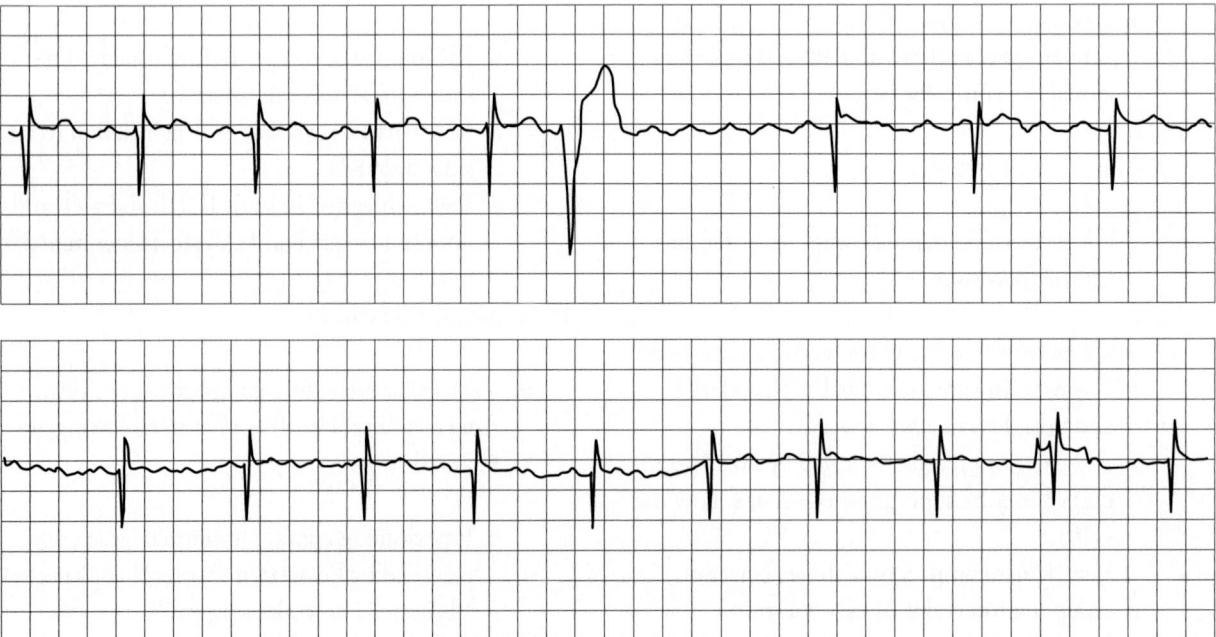

Fig. 8. Ventricular premature complex resulting in concealed retrograde conduction during atrial fibrillation.

septum near the normal conduction system may have a narrow QRS complex
- Rate >100 beats/min
- Regular or slightly irregular
- Abrupt onset and termination
- AV dissociation is common. On occasion, retrograde conduction and capture of the atria may occur
- Look for ventricular capture and fusion beats as a marker for ventricular tachycardia

Ventricular origin favored with the following:

- QRS complexes like those of ventricular premature complexes
- Tachyarrhythmia initiated by ventricular premature complexes
- AV dissociation
- Capture or fusion beats
- QRS ≥0.14 second if RBBB morphology and ≥0.16 second if LBBB morphology when QRS during sinus rhythm <0.12 second
- Left or northwest axis deviation
- All positive or all negative complexes in precordial leads
- In V_1, R > r′ (left rabbit ear taller than right)

Supraventricular origin favored with the following:

- QRS complex like aberrantly conducted atrial premature complexes or QRS in sinus rhythm
- Tachyarrhythmia initiated by atrial premature complexes
- RBBB configuration with rSR′ in V_1

g. Accelerated idioventricular rhythm—requires *all* of the following:

- Regular rhythm, rate 60-110 beats/min
- QRS complexes are abnormal and wide
- Usually AV dissociation
- Capture and fusion beats are common because of slower rate

Note: Also consider items **5a** and **5c**

h. Ventricular escape complexes or rhythm—requires *all* of the following:

- Rate is usually 30-40 beats/min (can be 20-50 beats/min)
- QRS complexes are abnormal and wide
- Occurs when the rate of supraventricular impulse arriving at the ventricle is slower

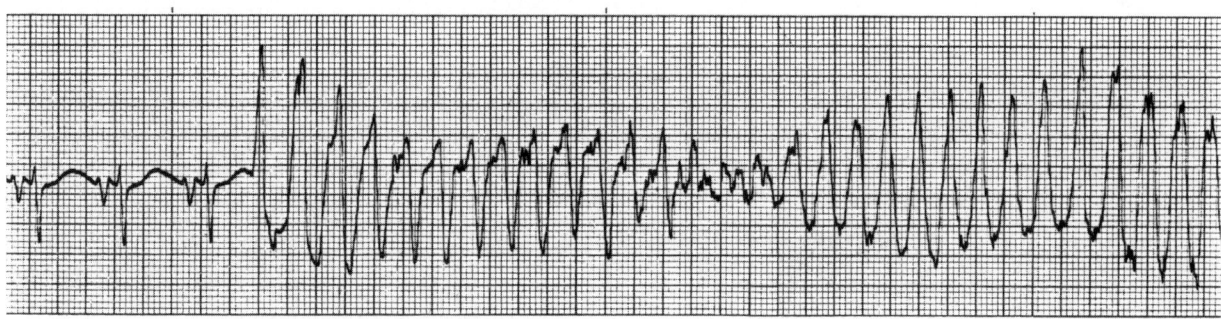

Fig. 9. Torsades de pointes in a patient with long QT syndrome.

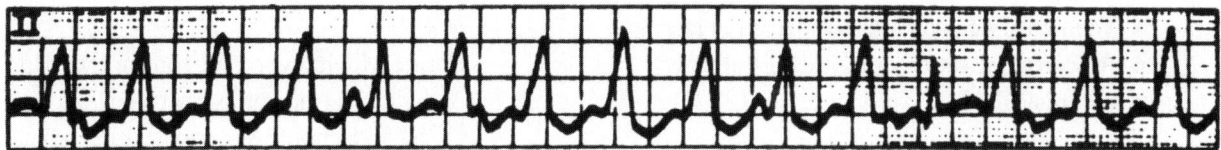

Fig. 10. Monomorphic ventricular tachycardia with fusion complexes.

than the inherent rate of the ectopic ventricular pacemaker

i. Ventricular fibrillation

- Chaotic and irregular deflections of varying amplitude and contour
- No P waves, QRS complexes, or T waves

5. Atrioventricular Interactions in Arrhythmias

a. Fusion complexes—caused by simultaneous activation of the ventricle from two sources and may occur with the following:

- Ventricular premature complexes
- Wolff-Parkinson-White syndrome
- Ventricular tachycardia
- Ventricular parasystole
- Accelerated idioventricular rhythm
- Paced rhythm

b. Reciprocal (echo) complexes

- The impulse activates a chamber (atrium or ventricle), returns, and reactivates the same chamber

c. Ventricular capture complexes

- Ventricular capture by conducted supraventricular impulses resulting in a fusion beat or a QRS morphology similar to that during sinus rhythm
- Strong but not infallible evidence for rhythm of ventricular origin

d. AV dissociation—requires *all* of the following:

- Atrial and ventricular activities that are independent
- Ventricular rate that is faster than atrial rate
- Always the result of some other disturbance of cardiac rhythm

e. Ventriculophasic sinus arrhythmia
- A PP interval containing a QRS complex is shorter than a PP interval without a QRS
- Common in presence of high-grade AV block

6. AV Conduction Abnormalities

a. AV block, first degree—requires *all* of the following:

- PR interval ≥0.20 second (usually 0.21-0.40 second, but may be as long as 0.80 second)
- Each P wave is followed by a QRS complex
- Usually a constant PR interval (Fig. 11)

b. AV block, second degree–Mobitz type I (Wenckebach) (Fig. 12 and 13)—requires *all* of the following:

- Progressive prolongation of PR interval until P wave fails to conduct to the ventricle
- Progressive shortening of RR interval until P wave is not conducted
- The RR interval containing the nonconducted P wave is shorter than the sum of two PP intervals
- Results in "group" or pattern beating

c. AV block, second degree–Mobitz type II (Fig. 14)—requires *all* of the following:

- There are intermittent nonconducted P waves with no evidence of atrial prematurity
- In conducted beats, PR intervals stay constant
- The RR interval containing the nonconducted P wave is equal to two PP intervals
- A 2:1 AV block can be Mobitz type I or II and cannot be distinguished without the following information:
  - Results of maneuvers used to increase heart rate and improve AV conduction (atropine and exercise typically decrease type I block and increase type II block) (Fig. 15), *or*
  - Classic Mobitz type I seen on another part of the ECG (then probably type I), *or*
  - QRS conduction is abnormal with bundle branch block or bifascicular block (then usually Mobitz type II)

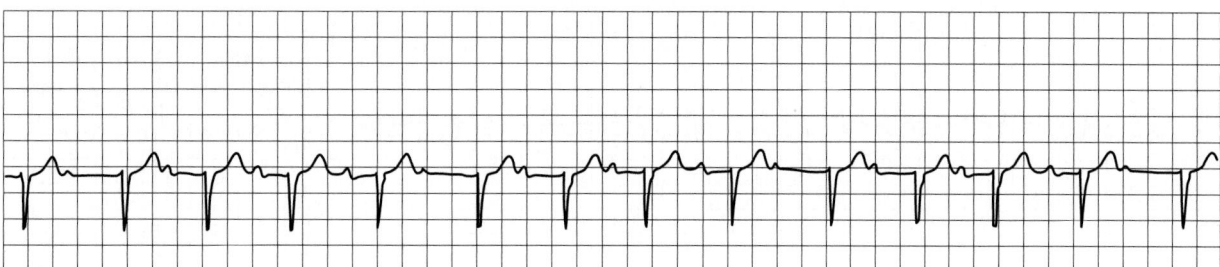

Fig. 11. Changing RP interval affecting the subsequent PR interval during sinus arrhythmia.

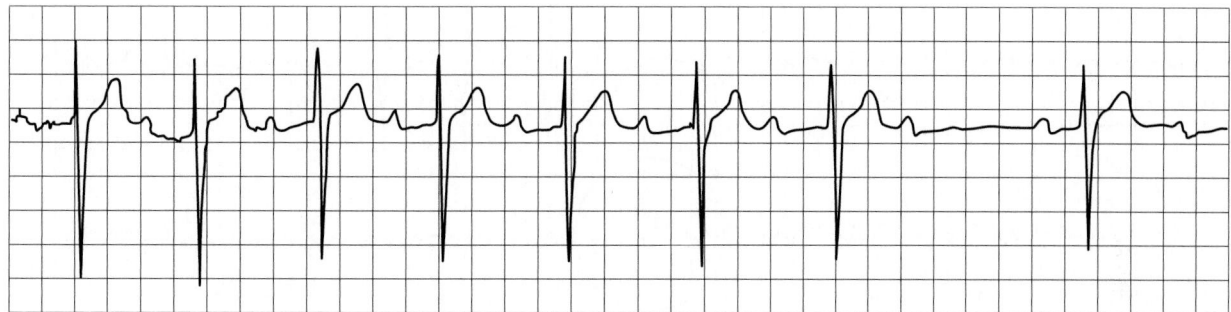

Fig. 12. Atrioventricular block, second degree–Mobitz type I (Wenckebach).

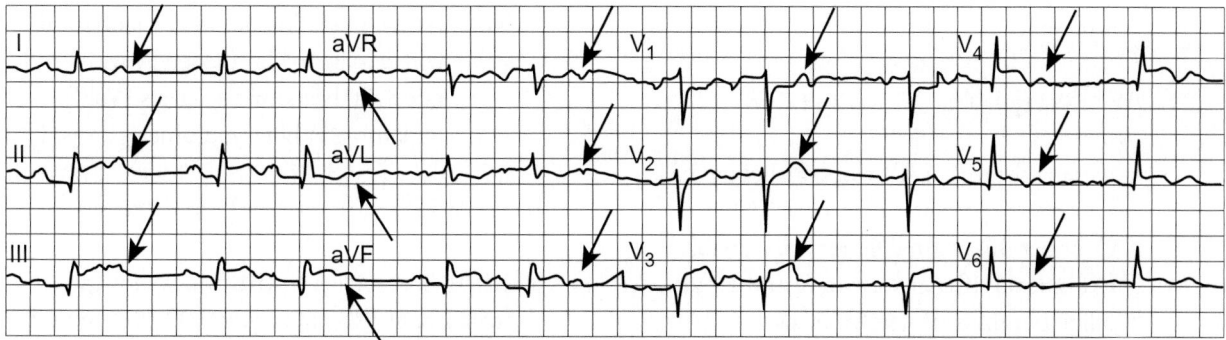

Fig. 13. Acute inferior myocardial infarction with atrioventricular block, second degree–Mobitz type I (Wenckebach), in a 69-year-old man. *Arrows* indicate P waves preceding dropped beats.

d. AV block, 2:1

- There are two P waves for each QRS complex (every other P wave is nonconducted)
  Note: Refer to item **6c**

e. AV block, third degree (Fig. 16)—requires *all* of the following:

- Independent atrial and ventricular activities
- Atrial rate faster than ventricular rate
- Ventricular rhythm maintained by a junctional or idioventricular escape rhythm or ventricular pacemaker
- Ventriculophasic sinus arrhythmia in 30% of cases (consider item **5e**)
- When the ventricular rate is faster than the atrial rate, AV dissociation (not AV block)

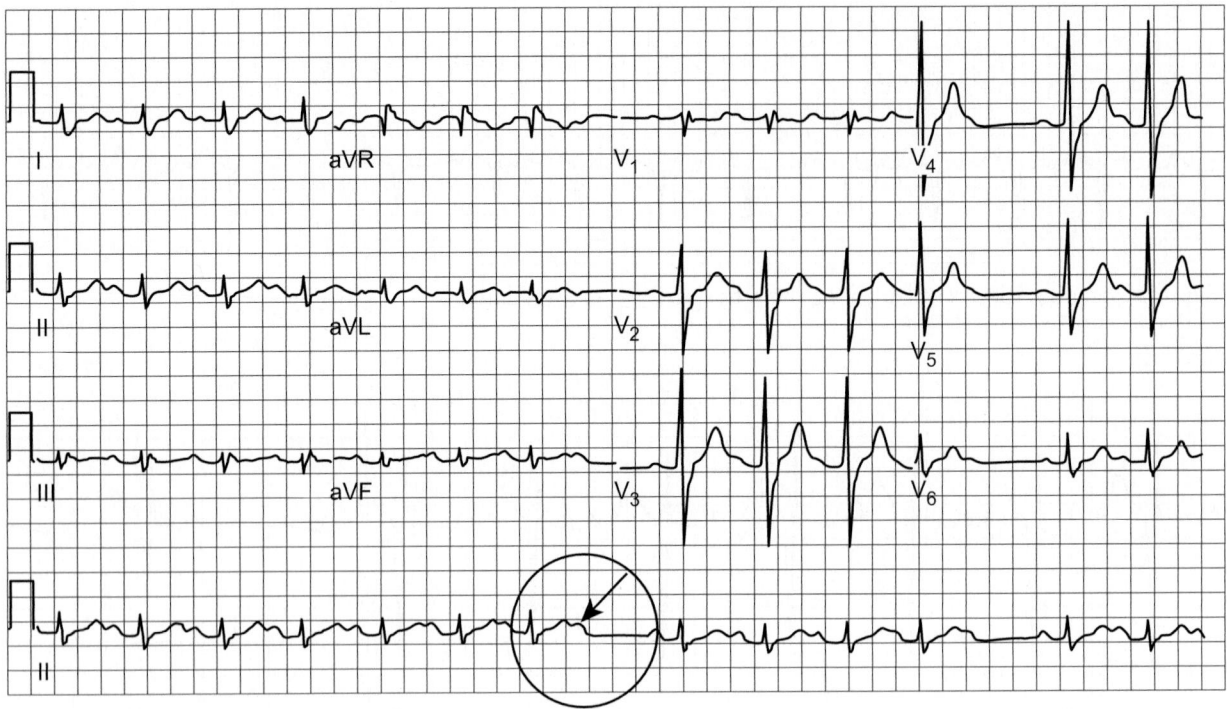

Fig. 14. Sinus rhythm with atrioventricular block, second degree–Mobitz type II, and right bundle branch block. *Arrow* indicates P wave before dropped beat.

is present

f. AV block, variable

- Varying degrees of AV block, including 3:2, 2:1, and 4:1 present on the same ECG
- Consider this in atrial flutter with variable RR intervals (flutter wave to R wave) after ruling out third-degree AV block

g. Short PR interval (with sinus rhythm and normal QRS duration)—requires the following:

- Sinus P wave
- PR interval <0.12 second

h. Wolff-Parkinson-White pattern (Fig. 17)— suggested by the following:

- Normal P wave with PR interval <0.12 second (rarely >0.12 second)
- Abnormally wide QRS >0.10 second
- Initial slurring of QRS (delta wave)
- PJ interval is constant and ≤0.26 second

Note: Atrial fibrillation or flutter that has QRS with varying width (generally wide) and rate >200 beats/min suggests Wolff-Parkinson-White syndrome

7.   Intraventricular Conduction Disturbances

a. RBBB, incomplete—RBBB morphology (rSR′), but QRS duration is 0.09-0.11 second
b. RBBB, complete—requires *all* of the following (Fig. 18):

- Prolonged QRS ≥0.12 second
- Secondary R wave (R′) in right precordial leads, usually with R′ > initial R
- Delayed intrinsicoid deflection in right precordial leads >0.05 second
- Wide S wave in I, V_5, and V_6
- Secondary ST-T changes in V_1 through V_3
- Axis as determined by initial 0.06 to 0.08 second of QRS should be normal unless concomitant left anterior fascicular block is present

Note: Consider item **12g**

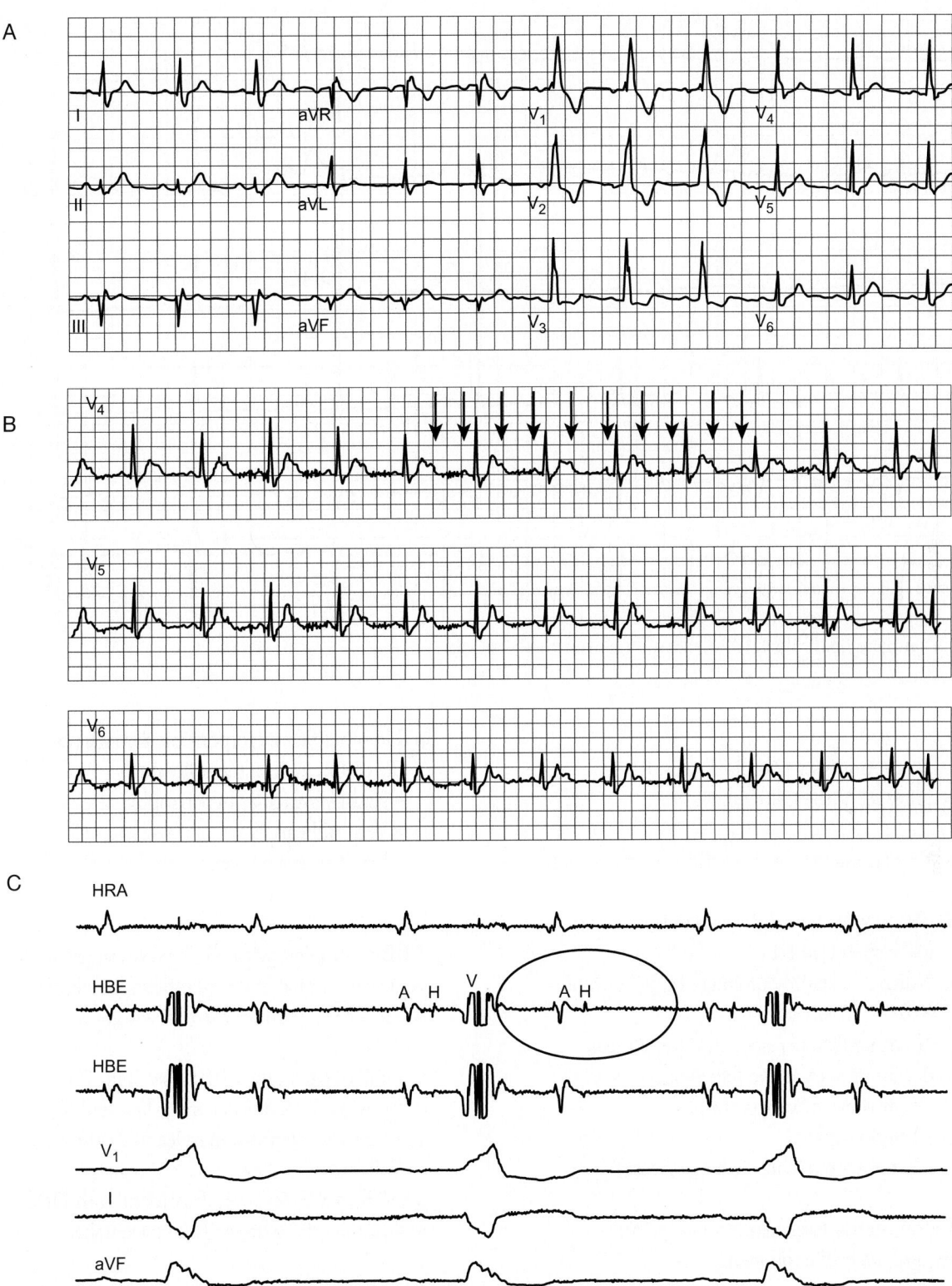

Fig. 15. *A* and *B*, Electrocardiograms (ECGs) in a 59-year-old man. *A*, Resting ECG with right bundle branch block. *B*, Exercise ECG with a 2:1 atrioventricular block. *Arrows* indicate P waves with conduction of every second beat. *C*, His bundle recording. Right bundle branch block and atrioventricular block distal to His. The highlighted complex shows an atrial (A) followed by a His (H) depolarization but no ventricular (V) depolarization. HBE, His bundle electrogram; HRA, high right atrium.

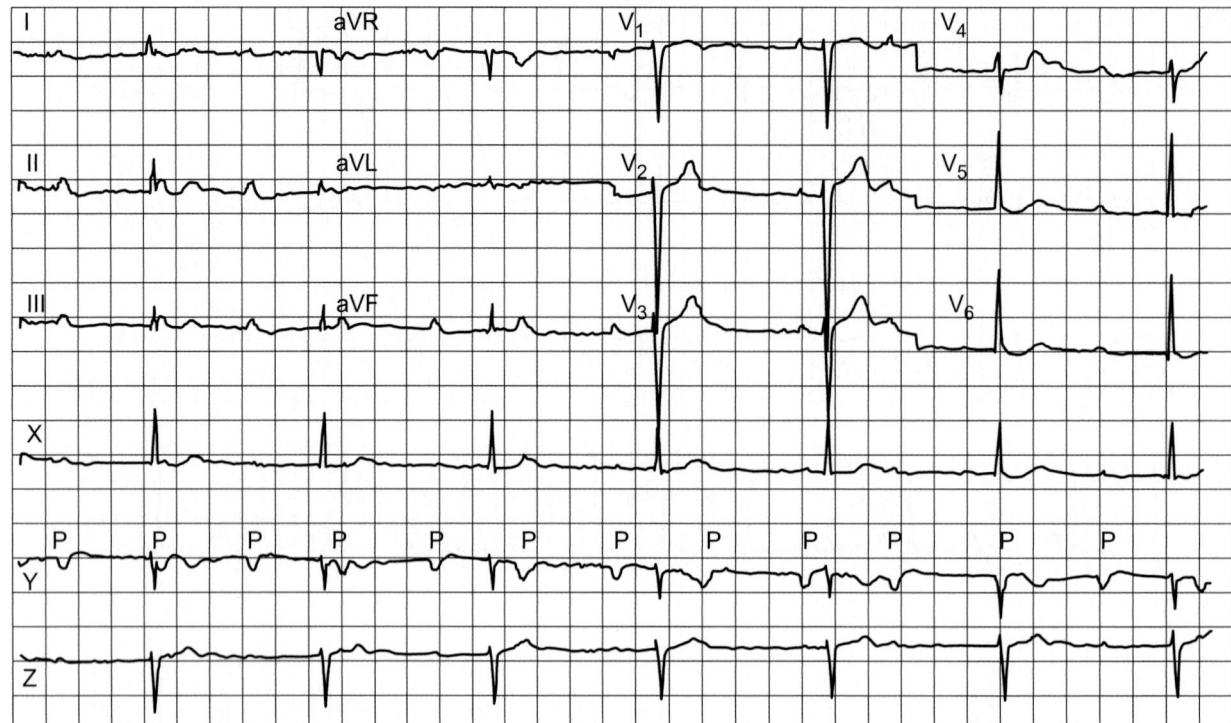

Fig. 16. Complete heart block (third-degree atrioventricular block).

c. Left anterior fascicular block (Fig. 19)—requires *all* of the following:

- Displacement of mean QRS axis to between −45° and −90°
- qR complex (or an R wave) in leads I and aVL; rS in lead III
- Normal or slightly prolonged QRS duration (0.08-0.10 second)
- No other factors responsible for left axis deviation, such as the following:
  - Left ventricular hypertrophy
  - Inferior infarct
  - Emphysema (chronic lung disease)

d. Left posterior fascicular block (Fig. 20)—requires *all* of the following:

- Frontal plane QRS axis of +100° to +180°
- S_1Q_3 pattern (deep S wave in lead I, with Q wave in lead III)
- Normal or slightly prolonged QRS duration (0.08-0.10 second)

- No other factors responsible for right axis deviation, such as the following:
  - Right ventricular hypertrophy
  - Vertical heart
  - Emphysema (chronic lung disease)
  - Lateral wall myocardial infarction

e. LBBB, complete with ST-T waves suggestive of acute myocardial injury or infarction (Fig. 21, 22, and 23)—requires the following:

- Fulfills criteria for LBBB (see item **7f**)
- ≥1 mm ST elevation concordant with QRS
- ≥1 mm ST depression in leads V_1 through V_3
- ≥5 mm ST elevation discordant with QRS
- Criteria valid with artificial pacemaker

f. LBBB, complete—requires *all* of the following:

- Prolonged QRS duration ≥0.12 second
- Delayed intrinsicoid deflection in left precordial leads and lead I >0.05 second
- Broad monophasic R in leads I, V_5, and V_6,

A

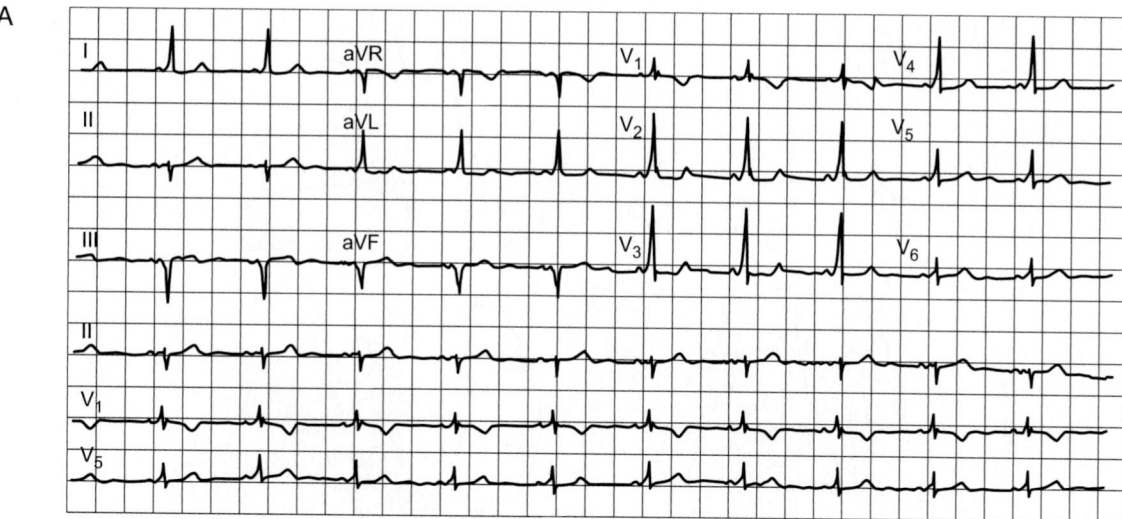

B

Location	V$_1$	aVF	aVL
Left lateral	+	+	-
Left posterior/septal	+	-	+
Right posterior/septal	-	-	+
Right lateral/anterior	-	+	+

Fig. 17. *A*, Wolff-Parkinson-White pattern. *B*, Pathway location in Wolff-Parkinson-White pattern based on the polarity of the delta wave.

which is usually notched or slurred
Note: Also consider items **9c** and **12g**

g. LBBB, intermittent—more common at high rates but also may be bradycardia-dependent

h. Intraventricular conduction disturbance, non-specific type

- QRS >0.11 second, but QRS morphology does not satisfy criteria for either LBBB or RBBB
- May also be used when there is abnormal notching of the QRS complex without prolongation
- May occur with antiarrhythmic drug toxicity,

hyperkalemia, and hypothermia
Note: Also consider items **12g**, **14d**, and **14e**

i. Aberrant intraventricular conduction with supraventricular arrhythmia (specify rhythm)
Note: See item **4f** for criteria of supraventricular vs. ventricular tachycardia

8.   P-Wave Abnormalities

a. Right atrial abnormality

- Amplitude >2.5 mm in leads II, III, or aVF with a normal P-wave duration (P pulmonale), *or*
- Positive amplitude >1.5 mm in V$_1$ or V$_2$, *or*

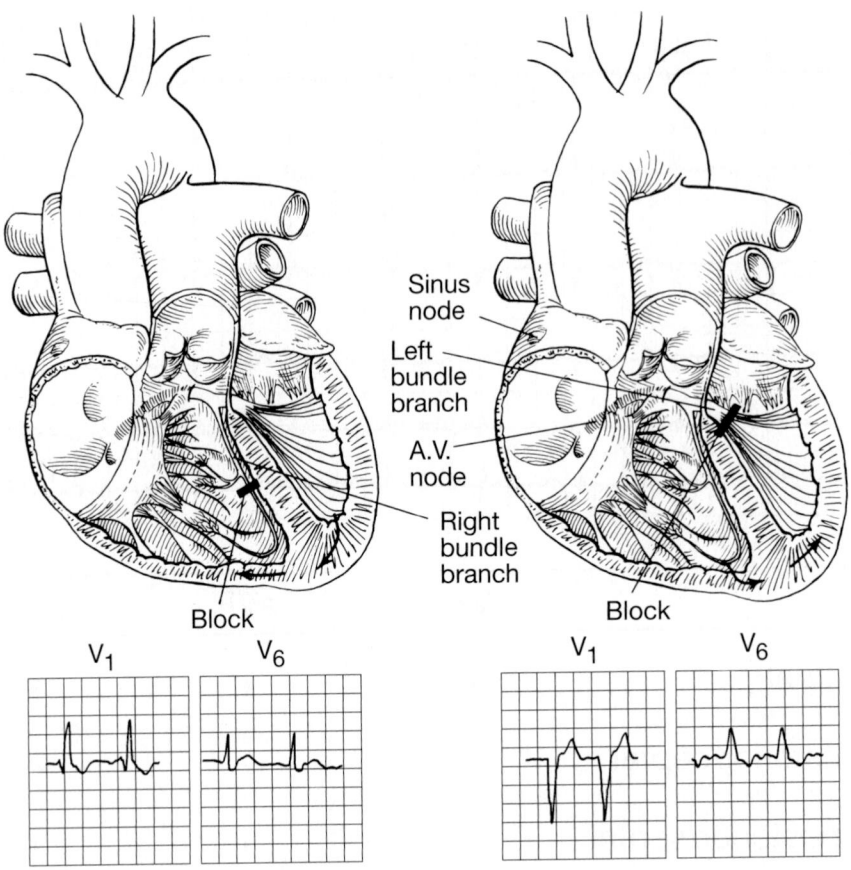

Fig. 18. Drawings of heart show location of right bundle branch block with the characteristic V₁ and V₆, scalar electrocardiographic (ECG) changes with RSR and terminal sagging of S wave (*left*) and left bundle branch block with the characteristic scalar ECG changes in V₁ and V₆, deep S waves, and broad, notched wide QRS (*right*). A.V., atrioventricular.

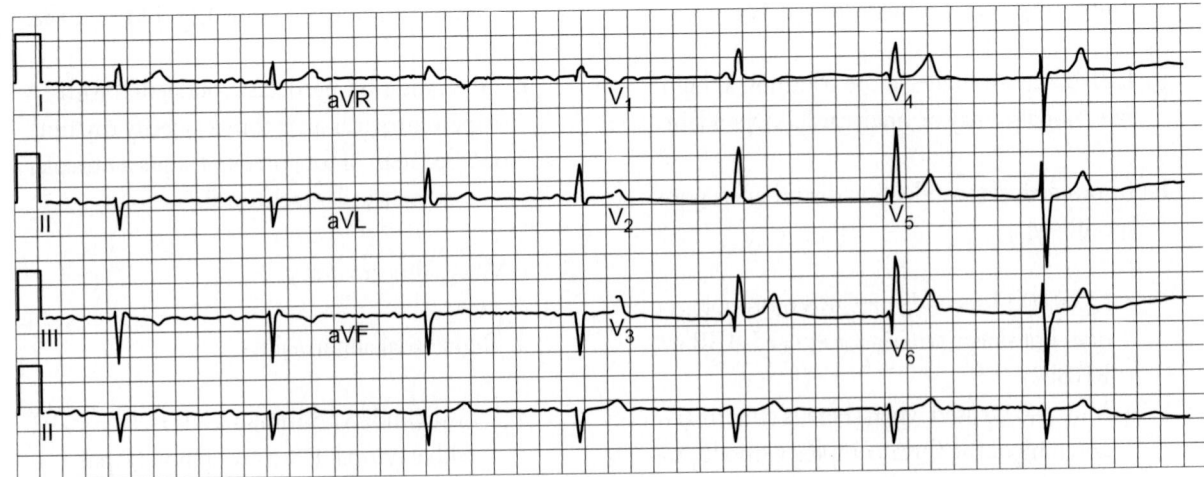

Fig. 19. Complete heart block with right bundle branch block and left anterior fascicular block.

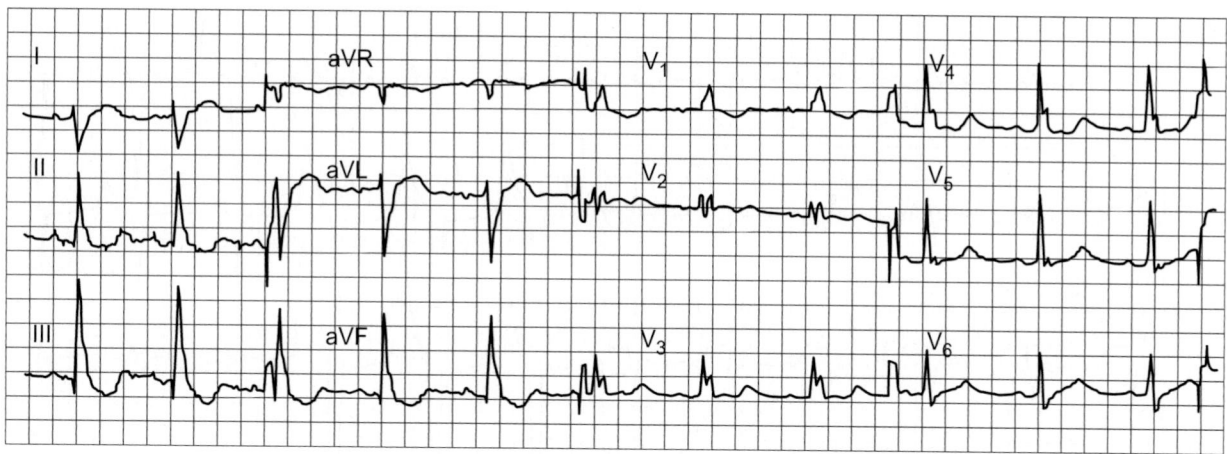

Fig. 20. Left posterior fascicular block and right bundle branch block in a 68-year-old man.

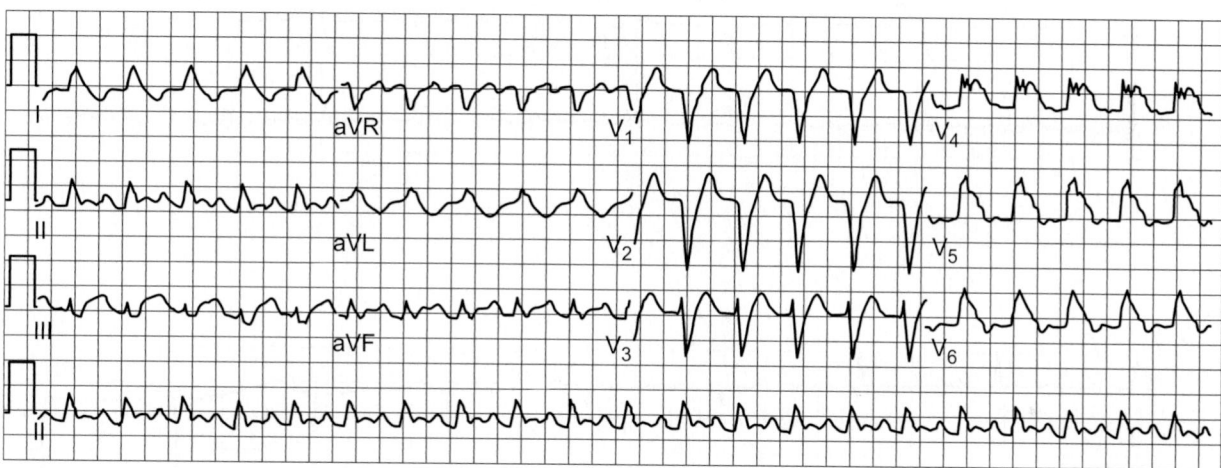

Fig. 21. Left bundle branch block with ST changes of acute anterior injury in a 76-year-old woman presenting with severe dyspnea.

- P-wave frontal axis ≥70° (rightward axis)

b. Left atrial abnormality

- Notched P wave with a duration ≥0.12 second in leads II, III, or aVF (P mitrale), *or*
- Downward terminal deflection of P wave in V_1 with a negative amplitude of 1 mm and with duration of 0.04 second (Fig. 24)

Biatrial enlargement suggested by any of the following:

- Large biphasic P wave in V_1 with initial

positive component of 1.5 mm and the P terminal force with a negative amplitude of 1 mm and a duration of 0.04 second

- Tall, peaked P waves (>1.5 mm) in right precordial leads (V_1 through V_3) and wide, notched P waves in left precordial leads (V_5 and V_6)
- P-wave amplitude ≥2.5 mm and duration ≥0.12 second in limb leads

c. Nonspecific atrial abnormality

- Abnormal P-wave morphology but not fulfilling criteria for right or left atrial enlargement

A

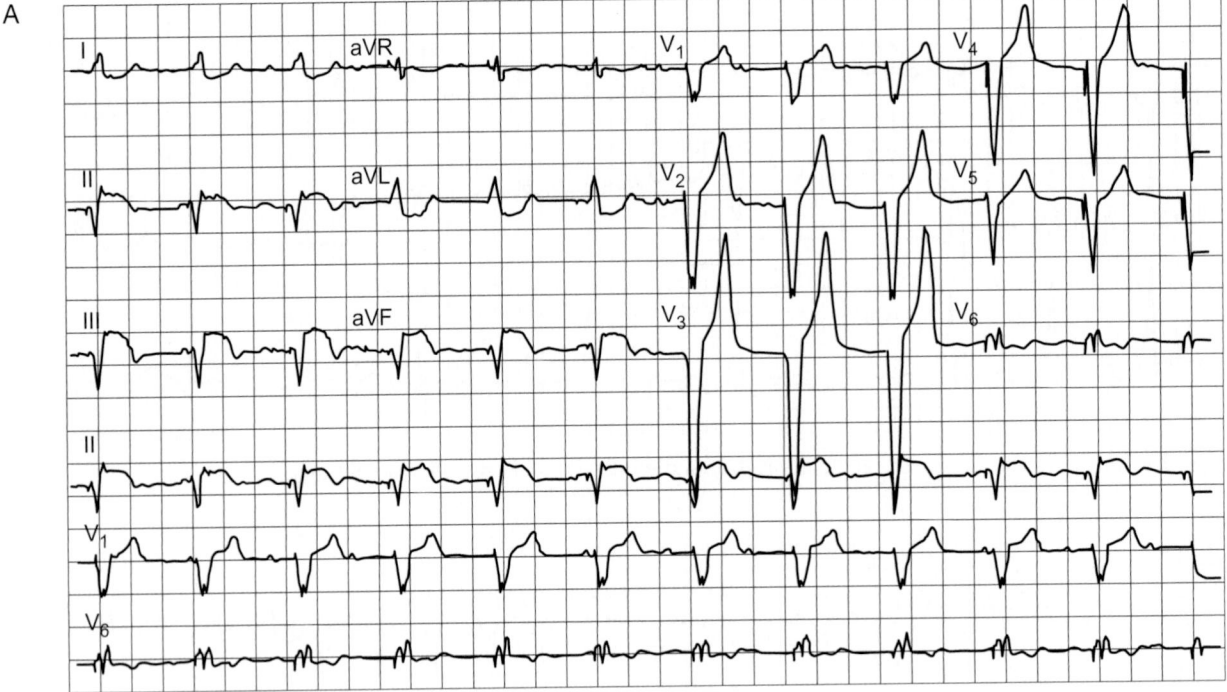

B

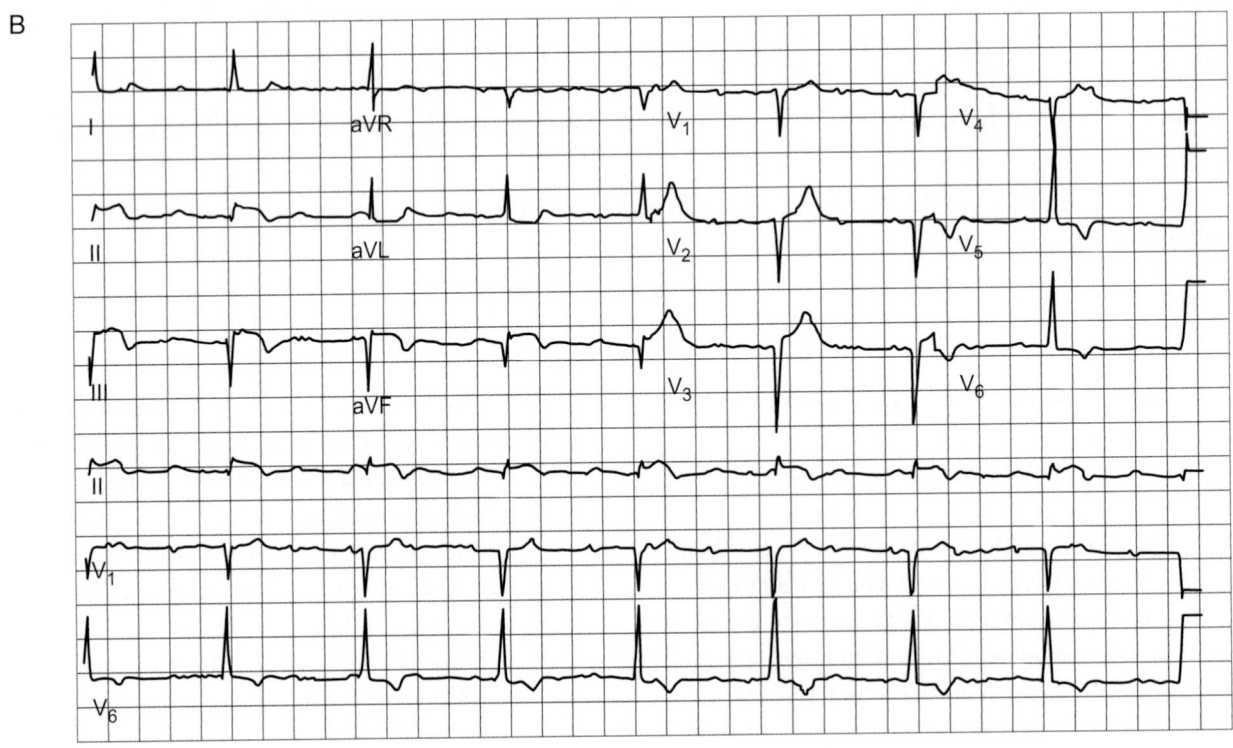

Fig. 22. *A,* Findings in a 78-year-old man presenting with severe chest pain, permanent ventricular pacemaker, and inferior ST elevation. *B,* Acute inferior myocardial infarction with complete heart block; pacemaker is off.

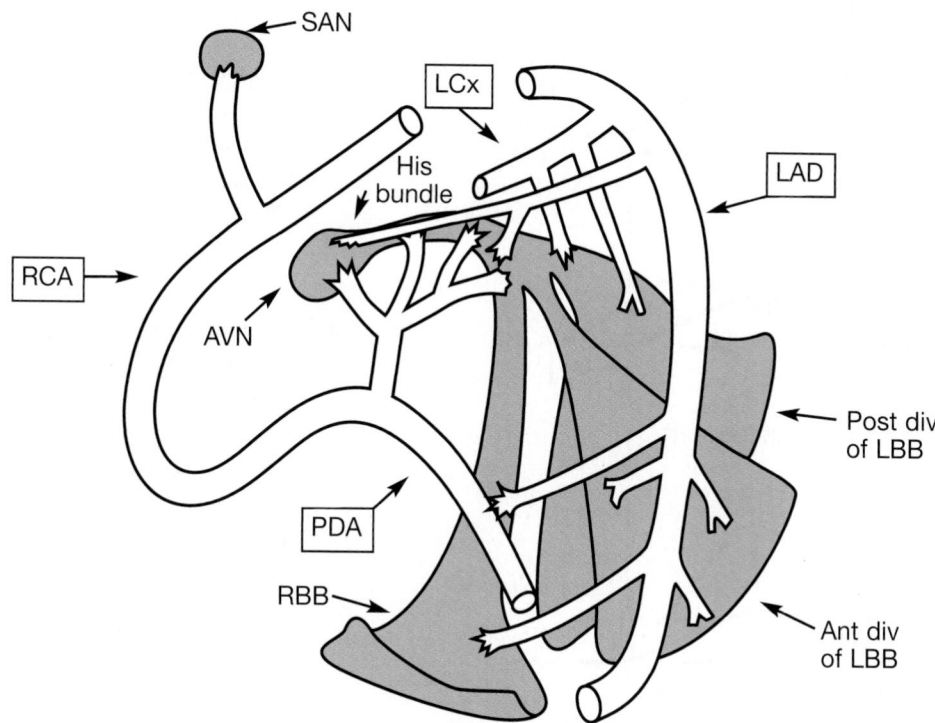

Fig. 23. Diagram of the conduction system and its blood supply. Ant div, anterior division; AVN, atrioventricular node; LAD, left anterior descending coronary artery; LBB, left bundle branch; LCx, left circumflex coronary artery; PDA, posterior descending branch of right coronary artery; Post div, posterior division; RBB, right bundle branch; RCA, right coronary artery; SAN, sinoatrial node.

9. Abnormalities of QRS Voltage or Axis

   a. Low voltage, limb leads only

      ■ Amplitude of the entire QRS complex (R + S) is <5 mm in all limb leads
      Note: Consider items **14m**, **14o**, and **14t**

   b. Low voltage, limb and precordial leads
      ■ Amplitude of the entire QRS complex (R + S) is <10 mm in each precordial lead
      ■ Amplitude of R + S in limb leads is <5 mm
      ■ Low voltage can also occur with obesity, pleural effusion, restrictive or infiltrative cardiomyopathies, and diffuse myocardial dis-ease
      Note: Consider items **14m**, **14o**, and **14t**

   c. Left axis deviation (>−30°)

      ■ Axis −30° to −90°
      ■ Be careful about diagnosing left axis deviation in the presence of an inferior infarct
      Note: Consider item **7c**

   d. Right axis deviation (>+100°)

      ■ Axis +101° to +270°
      ■ Pure right axis deviation (left posterior fascicular block) should have an S_1Q_3 pattern
      ■ Causes include the following:
        - Right ventricular hypertrophy (especially if axis >+100°); consider item **10c**
        - Vertical heart
        - Chronic lung disease; consider item **14m**
        - Pulmonary embolus; consider item **14n**
        - Left posterior fascicular block; consider item **7d**

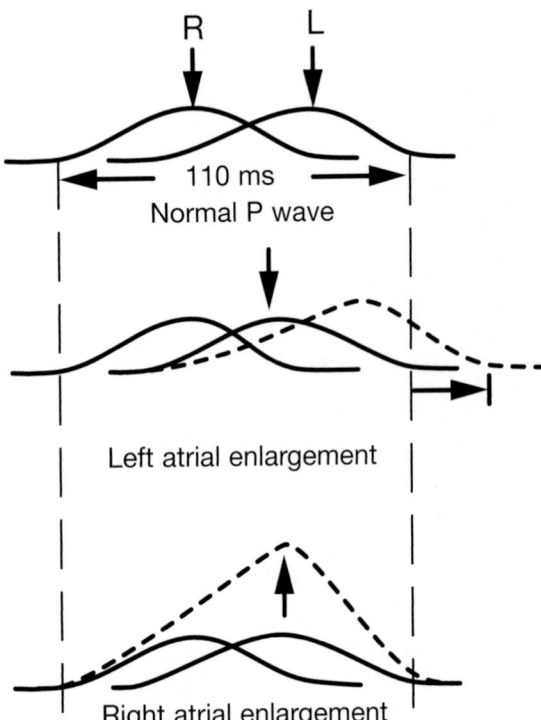

Fig. 24. *Top*, Normal surface P-wave morphology, illustrating right and left atrial activation sequence and normal duration. *Middle*, Left atrial enlargement (*broken line*), illustrating delayed peak and left atrial activation time, producing a prolonged P-wave duration and notched P-wave morphology. *Bottom*, Right atrial enlargement (*broken line*), illustrating effective combined right and left atrial voltage peaks occurring at the same time with resulting tall peaked P waves.

e. Electrical alternans (Fig. 25)

- Alternation of amplitude of the P, QRS, or T waves
- Causes include the following:
  - Pericardial effusion causes only a third of cases. But if electrical alternans involves the P wave, QRS complex, and T wave, significant effusion is usually present; 12% of simple pericardial effusions have electrical alternans.
  - Severe left ventricular failure
  - Hypertension
  - Coronary artery disease
  - Rheumatic heart disease
  - Supraventricular or ventricular tachycardia

10. Ventricular Hypertrophy

a. Left ventricular hypertrophy by voltage only

- Cornell criteria
  - R wave in lead aVL and S wave in lead V_3
  - >28 mm in males
  - >20 mm in females

- Precordial leads
  - The sum of the R wave in lead V_5 or V_6 and the S wave in lead V_1 is >35 mm in adults older than 30 years (40 mm in those 20-30 years old and 60 mm in those 16-20 years old), *or*
  - The sum of the maximal R and the deepest S waves in the precordial leads is >45 mm, *or*
  - The amplitude of the R wave in lead V_5 is >26 mm, *or*
  - The amplitude of the R wave in lead V_6 is >20 mm

- Limb leads
  - The sum of the R wave in lead I and the S wave in lead II is ≥26 mm, *or*
  - The amplitude of the R wave in lead I is ≥14 mm, *or*
  - The amplitude of the S wave in lead aVR is ≥15 mm, *or*
  - The amplitude of the R wave in lead aVF is ≥21 mm, *or*
  - The amplitude of the R wave in lead aVL is ≥12 mm (a highly specific, if insensitive, finding)

b. Left ventricular hypertrophy both by voltage criteria (refer to item **10a**) and by ST-T segment abnormalities, which include the following:

- ST-segment depression in any or all of the following leads: I, aVL, III, aVF, and V_4 through V_6
- Subtle ST elevation in V_1 through V_3
- Inverted T waves I, aVL, and V_4 through V_6
- Prominent or inverted U waves
- Nonvoltage-related criteria for left ventricular

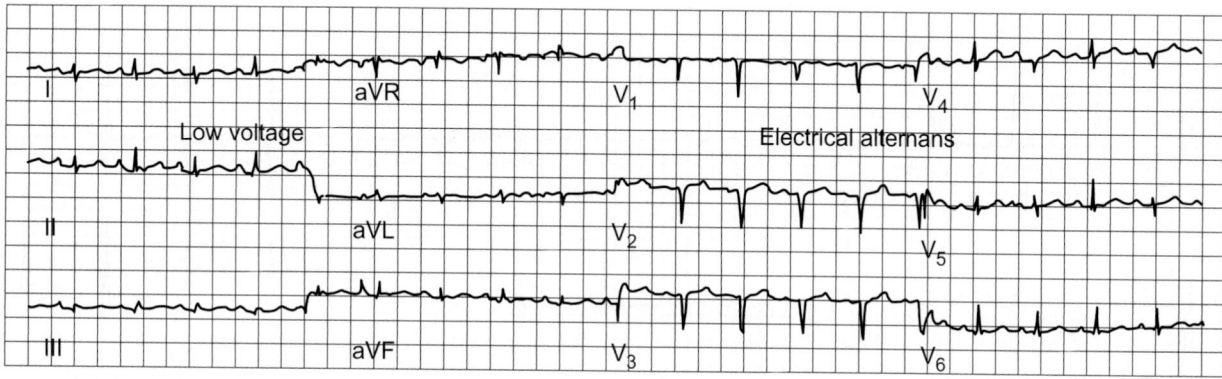

Fig. 25. Electrical alternans in a 51-year-old woman with pericardial tamponade. Note the low QRS voltage in the limb leads and the varying height of the QRS complex on consecutive beats. The RR interval and complex morphology are constant throughout, differentiating electrical alternans from a bigeminal rhythm.

hypertrophy (often with or without prominent voltage and ST-T changes in patients with left ventricular hypertrophy)
- Left atrial abnormality
- Left axis deviation
- Nonspecific intraventricular conduction delay
- Delayed intrinsicoid deflection
- Low or absent R waves in V_1, V_2, or V_3
- Absent Q waves in left precordial leads
- Abnormal Q waves in inferior leads due to left axis deviation
- Prominent U waves

■ Left ventricular hypertrophy should not be diagnosed in the presence of left axis deviation due to left anterior fascicular block when the only criterion for the hypertrophy is in lead aVL (Fig. 26)

c. Right ventricular hypertrophy—suggested by one or more of the following:

■ Right axis deviation ≥+100°
■ R/S ratio in leads V_1 or V_{3R} >1
■ R in V_1 + S in V_5 or V_6 >10.5 mm
■ Right atrial enlargement
■ R wave in V_1 ≥7 mm
■ qR in V_1
■ R/S ratio in V_5 or V_6 ≤1

■ rSR' in V_1 with R' >10 mm
■ Secondary ST-T changes in right precordial leads

To diagnose right ventricular hypertrophy, exclude the following:

■ Posterior wall myocardial infarction
■ Right bundle branch block
■ Wolff-Parkinson-White syndrome (type A)
■ Dextroposition
■ Left posterior fascicular block (lateral wall infarct)
■ Normal variant (especially in children)

Criteria to diagnose right ventricular hypertrophy in the presence of RBBB are the following (Fig. 27):

■ r' ≥15 mm in lead V_1
■ Right axis deviation of initial vector (unblocked forces)

d. Combined ventricular hypertrophy (Fig. 28)—suggested by any of the following:

■ ECG meets one or more diagnostic criteria for both isolated left and right ventricular hypertrophy
■ Precordial leads show left ventricular hyper-

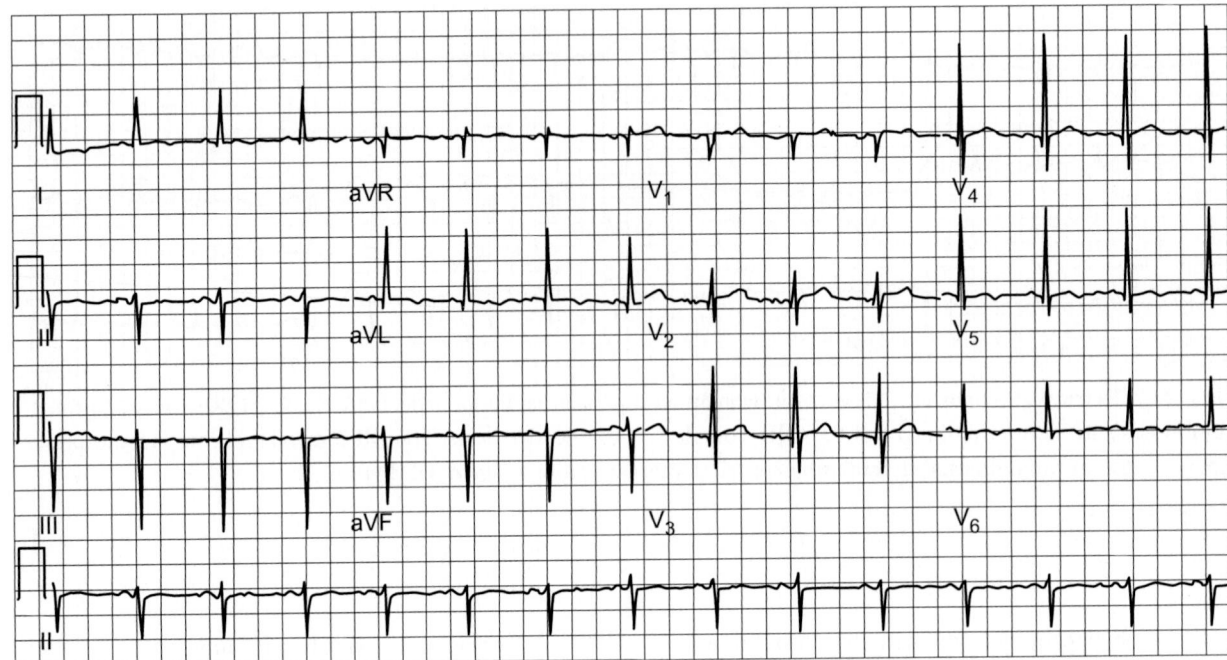

Fig. 26. Left axis deviation with increased voltage in lead aVL but not left ventricular hypertrophy. The left axis deviation is due to left anterior fascicular block.

trophy, but QRS axis in frontal plane >+90°

- R >Q in lead aVR, S >R in V₅, and T inversion in V₁ in conjunction with signs of left ventricular hypertrophy
- Kutz-Wachtel phenomenon—high-voltage equiphasic (R = S) complexes in mid-precordial leads
- Right atrial enlargement with left ventricular hypertrophy pattern in precordial leads

11. Transmural Myocardial Infarction

General considerations include the following:

- Acute myocardial infarction (MI): Q waves and ST elevation with or without reciprocal ST depression
- Recent MI: Q waves, isoelectric ST segments, and ischemic T waves
- Old MI: Q waves, isoelectric ST segments, nonspecific T-wave abnormalities, or normal ST and T waves
- Significant Q waves
  - Duration of Q wave ≥0.04 second

- Amplitude varies according to region of infarct

- ST elevation can persist 48 hours to 4 weeks after MI; >1 month suggests aneurysm
- T-wave inversions may persist indefinitely
- Watch for pseudoinfarctions, such as the following:

Condition	Pseudoinfarct
Wolff-Parkinson-White (Fig. 29)	Inferior, anteroseptal, posterior
Hypertrophic cardiomyopathy	Inferior, posterior, lateral, anteroseptal
LBBB	Anteroseptal, anterior, inferior
Left ventricular hypertrophy (Fig. 30)	Anteroseptal, anterior, inferior, lateral
Left anterior fascicular block	Inferior, anterior, lateral
Chronic lung disease or right ventricular hypertrophy	Inferior, posterior, anteroseptal, anterior

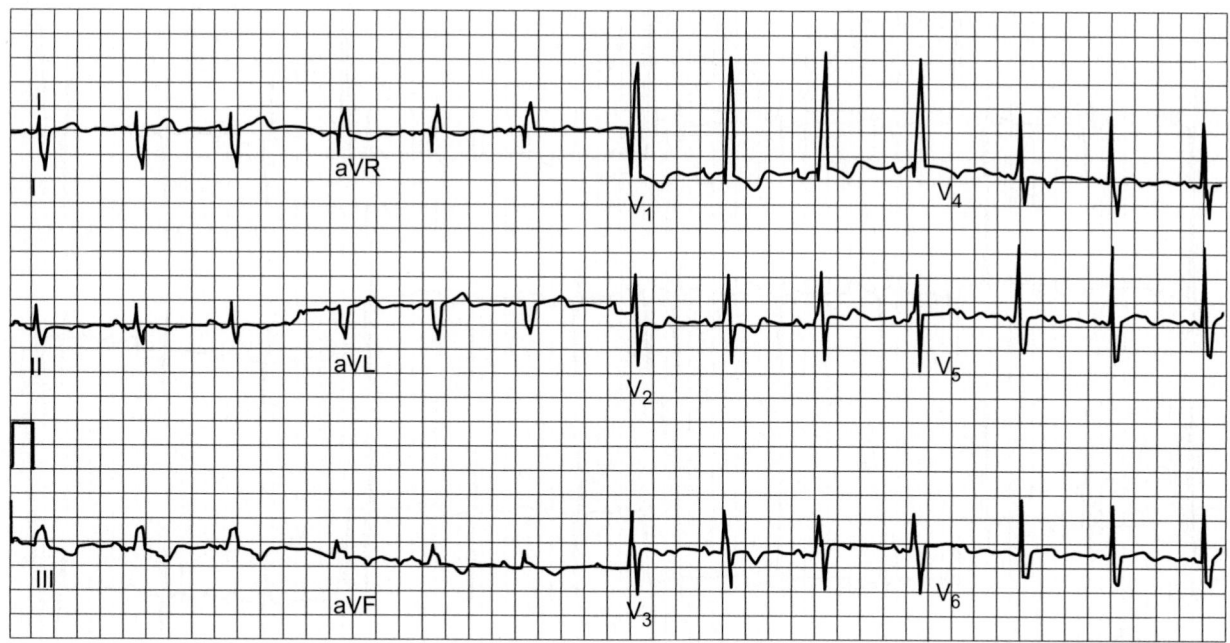

Fig. 27. Right bundle branch block with right ventricular hypertrophy (right axis deviation, r'≥15 mm in lead V_1).

Cardiomyopathy   Any
Chest deformity   Any
Normal variant   Posterior, anteroseptal,
                        anterior, lateral

- A Q wave may be present intermittently in lead aVF in the absence of MI as a result of respiratory effects and low voltage inferiorly (Fig. 31)
- In RBBB, Q-wave criteria apply for all infarcts (Fig. 32)
- It is difficult to diagnose any infarct in the presence of LBBB (Fig. 21 and 22)

a. Anterolateral infarction, probably acute or recent

- Abnormal Q waves in leads V_4, V_5, and V_6
- ST-segment elevation

b. Anterior infarction, probably acute or recent

- rS in V_1 followed by QS or QR in leads V_2 through V_4
- ST-segment elevation

c. Anteroseptal infarction, probably acute or

recent (Fig. 32)

- Q or QS deflection in leads V_1 through V_3 and sometimes in V_4
- Q in V_1 helps distinguish anteroseptal from anterior infarction
- ST-segment elevation

d. Lateral or high lateral infarction, probably acute or recent (Fig. 33)

- Q waves in leads I and aVL
- ST-segment elevation

e. Inferior (diaphragmatic) infarction, probably acute or recent

- Q waves in leads II, III, and aVF
- ST-segment elevation, often with reciprocal ST depression in leads I, aVL, V_1, and V_2

f. Posterior infarction, probably acute or recent (Fig. 34 and 35)

- Initial R wave in leads V_1 or V_2 ≥0.04 second with R ≥S and ST-segment depression and

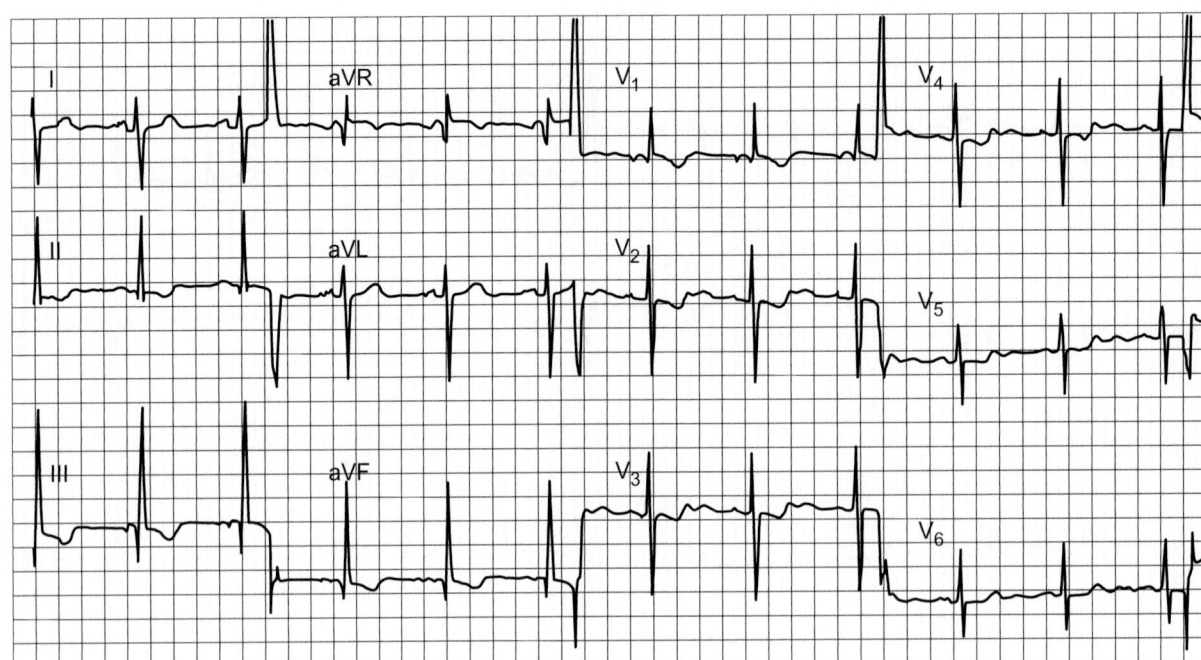

Fig. 28. Combined ventricular hypertrophy: right ventricular hypertrophy (right axis deviation and amplitude of R wave >S wave in lead V_1) and left ventricular hypertrophy (R wave amplitude >21 mm in lead aVF).

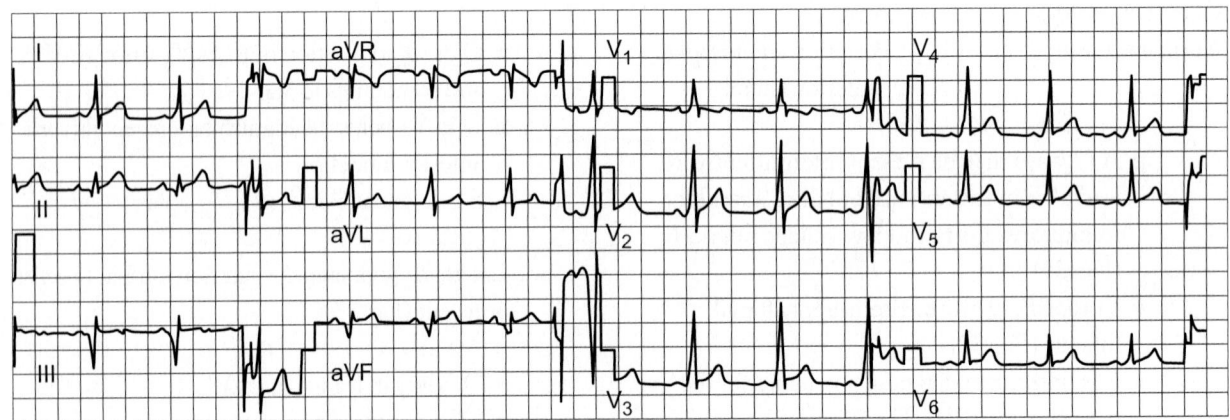

Fig. 29. Pseudo–inferior-posterior myocardial infarction due to Wolff-Parkinson-White pattern.

upright T wave in anterior precordial leads
■ Usually associated with inferior MI

g. Anterolateral infarction, probably old or age indeterminate

■ See above, no ST elevation

h. Anterior infarction, probably old or age indeter-

minate
■ See above, no ST elevation

i. Anteroseptal infarction, probably old or age indeterminate

■ See above, no ST elevation

j. Lateral or high-lateral infarction, probably old

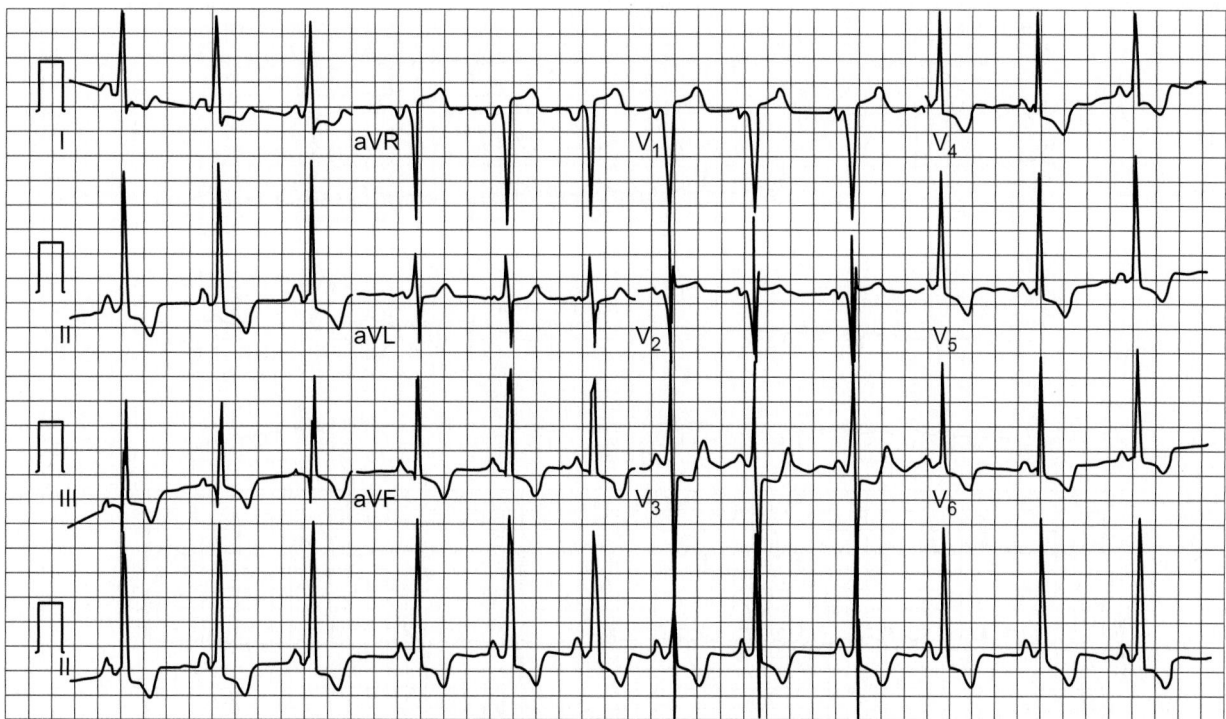

Fig. 30. Left ventricular hypertrophy simulating an anteroseptal myocardial infarction.

or age indeterminate

- See above, no ST elevation

k. Inferior (diaphragmatic) infarction, probably old or age indeterminate

- See above, no ST elevation

l. Posterior infarction, probably old or age indeterminate

- See above, no ST changes

m. Probable ventricular aneurysm

- Persistent ST-segment elevation of ≥1 mm in one or more leads with associated Q waves; timing must be ≥1 month after infarction to make this diagnosis on the basis of the ECG

12. ST-, T-, and U-Wave Abnormalities

a. Normal variant, early repolarization

- Some degree of ST-segment elevation is present in most young, healthy individuals, especially in the precordial leads—suggested by the following:
  - Elevated takeoff of ST segment at J junction with QRS
  - Distinct notch or slur on downstroke of R wave
  - *Upward* concavity of ST segment
  - Symmetrically limbed T waves, which are often of large amplitude
  - Most commonly involves leads V_2 through V_5, rarely V_6

- Sometimes also seen in leads II, III, and aVF
- No reciprocal changes

b. Normal variant, juvenile T waves—suggested by the following:

- Persistence of negative T wave in leads V_1 through V_3
- Most frequent in young, healthy females
- Usually not symmetrical or deep

A

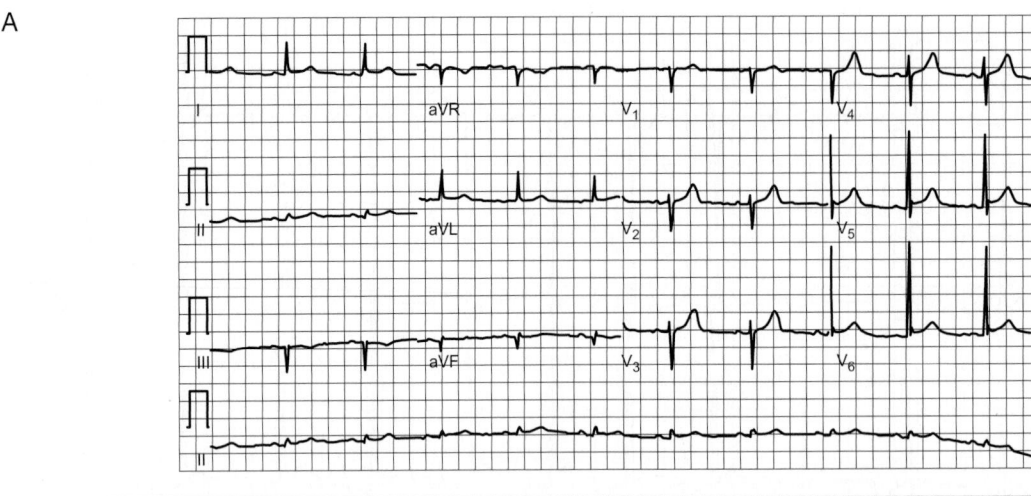

B

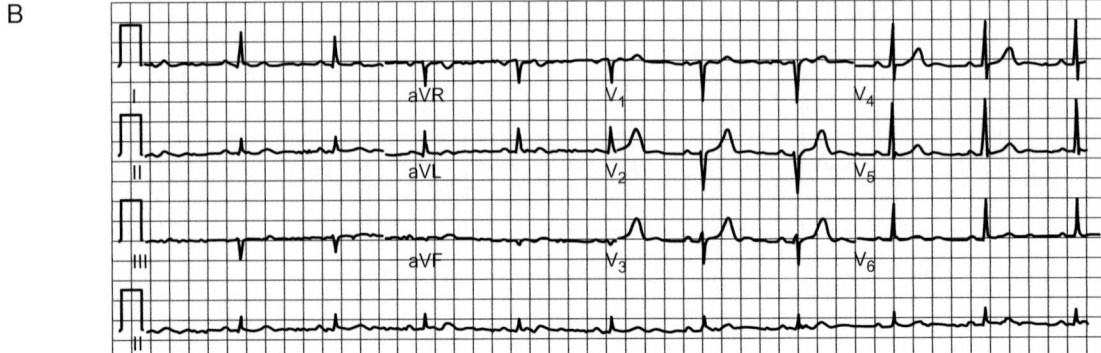

C

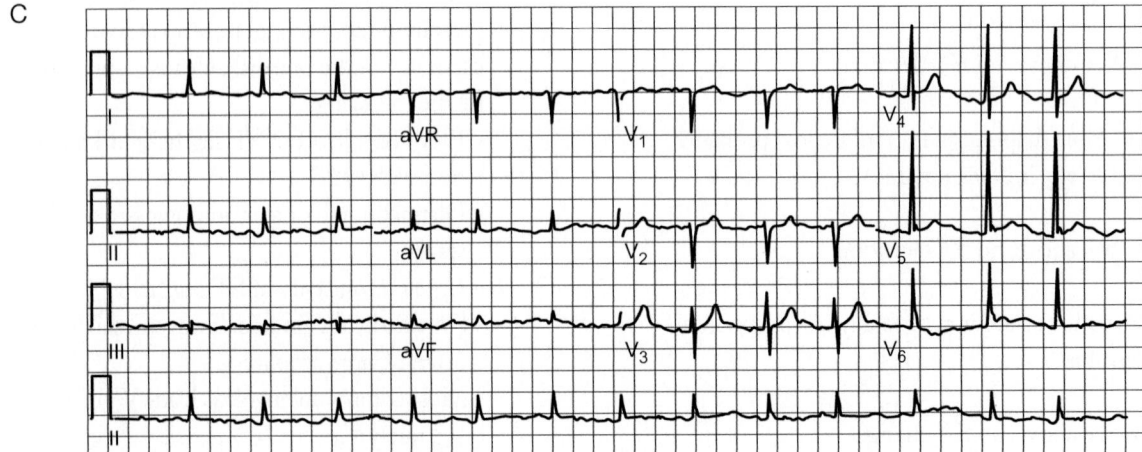

D Q-Wave Inconsistency:
1. Disappearance or reduction of Q waves in aVF on 2 consecutive daily ECGs: present on day 1, absent on day 2

2. Occurred in 33% of 167 patients

3. Due to respiratory effects on axis shift and low-voltage QRS inferiorly

Fig. 31. *A-C*, Electrocardiograms (ECGs) in a 73-year-old man. *A*, Asymptomatic, preoperative ECG on July 9. *B*, Asymptomatic, last prior ECG on January 14, 6 months before noncardiac operation. *C*, Asymptomatic, postoperative ECG on July 10. *D*, Inferior myocardial infarction: Q-wave inconsistency on ECG.

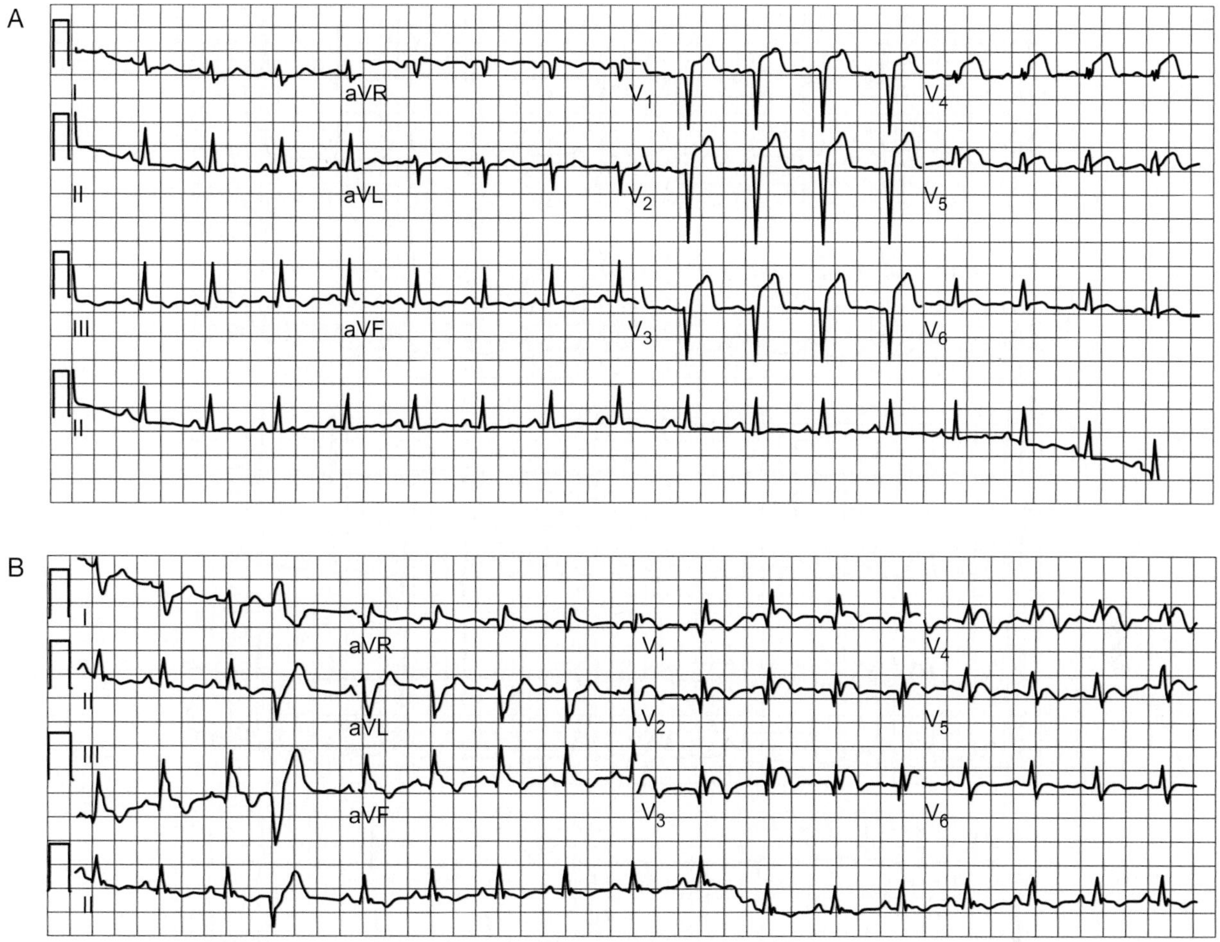

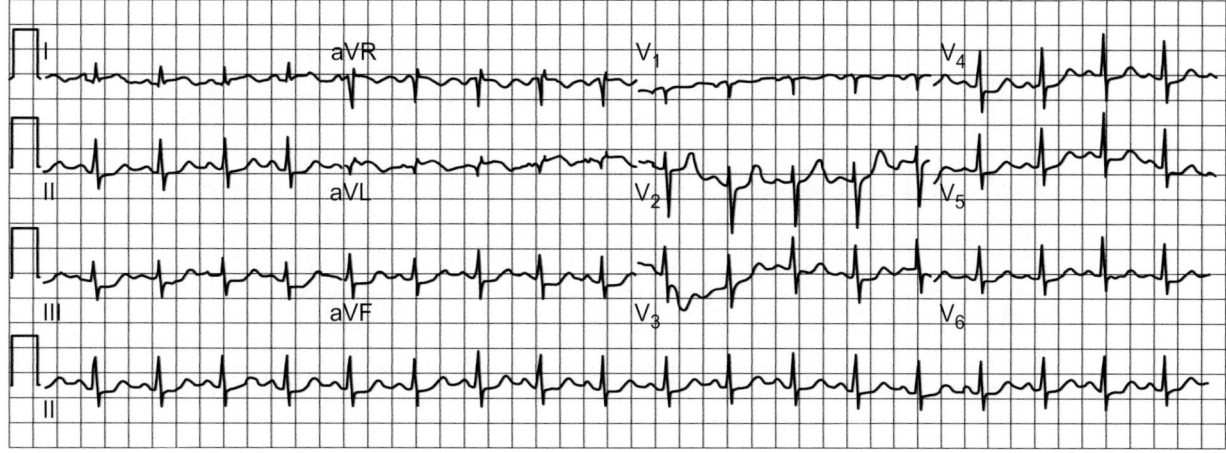

Fig. 32. Electrocardiograms in a 62-year-old man. *A*, Anteroseptal myocardial infarction. *B*, Anteroseptal myocardial infarction in the presence of right bundle branch block.

Fig. 33. Acute high lateral wall myocardial infarction in an 80-year-old woman which was interpreted as normal by a computer electrocardiographic reading program.

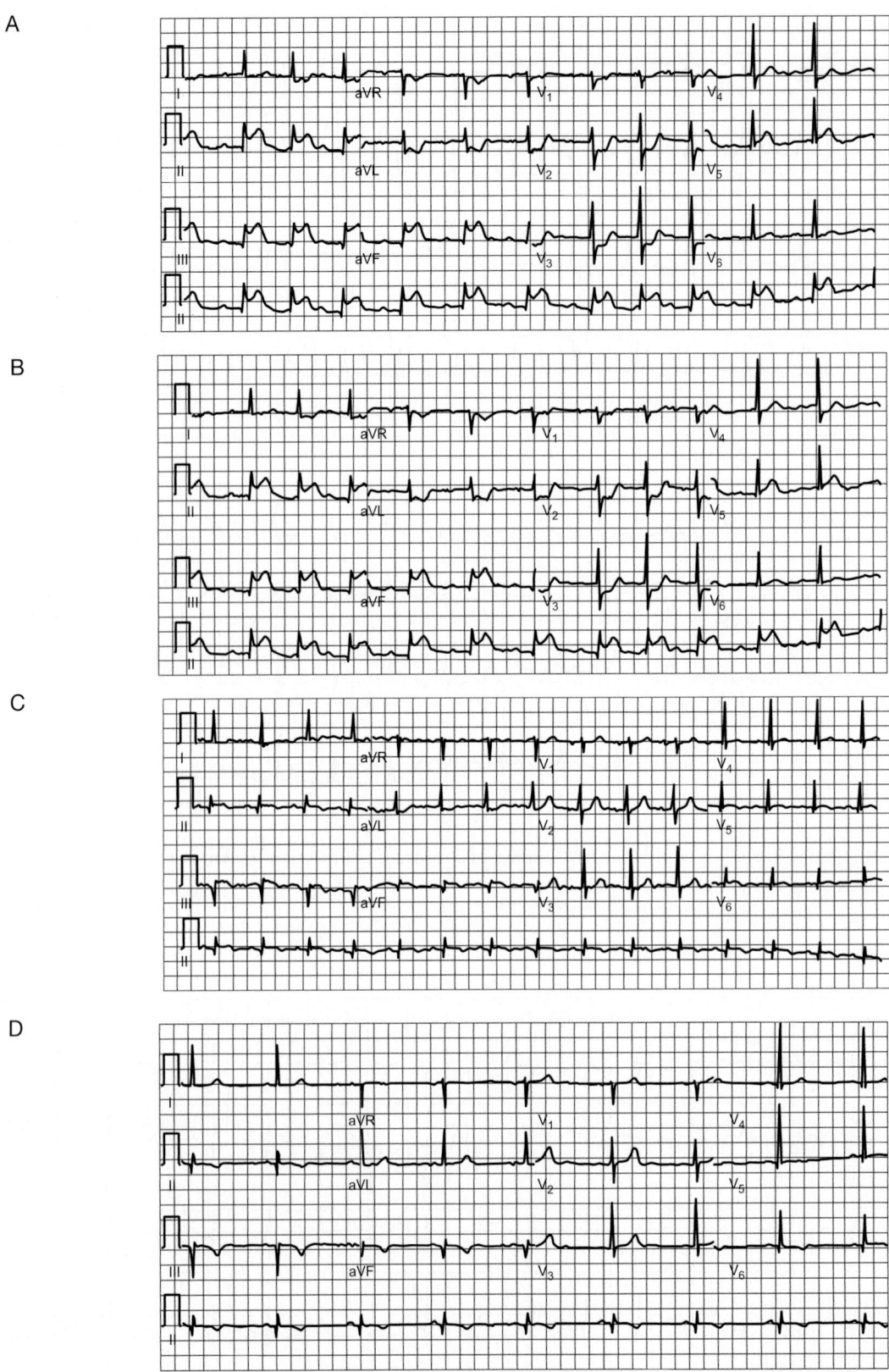

Fig. 34. Electrocardiograms in a 71-year-old man. *A*, With severe chest pain. *B*, Acute inferior-posterior myocardial infarction. ST changes in leads V_1 through V_3 represent posterior injury. *C*, Evolving inferior-posterior myocardial infarction 1 day after presentation. *D*, Inferior-posterior infarction 6 months after presentation.

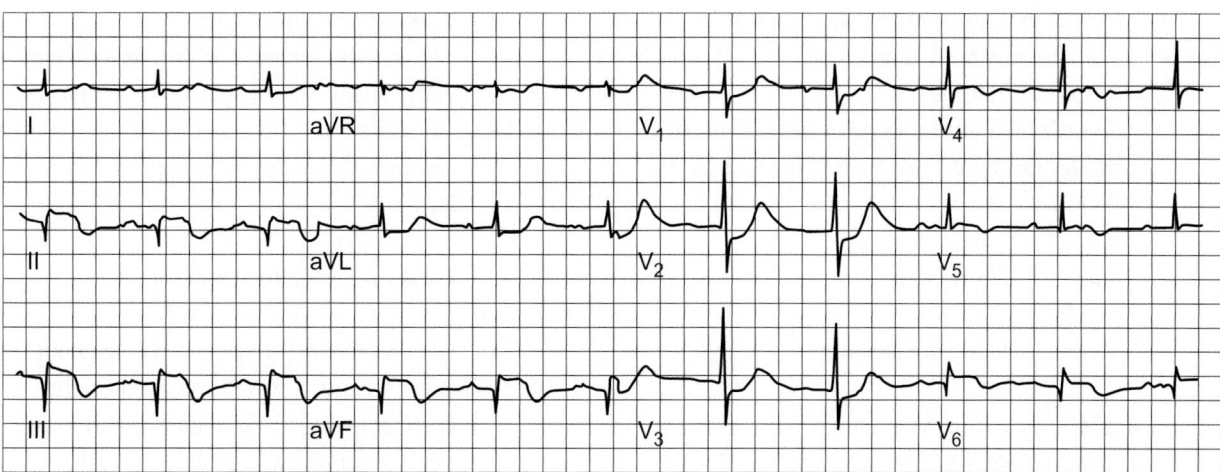

Fig. 35. Acute inferior-posterior-lateral myocardial infarction.

■ T waves still upright in left precordial leads I
and II

c. Nonspecific ST- or T-wave abnormalities—
suggested by any of the following:

■ Slight ST-segment depression or elevation
■ T wave flat, low, or slightly inverted; T wave
normally should be ≥0.5 mm in leads I and
II

d. ST- or T-wave abnormalities suggesting
myocardial ischemia—ischemic T-wave
changes:

■ Abnormally tall, symmetrical, upright T
waves; QT usually prolonged, and there may
be reciprocal changes
Differential diagnosis:
- Hyperkalemia—tall, peaked (tented), sym-
metrical (QT normal or short)
- Intracranial bleeding—QT long, prominent
U waves
- Normal variant

■ Symmetrically or deeply inverted T waves
Differential diagnosis:
- Giant T inversion from Stokes-Adams
attack
- Post-tachycardia T-wave inversion
- Apical hypertrophic cardiomyopathy

- Post-extrasystolic or pacemaker T-wave
inversion
- Central nervous system disease (e.g.,
intracranial hemorrhage)

■ Pseudonormalization of T waves during
exercise

Ischemic ST-segment changes:

■ Horizontal or downsloping ST-segment
depression with or without T-wave inversion
■ Prinzmetal angina typically manifests as ST-
segment elevation without Q waves

e. ST- or T-wave abnormalities suggesting
myocardial injury

■ Acute ST-segment elevation with upward
convexity in the leads representing the area of
infarction
■ Reciprocal ST-segment depression in the
opposite leads
■ Acute posterior injury often has horizontal or
downsloping ST-segment depression with
upright T waves in leads V$_1$ through V$_3$, with
or without a prominent R wave in these same
leads

f. ST- or T-wave abnormalities suggesting acute
pericarditis (Fig. 36)—four stages:

Stage 1: ST-segment elevation (upwardly concave) in almost all leads except aVR; no reciprocal changes

Stage 2: ST junction (J point) returns to the baseline and the T-wave amplitude begins to decrease

Stage 3: T waves are inverted

Stage 4: ECG resolution

Other clues include the following:

- PR-segment depression early
- Low-voltage QRS with pericardial effusion (consider item **14o**)
- Electrical alternans (consider items **9e** and **14o**)
- Sinus tachycardia
- Regional pericarditis after acute MI (Fig. 37 and 38)
  - T waves normally invert by 48 hours and slowly return to normal over several days to weeks
  - Abnormal T-wave evolution due to regional pericarditis is characterized by either persistently positive T waves or early reversal of normal T-wave inversion

Note: Also consider item **14p**

g. ST-segment or T-wave abnormalities due to intraventricular conduction disturbance or hypertrophy

- *Left ventricular hypertrophy*
  - ST-segment depression with upward convexity and T-wave inversion in left precordial leads
  - Reciprocal changes in right precordial leads
  - In limb leads, ST- and T-wave vectors are usually opposite the QRS vector

- *Right ventricular hypertrophy:* ST-segment depression and T-wave inversion in right precordial leads (V_1 through V_3) and sometimes in inferior leads (II, III, and aVF)
- *LBBB:* ST-segment and T-wave displacement are opposite the main QRS deflection
- *RBBB*
  - Uncomplicated RBBB has little ST displacement
  - T-wave vector is opposite terminal slowed portion of QRS: upright in leads I, V_5, and V_6 and inverted in right precordial leads

h. Post-extrasystolic T-wave abnormality—any alteration in contour, amplitude, or direction of T wave in sinus beat(s) after ectopic beat(s)

i. Isolated J-point depression

- Most frequent in exercise testing
- In normals, ST segment should be within 1 mm of the isoelectric line by 0.08 second

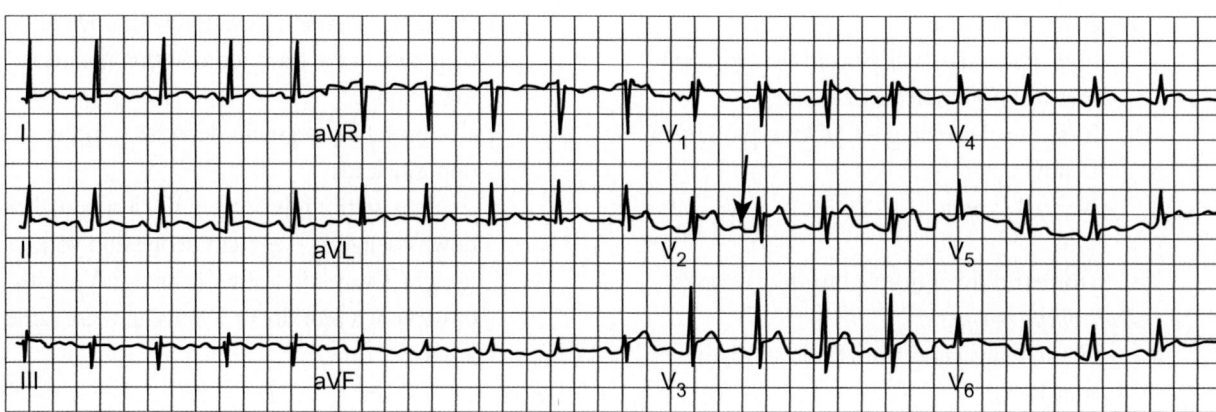

Fig. 36. Acute pericarditis with PR-segment depression (*arrow*).

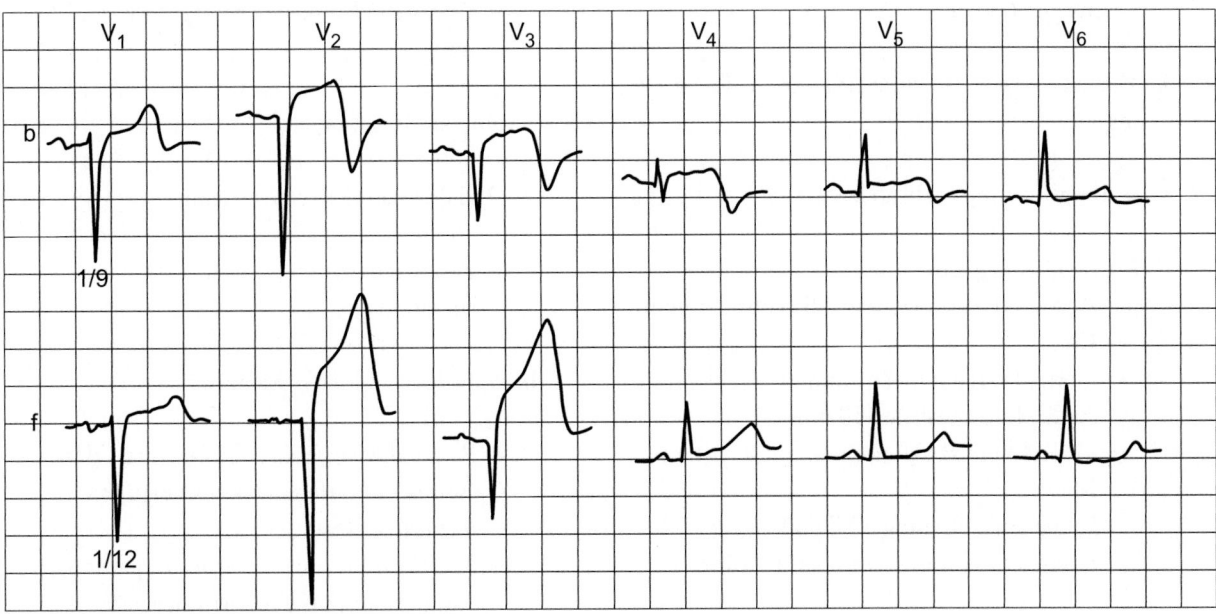

Fig. 37. Regional pericarditis after acute myocardial infarction. b, acute infarction; f, persistent ST elevation V_2-V_4.

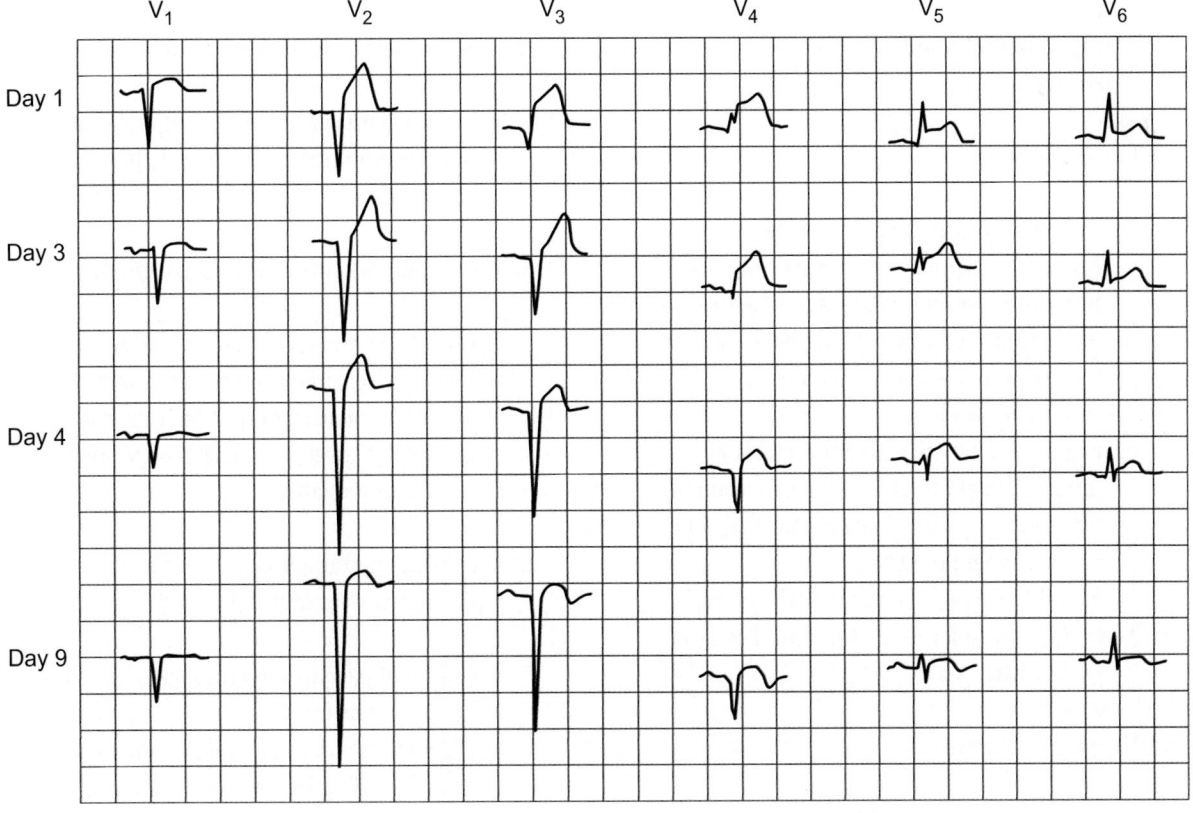

Fig. 38. Persistently positive T waves (leads V_2 through V_6) due to regional pericarditis after acute myocardial infarction.

after the J point

j. Peaked T waves—require either of the following:

■ T wave >6 mm in limb leads
■ T wave >10 mm in precordial leads
Differential diagnosis:
  - Acute MI. Also see item **12k**; consider item **12e**
  - Normal variant; most commonly mid-precordial leads; may be >10 mm
  - Hyperkalemia; QT normal; consider item **14e**
  - Intracranial bleeding; QT prolonged; prominent U waves; consider item **14r**

k. Prolonged QT interval (Fig. 39)

■ QT interval varies inversely with heart rate
■ Measure lead with a large T wave and distinct termination
■ Corrected QT interval = QTc = QT ÷ the square root of the RR interval (normal, <0.44 second in males and <0.46 second in females)

Easier methods:
  - Use 0.40 second as the normal QT interval for heart rate of 70 beats/min. For every 10-beats/min change in heart rate from 70 beats/min, adjust by 0.02 second appropriately. Measured value should be within 0.07 second of the calculated normal. (Example: For a heart rate of 100 beats/min, the calculated "normal" QT interval would be 0.34; for a heart rate of 50 beats/min, the calculated "normal" QT interval would be 0.44.)
  - Should be less than half the RR interval
Note: Also consider items **14c, 14d, 14h, 14s,** and **14u**

l. Prominent U waves

■ Largest in leads V_2 and V_3
■ Normally 5%-25% of T wave

■ Considered large when amplitude is ≥1.5 mm

13. Pacemaker Function and Rhythm

a. Atrial or coronary sinus pacing

■ Pacemaker stimulus followed by atrial depolarization

b. Ventricular demand pacing

■ Pacemaker stimulus followed by a QRS complex of different morphology than intrinsic QRS
■ Must demonstrate *inhibition* of pacemaker output in response to intrinsic QRS

c. AV sequential pacing

■ Atrial followed by ventricular pacing
■ Could be DVI, DDD, DDI, or DOO pacing mode

d. Ventricular pacing, fixed rate (asynchronous)

■ Ventricular pacing with no demonstrable output inhibition by intrinsic QRS complexes

e. Dual-chamber, atrial-sensing pacemaker

■ DDD and possibly VAT or VDD
■ For atrial sensing, need to demonstrate inhibition of atrial output or triggering of ventricular stimulus in response to intrinsic atrial depolarization

f. Pacemaker malfunction, not constantly capturing (atrium or ventricle) (Fig. 40)

■ Failure of pacemaker stimulus to be followed by depolarization
■ Rule out pseudomalfunction (e.g., pacer stimulus falling into refractory period)

g. Pacemaker malfunction, not constantly sensing

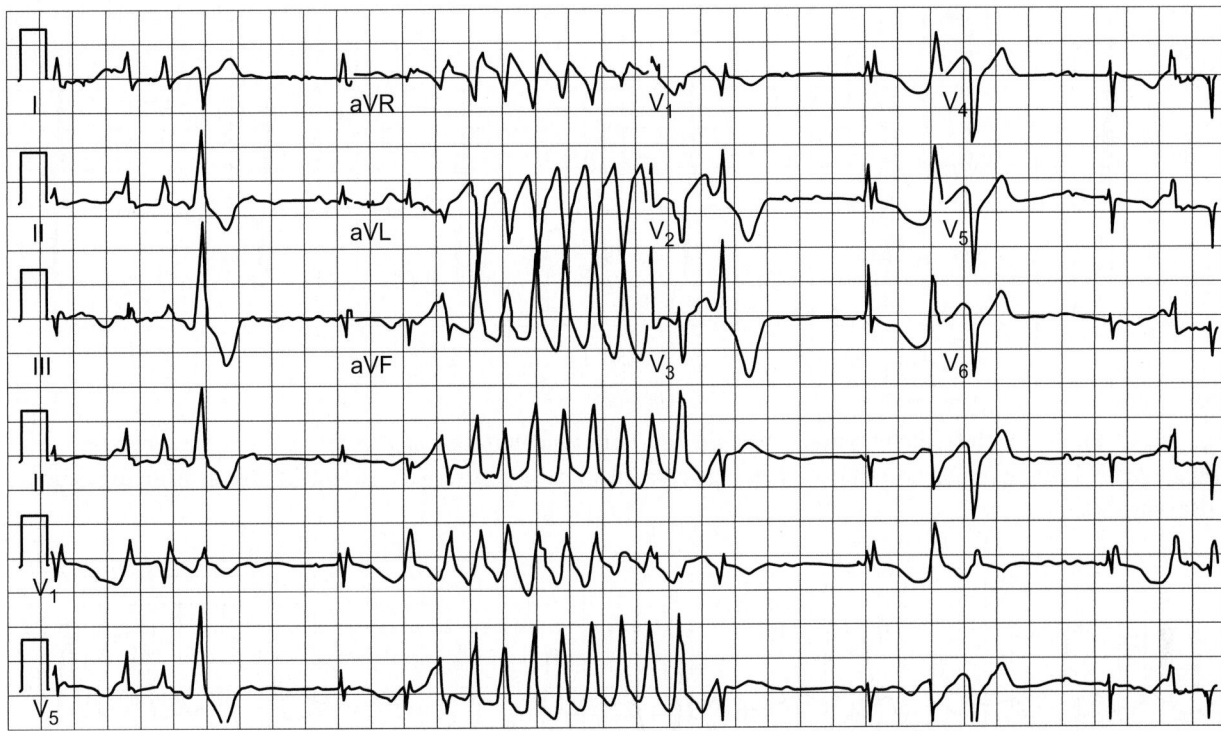

Fig. 39. Complete heart block, right bundle branch block, QT prolongation, and polymorphic ventricular tachycardia in a 76-year-old woman with acute myocardial infarction.

(atrium or ventricle) (Fig. 41)

- For pacemakers in inhibited mode, it is fail ure of pacemaker to be inhibited by an appro-priate intrinsic depolarization
- For pacemakers in triggered mode, it is failure of pacemaker to be triggered by an appropri-ate intrinsic depolarization
- Watch for pseudomalfunction

Premature depolarizations may not be sensed if the following are true:
  - They fall within the programmed refractory period of the pacemaker
  - They have insufficient amplitude at the sensing electrode site
Note: Any stimulus falling within the QRS complex probably does not represent sensing malfunction. Common with right ventricular electrodes in RBBB

h. Pacemaker malfunction, not firing (Fig. 42)
  - Failure of appropriate pacemaker output

i. Pacemaker malfunction, slowing

- An increase in stimulus intervals over the programmed intervals
- Usually an indicator of end of battery life
- Often noted first during magnet application

14. Suggested or Probable Clinical Disorders

a. Digitalis effect—suggested by the following:

- Sagging ST-segment depression with upward concavity
- Decreased T-wave amplitude; T wave may be biphasic
- QT shortening
- Increased U-wave amplitude
- Lengthened PR interval

In left or right ventricular hypertrophy or bun-dle branch block, ST changes are difficult to interpret, but if typical sagging ST segments are present and QT is shortened, consider dig-

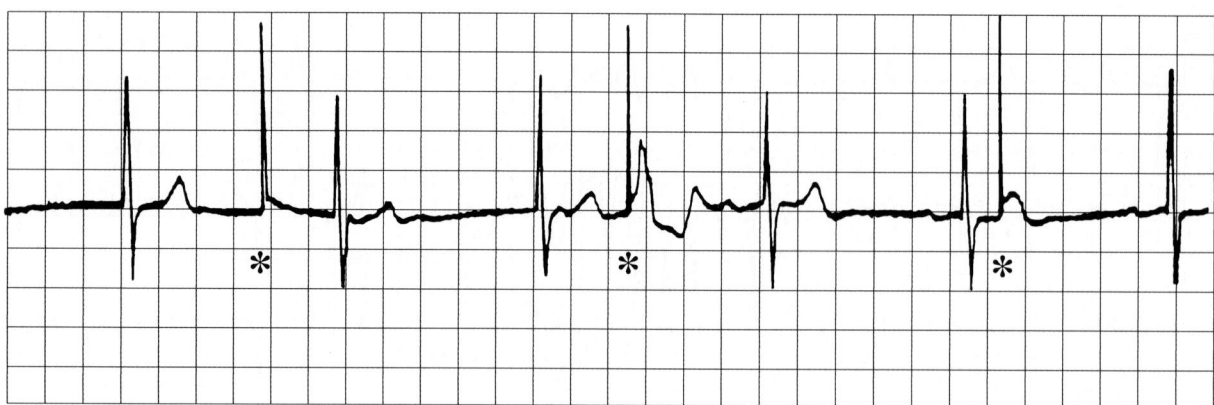

Fig. 40. VVI pacing with failure to capture (*first asterisk*), normal capture (*second asterisk*), and functional noncapture (*third asterisk*) because pacing artifact occurs during ventricular refractoriness. The pacemaker fails to sense the native QRS complexes.

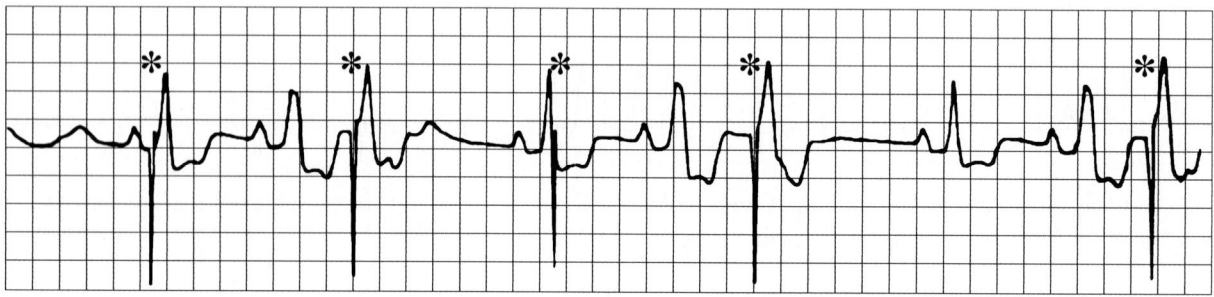

Fig. 41. VVI pacing with undersensing, which results in potentially undesirable competitive ventricular stimulation (*first and fourth asterisks*).

italis effect

b. Digitalis toxicity (Fig. 43)

- Almost any type of cardiac arrhythmia resulting from either a disturbance in impulse formation or an impairment of conduction, except bundle branch block
- Typical abnormalities include the following:
  - Paroxysmal atrial tachycardia with block
  - Atrial fibrillation with complete heart block
  - Bidirectional tachycardia
  - Second- or third-degree AV block with digitalis effect
  - Complete heart block with accelerated junctional or idioventricular rhythm

c. Antiarrhythmic drug effect—suggested by the

following:

- Decrease in the amplitude of the T wave or T-wave inversion
- ST-segment depression
- Prominent U waves—one of the earliest findings
- Prolongation of the QTc interval
- Notching and widening of the P waves
- Decrease in the atrial flutter rate

d. Antiarrhythmic drug toxicity—suggested by the following:

- Widening of the QRS
- Various degrees of AV block
- Ventricular arrhythmias—torsades de pointes
- Marked sinus bradycardia, sinus arrest, or sinoatrial block

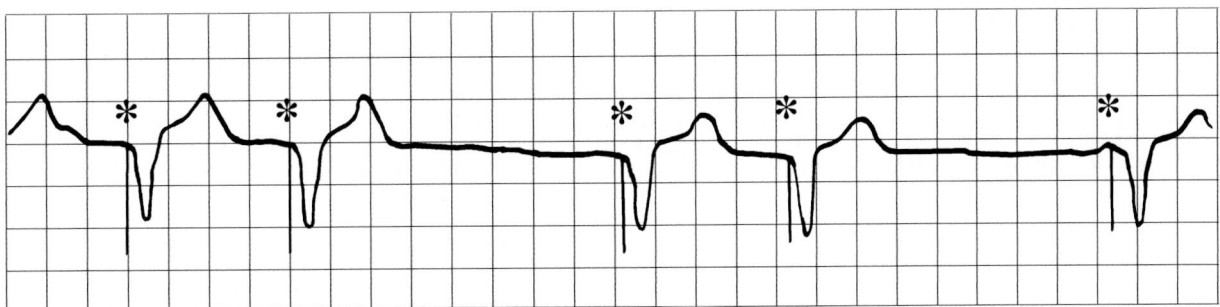

Fig. 42. Oversensing, resulting in an inappropriate, irregular pacemaker bradycardia. It is impossible to tell what is being oversensed in this electrocardiographic tracing.

e. Hyperkalemia (Fig. 44)

- *Potassium value 5.5–7.5 mEq/L*
  - Reversible left anterior fascicular block or left posterior fascicular block
  - Tall, peaked, narrow-based T waves
- *Potassium value >7.5–10.0 mEq/L*
  - First-degree AV block
  - Flattening and widening of P waves, later disappearance of P waves (sinoventricular conduction) or sinus arrest
  - ST-segment depression
- *Potassium value >10.0 mEq/L*

- LBBB, RBBB, markedly widened, diffuse intraventricular conduction delay
- Ventricular tachycardia or fibrillation, idioventricular rhythm

f. Hypokalemia—suggested by the following:

- Prominent U waves
- ST-segment depression, decreased T-wave amplitude
- Increase in amplitude and duration of the P wave
- Cardiac arrhythmias and AV block may be

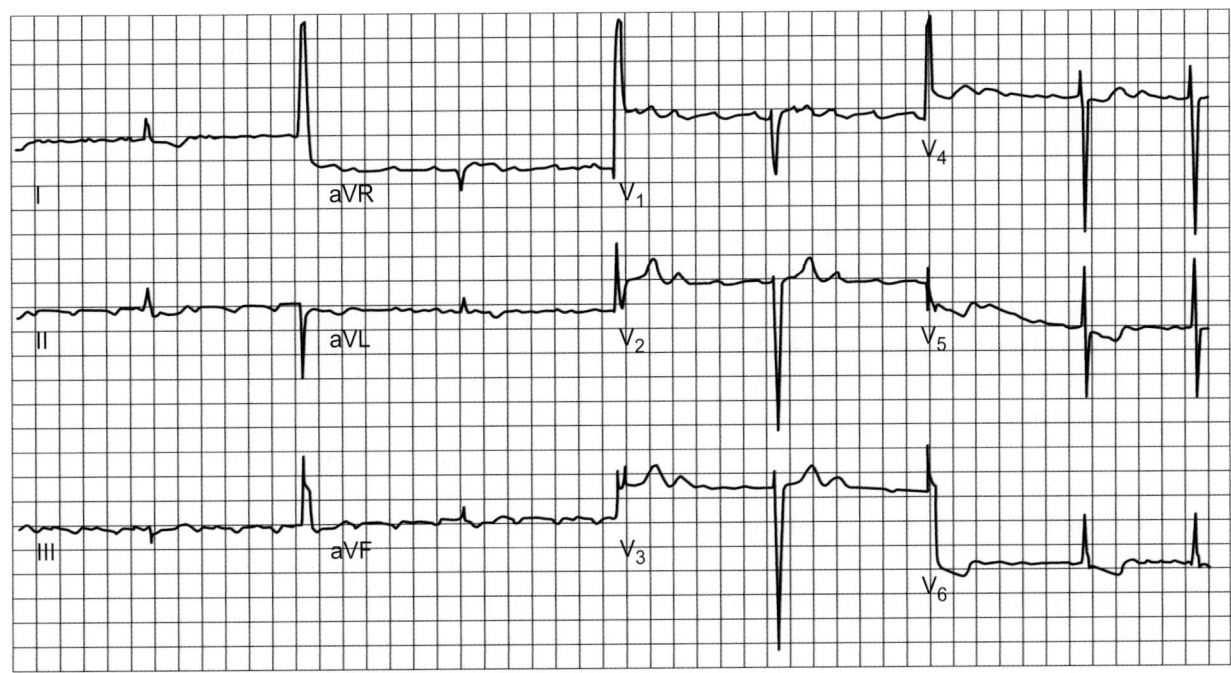

Fig. 43. Paroxysmal atrial tachycardia with atrioventricular block due to digitalis toxicity in a 79-year-old man.

digitalis related

g. Hypercalcemia

- Major ECG change is shortened QTc
- Little effect on QRS, P, and T waves; may see PR-interval prolongation

h. Hypocalcemia

- Earliest and most common finding is prolongation of QTc; results from ST-segment prolongation
- ST-segment prolongation occurs without changing the duration of the T waves; only hypothermia and hypocalcemia do this
- There can be flattening, peaking, or inversion of T waves

i. Atrial septal defect, secundum (Fig. 45)—suggested by the following:

- Typical RSR´ or rSR´ in V_1 with duration <0.11 second; right ventricular conduction delay in 90% (most are incomplete RBBB)
- Right axis deviation due to right ventricular hypertrophy
- Right atrial enlargement in 36%
- PR interval prolonged in <20%

j. Atrial septal defect, primum (Fig. 46)—suggested by the following:

- Most have left axis deviation (in contradistinction to right axis deviation in secundum atrial septal defect)
- PR-interval prolongation in 15% to 40%
- Far-advanced cases have biventricular hypertrophy

k. Dextrocardia, mirror image (Fig. 47)—suggested by the following:

- Decreasing R-wave amplitude from leads V_1 to V_6
- The P, QRS, and T waves in leads I and aVL are inverted, or "upside down"

- Be wary of lead malposition producing similar findings in leads I and aVL but not in V_1 through V_6

l. Mitral valve disease

- Mitral stenosis
  - No diagnostic findings
  - Combination of right ventricular hypertrophy and left atrial abnormality is suggestive
- Mitral valve prolapse—may see any of the following:
  - Flattened or inverted T waves in leads II, III, and aVF with or without ST-segment depression (sometimes left precordial leads); T-wave changes in the right precordial leads can be associated with prolapse of leaflets
  - Prominent U waves, QT prolongation

m. Chronic lung disease—suggested by any of the following:

- Right ventricular hypertrophy
- Right axis deviation
- Right atrial abnormality
- Shift of transitional zone counterclockwise
- Low voltage
- Pseudoanteroseptal infarct

Right ventricular hypertrophy in the setting of chronic lung disease:

- Rightward shift of QRS
- T-wave abnormalities in right precordia leads
- ST depression inferiorly
- Transient RBBB
- rSR' or QR in V_1

n. Acute cor pulmonale, including pulmonary embolus (Fig. 48)

- ECG abnormalities are frequently transient
- Sinus tachycardia most common
- Findings consistent with right ventricular pressure overload include the following:
  - Right atrial abnormality

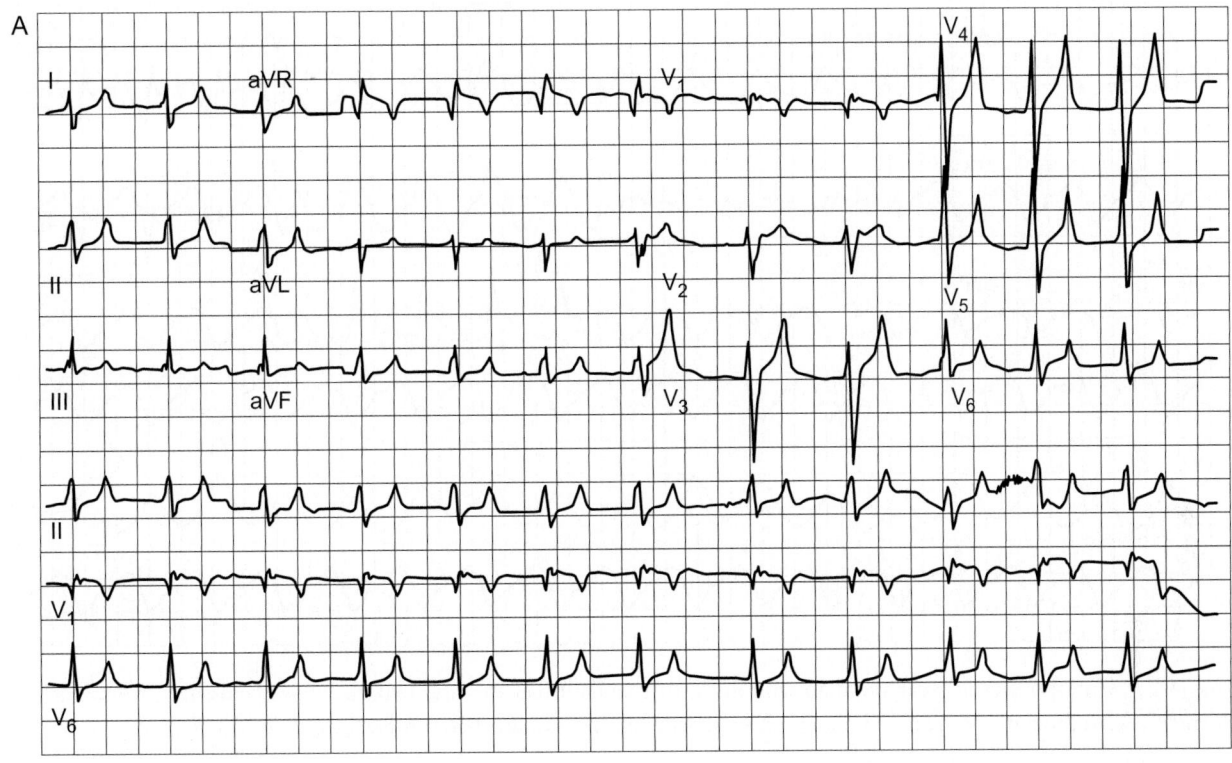

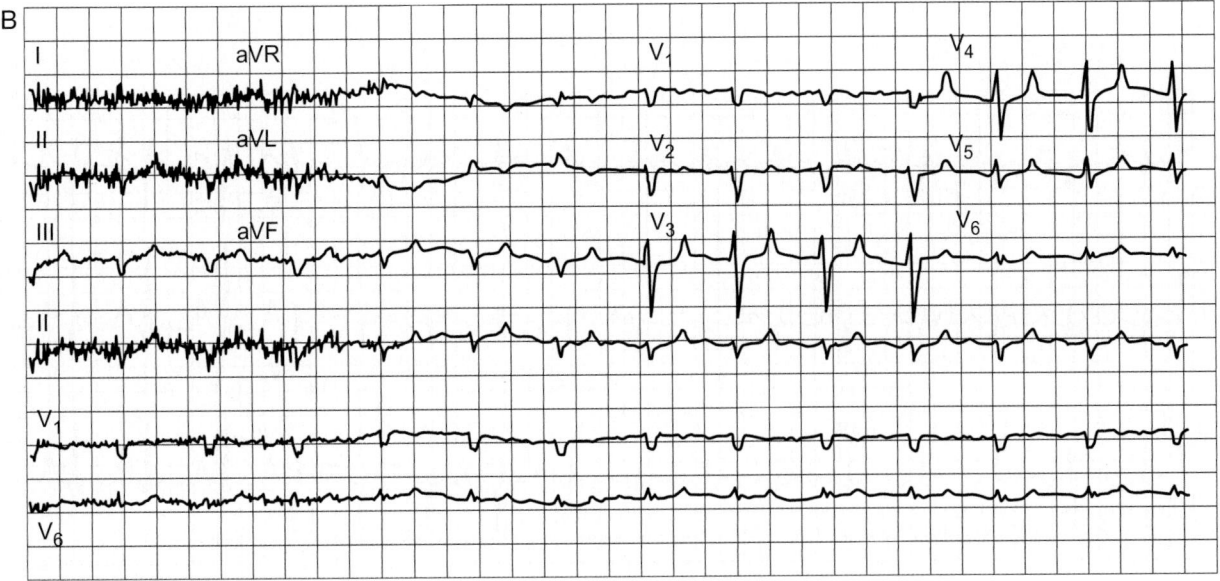

Fig. 44. continued on next page.

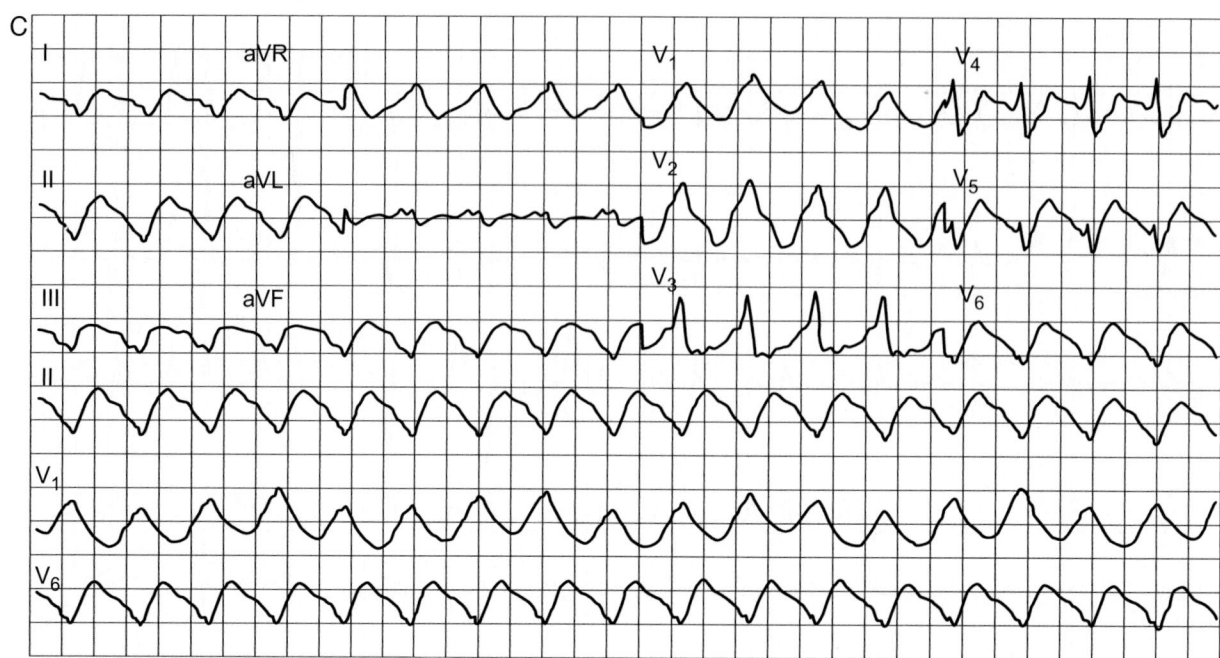

Fig. 44. *A*, Unresponsive 35-year-old man with insulin-dependent diabetes and hyperkalemia (potassium, 7.4 mEq/L). *B* and *C*, Asymptomatic 66-year-old man with hyperkalemia (potassium: *B*, 6.0 mEq/L; *C*, 9.2 mEq/L.)

- Inverted T waves in leads V_1 through V_3
- Right axis deviation
- S_1Q_3 and $S_1Q_3T_3$ patterns
- Pseudoinfarct pattern in inferior leads
- Transient RBBB
- Various supraventricular tachyarrhythmias

o. Pericardial effusion (Fig. 25)—suggested by either of the following:

- Low-voltage QRS (consider items **9a** and **9b**)
- Electrical alternans (consider item **9e**)

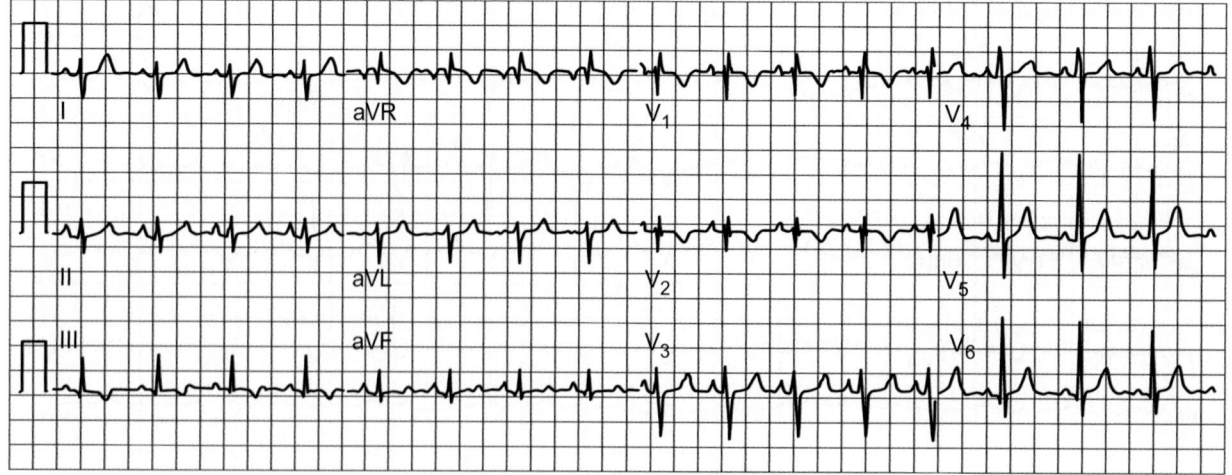

Fig. 45. Right axis deviation and RSR′ in lead V_1 with duration <0.11 second in a 6-year-old girl with secundum atrial septal defect.

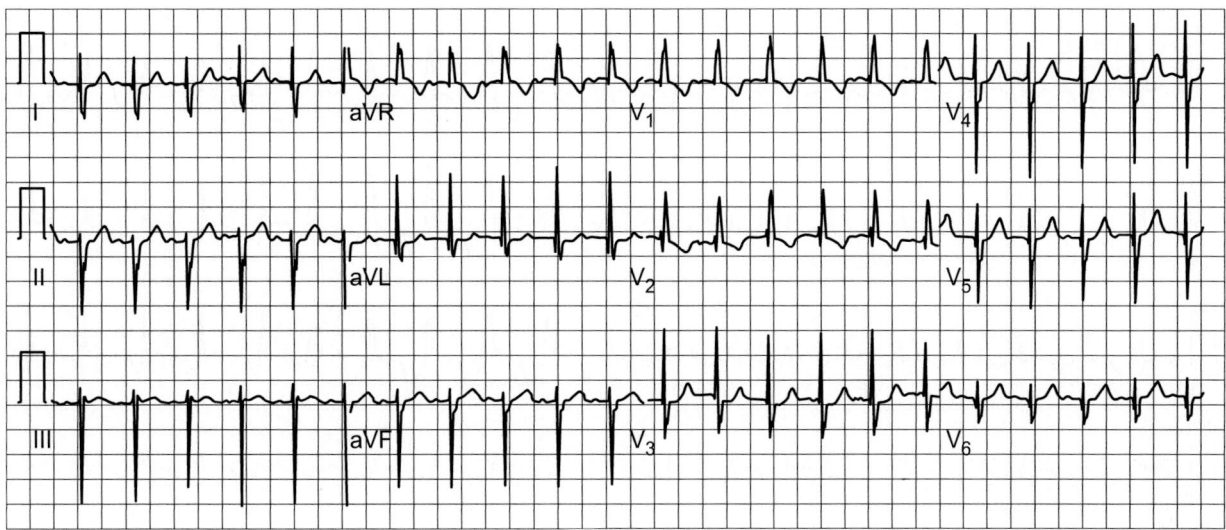

Fig. 46. Left axis deviation and RSR′ in lead V$_1$ with duration <0.11 second in a 1-year-old boy with primum atrial septal defect.

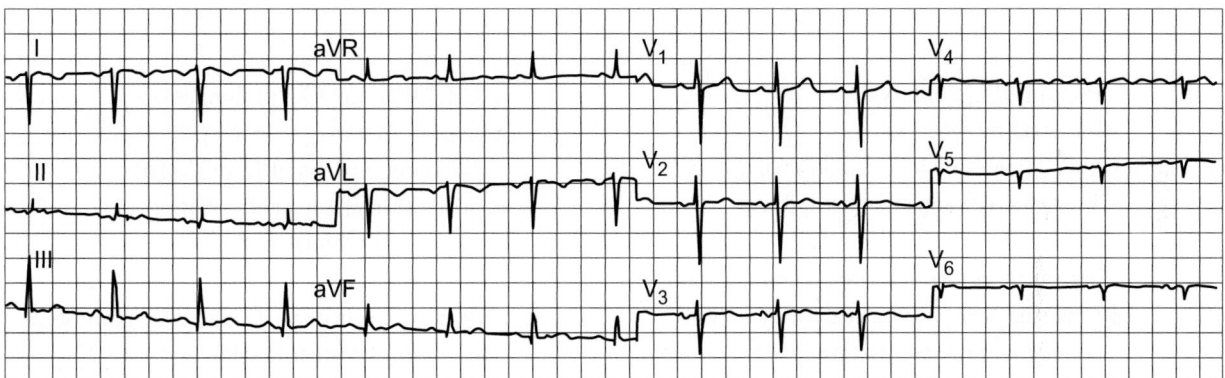

Fig. 47. Dextrocardia.

p. Acute pericarditis

■ Refer to item **12f** for criteria

q. Hypertrophic cardiomyopathy (Fig. 49 and 50)—suggested by the following:

■ Left atrial abnormality common
■ Majority of cases have abnormal QRS
 - Left axis deviation in 20%
 - High-voltage QRS
 - Large abnormal Q waves can give pseudo-infarct patterns in inferior, lateral, and precordial leads

 - Tall R wave in V$_1$ with inverted T waves simulating right ventricular hypertrophy
■ ST-T wave abnormalities common
 - ST-T wave changes due to ventricular hypertrophy or conduction abnormalities
 - Apical variants of hypertrophic obstructive cardiomyopathy have deep lateral, precordial T-wave inversions (Fig. 50)

r. Central nervous system disorder (Fig. 51)

■ "Classic changes," usually in precordial leads, include the following:
 - Large upright or deeply inverted T waves

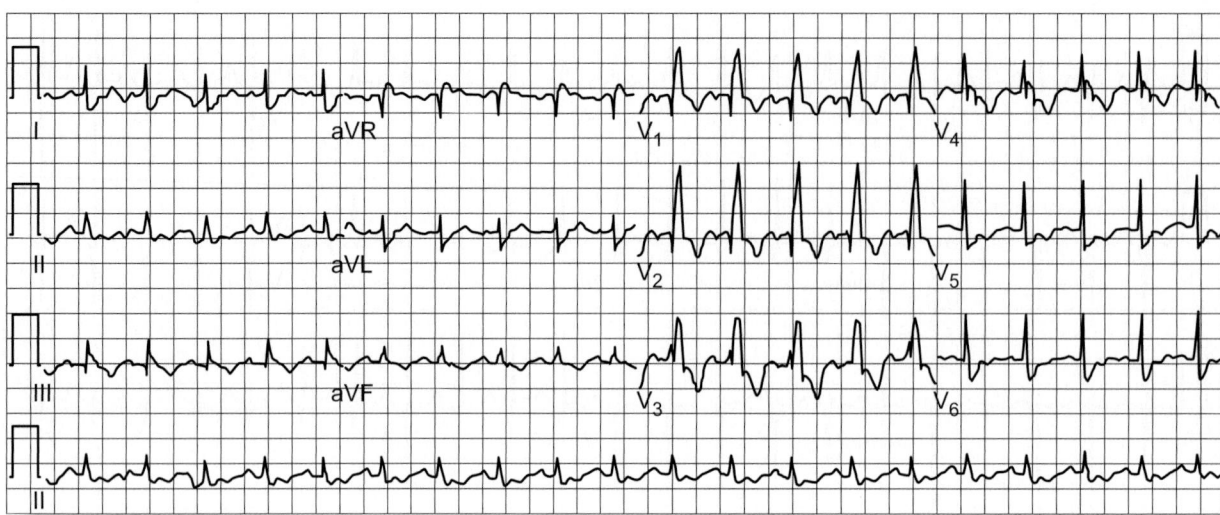

Fig. 48. Electrocardiogram in a 76-year-old man with massive pulmonary embolus.

- Prolonged QT interval
- Prominent U waves
■ Other changes include the following:
- T-wave notching, loss of amplitude
- Diffuse ST-segment elevation imitating pericarditis or focal ST-segment elevation imitating acute myocardial injury pattern
- Abnormal Q waves imitating MI
- Almost any rhythm abnormality
Differential diagnosis:
- Acute MI
- Acute pericarditis
- Drug effect

s. Myxedema (Fig. 52)

■ Low voltage of all complexes
■ Sinus bradycardia
■ Flattening or inversion of the T waves
■ PR interval may be prolonged
■ Frequently associated with pericardial effusion

t. Hypothermia (Fig. 53)

■ Sinus bradycardia

■ PR, QRS, and QT prolongation
■ J waves that may be quite prominent (Osborne, or "camel-hump" sign)
■ 50%-60% have atrial fibrillation
■ Other arrhythmias occur

u. Sick sinus syndrome—frequently manifests as one or more of the following:

■ Sinus bradycardia of marked degree
■ Sinus arrest or sinoatrial block
■ Bradycardia alternating with tachycardia
■ Atrial fibrillation with slow ventricular response preceded or followed by sinus bradycardia, sinus arrest, or sinoatrial block
■ Prolonged sinus node recovery time after atrial premature complex or atrial tachy-arrhythmias
■ AV junctional escape rhytm
■ Additional conduction system disease is often present

v. Ebstein anomaly (Fig. 54)

■ Characteristic RBBB with abnormal terminal forces (R' in lead V_1, S in I and aVL)

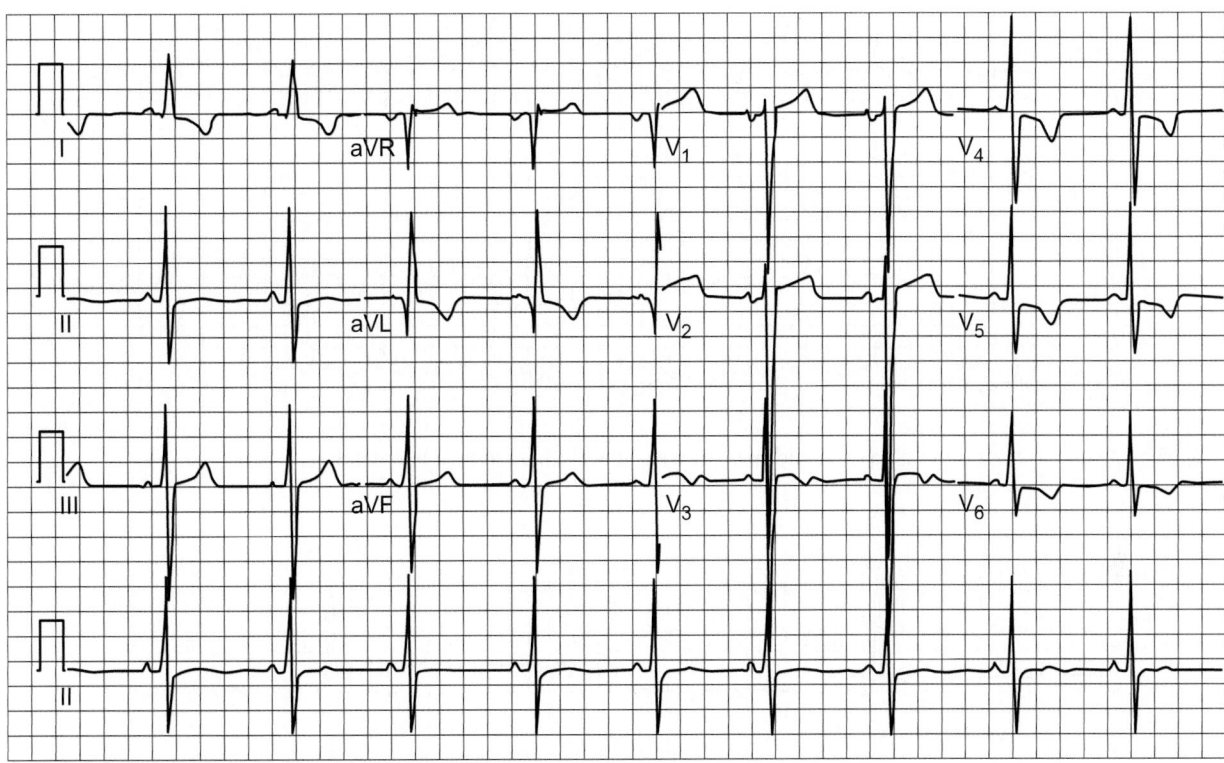

Fig. 49. Electrocardiogram in a 21-year-old man with hypertrophic cardiomyopathy.

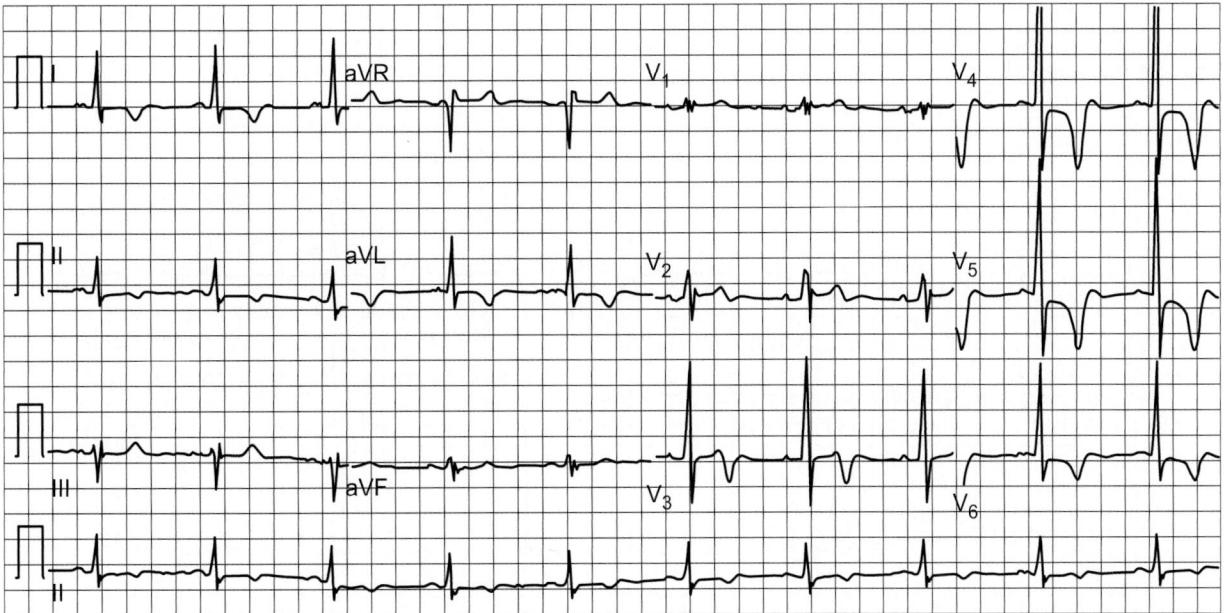

Fig. 50. Electrocardiogram in a 72-year-old man with apical hypertrophic cardiomyopathy. Note deep symmetrical T-wave inversion in leads V_3 through V_6.

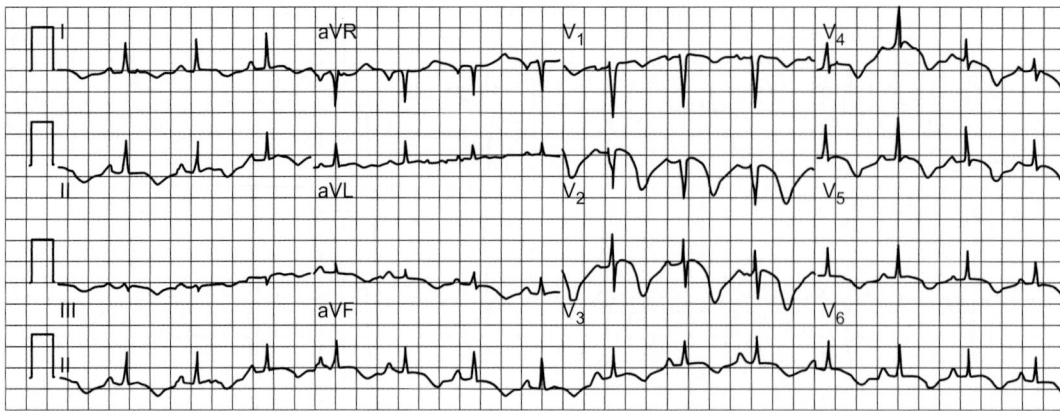

Fig. 51. Electrocardiogram in a 65-year-old woman with acute subarachnoid hemorrhage.

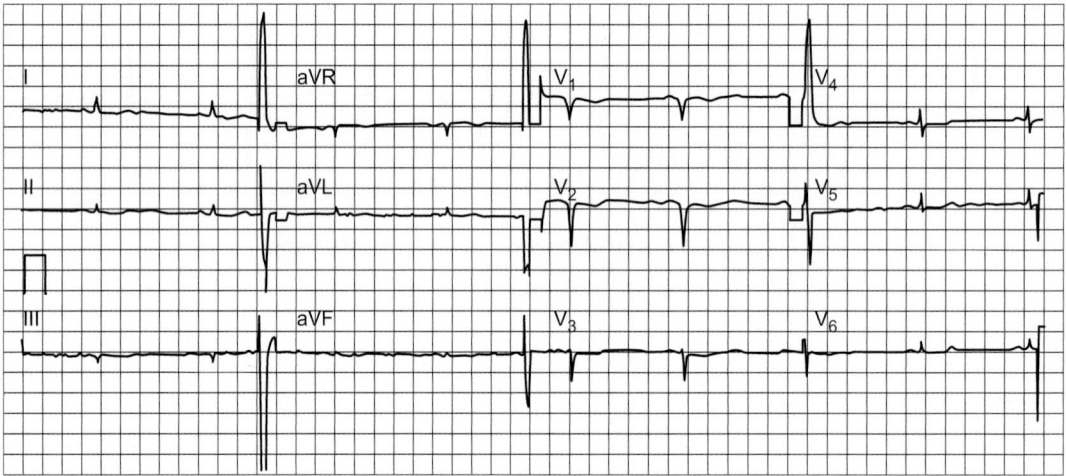

Fig. 52. Electrocardiogram in a patient with myxedema.

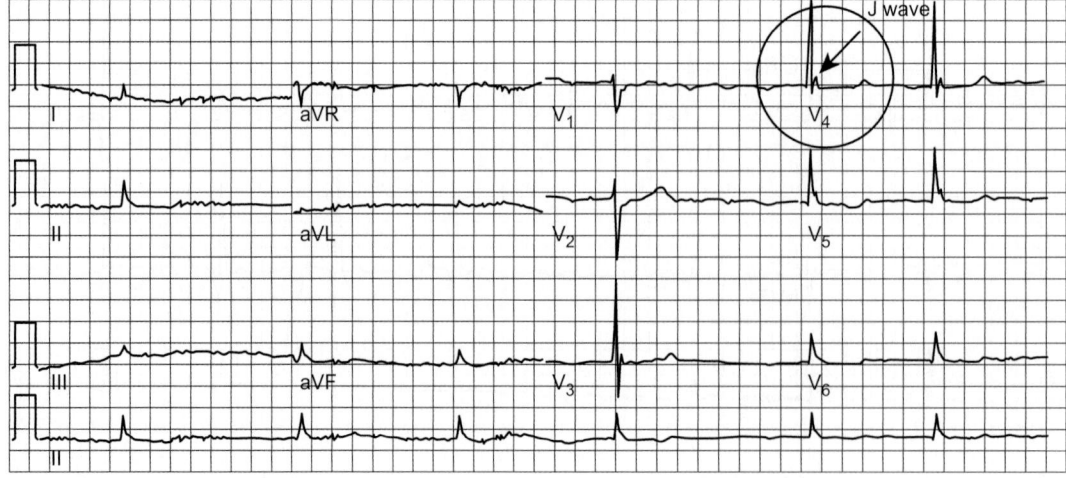

Fig. 53. Electrocardiogram in a 63-year-old woman with hypothermia.

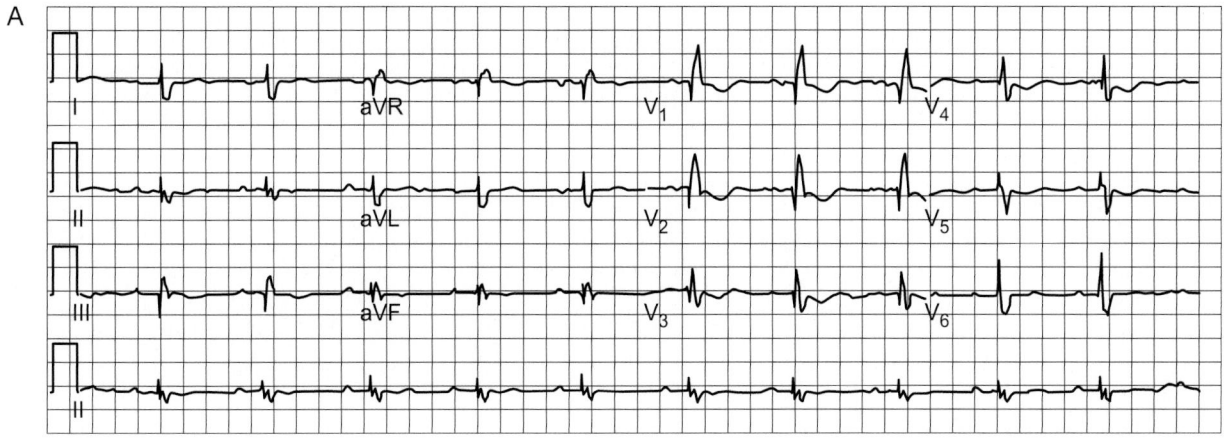

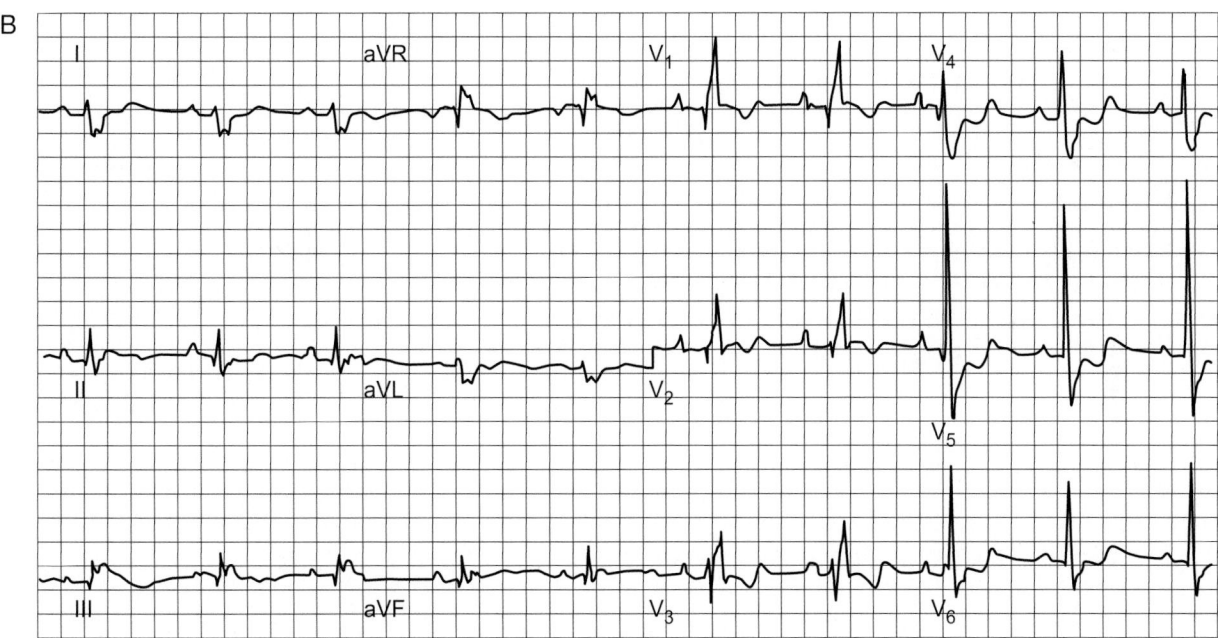

Fig. 54. Electrocardiograms from patients with Ebstein anomaly. *A*, A 25-year-old man. *B*, A 10-year-old boy.

19

CARDIAC CELLULAR ELECTROPHYSIOLOGY

Hon-Chi Lee, MD, PhD

This chapter provides an overview of cardiac cellular electrophysiology. A review of the structure and function of cardiac ion channels is followed by a discussion of the effect of ion channels on cardiac action potential, mechanisms of arrhythmia, and inherited and acquired channelopathies.

STRUCTURE AND FUNCTION OF CARDIAC ION CHANNELS

Cardiac ion channels are integral membrane proteins that regulate the traffic of ions in heart cells. They are determinants of the cardiac action potential, which in turn underlies cardiac impulse conduction, excitation-contraction coupling, automaticity, and arrhythmogenesis.

Structure of Ion Channels

In the heart, most of the important ion channels assume one of the following structural motifs, presented in increasing order of complexity:

1. The inward rectifier potassium (Kir) channels are proteins with two transmembrane segments that sandwich a channel pore loop (Fig. 1 *A*). Four of these subunits coassemble to form a functional channel. These channels are not voltage sensitive and are frequently gated by ligands. Examples include the adenosine triphosphate (ATP)-sensitive potassium (K_{ATP}) channels and the strong rectifier potassium channel that gives rise to the strong inward rectifier potassium current (I_{K1}).

2. Voltage-gated potassium channels are proteins that have six transmembrane segments (S1 to S6, Fig. 1 *B*) with cytoplasmic N- and C-termini. The voltage sensor is located in the fourth transmembrane segment (S4), which contains a high density of positively charged amino acids (lysine and arginine) that move according to changes in membrane potential. This movement causes the channel to open and close through allosteric and conformational changes in the ion channel structure. The fifth (S5) and sixth (S6) transmembrane segments sandwich a pore loop. Four of these pore-forming channel protein subunits coassemble to form a functional channel. Examples include the transient outward potassium channels and the delayed rectifier potassium channels.

3. Voltage-gated sodium and calcium channel proteins are the most structurally complex. The channel is a single peptide consisting of four homologous domains, each of which has six transmembrane segments that include a voltage sensing S4 and a pore loop between S5 and S6 (Fig. 1 *C*).

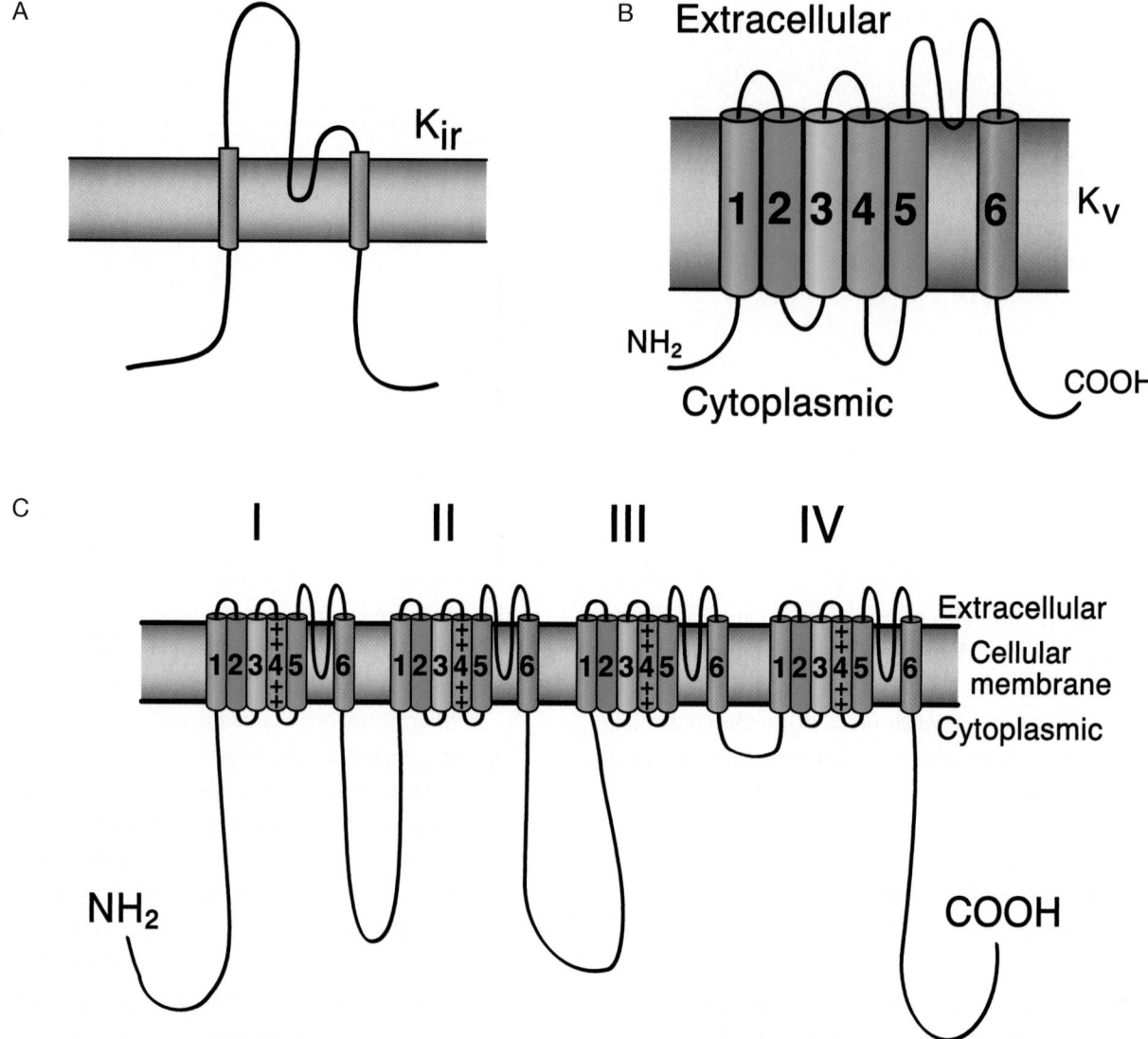

Fig. 1. *A*, Inward rectifier potassium channels have two transmembrane segments and an intervening pore loop. Four of these subunits coassemble to form a functional channel. *B*, Voltage-gated potassium channels have six transmembrane segments, including the voltage sensor S4 and the pore loop between S5 and S6. Four of these subunits coassemble to form a functional channel. *C*, Voltage-gated sodium and calcium channels consist of a single polypeptide containing four repeats of six transmembrane segments.

- Ion channels in the heart have a fourfold structural symmetry.
- The ion channel pore is lined by four pore loops.
- The voltage-gated channels contain the voltage-sensing S4.

Function of Ion Channels

The function of ion channels is defined by two basic properties: conductance and gating.

1. *Conductance* describes which ions are allowed to permeate the channel and at what rate. Ion channel conductance is determined by the selectivity filter in the pore loop that lines the narrowest portion of the channel pore. Sodium channels preferentially conduct sodium over potassium (12:1 ratio) and calcium (10:1 ratio), whereas potassium channels are selective for potassium over sodium (1,000:1 ratio).

Most cardiac ion channels show *rectification*, which refers to the preferential conduction of ions in the outward or inward direction. Ion channel rectification can be influenced by unequal ion concentration across the membrane, the range of voltages that open voltage-gated ion channels (e.g. transient outward potassium current [I_{to}] and pacemaker current [I_f]), or blockade of the channel by intracellular magnesium or polyamines at positive voltages (e.g., Kir channels).

2. *Gating* describes what governs the opening and closing of the channel. *Voltage-gated channels* open and close according to changes in membrane potential. The sodium current (I_{Na}), the L-type calcium current ($I_{Ca,L}$), the T-type calcium current ($I_{Ca,T}$), I_{to}, the rapid component of the delayed rectifier potassium current (I_{Kr}), and the slow component of the delayed rectifier potassium current (I_{Ks}) are all activated by membrane depolarization, whereas I_f is activated by membrane hyperpolarization. Voltage-gated ion channels all contain a voltage-sensing S4 in which every third amino acid is a positively charged lysine or arginine. *Ligand-gated channels* are activated or inactivated by the binding of chemical ligands: the acetylcholine (ACh)-sensitive potassium channel ($I_{K,ACh}$) is activated by ACh, whereas the ATP-sensitive potassium channel ($I_{K,ATP}$) is inhibited by ATP.

Open channels can be inactivated by different mechanisms, including the following:

1. Physical occlusion of the channel pore by cytoplasmic portions of the channel (e.g., "ball-and-chain" mechanism in I_{to} or "hinged-lid" mechanism in I_{Na})
2. Conformational changes in channel structure (e.g., C-type inactivation in I_{to}).
3. Increase in intracellular calciuim, which promotes calcium-calmodulin binding to the C-terminus of the channel (e.g., $I_{Ca,L}$).
4. Chemical ligand binding (e.g., $I_{K,ATP}$).

Some channels, such as the delayed rectifier potassium channels, are non-inactivating. In these channels, potassium conduction stops when membrane potentials are hyperpolarized, resulting in channel deactivation.

Cardiac Ionic Currents

I_{Na}

Atrial and ventricular myocytes, as well as Purkinje fibers, are densely populated with sodium channels. These channels open very briefly (≤1 ms) when the membrane is depolarized to −50 mV and require repolarization to −100 mV for complete recovery. Atrial and ventricular myocytes have normal resting potentials of −85 to −90 mV and on depolarization, I_{Na} produces a fast upstroke of 100-200 V/s. Depolarized resting potentials in injured or ischemic myocardium prevent complete recovery of sodium channels, resulting in reduced I_{Na} and action potential upstroke velocity. I_{Na} is inactivated by voltage with physical occlusion of the channel pore by the cytoplasmic linker between domains III and IV in a "hinged-lid" mechanism. Nodal cells are sparsely populated with sodium channels and have normal resting potentials of −50 to −70 mV; they have little I_{Na} and their action potential upstrokes are slow.

$I_{Ca,L}$

The L-type calcium channels are present in all cell types in the heart. $I_{Ca,L}$ is activated by membrane depolarization but has much slower inactivation than I_{Na}. In nodal cells, $I_{Ca,L}$ is responsible for impulse generation and conduction. In atrial and ventricular myocytes, $I_{Ca,L}$ is a critical determinant of the action potential plateau and plays a crucial role in cardiac excitation-contraction coupling. $I_{Ca,L}$ is enhanced severalfold by sympathetic stimulation. It is inactivated by voltage and by increases in intracellular calcium, which promote calcium-calmodulin binding to the C-terminus of the channel, inducing channel inactivation by conformational changes.

$I_{Ca,T}$

The T-type calcium channels are more highly expressed in atrial myocardium, the conduction system, and nodal cells than in ventricular myocytes. $I_{Ca,T}$ is activated at hyperpolarized potentials (positive to −70 mV) and is rapidly inactivated (−80 to −50 mV). $I_{Ca,T}$ is small compared with $I_{Ca,L}$ and negligible in ventricular cells. $I_{Ca,T}$ is thought to be responsible for impulse generation in nodal cells and automaticity in atrial myocytes, including pulmonary vein potentials.

I_{to}

The transient outward potassium current, I_{to}, is produced by several channels, including Kv1.4, Kv4.2, and Kv4.3. I_{to} is present in atrial, ventricular, and conduction system cells. The rapid activation and inactivation of I_{to} contributes to phase 1 of the cardiac action potential. In the ventricular myocardium, I_{to} is robust in the epicardium and modest in the endocardial layers, leading to a transmural gradient that gives rise to J waves (Osborne waves) and U waves on electrocardiograms (ECGs). I_{to} is inactivated by the physical occlusion of the channel pore by the N-terminal portion of the channel in a "ball-and-chain" mechanism.

I_K

Three components of the delayed rectifier potassium channels are identified: I_{Kur}, I_{Kr}, and I_{Ks}. The rapidly activating and slowly inactivating I_{Kur} is prominent in atrial myocytes, accounting for their shortened action potential duration. I_{Kr} and I_{Ks} are activated very slowly during the cardiac action potential and are responsible for phase 3 repolarization. I_{Kr} inactivates at depolarized potentials whereas I_{Ks} is noninactivating; potassium conduction stops when membrane potentials are hyperpolarized, resulting in channel deactivation. The slow deactivation of I_{Ks} contributes to the short action potential durations at high heart rates.

I_{K1}

The strong inward rectifier potassium current, I_{K1}, is robust in ventricular myocytes, weak in atrial myocytes, and absent in nodal cells. I_{K1} conducts very little outward current, is crucial for maintaining the resting potential near the potassium reversal potential at around −90 mV, and is responsible for the rapid terminal repolarization in phase 3. Damaged myocardium with weakened I_{K1} is susceptible to the development of abnormal automaticity.

$I_{K,ATP}$

$I_{K,ATP}$ is an inward rectifier potassium channel that is inhibited by physiologic intracellular concentrations of ATP, but is activated during ischemia, on depletion of ATP, or with a decrease in the ATP–adenosine diphosphate (ADP) ratio. Ventricular myocytes are endowed with high densities of these channels and activation of $I_{K,ATP}$ accounts for the ST-segment elevation seen on ECG during myocardial infarction. $I_{K,ATP}$ is also a crucial element in mediating cardiac ischemic preconditioning.

I_f

The "funny" current, I_f, is activated by membrane hyperpolarization. I_f, a nonselective cationic channel, is responsible for pacemaker activity and diastolic depolarization during phase 4 in the sinus node, the atrioventricular (AV) node, and the Purkinje fibers. Activity of I_f is tightly regulated by sympathetic activation and parasympathetic inhibition.

Electrogenic Membrane Pumps and Exchangers

The *sodium-potassium pump* is ubiquitous and is inhibited by digitalis. The pump extrudes three sodium ions in exchange for the entry of two potassium ions with hydrolysis of ATP; hence, the pump is electrogenic and contributes a hyperpolarizing outward current to the cardiac action potential. The *sodium-calcium exchange* facilitates the exchange of one calcium ion for three sodium ions. The direction of exchange depends on the membrane potential. At the resting potential, calcium is extruded, allowing the cell to maintain low intracellular calcium concentration. At the plateau, the exchanger facilitates calcium entry and contributes to cardiac excitation-contraction coupling. The exchanger is electrogenic and is thought to mediate the development of delayed afterdepolarizations and triggered activities.

In addition to the sarcolemmal voltage-gated ion channels mentioned above, two other ion channels are worth noting for their important roles in cardiac electrophysiology and the development of cardiac arrhythmias:

1. *Gap junction channels* are hexomeric complexes of connexin (connexin 40 and connexin 43) that form hemichannels on the cell surface. Two hemichannels from two different cells are united to form a functional gap junction. Opening and closing of the gap junction channels are regulated by several metabolic factors, including pH, intracellular calcium, and channel phosphorylation. Because intercellular transfer of currents can occur only where cells share gap junctions, activities and distribution of the gap junction channels can profoundly affect electrical impulse conduction, especially under conditions of ischemia.

2. *Ryanodine receptors* are intracellular ion channels located in the sarcoplasmic reticulum. They are responsible for releasing calcium from the sarcoplasmic reticulum and are crucial elements in the regulation of intracellular calcium homeostasis.

Opening of the ryanodine receptors is triggered by calcium entry through the sarcolemmal calcium channels in a process known as calcium-induced calcium release and is critical in regulating excitation-contraction coupling of the heart. In the normal heart, ryanodine receptors are closed during diastole. In disease states, however, these channels become "leaky," resulting in intracellular calcium overload and the development of arrhythmias.

Many ion channels in the heart contain *auxiliary subunits*, which modulate the expression and function of ion channels. Listed below are several notable examples.

1. The function and expression of sodium channels are regulated by β subunits.
2. The L-type calcium channels in the heart contain α_2, β, and δ subunits.
3. Kv1.4 and Kv4.3, which encode I_{to}, are modulated by the potassium channel interacting protein (KCHIP), which may be responsible for the transmural gradient of I_{to}.
4. K_{ATP} channels contain Kir6.2 and the sulfonylurea receptor SUR2A subunits. SUR2A confers channel sensitivity to sulfonylurea.
5. *KVLQT1*, which encodes I_{Ks}, is profoundly modulated by *MinK*.
6. *HERG*, which encodes I_{Kr}, is profoundly modulated by *MiRP*. Mutations in *MinK* and *MiRP* are known to cause long QT syndromes.

ION CHANNELS AND THE CARDIAC ACTION POTENTIAL

Conceptually, the configuration of the cardiac action potential is determined by the sum of ionic current activities at any given time point during the cardiac cycle. The upstroke of the action potential, phase 0, is associated with the opening of the sodium channels. Inactivation of the sodium currents and activation of the transient outward potassium currents, I_{to}, give rise to early rapid partial repolarization and phase 1. The balance between inactivation of I_{to} currents, activation of $I_{Ca,L}$ currents, I_K currents, and the sodium-calcium exchange currents constitutes phase 2, which is the plateau of the action potential. Phase 3 represents the final rapid repolarization of the action potential and is the result of further activation of the I_K currents and

inactivation of the calcium currents. Toward the end of phase 3, the strong inward rectifier potassium currents, I_{K1}, are activated, leading to rapid repolarization. During diastole or phase 4, atrial and ventricular myocytes are normally quiescent electrically. However, pacemaker tissues, such as the sinus node, AV node, and His-Purkinje fibers, show slow diastolic depolarization, indicating the presence of pacemaker activity caused by the activation of I_f, calcium currents, and inactivation of potassium currents. Activities of the different ionic currents during the cardiac action potential are shown in Figure 2.

■ The major currents activated at different phases of the cardiac action potential:
Phase 0—sodium currents
Phase 1—transient outward potassium currents, I_{to}
Phase 2—calcium currents, sodium-calcium exchange currents
Phase 3—delayed rectifier potassium currents, I_{K1} (late phase 3)
Phase 4—pacemaker currents, I_f

Different cardiac tissues have different ion channel compositions and thus have different configurations of action potentials (Fig. 3).

Sinus Node

The sinus node is characterized by its phase 4 depolarization, which gives rise to pacemaker activities. Phase 4 depolarization is due to the high density of pacemaker currents and the lack of I_{K1}, which also accounts for the relative depolarized state of the tissue. Sodium channels are sparse and the action potential upstroke is slow since it is mediated mainly by $I_{Ca,L}$. There is no discernible phase 1 owing to the lack of I_{to}. Action potential durations are short and the frequency of depolarization is determined by the sympathetic and parasympathetic modulation of I_f.

Atrium

The atrial action potential has rapid upstrokes, allowing rapid electrical impulse conduction from the right atrium to the left atrium and from the sinus node to the AV node. It has a discernible phase 1 followed by a short plateau phase and rapid repolarization. The short plateau may partially explain why an antiarrhythmic

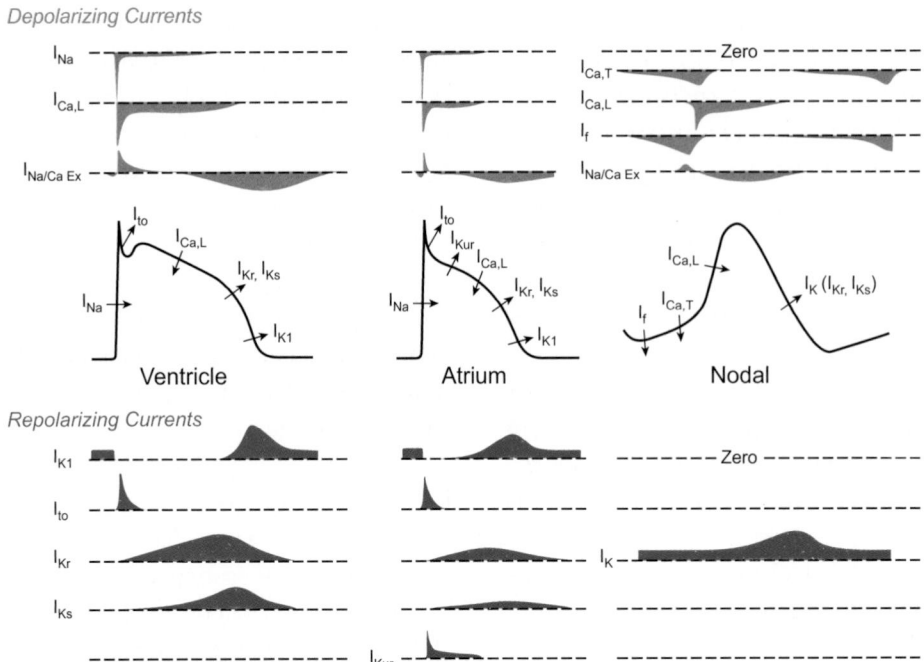

Fig. 2. Ionic currents that contribute to the cardiac action potentials. Depolarizing (red) and repolarizing (blue) currents contribute to the action potentials in the ventricle (*left panel*), atrium (*middle panel*), and nodal tissue (*right panel*). $I_{Ca,L}$, L-type calcium current; $I_{Ca,T}$, T-type calcium current; I_f, pacemaker current; I_K, delayed rectifier potassium current; I_{K1}, strong inward rectifier poteasium current; I_{Kr}, rapid component of the delayed rectifier potassium current; I_{Ks}, slow component of the delayed rectifier potassium current; I_{Kur}, rapidly activating and slowly inactivating potassium current; I_{Na}, sodium current; $I_{Na/CaEx}$, sodium-calcium exchange; I_{to}, transient outward potassium current.

drug like lidocaine, which exerts its effects during the plateau phase, is ineffective in the treatment of atrial arrhythmias. Normal atrial tissue has no phase 4 activity owing to the presence of I_{K1}.

Atrioventricular Node

The AV node is similar to the sinus node in its lack of I_{Na}. Conduction through the AV node is mediated by $I_{Ca,L}$ and propagation is slow, accounting for its decremental conduction properties. Activities of $I_{Ca,L}$ are activated by sympathetic stimulation and inhibited by parasympathetic influences; these are important determinants of impulse conduction through the AV node. Phase 4 depolarization is present but usually not as prominent as that in the sinus node.

His-Purkinje Fibers

His-Purkinje fibers have high densities of I_{Na} that facilitate rapid conduction of impulses so that ventricular myocytes can be activated synchronously. In addition,

the His-Purkinje fibers have strong I_{K1} and weak pacemaker currents. Hence, His-Purkinje tissue is characterized by a resting potential of −90 mV, which is close to the reversal potential of potassium, and slow diastolic depolarization.

Ventricle

Ventricular myocytes have densities of I_{Na} and I_{K1} that are higher than those in atrial myocytes; hence, these cells rest near −90 mV and are electrically quiescent. The configuration of the action potential varies according to location in the left ventricle. Myocytes in the *epicardial* layer have very strong I_{to}. This leads to marked repolarization in phase 1 followed by depolarization as calcium currents are activated, generating the characteristic "spike-and-dome" configuration. In contrast, the *endocardial* layer has much lower I_{to} density with reduced phase 1 amplitude and no spike-and-dome configuration. The mid-myocardial layer is endowed with the so-called *M cells*, which have strong I_{to} but

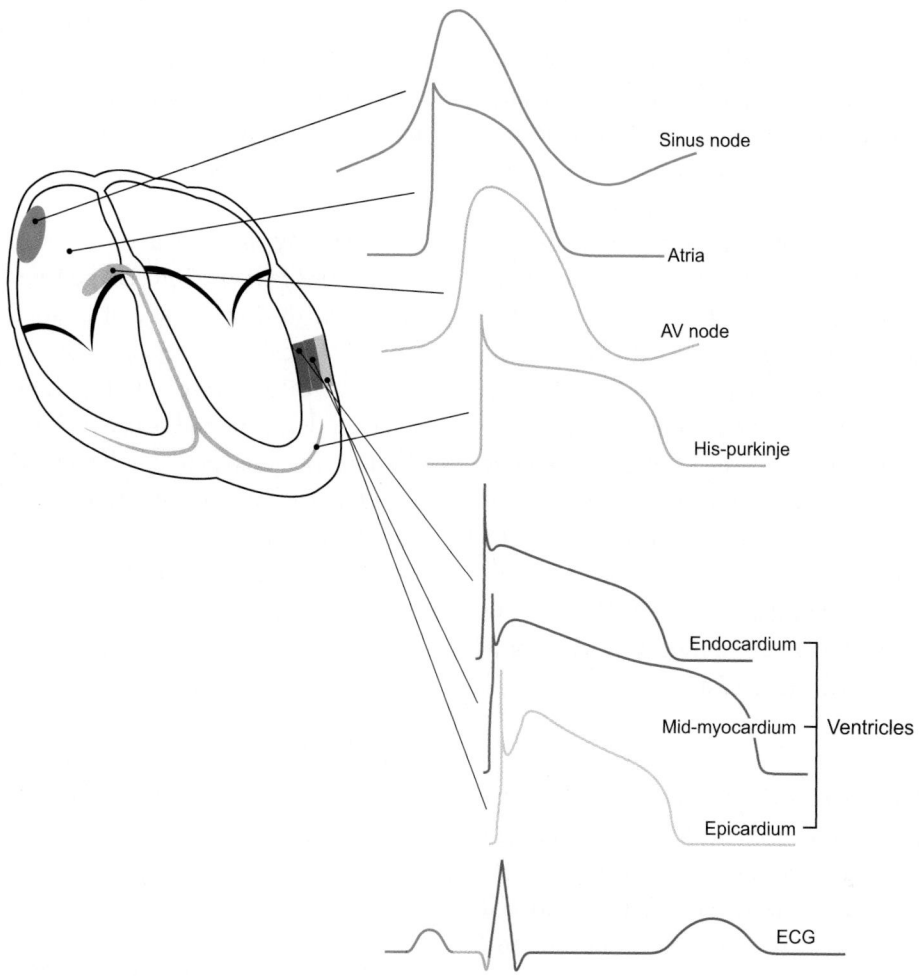

Fig. 3. Action potential waveforms in different heart tissues. Action potential configurations in different tissues of the heart vary according to their specific roles in impulse generation, conduction, and contraction. The sinus and atrioventricular (AV) nodes are important in impulse generation and have pacemaker activity. Atrial and ventricular myocardium are important for contraction. The His-Purkinje tissue has the fastest upstroke velocity for rapid conduction of electrical impulse to activate the ventricles synchronously. The ventricular epicardium, endocardium, and mid-myocardium have distinct action potential configurations. The contributions of the action potentials from various tissues to the surface electrocardiographic signals are displayed. ECG, electrocardiogram.

weak delayed I_K currents and an enhanced slow component of the voltage-gated sodium currents. Thus, the M cell action potential is characterized by a spike-and-dome configuration and lengthened action potential duration, exceeding those of epicardial and endocardial myocytes by 200 ms. This regional heterogeneity in the electrophysiology of the heart is thought to be the basis for development of U waves and triggered activities.

■ A favorite board exam question is to correlate action potential configurations with various cardiac tissues.

MECHANISMS OF ARRHYTHMIAS
There are three major mechanisms of arrhythmias: reentry, abnormal automaticity, and triggered activities.

Reentry
Reentry is the most common mechanism involved in many clinically important cardiac arrhythmias, including AV nodal reentry tachycardia, AV reentry tachycardia using an AV accessory connection, atrial flutter, and ventricular tachycardia in an infarcted heart. Reentry arises as a result of altered impulse conduction. The sine

qua non of reentry is unidirectional block. To occur, reentry must have a substrate with an area of slow conduction in the reentry circuit (Fig. 4 *A*). The premature beat that sets up reentry is blocked in the area of slow conduction, thereby allowing conduction in the reverse direction from the other end of the reentry circuit. By the time the impulse reaches the area of slow conduction, block has recovered, allowing reentry to occur. Conditions that decrease conduction velocity or refractoriness promote reentry. The wavelength of the reentry impulse is defined as the product of conduction velocity and refractoriness. These properties are important in determining the effectiveness of antiarrhythmic drugs and overdrive pacing in the termination of reentry arrhythmias. Reentry tachyarrhythmias usually exhibit the following properties: 1) they are inducible by programmed electrical stimulation, 2) they have abrupt onset and offset, and 3) during reentrant tachycardia, the RR intervals are regular.

Abnormal Automaticity

Abnormal automaticity is the spontaneous development of impulses independent of preceding impulses or stimulation. The underlying mechanism is due to abnormal diastolic depolarization in atrial or ventricular muscle, usually as a result of tissue damage or abnormal enhancement of pacemaker activities in subsidiary tissues such as nodal cells or His-Purkinje fibers (Fig. 4 *B*). Important automatic tachyarrhythmias include certain types of atrial tachycardias, pulmonary vein potentials in atrial fibrillation, acclerated junctional tachycardias, idioventricular rhythms, and inappropriate sinus tachycardias. Automatic tachycardias are usually not inducible by programmed electrical stimulation during electrophysiologic studies. They are characterized by 1) rate acceleration at the onset (warming up) and deceleration before termination (cooling down) and 2) response to sympathomimetics and to autonomic modulation.

Triggered Activities

Triggered activity is the development of abnormal impulses as a result of the preceding impulse or impulses. Triggered activities are involved in only a small portion of clinically observed arrhythmias but are important because they are frequently associated with life-threatening conditions. Unless a proper diagnosis is made and the underlying conditions that set up the triggered activities are removed, the ensuing arrhythmias are potentially lethal. There are two types of triggered activities: early afterdepolarizations and delayed afterdepolarizations.

Early Afterdepolarizations

Early afterdepolarizations (EADs) are depolarizations that occur during phase 2 or phase 3 of the cardiac action potential before repolarization is completed (Fig. 4 *C*). Conditions associated with prolonged action potential durations and hence prolonged QT intervals promote the development of EADs, which are thought to be the mechanism that underlies torsades de pointes (Table 1).

Torsades de pointes is characterized by following:
- Prolonged QT intervals
- Exacerbation by bradycardia (which prolongs QT)
- Short-long coupling intervals
- "Salvos" of nonsustained polymorphic ventricular tachycardias (VTs) before degeneration into sustained polymorphic VT and ventricular fibrillation (VF)

Table 1.   Conditions Known to Promote Torsades de Pointes

Condition	Mechanism
Hypokalemia	↓ K^+ channel activity
Hypomagnesemia	? ↑ Ca^{2+} channel activity
Antiarrhythmic drugs	
Class 1A antiarrhythmics	K^+ channel blockade
Class 3 antiarrhythmics:	
sotalol, dofetilide	K^+ channel blockade
Ibutilide	Na^+ channel activation, K^+ channel blockade
Antihistamines	K^+ channel blockade
Macrolide antibiotics:	
erythomycin	K^+ channel blockade
Congenital long QT syndrome	Channelopathies

Ca, calcium; K, potassium, Na, sodium.

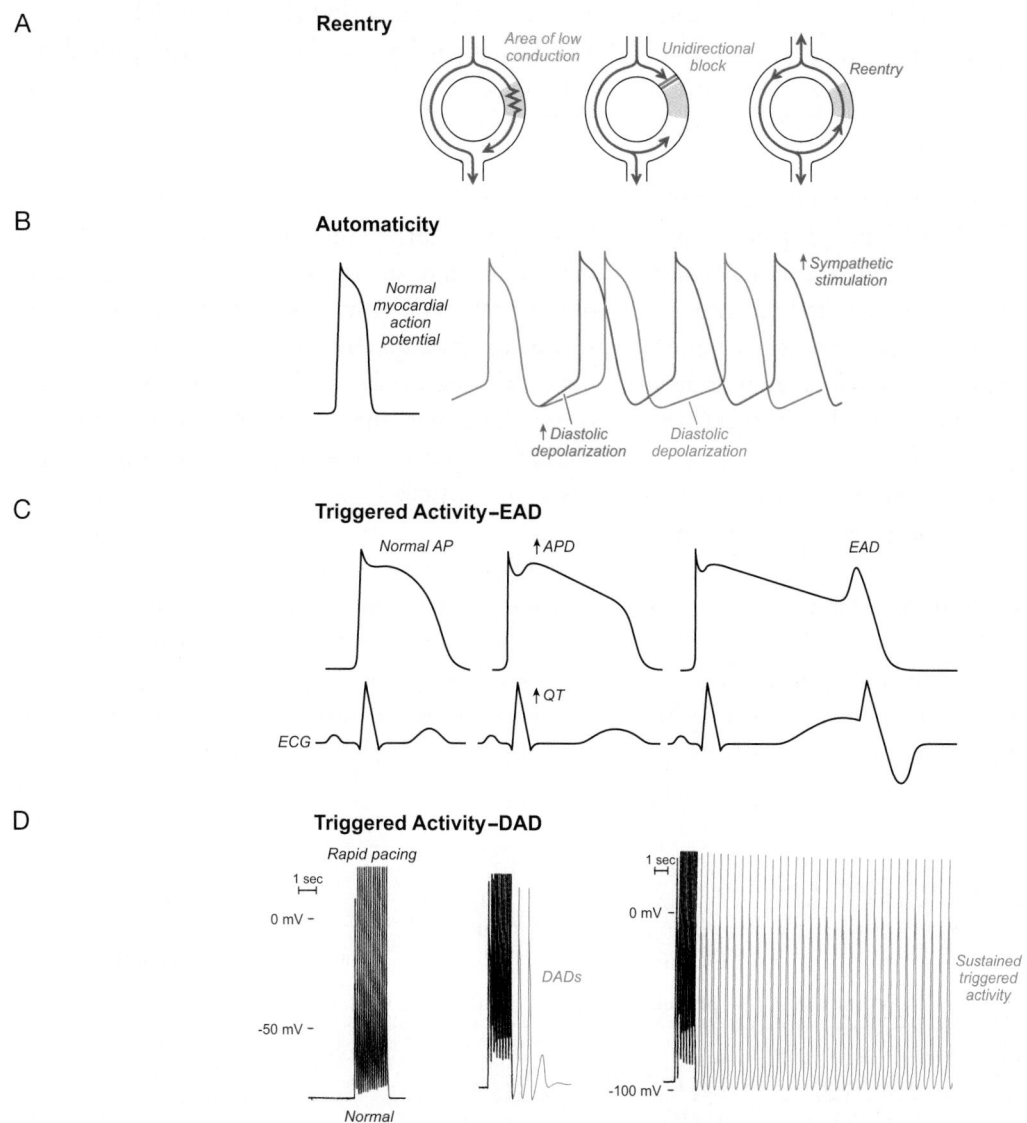

Fig. 4. *A*, Reentry arrhythmia requires the presence of a substrate and an area of slow conduction (*left panel*). Reentry is initiated by unidirectional block (*middle panel*). The electrical impulse travels from the opposite direction to the area of block when the area of block recovers, allowing reentry to occur (*right panel*). *B*, Automaticity is normally absent in atrial and ventricular myocardium (*left panel*). In injured or depolarized tissue, abnormal automaticity can occur with diastolic depolarization (*right panel*, red). Automaticity usually is augmented by sympathetic or adrenergic stimulation, which enhances the rate of diastolic depolarization (green). *C*, Triggered activity—early afterdepolarization (EAD). A normal action potential (AP) is associated with a normal QT interval (*left panel*). With an increase in action potential duration (APD) (for causes, see Table 1), QT is prolonged (*middle panel*). With further prolongation of the AP, a depolarization occurs in late phase 2 as EAD (*right panel*). Note that the depolarization occurs before complete repolarization of the AP. ECG, electrocardiogram. *D*, Triggered activity—delayed afterdepolarization (DAD). DAD in cardiac tissue is induced by rapid pacing. Normal tissue shows no afterdepolarizations (*left panel*). Under conditions of intracellular calcium overload, rapid pacing induces DADs (red, *middle panel*). Note that the depolarizations occur after complete repolarization of the action potential. Further calcium overload results in sustained triggered activity (red, *right panel*).

- Polymorphic VT with characteristic "twisting around the axis" morphology

Delayed Afterdepolarizations

Delayed afterdepolarizations (DADs) are depolarizations that occur after the action potential has completely repolarized (Fig. 4 *D*). The mechanism that underlies the development of DADs is intracellular calcium overload. DADs are thought to be associated with conditions such as digitalis toxicity, ischemic reperfusion arrhythmias, and ryanodine receptor dysfunction. Arrhythmias involving DADs are characterized by the following conditions:

1. Intracellular calcium overload
2. Exacerbation by tachycardia (which increases intracellular calcium)
3. Enhancement by sympathomimetics

Triggered activities are usually not inducible by programmed electrical stimulation. Burst pacing may be able to induce DADs and triggered activities, but current recording facilities in the electrophysiology laboratory cannot reliably record early or delayed afterdepolarizations.

INHERITED CARDIAC CHANNELOPATHIES

Conditions of arrhythmia can be inherited. Advances in molecular biology have yielded an explosive amount of information on primary ion channel abnormalities, known as *channelopathies*, that constitute the molecular basis of familial cardiac rhythm disturbances. Details of channelopathies are discussed in Chapter 22 ("Channelopathies"). Key features are highlighted below and in Table 2.

Long QT Syndrome

- Long QT syndrome is associated with mutations in membrane proteins that affect potassium channels (loss of function with decreased I_{Kr}, I_{Ks}, and I_{K1}), sodium channels (gain-of-function with incomplete inactivation during phase 2), calcium channels (gain-

Table 2. Inherited Cardiac Channelopathies

Condition	Mutation	Channel or protein affected	Effects of mutations	Relative frequency
Long QT syndrome				
LQT1	*KCNQ1*	KvLQT1	$\downarrow I_{Ks}$	+++
LQT2	*KCNH2*	hERG	$\downarrow I_{Kr}$	++
LQT3	*SCN5A*	Na+ channel	$\uparrow I_{Na}$ with noninactivating Na+ currents	+
LQT4	*ANK2*	Ankyrin B		Rare
LQT5	*KCNE1*	MinK	$\downarrow I_{Ks}$	Rare
LQT6	*KCNE2*	MiERP1	$\downarrow I_{Kr}$	Rare
LQT7 (Andersen syndrome)	*KCNJ2*	Kir2.1	$\downarrow I_{K1}$	Rare
LQT8 (Timothy syndrome	*CACNA1C*	Cav1.2	$\uparrow I_{Ca,L}$	Rare
Short QT syndrome	*KCNH2*	hERG	$\uparrow I_{Kr}$	Rare
	KCNQ1	KvLQT1	$\uparrow I_{Ks}$	Rare
	KCNJ2	Kir2.1	$\uparrow I_{K1}$	Rare
Brugada syndrome	*SCN5A*	Na+ channel	$\downarrow I_{Na}$	+
Catecholaminergic polymorphic VT	*RyR2*	Ryanodine receptor	$\uparrow$ Abnormal Ca2+ release from SR	Rare
	CASQ2	Calsequestrin		Rare

Table 2. (continued)

Condition	Mutation	Channel or protein affected	Effects of mutations	Relative frequency
Familial AF				
	KCNQ1	KvLQT1	↑ I_{Ks}	Rare
	KCNE2	MiRP1	↑ I_{Ks}	Rare
	KCNJ2	Kir2.1	↑ I_{K1}	Rare
	SCN5A	Na+ channel	↓ I_{Na}	Rare
Conduction disease				
	SCN5A	Na+ channel	↓ I_{Na}	Rare
Sinus node dysfunction				
	SCN5A	Na+ channel	↓ I_{Na}	Rare
	HCN4	Pacemaker channel	↓ I_f	Rare

Ca, calcium; $I_{Ca,L}$, L-type calcium current; I_f, pacemaker current; I_{K1}, delayed rectifier potassium current; I_{Kr}, rapid component of the delayed rectifier potassium current; I_{Ks}, slow component of the delayed rectifier potassium current; I_{Na}, sodium current; Na, sodium; SR, sarcoplasmic reticulum.

of-function), and nonchannel protein (ankyrin B).

- Mutations can occur at many different sites on the same channel protein, resulting in the loss of channel function and manifesting as the same phenotype.
- Loss-of-channel function (I_{Kr} and I_{Ks}) can be due to reduced channel expression, increased channel turnover, impaired channel maturation, and impaired channel trafficking.
- Ankyrin B mutations affect the function of the sodium-potassium pump, sodium-calcium exchange, and the inositol-1,4,5-triphosphate (IP3) receptor, resulting in abnormal calcium homeostasis and calcium overload, thereby promoting the development of DADs and EADs.

Short QT Syndrome

- Corrected QT intervals of <320 ms, high incidence of sudden cardiac death, syncope, atrial fibrillation, and frequently inducible ventricular fibrillation in structurally normal heart.
- Caused by gain-of-function mutations in potassium channels (I_{Kr}, I_{Ks}, and I_{K1}).
- Treatment with implantable cardioverter defibrillator is indicated in sudden death survivors and those with a history of syncope or a strong family history of sud-

den death.

- QT-prolonging drugs, such as sotalol and quinidine, have been used but long-term effectiveness has not been established.

Brugada Syndrome

- Autosomal dominant primary arrhythmia syndrome with male predilection (75%).
- Reduced peak I_{Na}: loss-of-function mutations of I_{Na} in 20% of patients.
- Abnormal ST in right precordial leads V_1 to V_3.
- Use of class I antiarrhythmic drugs to unmask and bring out ST abnormalities.
- Idiopathic VF, highly lethal, 40% 5-year survival in high-risk patients.
- The same mutation in I_{Na} can cause Brugada syndrome, short QT syndrome, or LQT3.
- It is the same disease as sudden unexplained death syndrome in Southeast Asia.

Catecholaminergic Polymorphic Ventricular Tachycardia

- Exercise- or stress-induced polymorphic VT, syncope, and sudden death.
- Catecholamine infusion produces polymorphic VT, bidirectional VT, and VF.

- Mutations in the cardiac ryanodine receptor (RyR2) gene (*RyR2*, autosomal dominant) and the calsequestrin (CASQ2) gene (*CASQ2*, autosomal recessive); RyR2 and CASQ2 are critical elements in intracellular calcium homeostasis and in the regulation of excitation-contraction coupling.
- RyR2 is regulated by binding to calstabin2, which keeps the channel in a closed state and prevents calcium leakage during diastole. RyR2 is activated by sympathetic stimulation, which causes the dissociation of RyR2 from calstabin2. The mutant RyR2 channels in patients with catecholaminergic polymorphic VT show decreased binding to calstabin2. Catecholamine stimulation significantly disrupts RyR2-calstabin2 interaction by increasing calcium release and producing polymorphic VT, possibly through triggered activity and DADs.

Familial Atrial Fibrillation

- Mutations causing an increase in I_{Ks} and I_{K1}.
- Mutations causing a decrease in I_{Na}.
- Atrial action potentials are shortened, with enhanced susceptibility to development of reentry and increased dispersion of refractoriness.

Other Arrhythmia Conditions

Other arrhythmias that are associated with inherited channelopathies include the following:

- *Isolated cardiac conduction disease*—a single mutation in I_{Na} (*G514C*) is manifested as cardiac impulse conduction abnormalities, including broad P waves, prolonged PR, and widened QRS in five families.
- *Congenital sick sinus syndrome*—autosomal recessive inheritance of I_{Na} mutations causes loss of function or impairment in inactivation gating with reduced cardiac excitability in 10 pediatric patients from 7 families.
- *Sinus node dysfunction*—a truncation mutation of I_f causes sick sinus syndrome in a patient with syncope.

ACQUIRED CARDIAC CHANNELOPATHIES

Abnormal ion channel expression, regulation, and function are associated with various cardiac pathologic conditions. These changes in cardiac electrophysiologic properties are thought to be the result of maladaptation to disease states, a process termed *electrical remodeling*. Some of the important examples are highlighted below and in Table 3.

Atrial Fibrillation

Atrial fibrillation is the most common sustained heart rhythm disturbance, having a prevalence of 0.4% in the general population and affecting 2.2 million Americans. Atrial fibrillation is a multifactorial disease, and its incidence increases with age. Sustained atrial fibrillation produces adaptive changes in the electrical properties of the heart or electrical remodeling, which in turn accommodates atrial fibrillation. This allows atrial fibrillation to stabilize and perpetuate—that is, atrial fibrillation begets atrial fibrillation. In the fibrillating atria, the action potential is shortened, with a loss of adaptation to rate. Contributing factors include the following:

1. Reduced functional expression of L-type calcium channels
2. Reduction in the I_{to} currents
3. Enhanced I_{K1}
4. Persistent activation of $I_{K,ACh}$

Persons who have polymorphisms involving connexin 40 have an increased susceptibility to atrial fibrillation because of slowing in impulse conduction. The overall net effect is a reduction in the atrial fibrillation wavelength, allowing more atrial fibrillation wavelets to exist simultaneously with more stable circuits. The increased spatial heterogeneity in refractoriness and conduction provides the substrate for reentry and fibrillation.

In addition to electrical remodeling, structural remodeling occurs in the atria with the development of atrial fibrillation. Atrial dilatation with a decrease in atrial contractility results from atrial fibrillation. This atrial "stunning" is probably a form of tachycardia-induced cardiomyopathy in the atria. These structural and functional changes provide further accommodation to the fibrillation wavelets, resulting in a vicious cycle.

Heart Failure

The prevalence of heart failure and the incidence of sudden death in patients with heart failure have increased steadily in the past 25 years. Currently, 5 million Americans live with heart failure and about 550,000 new cases are diagnosed annually. Patients

Table 3. Acquired Cardiac Channelopathies

Condition	Expression of channel or protein	Electrical activity	Effect
Atrial fibrillation	$\downarrow I_{Ca,L}$	$\downarrow$ AERP	Overall net effect: $\downarrow$ wavelength of tachycardia & loss of rate adaptation
	$\downarrow I_{to}$	$\uparrow$ AERP	
	$\uparrow I_{K1}$	$\downarrow$ AERP	
	$\uparrow I_{KACh}$	$\downarrow$ AERP	
	$\downarrow$ Connexin 40	$\downarrow$ Conduction	
Heart failure	$\downarrow I_{to}$	$\uparrow$ VERP	$\downarrow$ Rate adaptation
	$\downarrow I_{Kr}$	$\uparrow$ VERP	$\uparrow$ APD
	$\downarrow I_{Ks}$	$\uparrow$ VERP	$\uparrow$ EAD
	$\downarrow I_{K1}$	$\uparrow$ VERP	$\uparrow$ Automaticity
	$\uparrow$ Na$^+$/Ca^{2+} exchange		$\uparrow$ DAD
	$\uparrow I_{Ca,L}$ inactivation		$\downarrow$ APD
	Connexin-43 redistribution	$\downarrow$ Conduction	$\uparrow$ Reentry
Cardiac hypertrophy	$\uparrow I_{Ca,L}$	$\uparrow$ APD	$\uparrow$ EAD
	$\downarrow$ Na$^+$/Ca^{2+} exchange	Ca^{2+} overload	$\uparrow$ DAD
Myocardial infarction	$\downarrow$ Connexin 43	$\downarrow$ Conduction	$\uparrow$ Reentry
	$\downarrow I_{Na}$	$\downarrow$ Conduction	
	$\downarrow I_{to}$	$\uparrow$ VERP	
	$\downarrow I_{Kr}$	$\uparrow$ VERP	
	$\downarrow I_{Ks}$	$\uparrow$ VERP	
	$\downarrow I_{Ca,L}$	$\downarrow$ Plateau	

AERP, atrial effective refractory period; APD, action potential duration; Ca, calcium; DAD, delayed after depolarization; EAD, early afterdepolarization; $I_{Ca,L}$, L-type calcium current; I_{K1}, strong inward rectifier potassium current; $I_{K,ACh}$, acetylcholine-sensitive potassium current; I_{Kr}, rapid component of the delayed rectifier potassium current; I_{Ks}, slow component of the delayed rectifier potassium current; I_{Na}, sodium current; I_{to}, transient outward potassium current; VERP, ventricular effective refractory period.

with class III or IV heart failure have a 2-year mortality rate of 50%, and many of these patients die from arrhythmia. Electrical remodeling occurs in heart failure; the hallmark is prolongation of the ventricular action potential, resulting from: 1. down-regulation of repolarizing potassium currents, including I_{to}, I_{Kr}, I_{Ks}, and I_{K1}; and
2. altered intracellular calcium homeostasis.

Diminution in I_{to} leads to the loss-of-rate adaptation of the cardiac action potential. A decrease in I_{Kr} and I_{Ks} leads to prolongation of the action potential duration with an increase in propensity for developing EADs and triggered activity. Reduced I_{K1} leads to enhanced automaticity and prolongation of the termination portion of phase 3 of the action potential.

An increase in intracellular calcium may increase inactivation of the L-type calcium currents, enhance sodium-calcium exchange activities, and cause the development of DADs and triggered activity.

In addition, long-standing heart failure is associated with structural remodeling, which includes interstitial fibrosis, cardiac chamber dilatation, and connexin 43 redistribution. This results in reduced impulse conduction velocity and increased anisotropy, providing the substrate for reentry.

Cardiac Hypertrophy

Cardiac hypertrophy occurs in many pathologic conditions, including ischemic heart disease, hypertension, valvular heart disease, and heart failure. Cardiac hypertrophy is an independent predictor of morbidity and mortality and predisposes the heart to the development of arrhythmia, ischemia, and congestive failure. The ventricular action potential of the hypertrophied heart is prolonged. Unlike the situation in heart failure, the prolongation in cardiac hypertrophy is due to the following:

1. $I_{Ca,L}$ upregulation
2. No change in I_{to} and I_{K1}
3. Reduced sodium-calcium exchange activity with intracellular calcium overload
4. The prolongation of the action potential is more pronounced in the endocardial layers, where I_{to} is weak

The hypertrophied heart is susceptible to developing arrhythmia from triggered activity. EADs may result from prolonged action potential durations and DADs from an increase in intracellular calcium overload. Cardiac hypertrophy is also associated with interstitial fibrosis with myofibrillar disarray, leading to altered impulse conduction and dispersion of refractoriness.

Myocardial Infarction

Patients with previous myocardial infarctions have an increased risk of life-threatening ventricular tachycardia and ventricular fibrillation. The peri-infarct zone appears to be the main site where significant electrical remodeling takes place. In the human infarct border zone, connexin 43 is displaced from its usual location in intercalated disks to random locations over the cell surface. Also, I_{Na} density is reduced with altered channel kinetics, including enhanced current inactivation. These changes underlie reduced cardiac excitability, with slowing of the impulse conduction velocity, which contributes to reentry arrhythmias. In addition, the densities of $I_{Ca,L}$, I_{to}, I_{Kr}, and I_{Ks} have all been found to be reduced in the infarct border zone. The remodeling of ion channels alters action potential configuration and creates heterogeneity in repolarization, contributing to the development of arrhythmias.

20

NORMAL AND ABNORMAL CARDIAC ELECTROPHYSIOLOGY

Douglas L. Packer, MD

THE HEART'S ELECTRICAL SYSTEM

Sinus Node

The sinus node is a tapered cylindrical structure that lies subepicardially at the junction between the right atrium and the superior vena cava. Histologically, the sinus node consists of several cell types that are embedded within a connective tissue stroma. Round or ovoid P cells are probably the site of impulse formation, and transitional cells, which are considerably greater in number, serve as the link between the P cells and the remaining atrial tissue (Fig. 1).

Atrioventricular Node

The atrioventricular (AV) node is a dense structure positioned in the subendocardium of the low right atrium at the apex of the triangle of Koch (formed by the ostium of the coronary sinus, the tendon of Todaro, and the septal attachment of the tricuspid valve leaflet). Several cell types are present within the AV node, including P cells similar to those found in the sinoatrial node, N (or nodal) cells comprising the compact node, and transitional cells between atrial and nodal tissue (Fig. 2).

■ The P cells within the sinoatrial node are probably the site of formation of normal cardiac impulse.

Intra-atrial Pathways

There is evidence for the preferential spread of atrial activation between the sinus and AV nodes by way of intranodal pathways, but whether these are true tracts or simply preferential pathways of conduction remains unclear. These tracts are the anterior internodal tract, which curves leftward and anteriorly around the superior vena cava; the middle internodal tract, which crosses toward the interatrial septum to join the anterior internodal tract; and the posterior pathway, which exits posteriorly from the sinus node and courses toward the inferior vena cava. The Bachmann bundle may represent an alternative specialized tract for impulse propagation between atria (Fig. 3).

■ Intra-atrial pathways are less well defined than the His-Purkinje system and are likely facilitated by the electrophysiologic properties of those atrial fibers.

His-Purkinje System

The His bundle begins from the inferior portion of the AV node, penetrates the fibrous portion of the interventricular septum, and travels down across the muscular septum to the remainder of the ventricles. The right bundle branch is more discrete than the left bundle branch. Activation of the right ventricle spreads peripherally through specialized Purkinje fibers.

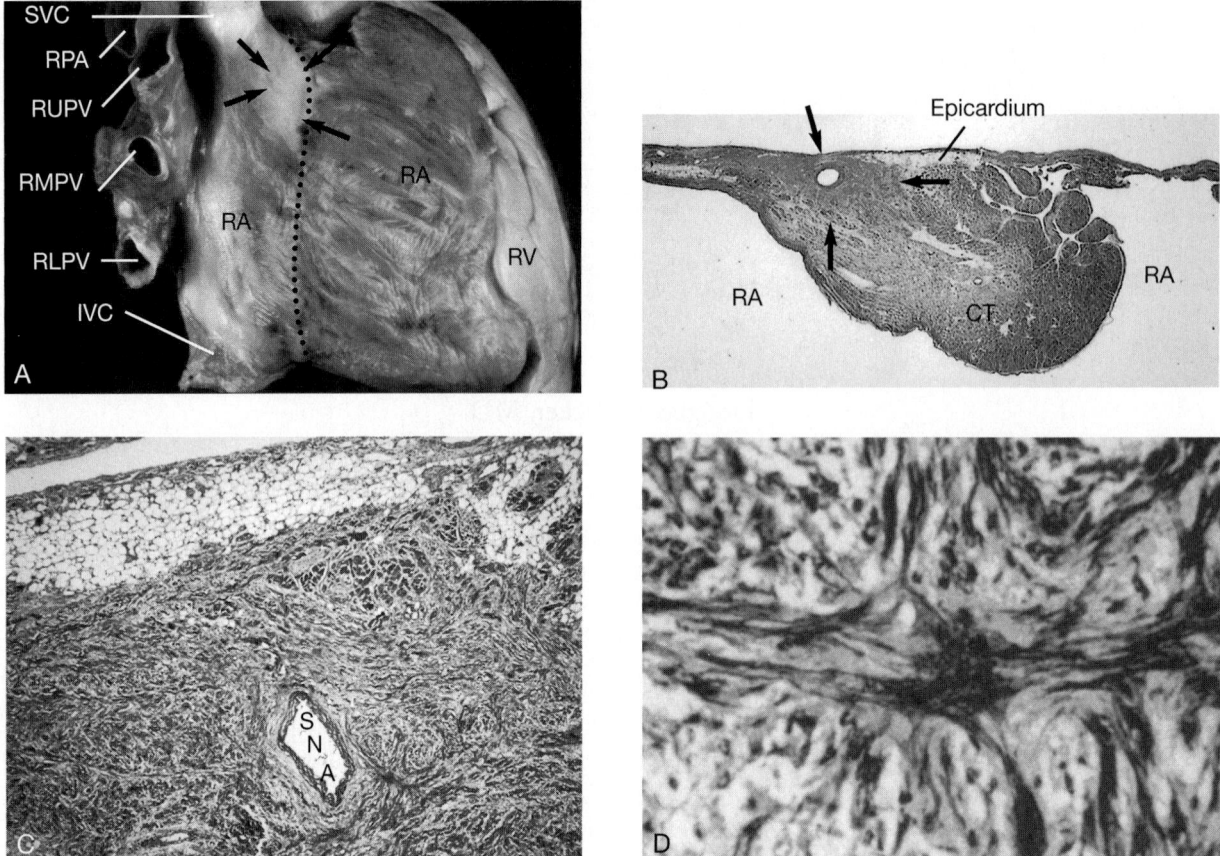

Fig. 1. Sinus node. *A,* The sinus node (*arrows*) lies in the sulcus terminalis (*dotted line*) near the cavoatrial junction. (Right lateral view from 32-year-old man.) *B,* The sinus node (*arrows*) is a subepicardial structure that overlies the superolateral portion of the crista terminalis. (Trichrome x5; from 61-year-old man.) *C,* The sinus nodal artery (SNA) courses through the center of the sinus node. (Trichrome x20; from 20-year-old man.) *D,* The specialized myocardial cells of the sinus node form an interlacing pattern. (Trichrome x100; from 20-year-old man.) CT, crista terminalis; IVC, inferior vena cava; RA, right atrium; RLPV, right lower pulmonary vein; RMPV, right middle pulmonary vein; RPA, right pulmonary artery; RUPV, right upper pulmonary vein; RV, right ventricle; SVC, superior vena cava.

Alternatively, the left bundle branch, which may be described in terms of the left anterior and left posterior hemifascicles, is less discrete, particularly proximally, where the left bundle proper is a sheet of specialized conducting tissue rather than a discrete bundle. Purkinje cells of the bundle and peripheral branches are large: 15 to 30 μm in diameter and 20 to 100 μm in length. These cells, in turn, arborize with actual myocardial cells to facilitate local ventricular activation. The vascular supply of the conduction system is shown in Figure 4.

TISSUE ELECTROPHYSIOLOGIC PROPERTIES

Fast Action Potentials

Atrial, ventricular, and His-Purkinje tissues show characteristic action potentials with rapid upstrokes (phase 0), as described by V_{max} (most rapid rate of increase of the upstroke of the action potential), the values of which range up to 300 V/s in atrial and ventricular tissue and up to 900 V/s in Purkinje tissue (Fig. 5). In these tissues, the upstrokes of the action potential are generated by inward sodium current, with calcium cur-

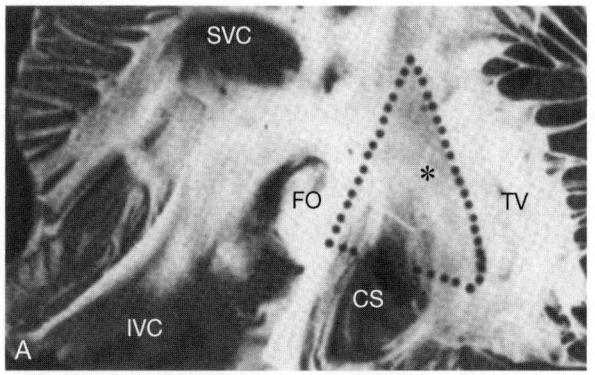

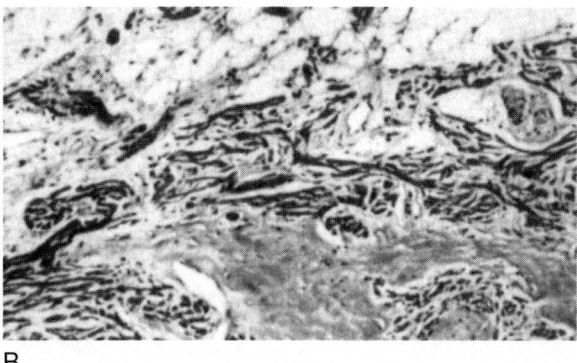

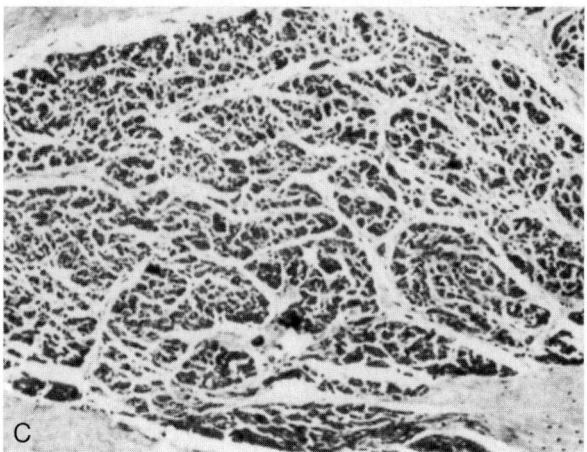

Fig. 2. Atrioventricular (AV) conduction system. *A*, The AV node (*) lies within the triangle of Koch (*dotted lines*), along the right atrial aspect of the AV septum. (Opened right atrium from 32-year-old man.) *B*, The node is characterized by an interlacing pattern of specialized myocardial cells. (Trichrome x50; from 20-year-old man.) *C*, The AV bundle consists of parallel bundles of specialized myocardial cells. (Trichrome x50; from 20-year-old man.) CS, coronary sinus; FO, fossa ovalis; IVC, inferior vena cava; SVC, superior vena cava; TV, tricuspid valve.

rents contributing to active sinoatrial and AV nodal tissue. The action potential durations are shortest in atrial cells, intermediate in ventricular myocytes, and longer in Purkinje cells. The duration of the action potential and the characteristic contours of repolarization are determined largely by outgoing potassium currents, although inward calcium currents contribute to a lesser degree (Fig. 6). These calcium currents are more responsible for phase 2 of the action potential. Resting membrane potentials typically range from –80 to –90 mV, and activation thresholds from –60 to –70 mV. The action potential amplitudes are large, ranging from 90 to 130 mV.

- Upstrokes of the action potential in atrial, His-Purkinje, and ventricular tissue are generated by inward sodium current.
- Action potential durations are shortest in atrial cells, intermediate in ventricular myocytes, and longer in Purkinje cells.

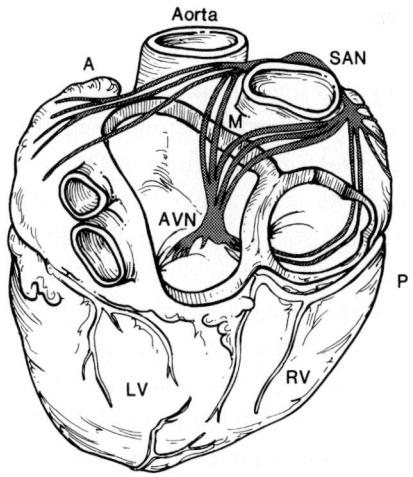

Fig. 3. Posterior schematic of the heart with internodal pathways connecting the sinoatrial node (SAN) and atrioventricular node (AVN). The anterior internodal tract (A) curves leftward and anteriorly around the superior vena cava. The middle internodal tract (M) crosses toward the interatrial system to join the anterior internodal tract. The posterior pathway (P) exits posteriorly and courses toward the inferior vena cava. LV, left ventricle; RV, right ventricle.

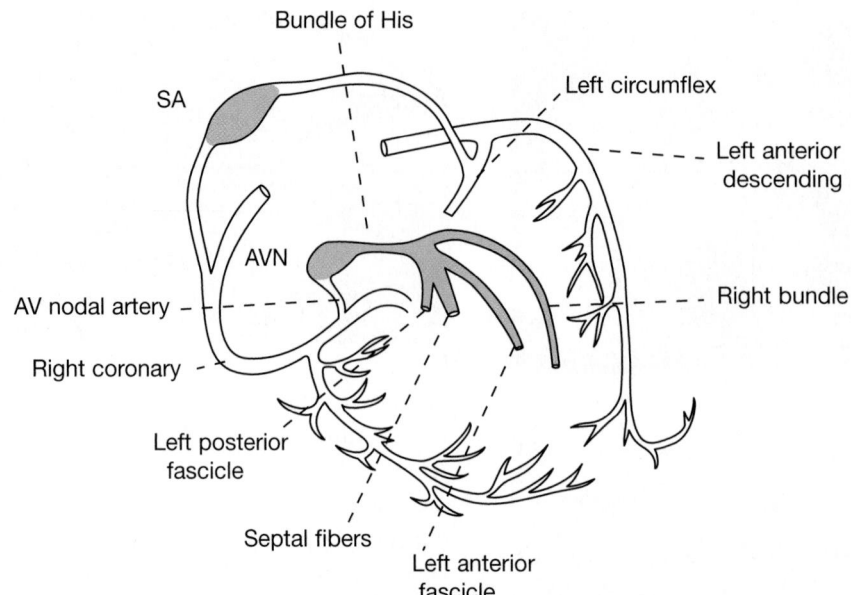

Fig. 4. Schematic of the vascular supply to the cardiac conduction system. The sinus node artery may arise from the right coronary artery (55%-65%) or as a branch of the left circumflex (35%-45%). The atrioventricular node (AVN) artery arises from the right coronary artery in 90% of patients. The right coronary artery also supplies the common His bundle and portions of the right bundle. The left anterior descending coronary artery also supplies blood to the His bundle by way of septal perforators and the left anterior fascicle. The left posterior fascicle usually receives a blood supply from both the right coronary artery (posterior descending) and the left anterior descending artery. SA, sinoatrial node.

Slow Action Potentials

In contrast, the sinoatrial nodal and AV nodal cells are activated by slow inward calcium-carried currents. As such, the rates of activation and inactivation are slower, membrane potentials range from −40 to −70 mV, activation thresholds range from −30 to −40 mV, and the V_{max} of the upstroke of action potentials is typically slow, less than 15 V/s (Fig. 7). In addition, cells of the sinus and AV nodal regions demonstrate phase 4 depolarization, in which there is a gradual reduction in the negativity of the membrane potential during the diastolic interval. These cells are also highly influenced by both sympathetic and parasympathetic nerve input, which increases or decreases the rate of phase 4 depolarization. Similarly, these cells may be modulated by catecholamines or acetylcholine. Because conduction is driven by the slow inward current, conduction velocities are more on the order of 0.01 to 0.1 m/s. In contrast, velocities in fast-current tissue range from 0.5 to 3.0 m/s.

Table 1 lists the features of fast and slow inward currents of the action potential.

■ Sinoatrial nodal and AV nodal cells are activated by slow inward calcium-carried currents.

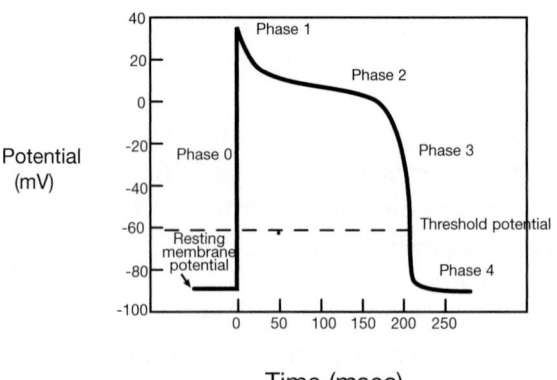

Time (msec)

Fig. 5. Action potential with five phases. The resting membrane potential is −90 mV. In spontaneously active cells, there is slow diastolic depolarization during phase 4, which returns the fiber toward the threshold potential.

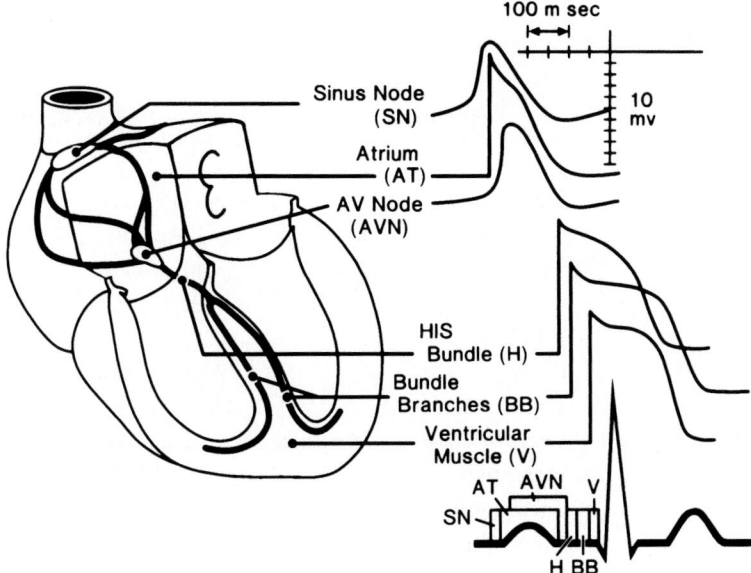

Fig. 6. Action potentials recorded from different regions of the heart. Action potentials from the sinus and certain cells in the atrioventricular (AV) node are similar and distinct from those from the rest of the heart.

Tissue Refractoriness

In addition to the action potential durations, all cardiac cells show refractoriness, which is the fundamental resistance to reexcitation after a previous electrical activation. This resistance can be described in terms of effective refractoriness, which can be measured by the introduction of an extrastimulus. In such testing, the effective refractory period is the longest paired S_1-S_2 (first heart sound-second heart sound) impulse coupling interval that does not activate the cell when introduced at twice the diastolic threshold during the diastolic interval.

■ The effective refractory period of the cell is the longest paired S_1-S_2 impulse coupling interval that does not activate the cell.

Tissue Innervation

All cardiac tissue is innervated by both sympathetic and parasympathetic nerves. In atrial tissue, parasympathetic nerve stimulation produces shortening of the duration of the action potential and slowing of conduction. Sympathetic nerve activation may also shorten the duration of the action potential, but it accelerates conduction. In AV nodal tissue, parasympathetic nerve stimulation, as mediated by acetylcholine release, results in the slowing of conduction and prolongation of refractoriness, whereas the opposite reaction occurs with sympathetic nerve stimulation. In contrast, refractoriness of ventricular tissue typically is decreased by

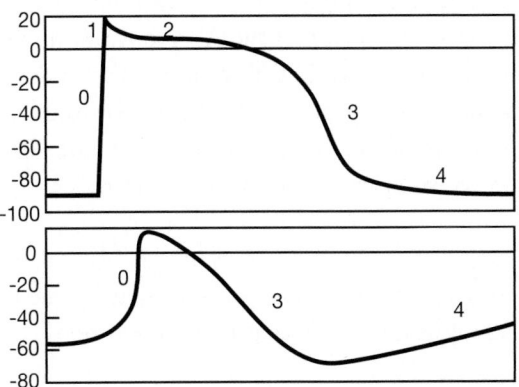

Fig. 7. Action potentials recorded by intracellular electrodes from two types of cardiac cells. *Top*, Action potential recorded from a cell that is dependent mainly on a rapid-current, fast-channel response. *Bottom*, Action potential recorded from a sinus node cell that is dependent on a slow inward current. The slow inward current is characterized by lower resting and activation potentials and slower conduction velocity. Numbers 0 through 4 refer to the phases shown in Figure 5.

Table 1. Distinguishing Features of Fast and Slow Inward Currents of the Action Potential

Characteristic	Fast current	Slow current
Main ion	Na$^+$	Ca^{2+}
Rates of activation and inactivation	Rapid	Slow
Activation threshold, mV	−60 to −70	−30 to −40
Resting membrane potential, mV	−80 to −90	−40 to −70
Conduction velocity, m/s	0.5-3.0	0.01-0.1
Action potential amplitude, mV	100-130	35-75
Recovery	Prompt	Delayed, outlasts full repolarization
Current decreased by	Tetrodotoxin Decreased resting membrane potential Local anesthetics	Manganese, verapamil, D600, nifedipine, diltiazem, perhexiline, acetylcholine
Current enhanced by	Veratridine	Catecholamines, cAMP
Role in nodal automaticity	Doubtful	Probable
Role in toxic or ischemic arrhythmias	?	Possible

cAMP, cyclic adenosine monophosphate.

sympathetic nerve activation but increased by parasympathetic nerve activation. Interestingly, both sympathetic and parasympathetic nerve stimulation have relatively little effect on ventricular conduction. These nerves follow a characteristic course to the individual myocardial cells. Both sets of fibers typically enter the ventricles in the region of the AV groove. Although sympathetic fibers may initially course in a subendocardial location, they penetrate the ventricular wall location to course along the epicardial surface. The opposite occurs with parasympathetic nerve fibers.

■ Sympathetic and parasympathetic nerve stimulation have major effects on sinus and AV nodal tissue but relatively little effect on ventricular conduction.

NORMAL RHYTHM GENERATION

Cardiac cells have the ability for spontaneous action potential formation (automaticity). This manifests itself in a hierarchical pattern: sinus nodal tissue tends to be more automatic than atrial tissue, which is, in turn, more automatic than AV nodal, His-Purkinje, or ventricular cells. This hierarchy is due to differences in the intrinsic automaticity of the cells, which is

dependent on 1) the slope and rate of phase 4 depolarization, which sets the rate of impulse formation; 2) the threshold potential, at which the action potential is initiated; and 3) the maximal diastolic potential, from which phase 4 spontaneous depolarization begins. Typically, normal sinus node rates range between 60 and 100 beats per minute. In contrast, junctional tissue produces rates in the range of 50 to 60 beats per minute, and ventricular automaticity, when observed in the absence of higher pacemakers, usually produces rates of only 30 to 45 beats per minute.

■ Sinus nodal tissue is more automatic than atrial tissue, which is, in turn, more automatic than AV nodal, His-Purkinje, or ventricular cells.

Sinus node function can be assessed in terms of *sinus node recovery time*, or the time required for repeat sinus node activation after prolonged overdrive suppression of the node by pacing the atria at rates of 100 to 175 beats per minute. Normal values of sinus node recovery times are usually less than 1,500 ms. The corrected sinus node recovery time provides a more accurate description of sinus node "normalcy." This is calculated by subtracting the baseline sinus rate from the sinus node recovery time. Normal values of the corrected sinus node recovery time are typically less than 550 to 600 ms. Because of sinus node automaticity, it is considerably more difficult to assess recovery times from overdrive suppression of AV nodal or junctional tissue. Nevertheless, in the absence of a functioning sinus node or after the creation of AV conduction system block, lower-level pacemakers can emerge, at the above-mentioned rates.

ABNORMAL RHYTHM GENERATION

Abnormal Automaticity

Abnormal automaticity may create impulse formation in regions other than the sinus node. Such automaticity may occur in ischemic or other diseased cardiac tissues. Spontaneous depolarization of affected cardiac fibers occurs, particularly when atrial or ventricular resting membrane potentials are reduced to values less than -60 mV. Abnormal atrial automatic rhythms typically arise from the region of the crista terminalis, around pulmonary veins, or in the pericoronary sinus orifice region. Some ventricular tachycardias, which also may be automatic in mechanism, are usually catecholamine-dependent.

Triggered Automaticity

An additional mechanism of abnormal arrhythmia generation is that of triggered automaticity. This term is used to describe arrhythmias originating from afterdepolarizations or oscillatory afterpotentials occurring during diastole which reach threshold and generate subsequent action potentials. These afterdepolarizations are typically dependent on prior activation of the heart and can be further classified as early afterdepolarizations if they occur during phase 2 or 3 of the action potential or as delayed afterdepolarizations if they occur after complete repolarization. The early afterdepolarizations are typically pause-dependent. Such a pause may be set up by a prior premature depolarization. Early afterdepolarizations are facilitated by low potassium level, low magnesium level, or potassium channel block with agents such as quinidine, N-acetylprocainamide, sotalol, dofetilide, or other class 1 or 3 antiarrhythmic agents (Table 2). Various other drugs may similarly prolong the action potential duration by modulation of constituent ionic currents. Some of these include erythromycin, pentamidine, and terfenadine. Early afterdepolarizations are probably responsible for torsades de pointes, which is polymorphic ventricular tachycardia with QRS morphologic features that appear to twist around an isoelectric baseline and

Table 2.   Factors That Influence Early Afterdepolarization

Factor	Increase	Decrease
Autonomic	↑ sympathetic tone	↓ sympathetic tone
	↑ catecholamines	↓ catecholamines
	↓ parasympathetic tone	↑ parasympathetic tone
Metabolic	↑ hypoxia	↑ O_2
	↑ acidosis	↓ acidosis
Electrolytes	$C_s{}^+$	K^+
	Hypokalemia	Mg^{2+}
Drugs and metabolites	Sotalol	Acetylcholine/adenosine
	N-acetylprocainamide	Lidocaine
	Quinidine	Procainamide
	Aconitine	Ca^{2+} channel blockers
	Veratridine	β-Blockers
		Tetrodotoxin
		K^+ channel openers
Heart rate	Slow	Fast

occurring in the setting of a prolonged QT interval. Similar abnormalities may occur in patients with the congenital long QT syndromes.

In contrast, delayed afterdepolarizations, which occur during phase 4 of diastole, are more likely to occur after rapid, repetitive pacing. These are thought to be related to accumulation of intracellular calcium and activation of a nonspecific cation channel. The most common cause of the delayed afterdepolarization type of arrhythmia is digitalis toxicity. With digitalis, the sodium-potassium pump is inhibited, producing an increase in intracellular sodium and subsequent acceleration of sodium for calcium exchange. Both abnormal atrial and ventricular arrhythmias may have triggered automaticity as an underlying mechanism. A potential clue to the presence of such a mechanism is the termination of arrhythmias with calcium channel blockers or adenosine, although reentrant arrhythmias under certain circumstances may be interrupted by these agents.

- Early afterdepolarizations are thought responsible for torsades de pointes.
- The most common cause of the delayed afterdepolarization type of arrhythmia is digitalis toxicity.

ARRHYTHMIAS RELATED TO ABNORMAL IMPULSE CONDUCTION

AV Conduction
Electrical impulse propagation through atrial, ventricular, or specialized tissues occurs with each cardiac activation. Purkinje tissue may have conduction velocities of 1 to 3 m/s, but conduction velocity in atrial or ventricular tissue is substantially slower, about 0.3 m/s. On the scale of the intact heart, conduction through the atrium can be expressed as the PA interval, taken as the onset of the surface P wave to the activation of the atrial tissue in the region of the AV node, as recorded on the His bundle electrogram. The normal PA interval is 20 to 50 ms.

In addition, conduction through the AV node is reflected by the AH interval, or the point of earliest rapid upstroke of the atrial deflection on the His bundle electrogram to the similar rapid onset of the deflection recorded from the His bundle. Under normal

conditions, the AH interval ranges between 60 and 120 ms. In some patients, enhanced AV nodal physiology may be observed, in which the AH interval may be less than 60 ms, prolongation of the AH interval which typically occurs with faster pacing is limited, and propagation by way of the AV node persists with atrial pacing rates in excess of 200 beats per minute (Fig. 8).

Conduction through the His-Purkinje system is reflected in the HV interval, which is taken as the onset of the His bundle deflection to the onset of the ventricular deflection recorded on the His bundle electrogram or the onset of the QRS. Normal HV intervals range between 35 and 60 ms. In patients with diseased His-Purkinje conduction, HV intervals are longer than 60 ms. The exact implication of HV intervals in the range of 60 to 80 ms is unclear. In patients with syncope, bifascicular conduction block on the surface electrocardiogram, and an HV interval longer than 70 ms, infra-His block is the likely cause of the syncopal episode. AV block below the His bundle during rapid atrial pac-

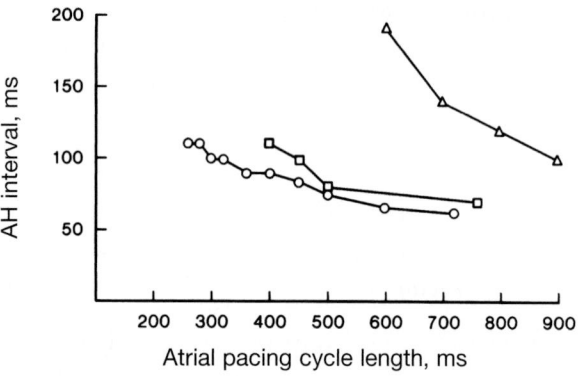

Fig. 8. Response of atrioventricular (AV) node to atrial pacing. Most common response is a gradual increase in the AH interval and then AV node block at less than 200 beats per minute. This is seen in patient □, in whom the resting AH is 70 ms at 80 beats per minute and increases to 110 ms at 150 beats per minute and then AV node Wenckebach periodicity. Patient ○ had accelerated AV node conduction with an initial AH of 60 ms, which increased to 110 ms with atrial pacing at 250 beats per minute (240 ms). Patient △ had abnormal AV node conduction and an initial AH of 100 ms, which increased to 190 ms with pacing at 100 beats per minute (600 ms). AV node Wenckebach periodicity then developed.

ing also suggests significant conduction system disease, which should be treated with permanent ventricular pacing.

In 0.1% of patients, normal activation of the ventricles by way of the AV conduction system can be short-circuited. This may result from the presence of an accessory pathway that bridges atrial and ventricular tissue. Because a portion of the ventricle may be activated before the onset of activation of the His-Purkinje system, ventricular tissue is said to be preexcited. This phenomenon is accompanied by the appearance of slurred upstrokes of surface QRS complexes (delta waves) and a very short or negative HV interval.

- Conduction through the atrium can be expressed as the PA interval.
- The normal PA interval is 20-50 ms.
- Conduction through the AV node is reflected by the AH interval.
- Under normal conditions, the AH interval ranges from 60-120 ms.
- Conduction through the His-Purkinje system is reflected in the HV interval.
- Normal HV intervals range from 35-60 ms.

Reentrant Arrhythmias

Conduction abnormalities in cardiac tissue may contribute to reentrant arrhythmias. The mechanisms of reentry involve three requisite conditions: 1) at least two functionally distinct conducting pathways, 2) unidirectional block in one pathway, and 3) slower conduction down a second conduction pathway, with return by way of the second pathway (Fig. 9). Initially, these mechanisms of reentry were observed in the setting of an anatomical obstacle around which a circulating impulse could propagate. Subsequent studies have clearly demonstrated that reentry also may occur in the absence of such an obstacle, strictly because of the properties of conduction and refractoriness in atrial or ventricular tissue. One form of such reentry is referred to as *functional*. In this type of reentry, a circulating impulse travels around an area of tissue rendered refractory by centripetal activation into the center of circuit. Although the anatomical obstacle form of reentry may be more likely to occur in the presence of atrial flutter or ventricular tachycardia in patients with islands of infarcted myocardium, functional reentry is undoubtedly operative in other forms of atypical atrial flutter or atrial fibrillation.

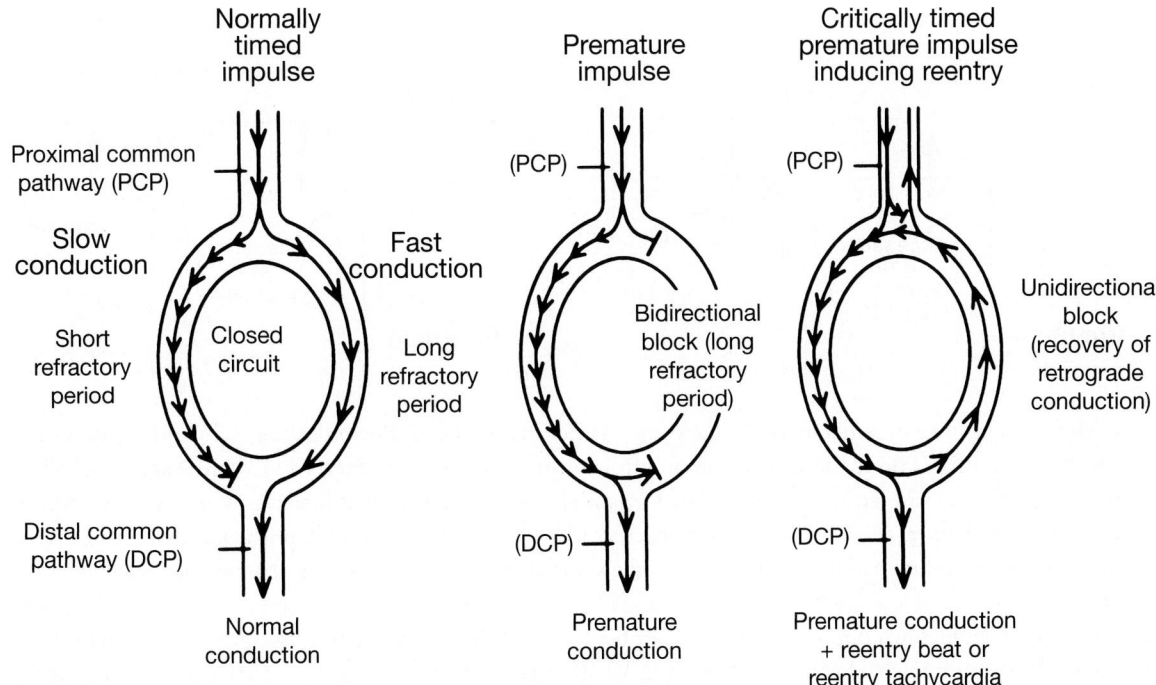

Fig. 9. Description of a reentrant circuit as a mechanism in initiating and sustaining tachycardia.

For understanding of the reentrant arrhythmias, it is often useful to consider the wavelength of a tachycardia, which is the minimal tachycardia circuit length that is necessary for the perpetuation of a reentrant arrhythmia, given the electrical properties of that circuit. The wavelength is the product of the functional refractory period and the conduction velocity. If conduction velocity is slowed or refractoriness is decreased, the minimal potential circuit length is similarly decreased, leading to an increased likelihood of an arrhythmia. However, when tissue refractoriness is significantly prolonged, as may be the case with an antiarrhythmic drug, the wavelength needed to perpetuate a reentrant arrhythmia increases. If the available circuits are of only limited size, that increase in refractoriness could produce a favorable elimination of the reentrant arrhythmia. In the case of atrial fibrillation, such an increase in refractoriness due to a drug results in the need for progressively larger tissue circuits for perpetuation of arrhythmia. Because the atria are of finite size in patients with atrial fibrillation, the five to seven circulating wavelets that typically compose atrial fibrillation increase in size and undergo coalescence to progressively fewer circuits and subsequent elimination of

atrial fibrillation. The mechanisms of reentry involve three requisite conditions:

- At least two functionally distinct conducting pathways.
- Unidirectional block in one pathway.
- Slower conduction down a second conduction pathway.

ARRHYTHMIAS ASSOCIATED WITH PREEXCITATION

Orthodromic Reciprocating Tachycardia
An additional form of macroreentry is that of orthodromic reciprocating tachycardia in patients with accessory pathways. In these patients, an electrical impulse propagates down the normal AV conduction system, inscribing a normal QRS complex on a surface electrocardiogram during tachycardia. The electrical impulse then propagates to an accessory pathway bridging between ventricular and atrial tissue, leading to retrograde atrial activation by way of the pathway (Fig. 10 *A*). If the accessory pathway is well removed from the region of the interventricular or atrial septum,

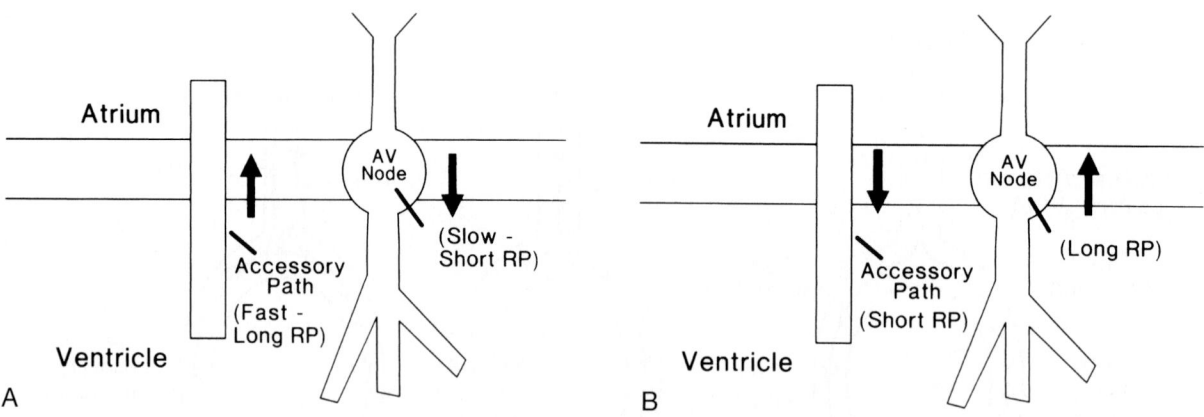

Fig. 10. Mechanisms of tachycardia in Wolff-Parkinson-White syndrome. *A,* Reciprocating tachycardia (also called orthodromic tachycardia). This is the most common mechanism of tachycardia observed in Wolff-Parkinson-White syndrome. In this form, tachycardia is often initiated by a premature atrial beat that blocks in the accessory pathway and then is conducted antegrade down the atrioventricular (AV) node. The impulse then is conducted retrograde to the atrium over the accessory pathway and returns to the ventricle over the AV node. In this manner, a reciprocating tachycardia is sustained. Unless functional bundle branch block is present, the QRS complex will be narrow, going to its antegrade conduction down normal AV conduction tissues. *B,* More unusual form of reciprocating tachycardia (sometimes called antidromic tachycardia) observed in Wolff-Parkinson-White syndrome in which the antegrade limb of the reentry circuit is the accessory pathway and the retrograde limb is the AV node. In this circumstance, the QRS complex is wide. RP, refractory period.

atrial activation as recorded on catheters positioned along the free-wall regions of the AV groove may show earlier atrial activation than that present in the septum. This is clearly distinctive from retrograde atrial activation by way of the normal VA conduction system. With return of the electrical impulse through the atria back down the normal AV conduction system, the cycle repeats itself.

Antidromic Tachycardia

In some patients, the pattern of excitation may reverse, yielding an antidromic tachycardia (Fig. 10 *B*). In such patients, activation of the ventricle proceeds by way of the accessory pathway, inscribing a maximally preexcited QRS complex on the surface electrocardiogram during tachycardia. Subsequent activation of the atria occurs by way of the normal VA conduction system, yielding activation of the atria in the center of the atrial septum and subsequent reactivation of the ventricles by way of the accessory pathway.

Dual AV Nodal Physiology

Some patients with dual AV nodal physiology may have AV nodal reentrant tachycardia. These patients may be viewed conceptually as having dual AV nodal pathways in which the electrical impulses activating the ventricle proceed by way of a fast pathway with a long refractory period or a slow pathway with shorter refractoriness. In these patients, an atrial premature complex may produce block in the fast pathway, resulting in delayed AV nodal propagation through the slow pathway. If this conduction is sufficiently slow to allow recovery of the fast pathway, retrograde return activation by way of the fast structure may lead to repeat atrial activation and subsequent conduction through the slow AV nodal pathway. Because an electrical impulse conducts through the His-Purkinje system into the ventricles with each circulating impulse, a tachycardia with a narrow QRS complex is observed.

Ventricular Tachycardia

In a similar but more microscopic fashion, ventricular tachycardia may occur in patients with diseased ventricular myocardium, such as that caused by a prior myocardial infarction. In these patients, the islands of infarcted tissue surrounded by some strands of tissue that continues to function may provide the requisite two or more potential conduction pathways. With a ventricular premature complex, block may occur in one pathway, with subsequent propagation occurring by way of a second conducting pathway. If this conduction is sufficiently slow, the impulse may return by way of the first pathway, leading to completion of the reentrant circuit.

- Orthodromic reciprocating tachycardia occurs when an electrical impulse propagates down the normal AV conduction system, inscribing a normal QRS complex on a surface electrocardiogram during tachycardia.
- Antidromic tachycardia occurs when activation of the ventricle proceeds by way of the accessory pathway, inscribing a maximally preexcited QRS complex on the surface electrocardiogram during tachycardia.

INDICATIONS FOR ELECTROPHYSIOLOGIC TESTING

Michael J. Osborn, MD

Electrophysiologic (EP) testing encompasses both invasive and noninvasive procedures that actively evaluate cardiac electrical function for diagnostic or therapeutic purposes, including the following studies: catheter-based diagnostic studies such as classic EP studies and esophageal stimulation and recording studies; noninvasive atrial and ventricular stimulation typically using implanted devices; head-up tilt testing with carotid sinus massage; drug infusion studies; and catheter mapping and radiofrequency ablation procedures.

It is important to appreciate when diagnostic electrophysiologic testing is indicated, what type of testing is appropriate in a given patient, what kind of information can be obtained from a particular test, and any risks associated with a test. Recently published clinical trials have altered our approach to many arrhythmias; therefore, one should clearly understand indications for invasive EP testing and for head-up tilt testing. One should also understand when additional testing is *not* appropriate, that is, the likely benefits do not outweigh the risks or device therapy is already indicated.

ELECTROPHYSIOLOGIC STUDY

A classic invasive EP study involves the insertion of multiple catheters into the femoral and jugular veins and occasionally the femoral artery. Once these catheters are in appropriate positions in the right atrium, at the tricuspid anulus, in the right ventricle, and in the coronary sinus os, resting intracardiac activity is assessed and recorded.

During resting rhythm, measurements of conduction through the atrium (PA interval), atrioventricular (AV) node (AH interval), and His-Purkinje system (HV interval) are recorded (Fig. 1). This assessment is followed by atrial pacing, which allows for assessment of sinus node function through the sinus node recovery time (Fig. 2). This is expressed as the longest return cycle after the cessation of atrial pacing and is corrected for the underlying sinus rate. Corrected sinus node recovery times in excess of 525 milliseconds are indicative of abnormal sinus node automaticity. This finding is highly specific for sinus node dysfunction, but this and other techniques are not sensitive predictors and identify only about 50% of cases of proven sinus node disease.

Conduction through the AV node and His-Purkinje system is also assessed with atrial pacing. AV node conduction should be maintained up to rates of 120 beats per minute followed by AV node block at rates between 120 and 200 beats per minute. During atrial pacing, AV block should occur at the level of the AV node. Block in the His-Purkinje system (distal to

HIS BUNDLE ELECTROGRAM

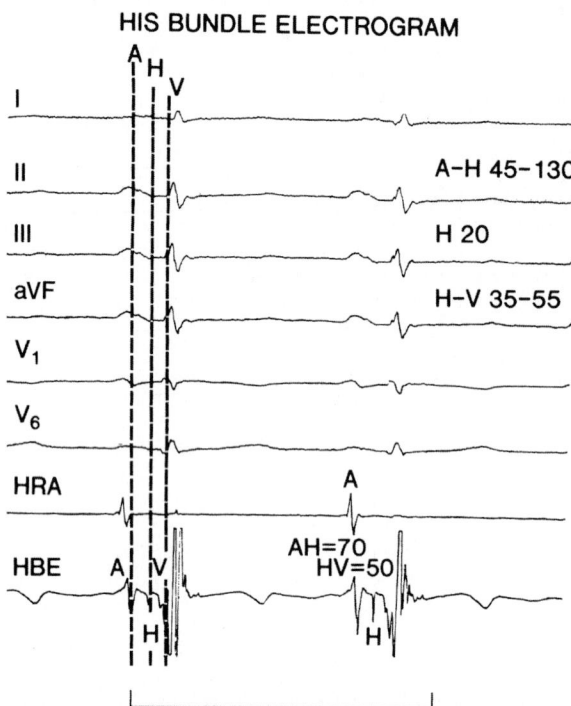

A–H 45–130

H 20

H–V 35–55

Fig. 1. Intracardiac His-bundle electrogram. Top six tracings are from surface electrogram leads I, II, III, aVF, V₁, and V₆. AH and HV intervals are shown. Normal values for AH and HV intervals and duration of H deflection are shown on the right. All numbers are in milliseconds. HBE, His-bundle electrogram (records low right atrial and ventricular activity sequentially); HRA, high right atrial electrogram. A, H, and V denote atrial, His-bundle, and ventricular deflections, respectively.

the His potential) indicates severe disease in this tissue (Fig. 3). Stimulation of the atrium with increasingly premature impulses allows further assessment of AV node and His-Purkinje function (Fig. 4). Significant

prolongation of the HV interval, prolongation of the His potential, and block distal to the His potential are highly specific and sensitive indicators of conduction system disease. Normal and abnormal conduction variables are summarized in Table 1.

Atrial and ventricular pacing also allows evaluation of atrioventricular and ventriculoatrial conduction pathways and identification of accessory atrioventricular connections. The conduction properties of these accessory pathways are assessed in the same manner as normal conduction tissue.

Atrial and ventricular pacing and premature stimulation have their greatest use in the initiation of supraventricular or ventricular tachycardias (Fig. 5). The catheters used for pacing and simple intracardiac recording also can be used to map induced arrhythmia or they can be exchanged for various mapping and ablation catheters, which allow more precise localization of tachycardia circuits and their treatment with ablation.

Medications such as isoproterenol, atropine, or procainamide often are used during these studies to facilitate identification of conduction abnormalities or enhance the ability to initiate tachycardia (Fig. 6).

Atrial and ventricular pacing and program stimulation also can be performed during tachycardia to assess the response (Fig. 7). Successful and consistent termination of tachycardia by these techniques can offer an alternative to drug or ablation therapy. This assessment is particularly important in patients with ventricular tachycardia in whom device therapy is planned. The ability to terminate arrhythmia by rapid pacing may eliminate the need for or reduce the frequency of shock therapy, which is often poorly tolerated (Fig. 8).

These same stimulation techniques can be

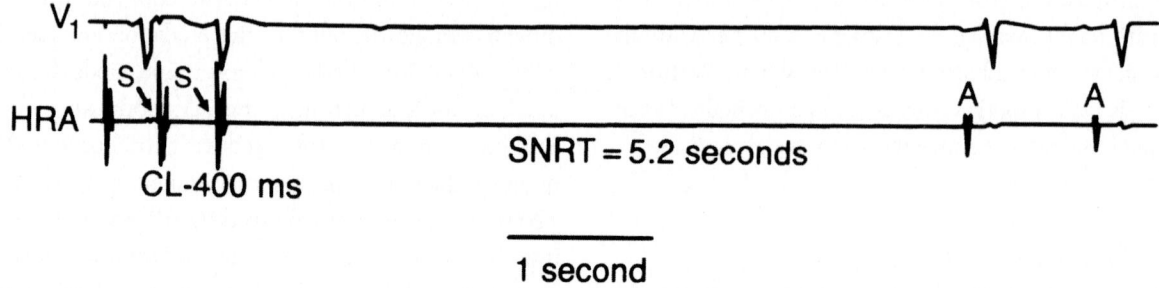

Fig. 2. Prolonged sinus node recovery time (SNRT) in a patient with two episodes of syncope. Results of noninvasive testing were nondiagnostic. The only abnormal finding during electrophysiologic testing was a markedly prolonged SNRT (5.2 seconds) that was associated with near syncope. A, atrial deflection; CL, cycle lengths; HRA, high right atrial electrogram; S, pacing stimulus.

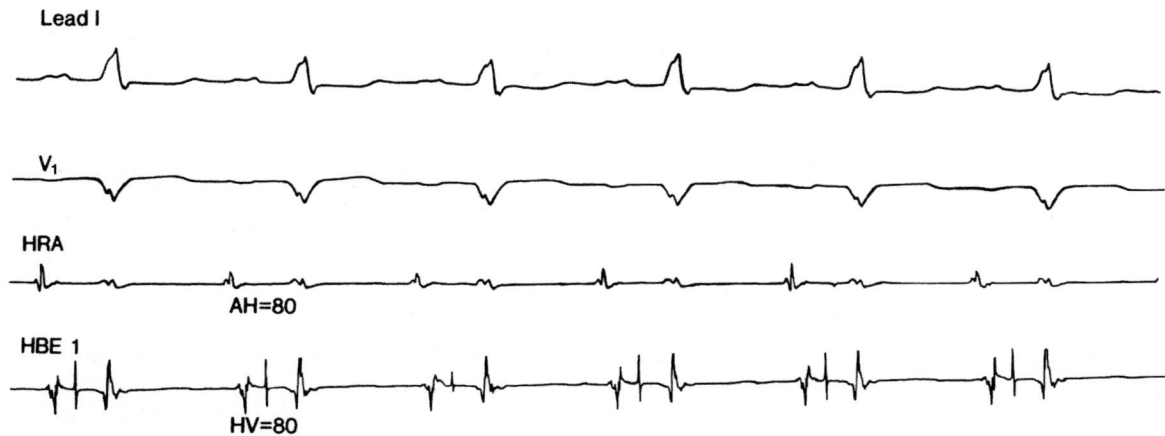

Fig. 3. Significant infranodal conduction system disease. A 12-lead electrocardiogram showed a left bundle branch block. A 24-hour ambulatory monitoring interval was nondiagnostic. During electrophysiologic testing, baseline HV interval was considerably prolonged (80 milliseconds). No other abnormalities were detected during atrial and ventricular programmed stimulation. HBE, His-bundle electrogram; HRA, high right atrial electrogram; A, H, and V denote atrial, His-bundle, and ventricular deflections, respectively.

performed through an implanted device (implantable cardioverter-defibrillator [ICD] primarily) and are done in various clinical situations: if there is concern about the stability of therapies over time (e.g., a high

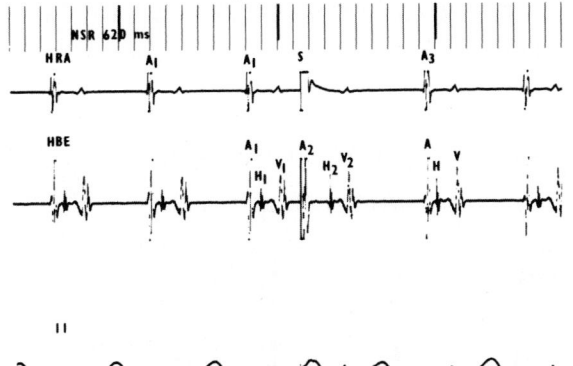

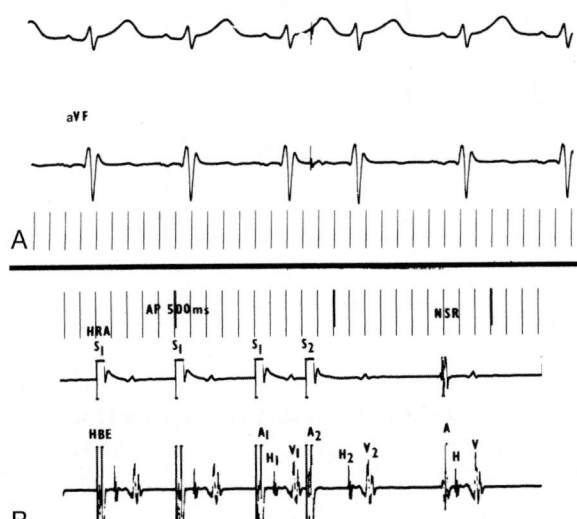

defibrillation threshold at device implantation), if there is a change in the frequency or rate of spontaneous tachycardia, or if there is a change in medication, which could affect either the tachycardia rate or the defibrillation threshold.

EP testing is not confined to invasive studies. Tilt-table testing has great utility in the evaluation of syncope, falls, and seizures unresponsive to therapy. This form of testing also may be useful for predicting the effects of proposed therapy in patients with neurocardiogenic syncope. Drug infusion studies are playing an increasingly important role in risk assessment and in the evaluation of syncope in the absence of heart disease.

Fig. 4. A, Recording during normal sinus rhythm (NSR, 620 milliseconds) from high right atrium (HRA), His bundle (HBE), and two surface electrocardiographic leads. Atrial, His bundle, and ventricular potentials of the sinus beats are A_1, H_1, and V_1, respectively. S, premature atrial beat is delivered. Atrial, His bundle, and ventricular potentials of the premature stimulated beat are A_2, H_2, and V_2, respectively. B, Recording during atrial-paced rhythm (AP, 500 milliseconds). Stimulation artifact and atrial, His bundle, and ventricular potentials of the paced rhythm are S_1, A_1, H_1, and V_1, respectively. S_2, premature atrial beat is delivered. Atrial, His bundle, and ventricular potentials of the premature stimulated beat are A_2, H_2, and V_2, respectively.

Table 1.   Normal and Abnormal Results of Invasive Electrophysiologic Tests

Test	Positive	Intermediate	Negative
		Results	
SNRT	>2 s	1.5-2 s	<1.5 s
CSNRT	≥525 ms		<525 ms
HV	100 ms	>55-99 ms	35-55 ms
	Infra-His block		
HP ERP	BDH		Block in AVN
SVT	Sustained hypotension	Nonsustained	No SVT
			Normal BP
VT	SMMVT*	PMVT/VF	No VT
		Nonsustained VT	
CSM	≥3-s pause		<3-s pause
	BP decrease >50 mm Hg		
	Symptoms or syncope		
HUT	>3-s asystole	Asymptomatic hypo-	No pause
	Hypotension <60 mm Hg	tension	Normal BP
	Syncope		

AVN, atrioventricular node; BDH, block distal to His; BP, blood pressure; CSM, carotid sinus massage; CSNRT, corrected sinus node recovery time; HP ERP, His-Purkinje effective refractory period; HUT, head-up tilt; HV, His-ventricle interval; PMVT, polymorphic ventricular tachycardia; SMMVT, single monomorphic ventricular tachycardia; SNRT, sinus node recovery time; SVT, supraventricular tachycardia; VF, ventricular fibrillation; VT, ventricular tachycardia.

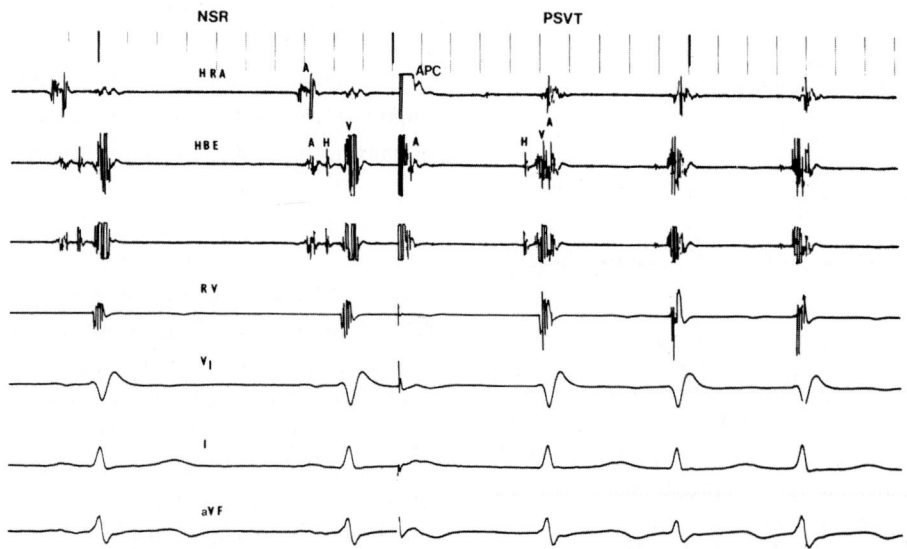

Fig. 5. Introduction of a critically timed atrial premature contraction (APC) results in induction of atrioventricular node reentry tachycardia. Left portion of figure shows recording from high right atrium (HRA), His bundle (HBE), right ventricle (RV), and three surface electrocardiographic leads during normal sinus rhythm (NSR). A critically timed atrial premature contraction results in prolongation of AH interval and induction of typical atrioventricular node reentry tachycardia (premature supraventricular tachycardia, PSVT).

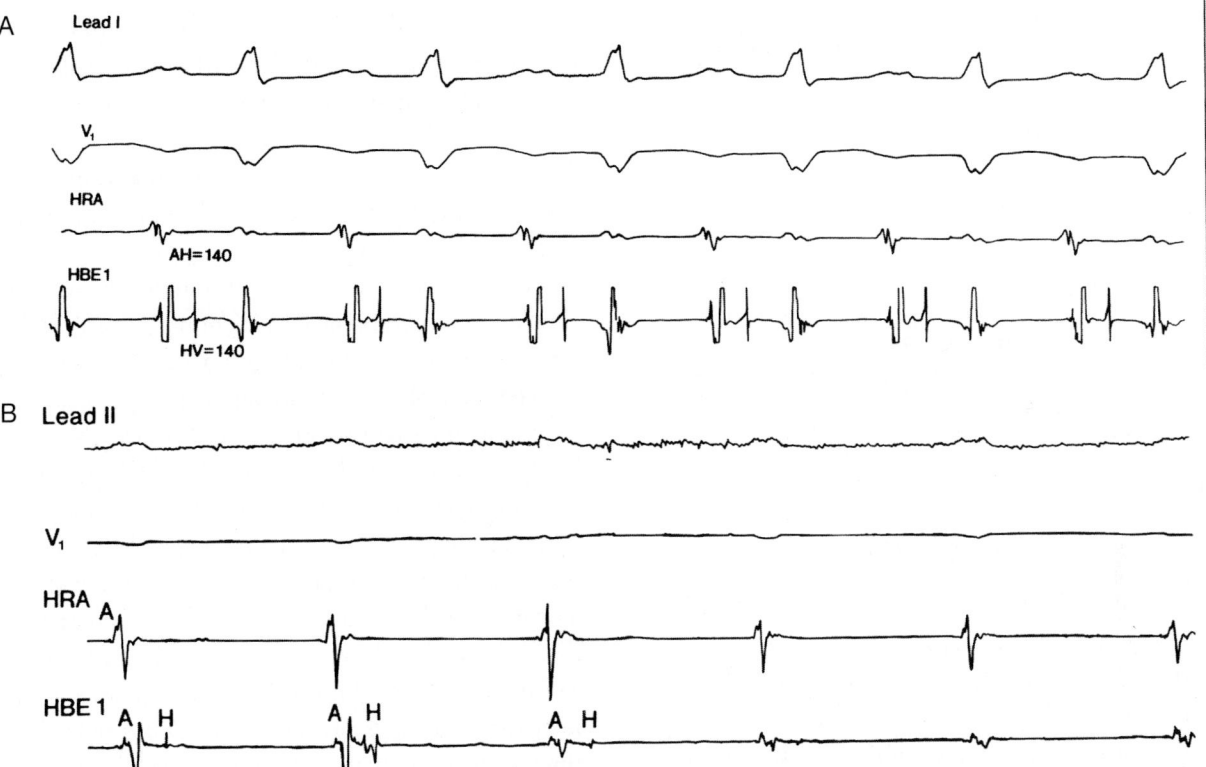

Fig. 6. Significant infranodal conduction system disease. Same patient as in Figure 3. *A*, After procainamide injection (50 mg/min, maximal dose of 15 mg/kg), HV interval increased further (140 milliseconds). *B*, This response was followed by spontaneous infrahisian block without any ventricular escape rhythm, which was associated with complete loss of consciousness. Temporary pacing was required for approximately 5 to 10 minutes before atrioventricular conduction was reestablished. HBE, His-bundle electrogram; HRA, high right atrial electrogram; A, H, and V denote atrial, His-bundle, and ventricular deflections, respectively.

INDICATIONS FOR ELECTROPHYSIOLOGIC STUDY

The indications for an EP study are evaluation of syncope (especially in the setting of heart disease), evaluation of wide or narrow QRS complex tachycardia (to determine mechanism and potential for ablation), assessment of the potential for life-threatening arrhythmia, and the evaluation of drug, ablation, or device therapy. The choice of an invasive or noninvasive method of assessment is determined by the clinical situation. For example, some patients with syncope (those with underlying heart disease) will require invasive studies, whereas others will be better served by a noninvasive approach.

An EP study (especially invasive) is not required or is inappropriate in various situations. Obviously, when the diagnosis is evident or can be established on the basis of a noninvasive evaluation, EP testing should be deferred. Certain forms of conduction disease (e.g., asymptomatic sinus bradycardia, sinoatrial block, bifascicular block, or first-degree AV block or Mobitz I second-degree AV block) are not associated with a poor prognosis and, therefore, require no further evaluation, whereas others (e.g., third-degree AV block) have obvious therapeutic implications. More controversy exists about the role of EP study for the assessment of risk of future arrhythmia. These indications are discussed in more detail subsequently in this chapter.

ELECTROPHYSIOLOGIC EVALUATION OF SYNCOPE

Invasive Study

Syncope has many potential causes; hence, the approach to identification of cause involves the systematic use of

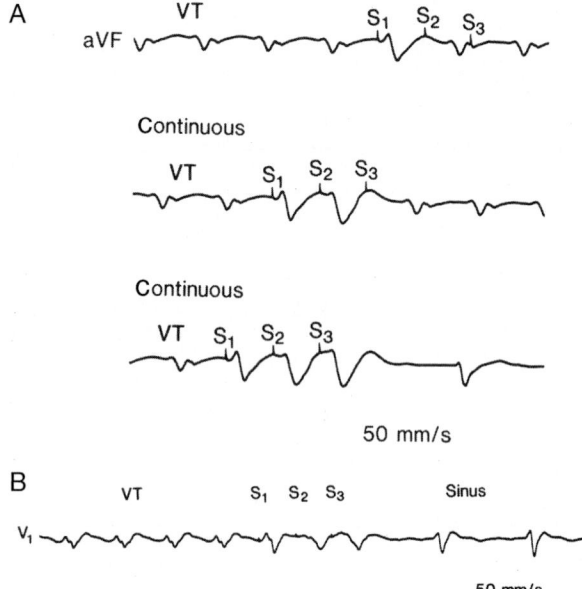

Fig. 7. Termination of ventricular tachycardia (VT) with critically timed premature extrastimuli. *A,* Three extrastimuli (S_1, S_2, S_3) are introduced during the tachycardia. S_1 captures the ventricle, but the tachycardia fails to terminate. Subsequently, S_1 and S_2 capture the ventricle, but again the tachycardia is not terminated. Finally, all three extrastimuli capture the ventricle and the tachycardia is terminated. *B,* Termination of ventricular tachycardia with triple extrastimuli.

various diagnostic procedures. The most common causes of syncope are cardiovascular in origin and are associated with a considerable rate of mortality in patients with underlying heart disease. The primary purpose of the evaluation is to determine whether the patient is at increased risk of death, and thus it involves identifying patients with substantial cardiac disease (e.g., cardiomyopathy, coronary artery disease) or potentially life-threatening genetic diseases such as the long QT syndrome. In many patients, the cause of

syncope can be determined from a thorough history, examination, and straightforward testing including electrocardiography and prolonged monitoring. More advanced and invasive procedures should be reserved for patients in whom the diagnosis remains in doubt and in whom there is a reasonable expectation of a meaningful test result.

Invasive EP study for the evaluation of syncope should be used primarily for patients at highest risk for cardiogenic syncope (Table 2). These patients have a considerable risk of mortality (up to 18% per year) and require aggressive assessment. Additionally, they are likely to have arrhythmias for which EP testing is designed. The factors that are most commonly associated with cardiogenic syncope include age older than 65 years, history of heart failure or myocardial infarction, an abnormal electrocardiogram (other than nonspecific ST-T changes), and a history of ventricular arrhythmias. With any of these abnormalities, the rate of spontaneous arrhythmia or death is 4% to 7% in 1 year. With three or more, the rate is 58% to 80%. These same factors predict a similar likelihood of abnormal results of EP study (any one, 6%; three or more, 60%). Other clinical conditions that should prompt an invasive assessment are syncope with injury, sudden syncope without relation to posture or activity, syncope during exercise, and syncope preceded by rapid palpitations. Syncope of short duration with rapid recovery also suggests cardiogenic rather than neurogenic syncope.

The true diagnostic accuracy of a positive EP study in syncope is not completely understood because of a lack of controlled randomized trials; however, it can be inferred from the results of many clinical studies based either on the incidence of device therapy or on freedom from symptom recurrence in response to study-directed therapy.

In patients with syncope, the induction of sustained monomorphic ventricular tachycardia is very predictive (Fig. 9). However, the predictive accuracy of

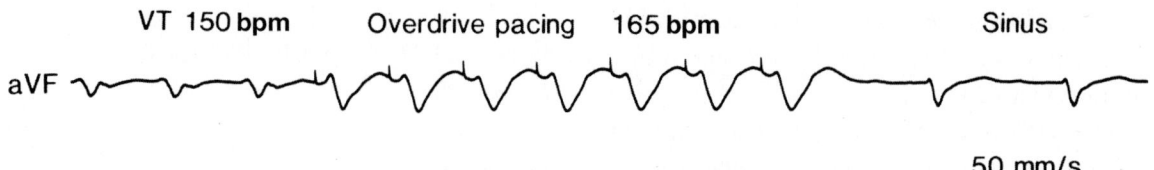

Fig. 8. Ventricular tachycardia (VT) at a rate of 150 beats per minute (bpm) is converted to sinus rhythm with overdrive pacing at 165 beats per minute.

Table 2.   Risk Factors for Cardiogenic Syncope*

1. Age >45 years (especially if >65 years)†‡
2. History of congestive heart failure or acute myocardial infarction†‡
3. Abnormal electrocardiographic results (other than nonspecific ST-T changes, especially bundle branch block)†‡
4. History of ventricular arrhythmias†‡
5. Injury
6. Sudden loss of consciousness without relation to posture or activity
7. Syncope during exercise
8. Short duration and rapid recovery
9. Syncope preceded by rapid palpitations

*Used as indications for electrophysiologic study.
†The rate of arrhythmia or death in 1 year is as follows:
   Numbers 1-4: with any, 4% to 7%; with three or more, 58% to 80%.
‡Electrophysiologic studies are positive in patients with organic heart disease or abnormal electrocardiogram as follows:
   Numbers 1-3: all three, 60%; with two, 40%; with one, 6%.

a study in which no ventricular tachycardia is induced has been called into question, particularly in patients with nonischemic left ventricular dysfunction. In these patients, the rate of recurrence of spontaneous episodes of ventricular tachycardia is similar to that in patients who have had previous documented spontaneous ventricular tachycardia or cardiac arrest. Therapy in this group of patients should be guided not only by the identification of abnormal findings but also by the potential for ventricular arrhythmia determined by the status of left ventricular function.

The identification of sinus node dysfunction and His-Purkinje conduction disease has a high degree of specificity (95%-99%) because pacing has resulted in suppression of syncope in almost all patients. However, studies have shown a lack of sensitivity (30%-50%) for identification of these abnormalities. Up to 40% of patients with negative invasive EP studies have had spontaneous abnormalities identified by prolonged monitoring, about half of which are significant sinus bradycardia or AV block. Most of these studies did not include head-up tilt testing or carotid sinus massage as part of the evaluation; therefore, the abnormalities noted by monitoring may have represented neurocardiogenic syncope or carotid sinus hypersensitivity which would not be identified by a catheter study alone. These findings reinforce the need for a complete evaluation of all patients with suspected cardiogenic syncope. The diagnostic yield for identification of His-Purkinje conduction disease can be increased by 15% with the addition of pharmacologic stress by infusion of class 1A antiarrhythmic agents, and this approach should be considered in patients with prolonged but nondiagnostic HV intervals.

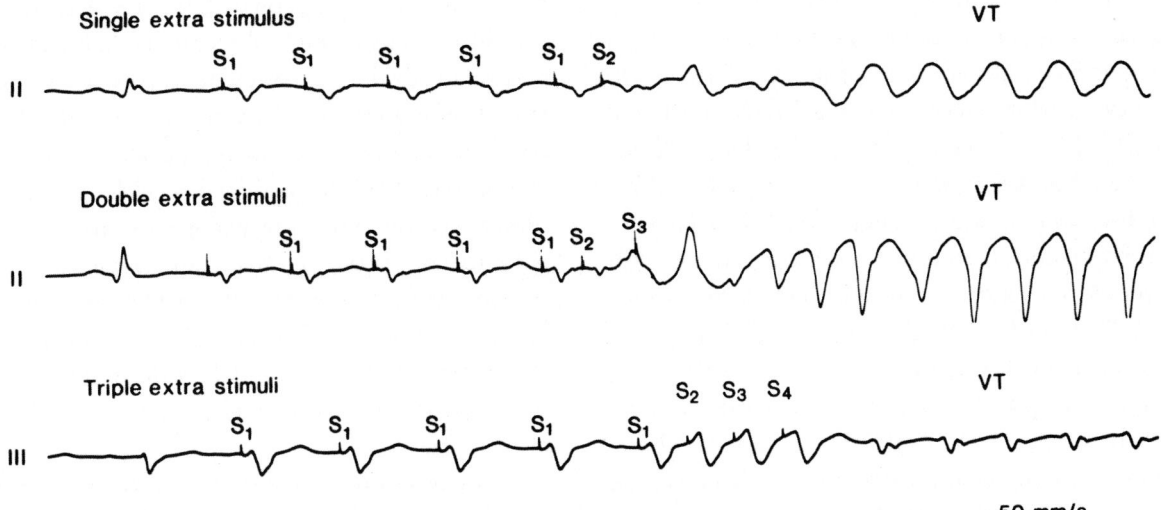

Fig. 9. Initiation of ventricular tachycardia (VT) in the electrophysiology laboratory with the use of single (S_2), double (S_2, S_3), and triple (S_2, S_3, S_4) extrastimuli introduced during ventricular pacing (S_1) at 120 beats per minute.

The significance of inducible ventricular fibrillation or polymorphic ventricular tachycardia is controversial. Among patients with coronary artery disease and syncope who have inducible ventricular arrhythmias other than monomorphic ventricular tachycardia, 13% to 30% have recurrent sustained ventricular tachyarrhythmias over 2 to 5 years. Most of these patients have considerable reduction in left ventricular function, and clinical trials support ICD therapy. In patients with normal left ventricular function, induction of these arrhythmias remains equivocal because it does not predict a risk of increased mortality.

Atrial stimulation can be accomplished with catheters inserted into the esophagus. In patients without evidence of heart disease, this technique has been used as an alternative to more invasive testing. The test has yielded positive results in up to 70% of patients, identifying supraventricular arrhythmias in most. Therapy based on test results has resulted in elimination of symptoms in more than 95% of patients.

An invasive EP study is indicated only in patients with probable or known heart disease in whom the diagnosis remains unknown after an initial evaluation. Echocardiography is an essential part of this evaluation, not only for the evaluation of causal structural heart disease but also for risk stratification.

The identification of significant left ventricular dysfunction (left ventricular ejection fraction less than 35% with at least New York Heart Association class II symptoms) indicates the need for ICD therapy in patients with or without coronary artery disease for primary prevention of sudden death. This guideline is based on the results of a series of controlled trials, most notably the Multicenter Unsustained Tachycardia Trial (MUSTT), Multicenter Automatic Defibrillator Implantation Trial (MADIT I and II), and Sudden Cardiac Death in Heart Failure Trial (SCD-HeFT). It is reasonable, therefore, to manage patients with depressed left ventricular function and syncope with a dual-chamber ICD rather than subject them to the rigor and risks of an invasive procedure. This approach, although adequate for some patients, may result in the lack of necessary clinical information in others. Ventricular tachycardia is not the only cause of syncope even in patients who have documented spontaneous episodes. Up to 10% to 15% of these patients will have syncope as a result of supraventricular tachycardia,

conduction system disease, sinus node dysfunction, carotid sinus hypersensitivity, or vasodepressor syncope.

The recent Dual Chamber and VVI Implantable Defibrillator (DAVID) trial showed the potential for significant exacerbations of heart failure resulting from right ventricular pacing in patients with significant ventricular dysfunction. Patients with an indication for pacing probably would benefit from biventricular rather than right ventricular pacing. EP evaluation in these cases could therefore result in very useful clinical information if sinus node, AV node, or His-Purkinje disease is discovered, findings thus indicating the potential need for pacing. Additionally, an understanding of the potential for supraventricular arrhythmia could assist in the tailoring of ICD therapy or lead to definitive therapy for supraventricular tachycardia (ablation) to minimize the potential for inappropriate device function.

Tilt-Table Testing With Carotid Massage

Neurocardiogenic or vasodepressor syncope is a common cause of loss of consciousness in all groups of patients, and thus tilt-table testing is an important tool in the evaluation of patients with syncope. In patients without evidence of structural heart disease, it can provide a diagnosis in approximately 60% of patients.

Tilt-table testing is definitely indicated in the following situations: unexplained recurrent syncope in the absence of heart disease, recurrent syncope in the setting of heart disease after cardiac causes are excluded, and a single episode of noncardiac syncope in a high-risk setting (e.g., occupation with the risk of injury).

Situations in which tilt-table testing may be of benefit are for differentiation of syncope with seizure from true seizure (especially in patients with current symptoms receiving medication), evaluation of repetitive unexplained falls in the elderly, and evaluation of recurrent highly symptomatic presyncope or dizziness. In patients with presumed neurocardiogenic syncope, tilt-table testing also may be of benefit when an understanding of the hemodynamic pattern of syncope may alter therapy. It is *not* indicated for the evaluation of a single episode of syncope without injury in the absence of heart disease.

Various testing protocols affect the sensitivity and specificity of the study. Patients are initially kept supine for 20 to 45 minutes and then passively tilted for 45 minutes at 60° to 80° of tilt (Fig. 10). Under these circumstances, the test results are positive in 8% to 50% of patients (greater sensitivity at higher degrees of tilt) and have a very high degree of specificity. The passive tilt is followed by the administration of medication by infusion, spray, or orally. Isoproterenol, nitroglycerin, clomipramine, and adenosine have all been used with benefit. The addition of these agents substantially increases the sensitivity (approximately 60%-80%) and maintains a high degree of specificity (Fig. 11). In general, there has been no substantial difference in the predictive accuracy of the test when these adjunctive agents have been compared in the same patients. The sensitivity of tilt-table testing is improved in patients with multiple episodes of syncope, especially if they have occurred over a long time in patients 12 to 25 years old (although neurocardiogenic syncope can occur at any age) and in patients whose syncope occurs under specific circumstances (e.g., stress, prolonged standing, or after exercise or with prodromal symptoms or signs such as pallor, light-headedness, or nausea). A positive test result is also more likely in syncope associated with trauma and episodes that occur in clusters.

Another important factor that affects the sensitivity of the test is the time from the last episode to the performance of the test. The longer the interval, the less likely the test result will be abnormal.

The three types of abnormal response to upright tilt are cardioinhibitory, vasodepressor, and mixed.

Cardioinhibitory response is characterized by asystole and profound bradycardia that coincides with or precedes a decrease in blood pressure. This type tends to be infrequent in older patients. A vasodepressor response is characterized by a profound drop in blood pressure with minimal change in heart rate, and it is most common in patients older than 60 years. The mixed type is a combination of heart rate and blood pressure reduction in which the blood pressure drop is the initial event. This type is most common in patients between the ages of 16 and 34 years. The patterns of response should be clearly identified because they have implications for therapy (i.e., pacing is most likely to be a benefit in patients with a cardioinhibitory-type response).

Because of its sensitivity and high degree of specificity, the diagnostic benefit of tilt-table testing is unquestionable. However, there are some potential limitations when the test is used to assess therapy. There is a lack of consistent reproducibility of a positive test result; estimates vary from 30% to 90% in a series of studies. Although some studies have reported that the same pattern of abnormality is found during repeat testing, frequently there is a mismatch between the findings identified during tilt-table testing with those of subsequent spontaneous syncopal episodes. Several studies have matched the clinical responses to acute interventions, including pacing, β-adrenergic blockers, midodrine, and selective serotonin reuptake inhibitors

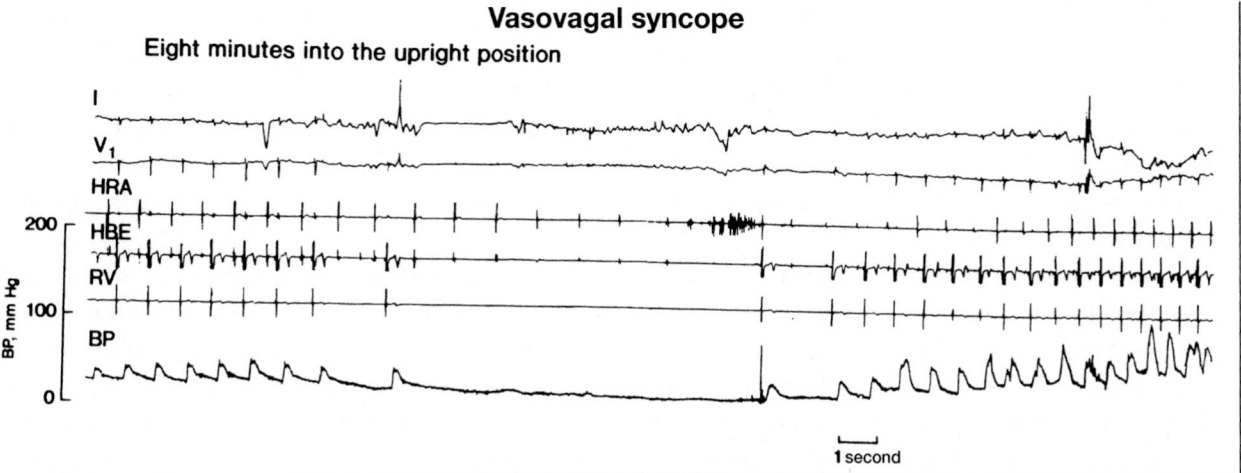

Fig. 10. Vasovagal reaction in patient with recurrent syncope. Bradycardia/asystole and significant hypotension associated with syncope occurred at 8 minutes in the tilted upright position. The patient spontaneously recovered immediately after being returned to the supine position. BP, blood pressure; HBE, His-bundle electrogram; HRA, high right atrial electrogram; I, surface lead I; RV, right ventricular electrogram.

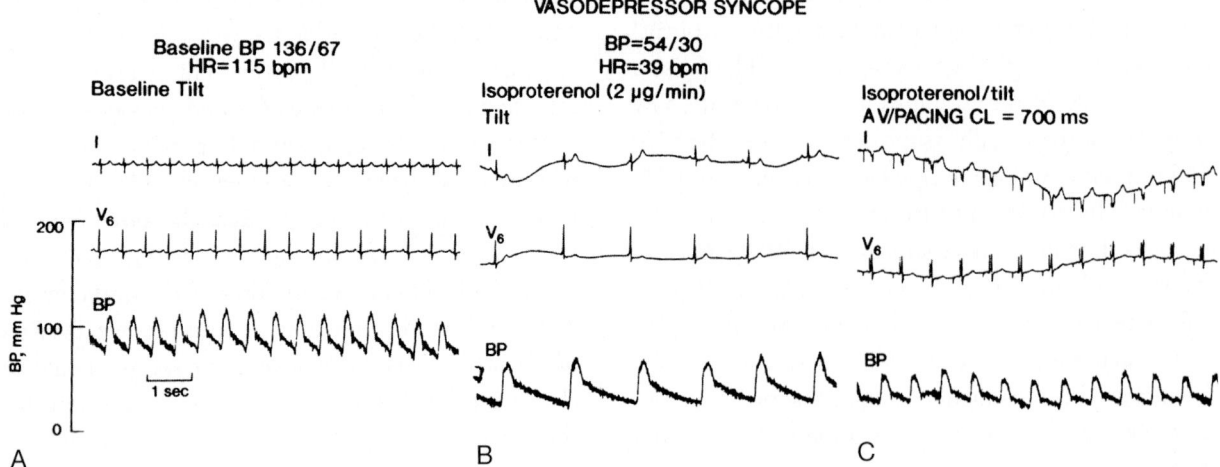

Fig. 11. Vasovagal reaction in patient with recurrent syncope. *A*, Results of tilt-table test at baseline were normal. The heart rate (HR) was 115 beats per minute (bpm), and blood pressure (BP) remained stable at 136/67 mm Hg in the upright position. *B*, During isoproterenol infusion (2 μg/min) in the upright position, the patient became nauseated, and this was followed by bradycardia (30 to 60 beats per minute), hypotension (54/30 mm Hg), and presyncope. *C*, Atrioventricular (AV) sequential pacing at three different cycle lengths (PCL; 800, 700, and 600 milliseconds) did not relieve the hypotension or the patient's symptoms. I, surface lead I.

to long-term therapy. Although some have been predictive, others have shown a poor correlation.

Carotid sinus hypersensitivity is a common form of syncope (especially in older patients) and accounts for 15% to 20% of the indications for pacemaker implantation in most series. Therefore, it should be part of every EP assessment of syncope and typically is included in a tilt-table study. There are three types: cardioinhibitory (asystole more than 3 seconds) (Fig. 12), vasodepressor (a pure decrease in blood pressure), and mixed (pause more than 3 seconds with persistence in hypotension after recovery of the heart rate). The mixed variety is the most frequent and occurs in 50% of patients, and the other two forms occur with equal frequency.

Carotid massage should be performed while the patient is upright because this position substantially increases the sensitivity of the test (specificity remains at approximately 100%) and allows the vasodepressor component to be assessed. As with neurocardiogenic syncope, an understanding of the pathophysiologic mechanisms of this condition can guide therapy.

There is a high degree of reproducibility of test results; the concordance between positive-positive and negative-negative test results is 93%. Additionally, the

test has high clinical relevance; multiple studies have indicated a recurrence of spontaneous pauses (determined during pacing therapy in patients with a positive response) and a considerable reduction in the frequency of syncopal spells as a result of pacing therapy.

Both tilt-table testing and carotid massage can be done with a high degree of safety. Carotid sinus massage should not be performed in patients with carotid bruits or a history of transient ischemic attack or stroke within the previous 3 months. Complications occur in 0.05% to 0.1% of patients and are typically transient.

Because syncope has many potential causes, the approach to the evaluation of patients varies. However, there is a need for a systematic and thorough approach because of the risks associated not only with cardiac syncope but with syncope that remains undiagnosed after an evaluation. There is debate about the relative benefits of prolonged monitoring (especially with the advent of implantable devices) compared with a more invasive approach. For patients at risk of cardiogenic syncope, an approach that involved an invasive EP study followed (if negative) by tilt-table testing and then by implantation of a recorder if the diagnosis was still in doubt led to the establishment of a diagnosis in 86% of patients. This seems to be a reasonable approach

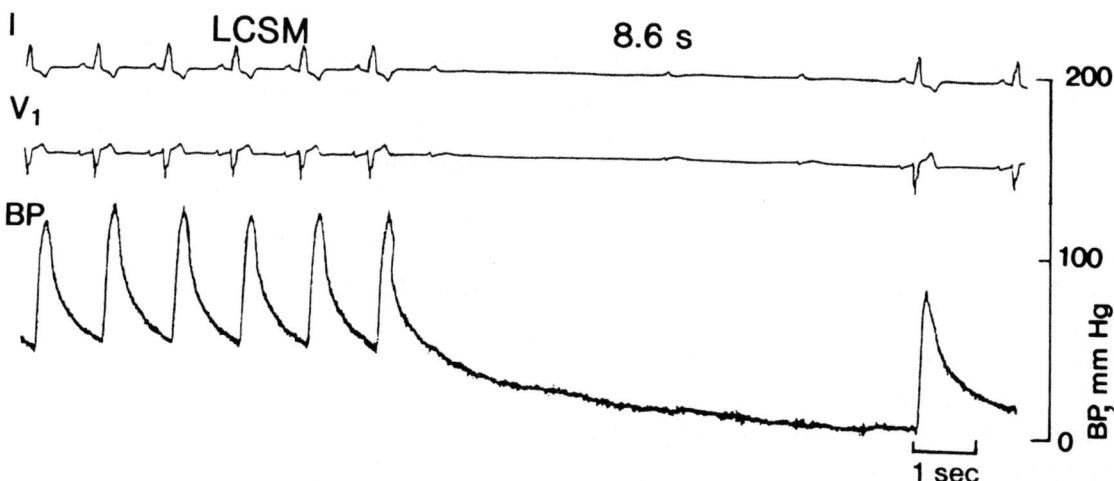

Fig. 12. Electrocardiographic tracing and blood pressure (BP) monitoring during left carotid sinus massage (LCSM), showing abrupt atrioventricular block, slowing of the sinus rate, and precipitous decline in the blood pressure for 8.6 seconds.

in these patients. For those without risk, tilt-table testing establishes the diagnosis in 60% to 70%. The efficacy of implantable loop recorders alone approaches this rate in many studies, but often many months are needed to establish the diagnosis. The combination of these two techniques seems to be reasonable.

ASSESSMENT OF RISK FOR FUTURE ARRHYTHMIC EVENTS

Cardiomyopathy

In the past, a major role of EP testing and of programmed ventricular stimulation in particular was the management of ventricular arrhythmias, initially after a spontaneous event and later in an attempt to identify populations of patients at risk of future events. Serial stimulation studies while patients were receiving antiarrhythmic agents led to noninducibility and chronic drug therapy, empiric amiodarone therapy, or ICD therapy.

A series of randomized clinical trials involving patients thought to be at the greatest risk for future events evaluated diagnostic and therapeutic interventions designed to provide the greatest reduction in total mortality of cardiac and arrhythmic cause. These studies identified the following: amiodarone therapy was better than any EP guided drug therapy, ICD therapy was superior to any drug therapy, EP-guided therapy was of limited clinical utility, and the status of left ventricular function was the most useful measure of arrhythmia risk. Hence, most patients with structural heart disease and associated ventricular dysfunction (ischemic or idiopathic cardiomyopathy) are managed by ICD therapy without EP testing.

Nonsustained Ventricular Tachycardia

EP testing, primarily programmed ventricular stimulation, still has a role in risk assessment for patients with coronary artery disease with a left ventricular ejection fraction between 35% and 40% in the presence of nonsustained ventricular tachycardia. In this group of patients, the induction of ventricular tachycardia indicates an increased risk of spontaneous arrhythmia and benefit from ICD therapy.

Other Heart Disease

EP study may be of benefit for risk assessment in selected populations of patients with conditions such as arrhythmogenic right ventricular dysplasia, sarcoid heart disease, and the Brugada syndrome, in whom there is a risk of spontaneous ventricular tachycardia or cardiac arrest. In these conditions, inducibility of ventricular tachycardia during EP study is an independent predictor of future life-threatening arrhythmia, but unfortunately it does not have 100% negative predictive accuracy. Use of the results of EP testing in combination with other clinical factors of arrhythmia-related mortality is the most appropriate approach to determination of the need for prophylactic therapy in these patients.

Cardiac Channelopathies

A group of patients with structurally normal hearts are at risk of lethal cardiac arrhythmia. Included in this group are patients with the long QT syndrome and Brugada syndrome (Table 3). These conditions frequently are associated with a family history of sudden death, but the first manifestation of the condition may be syncope or sudden death. Therefore, it is imperative that these patients are identified before spontaneous events. Each of these syndromes has a characteristic electrocardiographic finding; however, they are intermittently and transiently absent. These changes occur as a result of abnormalities in the transport of sodium or potassium across cell membranes, leading to prolongation and dispersion of cellular repolarization. The electrocardiographic changes can be enhanced by drugs that affect these channels, and these drugs have proved to be powerful tools to unmask silent carriers of mutant genes responsible for the abnormalities. Such findings allow for implementation of appropriate prophylactic measures, including ICD therapy. They should be considered in patients with a positive family history of sudden death, unexplained syncope in the absence of underlying heart disease, or abnormal electrocardiographic findings suggestive of or consistent with repolarization abnormalities.

Epinephrine infusion can be used to identify long QT syndromes 1 and 2. In long QT syndrome 1, a paradoxical increase in the QT interval occurs; in long QT syndrome 2, characteristic notching of the T wave may be enhanced. The test allows differentiation of the two syndromes and of both syndromes from normal results with a high degree of sensitivity and specificity. Because patients with long QT syndrome 3 do not respond abnormally to epinephrine, the test also can differentiate this syndrome from other prolonged QT syndromes. The use of sodium channel-stabilizing agents such as lidocaine also can assist in the identification of long QT syndrome 3. In this syndrome, drug infusion results in a decrease in the QT interval, which does not occur in the other syndromes.

Patients with the Brugada syndrome have abnormalities in sodium channel function and therefore can

Table 3.   Response to Pharmacologic Stress in Cardiac Channelopathies

Syndrome	Drug	Positive response
Brugada	Ajmaline, procainamide	Abnormal ST-T leads V_{1-2}
Long QT		
1	Epinephrine	Increased QT interval
2	Epinephrine	Increased notched T waves
3	Lidocaine	Decreased QT interval

be challenged with the use of sodium channel blocking agents such as procainamide and ajmaline. The classic electrocardiographic pattern in this condition can be induced with a high degree of sensitivity and specificity by drug infusion.

CONDITIONS IN WHICH ELECTRO-PHYSIOLOGIC EVALUATION IS OF NO OR LIMITED VALUE

Risk Assessment

ICD therapy is indicated in any patient with significant left ventricular dysfunction, and in the absence of symptoms EP study is of no added benefit. Patients with hypertrophic cardiomyopathy and Wolff-Parkinson-White syndrome have an increased risk of arrhythmic death, but EP study has not been proved to be of value in risk assessment. There are several well-established clinical criteria for risk assessment in hypertrophic cardiomyopathy. The results of programmed ventricular stimulation have not added to them, and therefore the decision to use an ICD for primary prevention is made on clinical grounds alone. The incidence of sudden death in Wolff-Parkinson-White syndrome is extremely low and is not a common presentation. The risk is increased in symptomatic patients (especially those with a history of atrial fibrillation) and in those with a positive family history. Currently, there is no indication for the routine invasive assessment of asymptomatic patients.

The clinical trials that have evaluated risk in patients with coronary artery disease have included only patients at least 1 month after an acute coronary event. Two recent trials evaluated patients within a short time (4-30 days) after myocardial infarction. Neither study found a significant survival benefit with either EP-guided or empiric ICD therapy.

Evaluation of Conduction System Disease
Symptomatic advanced AV block that develops in patients with underlying bifascicular and trifascicular block is associated with a high mortality rate and a significant incidence of sudden death. Therefore, anyone presenting with, for example, syncope or effort dyspnea in a setting of bifascicular or trifascicular block should be aggressively evaluated with EP study and treated accordingly. The cause of symptoms in this group of patients should not be assumed to be related to conduction system disease because most studies suggest that up to half of these patients have an inducible ventricular tachycardia. If the cause of syncope cannot be determined with certainty in these patients, prophylactic device therapy should be considered.

However, asymptomatic patients with bifascicular or trifascicular block should *not* be evaluated with invasive study. The incidence of progression with third-degree AV block in asymptomatic patients is low, and therefore the risk of death or injury as a result of high-grade block is too low to warrant EP study.

A decision about the management of second-degree AV block is most appropriately made on the basis of the type of block (Mobitz I or Mobitz II), the presence or absence of associated bundle branch block, and the presence or absence of accompanying symptoms. Invasive EP studies ordinarily do not add substantially to decision making.

EVALUATION OF TACHYCARDIA
EP studies are commonly used in the management of spontaneous tachycardia, both documented wide and narrow QRS complex arrhythmias and episodes of tachycardia that have not been recorded by electrocardiography or prolonged monitoring.

Wide Complex Tachycardia
Most episodes of spontaneous wide QRS complex tachycardia represent ventricular tachycardia. Although the usual approach to management in this group of patients is device therapy, EP testing can be of value, especially in patients with tachycardia not associated with hemodynamic instability or severe symptoms. Invasive study can determine the cause if the electrocardiogram is equivocal or the probability of ventricular tachycardia is low, especially if there is evidence of antegrade preexcitation on resting electrocardiography.

Mapping of the tachycardia circuit can help to determine the suitability of ablation therapy, especially in right ventricular outflow tract and ventricular tachycardia, idiopathic left ventricular tachycardia, bundle branch reentrant tachycardia, or monomorphic ventricular tachycardia due to coronary artery disease, in which the acute and long-term success rates with ablation therapy are high. The development of enhanced mapping techniques and technology has allowed mapping even during sinus rhythm in patients with unstable arrhythmias. The outcomes of ablation with all types of ventricular tachycardia could approach those expected for common types of supraventricular tachycardia.

Survivors of out-of-hospital cardiac arrest, however, generally are not considered candidates for EP testing. In patients without a reversible cause (myocardial infarction) before the arrest, an ICD has been established as the treatment choice in virtually all patients according to the results of many clinical trials. EP testing does not assist in clinical decision making.

If device therapy is chosen for the management of ventricular tachycardia, EP studies (primarily noninvasive studies with the implanted device) are often needed to assess the response to pacing or defibrillator therapy.

Narrow Complex Tachycardia
In patients with documented narrow complex tachycardia, invasive EP study is particularly useful for determination of the mechanism of arrhythmia, usually as an integral part of ablation therapy. Because ablation in supraventricular tachycardia is associated with acute success in more than 90% of patients, it has become the preferred therapy in many patients, especially in patients with severely symptomatic episodes, with tachycardias that are resistant to medication, or in whom drug therapy is either not wanted as long-term therapy or is associated

with significant symptoms. In patients with antegrade preexcitation, the potential for serious arrhythmias should prompt consideration of a more aggressive management approach with ablation.

PALPITATIONS

The use of invasive EP study in patients with palpitations (paroxysms of regular sustained tachycardia) is not as clear-cut, and prolonged monitoring might be preferred. However, EP studies should be considered if episodes elude detection by other means or are associated with severe symptoms, resting preexcitation, a family history of potentially lethal arrhythmias, or very rapid rates documented by a qualified observer.

COMPLICATIONS AND CONTRAINDICATIONS

EP testing can be of considerable benefit in the management of various patients. Invasive studies have inherent risk, however, and EP studies are no exception. In many cases, potentially lethal rhythms are provoked, and therefore these studies should be performed in laboratories with highly trained and skilled persons with every means of resuscitative support available. However, procedures performed in this type of environment by very experienced staff are still associated with the risk of serious complication. These include hypotension (1%); vascular problems, including arterial injury, hemorrhage, or thrombosis (0.7%); thromboembolism (0.2%); myocardial perforation (0.15%); and death (0%-0.6%).

For risk to be minimized, EP studies should not be performed in patients with acute coronary artery syndromes (unstable angina or myocardial infarction), severe left ventricular outflow obstruction (hypertrophic obstructive cardiomyopathy or aortic stenosis), decompensated heart failure, systemic infection, respiratory failure, significant electrolyte imbalance, or recent thromboembolic episodes.

22

CARDIAC CHANNELOPATHIES

T. Jared Bunch, MD

Michael J. Ackerman, MD, PhD

The discipline of cardiac channelopathies formally began in 1995 with the discovery of mutations in genes encoding critical ion channels of the heart as the pathogenic basis for congenital long QT syndrome (LQTS). Besides the classic autosomal dominant (Romano-Ward syndrome) and recessive (Jervell and Lange-Nielsen syndrome) forms of LQTS, the cardiac channelopathies now comprise Andersen-Tawil syndrome, Timothy syndrome, drug-induced torsades de pointes, short QT syndrome (SQTS), catecholaminergic polymorphic ventricular tachycardia (CPVT), Brugada syndrome, idiopathic ventricular fibrillation, progressive cardiac conduction disease or familial atrioventricular conduction block or Lev-Lenègre disease, and familial atrial fibrillation (FAF). Even primary cardiomyopathies such as dilated cardiomyopathy have been shown to stem from genetically mediated perturbations in ion channels, specifically the *SCN5A*-encoded cardiac sodium channel.

Cardiac channelopathies or heritable arrhythmia syndromes affect an estimated 1 in 2,000 to 1 in 3,000 persons. The conditions may lie dormant for decades or manifest as sudden death during infancy, they may or may not manifest signature electrocardiographic (ECG) features, and in general they represent treatable conditions when properly recognized and diagnosed. The clinical presentation generally consists of abrupt-onset syncope, seizures, or sudden death. Sudden cardiac death is uncommonly the sentinel event. It is estimated that nearly half of sudden cardiac deaths stemming from a cardiac channelopathy may have exhibited warning signs that went unrecognized (exertional syncope, positive family history of premature sudden death, etc.). An estimated 5% to 15% of sudden infant death syndrome cases and up to one-third of autopsy-negative sudden unexplained deaths in the young (younger than 40 years) may be precipitated by an underlying cardiac channelopathy.

In this chapter, the pathogenic basis, clinical evaluation and diagnosis, and therapeutic management of the QT syndromes, CPVT, Brugada syndrome, and FAF are reviewed.

QT CHANNELOPATHIES

Autosomal Dominant (Romano-Ward) LQTS
Congenital LQTS is the prototypical cardiac channelopathy affecting an estimated 1 in 3,000 persons. Clinically, LQTS is characterized by abnormal cardiac repolarization resulting in QT-interval prolongation (Fig. 1 *A*), which predisposes patients to its trademark dysrhythmia of torsades de pointes (TdP) (Fig. 1 *B*). If and when TdP occurs, the affected individual exhibits

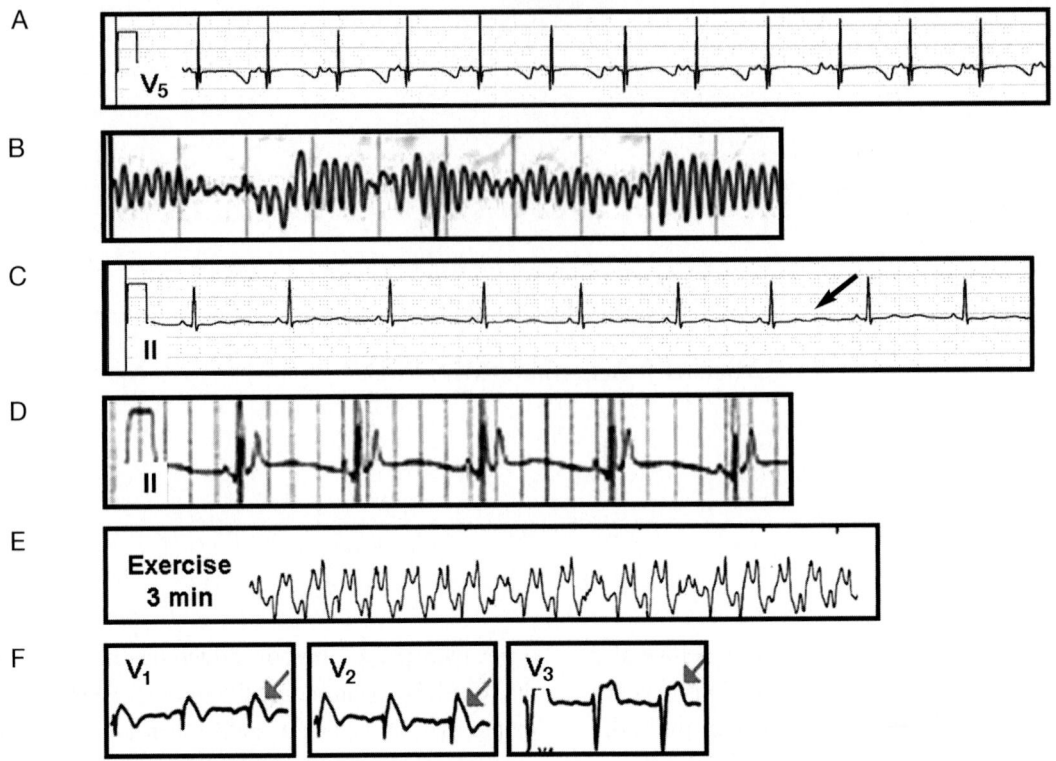

Fig. 1. Signature electrocardiographic (ECG) features of various channelopathies. *A,* QT prolongation is extreme in this example (heart rate–corrected QT interval [QTc] >650 ms). Note that the ST segment and T-wave morphology would predict type 3 long QT syndrome (LQT3), but the patient is among the 25% who are genotype negative. Also, the computer-calculated QTc was 362 ms, underscoring the mandate to independently compute the QTc. *B,* Torsades de pointes ("twisting of the points") is a hallmark dysrhythmia of long QT syndrome. *C,* Abnormal U wave in type 1 Andersen-Tawil syndrome (ATS1). Although the abnormalities are subtle in this lead II recording, they are quite abnormal: the QT interval is normal, but there is a long isoelectric segment from the end of the T wave to the beginning of the U wave and a long-duration U wave (*arrow*) in this female with an ATS1-associated mutation in *KCNJ2.* *D,* Short QT interval, with a QTc of approximately 250 ms. *E,* Exercise-induced bidirectional ventricular tachycardia in catecholaminergic polymorphic ventricular tachycardia. *F,* Coved ST-segment elevation (*arrow*) in Brugada syndrome (type I ECG pattern) in precordial leads V$_1$ and V$_2$ and a saddle back profile (*arrow*) (type II ECG pattern) in V$_3$.

the abrupt onset of either syncope or seizures or sudden death. The most common form of LQTS is autosomal dominant LQTS, previously known as Romano-Ward syndrome. Autosomal recessive LQTS, first described by Drs. Jervell and Lange-Nielsen, affects about 1 in 1 million persons and is characterized by a severe cardiac phenotype as well as by sensorineural hearing loss. LQTS can also occur as sporadic or spontaneous germline mutations (5%-10%).

Hundreds of mutations in nine distinct LQTS susceptibility genes have been identified so far and generally involve either loss-of-function potassium channel mutations or gain-of-function sodium channel mutations

(types 1 through 9 [LQT1 through LQT9] (Table 1). Except for two rare subtypes that stem from perturbations in key cardiac channel–interacting proteins or structural membrane scaffolding proteins (ankyrin B [LQT4] and caveolin-3 [LQT9]), LQTS is a pure channelopathy stemming from mutations in cardiac channel alpha and beta subunits. The vast majority of LQTS cases are due to mutations in the *KCNQ1*-encoded slow component of the delayed rectifier potassium current (I$_{Ks}$) channel (LQT1, 30%-35%), the *KCNH2*-encoded rapid component of the delayed rectifier potassium current (I$_{Kr}$) channel (LQT2, 25%-30%), or the *SCN5A*-encoded sodium channel (I$_{Na}$) (LQT3, 5%-10%).

Table 1.   Molecular Basis of Cardiac Channelopathies

Type	Locus	Gene	Mode of inheritance	Current	Frequency, %
QT channelopathies					
Romano-Ward syndrome—LQTS					
LQT1	11p15.5	*KCNQ1/KVLQT1*	AD	$I_{Ks(\alpha)}$	30-35
LQT2	7q35-36	*KCNH2/HERG*	AD	$I_{Kr(\alpha)}$	25-30
LQT3	3p21-p24	*SCN5A*	AD	I_{Na}	5-10
LQT4	4q25-q27	*ANKB*	AD	Na/Ca	<1
LQT5	21q22.1	*KCNE1/minK*	AD	$I_{Ks(\beta)}$	<1
LQT6	21q22.1	*KCNE2/MiRP1*	AD	$I_{Kr(\beta)}$	<1
CAV3-LQT (LQT9)	3p25	*CAV3*	Sporadic	Caveolin-3 (I_{Na})	<1
Jervell and Lange-Nielsen syndrome—LQTS					
JLN1	11p15.5	*KCNQ1/KVLQT1*	AR	$I_{Ks(\alpha)}$	>50
JLN2	21q22.1	*KCNE1/minK*	AR	$I_{Ks(\beta)}$	~5
Andersen-Tawil syndrome					
ATS1 (LQT7)	17q23	*KCNJ2*	AD	$I_{K1(\alpha)}$	50
Timothy syndrome					
TS1 (LQT8)	12p13.3	*CACNA1C*	Sporadic	$I_{Ca,L(\alpha)}$	50
Short QT syndrome					
SQT1	7q35-36	*KCNH2/HERG*	AD	$I_{Kr(\alpha)}$	?
SQT2	11p15.5	*KCNQ1/KVLQT1*	AD	$I_{Ks(\alpha)}$	?
SQT3	17q23	*KCNJ2*	AD	$I_{K1(\alpha)}$	?
Catecholaminergic polymorphic ventricular tachycardia					
CPVT1	1q42.1-q43	*RyR2*	AD	Calcium release channel	50-65
CPVT2	1p13.3	*CASQ2*	AR	Calsequestrin	<1
Brugada syndrome					
BrS1	3p21-p24	*SCN5A*	AD	I_{Na}	15-30
Familial atrial fibrillation					
FAF1	11p15.5	*KCNQ1/KVLQT1*	AD	$I_{Ks(\alpha)}$	<1
FAF2	21q22.1	*KCNE2/MiRP1*	AD	$I_{Kr(\beta)}$	<1
FAF3	17q23	*KCNJ2*	AD	$I_{K1(\alpha)}$	<1
FAF4	7q35-36	*KCNH2/HERG*	AD	$I_{Kr(\alpha)}$	<1
FAF5	3p21-p24	*SCN5A*	AD	I_{Na}	<1
FAFx	10q22	?	AD	?	?
FAFx	6q14	?	AD	?	?
FAFx	5p13	?	AR	?	?

AD, autosomal dominant; AR, autosomal recessive; Ca, calcium; $I_{Ca,L}$, L-type calcium channel; I_{K1}, delayed rectifier potassium channel; I_{Kr}, rapid component of the delayed rectifier potassium current; I_{Ks}, slow component of the delayed rectifier potassium current; I_{Na}, sodium channel; Na, sodium.

The past decade of LQTS research has identified numerous genotype-phenotype relationships. Genotype-ECG relationships include broad-based T waves in LQT1, low-amplitude or notched T waves in LQT2, and long ST isoelectric segment and normal T-wave morphology in LQT3. Gene-specific arrhythmogenic triggers have been identified, including exertion, particularly swimming, in LQT1; auditory triggers and the postpartum period in LQT2; and events during sleep in LQT3. Importantly, the response to standard LQTS pharmacotherapy (β-blockers) is strongly influenced by the underlying genotype. β-Blockers are extremely protective in LQT1, moderately effective in LQT2, and of no demonstrable protective benefit in LQT3. In May 2004, LQTS genetic testing became commercially available as a clinical diagnostic test involving a comprehensive open reading frame analysis of the translated exons for the genes associated with LQT1, LQT2, LQT3, LQT5, and LQT6. In the presence of a clinically robust presentation, the yield of LQTS genetic testing is about 75%. Indications for LQTS genetic testing are summarized in Table 2.

Electrocardiographically, individuals with LQTS may or may not show the hallmark repolarization abnormality of QT interval prolongation (Fig. 1 *A*). In fact, approximately 50% of patients with genotype-positive LQTS have a normal resting heart rate–corrected QT interval (QTc). This observation reinforces the critical role of genetic testing because the screening ECG has an unacceptable misclassification rate after the diagnosis of LQTS is established. In general, a QTc of more than 480 ms in *postpubertal* females or of more than 470 ms in *postpubertal* males should prompt a thorough investigation for LQTS because these values represent the top 1 percentile in the distribution of QTc values. Previously, a QTc greater than 440 ms (males) or greater than 450 ms (females) has been called *borderline QT prolongation*. Although 50% of patients with LQTS do show a QTc of less than 460 ms, these cut-off values would result in an unacceptably high rate of false-positives if used as part of a screening program. By the aforementioned cut-off values, an estimated 15% to 20% of the entire population has borderline QT prolongation (Fig. 2). These QTc-based assessments presume an accurate determination of the QTc. It is absolutely critical to independently determine the QTc manually because reliance on the instrument-derived QTc is unacceptable. Calculation of an average QTc from either lead II or lead V5 is recommended. Simply taking the beat yielding the maximal

---

Table 2. Indications for LQTS Genetic Testing

- Persons with unequivocal and unexplained QT prolongation (i.e., QTc >500 ms)
- Persons with clinically suspected LQTS regardless of 1) baseline QTc or 2) history of prior negative genetic testing in research laboratories or with commercially available targeted exon testing. (The rationale is that mutation detection methods over the past decade have changed significantly and false-negatives have been demonstrated. With respect to the targeted scan involving only 18 of the 60 translated exons comprising the comprehensive LQTS genetic testing, 35% of the LQTS-associated mutations detected in the Mayo Clinic Sudden Death Genomics Laboratory would have been missed.)
- All first-degree relatives of a genotype-positive index case. (Genetic testing is extended to more distantly related relatives in a concentric pattern as appropriate. For example, if confirmatory genetic testing demonstrates the index case's LQT1-associated mutation in the father, the father's parents and siblings—second-degree relatives to the index case—should be offered testing. Next, if the index case's paternal aunt tests positive, all the aunt's children—cousins or third-degree relatives to the index case—should be tested and so forth.)
- Persons with drug-induced torsades de pointes (debatable because estimated yield is 10%)
- Postmortem genetic testing in infant with sudden infant death syndrome (debatable because estimated yield is 5%-10%)

LQTS, long QT syndrome; QTc, heart rate–corrected QT interval.

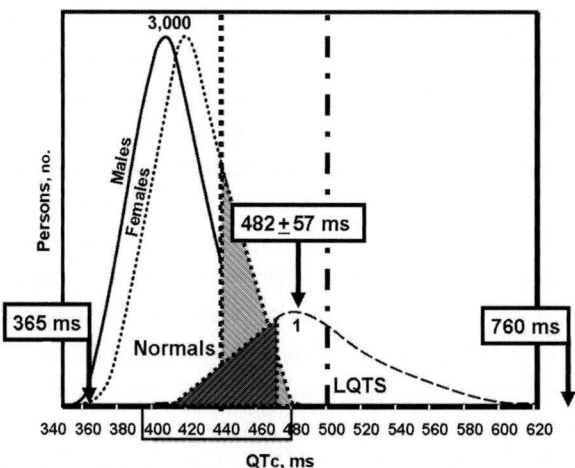

Fig. 2. Distribution of heart rate–corrected QT interval (QTc) in health and long QT syndrome (LQTS). Shown are the normal distribution of QTc values among healthy postpubertal males (solid line), postpubertal females (dotted line), and patients with genotype-positive LQTS from Mayo Clinic (dashed line). The shaded triangles indicate the proportion of the population with so-called borderline QT prolongation (>440 ms; the vertical broken line at 440 ms) and the proportion of patients with LQTS having QTc values that overlap with normals. The three annotated QTc values indicate the minimum, average, and maximum QTc values recorded in the Mayo Clinic Long QT Syndrome Clinic. The vertical broken line at 500 ms indicates increased torsadogenic potential for both congenital LQTS and drug-induced torsades de pointes.

QTc will yield too many false-positives. Further, these QT distributions do not apply to a 24-hour ambulatory ECG. In particular, the recording of a maximal QTc at, for example, 3 AM that happens to exceed 500 ms is not sufficient evidence for a diagnosis of LQTS.

To improve on the clinical diagnostic accuracy in the evaluation of LQTS, a composite clinical diagnostic scorecard (the Moss and Schwartz LQTS score) has been developed and is detailed in Table 3. This score includes ECG parameters (QT prolongation, torsades de pointes, T-wave alternans, notched T wave, and low heart rate for age), clinical history (syncope with stress, syncope without stress, and congenital deafness), and family history (LQTS and sudden death). A score of 4 or more indicates high clinical probability of LQTS and is associated with a 75% likelihood of a positive

LQTS genetic test result. Although this diagnostic scorecard helps with the evaluation of the index case, it will not identify many affected family members owing to incomplete penetrance and variable expressivity.

Efforts to identify individuals with concealed LQTS (genotype positive and resting ECG negative) include exercise stress testing and epinephrine QT stress testing. With exercise stress testing, failure to shorten the QT interval appropriately has been used to

Table 3.   Moss and Schwartz Score for the Clinical Diagnosis of LQTS

Variable	Points
Electrocardiogram	
QTc (at rest, not during Holter or exercise stress testing), ms	
≥480	3
460-470	2
450 (males)	1
Torsades de pointes	2
T-wave alternans	1
Notched T wave in 3 leads	1
Low heart rate for age	0.5
Clinical history	
Syncope	
With stress	2
Without stress	1
Congenital deafness	0.5
Family history	
Family member with LQTS	1
Sudden death in a family member younger than 30 years with no other identifiable cause	0.5

Congenital LQTS risk based on total score

Risk	Total score
Low	≤1
Intermediate	2-3
High*	≥4

LQTS, long QT syndrome; QTc, heart rate–corrected QT interval.
*The yield of LQTS genetic testing is 75% for patients with total score ≥4.

suggest LQTS. However, this failure to shorten during exercise is principally an LQT1-specific response. Therefore, the presence of normal QT-interval shortening during exercise does *not* rule out LQTS. Similarly, during infusion of low-dose epinephrine (≤0.1 μg/kg per minute), the presence of paradoxical lengthening (>30 ms) of the absolute QT interval is suggestive (75% positive predictive value) of concealed LQT1.

Annual mortality associated with LQTS is probably about 1% overall and 5% to 8% in the highest risk subset, which is similar to mortality in hypertrophic cardiomyopathy. Indicators of increased risk include QTc greater than 500 ms, history of LQTS-related symptoms, LQT2 or LQT3 genotype, and female sex. Both symptomatic and asymptomatic patients with LQTS must avoid concomitant exposure to medications that can lengthen the QT interval as an unwanted effect of the medication. In addition, patients should be alerted to maintain adequate hydration and electrolyte replenishment if they have vomiting and diarrheal illnesses, which could precipitate hypokalemia. Asymptomatic patients older than 40 years probably do not require active intervention, but this decision must be individualized.

In general, all symptomatic patients and all asymptomatic patients younger than 40 years at diagnosis should receive either medical or device-related therapy. β-Blockers, preferably nadolol or propranolol, should be considered standard therapy in all patients with either LQT1 or LQT2. In contrast, β-blockers are not protective and theoretically may be proarrhythmic in LQT3. Genotype-targeted therapy with late–sodium current blockers such as mexiletine should be considered in LQT3 instead. Indications for an implantable cardioverter-defibrillator (ICD) include 1) aborted cardiac arrest (regardless of genotype) as secondary prevention, 2) breakthrough cardiac event despite adequate medical therapy, 3) intolerance of primary pharmacotherapy, 4) symptoms with QTc greater than 550 ms (particularly in women with LQT2), and 5) LQT3 genotype (a debatable criterion).

In general, a single-lead ICD system is preferred unless pacing is required. Conversely, there is probably very little role for therapy with a pacemaker-only device. If a pacemaker is contemplated for therapy, then a dual-chamber pacemaker-ICD should be used instead. A left cardiac sympathetic denervation involving the surgical ablation of the lower half of the left stellate ganglion along with the left-sided thoracic ganglia T2 to T4 is indicated in patients receiving recurrent ventricular fibrillation (VF)-terminating ICD therapies. Radiofrequency ablation has been reported to eliminate a premature ventricular contraction trigger for TdP. According to the 2005 Bethesda Conference 36 guidelines, competitive sports are restricted (except class IA activities: golf, cricket, bowling, billiards, and riflery) in all patients with symptomatic LQTS (except possibly LQT3). This restriction may be loosened for patients with concealed LQTS (genotype positive but asymptomatic with QTc <480 ms in females and <470 ms in males).

Autosomal Recessive (Jervell and Lange-Nielsen) LQTS

In contrast to Romano-Ward LQTS, autosomal recessive LQTS (Jervell and Lange-Nielsen syndrome [JLNS]) is extremely rare, affecting 1 per million. The cardiac phenotype is generally more severe and, in fact, primary prevention ICD therapy is clinically indicated for JLNS. Pathogenetically, JLNS involves homozygous or compound heterozygous ("double hits") mutations in the I_{Ks} potassium channel (Table 1). Type 1 JLNS (JLN1) arises from such double mutations in *KCNQ1* (i.e., LQT1), whereas type 2 JLNS (JLN2) stems from double mutations in *KCNE1* (LQT5). These genes encode, respectively, the alpha subunit and the beta subunit of the critical phase 3 repolarizing potassium current, I_{Ks}. By definition, both parents of a child with JLNS are obligate affected individuals with either LQT1 or LQT5. That is, the cardiac phenotype in JLNS is a dominant trait, although the course in the parents is generally asymptomatic and the QT prolongation is minimal at most. In contrast, deafness is a recessive trait. This same I_{Ks} potassium channel is critical for potassium homeostasis of the endolymph in the inner ear. Again, β-blocker therapy and ICD therapy are the standard therapy in JLNS. Left cardiac sympathetic denervation should be considered for any patient with JLNS requiring recurrent VF-terminating ICD therapies.

Multisystem or Complex LQTS

Andersen-Tawil syndrome (ATS) is a multisystem disorder that affects skeletal and facial features, with periodic paralysis and abnormal cardiac repolarization. Loss-of-function mutations involving the *KCNJ2-*

encoded inwardly rectifying potassium channel (Kir2.1) are implicated in the pathogenesis of approximately 50% of ATS cases and are annotated as "ATS1" or "LQT7" (Table 1). Unlike the classic forms of LQTS, however, the abnormal repolarization in ATS1 is better characterized as normal QT intervals and prolonged QU intervals with long-duration U waves (Fig. 1 C). The incidence of sudden death is reportedly less in ATS1 than in LQT1, LQT2, and LQT3.

LQT8, also known as Timothy syndrome (TS), is a rare multisystem disorder that includes abnormal cardiac repolarization, syncope, and sudden death as well as syndactyly and significant learning disability. Mutations in the alpha subunit of the L-type calcium channel (Ca$_v$1.2) encoded by *CACNA1C*, particularly a specific missense mutation G406R, have been identified. The mutation results in nearly complete loss of voltage-dependent channel *inactivation* of Ca$_v$1.2, producing QT prolongation secondary to increased calcium influx (i.e., gain-of-function phenotype). Although extremely rare, LQT8 is associated with a very severe phenotype; primary prevention ICD therapy is probably indicated. Genetic testing for both ATS1 (LQT7) and TS1 (LQT8) remains largely confined to research laboratories.

Acquired LQTS

Besides mutant cardiac channels or cardiac channel–interacting proteins, abnormal cardiac repolarization, QT prolongation, and even TdP can result from numerous medical conditions (e.g., pheochromocytoma, anorexia, diabetes, and hypertrophic cardiomyopathy), electrolyte derangements particularly hypokalemia, and more than 50 Food and Drug Administration–approved medications that can affect the QT interval. In fact, QT liability and drug-induced TdP (DI-TdP) with sudden death have been among the most common reasons for withdrawing drugs from the market over the past 15 years (e.g., terfenadine, astemizole, cisapride, and grepafloxacin). Table 4 lists common medications that can precipitate QT prolongation and possibly DI-TdP and provides an Internet resource for an updated list of drugs with potential QT liability, which is maintained by the University of Arizona. The most potent QT-prolonging medications are the antiarrhythmic agents, particularly amiodarone, dofetilide, quinidine, and sotalol. Although QT prolon-

gation is extremely common with amiodarone, drug-induced TdP rarely occurs. In contrast, the drug with the most torsadogenic potential is probably quinidine.

The mechanism for the vast majority of potential QT-prolonging medications is inhibition of the *KCNH2*-encoded HERG potassium channel. Thus, DI-TdP and LQT2 are partially phenocopies stemming from either pharmacologically or genetically mediated perturbations in the I$_{Kr}$ potassium channel. In fact, an estimated 10% of patients with DI-TdP actually possess quiescent LQTS-susceptibility mutations. An adverse drug reaction could be the sentinel

Table 4. Common Medications* Known to Prolong the QT Interval and Potentially Cause Torsades de Pointes†

Antiarrhythmics
  Amiodarone (QT prolongation common, TdP extremely rare)
  Dofetilide
  Procainamide
  Quinidine (QT prolongation common, 5%-10% prevalence of drug-induced TdP)
  Sotalol
Antihistamines
  Astemizole (withdrawn from market)
  Terfenadine (withdrawn from market)
Antimicrobials
  Azithromycin
  Erythromycin
  Gatifloxacin
  Levofloxacin
  Moxifloxacin
Psychotropics
  Haloperidol
  Phenothiazine
  Thioridazine
  Tricyclic antidepressants
Motility agents
  Cisapride (withdrawn from market)
  Domperidone

TdP, torsades de pointes.
*Drugs are listed alphabetically.
†For a complete list, see www.torsades.org or www.qtdrugs.org.

event disclosing the presence of genetic LQTS. It is debatable whether clinical LQTS molecular genetic testing is indicated for all DI-TdP. At a minimum, a careful personal and family history should be obtained and consideration given for ECG screening of first-degree relatives. In DI-TdP, management includes discontinuation of the offending medication, intravenous magnesium sulfate, temporary transvenous overdrive pacing, and isoproterenol infusion. These strategies are aimed at preventing the pause-dependent or bradycardia-associated triggering mechanism for DI-TdP.

Short QT Syndrome

In contrast to LQTS, which was described clinically nearly 50 years ago, SQTS is a relative newcomer, with clinical descriptions first published in 2000. To date, there are 3 genetic subtypes of SQTS, each representing the antithesis of loss-of-function, potassium channel–mediated LQTS. Instead, the 3 SQTS subtypes stem from gain-of-function mutations in *KCNH2* (SQT1), *KCNQ1* (SQT2), and *KCNJ2* (SQT3) (Table 1). These mutant potassium channels accelerate cardiac repolarization.

The characteristic ECG findings are short QT intervals (QTc ≤320 ms) with tall, symmetrical, peaked T waves (Fig. 1 *D*). Clinically, these patients present with sudden death, syncope, and palpitations and sometimes paroxysmal atrial fibrillation. The age at which sudden death occurs varies greatly, from 3 months to 70 years. Most patients have a family history of sudden death, with probable autosomal dominant inheritance. The degree of incomplete penetrance, variable expressivity, and overall prevalence of SQTS are poorly understood. However, SQTS is felt to be much less common than LQTS, and examples have been reported of family members who are genotype positive for an SQTS-associated mutation but have a normal resting QT interval.

During electrophysiologic studies most of these patients have easily inducible VF with short atrial and ventricular refractory periods. The therapy of choice is implantation of an ICD. However, these patients are at increased risk of inappropriate therapies from T-wave oversensing. ICD detection algorithms may decrease the risk of inappropriate shocks. Adjunctive pharmacotherapy with propafenone or quinidine may help prolong the QT interval and decrease the potential for VF.

CATECHOLAMINERGIC POLYMORPHIC VENTRICULAR TACHYCARDIA

CPVT is characterized by exercise- or stress-induced syncope or sudden death in the setting of a structurally normal heart with a normal QT interval. CPVT clinically mimics concealed LQT1 (which has a normal QT interval) but is far more malignant. In fact, 3% to 4% of patients referred for LQTS genetic testing actually hosted CPVT-associated mutations. Initially, CPVT was described in children, but more recent studies suggest that the age at presentation varies from infancy to 40 years. One-third of patients with CPVT have a family history of juvenile sudden death. The hallmark ECG feature of CPVT is exercise- or isoproterenol-induced ventricular arrhythmias, particularly bidirectional ventricular tachycardia (Fig. 1 *E*). However, bidirectional ventricular tachycardia during exercise has been reported in ATS and LQTS. Nevertheless, a patient with a history of exertional syncope, normal QT interval at rest, and exercise-induced ventricular ectopy is far more likely to have CPVT than LQTS.

In contrast to the QT channelopathies, the pathogenic substrates for CPVT involve key components of intracellular calcium–induced calcium release from the sarcoplasmic reticulum (Table 1). Type 1 CPVT (CPVT1) stems from mutations in the *RyR2*-encoded cardiac ryanodine receptor or calcium release channel and accounts for an estimated 50% to 60% of CPVT. Mutations in *RyR2* confer a gain-of-function phenotype to the calcium release channel, resulting in increased calcium leak during sympathetic stimulation, particularly in diastole. In contrast to the autosomal dominant and sporadic CPVT1, CPVT2 is autosomal recessive and very rare and is due to mutations in *CASQ2*-encoded calsequestrin. Together, LQTS- and CPVT-producing mutations provide a potential explanation for approximately 10% to 15% of cases of sudden infant death syndrome and for 35% of autopsy-negative sudden death cases after the first year of life. CPVT genetic testing remains largely confined to research laboratories at this time.

All patients with symptomatic CPVT should receive an ICD because pharmacotherapy with either β-blockers or calcium channel blockers is not sufficiently protective.

BRUGADA SYNDROME

Brugada syndrome (BrS) is characterized by typical ECG findings of coved-type ST-segment elevation (type 1 BrS ECG; Fig. 1 *F*) in the right precordial leads (V_1 through V_3), in the presence or absence of incomplete or complete right bundle branch block morphology, and an increased risk of sudden death (Table 5). The prevalence of a spontaneous BrS ECG pattern in the general population is estimated to range from 0.05% to 0.6%. The characterization of a coved-type ST-segment elevation (type I ECG pattern) or saddle back ST-segment elevation (type II ECG pattern) may reflect distinct differences in the risk of sudden death. Overall, saddle back ST-segment elevation is more common in the general population and less specific for BrS. In contrast, the majority of patients who present with symptomatic BrS, both in Europe and in Japan, have a coved-type ST-segment elevation. The type I ECG pattern may be present at rest or when unmasked with class 1 sodium channel blockers, including ajmaline, flecainide, or procainamide. Provocative testing with class 1 agents is used strictly for diagnosis and is of little prognostic value. Superior performance with ajmaline during provocative testing has been demonstrated, but this medication is not available in the United States. Increased sensitivity with the resting ECG is achieved by placing the right precordial leads of V_1 through V_3 in the second intercostal space.

Patients are more often male, and they often present symptomatically with sudden cardiac death due to VF or with syncope due to polymorphic ventricular tachycardia. The age at diagnosis is variable, ranging from 2 months to 77 years, with a mean of approximately 40 years. In patients with idiopathic VF initially, up to 20% have BrS. An estimated 10% of patients with BrS also have atrial fibrillation (AF).

In contrast to LQT3, which is due to gain-of-function mutations involving the *SCN5A*-encoded cardiac sodium channel $Na_V1.5$, 15% to 30% of BrS is due to loss-of-function mutations in *SCN5A* (BrS1) (Table 1). To date, nearly 100 BrS-causing mutations have been identified in *SCN5A*, and this remains the only established BrS-susceptibility gene identified so far. There is no apparent difference in clinical outcome between patients with BrS1 and the approximately 80% with *SCN5A*-negative BrS. Patients with BrS1 tend to have longer HV intervals. Genetic testing is

Table 5. Diagnostic Criteria for Brugada Syndrome (European Society of Cardiology)

Appearance of type 1 ST-segment elevation (coved type) in >1 right precordial lead (V_1 through V_3) in the presence or absence of a sodium channel blocker

and

At least 1 of the following variables:
1. Documented ventricular fibrillation
2. Self-terminating polymorphic ventricular tachycardia
3. Family history of sudden death (younger than 45 years)
4. Type 1 (coved-type) ST-segment elevation in a family member
5. Inducible VT (electrophysiologic study)
6. Unexplained syncope suggestive of a ventricular tachyarrhythmia
7. Nocturnal agonal respiration

commercially available for BrS, but the a priori yield is approximately 20% and its principal role is in identifying asymptomatic carriers since it has no role in prognostic or treatment decisions.

The outcomes of BrS depend strongly on the presence or absence of symptoms and the spontaneous presence of a type I BrS ECG pattern. In patients who present with aborted sudden death, 62% had documented VF or sudden death in a 4.5-year follow-up period. In comparison, only 19% of patients who presented with syncope had VF or sudden death. This percentage further decreased to 8% in asymptomatic patients. Therefore, an ICD should be recommended for all symptomatic patients (either aborted cardiac arrest or syncope) with BrS.

The role of programmed electrical stimulation (PES) during an electrophysiologic study (EPS) in the risk stratification of asymptomatic individuals remains sharply debated. Proponents of PES-EPS recommend ICD therapy as primary prevention in the asymptomatic patient with inducible VF, whereas opponents suggest that there is little role for an EPS in the evaluation of BrS. Besides ICD therapy as secondary prevention, there may be a role for quinidine in the patient experiencing recurrent VF-terminating ICD therapies. Aggressive management of febrile illnesses is warranted since fever appears to be an arrhythmic trigger for patients with BrS.

FAMILIAL ATRIAL FIBRILLATION

AF is the most common sustained cardiac rhythm disturbance, affecting more than 2 million Americans. The prevalence increases rapidly with age. Traditionally, AF has been thought of as an acquired arrhythmia, with the majority of patients having coexistent structural heart disease and elevated ventricular filling pressures. However, recent discoveries have demonstrated a pivotal role for ectopic electrical beats within the pulmonary veins that contain myocytes for initiating AF. Maintenance of AF is associated with multiple cellular and tissue processes that are the phenotypic manifestation of genetic variation.

Some of the molecular underpinnings for AF have come to light recently. In 2003, a Mayo Clinic study demonstrated that 5% of patients with AF and 15% of patients with lone AF had a positive family history of AF. In 2004, the Framingham Offspring Study demonstrated an odds ratio of 2 to 3 for the development of AF if at least one parent had AF. In 1997, the first chromosome locus (10q22) for FAF was identified. Although that FAF susceptibility gene remains elusive, 5 FAF susceptibility genes have been discovered (Table 1). Consistent with the observation of AF as a frequent arrhythmic manifestation of SQTS and BrS, the pathogenic mechanism for FAF includes gain-of-function potassium channel mutations in *KCNQ1*, *KCNE2*, *KCNJ2*, and *KCNH2* and loss-of-function sodium channel mutations in *SCN5A*. Although these genes are part of the commercially available genetic test for LQTS, there is no clinical role presently for AF genetic testing. Overall, these genetic subtypes of FAF explain less than 1% to 2% of AF cases.

The clinical management of atrial fibrillation is discussed extensively in Chapter 25 ("Atrial Fibrillation: Management").

SUMMARY OF CLASS I AND CLASS II INDICATIONS FOR ICD IN CARDIAC CHANNELOPATHIES

Secondary Prevention

- History of aborted cardiac arrest (regardless of channelopathy).
- History of syncope in SQTS, CPVT, and BrS.

Primary Prevention

- Failed pharmacotherapy in LQTS (includes breakthrough syncopal episode or β-blocker intolerance).
- Jervell and Lange-Nielsen syndrome.
- Asymptomatic LQTS with QTc >550 ms (regardless of genotype).

Controversial or Debatable Indications

- LQT2 with QTc >500 ms (particularly females).
- LQT3.
- Asymptomatic or genotype-positive CPVT.
- Asymptomatic BrS with inducible VF during PES-EPS.

23

PEDIATRIC ARRHYTHMIAS

Co-burn J. Porter, MD

Although the mechanisms of dysrhythmias in pediatric and adult patients are usually the same, the clinical presentation and management plan vary considerably. Even such things as heart rate and PR interval are age-dependent; therefore, a table of normal values based on age is necessary when evaluating electrocardiograms from pediatric patients. This chapter reviews the salient features of most pediatric dysrhythmias, including their management. This chapter does not provide an extensive treatment of dysrhythmias in patients with complex congenital heart defects.

ACCESSORY PATHWAY-MEDIATED TACHYCARDIA IN STRUCTURALLY NORMAL HEARTS

Children have manifest or concealed accessory pathways; both participate in reciprocating tachycardias. *Orthodromic* reciprocating tachycardia occurs very often, and *antidromic* reciprocating tachycardia occurs very infrequently. Patients with manifest preexcitation are at risk of rapid atrioventricular conduction and sudden cardiac death if atrial flutter or fibrillation develops; however, both dysrhythmias are very rare in pediatric patients. Accessory pathway-mediated tachycardia

(APMT) can present at any time, from in utero to the teenage years, but patients who present when they are younger than 1 year tend to outgrow APMT. Because young children cannot register complaints about a rapid heart rate, parents have to be vigilant for subtle signs: pallor, rapid breathing, lethargy, irritability, and poor feeding. It is common for infants to have heart rates of 250 to 280 beats per minute ("too fast to count") during supraventricular tachycardia.

In patients with manifest preexcitation, echocardiography should be done to look for congenital heart defects; the incidence of associated congenital heart disease can be as high as 30%, most commonly Ebstein anomaly. Tumors of the atrioventricular ring (e.g., rhabdomyomas) also may cause preexcitation. Echocardiography is useful to assess ventricular dysfunction, which is frequently depressed after conversion of supraventricular tachycardia. Decreased ventricular function usually is temporary; however, in some cases it is permanent and part of a cardiomyopathy.

Conversion of supraventricular tachycardia depends on the clinical situation. For a fetus in utero, medication is administered intravenously or orally to the mother to convert the tachycardia and prevent progression to hydrops fetalis. It is much better for a premature baby to remain in utero. Control of the tachycardia is attempted by giving the mother medication. If a baby can be delivered at or near term, immature lungs can be prevented. The following medications have been given to mothers to convert and prevent recurrence of fetal tachycardia: digoxin, propranolol, procainamide, flecainide, and amiodarone.

For infants and children with hemodynamic compromise, direct-current cardioversion may be required even before an intravenous line is placed. For infants and children not in great distress, while materials for an intravenous line are being obtained, one can place a bag of ice slurry over the child's face to produce a strong vagal response to terminate supraventricular tachycardia. It is best to keep the ice bag over the eyes, nose, and mouth for only 5, 10, or 12 seconds (three separate tries) so as not to cause thermal injury to the tip of the nose. If the ice bag does not work, the intravenous line is placed and adenosine is administered. Once adenosine converts supraventricular tachycardia, it is best to give an intravenous medication (e.g., procainamide, propranolol, or amiodarone, but *not* verapamil) to prevent recurrence while determining which oral medication to use. Chronic therapy with oral digoxin is not used for patients with manifest preexcitation.

Any brief but sustained episode of supraventricular tachycardia in a pediatric patient warrants chronic daily medication or catheter ablation. For patients in whom APMT develops after the age of 8 to 10 years, the condition will be a lifelong problem and the risk of recurrent supraventricular tachycardia will not be outgrown. Orthodromic reciprocating tachycardia in a structurally normal heart is not a life-threatening problem, but it is a nuisance. Because it can occur at any time and place (e.g., on a family vacation, on a school field trip, or in isolated areas), it can be difficult to get emergency medical care. Thus, chronic daily medication (365 days a year) or catheter ablation is needed for APMT. Most centers prefer not to do an ablation until the patient is at least 4 years old. Currently, the success rate for ablations for pediatric APMT is 90% to 95% at the first attempt. Patients with appropriately evaluated and treated APMT should be able to participate in all activities. Generally, if a patient is substantially altering his or her lifestyle because of APMT, he or she is probably not receiving adequate or appropriate therapy.

ATRIOVENTRICULAR NODE REENTRANT TACHYCARDIA

Atrioventricular node reentrant tachycardia (AVNRT) occurs rarely in infants, but the relative incidence seems to increase in children 5 to 10 years old. By the teenage years, AVNRT and APMT account for about 95% of cases of supraventricular tachycardia in pediatric patients with a structurally normal heart, and they occur with equal frequency. AVNRT appears to be somewhat more common in females. More than 90% of clinical AVNRT episodes are of the typical form (slow-fast). The natural history of AVNRT is unknown, but some infants seem to have spontaneous resolution. Like most APMTs, AVNRT is a nuisance tachycardia and not life-threatening; tachycardia rates depend on the adrenergic state, sometimes with rates as low as 160 to 180 beats per minute. The key to diagnosis is a narrow QRS tachycardia and the absence of P waves, which are buried in the QRS complexes (RP interval <70 milliseconds).

Conversion of AVNRT can be attempted with an ice slurry while intravenous materials are being obtained. Because most patients with this tachycardia are older, carotid sinus massage can be attempted; it seems to work better in the more mature nervous system. Intravenous adenosine is very effective for conversion, and then intravenous propranolol or a calcium channel blocker can be given for a longer effect.

Sustained AVNRT generally indicates the need for chronic daily oral medication or catheter ablation. Currently, first-time ablation is successful in 95% to 98% of cases and is associated with complete heart block in less than 1% of cases.

ATRIAL ECTOPIC TACHYCARDIA

Atrial ectopic tachycardia (AET) is a rare dysrhythmia; only 5% to 10% of pediatric supraventricular tachycardias are AETs; however, it is the most common form of incessant supraventricular tachycardia in children. It is believed to be due to increased automaticity of nonsinus atrial focus or foci, has a high association with tachycardia-induced cardiomyopathy, is often refractory to medical therapy, and is not usually responsive to direct-current cardioversion. Ventricular function usually improves with control of ventricular rate or elimination of the atrial focus. AET occurs predominantly in infants and children with stucturally normal hearts. It occurs occasionally after open heart surgery. Most, if not all, patients are asymptomatic or only mildly symptomatic. Sometimes it is hard to distinguish AET with tachycardia-induced cardiomyopathy from a primary dilated cardiomyopathy with secondary sinus tachycardia. Almost all AETs have first-degree atrioventricular block. One must consider hyperthyroidism or pheochromocytoma in someone with apparent AET. AET is not abruptly terminated with ice or adenosine or other intravenous medication. Usually there is slowing of the atrial rate or evidence of atrioventricular block and the rapid atrial rate continues.

The three options for treatment of AET are 1) medication for rate control, 2) surgical ablation, or 3) catheter ablation of the focus. Radiofrequency catheter ablation is successful in 75% to 100% of patients. Unfortunately, some patients have multiple sites, which can result in failure to produce a stable sinus rhythm. Spontaneous remission of AET has been reported in both pediatric and adult patients.

Junctional Ectopic Tachycardia

Junctional ectopic tachycardia (JET) is a very rare form of supraventricular tachycrdia and occurs in two forms: 1) idiopathic chronic (usually *congenital*) JET, which occurs in the setting of a structurally normal heart, and 2) transient *postoperative* JET, which occurs after repair of certain types of congenital heart disease. The pathophysiology of JET is unclear, but it may be due to automatic or triggered activity. Congenital JET may go undetected for a while until signs of congestive heart failure develop; if the rate is very fast, affected newborns are brought to medical attention shortly after birth. Postoperative JET is more common in younger patients and usually occurs 6 to 72 hours after cardiopulmonary bypass for defects such as ventricular septal defect, tetralogy of Fallot, atrioventricular canal defect, truncus arteriosus, and single ventricle defects necessitating Fontan procedures. Electrocardiography can show junctional tachycardia with 1:1 retrograde conduction or retrograde ventriculoatrial dissociation with occasional sinus capture beats causing variation in the RR interval.

Treatment of the two forms of JET is different. Congenital JET usually is treated initially with antiarrhythmic medication, such as amiodarone or propafenone or cautious combinations of both. If medication is not successful in controlling the ventricular rate, then catheter ablation should be considered. For postoperative JET, a multiprong approach is taken: 1) minimizing inotropic infusions, 2) correcting electrolyte and other metabolic abnormalities, 3) using controlled hypothermia with paralysis and sedation, 4) infusing intravenous amiodarone or procainamide, 5) trying atrial or atrioventricular sequential pacing to restore atrioventricular sequence and improve cardiac output, and 6) considering use of extracorporeal membrane oxygenation.

Atrial Flutter

Atrial flutter is a rare condition in children with structurally normal hearts, but it can occur with some regularity in children with congenital heart defects either before or especially after surgical repairs. Atrial flutter even occurs in utero; however, many such atrial flutters are converted by the birth process and do not recur after delivery. A small number of fetuses with sustained atrial flutter may have associated morbidity or mortality; therefore, it is important to administer antiarrhythmic medication to the mother to obtain ventricular rate control at the very least. Once infants are delivered and undergo electrical conversion, long-term anti-arrhythmic medication is usually not required. Most fetuses and neonates with atrial flutter have structurally normal hearts, but some newborns and young children may have atrial septal aneurysms or restrictive cardiomyopathies. Thus, echocardiography is warranted. Many newborns with atrial flutter have 2:1 atrioventricular block and may not have any symptoms; however, they have a fixed ventricular rate without any normal variability, and this finding should be a tip-off to an abnormal heart rhythm.

Occasionally atrial flutter spontaneously develops in older children or teenagers with increased vagal tone. After direct-current cardioversion, these patients usually do not have a recurrence, but echocardiography is warranted to ensure that there is not a structural abnormality or ventricular dysfunction. Atrial flutter in the patient with a congenital heart defect, either before or after operation, can be a challenge to manage and may necessitate medication, ablation, operation, antitachycardia pacemaker, or any combination of these options.

VENTRICULAR ARRHYTHMIAS

Ventricular arrhythmias may be an isolated and completely benign finding, a marker of serious systemic disease or myopathy, or a mechanism for syncope and sudden cardiac death in pediatric patients. Isolated premature ventricular contractions are common. If they disappear with exercise testing and the results of electrocardiography and echocardiography are normal, they are usually of no consequence. They can occur with low daily frequency in as many as 40% of patients with apparently normal hearts. Sustained ventricular arrhythmias are much less frequent. Although sustained ventricular arrhythmias can occur in apparently normal hearts, approximately 50% of patients have either congenital heart disease or cardiomyopathy. The incidence of sudden cardiac death in pediatric patients is low; however, despite this, clinical decisions about management are difficult and generally require the expertise of a pediatric electrophysiologist. In large pediatric referral centers, only three to five patients with sustained ventricular tachycardia may be examined each year. The incidence of low-grade ectopy is notably higher in patients with congenital heart disease, especially in those who had repair many years previously, and cardiomyopathies such as hypertrophic cardiomyopathy and arrhythmogenic right ventricular dysplasia.

Symptomatic and asymptomatic patients with ion-channel abnormalities, such as long QT syndrome, catecholaminergic polymorphic ventricular tachycardia, and Brugada syndrome, are being recognized more frequently and providing greater management challenges, including consideration of implantation of a cardioverter-defibrillator. In the pediatric population, because neurally mediated syncope is common and life-threatening arrhythmias are rare, investigations of ventricular arrhythmias in patients with syncope often are uninformative. Details of the history, including medications or recreational drug use, and family history can direct more extensive investigation. Ventricular fibrillation is rare in the pediatric population. When it does occur, it is usually a degeneration of another malignant dysrhythmia. In a study of pediatric out-of-hospital cardiac arrests, ventricular fibrillation was the initial rhythm in 19% of cardiac arrests. Only 2 of 29 patients had a congenital heart defect. Fortunately, the outcome in patients with ventricular fibrillation is better than that in patients with asystole or pulseless electrical activity.

SINUS NODE DYSFUNCTION

Sinus node dysfunction is primarily manifested by sinus bradycardia, with heart rates less than the expected for age (a reference table of normal values is needed for evaluation) or sinus pauses of more than 3 seconds. The current approach to the diagnosis of sinus node dysfunction relies on noninvasive methods of testing (e.g., electrocardiography, 24-hour ambulatory monitoring, and exercise testing [chronotropic incompetence]). Invasive electrophysiologic testing can result in false-positive and false-negative results. Nonsurgical causes of sinus node dysfunction include genetic inheritance, certain types of congenital heart defects, inflammatory disease–like myocarditis, central nervous system disease, antiarrhythmic medications, hypothyroidism, and hypothermia. Unrecognized blocked premature atrial contractions concealed in the preceding T wave can appear to be sinus node dysfunction, especially true in newborns. Only *symptomatic* sinus node dysfunction should be treated with a permanent pacemaker. Occasionally, sinus node dysfunction can occur in concert with tachycardia, giving rise to the so-called bradycardia-tachycardia syndrome, which may require a pacemaker and antiarrhythmic medication.

SECOND-DEGREE ATRIOVENTRICULAR BLOCK

The implications of second-degree atrioventricular block depend on the underlying cause, its potential for progression to complete atrioventricular block, and the location and rate of the potential subsidiary pacemaker. Causes of second-degree atrioventricular block include mechanical (during catheterization), tumors (rhabdomyoma), myopathy (Duchenne muscular dystrophy), infection, immunologic (maternal systemic lupus erythematosus), genetic (long QT syndrome), metabolic, and drug-induced. A subgroup of newborns with congenital long QT syndrome may present with 2:1 atrioventricular block, related to His-Purkinje system or ventricular myocardial refractoriness. As in adults, heart block occurring above the His bundle (with a narrow QRS), and most commonly in a Wenckebach or Mobitz I pattern, is usually more benign than heart block occurring in or below the His bundle (Mobitz II pattern). Temporary or permanent pacing is dependent on symptoms and the likelihood of progression of the block.

THIRD-DEGREE ATRIOVENTRICULAR BLOCK

Third-degree atrioventricular block occurs in two forms, *acquired* and *congenital*. The acquired form has multiple causes: normal variations in vagal tone, associated congenital heart disease (L-transposition of the great arteries), direct injury to the conduction system, infections (Lyme disease), genetic causes (Kearns-Sayre syndrome), inflammatory disease (rheumatic fever), tumors (mesotheliomas, lymphomas), and medications. Postsurgical third-degree atrioventricular block, resulting from trauma to the atrioventricular node at operation, is the most common cause for acquired atrioventricular block in children. Generally, all patients with acquired third-degree atrioventricular block require permanent pacing.

Congenital third-degree atrioventricular block occurs in two forms. In one group, the fetus or newborn has bradycardia because of an embryologic disorder resulting in abnormal formation of the atrioventricular node–His-Purkinje axis in the setting of a complex structural congenital heart defect (e.g., L-transposition of the great arteries or ventricular inversion). In the other group, heart block develops in the setting of a structurally normal heart, but the mothers of affected infants form antibodies (anti-Ro) that pass through the placenta and affect the fetal atrioventricular conduction tissue. The mortality rate with autoimmune congenital atrioventricular block is estimated to be up to 50% in fetuses and may be 5% to 15% in newborns. Congenital third-degree atrioventricular block generally is identified during prenatal examinations. Occasionally bradycardia is found late in the third trimester and mothers are rushed to the delivery room unnecessarily for an emergency cesarean section. It is important that a fetal biophysical profile be obtained to avoid this unfortunate circumstance. Newborns with congenital heart block need to be monitored for congestive heart failure, the main indication for an early permanent epicardial pacing system. Occasionally third-degree atrioventricular block is found in an asymptomatic older child with a structurally normal heart, in which case the concern is that it is acquired; but in most cases the condition is congenital block that escaped detection in the newborn period. After the newborn period, the indications for permanent pacemaker include 1) pauses longer than 3 seconds on Holter monitoring, 2) progressive cardiomegaly with declining ventricular function, 3) junctional instability or wide QRS escape rhythm, 4) declining exercise performance on standardized testing, 5) QT prolongation, and 6) complex ventricular ectopy. Beyond the newborn period, a transvenous pacing system is a possibility to provide better long-term pacing thresholds. Currently there is discussion about the site of transvenous ventricular pacing and whether it contributes to late ventricular dysfunction.

ATRIAL FIBRILLATION: PATHOGENESIS, DIAGNOSIS, AND EVALUATION

Paul A. Friedman, MD

EPIDEMIOLOGY

Atrial fibrillation is the most common arrhythmia encountered in clinical practice, and its frequency increases with age (Fig. 1). Population-based studies have shown its prevalence to be 5% in patients 65 years or older. Atrial fibrillation is uncommon in young people, and its presence in individuals younger than 40 should prompt an assessment for secondary causes (see below).

■ In individuals younger than 40, look for secondary causes of atrial fibrillation.

MECHANISMS

Three broad mechanisms have been associated with the initiation and maintenance of atrial fibrillation: 1) rapidly discharging triggers or foci; 2) the autonomic nervous system, which may promote trigger activity and modify the substrate to facilitate arrhythmia; and 3) substrate abnormalities that permit and promote wavelet reentry. In a given individual, each of these mechanisms may have a varying role—atrial fibrillation is a heterogeneous disease.

Triggers

The thoracic veins that return blood to the heart are lined with smooth muscle that is electrophysiologically distinct from the endocardium proper (Fig. 2). The venous muscle has a shorter effective refractory period and is capable of more rapid discharge than the endocardium. Rapid discharge from the musculature lining the thoracic veins, most notably the pulmonary veins, leads to the initiation and maintenance of atrial fibrillation since the cardiac endocardium cannot keep up synchronously with the rapid discharge. A slower discharge rate may manifest as atrial tachycardia, and the coupling between venous and atrial muscle may

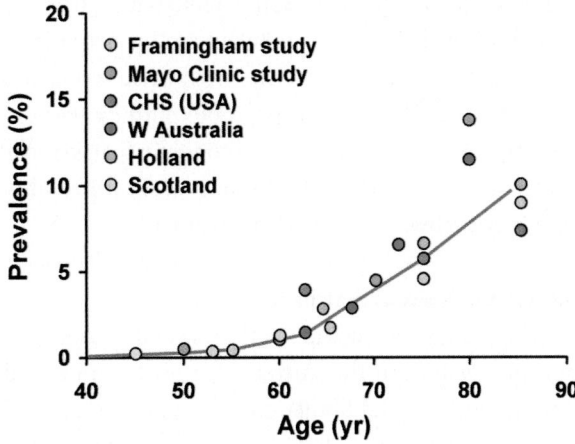

Prevalence of Atrial Fibrillation

Fig. 1. The prevalence of atrial fibrillation in six studies. W, western.

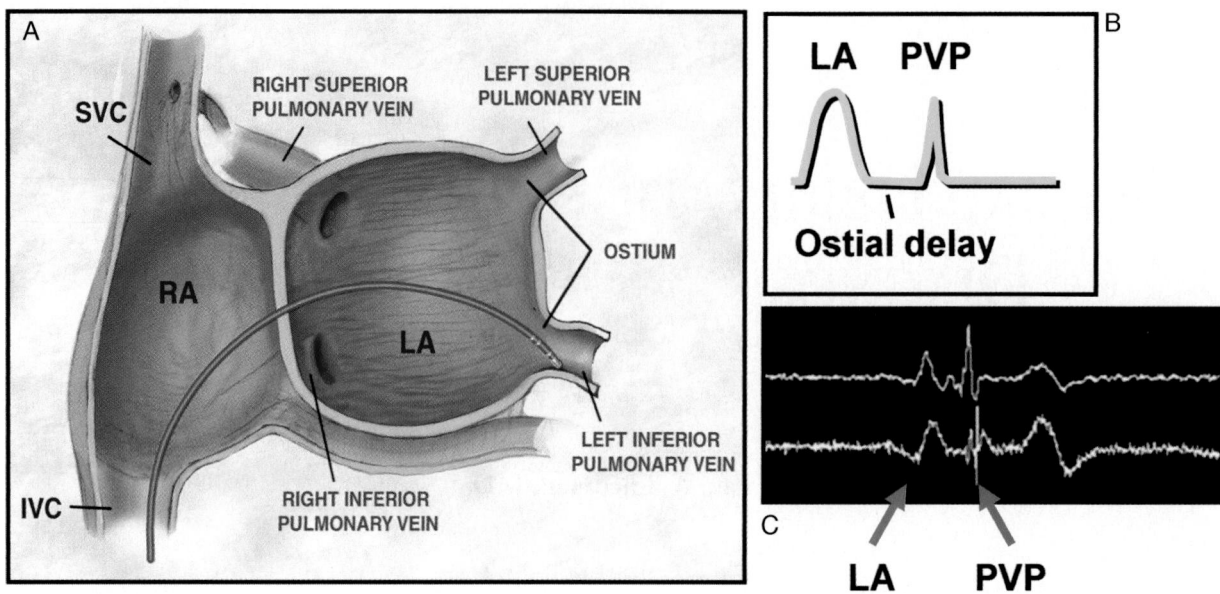

Fig. 2. *A*, A catheter is placed in the left inferior pulmonary vein to record the potentials. IVC, inferior vena cava; LA, left atrium; RA, right atrium; SVC, superior vena cava. *B*, Cartoon indicating the broad far field potential recorded from the LA and the sharp local pulmonary vein potential (PVP) generated by the musculature lining the vein. There is an ostial delay in propagation of the wave front from the LA into the vein. *C*, Actual recordings from a patient with atrial fibrillation.

determine which arrhythmia dominates. Ablation or isolation of pulmonary vein muscle sleeves isolates triggers and prevents arrhythmia in patients with this arrhythmia mechanism. Figures 3 and 4 demonstrate the presence of pulmonary vein potentials and their role in atrial fibrillation. This mechanism is particularly dominant in younger patients with little structural heart disease. Factors that promote pulmonary vein discharge include atrial stretch, autonomic (parasympathetic and sympathetic) stimulation, and possibly accessory pathway–mediated tachycardia.

Autonomic Nervous System

Numerous observations support the role of the autonomic nervous system in the initiation, maintenance, and termination of atrial fibrillation. The parasympathetic nervous system and enhanced vagal tone shorten the effective refractory period and increase its heterogeneity. Specific clinical entities associated with hypervagotonia and atrial fibrillation have been described (vagal atrial fibrillation) with characteristic onset at rest. Sympathetic stimulation, in contrast, tends to facilitate induction of

atrial fibrillation and automaticity in focal discharge. As seen in Figure 5, the autonomic components of the autonomic nervous system are in juxtaposition to cardiac structures. One of the proposed mechanisms for the effectiveness of catheter ablation for atrial fibrillation is modification of the autonomic nervous system.

Substrate

The third mechanism leading to atrial fibrillation is substrate abnormalities. Myocarditis and inflammation have been demonstrated in patients with lone atrial fibrillation. In patients with structural heart disease (such as congestive heart failure, valvular heart disease, coronary artery disease, and hypertension), abnormal hemodynamics, neurohormonal status, cellular connections, and other factors lead to atrial stretch and interstitial fibrosis. These in turn lead to heterogeneity in electrophysiologic cellular properties. This leads to a breakdown in waveform propagation and multiple wavelet reentry (Fig. 6).

It is important to recognize that the ventricular rate in atrial fibrillation in the absence of an accessory

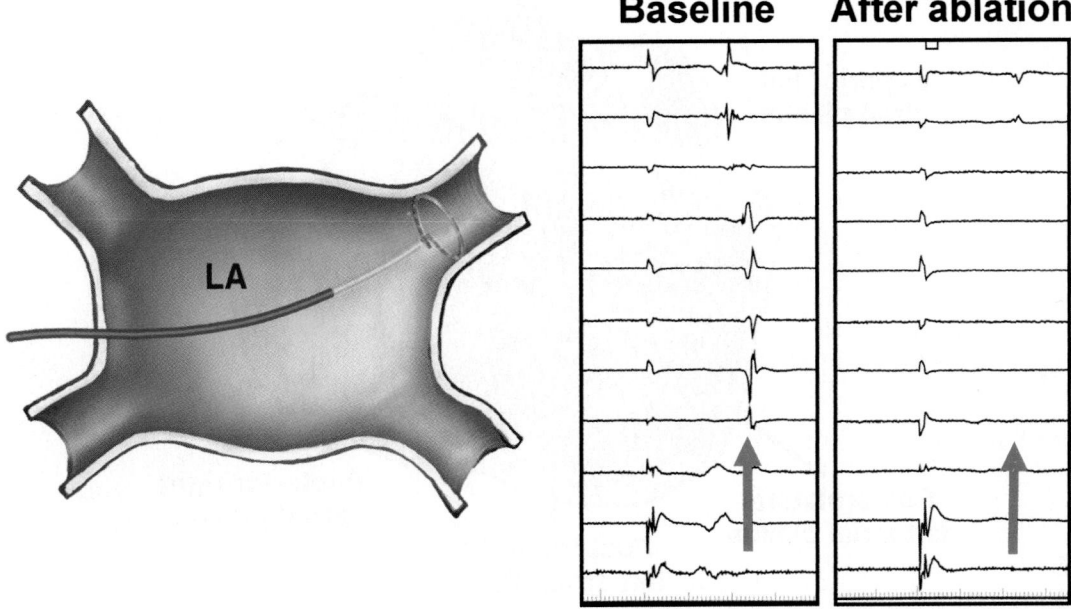

Fig. 3. *Left,* Use of a loop catheter to record potentials circumferentially around the pulmonary vein (left superior pulmonary vein shown). LA, left atrium. *Right,* In the baseline tracing, the pulmonary vein potentials are apparent (*arrow*). After ablation, these potentials are absent (*arrow*). Elimination of these potentials by catheter ablation has been associated with freedom from recurrence of atrial fibrillation, particularly in patients with lone atrial fibrillation.

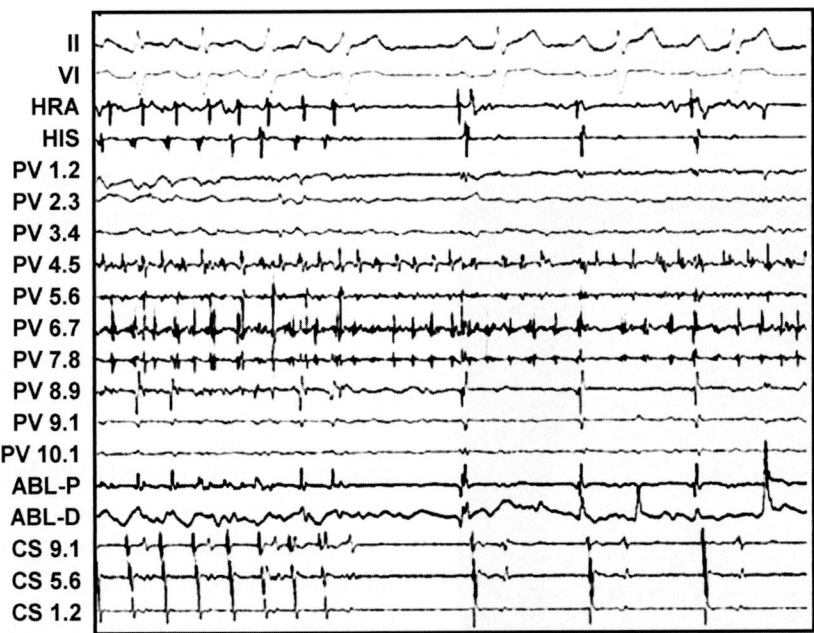

Fig. 4. Ablation during atrial fibrillation to isolate a pulmonary vein and restore normal rhythm. The top tracing is the surface electrocardiogram; note the termination of atrial fibrillation midway through the strip. The recordings labeled *PV* are from a loop catheter in the vein. Atrial fibrillation persists in the vein throughout the tracing. Ablation energy is delivered at the ostium of the vein. With vein isolation, the rapid vein discharges are "locked" within the isolated vein, so that normal rhythm is seen throughout the atria. CS, coronary sinus; HIS, His bundle region recording; HRA, high right atrium.

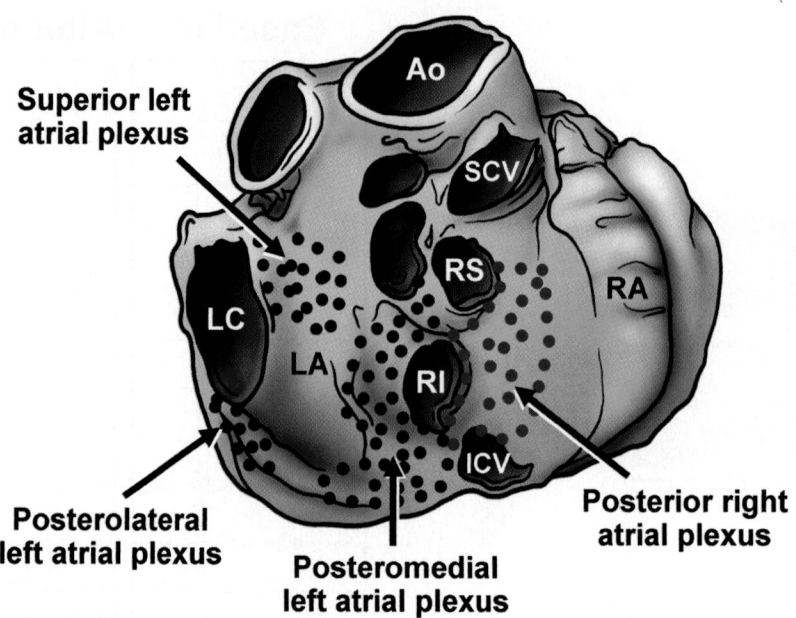

Fig. 5. Distribution of ganglionated plexuses (*circles*) around the epicardial surface of the heart. Ao, aorta; LA, left atrium; RA, right atrium.

pathway is determined by the conduction properties of the atrioventricular node (Fig. 7). The symptoms and effects of atrial fibrillation result from the loss of effective atrial contraction and from impaired ventricular function due to irregularity of a cardiac rhythm and elevated

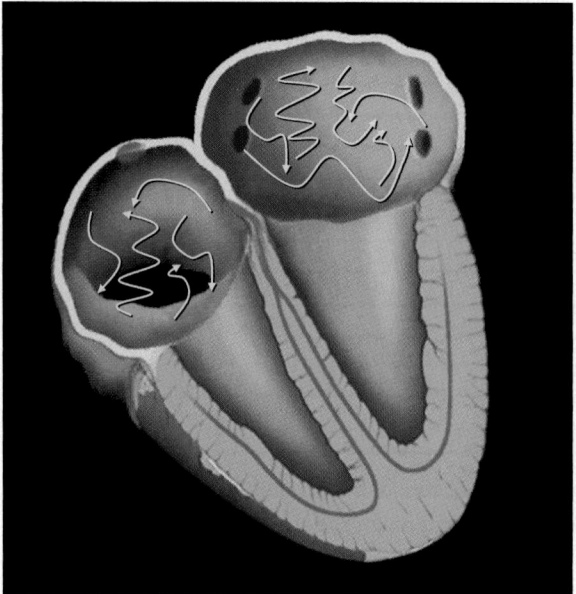

Fig. 6. Multiple wavelet reentry caused by substrate abnormalities in the atrial myocardium.

ventricular rate. Owing to its effect on overall ventricular function, atrial fibrillation has been associated with congestive heart failure, which in turn has been associated with atrial fibrillation (Fig. 8). Patients without symptoms of atrial fibrillation and with elevated ventricular rates (particularly resting heart rates >100 beats per minute) are at increased risk of tachycardia-induced cardiomyopathy because the arrhythmia may go untreated for a prolonged period.

■ Patients with asymptomatic arrhythmia are at increased risk of tachycardia-induced cardiomyopathy.

RISK FACTORS FOR ATRIAL FIBRILLATION
Atrial fibrillation is due to acutely reversible risk factors in a minority of cases. However, it is important to recognize reversible causes and treat them. This is particularly true in younger patients. Reversible risk factors include myocardial infarction, recent cardiac surgery, hypothyroidism, acute pulmonary disease, pericarditis, myocarditis, and toxin ingestion (in particular, alcohol). These are summarized in Table 1.

The ingestion of excessive alcohol has been well documented to be associated with atrial fibrillation.

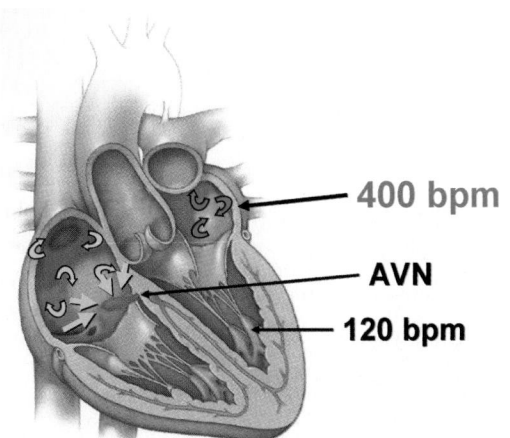

Fig. 7. The role of the atrioventricular node (AVN) in controlling the ventricular response. The atrial heart rate may be ≥400 beats per minute (bpm). Owing to variable conduction to the ventricle through the AVN, the ventricular rate is slower. Although atrial flutter has a slower atrial rate (typically 300 bpm), a higher percentage of the flutter beats may be conducted through the AVN, leading to a faster ventricular rate. This is particularly true with the administration of agents such as quinidine, which slow atrial conduction and enhance AVN conduction. This may paradoxically result in a faster ventricular heart rate.

Holiday heart syndrome refers to the occurrence of atrial fibrillation after heavy binge drinking. Ingesting more than three alcoholic beverages daily over the long-term is associated with a 33% increased risk of atrial fibrillation.

■ Binge drinking can lead to atrial fibrillation.

The minority of cases of lone atrial fibrillation have a strong genetic component. In the Mayo Clinic experience, 5% of the atrial fibrillation population has genetic atrial fibrillation.

It is also useful to divide atrial fibrillation risk factors into cardiac and extracardiac causes. These are summarized in Table 2. Common cardiac risk factors include valvular heart disease (mitral stenosis), sick sinus syndrome, cardiomyopathy, and Wolff-Parkinson-White syndrome. Common extracardiac causes include alcohol ingestion, hypertension, thyroid toxicosis, and advanced age. More recently recognized causes and factors include obstructive sleep apnea, obesity, and inflammation, as reflected in elevated C-reactive protein levels.

The role of sleep apnea warrants particular attention. Patients with obstructive sleep apnea have an increased

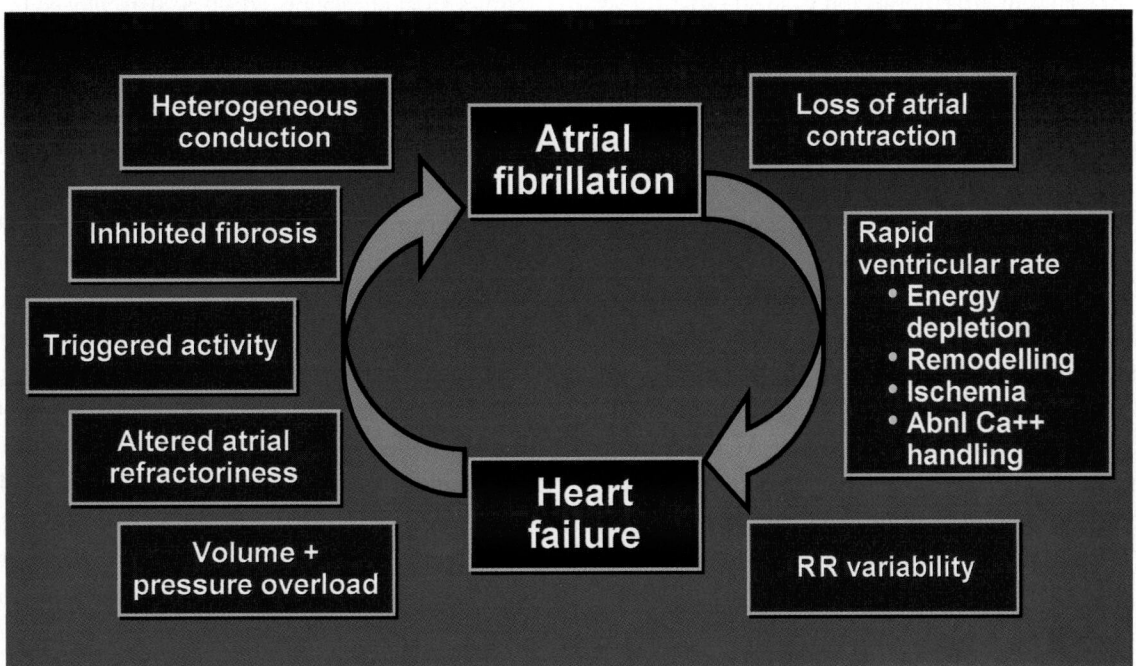

Fig. 8. Cycle of atrial fibrillation and heart failure. Atrial fibrillation propagates congestive heart failure, which in turn promotes atrial fibrillation. Abnl, abnormal.

Table 1.   Reversible Risk Factors for Atrial
            Fibrillation

Myocardial infarction

Recent cardiac surgery

Hypothyroidism

Acute pulmonary disease

Pericarditis

Myocarditis

Alcohol ingestion ("holiday heart")

Table 2.   Cardiac and Extracardiac Causes of
            Atrial Fibrillation

Cardiac	Extracardiac
Valvular heart disease (mitral stenosis)	Alcohol use ("holiday heart syndrome")
Sick sinus syndrome	Hypertension
Cardiomyopathy	Thyrotoxicosis
Wolff-Parkinson-White syndrome	Advanced age
	Sleep apnea
	Obesity
	Inflammation

risk of recurrence of atrial fibrillation after cardioversion. Evidence strongly suggests that treatment of sleep apnea with continuous positive airway pressure lowers the risk of recurrence.

The importance of inflammation and obesity is increasingly recognized. Postoperative elevations of C-reactive protein are associated with postoperative atrial fibrillation. In nonsurgical populations, an elevation of C-reactive protein has also been associated with atrial fibrillation. Therapies that reduce inflammation, as well as oxidative processes including statins, glucocorticosteroids, and vitamin C, have been shown to lower the risk of recurrent atrial fibrillation in small early studies, further highlighting the potential role of this form of therapy. Further studies are needed to support these therapies for atrial fibrillation; however, an aggressive stance toward the treatment of hyperlipidemia in atrial fibrillation patients appears warranted.

Hypertension is a particularly important risk factor for the development of atrial fibrillation. Among antihypertensive agents, angiotensin-converting enzyme (ACE) inhibitors and α_2 blockers may be particularly useful in preventing atrial fibrillation by mitigating cellular calcium overload and preventing interstitial fibrosis. Meta-analyses on the use of ACE inhibitors have demonstrated reduced atrial fibrillation. Use of β-adrenergic blockers may also be particularly useful to control the ventricular response.

Nutritional factors also appear to have a role in the pathogenesis. The consumption of broiled or baked fish was associated with a lower incidence of atrial fibrillation in a cardiovascular health study. This may be related to an anti-inflammatory effect.

DIAGNOSIS

Atrial fibrillation is diagnosed with the use of electrocardiography, which shows continuous and irregular activity of the electrocardiographic (ECG) baseline, caused by chaotic electrical currents in the atria. Atrial fibrillation is distinguished from atrial flutter, which is characterized by repetitive, stereotypical undulations in the baseline, resulting in a sawtooth pattern in the interior leads (Fig. 9). Multifocal atrial tachycardia (MAT) also mimics atrial fibrillation. MAT is characterized by premature atrial complexes with at least three different morphologic types that are distinguished from atrial fibrillation by the presence of an isoelectric baseline between complexes (Fig. 9). MAT therapy (calcium channel blockers and control of predisposing conditions) and atrial flutter therapy (medications or catheter ablation) can differ from atrial fibrillation therapy.

Typical atrial flutter results from a fixed reentrant wave front that propagates adjacent to the tricuspid valve anulus in the counterclockwise direction. Owing to the fixed circuit, a stereotypical pattern is seen with negative deflections in the inferior leads and positive deflections in lead V_1 (Fig. 10). This specificity of the flutter circuit is important because it permits catheter ablation at a localized site to eliminate the arrhythmia (Fig. 11). It is important to know that the same circuit can be activated in the opposite (clockwise) direction, resulting in a "reverse typical flutter" or clockwise isthmus-dependent flutter (Fig. 12). Both arrhythmias (clockwise and counterclockwise) use the same circuit and are treated with the same ablation procedure and medications, but they have different ECG appearances because of the direction in which the circuit is activated. In patients with previous left atrial ablation for atrial fibrillation (most commonly pulmonary vein isolation), the surface ECG may not be reliable for the diagnosis of typical atrial flutter since atrial activation is modified by the ablation process.

Several conditions can lead to a wide QRS complex in the setting of atrial fibrillation. These include the presence of a preexisting bundle branch block or aberrant conduction of a supraventricular impulse (Ashman phenomenon) or ventricular ectopy. In the Ashman phenomenon, after a long RR interval an early atrial impulse is conducted aberrantly because one bundle branch is not fully recovered from the previous impulse and is still partially refractory. Because the right bundle branch has a longer refractory period than the left bundle branch, aberrant conduction usually has a right bundle branch block (RBBB) morphology, classically with the right "rabbit ear" taller than the left (rsR'), as seen in "typical" RBBB (Fig. 13). Ashman phenomenon most commonly results in a small number of wide complex beats within an otherwise narrow complex rhythm, but

this can be variable.

Another cause for a wide QRS complex during atrial fibrillation is preexcitation, as seen in the Wolff-Parkinson-White syndrome. In the Wolff-Parkinson-White syndrome, atrial wave fronts may propagate to the ventricle through the atrioventricular node or an accessory pathway (Fig. 14). Variable activation by these two connections may lead to irregularly timed and variably wide complexes (Fig. 15).

- Atrial fibrillation must be distinguished from atrial flutter and MAT.
- In the presence of wide complexes, distinguish Ashman phenomenon (aberrant conduction) from the presence of an accessory pathway. Ashman phenomenon is characterized by long, short intervals and a typical RBBB pattern.

EVALUATION

History

Clinical patterns of atrial fibrillation are characterized in one of four ways: first episode, paroxysmal, persistent,

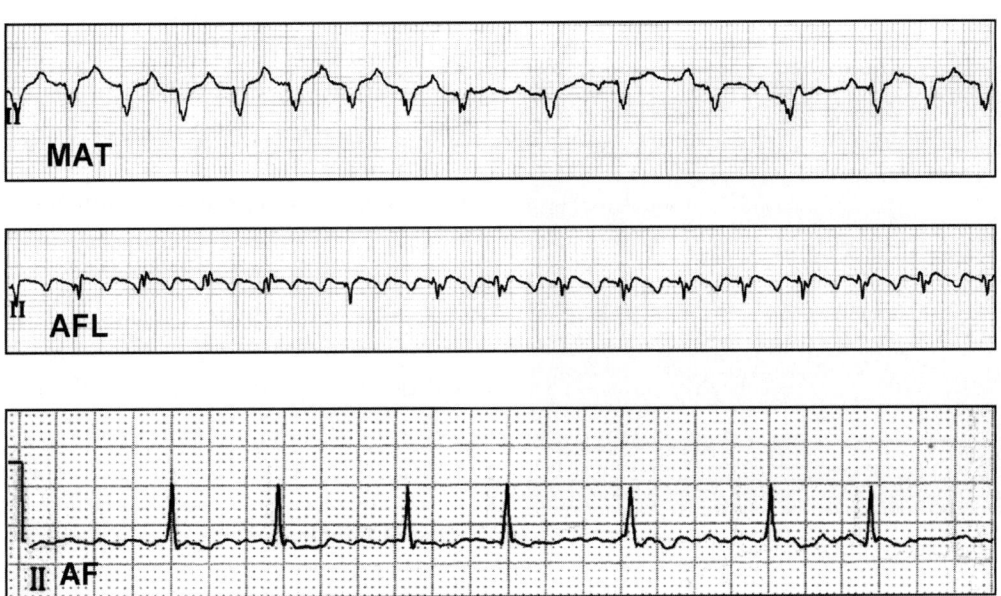

Fig. 9. Electrocardiographic identification of arrhythmias. *Top,* Multifocal atrial tachycardia (MAT) is characterized by premature atrial complexes of at least three different morphologic types with the presence of an isoelectric baseline. *Middle,* Atrial flutter (AFL) is characterized by repetitive monomorphic atrial activity. *Bottom,* Atrial fibrillation (AF) is distinguished by an irregularly and continuously undulating baseline tracing.

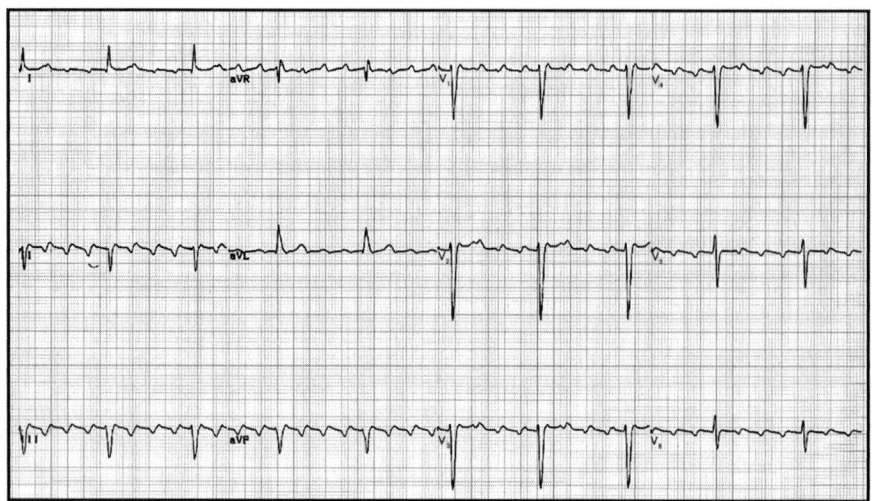

Fig. 10. Typical counterclockwise isthmus-dependent atrial flutter. Note that the atrial heart rate is typically 250 to 300 beats per minute and has negative sawtooth deflections in leads II, III, and F and positive deflections in lead V_1.

or permanent. Paroxysmal episodes are self-terminating, whereas persistent episodes require medical intervention for termination (pharmacologic or electrical cardioversion). Permanent atrial fibrillation is atrial fibrillation for which efforts to terminate either are not made or are not successful.

A key point of the history is to determine whether risk factors for complications of atrial fibrillation are present. Most importantly, these include symptoms of congestive heart failure, thromboembolism, and risk factors for thromboembolism (Table 3).

Patients with atrial fibrillation may be asymptomatic or they may present with palpitations, presyncope, dizziness, fatigue, or dyspnea. Frank syncope is less common and if present, specific causes should be considered. These may include pauses in patients with tachybrady syndrome (who may have a prolonged pause with the termination of atrial fibrillation), ventricular arrhythmias in patients who present with atrial fibrillation in the setting of cardiomyopathy, or, less commonly, hypotensive atrial fibrillation due to a rapid ventricular rate in the setting of cardiomyopathy.

- In a patient with atrial fibrillation and syncope, consider the tachybrady syndrome or underlying structural heart disease.
- Patients with asymptomatic atrial fibrillation are at greater risk of congestive heart failure owing to the possibility of prolonged, undetected rapid heart rates.

Physical Examination

On physical examination, there is an irregularly irregular heart rhythm and variable intensity of the first heart sound. This variability is from the changing interval between contractions, resulting in changes in filling of the ventricle and variation in the position of the mitral valve leaflet at the initiation of systole (Fig. 16).

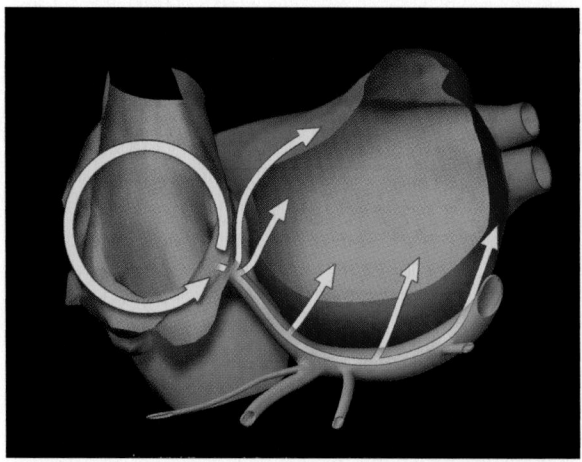

Fig. 11. The circuit responsible for atrial flutter. In this left anterior oblique view, the ventricles are cut away and the atria are seen. The *arrow* indicates the activation of the flutter circuit around the tricuspid valve anulus. The negative flutter waves in the inferior leads are seen because the wave front propagates from an inferior-to-superior direction in the left atrium.

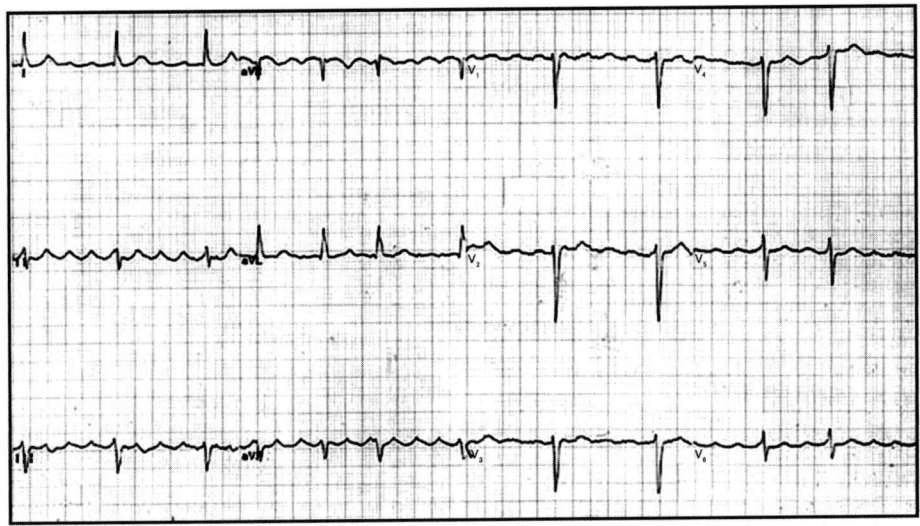

Fig. 12. Reverse typical or clockwise isthmus-dependent flutter. The electrocardiographic appearance of this arrhythmia may be more variable but typically has positive deflections in leads II, III, and F and negative or biphasic deflections in lead V_1. This arrhythmia uses the same circuit as typical atrial flutter but in the opposite direction.

A fourth heart sound is not present because of the lack of coordinated atrial contractions, and similarly an A wave is notably absent. If heart failure is present, the jugular venous pulsations may be increased, a third heart sound may be noted, and rales may be present. If atrial fibrillation is associated with valvular heart disease, physical examination findings associated with the valvular lesion may be present.

Investigations

All patients must have an ECG to identify the rhythm (verify atrial fibrillation). Additional important characteristics to look for on the ECG include the presence of left ventricular hypertrophy, absence or presence of preexcitation, bundle branch block, previous myocardial infarction, or abnormality of the RR, QRS, and QT intervals, which may be affected by antiarrhythmic drugs. Chest radiography is used to evaluate the lung parenchyma and to assess for the presence of pulmonary lung disease as well as to assess the vasculature for the absence or presence of congestive heart failure. An echocardiogram is of particular use to assess whether

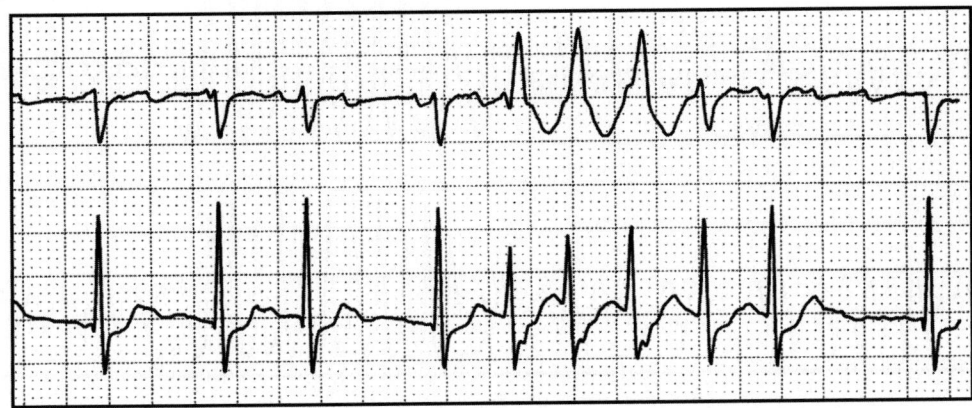

Fig. 13. An example of electrocardiographic findings in Ashman phenomenon.

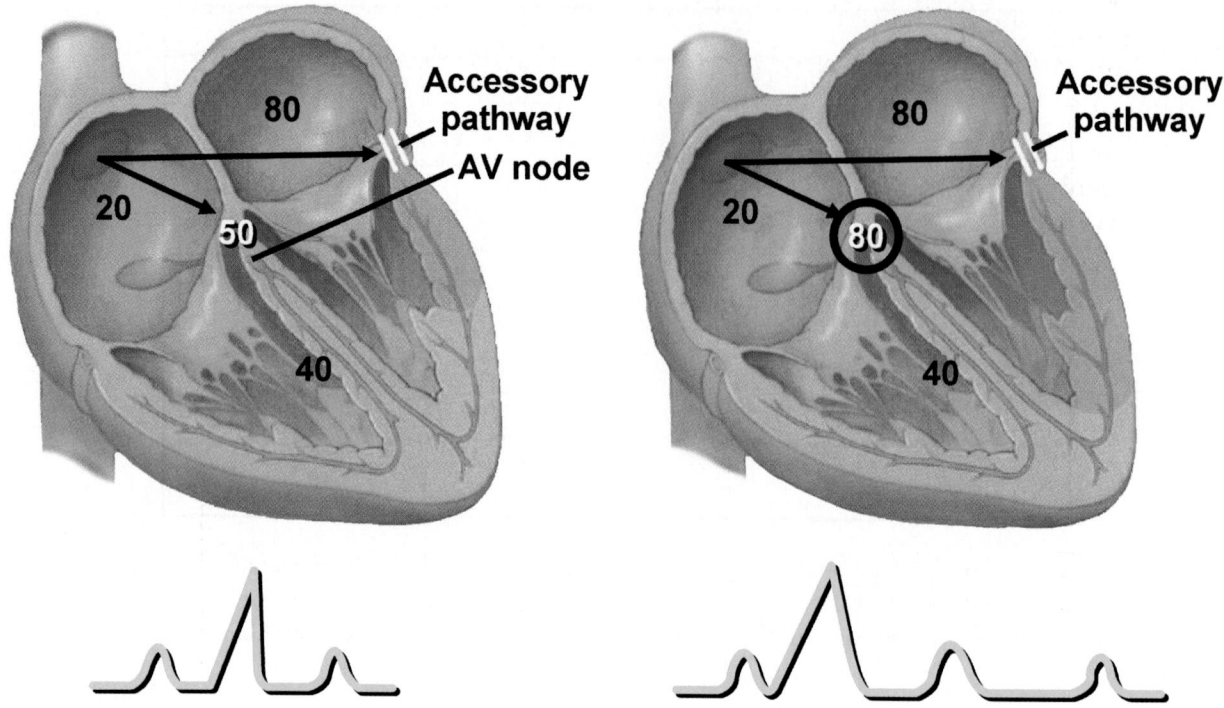

Fig. 14. Preexcitation. *Left*, An impulse simultaneously travels down the atrioventricular (AV) node and the accessory pathway with only modest preexcitation (region shown in purple). *Right*, There is greater delay in the AV node for a particular impulse. This allows for greater time for the wave front propagating through the accessory pathway to excite the ventricle, leading to a greater degree of preexcitation and a wider QRS complex. Varying degrees of propagation through the AV node and accessory pathway in atrial fibrillation lead to variably wide complexes.

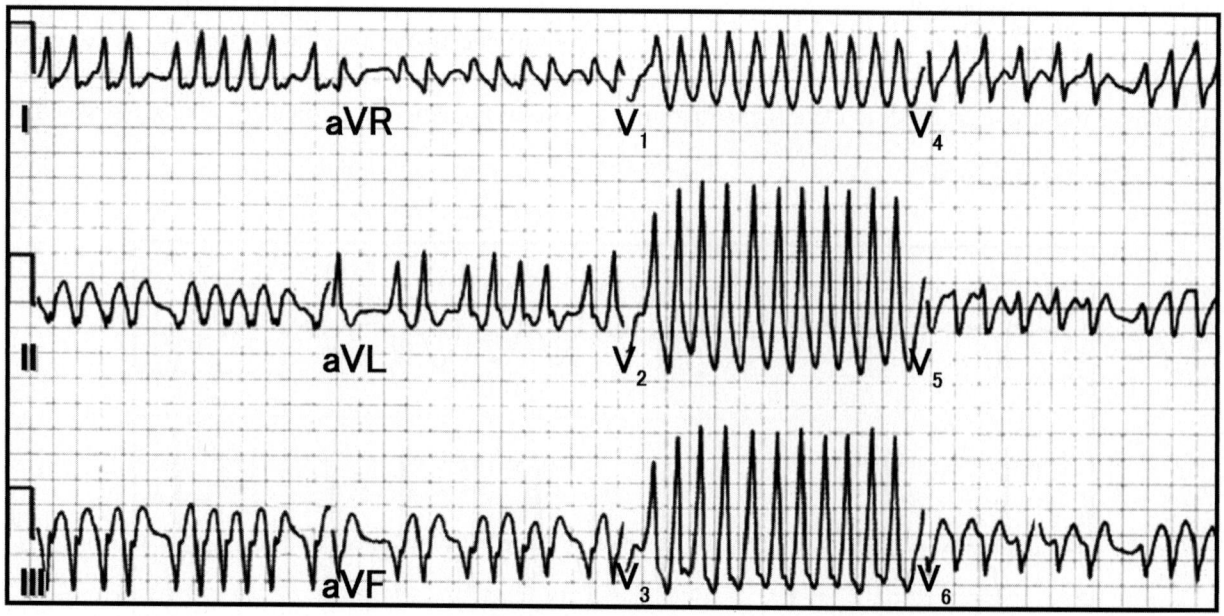

Fig. 15. The appearance of atrial fibrillation in the presence of an accessory pathway. The telltale features are variably wide complexes at irregular intervals.

valvular heart disease is present. Left ventricular size and function are assessed, as are pericardial disease and atrial sizes. Transesophageal echocardiography is warranted if cardioversion is planned and left atrial thrombus need be excluded. Screening blood tests, particularly electrolytes and thyroid function, are performed.

SUMMARY

A complete history and physical examination, with careful review of the ECG, screening blood test results, chest radiograph, and echocardiogram help in diagnosing atrial fibrillation, determining the risk of complications, and laying the groundwork for treatment.

Table 3.   Risk Factors for Ischemic Stroke and Systemic Thromboembolism in Nonvalvular Atrial Fibrillation

Risk factors (control groups)	Relative risk
Previous stroke or TIA	2.5
History of hypertension	1.6
Congestive heart failure	1.4
Advanced age (continuous, per decade)	1.4
Diabetes mellitus	1.7
Coronary artery disease	1.5

TIA, transient ischemic attack.

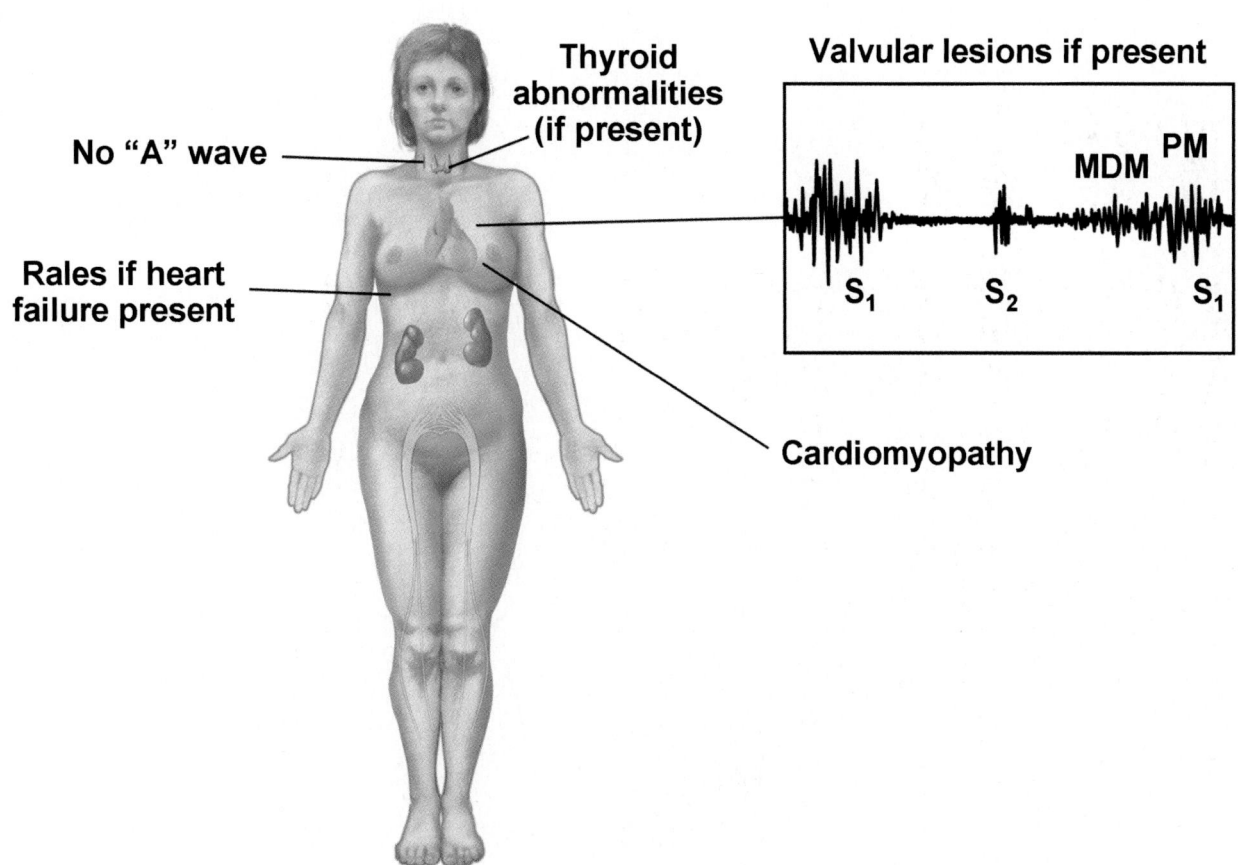

Fig. 16. Physical examination findings during atrial fibrillation. MDM, mid-diastolic murmur; PM, presystolic murmur; S_1, first heart sound; S_2, second heart sound.

ATRIAL FIBRILLATION: MANAGEMENT

David J. Bradley, MD, PhD

The major goals of treating atrial fibrillation are to minimize symptoms (chest pain, shortness of breath, palpitations, lightheadedness, fatigue, and malaise), prevent or reverse tachycardia-induced cardiomyopathy, and prevent thromboembolic complications, especially stroke. Whether treatment of atrial fibrillation in most patients improves survival is the subject of ongoing investigations. In general, atrial fibrillation treatment is individualized based on the patient's comorbidities, age, and symptoms and on the patient's preferences. Atrial fibrillation can be classified as 1) first-detected episode, 2) paroxysmal (self-terminating), 3) persistent (requires cardioversion for termination), or 4) permanent. The following discussion is derived from selected studies and from the American College of Cardiology (ACC)/American Heart Association (AHA)/European Society of Cardiology (ESC) atrial fibrillation guidelines.

SEARCH FOR REVERSIBLE CAUSES OF ATRIAL FIBRILLATION

The initial evaluation of a patient with atrial fibrillation includes not only a history, physical examination, and confirmation of the presence of atrial fibrillation by electrocardiography but also an effort to identify potentially reversible causes of atrial fibrillation. Reversible causes include myocardial infarction, cardiac surgery, pericarditis, alcohol use, pneumonia, pulmonary embolism, hyperthyroidism, atrial septal defect, caffeine use, pheochromocytoma, chest tumor, stroke, and Wolff-Parkinson-White syndrome.

Recognition of the relationship between Wolff-Parkinson-White syndrome and atrial fibrillation is important because episodes of atrial fibrillation in a patient with an accessory pathway can be associated with ventricular fibrillation and death (Fig. 1). Such a

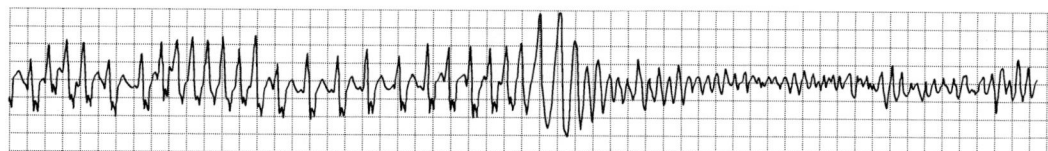

Fig. 1. Atrial fibrillation and accessory pathway–mediated, irregular wide complex tachycardia (*left half of tracing*) degenerating into ventricular fibrillation (*right half of tracing*).

patient may present with rapid, regular palpitations that become irregular later during an episode. The patient's electrocardiogram may show an irregular wide complex tachycardia with varying degrees of ventricular preexcitation (Fig. 1). Atrioventricular (AV) nodal blocking agents, such as β-blockers, diltiazem, verapamil, and digoxin, should generally be avoided under these circumstances because they may enhance accessory pathway conduction and thereby increase the risk of ventricular fibrillation. For patients who have atrial fibrillation and an irregular wide complex tachycardia and who are hemodynamically unstable, direct current cardioversion is recommended. In addition, intravenous procainamide or ibutilide can be administered to restore sinus rhythm. Ultimately, these patients should undergo radiofrequency ablation of the accessory pathway.

Another important, potentially reversible or transient cause of atrial fibrillation is cardiac surgery. Atrial fibrillation may occur in 20% to 50% of patients after cardiac surgery. It is most likely to occur on the second or third postoperative day, and it resolves in approximately 90% of patients within 2 months after surgery. Risk factors for atrial fibrillation after cardiac surgery include cessation of β-blocker therapy at surgery, chronic obstructive pulmonary disease, left atrial enlargement, advanced age, heart failure, and a history of atrial fibrillation. The risk of atrial fibrillation after cardiac surgery can be reduced substantially by treating the patient with a β-blocker before, during, and after cardiac surgery. Alternatively, amiodarone or sotalol may be administered prophylactically to decrease the risk. In addition, prophylactic biatrial pacing can be performed in patients shortly after surgery to decrease the likelihood of atrial fibrillation. In general, indications for pharmacologic rate control, cardioversion, antiarrhythmic drugs, and anticoagulation in patients with atrial fibrillation after cardiac surgery are similar to those for patients with atrial fibrillation not associated with surgery.

RATE CONTROL VERSUS RHYTHM CONTROL

For most patients with atrial fibrillation, a reversible cause cannot be found. Two general strategies, rate control and rhythm control, have arisen for the management of atrial fibrillation in these patients. *Rate control* refers to the use of drugs such as calcium channel

blockers and β-blockers and to procedures such as AV node ablation to control ventricular rate; no specific intervention is done to keep the patient in sinus rhythm. In contrast, *rhythm control* refers to an active attempt to keep the patient in sinus rhythm as much as possible through cardioversion, antiarrhythmic drug treatment, percutaneous ablation, and sometimes surgery. Regardless of whether a patient is treated with rate control or rhythm control, antithrombotic therapy for stroke prophylaxis needs to be strongly considered.

The relative merits of rate control versus rhythm control have been studied in several trials. The largest of these was the AFFIRM (Atrial Fibrillation Follow-up Investigation of Rhythm Management) trial. In the AFFIRM trial, 4,060 patients older than 65 years with a history of atrial fibrillation and additional risk factors for stroke or death were randomly assigned to receive therapy for either rate control or rhythm control. Mean follow-up was 3.5 years. Although patients assigned to the rhythm-control group were more likely to be in sinus rhythm than patients assigned to the rate-control group, there was no statistically significant difference in mortality, stroke, quality of life, or development of heart failure between the two treatment groups. Rhythm control was associated with a statistically nonsignificant trend toward higher mortality, and hospital admissions were more frequent in this group. A subsequent "on treatment" analysis of the AFFIRM trial showed that, although sinus rhythm was associated with improved survival, this benefit was offset by decreased survival associated with the use of antiarrhythmic drugs.

Trials such as AFFIRM have underscored the importance of individualizing therapy for atrial fibrillation. For example, elderly patients who are minimally symptomatic from atrial fibrillation will most likely benefit from rate control. In contrast, younger patients who are highly symptomatic from atrial fibrillation or who have no structural heart disease should be considered for rhythm control.

LONG-TERM PREVENTION OF THROMBOEMBOLIC COMPLICATIONS INCLUDING STROKE

One of the most important conclusions of the AFFIRM trial was that anticoagulation should be strongly considered in patients with a history of atrial fibrillation and risk factors for stroke. This is true even in patients in whom sinus rhythm has been restored. The reason is that silent episodes of atrial fibrillation may occur unbeknown to the patient or the physician. These silent episodes presumably contribute to the ongoing risk of thromboembolic complications in patients in whom sinus rhythm has been restored.

Risk factors for stroke in patients with atrial fibrillation can be conveniently remembered using the mnemonic *CHADS2*, which stands for "*c*ardiac failure, *h*ypertension, *a*ge 75 years or older, *d*iabetes mellitus, and *s*troke or transient ischemic attack." *CHADS2* also refers to a scoring system designed to estimate the risk of stroke among atrial fibrillation patients. This scoring system was designed from a study of 1,733 Medicare patients older than 65 years. To determine a patient's risk for stroke, one point is assigned for the presence of cardiac failure, hypertension, age 75 years or older, or diabetes, and two points are assigned for a history of stroke or transient ischemic attack (thus the *2* in *CHADS2*). As shown in Table 1, the annual risk of stroke is 1.2% among patients with a CHADS2 score of 0; the risk increases to 44% among patients with a CHADS2 score of 6. Patients are said to have low, intermediate, or high risks of stroke if their annual pre-

dicted risk of stroke is 2% or less, 3% to 5%, or 6% or more, respectively.

Which patients should receive aspirin and which patients should receive oral anticoagulant therapy (warfarin) for atrial fibrillation thromboembolism prophylaxis? Table 2 lists moderate- and high-risk factors for stroke among patients with atrial fibrillation. As shown in Table 3, aspirin is recommended for patients who have no risk factors for thromboembolism. For patients with one moderate-risk factor, therapy is individualized: aspirin (325 mg daily) or adjusted-dose warfarin with an international normalized ratio (INR) goal of 2.0 to 3.0. For patients with at least one high-risk factor or with more than one moderate risk factor, warfarin is recommended with an INR goal of 2.0 to 3.0. For example, a 47-year-old man with mitral stenosis and atrial fibrillation would receive warfarin with an INR goal of 2.0 to 3.0. In contrast, a 64-year-old woman with atrial fibrillation and no other moderate- or high-risk factors for stroke could receive aspirin.

As shown in Figure 2, maintaining the INR between 2.0 and 3.0 is important for minimizing stroke. An INR less than 2.0 is associated with an increased risk of ischemic stroke, and an INR greater than 3.0 is associated with an increased risk of hemor-

Table 1.   Risk of Stroke in National Registry of Atrial Fibrillation (NRAF) Participants Stratified by CHADS2 Score*

CHADS2 score	No. of patients (n = 1,733)	No. of strokes (n = 94)	NRAF crude stroke rate per 100 patient-years	NRAF adjusted stroke rate (95% CI)†
0	120	2	1.2	1.9 (1.2-3.0)
1	463	17	2.8	2.8 (2.0-3.8)
2	523	23	3.6	4.0 (3.1-5.1)
3	337	25	6.4	5.9 (4.6-7.3)
4	220	19	8.0	8.5 (6.3-11.1)
5	65	6	7.7	12.5 (8.2-17.5)
6	5	2	44.0	18.2 (10.5-27.4)

CI, confidence interval.
*See text for explanation of *CHADS2*.
†The adjusted stroke rate is the expected stroke rate per 100 patient-years from the exponential survival model, assuming that aspirin was not taken.

Table 2.   Risk Factors for Thromboembolism in Atrial Fibrillation

Moderate	High-risk factors
Age ≥75 years	Previous stroke, TIA, or
Diabetes mellitus	embolism
Hypertension	Mitral stenosis
Heart failure	Prosthetic heart valve
Ejection fraction	
≤35%	

TIA, transient ischemic attack.

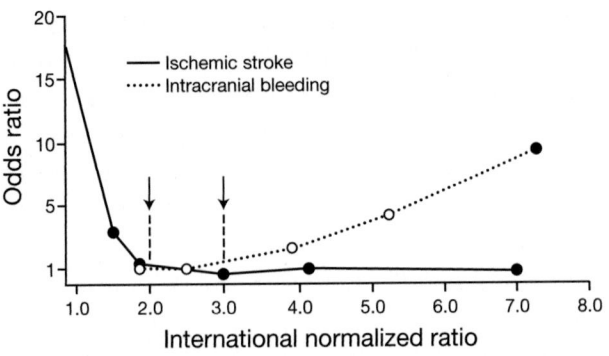

Fig. 2. Odds ratio of stroke according to the international normalized ratio (INR) in patients with atrial fibrillation. The risk of stroke increases with INR <2 and with INR >3 (*arrows*).

Table 3.   Antithrombotic Therapy for Patients With Atrial Fibrillation

Risk category	Recommended therapy
No risk factors	Aspirin, 81-325 mg daily
1 Moderate-risk	Aspirin, 81-325 mg daily
or	
factor	warfarin (INR 2.0-3.0)
Any high-risk factor	
or >1 moderate-risk	
factor	Warfarin (INR 2.0-3.0)

INR, international normalized ratio.

rhagic stroke. Overall, oral anticoagulation among patients with atrial fibrillation reduces the relative risk of stroke by approximately 60%. Warfarin is generally more efficacious than aspirin in reducing the risk of stroke. Among patients older than 75 years, a lower INR range of 1.6 to 2.5 can be used to minimize the risk of bleeding complications.

Several other nuances for anticoagulation in patients with atrial fibrillation should be kept in mind. Patients with thyroid toxicosis and atrial fibrillation are felt to be at increased risk of thromboembolic complications.

Likewise, patients with hypertrophic cardiomyopathy and atrial fibrillation have high rates of thromboembolic complications, and anticoagulation should be considered in these patients. In general, patients with atrial flutter should be treated like patients with atrial fibrillation for the prevention of thromboembolism. Patients without a mechanical heart valve may interrupt their anticoagulation for 7 days to facilitate invasive procedures that might otherwise increase the risk of bleeding. For procedures that require more than 7 days without anticoagulation therapy, treatment with unfractionated or low-molecular-weight heparin should be considered. Patients who have thromboembolic complications even though they have therapeutic INRs from 2.0 to 3.0 can be considered for higher intensity therapy with warfarin. An INR goal of 3.0 to 3.5 can be considered under these circumstances. For most patients with stable coronary artery disease, treatment with warfarin alone (no aspirin) is felt to be sufficient to minimize the risks of acute coronary syndrome or stroke. For patients undergoing percutaneous coronary intervention with stent placement, clopidogrel and warfarin can be combined without aspirin, although bleeding risks may be higher.

RATE CONTROL

Adequate rate control in patients with atrial fibrillation can be defined as a resting heart rate less than 80 beats per minute and a maximal heart rate of less than 110 beats per minute during a 6-minute walk. Controlling heart rate in atrial fibrillation may minimize symptoms by allowing adequate ventricular filling and by minimizing rate-related ischemia. Control of the ventricular rate may also reverse tachycardia-induced cardiomyopathy. For patients who present with hemodynamically unstable atrial fibrillation with rapid ventricular response, direct current cardioversion is indicated. The use of β-blockers, diltiazem, or verapamil is common to control ventricular rates in atrial fibrillation. Alternatively, amiodarone can be used for rate control. Digoxin alone is often insufficient to control heart rate, especially during exercise. It is important to remember that calcium channel blockers may exacerbate heart failure in patients with atrial fibrillation and low left ventricular ejection fraction.

For patients who have no response to drug therapy for rate control, AV node ablation combined with permanent pacemaker implantation can be considered. AV node ablation is a relatively low-risk procedure with very high success rates. By creating complete heart block, AV node ablation decreases symptoms and improves the quality of life for patients who have heart rates that are difficult to control. This procedure may also lead to an increase in left ventricular ejection fraction. AV node ablation does, however, generally leave the patient pacemaker dependent. Nonetheless, AV node ablation has been shown to have a neutral effect on survival. After AV node ablation, patients typically have their pacemakers programmed to a base rate of 90 beats per minute for 1 month to minimize the risk of ventricular arrhythmias and sudden death.

RHYTHM CONTROL

When restoration of sinus rhythm is the desired goal, patients can undergo direct current cardioversion. Young patients with atrial flutter and a short duration of atrial arrhythmias are more likely to have successful electrical cardioversions. In contrast, patients with cardiomegaly, including left atrial enlargement, are less likely to have successful electrical cardioversion. Biphasic shock is generally superior to monophasic shock for cardioversion of atrial fibrillation. Potential risks associated with direct current cardioversion include thromboemboli, sinus arrest, ventricular tachycardia, and ventricular fibrillation. Patients should have a normal serum potassium level and be free of elevated

digoxin levels before undergoing elective direct current cardioversion.

To increase the probability of restoring sinus rhythm and to maintain sinus rhythm for as long as possible, patients can be treated with antiarrhythmic medications in conjunction with direct current cardioversion. The choice of antiarrhythmic drug depends on the presence or absence of underlying cardiovascular disease (Fig. 3). For patients with no structural heart disease, flecainide, propafenone, or sotalol can be used. These treatment options are also available to patients with hypertension but no left ventricular hypertrophy. For patients with hypertension and left ventricular hypertrophy, amiodarone is generally recommended. For patients with coronary artery disease, options include dofetilide, sotalol, and, alternatively, amiodarone. For patients with heart failure, including those with depressed left ventricular ejection fractions, antiarrhythmic drug options include amiodarone and dofetilide. Note that amiodarone is a primary or secondary option for all the preceding patient categories. Amiodarone, however, has multiple potential side effects, including photosensitivity, thyroid abnormalities, pulmonary toxicity, hepatic toxicity, and bradycardia. Despite these side effects, amiodarone is generally at least as efficacious as other antiarrhythmic drugs in maintaining sinus rhythm. In the Canadian Trial of Atrial Fibrillation (CTAF), for example, patients were randomly assigned to receive 1) amiodarone or 2) propafenone or sotalol for maintenance of sinus rhythm after cardioversion. After 16 months of follow-up, 69% of patients in the amiodarone group were in sinus rhythm compared with 39% in the propafenone or sotalol group. However, 18% of patients in the amiodarone group stopped taking the medication (presumably because of side effects), and only 11% of patients in the propafenone or sotalol group stopped taking the medication.

Antiarrhythmic drugs can also be used without direct current cardioversion to restore sinus rhythm. Such pharmacologic cardioversion, however, is generally less effective than direct current cardioversion in combination with antiarrhythmic drugs. This is particularly true among patients who have had an episode of atrial fibrillation for more than 1 week. Pharmacologic cardioversion can be performed with dofetilide, flecainide, ibutilide, propafenone, or amiodarone. In contrast to its

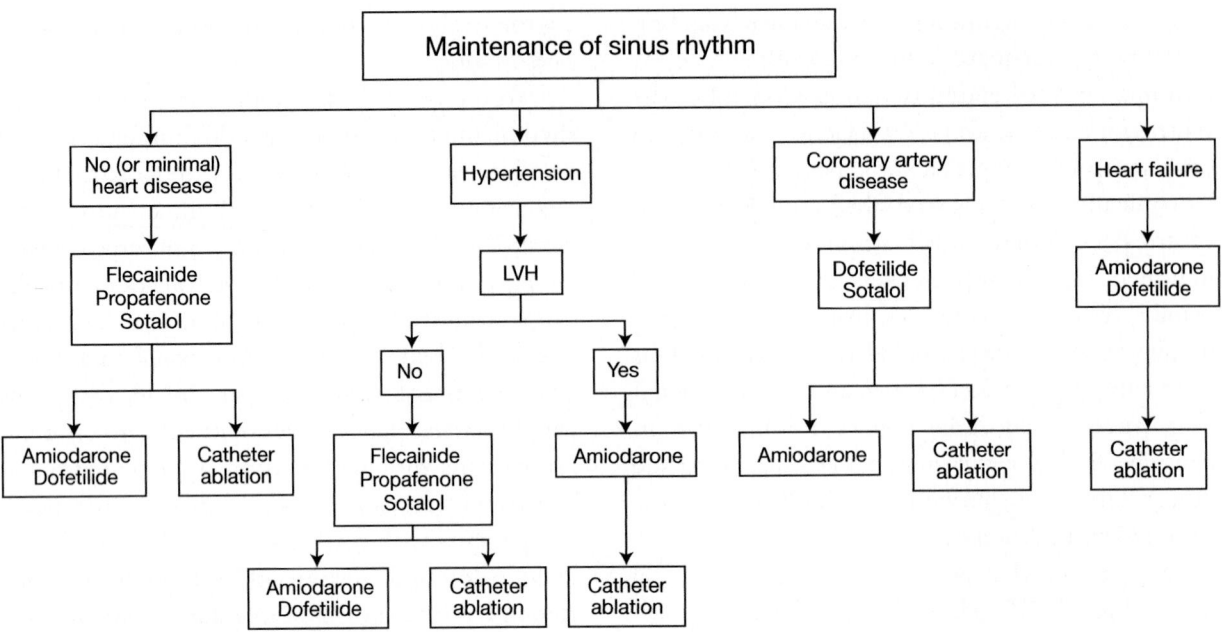

Fig. 3. Antiarrhythmic drug therapy to maintain sinus rhythm in patients with recurrent paroxysmal or persistent atrial fibrillation. Drugs are listed alphabetically and not in order of suggested use. The seriousness of heart disease proceeds from left to right, and selection of therapy in patients with multiple conditions depends on the most serious condition present. LVH, left ventricular hypertrophy.

ability to maintain sinus rhythm, sotalol is generally not recommended for pharmacologic cardioversion.

Regardless of which approach is taken to perform cardioversion, care must be taken to minimize the patient's associated risk of thromboembolism. After conversion from atrial fibrillation to sinus rhythm (spontaneously or by pharmacologic cardioversion, electrical cardioversion, or ablation), atrial stunning can occur, with recovery of mechanical atrial function occurring weeks after cardioversion. The early period after cardioversion is a high-risk time from the standpoint of thromboembolic complications. As a result, patients with atrial fibrillation for more than 48 hours or for an unknown duration should be anticoagulated (INR, 2.0-3.0) for 3 to 4 weeks before and after cardioversion. Alternatively, anticoagulation with heparin (to an activated partial thromboplastin time of 1.5-2.0 times the control value) can be initiated at the time of transesophageal echocardiography (TEE). If no intracardiac thrombus is identified with TEE, cardioversion can be performed with heparin bridging to warfarin therapy for 3 to 4 weeks with an INR of 2.0 to 3.0. For patients with atrial fibrillation for less than 48 hours, anticoagulation before and after cardioversion should be individualized based on the patient's risk of thromboembolic complications and bleeding. In general, patients with atrial flutter should be treated in a manner similar to patients with atrial fibrillation, with anticoagulation around the time of cardioversion. It is uncertain whether apparent maintenance of sinus rhythm after cardioversion justifies discontinuation of anticoagulation therapy, particularly in patients with a high risk of stroke.

Consider the following two special circumstances:
1. If atrial fibrillation is associated with heavy meals or sleep, vagally mediated atrial fibrillation should be considered. Such a patient may also present with worsening atrial fibrillation when treated with a β-blocker or a calcium channel blocker. These patients often respond to treatment with disopyramide.
2. In some patients, atrial fibrillation may develop only during exercise or stressful situations. These patients may respond well to treatment with β-blockers.

Some patients can be treated surgically to restore

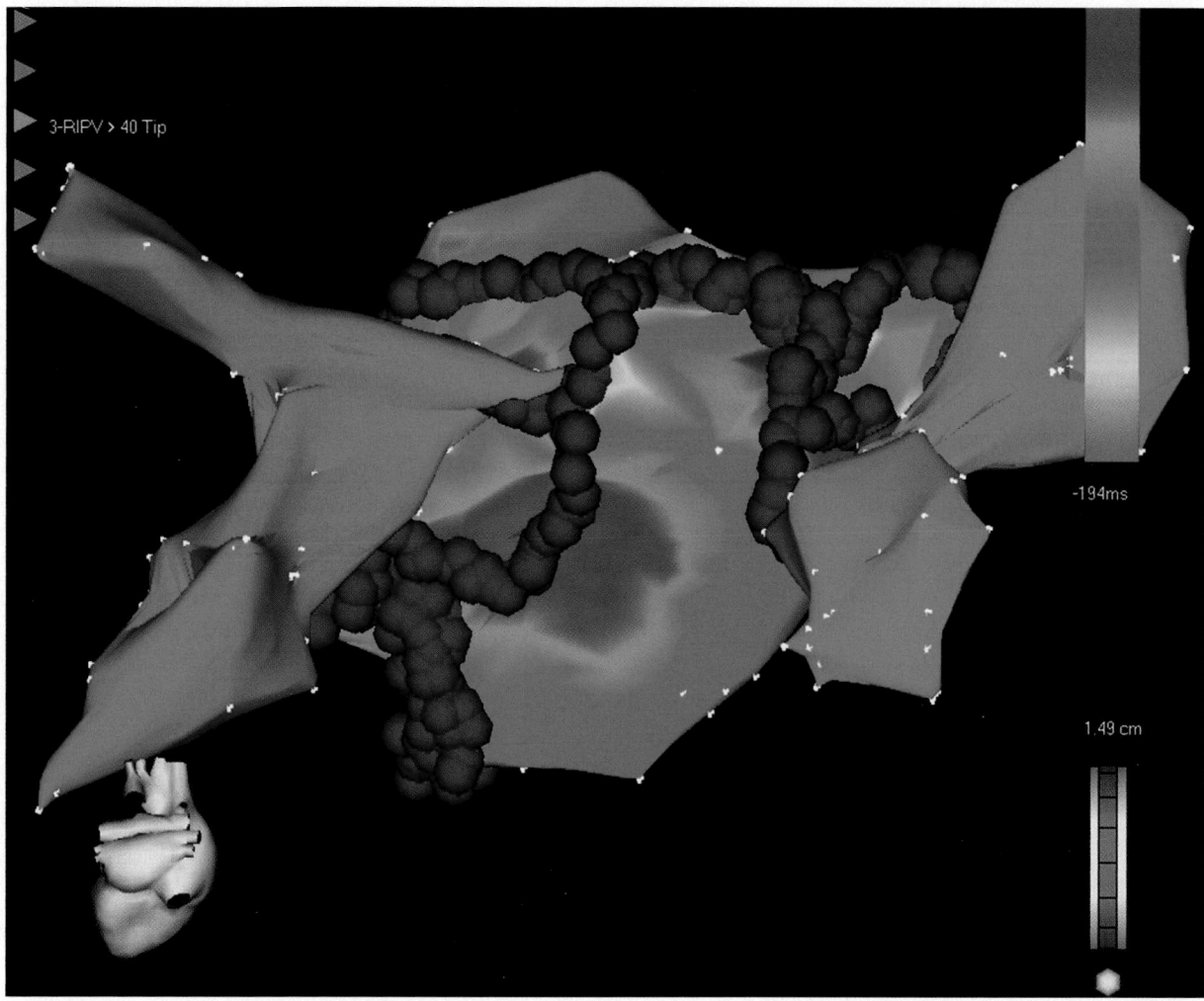

3-RIPV > 40 Tip

-194ms

1.49 cm

Fig. 4. Posterior view of the left atrium in the form of an electroanatomic map. Red circles indicate sites of ablation.

and maintain sinus rhythm. A surgical maze procedure involves the creation of linear lesions in the atria at cardiac surgery. This general approach has a high rate of success for maintenance of sinus rhythm. In addition, atrial function is maintained, and when combined with left atrial appendage closure, thromboembolic risk can be reduced. Surgical maze is generally reserved for patients who otherwise have an indication for cardiac surgery.

Left atrial ablation is an emerging alternative to traditional drug therapy for atrial fibrillation rhythm control (Fig. 4). The procedure continues to undergo rapid technical evolution, with improving success rates and decreasing complication rates. It is generally reserved for patients who remain symptomatic from atrial fibrillation despite treatment with at least one antiarrhythmic drug. With results from ongoing trials, left atrial ablation may become the primary therapy for atrial fibrillation. Complications from left atrial ablation include cardiac perforation, stroke, pulmonary vein stenosis, and atrial esophageal fistula formation.

ALTERNATIVE THERAPIES

Statin medications and angiotensin-converting enzyme (ACE) inhibitors have been associated with decreased rates of atrial fibrillation, and obstructive sleep apnea has been associated with atrial fibrillation. Further investigation is required, however, before statins, ACE inhibitors, and therapy for sleep apnea can be routinely recommended for patients with atrial fibrillation.

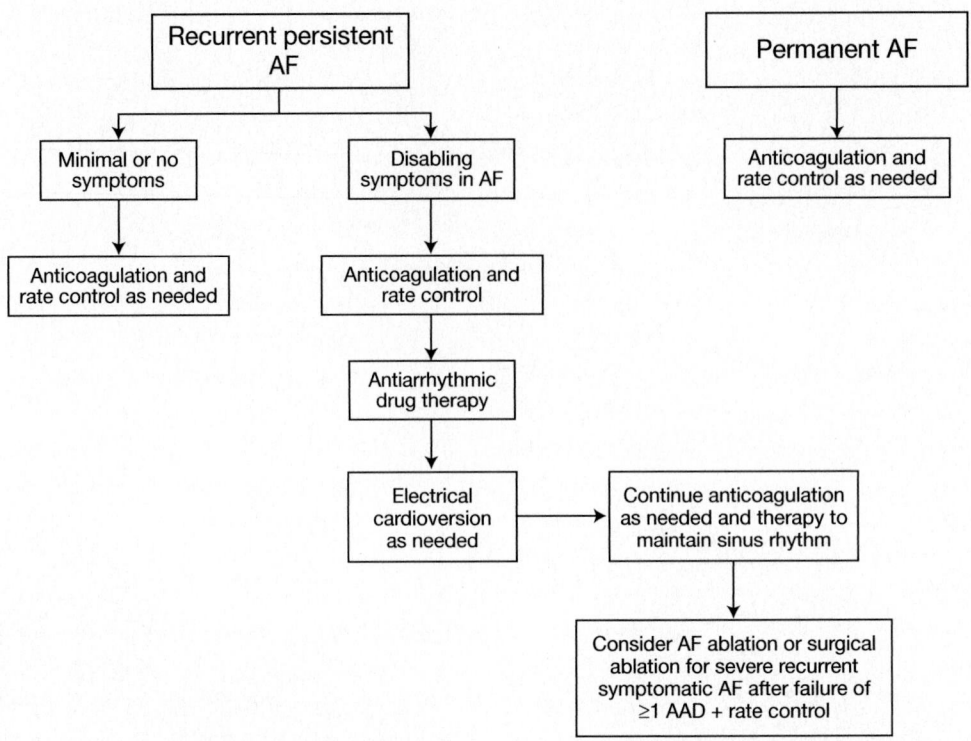

Fig. 5. General approach to management of patients with persistent and permanent atrial fibrillation. AAD, antiarrhythmic drug; AF, atrial fibrillation.

SUMMARY

Figure 5 summarizes the general approach to management of many patients with atrial fibrillation. For patients with persistent atrial fibrillation who have minimal or no symptoms, rate control with anticoagulation can be used. Other patients with persistent atrial fibrillation and pronounced symptoms or young patients with structurally normal hearts can receive anticoagulation and rate control medicines as well as antiarrhythmic drugs to maintain sinus rhythm. Electrical cardioversion can be used as an adjunct to these therapies to maintain sinus rhythm. If pharmacologic therapy fails to maintain sinus rhythm, left atrial ablation or a surgical maze procedure can be considered as alternatives to maintain sinus rhythm. For patients with permanent atrial fibrillation, rate control and anticoagulation can be used.

26

ATRIAL FLUTTER

Yong-Mei Cha, MD

DEFINITION

In 1906, Einthoven made the first electrocardiographic recording of atrial flutter. In the past century, experimental and clinical studies concurred that atrial flutter is an intra-atrial macroreentrant tachycardia involving a large area of atrial tissue with a critical slow conduction zone. An excitable gap in the macroreentry circuit allows the entrainment of the atrial flutter; the arrhythmia can be terminated by pacing at a rate faster than the flutter. On 12-lead electrocardiography, the atrial rhythm is typically regular at a rate of 250 to 350 flutter "beats" per minute with little or no isoelectric interval. Atrioventricular (AV) conduction is usually 2:1 if AV nodal conduction is intact.

EPIDEMIOLOGY

Atrial flutter is a common tachyarrhythmia, occurring in approximately 10% of patients presenting with supraventricular tachycardia. A population-based study found that it coexists in approximately 50% of patients who have atrial fibrillation. The estimated incidence of atrial flutter in the United States is 200,000 cases per year. Advanced age is an independent risk factor. The incidence of atrial flutter is 5 per 100,000 in persons younger than 50 years, and increases to 587 per 100,000 in persons older than 80 years. Men are more

prone to atrial flutter; it is 2.5 times more common in men than women. In addition to advanced age and male sex, other factors predispose to atrial flutter (Table 1). Mortality is 1.7 times greater among patients with atrial flutter than in those without it after adjustment for cardiovascular risk factors. Overall mortality is similar

Table 1. Factors Predisposing to Atrial Flutter

Advanced age
Male sex
Hypertension
Coronary artery disease
Valvular heart disease
Dilated or hypertrophic cardiomyopathy
Congestive heart failure
Sick sinus syndrome
Cardiac operation
Pericardial disease
Congenital heart disease
Thyroid toxicosis
Alcohol
Chronic lung disease

among patients with atrial fibrillation or atrial flutter or both arrhythmias.

CAVOTRICUSPID-DEPENDENT ATRIAL FLUTTER

Atrial flutter may use various reentry circuits in the right and left atria. The most common and classic type of atrial flutter (i.e., typical flutter) is dependent on the cavotricuspid isthmus (Table 2). The isthmus is bound anteriorly by the tricuspid valve and posteriorly by the inferior vena cava, the eustachian valve, and the eustachian ridge. In counterclockwise cavotricuspid isthmus-dependent flutter, there is a cranial caudal activation sequence along the right atrial lateral wall, across the cavotricuspid isthmus in a lateral-to-medial direction (Fig. 1 *A*). The wavefront then propagates superiorly in the right atrial septum. Morphologically, the flutter wave on 12-lead electrocardiography is characterized as negative sawtooth flutter waves in inferior leads II, III, and aVF and positive flutter waves in lead V_1 with transition to a negative deflection in lead V_6 (Fig. 2 *A*).

The activation sequence of atrial flutter is reversed in clockwise cavotricuspid isthmus-dependent flutter with a cranial caudal activation down the septum and a medial-to-lateral activation over the cavotricuspid isthmus (reverse typical flutter, Fig. 1 *B*). The sawtooth flutter waves are positive in inferior leads II, III, and aVF and negative in lead V_1 with a transition to positive waves in lead V_6. The conduction through the narrow isthmus is much slowed. Counterclockwise cavotricuspid isthmus-dependent atrial flutter makes up 90% of clinical cases.

Lower loop reentry is cavotricuspid isthmus-dependent flutter during which the reentry wavefront circulates around the inferior vena cava due to conduction across the crista terminalis (Fig. 1 *C*). Double wave reentry is defined as a circuit in which two flutter waves simultaneously occupy the usual flutter pathway because of a large excitable gap in the circuit.

NONCAVOTRICUSPID-DEPENDENT ATRIAL FLUTTER

This category includes the atrial flutter that does not use the cavotricuspid isthmus. Scar-related right atrial

Table 2.   Classification of Atrial Flutter

Cavotricuspid isthmus-dependent flutter
    Counterclockwise flutter (typical atrial flutter)
    Clockwise flutter
    Lower loop reentry
    Double wave flutter
Noncavotricuspid isthmus-dependent flutter
    Right atrium
        Incision or scar-related reentry
        Upper loop reentry
    Left atrium
        Mitral anular flutter
        Left septal flutter
        Scar- and pulmonary vein-related flutter

flutter occurs most often in patients with congenital heart disease and previous atriotomy. A narrow conduction zone between the incision scar and anatomical barrier, such as tricuspid valve or superior vena cava, is responsible for a reentry wavefront that circulates the incision scar. The appearance of the flutter waves on electrocardiography usually differs from cavotricuspid isthmus-dependent flutter, but it can resemble typical patterns. A linear ablation connecting from the scar to the inferior vena cava or tricuspid anulus eliminates the circuit.

Left atrial septal flutter indicates a macroreentry circuit rotating around the left septum primum. Characteristic electrocardiographic features include a dominant positive flutter wave in lead V_1 and low-amplitude waves in the other leads. Iatrogenic left atrial flutter has become more common in the era of ablation for eliminating pulmonary vein arrhythmogenic foci. After wide-area circumferential ablation of the left atrium, incomplete linear lesions connecting the left inferior pulmonary vein to the mitral anulus or an incomplete circular lesion around the pulmonary vein creates an arrhythmogenic slow conduction zone facilitating the development of atrial flutter. The flutter wave can rotate around the left atrial isthmus between the mitral anulus and the posterior wall of the left atrium or around any one of the pulmonary vein

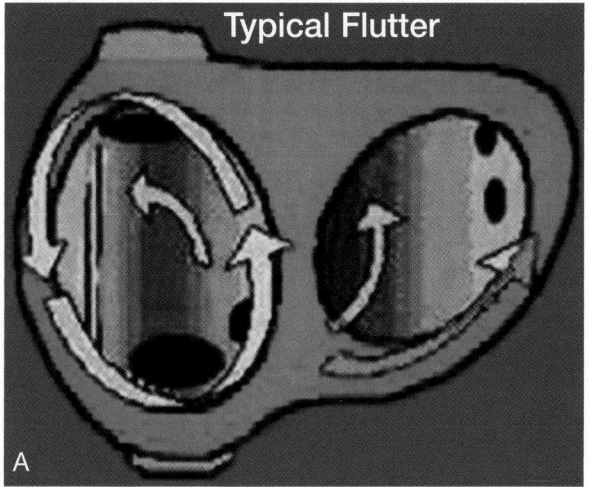

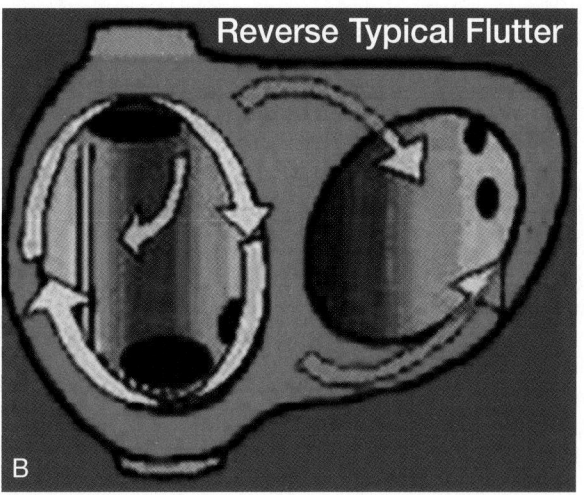

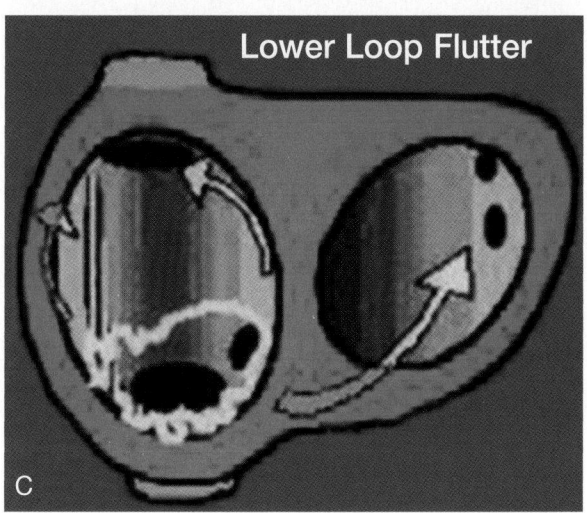

Fig. 1. Types of atrial flutter. *A*, Typical counterclockwise flutter. *B*, Reverse typical clockwise flutter. C, Lower loop flutter.

symptoms of congestive heart failure. Commonly, atrial flutter presents with 2:1 AV conduction with a ventricular rate at 150 beats per minute. Occasionally, patients present with tachycardia-induced cardiomyopathy. 1:1 AV conduction can occur when the flutter rate is slowed by class 1C antiarrhythmic agents or AV conduction is accelerated during exercise. Hence, an AV nodal-blocking agent, β-adrenergic blocker, or calcium channel blocker is necessary in combination with class 1C drugs to prevent 1:1 AV conduction. In the absence of an AV nodal blocking agent, 4:1 or higher AV conduction is suggestive of underlying nodal disease.

orifices. On 12-lead electrocardiography, left atrial flutter consistently presents positive flutter waves in lead V_1. Lead aVL is negative if the flutter wave breaks from the lateral wall of the left atrium or positive if the flutter wave is from the left atrial septum. The occurrence of left atrial flutter and atrial tachycardia ranges from 3% to 10%. Re-do ablation to complete the ablation line or circular ring around the pulmonary veins is usually successful. Atrial flutter classification is summarized in Table 2.

Clinical Presentation

Patients with new onset of atrial flutter often present with acute symptoms of palpitations, dyspnea, reduced effort tolerance, chest discomfort, and worsening

Management

Acute Treatment

When a patient is in atrial flutter with 2:1 or 1:1 AV conduction and hemodynamic instability, emergency direct-current cardioversion is necessary. Electrical cardioversion is safe and associated with a success rate of more than 90%. Usually, less than 50 joules is needed to resume sinus rhythm. Ibutilide is the most effective agent for chemical termination of atrial flutter, achieving a success rate up to 76%, which is higher than that with propafenone, sotalol, and amiodarone. The incidence of torsades de pointes is 1% in

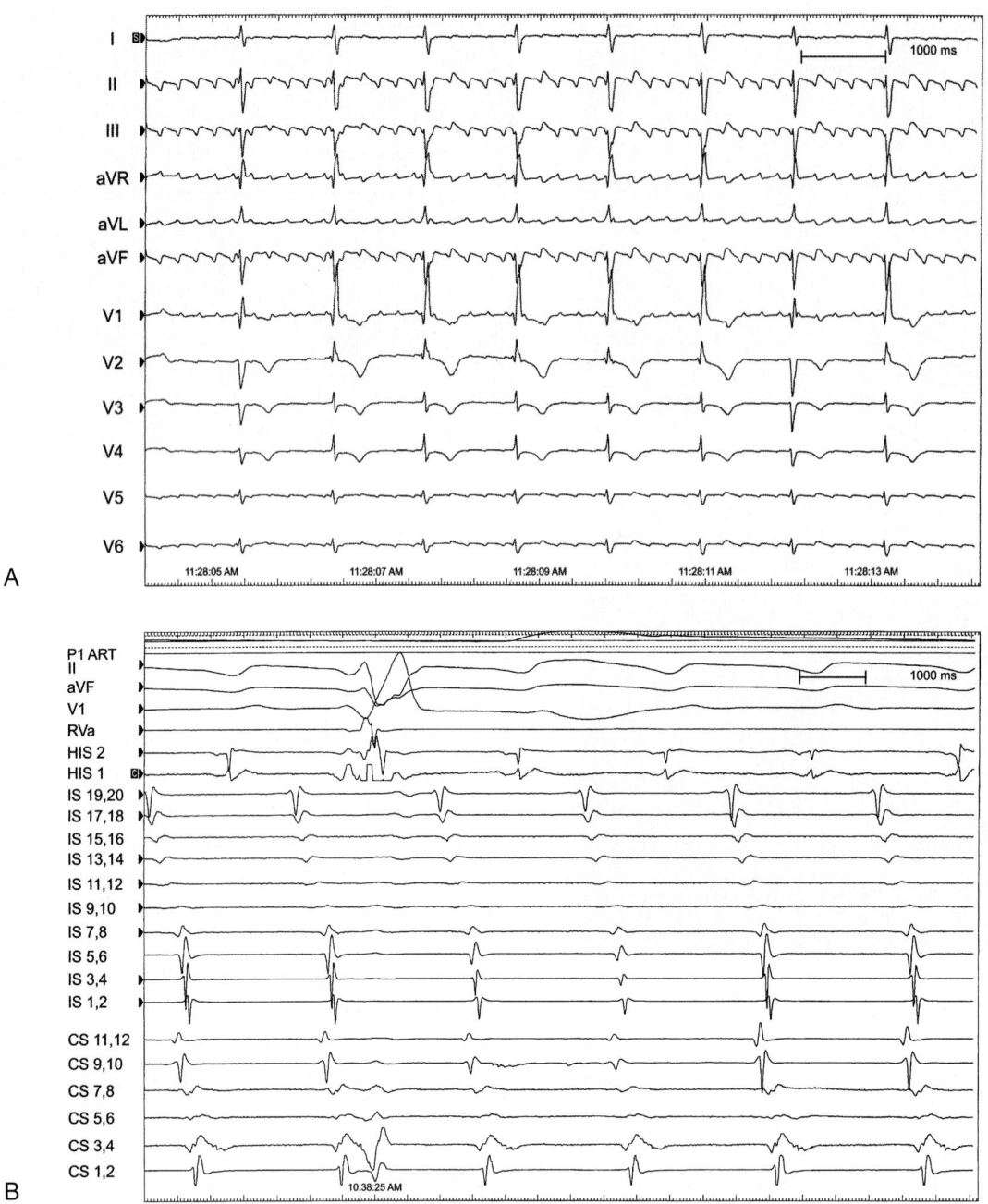

Fig. 2. *A,* Typical counterclockwise atrial flutter. Flutter waves are negative in inferior leads II, III, and aVF and positive in lead V_1. *B,* Intracardiac electrograms of counterclockwise flutter in same patient. A 20-pole bipolar catheter is placed in cavotricuspid isthmus with distal pole at orifice of coronary sinus. Activation sequence of atrial flutter is from proximal to distal (lateral right atrium to posterior septum). CS, coronary sinus; HIS, region of His; IS, isthmus; RVa, right ventricular apex.

patients with a structurally normal heart and up to 4% in the presence of organic heart disease, especially with reduced cardiac function. Ibutilide should be avoided in patients with prolonged QT interval, left ventricular dysfunction, a history of polymorphic ventricular tachycardia associated with class 1 or 3 antiarrhythmic drugs, or a significant electrolyte abnormality. The half-life of ibutilide is 3 to 6 hours. Patients should be monitored for 6 hours after administration. For acute chemical conversion, ibutilide or dofetilide is preferred rather than class 1C (flecainide, propafenone), class 1A (procainamide), and class 3 (sotalol, amiodarone) agents. In patients who have an implanted dual-chamber pacemaker or defibrillator or have temporary atrial epicardial wires after cardiac operation, overdrive atrial pacing is an alternative to terminate atrial flutter. The success rate is approximately 80%.

If a patient is hemodynamically stable, AV nodal blocking agents, including various β-blockers, verapamil, or diltiazem, can be administered to slow the ventricular response rate, although in practice ventricular rate control with these medications is often difficult to achieve. The efficacy of intravenous diltiazem and verapamil is comparable, achieving ventricular rate control within 30 minutes. The incidence of symptomatic hypotension, however, is higher for patients receiving verapamil. β-Blockers are equally effective for reducing ventricular rate. Digoxin alone is not an effective AV node blocking agent and is usually used in conjunction with other agents. Intravenous amiodarone is superior to digoxin, but it seems to be inferior to calcium or β-blockers in that it may require up to 6 hours to achieve adequate rate control. In patients with exacerbated congestive heart failure, restoration of sinus rhythm with direct-current cardioversion is preferable. Transesophageal echocardiography should be performed to confirm the absence of atrial thrombus and anticoagulation should be initiated before any type of cardioversion when atrial flutter has been present for more than 48 hours. Guidelines for anticoagulation in patients with atrial flutter are presented in Table 3.

Long-term Treatment

Pharmacologic Therapy

It is difficult to evaluate drug efficacy in patients with atrial flutter alone because most studies combine patients with atrial fibrillation and flutter. A small study showed that the long-term efficacy of flecainide was 50% for patients with atrial flutter only. Flecainide has no β-blockade effect, as does propafenone; therefore, it does not have β-blocker side effects such as bradycardia. Because of the marked sodium channel blocking effect of flecainide and propafenone, QRS duration should be closely monitored. The dose should be reduced when the increase in QRS duration reaches 25%. β-Blockers or calcium channel blockers always should be used in junction with a class 1C agent for treatment of atrial flutter because class 1C drugs slow flutter rate and may result in 1:1 AV conduction with an increase in ventricular rate. Randomized placebo-controlled trials have shown that the class 3 drug dofetilide has a 73% efficacy for maintaining sinus rhythm for more than 1 year in patients with atrial flutter compared with 40% of patients with atrial fibrillation. Contraindications for dofetilide are creatinine clearance less than 20 mL/min, hypokalemia, and prolonged baseline QT interval.

In light of the common coexistence of atrial flutter and atrial fibrillation, it is reasonable to apply the long-term outcome of antiarrhythmic drugs in patients with atrial fibrillation to those with atrial flutter. The efficacy of antiarrhythmic agents for

Table 3.   Guidelines for Anticoagulation in Atrial Flutter

Risk of thromboembolization is from 1.7% to 7%

Risk factors for development of embolic events are similar to those for atrial fibrillation, including hypertension, diabetes, coronary artery disease, prior cerebrovascular attack, congestive heart failure, and age older than 75 years

The guidelines for anticoagulation for patients with atrial fibrillation are extended to those with atrial flutter

Electrical or chemical cardioversion should be considered only if anticoagulation is adequate (international normalized ratio equals 2-3 for 3 weeks), the flutter is less than 48 hours in duration, or there is no evidence of atrial clots detected on transesophageal echocardiography

Chronic warfarin therapy is indicated for patients with any type of recurrent or persistent atrial flutter when risk factors for thromboembolic event are present

maintaining sinus rhythm in atrial fibrillation is, in descending order, amiodarone, sotalol, and class 1C and 1A agents. The Atrial Fibrillation Follow-up Investigation of Rhythm (AFFIRM) study indicated that amiodarone was more effective for maintaining sinus rhythm at 1 year (62%) than sotalol (38%) and class 1 agents (23%).

Nonpharmacologic Therapy

In 1992, a curative catheter-based *ablation for cavotricuspid isthmus-dependent atrial flutter* was developed. The circuit of macroreentrant atrial flutter can be identified from an endocardial activation map, show-ing a narrow cavotricuspid isthmus involved in the flutter circuit. A 20-pole Halo catheter is placed along the tricuspid anulus and the right atrial lateral wall to show the flutter activation sequence (Fig. 2 *B*). The ablation technique consists of placing a 2- to 4-cm linear lesion between the tricuspid anulus and inferior vena cava to disrupt the critical isthmus and block the atrial flutter circuit (Fig. 3). The end point of ablation is bidirectional block crossing the isthmus between the tricuspid anulus and inferior vena cava. The long-term success rate for cavotricuspid isthmus ablation, including counterclockwise, clockwise, and lower loop atrial flutter, is more than 90%. The overall frequency of serious complications is low, reported at 0.4%. In light of the high efficacy and low risks of procedural complications, catheter ablation is recommended as a class I therapeutic option for patients with recurrent atrial flutter and for patients who prefer curative ther-apy to pharmacologic therapy.

Atrial flutter develops in 15% to 20% of patients who receive propafenone, flecainide, or amiodarone for atrial fibrillation. These drug-induced flutter circuits are often cavotricuspid isthmus-dependent. A hybrid approach that combines catheter ablation of atrial flutter with continued antiarrhythmic drug therapy is often effective for preventing recurrent atrial fibrillation (class I indication for catheter ablation).

In catheter ablation for noncavotricuspid isthmus-dependent flutter, the reentrant circuits around an atri-otomy scar are carefully mapped with a three-dimen-sional mapping system to identify the critical slow conduction zone where radiofrequency ablation can eliminate the flutter. A line of ablation extending from the inferior margin of the scar to the tricuspid

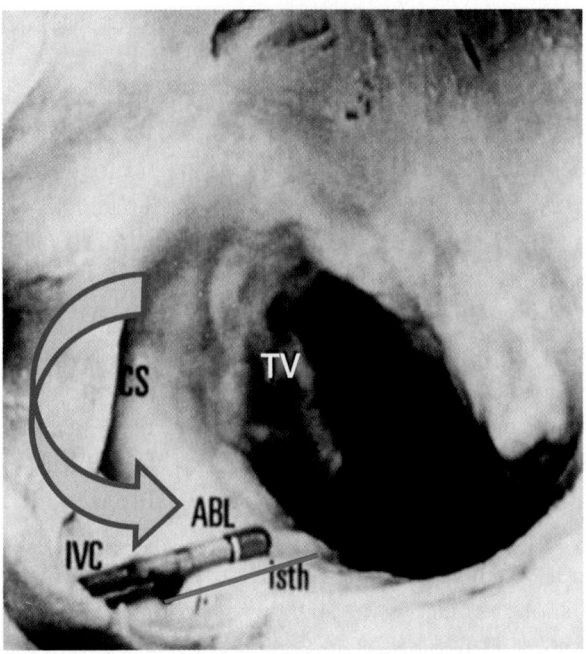

Fig. 3. A cavotricuspid isthmus ablation line (*red line*) is created with use of an ablation catheter to block isth-mus-dependent flutter circuit (*yellow arrow*).

anulus or superior margin of the superior vena cava often can disrupt the circuit. The success rate of ablation is up to 80%.

Macroreentry left atrial flutter is less common. It has been reported as an iatrogenic complication from left atrial catheter-based ablation for atrial fibrillation or from a prior maze operation. Left atrial flutter often uses the isthmus between the mitral anulus and the left inferior pulmonary vein. The flutter circuit can be elim-inated by creating a line of block in this isthmus.

AV node ablation and insertion of a permanent pacemaker is an option for patients who have persistent atrial flutter with rapid ventricular response and in whom pharmacologic management has failed, patients who are unable to tolerate antiarrhythmic agents, or patients who are not candidates for atrial flutter ablation.

Pregnancy

Atrial flutter may occur during pregnancy in patients with structural heart disease or a history of cardiac sur-gery. Guidelines for management during pregnancy are presented in Table 4. Atrial flutter is distinctly uncom-mon in pregnant patients without cardiac disease.

Table 4.   Management of Atrial Flutter During Pregnancy

Intravenous metoprolol is recommended to slow the ventricular rate. Intravenous verapamil may be associated
 with a greater risk of maternal hypotension and subsequent fetal hypoperfusion

Direct-current cardioversion is safe in all phases of pregnancy and can be used when necessary

All antiarrhythmic drugs cross the placenta barrier to some extent. The adverse effects on the fetus are teratogenic risk during the first trimester and retarded fetal growth and development during the second and third
 trimesters of pregnancy. All antiarrhythmic drugs should be avoided if possible, especially during the first
 trimester. Sotalol is a class B agent and is preferred to other antiarrhythmic agents

Catheter ablation is the procedure of choice for drug-refractory atrial flutter

27

SUPRAVENTRICULAR TACHYCARDIA: DIAGNOSIS AND TREATMENT

Samuel J. Asirvatham, MD

Supraventricular tachycardia is among the most common conditions encountered in cardiology. Supraventricular tachycardia includes atrial fibrillation and macroreentrant atrial arrhythmias such as atrial flutter (discussed in other chapters). The focus of this chapter is paroxysmal supraventricular tachycardias. Both automatic and reentrant mechanisms are responsible for these arrhythmias. The three most common types are atrioventricular node reentrant tachycardia (AVNRT), atrioventricular reentrant tachycardia (AVRT) using an accessory bypass tract, and atrial tachycardia (AT). The relationships of these arrhythmias with other cardiac diseases are discussed, and an approach to understanding these arrhythmias, with both the patient and the cardiovascular boards in mind, is provided.

DIFFERENTIAL DIAGNOSIS OF NARROW COMPLEX TACHYCARDIA

The most common presentation of patients with supraventricular tachycardia is palpitations, and electrocardiography shows a narrow QRS complex tachycardia. A careful analysis of the history and the 12-lead electrocardiogram often indicates the underlying disease process.

Clinical History

The typical patient with AVNRT or AVRT presents with paroxysms of palpitations that occur with a sudden onset and a sudden offset. Patients cannot usually identify a clear precipitating factor. The abruptness of the onset is often startling, and the patient feels regular thudding palpitations in the chest and often in the neck or head. During the palpitations, some patients describe light-headedness, anginal-type chest pressure, or an uneasy sensation in the neck. Frank syncope is rare but can occur in elderly patients, particularly those with coexisting cardiac and respiratory disease. Patients often describe an urge to micturate soon after termination of the arrhythmia.

With automatic AT, the symptoms are often of gradual onset and get more rapid over time (warm-up). The offset also may be gradual. Patients with AT sometimes find that a particular maneuver or position provokes the syndrome. In contrast to the irregular palpitations of atrial fibrillation or multifocal atrial tachycardia, patients can tap out of very regular rhythm with the forms of supraventricular tachycardia discussed in this chapter.

Physical Examination

The physical examination generally is not helpful for

elucidating the diagnosis of paroxysmal supraventricular tachycardia. Regular cannon *a* waves may occur during AVNRT and AVRT. With AT, particularly if associated with variable atrioventricular (AV) conduction, irregular cannon *a* waves occur. The absence of severe respiratory impairment, other cardiac conditions, infection, or bleeding is useful for excluding extreme forms of sinus tachycardia.

Electrocardiographic Differentiation With a Regular Narrow Complex Tachycardia

When a regular narrow complex tachycardia is found, the first determination should be whether the P wave can be visualized. It is useful to determine whether the P wave is closer to the preceding or succeeding QRS complex, giving rise to short RP tachycardias and long RP tachycardias. This classification is common, but there are numerous exceptions. A short RP tachycardia signifies relatively fast retrograde activation of the atrium (orthodromic AVRT) or near simultaneous activation of atrium and ventricle (AVNRT and junctional tachycardia). Similar to sinus tachycardia, AT has a long RP interval because there is no retrograde activation of the atrium from the ventricle. Thus, once the P wave has been visualized, if it is found to be occurring within the first half of the RR interval (short RP interval), AVNRT and orthodromic AVRT should be considered. Alternatively, if the PR interval is shorter than the RP interval, then AT is a likely possibility (Fig. 1). Further distinction is often possible between AVNRT and AVRT. In orthodromic AVRT, a finite interval has to elapse between activation of the ventricle by way of the AV node and travel of the electrical wave front through the ventricle and back to the atrium through the accessory pathway. This interval is almost never less than 100 milliseconds. Alternatively, with AVNRT from a common point near the AV node, there is near simultaneous activation of the atrium and ventricle. Thus, very short (sometimes 0 millisecond or negative) RP intervals are possible.

For the cardiovascular boards, this simple algorithm is useful:

1. P waves seen within or just after the QRS complex: AVNRT. Because of the very short RP interval with AVNRT, the P wave may give rise to a deflection at the end of the QRS complex, giving the appearance of incomplete right bundle branch block in lead V_1 (pseudo-R'). This is best seen in comparison with the QRS complex in sinus rhythm (Fig. 2).
2. Short RP tachycardia, but P waves 110 milliseconds or more after the QRS complex: orthodromic AVRT.
3. Long RP tachycardia: AT.

Important exceptions to these rules exist. For example, in certain types of retrograde conducting accessory pathways (Ebstein anomaly, previously damaged pathways), the retrograde conduction by way of the pathway is so slow that the resultant P wave is closer to the succeeding QRS complex (long RP tachycardia). Sometimes in AVNRT, the retrograde turnaround in the circuit to activate the atrium can be slow, also giving rise to a long RP tachycardia.

For the cardiovascular boards, it is important to recognize a very specific variant of slowly conducting retrograde pathways usually occurring in the posterior surface of the heart but present with incessant tachycardia from an orthodromic AVRT mechanism. A

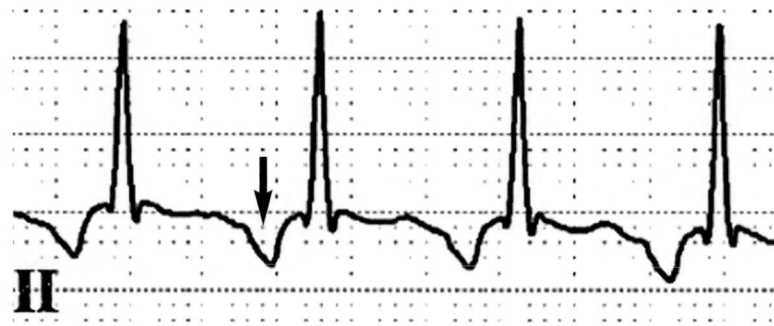

Fig. 1. Atrial tachycardia in lead II. *Arrow* is at P wave. This is a long RP tachycardia; the P wave is inverted.

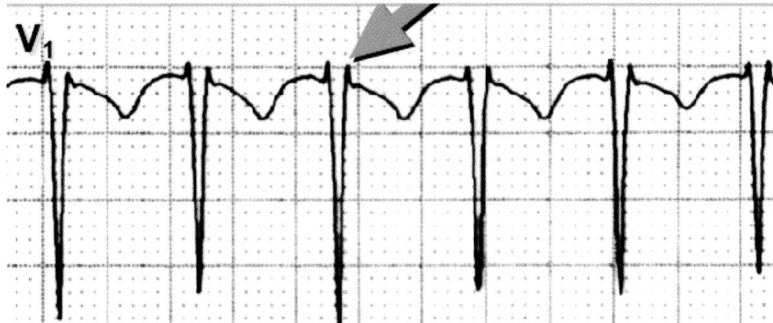

Fig. 2. Pseudo-R' configuration of lead V$_1$ in atrioventricular node reentrant tachycardia. *Arrow* is at P wave in terminal portion of QRS complex.

permanent form of junctional reciprocating tachycardia is incessant in this condition because the long retrograde conduction times allow for enough recovery of the atrial and antegrade AV nodal conduction to allow tachycardia to be easily initiated and sustained. This is a common cause for incessant tachycardia-related cardiomyopathy.

Conversely, AT may present as a short RP tachycardia. This occurs when antegrade AV nodal conduction is very slow (diseased or effective medication). Thus, depending on the cycle length of the tachycardia because of the long PR interval, the RP interval may be shorter than the PR interval.

During evaluation of the electrocardiogram in a patient presenting with regular narrow complex tachycardia (Table 1), the initiation and termination of the arrhythmia should be analyzed carefully. Tachycardia may terminate with or without a visualized P wave. When the terminal event is a P wave, this finding suggests that the tachycardia is dependent on antegrade conduction through the AV node. Thus, AVNRT and AVRT may terminate with a retrograde P wave. In contrast, it is very unusual for an AT to terminate with a P wave. For this to happen, the last beat from the tachycardia focus must coincidentally occur at the time of AV nodal block, which is rare. When the initiation of tachycardia is analyzed, if, during tachycardia, a premature atrial contraction of a different P wave than the subsequent P waves occurs and results in lengthening of the PR interval before initiation of tachycardia, an AVNRT or orthodromic reentry tachycardia is likely. Alternatively, if the first beat of tachycardia has little or no change in the PR interval and the P-wave morpho-

logic features of subsequent beats of tachycardia are identical, an automatic AT is likely. Often, automatic tachycardias have considerable irregularity soon after initiation or just before termination. This irregularity may present as a gradual increase in heart rate (warm-up phenomenon).

Supraventricular Tachycardia With a Wide QRS Complex

Because supraventricular arrhythmias typically conduct the ventricle through the usual AV node and His-Purkinje system, the QRS complex is narrow from simultaneous right and left ventricular conduction. Supraventricular tachycardias, however, may present with a wide QRS complex in two circumstances: 1) when bundle branch block exists during tachycardia,

Table 1.   Regular Narrow QRS Tachycardia for the Cardiovascular Boards

Short RP tachycardia: AVNRT, AVRT
Long RP tachycardia: AT
Pseudo-R'
Termination with a P wave: not AT
First beat similar to subsequent beats with warm-up: AT
Atypical AVNRT (often long RP tachycardia)

AT, atrial tachycardia; AVNRT, atrioventricular node reentrant tachycardia; AVRT, atrioventricular reentrant tachycardia.

and 2) because of antegrade conduction by way of an accessory bypass tract.

Wide QRS Complex Due to Bundle Branch Block

Patients with wide QRS may have an underlying bundle branch block or have development of bundle branch block during the rapid rates of tachycardia (rate-related aberrancy). The wider QRS may obscure the retrograde P wave in very short RP tachycardias, such as AVNRT. Differentiation of these arrhythmias from ventricular tachycardia is discussed in-depth in other chapters, but salient features are reviewed here. When the wide QRS complex is due to bundle branch block, typically the initial deflection of the QRS complex is rapid and normal, whereas the later part of the QRS complex reflecting intraventricular conduction is abnormal. Because the exit of the conducting bundle is located approximately midway between the base and apex, the frontal QRS axis shows a mixed vector. This means that in the chest leads (V_1 through V_6), concordance will not be seen; typically, there is a positive R wave in lead V_1 (right bundle pattern) but negative prominent S waves in leads V_4 through V_6. Finally, AV dissociation almost never occurs with AVRT reentry and is very rare with AVNRT, and when occurring with AT there are more P waves than QRS complexes. Thus, AV dissociation with more QRS complexes than P waves suggests ventricular tachycardia as the origin of the wide QRS rhythm.

The presence of rate-related aberration provides a useful observation that is important for the cardiovascular boards. When a change in the rate of the tachycardia occurs at the time of development of loss of a bundle branch block, AVRT is the likely diagnosis, because the AVRT circuit utilizes the ventricular myocardium (Fig. 3).

Wide QRS Complex Due to Antegrade Preexcitation

There are two situations in which supraventricular tachycardia presents with a wide QRS complex due to antegrade preexcitation. First, the "mirror image" of orthodromic AVRT may occur, called antidromic tachycardia. In this case, antegrade conduction is by way of the accessory pathway and retrograde conduction is by way of the AV conduction system. Because ventricular activation occurs directly into the ventricular myocardium, bypassing the specialized conduction tissue, the QRS complex is wide. Because most accessory pathways insert into the base of the heart (near the anulus), the QRS vector is from base to apex. Typically, the result is concordantly positive QRS complexes in

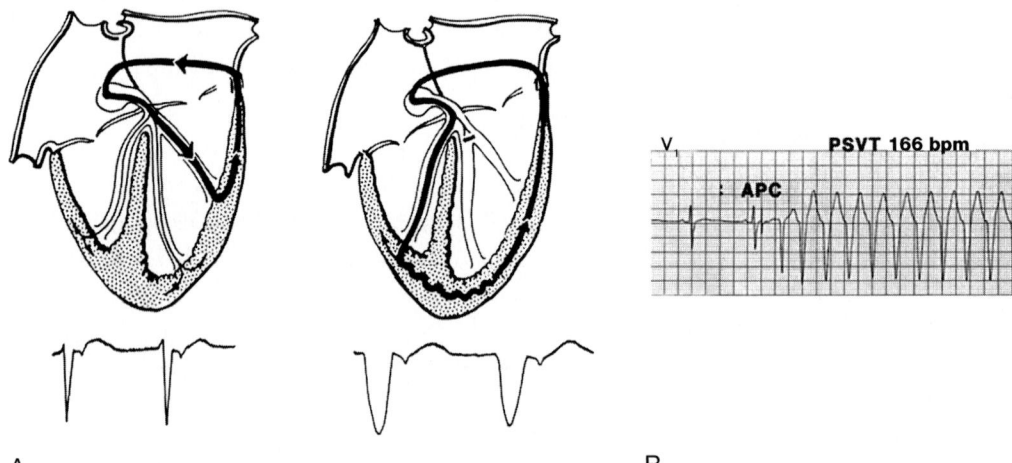

A   B

Fig. 3. *A*, Atrioventricular reentrant tachycardia (AVRT) with left-sided accessory pathway and normal conduction through the left bundle (on the left); AVRT with same left-sided accessory pathway and left bundle branch block (on the right). The circuitous conduction pathway results in a prolonged QRS complex. *B*, Paroxysmal supraventricular tachycardia (PSVT). Note that with the presence of left bundle branch block at the initiation of the tachycardia, the rate is 166 beats per minute (bpm). The block resolves, conduction through the normal conduction pathway resumes, and the tachycardia accelerates to 200 beats per minute with a narrow QRS complex. APC, atrial premature contraction.

the anterior chest leads. The tachycardia is regular, and AV nodal blocking agents that slow or limit conduction in the AV node terminate the arrhythmia. Second, the primary arrhythmia is not dependent on the accessory pathway but conducts to the ventricle by way of the accessory pathway. For example, an atrial tachycardia, atrial flutter, or atrial fibrillation may conduct to the ventricle by way of both the AV node and the accessory pathway. The result is a variably wide QRS complex during tachycardia. AV nodal blocking agents or maneuvers to slow AV node conduction will not terminate the arrhythmia and, in fact, will give rise to a greater degree of preexcitation (Table 2).

SPECIFIC FORMS OF SUPRAVENTRICULAR TACHYCARDIA

Atrioventricular Node Reentrant Tachycardia

Pathophysiology
The AV node is located in a relatively predictable position on the intra-atrial septum close to the tricuspid anulus. Atrial myocardium connects electrically to the AV node at distinct sites. Although initially all atrial fibers were thought to connect three dimensionally to

Table 2. Wide QRS Complex for the Cardiovascular Boards

Orthodromic AVRT: antegrade conduction over the AV node and retrograde conduction over the accessory pathway; narrow QRS complex unless bundle branch block exists during tachycardia
Antidromic AVRT: antegrade conduction over the accessory pathway and retrograde conduction through the AV node; wide QRS complex
Antidromic tachycardia is the opposite of orthodromic AVRT and is treated similarly
For preexcited tachycardias other than antidromic tachycardia, AV nodal blocking agents are contraindicated

AV, atrioventricular; AVRT, atrioventricular reentrant tachycardia.

the AV node, this is clearly now known not to be the case.

The sinus node impulse primarily travels superior to the fossa ovalis and posterior to the eustachian ridge in reaching the AV node. These fibers are referred to as the *fast pathway* to the AV node. A second method of atrial activation reaching the AV node is anterior (ventricular) to the eustachian ridge from the region of the coronary sinus, probably utilizing the musculature of the coronary sinus to reach the AV node. This inferior myocardial extension to the AV node in the region of the coronary sinus is referred to as the *slow pathway* to the AV node. Because of these two distinct atrial connections (pathways) to the AV node, a reentrant tachycardia becomes possible.

If a premature atrial beat occurs early enough to be in the refractory period of the fast pathway, conduction will not occur across this pathway, but conduction may still be possible by way of the slow pathway to reach the AV node. In this situation, a *sudden prolongation in the PR interval* is noted. Once the impulse reaches the AV node through the slow pathway, retrograde activation of the atrium by way of the fast pathway may occur if this structure has recovered from its state of refractoriness. This process now manifests as atrial premature contraction with sudden prolongation in the PR interval and an echo beat (second atrial activation from reentry). This echo beat (atrial activation) may now reenter the AV node through the slow pathway. This process of antegrade conduction down the slow pathway and retrograde conduction through the fast pathway represents the *typical form of AVNRT* (slow-fast reentry).

Clinical Presentation
The clinical and epidemiologic characteristics of AVNRT are summarized in Table 3. Repeated bouts of sudden-onset sudden-offset tachycardia occur; the episodes may terminate with Valsalva or other vagotonic maneuvers. Older patients or otherwise debilitated patients may have severe symptoms in addition to the palpitations, including angina and syncope. Persistent forms of this arrhythmia are very rare and should make the clinician consider alternative diagnoses.

Treatment
Therapy for AVNRT includes conservative, medical, and ablation approaches (Table 4). Patients with infrequent palpitations may need no specific therapy.

Table 3.   Clinical and Epidemiologic Characteristics of Atrioventricular Node Reentry Tachycardia

Age	Younger patients (average age 25-35 years)
Sex	Slightly more common in women (ratio of 1.2:1)
Structural heart disease	No
Induced cardio-myopathy	No
Mortality risk	No
Stroke risk	No
Association with atrial fibrillation	Usually not

Patients should be instructed on the use of Valsalva-like maneuvers to terminate the arrhythmia; if these are effective, no further therapy is required.

For patients with more frequent episodes, especially if visits to the emergency department are occurring regularly, medical therapy is warranted. AV nodal blocking agents (β-blockers, calcium channel blockers, or sometimes digoxin alone) are sufficient for greatly decreasing the frequency or eliminating the episodes of tachycardia altogether in many patients. If a patient presents to the emergency department in tachycardia and carotid sinus massage is not effective, adenosine invariably terminates the tachycardia. If adenosine fails to terminate the tachycardia or it immediately recurs, another diagnosis or an infiltrated intravenous line should be considered.

Some patients either continue to have frequent episodes despite medical therapy or are intolerant of the side effects associated with therapy. Young patients may prefer a curative approach at the outset to avoid long-term daily drug therapy. In these situations, radiofrequency ablation is an excellent option and has a success rate of more than 95% for eliminating tachycardia episodes in association with a 2% rate of serious complication. With long-term follow-up, recurrences are rare and repeated ablation is required in less than 2% of cases. Fast pathway ablation is no longer performed because of a high incidence of AV block.

Accessory Pathway-Related Tachycardias

Various arrhythmias are possible in patients who have an accessory pathway. The most common is reentrant tachycardia, either orthodromic or antidromic. The preexcited electrocardiogram and the common circuits of tachycardia in patients with accessory pathways are discussed with a specific emphasis on the cardiovascular boards.

The Preexcited Electrocardiogram

When accessory pathways conduct antegradely, the electrocardiogram is *preexcited*. Preexcitation consists of two findings: the PR interval is short, and the initial deflection of the QRS complex is abnormal and slurred. In sinus rhythm, every ventricular activation is a fusion between accessory pathway and AV nodal conduction. Because AV nodal conduction is usually slower, the initial portion of the QRS complex reflects the abnormal ventricular activation (delta wave). Again, because the AV node is being bypassed, ventricular activation is earlier than expected (preexcited) (Fig. 4).

The pattern of preexcitation on the 12-lead electrocardiogram is an important tool for finding the site of accessory pathway. For the cardiovascular boards, it is important to recognize that a right bundle branch block pattern (positive R wave in lead V_1) is seen in left-sided accessory pathways and a left bundle branch block pattern (QS complex in lead V_1) is seen in right-sided accessory pathways. Exact localization is beyond the scope of the cardiovascular boards.

Sometimes, even though there is antegrade conduction over an accessory pathway, the electrocardiogram does not show recognizable preexcitation. This

Table 4.   Atrioventricular Node Reentrant Tachycardia for the Cardiovascular Boards

Extremely short RP interval tachycardia
Valsalva-like maneuvers terminate the tachycardia
Radiofrequency ablation targets the slow pathway and is highly effective for eliminating future episodes
Junctional rhythm often occurs during successful ablation

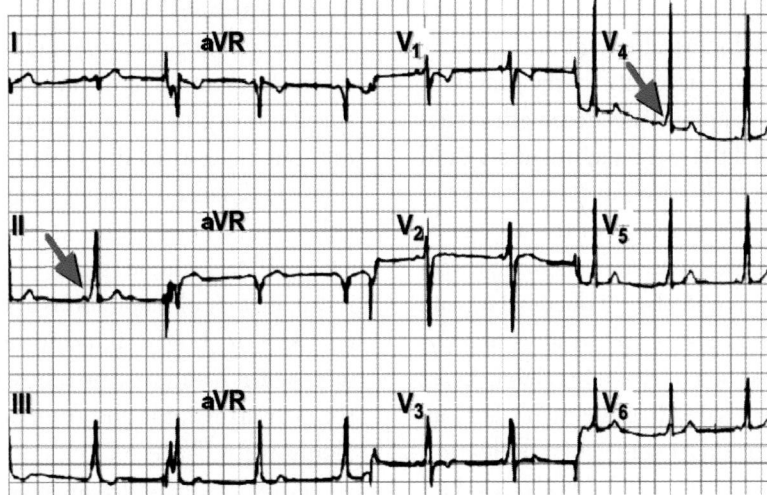

Fig. 4. Preexcited electrocardiogram. *Arrows* indicate delta waves.

can occur in decrementally conducting pathways, pathways located in the high lateral region of the left ventricular anulus, and a poorly conducting accessory pathway located far from the sinus node. This concept should not be confused with concealed accessory pathways (accessory pathways that conduct only retrogradely).

Reentrant Tachycardia Associated With Accessory Pathways

Orthodromic AVRT
This is the most common symptomatic arrhythmia associated with accessory pathways (Fig. 5 *A*). The antegrade limb of the circuit is made up of the AV node and the normal His-Purkinje system, and the accessory pathway conducts retrogradely. Either an atrial premature contraction or ventricular premature

contraction may incite the tachycardia, and once started it is usually symptomatic with palpitations. Termination may be a result of fatigue in the AV nodal conduction system, increased vagal tone from a vagal maneuver, or a premature extra systolic beat.

Antidromic AVRT
The antegrade limb of the circuit is the accessory pathway in this rare tachycardia. Because the earliest site of ventricular activation is ventricular myocardium rather than the normal conduction system, the QRS complex is wide and is maximally preexcited (Fig. 5 *B*). Drugs that inhibit AV nodal conduction and vagotonic maneuvers will terminate antidromic tachycardia, as in orthodromic tachycardia, because both circuits involve the AV node.

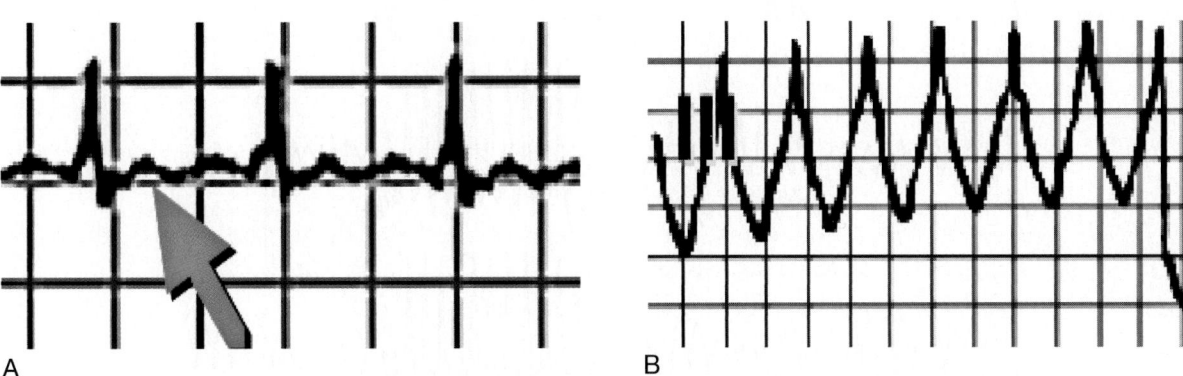

Fig. 5. *A*, Orthodromic reentrant tachycardia, lead III: narrow QRS complex and retrograde P waves. *B*, Antidromic reentrant tachycardia, lead III: wide QRS complex; P waves are not visible.

Preexcited Tachycardias

In this group of arrhythmias, although an accessory pathway is present, it is not necessary for the genesis of the tachycardia. For example, in a patient with preexcited atrial tachycardia, the atrial tachycardia would exist even if the patient did not have any accessory pathway. Because of the presence of the accessory pathway, however, the presentation of the arrhythmia is greatly changed. The ventricular conduction rates are much faster when an accessory pathway is present because these structures do not typically exhibit decremental conduction properties. Because each tachycardia beat represents fusion of ventricular activation between pathway conduction and AV nodal conduction, the QRS is often bizarre and varied. Depending on the degree of decrement through the AV node, varying degrees of fusion are present. Other examples of preexcited tachycardia include preexcited atrial fibrillation, preexcited AVNRT, preexcited sinus tachycardia, and preexcited orthodromic AVRT using a second bypass tract. Thus, the characteristic feature of preexcited atrial fibrillation is not only an irregularly irregular ventricular activation but also an irregularly irregular QRS duration. Although preexcited tachycardias may be regular (preexcited atrial tachycardia), the QRS morphologic variation is the important clue to the presence of a preexcited arrhythmia. With any preexcited tachycardia, if AV nodal conduction is slow, the degree of preexcitation increases and ventricular response rates can paradoxically increase, predisposing to ventricular fibrillation (Fig. 6) (Table 5).

Atrial Tachycardia

AT includes various conditions, such as automatic AT, macroreentrant AT, scar-related AT, atrial flutters, and specific forms of AT arising from venous structures that can incite atrial fibrillation. Most of these conditions are discussed in other chapters. Automatic AT is unlike AVNRT or AVRT in that it usually presents as a long RP tachycardia (Fig. 1). The clinical presentation is usually that of palpitations associated with exercise, emotion, or changes in position. Some patients have incessant AT and may present with fatigue both from the tachyarrhythmia and from possibly associated cardiomyopathy (Table 6).

A single site located anywhere in the atria exhibits inherent automaticity at a cycle length shorter than that of the sinus node. The P-wave morphologic pattern depends on the exact site of origin. AV nodal blocking agents will not terminate the arrhythmia but may control ventricular response rates. Sodium channel blocking agents and some potassium channel blocking agents may help uppress the arrhythmia. In highly symptomatic patients refractory to medical treatment, radiofrequency ablation of the tachycardia focus has a success rate of 95%.

SUMMARY

Recognition and management of paroxysmal supraventricular tachycardia are increasingly important components of the cardiovascular boards. *Symptoms* and *comorbid conditions* presented in each question should be carefully considered.

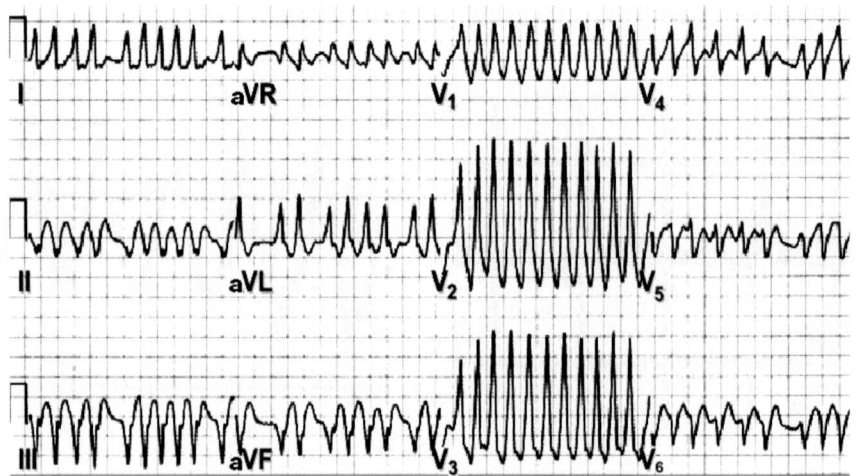

Fig. 6. Preexcited atrial fibrillation. Rate is irregular, and there are varying degrees of QRS preexcitation.

Table 5. Atrioventricular Reentry Tachycardia
for the Cardiovascular Boards

A preexcited electrocardiogram with a left bundle
branch block pattern indicates a right-sided
accessory pathway

A preexcited electrocardiogram with a right bundle branch block pattern indicates a left-sided
accessory pathway

Pathway-related tachycardias that are regular and
morphologically uniform can be safely treated
with AV nodal blocking agents (orthodromic or
antidromic AVRT)

Tachycardias associated with QRS morphologic
variation should never be treated with AV nodal
blocking agents

In patients with mild tachycardia (rates 100-130
beats per minute) but with an abnormal P wave
morphology and cardiomyopathy, permanent form
of junctional reciprocating tachycardia (inverted
P waves in leads 2, 3, aVF) should be suspected

AV, atrioventricular; AVRT, atrioventricular reentrant
tachycardia.

Table 6. Atrial Tachycardia for the
Cardiovascular Boards

Atrial tachycardia presents as a long RP tachycardia associated with exertion

Incessant atrial tachycardia may be associated
with tachycardia-related cardiomyopathy

Atrial tachycardia must be distinguished from
inappropriate sinus tachycardia

28

VENTRICULAR TACHYCARDIA

Thomas M. Munger, MD

INTRODUCTION

Ventricular tachycardia (VT) is a relatively common arrhythmia in the United States, being present in 1% to 2% of patients during the first year after myocardial infarction (MI). This is the largest subgroup of patients with VT who require treatment each year. Since the early 1980s, surgical as well as catheter ablative techniques—using direct current, and later, radiofrequency energy—have been used in an attempt to eradicate reentrant foci that are responsible for VT in patients with coronary artery disease (CAD). In addition to these patients, there are subsets of patients with VT that occurs in the absence of CAD (i.e., with dilated cardiomyopathy, arrhythmogenic right ventricular dysplasia [ARVD], hypertrophic cardiomyopathy [HCM], infiltrative diseases of the heart, and congenital heart disease). Additionally, VT can emerge in patients with structurally normal hearts; these patients may or may not have associated repolarization syndromes. VT is one arrhythmogenic cause for sudden death (Table 1), although in patients with normal repolarization and structurally normal hearts, sudden death is rarely a complication.

WIDE COMPLEX TACHYCARDIA AND VT

VT rhythms have rates between 100 and 280 beats per minute and can be monomorphic or polymorphic.

Monomorphic rhythms keep QRS morphology consistent from beat to beat and generally keep rates constant. Warm-up and cooldown changes in rate can occur, however, particularly in rhythms not due to myocardial reentry (triggered or automatic mechanisms). Polymorphic VT rhythms are most frequent in patients with repolarization abnormalities (long QT syndrome [LQTS], Brugada syndrome, acute myocardial ischemia, myocardial inflammation such as myocarditis, or drug toxicity); when the polymorphic form of VT turns about the isoelectric line in a regular pattern, the VT is termed *torsades de pointes*. VT generally has a wide QRS complex (fascicular VT rhythms are an exception, with QRS durations less than 120-140 ms) on the surface electrocardiogram (ECG).

Wide complex tachycardias encompass several different arrhythmias, including paroxysmal supraventricular tachycardia conducted aberrantly or anterogradely across an anomalous atrioventricular (AV) pathway ([e.g., in] Wolff-Parkinson-White syndrome or when Mahaim fibers are abundant), VT, drug or electrolyte toxicity–related arrhythmias, and device-related arrhythmias and artifacts (Table 2). Several clinical and ECG features have been identified that favor VT as the cause for wide complex tachycardia (Table 3).

In prior series of patients with undifferentiated, wide-QRS tachycardia, patients with a clinical history of structural heart disease had more than a 95% chance

Table 1. Cardiac Causes of Sudden Death

Coronary artery
  Atherosclerosis
  Embolism
  Dissection
  Spasm
  Coronary artery anomalies
Myocardial
  Dilated cardiomyopathy
  Hypertrophic cardiomyopathy
  Infiltrative (e.g., amyloid or sarcoid)
  Myocarditis
  Arrhythmogenic right ventricular dysplasia
  Tumors
Primary arrhythmias
  Wolff-Parkinson-White syndrome
  Long QT syndrome
  Catecholinergic polymorphic ventricular
    tachycardia
  Brugada syndrome
  Blunt chest trauma (commotio cordis)
  Primary atrial arrhythmias
  Bradycardias
Valvular
  Aortic stenosis
  Mitral valve prolapse
  Congenital (e.g., tetralogy of Fallot)
Vascular or pericardial
  Aortic aneurysm or dissection
  Marfan syndrome
  Pulmonary aneurysm or dissection
  Pulmonary embolism
  Tamponade
  Primary pulmonary hypertension
  Subarachnoid hemorrhage
  Massive gastrointestinal bleeding
  Drugs: torsades de pointes
  Toxins

Table 2. Wide Complex Tachycardias

Ventricular tachycardia
  Monomorphic
  Polymorphic
Aberrancy with PSVT (LBBB/RBBB/IVCD)
  Sinus tachycardia
  Junctional tachycardia
  Typical AVNRT
  Atypical AVNRT
  Orthodromic reciprocating tachycardia
  Antidromic reciprocating tachyardia
  Multiple pathway tachycardia
  Atrial fibrillation
  Atrial flutter
  Ectopic atrial tachycardia
  Reentrant atrial tachycardia
Accessory pathway with PSVT
  Sinus tachycardia
  Typical AVNRT
  Atypical AVNRT
  Orthodromic reciprocating tachycardia
  Antidromic reciprocating tachycardia
  Multiple pathway tachycardia
  Atrial fibrillation
  Atrial flutter
  Ectopic atrial tachycardia
  Reentrant atrial tachycardia
Toxicity related
  Electrolytes
  Drugs
Other
  Pacemaker-mediated tachycardia
  Artifacts

AVNRT, atrioventricular node reentry tachycardia; IVCD, interventricular conduction delay; LBBB, left bundle branch block; PSVT, paroxysmal supraventricular tachycardia; RBBB, right bundle branch block.

of having VT. A variable first heart sound (S₁), cannon *a* waves, and identification of AV dissociation on the ECG identify the presence of a ventricular rhythm independent of the atrial rhythm, which is indicative of VT. *Fusion beats*, which identify simultaneous activation of the ventricles through the normal conduction

system and an ectopic ventricular origin, are also indicative of VT; *capture beats* are normal sinus beats with a narrow QRS complex during VT in AV dissociation. With a criterion of QRS duration longer than 160 ms, VT discrimination achieves 97% specificity. ECG examples of wide complex tachycardias from

Table 3.   Features Favoring VT Over PSVT

Clinical

    History of coronary artery disease or heart
      failure

    Cannon *a* waves in jugular venous pulse
      contour

    Variable first heart sound on auscultation

ECG

    AV dissociation

    Fusion beats

    Capture beats

    QRS duration >140-160 ms

    Precordial concordance

    Northwest axis

    Lead V_1 RBBB with larger left peak

    Lead V_6 QRS with rS or S morphology

AV, atrioventricular; PSVT, paroxysmal supraventricular tachycardia; RBBB, right bundle branch block; VT, ventricular tachycardia.

various mechanisms are shown in Figures 1 through 4. The current American Heart Association (AHA) and advanced cardiac life support (ACLS) guidelines for the acute management of patients presenting with wide complex tachycardia, monomorphic VT, and polymorphic VT are shown in Figure 5.

Distinct Clinical Syndromes of VT

Ischemia and Acute Post–Myocardial Infarction VT

Initial case reports of ventricular fibrillation (VF) causing sudden death after the onset of MI appeared in the early 1900s. Wiggers, in the 1940s, noted that the VF threshold in dogs decreased after coronary occlusion. The incidence of VT and VF in the first 6 to 12 hours after MI was first described in the 1960s after the institution of the coronary care unit. The frequency of ischemic episodes actually increases in the early morning and decreases as evening approaches. A similar pattern is associated with the onset of MI and ventricular arrhythmias.

During the first 5 minutes of coronary occlusion, depolarization of the ventricular myocytes develops from approximately –90 mV to –60 mV because of an increase in intracellular calcium, as well as activation of the adenosine triphosphate–sensitive potassium channel (IK_{ATP}) (which causes an increase in extracellular potassium levels and subsequent membrane depolarization). The sodium-potassium pump also fails to function within the first 10 to 15 minutes after coronary occlusion, with subsequent excess accumulation of external potassium. The net rate of change of external potassium is 1 to 1.5 mEq/L per minute in the first 10 minutes of ischemia. Coincident with external augmentation of potassium is conduction slowing. At 15 minutes, myocytes at the central injury zone are electrically silent as necrolysis begins. Lysophosphoglycerides are released from cellular membranes. These agents electrically uncouple ventricular myocytes on the border zones of myocardial infarcts, thereby exacerbating further conduction slowing. Local acidosis exacerbates these effects. Catecholamines are released locally. Distal sympathetic fibers within the infarct zone undergo necrosis.

During the first 72 hours after MI, the incidence of premature ventricular contractions (PVCs), nonsustained VTs, and sustained VTs increases steadily. With sympathetic denervation in animals, ventricular ectopy can be decreased or eliminated in some cases. The excess ventricular ectopy during this time is due to increased automaticity. Ventricular ectopy (most often originating in the subendocardial Purkinje fibers of the left ventricle) can be altered by varying afterload, sheer stress on the infarct, collateral blood supply, and patency of the infarct artery. Border zone ischemic cells remain injured for several weeks after the healing phase of the myocardial infarct. These cells typically have depolarized resting membrane potentials, slowed conduction, and longer action potential phases. Complex ectopy and the presence of late potentials on the signal-averaged ECG become more frequent until 6 weeks after MI and then decrease thereafter. This time course correlates with the incidence of inducibility at electrophysiologic (EP) testing, and the incidence of sudden death following the very acute early phases after MI.

PVCs are absent in at least half of the patients who have VF in the acute phase after MI and are as frequent in patients who do not have VF. Because PVCs are not accurate predictors of VF occurrences, there is

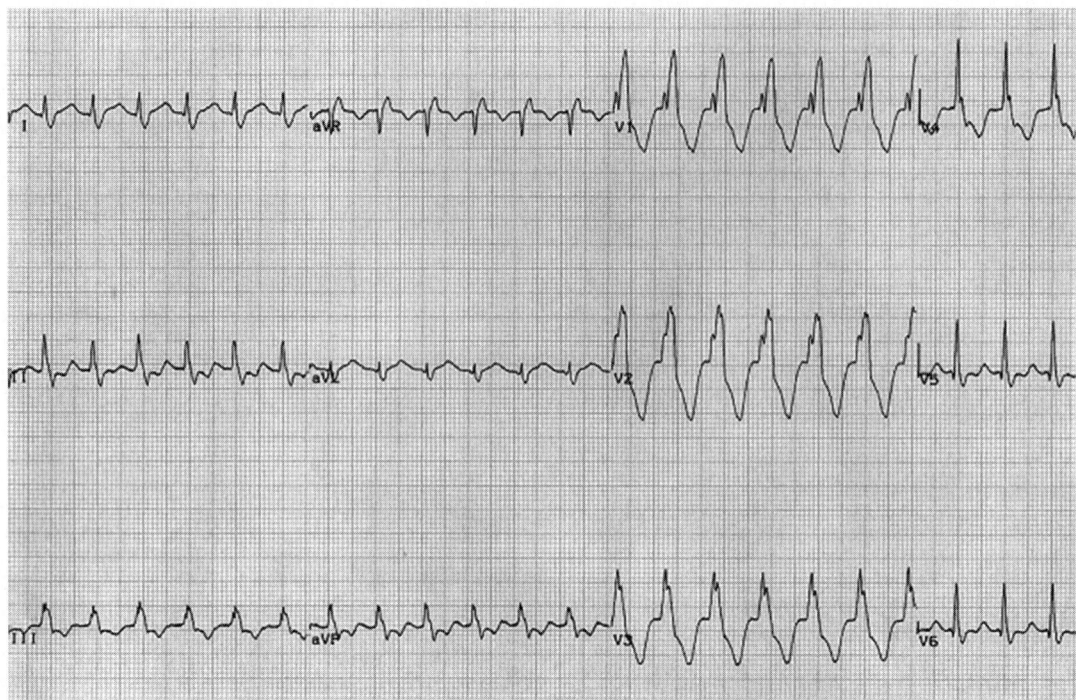

Fig. 1. Wide complex tachycardia due to aberrancy: orthodromic reciprocating tachycardia with right bundle branch block. Note the "typical" V_1 rSR′ right bundle branch block pattern and relatively narrow QRS complex.

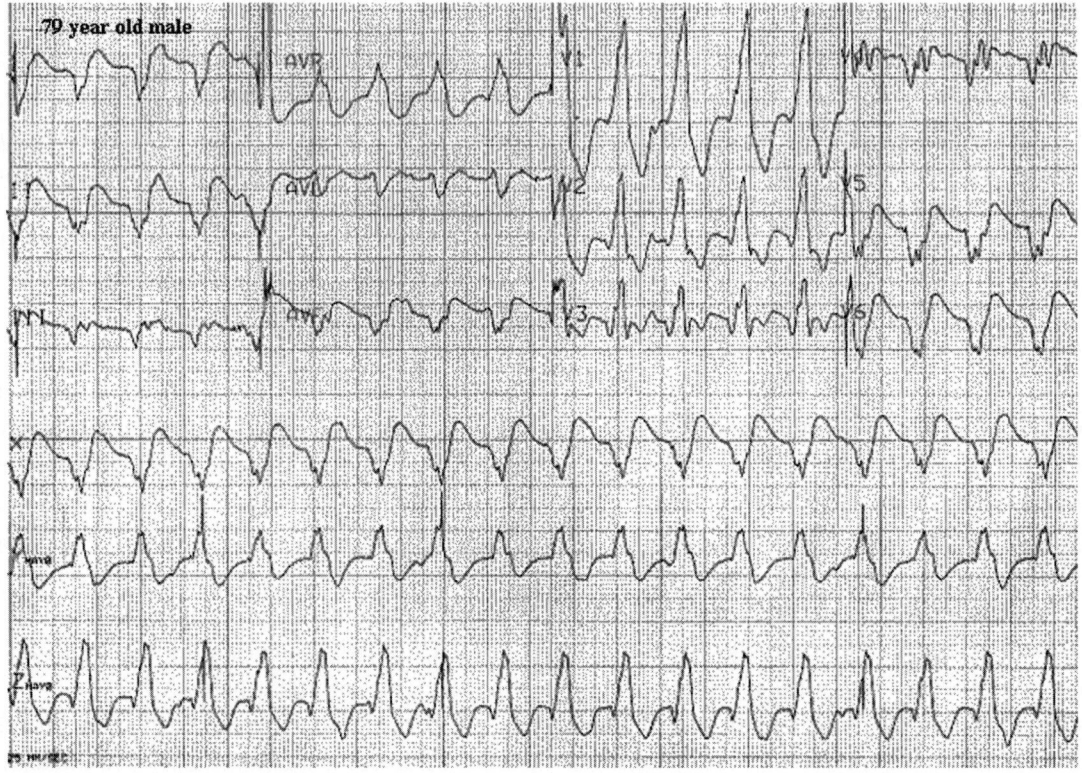

Fig. 2. Wide complex tachycardia due to slow ventricular tachycardia in a 79-year-old man. Note the northwest axis, wide QRS complex, single R wave in V_1, and prominent S wave in V_6.

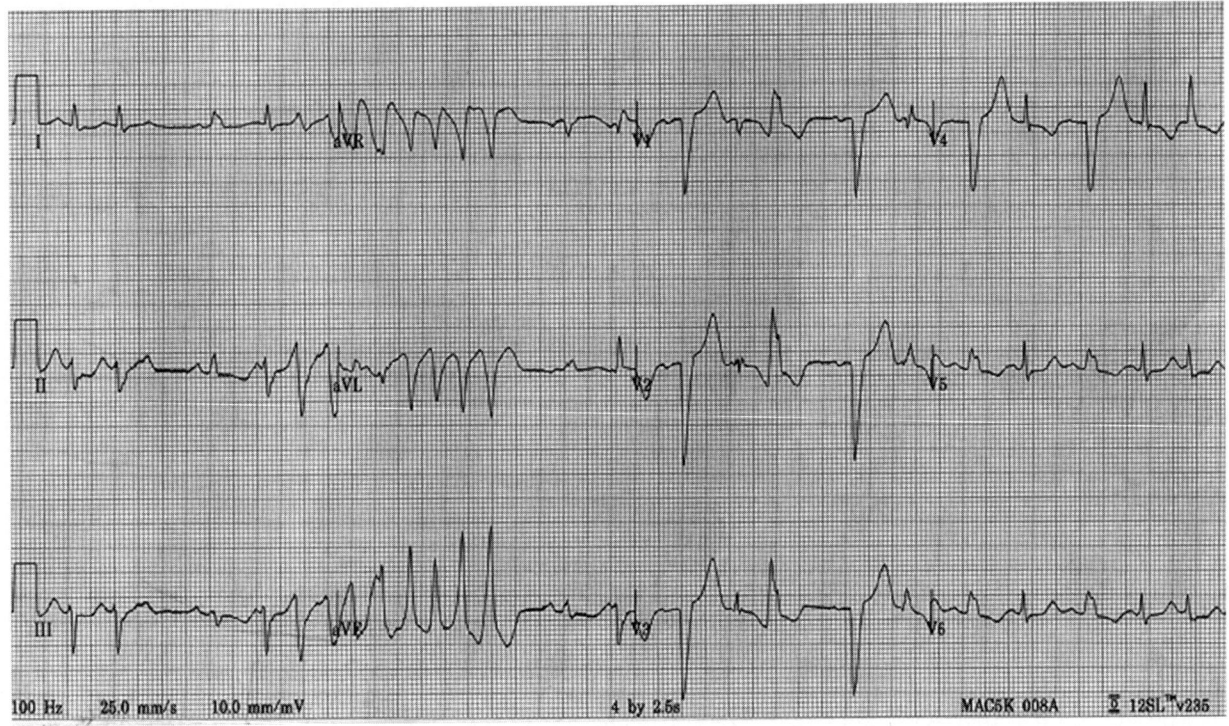

Fig. 3. Idiopathic polymorphic ventricular tachycardia from left ventricular Purkinje conduction system. This patient did not have long QT syndrome. Note the alternating left bundle branch block and right bundle branch block patterns to the premature ventricular contractions.

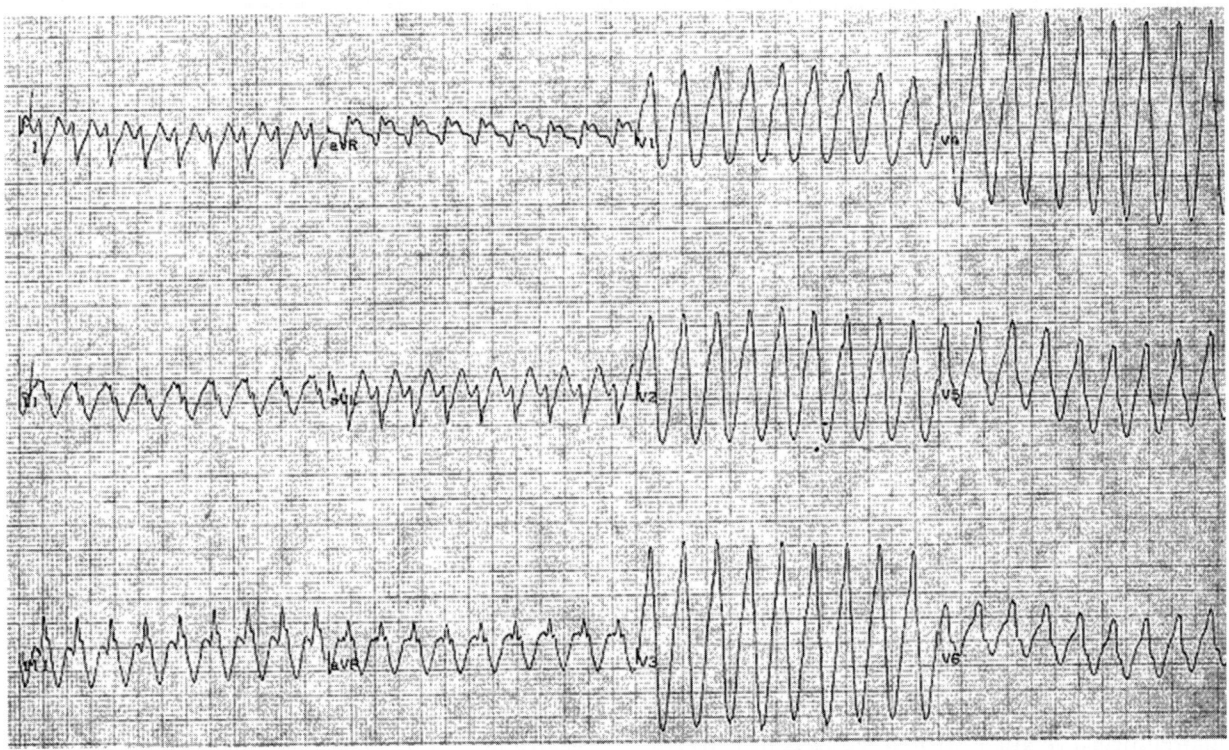

Fig. 4. Antidromic reciprocating tachycardia simulating ventricular tachycardia in a patient with a left-sided accessory bypass tract (Wolff-Parkinson-White syndrome). Note the northwest axis and the duration of the QRS complex.

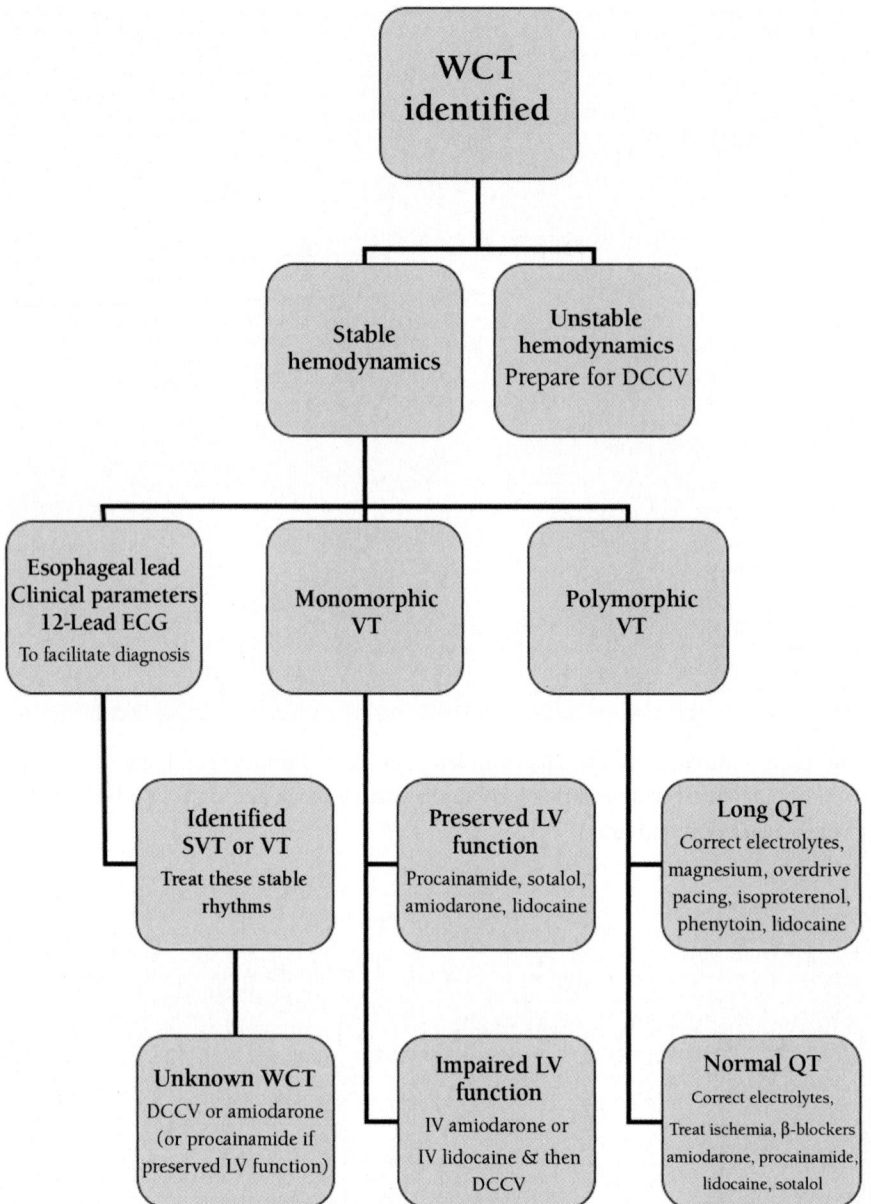

Fig. 5. American Heart Association and advanced cardiac life support guidelines for wide complex tachycardia (WCT). DCCV, direct current cardioversion; ECG, electrocardiogram; IV, intravenous; LV, left ventricular; SVT, supraventricular tachycardia; VT, ventricular tachycardia.

no role for prophylactic antiarrhythmics in these patients. Meta-analysis has demonstrated that intravenous lidocaine actually enhances mortality when given prophylactically to all post-MI patients. Revascularization strategies and β-blockers make more sense in the early acute phase after MI. Accelerated idioventricular rhythms occur at rates less than 100 to 120 beats per minute and are noted in more than 90% of patients who undergo successful revascularization.

These rhythms carry no adverse prognostic implications and do not require treatment.

Monomorphic VT is extremely uncommon during the first 48 hours after MI and is generally regarded as a triggered or automatic rhythm. However, after the first 48 hours, most monomorphic VTs are due to scar reentry and are associated with higher mortalities. The short-term treatment of VT depends on the status of the patient. If a patient is hemodynamically unstable—

with angina, shortness of breath, presyncope, syncope, and hypotension—immediate sedation and synchronized direct current cardioversion should be given. If the patient is stable, intravenous amiodarone or lidocaine is appropriate. The patient should be evaluated aggressively for residual CAD with coronary angiography and treated if feasible. Patients with late-onset VT should receive implantable cardioverter-defibrillators (ICDs). Catheter ablation or aneurysmectomy should be considered for continued VT despite medical and device therapies. The routine use of omega-3 fatty acids (fish oil) for suppression of post-MI VT remains controversial.

VT or Sudden Death in the Patient With Coronary Artery Disease or Heart Failure

Animal experimentation, surgical mapping data, and pacing interventions (e.g., resetting, manifest entrainment, and concealed entrainment) performed during VT have definitively shown that the VT of the patient with CAD is due to myocardial reentry. This reentry involves "slow zone" areas of conduction that are either adjacent to old MI scars or within the scars themselves. Most infarct scars are not homogeneous collections of connective tissue but rather areas of scar tissue intermixed with interdigitating surviving myocardial fibers, which are poorly coupled together electrically; the scars serve as excellent slow conduction zones (Fig. 6). When recording electrical signals from such areas during EP studies, the signals display low amplitude, complex fractionation, and increased duration of electrical activity. On occasion, such signals can appear biphasic or triphasic and can actually appear in the mid-diastolic interval. On the surface ECG, this is manifested as late potentials when analyzed using signal-averaged ECG.

These sites of slow conduction provide targets for ablative techniques. The surgical techniques of subendocardial resection and aneurysmectomy were used, particularly in the 1980s, for eradicating VT in patients with CAD. The overall mortality from the procedures was 5% to 8%, but cure rates were in excess of 70% to

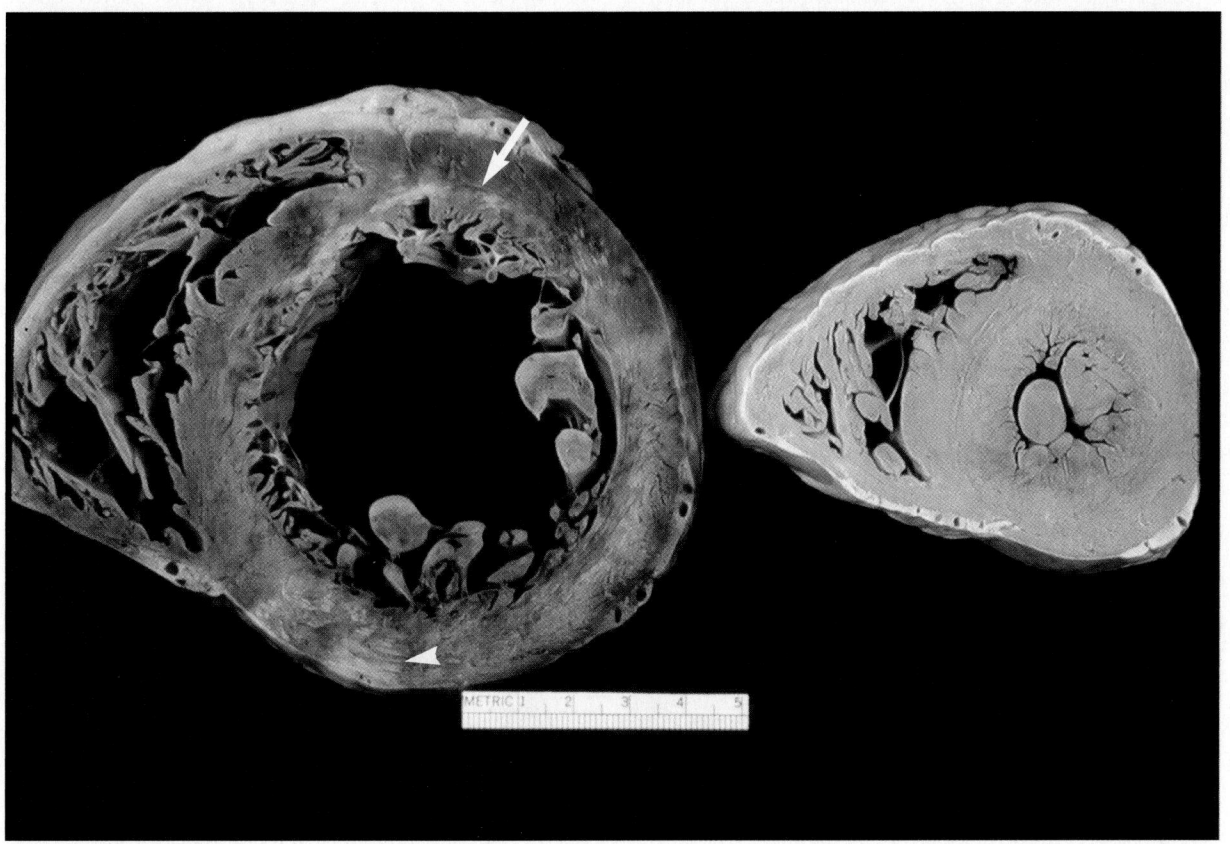

Fig. 6. Infarcted heart specimen (*left*) adjacent to normal heart specimen (*right*), showing nontransmural (*arrow*) and transmural (*arrowhead*) scarred areas, which are potential zones of slow conduction for reentry.

80%. As early as 1983, direct current catheter ablation was also used for treatment of VTs in patients with CAD; unfortunately, the success rate for abolishing VT in these patients was no better than 50%. Complications included pericardial tamponade, electrical mechanical dissociation, permanent heart block, and cardiac disruption. The procedure-related mortality rates among patients who underwent the procedure with direct current techniques in the 1980s was approximately 6%.

Because of the significant morbidity and mortality associated with direct current catheter ablation of VT in patients with CAD, radiofrequency catheter techniques were welcomed with open arms. In these patients, it is generally felt that ablation of VT with radiofrequency techniques (large tip or cool tip, at times supplemented with epicardial access) has a similar success rate (50%-70%) but with less risk to the patient. Ablation procedures should continue to be considered as palliative treatment and as an adjunct to the ICD in the symptomatic CAD patient with VT. Most patients undergoing VT radiofrequency catheter ablation in the setting of CAD are those who already have an ICD and who have had no response to multiple antiarrhythmic drugs (often including amiodarone) for

suppression of frequent antitachycardia pacing or shock therapies. Given the high recurrence of ventricular arrhythmias with different morphologies from the original VT, most of these patients cannot be considered cured after a successful radiofrequency ablation that was used as the primary therapy. Radiofrequency ablation remains the primary therapy for patients who present with incessant VT despite continuous antiarrhythmic therapy, recurrent antitachycardia pacing, or shock therapies from a device. Activation mapping can be done if the VT is reproducibly inducible, although noninducible and hemodynamically unstable VTs can be ablated using scar mapping (Fig. 7).

Several medical therapies that are appropriate after MI for prophylaxis of sudden death include aspirin, β-blockers, angiotensin-converting enzyme inhibitors, and statins. Multiple recent studies have documented the beneficial prophylactic effects of ICD use in CAD patients with impaired left ventricular function, positive EP studies, and clinical heart failure. These primary prevention trials are summarized in Table 4. Some trials required EP testing a priori (the Multicenter Automatic Defibrillator Implantation Trial [MADIT] and the Multicenter Unsustained Tachycardia Trial [MUSTT]), whereas the MADIT-II and the Sudden

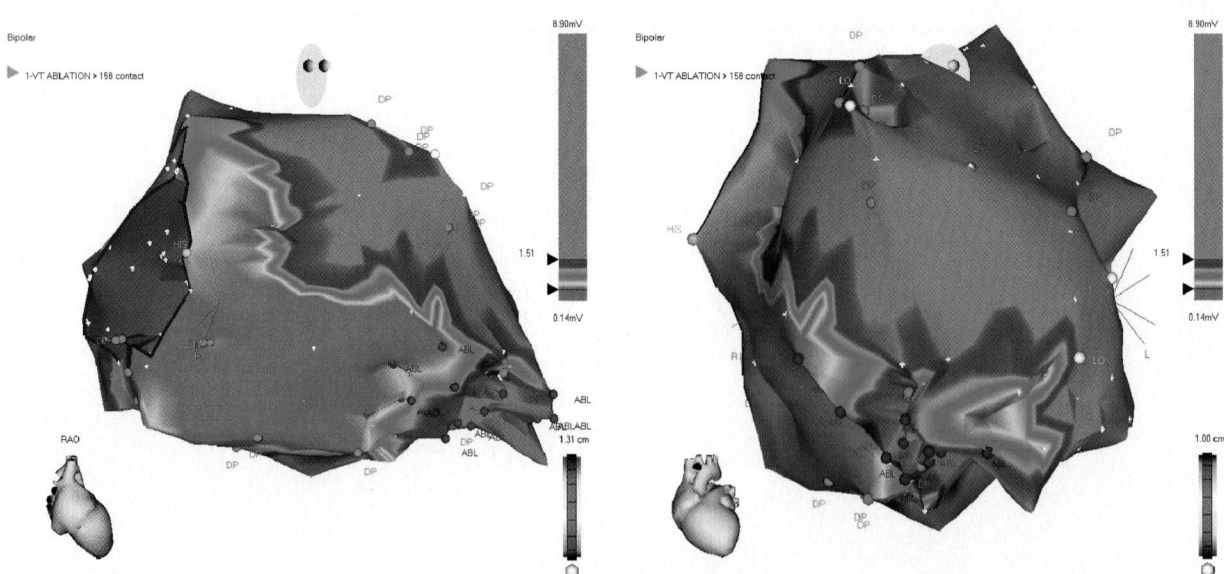

Fig. 7. Voltage map of infarcted myocardium (red) adjacent to normal myocardium (purple) in a patient with an antero-infero-septo-apical mycoardial infarction and reentrant ventricular tachycardia. *Left*, Right anterior oblique view. *Right*, Left anterior oblique view.

Cardiac Death in Heart Failure Trial (SCD-HeFT) required only ejection fraction impairment and clinical history (MI or heart failure). As lower-risk groups of patients have been investigated, the number needed to treat for a similar benefit has steadily increased. Recently, newer noninvasive risk stratification testing (e.g., T-wave alternans) has been advocated to further risk stratify prospective ICD candidates.

Bundle Branch Reentry VT

Bundle Branch Reentry VT is perhaps the easiest of all monomorphic VT rhythms to ablate using catheter techniques. The tachycardia is generally of left bundle branch morphology with a far left-axis deviation (Fig. 8). The rhythm can be replicated by pacing the right ventricle near the terminus of the right bundle at the apex. It is truly a macroreentrant tachycardia with activation proceeding anterogradely over the right bundle, transeptally to the left ventricular apex, returning retrogradely over the left bundle system, and then connecting back again at the junction of the bundles to proceed again anterogradely over the right bundle. The critical portions of the circuit include the left and right bundles and the ventricular septum. The His bundle is not part

of the circuit, although it is very common to note 1:1 retrograde His activation during this tachycardia. It is estimated that in perhaps 5% of patients with CAD and in up to 50% of patients with dilated cardiomyopathy, this is the mechanism for the clinical monomorphic VT. Typically, a patient presenting with bundle branch reentry VT has dilated cardiomyopathy, preexisting conduction disease (manifested on the ECG as left bundle branch block [LBBB] or nonspecific intraventricular conduction delay), a clinical history of either cardiac arrest or (more commonly) syncope, and an inducible, very rapid, monomorphic VT at EP testing. Usually there is an associated prolonged HV interval at baseline since conduction delay is critical to maintenance of the circuit. Ablation of the right bundle cures this VT, although most of these patients also require ICD placement for prophylactic indications.

VT in the Patient With Congenital Heart Disease

Late ventricular arrhythmias are a source of concern and late morbidity and mortality for patients with congenital heart disease. VT contributes to cardiac arrest in these patients. In particular, after repair of tetralogy of Fallot, patients have frequent ventricular

Table 4. Primary Prevention of Sudden Cardiac Death in Patients With Structural Heart Disease and an ICD

Study, year of publication	No. of patients	Inclusion criteria				3-Year mortality, %		Patients saved per 1,000 treated per year with ICD
		CAD	DCM	Other	%	LVEF, ICD	No ICD	
MADIT, 1996	196	+	−	VT$_{ns}$ + EP	≤35	41	16	83
MUSTT, 1999	704	+	−	VTns + EP Failed drug	≤40	35	16	63
MADIT II, 2002	1,232	+	−	Prior MI	≤30	31	22	30
SCD-HeFT, 2004	2,521	+	+	CHF	≤35	22	17	17

CAD, coronary artery disease; CHF, congestive heart failure; DCM, dilated cardiomyopathy; EP electrophysiologic study; ICD, implantable cardioverter-defibrillator; LVEF, left ventricular ejection fraction; MADIT, Multicenter Automatic Defibrillator Implantation Trial; MI, myocardial infarction; MUSTT, Multicenter Unsustained Tachycardia Trial; PCN, procainamide; ScD-HeFT, Sudden Cardiac Death in Heart Failure Trial; VT$_{ns}$, nonsustained ventricular tachycardia.

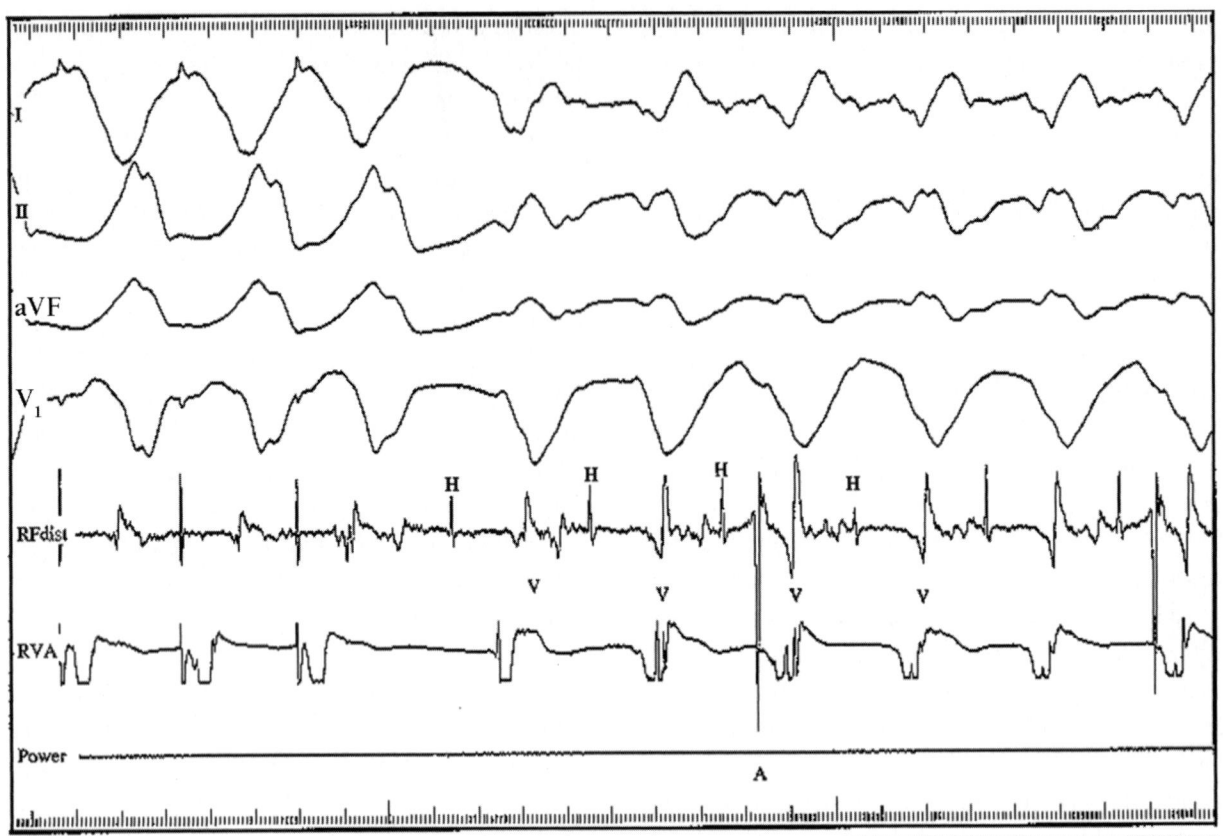

Fig. 8. Bundle branch reentrant ventricular tachycardia (VT) (paper speed, 100 mm/s) initiation with triple extrastimuli. Note tha 1:1 association of His activation to V activation (left bundle branch block with a left axis deviation VT).

arrhythmias that arise from either the ventriculotomy scar or the patch site in the right ventricular outflow tract (RVOT). The incidence of sudden death late in these patients ranges from 1% to 5% during mean follow-ups of 7 to 20 years postoperatively. Right ventricular failure, pulmonary hypertension, and number of years postoperatively are predictive factors for ventricular arrhythmias in these patients. Very limited data exist concerning the EP characteristics of this group or on the comparative efficacy of the treatments, including pharmacologic therapy, defibrillation, and ablation.

VT in Arrhythmogenic Right Ventricular Dysplasia, Hypertrophic Cardiomyopathy, and Infiltrative Diseases of the Heart

ARVD, HCM, and infiltrative diseases of the heart have distinctive underlying pathologic features, but they share a common mechanism for ventricular arrhythmias—myocardial reentry that is usually of

multiple sources. Lethal ventricular arrhythmias are a complication of all these disorders, including the infiltrative diseases and inflammatory diseases of the heart such as myocarditis, sarcoidosis, amyloidosis, and cardiac tumors.

ARVD is a special type of cardiomyopathy that chiefly affects the right ventricle and is present more often in younger patients with a familial pattern of inheritance. The right ventricle is generally large, baggy, and thin, with a depressed ejection fraction that often is not apparent in the left heart. Pathologically, the right ventricular walls are infiltrated with adipose tissue, providing a source for slow ventricular conduction and thus myocardial reentry (Fig. 9). The diagnosis can be made with echocardiography, computed tomography, magnetic resonance imaging, or endocardial biopsy. The VT is generally monomorphic with LBBB morphology, and it can be confused with the more benign RVOT VT variant. In these patients, the outcomes of surgical and ablative procedures, as

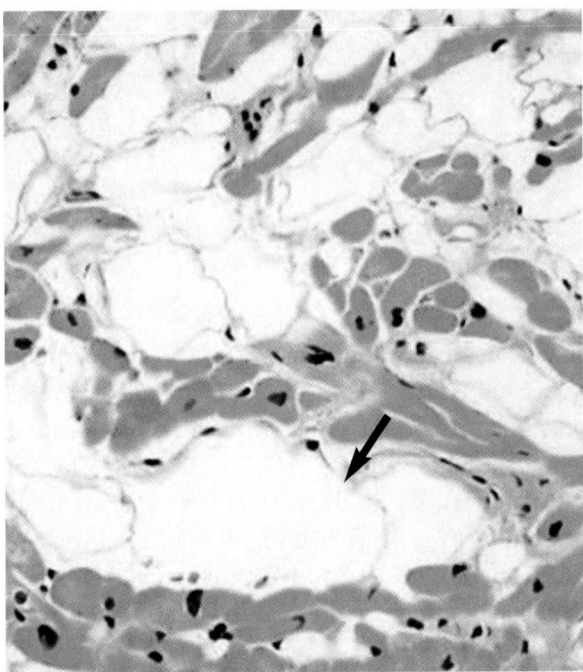

Fig. 9. Adipose replacement of right ventricular myocardium by arrhythmogenic right ventricular dysplasia in a 19-year-old with sudden cardiac dath. Fatty replacement (*arrow*) provides anatomical substrate for ventricular tachycardia.

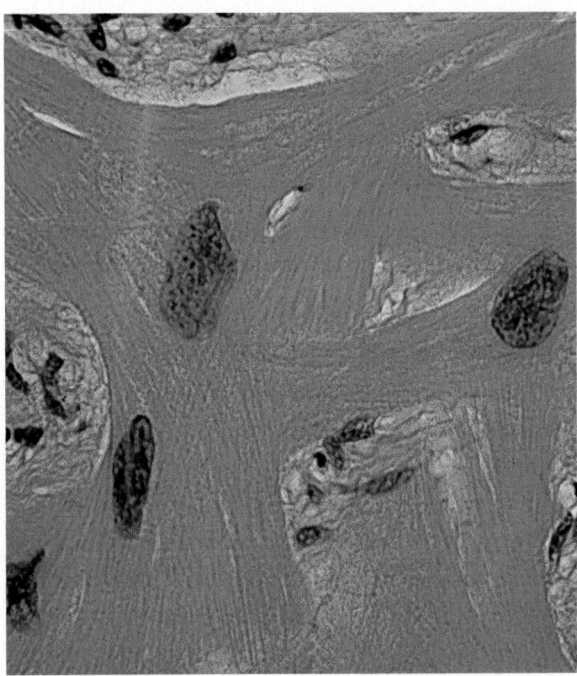

Fig. 10. Myocardial fiber disarray, which is characteristic of patients with hypertrophic cardiomyopathy and ventricular arrhythmias.

adjuncts to ICD and medical therapies, have been variable, with success rates no greater than 50% to 60% for a given patient.

HCM is characterized by myocardial fiber disarray (Fig. 10), which contributes to disorganized myocyte cellular electrical coupling, providing the substrate for myocardial reentry and lethal polymorphic ventricular arrhythmias. Nonsustained VT is present on Holter monitoring examinations 25% of the time. For sustained ventricular arrhythmias, amiodarone is the drug of choice. In general, for patients who have spontaneous ventricular arrhythmias that have caused cardiac arrest or syncope or for those with a positive family history of sudden cardiac death, ICD implantation is recommended and possibly adjunctive antiarrhythmic therapy.

Familial Channelopathy Syndromes and VT

Patients with familial channelopathy syndromes typically have hearts with morphologically normal structures, abnormalities of ion channel configuration, and poor repolarization reserves, making them susceptible to polymorphic VTs. The early afterdepolarization (EAD) (Fig. 11), which occurs during phase II/phase III of an action potential, is the cellular event common to these rhythms. EADs are easily produced experimentally by the inhibitor of the potassium channel (I_K) current, among others.

On the surface ECG, EADs produce polymorphic PVCs and, when regenerated, can produce polymorphic VT or torsades de pointes. Drugs that produce EADs experimentally clinically prolong the QT interval in animals and humans; these same agents also produce polymorphic VTs. Experimentally, EADs can be suppressed with increased extracellular potassium levels, acetylcholine (which hyperpolarizes the transmembrane potential), antiarrhythmic drugs such as lidocaine (which suppresses the sodium window current, a slow sodium current that is also responsible for prolongation of phase II), magnesium, β-blockers, pacing to increase heart rate, and potassium channel openers (which enhance potassium currents and thus hasten phase III). EADs represent the cellular cause for most proarrhythmia phenomena seen with antiarrhythmic drugs and other noncardiac drugs (e.g., terfenadine, pentamidine,

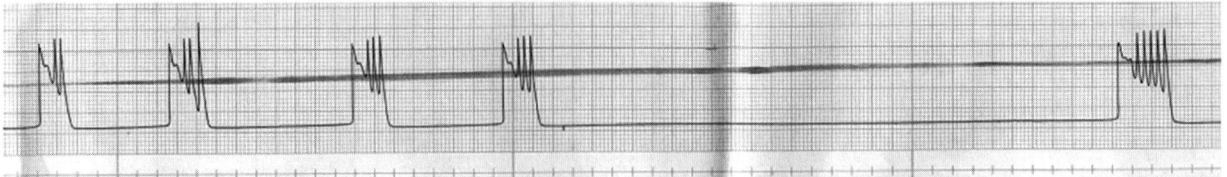

Fig. 11. Early afterdepolarizations (EADs) recorded from a canine Purkinje fiber under condtions of 10⁻⁷ M quinidine. Such activity on the surface electrocardiogram produces polymorphic ventricular ectopy in series.

and erythromycin). During EP testing, triggered rhythms can often be initiated and terminated with programmed stimulation, much like reentrant rhythms.

The congenital LQTS is characterized by long QT intervals and episodes of paroxysmal VT that can produce syncope and even cardiac arrest, particularly in younger individuals. Women are more affected than men with LQTS. Autosomal dominant (Romano-Ward syndrome) and recessive forms of the disease are recognized. Half of all deaths in association with LQTS occur in patients younger than 20 years, and a relationship to sudden infant death syndrome has been proposed. Recently, a molecular diagnosis of LQT1 was made post mortem after an infant died of sudden infant death syndrome. Higher-risk individuals include those who have family members who have died of sudden cardiac death and individuals who have syncope or QT interval in excess of 600 ms. Certain genotypes have been linked to particular clinical symptoms (e.g., drowning associated with sudden cardiac death with LQT1). β-Blockers, mexiletine, autonomic surgery, pacing, and ICD therapy have all been used in various groups of patients with this syndrome. Avoidance of medications that can aggravate this problem is imperative.

KVLQT1 mutations of the SCN5A sodium channel (diminished current, in contrast to LQT1) cause the Brugada phenotype and are also associated with polymorphic VT. Like LQTS patients, certain patients with asymptomatic Brugada syndrome have been identified with characteristics meriting prophylactic ICD implantation. (For further discussion see Chapter 22, "Arrhythmogenic Disorders: Cardiac Channelopathies.")

Idiopathic VT in the Patient With a Structurally Normal Heart and No Repolarization Abnormalities

Idiopathic VT causes less than 5% of VT cases in the general population, but nonetheless it is an important entity to identify since it is readily treatable. Unlike ventricular arrhythmias associated with myocardial scar (e.g., patients with CAD, cardiomyopathy, or myocarditis), VT in the patient with a structurally normal heart is overwhelmingly associated with an excellent prognosis. Sudden cardiac death in such patients is extremely rare, and thus the goal of treatment in these patients is relief of symptoms. The majority of patients present between the ages of 20 and 50 years, although children and the elderly can present with idiopathic VT as well. Presentation symptoms include palpitations in 80%, dizziness in 50%, and syncope in 10%. Idiopathic VT can be divided into two main groups: adenosine-sensitive and verapamil-sensitive intrafascicular.

Adenosine-Sensitive VT

Adenosine-sensitive VT accounts for more than 80% of all VT cases in patients with normal heart. This type of VT generally originates in the RVOT and manifests as two distinct subtypes: 1) repetitive monomorphic VT (or Parkinson-Papp VT), which occurs most frequently at rest, and 2) paroxysmal exercise-induced sustained VT. Both of these subtypes have LBBB morphology with a rightward (inferior) or normal axis (Fig. 12).

Repetitive monomorphic (RVOT VT), originally described in 1922, is associated with isolated PVCs, ventricular pairs, and salvos of nonsustained VT intermixed with episodes of sinus rhythm. Other patients have predominately the exercise-induced variant, which generally becomes sustained with catecholamine stimulation. Remission of symptoms over time can be expected in 5% to 20% of cases. Other LBBB tachycardias that should be considered include Mahaim (atriofascicular) tachycardia, antidromic reciprocating tachycardia or bystander tachycardias from right-sided accessory pathways, VT due to ARVD, VT associated with

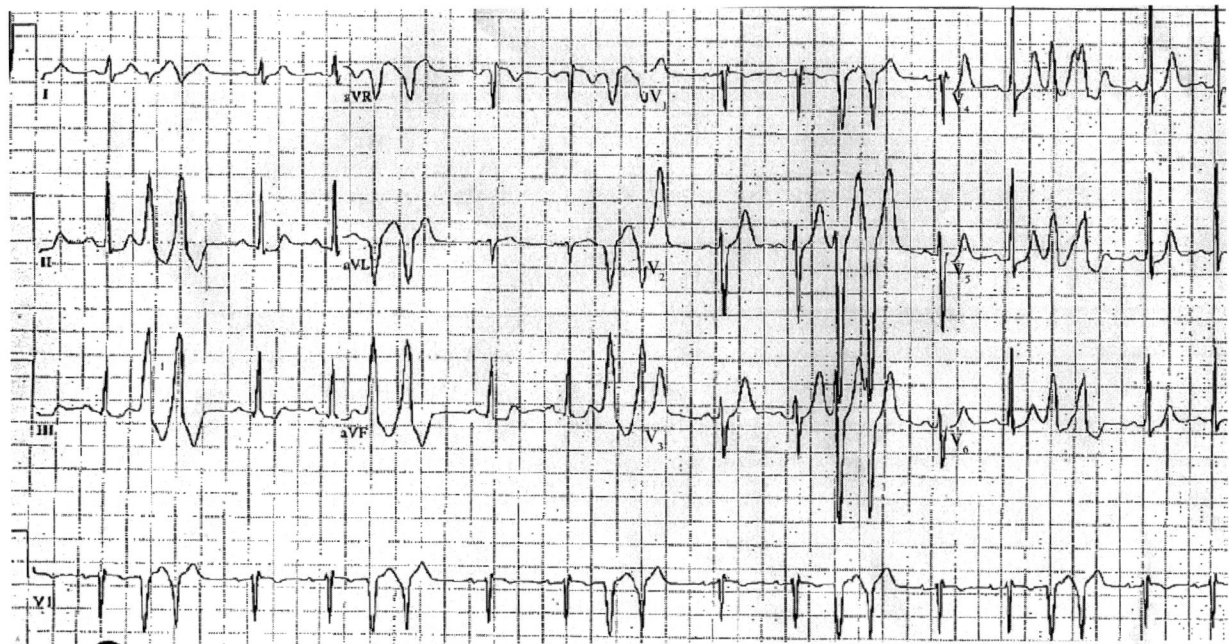

Fig. 12. RV outflow tract ventricular tachycardia (left bundle branch block—right-axis deviation variant). These tachycardias can be found in both the right ventricular outflow tract area and the left ventricular outflow tract.

tetrology of Fallot repair, and bundle branch reentry VT.

By echocardiography, the right ventricle is normal in more than 90% of patients; the minority of cases display tachycardia-induced cardiomyopathy changes, which are reversible. Occasionally, cases of ARVD can be confused with idiopathic RVOT VT by echocardiography and should be considered with additional imaging studies (computed tomography or magnetic resonance imaging) if indicated. Adenosine-sensitive RVOT tachycardias are most likely due to a triggered delayed afterdepolarization (DAD) mechanism. Experimentally, DADs can be produced or enhanced under conditions that augment intracellular calcium loading, such as rapid pacing, increased $[Ca^{2+}]_o$, digitalis glycosides, drugs that enhance $[Ca^{2+}]_i$, low $[K^+]_o$, or endogenous/exogenous catecholamines. Thus, DAD-dependent arrhythmias, such as RVOT VT, could be terminated at multiple levels of the β-receptor–adenyl cyclase cascade: muscarinic (vagal) activation, β-blockade, calcium blockade (with agents such as verapamil), the potassium channel opener nicorandil, and adenosine. Verapamil can terminate triggered ventricular arrhythmias, but it is not specific since the drug can also inhibit VT due to abnormal automaticity, intrafascicular reentry, and myocardial ischemia. In contrast, adenosine is very specific in its ability to terminate triggered ventricular arrhythmias. Adenosine binds to the A_1 adenosine receptor, which is coupled to adenyl cyclase through the inhibitory pertussis toxin–sensitive G-protein, G_i. Through this inhibitory effect of G_i, cyclic adenosine monophosphate (cAMP) is reduced, and the overall effect becomes antiadrenergic, thus reducing DAD activity. Adenosine is unable to terminate ventricular DAD activity due to cAMP-independent mechanisms, namely, digitalis, dibutyryl cAMP, or α_1 inosine triphosphate-dependent pathways. Also, adenosine does not suppress VT due to catecholamine-facilitated reentry in the presence of structural heart disease or VT due to EAD activity induced by quinidine or calcium agonists like Bay K8644.

At exercise testing, only 30% to 50% of patients display sustained VT, and a similar finding can be seen at EP testing. Signal-averaged ECG is generally negative and unhelpful. In most patients, VT is noninducible at EP testing in the sedated state. Triggered VT is generally induced with ventricular burst pacing or programmed ventricular stimulation and cannot be entrained (like reentry). To facilitate induction pharmacologically, isoproterenol, atropine, or aminophylline can be administered and used in conjunction with programmed stimulation. To support the diagnosis in a patient with LBBB VT, termination of the VT with adenosine, verapamil, edrophonium, vagal maneuvers, or β-blockers is suggestive.

Verapamil-Sensitive Intrafascicular VT

Verapamil-sensitive intrafascicular VT, described in 1979, originates from the posterior-inferior mid left ventricle (in the region of the left posterior hemifascicle) and produces right bundle branch block with left-axis deviation (Fig. 13). The ECG of this VT generally has a short RS interval (<60-80 ms) and a short QRS duration (<140 ms). Four features of this arrhythmia are the morphology, the induction with atrial pacing, the verapamil sensitivity, and the absence of structural heart disease. Akin to RVOT VT, this arrhythmia generally occurs in younger patients with normal ventricular function and no CAD; 80% are men. This VT can also be associated with tachycardia-mediated cardiomyopathy. Sudden death virtually never occurs in association with this form of VT, although the polymorphic form of this can cause syncope and VF. Presentation symptoms include palpitations, dyspnea,

dizziness, and syncope. The signal-averaged ECG is generally normal when analyzed in the time domain.

At EP testing, in the region of the left posterior hemifascicle, Purkinje fiber potentials that precede the earliest ventricular endocardial activation mapping site can be identified. Unlike RVOT VT, this rhythm is felt to be due to reentry and not to a triggered mechanism. The zone of slow conduction has been demonstrated to be between the late diastolic potential area (the common left bundle near the base of the left ventricular septum [the entrance]) and the more apically positioned posterior hemifascicle area (the exit). This area appears to depend on the slow inward calcium current since verapamil causes significant delay in this zone, whereas lidocaine has minimal effect. It is postulated that Purkinje potentials in the area of slow conduction are in a depolarized state, more dependent on the slow inward calcium current for maintenance of conduction. Entrainment is most easily demonstrated from the RVOT compared with RV apex. As the name implies, this type of VT is sensitive to verapamil but is generally unresponsive to vagal maneuvers or adenosine, although it can be adenosine sensitive if catecholamines are required for its initiation.

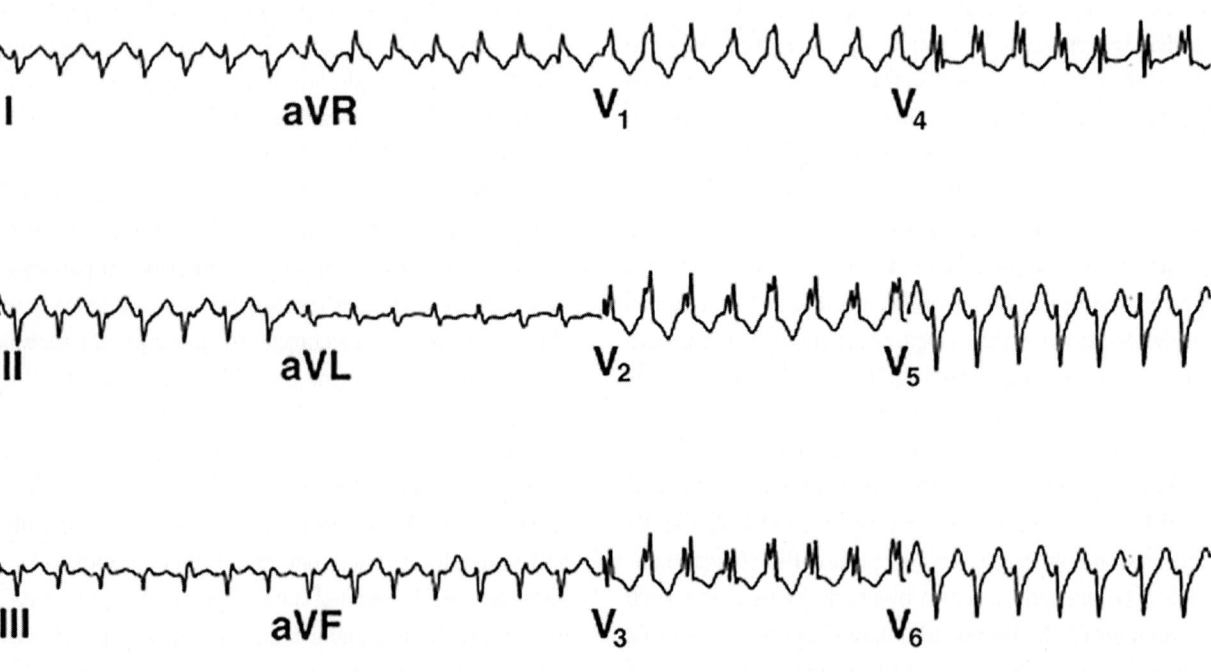

Fig. 13. Verapamil-sensitive ventricular tachycardia (right bundle branch block with left-axis deviation) typical of ventricular tachycardia originating from the left posterior fascicular area of the left ventricular septum. Note the relatively narrow QRS complex.

RVOT VT, if nonsustained and asymptomatic, requires no therapy. β-Blockers or calcium channel blockers inhibit the arrhythmia in 25% to 50% of cases and represent first-line medical therapies. Class 1 and class 3 antiarrhythmic drugs are effective in up to 50% of cases. Acutely, carotid sinus massage, adenosine, verapamil, and lidocaine facilitate termination. For verapamil-sensitive left ventricular VT, calcium channel blockers are the medical treatment of choice. Radiofrequency ablative therapy should be recommended for patients who experience side effects or inefficacy from drug therapy or for individuals who have arrhythmia-related symptoms (e.g., syncope or near syncope).

In RVOT VT, QRS duration greater than 140 ms with a triphasic QRS complex in the inferior leads suggests a free wall lateral origin, whereas QRS duration less than 140 ms with a monophasic QRS complex suggests a septal origin. During VT, precordial transition is generally seen in leads V_2 through V_4; for transition in V_2, a location just adjacent to the pulmonary valve or a left ventricular outflow origin is suggested. Successful ablation sites have been associated with activation times 10 to 45 ms ahead of the surface QRS, as well as pace map matches in 11 of 12 or in 12 of 12 ECG leads. Body surface potential mapping, electroanatomical three-dimensional mapping, and noncontact mapping have all been used to facilitate ablation of VT of RVOT origin. Successful ablation of RVOT VT occurs in 90% of cases, with 10% recurrence. Other unusual origins for adenosine-sensitive VT include the left ventricular outflow tract (where damage to the left main coronary artery, conduction system, or aortic valve must be monitored for), left fascicular conduction system, epicardial left ventricle, and RVOT diverticula.

For verapamil-sensitive left ventricular VT, the usual successful sites of ablation are sites of earliest ventricular activation. Success rates are approximately 85% to 90%. Pace mapping is not as useful as in RVOT VT, and the presence of Purkinje potentials is not a necessary requirement for successful ablation (the potentials can sometimes be recorded over a 2-3 cm² area of tissue). A similar region of targeting for ablation has recently been identified for "curing" patients with idiopathic VF (Fig. 14 and 15).

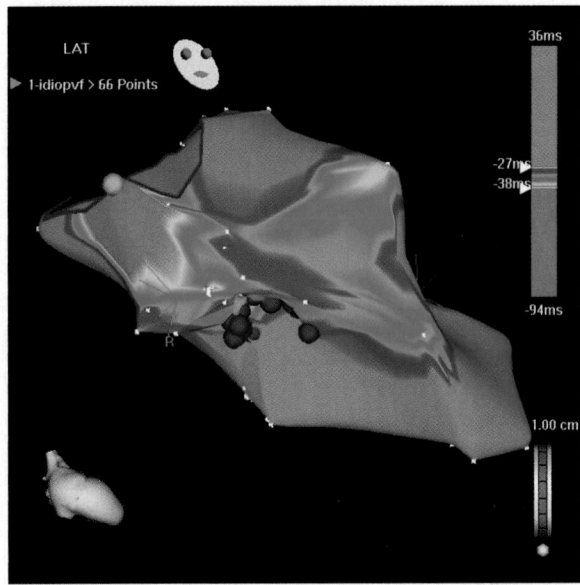

Fig. 14. Electroanatomical map (right anterior oblique view) left ventricle (LV) in same patient as in Figure 3, with idiopathic polymorphic ventricular tachycardia originating from the posterior LV hemifascicle. Map was displayed during normal sinus rhythm. The red area is the HIS bundle, and the more apical yellow areas are the anterior and posterior hemifascicles. The maroon dots are ablation sites corresponding to the electrograms in Figure 15.

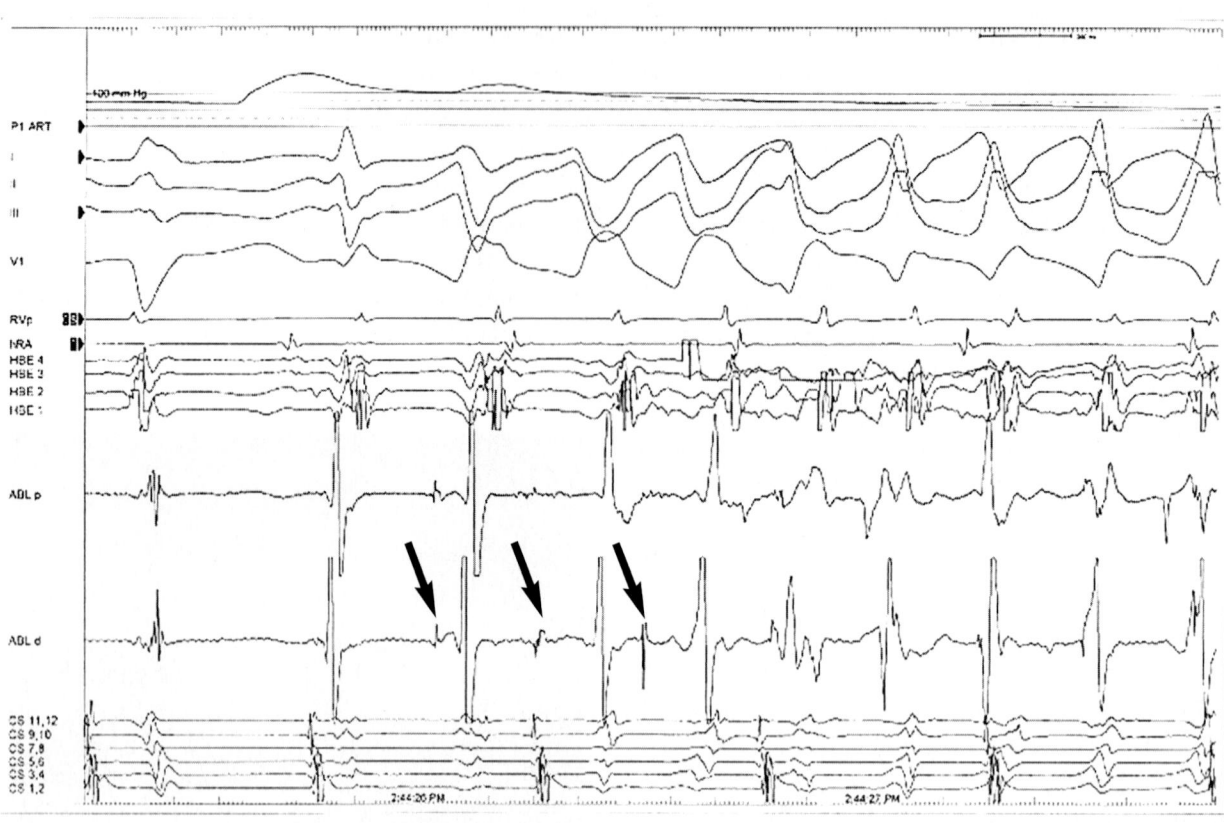

Fig. 15. Note the Purkinje potentials (*arrows*) preceding the local ventricular activations on the ABL channel on the first four beats of ventricular tachycardia.

29

ARRHYTHMIAS IN CONGENITAL HEART DISEASE

Peter A. Brady, MD

Patients with CHD comprise an increasingly prevalent population of patients presenting with symptoms due to arrhythmic syndromes and bradycardia. Due to reduced hemodynamic reserve, onset of arrhythmias in patients with complex CHD is a frequent cause of symptomatic deterioration or even sudden cardiac death. Effective arrhythmia management and risk stratification remains challenging due to limited data which in most cases are extrapolated from data in adults with ischemic heart disease. Important clinical markers that predict poorer outcome and increased risk of heart rhythm disorders include presence of uncorrected hemodynamic defects, surgical repair later in life, and older age (i.e., longer follow-up). Patients who present with new onset of an atrial or a ventricular arrhythmia require comprehensive hemodynamic and electrophysiological assessment.

Risk markers of arrhythmias in patients with CHD include:

■ Presence of residual hemodynamic defects.
■ Surgical repair later in life.
■ Older age (longer follow-up).

CLASSIFICATION

Although anatomic classification of congenital heart defects is complex, three major groups comprise the majority of patients with CHD presenting with arrhythmias and may be usefully classified into

1. Those that arise in the unoperated heart
2. Perioperative arrhythmias occurring immediately following surgical repair of a congenital heart defect
3. "Late" arrhythmias presenting remote from surgical repair of a congenital heart defect.

For CV boards you should be familiar with common arrhythmias in

■ Ebstein's anomaly of the tricuspid valve.
■ Arrhythmias following Mustard, Senning, and Fontan procedures and repaired tetralogy of Fallot.

ARRHYTHMIAS IN THE UNOPERATED HEART

Tachyarrhythmias

Paroxysmal Supraventricular Tachycardias (PSVT)

Accessory Pathway Mediated Tachycardias (Wolff-Parkinson-White Syndromes)
Because CHD and accessory pathways are relatively common (1 or 2% and 1% of live births respectively), the two may coexist by chance. However, certain types

of CHD are more frequently associated with accessory pathways in particular Ebstein's anomaly of the tricuspid valve (see below). Other defects associated with increased frequency of accessory pathways include L-transposition of the great vessels (ventricular inversion and congenitally corrected transposition), atrioventricular septal defect and hypertrophic cardiomyopathy.

Congenital heart defects associated with an increased likelihood of accessory pathways (WPW) include:

- Ebstein's anomaly of the tricuspid valve (most common for CV boards).
- Congenitally corrected transposition of the great vessels.
- Atrioventricular septal defect.
- Hypertrophic cardiomyopathy.

Atrial Arrhythmias (Including Atrial Tachycardia, Atrial Flutter and Fibrillation)

Atrial arrhythmias are common in patients both prior to and following surgical repair of CHD and should be suspected in previously stable patients in whom clinical status deteriorates even if heart rate is not increased (may have varying degrees of AV conduction due to concomitant AV nodal and/or His Purkinje disease). Atrial arrhythmias are most common in persons older than 40 years (younger patients are more likely to present with "ectopic" atrial and junctional rhythm disorders).

Terminology and classification of atrial arrhythmias in patients with CHD is often confusing. Three main types of atrial arrhythmia should be distinguished.

- Typical (isthmus-dependent or common) atrial flutter (Fig. 1).
- Atrial fibrillation (disorganized and irregular atrial rhythm without visible atrial activity) (Fig. 2).
- Intra-atrial reentrant tachycardia (IART). A common arrhythmia due to multiple circuits, most often within the right atrium and confined by anatomic and surgical boundaries. This rhythm is frequently difficult to distinguish from atrial flutter.

ATRIAL FLUTTER

Atrial flutter is often described as typical or atypical. The difference is that "typical" atrial flutter is characterized by a 'sawtooth' pattern in leads II, III and aVF, which are upright in V1 (Fig. 1). It is important to recognize this rhythm as it is amenable to catheter ablation with >95% likelihood of success and <2% likelihood of recurrence. Due to enlargement of either the right or left atrial chambers (or both), or surgical scar (atriotomy), the 'typical' appearance of typical atrial flutter may be distorted on the surface ECG. Any other sustained narrow complex tachycardia with a stable rate

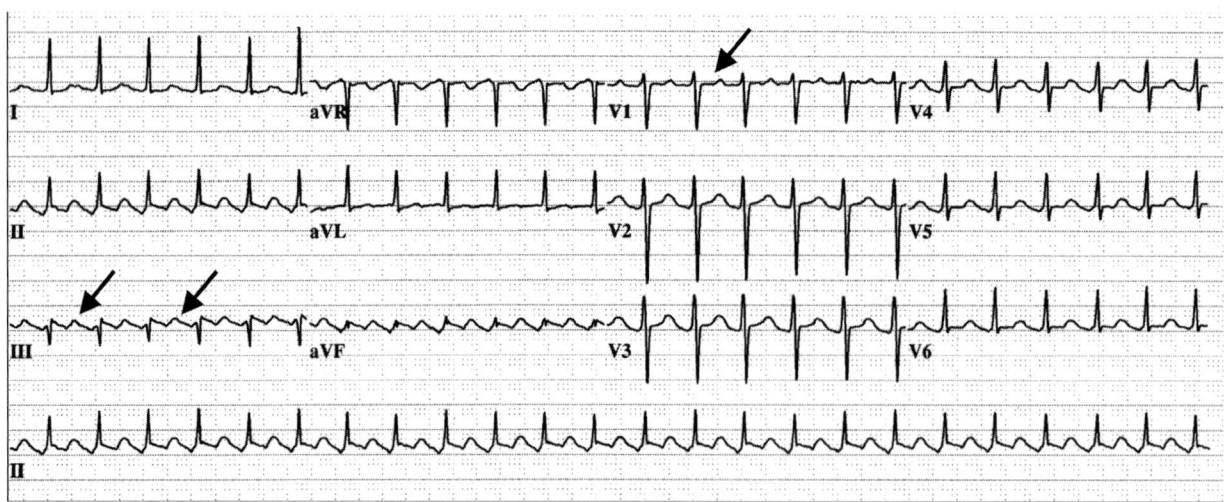

Fig. 1. Atrial flutter with 2:1 atrioventricular conduction. Note characteristic sawtooth pattern in leads II, III, and aVF, which are upright in V1. In patients with congenital heart disease, enlargement of atrial chambers or the presence of surgical scars may distort this pattern. In most cases, electrophysiologic study may be required to confirm the circuit of this atrial flutter. This is most commonly performed at the time of the planned ablation. *Arrows* indicate flutter waves.

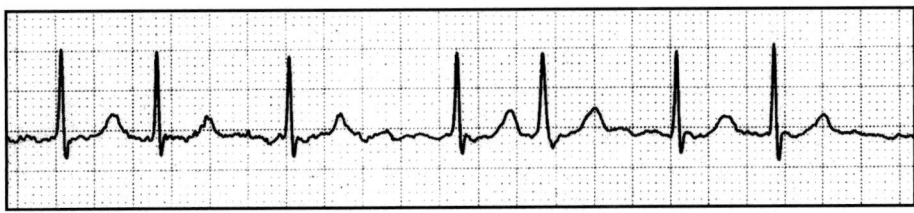

Fig. 2. Atrial fibrillation characterized by disorganized and irregular rhythm without visible atrial organization.

that is confined to the atria is termed atypical atrial flutter. In patients with CHD this rhythm is often termed IART.

IART

Like atrial flutter, intra-atrial reentrant tachycardia (IART) is characterized by uniform flutter wave morphology, constant cycle length, sudden onset and offset (due to reentrant mechanism) with variable AV conduction (may also conduct 1:1).

IART occurs most commonly in patients with atriotomy, or other surgical manipulation of the atrium, such as ASD repair (Fig. 3), Mustard and Senning palliation of transposition of the great arteries, construction of Fontan anastomosis for palliation of single ventricle physiology, TOF and repair of anomalous pulmonary venous connection.

Intra-atrial reentrant tachycardia is most common with

- ASD repair.
- Mustard/Senning procedure.
- Fontan.
- Tetralogy of Fallot.
- Repair of anomalous pulmonary venous drainage.

ATRIAL FIBRILLATION

AF may occur in up to 30% of patients with CHD, and is more common with residual left sided obstructive lesions or ventricular dysfunction causing left atrial pressure/volume overload. Similar to other atrial arrhythmias, loss of AV synchrony is particularly problematic and efforts to restore and maintain sinus rhythm (cardioversion, antiarrhythmic drugs and catheter ablation and pacing therapy) are usually necessary.

CV Board Point

- A narrow QRS complex tachycardia in a patient with CHD who is older than 40 years is most likely due to typical atrial flutter, IART (if previous repair involving atriotomy) or atrial fibrillation.

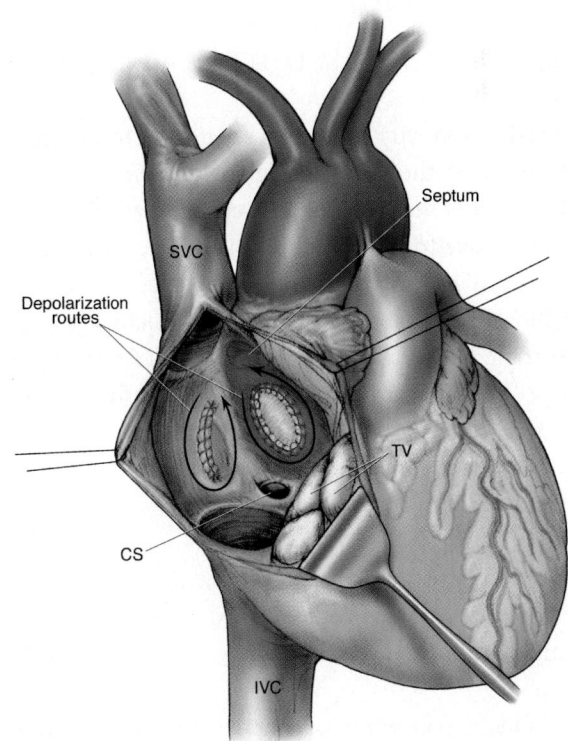

Fig. 3. Septal patch and atriotomy scar. The presence of these structures, which form a nonconductive boundary, allows re-entry circuits to develop within the atrium. These may lead to sustained atrial flutters that are non–isthmus-dependent and, therefore, in most cases have an atypical appearance. Ablation of these atrial flutters requires identification of these circuits and the use of linear ablation between scar and other nonconductive boundaries, such as the tricuspid valve anulus or the inferior vena cava. CS, carotid sinus; IVC, inferior vena cava; SVC, superior vena cava; TV, tricuspid valve.

ATRIAL SEPTAL DEFECT

Ostium secundum and sinus venosus atrial septal defects often result in dilatation of the right atrium and right ventricle due to chronic left to right shunting leading to delayed intra-atrial conduction that predisposes to reentrant arrhythmias and sinoatrial node dysfunction. This may present with palpitations, dyspnea, presyncope and syncope (due to bradycardia or sinus pauses). In the absence of surgical repair the most common arrhythmia is typical "isthmus-dependent" atrial flutter.

CV Board Point

- ASD is associated with "late" sinus node dysfunction and atrial arrhythmias (most commonly typical atrial flutter).

EBSTEIN'S ANOMALY OF THE TRICUSPID VALVE

Ebstein's anomaly comprises separation of the right atrium from the right ventricle with downward displacement of the posterior and septal leaflets of the tricuspid valve towards the right ventricle creating an "atrialized" portion of the right ventricle in which the right ventricle is morphologically and electrically right ventricle but functionally right atrium. Atrial septal defect or other cardiac anomaly is frequently associated; tricuspid regurgitation is common.

Two main arrhythmia mechanisms are important in patients with Ebstein's anomaly:

- Accessory pathway mediated tachycardia (PSVT).
- Atrial arrhythmias due to marked enlargement of the right atrium and ventricle.

Due to concomitant hemodynamic and anatomic abnormalities supraventricular arrhythmias are usually not well tolerated in patients with Ebstein's anomaly and frequently present with symptomatic deterioration or even presyncope, syncope or sudden cardiac death. In addition, mechanical stimulation of the "atrialized" ventricle may provoke ventricular arrhythmias.

Accessory Pathways and Ebstein's Anomaly

Accessory AV and atrio-fascicular pathways are present in around 25% of patients with Ebstein's anomaly. In situs solitus with AV concordance accessory pathways are almost exclusively right sided and often multiple. Accessory pathway mediated tachycardias (atrio-ventricular reentry) are most common in patients aged <35 years, whereas in older patients atrial flutter and fibrillation is more common.

Supraventricular arrhythmias in patients with Ebstein's anomaly of the tricuspid valve may be due to

- PSVT (accessory pathway mediated tachycardia—younger age; commonly right sided).
- Atrial flutter and fibrillation (age >35 years).

CV Board Point

- Most patients with Ebstein's anomaly have a RBBB pattern on the 12 lead ECG. Loss of RBBB may hint at the presence of a right-sided accessory pathway.

Preoperative Assessment of Ebstein's Anomaly

All patients with documented tachycardia or history of palpitations should undergo preoperative electrophysiologic testing regardless of the presence or absence of ventricular pre-excitation (WPW pattern). If an accessory pathway and inducible SVT is present either catheter ablation or surgical cryoablation should be performed.

VENTRICULAR DEFECT

Ventricular septal defect (VSD) is the most common congenital heart defect. Although defects occur in all portions of the interventricular septum, the effect on the cardiac conduction system and risk of arrhythmias in unoperated patients probably result mostly from hemodynamic effect rather than the precise location of the defect. Most moderate or large VSDs are associated with ECG findings of right and left ventricular hypertrophy and left atrial enlargement. Even when VSD is an isolated anomaly, associated arrhythmias are common in childhood and adults.

Independent predictors of arrhythmias in patients with VSD include

- Elevated pulmonary artery pressure at the time of surgery.
- Older age.

Although risk of ventricular arrhythmias and sudden cardiac death after VSD repair is low SCD may occur when ventricular hypertrophy and conduction system fibrosis are present. Late sudden death is observed in <5% of patients with surgically repaired VSD, depending upon length of follow-up. Risk factors for SCD include surgery after 5 years of age, increased pulmonary vascular resistance (especially Eisenmenger physiology) and untreated heart block.

ATRIOVENTRICULAR SEPTAL DEFECT

Atrioventricular septal defects are associated with postero-inferior displacement of the AV node and left bundle branch, a longer than normal penetrating bundle, and relative hypoplasia of the anterior portion of the left bundle branch which is associated with left axis deviation of the QRS complex (superior axis) along with evidence of chamber enlargement. In most cases of complete atrioventricular septal defect, the ECG shows biventricular hypertrophy and biatrial enlargement. In patients with an ostium primum ASD or with a complete atrioventricular septal defect but small VSD, the ECG is similar to that from a patient with an ostium secundum ASD plus QRS axis shift. Unoperated, AVSD may lead to Eisenmenger physiology right ventricular hypertrophy and risk of ventricular arrhythmias. Atrioventricular septal defect is also associated with accessory AV connections and PSVT most commonly located in the posteroseptal region.

TETRALOGY OF FALLOT

Tetralogy of Fallot comprises hyperplasia and anterior malalignment of the infundibular septum, infundibular and often valvular pulmonic stenosis, overriding aorta, and perimembranous outlet VSD. Right ventricular hypertrophy with normal pulmonary vascular resistance, arterial desaturation and secondary polycythemia are common prior to surgical repair. Typically, the preoperative ECG shows right ventricular hypertrophy and right axis deviation. Frequency of ventricular arrhythmias increases with age.

BRADYCARDIA

Sinus Node Dysfunction and AV Block

Sinus node dysfunction may present as profound bradycardia, asystole or pauses, or chronotropic incompetence. Loss of AV synchrony is often not well tolerated in patients with CHD and impaired ventricular function, therefore pacing is recommended if symptoms are present. Sinus node dysfunction is more common in patients with sinus venosus defects or heterotaxy syndromes, particularly left atrial isomerism. Risk of AV block is around 2% per year in patients with L-transposition (ventricular inversion and congenitally corrected transposition).

Congenital AV Block

Congenital AV block occurs most commonly in the absence of other cardiac disease. In most cases, block is proximal to the bifurcation of the His bundle or within the AV node. Therefore, the QRS is narrow (<100) and the ventricular rate is usually above 40 beats/min. In most cases, patients should undergo implantation of a permanent pacemaker even in the absence of symptoms.

PERIOPERATIVE ARRHYTHMIAS FOLLOWING CONGENITAL HEART SURGERY

Junctional tachycardia (junctional ectopic or His bundle tachycardia, [JT]) is most common in the 24 hours following repair of a congenital heart defect. Procedures associated with a higher likelihood of JT include repair of TOF, Mustard and Senning procedures for d-TGA, VSD closure, repair of total anomalous venous return and following Fontan operation.

ECG Characteristics

Typically, JT is regular with rates >200 bpm and a QRS morphology identical to that during sinus rhythm. In most cases, ventriculoatrial dissociation is present (ventricular rate faster than atrial rate) with occasional sinus capture. In some cases, it may be confused with atrial tachycardia with first degree AV block. The precise mechanism of JT is not well understood but may be due to surgical trauma to the conduction system, coupled with pulmonary arterial hypertension, inflammatory changes and hypoxia.

Overdrive suppression is common and typically the rhythm shows a 'warm-up' phenomenon following suppression increasing gradually up to the previous rate. Direct current cardioversion is *not* useful since the rhythm will rapidly recur.

Treatment

JT is associated with high mortality. If hemodynamic status can be stabilized the rhythm will resolve over time. The goal of therapy is to decrease the ventricular rate to less than 150 bpm. Some success has been reported with the use of both class I (flecainide and propafenone) and class III agents (mostly amiodarone). Restoration of AV synchrony with atrial pacing may be beneficial in some patients.

PERI- AND POSTOPERATIVE BRADYCARDIA

Postoperative sinus node dysfunction occurs most often following Fontan, Mustard and Senning procedures that involve extensive dissection and modification of the right atrium. In addition to "early" postoperative sinus node dysfunction, progressive ('late') loss of sinus node function may occur implying additional pathology such as chronic sinoatrial ischemia and fibrosis and/or the effects of chronic hemodynamic stress.

POSTOPERATIVE SINUS NODE DYSFUNCTION

Sinus node dysfunction is most common following:

- Senning and Mustard procedure.
- Fontan procedure.

POSTOPERATIVE AV BLOCK

AV block is most common following:

- Atrioventricular septal defect (canal or endocardial cushion).
- VSD closure involving the perimembranous region.
- Repair of subaortic stenosis.
- AV block after ASD repair is uncommon.

Patients who have persistent AV block following surgery should undergo permanent pacemaker implantation. In some cases spontaneous resolution of AV block may occur in the immediate postoperative period so a period of observation may be appropriate. However, since the duration of observation (typically >5 days) and the likelihood of 'late' recurrence of AV block is unknown, questions relating to the precise timing of pacemaker implantation are unlikely on the CV boards.

ARRHYTHMIAS IN SURGICALLY REPAIRED CHD

Atrial Septal Defect (ASD)

Although isthmus dependent flutter remains common, surgical incisions (atriotomy scar) increase the likelihood of a non-isthmus dependent IART although these two rhythms may also coexist in the same patient. The most common circuit for a macroreentrant atrial arrhythmia is along the lateral right atrial wall around atriotomy incision (Fig. 4). Complex double-loop circuits are also not uncommon increasing the complexity of the rhythm and attempted catheter ablation.

Risk factors for atrial arrhythmias in surgically repaired ASD include:

- Older age at repair.
- Longer duration of follow-up.

EBSTEIN'S ANOMALY

Following surgical repair of Ebstein's anomaly, enlargement of the right atrium and the presence of an atriotomy provide the substrate for IART (AFL). Freedom from occurrence of IART following surgery is improved with addition of right-sided maze or cryoablation procedure independent of corrective surgery and does not increase operative mortality.

MUSTARD, SENNING, AND FONTAN PROCEDURES

Sinus node dysfunction and atrial arrhythmias are common following **Mustard** and **Senning** procedures for D-transposition of the great arteries. Each involve creation of an intra-atrial baffle with a prosthetic material or pericardium (i.e. Mustard operation) or the atrial wall itself (i.e. Senning operation) associated with risk of damage to the sinus and perinodal structures as well as pacemaker tissue throughout the atrium. Late development of intra-atrial reentry and atrial flutter is also common.

The **Fontan procedure** directs systemic venous return to the pulmonary arteries in patients with a single ventricle and is associated with atrial arrhythmias due to myocardial scarring and chronic elevation of right atrial pressure. Repair of **ostium secundum, sinus**

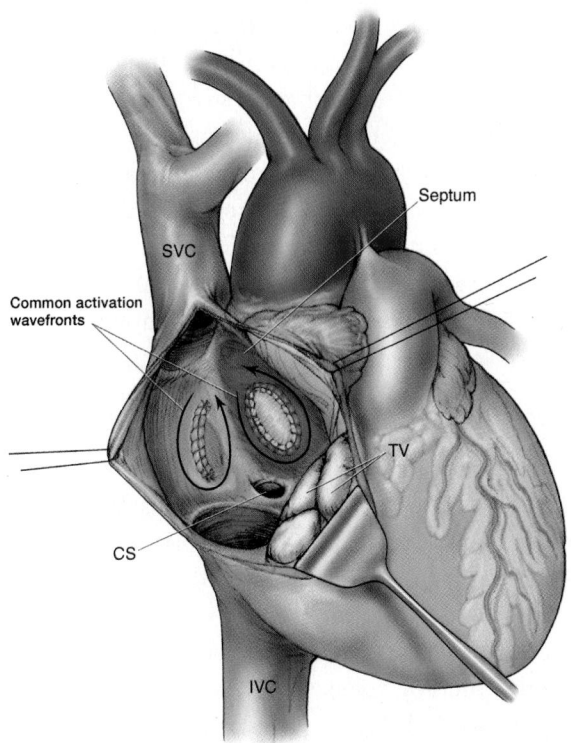

Fig. 4. Atriotomy scar and atrial septal patch. Wavefronts of activation are shown around the atriotomy and the atrial septal patches. These represent common pathways that form the substrate for reentrant atrial arrhythmias. CS, carotid sinus; IVC, inferior vena cava; SVC, superior vena cava; TV, tricuspid valve.

venosus ASD or partial or total anomalous pulmonary venous return may also result in sinus node dysfunction.

Risk factors for development of atrial arrhythmias following Mustard and Senning procedures include:

- Pulmonary hypertension.
- Right ventricular dysfunction.
- Persistent junctional rhythm.

Ventricular Arrhythmias and Tetralogy of Fallot

Ventricular tachycardia continues to be a management problem for patients who have previously undergone surgical repair of TOF. Postoperative TOF is the single most common condition associated with premature sudden cardiac death in patients with CHD.

Prior to repair, patients with TOF have a VSD which is usually severe and obstruction of the right ventricular outflow tract that leads to cyanosis. Correction of the defect involves patch closure of the VSD along with resection of a large amount of right ventricular muscle (which early on in surgical experience was performed via a ventriculotomy rather than atriotomy and retraction of the tricuspid valve) to relieve right ventricular outflow tract obstruction. A transanular patch is used to increase the size of the pulmonary valve anulus which may result in significant pulmonary regurgitation especially if significant pulmonary arterial stenosis is present. Although the precise mechanism of VT and SCD is unknown, there is a substrate for macro-reentry around the myocardial scar at the site of the right ventriculotomy or at the site of the VSD patch. Other contributing factors include chronic cyanosis and wall stress due to volume overload leading to myocardial fibrosis.

TREATMENT OF ATRIAL ARRHYTHMIAS IN PATIENTS WITH CHD

Pharmacologic Therapy

Acute

Rate control (AV nodal blocking agent) is the initial therapy in hemodynamically stable patients. However, drugs that block the AV node may not be well tolerated, especially in patients with IART, due to the relatively slow cycle length and concomitant sinus node dysfunction. Direct current cardioversion (DCCV) should be used if hemodynamic compromise is present.

ANTIARRHYTHMIC DRUG THERAPY

Vaughan Williams class I and III agents have been used to treat patients with CHD and atrial arrhythmias. However, no prospective studies have demonstrated the safety or efficacy of these agents in patients with CHD. Therefore, both class I and class III agents should be avoided in CV board scenarios. In highly symptomatic patients in whom catheter ablation is neither feasible nor desired, amiodarone may be used after consideration of risk and benefits.

CATHETER ABLATION

With development of more advanced mapping capability, the efficacy and safety of catheter ablation is increasing. Ablative therapy involves creation of nonconductive lesions based on understanding of anatomic barriers and critical circuits (isthmus) that form the circuit that sustains the arrhythmia.

Catheter ablation of typical (isthmus-dependent) atrial flutter is associated with a >95% likelihood of long-term success (defined as no recurrence of the atrial flutter) and should be considered early. One drawback of this approach is that even after successful ablation of this atrial flutter, other atrial arrhythmias such as atrial fibrillation, may supervene.

SURGICAL THERAPY OF ARRHYTHMIAS IN CHD

In general, attempts at preventing established arrhythmias by surgical revision of a conduit alone are of limited efficacy. In most cases, additional cryoablative therapy is necessary based upon knowledge of anatomical and surgically created barriers to conduction.

Modification of surgical techniques to *prevent* arrhythmias offers greater promise. These include: avoidance of the crista terminalis when performing atriotomy, creation of 'anchoring lesions' using cryoablation between surgical scar and anatomic boundaries (such as the tricuspid valve anulus or IVC/SVC) and primary performance of a lateral tunnel procedure or extracardiac repair which may be associated with a lower incidence of atrial arrhythmias.

SUDDEN CARDIAC DEATH

While annual mortality, even in "high risk" patients with CHD is low (<2%), the duration of risk exposure is extremely long given the younger age of this patient population and thus the potential for years of life saved is high. Sudden death risk increases with duration of follow-up, with greatest risk in patients more than 25 years from surgical repair.

SECONDARY PREVENTION OF SUDDEN CARDIAC DEATH

Patients who present with hemodynamically unstable ventricular tachycardia or cardiac arrest due to ventricular fibrillation, where no (*truly*) reversible cause is found should undergo ICD placement. However, such a presentation is uncommon with most sudden cardiac death events occurring in the absence of prior symptoms. Unfortunately, risk stratification of individuals with CHD is challenging since effective risk models are lacking and almost all prospective randomized data that drive clinical decision-making are extrapolated from adults with ischemic heart disease and ischemic cardiomyopathy.

EVALUATION AND RISK ASSESSMENT

Bradycardia or asystole associated with sinus or AV nodal disease or rapid conduction of atrial fibrillation or flutter over an accessory pathway (increased in the presence of multiple accessory pathways), such as in patients with Ebstein's anomaly should be excluded since these are correctable with pacemaker or catheter ablative therapy, respectively. Intra-atrial reentrant tachycardia (IART), after Mustard or Senning procedure, may present as a wide-complex tachycardia (mimicking VT) with hemodynamic symptoms and should also be excluded.

RISK MARKERS FOR SCD

Most data regarding SCD risk pertain to patients with repaired tetralogy of Fallot. Although prognosis in this population is generally excellent (~90% survival at 30 years with prevalence of around 4%) risk increases significantly beyond 25 years after repair.

Clinical
- Residual hemodynamic defect.
- Late surgical repair.
- Older age (i.e. longer follow-up).

Electrocardiographic
- QRS prolongation > 180 ms (suggesting slowed ventricular conduction).
- Nonsustained VT.
- "Dispersion" of repolarization (QT and JT dispersion).

Microvolt T-wave alternans, abnormal baroreceptor hypersensitivity and decreased heart rate variability have also been used for risk stratification but the sensitivity and specificity of these markers is unclear.

QRS Prolongation

Early lengthening of the QRS interval following repair of tetralogy of Fallot most often results from surgical injury to the right bundle branch and myocardium. "Late" broadening usually reflects progressive right ventricular dilatation.

Although quite specific, the sensitivity of this parameter is low and SCD is not uncommon in patients with normal QRS width.

Hemodynamic factors that increase risk of SCD include:

- Systemic ventricular dysfunction and/or dilation.
- Presence of a significant shunt.
- Pulmonary hypertension.
- Valve/conduit regurgitation.

Programmed Ventricular Stimulation for Risk Stratification in Patients With CHD

The utility of programmed ventricular stimulation for risk stratification in individual patients with CHD is unclear. Following repair of TOF, sustained monomorphic VT (usually arising from an anatomical circuit created between the right ventricular outflow tract patch and conal septum) is induced in up to 30% of patients who do not have documented clinical tachycardia and may not predict risk of SCD. Thus, both false positive and negative studies occur. Induction of sustained ventricular tachycardia at electrophysiologic study is however considered an independent risk factor for subsequent clinical ventricular tachycardia and sudden cardiac death.

Independent clinical predictors of inducible sustained ventricular tachycardia include:

- Age >18.
- Prior palliative surgery.

- Frequent ventricular ectopy.
- Increased cardiothoracic ratio.

CV Boards Points

In patients with repaired congenital heart disease:

- Onset of "late" arrhythmias (mostly atrial) is associated with significant morbidity.
- Patients who have stable systemic ventricular function and few symptoms and who are within 25 years of surgical repair have excellent survival and can be managed conservatively.
- Patients with "high-risk" clinical characteristics or symptoms of presyncope or syncope should undergo careful evaluation and risk-stratification (including hemodynamic and electrophysiological assessment) to determine the precise arrhythmia and risk of SCD.
- Patients with spontaneous sustained ventricular arrhythmias or high risk clinical profile and inducible VT should undergo ICD placement.

Summary

Arrhythmias in patients with CHD are summarized in Table 1.

CV board questions will most likely focus around common clinical scenarios

- In a previously stable patient with CHD who presents with clinical deterioration suspect onset of a supraventricular arrhythmia.
- Know broad treatment options and pacing indications.
- Avoid use of class I antiarrhythmic drugs because of the risk of proarrhythmia.
- Due to limited data regarding primary prevention of sudden cardiac death CV board questions on this topic are unlikely.

Table 1.   Arrhythmias in Patients With CHD

Surgery	Atrial arrhythmia*	Ventricular arrhythmia	SND	A-V block	PPM	SCD risk
Mustard/Senning	++++	++	++++	++	++	++
ASD closure	++++		++	+	+	
VSD closure		++++			+	++
Tetralogy of Fallot repair	++	+++			+	++
Fontan operation	++++	++	++	+	++	++
Aortic stenosis		+++				++

*Including atrial flutter, IART, and AF.

30

ARRHYTHMIAS DURING PREGNANCY

Peter A. Brady, MD

Arrhythmias that occur for the first time during pregnancy are uncommon and are usually due to exacerbation of a known rhythm disorder or an arrhythmic substrate (e.g., congenital heart disease). Appropriate management of the pregnant patient highlights several important issues that are frequently tested in cardiology examinations.

BASIC PRINCIPLES OF RHYTHM MANAGEMENT DURING PREGNANCY AND LACTATION

Evaluation and management of heart rhythm disorders during pregnancy and lactation are similar to those in nonpregnant patients. Special considerations for the pregnant patient include the following:

1. Heart rhythm syndromes affect both the mother and the fetus and continue throughout pregnancy, labor, and breast-feeding. Thus, the potential effect of the arrhythmia and the therapy on both maternal and fetal well-being need to be considered.
2. Pregnancy is accompanied by complex physiologic changes that alter drug efficacy and the risk of toxicity.
3. Almost all pharmacologic agents cross the placenta

and appear in breast milk, affecting the fetus and the newborn.
4. Patients with structural heart disease (most commonly congenital heart disease) represent a special population that requires coordination of care with a specialist in adult congenital heart disease.
5. In most instances, patients can be effectively evaluated noninvasively and treated conservatively.
6. Decisions about treatment of a heart rhythm disorder should be based on careful consideration of the severity of symptoms and the risks versus benefits.

PHYSIOLOGIC CHANGES DURING PREGNANCY

Physiologic changes associated with normal pregnancy include the following:

1. Increased total body water (approximately 5-8 liters) leading to a 40% increase in cardiac output beginning during the first trimester and continuing until mid pregnancy after which body water stabilizes and then begins to decline in the last week.
2. In parallel, peripheral vascular resistance decreases throughout pregnancy. Mean blood pressure

begins to decrease early in pregnancy, reaches a minimum in mid pregnancy, and returns to baseline levels at term.

For a comprehensive review of physiologic changes during pregnancy, see Chapter 80 ("Cardiac Disease in Pregnancy").

EVALUATION OF HEART RHYTHM SYMPTOMS

Accurate diagnosis and assessment of symptom severity (especially hemodynamic symptoms) is mandatory because of the potential for harm to both mother and fetus. Arrhythmias that result in hemodynamic compromise (usually in patients with structural heart disease) are of major concern—not only to the mother but also to the fetus through reduced placental blood flow—and should be evaluated and treated aggressively. Minor or minimal symptoms occurring in the patient with a normal heart should be treated conservatively. In all cases appropriate evaluation should include 1) correlation of symptoms and rhythm and 2) exclusion of structural cardiac disease.

■ Arrhythmias that result in hemodynamic compromise are of major concern.
■ Patients with minimal symptoms and a normal heart should be treated conservatively.

Electrocardiography

Normal electrocardiographic (ECG) changes that occur during pregnancy include a leftward shift in the frontal QRS axis and a small Q wave and inverted T wave in lead III, which results from a gradual shift in the position of the heart within the thorax. Although a 12-lead ECG obtained during symptoms helps in establishing a rhythm diagnosis, a "routine" 12-lead ECG (in the absence of symptoms) is helpful to exclude the following:

1. Ventricular preexcitation (short PR and delta wave)
2. Conduction system disease (bundle branch block and axis deviation, which is most common in patients with congenital heart disease and rare otherwise except in right bundle branch block)
3. Arrhythmogenic right ventricular dysplasia

associated with an epsilon wave
4. Prolongation of the QT interval

Echocardiography

Transthoracic echocardiography is useful especially in patients with hemodynamic symptoms to exclude structural heart disease, such as undiagnosed congenital or acquired cardiac defects as well as, for example, non-ischemic (peripartum) cardiomyopathy and arrhythmogenic right ventricular dysplasia.

Tilt Table Testing

Tilt table testing is generally safe during pregnancy. However, it is not frequently indicated in pregnant patients because of the apparent decrease in the frequency of neurocardiogenic syncope during pregnancy (perhaps owing to increased volume load).

Exercise Treadmill Testing

Exercise treadmill testing is generally safe to perform during early pregnancy and is most useful in patients with exertional symptoms, such as a right ventricular outflow tract tachycardia.

Ambulatory Monitoring (Holter and Event Recorder)

Ambulatory monitoring using either 24-hour or 48-hour Holter monitoring is helpful in patients who have frequent symptoms. If symptoms are less frequent an event recorder may be more appropriate.

Electrophysiologic Studies

Invasive electrophysiologic studies are rarely needed during pregnancy, and in most cases they should be avoided owing to the risks of radiation exposure to the fetus during the positioning of catheters and the use of contrast agents and heparin. If invasive electrophysiologic testing cannot be avoided, a lead apron placed under the abdominal area may reduce radiation exposure to the fetus. Alternative approaches, including using intracardiac echocardiography or electroanatomic mapping systems for guidance, may be helpful in minimizing radiation exposure if invasive testing is mandatory.

■ Risk of radiation exposure to the fetus is greatest during the first and second trimesters of pregnancy.
■ Increased exposure has been linked to congenital malformations, mental retardation and increased risk

of childhood malignancies, particularly leukemia.

DRUG THERAPY IN PREGNANCY

Risks of drug therapy for arrhythmias during pregnancy can be divided into maternal factors and fetal factors. Maternal factors include 1) alterations in absorption, distribution, and excretion of drugs (varies according to the stage of pregnancy) and 2) drug effects at the time of labor and delivery. Fetal factors include placental transfer of drugs during pregnancy and breast-feeding. In all cases, if drug therapy is initiated, the dosage should be the lowest possible effective dose, and it should be initiated only after review of all alternative drug options.

Pharmacologic Therapy of Arrhythmias During Pregnancy

Both pharmacokinetic and pharmacodynamic effects must be accounted for during pregnancy.

Pharmacokinetic Changes

Pharmacokinetic changes during pregnancy and the peripartum period are complex, leading to variable and unpredictable effects of drugs. Therefore, careful monitoring of drug dosage and effect is mandatory.

Absorption

Oral absorption of drugs, and thus bioavailability, is altered in unpredictable ways, decreasing or increasing, because of changes in gastric motility and secretion. In addition, unpredictable changes in gastric pH alter the rate and degree of absorption of drugs.

Distribution

Blood volume increases while plasma protein concentration decreases. Increased blood volume (i.e., increased volume of distribution) decreases the drug concentration in the central compartment and increases the elimination half-life, whereas decreased plasma protein concentration decreases the protein binding of medications and increases the drug effect.

Excretion

Renal blood flow is increased by 60% to 80%, which increases elimination of renally excreted drugs. Increased progesterone levels increase the hepatic clearance of hepatically metabolized drugs, decreasing the drug levels.

Effects on the Fetus

During the first 8 weeks after fertilization, the teratogenic risk is greatest. After that time, the risk decreases significantly.

Drug Safety During Pregnancy

Most drugs used in the treatment of heart rhythm disorders are classified in category C by the Food and Drug Administration (FDA) (Tables 1 and 2). For drugs in this category, risk cannot be ruled out. The drugs must be used with caution during pregnancy because data from adequate, well-controlled human studies are lacking and either animal studies have shown a risk to the fetus or data are lacking. Although the drug may harm the fetus, the potential benefits may outweigh the potential risks.

General Principles of Drug Therapy for Arrhythmias During Pregnancy

1. No drug is completely safe during pregnancy, although many are well tolerated with low risk.
2. Avoid drug therapy (unless absolutely necessary) in the first trimester.
3. Conservative treatment should always be used first when feasible.

SPECIFIC DRUGS

Atrioventricular Node Blocking Agents

Adenosine

Because of its rapid onset and short duration of action, adenosine appears to be safe for use during pregnancy, although it is a category C drug. On the basis of limited data, adenosine appears to have no direct effect on the fetus after bolus intravenous administration.

Verapamil

Verapamil is rapidly absorbed, but first pass metabolism is high, with only a small proportion of the drug excreted unchanged in the urine; 90% of the drug is bound to plasma proteins. Verapamil crosses the placenta and affects the fetal cardiovascular system, but there are no reports of congenital defects associated with its use.

Diltiazem

Diltiazem is newer than verapamil, so there has been

Table 1. Food and Drug Administration Classification of Drugs for Use During Pregnancy

Category	Interpretation
A	Adequate, well-controlled studies in pregnant women have failed to demonstrate a risk to the mother or fetus in any trimester
B	Adequate, well-controlled studies in pregnant women have not shown increased risk of fetal abnormalities despite adverse findings in animals, or in the absence of adequate human studies, animal studies show no fetal risk; the chance of fetal harm is remote but remains a possibility
C	Risk cannot be ruled out: Adequate, well-controlled human studies are lacking, and animal studies have shown a risk to the fetus or are lacking; fetal harm is possible if the drug is administerred during pregnancy, but the potential benefits may outweigh the risk
D	Positive evidence of risk: Studies in humans or investigational or post-marketing data have demonstrated fetal risk; however, the benefit may outweigh the potential risk (e.g., use of the drug may be acceptable in a life-threatening situation or serious disease for which safer drugs cannot be used or are ineffective)
X	Contraindicated in pregnancy: Studies in animals or humans or investigational or postmarketing reports have demonstrated clear evidence of fetal abnormalities or risk that outweighs possible benefit

less historical experience with use of diltiazem during pregnancy. Available data suggest that diltiazem is probably safe to use for rate control since it has been used in the treatment of premature labor without a report of congenital anomalies.

Digoxin

Digoxin is classified an FDA category C drug, but it is probably safe to use during pregnancy. It crosses the placenta readily; within 30 minutes, fetal plasma concentrations are similar to maternal values. Elimination is predominantly renal. Cardiac glycosides have a long history of use in pregnant patients and are frequently used in the management of supraventricular arrhythmias.

■ Adenosine, verapamil, diltiazem, and digoxin are probably safe to use during pregnancy.

β-Blockers

Like digoxin, β-blockers (in particular, propranolol) have been used extensively in pregnancy (Table 3). Adverse outcomes with β-blockers include fetal bradycardia, hypotonia, apnea, and hypoglycemia. No studies implicate β-blockers in fetal malformation.

Acebutolol and pindolol have recently been reclassified by the FDA as category B drugs and are therefore preferred as first-line agents. However, atenolol has recently been reclassified as category D, meaning that there is positive evidence of risk.

■ Avoid use of atenolol.
■ The best choices for β-blocker therapy are acebutolol (which is in category B and is cardioselective) and propranolol (which has a long history of safe use in pregnancy).

Vaughn Williams Class Drugs

Class 1A

Quinidine

Quinidine readily crosses the placenta and has been used to terminate fetal arrhythmias. It is generally considered safe, but fetal thrombocytopenia and cranial nerve VIII palsy have been reported.

■ Given the long history and safe use of quinidine in

Table 2. Antiarrhythmic Drugs During Pregnancy

Antiarrhythmic agent	Vaughan Williams classification	FDA category	Safety during lactation
Disopyramide	1A	C	S
Procainamide	1A	C	S
Quinidine	1A	C	S
Lidocaine	1B	B	S
Mexiletine	1B	C	S
Flecainide	1C	C	S
Moricizine	1C	B	?
Propafenone	1C	C	?
Amiodarone	3	D	NS
Azimilide	3	?	?
Dofetilide	3	?	?
Ebutilide	3	C	?
Sotalol	3	B	S
Adenosine	--	C	?
Verapamil	4	C	S
Diltiazem	4	C	S

FDA, Food and Drug Administration; NS, not safe; S, safe; ?, unknown.

pregnancy, it is the drug of choice among class 1A drugs.

Procainamide
Procainamide readily crosses the placenta and is also used to treat fetal arrhythmias. No adverse fetal outcomes have been reported.

Disopyramide
Disopyramide may cause uterine contractions; therefore, it is not desirable for use in the later stages of pregnancy.

Class 1C
Both flecainide and propafenone cross the placenta, yielding high drug levels in the fetal circulation. Although classified in category C, they have no reported teratogenic effects. Available data suggest that

flecainide is safe during pregnancy; therefore, it is a reasonable choice for treatment of atrial arrhythmias in patients without structural heart disease.

Class 3

Sotalol
There are reports of the use of sotalol in pregnant patients without adverse effects. Classified in category B, sotalol is therefore a good alternative to class 1 agents.

Amiodarone
Use of amiodarone should be avoided, even for a short duration, during pregnancy. Amiodarone has been associated with several problems involving the fetus, including the following:

Table 3. β-Blocker Therpay During Pregnancy

β-Blocker	FDA category	Safety during lactation	Cardioselectivity
Acebutolol	B	S	+
Atenolol	D	S	+
Bisoprolol	C	?	+
Esmolol	C	?	+
Inderal	C	S	−
Labetalol	C	S	−
Lopressor	C	S	+
Metoprolol	C	S	+
Nadolol	C	S	−
Pindolol	B	?	−
Propranolol	C	S	−
Timolol	C	S	−

FDA, Food and Drug Administration; S, safe; ?, unknown.

1. Bradycardia
2. Hypothyroidism
3. Congenital malformation
4. Premature labor
5. Death

ANTICOAGULATION IN PREGNANCY

Warfarin is a category X drug, which means that it is contraindicated in pregnancy since it crosses the placental barrier. Potential adverse effects include spontaneous abortion, fetal hemorrhage, mental retardation, and birth malformations. Table 4 lists advantages and disadvantages of anticoagulation therapy in pregnancy. See Chapter 80 ("Cardiac Disease in Pregnancy") for a full discussion of anticoagulation during pregnancy.

MANAGEMENT OF SPECIFIC ARRHYTHMIAS

Arrhythmias in the Normal Heart

Palpitations

Pregnancy is associated with an increase in "background" ectopic atrial and ventricular activity (most likely due to volume and hormonal changes) that may present as "palpitations." In patients with a structurally normal heart, these rhythm disorders are usually benign and well tolerated; appropriate management includes reassurance and avoidance of any identified triggers. Drug or invasive therapy should be avoided unless hemodynamic instability or intolerable symptoms occur.

Supraventricular Tachycardia

Occasionally episodes of previously diagnosed paroxysmal supraventricular tachycardia and atrial tachycardia increase in frequency and become more symptomatic during pregnancy. Although the precise mechanism for this is unclear, it probably relates to increased ectopy (secondary to volume, hormonal changes, etc.) causing more frequent initiation of sustained tachycardia.

In patients with structurally normal hearts, atrioventricular reentrant (Wolff-Parkinson-White syndrome and variants) and atrioventricular nodal reentrant tachycardia are the most common sustained arrhythmias. Atrial tachycardia and atrial fibrillation are less common. The risk of paroxysmal supraventricular tachycardia is equally distributed throughout pregnancy regardless of the mechanism; management strategies are shown in Figure 1.

Table 4. Anticoagulant Therapy During Pregnancy

Anticoagulant	Advantages	Disadvantages
Heparin	Does not cross placenta	Must be administered parenterally
	Easily and rapidly reversed	Bleeding risk to mother
	Short half-life	Maternal osteopenia and thrombocytopenia
		Risk of maternal valve thrombosis
		Systemic infection
Warfarin	Most effective for preventing thromboembolic events	Crosses the placenta
		Not easily reversed
		Teratogenic in first trimester
		Risk of hemorrhage during labor and delivery

Because of the increased frequency of arrhythmias during pregnancy and the problems with management, females with prior symptoms who are planning on pregnancy should be counseled about the benefit of definitive therapy (such as catheter ablation) before becoming pregnant.

Arrhythmias in Patients With Structural Heart Disease

In patients who have had congenital heart disease repaired, the most common arrhythmias are atrial tachyarrhythmias, such as atrial tachycardia, atrial flutter, and atrial fibrillation. Similar principles apply in management of these arrhythmias as in patients who are not pregnant. However, atrial arrhythmias are not dependent on the atrioventricular node, and therefore vagal maneuvers and adenosine are rarely effective. Risk factors for stroke in atrial fibrillation are the same as those in nonpregnant patients, although the risk may be increased in pregnancy. In all cases of refractory supraventricular tachycardia or hemodynamic instability, electrical cardioversion may be required (Fig. 1).

■ In patients with repaired congenital heart disease, narrow complex tachycardia is most likely due to atrial tachyarrhythmias, such as atrial tachycardia, atrial flutter, and atrial fibrillation.

Long-term management of arrhythmias is similar

to that for the nonpregnant patient. In pregnant patients without heart disease, β-blockers are a reasonable choice for initial therapy if symptoms warrant. Antiarrhythmic drugs that may be used with reasonable safety for refractory symptoms include flecainide, quinidine, procainamide, and sotalol.

Ventricular Tachycardia

Causes of ventricular tachycardia during pregnancy include arrhythmogenic right ventricular dysplasia, long QT syndrome, hypertrophic cardiomyopathy, peripartum cardiomyopathy, anomalous coronary artery and, rarely, coronary artery disease. In the absence of congenital heart disease and normal right and left ventricular function, the risk of ventricular tachycardia during pregnancy is low. In the presence of hemodynamically unstable ventricular tachycardia, immediate direct current cardioversion is appropriate. Intravenous antiarrhythmic drugs may also be used. For the pregnant patient, lidocaine is the drug of choice if an antiarrhythmic drug is considered. Most drugs used for the treatment of ventricular tachycardia are in FDA category C. Exceptions include atenolol and amiodarone which are in category D, and sotalol and lidocaine, which are in category B. Overall, procainamide and flecainide have been used in pregnancy with good effect and without adverse outcomes during long-term use. Since sotalol is now classified in

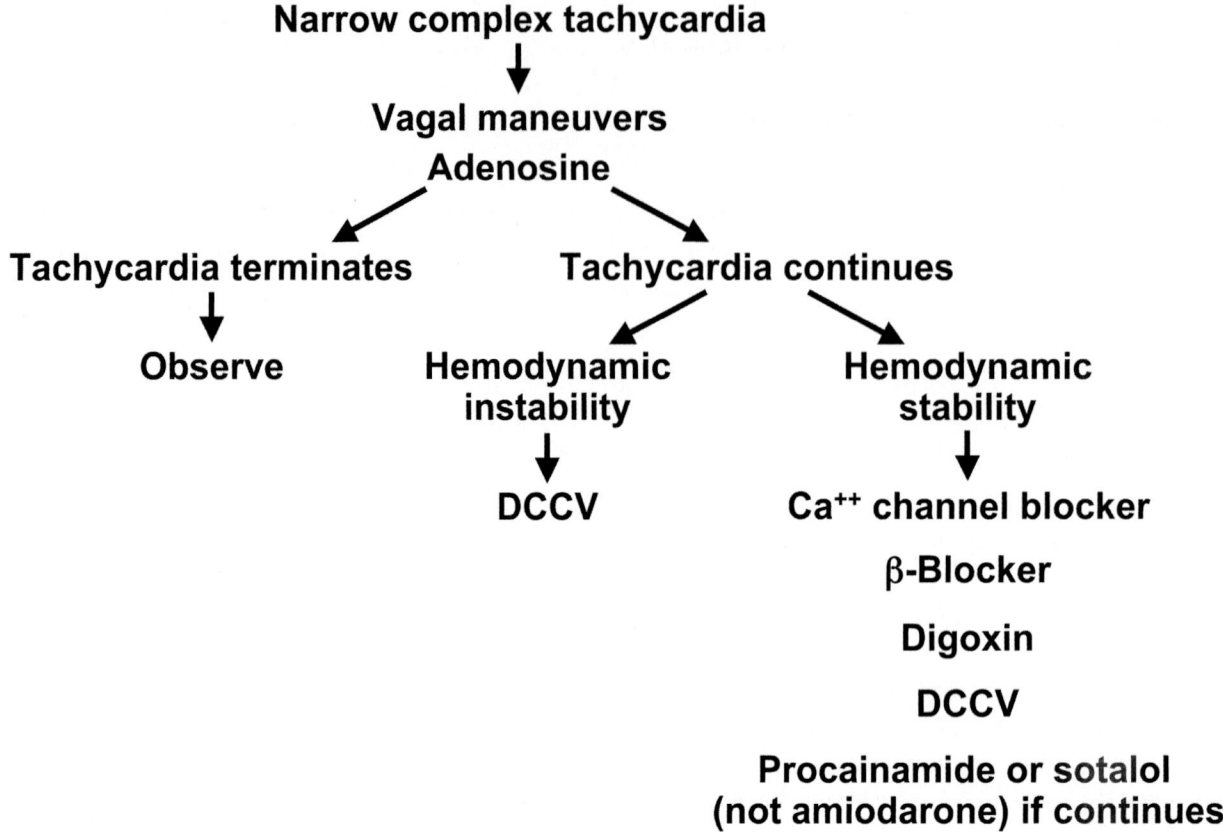

Fig. 1. Management of supraventricular tachycardia in pregnancy. DCCV, direct current cardioversion.

FDA category B, it may be a good choice for patients with normal renal function.

Bradycardia During Pregnancy

Congenital Complete Heart Block
Although most cases of congenital heart block are diagnosed during childhood, many are discovered incidentally during pregnancy. In patients who are asymptomatic, acute intervention is not required during pregnancy. For patients who are symptomatic in the first or second trimesters, no definite guidelines exist, but permanent pacemaker implantation is probably indicated, with avoidance of fluoroscopy if possible. For symptomatic patients who present at or near term, temporary pacing with induction of labor may be the procedure of choice.

Syncope During Pregnancy
Neurocardiogenic mechanisms are the most common cause of syncope in the younger nonpregnant female,

accounting for more than 20% of unexplained cases of syncope in women of childbearing age. Vasovagal syncope, however, is much less common during pregnancy (perhaps owing to increased volume load); therefore, evaluation of syncope in the pregnant female should focus on excluding other causes.

Cardiac Arrest
Cardiac arrest is rare in women of childbearing age, occurring in approximately 1 in 30,000 deliveries. Causes of cardiac arrest during pregnancy include the following:

1. Postpartum hemorrhage
2. Pulmonary/amniotic fluid embolism
3. Eclampsia
4. Anaphylaxis or drug toxicity
5. Peripartum cardiomyopathy
6. Aortic dissection

In general terms, advanced cardiac life support standard

guidelines apply for medications, intubation, and defibrillation except that amiodarone should be avoided because of the risk of adverse fetal effects. Lidocaine or procainamide should be substituted.

Special Issues in Resuscitation of the Pregnant Female

Until the fetus becomes viable, at approximately 25 weeks, resuscitation should be performed as in the nonpregnant patient. One problem with resuscitation during late-term pregnancy is aortocaval obstruction due to the gravid uterus that may reduce venous return and forward flow during chest compressions. Venous return may be facilitated by performing cardiopulmonary resuscitation with the patient tilted on her side or in the semirecumbent position. In addition, chest compressions should usually be performed higher on the chest to accommodate the shift of pelvic and abdominal contents toward the head.

After 25 weeks, if resuscitation is prolonged (>5 minutes) emergency cesarean section should be considered in order to save the fetus. In most cases, external defibrillation (up to 300 J) can be performed without significantly affecting the fetus, with a low risk of inducing fetal arrhythmias.

Patients With Previously Implanted Cardioverter-Defibrillator

Pregnancy in patients with a previously implanted cardioverter-defibrillator (ICD) is safe and should not be considered a contraindication. Pregnancy does not appear to increase the risk of ICD-related complications or result in increased ICD discharges.

Pregnancy and Long QT Syndrome

Risk of significant cardiac events in patients with congenital long QT syndrome is not increased during pregnancy. However, risk is increased in the postpartum period. Thus, syncope in the postpartum period should be evaluated very carefully to exclude a cardiogenic mechanism. In patients at higher risk, prolonged hospitalization or (rarely) consideration of ICD implantation during pregnancy may be necessary.

Hypertrophic Cardiomyopathy

Owing to the hemodynamic changes that occur during pregnancy, patients with hypertrophic cardiomyopathy usually experience symptomatic improvement during pregnancy. However, maternal and fetal deaths due to ventricular arrhythmias in patients with hypertrophic cardiomyopathy have been reported during pregnancy. One contributor may be aortocaval compression, particularly toward the end of pregnancy. It reduces venous return (and is exacerbated by blood loss during delivery), which can dramatically decrease preload and lead to hemodynamic collapse and difficulties in adequate resuscitation.

Labor and Delivery

Immediately after delivery, cardiac output increases but then declines, reaching a baseline level 2 weeks post partum. Supraventricular arrhythmias occurring in the peripartum period can be managed as for the nonpregnant patient. Adenosine is safe to use.

Lactation and Breast-feeding

Considerations for drug therapy, including antiarrhythmic drugs, during breast-feeding are similar to those during pregnancy. Most antiarrhythmic drugs and atrioventricular node–blocking agents are excreted in breast milk; thus, continued use while breast-feeding must be considered case by case. Warfarin and heparin are safe for use in nursing mothers.

SUMMARY

- In most cases, arrhythmias during pregnancy can be safely managed conservatively or with minimal medical therapy. Although a correct diagnosis is important with any patient, it is vital during pregnancy because of the risk of harm to the mother and the fetus.
- If an antiarrhythmic drug is needed, medications with a long history of use during pregnancy should be chosen.
- In all therapeutic considerations, use the least number of medications at the lowest effective dose.
- Cardioversion is safe during pregnancy and should be used as an early treatment option in arrhythmia management, particularly if hemodynamic compromise is present.

31

HERITABLE CARDIOMYOPATHIES

Shaji C. Menon, MD

Steve R. Ommen, MD

Michael J. Ackerman, MD, PhD

Cardiomyopathies are primarily the diseases of myocardium associated with cardiac dysfunction. According to the World Health Organization classification, cardiomyopathies can be classified as either primary or secondary. Heritable cardiomyopathies are primary myocardial diseases caused by inherited gene defects. Causes of secondary cardiomyopathies are diverse and include ischemia, infection, toxins, metabolic syndromes, arrhythmias, and congenital malformations associated with pressure or volume overload. Improvement in outcomes and prevention of coronary artery disease has led to the emergence of a new epidemic, the heart failure epidemic. Heart failure affects 4.5 million patients in the United States and is responsible for 300,000 deaths annually. Heritable cardiomyopathies constitute a substantial number of these cases. During the past decade, advances in molecular genetics have provided better insight into the molecular pathophysiology and genetic basis for heritable cardiomyopathies.

On the basis of morphologic and functional criteria, heritable cardiomyopathies are classified into four primary categories: hypertrophic cardiomyopathy (HCM), dilated cardiomyopathy (DCM), arrhythmogenic right ventricular cardiomyopathy (ARVC), and restrictive cardiomyopathy (RCM). Recently, left ventricular noncompaction (LVNC) syndrome was added as a category.

In developed countries such as the United States, sudden cardiac death (SCD) causes more deaths than any other medical condition. More than 300,000 SCDs occur each year in the United States. The majority of these SCDs stem from coronary artery disease in the elderly, and heritable cardiomyopathies such as HCM and ARVC are responsible for a substantial proportion of SCDs in the young. HCM is the most common cause of SCDs occurring on the athletic field, and ARVC is the most common cause of SCD in the young in Italy.

This chapter reviews the current understanding of molecular pathogenic mechanisms, molecular diagnostic and genetic testing, and the electrocardiographic/arrhythmic phenotype associated with these cardiomyopathies, and particular attention is given to risk stratification for and prevention and treatment of SCD.

GENERAL MECHANISM OF ARRHYTHMIA IN CARDIOMYOPATHIES

Histopathologically, cardiomyopathies are characterized by changes in myocardium consisting of areas of fibrosis, disruption of cellular architecture, and hypertrophied or dysplastic myocytes. These changes may create a non-homogeneous and unstable, proarrhythmic electrical milieu. The various mechanisms of arrhythmias in cardiomyopathies include the following:

1. Reentrant tachycardias—Localized areas of scarring, fibrosis, and unhealthy myocardium lead to conduction delay or block and substrate for reentry tachycardia.
2. Focal automaticity—Focal automaticity, as occurs in patients with DCM, may be responsible for monomorphic ventricular tachycardia. In ventricular dysrhythmias, it refers to an accelerated discharge rate of the His-Purkinje system.
3. Supraventricular arrhythmias—Patients with atrial enlargement due to valvular abnormality or abnormal loading conditions are prone to supraventricular arrhythmias, especially atrial fibrillation. In some patients, supraventricular tachyarrhythmias can trigger ventricular tachyarrhythmias.
4. Bradyarrhythmias—Sick sinus syndrome and bradyarrhythmias may occur in some of these patients.
5. Others causes—Associated conditions such as electrolyte imbalance due to diuretic treatment, prolongation of the QT interval, and proarrhythmia properties of antiarrhythmic drugs may precipitate arrhythmias.

SCD Substrates

There is no single electrocardiographic test, clinical marker, or biomarker for risk stratification and identification of SCD substrate. The presence of multiple risk factors is more specific. Various proposed tests and variables for recognition of substrates for SCD include electrophysiologic study, signal-averaged electrocardiography, microvolt T-wave alternans, QT dispersion, ejection fraction, nonsustained ventricular tachycardia, number of ventricular premature beats, heart rate variability, baroreceptor sensitivity, echocardiographic assessment of hypertrophy, and scoring of delayed myocardial enhancement (fibrosis) by cardiac magnetic resonance imaging. These tests and the clinical history should be repeated periodically to restratify risk as the disease progresses.

Hypertrophic Cardiomopathy

Definition of HCM

Hypertrophic cardiomyopathy (HCM) is a primary disorder of myocardium associated with an increase in cardiac mass and, typically, asymmetric but diffuse or segmental left (and right) ventricular hypertrophy. HCM is a complex disease with protean morphologic, functional, and clinical features affecting approximately 1 in 500 persons. On a genetic level, HCM is a heterogeneous disease with at least 21 HCM-susceptibility genes, permitting a genomics-based classification of HCM into myofilament HCM, Z-disc HCM, energetic or storage disease (metabolic) HCM, and mitochondrial HCM.

Nomenclature for HCM

HCM is known by confusing nomenclature such as hypertrophic obstructive cardiomyopathy and idiopathic hypertrophic subaortic stenosis. HCM is the preferred term because left ventricular outflow obstruction is not a prerequisite for the disease process.

Pathology of HCM

Histopathologic characteristics of HCM are unexplained, markedly enlarged, and bizarre-shaped myocytes, myocyte disorientation (myofibrillar disarray), and premature death of hypertrophic muscle cells and replacement with fibroblasts and extracellular matrix (replacement fibrosis). The areas of myocyte disarray vary from focal to extensive involvement of myocardium.

Molecular Basis of HCM

HCM is generally considered a disease of the sarcomere. HCM usually occurs with an autosomal dominant mode of inheritance, although autosomal recessive forms and spontaneous germline mutations have been identified (Table 1). A familial history of HCM is present in 33% to 50% of all index cases. The first gene (*MYH7*-encoded β-myosin heavy chain) for familial HCM was mapped to chromosome 14q11.2-q12 with genome-wide linkage analysis in a large Canadian family in 1989. Subsequently, mutations in genes encoding proteins composing the cardiac sarcomere, particularly the myofilaments and Z-disc architecture, were discovered. Hundreds of HCM-associated mutations (mostly missense mutations) scattered among at least 21 genes

Table 1. Summary of Hypertrophic Cardiomyopathy Susceptibility Genes

Subtype	Gene	Locus	Protein	Frequency, %
Myofilament HCM				
Giant filament	TTN	2q24.3	Titin	<1
Thick filament	MYH7	14q11.2-q12	β-Myosin heavy chain	15-25
	MYH6	14q11.2-q12	α-Myosin heavy chain	<1
	MYL2	12q23-q24.3	Ventricular regulatory myosin light chain	<2
	MYL3	3p21.2-p21.3	Ventricular essential myosin light chain	<1
Intermediate filament	MYBPC3	11p11.2	Cardiac myosin-binding protein C	15-25
Thin filament	TNNT2	1q32	Cardiac troponin T	<5
	TNN13	19p13.4	Cardiac troponin I	<5
	TPM1	15q22.1	α-Tropomyosin	<5
	ACTC	15q14	α-Cardiac actin	<1
Z-disc HCM				
	CSRP3	11p15.1	Muscle LIM protein	<1
	TCAP	17q12-q21.1	Telethonin	<1
	VCL	10q22.1-q23	Vinculin/metavinculin	<1
	ZASP, LBD3	10q22.2-q23.3	Z-band alternatively spliced PDZ-motif protein/LIM binding domain 3	1-5
	ACTN2	1q42-q43	α-actinin 2	<1
Calcium-handling HCM				
	RYR2	1q42.1-q43	Cardiac ryanodine receptor	<1
	JPH2	20q12	Junctophilin 2	<1
Storage disease HCM				
	PRKAG2	7q35-q3636	AMP-activated protein kinase	<1
	LAMP2	Xq24	Lysosome-associated membrane protein 2	<1
	GLA	Xq22	α-Galactosidase A	<1
Mitochondrial HCM				
	FRDA	9q13	Frataxin	<1

AMP, adenosine monophosphate; HCM, hypertrophic cardiomyopathy.

have been identified. The three most common genes are *MYH7* (15%-25% of all HCM cases), MYBPC3 (15%-25%), and TNNT2 (<5%). In a Mayo Clinic series derived from the largest reported cohort of unrelated patients with HCM, the overall yield was nearly 40%, MYBPC3 and MYH7 HCM being the leading genetic subtypes.

Role of Genetic Testing in HCM
Initial genotype-phenotype correlative studies suggested

the possibility of specific genotype-phenotype correlations, particularly specific mutations being associated with a malignant or benign natural history and SCD risk. However, subsequent studies suggested that HCM-associated mutations are not inherently good or bad, benign or malignant. Each HCM-associated mutation provides the fundamental pathogenetic substrate, but the degree of penetrance and expressivity varies based on gene modifiers, epigenetic factors, and environmental triggers. It is difficult to establish a prognosis on the basis of the genetic mutation. A decision to place an implantable cardioverter-defibrillator (ICD) should not be based on a patient's HCM-causing mutation.

Clinical genetic testing for HCM is now commercially available through Harvard Medical School-Partners Healthcare Center for Genetics and Genomics. The eight myofilament gene panel (panel A and panel B) is responsible for the majority of genetically identifiable HCM. The yield of genetic testing ranges from 30% to 70%, depending on the series. The overall yield associated with this genetic test was nearly 40% in the Mayo Clinic HCM cohort. However, the yield was markedly dependent on the underlying septal morphologic subtype, ranging from 8% for sigmoidal contour HCM to nearly 80% for reverse septal curvature HCM (Fig. 1). These two anatomical morphologic subtypes represent the two most common clinical subsets of HCM, suggesting a role for echocardiography-guided genetic testing.

Genetic testing will play a key role in screening for and identification of at-risk family members, even with preclinical HCM, and in guiding proper surveillance of those harboring an HCM-predisposing genetic substrate. In the future, predisease interventions with antifibrotic and myocardial remodeling agents such as aldactone, angiotensin-converting enzyme inhibitors, angiotensin receptor blockers, calcium channel blockers, or hydroxymethylglutaryl coenzyme A inhibitors may favorably alter the natural history of HCM.

Clinical Presentation of HCM

HCM is one of the most common causes of SCD in people younger than 30 years and is the most common cause of sudden death in athletes. Clinical presentation is underscored by extreme variability from an asymptomatic course to that of severe heart failure, arrhythmias, and premature and sudden cardiac death. Many patients are asymptomatic or only mildly symptomatic.

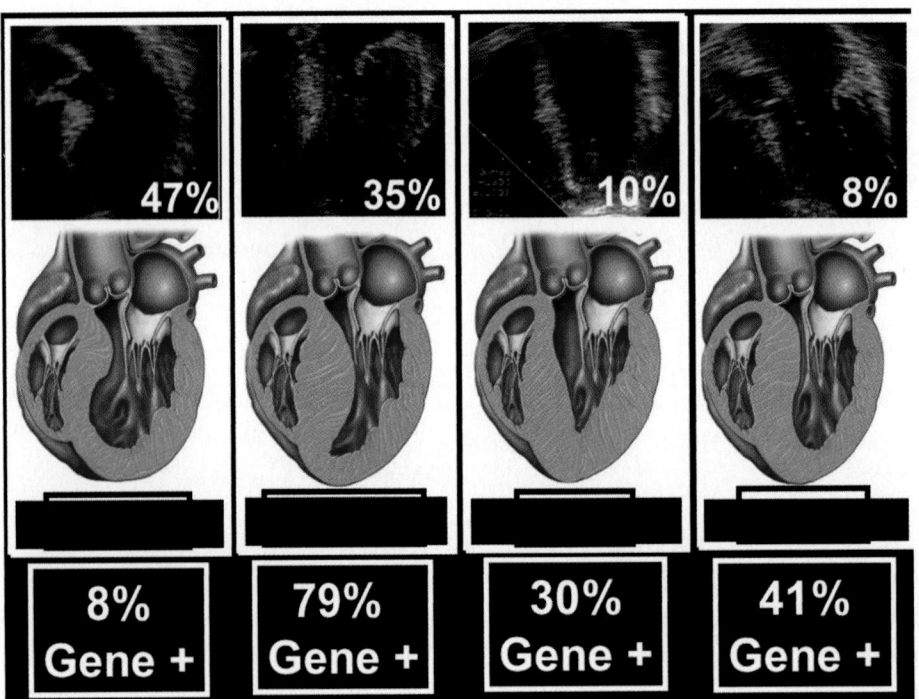

Fig. 1. Hypertrophic cardiomyopathy (HCM) septal morphologic subtypes and yield of myofilament (panel A and panel B) genetic testing. The morphologic subtype classifications (left to right) are sigmoid, reverse curve, apical, and neutral contour HCM on the basis of standard echocardiography long-axis views obtained at end-diastole. The percentage in each echocardiographic still frame indicates the relative frequency of that particular morphologic subtype at Mayo Clinic. The percentage at the bottom of each panel indicates the yield of the commercially available genetic test for each morphologic subtype of HCM. Gene, presence of myofilament mutation (positive panel A and B test).

HCM commonly manifests between the second and fourth decades of life but can present at the extremes of age. Rarely, infants and young children present with heart failure, and these patients have a poor prognosis. SCD can be the tragic sentinel event for HCM in children, adolescents, and young adults. Symptomatic patients may present with exertional dyspnea, chest pain, and syncope or presyncope. Progression to end stage disease with systolic dysfunction and heart failure occurs later in life. Five percent of patients with nonobstructive HCM have progression to left ventricular dilatation and heart failure necessitating cardiac transplantation. Other serious life-threatening complications include embolic stroke and arrhythmias. The general management of HCM is discussed in detail in the chapter on HCM.

Electrocardiographic Findings in HCM
The 12-lead electrocardiogram is abnormal in 75% to 95% of patients who have HCM. The results in HCM are nonspecific and do not predict clinical status, magnitude of hypertrophy, and degree of left ventricular outflow tract obstruction. In adults, a weak correlation can be shown between electrocardiographic voltages and the magnitude of left ventricular hypertrophy that is determined on echocardiography. Family members identified from pedigree screening and patients with localized hypertrophy usually have normal electrocardiographic results. Electrocardiography may show non-specific ST- and T-wave changes, abnormal Q waves, left ventricular hypertrophy, and, in a few patients, right ventricular hypertrophy. QT dispersion and prolongation of the QT interval may be found.

Arrhythmias in HCM
Ventricular arrhythmias are an important clinical feature in adults with HCM. On routine ambulatory (Holter) 24-hour electrocardiographic monitoring, 90% of adults have ventricular arrhythmias. These are often frequent or complex, including premature ventricular depolarizations (≥200 in 20% of patients), ventricular couplets (>40%), and nonsustained bursts of ventricular tachycardia (in 20%-30%). Older patients with chronic high left ventricular end-diastolic pressures and diastolic dysfunction are prone to chronic sustained atrial fibrillation due to dilating left atrium. Young patients with considerable outflow tract obstruction and dilated

left atrium also have a higher propensity for development of paroxysmal atrial fibrillation. Ultimately, paroxysmal episodes or chronic atrial fibrillation occurs in 20% to 25% of patients who have HCM, and these conditions are linked with left atrial enlargement and increasing age.

Atrial fibrillation in HCM is associated with progressive heart failure and embolic events. Because of the increased risk of systemic thromboembolization, the threshold for initiation of anticoagulant therapy should be low and can include patients who have had one or two episodes of paroxysmal atrial fibrillation. Warfarin is the anticoagulant of choice. In some patients, supraventricular tachyarrhythmias could trigger ventricular arrhythmias. Currently, there is insufficient evidence linking atrial fibrillation to SCD. Nevertheless, atrial fibrillation is independently associated with heart failure-related death and the occurrence of fatal and nonfatal stroke. There is no consensus on the various methods for treatment of atrial fibrillation, such as radiofrequency ablation, the surgical maze procedure, or implantable atrial defibrillators. Other arrhythmias include Wolff-Parkinson-White syndrome, supraventricular tachycardia, atrioventricular block, and sinus bradycardia. Some patients with bradyarrhythmias may require backup pacing.

Risk Stratification of SCD and ICD Therapy in HCM
HCM causes more than half of all cases of SCD in persons younger than 25 years. Overall, the annual mortality rate is less than 1%, but reaches 6% to 8% per year for the highest risk subset. Of the total population with HCM, only a small proportion have high-risk HCM. SCD is more frequent in adolescents and young adults (<35 years old) and could be the first presenting symptom. The ICD plays an important role in primary and secondary prevention of the arrhythmias. In many young patients, ICD use prolongs life substantially and could offer a near normal life expectancy. In a multicenter study of ICD use in patients with HCM, the device intervened appropriately at a rate of 5% per year for primary prevention and 11% per year for secondary prevention during an average follow-up of 3 years.

No single clinical, morphologic, genetic, or electrophysiologic factor has emerged as the single reliable predictor of risk in HCM. SCD risk stratification based on the genetic substrate must be made cautiously. A decision to intervene with an ICD should not be based on the HCM-causing mutation. There is general consensus that the patients at highest risk of SCD are those with 1) a prior history of cardiac arrest or aborted sudden death; 2) spontaneous ventricular tachycardia and sustained or unsustained ventricular tachycardia on ambulatory monitoring; 3) a family history of HCM-related sudden death involving at least two relatives younger than 45 years; 4) severe left ventricular hypertrophy (wall thickness ≥30 mm); 5) unexplained syncope, especially in young patients with exertion, or recurrent syncope; 6) an abnormal blood pressure response with exercise testing (higher specificity in patients younger than 50 years) and hypotension; and 7) increased delayed enhancement on cardiac gadolinium-enhanced magnetic resonance imaging. Minor risk factors associated with an increased risk of SCD include the presence of atrial fibrillation, myocardial ischemia, and left ventricular outflow tract obstruction and intense physical activity.

In general, secondary prevention ICD therapy is indicated for all patients with a history of aborted cardiac arrest. Primary prevention ICD therapy is generally advised if two major risk factors are present. In such cases, the relative risk for SCD is twofold more than the annual mortality rate attributed to HCM. Debate continues as to whether ICDs are indicated if only a single major risk factor is present. In addition, a single sudden death is most often considered indicative of a positive family history despite the published risk factor requiring at least two deaths.

Treatment of HCM

The pharmacologic, interventional, and surgical management of HCM is detailed in the chapter on HCM.

Follow-up and Sports Participation in HCM

Intense physical exertion potentially can trigger SCD in persons with HCM. According to the 36th Bethesda Conference (2005) recommendations, athletes with HCM should be excluded from participation in contact sports and most organized competitive sports, with the possible exception of low-intensity sports (class IA, golf, bowling, cricket, billiards, and riflery). According to the guidelines, the presence of an ICD does not alter these recommendations. This restrictive approach is loosened for patients with genotype-positive but phenotype-negative (including normal diastolic

function) HCM. All patients with HCM should undergo, on an annual basis, recording of a careful personal and family history, two-dimensional echocardiography, 12-lead electrocardiography, 24 to 48 hour ambulatory Holter electrocardiography, and exercise stress testing (for evaluation of exercise tolerance, blood pressure, and ventricular tachyarrhythmias). Peak oxygen consumption during exercise should be evaluated, as even asymptomatic patients with HCM have a decrease in oxygen consumption compared with normal patients.

Family Screening in HCM

All first- and second-degree relatives of an index case of HCM should be screened with electrocardiography and echocardiography. Annual screening is recommended for young adults (age 12-25 years) and athletes and thereafter every 5 years. If the HCM-causing mutation is known, first-degree relatives should have confirmatory genetic testing in addition to the screening electrocardiography and echocardiography. Depending on the established familial or sporadic pattern, confirmatory genetic testing should proceed in concentric circles of relatedness. For example, if the HCM-associated mutation is established in the patient's father, then the patient's paternal grandparents should be tested and, if necessary, then the paternal aunts and uncles and so forth.

DILATED CARDIOMYOPATHY

Definition of DCM

Idiopathic DCM is a heterogeneous group of primary heart muscle diseases characterized by biventricular dilatation and systolic dysfunction in the absence of any other identifiable cause. The ultimate prognosis is generally poor, heart failure being the final outcome in the end stages of the disease.

Epidemiology of DCM

DCM is a prevalent cardiomyopathy, affecting 36.5 per 100,000 persons in the United States. The mortality rate in patients with symptomatic DCM is 25% at 1 year and 50% at 5 years. Initially, most patients are asymptomatic or minimally symptomatic for years. At least 80% of gene carriers younger than 20 years are asymptomatic. With careful evaluation and echocardiographic screening, 20% to 35% of patients with DCM seem to have familial DCM.

Molecular Basis and Pathogenesis of DCM

Familial DCM is mostly inherited as an autosomal dominant trait (90%). X-linked DCM accounts for 5% to 10% of cases. A single autosomal recessive mutation involving cardiac troponin I has been reported. To date, more than 22 DCM susceptibility genes and 4 additional chromosomal loci have been implicated in the pathogenesis of DCM (Table 2). Unlike HCM, in which myosin-binding protein C and β-myosin heavy chain mutations are relatively common, none of the DCM-associated genes seem to contribute to more than 5% of cases. Penetrance in DCM is highly variable. In a single family, the presentation can vary from no symptoms to mild arrhythmia to SCD and severe heart failure and cardiac transplantation.

Role of Genetic Testing in DCM

Currently, there is no clinically available genetic test for DCM. Even in research laboratories, the only envisioned role of genetic testing is identification of persons with preclinical disease.

Pathology of DCM

Pathologically, DCM is characterized by biventricular and atrial dilatation with pale and mottled myocardium and a high incidence of mural thrombi. On microscopy, there is evidence of myocyte hypertrophy and degeneration, interstitial fibrosis, and occasionally small clusters of lymphocyte infiltration. If inflammatory cells are present, the primary diagnosis of myocarditis should be excluded.

Clinical Presentation of DCM

Patients usually present with decreasing exercise tolerance, dyspnea, tachypnea, failure to thrive (particularly in the pediatric age group), palpitations and syncope. The signs of DCM are due to heart failure leading to systemic and pulmonary venous congestion. Physical examination may show findings of heart failure; tachypnea, tachycardia, systemic venous congestion, hepatosplenomegaly, poor peripheral circulation, and peripheral edema. Cardiac examination is characterized by findings of a dilated and poorly functioning heart,

such as murmur of mitral regurgitation, muffled heart sound, lateral shifting of apical impulse, and gallop rhythm. On examination of the respiratory system, tachypnea with retraction and basal rales indicate pulmonary venous congestion.

Diagnosis of DCM

Echocardiography shows dilated ventricle and atrium with globally reduced systolic function. An increase in the ratio of preejection period to ejection time (index of myocardial performance) is an indicator of poor systolic function. Mitral anular dilatation, mitral regurgitation, and decreased aortic Doppler flow signals due to reduced cardiac output may be present. Doppler diastolic function studies may show an abnormal mitral inflow and pulmonary vein Doppler findings suggestive of increased left ventricular end-diastolic pressure and decreased tissue Doppler velocity. The incidence of thrombus formation is high in a dilated, poorly functioning heart. Anomalous coronary origins as a cause of ischemic DCM should be excluded.

Electrocardiographic Findings and Arrhythmias in DCM

Sinus tachycardia with nonspecific electrocardiographic changes, such as left ventricular hypertrophy, repolarization changes, inverted T waves, ST-segment changes, and axis shifts, are the most common electrocardiographic findings in DCM. Left ventricular hypertrophy is found in 45% to 75% of patients. Right ventricular hypertrophy and right and left atrial enlargement occur in 20% to 25% of patients. Paroxysmal supraventricular tachycardia, Wolff-Parkinson-White syndrome, sinus node dysfunction, complete heart block, intraventricular conduction abnormalities, and atrioventricular block may occur in patients with idiopathic DCM.

Ventricular arrhythmias are prevalent in DCM. Among all patients with DCM, ventricular ectopy occurs in 82% and nonsustained ventricular tachycardia, in 42%. Nonsustained ventricular tachycardia is usually asymptomatic and constitutes an important independent risk factor for total mortality in DCM.

Treatment of nonsustained ventricular tachycardia in DCM is controversial because it is often asymptomatic. Nonsustained ventricular tachycardia is linked to overall mortality, not simply mortality due to a fatal arrhythmia. Primary prevention strategies for sudden

Table 2.   Summary of Dilated Cardiomyopathy Susceptibility Genes and Loci

Locus	Inheritance	Gene	Protein	Other features
1p1-q21	AD	LMNA	Lamin A/C	Conduction disease, SND, AF, skeletal myopathy
1q32	AD	TNNT2	Cardiac Troponin T	None
2q14-q22	AD	?	?	Conduction disease
2q31	AD	TTN	Titin	None
2q35	AD	DES	Desmin	Skeletal myopathy
3p22-p25	AD	SCN5A	Cardiac sodium channel α subunit (hNav1.5)	Conduction disese, sinus node dysfunction, AF
5q33	AD	SGCD	Delta sarcoglycan	Skeletal myopathy
6p23-p4	AD	DSP	Desmoplakin	Woolly hair, keratoderma, recessive transmission
6q12-q16	AD	?	?	None
6q22.1	AD	PLN	Phospholamban	None
6q23-q24	AD	EYA4	Eyes absent homolog 4	Skeletal myopathy, sensorineural hearing loss
9q13-q22	AD	?	?	None
q22-q31	AD	?	?	None
10q22-q23	AD	VCL	Metavinculin	Mitral valve prolapse
10q22.3-q23.2	AD	ZASP, LBD3	Z-band alternatively spliced PDZ-motif protein/LIM binding domain 3	LVNC
11p11.2	AD	MYBPC3	Myosin-binding protein C	None
11p15.1	AD	CSRP3	Cardiac muscle LIM protein	None
12p12.1	AD	ABCC9	Sulfonylurea receptor 2A	Ventricular arrhythmias
14q1	AD	MYH6	α-Myosin heavy chain	
14q12	AD	MYH7	β-Myosin heavy chain	None
15q14	AD	ACTC	Cardiac actin	None
15q22	AD	TPM1	α-Tropomyosin	None
16p11	AD	CTF1	Cardiotrophin	None
19p13.2	AR	TNN13	Cardiac troponin I	Conduction disease
Xp21	X-linked	DMD	Dystrophin	Skeletal myopathy
Xq28	X-linked	TAZ	Tafazzin	Skeletal myopathy

AD, autosomal dominant; AF, atrial fibrillation; AR, autosomal recessive; LVNC, left ventricular noncompaction.

death in patients with DCM who have asymptomatic, nonsustained ventricular tachycardia include treatment of precipitating factors such as hypokalemia and optimizing heart failure therapy with angiotensin-converting enzyme inhibitors, β-adrenergic blockers, and aldosterone inhibitor therapies. Pacing therapy and chronic resynchronization therapy is useful in a select group of patients. Substantial improvement of left systolic function, (reverse remodeling) with associated improvement in mitral regurgitation and regression of the restrictive filling pattern occurs in almost 50% of patients treated with this regimen. The severity of mitral regurgitation is also an important risk factor for mortality with DCM.

Symptomatic patients with ventricular tachycardia should receive β-blockers; if symptoms persist, amiodarone therapy should be started. Combined use of amiodarone and β-blockers, if tolerated, seems to have some synergistic effects in these patients. Empiric treatment with amiodarone is preferred to the use of other drugs for secondary prevention of sustained ventricular tachycardia.

Routine electrophysiologic testing is not indicated in patients with DCM and has limited prognostic significance. There is a role for electrophysiologic testing and ablation in sustained ventricular tachycardia, if it has a mechanism that is amenable to ablation, such as focal-origin ventricular tachycardia or BBR. Other described risk factors of limited value include prolonged QRS duration, signal-averaged electrocardiography, T wave alternans, and B-type natriuretic peptide.

SCD and ICD Use in DCM

DCM is associated with a high mortality rate within 2 years of diagnosis; a minority of patients survive 5 years. SCD accounts for between 30% and 40% of all causes of death in patients with DCM.

The risk of sudden death is high, particularly in patients with long-term persistent or progressive left ventricular dilatation and dysfunction. The combination of poor left ventricular function and frequent episodes of nonsustained ventricular tachycardia in these patients is associated with an increased risk of sudden death. Antiarrhythmic drug therapy is of limited use in this group of patients. ICDs should be implanted in patients 1) who were resuscitated from cardiac arrest, 2) with syncope or presyncope, 3) with poorly tolerated and symptomatic ventricular tachycardia, or 4) with severe left ventricular systolic dysfunction (ejection fraction <35%).

Randomized trials of defibrillator use in DCM showed a considerable reduction in arrhythmic death and a strong trend toward a benefit of ICD therapy over medical therapy in patients who have DCM with reduced left ventricular ejection fractions and nonsustained ventricular tachycardia. Unexplained syncope is the most critical risk factor associated with sudden death in these patients with heart failure. These patients have a very high risk of subsequent ventricular arrhythmias and should be strongly considered for ICD therapy. The evidence is weak for the use of an ICD in patients with DCM presenting with sustained ventricular tachycardia and no severe left ventricular dysfunction or with hemodynamically tolerated sustained ventricular tachycardia.

Family Screening in DCM

A thorough family history and pedigree analysis is the best current surrogate for genetic testing in DCM and should be performed on every patient with DCM. The diagnosis of familial DCM is based on the diagnosis of DCM in two or more close relatives. All first-degree relatives of an index case should receive screening electrocardiography and echocardiography. The American Heart Association recommends that patients with familial HCM be referred to a cardiovascular genetic center. Skeletal muscle tests may be needed in specific forms of familial DCM. The disease can be asymptomatic because of the reduced and age-related penetrance. The profound genetic heterogeneity underlying DCM makes it difficult and impractical to perform routine genetic testing for DCM.

After a negative initial screening, subsequent surveillance should be performed every 3 to 5 years in all first-degree relatives of patients with DCM. Those with abnormal results on screening echocardiography should be evaluated yearly.

ARRHYTHMOGENIC RIGHT VENTRICULAR CARDIOMYOPATHY

Definition of ARVC

ARVC is a primary heart muscle disease characterized by progressive degeneration and fibrous-fatty replacement of total or partial right ventricular (with or without left ventricular) myocardium associated with arrhythmias of right ventricular origin. ARVC is characterized clinically by ventricular tachycardia or ventricular fibrillation of left bundle branch block configuration, and it is responsible for sudden cardiac arrest mostly in young people and athletes.

Epidemiology of ARVC

ARVC is a major cause of SCD in young people and athletes, particularly in certain regions of Italy (Padua, Venice) and Greece (island of Naxos), where the prevalence is 0.4% to 0.8%. In the United States, the estimated prevalence of ARVC is much lower, approximately 1 in 5,000 (0.02%-0.1%). In the Veneto region of Italy, ARVC is responsible for 12.5% to 25% of exercise-related sudden deaths in persons younger than 35 years. Although ARVC is less common in the United States, it remains an important cause of sudden death in the young and should be considered when evaluating patients with syncope, palpitations, and aborted sudden death. The annual mortality rate associated with untreated ARVC is around 3%.

Molecular Basis of ARVC

ARVC is viewed as a disease of the desmosome. ARVC is familial in 30% to 50% of cases, commonly having an autosomal dominant pattern of inheritance. In autosomal dominant ARVC, there are 10 ARVC disease genes or loci (Table 3). The most common subtype of ARVC is ARVC9, which is due to mutations in the PKP2-encoded type 2 plakophilin and accounts for approximately 25% of cases of ARVC. There are two forms of autosomal recessive ARVC, including Naxos disease caused by plakoglobin mutations.

There are two modes of inheritance in ARVC: autosomal dominant and autosomal recessive (Table 3). Two forms of autosomal recessive ARVC have been identified: Naxos disease (17q21) and ARVC/APC (14q24-q terminal). Naxos disease also is associated with palmoplantar keratosis and woolly hair, and, unlike the incomplete penetrance associated with autosomal dominant-ARVC, Naxos disease is essentially 100% penetrant.

Pathology of ARVC

In general, ARVC involves the so-called triangle of dysplasia (i.e., the right ventricular outflow tract, apex, and infundibulum). Later in the natural history, the right ventricle may become more diffusely involved and the interventricular septum and left ventricle are progressively affected, a process leading to biventricular heart failure. Histopathologically, ARVC is characterized

Table 3.   Summary of Arrhythmogenic Right Ventricular Cardiomyopathy Susceptibility Genes and Loci

Subtypes	Inheritance	Locus	Gene	Protein	Other features
ARVC1	AD	14q23-q24	*TGFB-3*	Transforming growth factor, β-3	
ARVC2	AD	1q41.2-q43	*RYR2*	Type 2 ryanodine receptor/calcium release channel	Catecholaminergic
ARVC3	AD	14q12-q22	?	?	
ARVC4	AD	2q32.1-q32.3	?	?	Localized LV involvement
ARVC5	AD	3p23	?	?	
ARVC6	AD	10p14-p12	?	?	Early onset, high penetrance
ARVC7	AD	10q22	?	?	Myofibrillar myopathy
ARVC8	AD/AR	6p24	*DSP*	Desmoplakin	A homozygous mutation-Carvajal syndrome, hair and skin disorders associated with cardiac disease
ARVC9	AD	12p11	*PKP2*	Plakophilin-2	Most common subtype (~24%)
ARVC10	Unknown	18q12.1	*DSG2*	Desmoglein-2	Frequent LV involvement
Naxos disease	AR	17q21	*JUP*	Junctional plakoglobin	Palmoplantar keratoderma and wooly hair

AD, autosomal dominant; AR, autosomal recessive; ARVC, arrhythmogenic right ventricular cardiomyopathy; LV, left ventricular; VT, ventricular tachycardia.

by loss of myocytes with fatty or fibrofatty replacement with frequent infiltration of inflammatory cells reminiscent of myocarditis, resulting in segmental or diffuse wall thinning in the right ventricular myocardium. On gross pathologic examination, right ventricular dilatation or segmental wall motion abnormalities, aneurysm formation, and fatty deposition in the right ventricular wall are identified. Left ventricular fibrofatty infiltration occurs in 20% of patients.

Clinical Presentation of ARVC

There are four phases of ARVC: 1) the concealed phase, 2) an overt electric disorder, 3) right ventricular failure, and 4) a biventricular pump failure. Patients with ARVC typically present between the second and fifth decades of life. However, the age at presentation ranges widely, between 2 and 70 years. Up to 25% of patients may present with heart failure, but 10% are asymptomatic. In some series, the mortality rate when ARVC is untreated, is approximately 3% per year and up to 19% after 10 years of follow-up. The most common presenting symptoms include palpitations, syncope, and death. Notably, half of patients with ARVC present with a malignant or potentially malignant ventricular arrhythmia. An additional 44% of the remaining patients experienced a sustained ventricular arrhythmia during the course of the disease. This fact emphasizes the importance of screening family members of patients with known ARVC.

Electrocardiographic Findings and Arrhythmias in ARVC

Patients with ARVC have a progressive disorder that is characterized by ventricular arrhythmias in 45% to 79% of cases. Sometimes they have inducible ventricular tachycardia with left bundle branch block. Other arrhythmias include supraventricular tachycardias, including atrial fibrillation, atrial flutter, or paroxysmal atrial tachycardia. Complete heart block occurs in 5% of cases. Electrocardiographic abnormalities occur in almost 90% of patients with ARVC.

Characteristic electrocardiographic features suggestive of ARVC include 1) T-wave inversions in leads V_1 through V_3 (excluding patients <12 years old and right bundle branch block) (54%), 2) QRS duration 110 milliseconds or more in leads V_1 through V_3 (up to 98%), 3) presence of an epsilon wave (23%) (small

upright electric potentials after the end of the QRS complex), 4) left bundle branch type ventricular tachycardia, and 5) frequent extrasystoles (>1,000/24 hours) (Table 4). Epsilon waves are abnormal electrical potentials along the terminal portion of the QRS, resulting from delayed RV depolarization. Late potentials are seen better on signal-averaged electrocardiography (31%). Complete (6%-15%) or incomplete (14%-18%) right bundle branch block may be present. Additional reported electrocardiographic markers of ARVC include 1) QRS and QT dispersion, QRS dispersion 40 milliseconds or more on 12-lead electrocardiography as an independent predictor of SCD in patients with ARVC; 2) parietal block, defined as a QRS duration in leads V_1 through V_3 that exceeds the QRS duration in lead V_6 by >25 milliseconds; and 3) a ratio of the QRS duration in leads $V_1+V_2+V_3/V_4+V_5+V_6$ of 1.2 or more. Patients are usually in sinus rhythm.

Clinical diagnosis relies largely on familial occurrence and ventricular tachyarrhythmias, particularly ventricular tachycardia of right ventricular origin elicited during exercise testing, which is (50%-60% of patients) characteristically monomorphic with a left bundle branch block pattern. Late potentials are more easily defined with signal-averaged electrocardiography and correlate with the extent of right ventricular involvement. Prolonged S-wave upstroke (≥55 milliseconds) in right precordial leads V_1 through V_3 in the absence of right bundle branch block is sensitive and specific for differentiating ARVC from right ventricular outflow tract ventricular tachycardia. An inferior QRS axis during ventricular tachycardia reflects the right ventricular outflow tract as the site of origin, whereas a superior axis reflects the right ventricular inferior wall as the site of origin. Several studies have shown a relation between ARVC and the Brugada syndrome.

Diagnosis of AVRC

Diagnostic evaluation of patients suspected of having ARVC includes 12-lead and signal-averaged electrocardiography, 24-hour Holter monitoring, exercise treadmill testing, echocardiography, magnetic resonance imaging, electrophysiologic testing, and cardiac catheterization that includes right ventricular angiography and right ventricular endomyocardial biopsy. Morphologic right ventricular changes in ARVC consist of ventricular dilatation, segmental wall

Table 4. Major and Minor Crtieria for Arrhythmogenic Right Ventricular Cardiomyopathy

Major criteria	Minor criteria
Global or regional dysfunction and structural alterations	
Severe dilatation and reduction of RV ejection fraction with no (or mild) LV involvement	Mild global RV dilatation or decreased ejection fraction with normal LV
Localized RV aneurysms (akinetic or dyskinetic areas with diastolic bulging)	Mild segmental RV dilatation
Severe segmental RV dilatation	Regional RV hypokinesia
Tissue characterization of walls	
Fibrofatty replacement of myocardium on endomyocardial biopsy	
Repolarization abnormalities	
	Inverted T waves in right precordial leads (V_1-V_3) (age >12 years) in the absence of right bundle branch block
Depolarization or conduction abnormalities	
Epsilon waves or localized prolongation (>110 milliseconds) of QRS complex in right precordial leads (V_1-V_3)	Late potentials on signal-averaged electrocardiography
Arrhythmias	
	Left bundle branch block VT (sustained or nonsustained) documented on electrocaqrdiography, Holter monitoring, or exercise testing
	Frequent premature ventricular contractions (1,000/24 hours) on Holter monitoring
Family history	
Familial disease confirmed at autopsy or surgery	Family history of premature sudden death (<35 years) presumed due to ARVD
	Family history of ARVD (based on these criteria)

LV, left ventricular; RV, right ventricular; VT, ventricular tachycardia.

motion abnormalities, aneurysm formation, and fibrofatty deposition can be identified with echocardiography, multislice computed tomography, or cardiac magnetic resonance imaging. Standard diagnostic criteria for ARVC based on the European Society of Cardiology and International Society and Federation of Cardiology task force include major and minor criteria proposed in 1994 (Table 4). These criteria are based on evaluation of genetic, electrical, anatomical, and functional status of the right ventricle. A diagnosis of ARVC requires the presence of two major criteria, one major criterion and two minor criteria, or four minor criteria (from separate categories).

Echocardiography is the initial imaging method of choice. It should be performed with particular attention given to right ventricular function, segmental dilatation, and wall motion abnormalities. The echocardiographic findings suggestive of ARVC are right ventricular dilatation, enlargement of the right atrium, isolated dilatation of the right ventricular outflow tract, increased reflectivity of the moderator band, localized aneurysms, and decreased fractional area change and akinesis or dyskinesis of the inferior wall and the right ventricular apex. Transesophageal echocardiography, intracardiac echocardiography, and contrast echocardiography may provide better visualization of the right ventricle, especially in adults with challenging transthoracic echocardiographic images. Analysis of regional right ventricular contractility with tissue Doppler imaging and strain rate imaging may help identify early changes in right ventricular function.

Currently, the preferred diagnostic imaging method for ARVC is magnetic resonance imaging. Cardiac magnetic resonance imaging is extremely effective for assessing structural and functional changes of the right ventricle in multiple planes. Caution should be exercised in diagnosing ARVC solely on the basis of the presence of fatty infiltration, particularly in elderly women and obese individuals. Better and more specific criteria for a magnetic resonance imaging-based diagnosis of ARVC are delayed signal enhancement, segmental right ventricular dyskinesia or hypokinesia, dilatation and aneurysm formation.

Cardiac catheterization is useful for assessment of intracardiac hemodynamics, right ventricular angiography, and right ventricular endomyocardial biopsy. Angiographic evidence of ARVC includes 1) akinetic or dyskinetic bulging in the triangle of dysplasia (diaphragmatic, apical, and infundibular areas), 2) localized aneurysms, and 3) right ventricular dilatation and hypokinesis. Caution should be exercised during right ventricular endocardial biopsy to localize the affected area using ultrasound guidance to avoid the typically favored interventricular septum during a blind procedure.

Invasive electrophysiologic testing may be useful for differentiating ventricular arrhythmias due to ARVC from right ventricular outflow tract ventricular tachycardia. In contrast to HCM, inducibility during electrophysiologic testing can guide, in part, treatment recommendations.

SCD and Indications for ICD in ARVC

It is estimated that ARVC causes up to a fifth of all episodes of SCD in persons younger than 35 years. Of all cases of sudden death, 40% occur with exercise, but a large proportion of patients have SCD during sedentary activity. In the United States, although SCD is a common presenting symptom, once it is diagnosed the incidence of SCD is rare because of the widespread use of ICDs. The occurrence of arrhythmic cardiac arrest due to ARVC is substantially increased in athletes. ICD implantation is clearly indicated for secondary prevention after a survived cardiac arrest or sustained

ventricular tachycardia. In contrast, the role of an ICD for primary prevention in patients with asymptomatic ARVC or their relatives remains controversial. Because of the paucity of scientific data, the decision must be based on individual risk assessment, physician judgment, patient preference, and economic considerations. ICDs are recommended for *primary prevention* in patients with 1) inducible ventricular fibrillation during programmed-stimulation electrophysiologic study, 2) sustained ventricular arrhythmia resistant to drug therapy, 3) extensive myocardial involvement, (left ventricular involvement with poor cardiac function), 4) syncope or presyncope, or a 5) family history of sudden death. ICDs are recommended for secondary prevention in patients with a previous cardiac arrest.

Patients with normal sinus node and atrioventricular nodal function should have a single-lead ICD. A dual-chamber ICD has the advantage of better discrimination and treatment of atrial arrhythmias. Physicians must be cognizant of the anticipated higher incidence of long-term complications associated with increased hardware (particularly in young patients), perforation of a thin, dysplastic right ventricle, inadequate sensing, and high pacing threshold in patients with ARVC.

Medical Therapy for ARVC

The five therapeutic considerations in patients with ARVC are 1) antiarrhythmic medications, 2) radiofrequency ablation, 3) ICD, 4) heart failure treatment, and 5) surgical treatment. Preferred antiarrhythmic agents are sotalol or amiodarone with or without β-blockers. Catheter ablation of ventricular tachycardia in ARVC has a success rate of 60% to 90%, but relapses are frequent as the disease progresses. Nonpharmacologic options for treatment of significant arrhythmias include catheter ablation of the sites of tachycardia, surgical disarticulation of the right ventricle, and ICDs. In patients with drug-refractory malignant arrhythmias, an ICD provides prophylaxis against syncope due to hemodynamically unstable ventricular tachycardia and sudden death.

In patients with right or biventricular systolic dysfunction, the mainstays of therapy are diuretics, angiotensin-converting enzyme inhibitors, β-blockers (carvedilol), digitalis, and anticoagulants. Patients with refractory heart failure and incessant ventricular tachycardia nonresponsive to therapy are candidates for cardiac transplantation.

Recommendation for Athletes With ARVC

Athletes with a probable or definite diagnosis of ARVC should be excluded from most competitive sports, with the possible exception of sports of low intensity (class IA).

Family Screening in ARVC

All first-degree relatives of an index case of ARVC should be screened with electrocardiography, echocardiography, and cardiac magnetic resonance imaging. Mutational analyses are performed in research laboratories. No clinical tests are available, and routine genetic testing is not indicated except for research purposes.

IDIOPATHIC RESTRICTIVE CARDIOMYOPATHY

Definition of RCM

Restrictive cardiomyopathy (RCM) is an idiopathic or systemic myocardial disorder characterized by impaired diastolic filling, reduced or normal biventricular volumes, normal or mildly abnormal biventricular systolic function, and normal myocardial thickness. Although it is most frequently due to diseases causing infiltration or fibrosis (e.g., constrictive pericarditis, amyloidosis), RCM also can be idiopathic or familial.

Epidemiology of RCM

The prevalence and incidence of RCM are not well known. It is estimated that RCM accounts for less than 5% of all cardiomyopathies in children.

Molecular Basis of RCM

Idiopathic RCM often occurs as a sporadic case, but familial RCM has been reported as an autosomal dominant trait. The two genes implicated thus far in RCM are *TNNI3* and *DES* (Table 5).

Clinical Presentation of RCM

The common presenting symptoms of RCM are dyspnea and fatigue due to pulmonary venous congestion and edema and ascites due to right heart failure. Clinical examination is characterized by jugular venous distention and prominent *y* descent with the Kussmaul sign. The jugular venous pulse fails to decrease during inspiration and may actually increase (Kussmaul sign). Peripheral edema and ascites are present in advanced cases, and the liver is enlarged and pulsatile.

Diagnosis of RCM

The challenge for diagnosis is accurate differentiation of incurable RCM from potentially treatable constrictive pericarditis. None of the single echocardiographic or hemodynamic variables of cardiac catheterization are diagnostic, and there is a considerable overlap.

The diagnosis of RCM should be considered in a patient presenting with heart failure and found by echocardiography to have 1) normal systolic function, 2) normal left and right ventricular size, but 3) severe atrial enlargement. On Doppler echocardiography, e′ is usually less than 8 cm/s and E/e′ is more than 15, findings of increased left ventricular pressure. Other features are short mitral deceleration time (<150 milliseconds), increased velocity and duration of atrial reversal in the pulmonary vein, pulmonary vein reversal duration longer than mitral A wave duration, increased reversal of diastolic flow after atrial contraction with inspiration in the hepatic and pulmonary veins, increased ratio of early diastolic filling (mitral E) to atrial filling (>2), and decreased isovolumic relaxation time (<70 milliseconds).

On cardiac catheterization, there is a deep *y* descent and rapid rise to a plateau in early diastole called the "square root," or "dip-and-plateau," pattern. Left ventricular end-diastolic pressure, right ventricular systolic end-diastolic pressure, pulmonary capillary wedge pressure, and both atrial pressures are increased. The left ventricular end-diastolic pressure is typically 5 mm Hg more than the right ventricular end-diastolic pressure.

Table 5.   Summary of Restrictive Cardiomyopathy Susceptibility Genes

Subtype	Locus	Gene	Protein
RCM with HCM	19q13	*TNNI3*	Cardiac troponin I
RCM with skeletal myopathies	2q35	*DES*	Desmin

HCM, hypertrophic cardiomyopathy; RCM, restrictive cardiomyopathy.

Electrocardiographic Findings and Arrhythmias in RCM

The most common electrocardiographic changes in RCM are atrial enlargement and nonspecific ST- and T-wave changes. Other electrocardiographic findings include intraventricular conduction abnormalities, sinus node dysfunction, and atrioventricular block. Increased left ventricular end-diastolic pressure and giant atria make them prone to atrial fibrillation. Maintenance of normal sinus rhythm is paramount. Atrial kick is extremely important in ventricular filling in these patients, and its absence can precipitate hemodynamic decompensation. RCM is associated with complete heart block, sinus node dysfunction and bradyarrhythmias necessitating pacemaker support.

Treatment of RCM

Treatment is aimed at symptomatic relief. Diuretics are used to treat venous congestion in the pulmonary and systemic circulation. Patients with RCM are preload-dependent, and excessive diuresis may lead to decreased cardiac output and hypotension. Patients with systolic dysfunction may benefit from adrenergics and phosphodiesterase inhibitors. Large atria, low cardiac output, and atrial fibrillation make patients susceptible to thrombus formation and thromboembolism; anticoagulation is recommended. Overall, the prognosis is poor, and cardiac transplantation should be considered for end-stage, refractory symptoms in RCM.

ICD Therapy in RCM

There are no standard recommendations for use of ICDs in RCM. Currently, there is no single test for SCD risk stratification.

Family Screening in RCM

All first-degree relatives of an index case of RCM should be screened with electrocardiography and echocardiography.

Isolated Left Ventricular Noncompaction

Definition

Isolated left ventricular noncompaction (LVNC) is a genetically heterogeneous congenital disorder characterized by a hypertrophied left ventricle with deep trabeculations (so-called spongiform myocardium), decreased systolic function, and possible left ventricular dilatation. LVNC can be isolated or can present with other congenital heart diseases.

Pathogenesis and Molecular Basis of LVNC

LVNC is a rare disorder and is thought to be due to an arrest of myocardial morphogenesis. This arrest leads to deep recesses that communicate only with the ventricular cavity, not the coronary circulation. LVNC occurs in the presence of other cardiac anomalies associated with pressure or volume overload lesions. LVNC in the absence of these associated lesions is a rare form of cardiomyopathy first described only a decade ago. LVNC is still an unclassified cardiomyopathy according to the World Health Organization classification of cardiomyopathies.

There is now enough evidence to suggest that LVNC is a distinct form of cardiomyopathy. The genetic basis of LVNC remains a mystery in many cases with both familial and sporadic occurrence. The prevalence of noncompaction on echocardiography in older populations ranges from 0.05% to 0.24%. Familial recurrence in pediatric LVNC initially was reported as approximately 40%. In a larger study of an adult population, the rate of familial recurrence was 18% to 25%. Autosomal dominant inheritance is the most common pattern, and there are fewer cases of X-linked and mitochondrial inheritance. Mutations in the genes encoding α-dystrobrevin (*DTNA*), G4.5 (*TAZ*), and LIM domain binding protein 3 (*LDB3* or *ZASP*) are the currently known genetic subtypes of LVNC. Mutations in G4.5 result in not only Barth syndrome but also other X-linked infantile cardiomyopathies, including LVNC, X-linked infantile cardiomyopathy, and X-linked endocardial fibroelastosis (Table 6).

Diagnosis of LVNC

In general, the diagnosis of LVNC is made with echocardiography. However, the correct diagnosis is often missed or delayed because of insufficient awareness by echocardiographers of this congenital cardiomyopathy or because of nonoptimal imaging of the lateral and apical myocardium. The two-dimensional echocardiographic image of LVNC is characterized by large, prominent trabeculation and deep intertrabecular recess in continuity with ventricular cavity, as seen on color Doppler. The following characteristic two-dimensional

Table 6.   Summary of Left Ventricular Noncompaction Hypertrophic Cardiomyopathy Susceptibility

Subtype	Inheritance	Locus	Gene	Protein	Other features
X-linked isolated LVNC	X-linked	Xp28	TAZ (G4.5)	Tafazzin	Isolated LVNC, Barth syndrome, endocardial fibroelastosis, Emery-Dreifuss muscular dystrophy, and myotubular myopathy
LVNC and left ventricular dysfunction	Unknown	10q22.2-q23.3	ZASP, LDB3	Z-band alternatively spliced PDZ-motif protein and LIM domain binding protein 3	
LVNC associated with congenital heart defects	Unknown	18q12	DTNA	α-Dystrobrevin	
LVNC with dilated cardiomyopathy and ventricular deptal defects	Unknown	20p13	FKBP1A (previously known as FKBP12)	FK506 binding protein 1A	LVNC and congenital heart disease in mice
LVNC and complex heart disease	Unknown	Distal 5q deletion, del(5)(q35.1q35.3)	CSX	Cardiac-specific homeo box	
LVNC and dilated dilated cardiomyopathy	Unknown	1q21	LMNA	Lamin A/C	DCM
LVNC	AD	22q11	?	?	DiGeorge syndrome
LVNC	AD	11p155	?	?	

AD, autosomal dominant; AR, DCM, dilated cardiomyopathy; LVNC, left ventricular noncompaction.

echocardiographic features are diagnostic of LVNC; 1) presence of exaggerated, numerous, coarse, and deep trabeculations, 2) prominent intertrabecular recesses, and 3) end-systolic noncompacted to compacted ratio of 2 or more. Unlike left ventricular hypertrophy due to volume or pressure overload lesions, LVNC is segmental with predominant apical and inferolateral left ventricular involvement. Magnetic resonance imaging may provide better visualization of these anatomical details. As in patients with HCM, patients with LVNC may present with initial signs of diastolic dysfunction progressing to systolic dysfunction, dilated ventricle, and heart failure in later life.

Clinical Presentation of LVNC
Clinical manifestations are highly variable, ranging

from no symptoms to disabling congestive heart failure, arrhythmias, systemic thromboembolism, cardiac transplantation, and death. Most reports of LVNC are in adults. However, the age at presentation ranges from prenatal (severe heart failure and hydrops recognized on fetal echocardiography) to old age (severe heart failure). Facial dysmorphism and neurologic abnormalities occur in a high proportion of patients with LVNC.

Electrocardiographic Findings and Arrhythmias in LVNC

Nonspecific electrocardiographic changes of left ventricular hypertrophy, repolarization changes, inverted T waves, ST-segment changes, axis shifts, intraventricular conduction abnormalities, and atrioventricular block are frequent. Arrhythmias are common in patients with ventricular noncompaction. Atrial fibrillation occurs in 25% of patients. Paroxysmal supraventricular tachycardia and complete heart block also have been reported in patients with LVNC. Wolff-Parkinson-White syndrome was reported in 15% of a pediatric population, but it is infrequent in adults. Left bundle branch block has been described in 44% of adults with LVNC, and ventricular tachyarrhythmias are found in 47% of patients with LVNC. SCD causes half of the deaths in patients with LVNC. The incidence of death at 5 years may approach 50%.

Indication for ICD in LVNC

There are no standard recommendations for use of ICDs in LVNC. Cases should be analyzed individually, but, given the high mortality rate, ICD implantation should be strongly considered. As in all cardiomyopathies, a presentation of aborted cardiac arrest necessitates ICD therapy for secondary prevention.

Treatment of LVNC

Treatment of LVNC focuses on the three major clinical manifestations: heart failure, arrhythmias, and systemic embolic events. Standard medical therapy is warranted for systolic and diastolic ventricular dysfunction and heart failure. Anticoagulants are indicated for a poorly functioning, dilated heart. Resynchronization therapy may be beneficial for patients with heart failure.

Cardiac Transplantation in LVNC

Cardiac transplantation is indicated for patients with refractory congestive heart failure.

Family Screening in LVNC

All first-degree relatives of an index case of LVNC should be screened with electrocardiography and echocardiography.

Recommendation for Athletes With LVNC

Few data are available regarding the relative risks of training and competition in athletes with LVNC. Until more information is available, it is most prudent to consider each case individually. The decision to restrict participation in competitive sports should be based on associated comorbidities of arrhythmias, heart failure, and possibly extrapolation of SCD risk factors from other cardiomyopathies. In general, patients with LVNC probably should be restricted from competitive sports, with the possible exception of class IA activities.

IMPLANTABLE CARDIOVERTER-DEFIBRILLATORS

In summary, the ICD indications for use of ICDs in heritable cardiomyopathies are as follows:

HCM

   Secondary prevention (aborted cardiac arrest):
      Prior cardiac arrest or aborted sudden death
   Primary prevention:
      Presence of two major risk factors
      Major risk factors:
         1. Spontaneous ventricular tachycardia and sustained or unsustained ventricular tachycardia on ambulatory monitoring
         2. Family history of HCM-related sudden death involving at least two relatives younger than 45 years
         3. Severe left ventricular hypertrophy, wall thickness of 30 mm or more
         4. Unexplained syncope, especially in young patients with exertion or recurrent
         5. Abnormal blood pressure response with exercise testing, higher specificity in patients younger than 50 years and hypotension
         6. Increased delayed enhancement on cardiac gadolinium-enhanced magnetic resonance imaging

If only one major risk factor is present, use of an ICD must be carefully individualized because the potential complications from the intervention may exceed its intended purpose.

DCM

Secondary prevention:

Patients who were resuscitated from cardiac arrest (no reversible cause)

Primary prevention:

1. Syncope or presyncope
2. Poorly tolerated and symptomatic ventricular tachycardia
3. Severe left ventricular systolic dysfunction (ejection fraction ≤ 35%)

ARVC

Secondary prevention:

Patients who were resuscitated from cardiac arrest (no reversible cause)

Primary prevention

1. Syncope or presyncope
2. Family history of sudden death
3. Sustained ventricular arrhythmia resistant to drug therapy
4. Extensive myocardial involvement (left ventricular involvement)

RCM and LVNC

No standard recommendations

Consider each case individually. The decision to offer ICD therapy should be based on associated comorbidities of arrhythmias, heart failure, and extrapolation of SCD risk factors from other cardiomyopathies

32

SYNCOPE: DIAGNOSIS AND TREATMENT

Win-Kuang Shen, MD

INTRODUCTION

This chapter on syncope is constructed differently from a standard textbook chapter. Instead of providing a detailed review on various conditions causing syncope, on the complex mechanisms of vasovagal syncope, or on how tilt table testing or an electrophysiologic study is performed, this chapter provides a synopsis of the approach to syncope evaluation according to the patient's presentation and patient management. It is expected that the reader has reviewed the indications for tilt table or electrophysiologic study after a syncopal event (Chapter 21, "Indications for Electrophysiologic Testing"). The reader should understand the role of syncope as a risk factor in determining prognosis and therapy in patients with various structural and familial conditions. It is also expected that the reader knows the available evidence for the efficacy of various treatment of vasovagal syncope, including the role of β-blocker therapy or pacemaker therapy. Pertinent information from guidelines pertaining to syncope is synthesized in this chapter.

DEFINITION

Syncope is a symptom. Syncope is defined as a transient, self-limited loss of consciousness associated with loss of postural tone. The onset of syncope is relatively rapid

and the subsequent recovery is spontaneous, complete, and relatively prompt. The underlying mechanism is a transient global cerebral hypoperfusion. Conceptually, one should distinguish syncope from other forms of transient loss of consciousness (TLOC) such as concussion due to trauma, epilepsy due to primary cerebral electrical abnormality, and "syncope-mimics" such as psychiatric problems. The conditions resulting in nonsyncopal TLOC or syncope-mimics are not caused by cerebral hypoperfusion. On cardiology examinations, one should expect questions about what syncope is, although one should be cognizant about the broader differential diagnosis for TLOC in clinical practice.

CLINICAL SPECTRUM AND DIAGNOSTIC STRATEGY

The population of patients with syncope is large and heterogeneous, ranging from infants to the very elderly. The spectrum of physiologic and pathophysiologic conditions that may cause syncope ranges from common, benign faints to severe, life-threatening cardiac structural or rhythm abnormalities. The prognosis for a patient with syncope depends on the presence or severity of any underlying organic disease and the severity of any traumatic injuries that may be sustained after syncope. Because syncope is often episodic and infrequent in occurrence, establishing a cause-and-effect relationship can be challenging.

Several key elements are critical to the formulation of a logical diagnostic strategy:

1. One must be familiar with the overall organization and broad categories of syncope and nonsyncopal conditions with or without TLOC (Table 1). In the evaluation of any patient presenting with syncope or syncope-like symptoms, the following differential scheme can be useful: neurally mediated conditions (most common, approximately 40%-60% of the entire syncope population), orthostatic hypotension, cardiopulmonary conditions, cerebrovascular disease, and nonsyncopal conditions such as seizures, metabolic or psychiatric disorders. A more detailed list of causes of syncope is provided in Table 2.

2. "Standard of care" initial evaluation includes a thorough history, physical examination, orthostatic blood pressure checks and a 12-lead electrocardiogram.

3. After initial evaluation, the presumed cause of syncope can be categorized as confirmed or certain, suspected or probable, or unexplained.

4. When the cause of syncope is suspected or unexplained after initial investigation, further evaluation should be individualized based on the frequency and severity of the patient's clinical presentation, presence or absence of underlying heart disease (including familial conditions), and anticipated prognosis.

HISTORY AND PHYSICAL EXAMINATION

The most important and fruitful elements of the evaluation are a detailed clinical history and a careful physical examination. When a diagnosis is eventually established, the diagnostic yield from the history and physical examination is high, ranging from 40% to 75% among patients during the initial evaluation. Impressions from an accurate history and physical examination are critical in further triaging patients for appropriate subsequent evaluation and management.

During acquisition of the clinical history and physical examination, the following components should be considered:

1. Age and sex—In elderly patients, clinical presentation is often less typical and potential causes of syncope can be multiple. Cardiac causes are more common in the elderly because cardiovascular diseases are more prevalent. Orthostatic intolerance is common in young women with syncope.

2. Position—Cardiac causes of syncope can occur in any position; neurally mediated syncope does not usually occur in the supine position.

3. Surrounding circumstances—Are there any obvious precipitants such as physical or emotional distress, pain, time relationship to meals, drugs, micturition, defecation, cough, swallowing, exercise, or neck turning?

4. Premonitory symptoms—Shortly before the syncopal event, were there symptoms of lightheadedness, tunnel vision, nausea, vomiting, abdominal discomfort, sweating, aura, chest pain, or palpitations? What was the duration of the symptoms?

5. The index event—Was the index event witnessed? If it was witnessed, was the fall or slumping abrupt? Was the patient breathing? Did the pateint have

Table 1.   Categories and General Causes of Real or Apparent Transient Loss of Consciousness

Syncope (cerebral hypoperfusion)	Nonsyncopal conditions
Neurally mediated syndromes	Transient loss of consciousness
	Seizures
Orthostatic hypotension	Metabolic conditions
	Trauma
Cardiac causes	No loss of consciousness
Arrhythmias	
Structural conditions	Psychogenic "syncope"
Cardiopulmonary	
Cerebrovascular	Transient ischemic attacks of anterior circulation

Table 2. Specific Causes of Syncope and Nonsyncopal Attacks

Causes of syncope
    Neurally mediated reflex syncopal syndromes
        Vasovagal faint (common faint)
        Carotid sinus syncope
        Situational faint
        Acute hemorrhage
        Cough, sneeze
        Gastrointestinal stimulation (swallow, defecation, visceral pain)
        Micturition (postmicturition)
        Postexercise
        Others (e.g., brass instrument playing, weight lifting, postprandial)
        Glossopharyngeal and trigeminal neuralgia
    Orthostatic
        Autonomic failure
            Primary autonomic failure syndromes (e.g., pure autonomic failure, multiple system atrophy, Parkinson disease with autonomic failure)
            Secondary autonomic failure syndromes (e.g., diabetic neuropathy, amyloid neuropathy)
        Drugs and alcohol
        Volume depletion
            Hemorrhage, diarrhea, Addison disease
    Cardiac arrhythmias as primary cause
        Sinus node dysfunction (including bradycardia-tachycardia syndrome)
        Atrioventricular conduction system disease
        Paroxysmal supraventricular and ventricular tachycardias
        Inherited syndromes (eg, long QT syndrome, Brugada syndrome, hypertrophic cardiomyopathy, arrhythmogenic right ventricular cardiomyopathy)
        Implanted device (pacemaker, implantable cardioverter-defibrillator) malfunction
        Drug-induced proarrhythmias
    Structural cardiac or cardiopulmonary disease
        Cardiac valvular disease
        Acute myocardial infarction or ischemia
        Obstructive cardiomyopathy
        Atrial myxoma
        Acute aortic dissection
        Pericardial disease or tamponade
        Pulmonary embolus or pulmonary hypertension
    Cerebrovascular
        Vascular steal syndromes
Causes of nonsyncopal attacks (commonly misdiagnosed as syncope)
    Disorders with impairment or loss of consciousness
        Metabolic disorders, including hypoglycemia, hypoxia, hyperventilation with hypocapnia
        Epilepsy
        Intoxication
        Vertebrobasilar transient ischemic attack
    Disorders resembling syncope without loss of consciousness
        Cataplexy
        Drop attacks
        Psychogenic "syncope" (somatization disorders)
        Transient ischemic attacks of carotid origin

pallor, cyanosis, or shaking or tonic-clonic movements? If the event was not witnessed, was there associated injury, urinary or fecal incontinence, or tongue biting? What was the estimated duration of unresponsiveness?

6. Recovery—Was the recovery immediate or prolonged? Did the patient have confusion or any recall of the event?

7. Past medical history—Was the index event isolated? Was it the first occurence or a recurrence? If recurrent, were previous episodes similar or different? A comprehensive review of coexisting medical and cardiovascular conditions is required.

8. Medications—A complete list of prescribed and over-the-counter medications should be documented. Pay particular attention to negative chronotropic or dromotropic drugs (β-blockers, calcium channel blockers, digoxin, and vagotonic agents), antihypertensive drugs or vasodilators (diuretics, α-antagonists, angiotensin receptor blockers, and angiotensin-converting enzyme inhibitors), and drugs prolonging cardiac repolarization or the QT interval (Table 3).

9. Family history—Family history should be highlighted when a young patient presents with *unexplained* syncope in the absence of any preexisting structural heart disease. The ethnicity of the patient's family should be reviewed. Brugada syndrome was first reported from Europe (Flemish and southern European countries) and South Asia. Arrhythmogenic right ventricular cardiomyopathy was reported from northern Italy and France. With the advancement of medical sciences and increased awareness of these conditions, international registries have been documenting accumulated experiences from around the world. Be aware of first-degree relatives with sudden, explained premature death (younger than 50 years). In conjunction with appropriate and diagnostic laboratory evaluation, a positive family history of premature, unexplained sudden death is a critical factor in the risk stratification for sudden death in a patient who presents with unexplained syncope.

10. Physical examination—Blood pressure and heart rate should be measured in the supine, sitting, and standing positions. A postural decrease in systolic blood pressure of more than 20 mm Hg is

Table 3.   Drugs and Metabolic Conditions That Prolong the QT Interval

Antiarrhythmics
   Class 1A: quinidine, procainamide, disopyramide
   Class 3: sotalol, ibutilide, dofetilide, azimilide, amiodarone,
   Class 4: bepridil

Antimicrobials
   Antibiotics: macrolides (erythromycin), trimethoprim-sulfamethoxazole
   Antifungals: itraconazole, ketoconazole
   Antimalarials: chloroquine
   Antiparasitic: pentamidine
   Antivirals: amantadine

Antihistamines
   Terfenadine, astemizole,

Antidepressants
   Tricyclics (amitriptyline, tetracyclics)

Psychotropics
   Haloperidol, droperidol, phenothiazines

Miscellaneous
   Cisapride, probucol, ketanserin, vasopressin, organophosphate poisoning, chloral hydrate overdose

Electrolyte abnormalities
   Hypokalemia, hypomagnesemia, hypocalcemia

Severe bradyarrhythmias
   Sinus node dysfunction, complete atrioventricular block

Intrinsic cardiac disease
   Myocarditis

Hypothyroidism

Intracranial pathology
   Head trauma, encephalitis, right radical neck dissection

Nutritional
   Starvation, anorexia nervosa, liquid protein diet

considered significant. Measuring blood pressure in both arms and listening for bruits in the carotid, subclavian, and temporal areas may identify patients with vascular disorders, such as cerebrovascular disease, Takayasu disease or subclavian steal syndrome. Cardiac examination should focus on identifying signs of overall cardiac function, valvular heart disease, hypertrophic cardiomyopathy, and pulmonary hypertension. Carotid sinus massage should be a mandatory part of the examination in older patients with syncope. It is imperative, however, to exclude carotid artery disease before performing carotid sinus massage. The presence of carotid bruits or a prior history of stroke or transient ischemic attacks is considered a contraindication for carotid sinus massage.

Pertinent clinical features associated with specific causes of syncope are summarized in Table 4. The specificity and sensitivity of these clinical features vary significantly in different patient populations and from time to time. Combinations of these characteristics, rather than a single feature, provide the basis for management strategies.

LABORATORY INVESTIGATION

Investigational testing is summarized in Table 5. Although "routine" tests for syncope evaluation have not been established, the general consensus is that results for a complete blood cell count, electrolytes, and fasting glucose and a standard electrocardiogram (ECG) should be obtained during the initial evaluation. The decision to pursue additional testing depends on the patient's clinical presentation and the ultimate diagnostic, therapeutic, and educational goals of the procedure. The risk-benefit ratio should be clearly defined. For cardiology examinations, be familiar with the published indications for tilt table testing and electrophysiologic evaluation.

Risk Stratification

Although the fundamental and comprehensive goal of syncope evaluation is to establish the cause of the patient's symptoms, mortality risk assessment in determining prognosis and guiding effective therapy is an important component of the overall objectives. Evidence suggests that syncope by itself is not an independent predictor of mortality. Syncope in individuals with coexisting cardiovascular diseases (thereby having an increased risk of cardiogenic causes of syncope) is associated with increased mortality. Factors associated

Table 4.   Clinical Features Associated With Specific Causes of Syncope

Neurally mediated syncope
  Absence of cardiac disease
  Long history of syncope
  After unpleasant sight, sound, smell, or pain
  After prolonged standing or being in crowded, hot places
  Nausea and vomiting associated with syncope
  During a meal or in the absorptive state after a meal
  With head rotation, pressure on carotid sinus (as in tumors, shaving, tight collars)
  After exertion
Syncope due to orthostatic hypotension
  After standing up
  After a meal
  Temporal relationship with beginning to take medication or changing the dosage
  Prolonged standing, especially in crowded, hot places
  Presence of autonomic neuropathy or parkinsonism
  After exertion
Cardiac syncope
  Presence of severe structural heart disease
  During exertion or while supine
  Preceded by palpitations or accompanied by chest pain
  Family history of sudden death
Cerebrovascular syncope
  With arm exercise
  Difference in blood pressure or pulse in the two arms

with cardiac and noncardiac causes of syncope are summarized in Table 6.

Selected Diagnostic Testing

Recommendations for specific additional diagnostic evaluation for syncope based on the initial evaluation have been provided in a recent update of the European Society of Cardiology (ESC) guidelines. A brief review of the indications and contraindications of tilt table testing, electrophysiologic study and implantable loop recorders follows.

Tilt Table Testing

The most common cause of syncope and neurally mediated syncope is vasovagal (common faint). Although the pathophysiology of vasovagal response is incompletely understood, it is generally accepted that certain physical or emotional distresses trigger a chain of events that culminate in vasodilation or bradycardia (or both). This in turn leads to the hypotension and loss of consciousness associated with vasovagal syncope.

It is generally thought that tilt table testing provokes a vasovagal response by venous pooling and orthostatic distress. Protocols for tilt table testing have not been standardized. Most recent guidelines suggest a tilt test duration of 20 to 45 minutes at 60° to 70°. Pharmacologic agents are often used to provoke a positive response if vasovagal syncope is not induced by a passive tilt table test alone. Intravenous infusion of isoproterenol and sublingual nitroglycerin are the two most frequently used provocative agents in conjunction with tilt table testing. Be aware that increased *sensitivity* (a positive response) from use of a pharmacologic agent during tilt table testing is inevitably associated with a decrease in the specificity of the test. Carefully seek a correlation of the symptoms induced during tilt table testing and the symptoms during the spontaneous clinical event.

The vasovagal response induced during tilt table testing can be classified into three subtypes: 1) mixed response (manifested by coexisting bradycardia and hypotension), 2) cardioinhibitory response (manifested by persistent bradycardia or prolonged pauses and an absence of significant hypotension when bradycardia is prevented by pacing or vagolytic agent such as atropine),

---

Table 5.   Laboratory Investigations for Syncope Evaluations

"Routine"
  CBC, electrolytes, glucose
  ECG
"Elective"
  Echocardiogram
  Holter monitor
  Ambulatory continuous blood pressure
    monitor
  Ambulatory event recorder
  Implantable event recorder
  Tilt table testing
  Electrophysiologic testing
  Neurologic testing–autonomic testing, EEG,
    OPG, carotid US, TCD, CT, MRI
  Endocrinologic testing–serum cate-
    cholamines, urine metanephrines
  Other cardiac testing–TMET, coronary
    angiography

CBC, complete blood cell count; CT, computed tomography; ECG, electrocardiogram; EEG, electroencephalogram; MRI, magnetic resonance imaging; OPG, ophthalmogram; TCD, transcranial Doppler ultrasonography; TMET, treadmill exercise test; US, ultrasonography.

Table 6.   Factors Associated With Syncope

Noncardiogenic syncope
  History and physical examination
    Isolated syncope without underlying
      cardiovascular disease
    Young age
    Symptoms consistent with a vasovagal
      cause
    Normal cardiovascular examination
  Laboratory findings
    Normal electrocardiogram
Cardiogenic syncope
  History and physical examination
    Coronary artery disease or prior
      myocardial infarction
    Congestive heart failure
    Older age
    Abrupt onset, during exertion, or when
      supine
    Serious injuries
    Abnormal cardiovascular examination
  Laboratory findings
    Abnormal electrocardiogram
    Presence of Q wave, bundle branch
      block, or sinus bradycardia
    Structural heart disease
    Left ventricular dysfunction

and 3) vasodepressor response (manifested by significant hypotension in the absence of bradycardia). The definitions of this classification are provided in Table 7. Examples of the three types of responses are shown in Figure 1.

It is generally agreed that tilt table testing is warranted in patients whose syncope is presumed (but not conclusively known) to be vasovagal and in patients with one or more of the following: 1) recurrent syncope after exclusion of organic heart disease, 2) a single syncopal episode associated with an injury or a motor vehicle accident, 3) a single event in a high-risk setting, or 4) syncope of another established cause whose treatment might be affected by vasovagal syncope. Tilt table testing is not warranted in patients who have a single episode without an injury in a low-risk setting and have no clinical features that clearly support a diagnosis of vasovagal syncope. Tilt table testing is contraindicated in patients with critical obstructive cardiac disease (e.g., critical proximal coronary artery stenosis, critical mitral stenosis, or severe left ventricular outflow tract obstruction) or critical cerebrovascular stenosis. Indications for tilt table testing from the ESC guidelines are summarized in Table 8.

Electrophysiologic Testing

When syncope is unexplained after the initial evaluation, an electrophysiologic study should be considered if the risk of an arrhythmic cause of syncope is high. During an electrophysiologic study for syncope evaluation, the following assessment should be made: 1) sinus node function, 2) atrioventricular node and His-Purkinje system conduction, and 3) inducibility of supraventricular and ventricular arrhythmias. Details of the programmed stimulation protocols during an electrophysiologic study are provided elsewhere in this book.

Indications for electrophysiologic testing are summarized in Table 9. Depending on the patient population studied and diagnostic end points, the yield from electrophysiologic testing varies significantly. An arrhythmic cause of unexplained syncope disclosed by an electrophysiologic study in patients without underlying heart disease or any abnormalities on ECG is uncommon (<10%-20%). In patients with underlying heart disease in association with left ventricular dysfunction and an abnormal ECG as a consequence of coronary artery disease or prior myocardial infarction (or both), the yield from an electrophysiologic study is higher. The value of electrophysiologic testing in patients with nonischemic cardiomyopathy undergoing syncope evaluation is less well established. Although an electrophysiologic study is indicated in this patient population with syncope, a negative study does not predict low mortality or low risk of sudden cardiac death in patients with low ejection fraction. As indications for implantable cardioverter-

Table 7.   Classification of Positive Responses to Tilt Testing

Classification	Interpretation
Type 1—mixed	HR decreases at syncope, but the ventricular rate does not decrease to <40 bpm, or it decreases falls to <40 bpm for <10 seconds with or without asystole of <3 seconds; BP decreases before HR decreases
Type 2A—cardioinhibition without asystole	HR decreases to a ventricular rate <40 bpm for >10 seconds, but a pause >3 seconds does not occur; BP decreases before the HR falls
Type 2B—cardioinhibition with asystole	A pause occurs for >3 seconds; the BP decreases with or occurs before the decrease in HR
Type 3—vasodepressor	HR does not decrease >10% from its peak at syncope

bpm, beats per minute; BP, blood pressure, HR, heart rate.

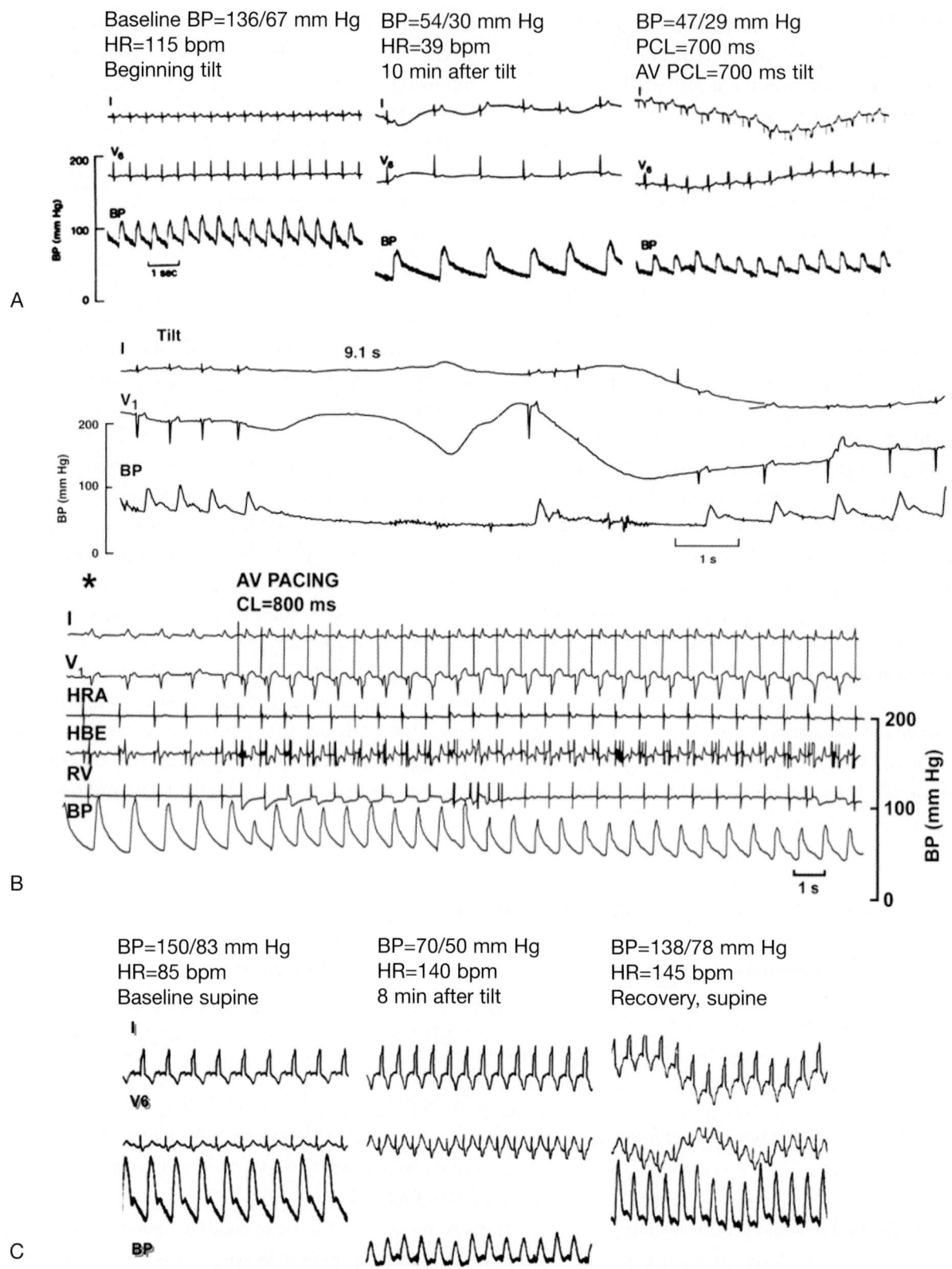

Fig. 1. Three subtypes of vasovagal response induced during tilt table testing. *A,* Mixed response. *B,* Cardioinhibitory response. *C,* Vasodepressor response. AV, atrioventricular; BP, blood pressure; bpm, beats per minute; CL, cycle length; HBE, His bundle electrogram; HR, heart rate; HRA, high right atrial electrogram; PCL, pacing cycle length; RV, right ventricular electrogram.

defibrillator (ICD) are rapidly expanding, indications for electrophysiologic testing are also rapidly evolving. The prophylactic use of ICDs for prevention of primary sudden cardiac death is now considered to be the standard of care for asymptomatic patients with an ejection fraction less than 35% with either an ischemic or a nonischemic cause and class II or III functional capacity. After patients in this population experience syncope, electrophysiologic testing is no longer deemed necessary since ICD implantation would provide appropriate therapy for syncope caused by intermittent bradycardia or ventricular tachycardia.

Implantable Loop Recorders

The implantable loop recorder has the capability of long-term (14-16 months) continuous rhythm monitoring in patients with infrequent episodes of syncope that may have an arrhythmic cause. The advantage of this approach is that the rhythm can be documented when the patient experiences a recurrent syncopal spell after the loop recorder is implanted. The potential disadvantage of this "wait-and-watch" approach is the uncertain risk of increased morbidity or mortality for the patient from waiting for another event to occur. Although several clinical studies have been conducted, the precise role of the implantable loop recorder in the evaluation of syncope has not been determined. In the ESC updated guidelines, implantable loop recorders *may* be indicated in the following circumstances:

1. In an initial phase of the work-up, instead of after completion of conventional investigations in patients with preserved cardiac function and clinical ECG features suggesting an arrhythmic syncope. (This was primarily deduced because of the low sensitivity of detecting intermittent bradycardia during an electrophysiologic study and the low risk of sustained ventricular tachycardia in patients with preserved ejection fraction and no palpitations or documented arrhythmias.)

2. To assess the contribution of bradycardia before embarking on cardiac pacing in patients with suspected or certain neurally mediated syncope who present with frequent or traumatic syncopal episodes.

In the Mayo Clinic practice, use of an implantable loop recorder is considered when infrequent episodes remain to be unexplained and when an arrhythmic cause cannot be excluded.

Table 8.   Indications for Tilt Table Testing

Class I

Unexplained single episode in a high-risk setting (occurrence of or potential risk for physical injury or occupational implications)

Recurrent, without organic heart disease

With heart disease, after cardiac causes have been excluded

When there is clinical value in demonstrating susceptibility to neurally mediated syncope to the patient

Class II

When an understanding of the hemodynamic pattern may alter the therapeutic approach

Differentiaton of syncope from jerking movements from epilepsy

Evaluation of patients with recurrent, unexplained falls

Assessment of recurrent presyncope or dizziness

Class III

Assessment of treatment

Single episode without injury and not in a high-risk setting

Clear-cut clinical vasovagal features leading to a diagnosis when demonstration of a neurally mediated susceptibility would not alter treatment

THERAPEUTIC MANAGEMENT

The appropriate treatment for syncope is usually quite obvious after the cause of syncope has been determined. Indications for pacemaker therapy in patients with documented bradycardia associated with syncope are discussed in Chapter 34 ("Cardiac Resynchronization Therapy"), appropriate therapy for symptomatic supraventricular arrhythmias (drugs or ablation) is discussed in Chapter 27 ("Supraventricular Tachycardia"), and therapy for ventricular arrhythmias (drugs, ablation, or ICD) is discussed in Chapter 28 ("Ventricular Tachycardia"). The following section provides a brief review of two areas related to syncope management that are challenging in clinical practice, namely 1) therapy for vasovagal syncope and 2) the role of ICDs after a syncopal event.

Table 9.   Indications for Electrophysiologic
           Testing

Class I

An invasive electrophysiologic procedure is
indicated when the initial evaluation
suggests an arrhythmic cause of syncope
(see Tables 4 and 6)

Class II

To evaluate the exact nature of an arrhythmia
that has already been identified as the cause
of the syncope

In patients with high-risk occupations, in
whom every effort to exclude a cardiac
cause of syncope is warranted

Class III

In patients with normal electrocardiograms,
no heart disease, and no palpitations an
electrophysiologic study is *not* usually
undertaken

Vasovagal Syncope (Common Faint)

The goals of therapy in patients with vasovagal syncope
are threefold: 1) educating patients on the causes,
prognosis, and management; 2) improving quality of
life; and 3) reducing recurrences and associated morbidity. Although most patients with vasovagal syncope
respond to conservative measures (patient education,
adequate hydration, liberalization of salt intake, compression stockings, and orthostatic training), some
patients continue to have recurrent syncope.
Pharmacologic therapy could be considered in this
group of patients.

Although the autonomic neurocardiogenic reflex
underlying the vasovagal response is complex and is
not fully understood, it is generally accepted that the
Bezold-Jarisch reflex is important in the pathogenesis
of vasovagal syncope. In this reflex, activation of
mechanoreceptors in the left ventricle (as a result of
increased cardiac contractility from sympathetic activation) stimulates C fibers, which in turn lead to vagal
activation and a withdrawal of sympathetic outflow.
Conceptually, the aim of most pharmacologic therapies
is to interrupt one or more components of this reflex
arc (Fig. 2).

One of the most challenging aspects of assessing
the efficacy of any therapeutic intervention for vasovagal
syncope is the sporadic, infrequent, and sometimes
clustering nature of this condition in a highly heterogeneous population. Most of the clinical trials with drug
therapy for vasovagal syncope have enrolled relatively
few patients and have had limited follow-up. β-
Blockers have been widely used for many years as therapy
for recurrent vasovagal syncope. However, evidence
from randomized, placebo-controlled, double-blind
clinical trials clearly does not support this widespread
practice. According to data from limited, randomized,
placebo-controlled, double-blind clinical trials, midodrine appears to be effective in selected patient groups.
When used under proper supervision, it is usually well
tolerated with minimal side effects.

One area of ongoing investigation is cardiac pacing
for vasovagal syncope. Although it was listed as a class
IIA indication for recurrent vasovagal syncope in the
2002 guidelines, recent data suggest that its efficacy is
equivocal and that it should be reserved only for severe
and refractory cases in patients with documented
bradycardia.

In summary, the treatment of vasovagal syncope
should be individualized. In some cases, reassurance
may suffice. In others, augmenting central blood volume
by increasing fluid or salt intake (or both) is effective.
The role of nonpharmacologic physical maneuvers is
increasingly recognized, given the recent clinical trial
data supporting their efficacy. Of the many pharmacologic
agents, the most promising is midodrine. Its use should
be reserved for patients with recurrent and refractory
syncope. Recommendations from the ESC guidelines
are summarized in Table 10.

ROLE OF ICD AND SYNCOPE MANAGEMENT

One should keep a clear perspective in the mortality
risk assessment of syncope patients. The vast majority
of syncope patients have disturbing or disabling conditions that are not life-threatening but may cause
injuries and a substantial decrease in quality of life.
However, syncope could be the first (and perhaps the
last) clinical event in patients with increased risk of
cardiac and arrhythmic death. These patients must be
recognized during the evaluation and therapy (i.e.,
ICD) must be implemented if appropriate. One also

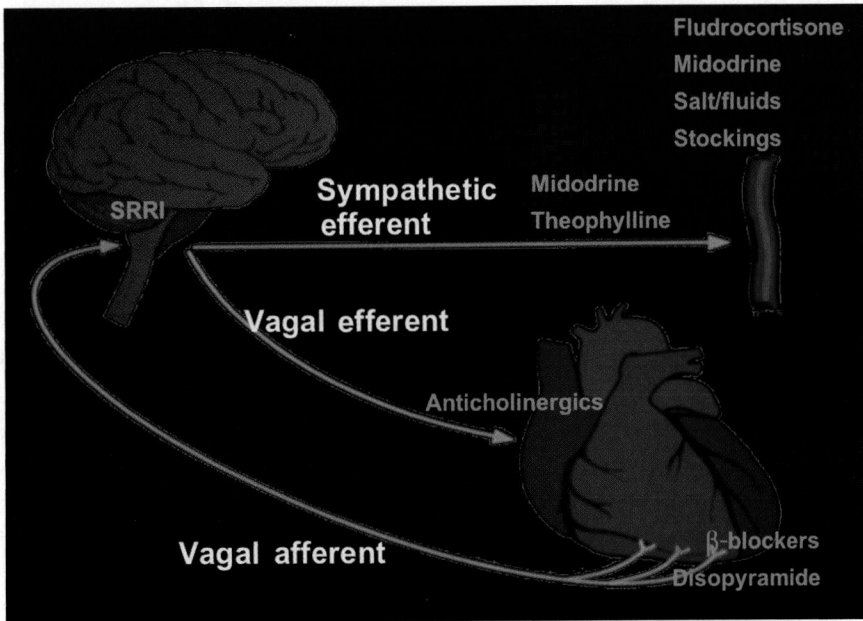

Fig. 2. Neurocardiogenic reflex and drug targets.

must be cognizant that although ICDs may prevent arrhythmic death, they may not alleviate syncope. This aspect of the treatment of the high-risk fainter is a common dilemma in ischemic heart disease and cardiomyopathy patients as well as in individuals with familial conditions such as long QT syndrome, Brugada syndrome, arrhythmogenic right ventricular cardiomyopathy, and hypertrophic cardiomyopathy.

Indications from the most recent guidelines for ICD implantation in patients with increased risk of sudden cardiac death are reviewed elsewhere in this book (Chapter 36, "ICD Trials and Prevention of Sudden Cardiac Death"). In brief, some of the key elements for ICD consideration in the context of syncope evaluation are the following:

1. When *unexplained* syncope occurs in patients who

Table 10. Treatment of Vasovagal Syncope

Class I
    Explanation of the risk and reassurance about the prognosis of vasovagal syncope
    Avoidance of potential triggers
    Modification or discontinuation of hypotensive drug treatment for concomitant conditions
    Cardiac pacing in patients with cardioinhibitory or mixed carotid sinus syndrome

Class II
    Volume expansion by salt supplements, an exercise program, or head-up tilt sleeping (>10°) in posture-
        related syncope
    Cardiac pacing in patients with cardioinhibitory type of vasovagal syncope with a frequency >5/year or
        severe injury or accident and age >40 years
    Tilt training in patients with vasovagal syncope

Class III
    Current evidence fails to support the efficacy of β-adrenergic blocking drugs. β-Adrenergic blocking drugs
        may aggravate bradycardia in some cardioinhibitory cases

meet the current criteria for ICD implantation for primary prevention of sudden cardiac death (ischemic or nonischemic cardiomyopathy with ejection fraction ≤35% and functional class II or III, or ejection fraction ≤30%), ICD implantation is indicated without an electrophysiologic study.

2. In syncope patients with ischemic or nonischemic cardiomyopathy with ejection fraction greater than 35%, ICD is indicated when sustained ventricular arrhythmia is inducible by electrophysiologic testing.

3. Among patients with primary arrhythmic congenital conditions without structural abnormalities (long QT syndrome or Brugada syndrome), *unexplained* syncope is recognized as a risk factor associated with increased sudden death. Data have been accumulated from international registries for these conditions. An ICD implantation is considered a class II indication in these patients. There is no proven role for electrophysiologic testing in long QT syndrome patients with syncope. The value of electrophysiologic testing in Brugada syndrome patients is evolving as a risk assessment tool for asymptomatic patients.

4. Among patients with primary congenital structural conditions (e.g., hypertrophic cardiomyopathy or arrhythmogenic right ventricular cardiomyopathy), *unexplained* syncope is also a risk factor associated with increased risk of sudden death. An ICD implantation is considered a class II indication in these patients. Although an electrophysiologic study could be considered (a class II indication), its role in risk stratification is also limited because of the uncertain negative predictive value of the test in both of these patient populations.

RESOURCES

Benditt DG, Ferguson DW, Grubb BP, et al. Tilt table testing for assessing syncope. J Am Coll Cardiol. 1996; 28:263-75.

Brignole M, Alboni P, Benditt D, et al. Guidelines on management (diagnosis and treatment) of syncope. Eur Heart J. 2001; 22:1256-1306.

Brignole M, Alboni P, Benditt DG, et al. Guidelines on management (diagnosis and treatment) of syncope – Update 2004. Europace. 2004;6:467-537.

Gregoratos G, Abrams J, Epstein AE, et al. ACC/AHA/NASPE 2002 guideline update for implantation of cardiac pacemakers and antiarrhythmia devices: summary article. Circulation 2002;106:2145-61.

Strickberger SA, Benson DW, Biagggioni I, et al AHA/ACCF scientific statement on the evaluation of syncope. J Am Coll Cardiol 2006; 47:473-84. Erratum in: Circulation. 2006;113:316-27.

Zipes DP, DiMarco JP, Gillette PC, et al. Guidelines for clinical intracardiac electrophysiological and catheter ablation procedures. J Am Coll Cardiol. 1995; 26:555-73.

33

Pacemakers

David L. Hayes, MD

Margaret A. Lloyd, MD

Indications for Permanent Pacing

Guidelines for permanent pacemaker implantation were established in 1984 by a joint task force of the American Heart Association and American College of Cardiology. The guidelines have been updated multiple times; the most recent were published in 2002. Indications for permanent pacing are divided into three classes: class I, pacing is acceptable and necessary; class II, pacing is probably acceptable and necessary; and class III, pacing is inappropriate. In some clinical situations, the subjective and objective data do not fit neatly into either class I or class II.

Class I

Class I indications include those in which pacing is considered necessary, provided that the indication is chronic or recurrent and is not due to transient underlying causes, such as drugs, electrolyte imbalance, or acute myocardial infarction. A single symptomatic episode is sufficient to establish the necessity for pacing. Symptoms must be clearly related to the rhythm disturbance. Indications are as follows:

1. Acquired complete (third degree) and advanced second degree atrioventricular (AV) block. Typical symptoms include syncope, seizures, dizziness, confusion, limited exercise tolerance, and congestive heart failure. Exercise testing may provide evidence of exercise intolerance. Symptoms may be subtle, especially in elderly patients. In asymptomatic patients, documented asystole of more than 3.0 seconds or a heart rate of less than 40 beats per minute during waking hours is also included as a class I indication.

2. Congenital complete (third degree) AV block with wide QRS escape complexes, complex ventricular ectopy, or left ventricular dysfunction. Another consideration for pacing is asymptomatic bradycardia with a rate less than 50 to 55 beats per minute in the awake infant or 70 beats per minute with associated congenital heart disease.

3. Second degree AV block at any level of the conduction system if associated with symptomatic bradycardia.

4. In patients with chronic bifascicular or trifascicular block with intermittent complete heart block, intermittent type II second degree AV block or alternating bundle branch blocks should be considered class I indications.

5. Symptomatic sinus bradycardia (heart rate <40 beats per minute) or symptomatic chronotropic incompetence. Symptoms include syncope or presyncope, confusion, seizures, or congestive heart failure, and they must be clearly related to the bradycardia. Pacing in patients with a heart rate

of more than 40 beats per minute may be considered; however, careful documentation of symptoms correlated with bradycardia is required.

6. Symptomatic sinus bradycardia secondary to drug treatment for which there is no acceptable alternative (e.g., amiodarone or β-blockers).

7. Sinus node dysfunction with life-threatening, bradycardiac-dependent arrhythmias (e.g., pause-dependent ventricular tachycardia). Bradycardia itself need not be symptomatic.

8. Recurrent syncope caused by carotid sinus stimulation; minimal carotid sinus pressure induces ventricular asystole of more than 3 seconds in the absence of any medication that suppresses the sinus node or AV node.

9. Neuromuscular disease, for example, myotonic muscular dystrophy, Kearns-Sayre syndrome, Erb dystrophy (limb-girdle muscular dystrophy), and peroneal muscular atrophy with AV block, with or without symptoms, because there may be an unpredictable progression of AV conduction disease.

Class II

Class II indications include those in which permanent pacing may be necessary, provided that the potential benefit to the patient can be documented. Indications are as follows:

1. Recurrent syncope caused by carotid sinus stimulation; minimal carotid sinus pressure induces ventricular asystole of more than 3 seconds in the absence of any medication that suppresses the sinus node or AV nodal conduction. Asymptomatic third degree AV block at any anatomical site with an average, awake ventricular rate of less than 40 beats per minute, especially if cardiomegaly or left ventricular dysfunction is present.

2. Asymptomatic third degree AV block with a narrow QRS complex and an average heart rate during waking hours of more than 40 beats per minute, especially if left ventricular dysfunction or cardiomegaly is present, and asymptomatic type II second degree AV block with a narrow QRS.

3. Asymptomatic type I second degree AV block at intra- or infra-His levels found at the electrophysiologic (EP) study.

4. First or second degree AV block with effective loss of AV synchrony and symptoms similar to pacemaker syndrome.

5. Neuromuscular diseases with any degree of AV block (including first degree AV block), with or without symptoms.

6. Syncope not demonstrated to be due to AV block when other likely causes have been excluded, specifically ventricular tachycardia.

7. Incidental finding at EP study of a markedly prolonged HV interval (≥100 ms) in asymptomatic patients.

8. Incidental finding at EP study of a pacing-induced infra-His block that is not physiologic.

9. Sinus node dysfunction with a heart rate less than 40 beats per minute, developing either spontaneously or as a result of necessary drug therapy, without documentation of a clear association between significant symptoms consistent with bradycardia and the actual presence of bradycardia.

10. Syncope of unexplained origin when major abnormalities of sinus node function are discovered or provoked in EP studies.

11. Prevention of symptomatic, drug-refractory, recurrent atrial fibrillation in patients with coexisting sinus node dysfunction.

12. Recurrent syncope without clear, provocative events and with a hypersensitive cardioinhibitory response.

13. Significantly symptomatic and recurrent neurocardiogenic syncope associated with bradycardia documented spontaneously or at tilt table testing.

14. Medically refractory, symptomatic hypertrophic cardiomyopathy with significant resting or provoked left ventricular outflow obstruction.

15. Biventricular pacing in medically refractory, symptomatic New York Heart Association (NYHA) class III or IV patients with idiopathic dilated or ischemic cardiomyopathy, prolonged QRS interval (≥130 ms), left ventricular end-diastolic diameter of 55 mm or more, and left ventricular ejection fraction of 35% or less.

Class III

Class III indications are those in which permanent pacing is unlikely to be of benefit; therefore, pacing is generally inappropriate. The following is an abbreviated list of such nonindications:

1. Asymptomatic sinus bradycardia
2. Asymptomatic sinus arrest or sinoatrial block
3. Asymptomatic first degree or Mobitz type I second degree AV block (Wenckebach block)

ACUTE MYOCARDIAL INFARCTION

Although the need for temporary pacing in the peri-infarct period has decreased as a result of acute coronary intervention and other aggressive approaches, various conduction disturbances may be seen in the peri-infarct period, including bradycardia and AV block. Disturbances are usually related to the site of infarction; they may be transient or permanent. Temporary pacing during the peri-infarct period is not necessarily an indication for permanent pacing. The guidelines for pacing after myocardial infarction are the following:

Class I

1. Persistent second degree AV block in the His-Purkinje system with bilateral bundle branch block or third degree AV block within or below the His-Purkinje system.
2. Transient, advanced (second or third degree) infranodal AV block and associated bundle branch block. If the site of the block is uncertain, an EP study may be necessary.
3. Persistent and symptomatic second or third degree AV block.

Class II

1. Persistent second or third degree AV block at the AV node level.

Inferior Myocardial Infarction

Conduction disturbances commonly seen in inferior myocardial infarction include sinus bradycardia, sinus arrhythmia, sinus arrest, atrial fibrillation or flutter, and AV block. First degree AV block and Mobitz type I second degree block (Wenckebach block) are more commonly seen; a minority of patients will have Mobitz type II second degree block or complete (third degree) AV block. Patients who are hemodynamically unstable may require temporary pacing. Conduction defects are usually transient and rarely require permanent pacing.

Anterior Myocardial Infarction

Patients with acute anterior myocardial infarction are more likely to have persistent conduction disturbances. Anterior myocardial infarction accompanied by AV block has an unfavorable prognosis and an increased incidence of sudden cardiac death, which are related to the large area of myocardium involved in this type of infarction. Temporary pacing is required in patients who have intermittent or persistent complete heart block, new-onset bifascicular block, or bilateral bundle branch block. Permanent pacing is usually required in these patients.

NONBRADYCARDIAC INDICATIONS FOR PACING

Pacing for medically refractory hypertrophic cardiomyopathy is a class II indication. Although enthusiasm was initially significant for pacing in hypertrophic cardiomyopathy, pacing is now used very selectively. When device therapy is used in patients with hypertrophic cardiomyopathy, it is most commonly implantable cardioverter-defibrillator (ICD) therapy for the prevention of sudden cardiac death.

Cardiac resynchronization therapy (CRT) is the term for reestablishing synchronous contraction between the left ventricular free wall and the ventricular septum in an attempt to improve left ventricular efficiency and subsequently improve functional class (see Chapter 34, "Cardiac Resynchronization Therapy"). CRT is now an accepted part of therapy for congestive heart failure. CRT has generally been used to describe biventricular pacing, but cardiac resynchronization can be achieved in some patients by left ventricular pacing only.

The Food and Drug Administration's labeling criteria for CRT are as follows: NYHA functional class III or IV; QRS complex more than 130 ms; left ventricular ejection fraction 35% or less; optimized medical therapy; and normal sinus rhythm. Devices combining CRT and ICD capabilities are also available.

PACING MODES AND NOMENCLATURE

The North American Society of Pacing and Electrophysiology and British Pacing and Electrophysiology Group (NASPE/BPEG) Generic Code is used to describe pacemaker function. The code has five positions (Table 1).

1. *Position I* indicates the chamber paced. Five letters are commonly used: *A* for atrium, *V* for ventricle, *D* if both chambers are paced, and *O* if no pacing is to occur. *S* is used by some manufacturers to indicate pacing capability in a single-chamber device.

2. *Position II* indicates the chamber sensed. Five letters are commonly used: *A* for atrium, *V* for ventricle, *D* if both chambers are sensed, and *O* if no sensing is present in any chamber and asynchronous pacing is to occur. S is used by some manufacturers to indicate sensing capability in a single-chamber device.

3. *Position III* indicates the response to a sensed signal. *I* indicates that output is inhibited by a sensed event, *T* indicates that a stimulus is triggered by a sensed event, and *D* indicates that a stimulus may be triggered or inhibited by a sensed event. For example, in dual-chamber devices, the atrial output may be inhibited by a sensed atrial event, and the ventricular stimulus triggered by a sensed atrial event (in the absence of a sensed ventricular event). The letter *O* indicates that there is no mode of response, mandating that there likewise be an *O* in the second (sensing) position.

4. *Position IV* reflects both programmability and rate modulation. An *R* in the fourth position indicates that the pacemaker incorporates a sensor to modulate the rate independently of intrinsic cardiac activity, such as with activity or respiration. From a practical standpoint, *R* is the only indicator commonly used in the fourth position.

5. *Position V* is now used to indicate whether multisite pacing is present in none of the cardiac chambers (*O*), one or both atria (*A*), one or both ventricles (*V*), or any combination of atria and ventricles (*D*). To describe a patient with a DDDR (dual-chamber rate-adaptive) pacemaker with biventricular stimulation, the code would be *DDDRV*.

When choosing the appropriate pacing mode for an individual patient one must consider the underlying rhythm abnormality, chronotropic status (i.e., whether the patient can mount an appropriate rate response for a given physiologic activity), and activity level. Table 2 summarizes available pacing modes and appropriate indications.

PERMANENT PACING LEADS

A few basic facts about permanent pacing leads warrant discussion. Pacing leads are either unipolar or bipolar. In a unipolar lead the distal electrode is the negative pole and the pulse generator "can" serves as the positive pole. In a bipolar lead the distal electrode is the negative pole and a more proximal electrode on the pacing lead is the positive pole. Bipolar leads are less susceptible to electromagnetic and electromechanical interference than unipolar leads. (Some pulse generators are polarity

Table 1.   The Revised NASPE/BPEG Generic Code for Antibradycardiac Pacing

Position I (chamber(s) paced)	Position II (chamber(s) sensed)	Position III (response to sensing)	Position IV (rate modulation)	Position V (multisite pacing)
O - None	O = None	O = None	O = None	O = None
A = Atrium	A = Atrium	T = Triggered	R = Rate modulation	A = Atrium
V = Ventricle	V = Ventricle	I = Inhibited		V = Ventricle
D = Dual (A + V)	D = Dual (A + V)	D = Dual (T + I)		D = Dual (A + V)
S* = Single (A or V)	S* = Single (A or V)			

NASPE/BPEG = North American Society of Pacing and Electrophysiology and British Pacing and Electrophysiology Group.
*Manufacturers' designation only.

Table 2. Indications for Various Pacing Modes

Mode	Generally agreed upon indications	Controversial indications	Contraindications
VVI	Atrial fibrillation with symptomatic bradycardia in the CC patient	Symptomatic bradycardia in the patient with associated terminal illness or other medical conditions from which recovery is not anticipated and pacing is life-sustaining only	Patients with known pacemaker syndrome or hemodynamic deterioration with ventricular pacing at the time of implant CI patient who will benefit from rate response Patients with hemodynamic need for dual-chamber pacing
VVIR	Fixed atrial arrhythmias (atrial fibrillation or flutter) with symptomatic bradycardia in the CI patient	As for VVI	As for VVI
AAI	Symptomatic bradycardia as a result of sinus node dysfunction in the otherwise CC patient and when AV conduction can be proved normal		Sinus node dysfunction with associated AV block either demonstrated spontaneously or during testing before implantation When adequate atrial sensing cannot be attained
AAIR	Symptomatic bradycardia as a result of sinus node dysfunction in the CI patient and when AV conduction can be proved normal		As for AAI
VDD†	Congenital AV block AV block when sinus node function can be proved normal		Sinus node dysfunction AV block when accompanied by sinus node dysfunction When adequate atrial sensing cannot be attained AV block when accompanied by paroxysmal supraventricular tachycardias
DDI	Need for dual-chamber pacing in the presence of significant PSVT in the CC patient	Sinus node dysfunction in the absence of AV block and in the presence of significant PSVT in the CC patient	CI patient with a demonstrated need or improvement with rate responsiveness
DDIR‡	AV block and sinus node dysfunction in the CI patient in the presence of significant PSVT	Sinus node dysfunction without AV block in the CI paient in the presence of significant PSVT	

Table 2 (continued)

Mode	Generally agreed upon indications	Controversial indications	Contraindications
DDD	AV block and sinus node dysfunction in the CC patient Need for AV synchrony, (i.e., to maximize cardiac output) in CC active patients Previous pacemaker syndrome	For any rhythm disturbance when atrial sensing and capture is possible for the potential purposes of minimizing future atrial fibrillation and improving morbidity and survival	Presence of chronic atrial fibrillation, atrial flutter, giant inexcitable atrium, or other frequent paroxysmal supraventricular tachyarrhythmias When adequate atrial sensing cannot be attained
DDDR	AV block and sinus node dysfunction in the CI patient	As for DDD	As for DDD

AV, atrioventricular; CC, chronotropically competent (i.e., able to achieve an appropriate heart rate for a given physiologic activity); CI, chronotropically incompetent (i.e., unable to achieve an appropriate heart rate for a given physiologic activity); PSVT, paroxysmal supraventricular tachycardia.

*DVI as a stand-alone pacing mode (i.e., a pacemaker capable of DVI as the only dual-chamber mode of operation) is obsolete. All primary uses of this mode should be considered individually.

†VDD as a stand-alone pacing mode (i.e., a pacemaker capable of VDD as the only dual-chamber mode of operation) is currently used primarily as a single-lead VDD system. If a dual-lead system is implanted, the capability of DDD pacing is desirable.

‡DDIR is being supplanted by DDD or DDDR pacemakers with the capability of mode-switching (i.e., the pacemaker automatically reprograms to a mode incapable of tracking the atrial rhythm in the presence of an atrial rhythm that the pacemaker classifies as pathologic). When the pacemaker recognizes the atrial rhythm as physiologic, the pacemaker reprograms to the previously programmed mode.

programmable. If a problem occurs when a bipolar lead is in service, reprogramming the pacemaker to unipolar pacing configuration may restore normal function. Likewise, if a bipolar pulse generator is in use and electromagnetic interference (EMI) is problematic when programmed to a unipolar sensing configuration, reprogramming to a bipolar sensing configuration may alleviate the problem.)

The outer insulation of pacing leads may by silicone rubber or polyurethane. There are advantages and disadvantages of each type of insulating material. All pacing leads have some mechanism of fixation, which is classified as either active or passive. Passive fixation leads usually have small tines that extend from the lead tip. The tines are designed to become entrapped in the endocardial trabeculae and stabilize the lead until scar tissue forms around the lead. Active fixation leads

usually have a screw that is screwed into the endocardium. The screw may be permanently extended or it may be extendable and retractable. Active fixation leads are currently the most commonly used variety.

Most leads are designed to maintain a low stimulation or capture threshold. Steroid-eluting leads characteristically have lower acute and chronic thresholds than non–steroid-eluting leads. In addition to steroid-eluting leads, there are other low-threshold design leads (e.g., carbon-tipped and platinized electrodes). Low thresholds are desirable to maximize the battery life of the device.

PACEMAKER SYNDROME

Pacemaker syndrome is a hemodynamic abnormality that can result when use of ventricular pacing is inappropriate or when ventricular pacing is uncoupled from the atrial contraction. This syndrome is most common when the VVI mode is used in patients with sinus rhythm, but it can occur in any pacing mode if AV synchrony is lost.

Although the most common clinical presentation is that of general malaise, patients may experience a sensation of fullness in the head and neck, syncope or presyncope, hypotension, cough, dyspnea, congestive heart failure, or weakness. Physical findings include cannon *a* waves and a lower blood pressure when pacing than when in normal sinus rhythm. If pacemaker syndrome occurs in the patient with a VVI or VVIR pacemaker, the only definitive treatment is conversion to a dual-chamber system. If the episodes of symptomatic bradycardia are rare, the symptoms of pacemaker syndrome may be alleviated by programming the pacemaker to a lower rate limit and programming hysteresis "on." This would minimize pacing and allow the patient to stay in normal sinus rhythm for longer periods. If pacemaker syndrome occurs in the patient with an atrial or dual-chamber pacing system, the cause of AV uncoupling

must be identified and corrected (e.g., in the patient with an AAIR pacing system and a very long AR interval and effective AV uncoupling, ventricular pacing may be required to allow a shorter AV interval); in the patient with a DDD system and noise sensed on the atrial lead with ventricular tracking and effective ventricular pacing and AV uncoupling.

If single-chamber ventricular pacing is considered, a trial of ventricular pacing should be performed at implantation and the blood pressure compared with that during sinus rhythm. If blood pressure decreases with ventricular pacing or if the patient experiences symptoms, dual-chamber pacing should be used; however, pacemaker syndrome may develop even without symptoms or a decrease in blood pressure (Fig. 1).

TROUBLESHOOTING

Pacemaker questions on cardiology examinations will most likely relate to troubleshooting. Most pacemaker problems are the result of inappropriate programming,

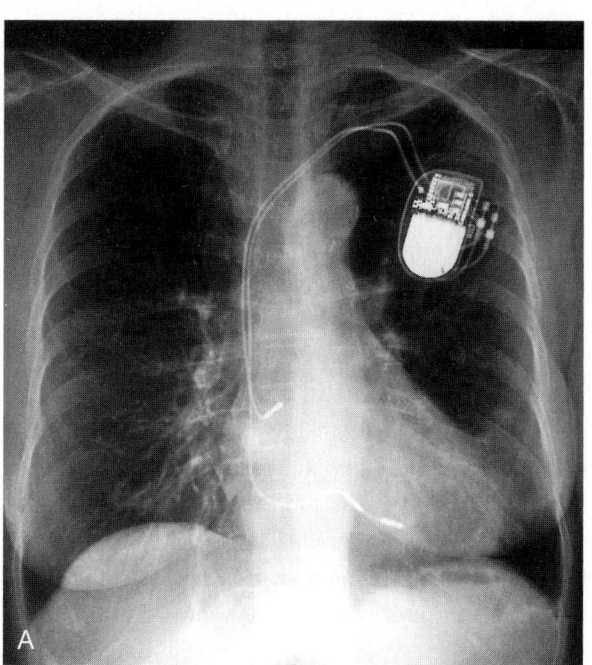
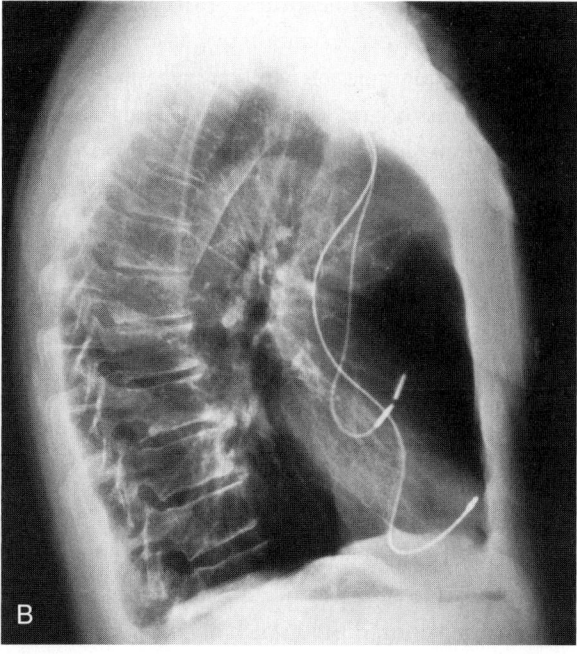

Fig. 1. *A,* Posteroanterior chest radiograph. Normal appearance of dual-chamber pacing system. Pacemaker generator is implanted in the upper left infraclavicular region. One atrial lead is present in right atrial appendage, and one ventricular lead is present in right ventricular apex. Gentle redundancy is present on both leads. Ventricular lead can be clearly visualized as bipolar. *B,* Lateral chest radiograph. Normal appearance of dual-chamber pacing system. Ventricular lead is clearly anterior; therefore it is in right ventricular apex and not in coronary sinus (in which case it would be pointing backward toward the spine). Atrial lead is clearly visualized as bipolar.

inappropriate mode selection, or lead malfunction. Initial troubleshooting should always include interrogation of the device and careful evaluation of electrocardiographic tracings. Pacing and sensing thresholds should be evaluated, and lead impedance should be noted. A chest radiograph should be obtained if lead impedances or electrocardiographic tracings suggest a potential lead problem (Fig. 1).

Failure to sense or capture in the immediate post-implantation period is most likely due to micro- or macrodislodgment of the lead or to a poor connection between the lead and the set screw within the connector block of the pulse generator (Fig. 2).

Failure to output is not synonymous with failure to capture and is usually the result of oversensing (Table 3). Failure to capture is characterized by a pacemaker artifact without subsequent depolarization of the chamber paced, and failure to output is characterized by a lack of pacemaker artifact at the appropriate point in the timing cycle.

Lead Abnormalities

Lead conductor fracture may manifest as high lead impedance, failure to capture, or oversensing with inappropriate output inhibition or muscle stimulation (Table 4). Lead insulation failure usually presents with low lead impedance, undersensing or oversensing, failure to capture, muscle stimulation, or early battery depletion. Every lead has a characteristic range of normal impedance. Lead impedance is most commonly 400 to 1500 ohms but there are exceptions. Steroid-eluting leads characteristically have lower acute and chronic thresholds than non–steroid-eluting leads.

Crosstalk

Crosstalk develops when an electrical event in one chamber is sensed in the other chamber, with inappropriate inhibition of the pacing stimulus in the second chamber (Fig. 3). An example is an atrial stimulus that is sensed by the ventricular lead as a ventricular event, with consequent inhibition of ventricular output and ventricular asystole. Crosstalk most commonly occurs when the stimulus field is large or the stimulus output is high. Although these conditions are more likely to develop when unipolar sensing or pacing is used, crosstalk can be seen in bipolar systems.

Crosstalk may be eliminated by altering the

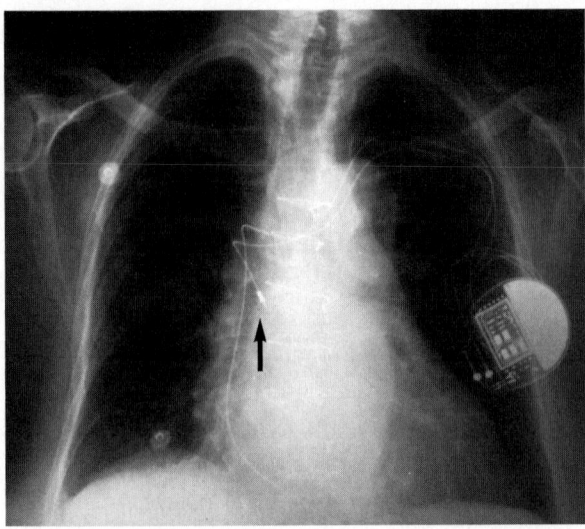

Fig. 2. Posteroanterior chest radiograph, demonstrating dislodgment of the atrial lead (*arrow*) the day after implantation of a permanent dual-chamber pacemaker. Position of the lead does not permit atrial sensing or pacing.

ventricular blanking period. The *blanking period* is a portion of the timing cycle that begins with the atrial pacing stimulus. During the blanking period the sensing circuit is "turned off" so that no electrical activity is sensed on the ventricular sensing circuit. The ventricular blanking period is almost always programmable. The adverse outcome of crosstalk (i.e., ventricular asystole) may be prevented by using safety pacing; however, it is important to understand that safety pacing does not correct crosstalk. With safety pacing, any event that is sensed immediately after the blanking period in the "crosstalk sensing window" is followed by a committed early ventricular stimulus, producing a shortened AV delay, usually from 100 to 110 ms (Fig. 4). This portion of the timing cycle is programmable in some pacemakers.

There are other ways to treat crosstalk in addition to lengthening the ventricular blanking period. One or both of the following approaches can be used: decrease the atrial output or program the ventricular sensitivity to a less sensitive value. (These approaches are predicated on the continued ability to achieve atrial capture and appropriate ventricular sensing, respectively.) Switching from unipolar pacing or sensing to bipolar pacing or sensing may eliminate crosstalk if the pacing system allows this programmable change in lead polarity configuration.

Table 3.   Causes of Pacemaker Malfunction

Failure to capture
    High thresholds with an inadequately pro-
       grammed output
    Partial conductor coil fracture
    Insulation defect
    Lead dislodgment or perforation
    Impending total battery depletion
    Functional noncapture
    Poor or incompatible connection at connector
       block
    Circuit failure
    Air in pocket (unipolar pacemaker)
Failure to output
    Circuit failure
    Complete or intermittent conductor coil frac-
       ture
    Intermittent or permanently loose set screw
    Incompatible lead or header
    Total battery depletion
    Internal insulation failure (bipolar lead)
    Far-field sensing or T-wave oversensing
    Oversensing any noncardiac activity
    Lack of anodal connector contact*
    Crosstalk
Undersensing
    Morphology of intrinsic event different from
       that measured at implantation
    Lead dislodgment or poor lead positioning
    Lead insulation failure
    Circuit failure
    Magnet application
    Malfunction of reed switch
    Electromagnetic interference
    Battery depletion
    Poor or incompatible connection at connector
       block
    Circuit failure
    Air in pocket (unipolar pacemaker)

*Examples include unipolar lead in bipolar generator, bipolar lead in pacemaker programmed as unipolar, air in the pocket of a unipolar device, and unipolar pacemaker not in the pocket.

Pacemaker-Mediated Tachycardia

Pacemaker-mediated tachycardia (PMT) can occur only with dual-chamber pacing systems with intact atrial sensing (i.e., DDD, DDDR, and VDD systems) (Fig. 5). Types of PMT include rapid tracking of atrial fibril-

Table 4.   Intraoperative Evaluation of Pacing System

Defect	Voltage threshold	Current threshold	Lead imped-ance
Wire fracture	High	High, normal, or low	High
Insulation break	Low	High	Low
Lead dis-lodgment	High	High	Normal
Exit block	High	High	Normal

lation or flutter or rapid ventricular triggering from electromagnetic interference. Endless-loop tachycardia refers to a specific type of PMT; intact VA conduction results in retrograde P waves, which trigger another ventricular stimulation, creating a loop. The situation can be corrected by lengthening the post-ventricular atrial refractory period (PVARP) beyond the retrograde P wave, so that the retrograde P wave is not sensed and therefore does not initiate an AV timing cycle. Most devices have a programmable option of PVARP extension after a premature ventricular contraction or some other algorithm to recognize and terminate PMT. Premature ventricular contractions are the most common initiator of endless-loop tachycardias.

Electromagnetic Interference

EMI can affect pacemaker performance. Devices are designed to filter out much EMI; however, some sources of EMI cannot be avoided.

EMI in the Hospital Environment

The hospital environment is a frequent source of EMI. Electrocautery, for example, inhibits pacemakers; therefore, the pacemaker should be programmed to an asynchronous mode before starting the surgical procedure, especially in pacemaker-dependent patients. The use of electrocautery, cardioversion, and defibrillation equipment can damage the pacemaker internal circuitry if used near the pacemaker; this equipment should be kept at

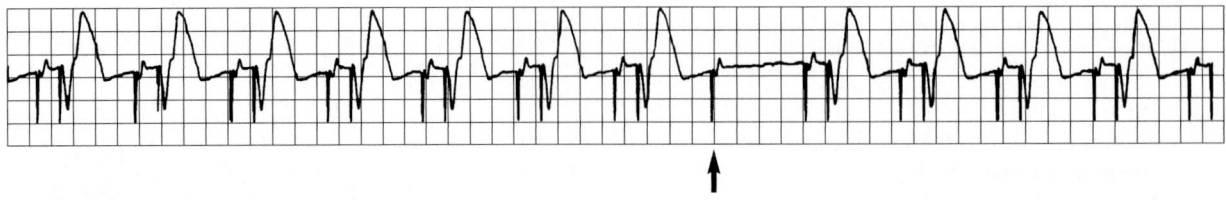

Fig. 3. Electrocardiographic strip demonstrating pacemaker crosstalk. In the eighth complex (*arrow*), the ventricular output is inhibited as a result of sensing of the atrial pacemaker artifact in the ventricular channel.

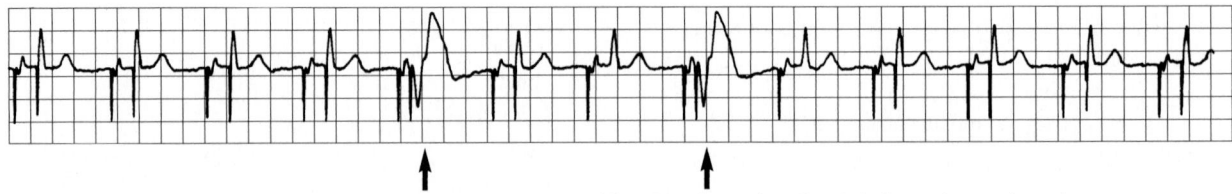

Fig. 4. Electrocardiographic strip demonstrating safety pacing. The fifth (*arrow*) and eighth (*arrow*) complexes have atrial pacing followed by ventricular pacing artifact at a fixed atrioventricular (AV) interval of 110 ms. At this interval, there is complete depolarization of the ventricle by the pacemaker. The remainder of the complexes on the strip reveal an AV delay of 200 ms and ventricular fusion complexes.

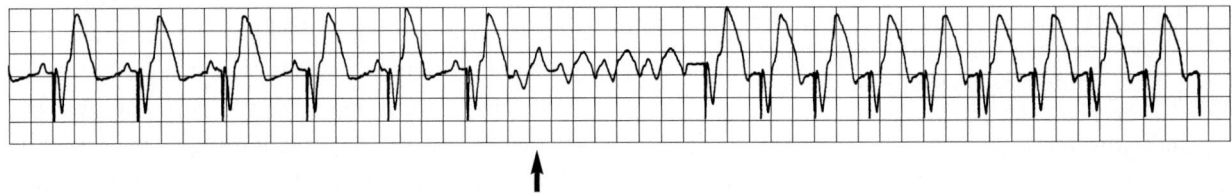

Fig. 5. Electrocardiographic strip demonstrating pacemaker-mediated tachycardia initiated by a ventricular triplet (*arrow*).

least 6 inches away from the pacemaker during surgical procedures.

Magnetic resonance imaging (MRI) uses magnetic and radiofrequency fields that cause all pacemakers to pace asynchronously by closing the reed switch. Additionally, the radiofrequency field theoretically has the potential to induce rapid, asynchronous pacing. Although it is recommended that patients with pacemakers avoid MRI, patients who are not pacemaker dependent have undergone MRI with the pacemaker output lowered below the capture threshold or programmed off. The patient must be carefully monitored throughout the procedure.

Radiofrequency ablation can result in pacemaker inhibition or reprogramming. The pacemaker programmer should be available during the procedure and the pacemaker interrogated at the end of the procedure to document programmed parameters.

Therapeutic radiation may damage the pacemaker components, resulting in damage to circuits or complete pacemaker failure. Radiation-induced failure may manifest as sudden "no output" or "runaway" pacemaker. This potential is of special concern in patients receiving therapeutic radiation for breast or chest malignancies. Damage is not related to the cumulative dose but rather may occur at any time during the course of therapy. If irradiation is being used for carcinoma of the breast or lung and the pacemaker is located on the same side as the malignancy, the pacemaker should be moved before initiating irradiation. For irradiation of any other portion of the body, the generator should be shielded.

Electroshock therapy for depressive disorders will not result in pacemaker malfunction but may cause significant electrocardiographic artifact and could potentially reprogram the pacemaker.

Extracorporeal shock wave lithotripsy may interfere

with pacemaker function. The lithotriptor is usually synchronized to the ventricular output or the pacemaker ventricular stimulus, so programming the pacemaker to fixed-rate ventricular pacing is safe. If the lithotriptor is synchronized to the atrial stimulus, loss of ventricular output may result and should be avoided. Therefore, before lithotripsy the pacemaker should be programmed to the VOO, VVI, or DOO modes. The focal point of the lithotriptor should be at least 6 inches away from the pulse generator to avoid damage to the device.

All pacemakers should be interrogated before and after procedures known to be capable of producing EMI to ensure that inadvertent reprogramming or damage to the pacemaker has not occurred. Appropriate programmers should be available during the procedures in the event that problems occur.

EMI in the Nonhospital Environment

Permanent damage to pacing systems by electrical equipment outside the hospital environment is unlikely; however, temporary interference may occur with exposure to certain devices and electromagnetic fields. Potential sources of exposure include heavy motors and arc welding. Devices such as airport metal detectors may cause single-beat inhibition, but should not cause significant clinical sequelae. Microwave ovens do not interfere with pacemaker function. Patients who work in an environment that may cause significant interference with pacemaker function may need to change occupations or at least avoid specific devices in the workplace. If there is a question of risk in the workplace, an engineer from the manufacturer can be consulted, or work site testing can be performed.

Commercially available cellular phones do not usually cause significant EMI. Pacemaker patients using cellular phones should avoid carrying an activated phone in a pocket directly over the pacemaker.

Antitheft devices and electronic article surveillance equipment can cause pacemaker interference. However, as long as the pacemaker patient does not linger near the antitheft device, there is little chance of significant interference.

Miscellaneous Considerations

Several physiologic conditions can affect pacemaker function and are sometimes interpreted as intrinsic pacemaker malfunction. Electrolyte and severe metabolic disturbances may result in failure to capture or sense. Severe hyperkalemia is the most common electrolyte disorder to cause pacing-related problems and is most commonly encountered in patients with severe renal insufficiency. Toxic levels of several antiarrhythmics raise pacing thresholds; however, no significant problems have been demonstrated at therapeutic levels of these drugs. Class 1C antiarrhythmics (flecainide, encainide, and propafenone) have consistently been shown to significantly increase pacing thresholds. This increase is sometimes dramatic, and these agents should be avoided or used with caution in pacemaker-dependent patients. Amiodarone does not consistently increase pacing thresholds but often increases defibrillation thresholds in the ICD patient. If amiodarone administration leads to hypothyroidism, pacing thresholds may be elevated as a result of the hypothyroid state.

Systemic steroids can lower pacing thresholds and have been used clinically for this purpose. Pacing thresholds usually increase to pretreatment levels when systemic steroid use is discontinued.

RISKS OF PACEMAKER IMPLANTATION

Patients should be advised that pacemaker implantation is a surgical procedure and is associated with procedural risks such as bleeding, infection, lead dislodgment, and pneumothorax (Fig. 6). Implantation should be avoided in patients with active infection. Coagulation test results should be normalized, although implantation can usually be accomplished with mildly elevated prothrombin times. Chest radiography should be performed after implantation to check for pneumothorax and to verify lead position. Patients should also be advised of the additional risk of coronary sinus dissection and phrenic nerve or diaphragmatic stimulation if a coronary sinus lead is being placed.

TEMPORARY PACING

Temporary pacing can be used in patients with symptomatic bradycardia, either transiently if the cause is reversible or as a bridge to permanent pacing. Common transvenous approaches include the internal jugular vein, the subclavian vein, the femoral vein, and, less commonly, the external jugular vein.

There are two major types of temporary ventricular

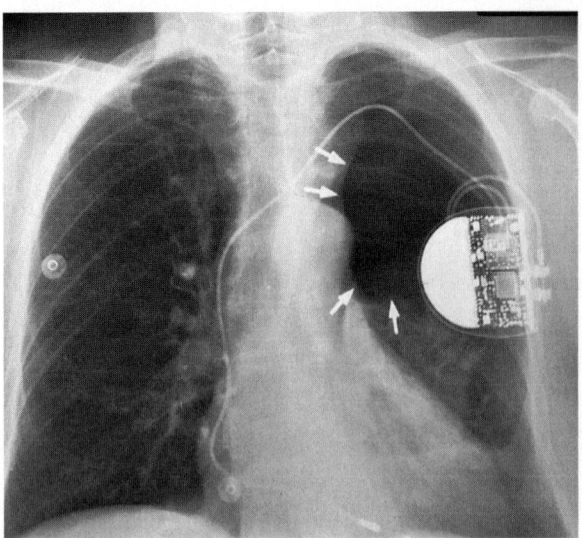

Fig. 6. Posteroanterior chest radiograph revealing pneumothorax the day after pacemaker implantation.

pacing catheters: 1) a rigid, firm catheter and 2) a more flexible, balloon-tipped catheter. Although the balloon-tipped catheter may be easier to advance into the right ventricular apex, the firmer catheter usually provides a more stable catheter position. Pulmonary artery catheters are available with an extra port through which a temporary pacing wire can be placed. These are advantageous in that they can be placed quickly without fluoroscopic guidance; however, the pacing wire is relatively unstable. Atrial "J" catheters are available

for those cases in which atrial pacing is required (e.g., atrial overdrive pacing or dual-chamber temporary pacing for patients who, hemodynamically, do not tolerate single-chamber ventricular pacing).

Potential complications of temporary pacing include complications of permanent pacing: bleeding, infection, lead dislodgment, and pneumothorax. There is a higher risk of cardiac perforation with temporary pacing catheters owing to the stiffness of the catheters.

External pacing systems are widely available and can be used in patients who have intermittent conduction disturbances or who need to maintain rhythm until a transvenous pacing catheter can be placed. Disadvantages of external pacing include occasional difficulty maintaining capture as well as potentially significant discomfort from the pacing stimulus for some patients.

RESOURCES

Pacing indications:

ACC Pacing Indications [cited 2006 Aug 6]. Available at: http://www.acc.org/clinical/guidelines/pacemaker/incorporated/index.htm

NASPE/BPEG nomenclature:

Bernstein AD, Daubert J-C, Fletcher RD, et al. The revised NASPE/BPEG generic code for antibradycardia, adaptive-rate, and multisite pacing. PACE. 2002;25:260-4.

34

Cardiac Resynchronization Therapy

David L. Hayes, MD

Cardiac resynchronization therapy (CRT) is the term applied to reestablishing synchrony between left ventricular free wall and ventricular septal contraction in an attempt to improve left ventricular efficiency and subsequently improve functional class. In some patients, this therapy may be biventricular pacing and in other patients, left ventricular pacing only may accomplish resynchronization.

The inclusion criteria for clinical trials have been relatively narrow. As a result, the data are convincing for the current U.S. Food and Drug Administration labeling criteria: New York Heart Association (NYHA) functional class III or IV, wide QRS, normal sinus rhythm, and biventricular pacing configuration. Clinical trial data have led to the following class IIa indication: biventricular pacing in patients with medically refractory, symptomatic NYHA class III or IV who have idiopathic dilated or ischemic cardiomyopathy, prolonged QRS interval ($\geq$130 milliseconds), left ventricular end-diastolic diameter 55 mm or more, and ejection fraction 35% or less.

To date, more than 4,000 patients have been included in completed randomized clinical trials of CRT. The majority of trials have relied on primary end points reflecting functional status, specifically, the 6-minute walk test, NYHA functional class, and quality of life. More recent trials have used composite end points, including outcomes such as cardiac mortality, all-cause mortality, and hospitalization for congestive heart failure.

Randomized clinical trials have been relatively consistent in finding improvement in the 6-minute walk test, NYHA functional class, and quality of life as assessed with the Minnesota Living With Heart Failure questionnaire (Table 1).

Relative consistency also has been found in some secondary end points. In studies assessing peak oxygen consumption ($\dot{V}O_2$) in patients in NYHA class III or IV, this end point has usually improved. The echocardiographic variable of left ventricular end-diastolic dimension has consistently shown a decrease, a finding suggesting reverse left ventricular remodeling. When mitral regurgitation has been assessed, it has often decreased after CRT (http://www.hrsonline.org/positionDocs/CRT_12_3.pdf).

IMPLANTATION TECHNIQUE

Implantation of a CRT device requires placing a lead in the coronary venous system, positioned in such a way that the left ventricular free wall is stimulated. There is marked variation in coronary venous anatomy, and lead placement is sometimes technically challenging (Fig. 1 and 2). With experience, the placement success rate in the left ventricle is more than 90%. When

Table 1. Randomized Clinical Trials of Cardiac Resynchronization Therapy

Trial	Design	No. of patients	End points		Results
			Primary	Secondary	
PATH-CHF	Crossover	41	Peak $\dot{V}O_2$ 6MW	Hospitalizations NYHA class QOL	Chronic improvement in 6MW, QOL, and NYHA class
MUSTIC-SR	Crossover	58	6MW	NYHA class QOL Peak $\dot{V}O_2$ Worsening CHF Pt preference Total mortality	Sustained improvement in 6MW, NYHA class, QOL, and peak $\dot{V}O_2$ Hospitalizations reduced with CRT at $P<.05$
MUSTIC-AF	Crossover	43	6MW	NYHA class QOL Peak $\dot{V}O_2$ Worsening CHF Pt preference Total mortality	Sustained improvement in 6MW, NYHA class, QOL, and peak $\dot{V}O_2$ Fewer hospitalizations with CRT
MIRACLE	Parallel arms	453	6MW NYHA class QOL	Peak $\dot{V}O_2$ Exercise time LVEF LVEDD MR QRS duration Clinical composite response	Sustained improvement in all three primary end points
MIRACLE-ICD	Parallel arms	555	6MW NYHA class QOL	Peak $\dot{V}O_2$ Exercise time Clinical composite response	Improvement in QOL and functional class; no improvement in 6MW
COMPANION	Parallel arms	1,520	Primary composite end point was time to death from or hospitalization for any cause	All-cause mortality Cardiac morbidity Maximal exercise	CRT and CRT-D reduced risk of primary end point

Table 1 (continued)

Trial	Design	No. of patients	End points		Results
			Primary	Secondary	
CARE-HF	Open label randomization to control vs. CRT device	813	All-cause mortality	All-cause mortality; All-cause mortality and unplanned hospitalizations for or with heart failure; Days alive and not in hospital for unplanned cardiovascular cause during minimum period of follow-up; Days alive and not in hospital for any reason during minimum period of follow-up; NYHA at 90 days; QOL at 90 days; Patient status at end of study	CRT (without defibrillation) improved symptoms and QOL and reduced complications and risk of death
PATH-CHF II	Crossover (no pacing vs. left ventricular pacing)	86	$\dot{V}O_2$ peak; $\dot{V}O_2$ anaerobic; 6MW	QOL; NYHA class	Exercise tolerance, 6MW, and QOL improved
MIRACLE ICD II	Parallel arms	186	$\dot{V}O_2$	$\dot{V}E/\dot{V}O_2$; NYHA class; QOL; 6MW; LV volumes; LVEF; Composite clinical response	Improvement in QOL, functional status, and exercise capacity
CONTAK-CD	Crossover and parallel controlled	490	6MW; NYHA class; QOL	Composite of mortality, CHF, hospitalizations, VT, and VF	Trend toward decreased morbidity and mortality end point; Improvement in exercise capacity, QOL, and NHYA class

Table 1 (continued)

| Trial | Design | No. of patients | End points | | Results |
			Primary	Secondary	
PATH-CHF II	Crossover (left univentricular pacing vs. biventricular pacing)	41	Peak $\dot{V}O_2$ 6MW	Hospitalizations NYHA class QOL	Chronic improvement in 6MW, QOL, and NYHA class when results pooled No significant difference between left univentricular and biventricular pacing
RD-CHF	Crossover of patients already paced with class III or IV CHF (right ventricular vs. biventricular pacing)	44	6MW NYHA class QOL	QRS width Hospitalizations	In previously paced patients, upgrading from RV to biventricular pacing significantly improved symptoms and exercise tolerance
MIRACLE ICD II	Parallel controlled trial. Patients with class II CHF randomized to ICD on and CRT activated or ICD on and CRT not activated	186	Quality of life NYHA class 6MW $\dot{V}O_2$, $\dot{V}E/CO_2$	LV volumes Ejection fraction Composite clinical response	CRT did not alter exercise capacity CRT did result in significant improvement in cardiac volumes and LVEF and composite clinical response over 6 mo

*The names of the trials are provided in the Appendix at the end of the chapter.

CHF, congestive heart failure; CRT, cardiac resynchronization therapy; ICD, implantable cardioverter-defibrillator; LVEDD, left ventricular end-diastolic diameter; LVEF, left ventricular ejection fraction; MR, mitral regurgitation; MW, mile walk; NYHA, New York Heart Association; Pt, patient; QOL, quality of life; RV, right ventricular; $\dot{V}E/\dot{V}CO_2$, ventilatory response to exercise; $\dot{V}O_2$, oxygen consumption.

an adequate position cannot be obtained, CRT can be achieved by placing an epicardial lead on the desired location of the left ventricle.

In addition to the risks normally quoted to any patient undergoing implantation of a pacemaker or cardioverter-defibrillator, the coronary sinus or coronary veins can be damaged (e.g., dissection or perforation) with implantation of a CRT device. In experienced hands, such complications are uncommon, but they should be discussed with the patient.

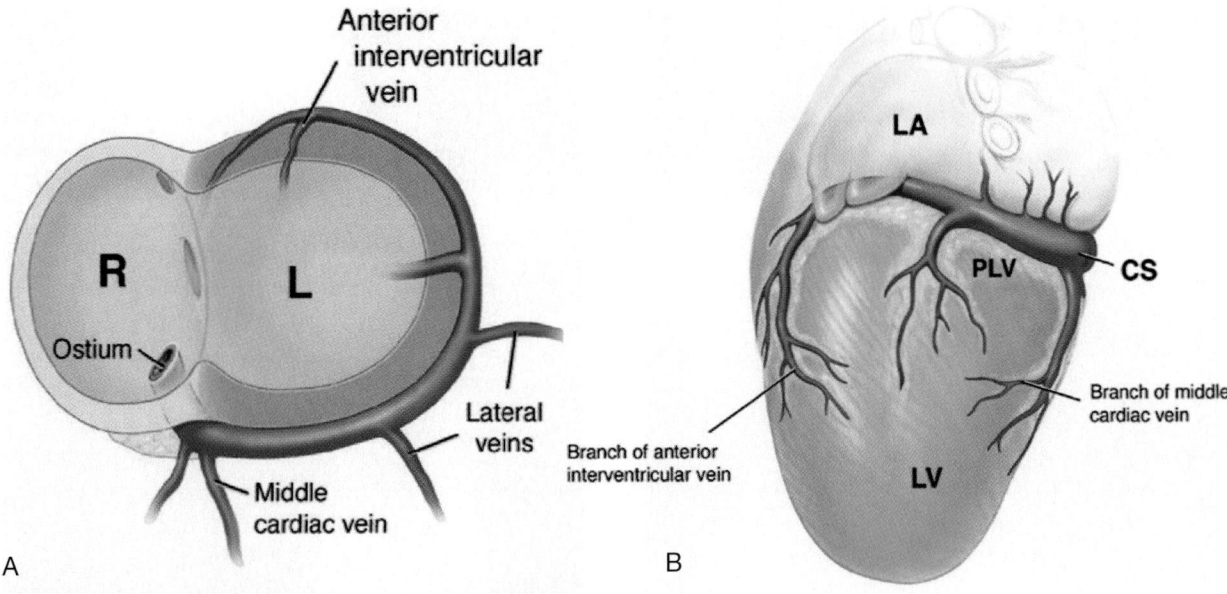

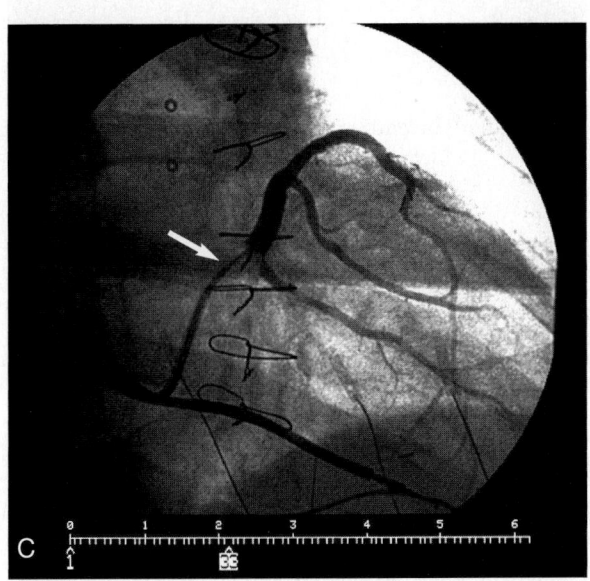

Fig. 1. *A*, Left anterior oblique cross-sectional view of heart at level of coronary sinus, showing most common location of cardiac veins in relation to left ventricle. L, left; R, right. *B*, Left lateral view of heart, showing cardiac veins and usual left ventricular epicardial location. CS, coronary sinus; LA, left atrium; LV, left ventricle; PLV, posterolateral vein. *C*, Fluoroscopic view of coronary sinus system. Inflated balloon-tipped catheter is occluding coronary sinus (*arrow*) while contrast material is injected, outlining the coronary venous system.

Leads positioned in the coronary venous system also have a higher potential to cause diaphragmatic stimulation. This complication must be assessed at the time of implantation. Even if diaphragmatic stimulation is absent at the time of testing, slight movement of the lead may cause this complication, which could subsequently require reprogramming or lead repositioning.

ASSESSMENT AFTER IMPLANTATION

There are different definitions for a "responder" to CRT. Functional response includes an improvement in NYHA functional class, 6-minute walk test, and the Minnesota Living With Heart Failure score compared with baseline. Other, more objective measurable end points were described above.

An emerging technique is to assess left ventricular dyssynchrony with various echocardiographic techniques. These techniques also are being used before implantation to determine that there is intraventricular dyssynchrony of the left ventricle before a CRT device is implanted. Many echocardiographic variables are available, and the superior ones have not yet been established with certainty.

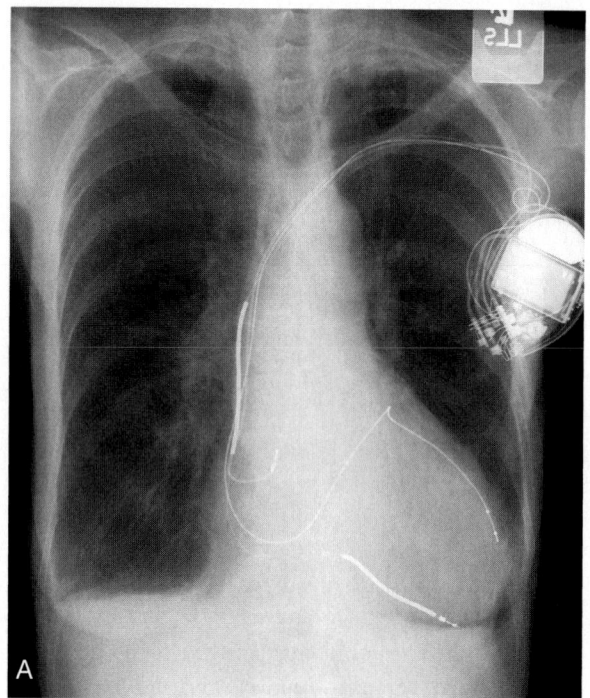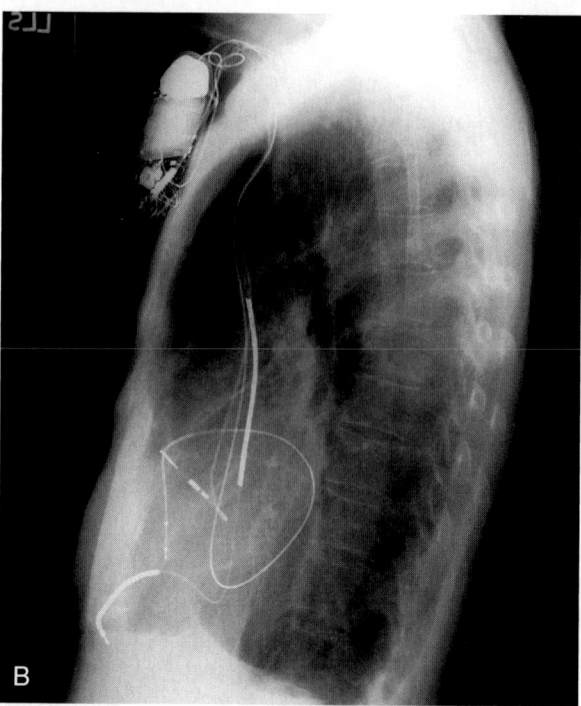

Fig. 2. Posteroanterior (*A*) and lateral (*B*) chest radiographs for patient with biventricular dual-chamber implantable cardioverter-defibrillator in place.

APPENDIX
NAMES OF CLINICAL TRIALS

CARE-HF	Cardiac Resynchronization in Heart Failure
COMPANION	Comparison of Medical Therapy, Pacing, and Defibrillation in Heart Failure
CONTAK-CD	Guidant CONTAK CD CRT-D System Trial
MIRACLE	Multicenter InSync Randomized Clinical Evaluation
MIRACLE-ICD	Multicenter InSync Randomized Clinical Evaluation Implantable Cardioverter-Defibrillator
MIRACLE-ICD II	Multicenter InSync Randomized Clinical Evaluation Implantable Cardioverter-Defibrillator II
MUSTIC-AF	Multisite Stimulation in Cardiomyopathy-Atrial Fibrillation
MUSTIC-SR	Multisite Stimulation in Cardiomyopathy-Sinus Rhythm
PATH-CHF	Pacing Therapies for Congestive Heart Failure
PATH-CHF II	Pacing Therapies for Congestive Heart Failure II

35

Technical Aspects of Implantable Cardioverter-Defibrillators

Robert F. Rea, MD

Implantable cardioverter-defibrillators (ICDs) have become increasingly complex and feature-laden, but, for the board examination in cardiovascular diseases, only a handful of concepts and pieces of technical information are critical.

Components of an ICD System

An ICD consists of a pulse generator, a ventricular shocking or sensing lead, and sometimes an atrial lead. The ICD lead differs from a standard pacing lead in that it has coil electrodes, typically two, one in the superior vena cava-right atrium and one in the right ventricle; in addition, one or two small electrodes used for pacing and sensing are near the tip of the lead (Fig. 1). Shocks are delivered between the electrodes and the pulse-generator canister in different pathways, but most commonly with the right ventricle as cathode (negative) and the superior vena cava-right atrium coil and the pulse-generator canister as anode (positive). The shock pathways are programmable in various ways in different manufacturers' devices. The most common variation is to reverse the polarity so that right ventricle is anode and the superior vena cava-right atrium–canister is cathode.

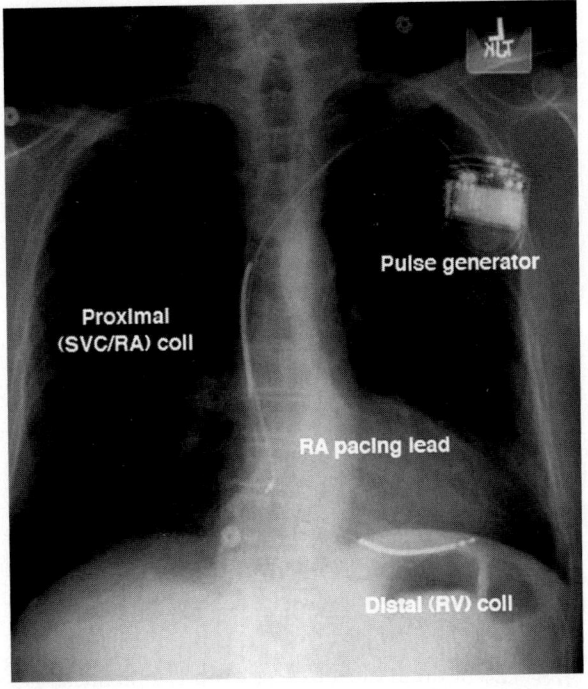

Fig. 1. Posteroanterior chest radiograph of a patient with an implantable cardioverter-defibrillator (ICD). Components of the system include pulse generator, an ICD lead with proximal and distal shocking coils, and a right atrial (RA) pacing lead. RV, right ventricular, SVC, superior vena cava.

473

DEFIBRILLATION THRESHOLD TESTING

Perhaps the most important assessment at the time of ICD placement is the defibrillation threshold. This is the amount of energy in joules required to terminate ventricular fibrillation. Different approaches have been advocated, but a common one is the step-down-to-failure algorithm, in which ICD shock energy is progressively reduced with each ventricular fibrillation induction until failure occurs. At that point, a high-energy rescue shock is delivered from the device or externally. The minimal requirement is two consecutive successful defibrillations at an energy output of 10 J or more below the maximal output of the device. For example, in a 35-J output ICD, two successful defibrillations at 25 J or less are required. It is important to understand that the relationship between shock energy and the likelihood of successful defibrillation is not linear but sigmoidal; that is, successful defibrillation is unlikely at very low energies and likely at high energies. In the middle range of energies, the relationship is roughly linear (Fig. 2).

Common reasons for high defibrillation thresholds at implantation include a shock pathway that does not traverse sufficient heart mass, use of certain membrane-active antiarrhythmic drugs (e.g., amiodarone), or massive cardiomegaly or hypertrophy.

Repositioning of the ICD lead, reversal of shock polarity, exclusion of one coil from the shock pathway, or addition of subcutaneous array electrodes can be used to improve the defibrillation threshold. Most modern ICDs incorporate biphasic shock waveforms that are substantially more effective than monophasic. In some manufacturers' ICDs, the shape of the biphasic waveform can be changed (i.e., the relative duration of the positive and negative components) and in some cases this adjustment can improve the defibrillation threshold. For the cardiovascular boards, it is most important to know 1) how drugs can affect the defibrillation threshold, 2) that a malpositioned ICD lead may cause an unacceptable defibrillation threshold, and 3) that reversing polarity can improve the defibrillation threshold.

BASICS OF PROGRAMMING AN ICD

ICDs can be programmed to function as single-zone "shock boxes" that respond to very rapid ventricular arrhythmias with high-energy defibrillating shocks.

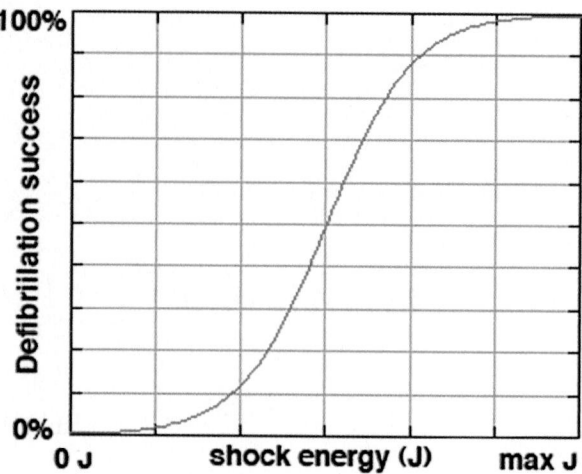

Fig. 2. Relationship between shock energy and likelihood of defibrillation success.

This type of programming is common in patients who receive the devices prophylactically (i.e., according to the criteria established by the Multicenter Automatic Defibrillator Implantation Trials, MADIT). Patients with an ICD who manifest sustained ventricular tachycardia that is not associated immediately with hemodynamic collapse may have multizone programming, in which antitachycardia pacing algorithms are used in an attempt to terminate ventricular tachycardia painlessly, or low-energy synchronized cardioversion is used, which may be less uncomfortable and more prompt than high-energy defibrillation. In general, with single zone shock box programming, antitachycardia pacing is not an option; one or more slower ventricular tachycardia zones must be programmed, and in these zones antitachycardia pacing may be programmed (Fig. 3).

HOW TO PREPARE A PATIENT WITH AN ICD FOR PROCEDURES

Electromagnetic interference with ICDs can occur with many medical and surgical procedures, including electrocautery of any kind, radiofrequency ablation, magnetic resonance imaging, lithotripsy, transcutaneous electrical nerve stimulation, and diathermy. High-frequency electrical interference commonly causes inappropriate tachyarrhythmia detection and shock delivery. Radiation therapy, if delivered close to the pulse generator, can damage the hybrid circuitry.

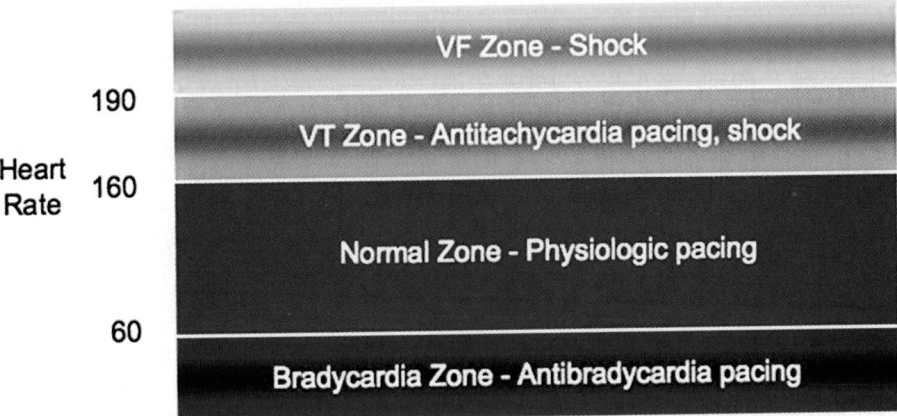

Fig. 3. Therapy zones in an implantable cardioverter-defibrillator. At less than 60 beats per minute, the device provides backup pacing support. Between the lower rate limit and the lower edge of the ventricular tachycardia (VT) zone, 160 beats per minute, physiologic pacing occurs. Heart rates between 160 and 190 beats per minute are operationally called ventricular tachycardia and can be treated with antitachycardia pacing or high- or low-energy shocks. Heart rates more than 190 beats per minute are operationally called ventricular fibrillation and are treated with shocks.

It is important to know the difference between ICDs and pacemakers with respect to their behavior with magnet application. Magnet application over a pacemaker causes asynchronous pacing (VOO, AOO, DOO), and this prevents inhibition of pacing output by electromagnetic interference. Magnet application over an ICD does not affect antibradycardia pacing (with the exception of one particular model of ICD uncommonly used in the United States). Rather, in ICDs, the effect is to inhibit tachyarrhythmia detection for the duration that the magnet is applied. Thus, in a pacemaker-dependent patient, electrocautery may inhibit pacemaker output from the ICD and produce symptomatic pauses or bradycardia. Delivery of cautery in short bursts may prevent this problem. It is always advisable to formally interrogate the ICD as soon as possible after any procedure during which a magnet has been applied.

If feasible, it is best to program ICD detections off before and reprogram them back on after potentially interfering procedures. Some ICDs also have a feature that provides for continuous antibradycardia pacing during electromagnetic interference, so-called "cautery mode." For the cardiovascular boards, it is important to know 1) how a magnet affects ICD function, 2) which procedures might interfere with ICD function, and 3) that disabling of tachyarrhythmia detection by using the programmer is the method of preparing a patient for a procedure.

TROUBLESHOOTING ICDS

The most common situation calling for troubleshooting an ICD is patient receipt of a therapy from the device. Asking a simple series of questions and analyzing stored data from the device usually provide an answer. In practice (but not, obviously, during the board examination) when this approach does not work the manufacturer can be called on for help.

Was Therapy Delivered Appropriately in Response to a Tachyarrhythmia?

In addition to obtaining a symptom inventory from the patient and performing a focused examination, the most important maneuver is interrogation of the ICD and review of information about the event. Most ICDs record intracardiac electrograms before and after an arrhythmic event triggering therapy. There are differences in the manner in which these recordings are displayed and annotated, but in general they follow the format outlined in Figure 4.

The two types of electrograms that can be displayed are near field and far field. Near-field electrograms are recorded from closely spaced bipoles on intracardiac leads just like those recorded with catheters in the electrophysiology laboratory. Far-field electrograms are recorded between small-mass tip electrodes and shocking coils on ICD leads or between tip electrodes-pulse generator canisters. These look much like surface electrocardiogram tracings.

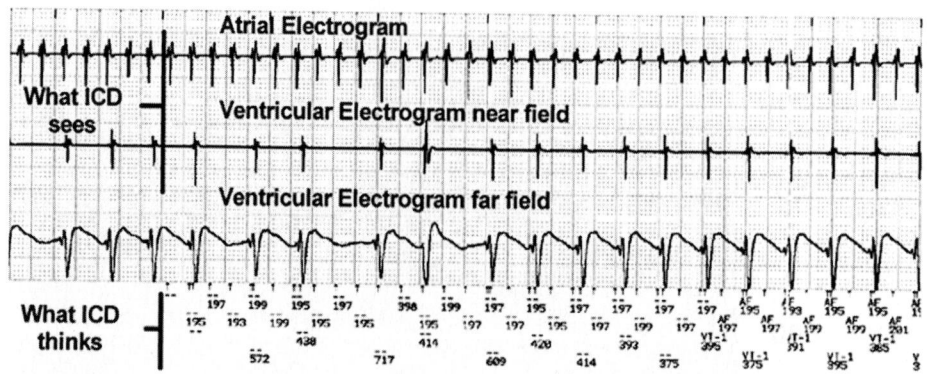

Fig. 4. Atrial, ventricular near-field, and ventricular far-field electrograms recorded during an atrial arrhythmia with variable atrioventricular conduction. Note the numerical and temporal relationship of atrial and ventricular events. Markers at bottom of tracing indicate how the implantable cardioverter-defibrillator (ICD) categorizes the arrhythmia (i.e., "what the ICD thinks") from the recorded information (i.e., "what the ICD sees"). AF, atrial fibrillation sense; VT-1, ventricular sense in ventricular tachycardia zone 1.

By comparing the relationship of atrial and ventricular events on these tracings, one can usually determine whether the arrhythmia is ventricular or supraventricular. The most common reason patients receive inappropriate therapy from a device designed to recognize and treat ventricular tachycardia and fibrillation is a rapidly conducted supraventricular arrhythmia (Fig. 5). This is normal device function but inappropriate therapy delivery.

There are two ways to solve this problem. One is to suppress the supraventricular arrhythmia with medications or ablation, and the other is to reprogram the ICD. Commonly, both are done. Raising the detection rate for ventricular tachycardia or ventricular fibrillation may avoid inappropriate recognition and treatment of slower supraventricular arrhythmias. Also, most ICDs incorporate algorithms by which supraventricular and ventricular arrhythmias can be distinguished (Table 1).

Was There Inappropriate Detection of Noncardiac Electrical Signals?

Analysis of recorded electrograms may show high-frequency signals in stored or real-time electrograms that do not correspond to cardiac activity. The most common sources are myopotentials, electromagnetic interference, and defects in lead integrity.

Myopotential sensing occurs when skeletal or diaphragmatic muscle electrical activity is picked up by the ICD sensing lead. This can result in inappropriate

detection of a tachyarrhythmia or inhibition of bradycardia pacing or both (Fig. 6).

Environmental electromagnetic interference with ICDs is uncommon but not rare. Patients should be cautioned regarding placement of digital cellular phones on the ear or in a breast pocket ipsilateral to the device, possible effects of metal detectors at airports,

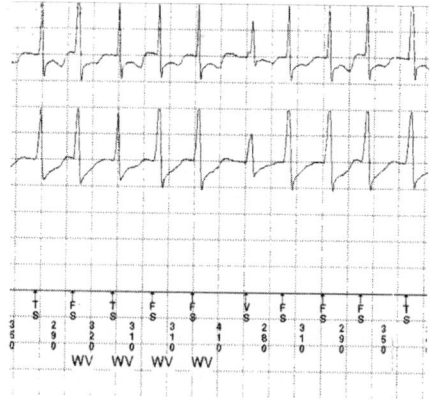

Fig. 5. Stored electrograms from an implantable cardioverter-defibrillator, showing a rapid narrow QRS tachycardia with cycle lengths between the ventricular tachycardia (TS, tachy-sense marker) and ventricular fibrillation (FS, fib-sense marker) zones. Therapy was not delivered because the device compared the morphologic pattern of the electrogram in tachycardia to baseline (WV, wavelet marker) and determined this was not ventricular in origin.

Table 1.   Distinguishing Supraventricular Arrhythmias From Ventricular Arrhythmias

Criterion	Rationale	Use
Sudden onset (value in milliseconds or beats per minute, programmable)	Paroxysmal arrhythmias abruptly increase heart rate	Distinguishes sinus tachycardia (gradual onset) from sudden arrhythmias
Stability (value in milliseconds, programmable)	Ventricular tachycardia usually varies less than 40-60 milliseconds cycle to cycle	Distinguishes supraventricular arrhythmias with variable atrioventricular conduction (atrial tachycardia/atrial fibrillation) from more regular arrhythmias such as ventricular tachycardia. Does not require atrial lead
Atrioventricular relationship	Supraventricular arrhythmias typically show ≥1:1 atrial to ventricular ratio, and ventricular arrhythmias may show atrioventricular dissociation. Timing of atrial and ventricular events may be compared to catalog of templates	More sophisticated mechanism for distinguishing supraventricular and ventricular arrhythmias. Requires atrial lead
Electrogram morphology	Intracardiac electrograms of ventricular arrhythmias show a change in morphology compared with baseline normal rhythm	Distinguishes activation of ventricles over normal conduction system from activation. Does not require atrial lead

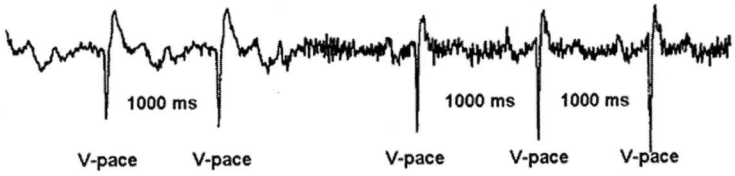

Fig. 6. High-frequency chatter in far-field electrogram which is associated with inhibition of pacing (device was programmed to VVI at 60 beats per minute) and inappropriate detection and treatment of an arrhythmia the device "thought" was ventricular fibrillation at a rate of 256 beats per minute.

and electronic theft-deterrent scanners in stores. In rural and agricultural areas, arc welding is common, and the radiofrequency signals generated with such welding can be intercepted by the ICD sensing circuit (Fig. 7.)

In pacemakers, lead fractures can result in failure of pacing output due to conductor discontinuity and high resistance. In ICDs, fractures also can cause inappropriate sensing of tachyarrhythmia. Conductor move-ment at the fracture site generates electrical signals sent back to the pulse generator which can trigger spurious detection (Fig. 8).

Was There Inappropriate Detection of Intracardiac Electrical Signals?

In addition to detection of noncardiac signals, ICDs can inappropriately detect cardiac electrical signals,

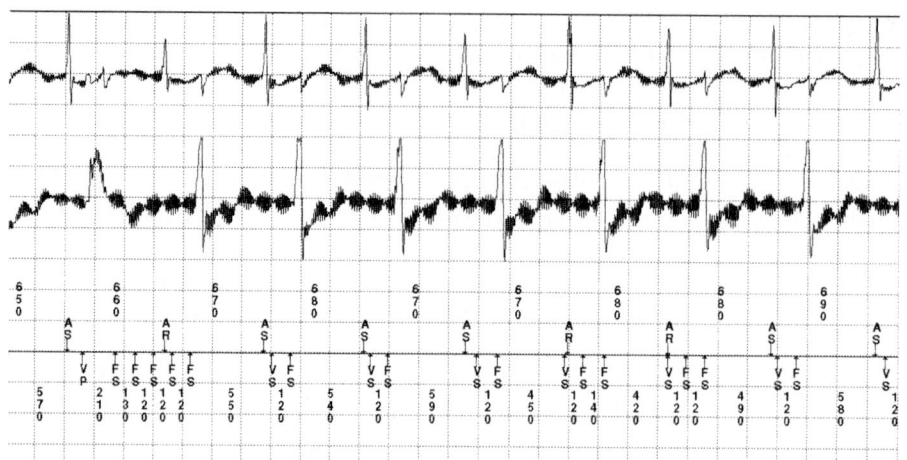

Fig. 7. From top to bottom, atrial near-field, ventricular near-field, and ventricular far-field electrograms from a patient with an implantable cardioverter-defibrillator who received a shock while close to high-amperage arc welding. Note the very high-frequency noise in both atrial and ventricular near-field electrograms. Marker annotations at bottom show that the device "thinks" both atrial and ventricular arrhythmias are present. The finding of noise on both atrial and ventricular channels suggests an environmental source of noise rather than something originating from the device or leads.

leading to incorrect delivery of therapy. The most common cause is T-wave sensing, in which the T wave is counted as an R wave, leading to intermittent or continuous double counting (Fig. 9).

The solution to T-wave oversensing includes 1) increasing the voltage threshold for detection of ventricular events (sensitivity) or 2) placing a new rate-sensing lead in a different position where the T-wave amplitude is attenuated. In either case, before hospital

discharge, testing of the ICD with induction of ventricular fibrillation is required to document appropriate detection of low-amplitude ventricular electrical activity during arrhythmias.

Was Therapy Delivered Appropriately for Multiple Episodes of Ventricular Tachycardia or Ventricular Fibrillation?

As more patients receive ICDs for both primary and

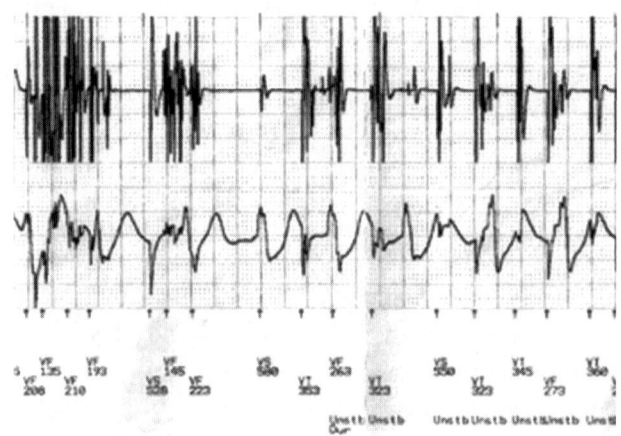

Fig. 8. Fracture of rate-sensing portion of an implantable cardioverter-defibrillator lead resulting in inappropriate detection of ventricular tachycardia. Large-amplitude high-frequency spikes are most prominent in near-field electrogram.

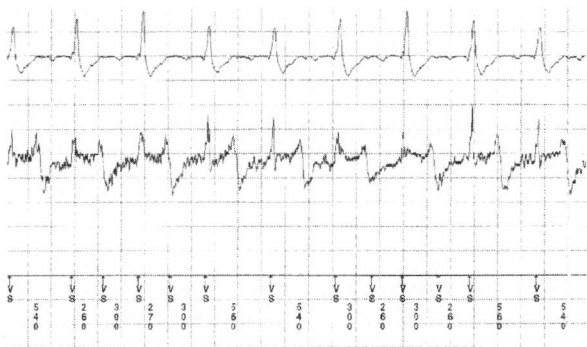

Fig. 9. From top to bottom, far-field and near-field intracardiac electrograms and marker channels. In the near-field recording are large-amplitude T waves that are registered in the marker channel as ventricular events. This strip was obtained at the end of a charging cycle during which the device marks all ventricular events as "VS" regardless of the cycle length. CD, delivery of a 35.4-J shock; CE, end of charge.

secondary prevention, more patients will receive appropriate shocks for ventricular arrhythmias. If a patient receives one or two shocks but feels otherwise well, hospitalization is not critical. If a patient receives a flurry of shocks over a period of time, or if cardiac symptoms persist after receipt of shocks, hospitalization is important. The psychological toll on the patient who receives multiple discharges is considerable, and prompt control of the triggering events is required.

Treatment options include drug therapy to suppress arrhythmias (commonly amiodarone, sotalol, β-adrenergic blockers), ablation of ventricular tachycardia foci, treatment of exacerbating factors such as ischemia, discontinuing use of proarrhythmic drugs, correction of electrolyte abnormalities, and surgical aneurysm resection. Programming of nonshock therapies for ventricular tachycardia (antitachycardia pacing) often reduces the shock burden.

If membrane-active antiarrhythmic drugs are given, it is important to test their effect on ICD function. Three variables need to be checked: 1) pacing threshold, 2) defibrillation threshold, and 3) ventricular tachycardia detection rate.

For the purposes of the board examination, the following should be noted: 1) potent sodium channel blockers (such as flecainide and propafenone) are likely to increase the defibrillation threshold and the pacing threshold, 2) amiodarone may increase the defibrillation threshold, and 3) relatively pure potassium channel blockers may lower the defibrillation threshold.

Implantable Cardioverter-Defibrillator Trials and Prevention of Sudden Cardiac Death

Margaret A. Lloyd, MD

Bernard J. Gersh, MB, ChB, DPhil

The development of implantable cardioverter-defibrillators (ICDs) during the past 25 years has revolutionized the approach to prevention of sudden cardiac death (SCD). Multiple clinical trials have defined the indications for ICD therapy in the prevention of primary and secondary SCD. Our current understanding of risk stratification is a victory for evidence-based medicine; perhaps no other area of cardiology has been so rigorously evaluated. As such, these fact-driven clinical trials are rich fodder for the cardiology board examination.

Approximately 450,000 people experience SCD each year in the United States. This number may be an overestimation because it is understood that perhaps 25% to 50% of deaths attributed to "cardiac arrest," when no other obvious cause is identified, are noncardiac. It has long been long recognized that patients who experienced SCD and survived were at risk for a second event. The challenge has been identifying patients at risk before the first event, because some studies suggest that less than 5% of patients survive neurologically intact. Furthermore, optimal treatment for persons at risk for a primary or secondary event needed to be identified.

Although clinical trials have provided much information about risk stratification and treatment, conclusions must be evaluated critically. In retrospect, some trials had flaws in design, were terminated too early to

clearly test the hypothesis, had unacceptable crossover rates, or used surrogate end points (syncope, death without autopsy, ventricular arrhythmia) that may or may not have been equivalent to SCD. Differences in trial design make direct comparison of results difficult (Table 1). Nevertheless, the accumulated data have allowed guidelines to be formulated which allow us to predict with more certainty patients at risk for SCD and patients who should be considered for ICD therapy. The bulk of evidence now suggests that ICDs are superior to antiarrhythmic drug therapy in most instances for the primary and secondary prevention of SCD in patients at risk; antiarrhythmic drug therapy is now mainly relegated to adjuvant therapy.

A summary of secondary prevention trials is presented in Table 2; primary prevention trials are summarized in Table 3. Recent important trials are summarized in the text that follows (the names of the trials are provided in the Appendix.

CARE-CHF (2005)

This nonblinded European trial compared the risk of death in patients randomized to standard medical therapy alone with the risk of patients receiving standard therapy and biventricular pacing (without an ICD). Inclusion criteria included New York Heart Association

Table 1.   Inclusion Criteria for Implantable Cardioverter-Defibrillator Trials

| Trial* | Criteria | |
	Ejection fraction, %	Other
Definite	<36	NSVT or PVCs
SCD-HeFT	≤35	NYHA class II, III CHF
MUSTT	<40	NSVT, inducible sustained VA
MADIT	≤30	Prior MI
MADIT II	≤30	Prior MI
DINAMIT	≤35	↓ HRV

*The names of the trials are provided in the Appendix. CHF, congestive heart failure; MI, myocardial infarction; NSVT, nonsustained ventricular tachycardia; PVCs, premature ventricular contractions; VA, ventricular arrhythmia.

(NYHA) class III or IV heart failure present for at least 6 weeks, ejection fraction less than 35%, QRS interval of at least 120 milliseconds, and an indexed left ventricular end-diastolic dimension more than 30 mm. Patients with atrial arrhythmias were excluded. Primary end points were unplanned hospitalization for a major cardiac event and death from any cause.

The study enrolled 813 patients; the mean duration of follow-up was 30 months. Among the patients randomized to device therapy, 95% had a biventricular pacing device successfully implanted. Thirty percent of the medical therapy alone group died, and 20% of the device therapy group died, a significant absolute and relative reduction.

This study importantly showed the beneficial effect of cardiac resynchronization alone on survival in patients with severe heart failure and has led some investigators to question the survival benefit of ICD therapy compared with biventricular pacing in these patients. Nevertheless, SCD caused 35% of the deaths in patients with a device in this trial, and likely some of these deaths would have been aborted with ICD therapy.

SCD-HeFT (2004)

This was a prospective, randomized, double-blind trial involving 2,521 patients at 148 sites from 1997-2001. The average age of patients was 60.1 years, average ejection fraction was 25%, and the numbers of patients with ischemic and nonischemic cardiomyopathy were nearly equal. Patients were randomized to receive amiodarone, ICD, or placebo. Medical management was optimized; blinding was imperfect because some patients receiving amiodarone had development of revealing side effects from the medication, and no sham devices were implanted. After at least 30 months of follow-up, ICD decreased mortality by 23% compared with placebo (Fig. 1). Amiodarone did not improve survival.

Surprisingly in subgroup analysis, mortality improved exclusively in the NYHA II group (46%) and *not* in the NYHA III group (0%). Subgroup analysis also did not show a benefit for women, blacks, or patients with diabetes. Nonetheless, the data have been extrapolated to include NYHA classes II and III heart failure as primary inclusion criteria, and the trial results were critical in formulating the most recent guidelines of the Centers for Medicare & Medicaid Services for ICD therapy.

DINAMIT (2004)

In this randomized, open-label trial comparing ICD therapy to optimal medical therapy, 674 high-risk patients (defined by an ejection fraction <35% and evidence of impaired cardiac autonomic function) were enrolled 6 to 40 days after myocardial infarction. The primary end point was death from any cause; death from arrhythmia was a secondary end point. There was no difference in baseline characteristics between the groups. During a mean follow-up of 30 months, there was no difference in overall mortality between the two treatment groups. A reduction in deaths due to arrhythmia was balanced by an increase in overall mortality (cardiac but nonarrhythmic) in the ICD group.

The reason for this surprising finding is unclear. There was a higher use of amiodarone in the medical therapy group, but given that prior trials have found no survival advantage with amiodarone use, this is unlikely to be responsible. The rate of revascularization was low, which also may have been a factor. More likely, it is related to the inclusion criteria of this trial, not included

Table 2. Trials of ICD Therapy for Secondary Prevention of SCD

Trial*	Inclusion criteria	End point	Treatment arms	Key results
CASCADE (1993)	Recent history of resuscitation for out-of-hospital VF No occurrence of an acute Q-wave MI at time of VF	Cardiac arrest from VF Cardiac mortality Syncope followed by ICD shock	Amiodarone (n=113) EP or Holter-guided conventional AA drug therapy, mostly quinidine or procainamide (n=115)	Amiodarone performed better than conventional AA drugs on all end points at the end of 6 years Percentage of patients with survival free of cardiac death, resuscitated VF, or syncope followed by ICD shock: 53% amiodarone group 40% conventional AA drug group
ESVEM (1993)	Documented episode of sustained (>15 s) VT Resuscitated SCD or syncope Inducible on EPS	All-cause mortality or survivor or SCD Overall cardiac death Arrhythmic death	EPS-guided AA drugs (n=242) Holter-guided AA drugs (n=244) Drugs evaluated: six class 1 AA drugs and sotalol	Both treatment arms provided similar accuracy of drug efficacy prediction Only sotalol was associated with a significant reduction in risk of arrhythmia recurrence
CIDS (1993)	Documented VF or Out-of-hospital cardiac arrest requiring defibrillation or Sustained VT ≥150 bpm causing presyncope or angina with LVEF ≤35% or Unmonitored syncope with spontaneous or inducible VT	All-cause mortality Arrhythmic death Nonfatal VF or VT Cause-specific mortality	ICD (n=328) Amiodarone (n=331)	ICDs provided a 20% relative risk reduction in all-cause mortality and a 33% reduction in arrhythmic mortality compared with amiodarone
CASH (1994)	SCD survivors	All-cause mortality	Propafenone (n=58) (this arm was stopped due to excess mortality compared with ICD arm) Amiodarone (n=92) Metoprolol (n=97) ICD (n=99)	ICD treatment arm had a 37% reduction in mortality at 2 years and a 23% reduction in mortality over long-term follow-up of 9 years compared with both amiodarone and metoprolol ICD arm had a 63% reduction in mortality compared with propafenone at 11 months

Table 2. (continued)

Trial*	Inclusion criteria	End point	Treatment arms	Key results
Wever et al (1995)	Post-MI survivors of cardiac arrest caused by documented VT or VF. Baseline inducibility of VT	All-cause mortality. Costs and cost-effectiveness	Early ICDs (n=29). Tiered therapy, starting with AA drugs (mainly class 3) (n=31)	Early ICD therapy reduced overall mortality by 66% at 2 years: ICD group: 14% deaths. Tiered-therapy group: 35% deaths. Early ICD therapy resulted in cost savings of $11,315 per life-year saved compared with tiered therapy
AVID (1997)	VF or Sustained VT with syncope or Sustained VT without syncope and LVEF ≤40 and SBP <80 mm Hg, chest pain or near syncope	All-cause mortality. Quality of life. Costs and cost-effectiveness	ICD therapy (n=507). EPS or Holter-guided sotalol or empiric amiodarone (n=509)	ICDs reduced total mortality 39% after 1 year, 27% after 2 years, and 31% after 3 years compared with AA drugs

AA, antiarrhythmic; bpm, beats per minute; EPS, electrophysiologic study; ICD, implantable cardioverter-defibrillator; LVEF, left ventricular ejection fraction; MI, myocardial infarction; SBP, systolic blood pressure; SCD, sudden cardiac death; VF, ventricular fibrillation; VT, ventricular tachycardia.
*The names of the trials are provided in the Appendix at the end of the chapter.

Table 3.   Trials of ICD Therapy for Primary Prevention of SCD

Trial*	Inclusion criteria	End point	Treatment arms	Key results
BHAT (1982)	Acute MI. ECG and enzyme changes	All-cause mortality. Secondary: CHD mortality, SCD mortality, CHD mortality with definite nonfatal MI	β-Blocker: Propranolol (n=1,916). Placebo (n=1,921)	Propranolol reduced SCD mortality by 28% and overall mortality by 26%. ≥90% of observed deaths were from cardiovascular causes. Both sudden and non-sudden arteriosclerotic heart disease mortality was less in propranolol group

Table 3 (continued)

Trial*	Inclusion criteria	End point	Treatment arms	Key results
CAST (1991)	6 days to 2 years after MI >6 PVCs per hour No VT ≥15 beats or ≥120 bpm LVEF: 　≤55% recruited within 90 days post-MI *or* 　≤40% if recruited ≥90 days after MI	All-cause mortality or survivor of SCD Overall cardiac death Arrhythmic death	Class 1 AA drugs: 　encainide (n=432) or flecainide (n=323) Placebo (n=743)	At 14 mo follow-up, total mortality for patients in the class 1 AA drug group was 3.6 times higher than that for patients in placebo arm. Study was stopped early
GESICA (1994)	NYHA advanced class II, III, and IV 2 or 3 indexes of systolic myocardial dysfunction: 　1. Chest x-ray, cardiothoracic ratio >0.55 　2. LVEF ≤35% 　3. LVEDD >3.2 cm/m^2 of body surface	All-cause mortality SCD Death due to progressive heart failure Hospital admissions	Amiodarone (n=260) Standard treatment (n=256)	Amiodarone reduced overall mortality at 2 years by 28%: 　Amiodarone: 33.5% mortality 　Placebo: 41% mortality
CHF-STAT (1995)	NYHA class II, III, or IV ≥10 PVCs/hour LVEF ≤40%	All-cause mortality SCD Suppression of ventricular arrhythmias LVEF Hospitalizations	Amiodarone (n=336) Placebo (n=338)	Amiodarone did not reduce total mortality, despite improved left ventricular function and suppressed ventricular arrhythmias
MADIT (1996)	Q-wave MI ≥3 weeks Asymptomatic, unsustained VT LVEF ≤35% Inducible, non-suppressible VT on EPS with procainamide NYHA class I-III	All-cause mortality Costs and cost-effectiveness	ICDs (n=95) Conventional therapy (n=101)	ICDs reduced overall mortality by 54% ICDs cost $22,800 per life-year saved versus conventional therapy, assuming transvenous devices were used

Table 3 (continued)

Trial*	Inclusion criteria	End point	Treatment arms	Key results
SWORD (1996)	LVEF ≤40% Recent MI (6-42 days) or remote MI (>42 days) with NYHA class II or III	All-cause mortality SCD	D-sotalol (n=1,549) Placebo (n=1,572)	Prophylactic oral D-sotalol had excessive mortality (5%) vs. placebo (3.1%)

DIAMOND (1997)	CHF study:
	  Hospital admission for CHF
	  EF ≤35%
	MI study:
	  Acute MI within past 7 days
	  EF ≤35%
		All-cause mortality	CHF (n=1,518)
			Dofetilide (n=762)
			Placebo (n=756)
			MI (n=1,510)
			Dofetilide (n=749)
			Placebo (n=761)
				Treatment with dofetilide in CHF group with left ventricular dysfunction and in post-MI patients did not result in any significant reduction in mortality compared with placebo

CAMIAT (1997)	Acute MI in past 6-45 days ≤10 VPDs/hour or any VT on Holter monitoring	All-cause mortality Arrhythmic death Resuscitated VF	Amiodarone (n=606) Placebo (n=596)	No difference in overall mortality between amiodarone and placebo groups. Amiodarone reduced cumulative risk of arrhythmic death or resuscitated VF by 48.5%
EMIAT (1997)	5-21 days after MI LVEF ≤40%	All-cause mortality Cardiac mortality Arrhythmic death	Amiodarone (n=385) Placebo (n=444)	No difference in overall mortality or cardiac mortality between amiodarone and placebo patients. Amiodarone reduced arrhythmic death by 35%
CABG Patch (1997)	Scheduled for elective CABG surgery LVEF ≤35% Abnormalities on SAECG	All-cause mortallity	ICD (n=446) Standard treatment (n=454)	Survival was not improved by prophylactic implantation of ICD at time of elective CABG
MUSTT (1999)	Coronary artery disease LVEF ≤40% Asymptomatic unsustained VT (≥3 beats)	Cardiac arrest or arrhythmic death All-cause mortality Cardiac mortality Spontaneous, sustained VT	EPS-guided therapy (n=351) No antiarrhythmic therapy (n=353)	EPS-guided antiarrhythmic therapy with ICDs, but not with AA drug; reduced the risk of SCD in high-risk patients with coronary disease (9% vs. 37% arrhythmic mortality at 5 years, respectively)

Table 3 (continued)

Trial*	Inclusion criteria	End point	Treatment arms	Key results
SCD-HEFT (2004)	Ischemic or non-ischemic NYHA class II and III CHF, EF ≤35%	Primary: overall mortality Secondary: sub-group analysis QOL Cost-effective-ness	Placebo (n=847) ICD (n=845) Amiodarone (n=829)	Shock-only ICD reduced mortality by 23% Amiodarone alone did not improve survival

AA, antiarrhythmic; bpm, beats per minute; CABG, coronary artery bypass grafting; CHD, coronary heart disease; CHF, congestive heart failure; ECG, electrocardiographic; EF, ejection fraction; EPS, electrophysiologic study; ICD, implantable cardioverter-defibrillator; LVEDD, left ventricular end-diastolic diameter; LVEF, left ventricular ejection fraction; MI, myocardial infarction; NYHA, New York Heart Association; PVCs, premature ventricular contractions; SAECG, signal-averaged electrocardiogram; SCD, sudden cardiac death; VPDs, ventricular premature depolarizations; VT, ventricular tachycardia.
*The names of the trials are provided in the Appendix at the end of the chapter.

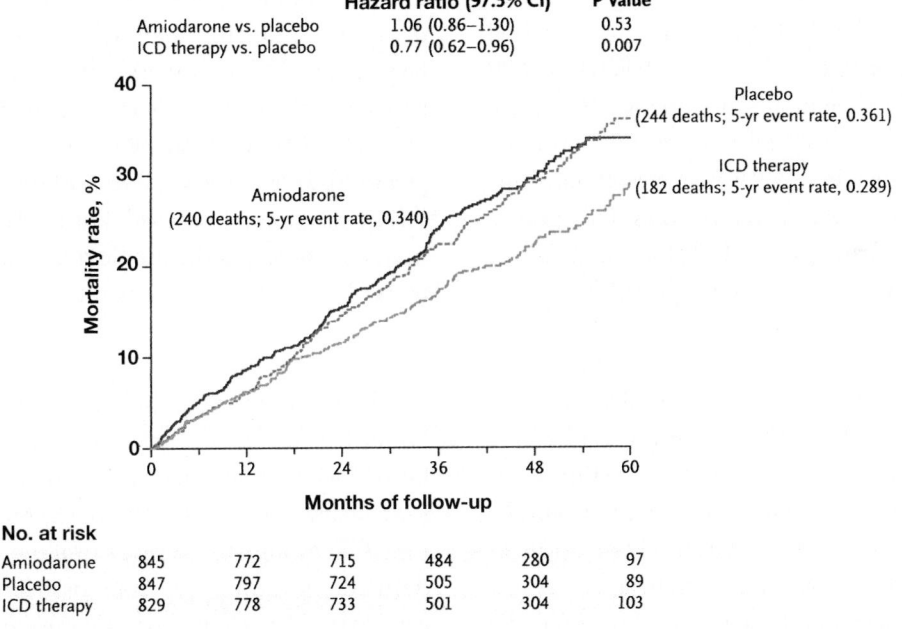

Fig. 1. Kaplan-Meier estimate of death from any cause, by study group, Sudden Cardiac Death in Heart Failure Trial. ICD, implantable cardioverter-defibrillator.

or specifically excluded in recent trials, namely, the patients were enrolled early after MI and had evidence of impaired cardiac autonomic function. The inclusion of autonomic dysfunction may have preselected patients with a poorer prognosis regardless of treatment strategy. The degree of cardiac autonomic dysfunction was not reevaluated during the study, and improvement or deterioration might have influenced the results.

Remodeling and infarct maturation, which may take months or years to become evident and are manifest by a reduced ejection fraction, are the critical determinants, and not left ventricular dysfunction, in the peri-infarct period. Orn and colleagues found that most deaths that occurred early after myocardial infarction were due to recurrent infarct. In this setting, device discharge may be related to myocardial infarction-induced arrhythmia. The MADIT database showed no ICD benefit until 18 months after infarct. The benefits of ICD therapy for the prevention of SCD may not become evident until years after myocardial infarction and may have not been captured in the mean 30-month follow-up of the DINAMIT study.

Current guidelines of the Centers for Medicare & Medicaid Services specifically exclude prophylactic use of an ICD immediately after acute myocardial infarction, although in some individual circumstances it may be considered (e.g., in patients with recurrent, sustained arrhythmias).

DEFINITE (2004)

This trial included 458 patients with nonischemic dilated cardiomyopathy and ejection fraction less than 36%, nonsustained ventricular tachycardia or premature ventricular contractions, and NYHA class I, II, or III who were randomly divided to receive standard medical therapy or ICD. After a mean follow-up of 29 months, ICD implantation substantially reduced the all-cause death rate (34% relative and 5.7% absolute reduction) and the rate of death from arrhythmia compared with optimal medical therapy only. The greatest benefit occurred in the NYHA III subgroup of patients (in contrast to the findings of SCD-HeFT). There was initial concern that women did not seem to benefit from ICD implantation in this trial, but further analysis suggests that the excess mortality was from causes unrelated to the ICD or underlying cardiac disease; there seemed to be an excess of malignancy, stroke, and other noncardiac, nonarrhythmic conditions. Another limitation is the relatively small size of this trial, making subgroup analysis difficult.

In part on the basis of the results of this trial, the Centers for Medicare & Medicaid Services expanded coverage for ICD implantation to patients with nonischemic cardiomyopathy of more than 9 months in duration who have NYHA class III or IV heart failure and ejection fraction of 35% or less. Describing the data as "less than compelling," the Centers for Medicare & Medicaid Services advised that reimbursement would be provided for ICD implantation in patients who had nonischemic cardiomyopathy for more than 3 months and less than 9 months only if included in U.S. Food and Drug Administration-approved ICD clinical trial or registry.

COMPANION (2004)

This was the first trial to test the effect of biventricular pacing (cardiac resynchronization) in combination with ICD on death from any cause and hospitalization. The 1,520 study patients had advanced heart failure (ischemic or nonischemic) and a QRS interval more than 120 milliseconds were randomized in a 1:2:2 ratio to receive optimal medical therapy alone or in combination with either biventricular pacing alone or in combination with an ICD.

Approximately 90% of patients randomized to device therapy had a left ventricular lead successfully placed, a remarkable feat given lead technology available at the time.

A statistical difficulty in this trial was the crossover from medical to device therapy. Patients with cardiomyopathies frequently require device therapy (pacing or ICD) as their disease progresses, and crossover into the device therapy arm has been an issue with many trials. During the COMPANION trial, the biventricular ICDs became commercially available, and patients in the medical therapy alone group thus were free to have device implantation. In the medical therapy group, 26% of the patients withdrew, and most of these patients eventually had devices placed outside the trial. In addition to the problem of crossover, the two parts of the combined end point of death or hospitalization for congestive heart failure are not equivalent clinical end points.

The risk of the combined end point of death or hospitalization for congestive heart failure was reduced by 34% with biventricular pacing compared with medical therapy alone and by 40% in the biventricular pacing-ICD group after 1 year of follow-up. Given the defined end point and the crossover, it is hard to extrapolate the relative contributions of biventricular pacing and ICD therapy to the mortality reduction compared with medical therapy alone (note the similarity of risk reduction compared with the CARE-CHF trial discussed previously).

MADIT II (2002)

This multicenter trial was the third major clinical trial to evaluate the effectiveness of ICD therapy compared with conventional therapy in high-risk patients who had had a myocardial infarction. The study enrolled

1,232 patients. Invasive testing for risk stratification was not required; inclusion criteria included prior myocardial infarction (>1 month) and an ejection fraction of 30% or less. The primary end point was death from any cause. At an average follow-up of 20 months, the mortality rate was 19.8% in the conventional therapy group and 14.2% in the ICD group.

This trial was novel in that there was no requirement for invasive electrophysiologic testing or prior ventricular arrhythmia. Survival benefit became apparent at 9 months after device implantation.

This trial expanded on the findings of MADIT I, which showed the superiority of ICD therapy in patients with coronary artery disease, nonsustained ventricular tachycardia on Holtor monitoring, and an ejection fraction of 35% or less who had inducible sustained ventricular tachycardia not suppressed by intravenous procainamide (subgroup analysis), and the MUSTT Trial, which showed ICD superiority in patients with an ejection fraction of 40% or less, coronary artery disease, and inducible arrhythmias regardless of whether or not arrthythmias were suppressible by drug therapy. These trials importantly showed the lack of any role for Holtor monitoring and invasive electrophysiologic study and the effect of antiarrhythmic drugs on inducibility status in predicting risk for SCD in patients with coronary artery disease and depressed ejection fraction.

fractions postoperatively may have had a survival advantage with ICD therapy. Also abnormalities on signal-averaged electrocardiography may preselect patients at higher risk, because both groups had relatively high mortality rates. Nevertheless, the results suggest that revascularization should be performed when feasible and that SCD risk stratification should be performed after revascularization.

SUMMARY

On the basis of the results of the accumulated evidence from clinical trials and professional advisory groups, the Centers for Medicare & Medicaid Services issued new guidelines for ICD implantation that went into effect in January 2005 (Table 4). Exceptions to the rule will occur, and clinical judgment may deem that an individual outside the guidelines may have risk sufficient to justify ICD placement. Additionally, even if a patient qualifies for an ICD on the basis of the guidelines, device placement may be deemed inappropriate by family and caregivers (e.g., a patient with severe dementia living in a nursing home). Notably, in all trials the patients had a mean age in the 60s or 70s; it is not at all clear that patients in their 80s or 90s will derive meaningful life extension from ICD placement.

CABG PATCH TRIAL (1997)

Although this trial was reported almost a decade ago, it is important in that it is the only trial to address the effect of revascularization on the risk of SCD. The 900 patients in the study had an ejection fraction less than 36%, abnormal signal-averaged electrocardiograms, and scheduled coronary artery bypass grafting. They were randomized to receive an ICD and standard medical care or standard medical care alone at the time of bypass surgery. At an average of 32 months follow-up, there was no difference in the primary end point, overall mortality, between the groups (Fig. 2). Of note, 88 patients enrolled were not randomized because they were deemed too unstable at the time of surgery for ICD placement. Additionally, ejection fractions and signal-averaged electrocardiograms were not assessed postoperatively. The patients with depressed ejection

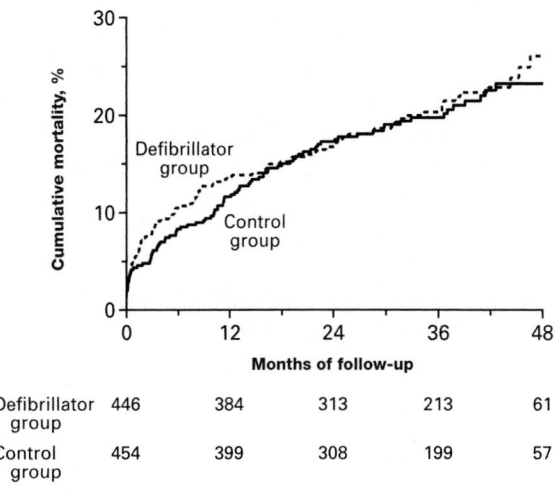

Fig. 2. Kaplan-Meier estimate of death, by study group, Coronary Artery Bypass Graft Trial.

Table 4.   Summary of Coverage for Implantable Cardioverter-Defibrillators: January 27, 2005

1. Documented episode of cardiac arrest due to VF, not due to a transient or reversible cause (effective July 1, 1991)
2. Documented sustained VT, either spontaneous or induced by an EP study, not associated with an acute MI and not due to a transient or reversible cause (effective July 1, 1999)
3. Documented familial or inherited conditions with a high risk of life-threatening VT, such as long QT syndrome or hypertrophic cardiomyopathy (effective July 1, 1999)
4. Coronary artery disease with a documented prior MI, a measured LVEF ≤35%, and inducible sustained VT or VF on EP study. (The MI must have occurred more than 4 weeks before defibrillator insertion. The EP test must be performed more than 4 weeks after the qualifying MI)
5. Documented prior MI and a measured LVEF ≤30%. Patients must not have:
   a. NYHA class IV
   b. Cardiogenic shock or symptomatic hypotension while in a stable baseline rhythm
   c. Had a CABG or PTCA within past 3 months
   d. Had an MI within past 40 days
   e. Clinical symptoms or findings that would make them a candidate for coronary revascularization
   f. Any disease, other than cardiac disease (e.g., cancer, uremia, liver failure), associated with a likelihood of survival of less than 1 year
6. Patients with ischemic dilated cardiomyopathy, documented prior MI, NYHA class II and III heart failure, and measured LVEF <35%
7. Patients with nonischemic dilated cardiomyopathy >9 months, NYHA class II and III heart failure, and measured LVEF ≤35%
8. Patients who meet all current Centers for Medicare & Medicaid Services coverage requirements for a cardiac resynchronization therapy device and have NYHA class IV heart failure

Indications #3 - #8 (primary prevention of sudden cardiac death) must also meet the following criteria:
   a. Patients must be able to give informed consent
   b. Patients must not have:
   - Cardiogenic shock or symptomatic hypotension while in a stable baseline rhythm
   - Had a CABG or PTCA within the past 3 months
   - Had an acute MI within the past 40 days
   - Clinical symptoms or findings that would make them a candidate for coronary revascularization
   - Irreversible brain damage from preexisting cerebral disease
   - Any disease, other than cardiac disease (e.g., cancer, uremia, liver failure), associated with a likelihood of survival less than 1 year
   c. Ejection fractions must be measured with angiography, radionuclide scanning, or echocardiography
   d. MIs must be documented and defined according to the consensus document of the Joint European Society of Cardiology / American College of Cardiology Committee for the Redefinition of Myocardial Infarction

CABG, coronary artery bypass graft; EP, electrophysiologic; LVEF, left ventricular ejection fraction; MI, myocardial infarction; NYHA, New York Heart Association; PTCA, percutaneous transluminal coronary angioplasty; VF, ventricular fibrillation; VT, ventricular tachyarrhythmia.

Generalizations to keep in mind for the board examination:

1. ICDs are more effective than antiarrhythmic drugs for reducing mortality.
2. β-Blockers reduce the risk of SCD and all-cause mortality.
3. Electrophysiology-guided antiarrhythmic therapy is generally ineffective for predicting the risk of SCD.
4. Ejection fraction is the best predictor of the risk for SCD. Nevertheless, it is a relatively "blunt instrument," and future trials to further refine the risk of SCD are needed.

Guidelines for ICD use in patients with high-risk disorders such as long QT syndromes, Brugada syndrome, arrhythmic right ventricular dysplasia, and hypertrophic cardiomyopathy are discussed in other chapters in this book.

RESOURCES
Center for Medicare/Medicaid Services: http://www.cms.hhs.gov/CoverageGenInfo/04_ICDregistry.asp#TopOfPage

Heart Rhythm Society: http://www.hrsonline.org/swAdvocacyFiles/advocacy103469847.asp

APPENDIX
NAMES OF CLINICAL TRIALS

AVID	Antiarrhythmics Versus Implantable Defibrillators
BHAT	β-Blocker Heart Attack Trial
CABG Patch	Coronary Artery Bypass Graft Patch
CAMIAT	Canadian Amiodarone Myocardial Infarction Arrhythmia Trial
CARE-CHF	Cardiac Resynchronization in Heart Failure
CASCADE	Cardiac Arrest in Seattle: Conventional vs. Amiodarone Drug Evaluation
CASH	Cardiac Arrest Study Hamburg
CAST	Cardiac Arrhythmia Suppression Trial
CHF-STAT	Survival Trial of Antiarrhythmic Therapy in Congestive Heart Failure
CIDS	Canadian Implantable Defibrillator Study
COMPANION	Comparison of Medical Therapy, Pacing, and Defibrillation in Heart Failure
DEFINITE	Defibrillators in Nonischemic Cardiomyopathy Treatment Evaluation
DIAMOND	Danish Investigations of Arrhythmia and Mortality On Dofetilide
DINAMIT	Defibrillator in Acute Myocardial Infarction Trial
EMIAT	European Myocardial Infarct Amiodarone Trial
ESVEM	Electrophysiology Study Versus Electrocardiographic Monitoring
GESICA	Grupo de Estudio de la Sobrevida en la Insuficiencia Cardiaca en Argentina
MADIT, MADIT II	Multicenter Automatic Defibrillator Implantation Trial, MADIT II
MUSTT	Multicenter Unsustained Tachycardia Trial
SCD-HeFT	Sudden Cardiac Death in Heart Failure Trial
SWORD	Survival With Oral D-Sotalol

Sudden Cardiac Death

Ravi Kanagala, MD

Sudden cardiac death (SCD) accounts for up to 50% of cardiovascular-related deaths in the United States and other developed countries. By definition, *SCD* refers to the acute and natural death from cardiac causes within a short period (often within an hour of onset of symptoms). The time and mode of death are unexpected, and often death occurs in patients without any prior potentially fatal conditions. Most cases of SCD are associated with underlying cardiac arrhythmias; however, other causes have been identified (Table 1).

EPIDEMIOLOGY
SCD causes an estimated 300,000 to 400,000 deaths annually. Structural coronary arterial abnormalities and their consequences cause 80% of the fatal arrhythmias associated with SCD. Recordings during episodes of SCD have shown an underlying rhythm of ventricular tachycardia (VT), ventricular fibrillation (VF), or VT degenerating into VF in 85% of cases. In other studies, bradyarrhythmia was the underlying rhythm in 16% of patients who died suddenly. Hypertrophic and dilated cardiomyopathies are the second most common causes of SCD. Other cardiac disorders that account for only a small portion of SCD cases include channelopathies, acquired infiltrative disorders, and valvular and congenital heart diseases. Several noncardiac conditions mimic SCD. They include cardiac tamponade, acute asthmatic attack, aortic dissection, massive pulmonary embolus, and stroke. Other nonatherosclerotic coronary artery abnormalities that can lead to SCD include coronary artery anomalies, coronary arteritis, and congenital malformations.

The incidence of SCD is higher among men than women. The incidence also increases with age. In older patients, SCD occurs most often with reduced left ventricular function and symptomatic heart failure. Only 5% to 15% of cardiac arrest patients are successfully resuscitated and discharged from the hospital without any associated neurologic deficits. Survival from SCD often depends on immediate cardiopulmonary resuscitation and the availability and use of automated external defibrillators (AEDs). The American Heart Association recommends the placement of AEDs in public locations, where an average of one cardiac arrest occurs every 5 years.

PATHOPHYSIOLOGY AND MECHANISM OF SUDDEN CARDIAC DEATH
The mechanism of SCD is complex and is often associated with an interplay between anatomical substrates, functional substrates, and transient events that lead to the initiation of ventricular arrhythmias (VT or VF).

Table 1. Causes of Sudden Cardiac Death

Electrophysiologic abnormalities
    Conduction system disease involving the His-
        Purkinje conduction system
    Primary ventricular arrhythmia associated
        with cardiac conditions
    Abnormalities of the QT interval
    Brugada syndrome
    Wolff-Parkinson-White syndrome
    Catecholaminergic ventricular tachycardia
    Idiopathic ventricular fibrillation
    Malignant ventricular arrhythmia resulting
        from metabolic abnormalities
    Commotio cordis
Coronary artery disease
    Atherosclerotic disease
    Congenital anomalies
    Spasm
    Arteritis
    Dissection
    Embolism
Primary cardiomyopathies
    Nonischemic dilated cardiomyopathy
    Hypertrophic cardiomyopathy
Myocarditis
Valvular heart disease
Arrhythmogenic right ventricular dysplasia
Pulmonary hypertension
Hypertensive heart disease
Congenital heart disease
Inflammatory and infiltrative disease of the
    myocardium
    Sarcoidosis
    Chagas disease
    Hemochromatosis
    Amyloidosis
    Hydatid cyst
Neuromuscular disease
    Muscular dystrophy
    Myotonic dystrophy
    Kearns-Sayre syndrome
    Friedreich ataxia
Intracardiac obstruction
    Primary cardiac tumors (e.g., myxoma)
    Intracardiac thrombus
    Massive pulmonary embolism
Acute aortic dissection

Figure 1 illustrates the many possible variations between the functional and anatomical substrates and the transient events that can occur, ultimately leading to SCD.

ISCHEMIC HEART DISEASE ASSOCIATED WITH SUDDEN CARDIAC DEATH

Atherosclerotic coronary artery disease is the leading cause of SCD. Studies have shown that 40% to 86% of patients who survived SCD, depending on the age and sex of the population, had coronary vessels with more than 75% cross-sectional stenosis. No specific distribution pattern of coronary artery lesions appears to favor the development of SCD. Overall, the extent of coronary artery stenosis appears to have a greater predictive value for predicting SCD than the specific location of the lesion. SCD does occur in the absence of acute myocardial infarction (MI), but it usually occurs in the presence of diffuse coronary artery disease. It has been reported that only 20% of SCD patients have evidence of acute MI at autopsy. In contrast, a healed MI is a more common finding among SCD patients, ranging in frequency from 40% to more than 70% in epidemiologic studies. Risk factors for SCD in this population include an ejection fraction of less then 40%, more than 10 premature ventricular contractions per hour, and nonsustained VT.

Several randomized, prospective trials have shown a significant benefit with use of an implantable cardioverter-defibrillator (ICD) in improving long-term survival in SCD patients who survived the initial event. Furthermore, recent trials such as MADIT, MUSTT, MADIT II, and SCD-HeFT (Appendix) demonstrated significant primary prevention benefits with implantation of an ICD in patients with reduced ventricular function. Patients with an ejection fraction of 35% or less derived the most benefit.

Results from major trials looking at benefits of antiarrhythmic medication for primary and secondary prevention of SCD have been disappointing. The use of class 1 and class 3 medications (D-sotalol, dofetilide) and calcium antagonists did not decrease but rather increased the incidence of SCD in some cases after MI. Of all the drugs evaluated, only β-blockers and amiodarone showed evidence for reduction of SCD after MI. However, evidence also demonstrated the

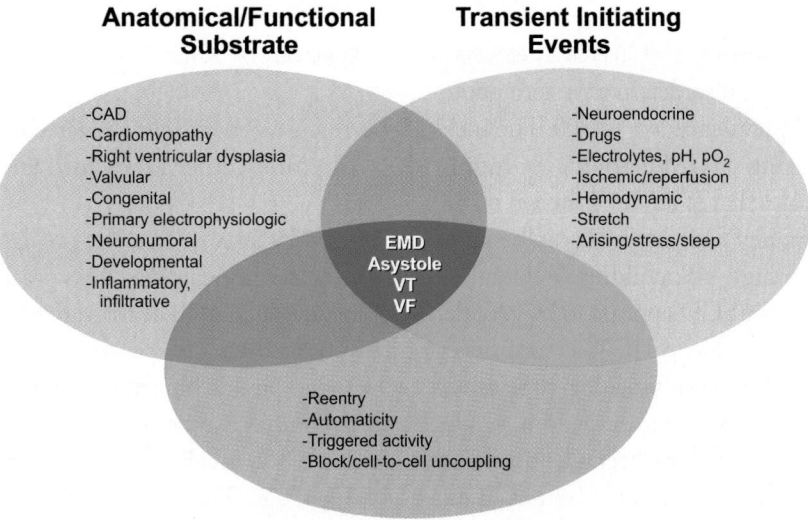

Fig. 1. Venn diagram showing interaction of various anatomical/functional and transient factors that cause sudden cardiac death. CAD, coronary artery disease; EMD, electromechanical dissociation; VF, ventricular fibrillation; VT, ventricular tachycardia.

clear benefit and superiority of ICDs over class 3 antiarrhythmics or β-blocker monotherapy in reducing mortality from life-threatening ventricular arrhythmias. All recent and major trials on the mortality benefits and effects of ICDs on SCD are covered in detail in Chapter 36 ("Implantable Cardioverter-Defibrillator Trials and Prevention of Sudden Cardiac Death").

- Atherosclerotic coronary artery disease is the leading cause of SCD.
- Randomized, prospective trials have shown a significant benefit with the implantation of an automatic ICD in improving long-term survival in SCD patients.
- The benefits of antiarrhythmic medications for primary and secondary prevention of SCD have been disappointing.

NONISCHEMIC HEART DISEASE ASSOCIATED WITH SUDDEN CARDIAC DEATH

Dilated Cardiomyopathy

Idiopathic dilated cardiomyopathy (DCM) accounts for approximately 10% of adult SCD patients. The overall mortality from idiopathic DCM ranges from 10% to 50% annually, depending on the severity of the disease. Subendocardial scarring and interstitial and perivascular fibrosis can be seen in DCM patients and are thought to be the culprits leading to reentrant ventricular arrhythmia in this group. In idiopathic DCM patients, SCD is usually associated with polymorphic and monomorphic VT. Among patients with DCM, those with functional class I or II have a lower mortality risk than those with poor functional capacity (class III or IV). High-risk predictors for sudden death in this population include syncope, heart failure symptoms, and nonsustained VT. There is very limited value in electrophysiologic testing for risk stratification in patients with nonischemic DCM.

- Idiopathic DCM accounts for approximately 10% of adult SCD patients.
- SCD is usually associated with polymorphic and monomorphic VT.
- Predictors of high risk for sudden cardiac death in this population include syncope, heart failure symptoms, and nonsustained VT.

Heritable Cardiomyopathies

Specific genetic abnormalities, indications for genetic testing, and additional diagnostic information are discussed in Chapter 31 ("Heritable Cardiomyopathies"). The clinical management of specific heritable cardiomyopathies is discussed below.

Hypertrophic Cardiomyopathy

Hypertrophic cardiomyopathy (HCM) is a heterogenous autosomal dominant disorder. In a western population, the estimated prevalence is 1 in 500. The incidence of SCD among HCM patients is highly variable. It approximates that of an age-matched population in older community patients, but it can be up to 4% to 6% per year in high-risk children and adolescents. The propensity for SCD appears to be genetic, and if a diagnosis of SCD due to HCM is confirmed, it is now recommended that all first-degree relatives receive periodic echocardiographic evaluation. High-risk clinical markers for SCD have been identified and are outlined in Table 2. HCM patients with one of the major risk factors or three or more of the minor risk factors may benefit from implantation of an automatic ICD, although the decision to proceed must be made on an individual basis. ICD is the treatment of choice to prevent sudden death in high-risk patients. Recent studies also suggest that septal myectomy reduces the likelihood of sudden death after myectomy. Electrophysiologic studies (EPSs) are not useful in identifying HCM patients at high risk of SCD.

- Hypertrophic cardiomyopathy is an autosomal dominant disorder.
- HCM patients with one of the major risk factors or three or more of the minor risk factors benefit from automatic ICD implantation.

Table 2. Clinical Risk Factors for Sudden Death in Hypertrophic Cardiomyopathy

Major risk factors
   Cardiac arrest
   Spontaneous sustained ventricular tachycardia
   History of sudden cardiac death in first-degree relatives
Minor risk factors
   Recurrent unexplained syncope
   Marked left ventricular hypertrophy (>30 mm)
   Nonsustained ventricular tachycardia
   Abnormal blood pressure response to exercise
   Perfusion defects on magnetic resonance imaging

- EPSs are not useful in identifying HCM patients at high risk of SCD.

Arrhythmogenic Right Ventricular Cardiomyopathy

Arrhythmogenic right ventricular cardiomyopathy (ARVC) is a myocardial disease, often familial, characterized by fatty or fibrofatty replacement of the right ventricular myocardium. This process can lead to thinning and dilatation of the right ventricle and can predispose patients to recurrent ventricular arrhythmias with left bundle branch morphologies. The ventricular arrhythmias can be precipitated by exercise. Patients with ARVC usually present after puberty but before 50 years of age. The pattern of inheritance is autosomal dominant in one-third of patients. The annual incidence for sudden death is estimated to be 2%. The course and prognosis of ARVC are highly variable and difficult to predict.

The diagnosis for ARVC is based on the major and minor criteria created by the Task Force of the Working Group of Myocardial and Pericardial Disease of the European Society of Cardiology and the Scientific Council on Cardiomyopathies of the International Society and Federation of Cardiology. These criteria are summarized in Table 3. The electrocardiographic (ECG) features during sinus rhythm include the presence of T-wave inversions in the right precordial leads (V_1-V_3), epsilon wave in V_1, and a widened localized QRS complex in V_1 through V_3. The ventricular ectopy usually has left bundle branch morphology (suggesting right ventricular origin) and a QRS axis usually between −90 and +110. ARVC should be considered if a patient presents with frequent premature ventricular beats with multiple left bundle branch block morphologies and left axis deviation. Common noninvasive modalities used to evaluate ARVC include two-dimensional echocardiography and radionuclide ventriculography. Recently, magnetic resonance imaging (MRI) and computed tomography (CT) have emerged as extremely useful tools in providing direct evidence for fatty infiltration and structural alterations of the right ventricle.

Management of patients who have a diagnosis of ARVC should include avoidance of competitive athletics, initiation of a β-blocker, and consideration for ICD implantation. Any ARVC patient who presents with a history of sustained VT or SCD should be considered

Table 3.   Diagnostic Criteria for Arrhythmogenic Right Ventricular Dysplasia or Cardiomyopathy*

Feature	Major criteria	Minor criteria
Structural or functional abnormalities	1. Severe dilatation and reduction of RVEF with mild or no left ventricular involvement	1. Mild global right ventricular dilation or RVEF reduction with normal left ventricle
	2. Localized right ventricular aneurysm (akinetic or dyskinetic areas with diastolic bulging)	2. Mild segmental dilation of the right ventricle
	3. Severe segmental dilatation of the right ventricle	3. Regional right ventricular hypo-kinesis
Tissue characterization	Infiltration of right ventricle by fat with presence of surviving strands of cardiomyocytes	
Electrocardiogram depolarizaion or conduction abnormalities	1. Localized QRS complex, duration >110 ms in V_1, V_2, or V_3	Late potentials in SAECG
Electrocardiogram repolarization abnormalities	2. Epsilon wave in V_1, V_2, V_3	Inverted T waves in right precordial leads (V_2-V_3 if older than 12 years in absence of RBBB)
Arrhythmias		1. LBBB ventricular tachycardia (sustained or nonsustained) on electrocardiogram, Holter or ETT
		2. Frequency PVCs (>1,000/24 h on Holter)
Family history	Family history of ARVD confirmed by biopsy of autopsy	1. Family history of premature sudden death (<35 years) due to suspected ARVD
		2. Family history of clinical diagno-sis based on present criteria

*The criteria state that an individual must have two major, one major plus two minor, or four minor criteria from different categories to meet the diagnosis of arrhythmogenic right ventricular dysplasia/cardiomyopathy.
ARVD, arrhythmogenic right ventricular dysplasia; ETT, exercise toleration test; LBBB, left bundle branch block; PVC, premature ventricular contraction; RBBB, right bundle branch block; REVF, right ventricular ejection fraction; SAECG, signal-averaged electrocardiogram.

for placement of an ICD. Because of the progressive nature of this disease, catheter ablation is not curative but rather palliative for patients with frequent ICD discharges from ventricular arrhythmias.

■ ARVC is a myocardial disease, often familial, characterized by fatty or fibrofatty replacement of the right ventricular myocardium.
■ ARVC patients are predisposed to recurrent and intractable ventricular arrhythmias with multiple left bundle branch block morphologies.

■ The annual incidence for sudden death is estimated to be 2%.
■ Management of patients who have a diagnosis of ARVC includes avoidance of competitive athletics, initiation of a β-blocker, and consideration for ICD implantation.

Long QT Syndrome

Long QT syndrome can be congenital or acquired. Studies of patients with congenital long QT syndrome have reported the mean age at presentation to be 24 years, with an annual incidence of 1.3% for SCD and 8.6% for recurrent syncope. Patients with this syndrome can present with variable symptoms, including seizures, syncope, or sudden death. These symptoms can be triggered by physical or emotional stress or loud noises. Symptoms usually appear in childhood, with males seeming to present earlier than females.

High-risk predictors for this population include female sex, prior cardiac arrest, recurrent syncope, long QT syndrome associated with deafness, siblings of patients with SCD, corrected QT interval exceeding 500 ms, prior VF episodes, and documented torsades de pointes. These patients should be considered for aggressive medical intervention or ICD implantation. Interestingly, high adrenergic states caused by defibrillator shocks may reinitiate torsades de pointes in patients with congenital long QT syndrome. Therefore, β-blocker therapy should be considered in addition to ICD therapy. Potentially life-threatening arrhythmias may be provoked by exercise-associated tachycardia. Therefore, patients with documented irreversible long QT syndrome should abstain from competitive sports. The degree of QT prolongation is weakly correlated with the risk of cardiac events.

- Long QT syndrome can be congenital or acquired.
- Patients with long QT are at risk of life-threatening ventricular arrhythmias, such as torsades de pointes.
- Patients with documented irreversible long QT syndrome should abstain from competitive sports.

Short QT Syndrome

Short QT syndrome is an inheritable electrical disorder first described in 1999. The disorder is characterized by a short QT interval (<300 ms) and presenting symptoms that can include syncope, paroxysmal atrial fibrillation, and life-threatening cardiac arrhythmias. Another characteristic of short QT syndrome is a short or even absent ST segment followed by a tall and narrow T wave. Any patient presenting with atrial or ventricular arrhythmias along with a short QT on an ECG, which is not associated with any underlying correctible, cause should be evaluated for short QT syndrome.

This syndrome typically affects young, healthy people with no underlying structural heart disease. Most patients with this syndrome have a family history of sudden death or atrial fibrillation. The best treat-

ment for this disorder is still unknown. Antiarrhythmics known to prolong the QT interval, such as sotalol or quinidine, may be a beneficial treatment for this disorder. Atrial fibrillation associated with short QT syndrome responds well to propafenone. The first line of therapy for this disorder, especially in SCD survivors or in those with a history of syncope, is an ICD.

- Short QT syndrome is characterized by a short QT interval (<300 ms), and presenting symptoms can include syncope, paroxysmal atrial fibrillation, and life-threatening cardiac arrhythmias.
- Short QT syndrome typically affects young, healthy people with no underlying structural heart disease.
- The best treatment for this disorder is still unknown; however, implantation of an ICD is first-line therapy in SCD survivors or those with a history of syncope.

Brugada Syndrome

Brugada syndrome is an autosomal dominant disorder known to cause SCD and syncope in young, healthy individuals who have structurally normal hearts. This syndrome is diagnosed on the basis of symptoms and the presence of an abnormal ECG with ST-segment elevations in the right precordial leads (V_1-V_3). The syndrome typically manifests during adulthood, with a mean age of 40 years for the appearance of arrhythmic events and sudden death.

Three clinical ECG repolarization patterns of the right precordial lead can be found with Brugada syndrome. Type 1 is diagnostic for Brugada syndrome. This pattern is characterized by a coved ST-segment elevation of 2 mm or more in the right precordial leads (V_1-V_3) associated with a negative T wave (Fig. 2). Typically, if type 1 ECG pattern is present in asymptomatic patients under baseline conditions, no further pharmacologic challenge is needed to diagnose this syndrome. Type 2 is associated with ST-segment elevation with a saddleback appearance and a high takeoff ST elevation of 2 mm or more with a trough of 1 mm or more. The T wave is either positive or biphasic (Fig. 2). Type 3 can have either a saddleback or a coved appearance, with an ST-segment elevation of less than 1 mm. All three patterns can be seen in the same patient; however, types 2 and 3 are not diagnostic for Brugada syndrome. The ECG manifestations of this syndrome may be concealed and can be unmasked by using sodium channel blockers.

Patients with Brugada syndrome may present with syncope and sudden death. Other presenting symptoms may include seizures, agitation, recent memory loss, and loss of bladder control. VF and sudden death with this syndrome usually occur at rest and at night. This syndrome has also been associated with supraventricular tachyarrhythmias. The prognosis and therapeutic approach in patients with a diagnostic ECG but without any previous history of sudden death are controversial. One approach to managing patients with type 1 ECG findings for Brugada syndrome is summarized in Figure 3. EPS is recommended only for symptomatic patients with Brugada syndrome who are suspected of having an underlying supraventricular arrhythmia or for asymptomatic patients with a type 1 ECG either spontaneously or with induction from a sodium channel blockade and with a family history of suspected SCD. EPS should also be considered in asymptomatic patients with no family history of SCD showing a type 1 ECG pattern spontaneously. Patients with no clinical symptoms and no family history of SCD who develop a type 1 ECG pattern only with

sodium channel blockade can be followed closely without immediate ICD implantation. All symptomatic and asymptomatic patients with a malignant family history should be considered for ICD implantation. ICD is the only proven, effective prevention strategy for SCD in patients with Brugada syndrome.

- Brugada syndrome is an autosomal dominant disorder known to cause SCD and syncope in young, healthy individuals with structurally normal hearts.
- Brugada syndrome has been linked to an inherited mutation in the *SCN5A* gene.
- All symptomatic and asymptomatic patients with a malignant family history should be considered for ICD implantation.

Wolff-Parkinson-White Syndrome

The risk of SCD in patients with Wolff-Parkinson-White (WPW) syndrome is less than 1 per 1,000 patient-years of follow-up. In 10% of patients, SCD is the first manifestation of the disease. The mechanism for SCD is thought to be associated with the develop-

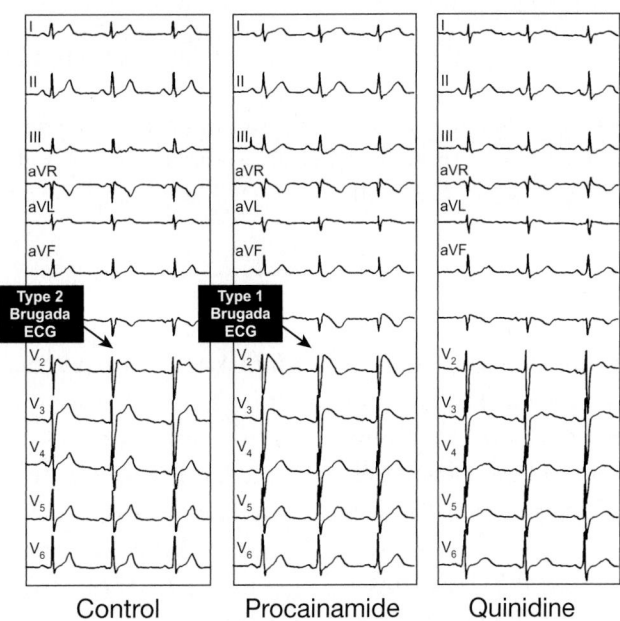

Fig. 2. Twelve-lead electrocardiographic (ECG) tracings in an asymptomatic 26-year-old man with Brugada syndrome. *Left*, Baseline-type 2 ECG (not diagnostic) displaying a saddleback-type ST-segment elevation is observed in V$_2$. *Center*, After intravenous administration of 750 mg procainamide, the type 2 ECG is converted to the diagnostic-type 1 ECG, which consists of a coved-type ST-segment elevation. *Right*, A few days after oral administration of quinidine bisulfate (1,500 mg/d; serum quinidine level, 2.6 mg/L), ST-segment elevation is attenuated displaying a nonspecific abnormal pattern in the right precordial leads. Ventricular fibrillation could be induced during control and procainamide infusion periods but not after quinidine.

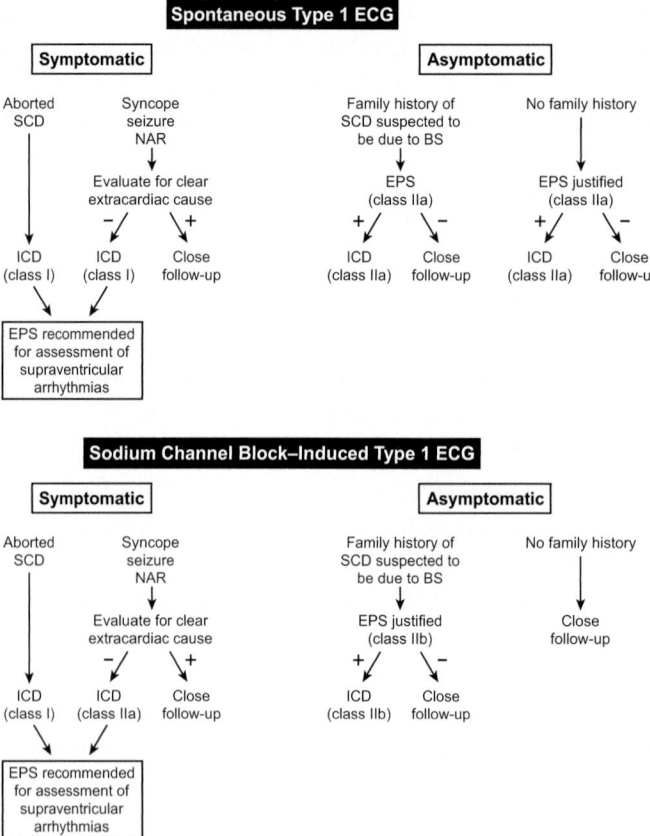

Fig. 3. Indications for use of implantable cardioverter-defibrillator (ICD) in patients with Brugada syndrome. Class I designation indicates clear evidence that the procedure or treatment is useful or effective; class II, conflicting evidence about usefulness or efficacy; class IIa weight of evidence is in favor of usefulness or efficacy; and class IIb, usefulness or efficacy is less well established. BS, Brugada syndrome; ECG, electrocardiogram; EPS, electrophysiologic study; NAR, nocturnal agonal respiration; SCD, sudden cardiac death.

ment of atrial fibrillation with rapid conduction to the ventricles over the accessory pathway, causing fast ventricular rates and degeneration into VF. The best predictor for development of VF during atrial fibrillation is the presence of spontaneous rapid conduction over the accessory pathway, leading to rapid ventricular rates of 250 ms or less.

Management of asymptomatic WPW patients is controversial. In general, patients with only intermittent ventricular preexcitation and those in whom the refractory period of the accessory pathway was determined to be long are considered to be at low risk for SCD. However, when the benign nature of the accessory pathway is in question by noninvasive evaluation, EPS with possible radiofrequency ablation should be considered. Prophylactic EPS with ablation should also

be considered in patients with high-risk occupations such as truck drivers and airplane pilots.

- SCD risk in patients with WPW syndrome is <1 per 1,000 patient-years of follow-up.
- Spontaneous rapid conduction over the accessory pathway, leading to rapid ventricular rates ≤250 ms during atrial fibrillation is the best predictor for development of VF.
- Prophylactic EPS with ablation should be considered in patients with high-risk occupations.

Valvular Heart Disease
Aortic stenosis has been associated with SCD. Patients with asymptomatic aortic stenosis have a lower incidence of SCD. Both ventricular and bradyarrhythmias

have been reported as possible underlying mechanisms for SCD in these patients. Patients with prosthetic or heterograft aortic valve replacement are at risk of SCD. This may be due to underlying prosthetic valve dysfunction, arrhythmias, or coexistent coronary artery disease. A high incidence of ventricular arrhythmias has also been observed at follow-up after valve replacement in patients who had multiple valve operations or cardiomegaly. SCD has been reported to peak 3 weeks after both aortic valve replacement and mitral valve surgery and plateaus after 8 months. Studies have shown that SCD is the second most common mode of death after valve replacement surgery. The incidence has been estimated at 2% to 4% during a 7-year follow-up.

Regurgitant lesions, including chronic aortic regurgitation and acute mitral regurgitation may also be associated with SCD; however, the risk is lower than that with aortic stenosis. Overall, the risk of SCD in patients with mitral valve prolapse is low.

Congenital Heart Disease

Increased risk of SCD has been identified with congenital conditions including tetralogy of Fallot, transposition of the great arteries, and aortic stenosis. SCD has also been described as a complication from surgical repair of complex congenital cardiac lesions. Potential risk markers for development of malignant ventricular arrhythmias in patients with tetralogy of Fallot include older age at surgical repair, wide QRS complex (>180 ms), and moderate or severe pulmonary regurgitation. Even with the identification of potential risk markers, the best way to identify patients who would benefit the most from ICD implantation is still clinically challenging.

Inflammatory and Infiltrative Heart Disorders

Any inflammatory disorder can be associated with SCD due to either ventricular arrhythmias or complete heart block. Viral myocarditis with or without left ventricular dysfunction can be associated with potentially lethal cardiac arrhythmias. This inflammatory condition is often the result of a viral infection from coxsackievirus or echovirus. Myocardial involvement in chronic granulomatous diseases and vascular and infiltrative disorders can also be associated with SCD. Common infiltrative disorders that have been associated with ventricular arrhythmias and SCD include amyloidosis, hemochromatosis, and sarcoidosis.

Idiopathic Ventricular Fibrillation

SCD from primary VF without evidence for any underlying structural heart disease can occur in approximately 5% of SCD patients. The diagnosis of idiopathic VF is made by exclusion of all other potential possibilities. Studies have shown that patients with primary VF can have a recurrence rate as high as 30% for syncope, VF, and cardiac arrest. For these patients, the current consensus is that drug therapy is ineffective and that ICD is most effective for secondary prevention but may be used to reduce frequency of shocks.

SUDDEN CARDIAC DEATH IN THE YOUNG AND ATHLETES

The overall annual incidence of SCD among young patients is 600; 19% of SCD in children occurs between 1 and 13 years of age and 30%, between 14 and 21 years. In more than 80% of cases in young athletes, SCD occurs either during or immediately after strenuous exercise. In the young population, in particular competitive athletes, the most common cause of sudden death is HCM and the second most common cause is congenital coronary artery anomalies. The most common coronary anomaly associated with SCD in athletes is left main artery originating from the right sinus of Valsalva. In mature athletes, older than 35 years, atherosclerotic coronary artery disease is the most common cause of SCD. In addition, commotio cordis (concussion of the heart from nonpenetrating blunt trauma to the anterior chest) can cause SCD in athletes.

The annual incidence of SCD during exercise is 1 per 200,000 to 1 per 250,000 healthy young people. Only 20 to 25 sports-related cases of SCD occur annually in United States. Any athlete presenting with a history of syncope or near-syncope with exercise should be excluded from participation in any sports until after a complete cardiac evaluation. Most patients who have a genetic cardiovascular disorder, including HCM, ARCV, Marfan syndrome, long QT syndrome, and Brugada syndrome, can still safely participate in most forms of low- or moderate-intensity recreational exercise. Table 4 summarizes the recommendations for noncompetitive recreational sports in patients with genetic cardiovascular disease. General screening programs for identifying rare cardiac conditions in large populations of asymptomatic athletes can be costly and inefficient.

Therefore, guidelines have been published outlining which athletes should be screened and which athletes with cardiac arrhythmias can participate in competitive sports (See Chapter 38, "Heart Disease in Athletes").

- The most common cause of sudden death in competitive athletes is HCM, and the second most common cause is congenital coronary artery anomalies.
- The most common cause of SCD in athletes older than 35 years is atherosclerotic coronary artery disease.
- General screening programs for identifying rare cardiac conditions in large populations of asymptomatic athletes can be costly and inefficient.

EVALUATION AND RISK STRATIFICATION

Evaluation of SCD survivors should always begin with a complete history and physical examination covering patient medications, family history, drug use, and risk factors. Common cardiac risk factors, including smoking, hypertension, and hyperlipidemia, can serve as easily identifiable markers of increased risk for underlying ischemic cardiomyopathy. These risk factors can help identify the risk of underlying disease that may be responsible for SCD; thereby active intervention in preventing these risk factors may ultimately help to reduce the number of fatal arrhythmic events. Other useful tools for evaluation, based on the clinical scenario, can include Holter monitor, echocardiogram, ECG, CT, MRI, and coronary angiogram. One of the most powerful predictors of primary and secondary cardiac arrest is left ventricular ejection fraction, and this should be assessed in all SCD survivors. More specific markers for identifying patients at risk of SCD have been researched and are summarized in Table 5. The usefulness of EPS for stratifying patients at risk of SCD is limited. Recent trials including MADIT II and SCD-HeFT have further reduced the need for an EPS. The sensitivity of EPS is better in patients with a previous history of MI than in those with nonischemic cardiomyopathy. Many tools are available for evaluating SCD survivors. The key is to focus the evaluation based on the clinical scenario. With the exception of patients with reversible causes, the majority of SCD survivors will ultimately require ICD implantation for prevention of future life-threatening arrhythmic episodes.

Table 4.   Recommendations for the Acceptability of Recreational (Noncompetitive) Sports Activities and Exercise in Patients With Genetic Cardiovascular Disease*

Intensity level	HCM	LQTS†	Marfan syndrome‡	ARVC	Brugada syndrome
High					
Basketball					
Full court	0	0	2	1	2
Half court	0	0	2	1	2
Body building§	1	1	0	1	1
Ice hockey	0	0	1	0	0
Racquetball/squash	0	2	2	0	2
Rock climbing	1	1	1	1	1
Running (sprinting)	0	0	2	0	2
Skiing (downhill)	2	2	2	1	1
Skiing (cross-country)	2	3	2	1	4
Soccer	0	0	2	0	2
Tennis (singles)	0	0	3	0	2
Touch (flag) football	1	1	3	1	3
Windsurfing‖	1	0	1	1	1

Table 4.   (continued)

Intensity level	HCM	LQTS†	Marfan syndrome‡	ARVC	Brugada syndrome
Moderate					
Baseball/softball	2	2	2	2	4
Biking	4	4	3	2	5
Modest hiking	4	5	5	2	4
Motorcycling	3	1	2	2	2
Jogging	3	3	3	2	5
Sailing	3	3	2	2	4
Surfing	2	0	1	1	1
Swimming (lap)¶	5	0	3	3	4
Tennis (doubles)	4	4	4	3	4
Treadmill/stationary bicycle	5	5	4	3	5
Weightlifting (free weights)§¶	1	1	0	1	1
Hiking	3	3	3	2	4
Low					
Bowling	5	5	5	4	5
Golf	5	5	5	4	5
Horseback riding§	3	3	3	3	3
Scuba diving	0	0	0	0	0
Skating#	5	5	5	4	5
Snorkeling	5	0	5	4	4
Weights (non-free weights)	4	4	0	4	4
Brisk walking	5	5	5	5	5

ARVC, arrhythmogenic right ventricular cardiomyopathy; HCM, hypertrophic cardiomyopathy; LQTS, long QT syndrome.

*Recreational sports are categorized with regard to high, moderate, and low levels of exercise and graded on a relative scale (from 0 to 5) for eligibility, with 0 to 1 indicating generally not advised or strongly discouraged; 4 to 5, probably permitted; and 2 to 3, intermediate and to be assessed clinically on an individual basis. The designation of high, moderate, and low levels of exercise are equivalent to an estimated >6, 4 to 6, and <4 metabolic equivalent, respectively.

†Assumes absence of laboratory DNA genotyping data; therefore, limited to clinical diagnosis.

‡Assumes no or only mild aortic dilatation.

§These sports involve the potential for traumatic injury, which should be taken into consideration for individuals with a risk of impaired consciousness.

//The possibility of impaired consciousness occurring during water-related activities should be taken into account with respect to the clinical profile of the individual patient. Barotrauma is a primary risk associated with the use of scuba apparatus in Marfan syndrome.

¶Recommendations generally differ from those for weight-training machines (non-free weights), based largely on the potential risks of traumatic injury associated with episodes of impaired consciousness during benchpress maneuvers; otherwise, the physiologic effects of all weight-training activities are regarded as similar with respect to the present recommendations.

#Individual sporting activity not associated with the team sport of ice hockey.

- Evaluation of SCD survivors should always begin with a complete history and physical examination covering medications, family history, drug use, and risk factors.
- The usefulness of EPS for stratifying patients at risk of SCD is limited.
- With the exception of patients with reversible causes, such as electrolyte abnormalities, the majority of SCD patients ultimately require ICD implantation for prevention of future life-threatening arrhythmic episodes.

Table 5.   Indicators of an Increased Risk of Sudden Death From Arrhythmia

Variable	Measure	Predictive power
Conventional coronary risk factors High cholesterol High blood pressure Smoking Diabetes	Risk of underyling disease	Low power to discriminate the individual person at risk of sudden death from arrhythmia
Clinical markers NYHA functional class Ejection fraction	Extent of structural disease	High power to predict death from cardiac causes; relatively low specificity as predictors of death from arrhythmia
Ambient ventricular arrhythmia Frequency of premature depolarization Nonsustained ventricular tachycardia	Presence of transient triggers	Low overall power if not combined with other variables
Sustained ventricular tachycardia		Higher predictive power, with low ejection fraction
Electrocardiographic variables Standard ECG Left ventricular hypertrophy Width of QRS complex QT dispersion	Presence of electrical abnormalities	Low power to predict death from arrhythmia
Specific abnormalities (e.g., prolonged QT interval, right bundle branch block plus ST-segment elevation in lead V_1 [Brugada syndrome], ST-segment and T-wave abnormalities in leads V_1 and V_2 [right ventricular dysplasia], delta waves [Wolff-Parkinson-White syndrome]		High degree of accuracy in identifying specific electrical abnormalities
High-resolution ECG Late potentials on signal-averaged ECG		High negative predictive value but low positive predictive value
T-wave alternans		Primary predictive value unknown
Markers of autonomic nervous function Heart rate variability Baroreflex sensitivity	Presence of conditioning factors	Exact predictive value unknown
Electrophysiological testing Inducibility of sustained tachy-arrhythmia by programmed electrical stimulation	Presence of permanent substrate for ventricular arrhythmias	High degree of accuracy in specific high-risk subgroups

ECG, electrocardiogram; NYHA, New York Heart Association.

Appendix
Names of Clinical Trials

MADIT	Multicenter Automatic Defibrillator Implantation Trial
MUSTT	Multicenter Unsustained Tachycardia Trial
SCD-HeFT	Sudden Cardiac Death in Heart Failure Trial

38

HEART DISEASE IN ATHLETES

Stephen C. Hammill, MD

The medical community, the public, and athletes all have concerns about identifying a priori individuals at risk for sudden cardiac death. Physicians are frequently asked to assess an individual's suitability to participate in a particular sport. Ideally, identification of individuals at risk and intervention should be aimed at younger athletes, who are at a stage in their lives when it is easier for them to alter their lifestyles and redirect their interests toward other activities.

In high school, the athlete is a minor, the activity is extracurricular, and the athlete is considered an amateur. As athletes age through college and gain independence as adults, their sport becomes a vocation and personal and institutional financial incentives to pursue athletic competition are considerable. Professional athletes may have devoted their entire lives to athletic training, and they have even stronger financial and organizational interests in playing.

Typically, compared with nonathletes, athletes have a slower minimal heart rate, higher percentage of sinus pauses longer than 2 seconds, and more Mobitz I atrioventricular block (Wenckebach) because of higher vagal tone that occurs with conditioning. The slower heart rate causes a compensatory increase in stroke volume to maintain cardiac output; therefore, athletes often have increased left ventricular size but not increased left ventricular wall thickness. Sports associated with the largest left ventricular size include rowing, cycling, and cross-country skiing.

The causes of sudden death in athletes depend on age. Among athletes younger than 35 years, approximately 50% who die suddenly are found at autopsy to have hypertrophic cardiomyopathy, 18% idiopathic left ventricular cardiomyopathy, 14% coronary artery abnormalities, 10% coronary artery disease, and 7% ruptured aorta. An additional 3% have an unexplained cause; presumably these persons had some type of an electrical abnormality such as long QT syndrome, Brugada syndrome, polymorphic ventricular tachycardia, or idiopathic ventricular fibrillation. In contrast, among athletes 35 years or older, 80% are found at autopsy to have severe coronary disease, 5% hypertrophic cardiomyopathy, 5% mitral valve prolapse, 5% acquired valvular disease, and 5% no identified cause.

Screening for heart disease is difficult because of the large number of persons who need to be screened to prevent just one sudden death. In asymptomatic persons younger than 35 years, approximately 200,000 athletes would need to be screened to identify 1 in whom sudden death could be prevented (Fig. 1). Screening is equally difficult in competitive athletes who are asymptomatic and older than 35 years (Fig. 2). In this group, 10,000 asymptomatic persons need to be screened to prevent 1 sudden death, but 4 sudden

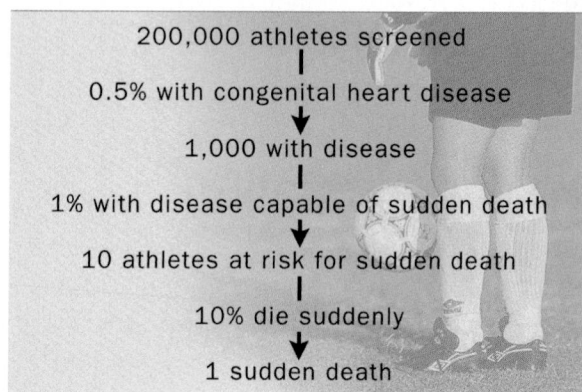

Fig. 1. Screening asymptomatic competitive athletes younger than 35 years for risk of sudden death.

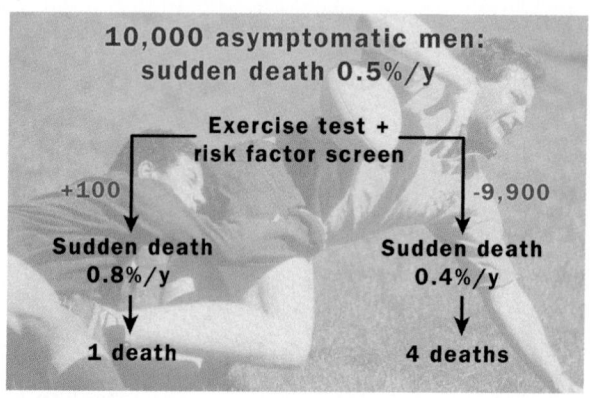

Fig. 2. Screening asymptomatic competitive athletes 35 years or older for risk of sudden death.

deaths would have occurred in the group with no risk factors and normal stress test. Obviously, intensive screening in both of these groups is not cost-effective. Furthermore, published studies have included almost exclusively male athletes; their applicability to female athletes is unknown.

Guidelines for determining athletic eligibility, formulated at the 26th Bethesda Conference, were published by the American College of Cardiology and the Heart Rhythm Society. These guidelines recommend that athletes be screened initially with a history and physical examination. If the history identifies an individual with previous near syncope, syncope, palpitations, or a family history of sudden cardiac death or if the physical examination identifies a serious heart murmur or other cardiac problem, the athlete should undergo electrocardiography, echocardiography, and stress testing. Depending on the results of these tests, electrophysiologic testing or long-term monitoring should be considered. Hypertrophic cardiomyopathy is the most common abnormality identified during pre-participation screening of athletes.

The athlete presenting with syncope or palpitations needs to undergo a history and physical examination, along with electrocardiography, stress testing, and echocardiography. If *no* heart disease is identified, further evaluation may include tilt testing and event recording; if heart disease *is* identified, further evaluation may include electrophysiologic studies followed by tilt testing or event recording if no serious abnormality is identified. In this population, an implantable loop recorder is extremely useful for capturing the

electrocardiographic findings during infrequent symptoms.

In summary:

1. It is common for athletes to have increased left ventricular size but not increased left ventricular wall thickness.
2. Hypertrophic cardiomyopathy is the most common abnormality identified during pre-participation screening of athletes.
3. Among athletes younger than 35 years, approximately 50% who die suddenly are found at autopsy to have hypertrophic cardiomyopathy.
4. Among athletes 35 years or older, 80% are found at autopsy to have severe coronary disease.

■ Patients should always be excluded from competitive athletics if they have the following conditions: hypertrophic cardiomyopathy, Brugada syndrome, arrhythmogenic right ventricular dysplasia, severe aortic stenosis.

RESOURCES

Extes NA III, Link MS, Cannom D, et al. Expert Consensus Conference on Arrhythmias in the Athlete of the North American Society of Pacing and Electrophysiology. J Cardiovasc Electrophysiol. 2001;12:1208-19.

26th Bethesda Conference: recommendations for determining eligibility for competition in athletes with cardiovascular abnormalities; January 6-7, 1994. J Am Coll Cardiol. 1994;24:845-99.

39

ATLAS OF ELECTROPHYSIOLOGY TRACINGS

Douglas L. Packer, MD

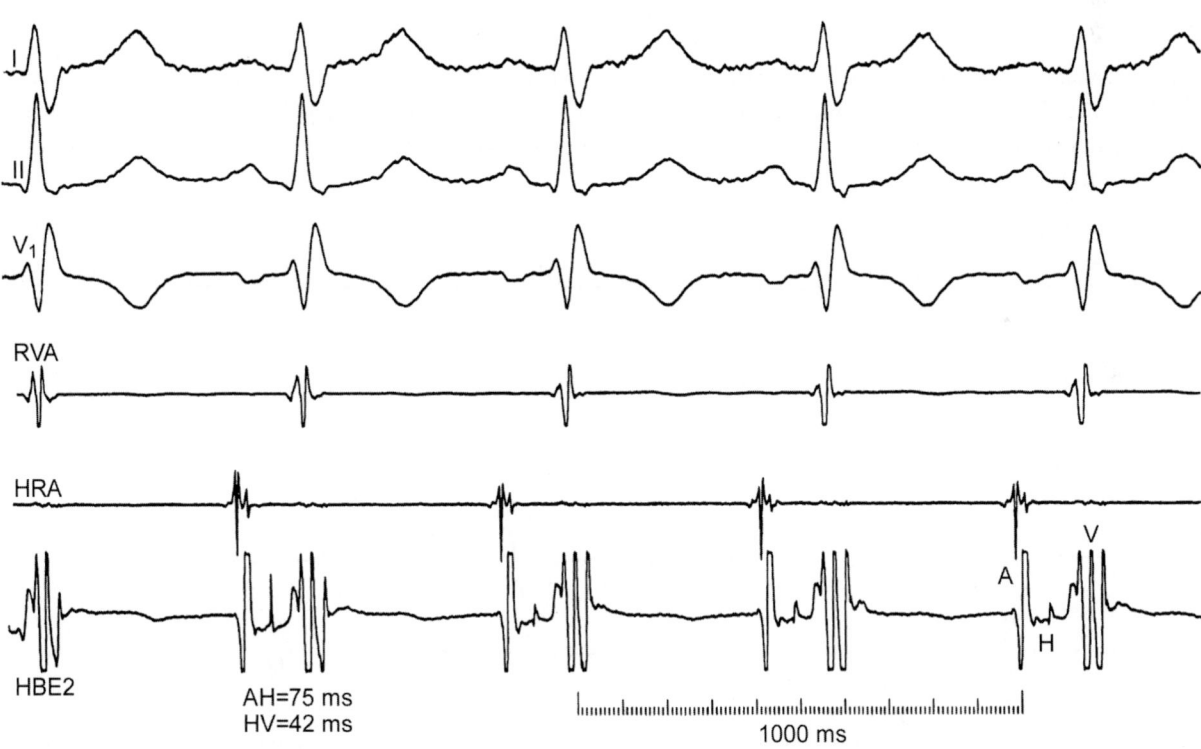

Fig. 1. *Normal sinus rhythm with normal conduction intervals.* Despite the presence of right bundle branch block, the AH interval of 75 ms and HV interval of 42 ms shown on the electrogram labeled HBE2 are normal. The AH interval is measured from the first discrete, rapid atrial deflection to the first deflection of the His bundle. The HV interval is taken from the first discrete, rapid His deflection to the onset of the surface QRS or ventricular deflection on the HBE2 channel, as indicated by the straight line. HBE, His bundle electrogram; HRA, high right atrium; RVA, right ventricular apex.

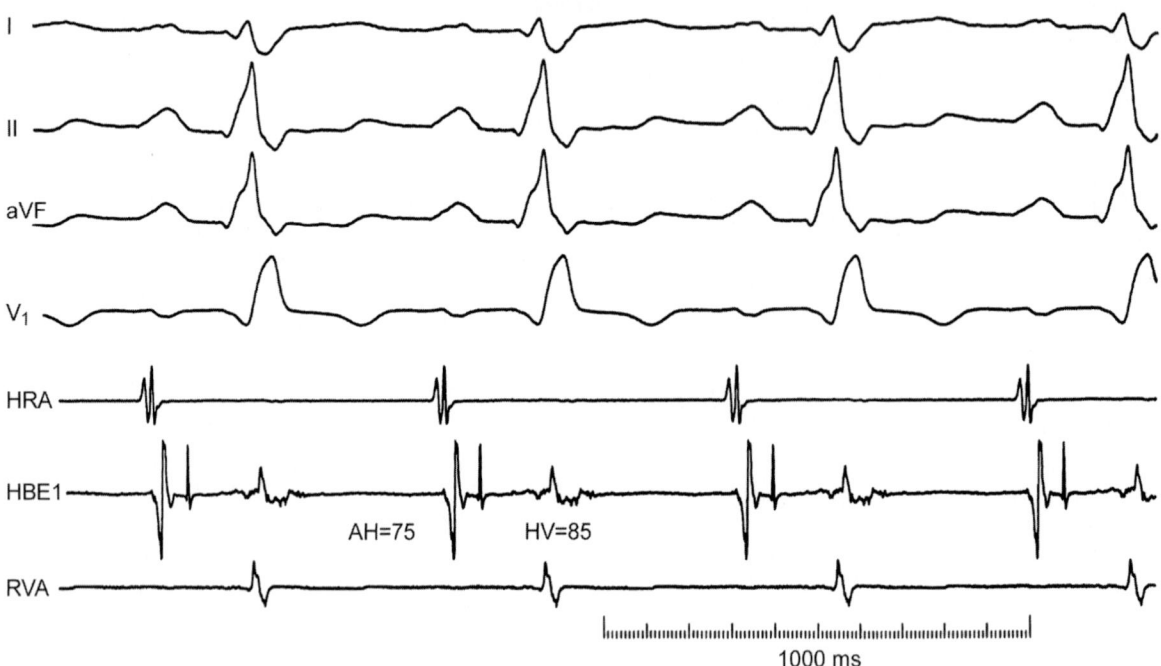

Fig. 2. *Normal sinus rhythm with infra-His conduction delay.* Here, the HV interval is grossly prolonged. In the setting of bifascicular block, this finding is accompanied by a 12% risk of progression to complete heart block. The HV interval is 85 milliseconds in duration. A normal HV interval is less than 60 milliseconds. See Figure 1 for explanation of abbreviations.

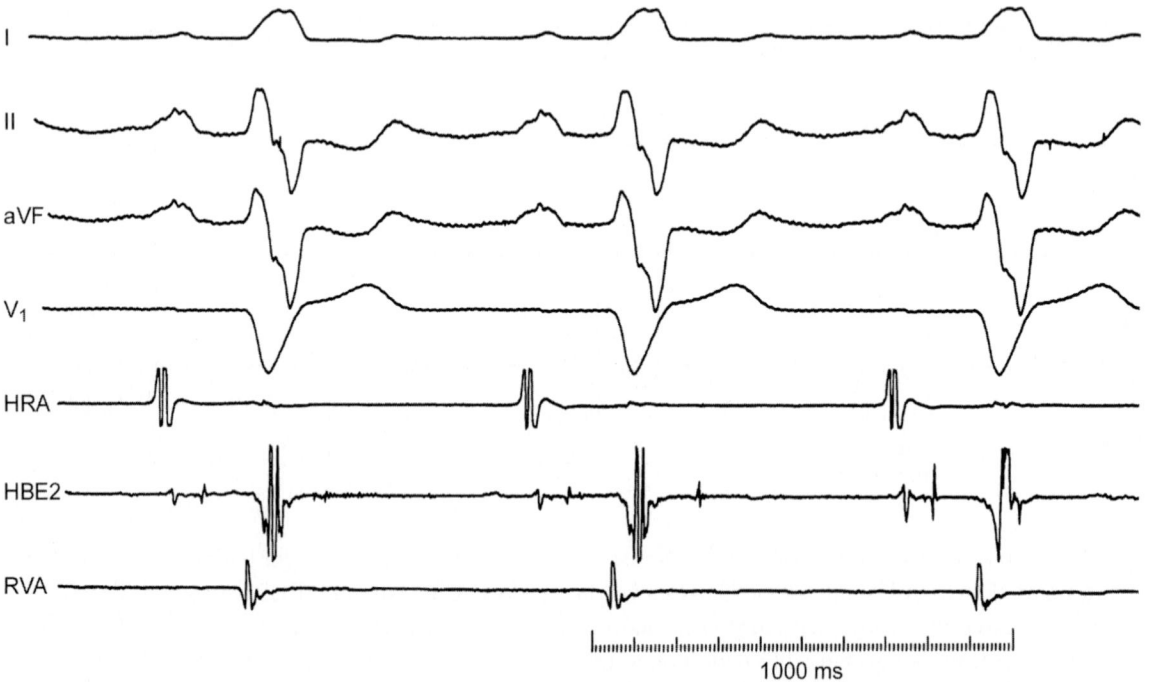

Fig. 3. *Normal sinus rhythm with left bundle branch block QRS morphology (negative deflection in V₁ lead) and a prolonged HV interval.* The infra-His conduction time is grossly prolonged at 100 milliseconds. In a patient with a history of syncope, this interval would be a sufficient indication for pacemaker implantation. See Figure 1 for explanation of abbreviations.

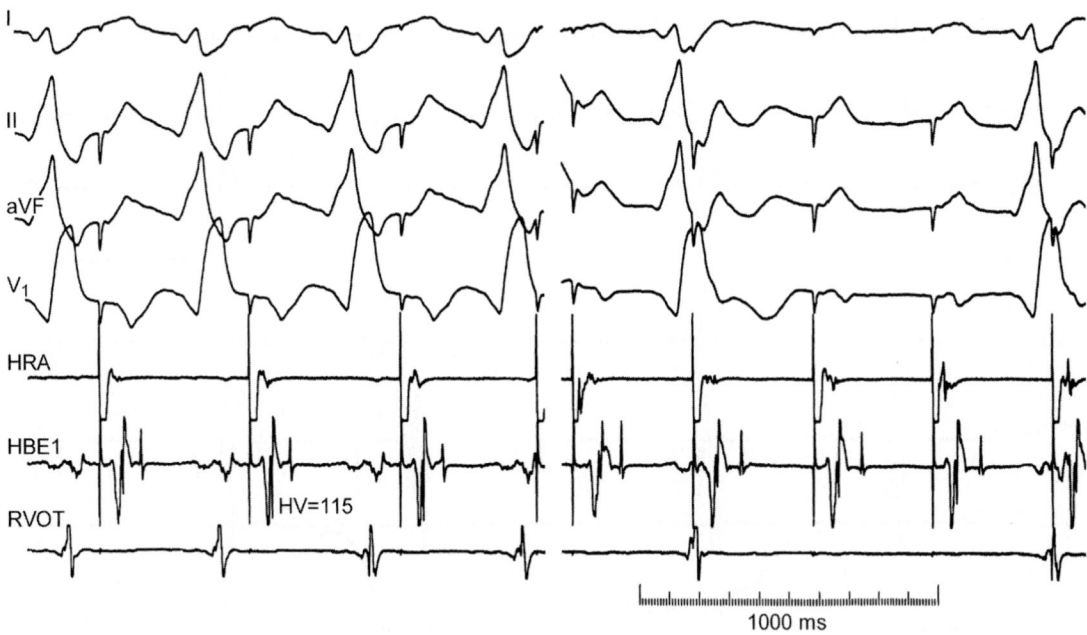

Fig. 4. *Atrial pacing with infra-His block.* The left panel shows atrial pacing (note sharp pacing spikes) at a rate of 100 beats per minute. The HV interval is 115 milliseconds. The right panel shows faster pacing at 150 beats per minute, which produced infra-His block (after the sharp His spike on the HBE1 tracing). Only two ventricular complexes are seen on the right ventricular outflow tract (RVOT) tracing. See Figure 1 for explanation of other abbreviations.

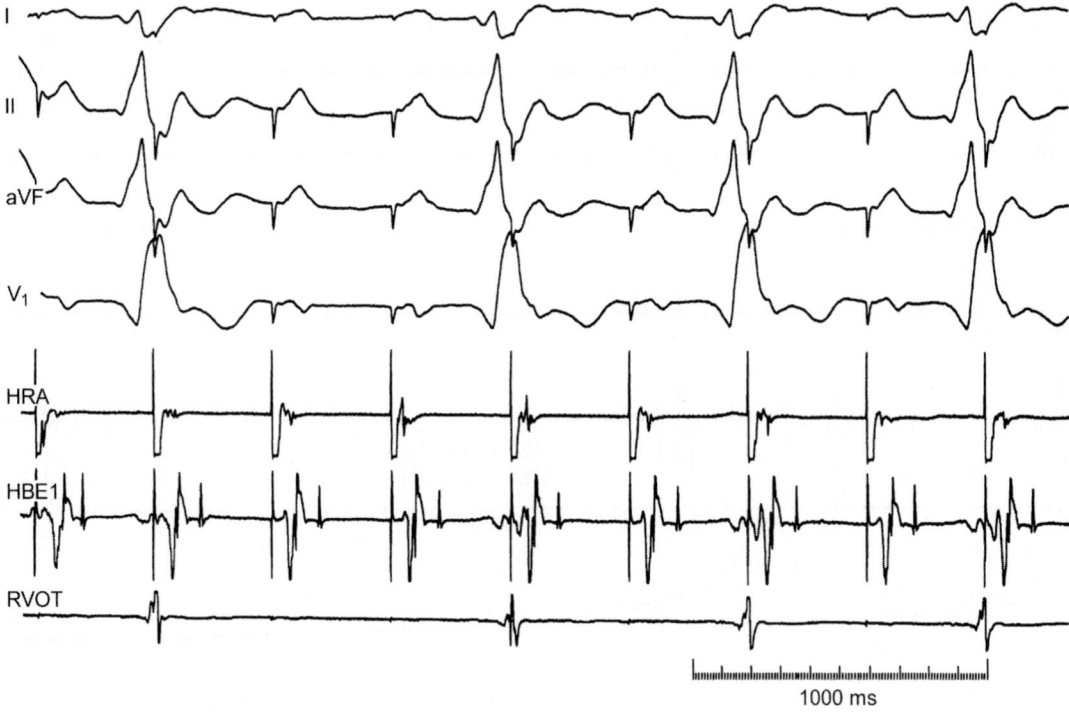

Fig. 5. *Longer recording during atrial pacing demonstrating block within or below the His bundle.* With atrial pacing at a rate of 150 beats per minute, recurrent conduction interruption at a level within or below the His bundle is noted. This is a type 1 indication for pacemaker implantation. Note that only four ventricular complexes are seen on the right ventricular outflow tract (RVOT) tracing. See Figure 1 for explanation of other abbreviations.

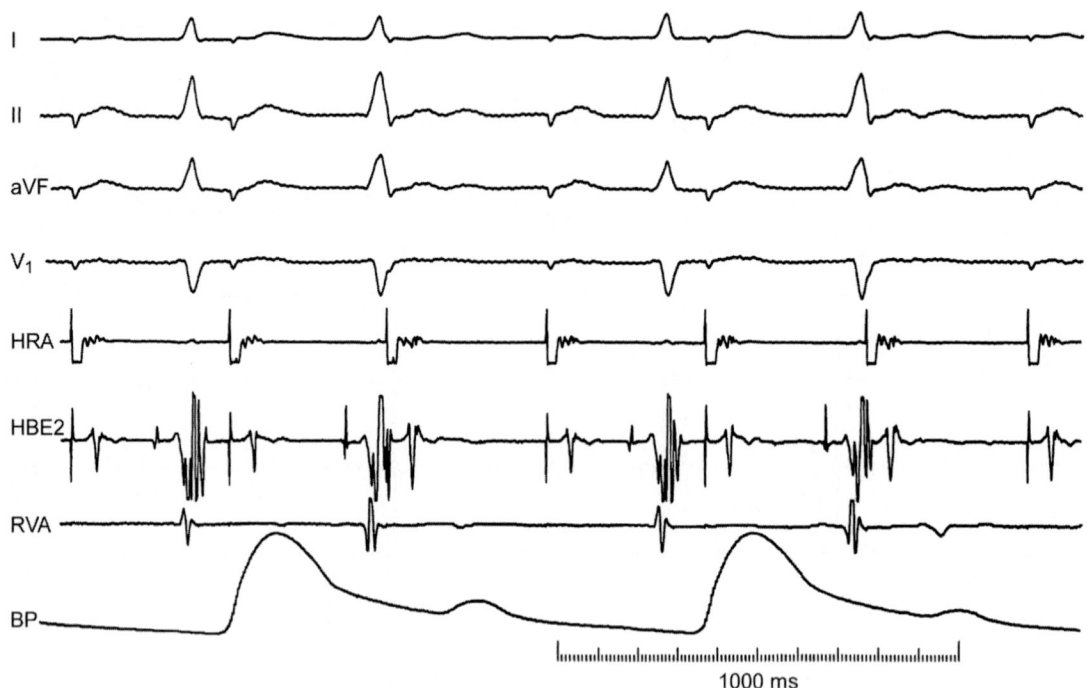

Fig. 6. *Atrial pacing with Wenckebach block in the atrioventricular node.* Note the gradual prolongation of the AH interval, as recorded on the HBE2 electrogram during atrial pacing at a rate of 150 beats per minute. BP, blood pressure. See Figure 1 for explanation of other abbreviations.

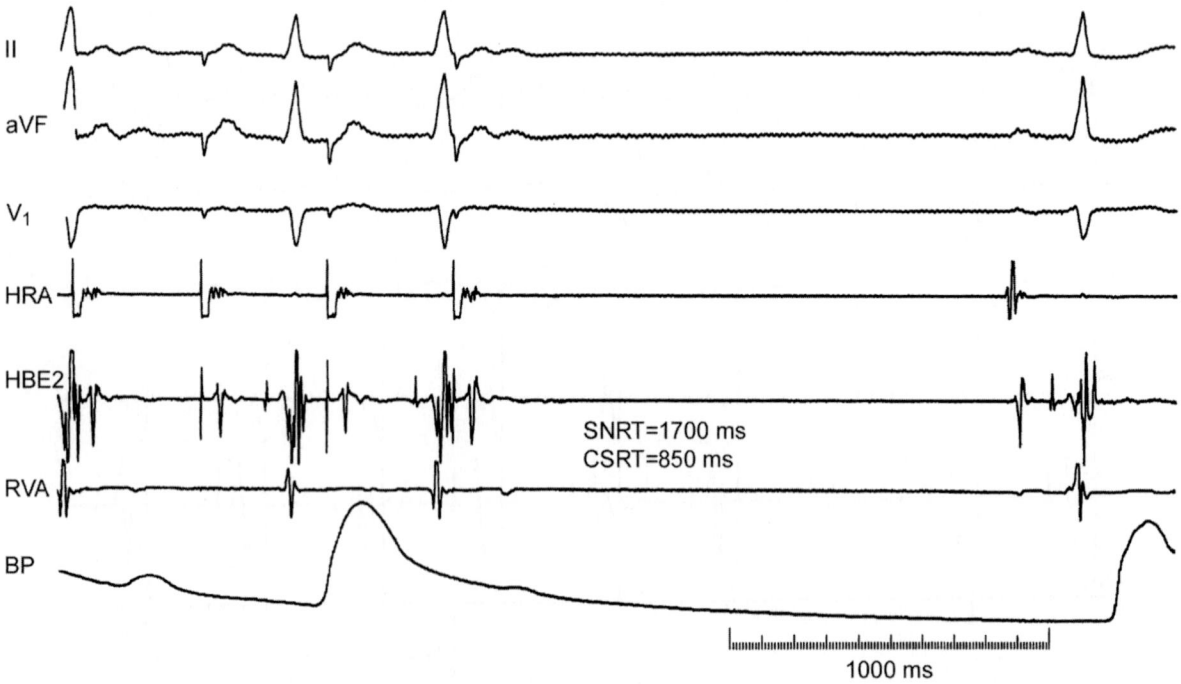

Fig. 7. *Abnormal sinus node recovery time (SNRT) after atrial pacing (150 beats per minute).* Here, 1,700 milliseconds was required to generate the next sinus node impulse. The corrected sinus node recovery time (CSRT), which equals the SNRT – sinus cycle length, also was prolonged at 850. A value more than 600 is abnormal. BP, blood pressure. See Figure 1 for explanation of other abbreviations.

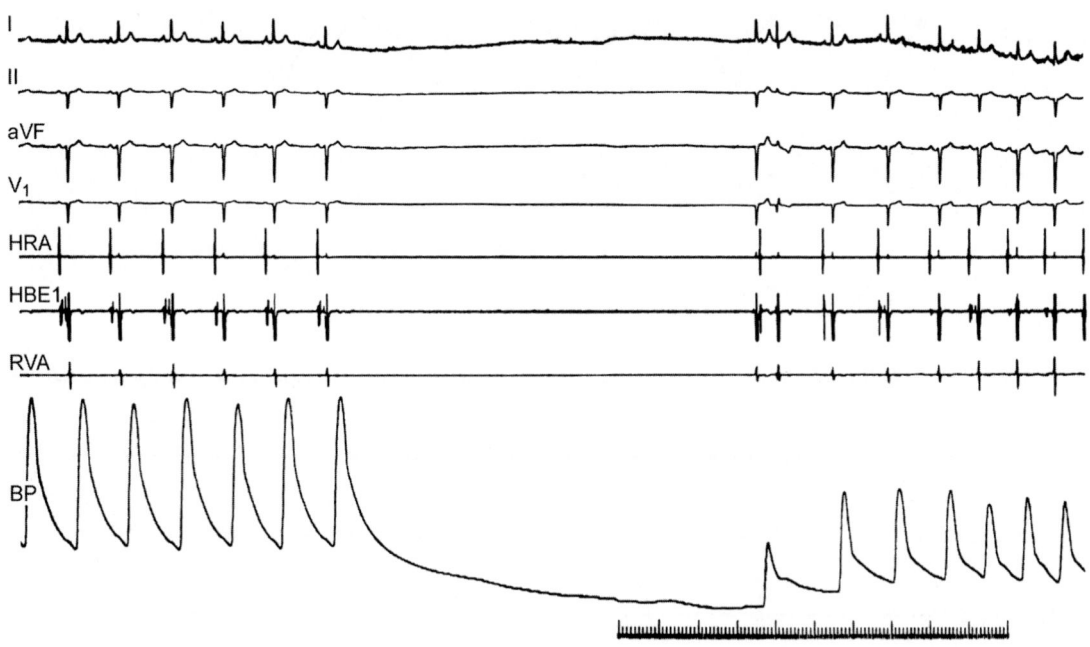

Fig. 8. *Response to right carotid sinus massage (RCSM) in the setting of carotid sinus hypersensitivity.* Note the 10-second pause precipitated by RCSM. BP, blood pressure. See Figure 1 for explanation of other abbreviations.

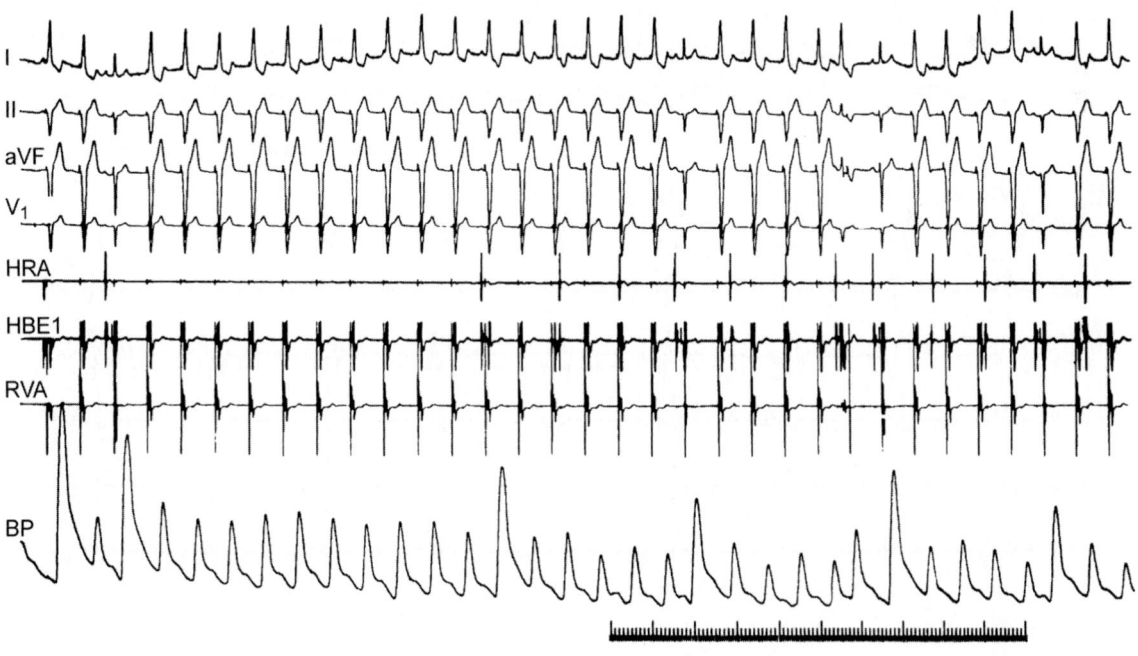

Fig. 9. *Partial recovery of blood pressure (BP) with ventricular pacing during right carotid sinus massage (RCSM).* Note the absence of atrial activity on the high right atrium (HRA) channel in the left half of the figure. BP recovers to a less than normal value during ventricular pacing. This suggests the presence of both cardioinhibitory and vasodepressor components of the carotid hypersensitivity. See Figure 1 for explanation of other abbreviations.

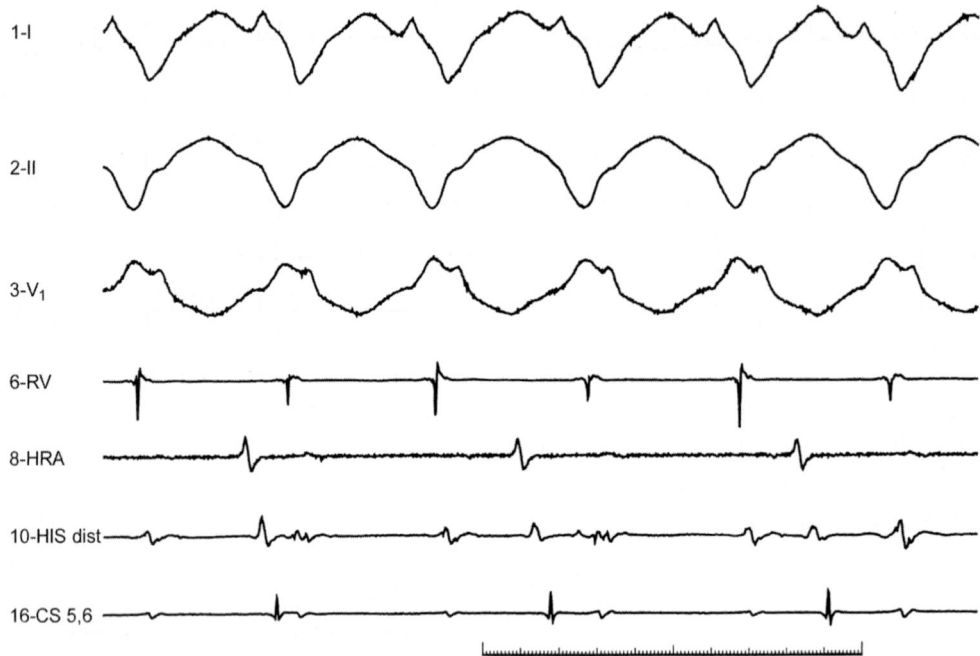

Fig. 10. *Wide complex tachycardia with right bundle branch block morphology.* Note the presence of a ventricular deflection on the right ventricular (RV) channel accompanying each QRS complex. In contrast, the presence of ventriculoatrial dissociation is indicated by the presence of only three atrial deflections on the high right atrium (HRA) or coronary sinus (CS) 5,6 tracings. This is consistent with the diagnosis of ventricular tachycardia. dist, distal electrode.

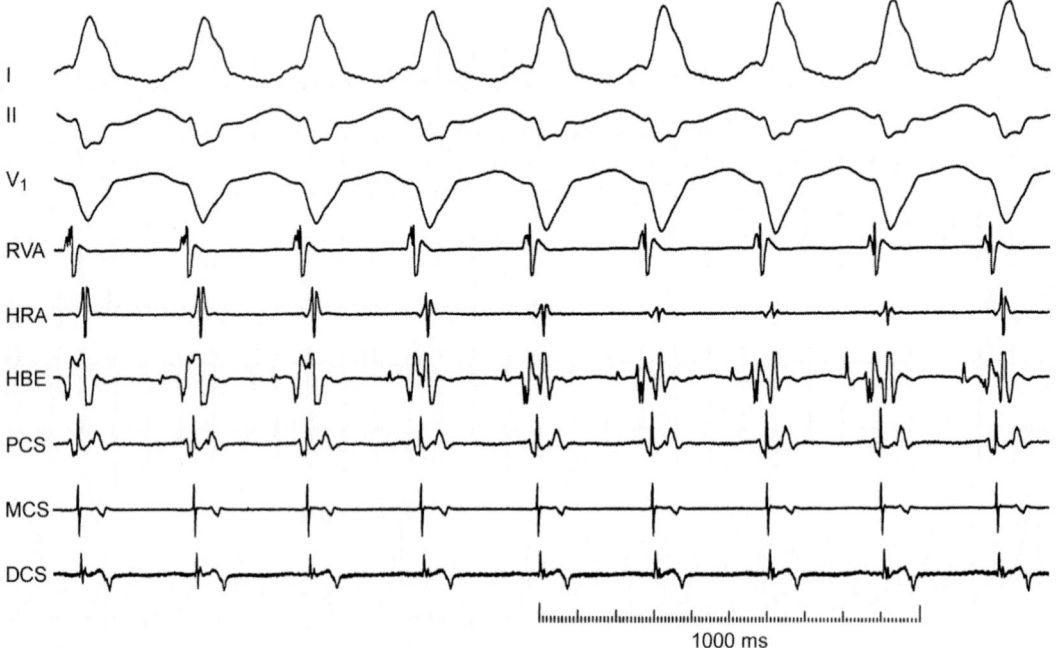

Fig. 11. *Left bundle branch block, left-axis deviation, wide complex tachycardia.* A discrete ventricular deflection (right ventricular apex [RVA] channel) is seen with each QRS complex. There is also an atrial deflection on the high right atrium (HRA) channel indicating a 1:1 atrioventricular relationship. Each ventricular deflection on the His-bundle electrogram (HBE) channel, however, shows a discrete high-frequency His-bundle deflection, indicating that this is a supraventricular tachycardia. DCS, distal coronary sinus; MCS, mid-coronary sinus; PCS, proximal coronary sinus.

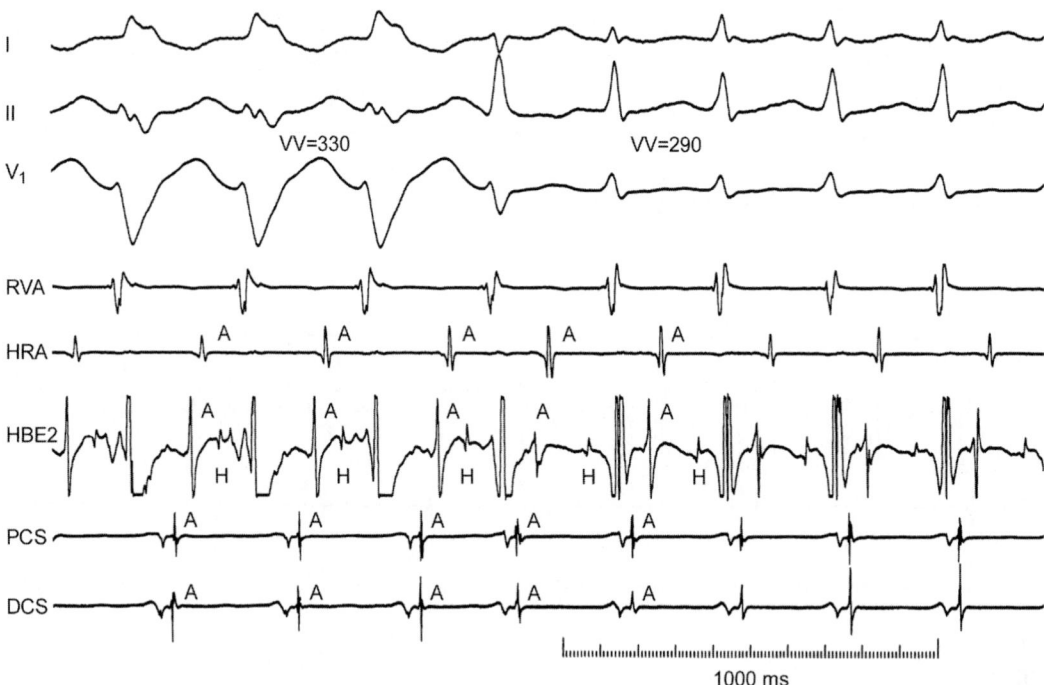

Fig. 12. *Conversion from left bundle branch block during atrioventricular reentrant tachycardia to normal QRS morphology tachycardia* in a patient with a left freewall accessory pathway. Importantly, the VV intervals shorten from 330 to 290 milliseconds with the loss of bundle branch aberrancy. This is diagnostic for a freewall accessory pathway on the same side as the bundle branch block. The atrial and ventricular deflections are clearly marked. DCS, distal coronary sinus; PCS, proximal coronary sinus. See Figure 1 for explanation of other abbreviations.

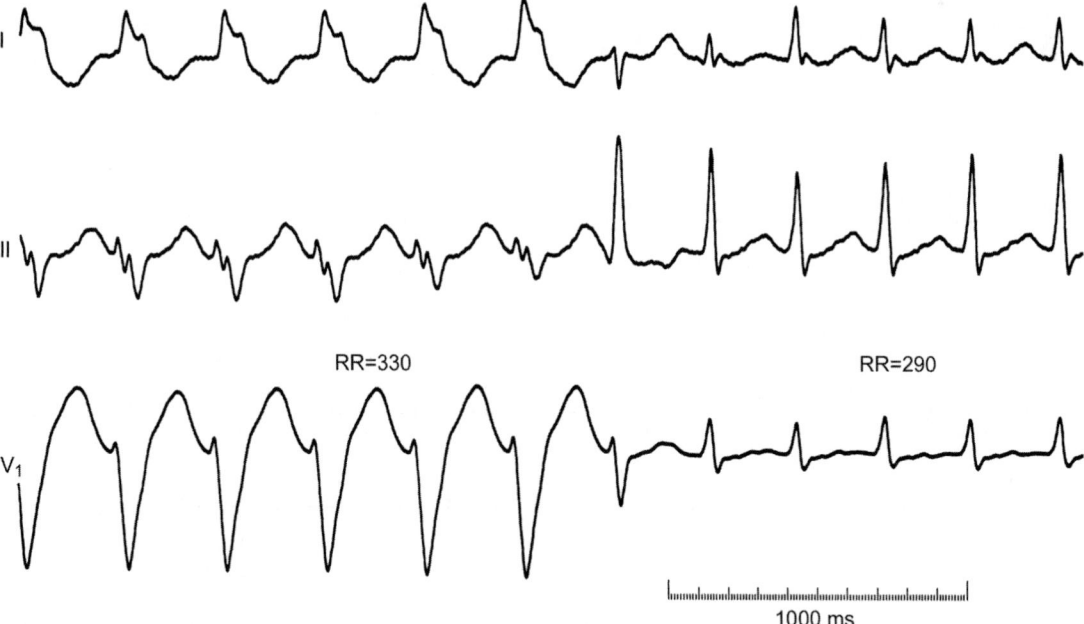

Fig. 13. *Surface electrocardiogram demonstrating conversion of left bundle branch block aberrancy during atrioventricular reentrant tachycardia to a normal QRS tachycardia.* The RR interval of 330 milliseconds during the left bundle branch block aberrant supraventricular tachycardia is longer than that during the narrow QRS complex. This provides sufficient information for making the diagnosis of a left freewall accessory pathway-mediated tachycardia.

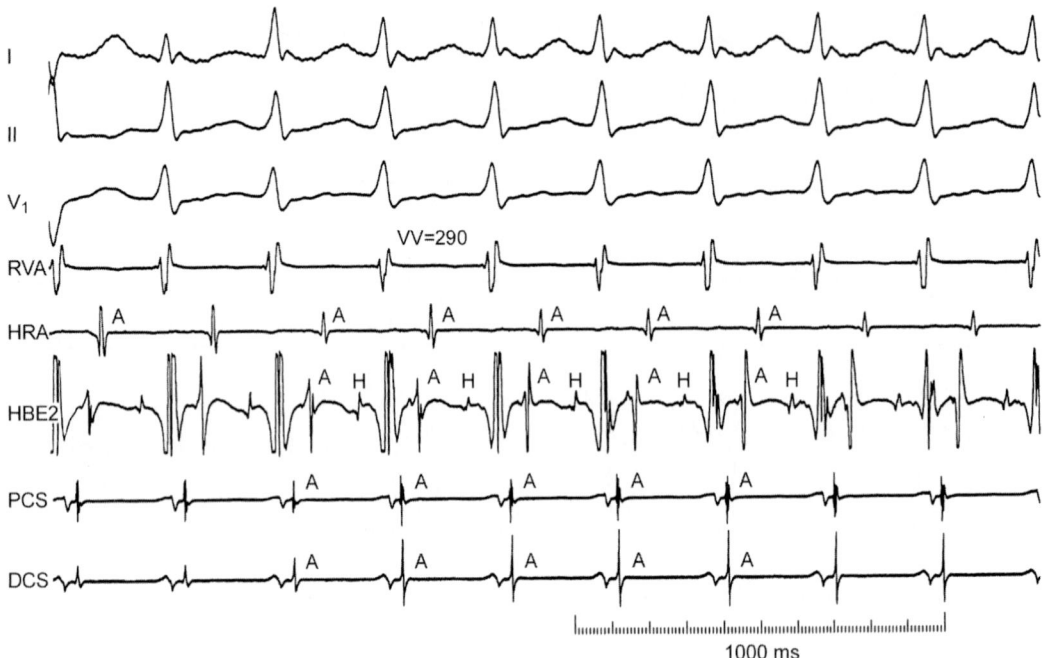

Fig. 14. *Atrioventricular reentrant tachycardia using a left freewall accessory pathway.* Note that the earliest retrograde atrial activation on the proximal (PCS) and distal (DCS) coronary sinus channels occurs before the atrial deflection on the His-bundle electrogram (HBE2) or high right atrium (HRA) channels. The distance from the onset of the surface QRS to the earliest retrograde atrial deflection is 75 milliseconds, which is also consistent with this diagnosis. RVA, right ventricular apex.

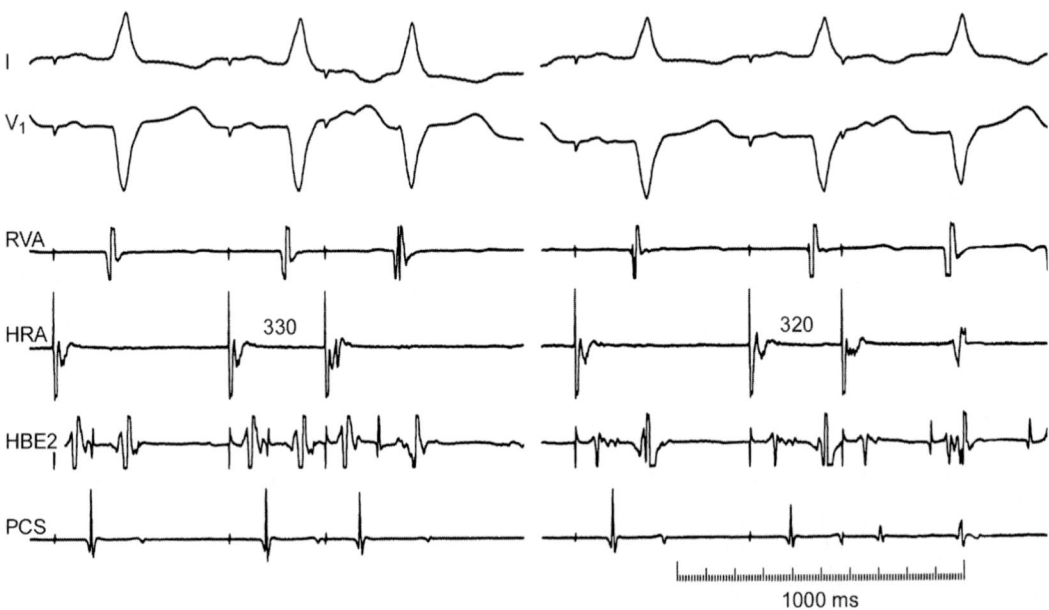

Fig. 15. *Introduction of a premature atrial complex during atrial pacing.* It is introduced 330 milliseconds after the last paced beat. Note that the AH interval generated is relatively short at 130 milliseconds. The right panel shows a premature atrial complex introduced 10 milliseconds earlier, at 320 milliseconds after the last paced atrial beat. Note the significant prolongation of the AH interval out to 230 milliseconds. PCS, proximal coronary sinus. See Figure 1 for explanation of other abbreviations.

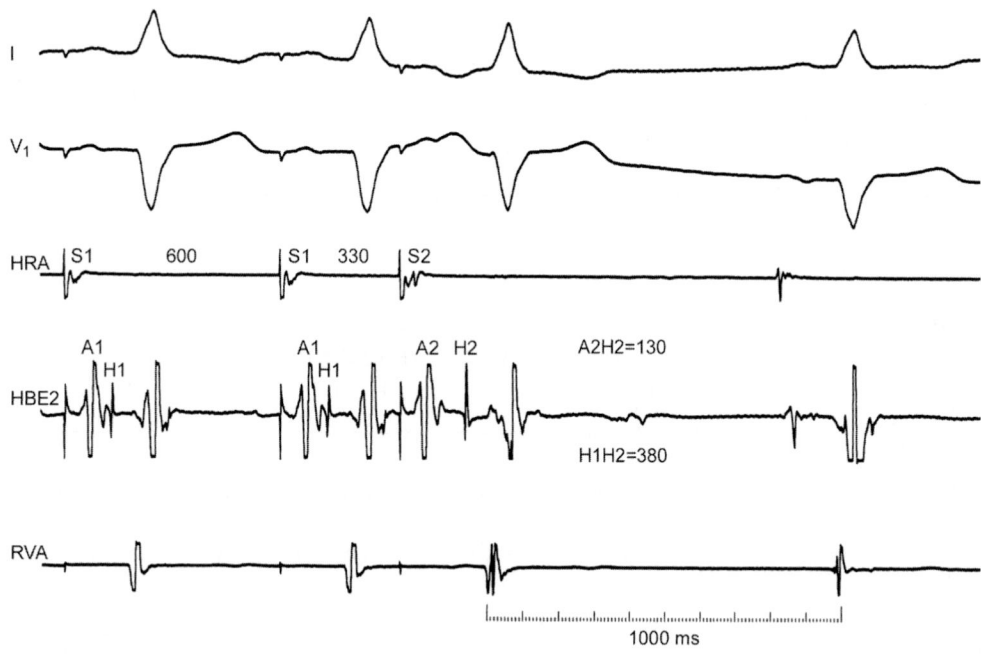

Fig. 16. *Expanded view of the impact of the timing of a premature atrial complex on the A2H2 interval.* The interval is 130 milliseconds. In this patient with dual atrioventricular nodal physiology and atrioventricular nodal reentrant tachycardia, the impulse is proceeding down the fast pathway. See Figure 1 for explanation of abbreviations.

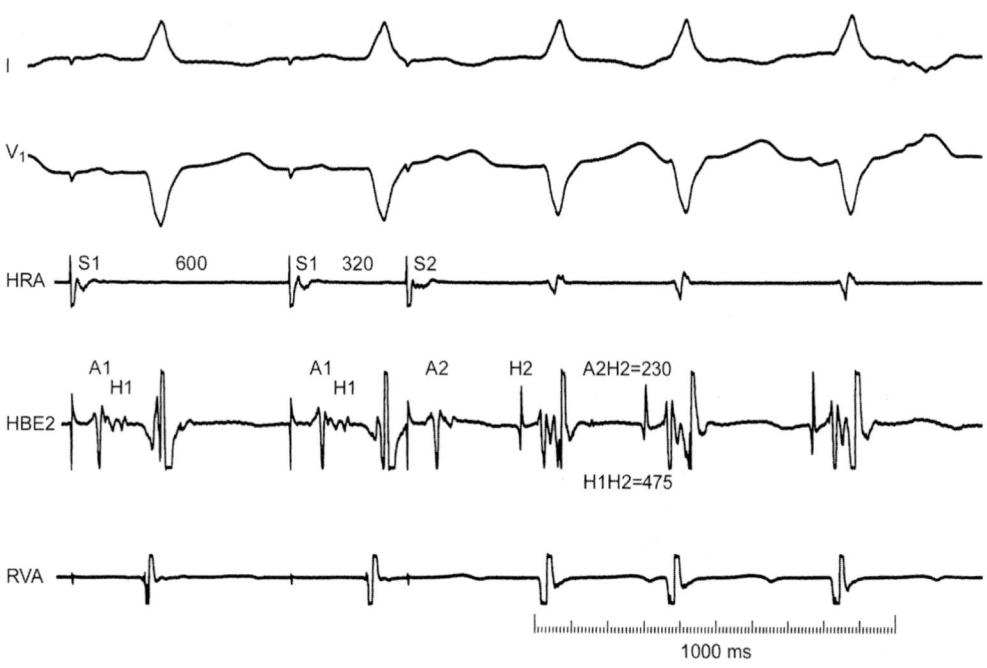

Fig. 17. *Jump in the A2H2 interval with introduction of a premature atrial complex.* A 10-millisecond decrease in the S1S2 coupling interval to 320 milliseconds results in a dramatic prolongation of the A2H2 interval to 230 milliseconds. This indicates that the premature atrial complex produced block in the fast pathway but conducted to the ventricle via the slow pathway. Note also the onset of atrioventricular nodal reentrant tachycardia. See Figure 1 for explanation of abbreviations.

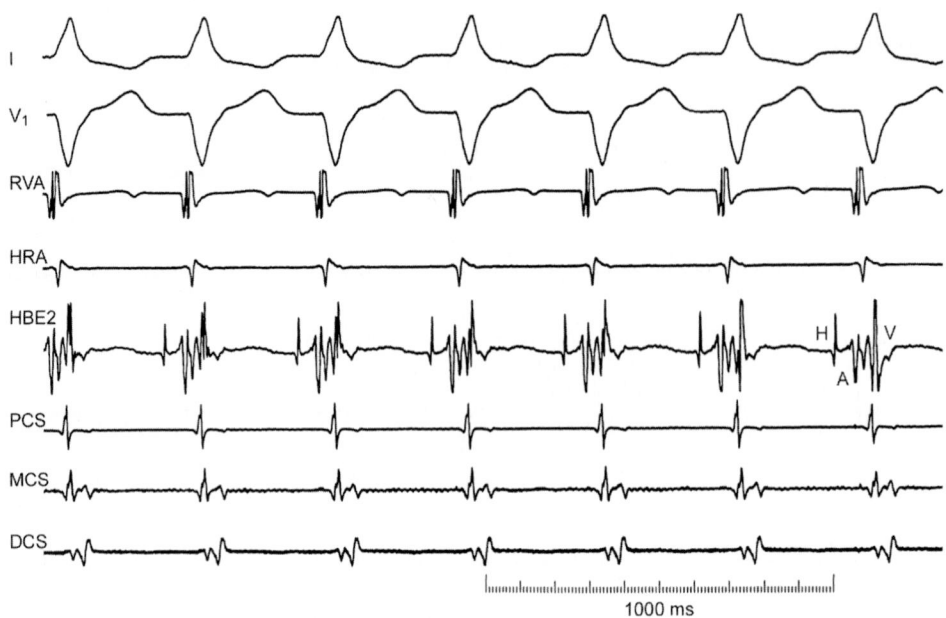

Fig. 18. *Intracardiac tracings of atrioventricular nodal reentrant tachycardia.* The QRS complex is narrow, and atrial deflections are seen with each QRS complex. This 1:1 atrioventricular relationship, with a sharp His-bundle deflection preceding the surface QRS, is consistent with a supraventricular tachycardia dependent on atrioventricular nodal conduction. The final complex shows the His-bundle deflection followed by a surface QRS complex and a normal HV interval. The retrograde atrial deflection, however, times with the onset of the surface QRS, giving a ventriculoatrial interval of zero. Usually, this interval is 10 to 55 milliseconds. In this case, it took an equal amount of time for the reentrant impulse to return back to the atrium as it did for one to proceed down the His-Purkinje system to yield a QRS complex. DCS, distal coronary sinus; MCS, mid-coronary sinus; PCS, proximal coronary sinus. See Figure 1 for explanation of other abbreviations.

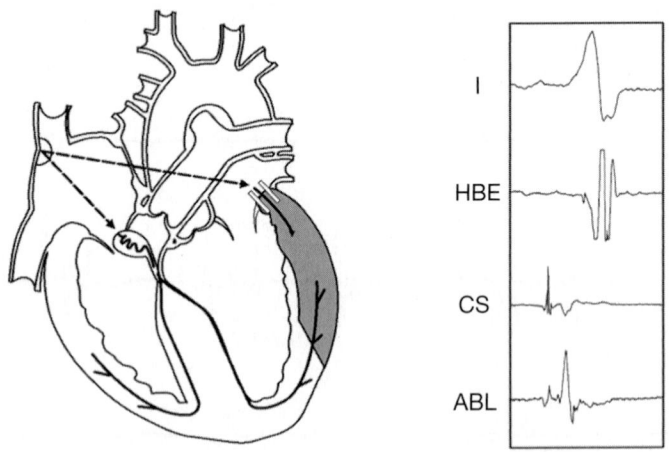

Fig. 19. *Ventricular preexcitation via an accessory pathway.* A characteristic delta wave is seen in limb lead I. This occurs well before the first sharp, discrete deflection on the His-bundle electrogram (HBE) channel, which is the "His deflection." An ablation catheter (ABL) placed near the accessory pathway shows that the local ventricular deflection actually occurs before the onset of the surface QRS. A line is drawn to reflect the timing from the onset of the surface QRS. Note that much of the ventricular deflection on the ablation (ABL) lead and a small Kent potential occur before the onset of the surface lead. The His-bundle spike on the HBE lead, however, is well after the onset of the surface QRS. CS, coronary sinus.

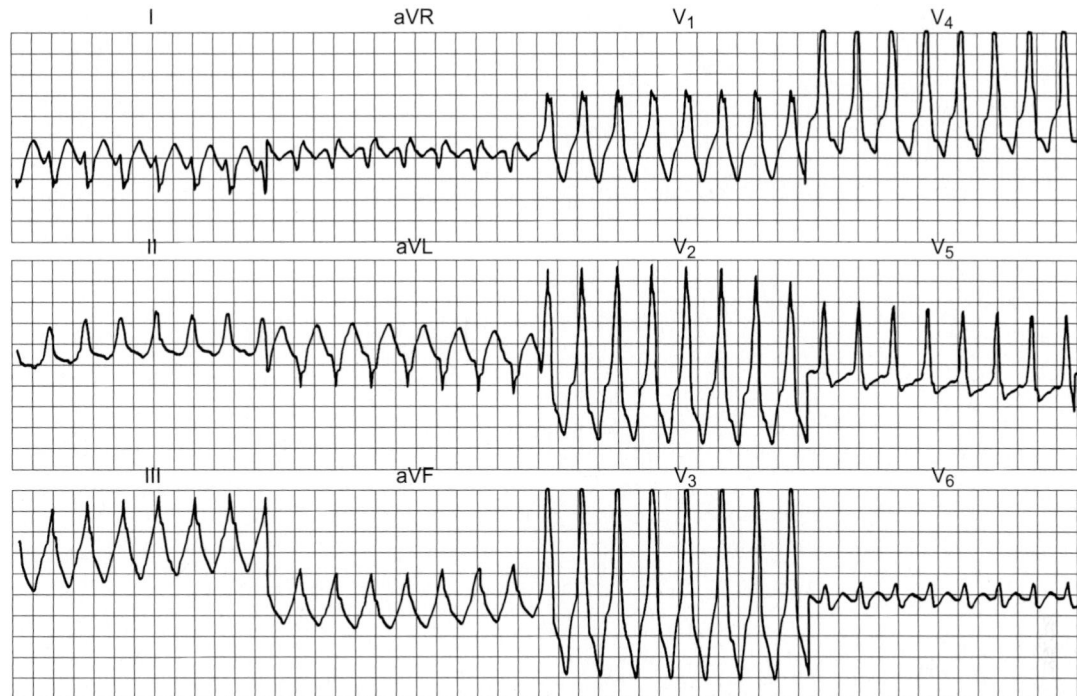

Fig. 20. *Electrocardiograms show antidromic reciprocating tachycardia.* Ventricular activation is via the accessory pathway. As a result, all of the QRS complexes show maximal preexcitation, with characteristic delta waves. Retrograde atrial activation occurs via the atrioventricular node.

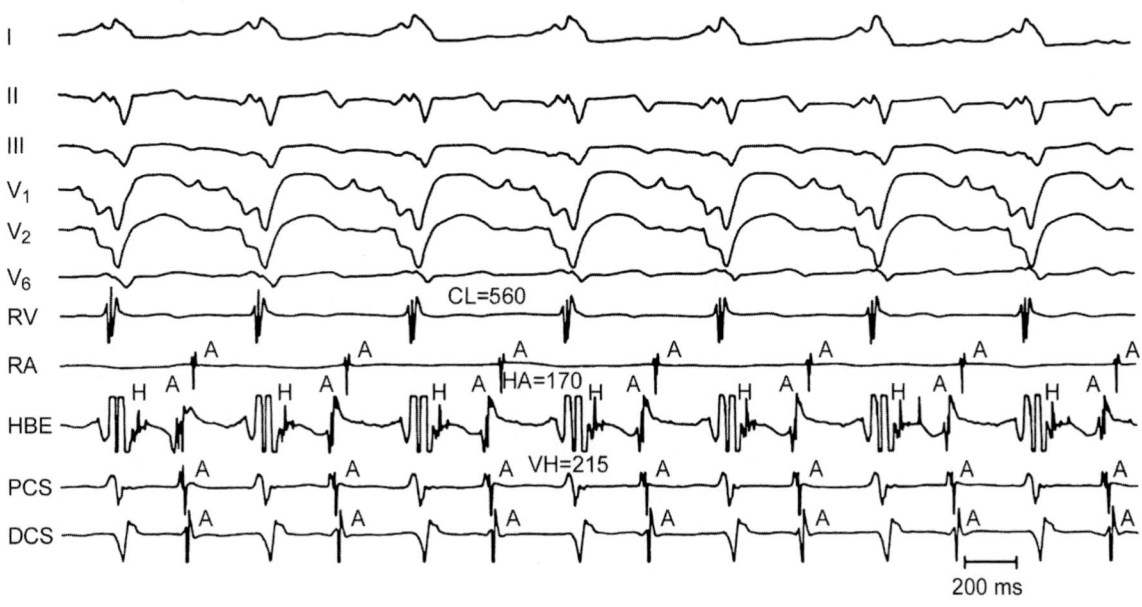

Fig. 21. *Intracardiac tracing of antidromic reciprocating tachycardia.* Note presence of a delta wave, particularly prominent on leads I and V₁. The His-bundle deflection occurs well after the local ventricular activation on the HBE lead. This is followed by retrograde atrial activation via the atrioventricular conduction system. Note that the atrial deflection (A) on the HBE channel precedes any of the other atrial depolarizations. DCS, distal coronary sinus; HBE, His-bundle electrogram; PCS, proximal coronary sinus; RA, right atrium; RV, right ventricle.

SECTION IV

Valvular Heart Disease

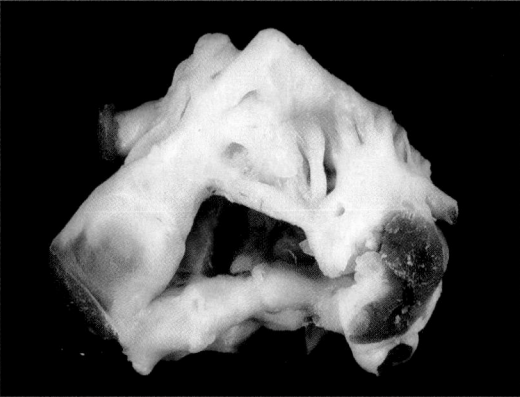

Ergot Valve Disease

40

Valvular Stenosis

Rick A. Nishimura, MD

Aortic Stenosis

Definition and Causes

Aortic stenosis is a disease in which progressive obstruction to left ventricular outflow results in the following: 1) pressure hypertrophy of the left ventricle; 2) symptoms of angina, dyspnea, and syncope; and 3) if untreated, death. The presentation, diagnosis, and eventual treatment of aortic stenosis depend on the cause and severity of the outflow obstruction. The causes can be divided into supravalvular aortic stenosis, fixed subvalvular aortic stenosis, and valvular aortic stenosis (Table 1). Valvular aortic stenosis has many causes, including congenital, unicuspid, or bicuspid aortic valves, rheumatic heart disease, and senile degenerative disease. Two-dimensional and Doppler echocardiography can be used to determine reliably the level of obstruction and to assess the severity of obstruction.

Supravalvular Aortic Stenosis

Supravalvular aortic stenosis is a congenital abnormality in which the ascending aorta superior to the aortic valve is narrowed. This is the rarest site of aortic stenosis. The stenosis is seen as either a single discrete constriction or a long tubular narrowing. Important associations with supravalvular aortic stenosis include elfin facies, hypercalcemia, and peripheral pulmonic stenosis. The diagnosis

of supravalvular aortic stenosis should be suspected in a young patient who has a left ventricular outflow murmur. Typically, a thrill is felt on palpation of the right carotid artery but not the left one, because the obstructive jet is directed toward the innominate artery. The diagnosis can be made on the basis of two-dimensional echocardiography (which allows visualization of the narrowed ascending aorta) and Doppler echocardiography (which provides information about the magnitude of the obstruction). Aortic root angiography, transesophageal echocardiography, or magnetic resonance angiography may be required to show the extent of narrowing of the ascending aorta if surgical intervention is contemplated.

Table 1. Causes of Aortic Stenosis

Supravalvular
Subvalvular
    Discrete
    Tunnel
Valvular
    Congenital (1-30 years old)
    Bicuspid (40-60 years old)
    Rheumatic (40-60 years old)
    Senile degenerative (>70 years old)

Subvalvular Aortic Stenosis

Discrete subvalvular stenosis is seen in approximately 10% of all patients with aortic stenosis. It can be secondary to a subvalvular ridge that extends into the left ventricular outflow tract or to a tunnel-like narrowing of the outflow tract. The obstruction is frequently accompanied by aortic regurgitation due to malformation of the aortic valve from the high-velocity jet emanating from the subvalvular obstruction. The diagnosis can be made at echocardiography by visualization of a narrowing or discrete subvalvular ridge extending into the left ventricular outflow tract and a high-velocity turbulence on continuous wave Doppler echocardiography. A discrete ridge may be difficult to visualize directly in older patients, but it should be suspected when there is high-velocity flow across the outflow tract in the presence of a structurally normal aortic valve with early systolic closure. If the site of obstruction is not visualized on the initial echocardiogram, transesophageal echocardiography should be performed to confirm the diagnosis.

The diagnosis of subvalvular aortic stenosis needs to be differentiated from the dynamic outflow obstruction of hypertrophic obstructive cardiomyopathy because their treatment differs. Some recommend resection of the discrete subvalvular stenosis in all patients with at least moderate obstruction who are candidates for operation, both to relieve the degree of left ventricular outflow obstruction and to prevent progressive aortic regurgitation. The treatment of patients with hypertrophic obstructive cardiomyopathy is discussed in Chapter 97.

- Supravalvular aortic stenosis is associated with elfin facies, hypercalcemia, and peripheral pulmonic stenosis.
- Supravalvular aortic stenosis should be suspected when there is a palpable thrill in the right carotid artery.
- Discrete subvalvular aortic stenosis presents with a high Doppler velocity across the aortic outflow tract and a structurally normal aortic valve on two-dimensional echocardiography.

Be alert for supravalvular or subvalvular aortic stenosis in a young person presenting with signs and symptoms of aortic stenosis but with a normal aortic valve on echocardiography.

Valvular Aortic Stenosis

Obstruction at the valvular level accounts for most cases of aortic stenosis. The cause of the valve abnormality depends on the age at presentation. In patients who have symptomatic aortic stenosis in their teens and early 20s, the cause is usually a congenitally unicuspid or fused bicuspid aortic valve. Patients in their 40s to 60s who have symptoms usually have a calcified bicuspid aortic valve or the stenosis may be the end result of rheumatic heart disease. Since the 1990s, the most common presentation has been an elderly patient who has senile degeneration of the valve, with calcific deposits at the base of the cusps in the absence of commissural fusion.

- The most common cause of aortic stenosis since the 1990s has been senile degenerative changes.
- In patients with aortic stenosis due to rheumatic disease, "silent" mitral stenosis should be ruled out.
- A bicuspid or rheumatic cause should be suspected in a patient with aortic stenosis who presents in the sixth decade of life.

Pathophysiology

Progressive left ventricular outflow obstruction results in concentric pressure hypertrophy of the left ventricle caused by an increase in left ventricular wall thickness. The increase in wall thickness is a compensatory mechanism to "normalize" wall stress. In most patients, the size of the left ventricular cavity remains normal and systolic function is usually well preserved. Failure of the left ventricle to compensate for the long-standing pressure overload, results in ventricular dilatation and a progressive decrease in systolic function.

The pathophysiology of aortic stenosis is due to the following: 1) an increase in afterload, 2) a decrease in systemic and coronary blood flow from obstruction, and 3) progressive hypertrophy. These mechanisms result in the classic symptom triad of dyspnea, angina, and syncope. Exertional dyspnea is common, even in the presence of normal systolic function. Abnormalities of diastolic function are common in patients with aortic stenosis and result in increased left ventricular filling pressures that are reflected onto the pulmonary circulation. Diastolic dysfunction occurs from prolonged ventricular relaxation and decreased compliance and is caused by myocardial ischemia, a thick noncompliant left ventricle, and increased afterload. Symptoms of exertional angina may be present in the absence of epicardial coronary artery obstruction. Myocardial ischemia results from a mismatch myocardial oxygen supply and demand due to high diastolic pressure, a decreased myocardial perfusion gradient, and an increased myocardial mass. The cause of exertional syncope is multifactorial and may include ventricular arrhythmias, a sudden decrease in systemic flow caused by the obstruction, or abnormal vasodepressor reflexes caused by the high left ventricular intracavitary pressure. As a progressive, long-standing pressure overload is placed on the left ventricle, systolic decompensation may occur from the afterload mismatch and lead to symptoms of both left-sided and right-sided heart failure.

A "death spiral" may occur in patients with critical aortic stenosis. With the onset of systemic hypotension (due to either drugs or a vasovagal reaction), perfusion of the coronary arteries may decrease. This increases the myocardial oxygen supply/demand mismatch and results in myocardial ischemia. The myocardial ischemia, in turn, reduces forward cardiac output, and aortic diastolic pressure decreases, further decreasing coronary perfusion pressure. Unless immediate steps are taken to increase perfusion pressure, progressive hemodynamic deterioration and death may occur.

- Diastolic dysfunction is due to abnormalities of relaxation and compliance and is one of the primary pathophysiologic processes present in patients with aortic stenosis.
- Myocardial ischemia occurs in patients with aortic stenosis despite normal epicardial coronary arteries, because of a mismatch in myocardial oxygen supply and demand.
- The most common cause of syncope in patients with aortic stenosis is vasodepressor syncope.
- Suspect critical aortic stenosis in a patient with syncope and an aortic murmur.

Clinical Presentation

The clinical presentation of aortic stenosis varies. Some patients are asymptomatic, but a heart murmur is detected on physical examination. Others have one or more symptoms from the classic triad of exertional dyspnea, angina, and syncope. Uncommonly, patients with end-stage aortic stenosis and concomitant left ventricular dysfunction present with anasarca and car-

diac cachexia. Albeit rare, sudden death may be the initial manifestation of aortic stenosis.

Physical examination of a patient with aortic stenosis reveals classic, characteristic findings. Severe aortic stenosis is diagnosed on the basis of a dampened upstroke of the carotid artery, a sustained bifid left ventricular impulse, an absent A_2, and a late-peaking systolic ejection murmur. A concomitant systolic thrill indicates the presence of aortic stenosis (mean gradient, >50 mm Hg). In some patients, the systolic ejection murmur may be heard with equal intensity at the apex and at the base. It is not necessarily the intensity of the murmur that corresponds to the severity of aortic stenosis but rather the timing of the peak and duration of the murmur. The murmur of aortic stenosis must be differentiated from that of hypertrophic obstructive cardiomyopathy or mitral regurgitation due to a flail posterior leaflet.

- Hypertrophic cardiomyopathy is distinguished from aortic stenosis on the basis of physical examination findings.

Laboratory Tests

Electrocardiography and Radiography
Electrocardiography usually shows normal sinus rhythm with left ventricular hypertrophy. If atrial fibrillation is present, concomitant mitral valve disease or thyroid disease must be suspected. Chest radiography shows left ventricular predominance, with dilatation of the ascending aorta. Aortic calcification is frequently seen on lateral chest radiographs.

Echocardiography
Two-dimensional and Doppler echocardiography are the imaging modalities of choice for diagnosing aortic stenosis and estimating its severity. The location of the obstruction (supravalvular, valvular, or subvalvular) can be identified with two-dimensional echocardiography. In patients with valvular aortic stenosis, the cause (bicuspid, rheumatic, or senile degenerative) may be assessed from the parasternal short-axis view. Although the presence or absence of aortic stenosis is readily diagnosed on two-dimensional echocardiography, the severity of the stenosis cannot be judged on the basis of the two-dimensional echocardiographic image alone.

Doppler echocardiography is excellent for assessing the severity of aortic stenosis. By using the modified Bernoulli equation ($\Delta P = 4v^2$), a maximal instantaneous and mean aortic valve gradient can usually be derived from the continuous wave Doppler velocity across the aortic valve. However, accurate measurement of the aortic valve gradient requires a detailed, meticulous study with multiple sites of interrogation to ensure that the Doppler beam is parallel to the stenotic jet. In laboratories with experienced echocardiographers, the Doppler-derived aortic valve gradients are accurate and reproducible and correlate well with those obtained with cardiac catheterization. The mean gradient from the integral of the aortic valve velocity curve should be used to determine the severity of aortic stenosis. If the mean gradient is greater than 40 mm Hg, severe aortic stenosis can be diagnosed with certainty. In a patient with clinical findings of severe aortic stenosis and a Doppler-derived mean gradient greater than 40 mm Hg, no other hemodynamic information is needed to assess the severity of stenosis.

Aortic valve gradients depend not only on the severity of obstruction but also on flow. In patients with low cardiac output, the stenosis may still be severe, with mean gradients less than 40 mm Hg. To overcome these problems, an aortic valve area (AVA) has been derived using the hydraulic equation of Gorlin and Gorlin. In the cardiac catheterization laboratory, the AVA is calculated from the pressure gradient and an independent measure of cardiac output.

$$AVA = \frac{1{,}000 \times CO}{44 \times SEP \times HR \times \sqrt{\Delta P}}$$

where CO = cardiac output, HR = heart rate, P = pressure difference across the valve, and SEP = systolic ejection period.

Two-dimensional and Doppler echocardiography can also provide reliable estimations of aortic valve area by the continuity equation:

$$AVA = \frac{LVOT_{area} \times LVOT_{TVI}}{AV_{TVI}}$$

where AV = aortic valve flow velocity, LVOT = left ventricular outflow tract, and TVI = time-velocity integral.

Severe aortic stenosis can be diagnosed if a patient has clinical findings consistent with severe aortic stenosis, a mean gradient greater than 40 mm Hg, and AVA less than 1.0 cm^2 (Table 2).

There are limitations to using Doppler echocardiography in estimating the severity of aortic stenosis. The biggest problem occurs when the Doppler beam is not parallel to the aortic stenosis velocity jet, because the mean gradient will be underestimated. Thus, in a patient with the clinical features of severe aortic stenosis but echocardiographic and Doppler findings of mild or moderate stenosis, further evaluation with either another Doppler echocardiographic study or cardiac catheterization is required. Doppler echocardiography will not overestimate the mean gradient, except in rare instances of severe anemia (hemoglobin <8.0 g/dL), a small aortic root, or sequential stenoses in parallel (coexistent left ventricular outflow tract and valvular obstruction). The calculation of AVA with echocardiography is highly dependent on accurate measurement of the diameter of the left ventricular outflow tract. Thus, special attention must be used when diagnosing severe aortic stenosis in patients with small valve areas but relatively low mean gradients. In these instances, correlation with clinical findings is essential.

If the clinical findings are not consistent with the Doppler echocardiographic results, cardiac catheterization is recommended for further hemodynamic assessment. Cardiac catheterization should consist of the simultaneous measurement of two pressures, one in the left ventricle and one in the aorta, from which a mean gradient can be calculated. A "pull-back" tracing from

Table 2.   Criteria for Determining Severity of Aortic Stenosis

Severity	Mean gradient, mm Hg	Aortic valve area, cm^2
Mild	<25	>1.5
Moderate	25-40	1.0-1.5
Severe	>40	<1.0
Critical	>80	<0.7

the left ventricle to the aorta may be used in patients with normal sinus rhythm but is not accurate in patients with irregular rhythms or low-output states. The use of simultaneous left ventricular and femoral artery pressures is not accurate for assessing aortic valve gradient because there may be a significant difference between central aortic pressure and femoral artery pressure. At cardiac catheterization, cardiac output should be assessed for calculation of valve area, preferably by the Fick method. Thermodilution or green dye curves are used, but these tests have inherent limitations in patients with irregular heart rhythms or low-output states. Coexistent mitral or aortic regurgitation may cause errors in the calculation of valve area by cardiac catheterization.

- If atrial fibrillation is present on electrocardiography, suspect mitral valve disease.
- A mean aortic valve gradient greater than 40 mm Hg on Doppler echocardiography is indicative of severe aortic stenosis.
- The biggest pitfall of Doppler echocardiography is underestimation of the aortic valve gradient.

Natural History and Treatment

The natural history of aortic stenosis is well known (Fig. 1). After symptoms occur in a patient with severe aortic stenosis, there is a rapidly progressive downhill course, with a 2- to 3-year mortality of 50%. Therefore, it has been recommended that aortic valve replacement be performed in all patients with severe aortic stenosis who have symptoms (Table 3). Aortic valve replacement has a low perioperative mortality of less than 1% to 2% in young, healthy patients and results in significant improvement of longevity.

Before aortic valve surgery, a complete hemodynamic assessment of the aortic valve with either Doppler echocardiography or cardiac catheterization is required. Left ventricular function and concomitant mitral valve disease should be assessed. Coronary angiography should be performed in older patients who have risk factors for coronary artery disease, but it usually is not required in men younger than 40 years or women younger than 50 years without risk factors. Aortic valve replacement should be performed in all patients with severely symptomatic aortic stenosis, regardless of concomitant left ventricular function. If

significant mitral regurgitation is present, the degree of regurgitation should be evaluated intraoperatively after replacement of the aortic valve to determine the need for mitral valve repair or replacement, unless there is intrinsic disease of the mitral valve apparatus.

Since the 1990s, an increasing number of elderly patients have presented with severe aortic stenosis. The risk of aortic valve replacement increases with age and concomitant medical problems. In patients older than 80 years, operative mortality can be as high as 30%. Percutaneous aortic balloon valvuloplasty was introduced in the 1980s as an alternative to valve replacement, avoiding the high operative mortality in elderly patients. By inflating one or more large balloons across the aortic valve from a percutaneous route, a modest decrease in gradient and a significant improvement in symptoms could be achieved in elderly critically ill patients. However, follow-up has demonstrated a high rate of restenosis (>60% at 6 months and nearly 100% at 2 years), with no decrease in mortality rate after the procedure. Therefore, percutaneous aortic balloon valvuloplasty is used only 1) for critically ill elderly patients who are not candidates for surgical intervention or 2) as a "bridge" in critically ill patients before aortic valve replacement.

- Aortic valve replacement is indicated for patients with symptoms of severe aortic stenosis, regardless of the left ventricular ejection fraction.
- Coronary angiography may not be required preoper-

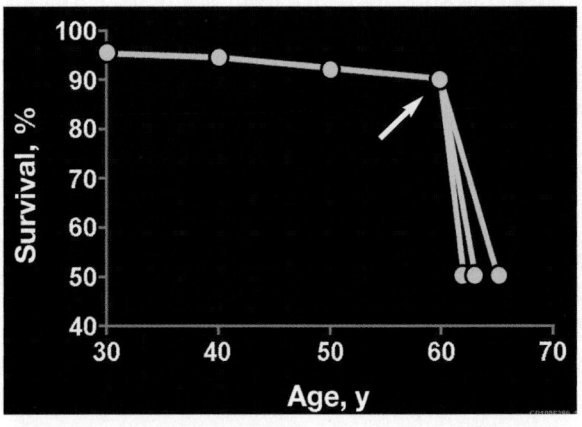

Fig. 1. Natural history of aortic stenosis. At the onset of symptoms (*arrow*), there is a rapid progression and survival is severely limited.

Table 3.   Recommendations for Aortic Valve
Replacement in Aortic Stenosis

Indication	Class
1. Symptomatic patients with severe AS	I
2. Patients with severe AS undergoing coronary artery bypass surgery	I
3. Patients with severe AS undergoing surgery on the aorta or other heart valves	I
4. Patients with moderate AS undergoing coronaryIIa artery bypass surgery or surgery on the aorta or other heart valves	IIa
5. Asymptomatic patients with severe AS and	
LV systolic dysfunction	IIa
Abnormal response to exercise (e.g., hypotension)	IIa
Ventricular tachycardia	IIb
Marked or excessive LV hypertrophy ($\geq$15 mm)	IIb
Valve area <0.6 cm^2	IIb
6. Prevention of sudden death in asymptomatic patients with none of the findings listed under indication 5	III

AS, aortic sttenosis; LV, left ventricular.

atively in younger patients without risk factors for coronary artery disease.

■ Percutaneous aortic balloon valvuloplasty is reserved only for critically ill patients as a "bridge" to surgery.

Controversial Issues in the Management of Patients With Aortic Stenosis

Asymptomatic Patients With Severe Aortic Stenosis

Treatment of asymptomatic patients with severe aortic stenosis remains controversial. Advocates of "prophylactic" aortic valve replacement in asymptomatic patients recommend that the procedure be done to prevent sudden death. However, longitudinal studies have shown that the incidence of sudden death in patients who are truly asymptomatic is low, probably less than 1% per year. It is thus reasonable to follow closely the asymptomatic patient as long as exercise tolerance is good and left ventricular systolic function is preserved. Exercise testing may be performed carefully to document exercise tolerance and the hemodynamic response to exercise; operation is considered for those with a reduced exercise tolerance or an abnormal hemodynamic response to exercise. If the patient with asymptomatic severe aortic stenosis undergoes close medical observation, surgery should be performed at the onset of symptoms or left ventricular systolic dysfunction.

Asymptomatic patients with very high gradients and critical aortic stenosis (gradients >80 mm Hg and valve areas <0.6 cm^2) may be at higher risk. In addition, 60% to 70% of asymptomatic patients with severe stenosis and calcified valves or rapid progression of the stenosis develop symptoms or die in 3 to 5 years. Thus, it is reasonable to offer surgical treatment in select subgroups of these patients with severe asymptomatic aortic stenosis if the operative risk is low (<1%) and the patient desires early operation.

Definition of "Severe" Aortic Stenosis

The definition of *severe aortic stenosis* varies. Valve areas less than 0.5, less than 0.7, and less than 1.0 cm^2 and a valve area indexed to body surface area less than 0.5 cm^2/m^2 have all been used as criteria for "severe" aortic stenosis. Valve area, especially from a single measurement, should not be used as the sole determinant for the severity of stenosis. The reproducibility of valve area may vary by as much as 0.4 to 0.6 cm^2. A valve area for a large man may have a different hemodynamic consequence than the same valve area for a small woman, supporting the concept that valve area should be corrected for body surface area. Studies have shown that the natural history of symptomatic patients with "moderate" aortic stenosis (valve area, 0.7-1.2 cm^2) is comparable to the classic natural history of symptomatic patients with "severe" aortic stenosis. The message is that patients should not be treated on the basis of a single determination of valve area in isolation from clinical signs and symptoms. Numerous factors, such as clinical presentation, exercise tolerance, mean gradient, and left ventricular function, should be considered when determining the need for aortic valve surgery.

Low-Output/Low-Gradient Aortic Stenosis

Patients may present with low-output/low-gradient aortic stenosis, that is, with a mean aortic valve gradient less than 30 mm Hg and the calculated valve area in the range of "severe" aortic stenosis (<1.0 cm2 or <0.5 cm2/m2). These patients may have critical end-stage aortic stenosis in which ventricular function has deteriorated because of progressive afterload on the left ventricle. Aortic valve replacement results in symptomatic improvement, increased longevity, and return of left ventricular systolic function. However, there may be other patients with a combination of mild calcific valvular aortic stenosis and concomitant left ventricular dysfunction due to another cause. In these patients, the "calculated aortic valve area" is low because the stroke volume is not sufficient to open completely the mildly stenotic aortic valve. It has been difficult to differentiate these two subsets of patients. The use of dobutamine stress testing has been recommended to select patients with true severe stenosis (the gradient increases to >40 mm Hg with dobutamine).

MITRAL STENOSIS

Cause

Most cases of mitral stenosis have a rheumatic cause. The rheumatic process causes "immobility" and thickening of the mitral valve leaflets, with fusion of the commissures. Leaflet calcification and subvalvular fusion occur in the late stages of the disease. In rare instances, the cause may be a congenital abnormality of the mitral valve or a parachute mitral valve. Cor triatriatum is an abnormality that simulates mitral stenosis. In this condition, a thin membrane across the left atrium obstructs pulmonary venous inflow. Left atrial myxoma and pulmonary vein obstruction may also present with signs and symptoms similar to those of mitral stenosis.

Pathophysiology

The pathophysiology of mitral stenosis is related to the increase in left atrial pressure from obstruction across the mitral valve. This increased pressure is reflected onto the pulmonary circulation, causing symptoms of dyspnea, orthopnea, and paroxysmal nocturnal dyspnea.

Unless mitral stenosis is severe, patients do not have symptoms at rest; however, with exercise or the onset of atrial fibrillation, left atrial pressure increases. This results from an increase in gradient and an increase in left atrial pressure, which occurs with a shortened diastolic filling period.

In long-standing severe mitral stenosis, secondary pulmonary hypertension may occur and lead to right ventricular failure and tricuspid regurgitation. Symptoms of angina pectoris are rare but may be due to right ventricular hypertrophy and ischemia of the right ventricle. The left ventricle is not affected in pure mitral stenosis.

Pathologically, rheumatic mitral stenosis results in commissural fusion. Secondary effects of the long-standing rheumatic process may involve progressive calcification and fibrosis of the mitral valve leaflets. The rheumatic process can also affect the subvalvular apparatus, leading to shortened and fibrotic chordae.

- The differential diagnosis of mitral stenosis should include cor triatriatum, atrial myxoma, and pulmonary vein obstruction.
- The hallmark of mitral stenosis is commissural fusion.
- The left ventricle is not affected in pure mitral stenosis.

Clinical Presentation

The presentation of mitral stenosis is related to the increase in left atrial pressure, which produces symptoms of dyspnea. The early course of the disease—before the development of symptoms—may last for decades, and symptoms then begin insidiously, with mild dyspnea only on exertion. Frequently, patients are not aware of progressive limitations in exercise because their activity level has decreased imperceptibly over the years. With a severe increase in left atrial pressure, paroxysmal nocturnal dyspnea and orthopnea occur. High pulmonary venous pressures may cause distention of the bronchial veins, and rupture of these veins may result in hemoptysis. Stasis occurs in the enlarged left atrium, especially in the presence of atrial fibrillation, and produces a nidus for thrombus formation. Systemic embolic events are seen in approximately one-third of patients with atrial fibrillation and mitral stenosis and may be the presenting event before the diagnosis of mitral stenosis is made.

Classically, the physical examination of a patient with mitral stenosis consists of a loud first heart sound, an opening snap, and a diastolic rumble. The interval between aortic valve closure and the opening snap (A_2-OS interval) is related to left atrial pressure and, thus, can be used to determine the severity of mitral stenosis. Patients with severe mitral stenosis have A_2-OS intervals shorter than 60 to 70 ms, and those with mild mitral stenosis have A_2-OS intervals longer than 100 to 110 ms. The intensity and duration of the diastolic rumble increase as the gradient across the mitral valve increases. However, because of differences in body habitus and chest cavity, severe mitral stenosis may be present with a barely audible diastolic rumble. If the mitral valve is pliable and noncalcified, the first heart sound is loud and snappy and the opening snap is very prominent. With progressive calcification and fibrosis of the leaflets, the first heart sound may diminish in intensity and the opening snap may disappear. The intensity of the pulmonic component of the second heart sound is important to note in determining the severity of coexistent pulmonary hypertension. In patients who do not have a diastolic rumble on initial auscultation, increasing heart rate by mild exercise (sit-ups or step-ups) may bring out a diastolic rumble.

Echocardiography

The standard for diagnosis and determination of the severity of mitral stenosis is two-dimensional/Doppler echocardiography. On two-dimensional echocardiography, the typical hockey-stick deformity of the mitral valve leaflets is easily visualized on the parasternal long-axis view. Commissural fusion and narrowing of the mitral valve opening area are seen on the short-axis view. In patients with adequate echocardiographic images, the area of the mitral valve can be determined planimetrically from the short-axis view if the plane of the two-dimensional view is at the tip of the mitral valve leaflets. Two-dimensional echocardiography is also important in identifying the morphology of the mitral valve leaflets and the subvalvular apparatus.

A grading system has been assigned to determine suitability for mitral valve valvotomy (surgical or percutaneous) based on two-dimensional features of the following: 1) leaflet thickening, 2) leaflet calcification, 3) leaflet mobility, and 4) subvalvular fusion. Each of the four morphologic features is assigned a score from 1 to 4, with 1 being the least involvement and 4, the most severe involvement. The mitral score is the sum of these four numbers. A score of 8 or less is indicative of a pliable noncalcified valve that should be suitable for balloon valvuloplasty or commissurotomy. Alternatively, a score of 12 or greater indicates a calcified fibrotic valve with subvalvular fusion that may not be appropriate for valve repair. Other factors must be taken into consideration when determining suitability for mitral valvotomy. Calcification of the commissures may preclude successful valvotomy. Isolated severe subvalvular fusion even with a pliable valve leaflet may preclude a successful valvotomy.

Determining the severity of obstruction across the mitral valve requires measuring the mean mitral valve gradient and calculating mitral valve area. By conventional criteria, mild mitral stenosis is present when the mean gradient is less than 5 mm Hg; moderate stenosis, 5 to 10 mm Hg; and severe stenosis, greater than 10 mm Hg. These values apply to patients with normal cardiac output and heart rates within the physiologic range of 60 to 90 beats per minute. Previously, cardiac catheterization was needed to determine the mitral valve gradient. However, Doppler echocardiography can be used to measure the mean mitral valve gradient accurately and reproducibly—it is more accurate than conventional cardiac catheterization when using pulmonary artery wedge pressure and left ventricular pressures.

The mean mitral valve gradient depends not only on the degree of obstruction but also on the flow and the diastolic filling period. A calculated mitral valve area (MVA) incorporates all these factors. By convention, an area less than 1.0 cm² indicates severe mitral stenosis; 1.0 to 1.5 cm², moderate stenosis; and greater than 1.5 cm², mild stenosis (Table 4). The hydraulic Gorlin equation has been the standard for calculating MVA in cardiac catheterization laboratories.

$$MVA = \frac{1{,}000 \times CO}{38 \times HR \times DFP \times \sqrt{\Delta P}}$$

where CO = cardiac output, DFP = diastolic filling period, HR = heart rate, and ΔP = pressured difference across the valve.

The Gorlin equation has limitations and is not applicable at low or high cardiac outputs. It is erroneous with concomitant mitral regurgitation. In addition, the determination of cardiac output by cardiac catheterization can be misleading, especially in the presence of atrial fibrillation and concomitant tricuspid regurgitation.

Doppler echocardiography uses the concept of a diastolic half-time to estimate MVA. The diastolic half-time, initially described at cardiac catheterization, is the time it takes for the maximal mitral gradient to decrease by 50%. It is inversely related to valve area. In most patients, an accurate measurement of MVA can be obtained from the rate of velocity decrease during early and mid-diastole, as assessed on the transmitral velocity curve.

$$t_{1/2} = DT \times 0.29$$

$$MVA = \frac{220}{t_{1/2}}$$

where $t_{1/2}$ = half-time and DT = deceleration time.

There are limitations to using the diastolic half-time, especially when abnormalities of left atrial and left ventricular compliance exist. In these instances, the MVA should be calculated with the continuity equation:

$$MVA = \frac{LVOT_{TVI} \times LVOT_{area}}{MV_{TVI}}$$

where LVOT = left ventricular outflow tract, MV = mitral valve, and TVI = time-velocity integral.

- Doppler echocardiography is more accurate than cardiac catheterization for determining the mean mitral valve gradient.
- Suitability for valvuloplasty should be assessed with two-dimensional echocardiography and based on the mitral score and appearance of the commissures.
- The continuity equation for MVA should be used when the area derived from the half-time does not correlate with the mean transmitral gradient.

Natural History and Treatment
Mitral stenosis is a disease of plateaus (Fig. 2). There is a period of 1 to 2 decades after the onset of rheumatic

Table 4. Criteria for Determining Severity of Mitral Stenosis

Severity	Gradient, mm Hg	Mitral valve area, cm2
Mild	<5.0	>1.5
Moderate	5.0-10.0	1.0-1.5
Severe	>10.0	<1.0

fever before signs of mitral stenosis appear. This is followed by another period of 1 to 2 decades before mild symptoms occur. Mild symptoms of dyspnea on exertion may be present for another 1 to 2 decades. During this time, the onset of atrial fibrillation may cause further decompensation, but this can be treated by rate control. Finally, severe New York Heart Association class III or IV symptoms develop. Indications for mitral valve replacement include a combination of severe mitral stenosis and New York Heart Association functional class III or IV symptoms, with significant limitation of lifestyle. With the advent of percutaneous mitral balloon valvotomy, it may be reasonable to perform balloon valvotomy earlier if the patient is a good candidate for this procedure from the morphologic standpoint.

In determining the need for intervention, it is necessary to correlate the symptoms with the gradient and, subsequently, the MVA. Some patients may have

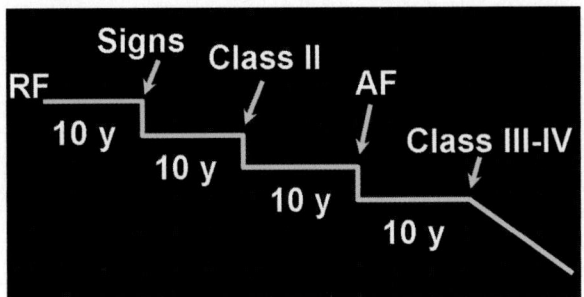

Fig. 2. Natural history of mitral stenosis, a disease of plateaus. After the onset of rheumatic fever (RF), the patient remains asymptomatic for 10 to 20 years but develops auscultatory signs of mitral stenosis. With the onset of mild symptoms, there is a long period before the development of atrial fibrillation (AF). After the onset of New York Heart Association class III or IV symptoms, a patient's condition rapidly deteriorates.

significant symptoms but a mitral valve gradient and an MVA that are consistent with only a mild or moderate degree of mitral stenosis (gradient <10 mm Hg or MVA >1.5 cm2). What may be a mild degree of obstruction for one patient may be a significant degree of obstruction for another.

In patients whose symptoms are out of proportion to the calculated mitral valve indices, the hemodynamic response to exercise should be measured. Previously, this was assessed at catheterization of the right and left sides of the heart with exercise. However, exercise Doppler echocardiography can provide all the information required. For this, the patient undergoes a treadmill or supine bicycle exercise test until symptoms occur. Mean mitral valve gradient and pulmonary artery systolic pressure should be measured at peak exercise. If the mean gradient increases more than 15 mm Hg with symptoms, the patient should be considered symptomatic on the basis of the mitral valve disease. Alternatively, if symptoms occur and the mitral valve gradient does not increase to those levels, another cause for the symptoms must be pursued. In patients with a mitral valve mean gradient that does not correlate with MVA, other Doppler estimates of MVA must be considered, including the continuity equation or proximal isovelocity surface area calculations.

The operations for mitral stenosis have consisted of closed commissurotomy, open commissurotomy, and mitral valve replacement. Closed commissurotomy was an effective procedure used before the institution of cardiopulmonary bypass. Through a lateral thoracotomy, the surgeon would attempt to split the commissural fusion with a finger or dilator. This was successful in most patients with noncalcified valves but was inadequate for those with calcified fibrotic valves and subvalvular fusion. With the advent of cardiopulmonary bypass, open commissurotomy became the procedure of choice. This requires a median sternotomy and cardiopulmonary bypass. The surgeon directly inspects the mitral valve apparatus and incises the commissures under direct vision, with chordal reconstruction if necessary. For patients with a mitral valve not believed to be suitable for commissurotomy, mitral valve replacement is performed.

Recently, percutaneous mitral balloon valvotomy has become an acceptable alternative to mitral valve surgery in selected patients (Table 5). Fused commissures can be split with one or more large balloons inflated across the mitral valve. This can produce hemodynamic improvement comparable to that of closed commissurotomy. Percutaneous mitral balloon valvotomy requires expertise, including the capability for performing a transseptal puncture. However, in experienced hands, the results are excellent and comparable to those of surgery, with the valve area typically increasing from 1.0 to 2.0 cm2. In several randomized trials comparing mitral balloon valvotomy with closed and open surgical commissurotomy, the acute results and long-term outcome have been comparable in young patients with pliable valves. Potential complications, such as systemic embolus, severe mitral regurgitation, and left ventricular perforation, can be avoided by preoperative assessment of mitral valve morphology and documentation of lack of atrial thrombus by transesophageal echocardiography. In selected patients with pliable valve leaflets, percutaneous mitral balloon valvotomy should be considered not only in those with New York Heart Association class III or IV symptoms but also in those with class I or II symptoms who have high resting gradients and pulmonary hypertension.

- Mitral stenosis is a disease of plateaus.
- Exercise hemodynamics should be performed in patients with symptoms out of proportion to calculated mitral valve gradient and MVA.
- Percutaneous mitral balloon valvotomy may be the procedure of choice for patients with mitral stenosis and a noncalcified pliable mitral valve.

Table 5.   Recommendations for Percutaneous
Mitral Balloon Valvotomy

Indication	Class
1. Symptomatic patients (NYHA functional class II, III, or IV), moderate or severe MS (MVA ≤1.5 cm^2),* and valve morphology favorable for percutaneous balloon valvotomy in the absence of left atrial thrombus or moderate or severe MR	I
2. Asymptomatic patients with moderate or severe MS (MVA ≤1.5 cm^2)* and valve morphology favorable for percutaneous balloon valvotomy who have pulmonary hypertension (pulmonary artery systolic pressure >50 mm Hg at rest or 60 mm Hg with exercise) in the absence of left atrial thrombus or moderate or severe MR	IIa
3. Patients with NYHA functional class III or IV symptoms, moderate or severe MS (MVA ≤1.5 cm^2),* and a nonpliable calcified valve who are at high risk for surgery in the absence of left atrial thrombus or moderate or severe MR	IIa
4. Asymptomatic patients with moderate or severe MS (MVA ≤1.5 cm^2)* and valve morphology favorable for percutaneous balloon valvotomy who have new onset of atrial fibrillation in the absence of left atrial thrombus or moderate or severe MR	
5. Patients in NYHA functional class III or IV, moderate or severe MS (MVA ≤1.5 cm^2), and a nonpliable calcified valve who are low-risk candidates for surgery	IIb
6. Patients with mild MS	III

MR, mitral regurgitation; MS, mitral stenosis; MVA, mitral valve area; NYHA, New York Heart Association. *The committee recognizes that there may be variability in the measurement of MVA and that the mean transmitral gradient, pulmonary artery wedge pressure, and pulmonary artery pressure at rest or during exercise should also be taken into consideration.

41

VALVULAR REGURGITATION

Rick A. Nishimura, MD

MITRAL REGURGITATION

The mitral valve is a complicated structure that requires the correct functioning of the valve leaflets, valve commissures, mitral anulus, papillary muscles, chordae tendineae, and left ventricle for competence. Mitral regurgitation results from failure of one or more of the components of normal mitral valve competence. The presentation and management depend on the underlying cause, duration, regurgitant severity, patient symptoms (including objective exercise tolerance), and left ventricular size and systolic function.

Anatomy

There are three basic mechanisms of mitral regurgitation.

Alteration of Mitral Leaflets, Commissures, or Anulus

Rheumatic Fever

Rheumatic mitral valve disease may deform valves, shorten chordae, or fuse commissures and lead to pure mitral regurgitation or predominant regurgitation in combination with stenosis.

Mitral Valve Prolapse

Mitral valve prolapse is the most common cause of isolated severe mitral regurgitation. The posterior leaflet is affected more frequently and severely than the anterior leaflet. Mitral anular dilatation and calcification and myxomatous changes of chordae tendineae may be associated. The likelihood of mitral valve prolapse resulting in significant mitral regurgitation increases with age and is greater in men than in women. Prolapse may occur alone or in association with other conditions, including Marfan syndrome, Ehlers-Danlos syndrome, and thoracic skeletal abnormalities.

Mitral Anulus Calcification

Isolated mitral anulus calcification is usually age-related and occurs in older patients with hypertension, hypertrophic obstructive cardiomyopathy, chronic renal failure, or aortic stenosis.

Infective Endocarditis

Infective endocarditis may damage valve leaflets by perforation or a vegetation that interferes with coaptation. Anatomical abnormalities may persist even after the active infection has been eradicated.

Congenital

A congenital cleft of the anterior mitral leaflet often is associated with primum atrial septal defect, but it can exist in isolation without other features of a persistent atrioventricular canal.

Rare Causes of Mitral Incompetence

Other, uncommon, causes of mitral leaflet abnormalities include endomyocardial fibrosis, carcinoid disease with right-to-left shunting or bronchial carcinoid-secreting adenomas, ergotamine toxicity, radiation therapy, trauma, rheumatoid arthritis, systemic lupus erythematosus (Libman-Sacks lesions), and diet-drug toxicity.

Defective Tensor Apparatus

Abnormal Chordae Tendineae

Ruptured chordae are responsible for a significant percentage of cases of mitral regurgitation. Rupture may be idiopathic, a complication of endocarditis, a result of myxomatous degeneration in the setting of mitral valve prolapse, or a result of blunt or direct penetrating thoracic trauma.

Papillary Muscle Dysfunction

Myocardial ischemia or infarction can cause papillary muscle dysfunction (without rupture). The posteromedial papillary muscle is more vulnerable to ischemia or infarction than the anterolateral papillary muscle because of its single end-artery vascular supply. Nonischemic causes of papillary muscle dysfunction include dilated cardiomyopathy, myocarditis, and hypertension.

Myocardial infarction (either transmural or subendocardial) can cause rupture of a papillary muscle. It usually occurs in the first week after infarction at a time when the inflammatory cell response is maximal and most frequently involves the posteromedial papillary muscle. Rarely, chest trauma can cause papillary muscle rupture, usually with coexistent myocardial or ventricular septal rupture.

Alterations of Left Ventricular and Left Atrial Size and Function

Global or regional left ventricular enlargement may alter the position and axis of contraction of the papillary muscles in addition to causing dilatation of the mitral ring. Progressive left atrial and ventricular enlargement associated with any type of chronic mitral regurgitation, in turn, leads to more mitral regurgitation by further altering the geometry of the chamber.

Mitral regurgitation in hypertrophic obstructive cardiomyopathy results both from the Venturi effect (systolic anterior motion of the mitral leaflets or chordae or both) and abnormal papillary muscle position.

- Understanding the mechanism of mitral regurgitation helps define the natural history and optimal treatment.
- Mitral prolapse is the most common cause of isolated severe mitral regurgitation.
- Ischemia can cause either dysfunction or rupture of papillary muscle. The posteromedial papillary muscle is affected most often because of its single end-artery blood supply.
- Left ventricular enlargement and abnormal contractile function are common causes of significant mitral regurgitation.

Pathophysiology of Mitral Regurgitation

Mitral regurgitation has three pathophysiologic stages.

Acute Stage

In acute severe mitral regurgitation, there is a sudden volume overload on an unprepared left ventricle and left atrium (Fig. 1). The left ventricle responds with increased sarcomere stretch and augmented left ventricular stroke volume via the Frank-Starling stretch mechanism. However, the larger volume increases left ventricular diastolic pressure, which in turn increases left atrial pressure. Because left atrial compliance is normal in the acute state, the large regurgitant volume markedly increases left atrial pressure, which causes pulmonary congestion, edema, and dyspnea.

The sudden opening of a new low-pressure pathway for systolic ejection decreases left ventricular afterload, permitting more complete volume ejection from the ventricle. Although total left ventricular stroke volume increases, forward stroke volume decreases. The combination of increased preload, decreased afterload, and increased left ventricular contractile function increases the measured ejection fraction to between 60% and 75%.

Chronic Compensated Stage

In the chronic compensated stage (Fig. 2), left ventricular volume overload elongates individual myocytes, causing compensatory eccentric left ventricular hypertrophy and increasing left ventricular end-diastolic volume. The Frank-Starling mechanism

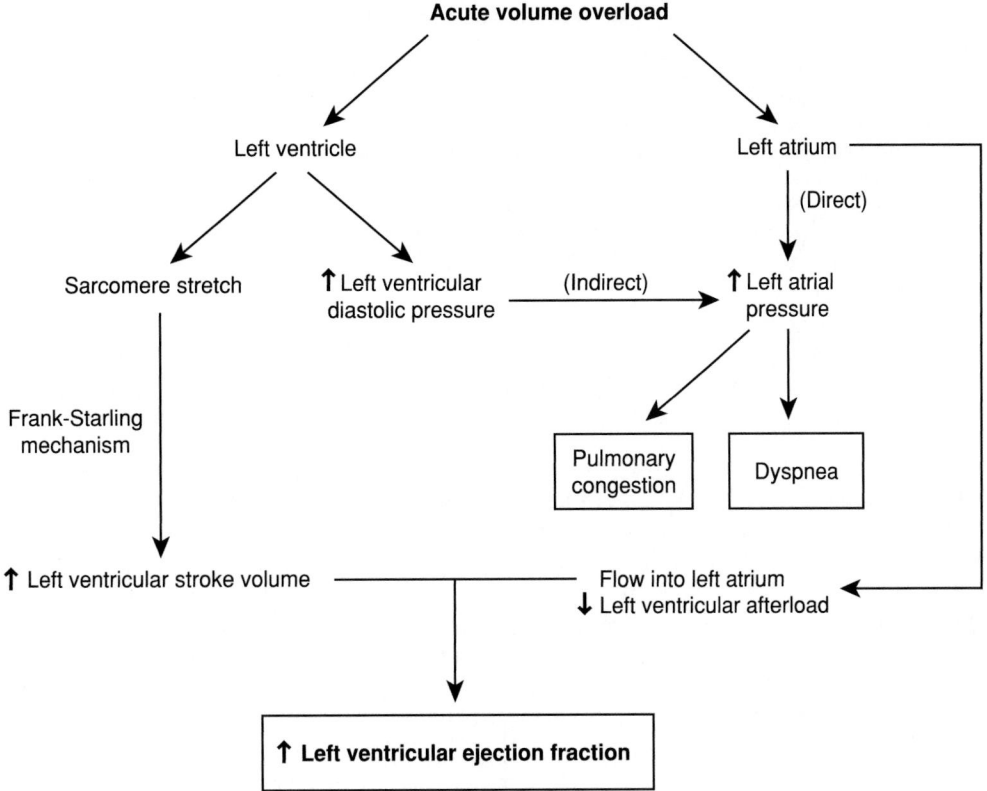

Fig. 1. Acute severe mitral regurgitation.

continues to augment total stroke volume. The left atrium dilates, thus increasing its compliance. There is an increase in preload from the volume overload and a decrease in afterload from ejection into the low impedance left atrium. The combination of increased end-diastolic volume, augmented contraction, and decreased afterload continues to result in a high ejection fraction. The dilated left ventricle and atrium allow the regurgitant volume to be accommodated at lower filling pressures, thereby minimizing symptoms of pulmonary congestion.

Chronic Decompensated Stage
Eventually, left ventricular contractile function declines, and the chronic decompensated stage of mitral regurgitation begins (Fig. 3). This downward spiral includes an increase in end-systolic volume as left ventricular function decreases. Left ventricular filling pressures increase and cause pulmonary congestion. Increased ventricular pressure further dilates the left ventricle, increasing systolic wall stress and afterload. The increased afterload further reduces ventricular systolic function, thus com-

pleting the downward cycle. As end-diastolic and end-systolic volumes increase, the ejection fraction may be in the 50% to 60% "normal" range. In patients with severe mitral regurgitation, an ejection fraction less than 60% is probably abnormal and indicative of ventricular dysfunction.

The time during which patients progress from compensated to decompensated mitral regurgitation depends on the severity of the regurgitation (which itself can change over time), variables that affect afterload and ventricular contractility, and individual, poorly understood, patient characteristics.

- Acute severe mitral regurgitation is characterized by normal-sized chambers, high ejection fraction, and pulmonary congestion.
- Chronic compensated severe mitral regurgitation is typified by few symptoms, enlargement of the left ventricle and atrium, and high ejection fraction.
- A "normal range" ejection fraction (50-60%) in the setting of severe mitral regurgitation usually implies left ventricular systolic dysfunction.

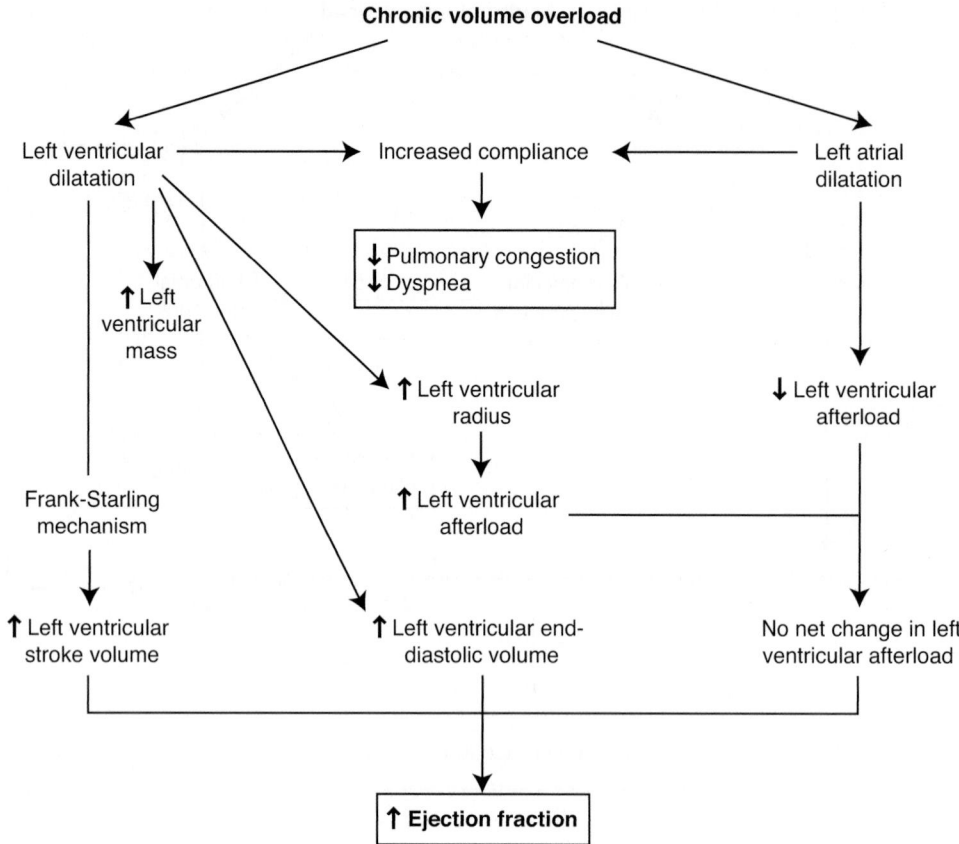

Fig. 2. Chronic compensated mitral regurgitation.

Clinical Syndrome of Mitral Regurgitation

Acute Mitral Regurgitation

Acute mitral regurgitation usually results from infective endocarditis, infarction, ischemic heart disease, trauma, or chordal rupture. If acute mitral regurgitation is severe, severe pulmonary congestion is expected. The high left atrial pressure and left ventricular end-diastolic pressure account for the third and fourth heart sounds. The systolic murmur of mitral regurgitation in this acute condition may be short, soft, or completely absent. Rarely, there may be only a small left ventricular-to-atrial pressure gradient (because left atrial pressure has increased close to that of the left ventricle). This may result in the absence of an audible murmur and Doppler color flow evidence of mitral regurgitation (indicating almost no turbulence in the regurgitant flow).

Chronic Mitral Regurgitation

Patients with chronic mitral regurgitation may have a prolonged asymptomatic interval. However, adverse ventricular changes may develop during this period. Once symptoms arise, the low cardiac output symptoms of fatigue and generalized weakness predominate early. As left ventricular function deteriorates, exertional dyspnea, orthopnea, and paroxysmal nocturnal dyspnea become more prominent.

Examination of the precordium in a patient with severe chronic mitral regurgitation reveals a brief, laterally displaced, and enlarged apical impulse. A ventricular filling impulse may be palpable. The presence of an apical thrill indicates severe mitral regurgitation. As ventricular systolic function deteriorates, the duration of the apical impulse increases.

Auscultation may reveal single or multiple nonejection clicks whose timing may be varied by maneuvers. An accentuated pulmonic component of the second heart sound indicates pulmonary hypertension. Aortic closure may be early because of decreased duration of forward flow, causing persistent wide splitting of the second heart sound (however, the duration of the murmur often obscures the second heart sound, mak-

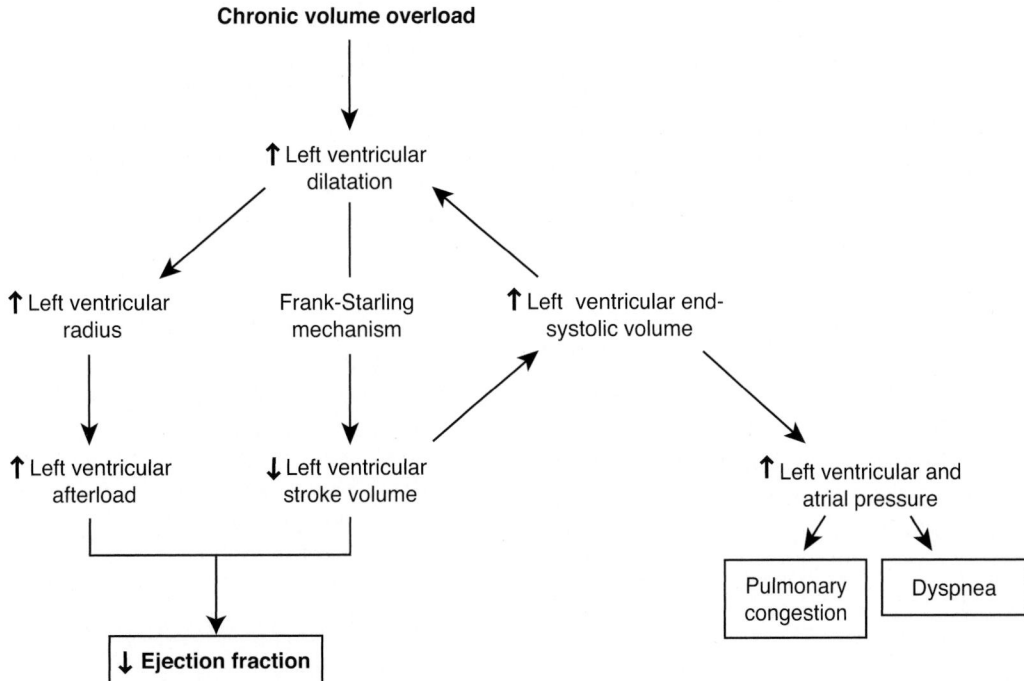

Fig. 3. Chronic decompensated mitral regurgitation.

ing the splitting hard to detect). An apical third heart sound is common, but fourth heart sounds are unusual.

A holosystolic murmur is the hallmark of mitral regurgitation. The intensity of the murmur does not necessarily correlate with the severity of the regurgitant flow. Although the murmur frequently radiates to the axilla, a primary posterior leaflet abnormality will direct the regurgitant flow anteriorly and the radiation may be toward the aortic area. Characteristically, the mitral regurgitant murmur is constant despite different cycle lengths; this feature helps, at the bedside, to distinguish it from aortic outflow murmurs. The presence of a short diastolic apical rumble in the absence of mitral stenosis implies high diastolic transmitral flow and severe mitral regurgitation.

- Acute severe mitral regurgitation may have a short or soft murmur because of the low left ventricular-to-atrial pressure gradient.
- Nonspecific fatigue and weakness may represent the early symptoms of chronic severe mitral regurgitation.
- A third heart sound in chronic mitral regurgitation is usually indicative of severe regurgitation.

- Posterior leaflet prolapse often produces a murmur that radiates to the aortic area.
- The failure of a mitral regurgitant murmur to change with variable cycle lengths distinguishes it from an outflow tract murmur.

Evaluation of Mitral Regurgitation

Electrocardiography
No electrocardiographic (ECG) findings are diagnostic of mitral regurgitation. The ECG may show atrial fibrillation; left atrial enlargement is expected if sinus rhythm persists. Left ventricular hypertrophy and nonspecific ST-segment and T-wave changes are also common.

Chest Radiography
Significant chronic mitral regurgitation causes the left ventricular and left atrial enlargement seen on chest radiographs. Left atrial enlargement might be recognized as straightening of the left border of the heart, an atrial double density, or elevation of the left mainstem bronchus. Pulmonary venous congestion may be present in any stage of mitral regurgitation.

Echocardiography

Echocardiography assesses the morphology of the mitral valve, anulus, commissures, and papillary muscles. Assessment of the severity of mitral regurgitation is performed with an integrated Doppler and two-dimensional echocardiographic examination (Table 1). A flail mitral valve leaflet usually is associated with severe mitral regurgitation. In some cases, trans-esophageal echocardiography is required to better assess the anatomy of the mitral valve and its supporting structures, to inspect the atria for thrombus, and to gather supplemental data used in qualitative and quantitative measures of regurgitation severity. Echocardiography also evaluates the impact of mitral regurgitation on left ventricular and atrial size and function, in addition to right ventricular function and hemodynamics.

Cardiac Catheterization

Left ventriculography is used primarily when noninvasive data are discordant or technically limited or differ from the clinical perception of the severity of mitral regurgitation or ventricular function. Angiographic grading of mitral regurgitation provides a semiquantitative measure of severity of regurgitation from the density of contrast going back into the left atrium (Sellan's criteria). However, it is dependent on the volume and injection rate of the contrast agent, catheter position, hemodynamics at the time of injection, and volume of the left atrium in addition to the severity of valve regurgitation. Calculations of the invasively derived regurgitant fraction are rarely used and dependent upon accurate measurement of left ventricular volume and cardiac output. The presence or absence of prominent "v" waves on a pulmonary wedge hemodynamic tracing depends not only on mitral regurgitant flow at the time of the study but also on the compliance of the left atrium.

- Echocardiography is invaluable for assessing the cause and severity of mitral regurgitation and its effects on the size and function of the left ventricle, left atrium, and right ventricle.
- Left ventriculography is most useful when noninvasive data are discordant or technically limited or differ from the clinical impression of the severity of mitral regurgitation or ventricular function.

Table 1. Doppler Indicators of Severe Mitral Regurgitation*

Color jet area (> 8.0 cm^2; > 1/3 LA area)
Wide vena contracta (color flow)
Regurgitant volume (> 60 mL)[†]
Regurgitant fraction (> 55%)[†]
ERO (> 0.35 cm^2)[†]
Pulmonary vein PW Doppler flow profile (systolic flow reversal)
CW Doppler signal intensity (dense)
Transmitral PW flow velocity (E >1.5 m/s)

CW, continuous-wave; E, early transmitral flow; ERO, effective regurgitant orifice area; LA, left atrium; PW, pulsed-wave.

*Measurements indicative of severe regurgitation are in parentheses.

†Can be measured by volumetric Doppler, proximal isovelocity surface area method, or a combination of these, including two-dimensional measures.

Mitral Valve Prolapse

In patients with mitral valve prolapse the systolic billowing of a portion of the mitral leaflet into the left atrium may cause an audible click. If the prolapse is significant, mitral regurgitation results. This condition is dynamic; the timing of the click and murmur varies with preload and afterload. Maneuvers that decrease the ventricular preload (Valsalva maneuver, standing) cause prolapse, and the click and murmur occur earlier in the cardiac cycle. The converse is true with maneuvers that increase preload.

The natural history of most cases of mitral valve prolapse is benign, although progression to severe mitral regurgitation is more prevalent in men than women and with advancing age. Rare complications of mitral valve prolapse such as endocarditis, severe rhythm disturbances, and strokes occur predominantly in patients with thickened valve leaflets.

Patients with mitral valve prolapse and severe mitral regurgitation are managed similarly to other patients with severe mitral regurgitation. If the regurgitation is mild, patients should be reassured and followed clinically for any changes in either symptoms or physical findings. Antibiotic prophylaxis is advised for patients with a click-and-murmur incompetence or a click and echocardiographic findings of significant leaflet thickening or regurgitation.

Patients with mitral valve prolapse and palpitations or increased adrenergic tone, atypical chest pain, anxiety, or fatigue should be counseled to minimize their use of exogenous stimulants and may benefit from β-adrenergic blocker therapy. Aspirin is advised for transient ischemic events in the setting of mitral valve prolapse if no other cause is found.

Natural History of Mitral Regurgitation

The natural history of *acute* mitral regurgitation is dependent on its cause and severity. Patients with papillary muscle rupture or severe regurgitation from an unstable mitral prosthesis have a poor short-term outlook without operation. Those with acute regurgitation from endocarditis have a variable course depending on the response to antibiotic treatment. Patients with abrupt chordal rupture have a natural history dependent primarily on the severity of regurgitation.

Patients with *chronic* mitral regurgitation have a clinical course characterized by an initial compensated phase followed by progressive left ventricular dysfunction. Patients with severe mitral regurgitation may go for years without symptoms. However, the long-standing volume overload causes progressive fibrosis and myocyte degeneration with eventual left ventricular dysfunction. This left ventricular dysfunction may occur before the onset of symptoms and portends a poor prognosis even if the regurgitation is surgically corrected. The natural history of severe mitral regurgitation is one of significant early mortality and morbidity if left untreated. In patients with severe mitral regurgitation due to a flail leaflet over 60% will develop heart failure by 10 years of follow-up.

Treatment of Acute Severe Mitral Regurgitation

Patients with *acute* severe mitral regurgitation may be hemodynamically stable or unstable at presentation. Any patient with hemodynamic instability requires rapid evaluation and therapy with intravenous vasodilators (usually sodium nitroprusside), intravenous inotropes, and, perhaps, intra-aortic balloon counterpulsation. Patients presenting with acute regurgitation often have a ruptured papillary muscle or an unstable mitral prosthesis, and repair or replacement of the mitral valve generally is indicated because long-term

medical therapy is ineffective.

Other therapies for mitral regurgitation include antibiotics if endocarditis is present and antianginal drugs or angioplasty or stenting in some cases of ischemic papillary muscle dysfunction. In endocarditis, operation is often delayed in the hope of sterilizing the mitral valve bed because ongoing active infection puts the new valve at peril of prosthetic endocarditis. Patients with endocarditis should be considered for urgent surgical intervention if progressive heart failure, infection unresponsive to antibiotics, intracardiac abscess, or recurrent systemic embolization develops despite therapy.

Treatment of Chronic Mitral Regurgitation

All patients with mitral regurgitation should be instructed in dental hygiene and infective endocarditis prophylaxis. Treatment of hypertension myocardial ischemia (in patients with coronary disease) and prevention of ventricular dilatation (in patients with cardiomyopathy) may be helpful in prevention of progression of severity of mitral regurgitation. There is no data to support the use of vasodilators or ACE inhibitors in patients with mitral regurgitation unless there is left ventricular dysfunction or hypertension.

Timing of operation is difficult. Early operation with a prosthetic mitral valve has its own short- and long-term complications and thus should not be performed prematurely. However due to the insidious progressive left ventricular dysfunction which occurs from the long-standing volume overload, by the time symptoms occur the golden opportunity for operation may have been missed.

Overall, operation is indicated for patients which chronic severe mitral regurgitation with the onset of any symptoms. Although left ventricular dysfunction may have already occurred, survival and outcomes are still better with operation than with medical management.

In asymptomatic patients, measure of left ventricular size and function determine the need for operation. An EF <60% or end-systolic dimension >40 mm indicate systolic function. Patients who exceed these parameters should be considered for operation. There is a subgroup who present with heart failure and EF <35% in whom the risk of operation is high as systolic function is severely reduced. In these patients, operation should only be considered if valve repair instead of valve replacement can be performed because of its better preservation of ventricular function.

In the above patients with symptoms of left ventricular dysfunction, operation should be considered irrespective of the type of operation (replacement or repair). However in any patient, repair is preferred over replacement due to better long-term outcome. The better outcome with mitral valve repair is due to better preservation of left ventricular dysfunction, durability of the repair, and avoidance of the potential complications of a valve prosthesis (and long-term anticoagulation).

There are some centers now advocating earlier operation in the asymptomatic patient with severe mitral regurgitation despite preserved ventricular function. This early operation is to avoid the onset of ventricular dysfunction, which, if it occurs, portends a poorer prognosis. However due to the attendant risks of a prosthetic valve, this early operation should only be done if there is a high chance of successful mitral valve repair (>90%) and a low operative risk.

- Patients with acute severe mitral regurgitation and hemodynamic instability require rapid evaluation, aggressive stabilization, and early valve operation.
- Patients with acute severe mitral regurgitation who are hemodynamically stable should have semielective cardiac operation.
- Indications for valve operation in endocarditis include progressive heart failure, resistance to antibiotics, intracardiac abscess, or recurrent systemic embolization despite therapy.
- Patients with severe chronic mitral regurgitation who are in New York Heart Association class II, III, or IV, have an ejection fraction less than 60%, have an end-diastolic diameter more than 40 mm, or have an end-systolic volume more than 50 mL/m^2 should undergo valve surgery, if not otherwise contraindicated.
- Emerging indications for mitral valve replacement include flail leaflet, paroxysmal or recent-onset atrial fibrillation, and pulmonary hypertension.
- Patients with impaired ventricular function are better served by valve repair than replacement.
- Successful valve repair is less likely in cases that are rheumatic, ischemic, or due to infection, when prolapse is anterior or bileaflet, or when significant calcification is present.

AORTIC REGURGITATION

Aortic regurgitation may result from intrinsic structural abnormalities of the aortic valve or the ascending aorta or both.

Anatomy

Intrinsic Valvular Disease

Rheumatic fever causes mild aortic regurgitation during the first episodes, but with time the leaflets fibrose, shorten, and contract, resulting in malalignment and loss of coaptation. There usually is associated aortic stenosis due to commissural fusion. It is uncommon to have rheumatic aortic disease without coexistent mitral disease.

The most common congenital cause of aortic regurgitation in adults is a bicuspid valve with malcoaptation or diastolic prolapse of a cusp or both. In addition, chronic progressive aortic regurgitation also may be associated with ventricular septal defects (due to weakening of the neighboring supporting aortic anulus) or subaortic stenosis (causing turbulent high-velocity jets that hit and damage the aortic leaflets).

Infective endocarditis usually involves previously abnormal valves and leads to tissue destruction, vegetation interference with proper alignment of the commissures during closure, or invasion and structural distortion of the aortic valve anulus. Even after medical eradication of infection, regurgitation may progress because of contracture of healing cusps.

Collagen vascular diseases usually affect the aortic root, but they also can affect the cusps themselves. The associated valvulitis leads to contracture of leaflets, with central regurgitation. Perforation of leaflets is less common.

Senile degenerative aortic valve disease is usually important clinically because of aortic stenosis, but some degree of aortic regurgitation, especially in early stages, is often seen. Significant regurgitation often occurs after either operative decalcification or percutaneous balloon valvuloplasty for aortic stenosis.

Diseases of the Ascending Aorta

Acute destruction of the aortic root disrupts the supporting structures of the valve and results in regurgitation. Aortic dissection longitudinally cleaves the aortic intima or media with a dissecting column of blood and occurs most often in patients with idiopathic dilatation of the ascending aorta, hypertension, or Marfan syndrome. It also can be associated with pregnancy, result from blunt chest trauma, or follow acute aortitis complicating aortic valve infective endocarditis.

Many diseases are associated with chronic dilatation of the aortic root, and they cause regurgitation by stretching the valve cusps. These diseases include 1) Marfan syndrome, usually associated with progressive aortic dilatation as a result of cystic medial necrosis; 2) progressive idiopathic aortic dilatation with cystic medial necrosis; 3) senile dilatation and anuloaortic ectasia of unknown cause; 4) syphilitic aortitis developing 15 to 25 years after the initial infection and sparing the sinuses of Valsalva; and 5) connective tissue disorders (rheumatoid arthritis, ankylosing spondylitis, Reiter syndrome, relapsing polychondritis, giant cell arteritis, and Whipple disease). Marfan syndrome, progressive idiopathic aortic dilatation, and some of the connective tissue disorders also can affect the mitral leaflets as well as the proximal conducting system.

- It is essential to know whether a patient's aortic regurgitation is due to valvular disease or proximal aortic disease or both.
- Many causes of aortic regurgitation often have associated mitral valve abnormalities: endocarditis, rheumatic fever, collagen vascular disease, or Marfan syndrome.

Pathophysiology of Aortic Regurgitation

Acute or subacute significant aortic regurgitation causes the abrupt introduction of a large volume of blood into a noncompliant left ventricle, thus increasing left ventricular end-diastolic and pulmonary venous pressures and leading to dyspnea or pulmonary edema.

In chronic aortic regurgitation, compensatory left ventricular changes occur over time. The excess volume load causes stretching and elongation of myocardial fibers, which in turn increase wall stress. Wall stress is normalized by sarcomere replication and hypertrophic thickening of the ventricular walls. Thus, although the ratio of wall thickness to cavity radius remains essentially normal, left ventricular mass increases (eccentric hypertrophy).

Initially, ventricular enlargement increases the ejection fraction through the Frank-Starling mechanism.

However, further enlargement exhausts preload reserve, and the ejection fraction decreases to the "normal" range. Eventually, ejection fraction decreases further, whereas end-systolic volume increases. This end-systolic volume increase is a sensitive index of myocardial dysfunction. When the ventricle can dilate no further, diastolic pressure increases and results in dyspnea, another sign of decompensation.

During exercise, the volume of aortic regurgitation tends to decrease because of decreased systemic vascular resistance and shortened diastolic period. However, there also are increases in venous return that the enlarged left ventricle may not be able to handle, thus causing a relative decrease in output (exertional fatigue) or increase in end-diastolic pressure (dyspnea) or both.

Patients with chronic aortic regurgitation may experience anginal symptoms despite normal coronary arteries. Mechanisms include increase in total myocardial oxygen consumption (increased left ventricular myocardial mass and wall tension), decreased subendocardial perfusion gradient due to compressed intramyocardial coronary arterioles, decreased central aortic diastolic driving pressure, and diminished coronary arteriolar vasodilatory reserve.

- Acute severe aortic regurgitation is characterized by normal left ventricular size, high ejection fraction, and dyspnea or pulmonary edema.
- Chronic compensated aortic regurgitation is typified by minimal symptoms and left ventricular enlargement.
- Decompensation is characterized by symptoms (initially with exertion) and decreasing ejection fraction.

Clinical Syndrome of Aortic Regurgitation

Acute aortic regurgitation usually is due to aortic dissection or infective endocarditis. In these circumstances, the manifestations of the underlying process usually predominate. Because compensatory cardiac mechanisms cannot develop, significant dyspnea occurs as a consequence of high left ventricular end-diastolic and pulmonary venous pressures. A murmur may be minimal because of the abrupt increase in left ventricular end-diastolic pressure and rapidly diminishing aortic-left ventricular diastolic pressure gradient. Peripheral manifestations (which are caused by rapid volume runoff into the left ventricle) may be absent because of acutely high ventricular diastolic pressures.

In chronic aortic regurgitation, the first symptom the patient often notices is an uncomfortable awareness of overactivity of the heart and neck vessels because of the forceful heartbeat associated with the high pulse pressure. Exertional dyspnea is a symptom of left ventricular failure.

Inspection of the patient may reveal nodding of the head (de Musset sign), visible capillary pulsation in the nail beds during gentle pressure on the edge of the nail (Quincke sign), features of Marfan syndrome, or stigmata of infective endocarditis.

Hemodynamically severe aortic regurgitation generally causes a widened pulse pressure more than 100 mm Hg with a diastolic pressure less than 60 mm Hg. Pulse pressure may not accurately reflect the severity of aortic regurgitation in young patients with compliant vessels or in patients with accompanying left ventricular failure and increased left ventricular end-diastolic pressure. Other signs of high-volume systolic ejection of blood with rapid diastolic runoff include a sharp, rapid carotid upstroke, followed by abnormal collapse (Corrigan pulse), a "pistol-shot" sound heard over the femoral artery (Duroziez murmur), or a biphasic bruit heard during mild compression of the femoral artery with the stethoscope. The jugular venous pulse and pressure are generally normal in isolated aortic regurgitation unless a dilated ascending aorta compresses the superior vena cava.

The apical impulse in chronic aortic regurgitation is diffuse, hyperdynamic, and displaced inferiorly and leftward. A third heart sound may be palpated. A diastolic thrill at the base of the heart signifies severe aortic regurgitation, whereas a systolic thrill at the base signifies a large systolic stroke volume.

Severe aortic regurgitation may cause partial diastolic closure of the mitral valve, decreasing the intensity of the first heart sound. An early systolic ejection click can signify either a bicuspid aortic valve or a large stroke volume entering a dilated aortic root. The second heart sound may be normal or abnormal (if the aortic valve does not close properly). A third heart sound may be present even without significant ventricular dysfunction, because of the rapid early diastolic filling of the ventricle by the sum of the transmitral and aortic regurgitant blood flow.

The characteristic auscultatory finding is a high-pitched diastolic decrescendo murmur best heard along the left sternal border. If it is most audible at the right sternal border, significant aortic root dilatation is suggested. The murmur is heard best with the diaphragm of the stethoscope, with the patient leaning forward with breath held in full expiration. The duration of the murmur, rather than its loudness, correlates best with the severity of regurgitation. When the murmur is musical or cooing, a cusp fenestration or perforation is suspected. A coexistent aortic systolic murmur does not necessarily imply the presence of aortic stenosis and may be a functional flow murmur due to the ejection of an abnormally high volume of blood during systole. The carotid upstroke helps define coexistent aortic stenosis. In significant aortic regurgitation, an additional diastolic apical rumbling (Austin Flint) murmur may be detected. Amyl nitrite inhalation softens an Austin Flint murmur but makes the rumbling murmur of mitral stenosis louder. Late in the course of disease, ventricular dilatation causes mitral anular dilatation and resultant mitral regurgitation.

- There may be few typical physical findings in acute aortic regurgitation.
- In patients with aortic regurgitation, "wide pulse pressure" implies low diastolic pressure in addition to the large difference between systolic and diastolic pressures.
- Physical findings in severe aortic regurgitation include a long diastolic murmur, apical diastolic rumble, enlarged and displaced apex, and peripheral findings of high output and rapid runoff.

Evaluation of Aortic Regurgitation

Acute, subacute, and mild chronic aortic regurgitation are not necessarily associated with ECG abnormalities. Chronic moderate or severe aortic regurgitation usually causes features of left ventricular hypertrophy, but a significant minority of such patients may not have ventricular hypertrophy by voltage criteria.

Chronic significant aortic regurgitation, with its associated enlargement of the left ventricle, increases the radiographic cardiothoracic ratio. The ascending aorta may be dilated, but it can appear normal because the most proximal portion of the ascending aorta is hidden within the cardiac silhouette

Echocardiography visualizes the ascending aorta and the aortic valve and measures left ventricular size and function. Findings may include aortic leaflet prolapse, diastolic vibration of the anterior mitral leaflet, or premature closure of the mitral valve. Assessment of the severity of aortic regurgitation involves an integrated assessment of left ventricular size in conjunction with a comprehensive Doppler investigation. Transesophageal echocardiography images the thoracic aorta more completely and may better assess aortic valvular vegetations or infectious complications involving the aortic leaflets or anulus. Often, however, it adds little information about the severity of regurgitation.

There are other noninvasive methods which can examine ventricular dimensions and myocardial function. Radionuclide angiography is the one which has been studied the most and provides accurate measurements of left ventricular volume and ejection fraction. Computed tomography and MRI scanning may also provide accurate measurements of volumes and ventricular function. The advantage of MRI scanning and cine computed tomography scanning is one can also get additional information about the thoracic aorta. Especially in patients with bicuspid aortic valve, it is necessary to examine the thoracic aorta for aortic aneurysm, dissection, and coarctation.

Noninvasive assessment of the cause and severity of aortic regurgitation is usually sufficient. Aortic root angiography is still appropriate, however, in patients in whom noninvasive testing was technically inadequate or gave results discordant with clinical findings. Exercise testing also may be valuable for determining functional capacity.

- Echocardiography assesses the cause and severity of aortic regurgitation in addition to left ventricular size and function.
- Transesophageal echocardiography is a useful adjunct for anatomical assessment but does not add to the quantitative assessment of aortic regurgitation.
- Echocardiographic assessment of the severity of regurgitation should not rely exclusively on color flow data.
- Aortography is indicated when noninvasive data are discordant, technically limited, or differ from the clinical impression of regurgitant severity.

Natural History and Treatment of Acute Aortic Regurgitation

In patients with severe acute aortic regurgitation, dyspnea and heart failure develop rapidly, due to the large volume of blood flowing backwards into an "unprepared" ventricle. This results in a rapid rise of left ventricular diastolic pressure and a rapid fall of aortic diastolic pressure. In these patients, the diastolic murmur may be short or even inaudible. There will be a shortened half-time on the aortic regurgitation Doppler velocity signal. One of the older indicators of severe aortic regurgitation is premature closure of the mitral valve on M-mode echocardiography. On the Doppler mitral inflow, the deceleration time will be very short.

In patients with severe acute aortic regurgitation due to an aortic dissection, emergency surgery is indicated. This is both to replace the aortic valve and to replace the ascending aorta from the dissection. This is a surgical emergency and must be performed as soon as possible.

In patients with acute severe aortic regurgitation due to infective endocarditis, early surgery is indicated. These patients will rapidly deteriorate from heart failure and cardiogenic shock. Even if there has not been a prolonged course of antibiotics, early surgery should be performed after bolus infusion of antibiotics. If possible, aortic valve homografts should be considered, since they seem to be most resistant to superimposed intraoperative and perioperative infection. In the patient with hemodynamically significant mild to moderate aortic regurgitation and active infective endocarditis, continued antibiotic therapy is indicated with close observation. However, surgical standby should be maintained, as acute severe aortic regurgitation may rapidly develop and require urgent surgery.

Natural History of Chronic Aortic Regurgitation

Patients with severe chronic aortic regurgitation may go on for years without symptoms. However, as with mitral regurgitation, the long-standing volume overload does cause progressive fibrosis and myocyte degeneration with subsequent left ventricular dysfunction (Fig. 4). Since exercise results in a shortening of the diastolic filling, and thus a decrease in the regurgitant volume, patients may not develop symptoms with exertion for decades.

In patients with aortic regurgitation, there is an increase in ventricular volume as well as an increase in ventricular mass. This is all in an attempt to normalize left ventricular wall stress imposed upon the ventricle by the large regurgitant volume. There will be both an increase in afterload as well as an increase in preload on

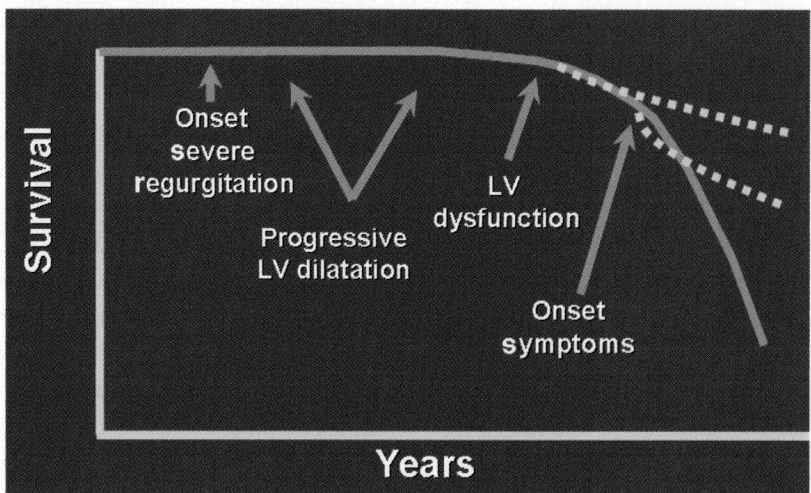

Fig. 4. Figure demonstrating a natural history of regurgitant lesions. Survival is on the "Y" axis and years are on the "X" axis. After the onset of severe regurgitation, patients remain asymptomatic for years during which progressive left ventricular dilatation occurs. Incipient left ventricular dysfunction may occur before the onset of symptoms. If operation is performed at the onset of symptoms (dotted line), the survival will be better than no operation. However, since incipient left ventricular dysfunction may have already occurred, there is a decreased survival as opposed to what would have occurred with earlier operation. Similarly, even if operation is performed at the onset of left ventricular dysfunction (dotted line), survival is still poorer than what may have occurred if operation had been performed earlier.

the left ventricle. Therefore, both the preload and the afterload on the left ventricle is increased in patients with aortic regurgitation. The ejection fraction, therefore, is an accurate assessment of ventricular function, as opposed to patients with mitral regurgitation.

Since the ventricle is able to compensate for aortic regurgitation with both an increase in ventricular volume and an increase in wall thickness, patients may go on for decades with severe asymptomatic aortic regurgitation and maintain normal ventricular function. In most patients, ventricular function begins to deteriorate before the onset of symptoms. Therefore, it is very important to continue to follow patients every 6 to 12 months with serial measurements of ventricular volume and ejection fraction. Overall, the outlook of patients with severe aortic regurgitation is much better than that of patients with severe mitral regurgitation, due to the very long period of time before ventricular dysfunction occurs.

Treatment of Severe Chronic Aortic Regurgitation

All patients with aortic regurgitation should be instructed in dental hygiene and infective endocarditis prophylaxis. Although initial studies had suggested that vasodilators such as calcium channel blockers or ACE inhibitors may be effective in halting the progression of

left ventricular dilatation, subsequent studies have shown that these medications are not effective in the patient with normal blood pressure. Therefore, afterload reduction is indicated only in patients who have severe aortic regurgitation and concomitant hypertension.

The timing of operation for aortic regurgitation is better understood than the timing for mitral regurgitation. Early operation with a prosthetic aortic valve has its own long- and short-term complications and, therefore, should not be performed prematurely. Since the ejection fraction is an accurate measurement of ventricular function, it is safe to continue to observe patients with periodic measurements of ventricular volume and function.

Overall, operation is indicated for patients with chronic severe aortic regurgitation with the onset of any symptoms. As with mitral regurgitation, although left ventricular dysfunction may have already occurred, survival and outcomes are better with operation than with medical management.

In asymptomatic patients with severe aortic regurgitation, measurements of left ventricular size and function determine the need for operation. An ejection fraction of less than 50-55 percent or an end-systolic dimension of greater than 55 mm, indicates the presence of left ventricular systolic dysfunction. Patients who exceed these parameters should be considered for operation with aortic valve replacement.

In those patients who have end-systolic dimension between 50 and 55 mm, it is also reasonable to consider earlier operation, especially if there has been a rapid progression of ventricular size. In patients with an end-systolic dimension of less than 50 mm in whom ventricular function with ejection fraction is maintained, serial follow-up should be performed. The follow-up should be performed initially at three months to make sure there is not rapid progression. Following that, the evaluation should be performed every six months if there is moderate to severe dilatation, (end-systolic dimension of 45-50 mm) or every year if there is mild to moderate dilatation (end-systolic dimension of less than 45 mm). Exercise testing is indicated in the initial screening, to determine whether or not the patient truly is asymptomatic, as this provides an objective measurement of exercise tolerance. The ventricular response to exercise is not a clear-cut indication for operation.

In considering operation, it is necessary to also examine the size of the ascending aorta. In patients with a dilated aorta greater than 5.0 cm, concomitant aortic replacement as well as aortic valve replacement is indicated. There are some patients in whom there is rapid dilatation of the ascending aorta and even if the aortic regurgitation is not severe, operation is indicated for the ascending aorta of greater than 5.5 cm.

RESOURCES

ACC/AHA guidelines for the management of patients with valvular heart disease. A report of the American College of Cardiology/American Heart Association Task Force on Practice Guidelines (Committee on Management of Patients with Valvular Heart Disease). J Am Coll Cardiol 32:1486-1588, 1998. *This is a comprehensive, referenced summary of regurgitant valvular lesions and many issues related to valvular heart disease.*

42

RHEUMATIC HEART DISEASE

Andrew G. Moore, MD

INTRODUCTION

Rheumatic heart disease is the most serious manifestation of acute rheumatic fever and is the end result of carditis, which affects 30% to 45% of patients with acute rheumatic fever. Damage to the cardiac valves, which is the hallmark of rheumatic heart disease, may be chronic and progressive and, in conjunction with left ventricular dysfunction, can lead to congestive heart failure and death. Although both acute rheumatic fever and rheumatic heart disease are rare in more affluent populations in North America and Europe, where valvular disease is now largely degenerative, pockets of resurgence have occurred in these regions in recent years. Acute rheumatic fever continues essentially unchecked in many developing countries, where it is an important public health problem.

ACUTE RHEUMATIC FEVER

Epidemiology

Although there has been no documented decrease in the incidence of group A streptococcal pharyngitis in industrialized countries over the past 100 years, the incidence of acute rheumatic fever has decreased during this period in those countries. This decrease, which began in the late 1800s, was accelerated by the development of antibiotics in the 1950s. In Denmark, for example, the incidence was approximately 250 per 100,000 in the 1860s, but by 1980, it was between 0.23 per 100,000 and 1.88 per 100,000. This contrasts with much greater incidence rates reported in some developing countries and specific populations. In Sudan, for example, the incidence exceeds 100 per 100,000, and the highest reported rates occur in indigenous populations in certain Pacific islands, Australia, and New Zealand. Rates as high as 374 per 100,000 have been documented in Aboriginal school-age children in parts of Australia. Interestingly, the medical literature contains several reports of more recent pockets of resurgence of acute rheumatic fever in isolated, intermountain populations in the United States, such as in West Virginia and Tennessee. Overcrowding, close person-to-person contact, and poor health care facilities seem to be consistent predisposing conditions for the high incidence of acute rheumatic fever in all these populations. An association with ethnic origin has not been identified.

Acute rheumatic fever is a disease of the young, occurring most commonly in preadolescent children. It is much rarer in children younger than 5 years and adults older than 35 years. Quite frequently, recurrent episodes occur through adolescence and into early adulthood, and it is thought that the cumulative effect of recurrent episodes of acute rheumatic fever leads to the development of rheumatic heart disease. Both acute rheumatic fever and rheumatic heart disease are more common in females in many populations for various reasons, including increased exposure to group A streptococcus through child rearing as well as less access to preventive medical care for females in some cultures.

Pathogenesis

The pathogenesis of acute rheumatic fever is incompletely understood. Although streptococci have not been found in the heart tissues of patients with acute rheumatic fever, there is strong circumstantial evidence that acute rheumatic fever is the result of an exaggerated immune response to pharyngeal infection with group A streptococcus. Outbreaks of acute rheumatic fever closely follow epidemics of streptococcal pharyngitis or scarlet fever, and adequate treatment of documented pharyngeal streptococcal infection clearly decreases the incidence of subsequent rheumatic fever. In addition, appropriate prophylaxis with antibiotics can prevent recurrence in patients with prior episodes of acute rheumatic fever. Tellingly, most patients with acute rheumatic fever also have elevated titers to one or more of the three antistreptococcal antibodies (streptolysin O, hyaluronidase, and streptokinase). It is noteworthy that group A streptococcal infection of the pharynx is a necessary element for the subsequent development of acute rheumatic fever. Documented outbreaks of impetigo can cause glomerulonephritis, but they have not been shown to cause acute rheumatic fever.

Clinical Features

Onset of acute rheumatic fever is typically characterized by an acute febrile illness 2 to 4 weeks after an episode of pharyngitis. Diagnosis is primarily clinical and is based on a constellation of signs and symptoms, which were initially established as the Jones criteria in 1944 (Table 1). Although the clinical usefulness of the Jones criteria has been recently reaffirmed, the main features have been modified or updated several times in order to increase the specificity of the criteria. The World Health Association (WHO) has more recently developed criteria that favor sensitivity over specificity (Table 2); they may be the preferred guidelines in countries with populations at high risk for acute rheumatic fever.

Table 1. Jones Criteria (1992 Revision) for Diagnosis of Acute Rheumatic Fever*

Major manifestations
1. Carditis
2. Polyarthritis
3. Chorea
4. Erythema marginatum
5. Subcutaneous nodules

Minor manifestations
1. Fever
2. Arthralgias
3. Previous rheumatic fever or rheumatic heart disease
4. Increased C-reactive protein concentrations or erythrocyte sedimentation rate
5. Prolonged PR interval on electrocardiogram

Evidence of antecedent group A streptococcal infection
1. Positive throat culture or rapid antigen test positive for group A streptococcus
2. Increased or increasing streptococcal antibody titer

*A firm diagnosis requires 1) 2 major manifestations *or* 1 major and 2 minor manifestations *and* 2) evidence of a recent streptococcal infection. However, when chorea or carditis is clearly present, evidence of an antecedent group A streptococcal infection is not necessary.

Table 2. World Health Association for Diagnosis of Acute Rheumatic Fever

1. First episode—same as the Jones criteria (see Table 1)
2. Recurrent episode in a patient *without* established RHD—same as for first episode
3. Recurrent episode in a patient *with* established RHD—requires 2 minor Jones criteria manifestations (see Table 1) *and* evidence of an antecedent group A streptococcus infection

RHD, rheumatic heart disease.

Beyond fever, arthritis is typically the earliest manifestation of acute rheumatic fever. In untreated patients, the arthritis is classically described as "migrating" from joint to joint in quick succession. The knees and ankles are often the first affected. The duration of joint inflammation is short (≤ 1 week), and the synovial fluid is generally sterile when examined.

Chorea, also known as Sydenham chorea or St. Vitus dance, is a neurologic movement disorder characterized by abrupt, purposeless involuntary movements of the muscles of the face, neck, trunk, and limbs. Muscular weakness (hypotonia) and behavioral disturbances such as obsessive-compulsive behaviors are considered to be additional findings of chorea. The course of the syndrome is variable. Symptoms tend to develop subtly, progressively worsen over 1 to 2 months, and spontaneously resolve gradually after 3 to 6 months. Residual waxing and waning of symptoms may occur for a year or more, and 20% of patients have recurrences within 2 years.

Two classic skin lesions with well-described identifying characteristics occur in acute rheumatic fever. Subcutaneous nodules ranging from several millimeters to 2 cm occur for approximately 2 weeks over bony surfaces or near tendons. The nodules are described as firm and painless, and the overlying skin is not inflamed. They are typically smaller and shorter lived than nodules of rheumatoid arthritis. Erythema marginatum is a classic skin rash that occurs early in the course of acute rheumatic fever. The rash is evanescent, pink to red, and nonpruritic. It typically occurs on the trunk or the proximal limbs. The rash appears as a ring that extends centrifugally, while the skin in the center of the ring returns to normal. The rash can persist or recur after other symptoms of acute rheumatic fever have passed. Interestingly, erythema marginatum and the subcutaneous nodules usually occur only in patients with carditis.

CARDITIS AND RHEUMATIC HEART DISEASE

According to the WHO, at least 15.6 million people have rheumatic heart disease. Of the 500,000 people who develop acute rheumatic fever every year, nearly half develop carditis, the most serious manifestation of the disease. Carditis, which leads to valvular lesions and eventually chronic rheumatic heart disease, is directly responsible for 233,000 deaths annually.

The term *carditis* refers to diffuse inflammation of the pericardium, epicardium, myocardium, and endocardium. Valvular involvement, with leaflet thickening, occurs as a rule. In addition to thickening, the valve leaflets frequently display small rows of vegetations called verrucae along their apposing surfaces. Symptoms include tachycardia and mild or moderate chest discomfort that is commonly pleuritic in nature. The cardiac physical examination is often noteworthy for the presence of a pericardial friction rub and, typically, new or changing murmurs. In young patients, mitral valve regurgitation is the predominant cardiac lesion; a new apical systolic murmur is characteristic. Aortic regurgitation is less common but can develop and present with a new basal diastolic murmur. The pulmonary and tricuspid valves are rarely involved. Mitral stenosis becomes progressively more common in early to mid adulthood. Heart block of all degrees is seen on the electrocardiogram, and the most common radiologic finding is cardiomegaly. Myocarditis is characterized by infiltration of mononuclear cells, vasculitis, and degenerative changes of the interstitial connective tissue. The pathognomonic lesion is the Aschoff body in the proliferative stage, which is present in 30% to 40% of biopsy samples from patients with acute rheumatic fever.

The use of echocardiography has contributed much toward understanding the pathogenesis of valvular regurgitation in rheumatic carditis. At least initially, the regurgitation appears to result from geometric changes and stresses affecting the left ventricle rather than from the rheumatic process directly involving the valve leaflets. Prolapse of the anterior leaflet of the mitral valve is the most common feature and is invariably associated with a posteriorly directed jet of mitral regurgitation as seen on color Doppler imaging. An increase in the mitral anular diameter, especially around the posterior anulus, appears to be the primary cause for leaflet prolapse. The typical mean anular diameter in a patient with carditis and mitral regurgitation is 37 mm, compared with 23 mm in a healthy individual. Elongated chordae to the anterior mitral valve leaflet is another feature present in severe mitral regurgitation associated with rheumatic carditis. The elongation is thought to be due to both involvement by the primary rheumatic process and secondary exposure to increased tensile stresses occurring during ventricular systole. The two-dimensional echocardiographic appearance of the rheumatic mitral valve early in the course of the disease shows some important differences compared with mitral valve prolapse associated with degenerative or myxomatous mitral valve disease. Myxomatous prolapse tends to affect the posterior leaflet, and myxomatous leaflets are thickened, voluminous, and redundant, with significant billowing toward the left atrium. The leaflets in rheumatic carditis have minimal thickening, redundancy, and billowing.

Acute rheumatic fever is also the predominant cause of mitral stenosis. Some degree of rheumatic involvement is present in nearly all stenotic mitral valves excised at valve replacement. Approximately 25% of patients with rheumatic heart disease have pure mitral stenosis. Mitral stenosis is characterized by progressive thickening, fibrosis and calcification of the leaflets and chordae tendineae (Fig. 1): 30% of patients have thickening of the commissures alone, 15% have thickening of the cusps, and 10% have isolated thickening of the chordae tendineae. The leaflets show fibrous obliteration, and the mitral valve orifice becomes funnel-shaped, like a fish mouth (Fig. 2). This feature and the classic hockey-stick appearance of the anterior mitral valve leaflet in diastole are well seen on two-dimensional echocardiography. (Fig. 3 and 4). A more detailed discussion of the evaluation of valvular heart disease with echocardiography is in Chapters 8 ("Principles of Echocardiography"), 40 ("Valvular Stenosis"), and 41 ("Valvular Regurgitation"). It is not

certain whether the progressive fibrosis of rheumatic mitral stenosis is the end result of a smoldering rheumatic process or the result of constant trauma from turbulent blood flow after initial deformation of the valve.

LEFT VENTRICULAR DYSFUNCTION

The development of left ventricular dysfunction is common in long-standing, untreated rheumatic heart disease. The course of left ventricular dysfunction can be slow and insidious or, sometimes, very rapid and

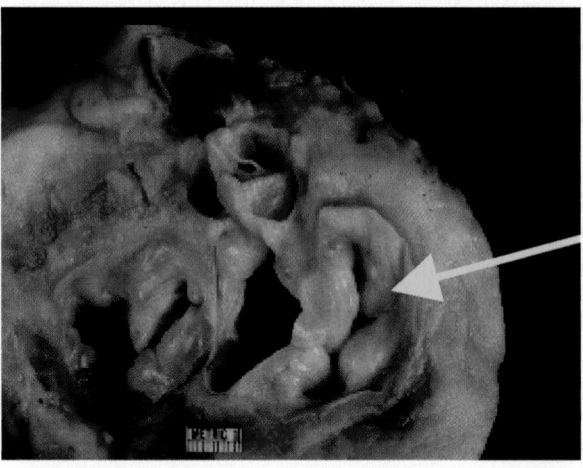

Fig. 2. Fish-mouth appearance of a mitral valve affected by chronic rheumatic heart disease (*arrow*).

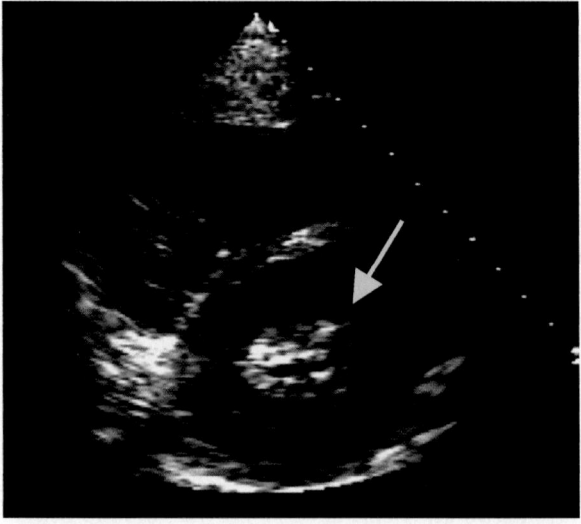

Fig. 3. Two-dimensional echocardiographic parasternal short-axis view of the stenotic mitral valve in rheumatic heart disease, showing the fish-mouth appearance (*arrow*).

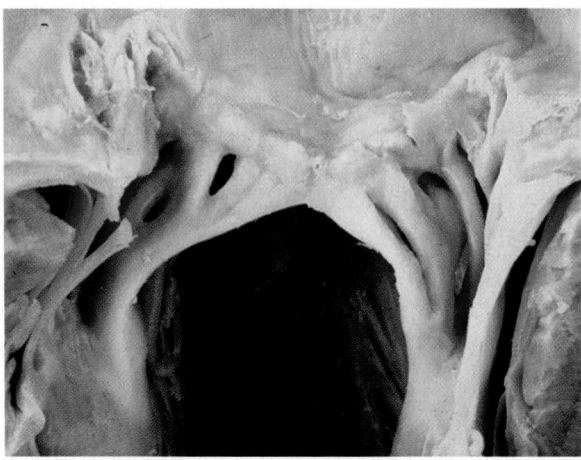

Fig. 1. Thickened mitral valve leaflets and subvalvular apparatus in rheumatic mitral stenosis.

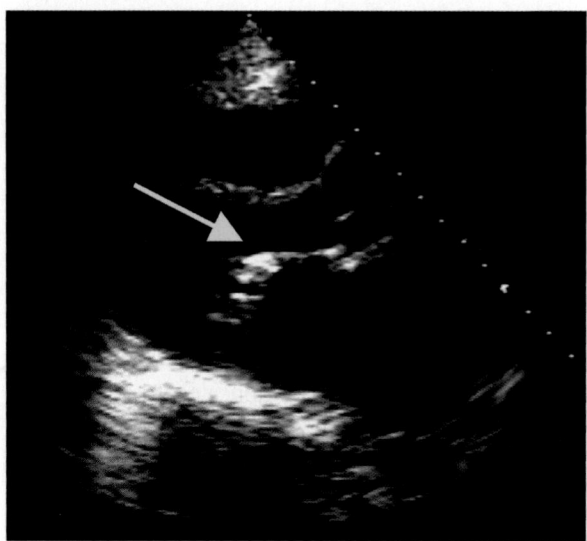

Fig. 4. Two-dimensional echocardiographic parasternal long-axis view of the mitral valve during diastole, showing the classic hockey-stick appearance of the anterior mitral valve leaflet (*arrow*).

fulminate, mimicking viral myocarditis. The associated development of congestive heart failure is the most life-threatening clinical syndrome of acute rheumatic fever, often requiring aggressive management. Rheumatic myocarditis in the absence of rheumatic valvular disease is rare. Although histologic evidence of myocarditis is frequently present at autopsy, left ventricular dilatation and heart failure rarely occur in the absence of hemodynamically significant mitral regurgitation. Recent studies of the development of left ventricular systolic dysfunction have attempted to clarify the relative contributions of 1) volume overload from valvular regurgitation and 2) the direct effect on the cardiac myocytes from the rheumatic process. Prompt reduction in the left ventricular dimensions and preservation of fractional shortening after isolated mitral or combined mitral and aortic valve replacement seem to provide reasonable evidence that, to a large degree, rheumatic carditis is not accompanied by myocardial contractile dysfunction.

TREATMENT OF ACUTE RHEUMATIC FEVER

Treatment of acute rheumatic fever consists of relieving symptoms, eradicating group A streptococcus, and providing prophylaxis against further infections to prevent long-term cardiac disease.

Relief of Symptoms

Salicylates lead to rapid resolution of fever and arthritis, thus relieving symptoms, and so are very useful as initial treatment of acute rheumatic fever. Salicylates should not be used for treatment of carditis, however. Results of comparisons of salicylates versus no treatment or bed rest alone suggest that they do not decrease the incidence of residual rheumatic heart disease.

Congestive heart failure associated with severe carditis should be treated with conventional therapy for heart failure. Many physicians also treat carditis with corticosteroids, believing that their use can result in a more rapid resolution of myocardial dysfunction. Results of randomized trials performed before the development of echocardiography have not shown a benefit of corticosteroids compared with placebo or salicylates, but with newer imaging modalities and steroid preparations, the outcome of these trials might have been different. The typical dosage of oral prednisone is 2 mg/kg per day for 1 to 2 weeks, with a tapered dosage thereafter.

Antibiotic Therapy

Penicillin is considered mandatory treatment to eradicate group A streptococcus infection from the upper respiratory tract. Antibiotics should be continued for at least 10 days, even if pharyngitis is not present at the time of diagnosis. Penicillin V is recommended in a dosage of 250 mg two to three times daily for children and 500 mg two to three times daily for adults. If compliance is a concern, a depot penicillin such as benzathine penicillin G, can be given as one intramuscular (IM) dose. Children should receive 600,000 units IM if they weigh less than 27 kg. The common dosage for children who weigh more than 27 kg and for adults is 1.2 million units IM.

Antibiotic Prophylaxis

Secondary prophylaxis for acute rheumatic fever is defined as the long-term administration of antibiotics to people with a history of acute rheumatic fever or rheumatic heart disease to prevent recurrences and the development or deterioration of rheumatic heart disease. Compared with primary prophylaxis, such as sore throat screening programs in school-age children, secondary prophylaxis has been a cost-effective, practical intervention against acute rheumatic fever. Recurrence is most common within 2 years of the original infection but can occur at any time. Prophylaxis should be initiated at the time of resolution of the acute episode. The best drug for prophylaxis has been shown to be intramuscular benzathine penicillin G administered IM every 3 to 4 weeks. This regimen has been more efficacious than oral treatments in direct comparisons. The recommended dose for adults is 1.2 million units IM. For children who weigh less than 27 kg, the WHO recommends 600,000 units IM.

Oral regimens include 1) penicillin V 250 mg twice daily or 2) sulfadiazine 500 mg daily for children who weigh less than 27 kg and 1,000 mg per day for children who weigh more than 27 kg and for adults. Patients allergic to either penicillin or sulfadiazine can take oral erythromycin 250 mg twice daily.

The duration of prophylaxis depends on several variables, including the age of the patient, the time since the last attack, the number of attacks, the severity of existing heart disease, and the risk of exposure to streptococcal infections. General WHO guidelines recommend that if no carditis has developed, prophylaxis should be continued for 5 years after an acute attack or until the age of 18 years (whichever is longer). In cases of mild or healed carditis, treatment should continue for 10 years past the last attack or until age 25 years (whichever is longer). In cases of more severe carditis or valve surgery, treatment should be lifelong. For additional discussion of antibiotic treatment and prophylaxis, see Chapter 82 ("Infective Endocarditis").

MANAGEMENT OF RHEUMATIC VALVULAR DISEASE

The management of significant mitral regurgitation associated with rheumatic heart disease differs somewhat from degenerative mitral regurgitation, which is much more common in the developed world. For the past decade, there has been a strong push to intervene surgically with mitral valve repair earlier in the course of degenerative mitral regurgitation to preserve left ventricular dimensions and systolic function. The benefits of mitral valve repair are not nearly as clear in patients with mitral regurgitation from a rheumatic cause. In active carditis, progressive fibrosis and leaflet deformity may preclude a durable long-term result. The results of mitral valve repair have also been disappointing in patients with chronic rheumatic mitral regurgitation and no evidence of active infection. Reoperation is frequently required, and in one study, overall freedom from valve failure was only 66% after a mean follow-up of 5 years. The situation is complicated by other associated problems in developing countries, such as a lack of adequate health care facilities and cardiac surgeons skilled in the repair of the mitral valve. It is well documented that mitral valve replacement results in a consistent reduction in left ventricular systolic function. However, if replacement is timed to occur when the end-systolic diameter of the left ventricle is between 40 and 50 mm, the long-term durability and success of the procedure may be a reasonable compromise.

Of all the rheumatic valvular lesions, mitral stenosis is the one most likely to lead to a potentially serious outcome. In developing nations, it is not unusual for occult mitral stenosis to be first diagnosed at pregnancy. In the past, surgical commissurotomy has been used frequently to treat mitral stenosis. Valve replacement is more common now, and mitral balloon valvuloplasty is a reasonable option, especially as a palliative therapy during pregnancy.

CONCLUSION

Before the development of antibiotics, acute rheumatic fever was the single largest cause of valvular heart disease. Although incidence rates have declined dramatically in most developed countries, acute rheumatic fever and, as a consequence, rheumatic heart disease continue to flourish in developing countries. Given the significant potential for severe morbidity and mortality associated with this disease, it is important that all physicians be familiar with the diagnosis.

43

CARCINOID AND DRUG-RELATED HEART DISEASE

Heidi M. Connolly, MD

Patricia A. Pellikka, MD

CARCINOID DISEASE

Progress in the medical and surgical management of patients with carcinoid disease has resulted in improved symptoms and survival, although carcinoid heart disease remains a major cause of morbidity and mortality among patients with carcinoid syndrome. Limited medical treatment options are available for patients with carcinoid valvular disease; for those with severe valvular heart disease, valve replacement has been increasingly utilized.

Introduction and Diagnosis

Carcinoid tumors are rare, occurring in 1.2-2.1/100,000 people in the general population per year. The tumors arise from enterochromaffin cells, and are usually located in the gastrointestinal tract, but may also originate in the lungs or ovary. In 20-30% of patients, the initial presentation is that of carcinoid syndrome. Malignant carcinoid syndrome consists of flushing, gastrointestinal hypermotility (secretory diarrhea), bronchospasm and carcinoid heart disease, caused by the release of the vasoactive substances 5-hydroxytryptamine (serotonin), 5-hydroxytryptophan, histamine, bradykinins, tachykinins and prostaglandins. The urinary 5-hydroxy indole acetic acid (HIAA) (24-hour collection) is a specific and reproducible test, which also provides a reliable biological marker for the assessment of tumor activity and the response to treatment. Measurement of circulating plasma chromogranin A, a protein product produced by neuroendocrine cells, may also be used as a marker for diagnosis and follow-up in select cases.

Systemic and Regional Therapy for Metastatic Carcinoid Disease

The somatostatin analog, octreotide acetate (Sandostatin), is a synthetic octapeptide that binds to subtypes of somatostatin receptors and inhibits the secretion of bioactive substances responsible for the carcinoid syndrome. Treatment relieves symptoms in more than 70% of patients, and is now available as a long-acting once a month intramuscular injection, Sandostatin LAR Depot. This micro-encapsulated depot formulation gives longer steady state levels, and provides similar therapeutic benefit with less discomfort and inconvenience.

Patients presenting with bulky metastatic liver disease and no other metastatic disease are candidates for surgical debulking (partial hepatectomy). Alternatively, tumors that cannot be surgically debulked may be debulked by catheter-based hepatic artery embolization. The use of a Somatostatin analog is recommended in conjunction with debulking because of its static effect on the tumor.

Carcinoid Heart Disease

Carcinoid heart disease eventually occurs in over 50% of patients with carcinoid syndrome, and may be the initial presentation of carcinoid disease in as many as 20% of patients (Fig. 1). Deposition of a matrixlike material on the valves and endocardium of the right side of the heart result in retraction and fixation of the tricuspid leaflets, reduced leaflet motion, and lack of central coaptation. Clinically, these changes produce severe tricuspid valve regurgitation and less commonly, tricuspid valve stenosis. The pulmonary valve is likewise affected, with thickening and retraction of the leaflets resulting in a combination of valvular regurgitation and stenosis. Patients with advanced carcinoid heart disease may develop right-sided endocardial lesions.

The mechanism of valve injury in carcinoid heart disease is incompletely understood. Circulating serotonin levels are higher among patients with carcinoid heart disease compared to carcinoid patients without cardiac involvement, implying that serotonin directly contributes to the development and progression of valvular disease. Bulky hepatic metastases allow large quantities of vasoactive tumor products to reach the right heart without being inactivated.

Rarely, carcinoid tumor may originate in the ovary. Because the ovarian veins bypass the portal circulation and enter the systemic venous circulation directly, cardiac involvement can occur without liver metastases.

The preferential involvement of right-sided cardiac structures in carcinoid heart disease is likely related to inactivation of the humoral substances by the pulmonary circulation. Left-sided valvular pathology occurs in 10-15% of carcinoid patients with cardiac involvement and is typically found in patients with an intracardiac shunt or with primary bronchial carcinoid. Presumably serotonin-rich blood enters the left heart chambers without pulmonary deactivation. Left-sided valve disease may rarely be seen in patients with severe, poorly controlled carcinoid syndrome. Left-sided carcinoid valve disease typically consists of valve thickening and regurgitation.

Unfortunately, treatment of the carcinoid tumor does not appear to result in regression of valvular disease. However, the posttreatment levels of 5-HIAA seem to predict the development or progression of valvular abnormalities, with a threshold of about 100 mg/day. In a report of 71 patients from Mayo Clinic Rochester who had serial echocardiograms, treatment with a somatostatin analog, hepatic dearterialization, and/or chemotherapy was not associated with a reduced risk of progressive valvular disease. In fact, chemotherapy was statistically correlated with a higher rate of progressive valvular disease, perhaps because this form of therapy is usually reserved for patients with more aggressive carcinoid tumors.

Clinical Features of Carcinoid Heart Disease

Early in the course of the disease, symptoms are insideous and include fatigue and dyspnea on exertion. Severe tricuspid and pulmonary valve disease may be asymptomatic for months. Right-sided heart failure eventually develops with progressive cardiac disease. Without treatment, the median duration of survival with malignant carcinoid syndrome is 38 months from the onset of systemic symptoms. Clinical evidence of carcinoid heart disease with NYHA class III or IV symptoms is associated with a median survival of only 11 months.

The physical findings among patients with carcinoid heart disease likewise may be subtle early in the course of the disease. The murmurs of tricuspid and pulmonary valve disease are typically difficult to detect due to the low pressure in the pulmonary circulation. Elevation of the jugular venous pressure with a prominent "v" wave is often the earliest finding on physical examination. As the valve disease worsens, peripheral edema, ascites and pulsatile hepatomegaly occur. In addition to the murmurs of tricuspid and pulmonary valve regurgitation, cardiac findings include a palpable right ventricular impulse.

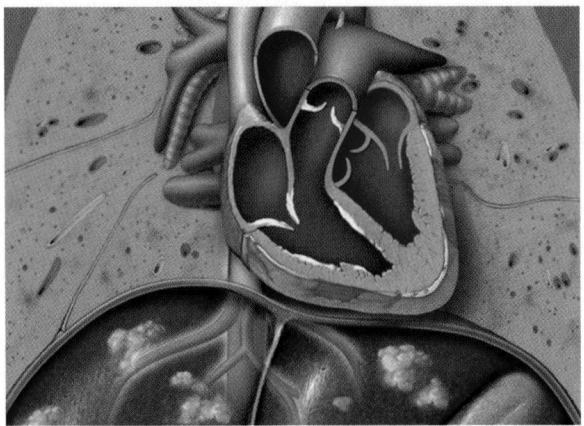

Fig. 1. Schematic demonstrating tricuspid and pulmonary valve disease as well as endocardial plaque deposition in carcinoid heart disease.

Less frequently murmurs of pulmonary stenosis and tricuspid stenosis may be noted.

For unknown reasons the electrocardiogram in advanced carcinoid heart disease demonstrates low voltage QRS. The chest x-ray demonstrates cardiomegaly with prominence of the right-sided cardiac chambers.

Echocardiographic Features of Carcinoid Heart Disease

Thickening and retraction of immobile tricuspid valve leaflets with associated severe tricuspid valve regurgitation are characteristic echocardiographic features (Fig. 2). Early in the course, the tricuspid valve leaflets may maintain some mobility; less commonly, tricuspid valve stenosis is noted. Pulmonary valve involvement usually coexists; the characteristic pulmonary valve features include immobility of the valve cusps that may be difficult to visualize due to cusp retraction (Fig. 3). Tricuspid and pulmonary valve regurgitation eventually results in progressive right ventricular volume overload and right ventricular diastolic pressure elevation. Other echocardiographic findings among patients with carcinoid heart disease include left-sided valvular pathology occurring in approximately 10% and myocardial metastases in less than 5%. Pericardial effusions are commonly noted but these are rarely hemodynamically significant.

Pathology of Carcinoid Valve Disease

The affected tricuspid and pulmonary valves in carcinoid heart disease have a white appearance with thickened leaflets and chordal structures (Fig. 4 and 5). The carcinoid plaque is composed of smooth muscle cells and myofibroblasts surrounded by an extracellular matrix and an overlying endothelial cell layer. The morphology of the valve leaflet is not disrupted and the carcinoid plaque generally affects the ventricular aspect of the tricuspid valve leaflets and the arterial aspect of the pulmonic valve cusps. Plaques may exhibit neovascularization and chronic inflammation.

Management of Carcinoid Heart Disease

Limited medical therapeutic options are available for patients with symptomatic right heart failure related to carcinoid heart disease. Cardiac surgery is the only effective treatment for carcinoid heart disease and should be considered for symptomatic patients whose metastatic carcinoid disease and carcinoid syndrome are well controlled. Patients with severe carcinoid heart disease should be considered for cardiac operation when they develop any of the following: 1) symptoms of right heart failure, 2) impaired exercise performance, 3) progressive right heart enlargement, or 4) right ventricular systolic dysfunction. Surgery is also rarely performed in minimally symptomatic patients with severe carcinoid heart disease in anticipation of hepatic surgery.

Patients with severe valvular disease are not candidates for partial hepatic resection or liver transplantation due to the risk of hepatic hemorrhage, induced by the elevated right-sided pressures, at the time of surgery.

Cardiac surgery has been successful in reducing or

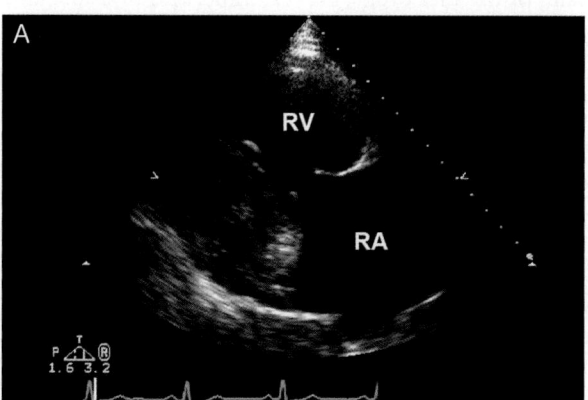
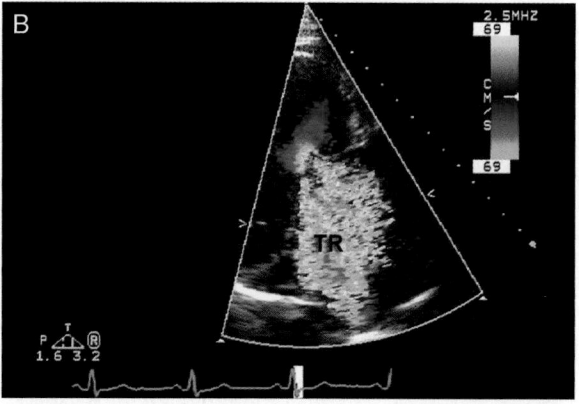

Fig. 2. Transthoracic echocardiographic right ventricular inflow view demonstrating advanced carcinoid tricuspid valve disease. *A*, The septal and anterior tricuspid leaflets are severely thickened and retracted, and fixed in a semiopen position, resulting in marked deficiency of central systolic coaptation. *B*, Color-flow Doppler imaging demonstrates severe central tricuspid valve regurgitation passing through the fixed open tricuspid orifice. RA, right atrium; RV, right ventricle; TR, tricuspid regurgitation.

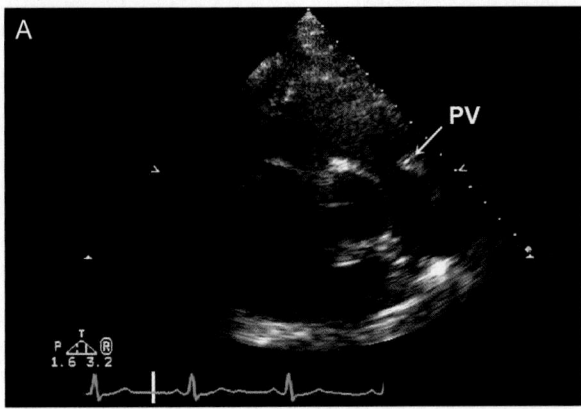
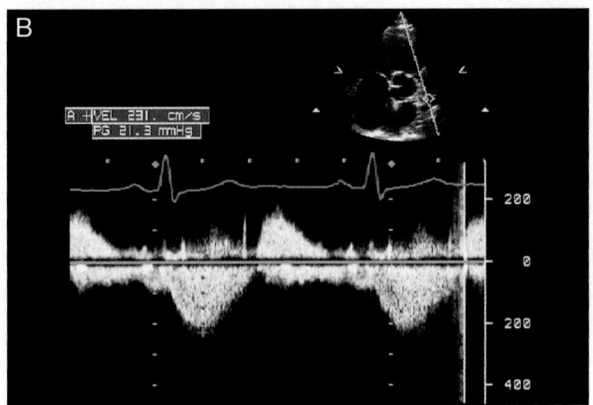

Fig. 3. *A*, Transthoracic echocardiogram demonstrating carcinoid involvement of the pulmonary valve. The pulmonary valve is difficult to visualize (*arrow*) which is characteristic of carcinoid pulmonary valve involvement. The pulmonary anulus is narrowed. *B*, Doppler examination demonstrates pulmonary stenosis and regurgitation. PV, pulmonary valve.

relieving the cardiac symptoms of many patients with carcinoid heart disease. Data from our institution suggest that early and regular cardiac evaluation of patients with metastatic carcinoid syndrome and cardiac surgical intervention prior to the development of advanced right heart failure may result in a reduction in surgical mortality, currently less than 10%, and an improvement in prognosis.

Choice of Valve Prosthesis
In the past, tricuspid valve replacement with a mechanical prosthesis was recommended for patients with carcinoid heart disease based on the assumption that the bioprosthetic valve could be damaged by vasoactive tumor substances. Treatment with synthetic somatostatin and hepatic artery interruption by embolization or ligation may potentially protect prosthetic valve tissue from the adverse effects of serotonin and other vasoactive peptides. Premature bioprosthesis degeneration may occur among carcinoid patients.

Mechanical tricuspid prostheses demonstrate a more favorable hemodynamic profile than most bioprostheses; however, mechanical prostheses are not ideal for patients with carcinoid heart disease as subsequent surgical procedures for tumor control are often required and are complicated by anticoagulation management. In addition, the risk of mechanical tricuspid prosthesis thrombosis is around 4% per year.

Anesthesia Management
Anesthesia can precipitate carcinoid crisis, characterized

by profound flushing, extreme changes in blood pressure, bronchoconstriction, and arrhythmias, and can be fatal. Thus, control of carcinoid symptoms by an octreotide analog should be attained prior to anesthesia; large doses of somatostatin are often required in the perioperative and postoperative periods.

DRUG-RELATED HEART DISEASE

Anorexigens and Valvular Heart Disease
Due in part to the increasing prevalence of obesity in the United States as well as the altered perception of desired body habitus and an effective advertising campaign, the sales of the diet drugs, phentermine, fenfluramine and

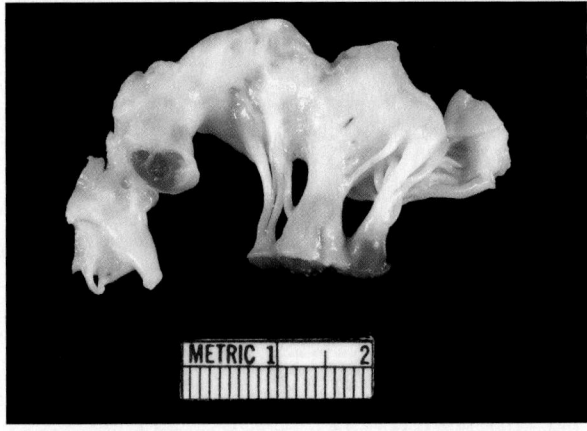

Fig. 4. Gross pathologic specimen of the tricuspid valve in a patient with carcinoid heart disease. The tricuspid valve leaflets are thickened, retracted and shortened.

dexfenfluramine increased exponentially in the United States between 1994 and 1996. Fenfluramine and dexfenfluramine act by increasing the release and decreasing the reuptake of the neurotransmitter serotonin.

In August 1997 a report was published describing 24 women with valvular heart disease that was atypical for degenerative or rheumatic etiologies; 5 required valve surgery. All of these women were treated with fenfluramine and phentermine for an average of 11 months. The Food and Drug Administration (FDA) requested reporting of similar cases, and by September 1997, over 100 spontaneous reports meeting a "case" definition had been reported to the FDA. A "case" of diet-drug related valve disease was described as an individual with no prior known valve disease who had used appetite suppressants and subsequently was found to have mild or more aortic valve regurgitation and/or moderate or more mitral valve regurgitation noted by echocardiography. This degree of valvular heart disease is expected in less than 1% of young healthy individuals.

The prevalence of valvular disease meeting the case definition was similar across all five groups, ranging from 30 to 38%. An important additional finding was that the prevalence of valve disease was time-dependent; 35% of patients treated for longer than 6 months had valve disease whereas only 22% of those treated for less than 3 months exhibited valve damage by echocardiography. In addition, 30% of patients taking dexfenfluramine (with or without phentermine) were found to have valvular regurgitation. Among these patients with valvuloplasty, 83% had mild or more aortic valve

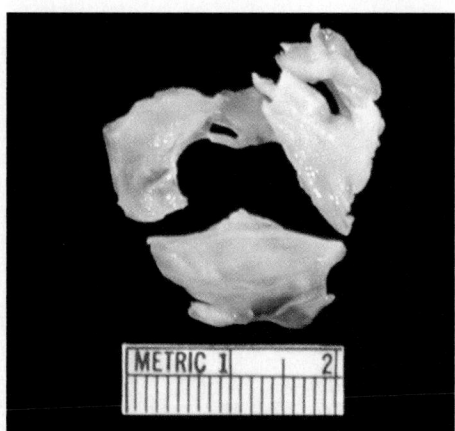

Fig. 5. Gross pathologic specimen of the pulmonary valve in a patient with carcinoid heart disease. The pulmonic valve cusps are thickened, retracted and shortened.

regurgitation and 21% had moderate or more mitral valve regurgitation either alone or in combination with other valve disease.

The 32% overall prevalence of valvular lesions meeting the FDA case definition in exposed persons was markedly higher than what would be expected in the general population (2 to 5%). A fifteenfold increased risk of valvuloplasty was noted in diet-drug-treated individuals compared to a normal population. Based on the FDA prevalence data, fenfluramine and dexfenfluramine were withdrawn from the United States market in 1997. Subsequent reports supported the association between the use of fenfluramine or dexfenfluramine and valvular regurgitation but differed with regard to the strength and clinical significance of this association. The duration and dose of appetite suppressant use appeared to be related to the incidence of valve disease; clinically important disease was not likely to develop after short-term exposure.

The American College of Cardiology and American Heart Association included a section on management of patients exposed to anorexigens in their 1998 Guidelines for the Management of Patients with Valvular Heart Disease. These recommendations include: 1) all exposed individuals should have a history and physical examination, 2) an echocardiogram is suggested for symptoms or signs of cardiovascular disease or an unreliable physical examination, 3) follow-up is dependent on the type of valve disease, and 4) endocarditis prophylaxis and clinical follow-up is recommended for patients with valvular heart disease. The optimal timing of cardiac surgery for patients with diet-drug-related valvular disease remains uncertain

The echocardiographic appearance of valve disease related to anorexigen use is characterized by thickening of one or more valves with associated valvular regurgitation. The features are similar to rheumatic valve disease, but the predominant valve lesion is *regurgitation* rather than *stenosis*.

There is unequivocal evidence that the diet drugs fenfluramine and dexfenfluramine cause valvular heart disease and pulmonary hypertension, although the mechanism remains uncertain. Due to the pathologic similarity of the valve disease in patients treated with diet drugs and those treated with ergot alkaloid derivatives or those with carcinoid heart disease, it is postulated that serotonin plays a role in valvular injury.

Fenfluramine and dexfenfluramine may cause direct valve injury or may alter serotonin metabolism in the circulation or in the platelets. The explanted valve pathology demonstrated intact leaflet and cusp architecture with a layer which appeared "stuck-on" to the valve (Fig. 6 *A* and 6 *B*). The adherent layer consisted of abundant myofibroblasts in an extracellular matrix. Although regression of valve disease after cessation of diet-drug therapy has been reported, the natural history remains uncertain.

Ergot Alkaloids and Valvular Heart Disease

Methysergide and ergotamine are used in various preparations for the prophylaxis and treatment of migraine headaches. The chemical structures of ergotamine, methysergide, and serotonin are similar. Ergotamine is a naturally occurring ergot alkaloid. Methysergide is a semisynthetic derivative of the ergot alkaloids. Ergotamine is a partial serotonin receptor antagonist in various smooth muscles and a partial agonist in certain blood vessels. Chronic ingestion of methysergide or ergotamine can produce endocardial thickening which can involve the valve structures and cause regurgitant or stenotic lesions.

Ergot alkaloid-associated heart disease refers to valvular lesions caused by endomyocardial fibrosis which extends onto the valve structures and distorts the anatomy of the valves, producing either stenosis, regurgitation or combined lesions. All described patients with ergot alkaloid valve disease used preparations of ergotamine suppositories or methysergide for over 6 years and usually up to 20 years. Chronicity of exposure seems to be the most important factor in producing valve disease. Methysergide and ergotamine use have been associated with lesions of all four valves; however, mitral and aortic valve regurgitation are the most common valve lesions.

Echocardiography in ergot-related valve disease typically shows thickening of one or more valves with associated regurgitation and stenosis; the features are similar echocardiographically to rheumatic valve disease.

The structural similarity of ergotamine, methysergide and serotonin, and the similarity of the valvular lesions in ergot alkaloid valve disease and carcinoid syndrome suggests a common pathophysiologic mechanism. However, ergot-alkaloid valve disease commonly produces left-sided valvular lesions, whereas carcinoid-associated valve disease is usually restricted to the right side. Presumably the altered chemical structure of methysergide and ergotamine allows these structures to be resistant to metabolism in the lungs. The macroscopic and histopathologic features of ergot alkaloid-related valve disease are identical to carcinoid and diet-drug-related valve disease.

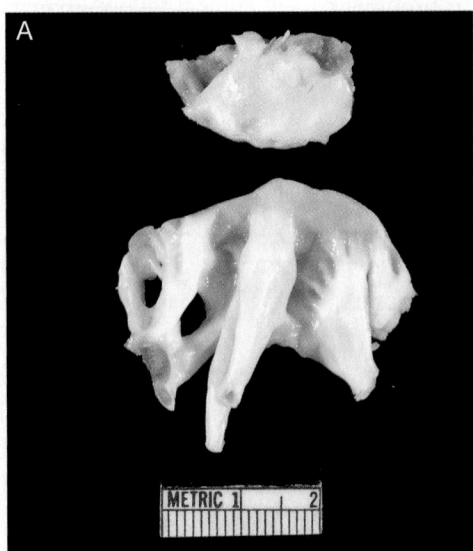

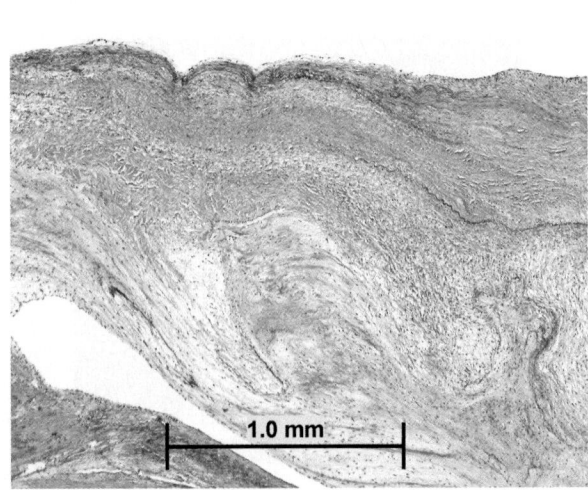

Fig. 6. *A*, Gross pathologic specimen of regurgitant mitral valve from patient taking fenfluramine/dexfenfluramine. *B*, Microscopic view of same valve.

Regression of valve disease has never been documented; however, diminution of murmurs has been reported. Surgical intervention is required in patients with advanced, symptomatic valve disease.

Pergolide-Related Valve Disease

Pergolide is an ergot-derived dopamine receptor agonist used to treat Parkinson's disease and restless legs syndrome. Chronic use has been associated with retroperitoneal, pleural, and pericardial fibrosis. Recently, drug-induced restrictive valvular heart disease has also been described.

Echocardiography and histology of surgically explanted valves revealed abnormalities suggestive of carcinoid involvement, ergot alkaloid or anorexigen treatment. The echocardiographic appearance of pergolide-related valve disease is notable for thickening of one or more valves with associated regurgitation. The initial estimate of the frequency of valvular heart disease in patients taking pergolide was very low (one in 20,000), although researchers later suggested a higher incidence. Any patient in whom pergolide therapy is being considered should be informed of the possible risk of restrictive valvular heart disease and pulmonary hypertension.

RESOURCES

Connolly H, Schaff H, Mullany C, et al. Carcinoid heart disease: tricuspid prosthetic choice and durability (abstract). Circulation Suppl 2002;106:II673.

Moller J, Pellikka P, Bernheim A, et al. Prognosis of carcinoid heart disease: analysis of 200 cases over two decades. Circulation. 2005;112:3320-7. *This article describes the improved expected survival of patients with carcinoid heart disease in the current era and outlines possible reasons for improved survival, including valve replacement surgery.*

44

PROSTHETIC HEART VALVES

Martha A. Grogan, MD

Fletcher A. Miller, Jr, MD

Prosthetic valves only approximate normal human valve hemodynamics and carry the risk of unique complications, such as structural failure, thrombosis, hemolysis, and infections.

VALVE TYPES

Valvular prostheses are classified as mechanical and bioprosthetic valves. Mechanical valves are subdivided into caged-ball, tilting-disk, and bileaflet. Bioprosthetic valves are subdivided into stented heterografts, homografts, and stentless heterografts (Fig. 1). The homograft and stentless heterograft valves are designed for implantation in the aortic or pulmonic positions. All the other valve types can be implanted in any valve position. Specific types of prosthetic valves are listed in Table 1.

Each different type of prosthesis is manufactured in several different sizes, ranging from 19 to 33 mm in diameter. Aortic prostheses are generally available in odd-numbered sizes from 19 through 31 and mitral and tricuspid prostheses, in odd-numbered sizes from 23 through 33. The size refers to the external diameter of the sewing ring in millimeters. The size of the prosthetic valve greatly influences its hemodynamics, particularly in the aortic position.

Starr-Edwards Valve

The currently available Starr-Edwards valves have a cage that is constructed from the alloy Stellite 21 and a Silastic poppet (ball) that is specially cured to prevent lipid accumulation (which can result in ball variance). The struts of the modern Starr-Edwards prosthesis are not covered with cloth.

Medtronic-Hall Valve

The Medtronic-Hall valve has a tilting disk made of pyrolytic carbon. The valve housing is machined from a single block of titanium and is composed of the valve ring with a sigmoid strut, which projects into the center of the ring and passes through a hole in the center of the disk. The tilting disk is supported by a smaller strut and two lugs, which also project from the ring. The disk tilts to an opening angle of 75° for aortic prostheses and 70° for mitral prostheses.

Björk-Shiley Valve

The Björk-Shiley valve also has a disk made of pyrolytic carbon. The standard disk is planar on one side and convex on the other. This disk is restrained by an inlet and an outlet strut. In 1978, the struts were modified and the disk was changed to a convexoconcave profile (the C-C model). This new model was available

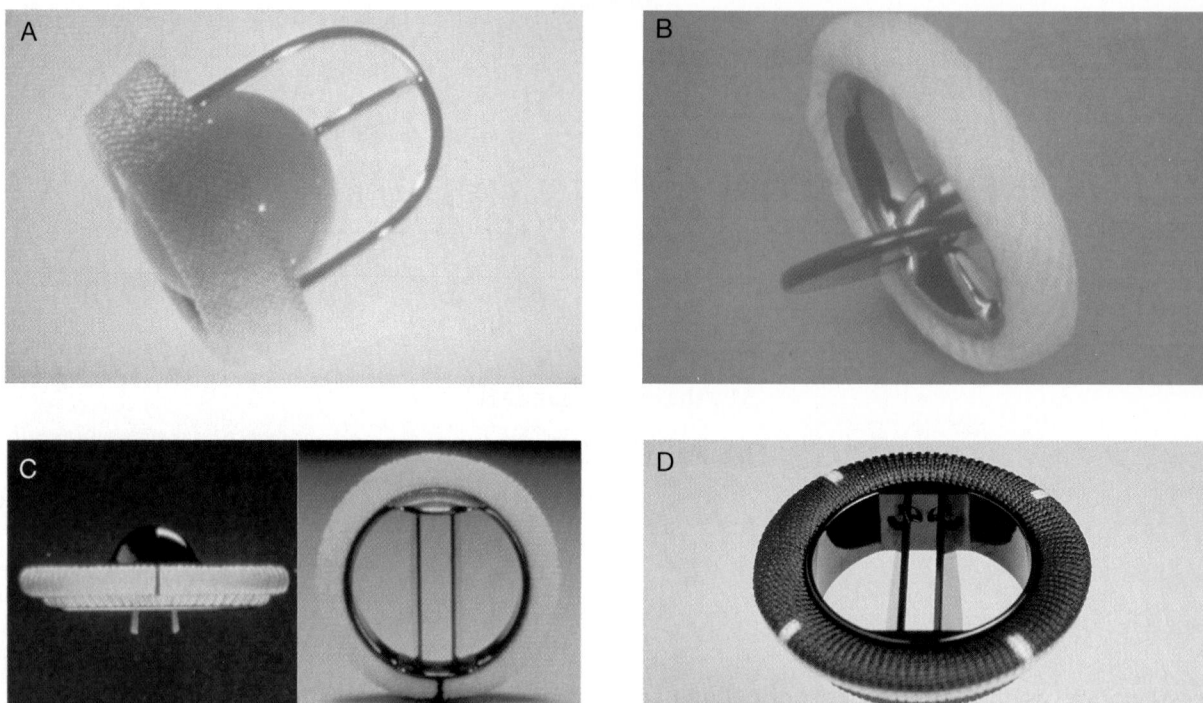

Fig. 1. Mechanical prostheses. *A*, Starr-Edwards prosthesis in closed position. *B*, Medtronic-Hall prosthesis in fully open position (central strut fits through hole in disk; open disk creates major and minor orifices). *C* and *D*, St. Jude Medical and Carbomedics bileaflet prostheses in fully open position (there are two large orifices and a smaller central orifice).

in versions that tilted to 60° and to 70° of opening angle. Only 60° valves have been implanted in the U.S. Subsequently, the Björk-Shiley C-C model was found to be subject to fractures of the outlet strut, with disk escape (see below). Later, a model with a modified outlet strut was developed. With this model, the entire ring and struts are machined from one piece (i.e., there are no welds). This is referred to as the "monostrut valve."

St. Jude Medical Valve

The most widely used mechanical prosthesis is the St. Jude Medical valve, a bileaflet valve. The housing and the leaflets are manufactured entirely from pyrolytic carbon. The leaflets move in a slot with complex opening and closing motions that are a combination of sliding and tilt. The leaflets open to a nearly parallel position (85°). The closing angle varies from 120° to 130°, depending on valve size, with valves ≤25 mm having the smaller closing angle. Other examples of bileaflet prostheses include Carbomedics and Duromedics valves.

Heterograft Valves

For all porcine heterograft prostheses, a pig aortic valve is used whether the valve is implanted in the aortic, pulmonic, mitral, or tricuspid position. The pig aortic valve is mounted on flexible stents, which are covered with Dacron. The leaflets are fixed with glutaraldehyde. For earlier-generation valves, a high-pressure technique was used for applying the glutaraldehyde fixative. This resulted in compression of the leaflets, which theoretically would provide better hemodynamics. Electron microscopy has shown that this high-pressure fixation results in destruction of the natural collagen architecture of the leaflets and likely contributes to valve degeneration. Therefore, with modern porcine valves, the glutaraldehyde is applied at low or no pressure. Currently, efforts are under way to treat tissue prostheses with chemicals that will delay calcification. An example is the Medtronic Intact porcine valve, which is treated with toluidine blue. The blue dye occupies sites that normally would be occupied by calcium. It is hoped

Table 1.   Types of Prosthetic Heart Valves*

Bioprostheses
   Porcine (stented)
      Hancock I
      Hancock II
      Hancock MO (modified orifice)
      Carpentier-Edwards
      C/E Duraflex
      Medtronic Intact
      Bioimplant
   Pericardial
      Ionescu-Shiley
      Carpentier-Edwards pericardial
      Mitroflow
   Homograft
   Porcine (stentless)
Mechanical prostheses
   Caged-ball
      Starr-Edwards
      Braunwald-Cutter
      Smeloff-Cutter
      Magovern-Cromie
   Tilting-disk
      Björk-Shiley
      Björk-Shiley convexoconcave
      Medtronic-Hall
      Lillihei-Kaster
      Omniscience
      Sorin
   Bileaflet
      St. Jude Medical
      Carbomedics
      Duromedics

*Boldface indicates valves most likely to be used in modern practice.

that this will delay calcification. Experience has shown that toluidine blue leeches out with time. Newer anticalcification agents, which bond irreversibly, are being intensely investigated.

   Heterograft valves have also been constructed from pericardium sutured to flexible, cloth-covered stents. The Ionescu-Shiley valve was one of the original pericardial valves. A design flaw predisposed this valve to sudden rupture of the cusps. Currently, the Carpentier-Edwards pericardial valve is being used and long-term studies are ongoing comparing durability to that of porcine heterografts.

Homograft Valves

Homografts are valves harvested from cadavers and cryopreserved. They frequently are used in the setting of infective endocarditis. Homografts have a low thromboembolic potential and superb hemodynamics; however, their durability is less than that of native valves. The original homograft valves were fixed with glutaraldehyde. A disastrous rate of degenerative calcification was observed with these valves. The current variety of homograft valve is fresh frozen and has proved to be very durable, with outstanding hemodynamic performance (Fig. 2). Homografts are prepared with the valve and entire ascending aorta or with the valve and pulmonary artery (Fig. 3). The surgeon can trim the homograft specimen, using as much of it as necessary (i.e., the entire ascending aorta can be used along with the valve in cases that involve significant root abnormality). As with all human donor tissue, availability of homograft valves is a limiting factor.

   Stentless porcine aortic prostheses are available and are reported to have superior hemodynamics, although long-term results are not available. As with homografts, the Medtronic Freestyle porcine prosthesis includes not only the valve but also the pig ascending aorta (Fig. 3). The surgeon trims the specimen as indicated for each case. This stentless aortic porcine prosthesis may be fashioned so that the porcine aortic sinuses are sutured inside the recipient aortic sinuses (the "cylinder within a cylinder" technique). In this case, the prosthesis is sutured both proximally and distally. This implantation technique, which can also be used with homografts, creates a unique echocardiographic appearance. The Toronto SPV, manufactured by St. Jude Medical, is already trimmed for subcoronary implantation (Fig. 3).

PRINCIPLES OF PROSTHETIC VALVE SELECTION

Similar early and late mortality rates have been reported for mechanical and tissue valves. Because valve durability is less with bioprostheses, the need for reoperation is

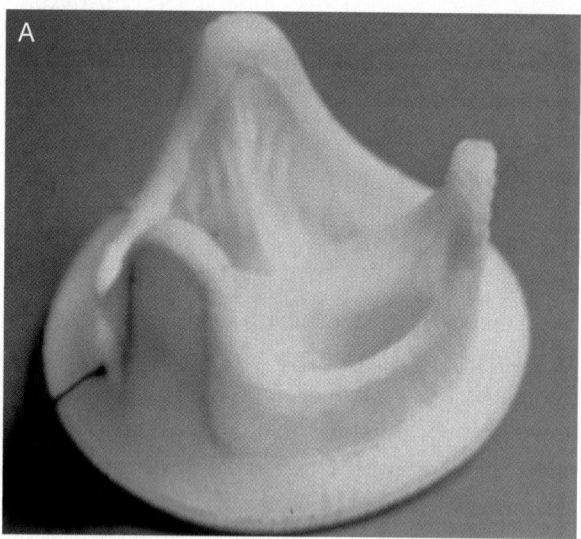

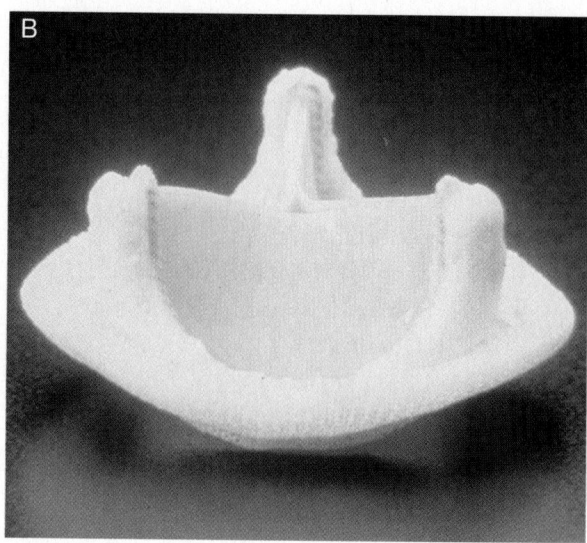

Fig. 2. Stented heterograft prostheses. *A*, Carpentier-Edwards standard valve. Porcine aortic valve is frame-mounted and glutaraldehyde-preserved. *B*, Carpentier-Edwards pericardial valve.

higher than with mechanical valves. Mechanical valves have higher thrombogenicity and a higher anticoagulation-related bleeding rate than tissue valves.

■ Mechanical valves should be used in patients requiring long-term anticoagulation for other reasons, such as atrial fibrillation.

Mechanical valves are the prosthesis of choice for individuals less than 65 years old undergoing aortic valve replacement and less than 70 years undergoing mitral valve replacement with the following exceptions:

1. Patients with a history of bleeding disorders should receive tissue valves.
2. Patients unwilling or unable to take warfarin or to comply with long-term monitoring.
3. Women with critical valve disease who desire pregnancy pose a therapeutic problem. Warfarin increases the risk of fatal fetal bleeding and is teratogenic, but heparin anticoagulation is problematic due to the hypercoagulable state of pregnancy. Bioprostheses have a lower durability in young women and a second valve operation will almost always be required if a tissue valve is implanted. The choice of prosthesis in women of child-bearing age needs to be individualized based on the overall clinical situation and an informed

discussion of the therapeutic challenges.
4. Patients with chronic renal failure (especially those receiving hemodialysis), hypercalcemia, and adolescents who are still growing should receive a mechanical prosthesis due to the high failure rate of biological prostheses in these subgroups.

■ Patients with hypercalcemia, chronic renal failure, and adolescents still growing should receive a mechanical prosthesis

Ross Procedure

A pulmonary autograft is the transplantation of a patient's own pulmonary valve and main pulmonary artery to the aortic position, with reimplantation of the coronary arteries. A homograft is placed in the pulmonary position (Ross procedure). This procedure usually is performed in children and adolescents. The advantages of the procedure are 1) durability is better than with tissue valves, 2) anticoagulation is not required, and 3) the valve and root continue to grow if the patient is a child or adolescent. The procedure is technically demanding.

COMPLICATIONS OF PROSTHETIC VALVES

Accurate diagnosis and management of prosthetic

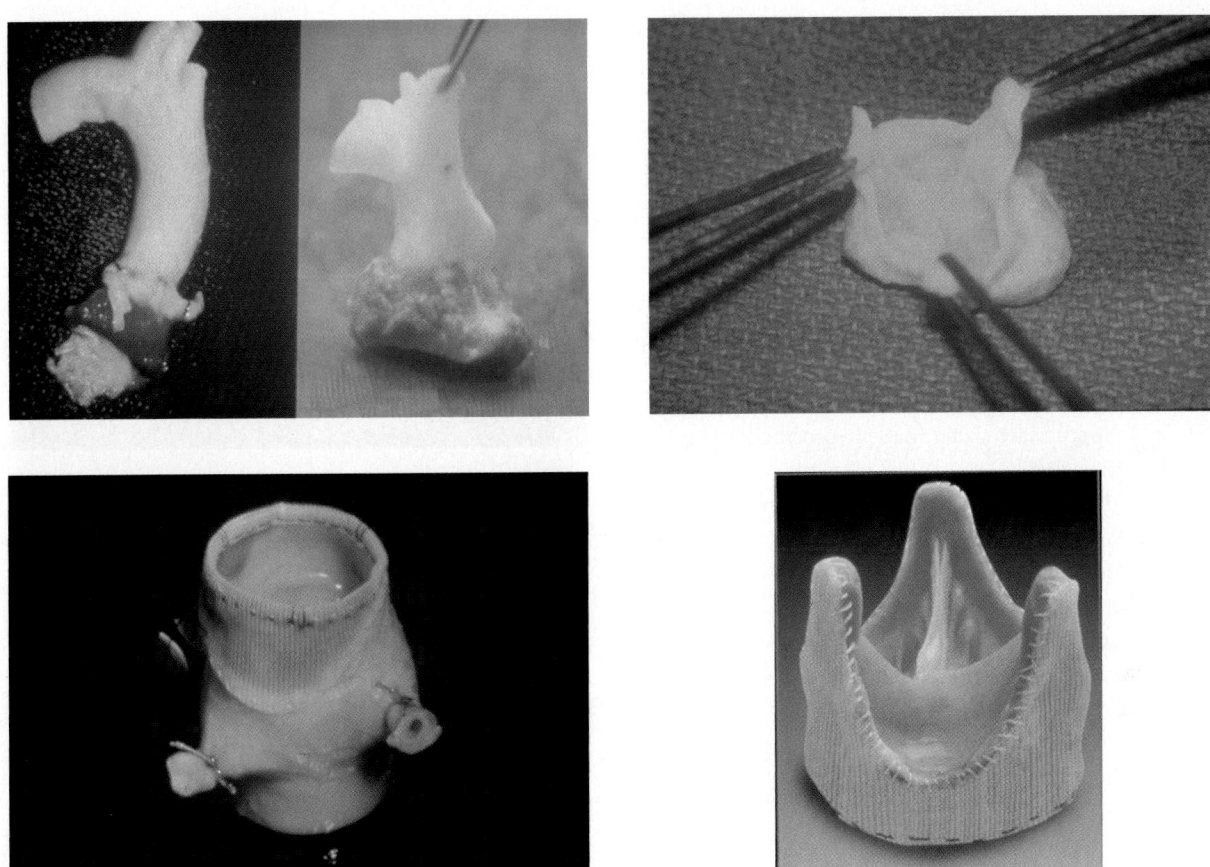

Fig. 3. Stentless bioprostheses. *A*, Aortic (left) and pulmonary (right) homografts. *B*, Aortic homograft scalloped for subcoronary implantation. *C*, Medtronic Freestyle porcine aortic prosthesis. It may be used as root replacement or root inclusion or trimmed for subcoronary implantation. *D*, Toronto SPV valve (St. Jude Medical) is manufactured for subcoronary implantation.

valve dysfunction are expected. Specific complications of prosthetic valves are outlined in Table 2.

Perivalvular Leak

Perivalvular regurgitation is always abnormal (Fig. 4). The clinical significance is determined by the volume of regurgitation or the presence of mechanical hemolysis (or both). Pathologic transvalvular regurgitation must be distinguished from the normal regurgitation that is "built into" various prosthetic valves. All prosthetic valves have associated closing volume regurgitation. This is the volume of blood displaced by the occluder when it closes (Fig. 5). Tilting-disk and bileaflet prostheses also have a built-in leakage volume, true transvalvular regurgitation that travels between the disk or leaflets and the housing and also between closed

bileaflets (Fig. 6). This leakage volume serves to wash the surface of the disk or leaflets. Earlier models that were designed without any leakage volume have an unacceptably high incidence of valve thrombosis. Closing volume depends on occluder size, length of travel, and speed of closure. Leakage volume depends on the size of the gap between the occluder and the rim of the housing. It increases with valve size and with decreasing heart rate. In the extreme, the sum of closing and leakage volumes may be as great as 10 mL per beat.

■ Perivalvular leak is always abnormal.

Structural Failure of Prosthetic Valves

Structural deterioration is most common for bioprostheses. Degenerative calcification most often results in

Table 2. Complications of Prosthetic Valves

1. Structural deterioration of the valve leading to
   stenosis and/or regurgitation
2. Nonstructural dysfunction—an abnormality,
   not intrinsic to the valve, resulting in stenosis
   and/or regurgitation (exclusive of infection and
   thrombosis)
   > Pannus
   > Suture entrapment
   > Parivalvular leak
   > Inappropriate sizing (patient-prosthesis
   >   mismatch)
   > Clinically important hemolytic anemia
3. Thromboembolism
   > Neurologic deficit
   > Peripheral emboli
   > Acute myocardial infarction after operation,
   >   if coronary arteries are known to be normal
4. Valve thrombosis
5. Anticoagulation-related hemorrhage
6. Prosthetic valve endocarditis

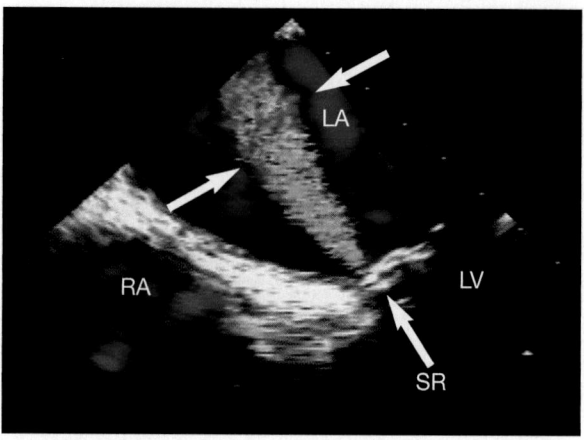

Fig. 4. Transesophageal echocardiography, horizontal plane view from a patient with a Starr-Edwards mitral prosthesis who had symptoms of congestive failure and a murmur of mitral regurgitation. Soon after the transducer was introduced into the esophagus, a relatively narrow periprosthetic jet (*arrows*) originating around the medial portion of the sewing ring (SR) was identified. Note the mosaic appearance. This jet would certainly explain the systolic murmur, but its size seems insufficient to explain the patient's congestive symptoms. LA, left atrium; LV, left ventricle; RA, right atrium.

leaflet tears with transvalvular regurgitation, but it may also result in stenosis. Nonstructural lesions such as pannus and suture entrapment are most common with mechanical prostheses, whereas perivalvular leaks are common with either mechanical valves or bioprostheses. Clinically important hemolytic anemia is usually the result of perivalvular regurgitation, particularly if the regurgitant jet is directed against prosthetic material.

Currently, the most common structural dysfunction of mechanical prostheses is fracture of the outlet strut of the Björk-Shiley Convexo-Concave prosthesis. The risk of outlet strut fracture is significantly higher for 70° C-C valves than for 60° C-C valves. Only 60° C-C valves were implanted in the U.S. The risk of strut fracture is highest for large valve sizes (29, 31, and 33 mm). The largest valves are estimated to have a potential strut fracture rate as high as 280/10,000 valves implanted.

Thromboembolism

Thromboembolism is a common problem of all prostheses, although it is significantly more common with mechanical valves than with bioprostheses and with mitral than with aortic prostheses. Thromboembolism

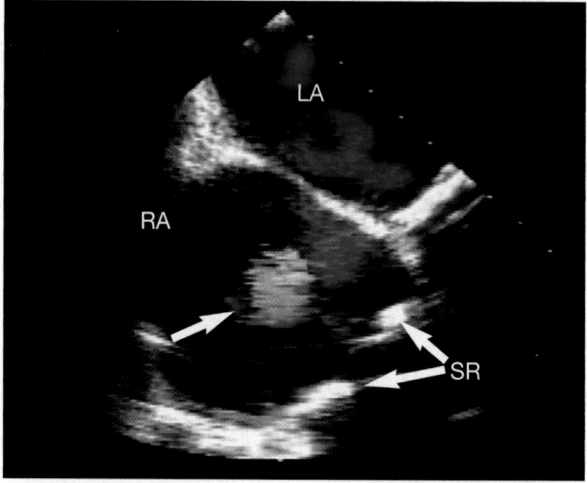

Fig. 5. Transesophageal echocardiography, horizontal plane, four-chamber view. Normal Starr-Edwards tricuspid prosthesis. In this systolic frame, the poppet and cage are not visible in the right ventricle. The ball-shaped, low-velocity color map (*arrow*) in the right atrium (RA) represents the volume of blood that is displaced as the poppet moves to its closed position against the sewing ring. This color array is therefore referred to as the prosthetic "closing volume." LA, left atrium; RV, right ventricle; SR, sewing ring.

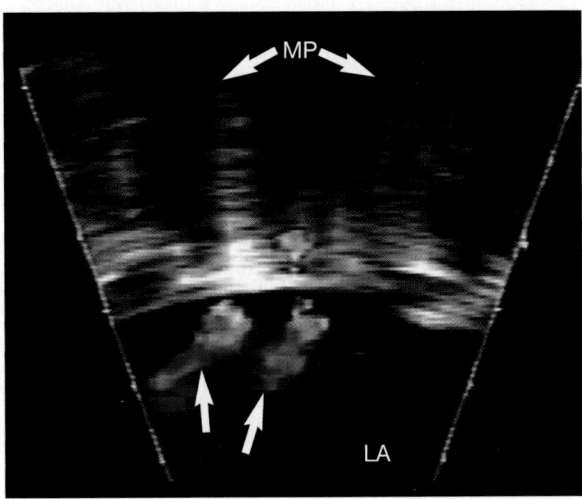

Fig. 6. Omniplane transesophageal echocardiographic evaluation, with color flow imaging, of a normal Lillihei-Kaster mitral prosthesis (MP). This tilting-disk valve has a normal, small amount of transvalvular regurgitation. Note the two separate jets (*arrows*) in the left atrium (LA). Besides their small size, these jets clearly represent very mild regurgitation, because they are uniformly red (nonturbulent). Very few blood cells are traveling at higher velocities (i.e., above the Nyquist limit); therefore, minimal color aliasing is seen within these jets.

should be clearly distinguished from valve thrombosis. The latter can result in thromboembolism, but it also has the potential for acute and severe hemodynamic disturbance due to entrapment of the moving parts with either severe stenosis or severe regurgitation.

■ The risk of thromboembolism is increased with mitral versus aortic prostheses

Prosthetic Valve Endocarditis
Prosthetic valve endocarditis can occur with any of the various prostheses. With mechanical prostheses, vegetations form on the sewing ring. With bioprostheses, vegetations can occur on the ring or on the cusps. In either case, the infection is difficult to eradicate without replacing the prosthesis. Perivalvular extension of infection, such as valve-ring abscess formation, is a dreaded and all-too-common complication of prosthetic valve endocarditis. Staphylococci are the most common isolate from patients with early-onset prosthetic valve infection, with *Staphylococcus epidermidis* accounting for a substantial

percentage of the cases. Streptococci are the predominant microorganism causing late-onset prosthetic valve infection.

■ Valve-ring abscess is a common complication of prosthetic valve endocarditis.

Prosthesis-Patient Mismatch
Prosthesis-patient mismatch is defined as an effective orifice area (EOA) which is too small for the patient's body surface area and results in abnormally high transvalvular gradients. An aortic prosthesis EOA of <0.85 cm^2/m^2 is generally considered indicative of prosthesis-patient mismatch, with <0.6 cm^2/m^2 considered severe. The frequency and clinical significance of prosthesis-patient mismatch is controversial, however several studies have shown reduced survival in these patients. In patients undergoing AVR it is recommended that the EOA be estimated. If the patient is found to be at risk for prosthesis-patient mismatch then strategies to reduce mismatch should be considered, including aortic root enlargement and alternate choice of prosthesis.

DIAGNOSIS OF PROSTHETIC VALVE DYSFUNCTION

Patient History
When evaluating a patient who has a prosthetic valve, the exact valve type, size, and model should be noted. If the patient is unaware of this information, it is contained on the identification card. The valve size, in millimeters, usually precedes an A or M (which indicates aortic or mitral models, respectively) in the serial number.

Ask whether patients with prosthetic valves are taking antiplatelet agents and/or receiving anticoagulation. If they are taking warfarin, the adequacy of anticoagulation should be assessed by checking their International Normalized Ratio (INR) over a period of months. Ask about bleeding, symptoms consistent with embolic events, and symptoms suggesting endocarditis. If a patient has been aware of valve clicks, ask about any sudden changes, because the loss of valve clicks may indicate valve thrombosis.

Establish whether the patient is in sinus rhythm or atrial fibrillation, because the latter increases the incidence of thromboembolic events. Ask about the patient's functional status, and look for symptoms of left-sided and right-sided heart failure. Patients with aortic prostheses should also be questioned about angina and exertional syncope or near-syncope, just as patients with native aortic stenosis would be questioned.

Physical Examination

Typically, there is a brief systolic ejection murmur across normal aortic prostheses. Normal mitral prostheses may create a brief and low-grade apical rumble (Table 3). This is particularly true for mitral bioprostheses. The bioprostheses create normal closing sounds (i.e., normal-sounding heart sounds). They do not create opening clicks. Caged-ball mechanical prostheses have prominent opening and closing clicks, whereas tilting-disk and bileaflet prostheses have prominent closing clicks, but muffled hard-to-hear opening sounds.

■ Loss of expected valve sounds is an important sign of mechanical valve thrombosis.

The examination of patients with prosthetic valve stenosis or regurgitation is similar to that of patients with corresponding native-valve lesions. This includes a decreased aortic-closure-to-mitral-opening interval in patients with prosthetic mitral valve stenosis. This finding is singled out because it is particularly easy to elicit in patients with certain types of prostheses, particularly those with the caged-ball variety of mitral prosthesis.

Radiography

The sewing ring of most prostheses can be visualized on standard posterior-anterior and lateral chest radiographs. Heterograft stents are radiopaque, as are many of the mechanical valve occluders. For patients with valvular prostheses, however, the standard chest radiograph is most useful in demonstrating signs of heart failure, such as pulmonary venous hypertension.

For valves with radiopaque occluders, fluoroscopy can be used to measure the opening and closing angles. Valve thrombosis will result in a significantly reduced opening or closing motion (or both). The fluoroscopic appearance is useful not only for diagnosing prosthetic valve thrombosis but also for assessing the efficacy of thrombolytic therapy.

■ Fluoroscopy is an excellent tool for visualizing

Table 3.   Auscultatory Findings in Patients With Normally Functioning Prosthetic Heart Valves

Prosthesis	Aortic	Mitral
Starr-Edwards ball valve	Sharp opening sound at S_1* Sharp closing sound at S_2 Ball "rattles" during systole SEM	Sharp opening sound 70-150 ms after S_2 Sharp closing sound at S_1 Ball "rattles" during diastole SEM
St. Jude	Sharp closing sound at S_2 SEM	Sharp closing sound at S_1
Heterograft	SEM	Diastolic rumble†

S_1, first heart sound; S_2, second heart sound; SEM, systolic ejection murmur.

*Absence of opening or closing sounds with mechanical prosthesis usually signifies severe prosthesis dysfunction.

†Should be brief; if prolonged, indicates bioprosthetic obstruction or prosthesis-patient mismatch.

prosthetic leaflet motion

Currently, fluoroscopy is the only method available for diagnosing strut fracture of the Björk-Shiley C-C prosthesis. However, once the fracture has occurred—and thus is identifiable on fluoroscopy—the patient's condition is extremely serious.

Echocardiography

Echocardiography provides a complete hemodynamic assessment of valvular prostheses in most clinical situations. This has revolutionized the diagnostic approach to patients with suspected prosthetic valve dysfunction.

Aortic Prostheses

Complete echocardiographic assessment of prosthetic aortic valves includes measurement of peak systolic velocity, mean gradient and effective orifice area (EOA). In addition, the presence or absence of regurgitation is noted, and the regurgitation is characterized as normal (i.e., closing volume and/or leakage volume) or pathologic. An attempt is made to separate pathologic regurgitation into perivalvular or transvalvular, according to the origin of the jet. Semiquantitative and quantitative measures are used to characterize the amount of regurgitation.

Gradients across prosthetic valves are determined by the simplified Bernoulli equation (see the chapter on echocardiography). It is crucial to ensure that the highest velocity of the aortic prosthesis has been obtained which requires interrogation from multiple windows, identical to the Doppler assessment of native aortic stenosis. The EOA for prosthetic valves is determined with the continuity equation and should be commonly performed for aortic and mitral prostheses. The prosthesis sewing ring must be visualized clearly to measure LVOT diameter. In rare cases in which this measurement cannot be made confidently, it is acceptable to approximate the measurement with the external diameter of the sewing ring (i.e., the valve size). It has been shown that this approximation will slightly overestimate the actual EOA.

In our experience, the average mean gradient was 13 to 15 mm Hg for heterograft, Björk-Shiley, St. Jude Medical, and Medtronic-Hall prostheses. The average mean gradient was significantly greater for Starr-Edwards aortic prostheses (23 mm Hg) and was significantly lower for homograft prostheses (8 mm Hg). However, it is important to be aware of patient-to-patient variability. With all valve types, except homografts, there are individuals with normally functioning prostheses with mean gradients as high as 35 to 45 mm Hg. In general, these patients have small prostheses, and these high gradients are due to prosthesis-patient mismatch. Because of this variability in mean gradient and EOA among patients with normal prosthetic valve function, it is mandatory that a baseline echocardiographic and Doppler examination be performed on each patient soon after implantation. This effectively "fingerprints" the individual prosthesis and serves as a baseline for comparison, should symptoms develop consistent with prosthetic valve dysfunction.

Assessment of Prosthetic Aortic Valve Incompetence
Semiquantitation of aortic regurgitation is performed by using information from two-dimensional imaging, spectral Doppler, and color flow imaging. The degree

to which color flow signals of regurgitation fill the LVOT in diastole is determined. In addition, the intensity of high-velocity signals in the continuous-wave spectrum of aortic regurgitation, the pressure half-time of the continuous-wave signal, the amount of diastolic flow reversal in the descending thoracic aorta (obtained by pulsed-wave Doppler), and the size of the left ventricle (from two-dimensional imaging) are assessed. If a patient has a native mitral valve that is competent, the aortic regurgitant volume and regurgitant fraction can be calculated by comparing forward flow through the LVOT with forward flow across the mitral anulus.

Assessment of Prosthetic Mitral and Tricuspid Valves
Mitral and tricuspid prostheses are assessed more easily by Doppler hemodynamics because the optimal window for interrogation is always apical or periapical. Complete assessment requires measurement of the peak early velocity (E velocity), the velocity with atrial contraction (A velocity) for patients in sinus rhythm, the pressure half-time, EOA, and the presence and degree of regurgitation. The velocities and mean gradient are measured from the continuous-wave Doppler signal. Although the EOA can be calculated from the pressure half-time for obstructed prostheses, this method tends to overestimate the EOA for normally functioning prostheses. Therefore, it is preferable to report the pressure half-time independently and to calculate the EOA by the continuity method. As with aortic prostheses, the LVOT stroke volume is divided by the prosthesis TVI to obtain the EOA. However, this method cannot be used with mitral or tricuspid prostheses if there is significant aortic regurgitation or significant prosthesis regurgitation; under these circumstances, continuity of flow will no longer exist. In such cases, the pressure half-time should be reported and the EOA should not be calculated.

Because mitral and tricuspid prostheses create reverberations and acoustic shadowing within the atria, visualization of regurgitant jets by surface echocardiography is always suboptimal. However, important clues to significant regurgitation may be found on the surface examination. These include an increased E velocity with normal pressure half-time, a dense continuous-wave regurgitant signal, and color Doppler signals of flow convergence on the ventricular side of the regurgitant orifice. Transesophageal echocardiography provides complete visualization of color jets due to prosthetic mitral or tricuspid regurgitation. It also allows sampling of the left and right upper pulmonary veins for systolic flow reversal.

The average mean gradient of a mitral prosthesis is 4- to 5-mm Hg for heterograft, tilting-disk, bileaflet, and caged-ball prostheses. There are occasional normal valves with mean gradients as high as 10 mm Hg. For normal tricuspid prostheses, the mean gradient averages 2 to 3 mm Hg, with mean gradients of outliers as high as 6 mm Hg. For all Doppler hemodynamic calculations, at least three cardiac cycles should be averaged for patients in sinus rhythm and at least five cycles for those in atrial fibrillation. For tricuspid prostheses, 10 cycles must be averaged, even for patients in sinus rhythm, because of significant variation in mean gradient with the respiratory cycle.

Transesophageal Echocardiography

Most prosthetic valve hemodynamic information is available from surface echocardiography. Similarly, the amount of prosthetic aortic regurgitation usually can be assessed by the surface examination. Complete visualization of mitral and tricuspid prosthesis regurgitant jets requires transesophageal echocardiography, which is also indicated if it is necessary to determine the mechanism of regurgitation or stenosis. Because transesophageal echocardiography is sensitive enough to detect normal closing volume and leakage volume, the echocardiographer must be aware of the normal patterns for each type of prosthesis.

For patients with clinically significant prosthetic valve dysfunction, an echocardiographic examination usually can obviate the need for invasive hemodynamics before surgical replacement.

Laboratory Tests and Hemolysis

For patients with prosthetic valves who are receiving long-term anticoagulation therapy, the INR should be checked at least monthly. Also, the hemoglobin value should be checked periodically, because a decrease could be due to bleeding or from significant hemolysis. Sheared red blood cells will appear as schistocytes on a peripheral blood smear. The level of serum haptoglobin will approach zero, and the level of lactate dehydrogenase will increase. There usually is a compensatory increase in reticulocytes. The loss of iron in the urine, in the form of hemosiderin, produces iron deficiency.

■ Hemolysis is a potential complication of prosthetic valves and leads to decreased serum haptoglobin and increased LDH

Invasive Hemodynamics

The diagnosis of prosthetic valve dysfunction seldom requires an invasive procedure. Catheters should not be passed across mechanical aortic prostheses; thus, measurement of aortic prosthesis gradients requires a transseptal approach. If both mitral and aortic prostheses are present, measurement of the gradients requires not only transseptal puncture but also left ventricular puncture. For mitral prostheses, it is always necessary to measure the gradient using a transseptal approach, with direct measurement of left atrial pressure, rather than depending on pulmonary artery wedge pressure. The latter nearly always results in significant overestimation of the gradient, even when the phase delay is taken into account.

PRIMARY PREVENTION OF VALVE DYSFUNCTION

Antithrombotic Therapy

Aspirin therapy (81 mg/day) should be used in all patients with prosthetic heart valves, both mechanical and biological, unless contraindicated, All patients with mechanical prostheses require anticoagulation with warfarin. The recommendations for target INR for long-term anticoagulation (greater than three months after valve implantation) are outlined in Table 4. The intensity of anticoagulation must be tailored for each patient, taking into account age, bleeding risk, gait stability, and risk factors for thrombosis and thromboembolism.

■ All patients with prosthetic valves (biologic and mechanical) should receive aspirin, unless contraindicated

Patients with bioprostheses generally receive anticoagulation treatment with warfarin for the first 3 months, although aspirin alone is used in some centers. The recommended target INR for both aortic and mitral bioprostheses is 2.0 to 3.0 during the initial 3 months after implantation. In patients with chronic atrial fibrillation, warfarin treatment should be continued indefinitely, which removes the major advantage for bioprostheses.

Table 4.   Recommendations for Long-term
           Anticoagulation With Mechanical
           Prosthetic Valves*

Target INR†	
2-3	**2.5-3.5**
AVR and no risk‡	AVR
Bileaflet	Other disk valves
Metronic-Hall	AVR with risk factor‡
	All MVR

AVR, aortic valve prosthesis; MVR, mitral valve prosthesis.
*Aspirin (81 mg/day) is recommended for all patients
with prosthetic heart valves.
†More than 3 months after valve replacement.
‡Risk factors: atrial fibrillation, left ventriclar systolic
dysfunction, previous thromboembolism, and hypercoagulable conditions.

Most patients with prosthetic valves will at some
time require short-term discontinuation of anticoagulation for invasive procedures. Management options for
"bridging" anticoagulation are based on individual risk
(including type and position of prosthesis), the nature
of the procedure, risk of bleeding, and the expected
duration of interruption of warfarin therapy. Short-
term discontinuation of warfarin without heparin coverage is appropriate for low risk patients, such as those
with a bileaflet aortic prosthesis, normal LV function,
and no additional risk factors. Risk factors for thromboembolism during discontinuation of anticoagulation
include atrial fibrillation, previous thromboembolism,
LV dysfunction, hypercoagulable conditions, older
generation thrombogenic valves, mechanical mitral
valves, or more than 1 mechanical valve (Table 5).

Warfarin should be resumed as soon as possible
after the procedure for all patients with and without
heparin therapy. Recommendations for management of
periprocedural anticoagulation are outlined in Table 6.
The use of low-molecular-weight heparin for periprocedural anticoagulation of prosthetic valves is controversial and currently not FDA approved. Guidelines
favor the use of unfractionated heparin; however, studies
are ongoing to address the safety and efficacy of
low-molecular-weight-heparin for "bridging" therapy
of prosthetic valves.

■ Patients with a bileaflet aortic prosthesis and no risk
  factors do not need heparin coverage during short-
  term warfarin discontinuation

In patients with mechanical valves requiring interruption
of warfarin therapy for noncardiac surgery, invasive procedures or dental care, high-dose vitamin K_1 should not
be given routinely, as this may create a hypercoagulable
condition.

Endocarditis Prophylaxis
All patients with prosthetic valves should receive
antibiotics for endocarditis according to the
AHA/ACC guidelines (see the chapter on infections of
the heart).

MANAGEMENT OF PROSTHETIC VALVE COMPLICATIONS

Replacement of a dysfunctional prosthetic valve carries
a significantly higher surgical risk in comparison with
initial valve replacement. Therefore, with most chronic
or subacute problems, one should be conservative when
deciding whether to replace a dysfunctional prosthesis.
Definite indications for surgery include 1) severe
prosthetic stenosis or regurgitation with resultant
symptoms and/or ventricular dysfunction, 2) transfusion-
dependent hemolysis, 3) recurrent emboli despite
adequate anticoagulation/antiplatelet therapy, and 4)
prosthetic valve endocarditis with hemodynamic compromise, persistent fever despite adequate antibiotic therapy, perivalvular extension of infection, or large mobile
vegetations seen on transesophageal echocardiography.

Table 5.   Risk of Thrombosis or
           Thromboembolism With Interruption
           of Anticoagulation in Prosthetic Valves

High risk	Other risk factors
Recent thrombus or embolus (1 year)	Atrial fibrillation
Previous event when "off" warfarin	History of thromboem-bolism
Björk-Shiley valve	Hypercoagulable state
	Decreased ejection fraction

Table 6.   Recommendations for Periprocedural Anticoagulation in Patients With Mechanical Valves

No heparin	Heparin
Newer AVR	Björk-Shiley valve
No risk factors	AVR: 1 risk factor*
	MVR

AVR, aortic valve prosthesis; MVR, mitral valve prosthesis.
*Risk factors: atrial fibrillation, previous thromboembolism, left ventricular systolic dysfunction, and hypercoagulable condition.

Valve thrombosis is a life-threatening and dreaded complication of mechanical valves. Treatment options include thrombolysis and surgery. In patients with small clots and stable hemodynamics a trial of heparin therapy may be considered. There is debate concerning the choice of thrombolytic therapy versus cardiac surgery. Thrombolysis is considered to be the first-line treatment for thrombosis of right-sided prostheses in most situations. For left-sided prostheses, thrombolytic therapy carries a significant risk of embolism and stroke. Nevertheless, many patients with thrombosed left-sided valves will also have a very high operative mortality. In these cases, it is best for the cardiologist and cardiac surgeon to arrive jointly at a decision, which will depend heavily on the estimated risk of cardiac surgery.

45

SURGERY FOR CARDIAC VALVE DISEASE

Thomas A. Orszulak, MD

The decision to perform an operation for valve disease is quite complex and requires a melding of many disciplines and diagnostic achievements. Obviously, the history and physical exam is tantamount to everything else in terms of deciding what the diagnosis is and the appropriate treatment. In this chapter, we will discuss the approach to valve correction for valvular heart disease.

Initially, a major statement that needs to be made is that repair of any valve is always preferable to replacement if it can be done safely and durably. We will discuss the application of this to each valve in the following paragraphs.

The indications for operation come based on historic events in cardiac surgery, natural history studies, and current literature studies.

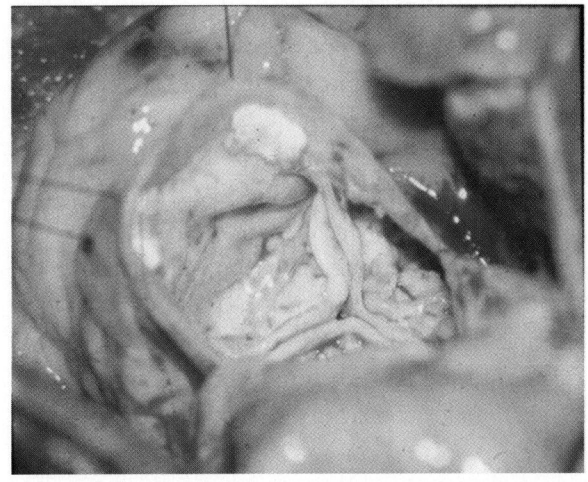

Fig. 1. Rheumatic aortic valvular disease. Valve cusps are thickened and fused.

AORTIC VALVE

If we examine aortic valve disease, predominantly aortic stenosis (Fig. 1), the indications for operation are dictated by severity of disease and symptoms produced. The most common symptoms include dyspnea on exertion, chest pain, and light-headedness or dizziness usually with sudden change of position, such as standing quickly. Although patients with symptoms certainly require correction, there are indications for valve replacement or repair for aortic stenosis in patients who are asymptomatic. This situation requires close scrutiny and is seen most frequently in patients who have excessively high gradients or valve areas below 0.75 cm^2. When this situation exists, a very carefully performed treadmill or exercise test can be done to evaluate the patient's myocardial response to a light form of exercise. The specific abnormality looked for is a fall in ejection fraction with exercise especially without symptoms. If this occurs at a very low work level, then we realize that the patient is on the edge of deterioration and, despite a claim of being asymptomatic, an operation can be performed. An exercise test will also determine what level of exercise a patient actually does at home that leads to a claim of no symptoms.

For aortic valve disease, repair is not nearly as frequent as mitral valve repair. The repair predominantly occurs with regurgitant lesions from healed endocarditis with perforated leaflet that can be patched or with some forms of commisural dilatation. Occasionally with aortic regurgitation due to aneurysms limited to the ascending aorta distal to the sinotubular junction, splaying of the commissures at the sinotubular junction can cause regurgitation that, by repairing the aneurysm and returning the sinotubular junction and commissures to their original or natural relationship, can preserve the valve. More direct approaches to valve lesions can be performed with a technique forwarded by both Yacoub and David where the valve leaflets are preserved, the aneurysm or ascending aorta is removed, and the valve resuspended within a graft (Fig. 2). These procedures are technically quite demanding and are limited to those patients who have Marfan's disease or ascending aortic aneurysm and still a minimal or mild amount of aortic valve regurgitation.

Endocarditis creates a situation where repair in the aortic position is impossible in the acute stage. Surgical principles for infection dictate removing and/or sterilizing all infected tissue before reconstruction (Fig. 3). When the infection is limited to the leaflets alone, the

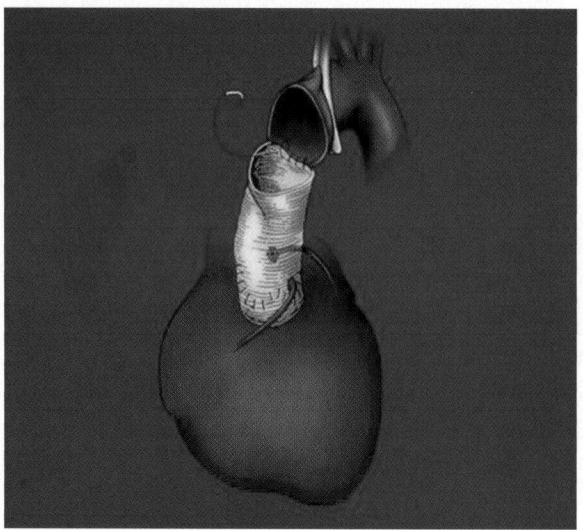

Fig. 2. Diagram of surgical repair as described by Yacoub and David. See text for discussion.

débridement mimics a normal valve replacement. The difficulty arises when an aggressive organism is present or there is delay in diagnosis or antibiotic treatment that allows the infection to breach the boundaries of the leaflets and destroy anular tissue with abscess formation. This requires broader debridement and reconstruction with autologous pericardium and/or homograft implantation. The autologous tissue and homograft have the lowest reinfection rate in the aortic root with extensive acute infection.

For aortic valve regurgitation, obviously echocardiographic findings and symptoms help determine the timing of the operation. If a patient's left ventricular function starts to fail or becomes dilated, it is appropriate to recommend an operation. For aortic stenosis, similar events are tantamount to recommending valve replacement.

Repair of aortic stenosis has been tried with various forms of decalcification and are only of historic interest. A fairly recent series from this institution showed a follow-up of patients who had decalcification of their leaflets with ultrasonic débridement with excellent early results (Fig. 4); however, fulminant scarring took place which caused the leaflets to retract, and these patients then returned with rather significant and severe aortic regurgitation requiring reoperation and valve replacement.

MITRAL VALVE

Mitral regurgitant pathologies, especially from myxomatous disease or ruptured chordae, are ideal situations for valve repair. Figure 5 shows generally the techniques that are involved in mitral valve repair. The indications, at least based on information from Mayo Clinic, have advanced the time frame for valve repair beyond those patients that are symptomatic. The presence of severe mitral regurgitation alone has become the indication for valve repair because of the late effects on survival and left ventricular function if the regurgitation is left to progress until symptoms or severe cardiomegaly develops. Repairs are quite durable. The most durable repair and results are found in the posterior leaflet, which has an approximately 0.5% per year chance of recurrent regurgitation requiring operation (Fig. 6). The anterior leaflet has a 1% per year chance of recurrent regurgitation requiring subsequent operation. The true advantage of the valve repair for patients is

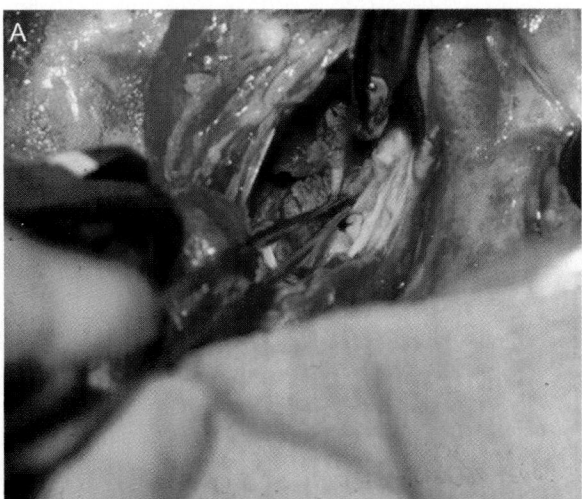 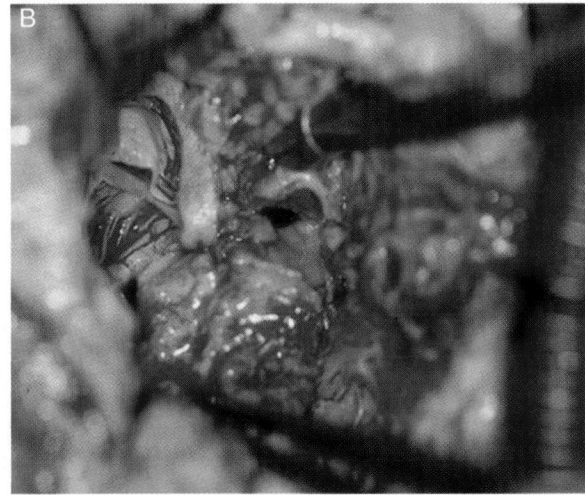

Fig. 3. *A*, Endocarditis of native aortic valve. *B*, Endocarditis of aortic tissue prosthesis.

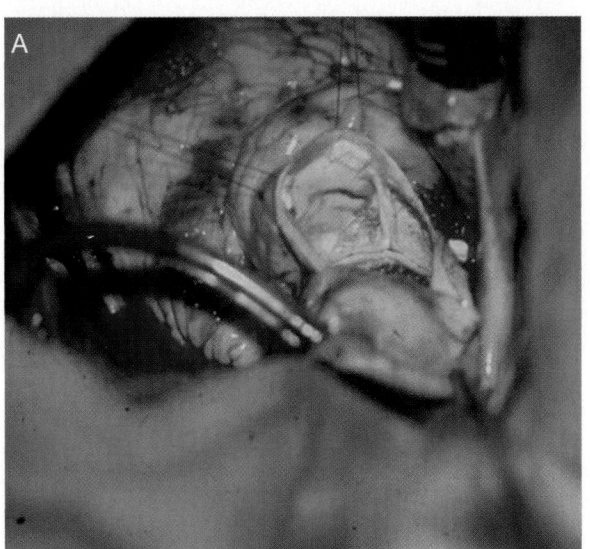 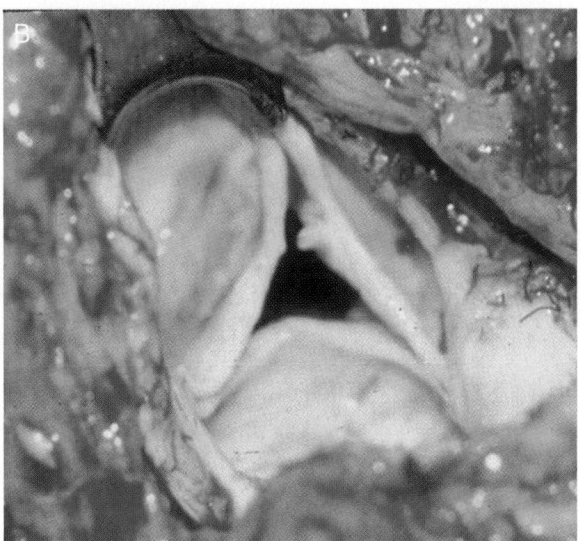

Fig. 4. *A*, Repair of calcified aortic valve at initial operation. *B*, Same patient at reoperation 8 months later. Valve leaflets are scarred and retracted, resulting in severe aortic regurgitation.

the elimination of a prosthesis and the preservation of left ventricular morphology and function. With repair, long-term anticoagulation (except the 6-8 weeks to allow endothelialization of the anuloplasty ring) is avoided. The long-term results with repair match those of a normal age-matched population.

Repair is also possible in some cases of endocarditis, if the operation is done in the early phases of the disease or in the healed state (Fig. 7). The principles of repair are basically the same, but additional features are present

with acute endocarditis. Any acute infection requires the removal of all infected tissue which limits repair when there is a large area of valve replaced with vegetations. When the infection is associated with abscess formation, the débridement almost always eliminates the chance of repair. It is frequently a cooperative balance between what can and should be done with antibiotic treatment and operative intervention to preserve valve tissue.

Mitral stenosis will require replacement more frequently from the surgical perspective. Any valve that

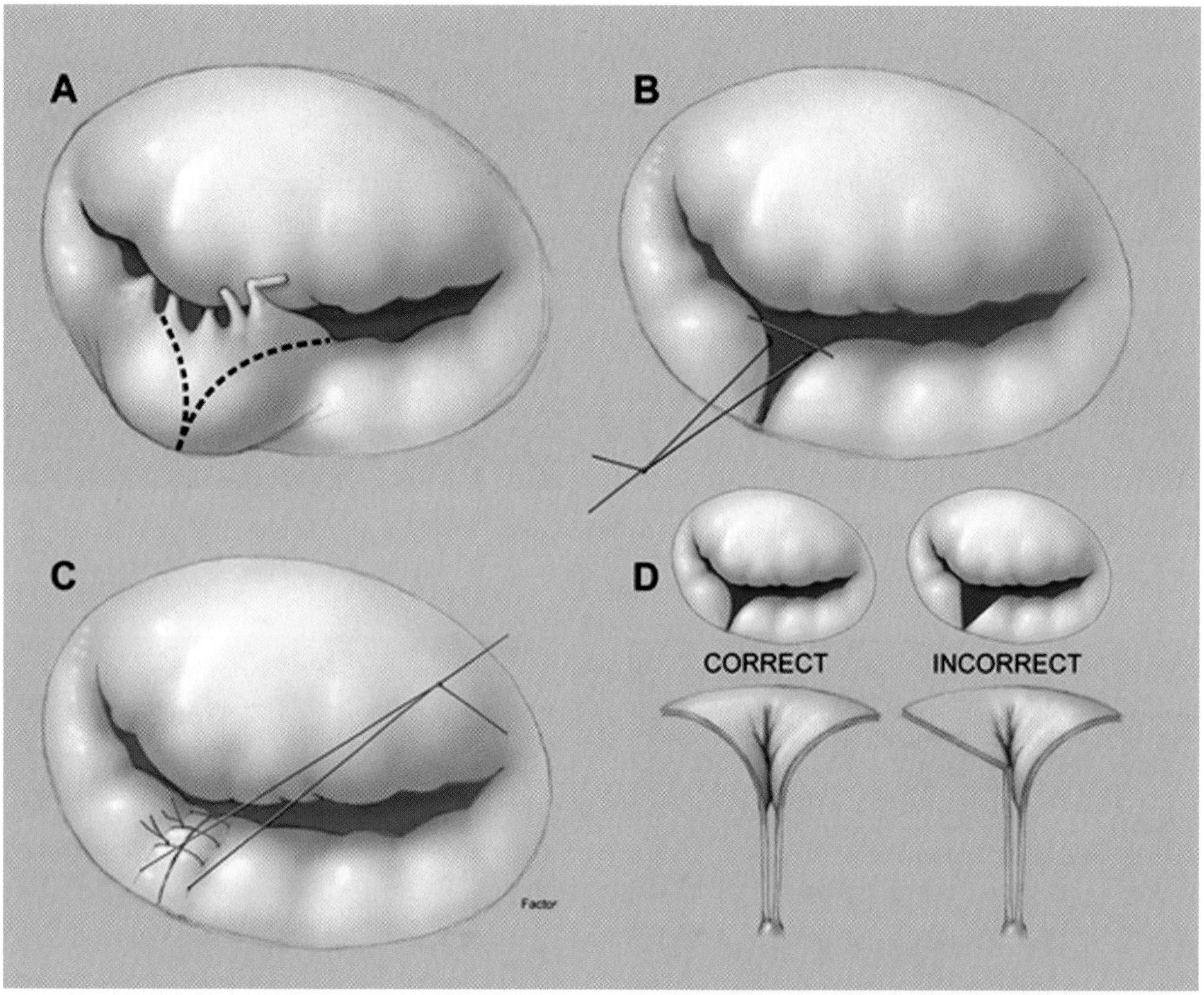

Fig. 5. Stages of mitral valve repair.

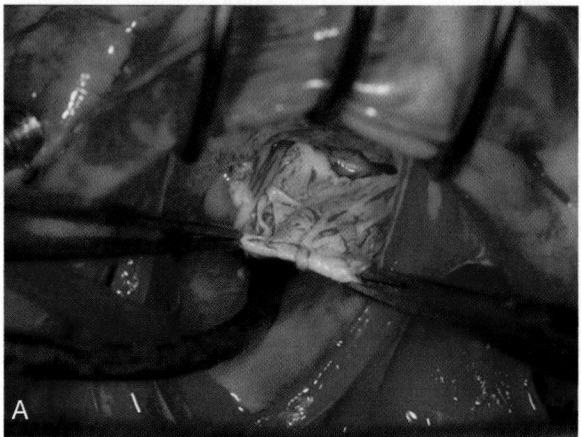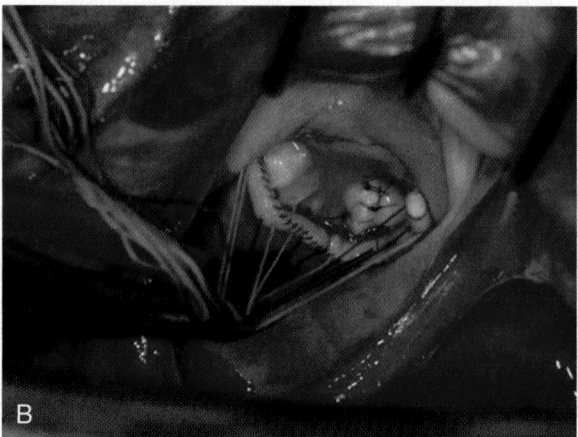

Fig. 6. Posterior leaflet repair. *A*, Before repair. *B*, After repair.

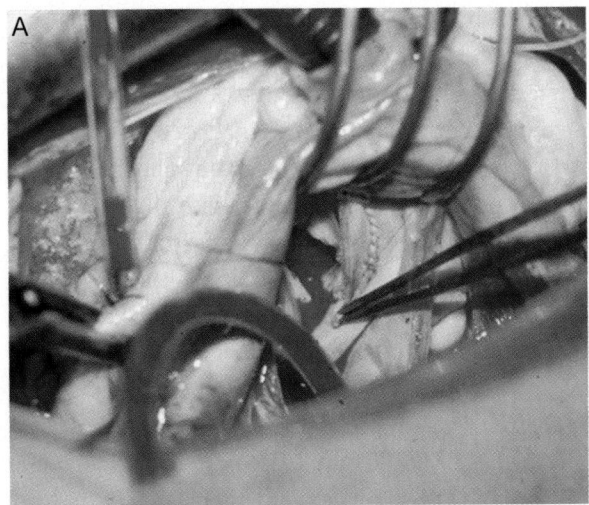
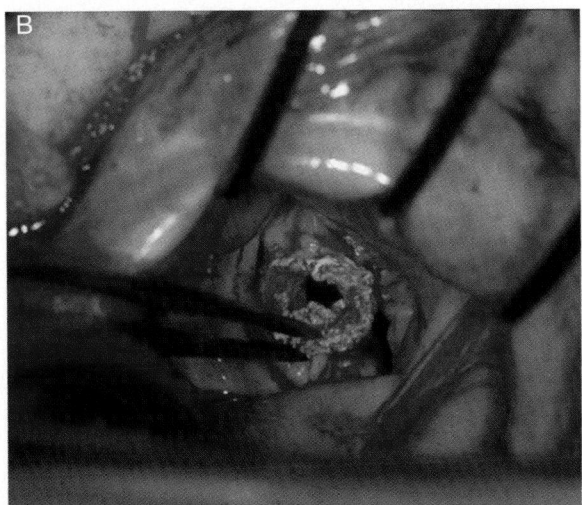

Fig. 7. *A*, Repaired mitral valve after acute endocarditis. *B*, Chronic endocarditis of the mitral valve. Scarring and calcification of the valve make repair impossible and valve replacement necessary.

would have been treated with an open or closed commissurotomy previously is now handled with a percutaneous balloon dilatation. Once a patient comes to operation for mitral stenosis that cannot be dilated, the valve generally will require replacement. This series differs in the United States compared to other developing countries because most patients in the United States that have mitral stenosis had their rheumatic fever years previously and the scarring is quite established and replete with calcium that prohibits or limits any form of reparative techniques (Fig. 8). This is, however, different from developing countries where young patients with fairly acute or recent rheumatic fever may have pliable valves that can be repaired quite effectively. Also, the patients in the United States coming to mitral valve replacement for rheumatic disease are generally older patients in whom a valve replacement is not as limiting as it would be in a patient in the adolescent or young adult years.

TRICUSPID VALVE

Today, the tricuspid valve rarely requires replacement except in several extenuating circumstances. Carcinoid involvement and endocarditis are probably the two most common situations where replacement of the tricuspid valve is required. Rheumatic fever involving the tricuspid valve in the United States is quite rare. Most tricuspid lesions are regurgitant. They are functional,

secondary to left-sided lesions, and respond very well to anuloplasty. The anuloplasty reduces the dilated anulus to a more normal diameter recreating leaflet coaptation. There are several techniques for this and the importance is to recreate the leaflet overlap to achieve competence.

Ruptured chordae do occur in the tricuspid valve but are quite infrequent, and the repair in this situation is identical to the mitral repair.

Another situation that is becoming more frequent for tricuspid valve surgery and requires replacement is significant dilatation from long-standing tricuspid regurgitation and even more frequently from device trapping or tethering of the leaflets. More frequently

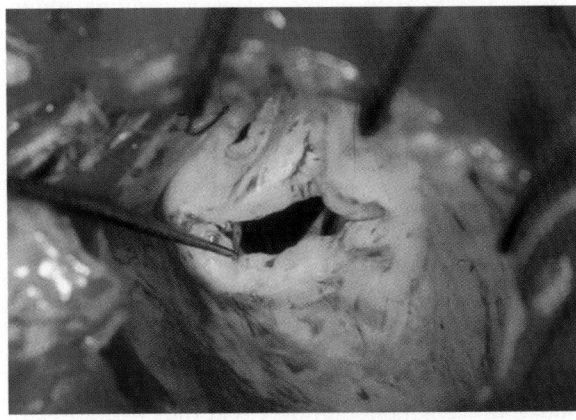

Fig. 8. Rheumatic mitral valve disease. Extensive scarring and deformity preclude surgical repair.

patients with pacemakers or ICDs that have leads crossing the tricuspid valve will cause limitation of motion of the leaflets and lead to severe tricuspid regurgitation. Occasionally, these leads can be positioned at the commissures without causing regurgitation; however, occasionally the leaflets become fused to the lead and require valve replacement. In this situation, the leads are exteriorized outside the prosthesis at the time of valve replacement. More frequently, tissue valves are used for this location as they have a much lower incidence of thrombosis and they also will allow a pacemaker lead to be passed through them should the need arise.

A general statement can be made about today's cardiology practice. Echocardiography has provided a window through which valvular disease can be accurately evaluated to provide patients with an earlier surgical treatment especially when the valve is repairable. When a valve is less likely repairable, further medical treatment is a better option than implanting a prosthesis unless the symptoms warrant intervention.

VALVE CHOICE

Discussions about valve choice can be distilled into two basic categories: mechanical valve vs. bioprosthesis. Both types are extremely functional; neither is perfect. The choice basically is life-long anticoagulation with warfarin with a mechanical valve vs. the greater need for repeat operation with a bioprosthesis. The latest generation of bioprostheses can effectively last 12-15 years in adults and longer in patients greater than 65 years of age. There is still a progressive or more rapid rate of deterioration in adolescents and young adults. Although there are many types of mechanical valves, the bileaflet valve has become the best mechanism for replacement. There is bioprosthetic data that, in the aortic position, the bovine pericardial valve is more durable than the porcine although the latest generation of valves is being studied with a randomized study to asses any real difference.

Today, it is critical to involve the patient in choices of valve prostheses. It has historically been said that the younger patients should have a mechanical prosthesis due to the long period of time that they look forward to life and that tissue valves or bioprosthesis should be reserved for the elderly population. Today, people have

much more information when coming for valve surgery, predominantly from the Internet and personal interest, and many patients' lifestyles are very active or involve activities that have an increased risk of injury which these patients are unable or unwilling to give up. This situation provides patients with the choice of a bioprosthesis that allows them to have the most normal life possible. Knowing that they will need a repeat operation is critical in the decision making. In patients who are elective and come to reoperation for deterioration of a bioprosthesis without coronary bypass grafts, operative risk is similar to the initial operation.

In general, aortic valve bioprostheses do not require any form of anticoagulation other than an aspirin a day. The mitral valve prostheses require anticoagulation for at least 6-8 weeks because of the lower rate of blood flow across the prosthesis and the possibility of thrombus forming on the sewing ring. Once the 6-8 weeks period has passed, the anticoagulation can be stopped. Frequently atrial fibrillation will occur post- operatively and anticoagulation needs to be continued until sinus rhythm returns. When patients are in chronic atrial fibrillation a mechanical valve is usually recommended, although this needs to be given thought in the elderly. Aging increases the chance of other illness and possible operative procedures; unsteadiness leads to falls and warfarin may be a double-edged sword in this situation. It is also important for the surgeon to ligate the atrial appendage in these patients to minimize the chance of thrombus formation. Obviously, mechanical valves in either position require early and indefinite anticoagulation. There are several situations that require a bioprosthesis over mechanical prosthesis: any patient who has easy bruising, ulcer disease, or a bleeding dyscrasia for which warfarin is contraindicated. An additional category is women of child-bearing age. A full discussion of anticoagulation in pregnancy is presented in Chapter 79 ("Pregnancy and the Heart"), but suffice it to say that it is easier to carry a pregnancy to delivery with a tissue prosthesis that does not require warfarin.

REOPERATION

In general, the indications for reoperation are similar to primary operation; however, there are some special presentations that need mention. Bioprostheses fail either by calcification of the leaflets and stenosis or by leaflet fatigue and regurgitation. These usually will be diagnosed by yearly surveilence echos. Occasionally, a bioprosthetic leaflet will tear and cause sudden severe regurgitation, an urgent need for reoperation.

Mechanical prostheses have the innate ability to function indefinitely. There are external factors that may cause failure. Thrombosis, endocarditis, and perivalvular leak are the most common failure modes of mechanical prostheses. Patients with valve thrombosis have almost invariably not been adequately anticoagulated for some period of time prior to thrombosis. Some are iatrogenic, stopping warfarin for noncardiac procedures or operations and delaying the reinstitution of anticoagulation. These patients usually present with valve obstruction and are surgical emergencies. Rarely, thrombolysis may be used but is complicated by strokes and recurrences. Other modes of presentation are thromboemboli, which may also occur without valve obstruction.

Endocarditis equally involves mechanical and bioprosthetic valves. Indications for operation in this group include valve dehiscence, valve obstruction due to vegetations, multiple emboli, persistent sepsis despite antibiotic treatment, and staphylococcus or fungal organisms. The recurrence rate is significant in this situation and is higher with early postoperative endocarditis (within 6 weeks).

SECTION V

Aorta and Peripheral Vascular Disease

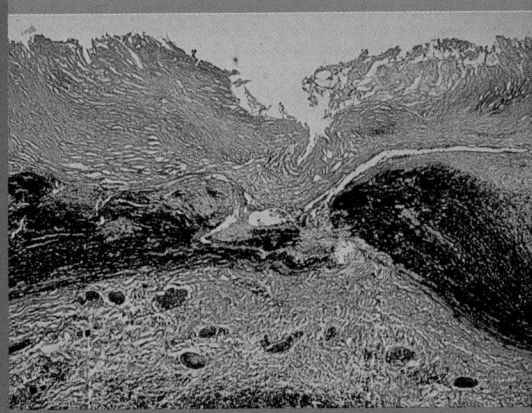

Syphilitic Aortitis

46

PERIPHERAL VASCULAR DISEASE

Peter C. Spittell, MD

CLAUDICATION

The clinical presentation of lower extremity arterial occlusive disease is variable, and includes asymptomatic patients (or patients with atypical symptoms), intermittent claudication, and critical limb ischemia (rest pain, ulceration, gangrene). The degree of functional limitation varies depending on the degree of arterial stenosis, collateral circulation, exercise capacity, and comorbid conditions. The discomfort of intermittent claudication (aching, cramping, or tightness) is always exercise-induced, may involve one or both legs, and occurs at a fairly constant walking distance. Relief is obtained by *standing still*. Supine ankle:brachial systolic pressure indices (ABI) before and after treadmill exercise testing can confirm the diagnosis (Table 1). Furthermore, a low ABI is associated with an increased risk of stroke, cardiovascular death, and all-cause mortality.

PSEUDOCLAUDICATION

Pseudoclaudication is caused by lumbar spinal stenosis and is the condition most commonly confused with intermittent claudication. Pseudoclaudication is usually described as a "paresthetic" discomfort that occurs with standing and walking (variable distances). Symptoms almost always are bilateral and relieved by sitting and/or leaning forward. The patient often has a history

Table 1. Grading System for Lower Extremity Occlusive Arterial Disease*

Grade	Supine resting ABI	Post-exercise ABI
Normal	> 1.0	No change or increase
Mild disease	0.8-0.9	> 0.5
Moderate disease	0.5-0.8	> 0.2
Severe disease	< 0.5	< 0.2

ABI, ankle:brachial systolic pressure index.
*After treadmill exercise (1-2 mph, 10% grade, 5 minutes or symptom-limited) or active pedal plantar-flexion (50 repetitions or symptom-limited).

of chronic back pain or previous lumbosacral spinal surgery. The diagnosis of lumbar spinal stenosis can be confirmed by characteristic findings on computed tomography (CT) or magnetic resonance imaging (MRI) of the lumbar spine and electromyography (EMG) (Table 2), together with normal or minimally abnormal ABIs before and after exercise.

■ The discomfort of intermittent claudication is always exercise-induced.

585

Table 2. Differential Diagnosis of True Claudication and Pseudoclaudication

Feature	Claudication	Pseudoclaudication
Onset	Walking	Standing and walking
Character	Cramp, ache	"Paresthetic"
Bilateral	+/-	+
Walking distance	Fairly constant	More variable
Cause	Atherosclerosis	Spinal stenosis
Relief	Standing still	Sitting down, leaning forward

■ Pseudoclaudication is usually described as a "paresthetic" discomfort that occurs with standing as well as walking.

NATURAL HISTORY OF PERIPHERAL VASCULAR DISEASE

Peripheral arterial occlusive disease is associated with considerable mortality because of its association with coronary and carotid atherosclerosis. The 5-year mortality rate in patients with intermittent claudication is 29%, and the overall amputation rate over 5 years is 4%. More than half of patients have stable or improved symptoms over this same period. Continued use of tobacco results in a 10-fold increase in the risk for major amputation and a more than 2-fold increase in mortality. The effect of diabetes mellitus on patients with intermittent claudication deserves special mention, as it accounts for the majority of amputations in a community (12-fold increased risk of below-knee amputation and a cumulative risk of major amputation exceeding 11% over 25 years). Other clinical features that predict an increased risk of limb loss in lower extremity arterial occlusive disease include ischemic rest pain, ischemic ulceration, and gangrene.

The location of occlusive arterial disease also affects overall prognosis. Patients with aortoiliac disease have a lower 5-year survival rate (73%) than those with predominantly femoral artery disease (80%). The increased mortality is attributable primarily to complications of coronary artery disease. Diabetes mellitus in combination with femoral artery disease results in a further decrease in overall survival and an increased incidence of major amputation. Patients with diabetes mellitus, particularly type II diabetes mellitus, have a distinct pattern and distribution of atherosclerosis in the lower extremity arteries. Compared to nondiabetics, there is less involvement of the aortoiliac segment, equal occurrence in the femoropopliteal segments, and more extensive disease in the infrapopliteal segments (tibial and peroneal arteries) (Fig. 1).

Occlusive arterial disease in other locations (e.g., the subclavian artery) is also important, especially in patients being considered for a coronary artery bypass graft and in those who have recurrent angina after having a left internal mammary artery-left anterior descending coronary artery bypass. Stenting of subclavian stenoses may improve myocardial perfusion in patients with internal mammary artery grafts and flow-limiting proximal subclavian stenoses (i.e coronary steal).

■ The 5-year mortality rate in patients with intermittent claudication is 29%, predominantly due to associated coronary atherosclerosis.

■ Tobacco use, diabetes mellitus, and critical limb

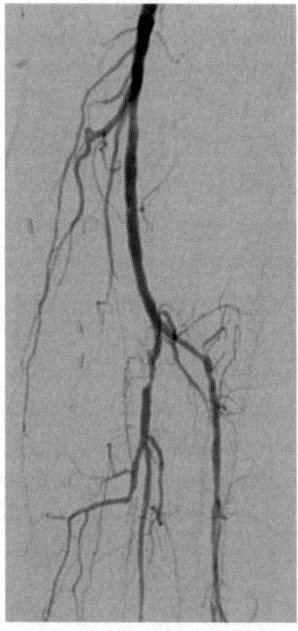

Fig. 1. Angiogram demonstrating the characteristic infrapopliteal location of arterial disease in a diabetic patient.

ischemia (ischemic rest pain, ulceration, and gangrene) are associated with an increased risk of limb loss in patients with intermittent claudication.

DIAGNOSIS OF PERIPHERAL VASCULAR DISEASE

Peripheral angiography is not needed to diagnose intermittent claudication. The diagnosis is made clinically and confirmed by noninvasive testing (ABI before and after exercise). A ratio of the ankle systolic pressure to the brachial systolic pressure (ABI) at rest provides a measurement of disease severity in patients with lower extremity arterial occlusive disease: normal 1.0-1.4, mild disease 0.8-0.9, moderate disease 0.5-0.8, severe disease <0.5. Angiography is indicated for 1) defining vessel anatomy preoperatively, 2) evaluating therapy, and 3) documenting disease (medicolegal issue). It is also indicated when an "uncommon type" of arterial disease is suspected. Magnetic resonance angiography and CT angiography are alternatives to standard angiography; MR angiography is also useful in preoperative planning in patients with contraindications to invasive angiography (i.e., renal insufficiency and/or allergy to contrast media) (Fig. 2).

■ The diagnosis of intermittent claudication is made clinically and confirmed by noninvasive testing (ABI before and after exercise).

TREATMENT OF PERIPHERAL VASCULAR DISEASE

Initial medical management of intermittent claudication involves three modalities: risk factor reduction, exercise training, and pharmacologic therapy. In addition, weight reduction (if obese), foot care and protection, and avoidance of vasoconstrictive drugs are of benefit. Foot care and protection are of paramount importance in diabetic patients with peripheral arterial disease. The combination of peripheral neuropathy, small vessel disease, and/or peripheral arterial disease in diabetic patients make foot trauma more likely to be associated with a nonhealing wound or ulcer.

All patients with peripheral arterial disease should be prescribed an antiplatelet agent. Aspirin (81-325

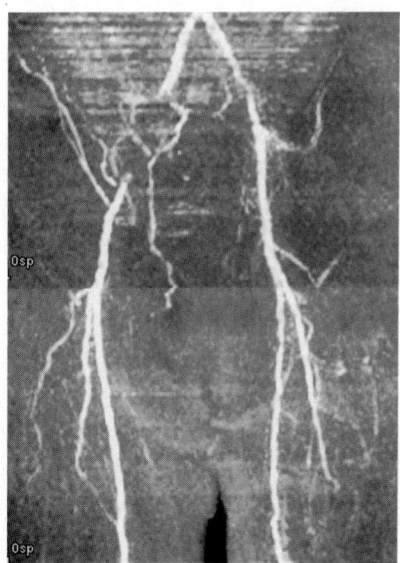

Fig. 2. Magnetic resonance angiography demonstrating high-grade stenosis of left common iliac artery and occlusion of right external iliac artery, with collateral formation.

mg/d) is effective in peripheral arterial disease, resulting in a decreased risk of limb loss and reduced need for vascular surgery, as well as a decreased incidence of major coronary and cerebrovascular events. Clopidogrel (75 mg/d) has been shown to be more effective than aspirin in preventing major atherosclerotic vascular events.

Exercise training is effective in intermittent claudication. A regular walking program (level ground, walking the distance to claudication, stopping to rest for relief, repeatedly for 45-60 minutes per session, four or more days a week, continued for 6 months) can result in a significant (often greater than 180%) improvement in initial claudication distance in many patients. For those who do not adequately respond to a walking program, cilostazol may be useful. Cilostazol, a phosphodiesterase III inhibitor, results in a more significant improvement in walking ability (an approximate doubling of initial and absolute claudication distance), compared to placebo and pentoxifylline. Statins should be considered in patients with peripheral arterial disease and may improve the symptoms of intermittent claudication, as well as reduce the incidence of adverse cardiovascular and cerebrovascular events. Angiotensin-converting enzyme inhibitors also reduce the risk of ischemic cardiovascular events in patients with peripheral arterial disease, in addition to their nephroprotective effects in diabetic patients.

Indications for revascularization (endovascular or surgical) in a patient with peripheral occlusive arterial disease are "disabling" (lifestyle-limiting) symptoms, diabetes mellitus with progressive symptoms, or critical limb ischemia (rest pain, ischemic ulceration, or gangrene).

Revascularization is elective in nondiabetic patients with intermittent claudication because 1) it does not improve coronary artery or cerebrovascular disease, the major causes of mortality, and consequently does not affect overall long-term survival and 2) the incidence of severe limb-threatening ischemia is relatively low because distal runoff is usually adequate.

Revascularization in patients with rest pain or ischemic ulceration or in those with diabetes mellitus with progressive symptoms is indicated because 1) the incidence of limb loss is increased without revascularization, 2) surgery may permit a lower anatomical level of amputation, and 3) the risks of the procedure are generally less than the risk of amputation.

Percutaneous transluminal angioplasty (PTA) is an effective alternative to surgical therapy in patients with short, partial occlusions and good distal runoff. The "ideal" lesion for PTA is an iliac stenosis less than 5 cm or a femoropopliteal occlusion or stenosis less than 10 cm in total length (excluding lesions involving the origin of the superficial femoral artery and those affecting the distal 2 cm of the popliteal artery). Advantages of PTA over surgery include less morbidity, shorter convalescence, lower cost, and preservation of the saphenous vein for future use. PTA in aortic or iliac disease may also allow for an infrainguinal surgical procedure to be performed at reduced perioperative risk (as compared with intra-abdominal aortic surgery).

Placement of an iliac stent when the hemodynamic results of PTA are inadequate or primary stent placement at the time of initial PTA is being used as treatment in an increasing number of patients (Fig. 3). A randomized trial of 279 patients with intermittent claudication with an iliac artery stenosis greater than 50% (proven by angiography) compared direct stent placement to primary angioplasty, with subsequent stent placement only in cases of residual gradient. The difference in the clinical outcomes between the two treatment

strategies was not significant at either short-term or long-term follow-up.

■ Diabetes mellitus with progressive symptoms, rest pain, ischemic ulceration, and gangrene are all associated with an increased risk of limb loss in patients with lower extremity arterial occlusive disease. The presence of these features warrants angiography followed by revascularization (endovascular or surgical).

Renal artery stenosis is discussed in the chapter on hypertension.

ACUTE ARTERIAL OCCLUSION

The symptoms of acute arterial occlusion are sudden in onset (<5 hours) and include the "5 Ps": pain, pallor, paresthesia (numbness), poikilothermy (coldness), and pulselessness (absence of peripheral pulses).

Features that suggest a *thrombotic* cause of acute arterial occlusion include previous occlusive disease in the involved limb, occlusive disease involving other extremities, acute aortic dissection, hematologic disease, arteritis, inflammatory bowel disease, neoplasm, and ergotism.

An *embolic* cause of acute arterial occlusion is suggested by the presence of ischemic or valvular heart disease, atrial fibrillation, proximal aneurysm, or atherosclerotic disease.

After confirmation by angiography, the initial therapeutic options for acute arterial occlusion include intra-arterial thrombolysis and surgical therapy (thromboembolectomy). If thrombolytic therapy is used, PTA or surgical therapy is often required subsequently to treat the underlying stenosis (if present) to improve long-term patency rates.

■ The "5 Ps" suggestive of acute arterial occlusion include pain, pallor, paresthesia, poikilothermy, and pulselessness.

ANEURYSMS

Because aneurysms are caused most commonly by atherosclerosis, they are more common in men 60 years or older. Coronary artery and carotid artery occlusive disease are frequent comorbid conditions. Other predisposing

A
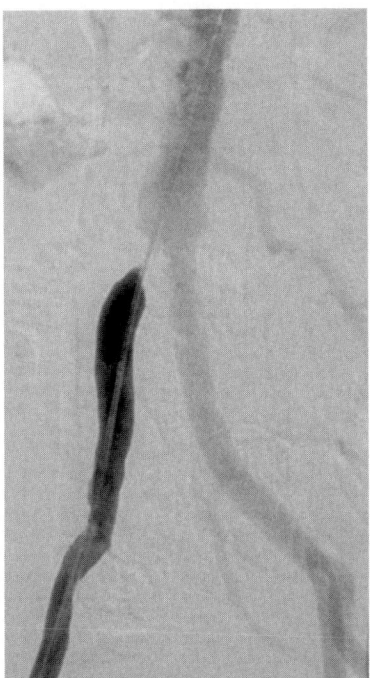

B
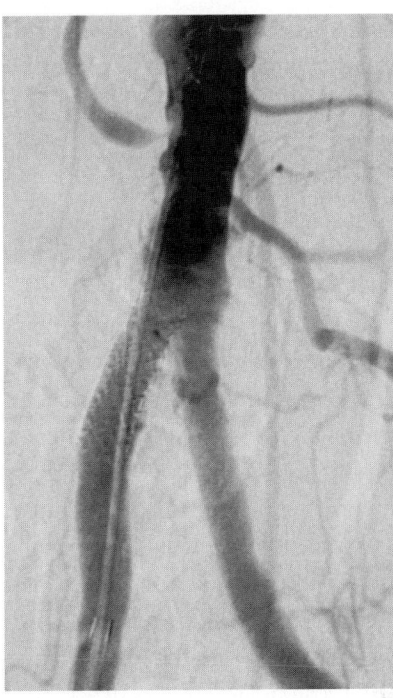

Fig. 3. Angiogram demonstrating >95% stenosis of right common iliac artery before (*A*) and after (*B*) percutaneous transluminal angioplasty and stent placement.

factors for aneurysmal disease include hypertension, familial tendency, connective tissue disease, trauma, infection, and inflammatory disease.

Most aneurysms are asymptomatic. Complications of aneurysms include embolization, pressure on surrounding structures, infection, and rupture. Aneurysms of certain arteries develop specific complications more often than other complications. For example, the most common complication of aortic aneurysms is rupture, and a common complication of femoral and popliteal artery aneurysms is embolism. Aortic aneurysms are discussed in the chapter on the aorta.

An iliac artery aneurysm usually occurs in association with an abdominal aortic aneurysm, but it may occur as an isolated finding. Iliac artery aneurysms may cause atheroembolism, obstructive urologic symptoms, unexplained groin or perineal pain, or iliac vein obstruction. CT with intravenous contrast agent or MRI is the preferred diagnostic procedure. Surgical resection is indicated when an iliac artery aneurysm is symptomatic or larger than 3 cm in diameter.

Popliteal artery aneurysms can be complicated by

thrombosis, venous obstruction, embolization, popliteal neuropathy, popliteal thrombophlebitis, rupture, and infection. They are bilateral in 50% of patients, and 40% of patients have one or more aneurysms at other sites, usually of the abdominal aorta. The diagnosis is readily made with ultrasonography, but angiography is necessary before surgical treatment to evaluate the proximal and distal arterial circulation. When a popliteal aneurysm is diagnosed, surgical therapy is the treatment of choice to prevent serious thromboembolic complications.

UNCOMMON TYPES OF OCCLUSIVE ARTERIAL DISEASE

The clinical features that suggest an uncommon type of peripheral occlusive arterial disease include young age, acute ischemia without a history of occlusive arterial disease, and involvement of only the upper extremity or digits. Uncommon types of occlusive arterial disease include thromboangiitis obliterans, arteritis associated with connective tissue disease, giant cell arteritis (cranial and Takayasu disease), and occlusive arterial disease due to blunt trauma or arterial entrapment.

THROMBOANGIITIS OBLITERANS (BUERGER DISEASE)

The diagnostic clinical criteria for thromboangiitis obliterans (Buerger disease) are listed in Table 3. More definitive diagnosis of thromboangiitis obliterans requires angiography, which usually reveals multiple, bilateral focal segments of stenosis or occlusion with normal proximal vessels (Fig. 4). Treatment of thromboangiitis obliterans is the same as for other types of occlusive peripheral arterial disease, but particular emphasis is placed on the need for permanent abstinence from all forms of tobacco. Smoking cessation ameliorates the course of the disease but does not invariably stop further exacerbations. Abstinence from tobacco also substantially reduces the risk of ulcer formation and amputation. Because the arteries involved are small, arterial reconstruction for ischemia in patients with Buerger disease is technically challenging. Distal arterial reconstruction, if necessary, is indicated to prevent ischemic limb loss. Collateral artery bypass

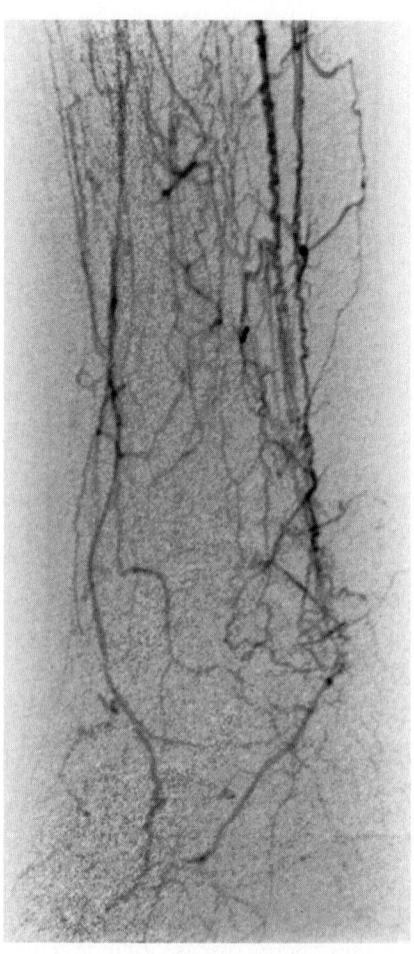

Fig. 4. Angiogram of patient with thromboangiitis obliterans showing characteristic abrupt occlusions, segmental stenoses, and "corkscrew" collaterals of infrapopliteal arteries.

is an option when the main arteries are affected by the disease. A patent but diseased artery should be avoided as a target for reconstruction. Sympathectomy may be useful in severe digital ischemia with ulceration to control pain and to improve cutaneous blood flow. Therapeutic angiogenesis with VEGF gene transfer may be beneficial in patients with advanced Buerger disease that is unresponsive to standard medical or surgical treatment methods.

POPLITEAL ARTERY ENTRAPMENT

Popliteal artery entrapment (PAE) occurs most often in young men and produces intermittent claudication in the arch of the foot or calf. If the popliteal artery is

Table 3.   Diagnostic Criteria for Thromboangiitis Obliterans

Age	<40 years (often <30 years)
Sex	Males most often
Habits	Tobacco
History	Superficial phlebitis
	Claudication, arch or calf
	Raynaud phenomenon
Examination	Small arteries involved
	Upper extremity involved (positive Allen test)
Laboratory results	Normal glucose, blood cell count, erythrocyte sedimentation rate, lipids, and screening tests for connective tissue disease
Radiography	No arterial calcification

not already occluded, the finding of diminished pedal pulses with sustained active pedal plantar flexion should increase suspicion of the disorder. Diagnosis is made by demonstrating with contrast or magnetic resonance angiography medial displacement of the popliteal artery from its normal position in the popliteal space. MRA is particularly useful when the popliteal artery is occluded, in which case angiography is of limited value. Angiographic findings in PAE include irregularity of the wall of the popliteal artery in an otherwise normal arterial tree, often associated with prestenotic or poststenotic dilatation. If the artery is still patent, medial displacement of the popliteal artery from its normal position in the popliteal space and popliteal artery compression with extension of the knee and dorsiflexion of the foot are diagnostic angiographic findings. If the mechanism of compression is by the plantaris or popliteal muscle, the position of the artery may appear normal on angiography. If PAE has been diagnosed in one limb, the contralateral limb should be screened because bilateral disease occurs in more than 25% of patients.

Management of PAE depends on the clinical presentation and anatomical findings. Surgery (release of the artery from the entrapping muscle and appropriate reconstruction of an occluded or aneurysmal popliteal artery) has been advocated to prevent progression of the disease from repetitive arterial trauma; furthermore, detection and treatment of PAE at an early stage appear to permit better long-term results.

THORACIC OUTLET COMPRESSION SYNDROME

Compression of the subclavian artery in the thoracic outlet (thoracic outlet compression syndrome) can occur at several points, but the most common site of compression is in the costoclavicular space between the uppermost rib (cervical rib or first rib) and the clavicle. If the person is symptomatic, the presentation may be any of the following: Raynaud phenomenon in one or more fingers of the ipsilateral hand, digital cyanosis or ulceration, and "claudication" of the arm or forearm. Occlusive arterial disease in the affected arm or hand is readily detected on examination of the arterial pulses and by the Allen test. Compression of the subclavian artery in the thoracic outlet can be demonstrated by

noting a decreased or absent pulse in the ipsilateral radial artery during performance of thoracic outlet maneuvers. The diagnosis is confirmed by duplex ultrasonography, magnetic resonance angiography, or angiography, with the involved arm in the neutral and hyperabducted position. Treatment of symptomatic or complicated thoracic outlet compression of the subclavian artery includes surgical resection of the uppermost rib.

■ Compression of the subclavian artery in the thoracic outlet can be demonstrated by noting a decreased or absent pulse in the ipsilateral radial artery during performance of the thoracic outlet maneuvers.

It is important to remember that all the connective tissue disorders and giant cell arteritides can involve peripheral arteries, and symptoms of peripheral arterial involvement may dominate the clinical picture. Other than the conservative measures already discussed for ischemic limbs, therapy is directed mainly at the underlying disease. Only after the inflammatory process is controlled should surgical revascularization of chronically ischemic extremities be performed.

HEPARIN-INDUCED THROMBOCYTOPENIA

Heparin-induced thrombocytopenia affects between 5% and 10% of patients who receive heparin therapy, but the incidence of arterial and/or venous thrombosis is less than 1% or 2%. Heparin-induced thrombocytopenia (type II) typically occurs 5 to 14 days after heparin exposure and is associated with arterial thrombosis (arterial occlusion, ischemic strokes, myocardial infarction) and venous thrombosis (pulmonary embolism, phlegmasia cerulea dolens [venous gangrene], and sagittal sinus thrombosis). The diagnosis of heparin-induced thrombocytopenia is primarily clinical—occurrence of thrombocytopenia during heparin therapy, resolution of thrombocytopenia when heparin therapy is discontinued, and exclusion of other causes of thrombocytopenia—and can be confirmed by demonstration in vitro of a heparin-dependent platelet antibody. Treatment of type II heparin-induced thrombocytopenia includes discontinuation of all forms of heparin exposure (subcutaneous, intravenous, or heparin flushes and heparin-coated catheters) and institution of alternative anticoagulation (thrombin inhibitors or heparinoids).

VASOSPASTIC DISORDERS

Vasospastic disorders are characterized by episodic color changes of the skin resulting from intermittent spasm of the small arteries and arterioles of the skin and digits. Vasospastic disorders are important because they frequently are a clue to another underlying disorder, such as occlusive arterial disease, connective tissue disorders, neurologic disorders, or endocrine disease. Vasospastic disorders also can appear as side effects of drug therapy, specifically of ergot preparations, estrogen replacement therapy, and certain β-blockers.

RAYNAUD PHENOMENON

When Raynaud phenomenon is present, several clinical features can help differentiate primary Raynaud disease from secondary Raynaud phenomenon, as indicated in Table 4.

Primary Raynaud disease is more common in women than men, and its onset usually is before age 40 years. Episodes are characterized by triphasic color changes (white, blue, red). Symptoms are usually bilateral and often symmetric and precipitated by emotion or exposure to cold. Ischemic or gangrenous changes are not present. The absence of any causal condition and the presence of symptoms for at least 2 years are also required for the diagnosis. Raynaud disease is a benign condition, with treatment emphasizing protection from cold exposure and other vasoconstrictive influences. Occasionally, a patient with severe symptoms not controlled by local measures may benefit from a low dose of nifedipine or a β-blocker.

Secondary Raynaud phenomenon affects men more often than women, and in most patients the onset is after age 40 years. It is usually unilateral or asymmetric at onset. Associated pulse deficits, ischemic changes, and systemic signs and symptoms are often present. Identification of the underlying cause is basic to appropriate treatment for secondary Raynaud phenomenon.

The initial laboratory evaluation in a patient with Raynaud phenomenon includes complete blood count, erythrocyte sedimentation rate, urinalysis, serum protein electrophoresis, and antinuclear antibody test and tests for cryoglobulin, cryofibrinogen, and cold agglutinins and chest radiography to detect disorders not identified by the medical history and physical examination.

- Primary Raynaud disease is more common in women than men, and its onset usually is before age 40 years.
- Secondary Raynaud phenomenon affects men more often than women, and, in most patients, the onset is after age 40 years.

LIVEDO RETICULARIS

Livedo reticularis, the bluish mottling of the skin in a lacy reticular pattern, is caused by spasm or occlusion of dermal arterioles. Primary livedo reticularis is idiopathic and not associated with an identifiable underlying disorder. Secondary livedo reticularis is suggested by an abrupt severe onset of symptoms, ischemic changes, and systemic symptoms. Most commonly, it is the result of embolism of atheromatous debris from a proximal aneurysm or from proximal atheromatous plaques. The appearance of livedo reticularis in a patient older than 50 years should suggest the possibility of atheroembolism. Other causes of secondary livedo reticularis include connective tissue disease, vasculitis, myeloproliferative disorders, dysproteinemias, reflex sympathetic dystrophy, cold injury, and as a side effect of amantadine hydrochloride (Symmetrel) therapy.

Table 4.   Comparison of Primary and Secondary Raynaud Phenomenon

Feature	Raynaud phenomenon	
	Primary	Secondary
Age at onset	<40 yr	>40 yr
Sex	Women	Men
Bilateral	+	+/-
Symmetric	+	+/-
Toes involved	+	-
Ischemic changes	-	+
Systemic manifestations	-	+

■ The appearance of livedo reticularis in a patient older than 50 years should suggest the possibility of atheroembolism.

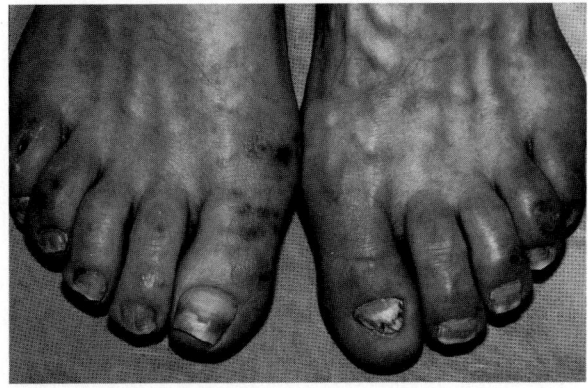

Fig. 5. Characteristic lesions of chronic pernio.

CHRONIC PERNIO

Chronic pernio is a vasospastic disorder characterized by sensitivity to cold in patients (usually women) with a past history of cold injury. Chronic pernio presents with symmetric blueness of the toes in the autumn and clearing in the spring (Fig. 5). Without treatment, the cyanosis may be accompanied by blistering of the skin of the affected toes. The cyanosis is relieved within a few days after initiating treatment with an α-blocker, which can then be used to prevent recurrences.

ERYTHROMELALGIA

Erythromelalgia is the occurrence of red, hot, painful burning fingers or toes (or both) on exposure to warm temperatures or following exercise. It is not a vasospastic disorder but is associated with color change of the skin. It may be primary (idiopathic) or be secondary to an underlying disorder, most commonly myeloproliferative disease, diabetes mellitus, or small fiber neuropathy. Treatment of the primary form includes avoidance of exposure to warm temperatures, aspirin, and a β-blocker (nonselective), which is helpful in some patients. In persons with secondary erythromelalgia, treatment of the underlying disorder usually relieves the symptoms.

RESOURCES

Hirsch AT, Haskal ZJ, Hertzer NR, et al. ACC/AHA 2005 Guidelines for the Management of Patients With Peripheral Arterial Disease (Lower Extremity, Renal, Mesenteric, and Abdominal Aortic): Executive Summary. J Am Coll Cardiol. 2006;47: 1239-1312.

47

Cerebrovascular Disease and Carotid Stenting

Peter C. Spittell, MD

David R. Holmes, Jr, MD

Carotid Artery Disease

Carotid artery disease is common in patients with coronary artery disease and has a wide spectrum of clinical presentations (asymptomatic carotid bruit, transient ischemic attack, or stroke). Stroke is the leading cause of disability in adults in the United States and is the third leading cause of death. There are approximately 750,000 new or recurrent strokes each year and 150,000 deaths and population-based studies have indicated an increase in incidence over the past 20 years as the population continues to age.

An asymptomatic carotid bruit is present in approximately 13% of the population and increases in population occurrence with age. Patients with asymptomatic carotid bruits are at greater risk for cerebral ischemic events than the general population and have a higher overall mortality, *primarily due to complications of coronary artery disease*. In asymptomatic patients, the annual risk of stroke is strongly related to the severity of stenosis, being <1% for stenoses <60% and increasing to 3-5% for stenoses >80%. For symptomatic patients, the annual stroke risk is higher than for asymptomatic patients but is also dependent upon stenosis severity. In addition, stroke risk is highest immediately after an initial ischemic event.

TIA is defined as a focal loss of brain function attributed to cerebral ischemia lasting less than 24 hours and localized to a limited region of the brain (Tables 1-3). Stroke is a permanent neurologic deficit. Generally, only 40% of thrombotic strokes are preceded by a TIA. Among patients with a TIA who do not die of another cause within 5 years, one-third will have a stroke, 20% of which occur within the first month after the TIA and 50% within the first year.

- An asymptomatic carotid bruit is present in approximately 13% of the population and increases in population occurrence with age.
- Carotid stenosis severity   1-year risk of TIA/stroke
  <60%   <1%
  >80%   3-5%

Table 1. Clinical Features of Transient Cerebral Ischemia (Transient Ischemic Attack)

Short-term symptoms—minutes to <24 hours
Rapid onset
Spontaneous occurrence
Focal neurologic signs
Patient is conscious
Patient has normal examination between attacks

Table 2. Features of a Transient Ischemic
Attack in the Territory of the Carotid
Artery

Monoparesis or hemiparesis
Numbness (unilateral)
Impaired vision (unilateral)
Aphasia, dominant hemisphere
Carotid bruit
Retinal findings (cholesterol emboli)

Table 3. Features of a Transient Ischemic
Attack in the Territory of the
Vertebrobasilar Arterial System

Limb paresis
Drop attacks
Numbness (limbs and face)
Impaired vision (diplopia or bilateral visual field
  defects)
Vertigo, nausea
Dysarthria
Ataxia

CAUSES OF STROKE

Cardioembolic causes of stroke include intracardiac thrombus, intracardiac mass lesions, valvular heart disease, infectious endocarditis, and paradoxic emboli. Other common causes of stroke are large vessel occlusive disease (ascending aorta, aortic arch, major branches of the cerebrovascular circulation) and small vessel disease (diabetes mellitus, hypertension, arteritis). Carotid atherosclerosis can produce symptoms by either embolization of thrombus or plaque debris or because of hypoperfusion. Less common causes include hematologic disease (polycythemia vera, thrombocytosis, leukemia, thrombophilia, antiphospholipid antibody syndromes, cryoglobulinemia, paraproteinemia), and rare causes are air and fat emboli, cortical vein thrombosis, and global hypoperfusion. Risk factors for stroke include hypertension, diabetes mellitus, hyperlipidemia, cigarette smoking, and excessive use of alcohol.

NONINVASIVE IMAGING

Given the dire consequences of stroke and the fact that stroke may not be preceded by warning symptoms or signs such as transient ischemic attack, there has been great interest in predicting and identifying patients at risk. Identification of carotid artery stenosis has been an important component of this process.

Noninvasive evaluation of a carotid bruit includes oculoplethysmography (OPG) or duplex ultrasonography. OPG measures ocular arterial pressure and is an indirect method of determining whether a hemodynamically significant stenosis is present in the ipsilateral carotid artery. Persons with an asymptomatic carotid bruit and abnormal oculoplethysmographic result have a twofold greater risk of stroke over 3 years compared to an age-matched normal population. Limitations of oculoplethysmography include its inability to further localize disease and contraindications in patients with glaucoma or previous ophthalmologic surgery.

Duplex ultrasonography (two-dimensional, pulsed-wave Doppler and color flow Doppler imaging) is able to provide both anatomic and hemodynamic information about the extracranial carotid artery and is the noninvasive test of choice in the initial evaluation of a patient with a carotid bruit or cerebral ischemic symptoms. Duplex ultrasonography can be used to quantify the severity of a carotid artery stenosis into categories of diameter reduction and also permits qualitative estimates of the degree of plaque and its location. Evaluation of the subclavian arteries for evidence of occlusive disease or aneurysmal disease and of the vertebral arteries for vessel patency and direction of flow is also possible with ultrasonography.

ANGIOGRAPHY

Magnetic resonance angiography (MRA) can accurately diagnose extracranial carotid artery disease and provide details about intracerebral arterial anatomy. MRA is primarily indicated for patients with symptomatic carotid artery disease to further characterize the internal carotid disease as well as to exclude intracerebral and arterial occlusive disease before carotid endarterectomy. Standard angiography is generally indicated before carotid endarterectomy to define precisely the extent of the extracranial carotid artery disease as well as to determine whether there is associated intracerebral arterial occlusive disease when the results of the MRA are inconclusive (Fig. 1). Angiography is associated with a stroke risk of about 1%.

CAROTID ENDARTERECTOMY

Carotid endarterectomy is superior to medical therapy for patients with symptomatic carotid artery disease and a high-grade stenosis. This includes carotid territory or retinal TIAs or nondisabling stroke with an ipsilateral high-grade carotid artery stenosis (70% to 99%). Medical therapy is better for persons with mild carotid artery stenosis (0% to 29%), even when symptomatic. The treatment of patients with moderate carotid artery stenosis (30% to 59%) is controversial and must be individualized.

VETERANS ADMINISTRATION TRIAL

The Veterans Administration study of 444 males with asymptomatic carotid stenosis greater than 50% on angiography demonstrated that carotid endarterectomy in combination with medical therapy reduced the incidence of ipsilateral neurologic events to 8% (over a

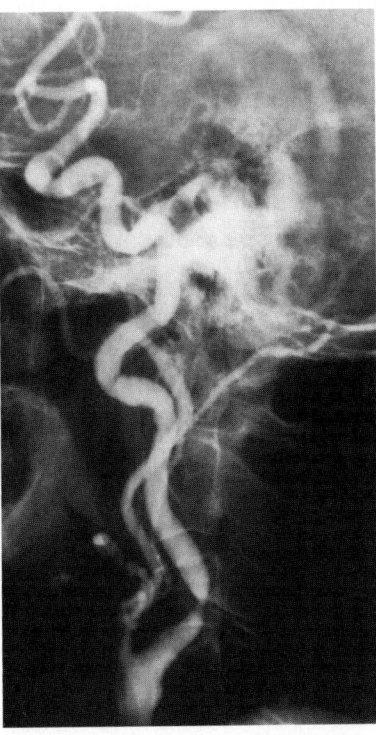

Fig. 1. Cerebral angiogram demonstrating severe stenosis of proximal right internal carotid artery.

mean follow-up of 4 years) in comparison with a 21% event rate with medical therapy alone. However, the combined end point risk of stroke and death was not statistically reduced in this study, emphasizing the need for individualized patient management, because most persons die of their associated coronary artery disease. It should be noted that lowering low-density lipoprotein cholesterol levels with statin medication reduces the stroke risk in patients with coronary artery disease.

- Carotid endarterectomy is superior to medical therapy for patients with symptomatic carotid artery disease and a high-grade stenosis.
- Medical therapy is better for persons with mild carotid artery stenosis even when symptomatic.
- Lowering low-density lipoprotein cholesterol levels with statin medication reduces the stroke risk in patients with coronary artery disease.

ASYMPTOMATIC CAROTID ATHEROSCLEROSIS STUDY TRIAL

The Asymptomatic Carotid Atherosclerosis Study (ACAS) demonstrated that carotid endarterectomy is superior to medical therapy (aspirin and reduction of risk factors) in persons with asymptomatic carotid stenosis greater than 60% if their general health is good and the medical center has a documented combined perioperative morbidity and mortality of less than 3%. When the above criteria were met, the aggregate risk for stroke or death over 5 years was 5% in the surgical group and 11% in the medical group. There was a marked gender effect in this study: the resultant 66% relative risk reduction in men was statistically significant, but the comparable risk reduction of 17% in women was not statistically significant.

Currently, the approach to a patient with a symptomatic carotid artery stenosis less than 60% is oral anticoagulation for 3 months, followed by antiplatelet therapy (aspirin, clopidogrel) indefinitely. If warfarin is contraindicated, aspirin should be used throughout.

In a patient requiring coronary artery bypass grafting who has significant carotid artery disease, management needs to be individualized. Available data on this group of patients suggest that carotid endarterectomy (when indicated according to the aforementioned conditions) performed simultaneously with coronary artery bypass grafting results in a lower stroke rate than delayed carotid endarterectomy performed within 2 weeks after the coronary artery surgery.

In summary, carotid endarterectomy is beneficial for symptomatic patients with recent nondisabling carotid artery ischemic events and ipsilateral 70% to 99% carotid artery stenosis. Carotid endarterectomy is not beneficial for symptomatic patients with 0% to 29% stenosis. The potential benefit of carotid endarterectomy for symptomatic patients with 30% to 69% stenosis is uncertain. For asymptomatic patients, guidelines for carotid endarterectomy include surgical risk less than 3% and a life expectancy of at least 5 years in the presence of a carotid artery stenosis greater than 60% or a carotid artery stenosis greater than 60% in patients scheduled to undergo coronary artery bypass grafting. There are no proven indications for carotid endarterectomy for patients with a surgical risk of 3% of more. However, for patients with a surgical risk of 3% to 5%, an acceptable indication for ipsilateral carotid endarterectomy is stenosis of 75% or greater in the presence of contralateral internal carotid artery stenosis of 75% of greater.

Carotid endarterectomy is superior to medical therapy for persons with: symptomatic carotid territory or retinal TIAs or nondisabling stroke and ipsilateral high-grade carotid artery stenosis (70% to 99%). Asymptomatic carotic stenosis greater than 60% if their general health is good and the medical center has a documented combined perioperative morbidity and mortality of less than 3%.

CAROTID ARTERY STENTING

Although the average risk for stroke or death with carotid endarterectomy is 2% to 5%, in high-risk patients it may be as high as 18%. The increased morbidity and mortality of carotid endarterectomy in high-risk patients formed the rationale for the application of carotid arterial stenting. If carotid artery stenting is considered, diagnostic angiography of both carotids is performed with attention to details of the common carotid, external carotid, and internal carotid artery and then evaluation of the intracranial vessels. In some centers, selective vertebral angiography is performed at the same time. During angiography, careful attention must be paid to the ease of access, tortuosity both in the common carotid as well as in the internal carotid, the presence or absence of calcification in the lesion, the presence or absence of a satisfactory landing zone for embolic protection devices. The goals of the procedure are to deliver and then retrieve embolization protection devices, balloon dilatation catheters used to pre-dilate and then post-dilate the stent, and the delivery system itself without the development of neurologic complications.

Access to the common carotid artery is obtained with a variety of long sheaths, usually 6 French or 7 French. A variety of embolic protection devices are available: both proximal and distal protection devices have been tested. The latter are easier to use and accordingly are used more widely. Data suggest that if an embolic protection device cannot be used for any reason, such as lack of a landing zone or severe tortuosity, then carotid artery stenting should not be performed. Typically, after placement of the embolic protection device, pre-dilatation is performed with a small 3.0 to 3.5-mm, 0.014 compatible coronary balloon. Following this, a stent is placed—most commonly a self-expanding stent which typically covers the origin of the external carotid artery. Compromise of this artery is almost always of no clinical consequence. Usually following stent implantation, post-dilatation is performed again using a coronary balloon, usually 5.0 or 5.5 mm, and matching the size to the internal carotid artery distal to the stent site. After this, the embolic protection device is retrieved. Minimizing trauma to the vessel wall and minimizing the duration of the procedure is important to minimize complications. Repeat angiography of the stent and the intracranial vessels is performed prior to termination of the procedure.

Adjunctive therapy is similar to that used for coronary interventions. Anticoagulation is administered in the form of heparin. An ACT of approximately 300 seconds is the target. Pretreatment with aspirin and clopidogrel is routine. If clopidogrel is not given prior to the procedure, 600 mg should be administered. A IIb/IIIa agent is infrequently used. Following the procedure, aspirin and clopidogrel are given orally, the latter for 1-2 months in a dose of 75 mg a day, and aspirin is continued indefinitely. It is important to avoid wide swings in blood pressure during the procedure. Typically, antihypertensive medications are withheld the day of the procedure to avoid significant hypotension.

Multiple registry data sets of carotid stenting have been published indicating a success rate of approximately 96-99%. The SAPPHIRE trial is the only published randomized trial that compares modern carotid endarterectomy with carotid arterial stenting. This trial included a >50% symptomatic carotid stenosis or >80% asymptomatic carotid stenosis. Patients had to have at least one high risk carotid endarterectomy criterion. The 30-day end point of stroke, myocardial infarction, and death was 4.8% with carotid arterial stenting and 9.8% with carotid endarterectomy (p = 0.09). The primary end point of this trial was complex and included a composite of stroke, myocardial infarction, and death within 30 days plus death from neurologic causes or perhaps lateral stroke with 31-100 in 360 days. This was seen in 12.2% of the carotid artery stent group versus 20.1% of the carotid endarterectomy group. A meta-analysis of clinical trials of 1,269 patients treated with either endovascular therapy or carotid endartectomy has documented no difference in stroke or mortality at 30 days, and at one year, no difference between the two treatment strategies in preventing stroke or death.

An important ongoing trial is the carotid revascularization endarterectomy versus stent trial (CREST) which randomizes 1,400 symptomatic patients with carotid stenosis >50% and 1,100 asymptomatic patients with stenosis >60% by angiography or >70% by ultrasound. The primary end point will be stroke, myocardial infarction, death at 30 days, and ipsilateral stroke during follow-up out to 4 years.

Patient selection criteria for carotid artery stenting continue to evolve. At the present time, Medicare reimburses qualified institutions and physicians in symptomatic high-risk surgical patients with ≥70% stenosis or patients enrolled in FDA-sponsored clinical trials.

CEREBRAL EMBOLISM

The identification of atherosclerotic plaque in the thoracic aorta by transesophageal echocardiography is an important finding in patients with cerebral (or systemic) embolic events (Fig. 2). Atherosclerotic plaque thickness greater than 4 mm or mobile thrombus (any size), or both, predicts a high incidence of recurrent embolic events. Many patients with cerebral ischemic events and protruding and mobile atheromas of the thoracic aorta have coexistent carotid artery disease (>70% stenosis), making precise identification of the source of embolism difficult. Treatment in symptomatic patients with no other identifiable source of embolism is surgical resection of the involved aorta, if the patient's general medical condition permits. Oral anticoagulation treatment for 3 months on the presumption that the friable components will have organized, followed by antiplatelet therapy, is an alternative.

■ Many patients with cerebral ischemic events and protruding and mobile atheromas of the thoracic aorta have coexistent carotid artery disease.

SPONTANEOUS DISSECTION OF CEPHALIC ARTERIES

Spontaneous dissection of the cervical cephalic arteries is uncommon but important for two reasons: 1) the clinical presentation is characteristic—either hemicrania with oculosympathetic paresis (Horner's syndrome) or hemicrania with delayed focal cerebral ischemic symptoms and 2) the prognosis is good for recovery, and recurrences are rare.

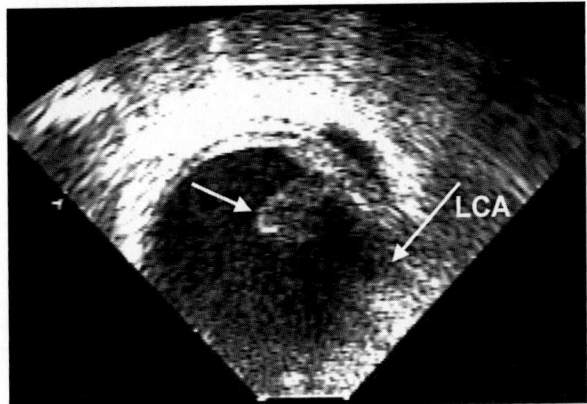

Fig. 2. Transesophageal echocardiography in a patient with recurrent left hemispheric transient ischemic attacks. Transverse view of the distal transverse aortic arch demonstrates large mobile thrombus (*short arrow*) adjacent to origin of the left common carotid artery (LCA).

48

THE AORTA

Peter C. Spittell, MD

AORTIC ATHEROEMBOLISM

Microemboli or macroemboli from atherosclerotic plaque and thrombus in the aorta are important causes of cerebral and systemic embolization. Cerebral atheroembolism suggests the source of embolic material is intracardiac or is in the ascending aorta and/or transverse aortic arch. Lower extremity atheroembolism is caused most commonly by abdominal aortic aneurysm or diffuse atherosclerotic disease. Unilateral blue toes suggest that the embolic source is distal to the aortic bifurcation. Atheroembolism is characterized by livedo reticularis, blue toes, palpable pulses, hypertension, renal insufficiency, increased erythrocyte sedimentation rate, and eosinophilia (transient) (Fig. 1). Atheroembolism can occur spontaneously or be due to medication (warfarin or thrombolytic therapy), or to angiographic or surgical procedures. Thoracic aortic atherosclerotic plaque is most accurately assessed with TEE. Plaque thickness more than 4 mm or mobile thrombus (of any size) are associated with an increased risk of embolism (Fig. 2). Severe aortic atherosclerosis is present in approximately 27% of patients with previous embolic events and is also a strong predictor of coronary artery disease.

Antiplatelet agents and a statin medication should be used in all patients with aortic embolic events unless there are absolute contraindications. Warfarin therapy

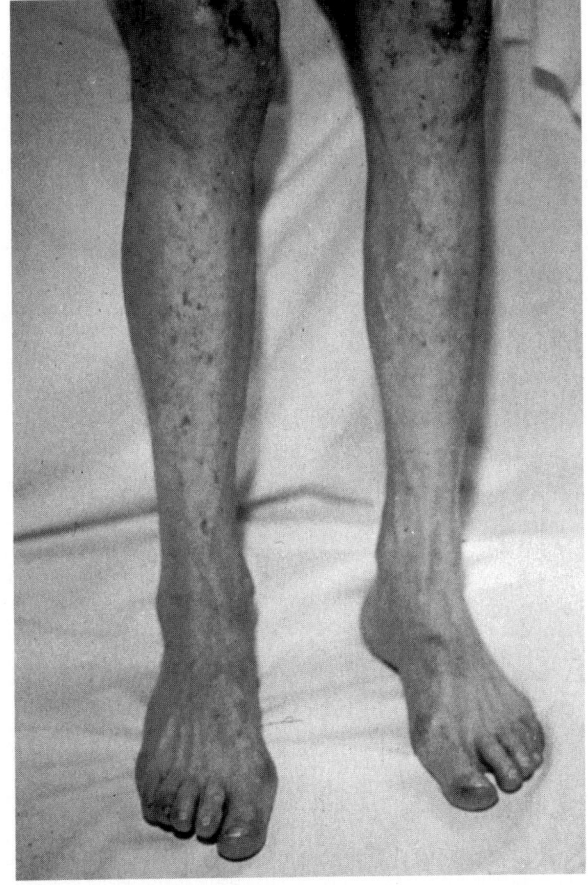

Fig. 1. Livedo reticularis over both patellae and multiple blue toes in a patient with atheroembolism from an abdominal aortic aneurysm.

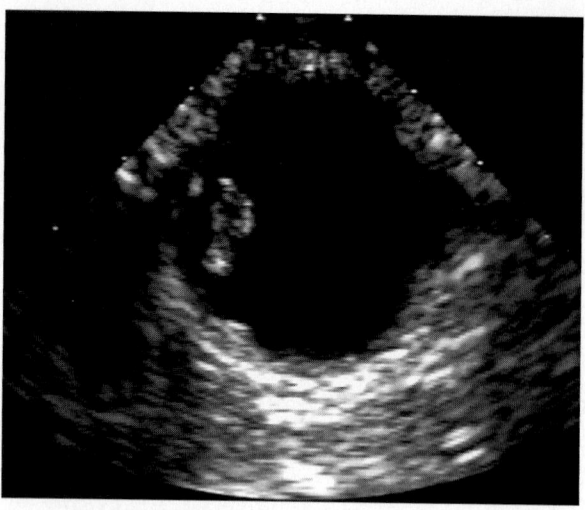

Fig. 2. Transesophageal echocadiography demonstrates advanced immobile atherosclerosis in the descending thoracic aorta.

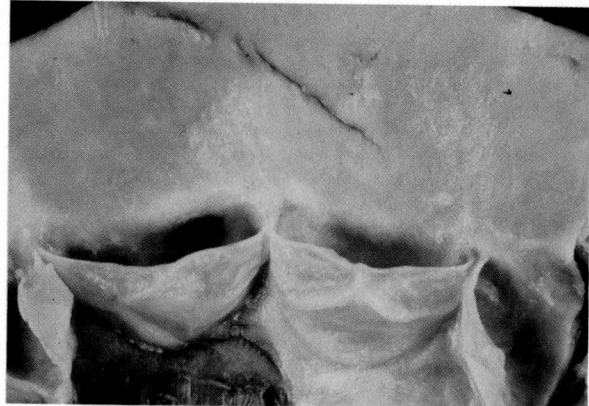

Fig. 3. Gross specimen showing isolated intimal tear of ascending aorta in giant cell aortitis.

may be beneficial for reducing subsequent embolic events, but may also exacerbate embolism in some patients, and further randomized trials are required. The treatment of choice is to identify the source of embolism and, if possible, to surgically resect it.

- Emboli from atherosclerotic plaque and thrombus in the thoracic aorta are important causes of stroke and peripheral emboli.
- Atheroembolism is characterized by livedo reticularis, blue toes, palpable pulses, hypertension, renal insufficiency, increased erythrocyte sedimentation rate, and eosinophilia (transient).

THORACIC AORTIC ANEURYSMS

Thoracic aortic aneurysms are caused most commonly by atherosclerosis, but they also occur in patients with systemic hypertension, Marfan syndrome, bicuspid aortic valve, giant cell arteritis (Fig. 3 and 4) (cranial and Takayasu disease [Fig. 5]), and infections (syphilis), and as a result of trauma. Most thoracic aortic aneurysms are asymptomatic and are discovered incidentally on chest radiography. Computed tomography (CT), magnetic resonance imaging (MRI), and transesophageal echocardiography (TEE) are all accurate noninvasive techniques for imaging thoracic aortic aneurysms (Fig. 6). Indications for surgical resection

include the presence of symptoms attributable to the aneurysm, an aneurysm rapidly enlarging under observation (particularly if the patient has hypertension), posttraumatic aneurysm, pseudoaneurysm, and an aneurysm 6 cm or greater in diameter (5.5-6 cm in low-risk patients). In patients with Marfan syndrome, surgery is usually indicated when the ascending aortic diameter is between 4.5 and 5 cm.

ABDOMINAL AORTIC ANEURYSM

Abdominal aortic aneurysm can be diagnosed reliably with ultrasonography, CT, or MRI (Fig. 7 and 8). Angiography is not required unless the renal or peripheral arterial circulation needs to be visualized to plan treatment. Because physical examination in the detection of AAA lacks sensitivity, screening tests are indicated in high-risk subsets of patients. It has been shown that early detection of abdominal aortic aneurysm can reduce mortality, furthermore, a single screening ultrasound of men >65 years of age can identify the majority of abdominal aortic aneurysms. The United States Preventive Services Task Force recommends a one-time screening ultrasound in men age 65 to 75 years who have ever smoked. Screening of siblings and first-degree relatives of patients with aneurysm generally begins at age 50 years. In a good-risk patient, elective surgical treatment of an abdominal aortic aneurysm should be considered for aneurysms greater than 54 cm in diameter. Elective surgical repair is definitely indicated when the aneurysm diameter is

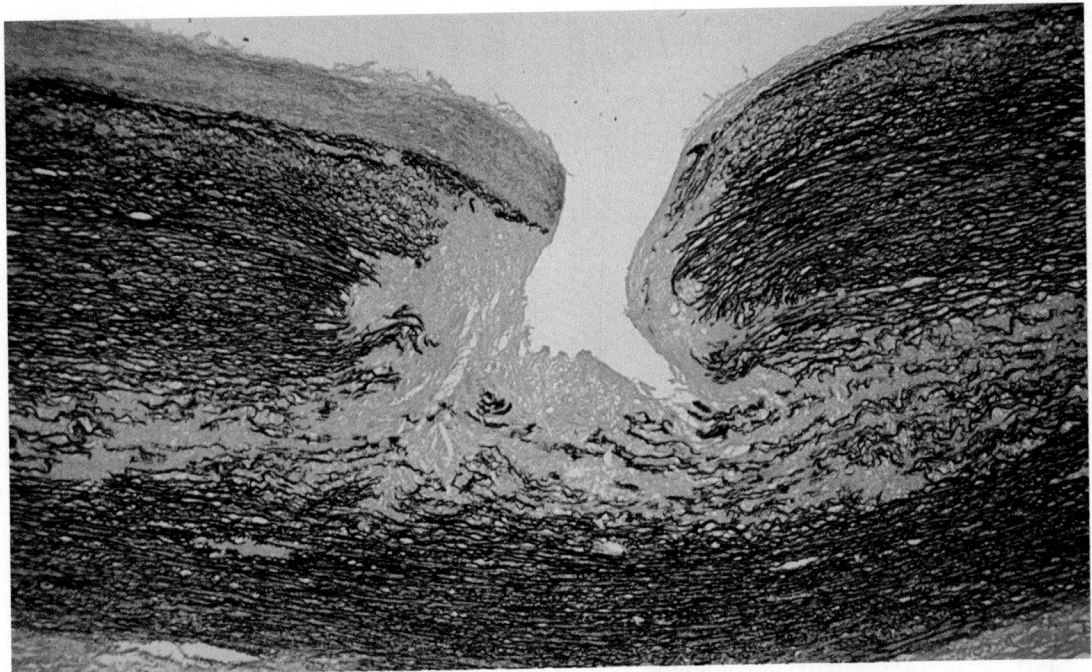

Fig. 4. Histologic specimen showing isolated intimal tear of ascending aorta in giant cell aortitis.

between 5.5 cm and 6.0 cm in good-risk patients. In patients with significant comorbid conditions (pulmonary, cardiac, renal, or liver disease), surgical therapy is individualized. In persons with a large and/or symptomatic abdominal aortic aneurysm whose comorbid condition makes them poor surgical candidates, exclusion of the aneurysm by an endovascular approach (placement of an intraluminal stent-anchored polyethylene terephthalate fiber [Dacron] prosthetic graft via retrograde transfemoral cannulation under local anesthesia) has given encouraging results. Percutaneous abdominal aortic aneurysm repair is a safe and effective treatment compared with open surgical repair for infrarenal abdominal aortic aneurysms with appropriate anatomy. Results are comparable to surgical repair with regard to mortality and may have improved short-term and long-term morbidity rates. All patients treated with endovascular repair need continued lifelong follow-up with tomographic imaging.

- Elective surgical repair is definitely indicated when aneurysm diameter is greater than 5.0 cm in good-risk patients.

An inflammatory abdominal aortic aneurysm is suggested by the triad of back pain, weight loss, and increased erythrocyte sedimentation rate. Obstructive uropathy may occur with ureteral involvement. The findings on CT are diagnostic (Fig. 9). The treatment is surgical resection.

Surgery is also indicated for abdominal aortic

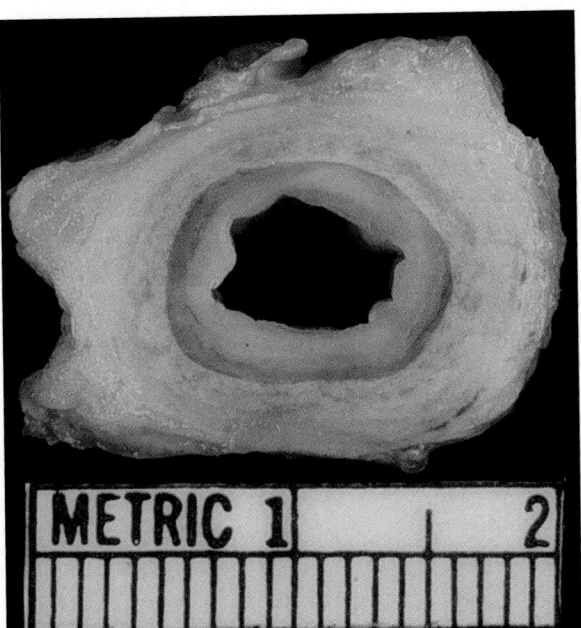

Fig. 5. Takayasu arteritis in descending thoracic aorta.

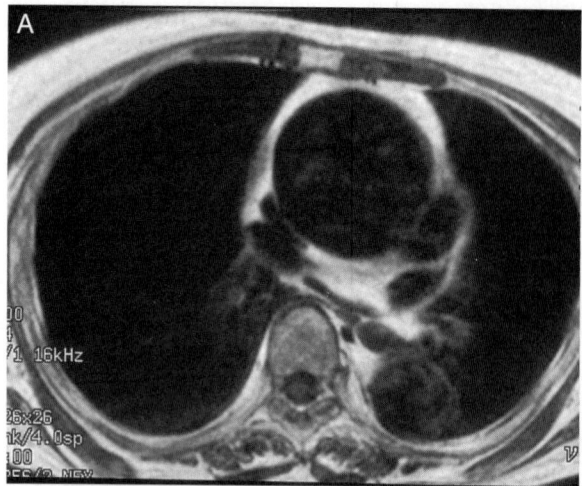

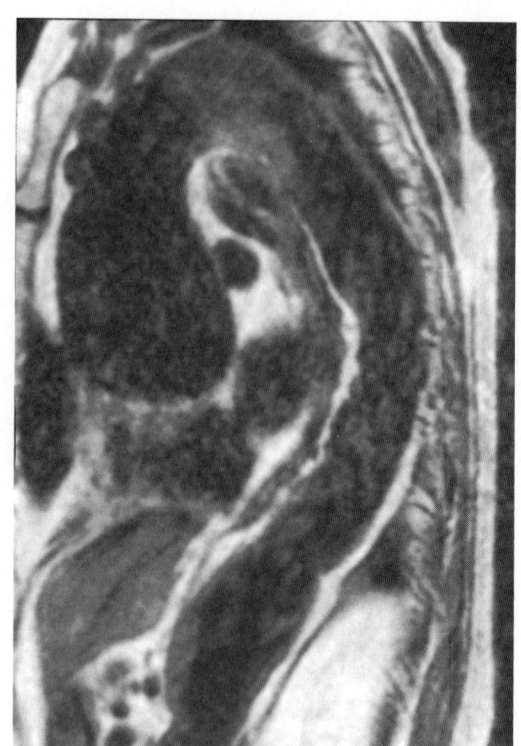

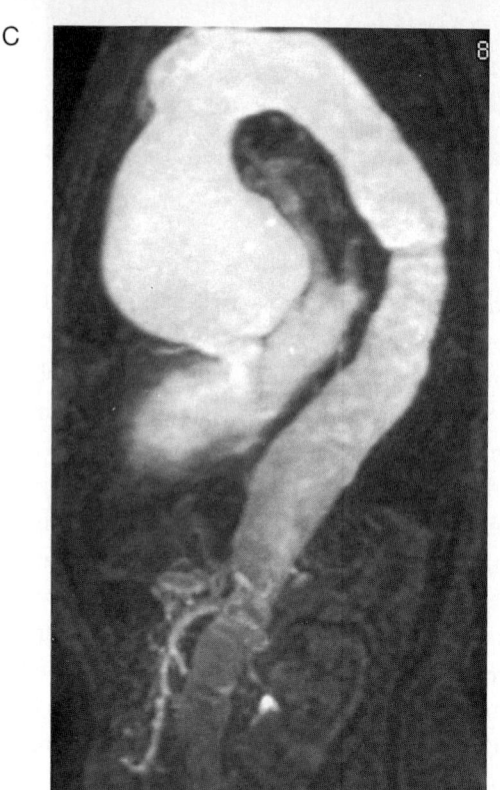

Fig. 6. Magnetic resonance imaging/angiography in a patient with asymptomatic thoracic aortic aneurysm. Images in the transverse, *A*, and longitudinal, *B*, planes demonstrate a large aneurysm of the ascending aorta (7.8 cm) and moderate dilatation (4.5 cm) of the descending thoracic aorta. Moderate aortic regurgitation is also demonstrated, *C*.

aneurysms that are symptomatic, traumatic or infectious in origin, or are rapidly expanding (>0.5 cm/year).

- An inflammatory abdominal aortic aneurysm is suggested by the triad of back pain, weight loss, and increased erythrocyte sedimentation rate.
- Surgery is indicated for abdominal aortic aneurysms that are greater than 5 cm in diameter, symptomatic, traumatic, or infectious in origin or are rapidly expanding (>0.5 cm/year).

AORTIC DISSECTION

Etiology

The most common predisposing factors for aortic dissection are advanced age, male gender, hypertension, Marfan syndrome, and congenital abnormalities of the aortic valve (bicuspid or unicuspid valve). When aortic dissection complicates pregnancy, it usually occurs in the third trimester. Iatrogenic aortic dissection, as a result of cardiac surgery or invasive angiographic procedures, can also occur.

Classification

Aortic dissection involving the ascending aorta is designated as *type I* or *type II* (proximal, type A), and dissection confined to the descending thoracic aorta is designated as *type III* (distal, type B) (Fig. 10 and 11).

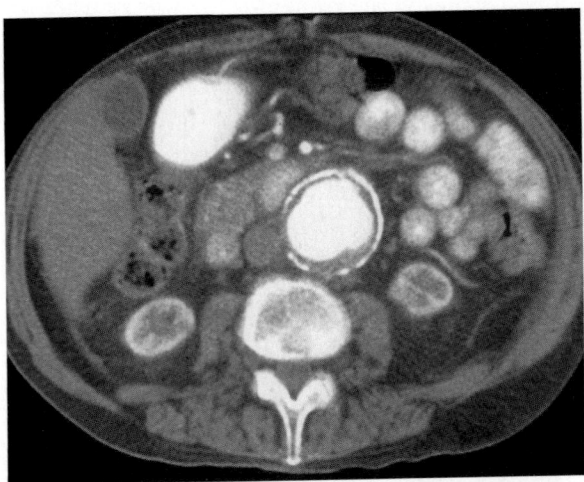

Fig. 7. Computed tomography with intravenous contrast demonstrating a large aneurysm of the infrarenal abdominal aorta. There is a small amount of laminated thrombus within the aneurysm and dense peripheral calcification.

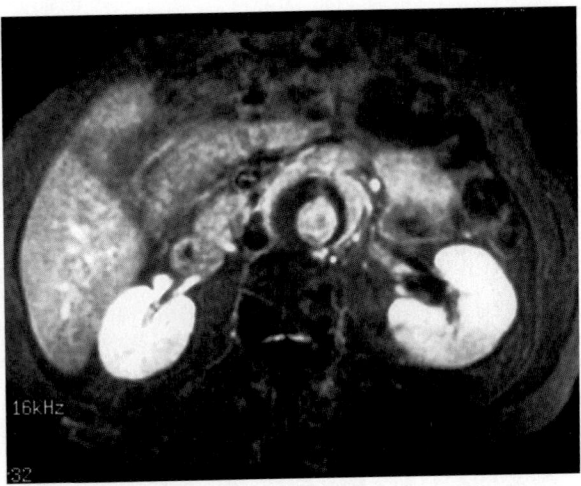

Fig. 9. Computed tomography scan of abdomen of patient with inflammatory abdominal aortic aneurysm. Note the high attenuation change surrounding the aorta, representing inflammatory change in periaortic retroperitoneal tissue.

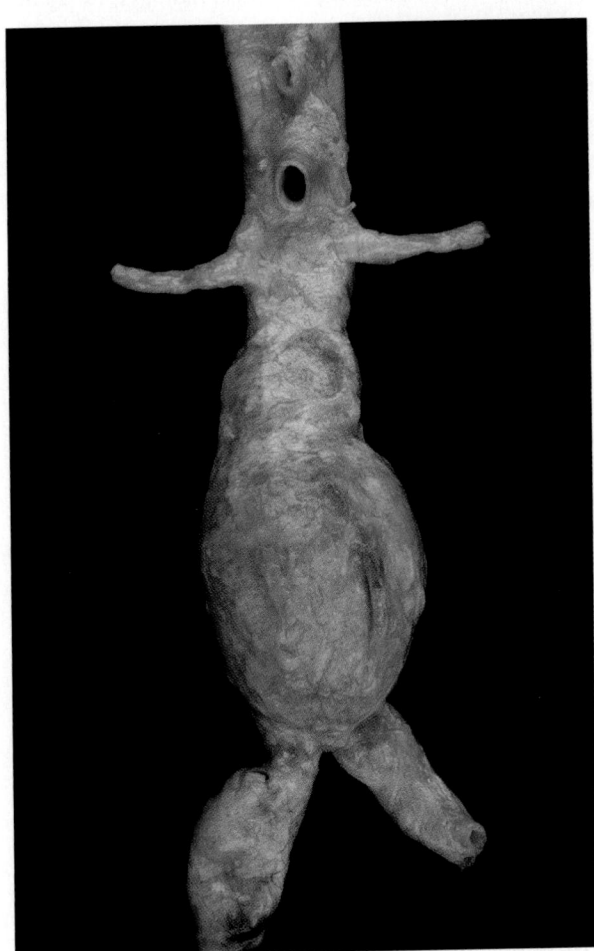

Fig. 8. Aneurysms of abdominal aorta and iliac artery.

Clinical Features

The acute onset of severe pain (often migratory) in the anterior chest, back, or abdomen is the most suggestive clinical finding (sensitivity of 90% and specificity of 84%). Additional findings include hypertension (49% of patients), an aortic diastolic murmur (28% of patients), pulse deficits or blood pressure differential (31% of patients), and neurologic changes (17% of

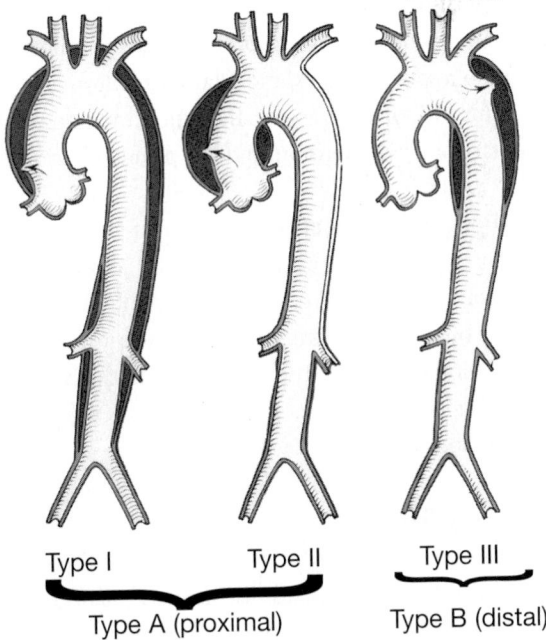

Type I   Type II   Type III

Type A (proximal)   Type B (distal)

Fig. 10. Classification of aortic dissection.

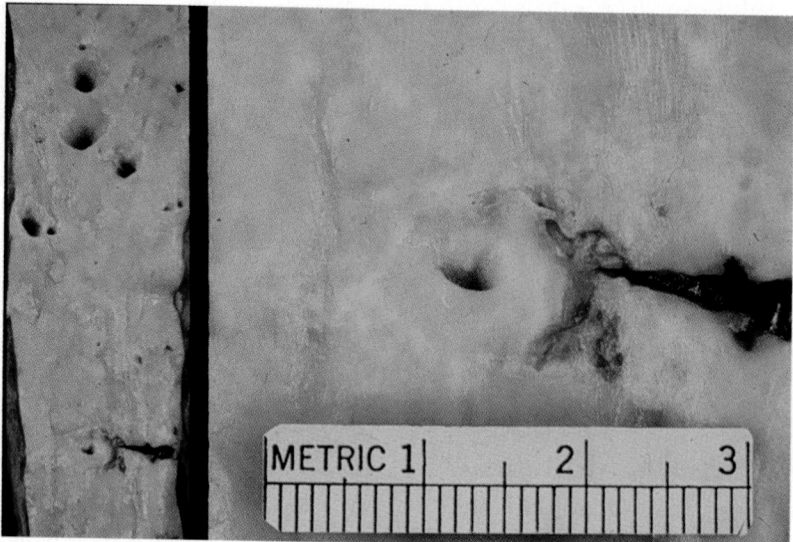

Fig. 11. Type III aortic dissection involving the abdominal aorta.

patients). Syncope in association with aortic dissection occurs when there is rupture into the pericardial space, producing cardiac tamponade. Congestive heart failure is due most commonly to severe aortic regurgitation. Acute myocardial infarction (most commonly inferior infarction due to right coronary artery ostial dissection) and pericarditis are additional cardiac presentations.

Clues to type I aortic dissection include substernal pain, aortic valve incompetence, decreased pulse or blood pressure in the right arm, decreased right carotid pulse, pericardial friction rub, syncope, ischemic electrocardiographic changes, and Marfan syndrome.

Clues to type III aortic dissection include interscapular pain, hypertension, and left pleural effusion.

■ In a patient with a catastrophic presentation, systemic hypertension, and unexplained physical findings of vascular origin—especially in the presence of chest or back pain and an aortic murmur—aortic dissection should always be included in the differential diagnosis, and an appropriate screening test should be performed emergently.

Laboratory Tests

Chest radiography may reveal widening of the mediastinum and supracardiac aortic shadow, deviation of the trachea to the right, a discrepancy in diameter between the ascending and descending aorta, and pleural effusion

(Fig. 12). Normal findings on chest radiography do not exclude aortic dissection.

Diagnosis

Definitive diagnosis of aortic dissection can be made using any of the following imaging modalities: echocardiography, CT, MRI, and aortography.

Echocardiography

The combination of transthoracic echocardiography (TTE) and TEE can be used to identify an intimal flap, communication between the true and false lumina, a dilated aortic root (>4.2 cm), thrombus formation, widening of the aortic walls, aortic regurgitation, and pericardial effusion/tamponade. Multiplane techniques have markedly improved the accuracy of TEE (Fig. 13). Advantages of TEE include portability, safety, accuracy, rapid diagnosis, use in patients with hemodynamic instability, and use intraoperatively.

CT

CT can accurately detect the intimal flap, identify two lumina, demonstrate displaced calcification, pericardial effusion, pleural effusion, and abdominal aorta involvement, and provide accurate aortic diameters (Fig. 14). The disadvantages include nonportability (limiting its use in patients with hemodynamic instability) and the need for intravenous contrast agents.

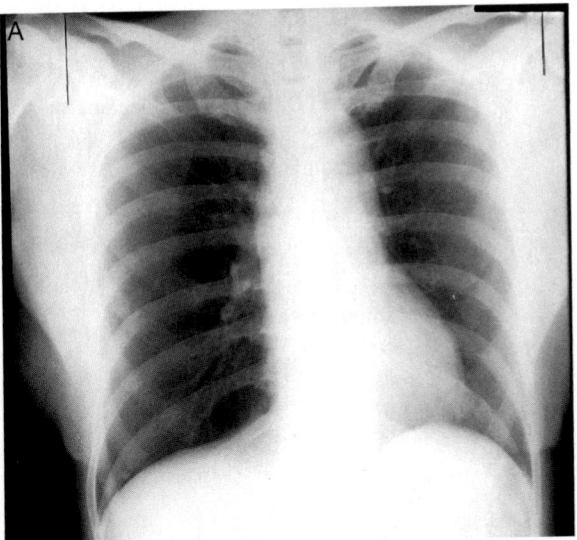
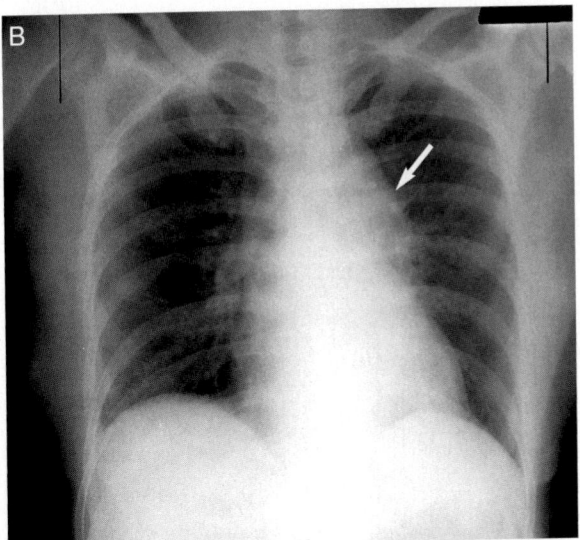

Fig. 12. Chest radiographs of patient before (*A*) and after (*B*) aortic dissection. Note widening of superior mediastinum after aortic dissection (*arrow*).

MRI

MRI is as accurate as CT in the diagnosis of aortic dissection, although MRI, with its inherent multiplanar imaging capability, can be used with or without contrast enhancement. Demonstration of the intimal flap, entry/exit sites, thrombus formation, aortic regurgitation, pericardial effusion, pleural effusion, and abdominal aorta and branch vessel involvement is possible (Fig. 15). Disadvantages of MRI include cost and nonportability.

Aortography

Aortography can accurately diagnose aortic dissection by showing the intimal flap, opacification of the false lumen, and deformity of the true lumen. Also, associated aortic regurgitation and coronary artery anatomy can be visualized. The disadvantages include invasive risks, exposure to intravenous contrast agents, delay in diagnosis, and nonportability.

The choice of test (TTE, TEE, CT, MRI, or aor-

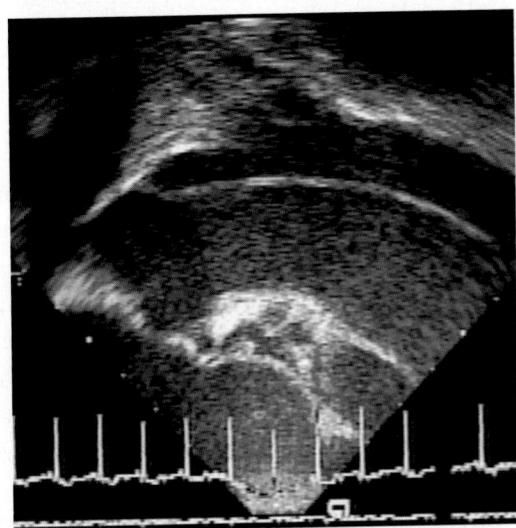

Fig. 13. Transesophageal echocardiographic view of ascending aorta in the longitudinal plane demonstrating an intimal flap originating in right coronary sinus.

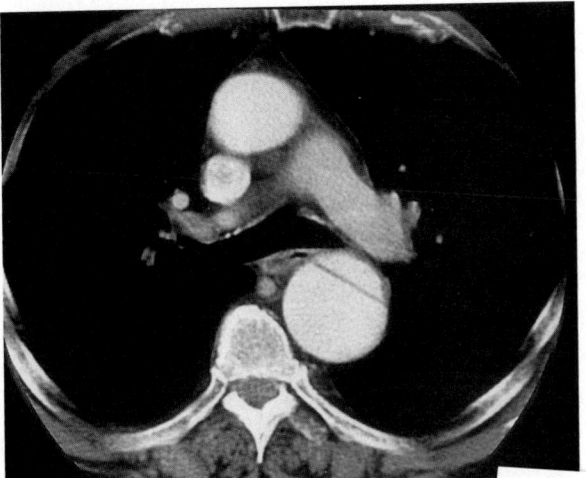

Fig. 14. Computed tomography with intravenou trast demonstrating dilatation of descending tho aorta and an intimal flap. Note the relatively equ opacification of true and false lumina.

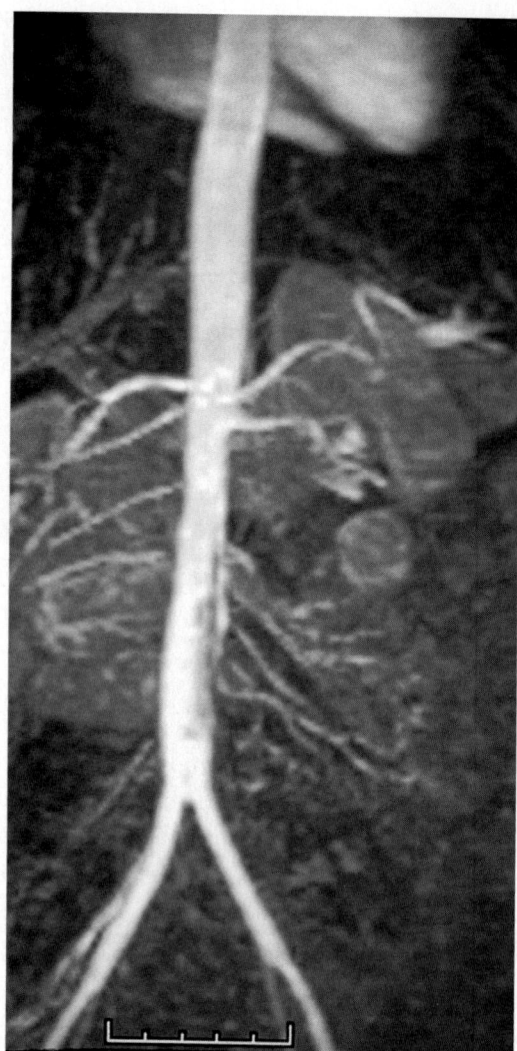

Fig. 15. Magnetic resonance angiography demonstrating dissection of mid and distal abdominal aorta in patient with a remote history of sudden deceleration injury.

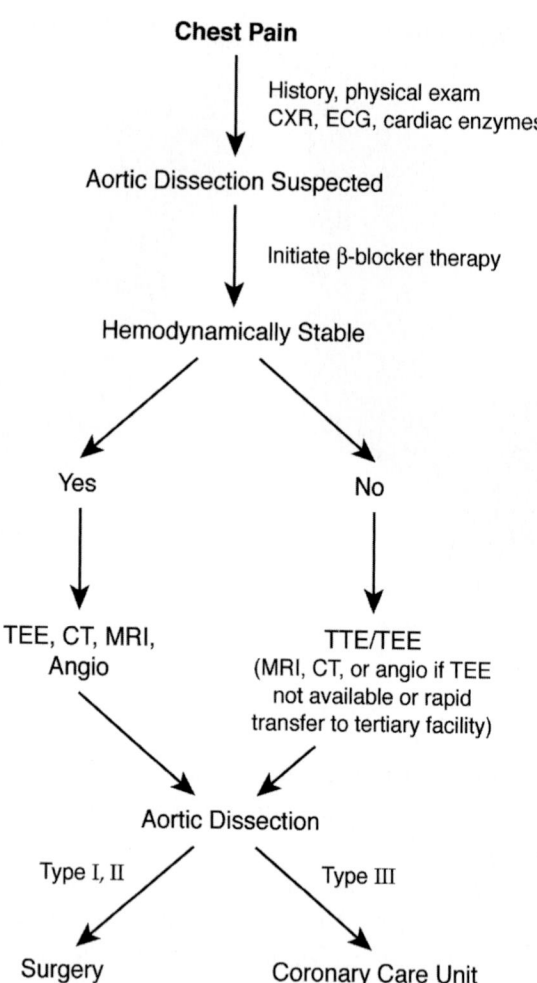

Fig. 16. Initial management of suspected acute aortic dissection. Angio, angiography; CT, computed tomography; CXR, chest radiography; ECG, electrocardiography; TEE, transesophageal echocardiography; TTE, transthoracic echocardiography.

tography) in a patient with suspected acute aortic dissection depends on which is most readily available and the hemodynamic stability of the patient. Currently, our test of choice in suspected acute aortic dissection is the combination of TTE and TEE. The initial management of suspected acute aortic dissection is shown in Figure 16.

The most common cause of death in aortic dissection is rupture into the pericardial space, with cardiac tamponade. Echocardiographically guided pericardiocentesis is associated with an increased risk of aortic rupture and death. Cardiac tamponade due to aortic dissection is a surgical emergency, and generally peri-

cardial fluid should be removed only in the operating room after cardiopulmonary bypass has been instituted. Other causes of death include acute congestive heart failure due to severe aortic regurgitation, rupture through the aortic adventitia, rupture into the left pleural space, and occlusion of vital arteries. Factors that propagate dissection include *impulse* pulsatile flow and increased mean arterial pressure.

■ Cardiac tamponade due to aortic dissection is a surgical emergency, and pericardial fluid should be removed only in the operating room after cardiopulmonary bypass has been instituted.

Treatment

Pharmacologic therapy should be instituted as soon as the diagnosis of aortic dissection is suspected (see below). Emergent surgery is indicated for types I and II (proximal, type A) aortic dissection. Coronary angiography prior to surgery is not indicated as it does not improve survival. Pharmacologic therapy in the coronary care unit is the preferred initial treatment for type III (distal, type B) aortic dissection, with delayed surgical therapy (2 to 3 weeks) for selected patients whose general medical condition permits operation.

The initial pharmacologic therapy is outlined in Table 1. When long-term pharmacologic therapy is used for type III aortic dissection, indications for surgery include development of saccular aneurysm, increasing aortic diameter, or symptoms related to chronic dissection.

Table 1. Initial Pharmacologic Therapy for Aortic Dissection

Hypertensive patients

Sodium nitroprusside intravenously, 2.5 µg/kg per minute

with

Propranolol intravenously, 1 mg every 4 to 6 hours (The goal is to have systolic blood pressure <110 mm Hg—a lower pressure is acceptable if urine output is maintained at least at 25 to 30 mL/hr—until oral medication is started)

or

Intravenous esmolol, metoprolol, or atenolol (in place of propranolol)

or

Intraveous labetalol (in place of sodium nitroprusside and a β-blocker)

Normotensive patients

Propranolol, 1 mg intravenously every 4 to 6 hours

or

20 to 40 mg orally every 6 hours (Metoprolol, atenolol, or labetalol may be used in place of propranolol)

PENETRATING AORTIC ULCER

Penetrating aortic ulcer occurs when an atherosclerotic plaque undergoes ulceration and penetrates the internal elastic lamina. It results in one of four possible consequences: 1) formation of an intramural hematoma, 2) formation of a saccular aneurysm, 3) formation of a pseudoaneurysm, or 4) a transmural rupture (Fig. 17). Penetrating aortic ulcer most commonly involves the mid or distal descending thoracic aorta, less often the ascending or abdominal aorta (Fig. 18). The clinical features of penetrating aortic ulcer are similar to those of aortic dissection and include acute onset of pain in the anterior or posterior chest (or both) and hypertension. Pulse deficits, neurologic signs, and acute cardiac disease (aortic regurgitation, myocardial infarction, pericardial effusion) are not seen in penetrating aortic ulcer as they are in classic aortic dissection. The diagnosis of penetrating aortic ulcer can be established with CT, MRI, TEE, or aortography (Fig. 19).

The treatment for penetrating aortic ulcer is usually nonoperative if only an intramural hematoma is present. With control of hypertension, the intramural hematoma tends to resolve spontaneously over time. Surgical therapy is indicated for patients who have ascending aortic involvement or develop a saccular aneurysm or a pseudoaneurysm or for patients with intramural hematoma who have persistent symptoms, increasing aortic diameter, or poorly controlled hypertension.

- Penetrating aortic ulcer occurs when an atherosclerotic plaque undergoes ulceration and penetrates the internal elastic lamina.
- The treatment for penetrating aortic ulcer is similar to that of aortic dissection (ascending aortic involvement is treated surgically, initial medical management is preferred when there is descending thoracic aortic involvement).

INCOMPLETE AORTIC RUPTURE

Incomplete rupture of the thoracic aorta (in the region of the aortic isthmus) results from a sudden deceleration injury. It is seen most often in motor vehicle accident victims and should be suspected when there is evidence of trauma to the chest wall, decreased or absent leg pulses, left-sided hemothorax, or widening of the superior mediastinum on chest radiography. These

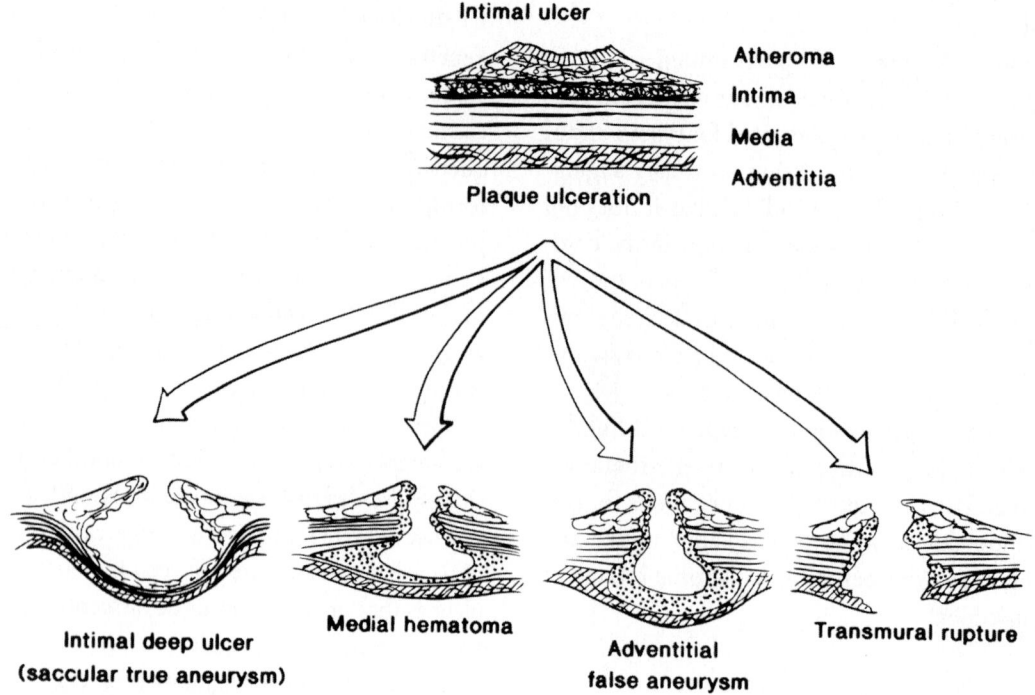

Fig. 17. Possible consequences of penetrating aortic ulcer.

patients usually are hypertensive at initial presentation. The diagnosis can be confirmed with TEE, CT, MRI, or angiography. Treatment is emergent surgical repair in patients who are suitable surgical candidates. At initial presentation, the condition of 40% to 50% of the patients is unstable. No clinical or imaging criteria accurately predict future complete rupture, so even if a patient presents with a chronic incomplete rupture, surgery is still indicated. Most of the patients are young, and the risk of elective surgical repair is low, with an otherwise good prognosis for long-term survival if aortic repair is successful.

■ Incomplete rupture of the thoracic aorta (in the region of the aortic isthmus) results from a sudden deceleration injury, frequently a motor vehicle accident.

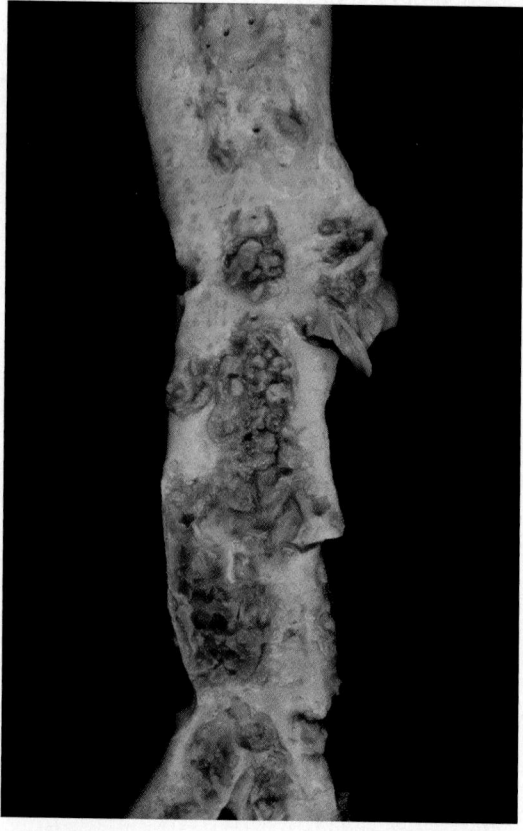

Fig. 18. Grade 4 ulcerocalcific disease of the abdominal aorta.

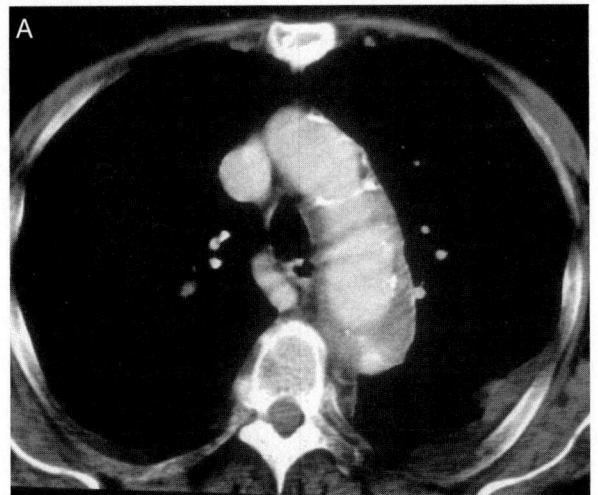

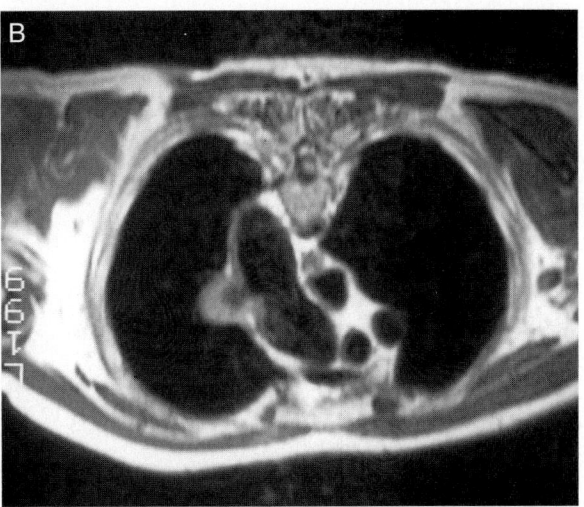

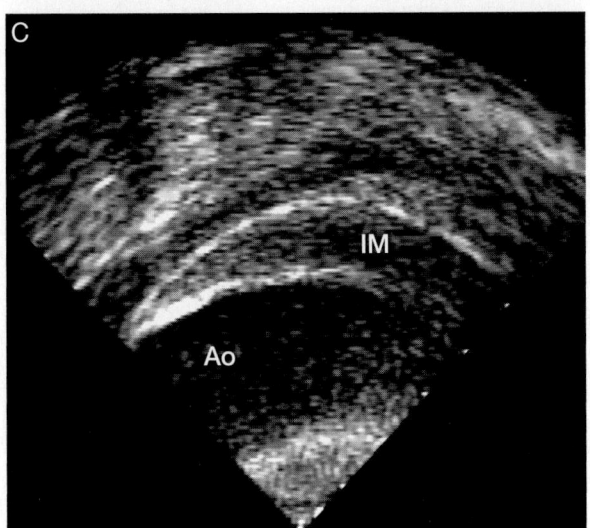

Fig. 19. *A,* Computed tomography with intravenous contrast demonstrating intramural hematoma of transverse aortic arch caused by a penetrating aortic ulcer. *B,* Magnetic resonance image scan demonstrating a penetrating aortic ulcer of transverse aortic arch. *C,* Transesophageal echocardiographic view of transverse aortic arch (transverse plane) demonstrating intramural hematoma (IM).

49

RENOVASCULAR DISEASE AND RENAL ARTERY STENTING

Verghese Mathew, MD

RENAL ARTERY DISEASE

Obstructive disease of the renal arteries can be categorized as either atherosclerosis (the majority of recognized renal artery stenosis) or fibromuscular dysplasia (FMD).

Renal FMD occurs in younger patients with a female preponderance and often involves secondary or distal branches; FMD may also coexist in other vascular beds including the coronary circulation. Renal artery revascularization for patients with renal FMD can often be curative with respect to hypertension control. Historically, surgical revascularization or percutaneous transluminal angioplasty (PTA) has been utilized; stenting has not been felt to have a beneficial role in percutaneous treatment of FMD above and beyond the benefit observed with PTA alone (Fig. 1).

The true prevalence of atherosclerotic renal disease in the general population is unknown, although the prevalence in selected populations of patients with identified atherosclerosis in other vascular beds has been reported to be 10-30%. Within the population of patients with identified renal artery stenosis (RAS), there are patients with significant as well as non-clinically significant renal stenosis, and those with physiologically important stenosis and those without. Despite the existence of noninvasive as well as invasive diagnostic modalities to define RAS, the true natural history of RAS, outcomes after renal revascularization and identi-

fication of those most likely to benefit from revascularization still require clarification. It may well be that the heterogeneous clinical outcome data after renal revascularization is due to our inability to accurately define *physiologically important* renal artery stenosis (Fig. 2).

CLINICAL CLUES TO DETECTING RENAL ARTERY STENOSIS

Acknowledging the possible limitations of accurate diagnosis of physiologically significant RAS, a number of clinical parameters have been proposed in which renovascular disease should be considered in the clinical differential diagnosis.

- Known atherosclerosis in other vascular beds is significantly associated with the presence of atherosclerotic RAS.
- Onset of hypertension prior to age 30 (consider FMD) or after age 55.
- Worsening of previously controlled hypertension.
- Malignant or resistant hypertension.
- Abdominal/flank bruit is not highly predictive but is supportive.
- Discrepancy of renal size (small kidney) is likely a later stage of renovascular disease.
- Azotemia not otherwise explained, or worsened by

613

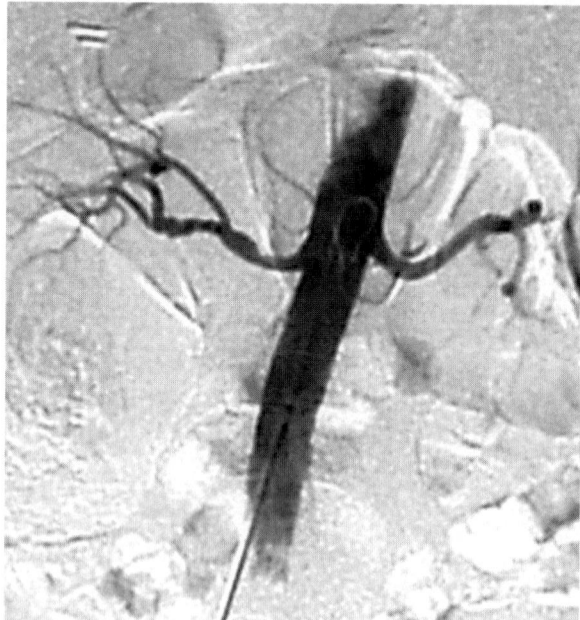
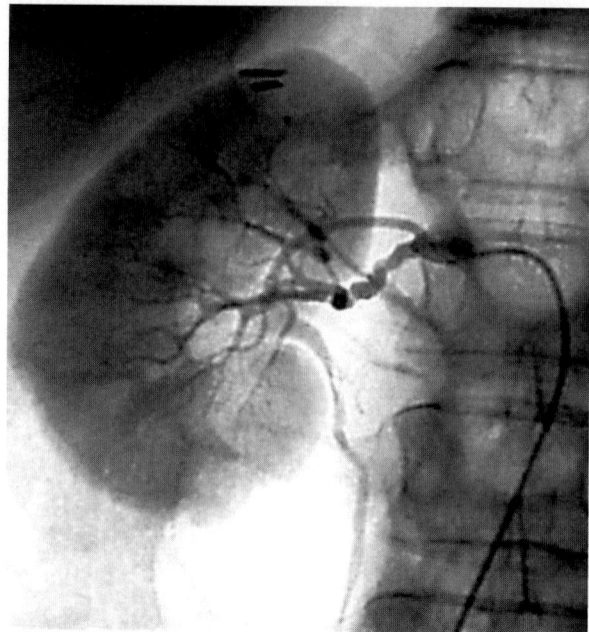

Fig. 1. Aortography demonstrates characteristic beaded, "string of pearls" appearance of renal FMD. Note that the lesion location is generally not the proximal aspect of the renal artery.

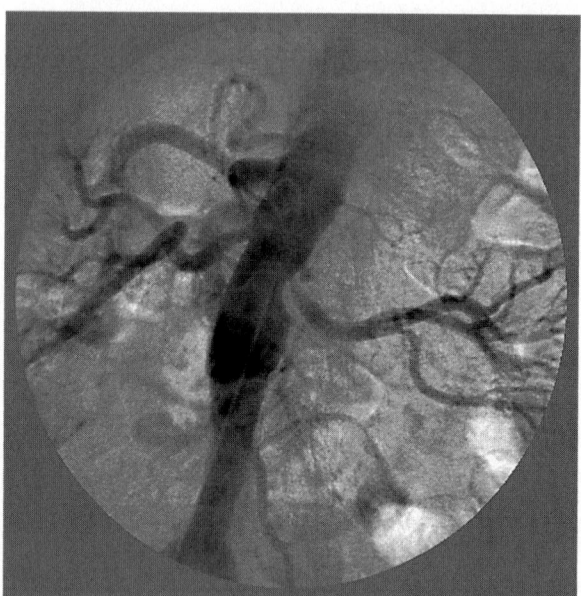

Fig. 2. Significant left renal artery stenosis in a 65-year-old male with poorly controlled hypertension on 4 medications. This was identified at the time of coronary angiography when the patient presented with unstable angina; screening aortography was requested by the referring cardiologist due to refractory hypertension. Note atheromatous disease of the aorta adjacent to the left renal artery origin.

angiotensin-converting enzyme inhibitors (ACE-I) or angiotensin receptor blockers (ARB).

■ Recurrent congestive heart failure/flash pulmonary edema in a hypertensive patient, particularly with preserved systolic LV function.

■ Angina without significant coronary artery disease in a hypertensive patient.

DIAGNOSTIC TESTING FOR RENAL ARTERY STENOSIS

A number of diagnostic tests are available for the evaluation of renal artery stenosis, assessing anatomic parameters (parenchyma, arterial imaging and flow information) and/or physiologic effect of presumed RAS. Intravenous pyelography, one of the earliest modalities used for the diagnosis of RAS, was associated with poor sensitivity and a high false-positive rate, and is no longer considered a useful or appropriate test for evaluation of RAS. Similarly, the use of plasma renin activity has low predictive value; with ACE-I administration (conventionally captopril is utilized), specificity rises, although the value of the test diminishes in bilateral RAS and the need to discontinue most antihypertensive agents is a practical limitation of the test. Captopril scintigraphy is useful for diagnosis of unilateral RAS in patients with preserved renal function, although it is of limited utility in patients with bilateral RAS and renal dysfunction; antihypertensive agents also need to be withheld for this test.

In clinical practice, the more frequently utilized noninvasive diagnostic modalities include ultrasound, computed tomographic imaging/angiography (CTA), and magnetic resonance imaging/angiography (MRI/MRA); arteriography is considered the gold standard for the diagnostic evaluation of RAS, although its invasive nature practically preludes its widespread application as a screening modality.

Duplex ultrasound is relatively inexpensive, and has a high sensitivity and specificity. Limitations include operator-dependent variability and technical difficulties with large patients (difficulty imaging through significant abdominal adipose tissue). In addition, accessory renal arteries, in which stenosis may still lead to renovascular hypertension, may be difficult to identify. In patients in whom FMD is suspected clinically, a negative ultrasound should be followed with an alternate imaging modality. In general, for the evaluation of suspected atherosclerotic RAS, ultrasound is a reasonable screening modality. A ratio of renal artery velocity to aortic velocity of >3.5 supports the diagnosis of significant RAS. The calculated resistive index is one variable that has often been used to determine the likelihood of benefit with renal revascularization: a resistive index of >0.8 suggests renal parenchymal disease which would not be expected to improve with revascularization. Additionally, the literature suggests the kidneys <8 cm in size are unlikely to benefit with revascularization, although these parameters should be taken in isolation to determine whether or not revascularization should be offered.

MR angiography has evolved into a useful imaging modality for the evaluation of RAS. Advantages include images that can be presented with a visual appearance similar to aortography with 3-dimensional capabilities, although image processing may introduce image inaccuracies in inexperienced hands. Additionally, iodinated contrast is not utilized, which is a clear advantage in patients in whom renal function is already compromised. MR interpretation may be hampered in arterial segments that have previously been stented due to signal dropout. The usual limitations/contraindications for MR examinations would apply (i.e., claustrophobic patients, indwelling metal hardware such as cardiac pacemakers, etc.). MR can also be utilized to ascertain regional renal perfusion and assess blood oxygenation, although these variables would not generally be part of routine clinical examinations at most centers, but have the potential to add to our understanding of renal physiology (Fig. 3).

CT angiography also is an excellent imaging modality for RAS. Though CTA is not limited by some of the patient factors that preclude MR examination (i.e., cardiac pacemakers), CTA does require radiation, as well as iodinated contrast, the latter of which makes it a less attractive option in patients with renal dysfunction.

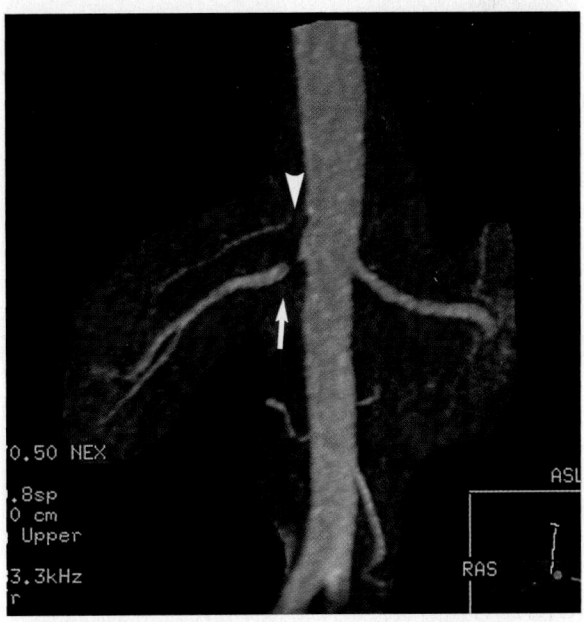

Fig. 3. A 75-year-old female with a prior history of diabetes mellitus and coronary revascularization of the left anterior descending artery 2 years previously (BARI IID Trial) who presents with poorly controlled hypertension on 3 agents and insidious worsening of her serum creatinine level from 1.4 mg/dL to 1.7 mg/dL over 2 years. MRA demonstrates a single left renal artery without significant stenosis. The main right renal artery has a high grade proximal stenosis (*arrow*); an accessory right renal artery to the superior pole may have a proximal stenosis (*arrowhead*), although this was difficult to characterize with certainty.

Calcification may hamper the assessment of stenosis severity, as may the presence of stents, although CTA would be preferred to MR for the latter issue. Similar to MR, CT has the ability to measure renal perfusion and flows, though this is not performed in standard clinical practice. Ultimately however, modalities such as MR and CTA may be useful to simultaneously assess for the anatomic presence of RAS and also assess the physiologic impact of RAS on the kidney (Fig. 4).

Invasive arteriography has long been considered the gold standard for renal artery imaging. Potential limitations include its invasive nature, making it less attractive

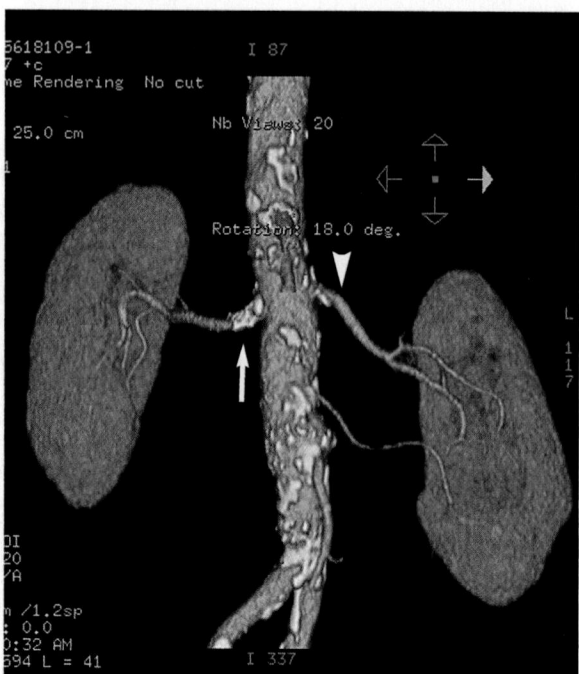

Fig. 4. A 66-year-old male with diabetes mellitus, multiple prior percutaneous coronary interventions, and carotid endarterectomy, with a recent right renal artery stent. CTA demonstrates a dominant superior left renal artery stenosis (*arrowhead*); calcification confounds the assessment of stenosis severity, but a pressure gradient performed in this vessel using a 0.014" pressure wire at the time of right renal stenting demonstrated no significant pressure gradient. Additionally, a left lower pole accessory renal artery is also identified. Note the stent in the proximal right renal artery (*arrow*) which could confound assessment of in-stent restenosis, although the cross-sectional images suggested absence of significant restenosis.

as a screening test, and the use of iodinated contrast (although CO_2 angiography and, more commonly, gadolinium angiography can also be performed with diagnostic image quality). The limitations of coronary angiography in assessing coronary lesion severity are well known; angiography can underestimate or overestimate lesion severity. Utilizing 0.014" flow/pressure wires, it has been clear for a number of years that angiographically mild-appearing coronary lesions may be physiologically significant, while angiographically significant lesions may not be flow-limiting. This issue of indeterminate angiography, or misdiagnosing the severity of stenosis based on angiographic assessment, has not been appreciated or evaluated to the same degree in the renal arterial bed. Translesional pressure gradients using 4 French catheters have been performed in the renal arterial vasculature for many years, the impact of the catheter diameter itself may overestimate the translesional gradient; conventionally, a 20-mm Hg peak-to-peak gradient or a 10-mm Hg mean gradient across a renal artery stenosis has been felt to be important, although these values are relatively arbitrary and have not been correlated with a measure of renal function or physiology. Recently, 0.014" pressure/flow wires from the coronary practice have begun to be utilized to assess renal artery stenosis. It is likely that a role for renal flow and pressure reserve assessments will emerge. The complexities of renal autoregulation make it unlikely that simply measuring resting or even inducible gradients across renal lesions will reveal completely the physiologic significance of a renal artery stenosis.

REVASCULARIZATION FOR RAS

Revascularization should be considered in patients with hypertension and/or renal insufficiency due to renal artery stenosis, although the ability to predict which patients will benefit is problematic. With respect to hypertension control and renal intervention, the blood pressure improvement with percutaneous angioplasty for FMD is generally good. For atherosclerotic RAS, however, our ability to predict blood pressure improvement or improvement or stabilization of renal function after revascularization is limited; an obvious shortcoming is our understanding of the relationship between anatomic renal artery stenosis and renal physiology and function. Renal revascularization may be considered in patients with "difficult to control" hypertension on multiple antihypertensive agents, or even when blood pressure is controlled on multiple drugs in an effort to reduce the need for medications. The ability to achieve an excellent procedural result with percutaneous stent placement for RAS has lowered the threshold at which revascularization may be considered or recommended. The NIH-sponsored Cardiovascular Outcomes in Renal Atherosclerotic Lesions (CORAL) trial randomizes patients with renal artery stenosis with significant hypertension on 2 or more antihypertensive agents to medical therapy versus renal stenting utilizing embolic protection and will shed light on the role of percutaneous renal revascularization for management of hypertension (Fig. 5).

Similarly with respect to renal artery revascularization for the indication of preservation or improvement of renal function, the *a priori* ability to predict when revascularization would be most beneficial is poor; a portion of patients will improve or stabilize their renal function with revascularization, while a significant minority will have deterioration of renal function. Whether these observations of renal function over the long term are related to renal revascularization or represent a natural history of disease is unknown. Current accepted indications for renal revascularization include patients with renal dysfunction with bilateral RAS or RAS involving a solitary kidney; this is particularly true in cases of worsening renal function. The value of revascularization for unilateral renal artery stenosis purely for renal dysfunction is debated but may be reasonable depending on the clinical scenario (Fig. 6).

The availability of low-profile catheters and stent delivery systems as well as better equipment in general has broadened the horizons for percutaneous renal revascularization. More complex lesion subsets, such as bifurcation lesions and small-caliber renal arteries, can be safely treated with excellent procedural results. The main limitation of percutaneous intervention has been felt primarily to be the issue of restenosis; 1-year

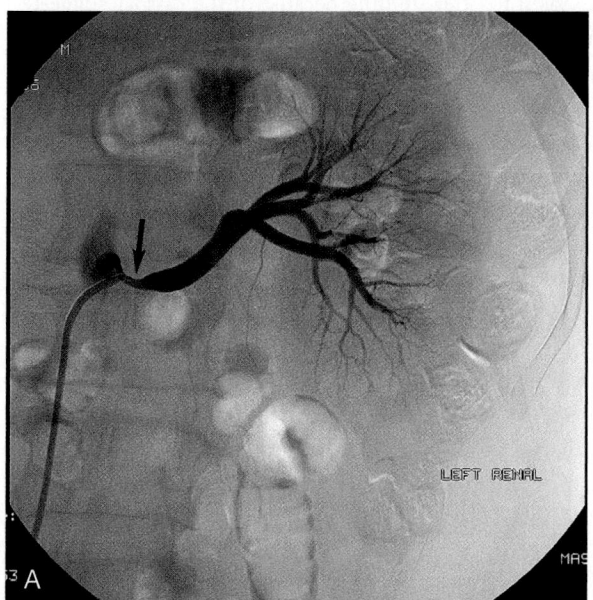
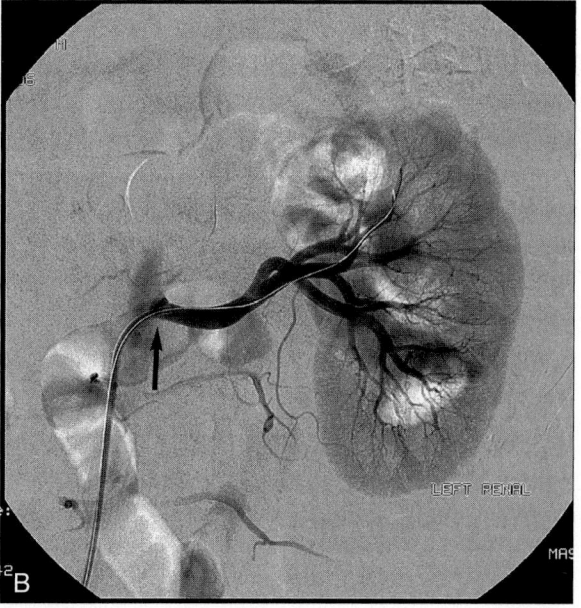

Fig. 5. *A*, A 52-year-old male with coronary disease and cerebrovascular revascularization presents with labile, uncontrolled hypertension on multiple medications. Evaluation for metabolic causes of hypertension was negative. An MRA had suggested left renal artery stenosis and the patient was referred for percutaneous revascularization. A selective injection through a 6 French mammary guide catheter demonstrates a high-grade ostial left renal artery stenosis (*arrow*). *B*, A 0.014" wire was used to cross the lesion easily and a 7 x 15 mm Guidant Herculink stent was directly deployed with an excellent angiographic result (*arrow*). The patient maintains excellent blood pressure control 2 months after the procedure on a tapering regimen of antihypertensive agents.

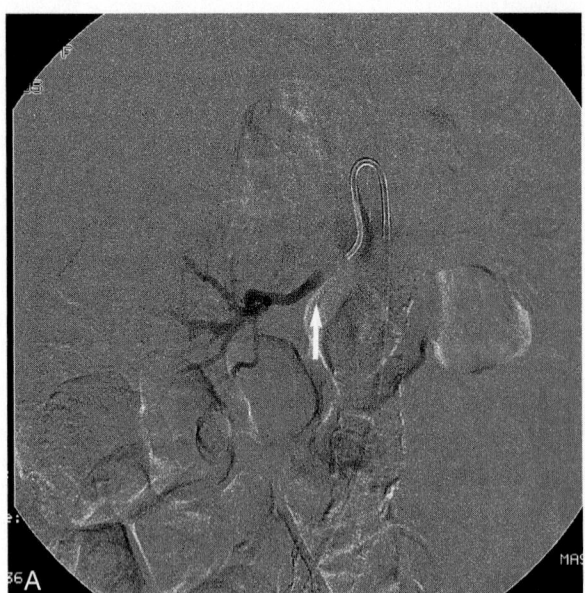 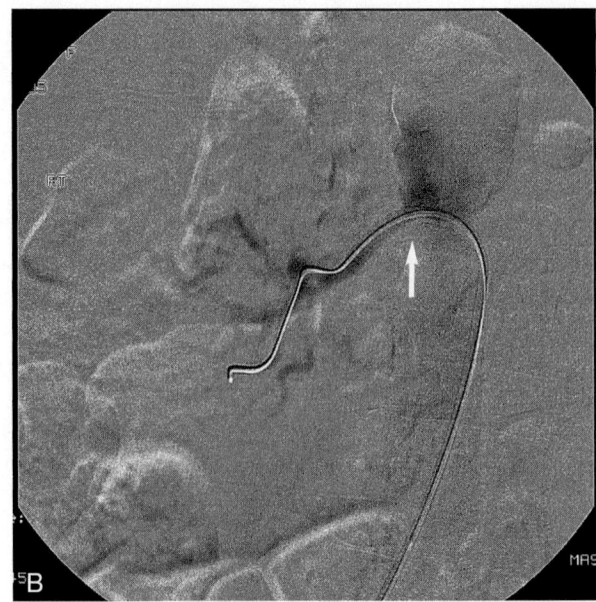

Fig. 6. An 82-year-old female with extensive vascular disease, severe COPD and unevaluated anemia presented with a subacute progression of chronic renal failure; baseline creatinine had been 1.7-2.0 mg/dL a year earlier; upon presentation her creatinine was 4.8 mg/dL and rose to 5.6 mg/dL within 48 hours. An ultrasound of the kidneys demonstrated mildly atrophic parenchyma; the right kidney measured 8 cm and the left 9.2 cm with single renal arteries bilaterally with significantly elevated velocities in both. The resistive indices were 0.7-0.8. The patient was initiated on hemodialysis and we were asked to evaluate her for the possibility of renal revascularization. Although the kidneys appeared small with borderline resistive indices of both renal arteries, we opted to offer stenting because of the history suggesting a recent decline in renal function and since the patient would be committed to dialysis in any case. Our practice in such a case is to perform an MRA to aid in procedure planning; the patient was unable to tolerate an MR scan due to restlessness and claustrophobia. Thus, the patient was brought to the angiographic suite, and accessed with difficulty through the left common femoral artery; the right femoral artery was occluded. The aorta was extremely tortuous and calcified; a 6 French 45-cm sheath was used, and an internal mammary (IM) catheter could not be manipulated sufficiently close to the right renal artery safely (without a risk of scraping the severely atherosclerotic aorta). Therefore, a Sos omni catheter was used with a 0.035" Benson wire to cannulate the right renal artery; gadolinium injection demonstrated a critical ostial stenosis (*A*) (*arrow*). The stenosis was crossed with a 0.014" Cordis Supersoft Reflex wire and the Sos omni was exchanged over this wire for a 6 French IM guide. Predilation was performed with a 3.0-mm Powersail (coronary) balloon, and a 3.5 x 18-mm Guidant Vision (coronary) stent was placed with an excellent result (*B*) (*arrow*). Similarly, the left renal artery was identified to have a high-grade ostial stenosis, and was stented with a 3.0 x 13-mm Guidant Vision stent. 60 cc of gadolinium was used for the case; no iodinated contrast was utilized. Serum creatinine decreased to 2.5 mg/dL within 72 hours, and hemodialysis was ceased. 4 months later, the creatinine remains at 1.4 mg/dL. Although visualization was somewhat compromised due to gadolinium use, the images were diagnostic; the avoidance of iodinated contrast, thus avoiding the added risk of contrast nephropathy in this case, was an important component of the procedural plan in this case.

freedom from restenosis is generally accepted to be 80-85%. The restenosis rates may be lower in large-diameter renal arteries (6 mm or greater), but may be higher in smaller (≤4 mm) arteries. Studies evaluating the role of drug-eluting stents (DES) in renal arteries have not been designed with sufficient numbers of patients to draw meaningful conclusions. We have utilized DES in smaller renal arteries (≤4 mm) with good success; large randomized trials are required to test the concept in the renal arterial vasculature (Fig. 7 and 8).

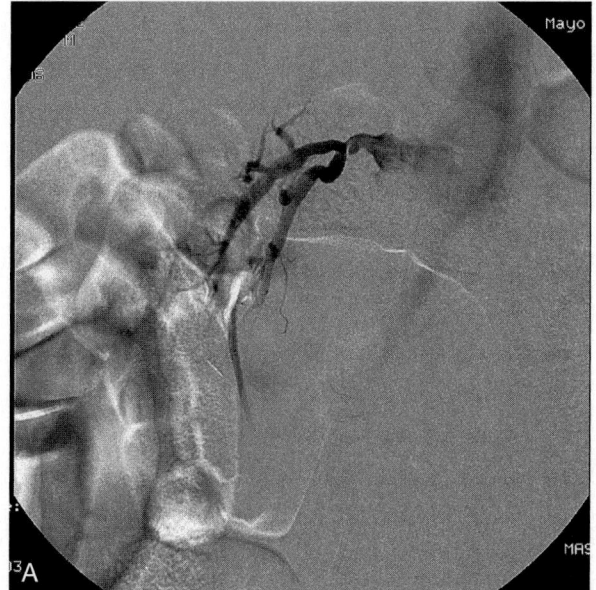

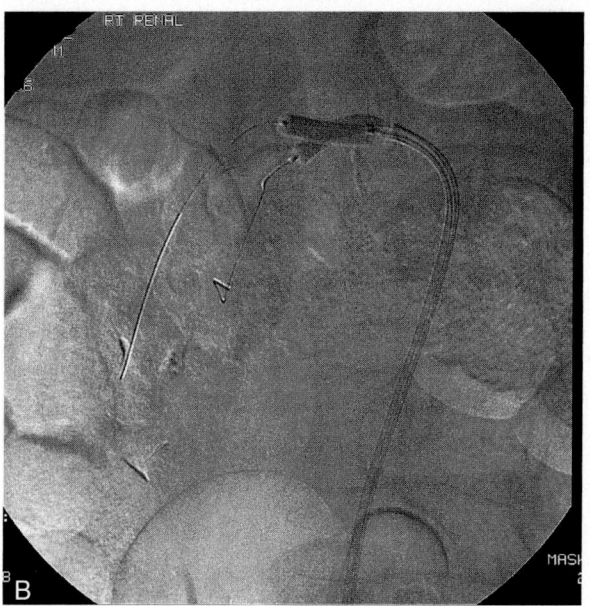

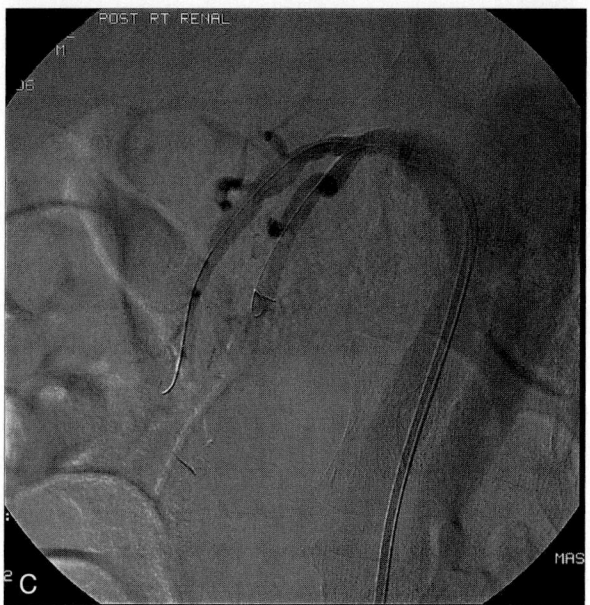

Fig. 7. A 59-year-old male with extensive vascular disease presents with a non-ST elevation myocardial infarction and uncontrolled hypertension on 5 antihypertensive agents. Successful percutaneous coronary intervention was performed on a protected left main artery; abdominal aortography demonstrates a high-grade right renal artery stenosis. *A,* Selective angiography demonstrated a complex lesion in an early bifurcating renal artery (*arrow*). Certainly such a lesion would be difficult to treat using 0.035" systems, with a significant risk of compromising at least one of the main branches. However, using a 6 French IM guide, a pair of 0.014" Cordis Supersoft Reflex wires were advanced into the upper and lower branches, respectively. *B,* A pair of 3.5 x 16-mm Boston Scientific Express (coronary) stents were placed simultaneously in a "kissing" fashion (*arrow*). *C,* The angiographic result was excellent.

Surgical revascularization (endarterectomy, renal bypass, or renal reimplantation) can be performed with very good intermediate-term patency (90-95% at 5 years) although reliable predictors of initial blood pressure improvement and/or renal function improvement with revascularization and the correlation between long-term patency and sustainability of hypertension control and renal function stability/improvement would ideally be better defined. Regardless of whether percutaneous or surgical revascularization is contemplated, predicting short- and long-term benefit (hyper-

tension and or renal function) is problematic, and will require further evaluation.

TECHNIQUES OF RENAL ARTERY STENTING

As with any percutaneous interventional procedure, the importance of optimal diagnostic angiography cannot be underestimated. Initial aortography is appropriate to define the aortic anatomy, the origins of the renal arteries, and assess for the possibility of accessory renal arteries. Abdominal aortography might be considered

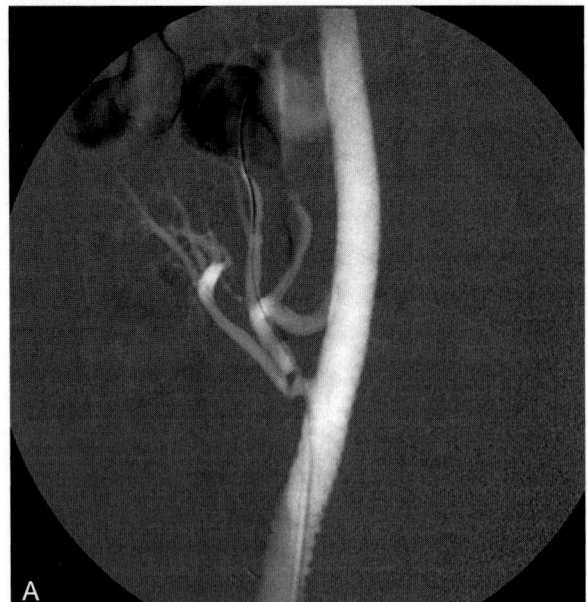

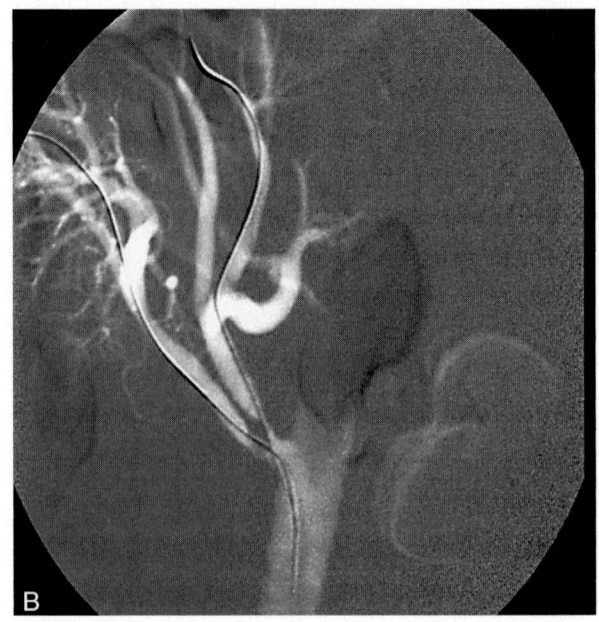

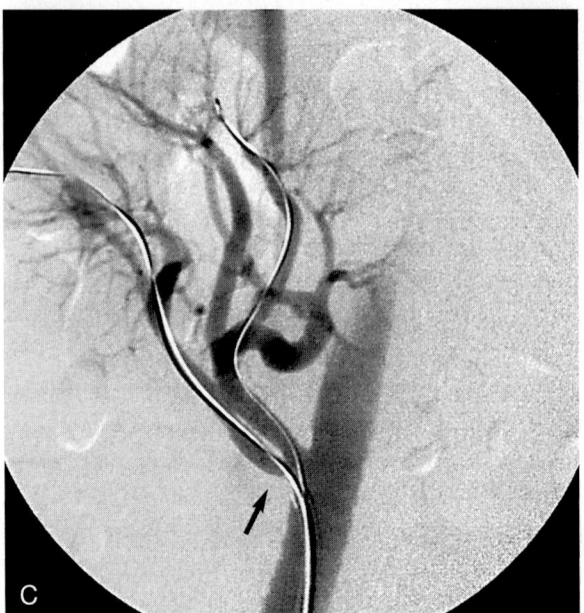

Fig. 8. A patient with a prior aortobifemoral graft underwent a recent cadaveric renal transplant. Within a few months, renal allograft dysfunction occurred, with an ultrasound revealing elevated velocities in the allograft renal artery. *A*, Angiography with a mixture of gadolinium and Visipaque demonstrated an early bifurcating allograft renal artery with stenoses in both branches (*arrow*), possibly due to injury at the time of organ harvest and/or anastomosis. The allograft had been anastomosed to the existing aorto-bifemoral graft (with a 0.014" wire in the superior limb). *B*, A pair of 0.014" coronary wires was advanced across the stenoses through a 6 French IM guide from the right femoral approach (*arrow*). *C*, A pair of 3.5 x 13-mm Cordis Cypher (sirolimus-eluting coronary) stents was simultaneously deployed in a "kissing" fashion, with an excellent angiographic result (*arrow*). Allograft function normalized subsequently.

optional if the patient has had an MRA or CTA prior to coming for the invasive procedure. Indeed, in patients with baseline renal dysfunction, we opt to perform MRA preprocedure to address the above issues and reduce iodinated contrast exposure.

Aortography can be performed with a number of different catheters including a pigtail, omni flush, or tennis racquet catheter; the advantage of the latter two catheters is that contrast is emitted laterally, thus avoiding opacification of the superior mesenteric artery aris-

ing above the renal arteries which may in turn obscure renal artery pathology. Generally, the origins of the main renal arteries will be around the L1-L2 vertebral interspace, but may exist between T12-L2. Ten to fifteen degrees of left anterior oblique projection is generally recommended for nonselective imaging of the renal arteries (Fig. 9).

Selective angiography can be performed using a number of catheters as well, including a Judkins right, mammary, renal double curve, Sos omni, Berenstein,

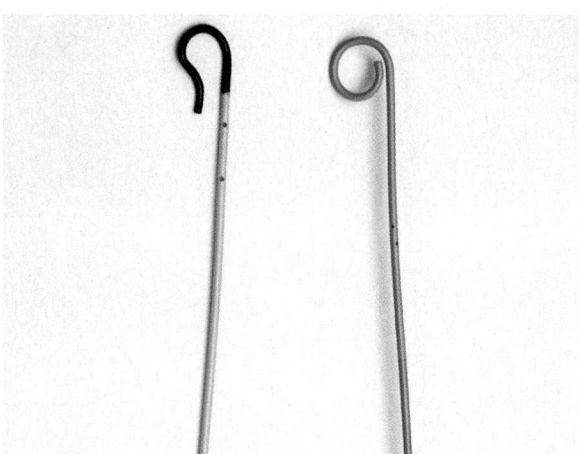

Fig. 9. An omni flush (*left*) and a pigtail (*right*) catheter are often used for nonselective imaging of the renal arteries.

and Simmons 1 or 2 (Fig. 10). Many operators advocate a "no-touch" technique, utilizing a 0.035" wire such as a Benson wire protruding 2-3 cm out of the catheter tip, thus keeping the tip of the catheter away from the aorta, and carefully and gently manipulating the catheter/wire until the catheter will fall into the renal artery orifice as the wire is withdrawn. When utilizing the shepherd's crook style catheters (Sos omni or Simmons), the renal artery can be cannulated with the wire using the "no-touch" technique, and the catheter is then pulled down into the renal artery. The important point of course is to avoid scraping and dislodging

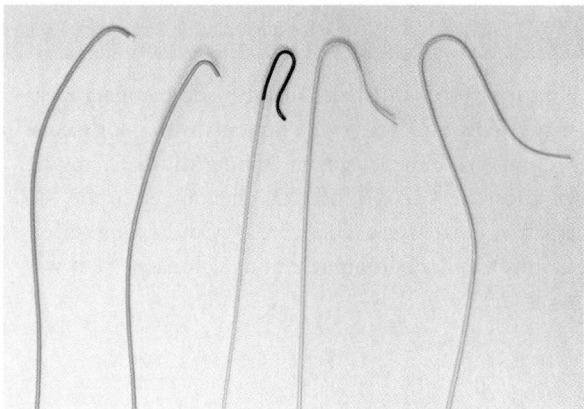

Fig. 10. Judkins right, mammary, Sos omni, and Simmons 1 and 2 (left to right) catheters are useful for selective renal artery cannulation.

atheromatous disease from the aortic wall into the renal arteries or peripherally. A 15-25 degree left anterior oblique projection often is best to lay out the origin of the left renal artery, and a 15-25 degree right anterior oblique projection for the right renal artery, although the exact angles may of course vary from patient to patient.

Historically, renal interventions have been performed with 0.035" wires, balloon catheters, and hand-crimped stents using a sheath without a guiding catheter. Cardiologists who perform renal intervention often use guide catheters and 0.014" wires, balloon catheters, and premounted stents similar to the designs available for coronary interventions, which is our preference. In general, use of lower profile equipment for renal artery interventions appears to be increasing, regardless of the specialty background of the operator. Our belief is that lower-profile equipment may be less traumatic to the renal artery and less likely to result in atheroembolism into the distal renal arterial bed, although this is not proven.

Guide catheter engagement is performed similar to what has been described above for selective renal angiography. A 0.014" wire is utilized to cross the stenosis, and generally we opt to directly stent the lesion with a 1:1 stent:artery sizing ratio. Occasionally, predilation will be required, which is performed with a relatively undersized balloon to just allow passage of the stent. Similarly, postdeployment inflations may be required as well with a noncompliant balloon or larger balloon size to optimally match the stent size to the vessel. Intraprocedural heparin, often arbitrarily given as a fixed dose of 5,000 U of heparin, or weight adjusted at approximately 70 U/kg, is given. Patients are generally pretreated with aspirin and clopidogrel, and we generally recommend at least 30 days of dual antiplatelet therapy following stenting (Fig. 11).

As the role of embolic protection devices have increased in coronary interventions (primarily saphenous vein graft disease) and carotid interventions, the concept of renal atheroembolism and its potential consequences has raised an interest in embolic protection devices for renal arterial interventions (Fig. 12).

The PercuSurge balloon occlusion device (Medtronic, Minneapolis, MN), the Filter Wire (Boston Scientific, Natick, MA) and now more recently the SpideRx (eV3, Minneapolis, MN) have all been

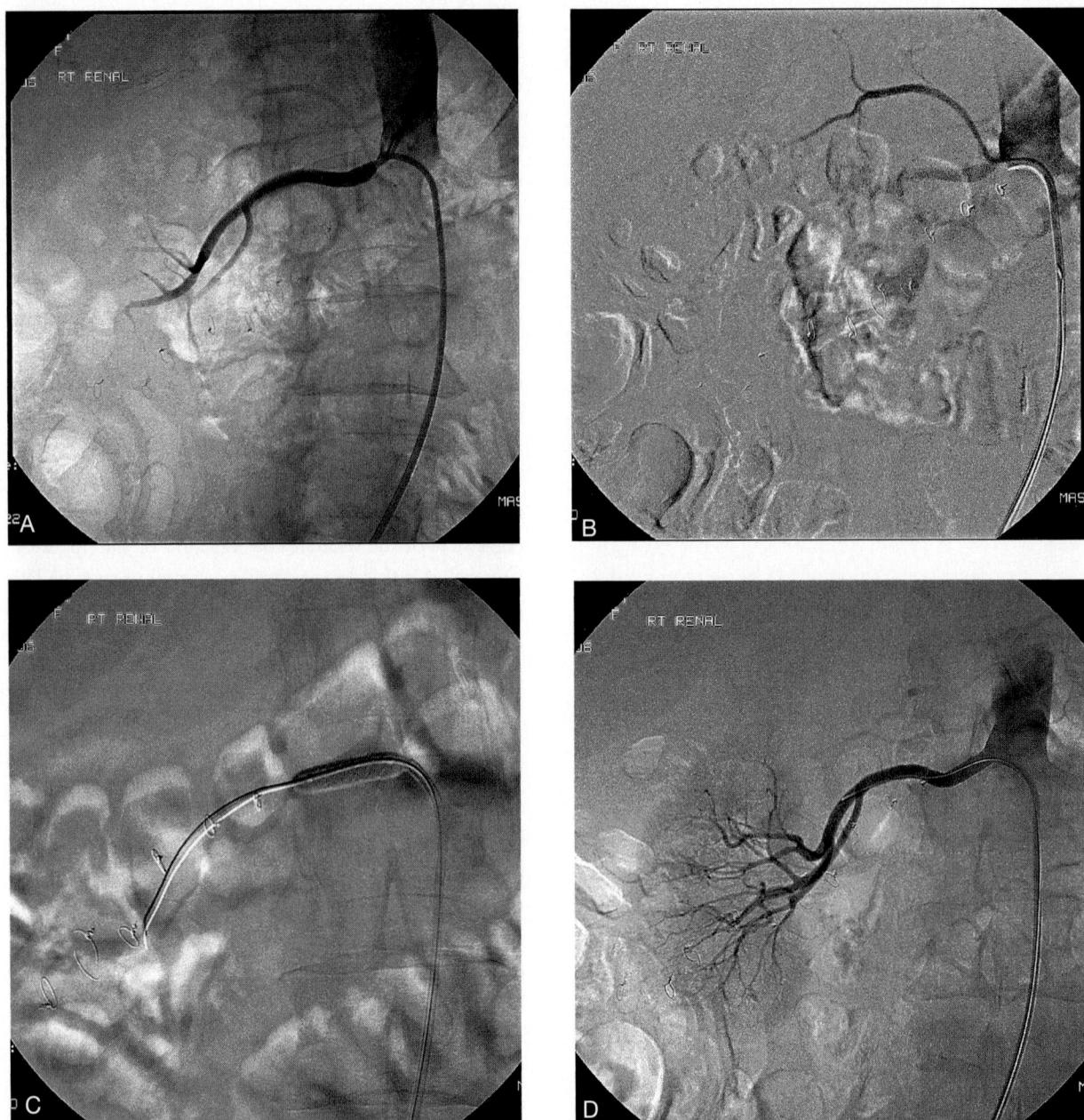

Fig. 11. A 75-year-old female (MRA shown in Figure 3) with a prior history of diabetes mellitus and coronary revascularization of the left anterior descending artery 2 years previously (BARI IID Trial) who presents with poorly controlled hypertension on 3 agents and insidious worsening of her serum creatinine level from 1.4 mg/dL to 1.7 mg/dL over 2 years. Angiography confirms a high-grade main right renal artery stenosis (*A*); note that in contrast to the MR scan, the accessory right renal arises immediately adjacent to the parent renal artery (*B*). A 0.014" Cordis Supersoft Reflex (coronary) wire was advanced easily, and a 3.5 x 13-mm Cordis Cypher (sirolimus-eluting coronary) stent was advanced and deployed (*C*), with an outstanding angiographic result (*D*).

utilized for renal protection in an off-label fashion, although the ideal renal embolization protection system has yet to be marketed; anatomic issues that vary from patient to patient, including short parent renals/early bifurcations which preclude complete protection and insufficient landing zone for the protection device, have yet to be addressed to allow the technology to be applied widely to renal interventions. We consider use of a distal protection device in patients with severe baseline renal dysfunction, solitary kidneys, or if, angiographically, the lesion volume appears large. Although nonrandomized series have reported capture of atheroembolic material using protection devices, a randomized comparison of percutaneous renal intervention with versus without embolic protection has not been done. Interestingly, the CORAL trial (randomized between medical therapy and stenting for RAS associated with hypertension) mandates the use of distal protection in the stent arm.

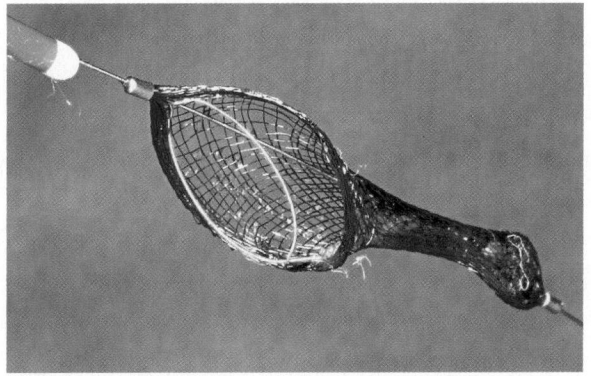

Fig. 12. An eV3 SpideRx embolic protection filter device that had been utilized for a renal stent case contains atherothrombotic material that otherwise would have likely showered distally into the renal parenchyma. The relative occurrence of renal atheroembolism during renal stenting is not clear but may be more common than initially appreciated. The role of such devices in modifying the outcome of percutaneous renal intervention merits investigation.

50

PATHOPHYSIOLOGY OF ARTERIAL THROMBOSIS

Robert D. McBane, MD

Waldemar E. Wysokinski, MD

Atherosclerosis is the most common cause of major disability and death in the United States. The most devastating complication of this disease occurs when a platelet-rich thrombus abruptly occludes arterial blood flow resulting in acute myocardial infarction (MI), stroke, or sudden cardiac death (SCD). Each year, 1.1 million Americans suffer from MI and 700,000 Americans suffer from a new or recurrent stroke. This chapter reviews the basic pathophysiology of arterial thrombosis.

The pathophysiology of arterial thrombosis involves platelet-rich thrombus formation over a ruptured atherosclerotic plaque. This process can be partitioned into platelet adhesion, coagulation factor activation and thrombus propagation through platelet accretion.

ENDOTHELIUM

The endothelial lining presents an inert interface between the vessel wall and circulating blood. More than just an inert surface, endothelium synthesizes nitric oxide (NO or EDRF) and prostacyclin (PGI2) which are potent vasodilators and inhibitors of platelet adhesion and aggregation. The endothelial glycocalyx is a rich source of proteoglycans such as heparan sulfate which in combination with antithrombin III provides a local source of anticoagulant. Endothelium also expresses thrombomodulin, a specific receptor which binds thrombin, changing its activity from prothrombotic to anticoagulant through the protein C activation pathway. The endothelium is therefore more than a passive barrier but rather an active participant in maintaining luminal patency by inhibiting local thrombosis.

PLATELET ADHESION

Following endothelial injury, exposed collagen binds von Willebrand factor (VWF) which serves as an initial tether to which the platelet receptor, glycoprotein (GP) Ib-IX-V, binds (Fig. 1 *A* and 1 *B*). The platelet, tethered by VWF, translocates along the injured surface in the direction of blood flow. A second platelet receptor, GP IaIIa (integrin $\alpha_2\beta_1$) then engages collagen thus arresting further translocation. A third receptor, GP VI also engages collagen and serves as a signal transducing receptor stimulating platelet activation, activation of platelet GP IIbIIIa (integrin $\alpha_{IIb}\beta_3$) and dense granule ADP secretion. ADP stimulates adjacent platelets and promotes further platelet recruitment to the growing thrombus. This sequence of platelet adhesion and receptor transduction mediated platelet activation is sufficient for the initial stages of platelet plug formation necessary for hemostasis.

1A. Arterial Injury

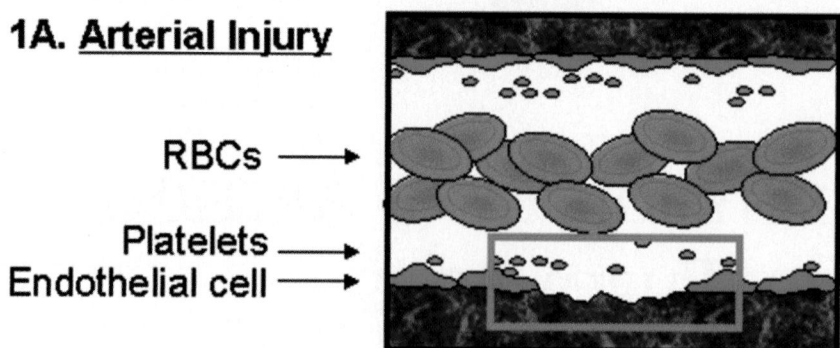

RBCs ⟶

Platelets ⟶
Endothelial cell ⟶

1B. Platelet adhesion

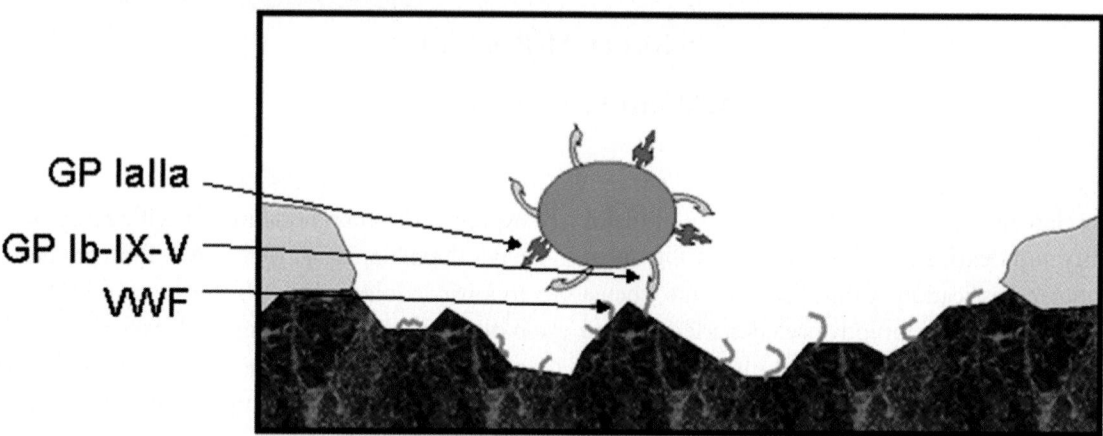

GP Ialla

GP Ib-IX-V

VWF

Fig. 1. **Platelet adhesion**. Von Willebrand Factor (VWF) binds exposed collagen following endothelial injury. Platelet glycoprotein (GP) Ib-IX-V then binds VWF to initiate platelet adhesion to the injured arterial surface.

COAGULATION FACTOR ACTIVATION

Pathologic arterial thrombosis is a thrombin mediated process and thus requires activation of the coagulation cascade. Coagulation factor activation occurs as a "cascade" of proenzymes are cleaved to their active form. This cascade of enzyme activation and amplification requires the assembly of activation complexes on the phospholipid membrane of activated platelets (Fig. 2). These activation complexes include activated platelet phospholipid membrane, activating enzyme and proenzyme, an activated cofactor, and calcium. Exposed tissue factor within the vessel wall initiates the cascade by binding circulating factor VIIa which in turn cleaves factors IX and X to their active forms (IXa and Xa respectively). Factor Xa then combines with factor Va on the platelet phospholipid membrane to form the prothrombinase complex, which cleaves prothrombin to thrombin.

THROMBUS PROPAGATION

Thrombin stimulation leads to further activation of GP IIbIIIa, which binds fibrinogen, crosslinking adjacent platelets to form aggregates (Fig. 3). Thrombin then orchestrates thrombosis by inducing further platelet granule secretion, cleaving fibrinogen to fibrin, and activating factor XIII which crosslinks fibrin strands to form a stable thrombus. Thrombin generation is therefore necessary for thrombus propagation sufficient for arterial occlusion.

ANTICOAGULANT SYSTEM

Thrombin activates an endogenous anticoagulant system, the central components of which include protein C, protein S, and antithrombin (Fig. 4). Thrombin binds to thrombomodulin on the luminal surface of endothelial cells and activates protein C to activated

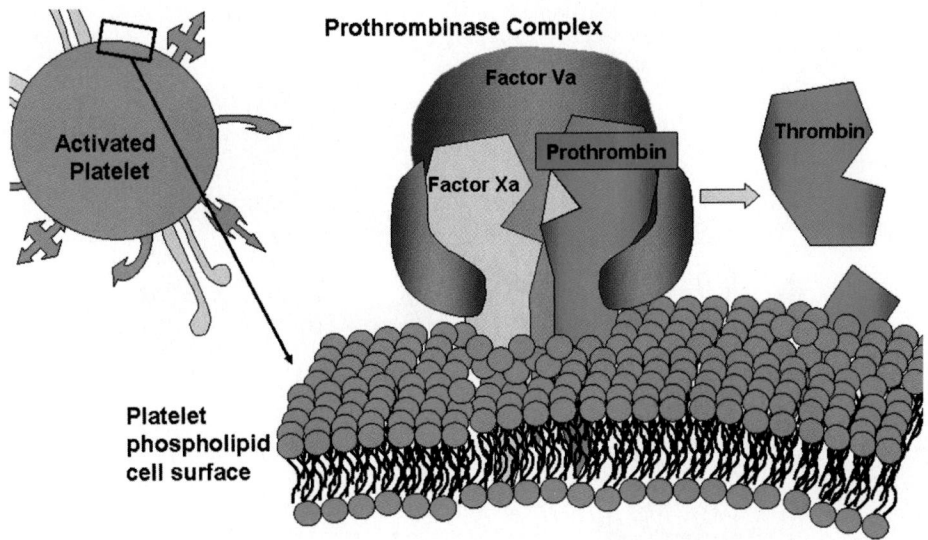

Fig. 2. Coagulation factor activation. Activation of vitamin K dependent factors (factors II, VII, IX and X) occur with factor complex assembly on the surface of activated platelets. This process is calcium dependent.

protein C (APC). APC (along with the cofactor, protein S) down-regulates the procoagulant pathway by inactivating the procoagulant proteins factor (f)VIIIa and fVa. Ultimately, antithrombin binds irreversibly to thrombin, and the complex is cleared by the liver (Fig. 5).

FIBRINOLYTIC SYSTEM

Thrombin also stimulates endothelial cells to release tissue-plasminogen activator (tPA), which activates plasminogen to plasmin, the central component of the fibrinolytic system. The fibrinolytic pathway removes (lyses) the arterial thrombus as part of the healing process of the arterial wall. Plasmin cleaves fibrin within the thrombus thus dissolving the thrombus. Plasmin also inactivates several important components of the procoagulant pathway, including factor V, factor VIII, and platelet glycoprotein (GP)-Ib-IX-V and GP IIbIIIa. Consequently, the overall action of plasmin is to promote thrombus dissolution and down-regulate ongoing thrombus formation.

PLATELETS

Platelets participate in every stage of arterial thrombosis, from the initial hemostatic plug formation to leukocyte recruitment necessary for wound healing. Platelets are

therefore not merely passive bystanders in this process. The platelet has four well-recognized storage granules, the α-granule, the dense body, lysosomal granule, and microperoxisome. These storage granules contain a large number of vasoactive amines, receptors, procoagulant and anticoagulant factors, and growth hormones (Table 1).

Platelet glycoprotein (GP) receptors mediate both platelet adhesion to the arterial wall and aggregation (Table 2). Three receptors play an important role in the initiating steps of platelet adhesion: GP Ib-IX-V, GP IaIIa, and GP VI. A fourth receptor, GP IIbIIIa, is principally involved in platelet aggregate formation, essential for the later stages of thrombus growth. Platelet glycoprotein (GP) receptors are highly polymorphic. These platelet receptor polymorphisms alter platelet function and have each been implicated in arterial thrombosis. Platelet receptor quality, quantity, function and polymorphism status have been studied extensively from basic science to large epidemiology studies. Whereas the family history contributes importantly to the risk of MI, interindividual differences in arterial thrombus formation may therefore in part be explained by a genetic basis. The following paragraphs will briefly review each of the platelet receptors relevant to arterial thrombosis.

GP Ib-IX-V initiates platelet adhesion by binding

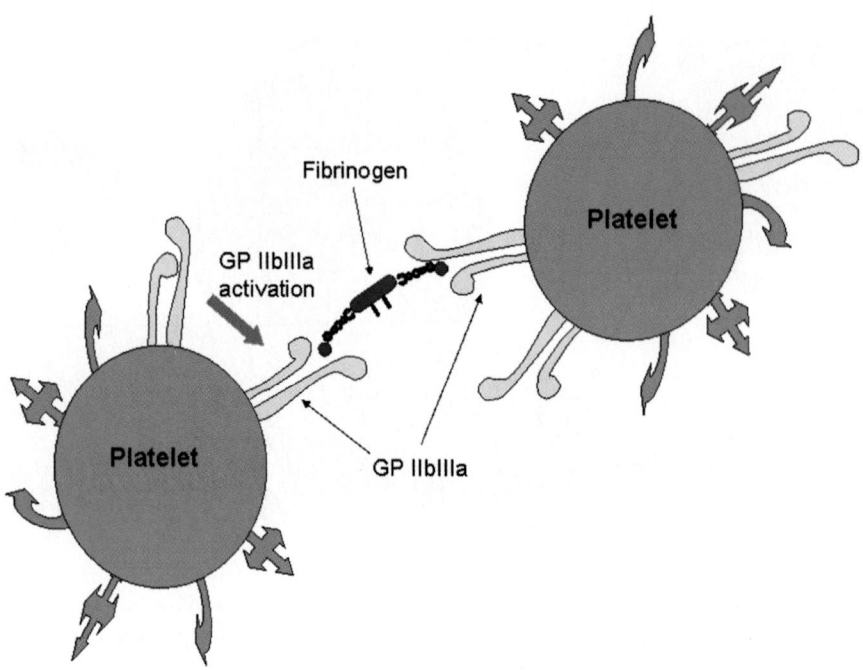

Fig. 3. Platelet aggregation. Platelet activation results in conversion of GP IIbIIIa from the inactive to the active form of the receptor. Binding of fibrinogen to this receptor facilitates platelet aggregation.

tethered von Willebrand factor (VWF) at the site of endothelial injury. There are approximately 25,000 copies of the receptor per platelet. The GPIb-IX-V complex is comprised of four polypeptide subunits, GP Ibα, GP Ibβ, GP IX, and GP V. Each polypeptide is present in duplicate in the complex except GP V. The VWF binding domain is found on the GP Ibα subunit. There are two polymorphisms in the coding sequence of the gene encoding the Ibα-subunit of the receptor. These polymorphisms lower the threshold for shear-induced platelet adhesion and shown to have a significant association with either stroke or MI.

Following the initial tether of GP Ib-IX-V to von Willebrand factor, a second platelet receptor, **GP IaIIa** (integrin $\alpha_2\beta_1$) binds fibrillar (type I-III, V) and non-fibrillar (IV, VI-VIII) collagen thereby arresting further translocation. This receptor, comprised of an α and β subunit, exists on the platelet cell surface in a low number of copies (n=3,000) compared to the more abundant fibrinogen receptor (GP IIbIIIa; n=50-80,000). The number of receptors, however varies considerably among individuals spanning a 10 fold range. There is a direct relationship between receptor density and platelet adhesion whereby type I collagen adhesion varies over a 20 fold range and type III collagen adhesion varies over

a 5 fold range respectively depending on the number of platelet receptors present. Receptor density is directly proportional to platelet adhesion to type I collagen under high shear conditions typical of stenosed arteries. Increased receptor density has been associated with both MI and stroke especially in the young. In contrast, in patients with mild type I von Willebrand disease characterized by a mild reduction of normally functioning VWF, GP IaIIa receptor density correlates with platelet adhesion under high shear conditions. Individuals who are both deficient in this receptor and have mild von Willebrand disease experience more clinical bleeding compared to those individuals with von Willebrand disease and normal receptor density.

Glycoprotein VI is a collagen receptor and member of the immunoglobulin superfamily of proteins. GP VI is important in signal transduction for collagen induced platelet activation and therefore plays a pivotal role in the initial stages of platelet adhesion. Optimal activity of GP VI requires a coreceptor, the FC receptor γ-chain. In genetically altered mice deficient in the FC receptor, collagen induced platelet activation is impaired. A direct relationship exists between GP VI receptor content and platelet dependent prothrombi-nase activity and thrombin generation. In platelets with

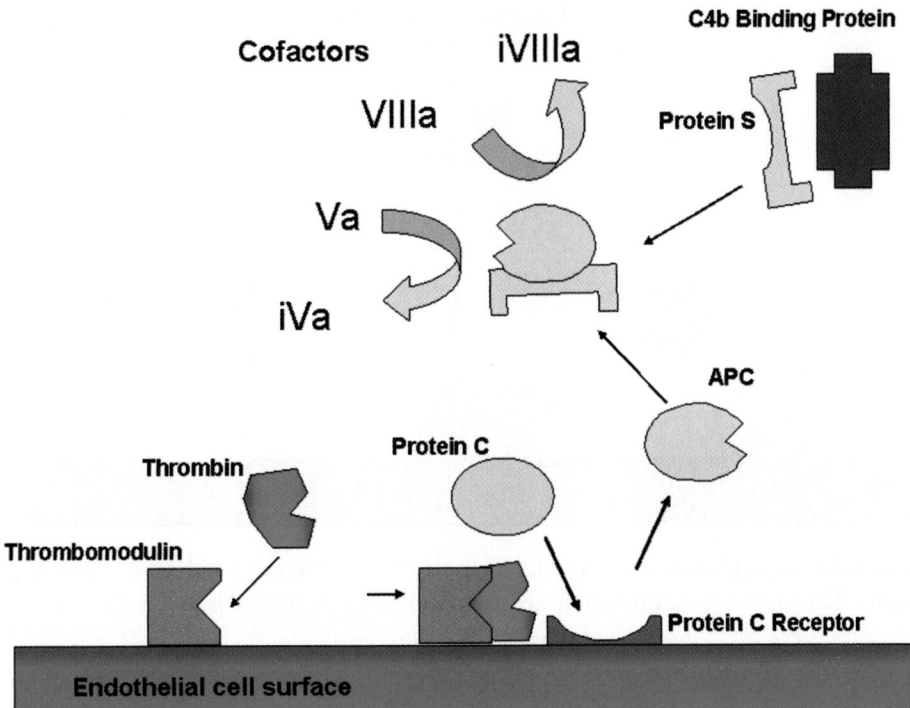

Fig. 4. Protein C anticoagulant system. The endogenous anticoagulant system turns off the coagulation cascade by cleaving cofactors Va and VIIIa to their inactive forms.

a high GP VI receptor density, prothrombin activation to thrombin is 3 fold greater than platelets with lower receptor content.

The **glycoprotein IIbIIIa** receptor (integrin $\alpha_{IIb}\beta_3$) plays a central role in platelet thrombus propagation. This receptor is abundant with 50-80,000 copies per cell, and requires activation before binding its primary ligand, fibrinogen. Activation of the platelet results in a conformational change of the receptor from the low affinity to the high affinity state. Binding fibrinogen to the activated receptor allows platelets to bind each other in the process of platelet aggregate formation. The PLA2 polymorphism results from a T – C nucleotide substitution at position 1565 and a Leu/Pro dimorphism at residue 33 of the β_3 chain. The PLA2 polymorphism results in a lower threshold of platelet activation, with increased P-selectin expression and fibrinogen binding. Platelets with this polymorphism bind fibrinogen more tightly and exhibit increased adhesion to immobilized fibrinogen with greater cell spreading, actin reorganization, and clot retraction. Furthermore, these platelets have a greater sensitivity to inhibition by therapeutic aspirin or abciximab

(Reopro; a chimeric monoclonal antibody against GP IIbIIIa). This polymorphism is common, occurring on at least one allele in 25% of northern Europeans.

P-selectin is expressed on the platelet cell membrane and mediates the binding of activated platelets to leukocytes. P-selectin is a component of platelet α-granules and is expressed on the cell surface following platelet activation. Binding of platelets to leukocytes by this receptor is mediated by p-selectin binding ligand (PSBL).

TISSUE FACTOR (EXTRINSIC) PATHWAY

Tissue factor is an integral surface membrane glycoprotein located in the wall of blood vessels (Fig. 6). The blood procoagulant system is initiated when vascular injury exposes tissue factor to flowing blood at the site of injury. Vascular injury results in rapid induction of tissue factor mRNA and a 10 fold augmentation of procoagulant activity. In both animal and human studies, inhibitors of tissue factor effectively prevent arterial thrombosis. Once the site of vascular injury has been covered by platelets and fibrin, exposure of flowing

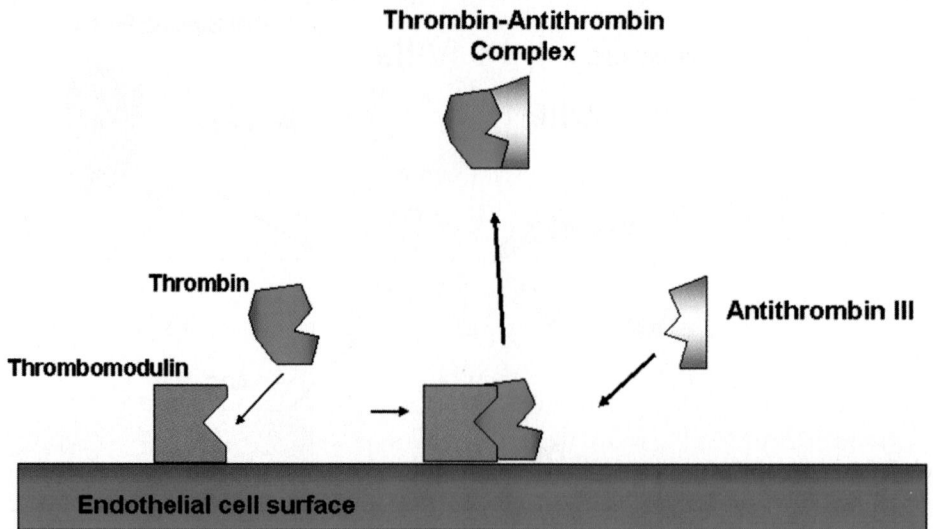

Fig. 5. Antithrombin III anticoagulant system. Antithrombin III captures thrombin and removes the inhibited enzyme from thrombomodulin. This thrombin-antithrombin complex is essentially irreversible and is cleared by the liver.

blood to the underlying vascular tissue factor is restricted. Recent work has shown that diffusion of procoagulant factors from the blood to vascular tissue factor exposed by injury is effectively blocked when the initial adherent platelet-fibrin thrombus reaches a thickness of just a few microns. Thus, vascular TF cannot support continued thrombus growth beyond a few microns thick. Additional studies have shown that TF also "circulates" within blood. Circulating TF appears to be "encrypted" within phospholipid microparticles that "bud" off monocytes stimulated by cytokines (e.g., TNF-α, IL-1). Circulating TF is essential for continued activation of the procoagulant system, accretion of fibrin and activated platelets, and thrombus growth. Levels of circulating tissue factor are elevated in patients with traditional risk factors for atherosclerosis such as diabetes, hyperlipidemia and tobacco exposure. Improved glycemic control in diabetic patients is associated with a reduction of circulating tissue factor and blood thrombogenicity assessed by ex vivo perfusion chamber platelet deposition.

Table 1. Platelet Storage Granule Content

Alpha granule	Dense body
• P-Selectin	• Adenosine nucleo-
• Growth factors	tides (ADP, ATP)
(PDGF, TFFβ)	• Serotonin
• Fibrinogen	
• Factor V	**Lysosome**
• Receptors (GP IIbIIIa;	• Hydrolases
GPIbIX; GPIV; GpV)	• LAMP 1/2
• Platelet factor 4	
• vWf	**Microperoxisome**
• Fibronectin	• Catalase
• Vitronectin	
• Osteonectin (SPARC)	

Table 2. Platelet Receptors, Receptor Ligands, and Shear Stress

Receptor	Ligand	Optimal shear stress
GP Ib-IX-V	VWF	High
GP Ia-IIa	Collagen	Low
GP VI	Collagen	Low
GP IIb-IIIa	Fibrinogen, VWF	Low
P-selectin	P-selectin binding ligand	

CONTACT ACTIVATION (INTRINSIC) PATHWAY

Both the extrinsic (tissue factor) and intrinsic (contact activation) coagulation factor activation pathways converge on prothrombin activation to thrombin (Fig. 6). The intrinsic pathway is initiated when factor XII comes into contact with negatively charged surfaces. Neither the mechanism for factor XII activation nor its relevance to *in vivo* coagulation activation is known. In contrast to factor VII deficiency for example, patients with factor XII deficiency do not experience excessive bleeding. From this, many have assumed that thrombin generation *in vivo* is largely the result of activation of the extrinsic (tissue factor) pathway with little input from factor XII activation. This hypothesis has been recently challenged by experiments with factor XII deficient mice. These mice did not bleed spontaneously and the bleeding times were normal. Following arterial injury, platelet adhesion occurred normally however both the formation and stabilization of thrombi in these mice was severely impaired. Thrombi did not occur at all in half of mice injured. In the remaining half, thrombi formed were unstable and detached from the vessel wall within 1 minute of formation. Similar results were noted in factor XI deficient mice following arterial injury.

VON WILLEBRAND FACTOR

Functional domains of von Willebrand factor (VWF) subunits include binding of platelet receptors GP Ib and GP IIbIIIa, coagulation factor VIII, heparin and collagen types I, III, and VI. VWF is synthesized in endothelial cells and megakaryocytes with the former being the principal source of circulating plasma protein content. In endothelial cells, newly synthesized VWF is either secreted constitutively or stored in Weibel-Palade bodies where polymerization of the protein occurs. This polymerization process can be extensive. Circulating VWF exists in plasma as multimers containing a variable number of subunits with molecular weights ranging from 500 kDa to more than 20,000 kDa. The ultra large VWF multimers when released form high-strength bonds with the platelet GP Ib–IX-V complex spontaneously, resulting in platelet adhesion, aggregation, and thrombus formation. Under normal circumstances, thrombosis is prevented by rapid (although partial) proteolysis by a metalloprotease called ADAMTS-13 (A Disintegrin And Metalloprotease with ThromboSpondin motif). ADAMTS-13 cleaves the Y842/M843 peptide bond in the VWF A2 domain releasing 176-kDa and 140-kDa fragments which are only active in the presence of modulators (ristocetin, botrocetin, high shear stress).

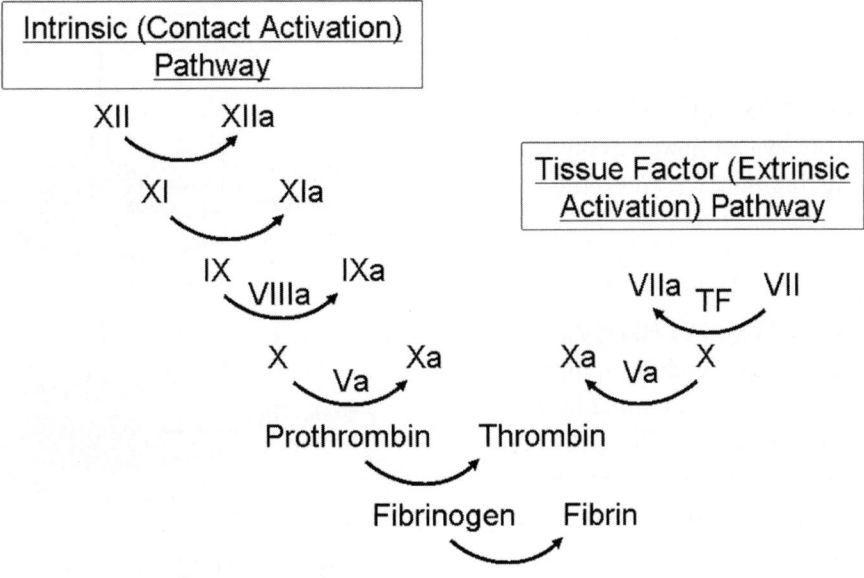

Fig. 6. **Coagulation cascade**. Both the intrinsic and extrinsic pathways converge on the prothrombinase complex which activates prothrombin to thrombin.

Disturbances in proteolysis have devastating outcome: increased cleavage causes severe bleeding (von Willebrand disease, type 2A) while decreased proteolysis induces multiorgan thrombosis (thrombotic thrombocytopenic purpura, TTP). Patients with stable angina not only have increased VWF antigen concentration, but significant decrease in ADAMTS-13 activity.

FIBRINOGEN

Plasmatic factors have been extensively studied for their contribution to arterial thrombosis. Elevated fibrinogen has been shown in a number of studies to be an independent risk variable for fatal or nonfatal cardiovascular events. In the Northwick Park Heart Study of 1511 men, high fibrinogen levels were associated with an 84% increased risk for fatal or nonfatal cardiovascular events. In the ARIC study of 14,477 individuals free of prevalent coronary atherosclerosis, fibrinogen was the only hemostatic variable to contribute beyond traditional risk factors to the prediction of coronary events though this contribution was modest. In another study, C reactive protein (CRP), fibrinogen and von Willebrand factor were compared in 150 patients with either recurrent myocardial infarction, stable coronary disease or matched controls. All three variables were elevated in both patient groups relative to controls. Compared to patients with stable coronary disease, those with recurrent MI had higher values of CRP (5.7±5.4 vs. 1.25±0.36 U/ml, p=0.003), fibrinogen (3.38±0.75 vs. 2.92±0.64 g/L, p=0.001) and von Willebrand factor (1.60±0.55 vs. 1.25±0.36 U/mL, p=0.0003). By multivariate analysis however, only CRP was predictive of future thrombotic events (odds 5.9, 95% CI 2.0 – 17.9, p=0.002).

OLD PARADIGM OF ARTERIAL THROMBOSIS

Acute arterial luminal thrombosis resulting in myocardial infarction is widely viewed as an unpredictable event governed predominantly by the rupture of an atherosclerotic plaque (Fig. 7). Observations of autopsy specimens have identified specific features associated with atherosclerotic plaques more likely to rupture. Plaques exhibiting these features are referred to as "vulnerable plaques." Features associated with plaque vulnerability include a lipid-rich core with abundant

lipid-laden macrophage foam cells enclosed within a thin friable fibrous cap typically less than 65 μm thick. The site of rupture is typically at the shoulder of the plaque and is histologically characterized by an inflammatory infiltrate of activated macrophages and T-lymphocytes. These inflammatory cells secrete cytokines and matrix metalloproteinases which proteolytically degrade the extracellular matrix thus weakening the structure of the thin fibrous cap. The plaque may rupture spontaneously or may be triggered by a surge of sympathetic activity associated with emotional stress or physical activity. Sudden increases in blood pressure and the force of cardiac contractility may result in critical

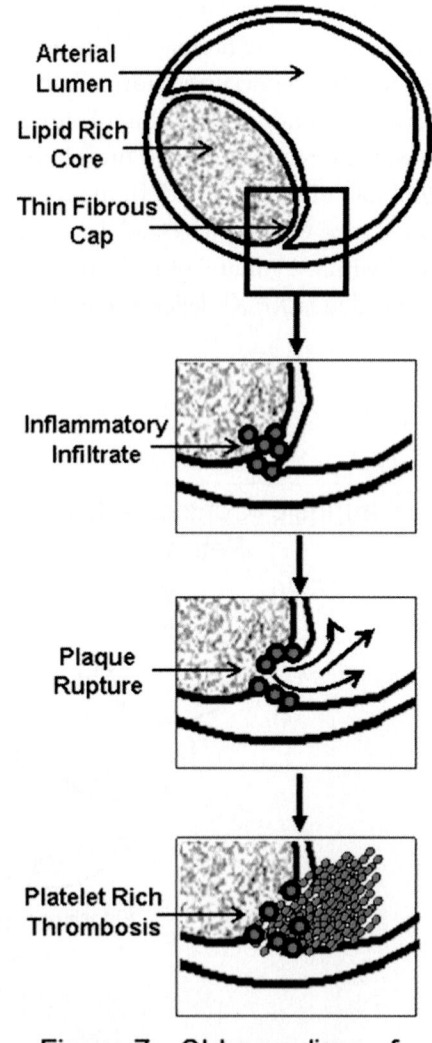

Figure 7. Old paradigm of arterial thrombosis

Fig. 7. Old paradigm of arterial thrombosis.

elevations of wall tension along the coronary arterial wall. Increases in wall tension with mechanical stress on the thin fibrous cap which lacks sufficient structural strength may then lead to plaque rupture. Following plaque rupture, exposure of the lipid rich core to flowing blood provides a potent stimulus for platelet-rich thrombus formation.

Although atherosclerotic plaque rupture is held to be the initiating event in most cases of acute MI, not all ruptured plaques result in thrombosis. Furthermore, many coronary thrombi occur without demonstrable plaque disruption and between 4% to as many as 30% of events occur in 'angiographically normal' coronary arteries. "Plaque erosion" defined as endothelial cell loss overlaying a smooth muscle and proteoglycan rich fibrous plaque may account for 15-44% of acute coronary thrombotic events. These latter coronary lesions lack the features typical of the vulnerable plaque including the lipid rich core. Endothelial denudation central to the plaque erosion hypothesis may be a very

common phenomenon in the general population and infrequently resulting in acute luminal thrombosis. This poor correlation between atherosclerosis and thrombosis suggests that additional factors other than simply the extent of atherosclerosis are important in determining *in situ* thrombosis. Acute arterial luminal thrombosis could be a random process or could arise from histologic or biochemical differences in atherosclerotic plaque composition, geometry, or stability. Alternatively, interindividual differences in the propensity for forming arterial thrombi could govern this process. These differences may arise from blood borne cellular or plasmatic factors and may be constitutive for the individual or constantly evolving in response to neuroendocrine, inflammatory or metabolic influences.

NEW PARADIGM OF ARTERIAL THROMBOSIS

The new paradigm for arterial thrombosis suggests that the clinical outcome is governed by both atherosclerotic

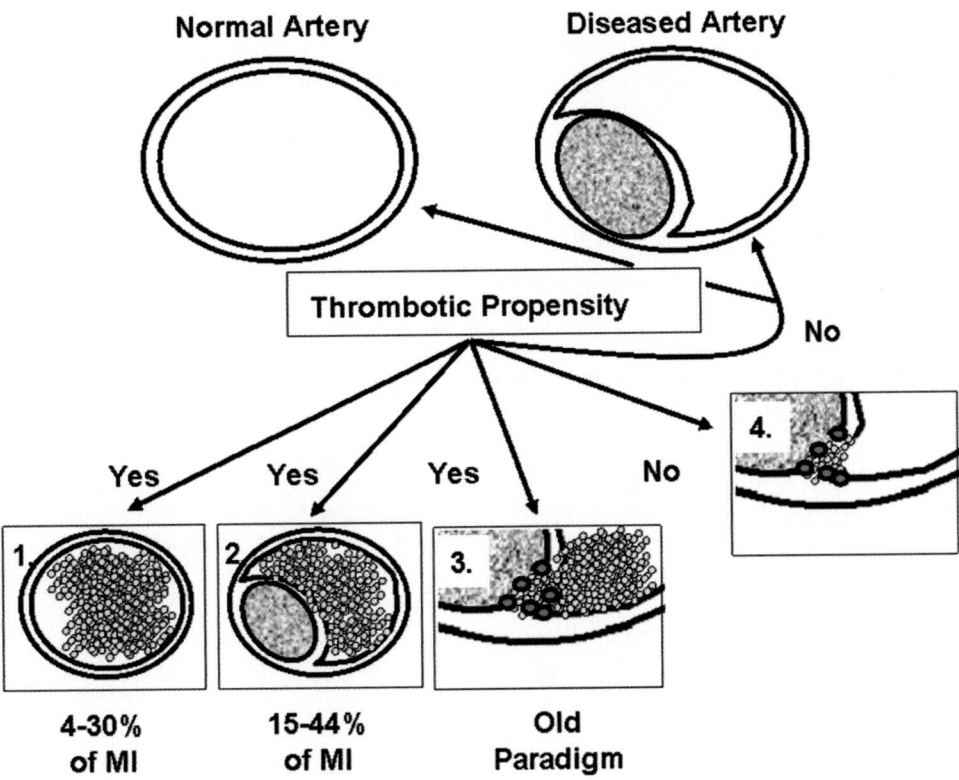

Fig. 8. **New paradigm of the vulnerable patient**. This paradigm combines the old paradigm of vulnerable plaque with the individual's thrombotic propensity.

plaque morphology, composition and stability and the propensity of the individual to form platelet-rich arterial thrombi. Under this new model (Fig. 8), individuals may be classified into one of four categories based on the presence or absence of variables increasing the propensity for thrombosis and presence or absence of atherosclerotic disease and plaque rupture. Within this new paradigm, individuals will range from very high risk for thrombosis when both atherosclerotic plaque rupture and an increased propensity for arterial thrombosis are present to very low risk when both variables are absent. The relative frequency of developing an acute MI within this paradigm would be low in the absence of atherosclerosis however between 4 and 30% of MIs occur in the setting of angiographically normal coronary arteries (scenario 1; "Acute Thrombosis/Normal Coronary Artery"). Whether these individuals harbor

cryptic atherosclerosis as a substrate for acute thrombosis is not known. The reported 15-44% prevalence of plaque erosion rather than rupture in MI cases may in actuality reflect scenario 2 ("Acute Thrombosis/Coronary Plaque without Rupture") whereby the major stimulus lies with the thrombotic propensity rather than the arterial substrate. Although scenario 3 ("Acute Thrombosis/Coronary Plaque Rupture") depicts the old paradigm, the contribution of the thrombotic propensity to this clinical outcome is poorly understood. Scenario 4 ("Plaque Rupture without Thrombosis") may be relatively prevalent in the general population of asymptomatic individuals and has been hypothesized to lead to plaque progression or growth. In summary, this thrombotic propensity may be governed by platelet variables, plasmatic variables or synergistic interaction between the two.

51

TREATMENT AND PREVENTION OF ARTERIAL THROMBOSIS

Robert D. McBane MD

Waldemar E. Wysokinski, MD

Each year, 1.1 million Americans suffer from MI and 700,000 Americans suffer from a new or recurrent stroke. These events are thrombotic in nature and therefore potentially both treatable and preventable with the appropriate use of antithrombotic agents. Current antithrombotic therapy targets three of four stages of thrombus formation including platelet activation, platelet aggregation, and coagulation cascade activation. There are no effective means to prevent the initial stage of platelet adhesion to injured arterial walls. This chapter reviews the mechanism of action, pharmacology and clinical use of agents for the prevention and treatment of arterial thrombosis. The current guidelines of the Seventh ACCP Conference on Antithrombotic and Thrombolytic Therapy are a valuable resource for anyone seeing cardiovascular patients and can be accessed online (www.chestjournal.org/content/vol126/3_suppl/).

- 4 stages of thrombus formation:
    - Platelet adhesion
    - Platelet activation
    - Platelet aggregation
    - Coagulation cascade activation

PLATELET INHIBITORS

Antiplatelet therapy is effective in preventing and treating arterial thrombotic events. Large clinical trials have documented a morbidity and mortality benefit with antiplatelet agents for coronary, cerebral, and peripheral arterial circulations. The three major classes of antiplatelet agents are cyclooxygenase inhibitors, ADP receptor antagonists, and finally platelet glycoprotein IIb/IIIa receptor inhibitors. The first two of these classes block platelet activation by agonist inhibition while the latter interferes with the final common pathway of platelet aggregation. Cyclooxygenase inhibitors and ADP receptor antagonists are well suited for both primary and secondary prevention of both myocardial infarction and stroke. As they are relatively weak platelet inhibitors their efficacy in acute arterial occlusion is somewhat limited. The latter class of agent, GP IIb/IIIa inhibitors, is much more effective in acute arterial thrombosis.

- Three major classes of antiplatelet agents:
    - Cyclooxygenase inhibitors
    - ADP receptor antagonists
    - Platelet glycoprotein IIb/IIIa receptor inhibitors

Platelet Activation

Aspirin (Table 1)

Aspirin permanently inhibits cyclooxygenase activity in the platelet. Cyclooxygenase (COX) exists in two isozyme forms (COX-1 and COX-2) and in the platelet is responsible for the first step in the conversion of arachidonic acid to its ultimate product, thromboxane A_2 (TxA_2). Thromboxane A_2 induces platelet activation and aggregation and promotes vasoconstriction (Fig. 1). Cyclooxygenase is also responsible for the production of endothelial cell-derived prostacyclin (PGI_2). In contrast to TxA_2, PGI_2 inhibits platelet aggregation and induces vasodilation. At doses of aspirin used for thromboprophylaxis, platelet COX-1 is preferentially inhibited and vascular PGI_2 production continues relatively unabated.

Aspirin is rapidly absorbed from stomach mucosa with peak plasma levels achieved within 30 minutes of ingestion. Enteric coating, however, may delay the absorption by 3-4 hours. In the urgent setting, therefore, chewing enteric coated aspirin is advisable. The plasma half-life of aspirin is short ranging from 15-20 minutes.

Table 1.   Aspirin

Settings with the greatest benefit-to-risk ratio
  Lone atrial fibrillatiion (without additional
    risk factors)
  Chronic stable angina
  Prior myocardial infarction
  Unstable angina
  Acute myocardial infarction or stroke
Risk of major hemorrhage is approximately 0.7%
  per year
No proven benefit for venous thrombosis prophy-
  laxis

In healthy subjects, a single dose of 100 mg of aspirin results in 98% inhibition of thromboxane production within one hour of ingestion. This same inhibition is seen with 0.45 mg/kg/day (ie, 40 mg) given over 4 days. With discontinuation of aspirin use, cyclooxygenase recovery occurs as new platelets enter the circulation. Platelet lifespan averages 9-11 days, therefore sensitive assays of platelet aggregation may be abnormal for up to

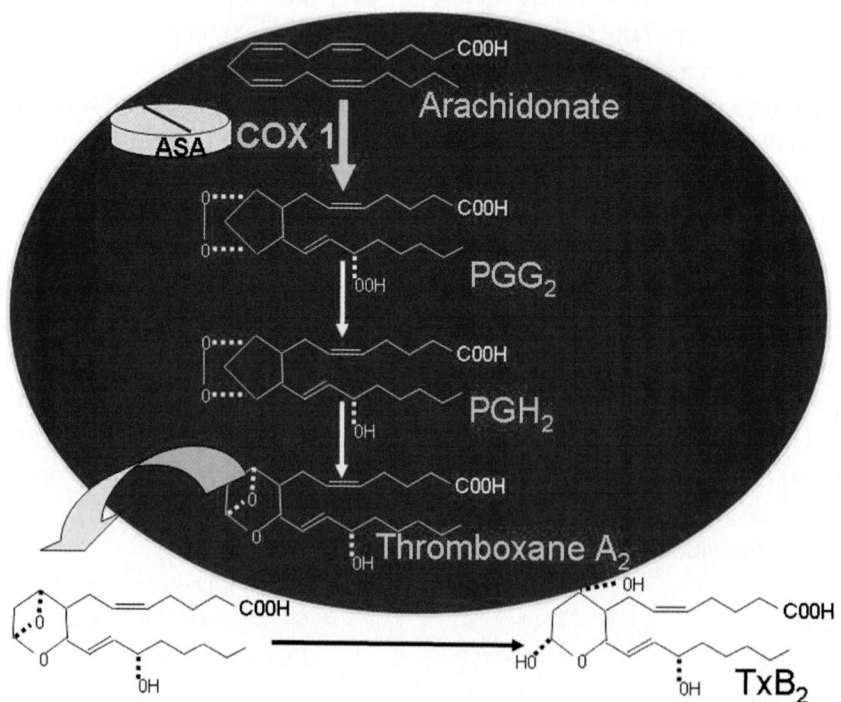

Fig. 1. Platelet arachidonate metabolism. Arachidonate is sequentially metabolized to thromboxane A_2 within the platelet. Thromboxane A_2 is the metabolite which ultimate accomplishes platelet activation before being converted to thromboxane B_2 for renal excretion.

10 days after a single dose of aspirin. Each day, 10% of the circulating platelet population is renewed.

Aspirin therapy in patients with coronary artery disease is associated with a 23% reduction in vascular events. As such, Americans consume 35,000 kg of aspirin daily. The search for the optimal dose of aspirin has led to the performance of multiple randomized controlled trials with aspirin doses ranging from 30 mg to 1,500 mg/day. These trials have demonstrated the efficacy of low-dose aspirin for both primary and secondary cardiovascular protection. For patients at high risk of developing arterial thrombosis, the lowest effective dose has been shown to be 75 mg. For patients suffering either an acute myocardial infarction or an acute stroke, the lowest effective dose is 160 mg. Although aspirin is an effective antithrombotic agent over a large dose range, the lower doses appear to be more effective than higher doses and produce fewer gastrointestinal side effects and lower bleeding rates. The risk of major bleeding on low-dose aspirin is less than 1%. Neither enteric-coated nor buffered preparations have been shown to reduce this risk.

More than 70 trials enrolling more than 100,000 patients have been completed assessing the efficacy of aspirin therapy. The biggest relative benefit is seen in those patients suffering acute arterial thrombotic events. In the ISIS-2 trial for example, patients receiving aspirin 162 mg/day experienced nearly 25% reduction in mortality and nearly 50% reduction of recurrent MI or stroke. In moderate to high-risk patients from other trials (those with remote history of MI, unstable angina, prior TIA or stroke), aspirin use was associated with 25% risk reduction. Primary prevention trials of aspirin have shown mixed results largely depending on the degree of cardiovascular risk of the population studied. In very low-risk individuals, it has been difficult to demonstrate an advantage of aspirin over placebo for primary prevention. In the setting of atrial fibrillation, the consensus is that anticoagulant therapy with coumarin derivatives reduces the risk of thromboembolism more effectively than antiplatelet therapy. This average risk reduction is 68% (range 45%-82%) for warfarin compared to 20% (range 0-42%) for aspirin. Protection from cardioembolic events with aspirin is therefore inferior to the use of warfarin in atrial fibrillation. Moreover, aspirin does not provide effective venous thromboembolism prophylaxis.

Some patients however will suffer a thrombotic event despite daily aspirin therapy. One in eight patients treated with aspirin will experience an arterial thrombotic event in 2-3 years of follow-up. One proposed explanation for these "aspirin failures" is that platelets from these individuals are not effectively inhibited and therefore "aspirin resistant." Aspirin resistance has been defined as the failure of aspirin to produce the anticipated inhibition of platelet function by in vitro testing or in vivo thrombotic outcomes. The prevalence of aspirin resistance varies from 5.2%-60% depending on the patient population studied and criteria used for defining the condition. Of more than academic interest, aspirin resistance has been shown to increase the risk of thrombosis. In a nested case-control substudy of the HOPE trial, aspirin-resistant patients had a 2-fold increased risk of MI (95% CI, 1.2-3.4) and a 3.5-fold increased risk of cardiovascular death (95% CI, 1.7-7.4) compared to aspirin-sensitive individuals. In an additional study of 326 stable patients taking aspirin undergoing elective coronary angiography, the annual event rate in aspirin-resistant patients was 12.9% compared to 5.4% in those patients sensitive to aspirin (HR 3.12, 95% CI, 1.10-8.90; P=0.03). The prevalence of aspirin resistance in 100 patients with peripheral arterial disease undergoing elective angioplasty was nearly 60%. During the one-year follow-up period following angioplasty, 8 arterial occlusions were confirmed, all of which occurred in aspirin-resistant patients. In 174 stroke survivors followed for 2 years, major thrombotic end points were nearly 10-fold higher in aspirin-resistant compared to aspirin-sensitive patients (4.0% vs. 4.4% respectively; P<0.0001). The exact mechanism of aspirin resistance is not known. Screening for aspirin resistance has not been widely endorsed. When present, it remains unclear what therapeutic adjustments should be instituted.

- At doses of aspirin used for thromboprophylaxis, platelet COX-1 is preferentially inhibited
- Platelet lifespan averages 9-11 days, therefore sensitive assays of platelet aggregation may be abnormal for up to 10 days after a single dose of aspirin.
- For patients at high risk of developing arterial thrombosis, the lowest effective dose of aspirin has been shown to be 75 mg.
- For patients suffering either an acute myocardial

infarction or an acute stroke, the lowest effective dose of aspirin is 160 mg.

■ Aspirin resistance has been shown to increase the risk of thrombosis.

Thienopyridines (Table 2)

ADP, a weak but important platelet agonist, stimulates platelets through the binding of the ADP receptor, P2Y12. Upon activation, ADP is released from platelet-dense granules and from endothelial cells. ADP release amplifies recruitment and aggregation of adjacent platelets thereby promoting arterial thrombus formation. There are two structurally similar ADP receptor antagonists currently available, clopidogrel and ticlopidine. Both agents require in vivo hepatic transformation to the short-lived active metabolite. Both agents inhibit platelet function by the irreversible modification of the P2Y12 (ADP) receptor. Steady-state platelet inhibition occurs 4-7 days after drug initiation. With clopidogrel, the inhibitory effect is achieved more rapidly if a 300-mg loading dose is given. Higher loading doses of clopidogrel (450-600 mg) prior to PCI may provide additional and earlier inhibitory effect compared to 300 mg.

Ticlopidine

Ticlopidine has been shown to be effective in secondary prevention trials of myocardial infarction and may be superior to aspirin in stroke. As compared with warfarin plus aspirin, combined antiplatelet therapy with ticlopidine and aspirin following coronary artery stenting reduced the incidence of MI, stent thrombosis, or the need for repeat PTCA, with fewer vascular access and hemorrhagic complications. In one study of more than 500 high-risk patients undergoing PCI with bare metal stents, this composite end point was 1.5% for those receiving ticlopidine plus aspirin compared to 6.2% for those randomized to warfarin plus aspirin. Stent thrombosis was reduced from 5.4% to 0.8% for patients receiving antiplatelet therapy. In another study of 1,653 moderate-risk patients, the use of ticlopidine plus aspirin reduced the composite end point from 3.7% to 0.5% compared to warfarin plus aspirin. These antithrombotic benefits were durable throughout the first year following the procedure. Based on this early experience with a thienopyridine plus aspirin following coronary stent placement, this combination of agents

Table 2.   Thienopyridines

Inhibit platelet ADP (P2Y12) receptor
Settings with the greatest benefit-to-risk ratio
    Peripheral arterial occlusive disease
    Non ST segment myocardial infarction
    (combined with aspirin)
    Coronary stent implantation (particularly if
    stent is drug eluting)
Risk of major hemorrhage
    1.4% per year (clopidogrel alone)
    2.0%-3.7% per year (combined with aspirin)
No proven benefit for venous thrombosis prophylaxis

has become the standard of care for this setting. The STIMS trial comparing ticlopidine to placebo in 687 patients with intermittent claudication found a relative risk reduction of 30% for all-cause mortality and a 50% reduction of fatal vascular events. Ticlopidine significantly improves long-term patency of saphenous vein bypass grafts to the lower extremity as compared to placebo. Diarrhea and neutropenia are potential adverse effects which require monitoring and drug discontinuation in 2% and 1% of patients respectively.

Clopidogrel

The efficacy of clopidogrel has been studied extensively in several randomized, controlled trials. The **CAPRIE** (Clopidogrel vs. Aspirin in Patients at Risk of Ischemic Events) trial randomly assigned 19,185 high-risk atherosclerosis patients to receive clopidogrel (75 mg/day) or aspirin (325 mg/day) to determine which therapy resulted in the greatest reduction in vascular events. Participant inclusion was nearly equally distributed into three patient subgroups: stroke, myocardial infarction, or symptomatic atherosclerotic peripheral arterial disease. After a mean follow-up of 1.91 years, patients treated with clopidogrel experienced fewer annual events (stroke, myocardial infarction, or vascular death) relative to aspirin (5.32% vs. 5.83%; $P=0.043$). The biggest risk reduction was seen in patients with peripheral arterial disease. For these patients, the average event rate per year in the clopidogrel group was 3.71% compared with 4.86% in the aspirin group

(*P*<0.005). In post-hoc analysis of the CAPRIE database, the likelihood of vascular events was assessed after excluding patients with asymptomatic atherosclerotic disease. In the remaining symptomatic individuals, clopidogrel therapy was associated with an absolute risk reduction of 3.4% for the combined end point of stroke, MI, or vascular death (yearly absolute risk reduction = 1.13%). The rates at 3 years were 20.4% with clopidogrel and 23.8% with ASA (number needed to treat, 29; *P*=0.045).

The **CURE** investigators randomly assigned 12,562 patients with recent onset non-ST-segment elevation myocardial infarction to receive clopidogrel or placebo in addition to aspirin for 3 to 12 months. Patients receiving clopidogrel plus aspirin experienced significantly lower composite end point (vascular death, nonfatal myocardial infarction, or stroke) compared to patients receiving placebo plus aspirin (9.3% vs. 11.4%; *P*<0.001). Clopidogrel therapy however was associated with a significantly greater risk of major bleeding (3.7% vs. 2.7%; *P*=0.001). Patients requiring cardiac surgery were required to wait for 5 days after stopping clopidogrel because of the increased risk of major hemorrhage when taking this drug. In an important substudy under the acronym **PCI-CURE**, the hypothesis was expanded to address whether clopidogrel was more effective than aspirin alone in preventing major ischemic events after PCI sustainable up to 1 year. In this substudy, 2,658 patients were pretreated for 6 days with either clopidogrel or placebo prior to undergoing PCI for their acute coronary syndrome. The primary end point (composite of cardiovascular death, myocardial infarction, or urgent target-vessel revascularization within 30 days) was achieved in significantly fewer patients in the clopidogrel group (4.5%) compared to the placebo group (6.4%). At one year, the rate of cardiovascular death or myocardial infarction was lower in the clopidogrel group (3.1%) compared to the placebo group (3.9%) [adjusted relative risk 0.72 (95% CI 0.53-0.96) *P*=0.030].

The **CREDO** trial sought to determine both the benefit of a preprocedure loading dose of clopidogrel and the efficacy of long-term clopidogrel therapy after PCI. Patients (n=2,116) were first randomly assigned to receive either a 300-mg clopidogrel loading dose or placebo 3 to 24 hours prior to PCI. After PCI, all patients received clopidogrel for one month. After one

month, those patients assigned to receive the loading dose were also assigned to continue clopidogrel therapy for 1 year. After one month of clopidogrel therapy, the non-loading dose group received placebo for one year. These investigators were able to show that at 1 year, clopidogrel therapy resulted in a 3% absolute risk reduction of the combined end points (death, MI, or stroke). A pretreatment loading dose however did not significantly reduce these endpoints.

The **MATCH** investigators randomized 7,599 patients with recent stroke or TIA to clopidogrel 75 mg/day or clopidogrel plus aspirin. Twelve patients were followed for 18 months to assess the composite end point of stroke, myocardial infarction, vascular death, or re-hospitalization for acute ischemia. End points were comparable for the clopidogrel plus aspirin (15.7%) vs. clopidogrel alone (16.7%) groups. Life-threatening bleeding however was significantly higher in the group receiving combination therapy (2.6% vs 1.3%; *P*<0.0001). Major bleeding occurred in 2% in the clopidogrel/aspirin group compared to 1% for clopidogrel/placebo patients. The rate of intracranial hemorrhage was 1% for both groups.

The combination of clopidogrel and aspirin has become standard therapy following coronary stent implantation, particularly if the stents are drug eluting. A thienopyridine combined with aspirin has been shown in several studies to be superior to warfarin plus aspirin for the prevention of thrombotic complications in this setting. The composite cardiovascular end points of death, MI, bypass surgery, and repeat angioplasty are reduced from 5.4%-6.2% to between 0.8%-1.5% with combined antiplatelet therapy. Furthermore, the long-term clopidogrel given up to 12 months reduced composite end points by 26.9% relative to short term therapy of 4 weeks.

Although the main side effect of clopidogrel therapy is hemorrhagic complications, there is clinical evidence that clopidogrel does more than inhibit the platelet ADP receptor. Indeed, the hemorrhagic complications of clopidogrel are not corrected simply by platelet transfusion. An additional adverse reaction of this drug includes thrombotic thrombocytopenic purpura (TTP). TTP is a rare, potentially fatal multisystem disease characterized by thrombocytopenia, microangiopathic hemolytic anemia, fever, neurologic deficits, and renal failure. Both clopidogrel and ticlopidine have been shown to cause TTP in about 0.02% of patients taking these drugs. In the original report of the association of TTP with clopidogrel, all but one of 11 patients developed the disease within 14 days of drug initiation. The pathophysiologic mechanism underlying clopidogrel-associated TTP appears to be related to impaired proteolysis of von Willebrand factor by ADAMSTS-13 metalloprotease. Ultra-large VWF multimers bind platelets resulting in platelet microthrombi that characterize the syndrome. Immune-mediated deficiency of ADAMSTS-13, possibly by an autoantibody (IgG) against the protease, has been suggested. In 2 patients tested, IgG inhibitors of the protease were not demonstrated in plasma samples. Most patients responded to plasma exchange therapy (91%); however, 2 required more than 20 treatments.

- Both ticlopidine and clopidogrel require in vivo hepatic transformation
- The combination of clopidogrel and aspirin has become standard therapy following stent implantation
- TTP may be a complication of clopidogrel or ticlopidine therapy

Dipyridamole (Table 3)

Phosphodiesterase is the principal enzyme responsible for the metabolism of cyclic adenosine monophosphate (cAMP) to AMP for regeneration ATP. Dipyridamole, by inhibiting phosphodiesterase, leads to an intracellular accumulation of cAMP. This accumulation inhibits platelet aggregation. Dipyridamole (200 mg) combined with aspirin (25 mg) is sold under the trade name of Aggrenox and is given orally twice daily. It is currently FDA approved for the prevention of stroke. Metabolism is primarily by the liver. This drug should be used with caution in patients with liver failure, renal failure and congestive heart failure. Available data are either insufficient or do not support the use of dipyridamole (alone or in combination with aspirin) for the prevention or treatment of arterial thrombosis in the setting of acute myocardial infarction, unstable angina, atrial fibrillation, mechanical heart prosthesis, or venous thrombosis. The combined use of aspirin plus dipyridamole has been used successfully in the prevention of neurovascular thrombotic events.

The first European Stroke Prevention Study (**ESPS-1**) randomized 2,500 patients with a recent

Table 3.   Dipyridamole

Phosphodiesterase inhibitor
Settings with the greatest benefit to risk ratio
    Stroke prophylaxis (when combined with aspirin)
Risk of major hemorrhage
    1.8% per year (when combined with aspirin)
No proven benefit for venous thrombosis prophylaxis

stroke, TIA or RIND of "atherosclerotic origin" to receive either dipyridamole 75 mg plus ASA 325 mg or placebo TID. After 24 months of follow-up, the predetermined end point (stroke or death from any cause) was significantly lower in the treatment arm (15.8%) compared to the placebo arm (22.6%). Although demonstrating statistical superiority to placebo, this study was criticized for not using aspirin alone as the comparator.

In the second European Stroke Prevention Study (**ESPS-2**), aspirin plus extended-release dipyridamole (ASA 25mg plus dipyridamole 200 mg given twice daily) was compared to aspirin alone (50 mg daily) or dipyridamole alone (400 mg daily) in patients with stroke or TIA within the preceding 3 months. In this study, 6,602 patients were randomized and followed for 2 years. The primary end points of this trial were stroke, death from all causes, or both. Compared to placebo, stroke risk was reduced by 18% with ASA alone, 16% with dipyridamole alone, and 37% with combination therapy. Combined risk of stroke or death was reduced by 13% with ASA alone, 15% with dipyridamole alone, and 24% with the combination. Based on these data, it was concluded that the combination of aspirin and dipyridamole result in additive protective effects against stroke and TIA.

GP IIb/IIIa Inhibitors

The final common pathway in arterial thrombosis, platelet aggregation, involves the binding of fibrinogen by activated GP IIb/IIIa receptors on adjacent platelets. Receptor blockade, by inhibiting fibrinogen binding, prevents aggregation regardless of the initiating agonist (Fig. 2). As there are a number of potential agonists, this strategy is particularly attractive. Numerous natural and synthetic peptides have been evaluated for their potential of blocking this receptor. These inhibitors can be subdivided into anti-GP IIb/IIIa monoclonal antibodies, viper venoms, RGD peptides, and nonpeptide analogs.

Abciximab (Table 4)

Abciximab (Reopro, c7E3), is the chimeric FAB fragment of a murine monoclonal antibody against the activated GP IIb/IIIa receptor. Infusion of this antibody produces prolonged and extensive receptor blockade with marked inhibition of platelet aggregation and bleeding times. Successful treatment with abciximab requires that the majority (90%) of the GP IIb/IIIa receptors are occupied by the antibody. Clinical efficacy has been documented in unstable angina, with a significant reduction in ischemic events and angiographic improvement of the coronary lesions. In combination with rt-PA for the treatment of acute MI, abciximab improved patency rates. Three trials, EPIC, EPILOG, and EPISTENT involving patients undergoing high-

risk angioplasty comprise the largest clinical experience with this drug. In the **EPIC** trial, 2,099 patients were randomized to receive abciximab or placebo prior to undergoing high-risk PCI. Abciximab resulted in a 35% reduction in the rate of the combined primary end point of death, nonfatal MI, surgical revascularization,

Table 4.   Summary: Abciximab

Antiplatelet glycoprotein IIb/IIIa murine monoclonal antibody
Settings with the greatest benefit-to-risk ratio
    High-risk angioplasty and stenting
    PCI for acute myocardial infarction
    Not recommended as a fibrinolytic adjunctive agent
Risk of major hemorrhage 1.4%-3.3%
Thrombocytopenia limits use in 1%-2% of patients
Anti-abciximab antibody which forms in a minority of patients is of unclear significance

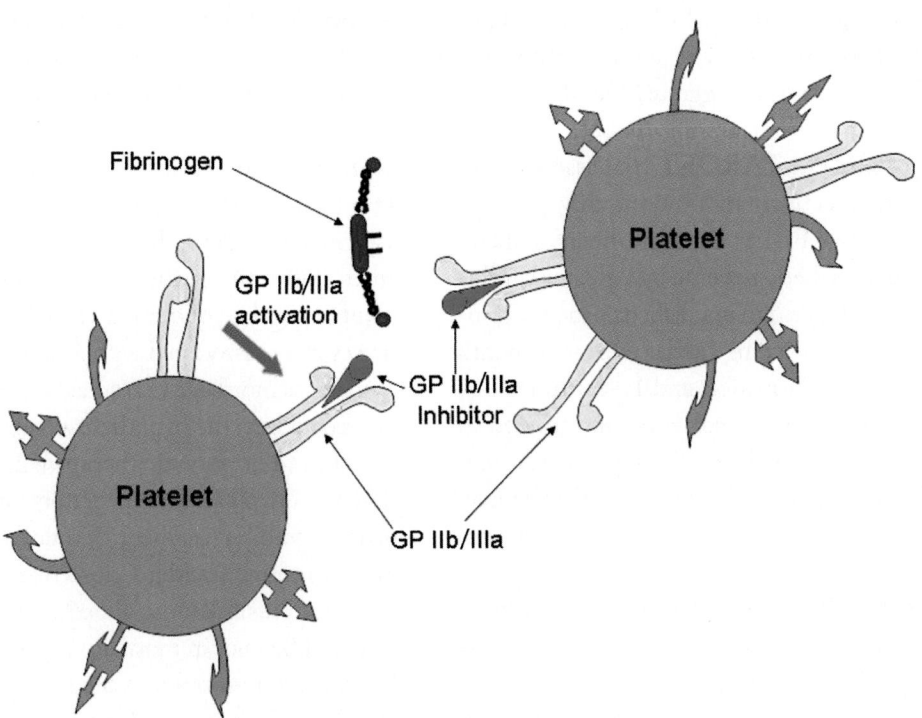

Fig. 2. Glycoprotein IIb/IIIa inhibitors. Platelet activation results in converson of GP IIb/IIIa from the inactive to the active form of the receptor. GP IIb/IIIa inhibitors block the binding of fibrinogen to this receptor and thus prevent platelet aggregation.

repeat PCI, unplanned implantation of a coronary stent, or insertion of an intra-aortic balloon pump for refractory ischemia. Initial trials in which abciximab was given in conjunction with standard doses of heparin and aspirin resulted in significantly increased bleeding complications and transfusion requirements.

In the subsequent **EPILOG** study, which included patients undergoing both urgent and elective PTCA, concomitant heparin therapy was significantly reduced in an attempt to improve clinical safety. This combination of abciximab plus reduced dose of heparin resulted in a 68% reduction in 30-day mortality and myocardial infarction with bleeding complication rates similar to placebo.

Six-month follow-up data from the **EPIC** trial revealed that treatment with abciximab reduces the rate of clinical restenosis. The mechanism behind this finding is unclear yet may related to the antibody cross reactivity with a second receptor, $\alpha v \beta III$, the vitronectin receptor. In addition to providing a scaffold for coagulation factor activating complex assembly, platelet storage granules contain rich stores of growth factors. By limiting platelet content at the site of injury, this agent may reduce platelet growth factor release and thrombin generation, both of which have been implicated in the pathogenesis of restenosis. Subgroup analyses of abciximab trials suggested that this benefit was particularly evident among diabetic patients undergoing PCI. The **TARGET** trial assessed this hypothesis prospectively by randomizing patients undergoing elective PCI to either tirofiban or abciximab. Although diabetic patients had greater cardiovascular events compared to nondiabetic patients, comparable event rates, including similar rates of 6-month target vessel revascularization and 1-year mortality, were seen among diabetic patients randomized to either of the two agents. These findings suggest that the non-glycoprotein IIb/IIIa properties of abciximab do not translate into a discernible long-term clinical benefit among diabetic patients

The **EPISTENT** trial randomized 2,399 patients to coronary stenting plus placebo, stenting plus abciximab, or angioplasty plus abciximab. The primary end point, combination of death, myocardial infarction, or need for urgent revascularization, was lowest in those patients assigned to coronary stenting plus abciximab (hazard ratio 0.48 [95% CI 0.33-0.69] P<0.001).

Major bleeding complications were not different between groups.

The **CAPTURE** study assessed the efficacy of abciximab in patients with refractory unstable angina undergoing PCI. Twelve hundred sixty five patients were randomized to receive intravenous abciximab or placebo for 18-24 hours prior to PTCA and continuing for 1 hour afterwards. By 30 days, there was a significant reduction in ischemic events in the abciximab group. After 6 months of follow up, however, death, myocardial infarction, or need for repeat intervention was equivalent in the two groups.

In the larger **CADILLAC** study, 2,082 patients with STEMI were randomized to undergo PTCA alone, PTCA plus abciximab, stenting alone, or stenting plus abciximab therapy. At six months, there were no significant differences among the groups in the rates of death, stroke, or reinfarction. The rates of target-vessel revascularization were significantly lower in patients undergoing stenting with abciximab (5.2%) compared to PTCA alone (15.7%). The rate of angiographically established restenosis was nearly 50% lower in those patients receiving a stent. The rates of reocclusion of the infarct-related artery were 11.3 percent and 5.7 percent (P=0.01), both independent of abciximab use.

The **GUSTO IV ACS** trial randomized 7,825 MI patients to receive either placebo, abciximab bolus plus 24 hour infusion, or abciximab bolus plus 48 hour infusion in addition to standard therapy of heparin and aspirin. At 30 days, there were no significant differences among the treatment groups for the primary end point (composite of death and MI). Abciximab therapy however was associated with a significantly higher risk of major hemorrhage (1.0% versus 0.2%).

To address the hypothesis combining GP IIb/IIIa inhibitor to fibrinolytic therapy will improve reperfusion, the **GUSTO V** investigators randomized 16,588 patients with ST-segment elevation myocardial infarction to receive standard-dose reteplase or half-dose reteplase plus full-dose abciximab. At 30 days, there was no difference in mortality between the two groups. Patients randomized to receive reteplase alone experienced less frequent need for urgent revascularization, fewer major nonfatal ischemic complications of their MI and less frequent major hemorrhage compared to the combined group. In a similar study, the **ASSENT 3** investigators randomized 6,095 patients with acute myocardial infarction to one of three regimens: full-dose tenecteplase plus enoxaparin; half-dose tenecteplase, abciximab, and unfractionated heparin; or full-dose tenecteplase plus unfractionated heparin. The efficacy outcomes were nearly identical for enoxaparin and abciximab groups. Based on these combined data, it is recommended that abciximab *not* be used as an adjunctive agent to fibrinolytic therapy.

Thrombocytopenia is one of the primary side effects of abciximab therapy and may contribute to hemorrhagic complications of this drug. It is therefore recommended that a platelet count be assessed 2-4 hours after initiating therapy. The platelet count decrement is often mild, with a nadir above 75 x 10³/µL. Marked thrombocytopenia may require abrupt abciximab cessation and platelet transfusion in 1%-2% of patients. True thrombocytopenia must be distinguished from pseudothrombocytopenia which results from platelet agglutination *in vitro* when blood is sampled in EDTA. This accounts for 1/3-2/3 of thrombocytopenia occurring after abciximab administration. Distinguishing thrombocytopenia from pseudothrombocytopenia is clinically important and must be completed rapidly as not to interrupt the delivery of this important antiplatelet therapy.

An additional potential side effect is the development of antibodies to abciximab which occurred in approximately 6% of patients enrolled in the **EPIC** trial. These antibodies form against the variable region of abciximab. The potential risk of abciximab reexposure in these patients is unclear but could include anaphylaxis or drug neutralization or thrombocytopenia.

- Abciximab should not be used as an adjunctive agent to fibrinolytic therapy.
- Thrombocytopenia is one of the primary side effects of abciximab therapy.
- The potential risk of abciximab reexposure in these patients with antibody formation is unclear but could include anaphylaxis or drug neutralization.

Tirofiban (Table 5)
The GP IIb/IIIa receptor recognition of the amino acid sequence RGD (arginine, glycine, aspartic acid) on the fibrinogen molecule permits binding of the receptor to this protein. Synthetic RGD peptides, by occu-

pying these receptor sites, competitively inhibit fibrinogen interaction with the receptor and thereby prevent aggregation. Tirofiban (Aggrastat) is a nonpeptide derivative of tyrosine which selectively inhibits the RGD binding site of the platelet GP IIb/IIIa receptor. Tirofiban is delivered intravenously with a rapid onset of action (5 minutes). The recommended dosage of tirofiban is 0.4 mcg/kg/min for 30 minutes followed by a continuous infusion of 0.1 mcg/kg/min for 12 to 24 hours. In most patients, platelet aggregation studies return to pretreatment levels within 4 to 8 hours after discontinuation. The clearance of tirofiban is primarily renal (65% with 35% fecal elimination), and therefore a dose reduction should be considered in patients with severe renal impairment (creatinine clearance <30 mL/min).

In a study of 2,139 patients with acute coronary syndromes undergoing PTCA, the **RESTORE** investigators assessed the efficacy of tirofiban in the reduction of composite end points including all-cause mortality and recurrent ischemic events. Within 2 days of intervention, a highly significant 38% relative risk reduction of composite end points were noted in the tirofiban group. By 7 days, the relative reduction was 27% and at 30 days this reduction had fallen to 16%, still in favor of tirofiban though no longer statistically significant. Major bleeding was not different between the two groups. In general, the rate of major bleeding with tirofiban varies from 1.4% to 2.2%. Bleeding complications appear to be higher in female and elderly patients.

Two trials have assessed tirofiban in the setting of non-ST segment elevation myocardial infarction, the PRISM and PRISM-PLUS trials. The **PRISM** trial randomized 3,231 patients to receive either tirofiban or

Table 5. Tirofiban

Synthetic platelet glycoprotein IIb/IIIa inhibitor
Settings with the greatest benefit-to-risk ratio
   Non-ST segment myocardial infarction
   Not recommended as a fibrinolytic adjunctive agent
Risk of major hemorrhage 0.4%-1.4%

heparin administered for 48 hours. Coronary angiography was deferred until study drug administration was complete. The primary end point assessed at the completion of drug infusion (death, MI, or refractory ischemia) was significantly lower in patients receiving tirofiban (3.8%) compared to heparin (5.6%). Furthermore, this benefit was maintained at 30 days. Major hemorrhage was the same for both groups (0.4%).

The second trial, **PRISM-PLUS**, randomized 1,915 patients to receive either tirofiban alone, tirofiban plus heparin, or heparin alone. At an interim analysis, the tirofiban-alone arm was discontinued by the Data Safety and Monitoring Board, due to excess mortality. At the final analysis, tirofiban plus heparin was associated with a significant reduction in the primary composite end point (death, MI, or refractory ischemia at 7 days) compared with heparin alone (12.9% vs 17.9%). This benefit was maintained at 30 days and 6 months. Major bleeding was similar between the tirofiban plus heparin group (1.4%) compared to the heparin alone group (0.8%).

To compare GP IIb/IIIa inhibitors in unstable angina and myocardial infarction, 4,809 patients undergoing PCI were randomly assigned to receive either tirofiban or abciximab initiated prior to angiography. The primary end point, a composite of death, nonfatal myocardial infarction, or urgent target-vessel revascularization at 30 days, occurred more frequently among patients in the tirofiban group (7.6%) than among patients in the abciximab group (6.0%). This study demonstrated superiority of abciximab over tirofiban in these clinical settings. The difference in the incidence of myocardial infarction between the tirofiban group (6.9%) and the abciximab group (5.4%) was significant. There were no significant differences in the rates of major bleeding complications between the two groups.

Eptifibatide (Table 6)

Eptifibatide (Integrilin) is a cyclic heptapeptide containing a modified KGD sequence in which arginine (R) has been replaced by lysine (K). This short-acting inhibitor was modeled after the venom of the southeastern pigmy rattlesnake, *Sistrurus m. barbouri*. The lysine substitution provides more inhibition specificity for GP IIb/IIIa compared to other integrins containing the RGD sequence. Eptifibatide is given intravenously (180 mg/kg bolus followed by 2 μg/kg per

minute infusion) for up to 72 hours for the indication of unstable angina or PCI. Plasma half-life is 2.5 hours and antiplatelet effects persist for 4 hours after infusion discontinuation. Eptifibatide is primarily cleared by the kidney and should be avoided in patients with renal impairment (creatinine clearance <30 mL/min).

The **IMPACT II** trial compared two doses of Integrilin to placebo in 4,010 patients undergoing elective, urgent or emergent coronary intervention. The lower of the two doses reduced rates of early abrupt closure and ischemic events at 30 days compared to placebo. This effect was not statistically significant at the higher dose.

The **ESPRIT** trial randomized 2,064 patients undergoing coronary stenting to receive eptifibatide (two 180 μg/kg boluses 10 min apart followed by an infusion of 2.0 μg/kg/min for 18-24 hours) or placebo in addition to aspirin, heparin, and a thienopyridine. The primary end point in this trial (the composite of death, myocardial infarction, urgent target vessel revascularization, and thrombotic bailout glycoprotein IIb/IIIa inhibitor therapy within 48 h after randomization) was significantly lower in the treatment arm (6.6%) compared to the placebo arm (10.5%). Major bleeding was more common in patients receiving eptifibatide (1.3%) compared to placebo (0.4%). These benefits were maintained at the six month follow-up assessment.

The **PURSUIT** investigators tested the hypothesis that eptifibatide would be more effective than heparin and aspirin in reducing adverse outcomes in patients with non ST-segment elevation acute coronary syndromes. In this study, 10,948 patients were randomly assigned to receive eptifibatide or placebo, in addition to standard ACS therapy. The primary end

---

Table 6.   Eptifibatide

Synthetic platelet glycoprotein IIb/IIIa inhibitor
Settings with the greatest benefit-to-risk ratio
   Non-ST segment myocardial infarction
   Not recommended as a fibrinolytic adjunctive agent
Risk of major hemorrhage 1.1%-3.0%

point, a composite of death and nonfatal myocardial infarction occurring up to 30 days, was significantly lower in the eptifibatide group (14.2%) compared to the placebo group (15.7%; *P*=0.04). The benefit was apparent by 96 hours and persisted through 30 days. In subgroup analysis however, the beneficial effects of eptifibatide was not evident in women (OR 1.1; 95% CI, 0.9-1.31).

Eptifibatide has also been assessed as an adjunct to thrombolysis in the setting of MI. The **INTRO-AMI** investigators tested the hypothesis that eptifibatide and reduced-dose tissue plasminogen activator (t-PA) will enhance infarct artery patency compared to standard t-PA alone. Although the early patency rates (TIMI grade III flow) were improved in those receiving eptifibatide, the incidence of death, reinfarction, or revascularization at 30 days were similar among treatment groups.

- Eptifibatide is primarily cleared by the kidney and should be avoided in patients with renal impairment (creatinine clearance <30 mL/min).

THROMBIN INHIBITORS

Thrombin, the most potent known platelet agonist, is directly involved in both aggregation and thrombus propagation. Thrombin has two sites important for enzymatic activity, the anion binding exosite which provides substrate recognition and interaction and the catalytic active site which cleaves the substrate. Direct thrombin inhibitors bind directly to thrombin and block its interaction with substrates. Parenteral direct thrombin inhibitors (hirudin derivatives and argatroban) and one oral direct thrombin inhibitor (ximelagatran) have been evaluated in phase 3 clinical trials. Specific antidotes are not available to neutralize these compounds. The parenteral thrombin inhibitors have been licensed in the USA for limited indications; hirudin and argatroban are approved for treatment of patients with heparin-induced thrombocytopenia, whereas bivalirudin is licensed as an alternative to heparin in patients undergoing percutaneous coronary interventions (PCI). Ximelagatran is still under investigation.

Lepirudin (Table 7)
Lepirudin (recombinant hirudin) is a specific and ***irreversible*** thrombin inhibitor derived from leech saliva.

Its aminoterminal domain interacts with the active site of thrombin and its carboxyterminal tail binds to exosite 1. The terminal half-life of hirudin is 60 minutes after intravenous injection and 120 minutes after subcutaneous injection. Hirudin is renally excreted and thus must be used with caution in patients with renal impairment. Careful dose adjustment based on creatinine clearance must be observed. Inhibition of thrombin by hirudin blocks platelet aggregation and limits platelet deposition at the injury site to a monolayer. Clot-bound thrombin, an important thrombotic risk factor inaccessible to ATIII-heparin, is effectively inhibited by hirudin. Hirudin therapy is monitored using standard aPTT assay. The recommended aPTT target range for patients receiving this drug is 1.5–2.5 times basal values. Three trials, the **OASIS** pilot study, **GUSTO IIb** and **TIMI 9b** compared hirudin to heparin in patients with either unstable angina or MI. Within the first week of randomization, the results were promising in favor of hirudin therapy however the benefits did not persist in either the **TIMI 9b** or the **GUSTO IIb** trials. Moderate bleeding was consistently more common in the hirudin-treated patients of the **OASIS** and **GUSTO** trials. The **Helvetica** trial compared heparin to hirudin in the prevention of restenosis following coronary angioplasty. Hirudin resulted in significant reduction in early cardiac events, however at 6 months there was no difference in angiographic restenosis rates. Several hirudin analogues have been developed including hirulog (bivalirudin) and hirugen.

Direct thrombin inhibitors have been assessed as adjunctive agents to fibrinolytic therapy in myocardial

Table 7.   Lepirudin

Recombinant hirudin—direct thrombin inhibitor
Settings with the greatest benefit-to-risk ratio
  Heparin-induced thrombocytopenia (FDA approval)
  Non-ST segment myocardial infarction (not FDA approved)
aPTT target range is 1.5-2.5 times basal values
Approximately 40% of patients develop antibodies which reduce renal clearance
Risk of major hemorrhage 1.2%-3.3%

infarction. The **HIT-4** trial randomized 1,208 patients receiving streptokinase for acute myocardial infarction to either lepirudin or heparin as adjunctive anticoagulant therapy. Lepirudin therapy resulted in significantly greater ST-segment resolution at 90 minutes (28%) relative to heparin treatment group (22%) yet 30-day mortality, reinfarction, stroke, cardiogenic shock, recurrent or refractory angina, rescue angioplasty or a composite clinical end point were similar between groups. The rates of major bleeding did not differ significantly between groups. Based on these data, it is not recommended that lepirudin be given as adjunctive therapy for patients with acute MI unless there is concomitant heparin induced thrombocytopenia (HIT).

Approximately 40% of patients treated with lepirudin will form antibodies to the drug. These antibodies do not block the thrombin inhibitory activity of lepirudin but rather delay renal excretion. In vivo drug concentrations may become dangerously high in these patients and precipitate major hemorrhage. For this reason, the aPTT must be followed closely with careful dose adjustment to keep the aPTT within the therapeutic range. The recommended aPTT target range for patients receiving this drug is 1.5-2.5 times basal values.

■ It is not recommended that lepirudin be given as adjunctive therapy for patients with acute MI unless there is concomitant heparin induced thrombocytopenia (HIT).

Bivalirudin (Table 8)

Bivalirudin (Hirulog), a 20-amino acid synthetic polypeptide analog of hirudin, has a terminal half-life of 25 minutes after intravenous injection and only a fraction is excreted via the kidneys. It has been evaluated in patients undergoing PCI and as an adjunct to streptokinase in patients with ST-elevation MI. Bivalirudin approval for use in high-risk patients undergoing PCI was based on data from several randomized clinical trials. Among 4,312 patients undergoing PCI, a 22% reduction in death, MI, or urgent revascularization in those receiving bivalirudin compared with UFH (6.2% vs 7.9%; P=0.03) was observed at 7 days and benefit was maintained at 90 days. There was a 62% relative risk reduction in bleeding complications among bivalirudin-treated patients compared with those treated with UFH.

Bivalirudin has been evaluated in a phase 3 clinical trial (**REPLACE-2**) of 6,010 PCI patients randomly assigned to either bivalirudin plus provisional glycoprotein (GP) IIb/IIIa antagonist (either abciximab or eptifibatide), or heparin plus a GP IIb/IIIa antagonist. The primary outcomes (death, MI, urgent revascularization, or major bleeding at 30 days) were similar, while rates of major bleeding were significantly lower in patients given bivalirudin than in those treated with heparin.

Bivalirudin also has been compared with heparin as an adjunct to thrombolytic therapy with streptokinase in a phase 3 randomized trial (**HERO-2**) of 17,073 patients with acute ST-elevation MI. Mortality at 30 days was similar between groups. In contrast to the results of **REPLACE-2** trial, there was a trend for higher major bleeding rates (including severe bleeding) with bivalirudin. For these reasons, bivalirudin is not recommended as adjunctive therapy with fibrinolytic agents for the treatment of acute coronary syndromes.

■ Bivalirudin is not FDA approved for use in patients with heparin induced thrombocytopenia.

Argatroban (Table 9)

Argatroban is a peptidomimetic arginine derivative that binds noncovalently to the active site of thrombin to form a reversible complex. The plasma half-life of argatroban is 45 minutes and the drug is metabolized in the liver in a process that generates several active intermediates. Although this drug is safely used in patients with renal insufficiently, it should be used very cautiously (if at all) in those with hepatic insufficiency. Relatively small trials have evaluated argatroban for

---

Table 8. Bivalirudin

Engineered hirudin—direct thrombin inhibitor
Settings with the greatest benefit-to-risk ratio
    PCI (FDA) approval—with provisional GP
    IIb/IIIa inhibitors)
    PCI for unstable angina
    Not recommended for routine use with
    fibrinolytic agents
Risk of major hemorrhage 3.7%-5.4%

treatment of unstable angina, as an adjunct to thrombolysis, and as an alternative to heparin in patients undergoing coronary angioplasty, and none has shown definitive advantages of argatroban over heparin. In the more recent **ARGAMI-2** trial, 1,001 patients treated with streptokinase or alteplase were randomized to receive either UFH or argatroban (120 μg bolus and 4 μg/kg/minute infusion) for 72 hours. An additional half-dose argatroban treatment limb was stopped early because of lack of efficacy after 609 patients had been enrolled overall. There was no difference in 30-day mortality (5.5% v 5.7%) and no difference in clinical event rates. There was a trend towards less bleeding in patients randomized to receive argatroban.

Ximelagatran

Ximelagatran is the first orally active thrombin inhibitor that, after absorbtion from the small intestine, undergoes rapid biotransformation to melagatran, the active agent. Melagatran is renally excreted with a terminal half-life of 4 to 5 hours. It therefore needs to be administered orally twice daily. Ximelagatran has been evaluated for thromboprophylaxis in high-risk orthopedic patients, treatment of VTE, and prevention of cardioembolic events in patients with nonvalvular atrial fibrillation. Based on its predictable anticoagulant response, ximelagatran was administered in fixed doses without coagulation monitoring. Although the data are promising, the FDA has not approved this drug for use in the United States.

ESTEEM was a dose-finding study comparing four doses of ximelagatran (24 mg, 36 mg, 48 mg, and 60 mg bid) plus aspirin, with aspirin alone for 6 months in 1,883 patients with ST-elevation or non–ST-elevation MI; it was the first trial of >7 days of direct thrombin inhibition in patients after ACS. This pilot study showed a 24% reduction (P=0.036) in the primary end points of death, MI, and severe recurrent ischemia for the combined ximelagatran groups vs placebo. Major bleeding was infrequent in both groups and was not significantly increased with ximelagatran.

Between 6% and 9.6% of patients treated with long-term ximelagatran develop a 3-fold or greater increase in alanine aminotransferase between 6 weeks and 6 months of treatment. This increase is usually asymptomatic and reversible, even if the medication is continued. Based on data from clinical trials, the increase in transaminases with ximelagatran has been benign. However, this side effect is of potential concern and, if the drug is approved, its long-term impact on liver function will need to be carefully monitored in clinical practice after the drug is marketed. It is likely that liver function tests will need to be monitored, at least during the initial 6 months of ximelagatran therapy.

The meta-analysis of 11 trials with direct thrombin inhibitors enrolling a total of 35,970 patients with acute coronary syndromes showed reduced rate of reinfarction at 30 days compared to UFH (3.9% versus 4.8%; P<0.001), but did not reduce mortality (9.1% versus 9.0%) or the combined incidence of death/reinfarction at 30 days (11.8% versus 12.4%). There was no increase in major bleeding or intracerebral bleeding with direct thrombin inhibitor therapy.

■ In summary, direct thrombin inhibitors reduce reinfarction, but not mortality, in patients with ST-elevation MI treated with fibrinolytic therapy. The major benefit of direct thrombin inhibitors appears to be in patients undergoing PCI, particularly after ST-elevation MI.

Heparinoids

Unfractionated Heparin (Table 10)

A mainstay of therapy for any thrombotic disorder, the anticoagulant properties of heparin are through its interaction with antithrombin III (Fig. 3). By inducing a conformational change in the protein, the affinity of

---

Table 9. Argatroban

Synthetic direct thrombin inhibitor
Settings with the greatest benefit-to-risk ratio
    Heparin induced thrombocytopenia (HIT)
    (FDA approved)
    Acute coronary syndromes (those with or at
    risk of developing HIT)
    Not recommended for routine use with
    fibrinoltic agents
Risk of major hemorrhage 0.5%-2.3%

ATIII for thrombin is enhanced by 1,000-fold. Once formed, the thrombin-antithrombin III complex is essentially irreversible and inhibits the actions of thrombin and factors IXa, Xa and XIa. Heparin is a highly negatively charged proteoglycan extracted from either porcine or bovine intestinal mucosa. Nonspecific binding to a variety of cells and plasma proteins neutralizes the anticoagulant activity of heparin. Unfractionated heparin (UFH) preparations are heterogeneous-containing heparin chains of variable lengths and molecular weights ranging from 5,000 to 50,000. Unpredictable volume of distribution and elimination kinetics requires that therapy with unfractionated heparin be strictly monitored by serial aPTT for both safety and efficacy. Using a weight-adjusted nomogram, only 82% of patients will reach the therapeutic range within 24 hours with a 5%-7% risk of major hemorrhage. Despite these imperfections, the efficacy of heparin in acute arterial occlusive syndromes has been well established. Combined results of the Antithrombotic Therapy in Acute Coronary Syndromes study, Research on Instability in Coronary Artery Disease, and Théroux et al studies yielded 0.44 (95% CI, 0.21 to 0.93) risk reduction for death/MI with combination aspirin and UFH therapy compared with aspirin alone. In the prethrombolytic era, unfrac-

tionated heparin reduced both the rate of reinfarction and mortality following acute MI. As an adjuvant to thrombolytic therapy, heparin improves early patency and may improve survival.

Low-Molecular-Weight Heparin (Table 11)

Low-molecular-weight heparin (LMWH) is produced by depolymerizing unfractionated heparin using either chemical or enzymatic methodologies (Fig. 4). This yields a preparation of small heparin fragments of a more uniform molecular weight (4-6,000 kD). LMWH requires AT-III for activity yet, unlike its parent compound, has a higher specificity for factor Xa as compared to thrombin. Because of its uniformity of size and less negative charge, it has much less nonspe-

Table 10. Heparin

Inhibitory action through activation of antithrombin III
Settings with the greatest benefit-to-risk ratio
    Acute coronary syndromes
    Acute venous thromboembolism
Risk of major hemorrhage 5%-7%

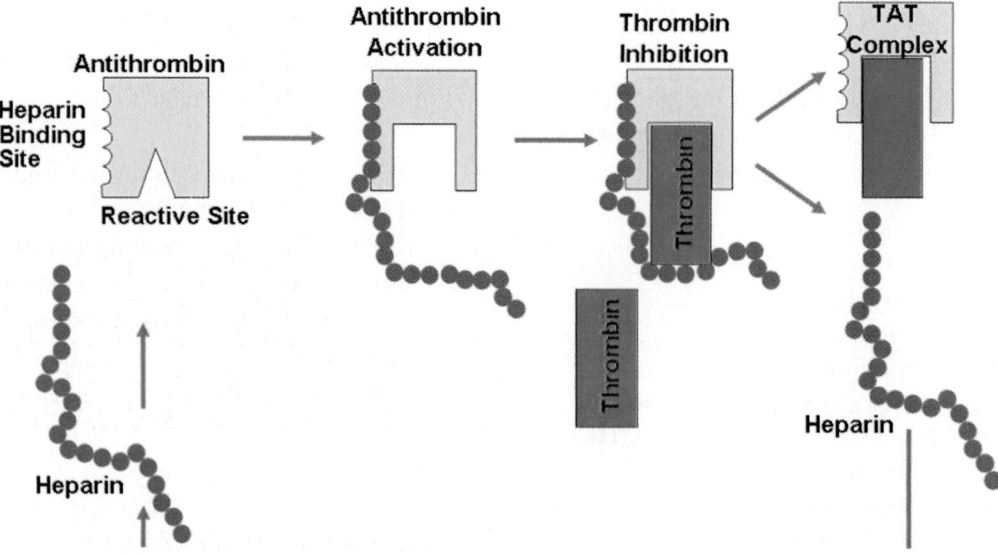

Fig. 3. Heparin interaction with antithrombin III. Heparin binds antithrombin III through the interaction of a specific pentasaccharide sequence within the molecule. This interaction then transforms antithrombin III into an active inhibitor. Bound to antithrombin III, heparin forms a scaffold promoting the interaction between thrombin and antithrombin. Once the complex has been formed, heparin is free to participate in another round of inhibition.

cific binding, improved bioavailability, and more predictable pharmacology. Insensitive to aPTT, dosing is safe and effective based on patient body weight. Several potential anticoagulant advantages also favor LMWH over UFH. Platelet factor 4 secreted by activated platelets blocks the interaction between ATIII and heparin but not LMWH. Secondly, factor Xa bound to the platelet surface within the prothrombin activation complex is inaccessible to ATIII-heparin whereas LMWH-ATIII can inhibit factor Xa under these circumstances.

By far the greatest experience with LMWH has been in the arena of DVT prophylaxis and venous thromboembolism treatment. Studies have provided efficacy data for the treatment of DVT, PE, and arterial thrombosis.

In the **ESSENCE** study, 3,171 patients with unstable angina or non-Q wave MI were treated with either LMWH (enoxaparin) or UFH. Enoxaparin therapy resulted in a significant reduction of angina, MI, or death as compared to UFH with fewer bleeding complications. This benefit persisted for 30 days with

Table 11. Low-Molecular-Weight Heparin

Inhibitory action through activation of anti-
    thrombin III
Settings with the greatest benefit-to-risk ratio
    Acute coronary syndromes
    Acute venous thromboembolism
Risk of major hemorrhage 3%-5%
Weight-adjusted dosing
Renal excretion
No monitoring necessary

fewer enoxaparin-treated patients requiring revascularization. In contrast, the FRIC study which compared LMWH (dalteparin) to UFH in patients with unstable angina, showed no difference between the two groups in terms of composite cardiac end points. The different outcomes of these two trials is difficult to explain, however, and may reflect efficacy differences between these two LMWH preparations. Nonetheless, it can be con-

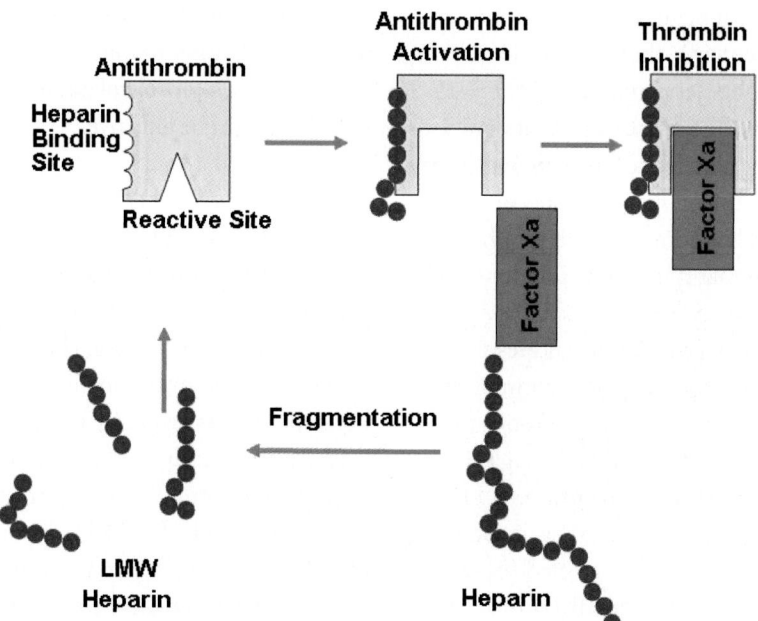

Fig. 4. Low molecular weight (LMW) heparin interaction with antithrombin III. The enzymatic or chemical fragmentation of heparin yields fragments of uniform size, "LMW-heparin." LMW heparin also binds antithrombin III through the interaction of a specific pentasaccharide sequence. This interaction then transforms antithrombin III into an active inhibitor. Unlike unfractionated heparin, LMW heparin is not able to form a scaffold with thrombin and therefore the specificity of antithrombin III is for factor Xa.

cluded that LMWH is at least as effective as standard heparin in the management of arterial occlusive syndromes. The dose of LMWH is weight adjusted, given once or twice daily subcutaneously depending on the formulation, and does not require laboratory monitoring.

Heparin-induced-thrombocytopenia (HIT) is an antibody-mediated, adverse effect of heparin that is important because of its strong association with venous and arterial thrombosis (heparin induced thrombocytopenia with thrombosis [HITT]). The neoepitopes recognized by HIT antibodies are located on platelet factor 4 (PF4), and are formed when PF4 binds to heparin. Only a subset of high-titer, IgG anti-PF4 antibodies activate platelets, which probably explains the greater diagnostic specificity of certain platelet activation assays (eg, platelet serotonin release assay for HIT compared with PF4-dependent enzyme immunoassay. HIT is a clinicopathologic syndrome; therefore, it should be diagnosed based on both clinical and serologic grounds. Consequently, HIT antibody seroconversion without thrombocytopenia or other clinical sequelae is not considered HIT. In patients receiving heparin, HIT should be suspected when the platelet count drops to less than 100,000/μL, or by more than 40% of the basal platelet count. This occurs in 1.3% of patients receiving therapeutic doses of porcine heparin. Thrombocytopenia may occur 3-15 days after the initiation of heparin. In patients previously exposed, however, platelet counts can begin to drop within hours of treatment. HIT is more common with bovine heparin and less common with prophylactic doses or LMWH preparations. The incidence of thrombosis in HIT ranges from 0.2 to 20%, may involve the arterial or venous circulation, and results in mortality rates as high as 30%. Current recommendations of the Seventh ACCP Conference on Antithrombotic and Thrombolytic Therapy regarding the recognition, treatment, and prevention of HIT include platelet count monitoring (at least every-other-day) and, for patients with strongly suspected (or confirmed) HIT or HITT, use of an alternative anticoagulant, such as lepirudin, argatroban, bivalirudin, or danaparoid. Moreover, patients with strongly suspected (or confirmed) HIT should have routine ultrasonography of the lower-limb veins for investigation of deep venous thrombosis. Vitamin K antagonist (coumarin) therapy should not be used until after the platelet count

has substantially recovered and only during overlapping alternative anticoagulation (minimum 5-day overlap) and begun with low, maintenance doses. UFH can be used for patients who require cardiac surgery and have a history of HIT but HIT antibody currently negative. Due to significant cross-reactivity, LMWH is not an acceptable alternative in these patients, but fondaparinux that does not bind to platelet factor 4 (PF4) should not cause heparin-induced thrombocytopenia.

- HIT antibody seroconversion without thrombocytopenia or other clinical sequelae is not considered HIT.
- Fondaparinux that does not bind to platelet factor 4 (PF4) should not cause heparin-induced thrombocytopenia.

Pentasaccharides

Fondaparinux and idraparinux, new indirect inhibitors, are synthetic analogs of the unique pentasaccharide sequence of heparin that mediates its interaction with antithrombin. Once the pentasaccharide/antithrombin complex binds factor Xa, the pentasaccharide dissociates from antithrombin/Xa complex and can be reutilized. Unlike heparin, there is no antidote for fondaparinux. If uncontrolled bleeding occurs with fondaparinux, a procoagulant, such as recombinant factor VIIa, might be effective.

Fondaparinux (Table 12)

Fondaparinux can be thought of as ultra-low-molecular-weight heparin. This drug is a synthetic pentasaccharide analog specific for the sequence necessary for antithrombin III activation (Fig. 5). It is given subcutaneously and has an elimination half-life is 17-21 hours. Fondaparinux is primarily renally excreted and as such is likely contraindicated in patients with severe renal impairment (creatinine clearance <30 mL/min). Fondaparinux, like LMWH, does not require monitoring. Routine coagulation tests such as PT and aPTT are relatively insensitive measures and unsuitable for monitoring. Like LMWH, the anti-factor Xa activity of fondaparinux can be measured if necessary. Because of its very low molecular weight and essentially neutral net charge, this drug does not bind significantly to other plasma proteins and specifically does not bind platelet factor 4 (PF-4). Therefore, the risk of develop-

Table 12. Fondaparinux

Synthetic pentasaccharide with actions through antithrombin III
Settings with the greatest benefit-to-risk ratio
    ST-segment elevation myocardial infarction
    Unstable angina
    Non ST-segment elevation myocardial infarction
    Acute venous thromboembolism
    Venous thromboembolism prophylaxis
Risk of major hemorrhage 2%-3%
Renal excretion with long half-life (17-21 hours)
No monitoring necessary

ing heparin induced thrombocytopenia is negligible. This net neutral charge however also means that this drug is not inhibited by protamine like unfractionated heparin or LMWH. Of note, there is no specific antidote for patients bleeding while receiving this drug. Recombinant factor VIIa has been suggested as a possible therapy if major bleeding complicates fondaparinux therapy.

Fondaparinux has been evaluated for prevention and treatment of VTE and for treatment of arterial thrombosis. It is currently approved for DVT prophylaxis for hip fracture, hip replacement, or knee replacement surgery. The Pentasaccharide in Unstable Angina study, a phase II trial of 1,147 patients, assess the efficacy of fondaparinux in acute coronary syndromes. Patients were randomized to receive either enoxaparin or fondaparinux for up to one week. The primary efficacy end point (composite of death, MI, or recurrent ischemia at 9 days and 30 days) was similar in each group.

The **OASIS-5** trial was designed to assess the efficacy of fondaparinux compared to enoxaparin in patients with unstable angina or myocardial infarction without ST-segment elevation. In this trial, 20,078 patients were randomized to receive either fondaparinux (2.5 mg daily) or enoxaparin (1 mg twice daily). The primary-outcome events were similar in the two groups. The rate of major bleeding however was significantly lower with fondaparinux (2.2%) compared to enoxaparin (4.1%). Furthermore, mortality outcomes at 30 days and 180 days were significantly lower with fondaparinux therapy.

The **OASIS-6** trial evaluated the efficacy of fondaparinux in the setting of acute ST segment elevation

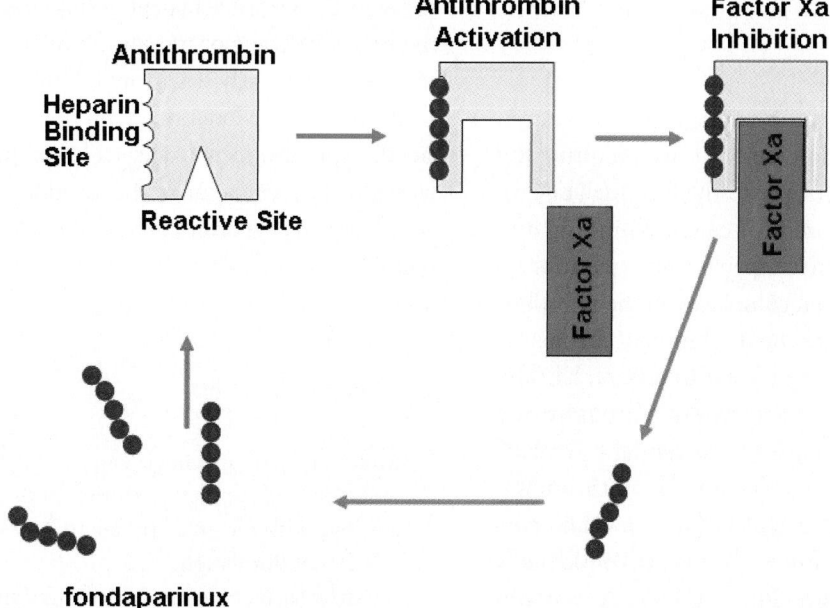

Fig. 5. Pentasaccharide interaction with antithrombin III. Whereas a specific pentasaccharide sequence is required for antithrombin III activation, a new class of agents exploiting this requirement have been introduced. These synthetic pentasaccharide molecules are not able to form a scaffold with thrombin and therefore the specificity is for factor Xa inhibition.

myocardial infarction. In this international multicenter study, 12,092 patients with STEMI were randomly assigned to receive either fondaparinux or unfractionated heparin for up to 8 days. The composite outcome of death or reinfarction at 30 days was significantly reduced in patients assigned to fondaparinux (9.7%) compared to heparin (11.2%). These benefits were not seen in those patients who underwent primary PCI. Furthermore, there was no difference in major hemorrhage between groups.

- Fondaparinux is not inhibited by protamine like unfractionated heparin or LMWH.
- There is no specific antidote for patients bleeding while receiving this drug.

Idraparinux

Idraparinux is a second-generation synthetic pentasaccharide analogue similar to fondaparinux. It has a very high affinity for antithrombin III. Idraparinux is given as a subcutaneous injection, has a very long half-life of 80 hours, and thus is administered once weekly. Unlike fondaparinux, which competes with UFH and LMWH, idraparinux has been developed to compete with warfarin because of its long half-life. It has not yet been FDA approved. A phase 3 trial with this dose of idraparinux is under way.

Warfarin (Table 13)

Warfarin blocks the hepatic carboxylation of vitamin K-dependent coagulation factors, thus inhibiting the activation of the proenzyme to the enzyme (Fig. 6). Carboxylation is required for calcium binding and shape reconfiguration necessary for incorporation of the protein into activation complexes on the phospholipid bilayer. With either the inhibition of carboxylation or calcium sequestration (with citrate, EDTA, etc.), coagulation factor activation is brought to a standstill. Relevant vitamin K-dependent proteins include both procoagulant (factors II-prothrombin, VII, IX, and X) and anticoagulant (protein C and protein S) proteins. Each of these factors has considerably different terminal half-lives in vivo (Fig. 7). As warfarin is initiated, there is a theoretic hypercoagulable state when protein C stores are depleted in the face of normal prothrombin (factor II) levels. The prothrombin time INR is very sensitive to factor VII depletion. INR

prolongation may occur despite more than adequate factor X and prothrombin levels necessary to form thrombi. For this reason, warfarin and heparin are given concordantly for at least 5 days or a therapeutic INR whichever is *longer*.

The clinical efficacy of warfarin in the setting of venous thromboembolism and atrial fibrillation is universally acknowledged. Its role in the treatment of acute and chronic coronary arterial occlusive syndromes is however less clear. In the prethrombolytic era, several post-myocardial infarction studies documented a significant reduction in recurrent MI, stroke, and mortality in those treated with warfarin anticoagulation. The **ASPECT** trial randomized patients with recent MI to warfarin at a goal PT-INR of between 2.8-4.8 or placebo. At 37 months of follow-up, there was a statistically significant reduction in the rate of recurrent MI and stroke however no mortality benefit was shown between the two groups. The **ATACS** study compared warfarin plus aspirin to aspirin alone in 214 patients with unstable angina or non-Q MI. At the end of the trial, there was a trend favoring the warfarin/aspirin group in the reduction of recurrent angina, MI or death. The **CARS** investigators hypothesized that the addition of a small, fixed dose of warfarin added to aspirin would add the benefit of an antithrombotic agent to an antiplatelet agent without increasing either the risk of bleeding or the complexity of the treatment regimen. The study was stopped prematurely by the Data and Safety Monitoring Committee based on similar efficacy of treatment strategies. In summary, the role of warfarin anticoagulation in the secondary prevention of acute coronary syndromes remains unclear and controversial.

Table 13. Warfarin

Inhibitory action through blockade of hepatic
  vitamin K-dependent γ-carboxylation
Settings with the greatest benefit-to-risk ratio
    Atrial fibrillation
    Mechanical heart valve prophylaxis
    Acute venous thromboembolism
    Venous thrombosis prophylaxis
Risk of major hemorrhage 1%-8%

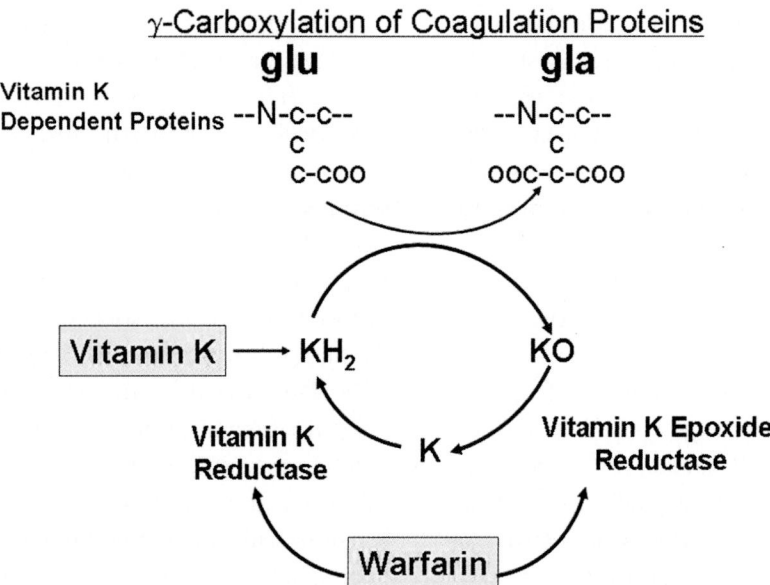

Fig. 6. Mechanism of warfarin anticoagulant effect. Posttranslational γ-carboxylation of vitamin K-dependent proteins occurs in the liver. Warfarin inhibits vitamin K reduction thus halting this process. Non-carboxylated proteins cannot bind calcium, cannot be activated, and thus are cleared more rapidly from the circulation. Warfarin anticoagulation represents a balance between this inhibition and exogenous vitamin K intake. Exogenous vitamin K (KH$_2$) is the reduced form.

Warfarin prophylaxis has been shown in many trials to provide effective prophylaxis against stroke in atrial fibrillation, recurrent venous thromboembolism, and both cardioembolic and valve thrombotic complications in patients with mechanical heart valve prosthesis.

Bleeding complications have limited the enthusiasm for warfarin use, especially in the elderly patient. In the SPAF II study, at an approximate PT-INR of between 2.0 to 4.5, major hemorrhage occurred at a rate of 2.3% per year as compared to 1.1% per year for aspirin. Age, increasing number of prescribed medications, and intensity of anticoagulation were independent risks for bleeding. In patients under age 75, the rate of major hemorrhage was 1.7% per year as compared to 4.2% per year in older patients. Other variables associated with excessive anticoagulation include advanced malignancy, potentiating medications such as antibiotics or acetaminophen, anorexia or diarrheal illnesses.

Fibrinolytic Agents

The mainstay of medical treatment for acute arterial thrombosis is the plasminogen activating agents: streptokinase, rt-PA, urokinase, and their derivatives. Unlike endogenous fibrinolysis which is marked by clot specificity, pharmacological plasminogen activation is indiscriminate in substrate preference degrading fibrin, fibrinogen, platelet receptors and coagulation factors. Streptokinase, unique from the endogenous activators, is not an enzyme and therefore cannot activate plasminogen directly. Purified from β-hemolytic strepto-

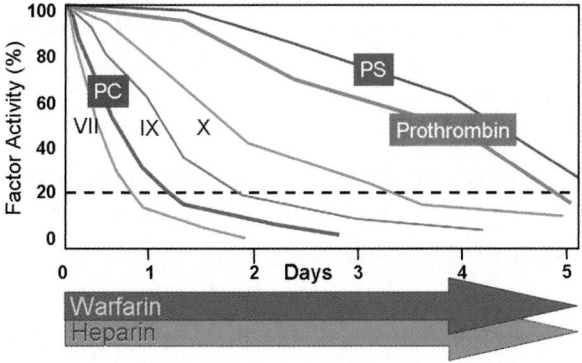

Fig. 7. Dynamics of vitamin K-dependent factor depletion with warfarin initiation. Effective anticoagulation is achieved once factor levels are reduced to approximately 20%. Despite depletion of factors VII and IX, thrombosis may still occur if prothrombin and factor X levels are normal.

cocci, streptokinase promotes fibrinolysis by inducing a conformational change of plasminogen exposing the enzymatic active site. The SK-plasminogen complex then cleaves a second plasminogen molecule to active plasmin. Although streptokinase does not possess a fibrin binding site, this process is accelerated in the presence of fibrin and is somewhat clot specific.

Anisoylated plasminogen streptokinase activator complex, APSAC, is a complex of streptokinase already bound to plasminogen. This complex has increased specificity for fibrin and is not inhibited by endogenous inhibitors of plasminogen systems. APSAC has a plasma half-life 2-3 times longer (70 minutes) than streptokinase (25 minutes) and therefore can be given as a single bolus rather than prolonged infusion. As these are foreign proteins, repetitive SK or APSAC use is hindered by neutralizing antibodies which limit their efficacy.

Staphylokinase, a protein produced by *Staphylococcus aureus*, activates plasminogen in much the same manner as streptokinase. Staphylokinase is fibrin specific and has reduced inhibition by α_2 antiplasmin. Although effective in the treatment of patients with acute MI, it has been associated with the induction of high titers of neutralizing antibody formation. Like streptokinase, its use will therefore be limited to a single infusion.

Purified and recombinant forms of the endogenous plasminogen activators have become widely used for local delivery and systemic fibrinolysis in a variety of both arterial and venous thrombotic disorders. These endogenous agents including recombinant t-PA, urokinase, single chain urokinase (scu-PA or pro-urokinase), have direct enzymatic activity toward plasminogen. The debate continues as to agent superiority and clinical indication, however *in vivo* plasminogen activation is likely comparable with minimal differences in clot specificity between agents. In contrast to bacterial proteins, these agents are nonimmunogenic and therefore can be reinstituted. Although effective in thrombolysis,

endogenous inhibitors of plasminogen activation such as PAI-1, have richest concentrations in platelet α-granules. This may explain the 20 to 50% failure rate of pharmacological fibrinolytic therapy.

One of the most devastating complications of thrombolytic therapy is stroke. The overall risk in the **GUSTO** trial was 1.4%, lower in patients treated with streptokinase (1.19%) as compared to rt-PA (1.55%). Forty five percent of all strokes were fatal and 31% were disabling. Of those patients who suffered from stroke, 45% were associated with primary intracranial hemorrhage resulting in a 60% mortality. Hemorrhagic conversion occurred in only 10% of the remaining stroke patients, with a 32% fatality rate. Advanced age, prior cerebrovascular disease, and hypertension were found to be significant predictors of intracranial hemorrhage. Severe or life-threatening hemorrhage, defined as either intracranial hemorrhage or hemodynamic compromise requiring treatment, occurred in 0.3%-0.5% of patients, and was similar in all groups. Moderate hemorrhage occurred with an overall frequency of 5%-6%, and was statistically less frequent for rt-PA treated patients.

The current recommendations are for the administration of any approved fibrinolytic agent (streptokinase, anistreplase, alteplase, reteplase, or tenecteplase) for patients with acute coronary syndrome of <12 h in duration. For patients with symptom duration <6 h, the administration of alteplase is preferred over streptokinase. Alteplase, reteplase, or tenecteplase should be used for patients with known allergy or sensitivity to streptokinase. In patients with any history of intracranial hemorrhage, closed head trauma, or ischemic stroke within past 3 months, fibrinolytic therapy is contraindicated.

■ Streptokinase, unique from the endogenous activators, is not an enzyme and therefore cannot activate plasminogen directly.

52

VENOUS AND LYMPHATIC DISORDERS

Raymond C. Shields, MD

INTRODUCTION

Venous disease is common in prevalence with significant complications worldwide and is a frequent part of a cardiovascular practice. Understanding the impact of venous and lymphatic diseases is important in the evaluation and management of these compelling peripheral vascular disease manifestations.

VENOUS THROMBOEMBOLISM

Venous thromboembolism (VTE) is the third most common cardiovascular disease, after acute coronary syndromes and stroke. The annual incidence exceeds 1 per 1,000 with more than 200,000 new cases in the United States annually. Virchow's triad of stasis, hypercoagulability, and vascular endothelial damage contribute in varying degrees to the development of venous thrombosis. Independent acquired risk factors for VTE include immobility, paralysis, recent surgery, trauma, malignancy, advanced age, prior history of superficial thrombophlebitis, central venous catheter/transvenous pacemaker, pregnancy, and estrogen use. An identifiable risk factor is present in up to 80% of patients with confirmed VTE. Patients undergoing total hip or knee replacement surgery have a 40% to 60% risk of VTE without prophylactic therapy. The major inherited thrombophilias are discussed below. Population-based risks of recurrent VTE are as outlined in Table 1.

PREGNANCY-RELATED VENOUS THROMBOEMBOLISM

The risk of venous thromboembolism during pregnancy is increased fivefold compared to nonpregnant women of similar age with an incidence of 1 in 1,000 to 1 in 2,000 pregnancies. More importantly, pulmonary embolism is the leading cause of pregnancy-related death in the United States. Congenital thrombophilias

Table 1. Population-Based Risks for Recurrent VTE

Antithrombin III deficiency
Protein C deficiency
Protein S deficiency
Hyperhomocysteinemia
Lupus anticoagulant
Antiphospholipid antibody
Homozygous factor V Leiden or prothrombin G20210A mutation
Double heterozygous with factor V Leiden and prothrombin G20210A
Active malignant neoplasm
Increased factor VIII level
Increased factor IX level

are associated with an increased risk for venous thromboembolism during pregnancy. Generalized screening for thrombophilia has not been supported; however, pregnant women with a personal or family history of venous thromboembolism should undergo screening along with genetic counseling.

Unfractionated and low-molecular-weight heparins do not cross the placenta and are recommended choices for treatment of venous thromboembolism during pregnancy. Coumarin derivatives have been traditionally contraindicated during pregnancy due to associated embryopathy, and the package insert specifically states that warfarin is contraindicated during pregnancy. However, coumarin derivatives may be considered during certain stages of pregnancy in patients with mechanical valve prosthesis (for a more complete discussion, please see Chapter 79, "Pregnancy and the Heart"). For nonpregnant women of childbearing age who require oral anticoagulation therapy, emphasis must be placed on ensuring adequate and appropriate contraceptive therapy.

Venous thromboembolism in pregnancy:

- Risk of VTE is increased by fivefold during pregnancy compared to nonpregnant women.
- Pulmonary embolism is the leading cause of pregnancy-related death in the United States.
- Coumarin derivatives have been contraindicated during pregnancy due to associated embryopathy.
- Screening for thrombophilia is warranted with a personal or family history of VTE.

CLINICAL EVALUATION OF PATIENTS WITH VTE

A complete patient and family history, physical examination, and general laboratory evaluation are indispensable in the initial evaluation of acute venous thromboembolism. Typical symptoms of deep venous thrombosis (DVT) include pain, redness, and swelling of a limb; although many patients may be asymptomatic. Signs of DVT include pitting edema, warmth, erythema, tenderness, and a dilated superficial venous pattern in the involved extremity. Although lower limbs are the most common site of DVT, upper extremity DVT may occur, especially in patients with a central venous catheter or transvenous permanent pacemaker.

Extensive DVT involving an entire extremity may lead to venous gangrene (phlegmasia cerulea dolens), most commonly in association with an underlying malignancy. DVT in an unusual site (e.g., cerebral, mesenteric, or renal vein) raises the probability of a hypercoagulable state. The clinical diagnosis of DVT is neither sensitive (60%-80%) nor specific (30%-72%), and three-fourths of patients who present with suspected acute limb DVT have other causes of leg pain such as cellulitis, leg trauma, muscular tear or rupture, postthrombotic syndrome, or Baker cysts. Objective noninvasive tests generally are required to establish a diagnosis of DVT.

Venography is the reference standard for the diagnosis of DVT and is highly accurate for both proximal and calf DVT; however, it is invasive, expensive, technically inadequate in about 10% of patients, and may precipitate DVT in approximately 3% of patients. Noninvasive tests for diagnosing DVT are accurate for diagnosing proximal but not calf vein thrombosis. If the results of noninvasive testing are nondiagnostic or are discordant with the clinical assessment, venography is indicated.

D-Dimer, a degradation product of cross-linked fibrin, is sensitive but not specific for acute DVT. In the presence of high clinical suspicion for DVT, a negative D-dimer alone is inadequate to rule out acute DVT.

Continuous Wave Doppler

Doppler assessment at the bedside, which evaluates each limb systematically for spontaneous venous flow, phasic flow with respiration, augmentation with distal compression, and venous competence with Valsalva and proximal compression, is useful in the diagnosis of proximal DVT. Doppler examination is relatively insensitive to calf vein thrombosis.

Impedance Plethysmography and Strain-Gauge Outflow Plethysmography

Impedance plethysmography and strain-gauge outflow plethysmography both reliably detect occlusive thrombi in the proximal veins (popliteal, femoral, and iliac veins) but are less reliable in detecting nonocclusive thrombi and are insensitive to calf DVT.

Compression Ultrasonography

Compression ultrasonography (venous noncompressibility is diagnostic of DVT, venous compressibility excludes DVT) is highly sensitive and specific for detecting proximal DVT even when compared to venography (Fig. 1 and 2).

Treatment of Deep Venous Thrombosis

Acute DVT is recommended to be treated with an initial course of unfractionated heparin or low-molecular-weight heparin overlapping with at least 5 days of oral vitamin K antagonist therapy (e.g., warfarin sodium). This initial course is then followed by at least 3 months of standard warfarin therapy with a goal INR range of 2 to 3. A longer period of anticoagulation therapy (i.e., 12 months) has been suggested for idiopathic or unprovoked DVT. Catheter-directed thrombolytic therapy should be considered in selected cases, such as younger patients, with acute ileofemoral DVT. Vena cava filter placement is indicated when there is a contraindication to or a complication of anticoagulation therapy; however, anticoagulation therapy should be started as soon as possible after filter placement. Catheter-based or surgical thrombectomy may be indicated in selected patients but routine use is not advocated due to the frequent need for reintervention.

Reduction of limb edema, initially by leg elevation and woven elastic wrapping, is an integral part of the initial therapy for acute DVT. When edema reduction is achieved, a graduated compression elastic support stocking (30- to 40-mm Hg) is recommended, both to control edema and to reduce the risk of post-thrombotic syndrome with venous stasis and ulceration. Additional

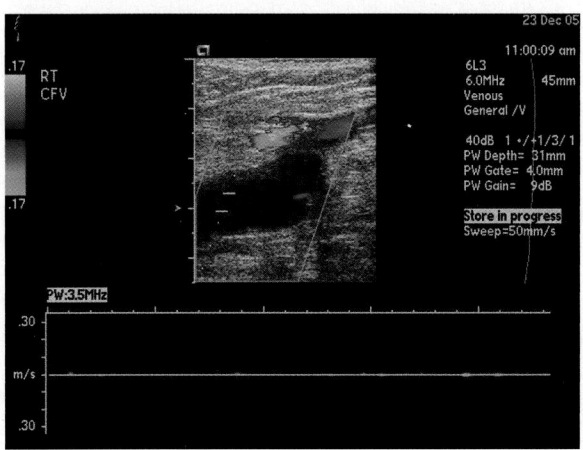

Fig. 2. Doppler evaluation of an acute occlusive thrombus in the common femoral vein demonstrating no flow.

details of the diagnosis and treatment of DVT, and DVT prophylaxis are included in the chapter on pulmonary embolism.

SUPERIOR VENA CAVA SYNDROME

Superior vena cava (SVC) syndrome is most commonly caused by lung carcinoma, mediastinal lymphadenopathy, and primary mediastinal malignancy. Indwelling central venous catheters, cardiac pacing, and cardiac defibrillator leads are increasingly associated with this syndrome with increased application and revision of these devices. Mediastinal fibrosis, granulomatous disease, and prior radiation therapy are also important contributors.

SVC syndrome classically presents with head and neck fullness which is exacerbated by supine position or head dependency. Venous hypertension often results in dizziness, visual disturbance, headache, and syncopal spells. Patients may also report impaired mentation, dyspnea, orthopnea, and cough. Computed tomography effectively demonstrates the location and extent of potential obstructing structures, and collateral venous routes.

Initiation of standard anticoagulation therapy is advocated for an acute thrombotic obstruction of the SVC. Thrombolytic therapy may be considered in patients with benign acute SVC syndrome. Endovascular stenting of the SVC currently is recommended as primary therapy for SVC obstruction due to malignant disease. Stenting results in prompt relief of

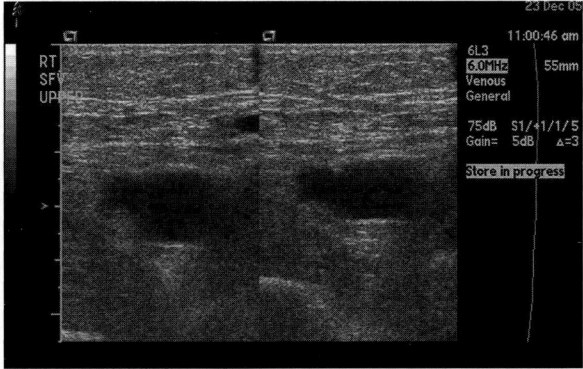

Fig. 1. Compression ultrasonography in a patient with suspected deep venous thrombosis demonstrates noncompressibility of right superficial femoral vein as evidence of intraluminal thrombus. Echogenic thrombus is visible in the superficial femoral vein.

symptoms with a high rate of prolonged efficacy.

Superior vena cava syndrome:

- Clinical manifestations include dizziness, visual disturbance, headache, and syncopal spells.
- Endovascular stenting of the SVC is recommended in selected patients.

POSTTHROMBOTIC SYNDROME

Postthrombotic syndrome occurs in as many as 80% of DVT patients and is associated with significant economic costs and physical disability. Postthrombotic syndrome encompasses the clinical and pathological findings of chronic venous insufficiency (CVI) as a result of DVT. CVI commonly results in swelling, pain, fatigue, and heaviness in the involved extremity. Secondary varicose vein formation, hyperpigmentation, brawny induration, and cutaneous ulceration can occur if untreated. Venous claudication in the setting of previous iliofemoral or vena caval thrombosis causes discomfort, fullness, tiredness, and aching of the extremity during exercise. Unlike intermittent claudication, patients with venous claudication prefer to sit down and elevate the extremity for relief. Postthrombotic syndrome due to chronic deep venous incompetence is frequently misdiagnosed as recurrent DVT. The correct diagnosis is suggested by the clinical findings of chronic venous insufficiency and confirmed by exclusion of new thrombus formation by compression ultrasonography. The *side-by-side* comparison of current ultrasonographic studies with previous ultrasonographic or venographic studies is invaluable in documenting new venous thrombosis. Treatment of postthrombotic syndrome initially includes aggressive efforts at edema reduction with woven elastic wrapping and pumping devices until edema is reduced, followed by fitting with a graduated compression elastic support stocking (30-40 mm Hg). Periodic leg elevation during the day and weight reduction in obese patients are also beneficial.

FAMILIAL THROMBOPHILIA

Protein C Deficiency

Protein C deficiency is characterized by recurrent venous thrombosis and is inherited in an autosomal

dominant fashion. Episodes of thrombosis are generally spontaneous and usually begin before the age of 30 years. Protein C levels are about 50% of normal. Treatment is lifelong oral anticoagulation, and there **is** a potential risk of warfarin necrosis. Acquired protein C deficiency can develop postoperatively and in patients with liver disease or disseminated intravascular coagulation. Purpura fulminans occurs in persons homozygous for this condition.

Protein S Deficiency

Protein S deficiency also causes recurrent venous thrombosis and is inherited as an autosomal dominant trait. Onset of episodes usually begins before the age of 35 years, and the episodes are generally spontaneous. Protein S levels are about 50% of normal. Treatment is lifelong oral anticoagulation, and there **is not** an increased risk of warfarin necrosis. Acquired protein S deficiency can occur in association with the nephrotic syndrome, warfarin therapy, pregnancy, antiphospholipid antibody syndrome, and disseminated intravascular coagulation.

Antithrombin III Deficiency

Antithrombin III deficiency, characterized by recurrent venous and arterial thrombosis, is also inherited in an autosomal dominant fashion. The first thrombotic episode is usually after age 20 years and is usually provoked by infection, trauma, surgery, or pregnancy. Antithrombin III levels are usually 40% to 60% of normal. An acquired form of antithrombin III deficiency can occur in patients with nephrotic syndrome or severe liver disease and in those receiving estrogen therapy.

Factor V Leiden Mutation

Heterozygous carriers of a mutation in factor V that destroys an activated protein C cleavage site (factor V Leiden) are at increased risk for venous thrombosis (i.e., activated protein C resistance). This mutation may occur in 5% to 10% of the general population and may account for as many as 50% of patients with recurrent venous thromboembolism.

Prothrombin G20210A Mutation

Heterozygoes carriers of this autosomal dominant prothrombin G20210A mutation are at an increased risk of deep venous and cerebral venous thrombosis.

These carriers have an increased plasma prothrombin level compared to normal. The prevalence is 0.7% to 6.5% in Caucasians and is rare in non-Caucasian populations.

Hyperhomocystinemia

Hyperhomocystinemia, a disorder of methionine metabolism, is a risk factor for premature atherosclerosis and recurrent DVT. Inherited forms (disorders of transsulfuration and remethylation) and acquired forms (chronic renal failure, organ transplantation, acute lymphoblastic leukemia, psoriasis, vitamin deficiencies [vitamins B_6 and B_{12} and folate], and medications [carbamazepine, phenytoin, theophylline]) can occur. Hyperhomocystinemia is an independent risk factor for stroke, coronary artery disease, peripheral vascular disease, and DVT. Folic acid 0.4 mg/day reduces homocysteine levels, but higher doses of folate are required in patients with chronic renal failure. Screening for hyperhomocystinemia should be considered in patients with premature atherosclerotic disease, a strong family history of premature atherosclerosis, idiopathic DVT, chronic renal failure, systemic lupus erythematosus, or severe psoriasis and in organ transplant recipients.

HEPARIN-INDUCED THROMBOCYTOPENIA

Thrombocytopenia is a known complication of heparin therapy. Heparin-induced thrombocytopenia (HIT) is generally separated into two categories. *HIT type I*, also known as heparin-associated thrombocytopenia, is not immune mediated and results in a transient drop in platelet count usually within the first two days following initiation of heparin. The platelet count will generally normalize despite continued administration of heparin and is otherwise of minimal clinical significance.

In *HIT type II*, antibodies to complexes of heparin and platelet α-granule protein, platelet factor-4 (PF-4), appear to further augment platelet activation by binding to the platelet FcγIIa receptor. Additional procoagulant platelet microparticles are then released stimulating endothelial cells which can lead to increased thrombin generation.

HIT type II is characterized by a 50% decline in platelet count beginning 5 to 10 days after heparin is started in 70% of patients with HIT. Rapid onset (<24 hours after heparin reexposure) may be seen in 30% of HIT patients with a prior exposure within the preceding 3 months. Although HIT is a clinical diagnosis, laboratory confirmation is generally recommended. The *gold standard* test for HIT is the ^{14}C-serotonin release assay (SRA) with positive predictive value nearing 100% and a negative predictive value approximating 20%. Approximately 50% of HIT patients develop thrombosis; venous manifestations include DVT, PE, limb gangrene, and cerebral sinus thrombosis. Arterial thrombosis is most commonly in peripheral arteries (particularly in synthetic grafts). Less frequently HIT is complicated by stroke, myocardial or mesenteric infarction, adrenal gland infarction, and skin necrosis. Mortality for HIT approximates 20% and limb loss rate is about 10%.

HIT is best managed with immediate and complete withdrawal of all forms of heparin followed by alternative anticoagulation therapy. Although the incidence of LMWH-associated HIT is much less, known cross-reactivity with HIT antibodies prohibits its use as an alternative to unfractionated heparin. Two direct thrombin inhibitors, lepirudin and argatroban, are approved for management of HIT. Warfarin can be initiated once adequate anticoagulation is achieved with a thrombin-specific inhibitor and the platelet count is above 100,000/μL. Fondaparinux, a pentasaccharide, has no demonstrated PF-4 cross reactivity and may be used for HIT prevention but is not approved for management of HIT.

Heparin-induced thrombocytopenia:

- Type II is immune-mediated.
- 50% of patients with HIT develop thrombosis.
- Withdrawal of all heparin and initiation of a thrombin-specific inhibitor is recommended for management.

ANTIPHOSPHOLIPID ANTIBODY SYNDROME

Antiphospholipid antibodies (APA) are a group of heterogeneous autoantibodies, including anticardiolipin and lupus anticoagulant antibodies, against phospholipid binding proteins. Clinical presentation is more commonly deep venous thrombosis of the legs; up to 50% of these patients will also have pulmonary emboli. Arterial thrombotic events are comparatively less common but up to 50% are stroke and transient ischemic attacks. Coronary occlusions account for 23%; the remaining 27% involve various other vascular regions. Cardiac manifestations also include valvular vegetations, intracardiac thrombi, and nonbacterial thrombotic (Libman-Sacks) endocarditis.

The diagnosis of antiphospholipid antibody syndrome (APS) requires one clinical criterion and one laboratory criterion to be present. Clinical criteria include objectively confirmed arterial, venous, or small-vessel thrombosis, or pregnancy morbidity consisting of recurrent fetal loss before the 10th week of gestation, one or more unexplained fetal deaths at or beyond 10th week of gestation, or premature birth due to placental insufficiency, eclampsia, or preeclampsia. Laboratory criteria consist of medium to high titers of IgG or IgM anticardiolipin antibodies or lupus anticoagulant on 2 or more occasions at least 6 weeks apart. Of note, acquired APA secondary to certain infections (HIV, Lyme disease, adenovirus, rubella, *Varicella*, *Klebsiella*, syphilis) and medications (procainamide, hydralazine, chlorpromazine, quinidine, isoniazid, methyl-DOPA) are generally not associated with thrombosis.

Antiphospholipid antibody syndrome:

- Clinical presentation includes venous and arterial thrombosis.
- Diagnosis requires one clinical criterion and one laboratory criterion.
- Acquired APA are generally not associated with thrombosis.

LYMPHEDEMA

Lymphedema can be primary (idiopathic) or secondary to an underlying disorder. Primary lymphedema, such as lymphedema praecox, usually affects young women (9 times more frequently than men) and begins before the age of 40 years (often before age 20 years). In women, lymphedema often first appears at the time of menarche or with the first pregnancy. Edema is bilateral in about half the cases and is usually painless (Fig. 3). The initial evaluation of a young woman with lymphedema should include a complete history and physical examination (including pelvic examination and Pap smear) and computed tomography of the pelvis to exclude a neoplastic cause of lymphatic obstruction.

Secondary lymphedema is broadly classified into obstructive (postsurgical, postradiation, neoplastic) and inflammatory (infectious) types. Obstructive lymphedema due to neoplasm typically begins after the age of 40 years and is due to pelvic neoplasm or lymphoma. The most frequent cause in men is prostate cancer.

Infection-related lymphedema frequently occurs as a result of chronic or recurring lymphangitis or cellulitis. The portal of entry for infection is usually dermatophytosis (tinea pedis) (Fig. 4). The diagnosis of lymphedema can be confirmed by lymphoscintigraphy. Medical management of lymphedema includes edema reduction therapy, followed by daily use of custom-fitted, graduated compression (usually 40-50 mm Hg compression) elastic support. Antifungal treatment is essential if dermatophytosis is present. Weight reduction in obese patients is also beneficial. Surgical treatment of lymphedema (lymphaticovenous anastomosis, lymphedema reduction surgery) is indicated in highly selected patients.

EDEMA

Lower extremity edema is commonly encountered in cardiology practice. Aside from edema due to cardiac disease, other causes of regional edema usually can be identified from characteristic clinical features as are outlined in Table 2.

LEG ULCERS

The etiology of lower extremity ulceration can usually be determined by clinical examination. Clinical features of the four most common types of leg ulcers are summarized in Table 3 and Figure 5.

RESOURCE

Creager MA, Loscalzo J, Dzau VJ. Vascular medicine: a companion to Braunwald's heart disease. Philadelphia: WB Saunders; 2006.

Hirsh J, Albers GW, Guyatt GH, et al (Co-Chairs). The Seventh ACCP Conference on Antithrombotic and Thrombolytic Therapy: evidence-based guidelines. Chest. 2004;126 Suppl:163S-696S.

Rutherford RB. Vascular surgery. 6th ed. Philadelphia: Saunders; 2005.

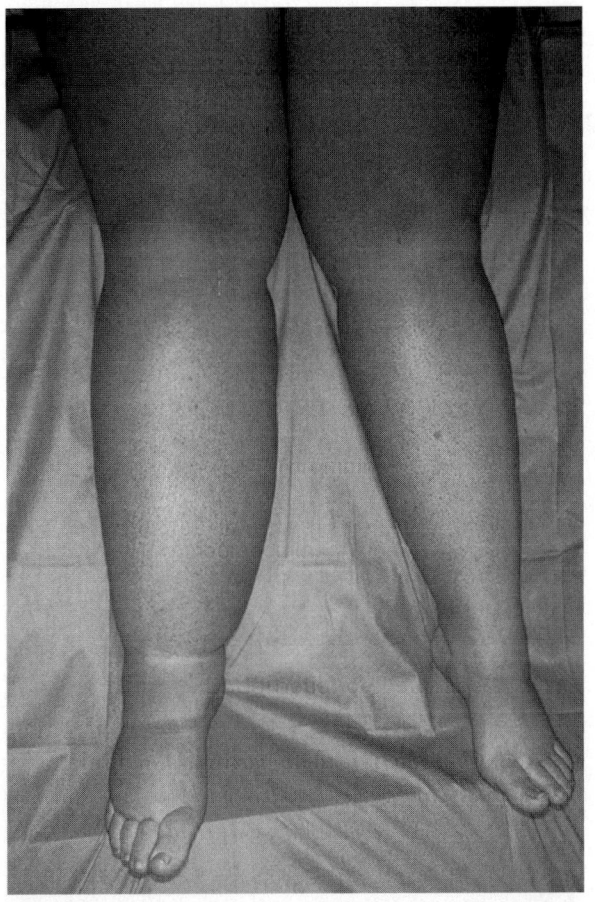

Fig. 3. Young woman with lymphedema praecox of right lower extremity. Note that the edema involves the toes.

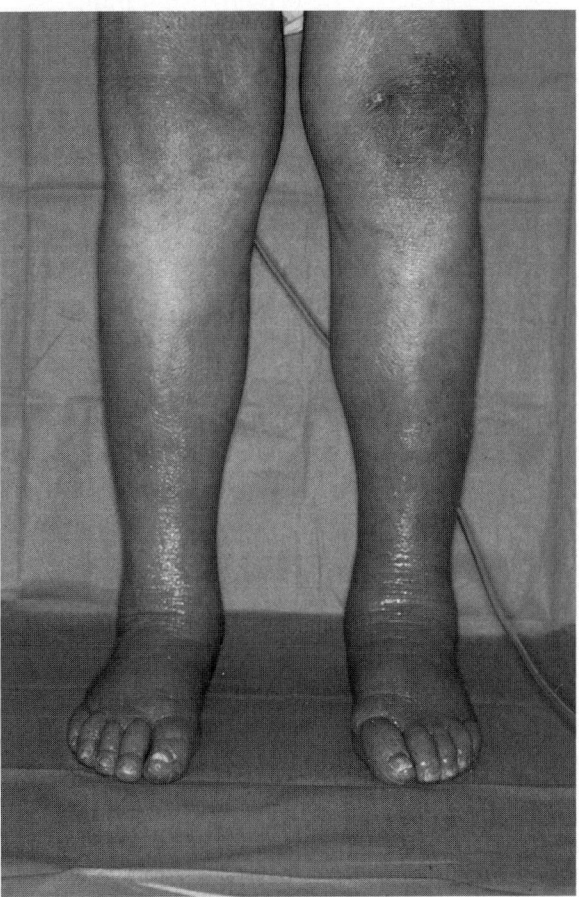

Fig. 4. Inflammatory lymphedema and cellulitis in a man with chronic tinea pedis as portal of entry for bacterial infection.

Table 2.   Characteristic Clinical Features of Regional Edema

Feature	Venous	Lymphedema	Lipedema
Bilateral	Occasional	Maybe	Always
Foot involved	Yes	Yes	No
Toes involved	No	Yes	No
Thickened skin	No	Yes	No
Stasis changes	Yes	No	No

Table 3.   Clinical Features of the Four Most Common Types of Leg Ulcer

Feature	Venous stasis	Arterial	Arteriolar	Neurotrophic
Onset	Trauma	Spontaneous	Trauma	
Course	Chronic	Progressive	Progressive	Progressive
Pain	No (unless infected)	Yes	Yes	No
Location	Medial leg	Toe, heel, foot	Lateral, posterior leg	Plantar
Surrounding skin	Stasis changes	Atrophic	Normal	Callus
Ulcer				
Edges	Shaggy	Discrete	Serpiginous	Discrete
Base	Healthy	Eschar, pale	Eschar, pale	Healthy or pale

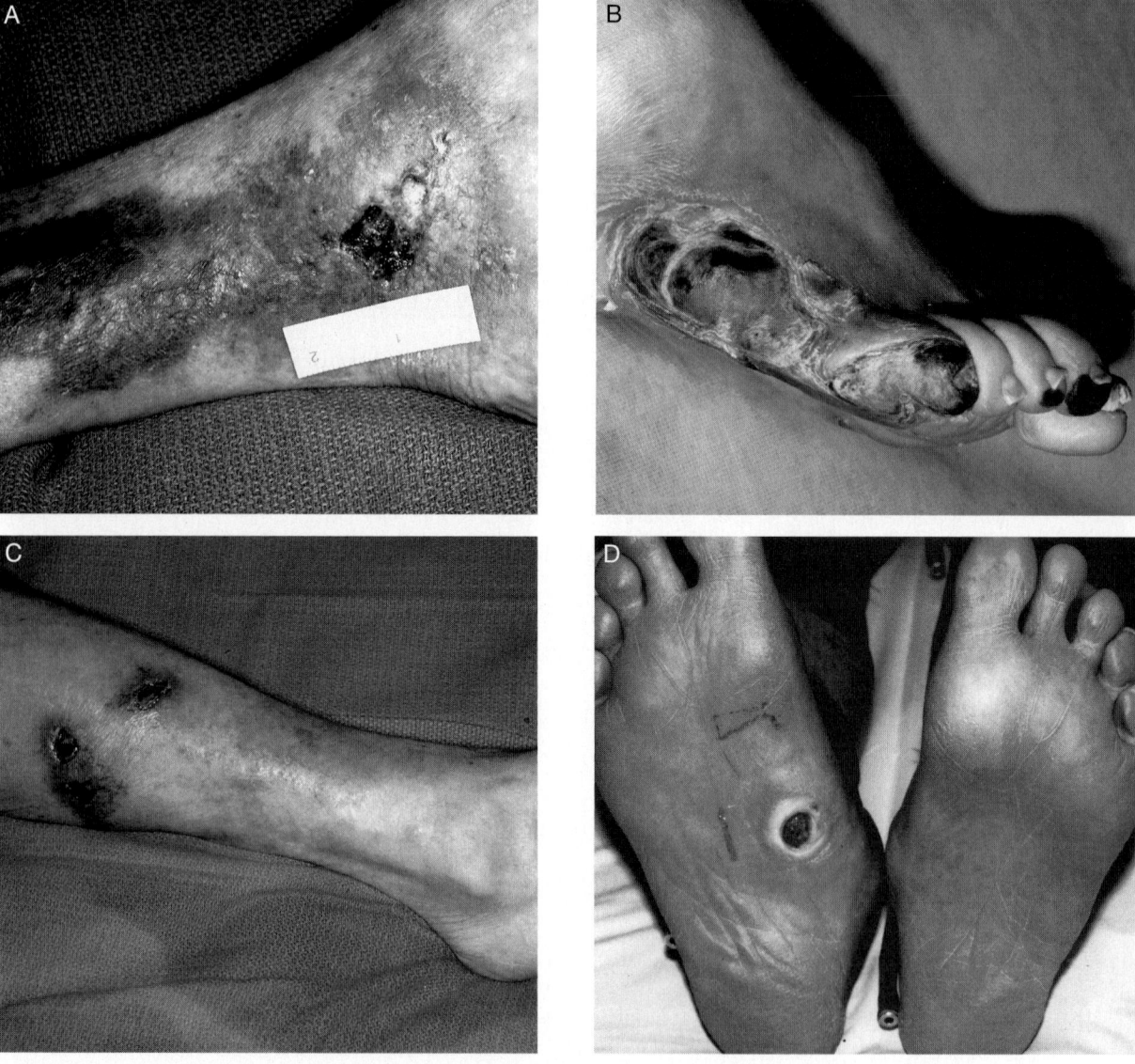

Fig. 5. Types of leg ulcer. *A*, venous; *B*, arterial; *C*, arteriolar; and *D*, neurotrophic.

53

VASCULITIS

Paul W. Wennberg, MD

DEFINITIONS AND PATHOGENESIS

By definition, vasculitis is inflammation of a vessel; any arteritis, capillaritis or phlebitis fulfills this definition. In fact it can be argued that atherosclerosis is in fact nothing more than an indolent, diffuse vasculitis. Practically, vasculitis is a diverse group of diseases that are as difficult to classify as they are to diagnose and treat. Large, medium and small arteries, capillaries and venules may be involved with presenting symptoms varying by the organ system or systems compromised (Table 1). Histopathology may be necrotizing or granulomatous. Both primary and secondary causes of vasculitis exist (Table 2) as well as a number of conditions that mimic vasculitis (Table 3). This review is arranged on the vessel size classification system, with cardiovascular pathology emphasized where appropriate.

In general, a humoral and or cell-mediated immune-mediated response to a noxious stimulus occurs. The inflammatory response is inappropriately sustained and inflammatory response to the vessel continues. The inflammation may be contained within the vessel wall or through the vessel wall. In either case, what sustains the process is often not known. Often the injury is nonspecific, due to immune-complex deposition. At times there is direct immune response to the vessel—such as the basement membrane in Henoch-Schönlein purpura.

Classification and Pathogenesis

- Vasculitis is commonly classified by the anatomic size of the vessel(s) affected.
- Pathogenesis is causes by a sustained inappropriate humoral and/or cellular mediated immune response.

GENERAL PRINCIPLES OF EVALUATION

Symptoms and Signs

Nonspecific systemic symptoms usually precede the diagnosis of a vasculitis by weeks to months. Fatigue, malaise, loss of stamina, fevers, unintentional weight loss, and night sweats are all common. New-onset or markedly worse vasospasm (Raynaud's phenomenon) in this setting is significant and should raise suspicion for medium and small-vessel changes. If an underlying disease is present, such as rheumatoid arthritis or fibromyalgia, the symptoms may be attributed to this rather than a vasculitis. Jaw or limb claudication is often overlooked by a patient due to an unconscious adaptation to the arterial compromise caused by the inflammatory narrowing or occlusion of the artery. Ischemic ulceration, a painful limb or visceral pain may occur later in the course. Erroneous diagnoses are often made and arguably the norm until more specific symptoms of muscle fatigue, weakness and pain are present.

Table 1. Vessel Segment Involvement and Clinical Location of Vasculitis Syndromes*

Aorta	Large and great vessels (major branches, carotids, subclavians, iliacs)	Medium-sized arteries (named major coronary mid-distal limb renal, mesenteric)	Small arteries (small named CNS, digital, unnamed intra-organ)	Arterioles, capillaries, venules (skin, mucosa alveoli, glomeruli)
Takayasu's arteritis	Takayasu's arteritis	Takayasu's arteritis		
Temporal arteritis	Temporal arteritis	Temporal arteritis		
Cogan's syndrome	Cogan's syndrome	Cogan's syndrome	Cogan's syndrome	
	Kawasaki's disease	Kawasaki's disease	Kawasaki's disease	
	Behçet's disease	Behçet's disease	Behçet's disease	
		Polyarteritis nodosa	Polyarteritis nodosa	
		Buerger's disease	Buerger's disease	
			Microscopic polyangiitis	Microscopic polyangiitis
		Churg-Strauss vasculitis	Churg-Strauss vasculitis	
		Wegener's granulomatosis	Wegener's granulomatosis	Wegener's granulomatosis
			Arteriopathy of CTD	Arteriopathy of CTD
			Hypersensitivity vasculitides:	
			Henoch-Schönlein purpura	Henoch-Schönlein purpura
			Leukocytoclastic vasculitis	Leukocytoclastic vasculitis

*The most commonly affected segment is in bold.

A thorough physical examination should be done with careful attention to the vessels, skin, and mucous membranes. A rash, localized pain over an organ, hemoptysis, or blood in the urine may be noted. Specific signs such as a pulseless limb or ischemic wound may allow one to consider vascular involvement early. Pain directly over an artery (such as pain over the temporal arteries in giant cell arteritis) is classic but rarely seen. Localized tenderness in the abdomen may indicate mesenteric artery involvement, especially if gastrointestinal symptoms have been present.

Signs and Symptoms
- Unexplained systemic illness with fever, malaise, and weight loss are due the systemic inflammatory syndrome.
- New-onset claudication, rash, Raynaud's phenomenon, arterial tenderness, and decrease or loss of pulses are signs suggestive of vasculitis.

Testing
There is no one "best test" for vasculitis. The goal of testing is twofold, to determine the extent of involvement—

Table 2.   Causes of Secondary Vasculitis

Connective tissues diseases	Infections
Scleroderma	Parvovirus B19
Rheumatoid arthritis	*Streptococcus*
Systemic lupus erythematosis	*Staphylococcus*
Sjögren's syndrome	Hepatitis B
Systemic sclerosis	HIV
Antiphospholipid antibody syndrome	Malaria
Dermatomyositis	Tuberculosis
Drugs	Other
Penicillin	Inflammatory bowel disease
Sulfonamide	Foreign proteins (immunizations)
Hydroxyurea	Insecticides
Methotrexate	Organ transplantion
Allopurinol	Malignancy-related vasculitis
Dilantin	
Tetracycline	
Quinidine	
Interferon alfa	

that is what arterial segments and organs systems are involved—and to establish the diagnosis. Testing to determine the extent of involvement should be guided by physical exam and symptoms (Table 4). Serologic evaluation typically begins at the same time and in many cases is diagnostic. Both avenues of testing are typically needed to make the diagnosis, however (Table 5).

Imaging of the arterial system is needed to determine the extent and severity of arteritis. Ultrasound may also be useful especially for the carotid arteries or when an aortic or mesenteric aneurysm is suspected. CT and MR angiography may be indicated and adequate in some cases, but lack the fine resolution of conventional contrast angiography. Angiography must be carefully planned to include selective injections of the involved, and sometimes uninvolved, arterial segments.

Biopsy of an affected vessel is the most specific test for making the diagnosis. In some cases, such as temporal arteritis, the vessel is easily accessible but this is more of the exception than the rule.

Treatment

Treatment of vasculitis is primarily by immunosuppre-sion, most often with corticosteroids. Dosing and duration of treatment are variable. Additional agents such as methotrexate, cyclosporine, azathioprine, and mycophenolate may be used in conjunction with or in

Table 3.   Conditions Mimicking Vasculitis

Cholesterol emboli
Bacterial endocarditis
Atrial myxoma
Pernio*
Leprosy
Vasoconstrictor use (e.g., ergot, cocaine)
Insect venom (e.g., brown recluse spider)
Thoracic outlet syndrome
Complex regional pain syndrome (reflex sympa-thetic dystrophy)
Malignancy
    Cutaneous lymphoma
    Basal cell carcinoma
Sneddon's syndrome
Factitious

*Some consider pernio to be a limited form of vasculitis.

Table 4.   Work-up of Vasculitis: Extent of Involvement

Renal
    Urinalysis, creatinine, biopsy
Respiratory
    PFTs, CXR, CT
Cardiac
    EKG, Holter monitoring, echocardiography
Muscular
    CK, aldolase, EMG
CNS
    EMG, CSF analysis, MRI, CT
Vascular
    Segmental pressures, conventional angiography, CTA, MRA, duplex ultrasound

Table 5.   Work-up of Vasculitis: Serologic Assessment

ANA (with extractable antigens)
ANCA
Rheumatoid factor
Cryoglobulins
Anti Scl-70 antibodies
Anticentromere antibodies
SPEP/UPEP
CH_{50}
HIV
Hepatitis serologic tests
Parvovirus B19
Blood cultures

place of steroids. While treatment for long duration is best managed by those do it frequently, immediate treatment with high-dose oral or intravenous corticosteroids must be started in situations where organ or limb ischemia is critical. This is most commonly required for visual loss in suspected giant cell arteritis.

Testing and Treatment

■ Testing should define the organ systems involved and location of stenosis and occlusion.
■ Serologic testing may be diagnostic, but not in all cases. Even when diagnostic, the extent and severity of arterial compromise must be defined.
■ Arterial of organ biopsy is the best test for diagnosis.
■ Conventional contrast angiography is frequently required for diagnosis and or determining extent and severity of arterial compromise.

LARGE VESSEL ARTERITIS

The two most commonly occurring large vessel arteritides are temporal arteritis (often referred to as giant cell arteritis) and Takayasu's arteritis. Both of these are giant cell arteritides with histopathology demonstrating multinucleated giant cells. There is significant overlap between temporal arteritis (TmA) and Takayasu's arteritis (TkA) in both pathology and distribution of disease and in practice they present as a spectrum of disease.

Temporal Arteritis

Epidemiology

TmA by definition occurs in those over the age of 50. Frequency increases with age. Women are affected twice as often as men. Caucasians, specifically those of northern European ancestry, show the highest prevalence. There is a strong association with polymyalgia rheumatica with up to 50% of patients diagnosed with TmA having had previous diagnosis of polymyalgia.

Anatomy and Pathology

The ophthalmic, temporal, vertebral and carotid arteries are the segments most commonly involved. The other intracranial arteries are typically spared. Disease involvement is patchy with normal segments present between those affected. Involvement of arteries below the diaphragm is rare. Pathology shows granulomatous changes with disruption of the internal elastic lamina with T-lymphocyte infiltrates and multinucleated giant cells (Fig. 1).

Symptoms and Signs

Headache is the most common symptom at presentation. Nonspecific fatigue, weight loss and myalgias are also common. Jaw claudication, scalp tenderness, facial pain and earache occur with decreasing frequency. Ischemic events most commonly present as transient ocular changes, although permanent blindness can occur.

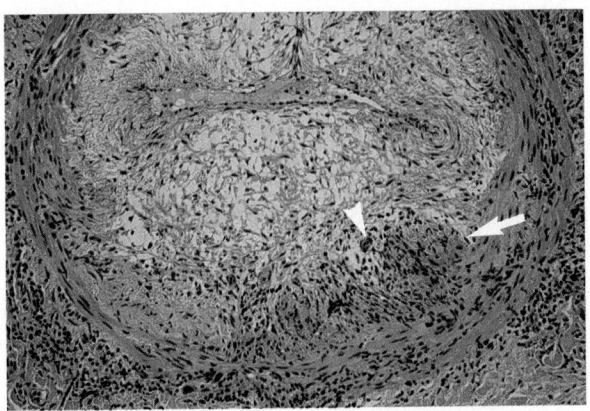

Fig. 1. Giant cell arteritis of left temporal artery. Granulomatous change disrupting internal elastic lamina (*arrow*) and lymphocytic infiltrate. Multinucleated giant cell (*arrowhead*).

Coronary artery involvement is uncommon but should be considered if typical angina occurs in the setting of a high sedimentation rate and other symptoms suggestive of TmA. Tenderness over the temporal arteries is commonly present but if not present it does not rule out the diagnosis. The temporal arteries are best palpated at the proximal portion, just anterior to the pinnae of the ear.

Diagnosis and Treatment

A sedimentation rate of 50 mm/hour or greater is expected, but frequently a sedimentation rate greater than 100 mm/hour is found. Rarely (1%-2%) patients with TmA have a normal ESR. If the ESR is negative and the rest of the clinical picture is suggestive the diagnosis should still be considered. C-reactive protein is usually elevated. Bilateral biopsy of the temporal arteries provides definitive diagnosis. A 2-3 cm segment is taken and multiple sections examined. Histopathologic changes do not change for several days so biopsy several days after initiation of treatment does not negate the need for confirmatory biopsy.

Treatment by immediate initiation of moderate to high-dose corticosteroid (40 to 60 mg/day or greater) should occur in an effort to minimize permanent ocular changes. If severe ocular symptoms or blindness are present, high-dose intravenous steroid therapy is recommended. The ESR is usually a good marker of disease activity. Surgical or endovascular intervention is rarely indicated in the acute setting but may be required late.

Giant Cell Arteritis

- Age greater than 50, women affected more often than men.
- Prior history of polymyalgia rheumatica in about 50%.
- Temporal artery biopsy is diagnostic. Should be done bilaterally, within several days of starting steroids, and multiple sections examined for best sensitivity.
- Treatment should begin as soon as diagnosis is entertained. High-dose intravenous steroids are appropriate when ocular symptoms are present.
- Sedimentation rate elevated in greater than 95% and serves as a good marker for disease activity.

Takayasu's Arteritis

Epidemiology

Unlike TmA, TkA affects women much more often than men with studies ranging from 2:1 to 9:1. Women are typically of child-bearing age. Those of Asian and Indian ancestry appear to be at greater risk than European ancestry.

Anatomy and Pathology

The aorta is affected in all patients. The great vessels, subclavian arteries, renal arteries and mesenteric arteries are frequently involved. The histopathology is varied with granulomatous changes and multinucleated giant cells early, followed by a diffuse inflammatory infiltrate, then fibrosis with accelerated atherosclerotic changes. The aggressive inflammation can result in stenosis and occlusion early and aneurysmal degeneration later (Fig. 2).

Symptoms and Findings

The classic finding on physical exam is discrepant pulse exam of blood pressure in a young woman. Symptoms may or may not be present depending on the activity level of the patient. Nonspecific symptoms such as fever, fatigue, and weight loss may occur. Specific symptoms reflect the anatomic site(s) of involvement. Arm or leg claudication and cerebrovascular symptoms (TIA, visual disturbances, and syncope) are the most common symptoms on presentation.

Cardiac manifestations may be very significant. Angina, arrhythmia, and dyspnea are common reflecting coronary inflammation in the acute setting and accelerated

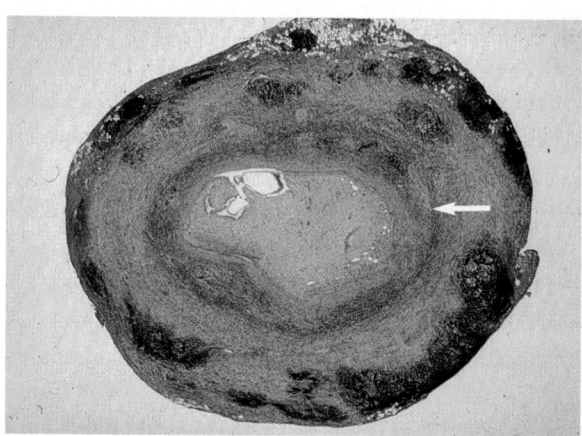

Fig. 2. Takayasu's arteritis of right carotid artery in 29-year-old female. Accelerated atherosclerosis with thickened intima (*arrow*) and vessel obliteration.

atherosclerosis in the chronic setting. Congestive heart failure due to acute aortic insufficiency with or without valve rupture affects up to 10% of patients in several series. Pulmonary symptoms include dyspnea, hemoptysis or pleurisy, are common and reflect pulmonary artery involvement. Renal involvement usually manifests as hypertension. Assessment of blood pressure can be problematic since stenosis may be present at the great vessels. All four limbs should be assessed and the highest pressure used to guide anti-hypertensive therapy.

Diagnosis and Treatment
Diagnosis is made with imaging in the majority of cases. Histology is rarely available or required. CT and MR angiography are usually adequate to define the location of disease and degree of stenosis. Segmental pressures and duplex ultrasound are good for chronic assessment of disease. Echocardiography is needed to assess severity or presence of aortic insufficiency. Conventional angiography is needed when coronary artery involvment is considered. An elevated sedimentation rate is absent in 10% to 30% of cases. C-reactive protein may not be elevated either. Other markers such as interleukin-6 are used in some centers. Because of the variability in markers for disease activity, symptoms and imaging studies must be relied on in many cases for long-term assessment.

Treatment is based on corticosteroids, frequently with the addition of cyclosporine. Antiplatelet therapy is indicated in all patients. Aggressive treatment of

blood pressure and optimizing lipids to decrease atherosclerosis is reasonable. Revascularization of symptomatic arteries by endovascular or surgical techniques is appropriate in the chronic setting. In the setting of acute inflammation, manipulation of the vessel should be done only in the presence of severe cerebral, coronary or organ ischemia or critical limb ischemia.

- Affects women of child-bearing years
- Nonspecific symptoms may be present for months prior to arterial symptoms
- Unilateral weakness or loss of pulse, discrepant blood pressures, or onset of claudication in a young woman with systemic symptoms are suggestive
- Cardiac involvement common
    Coronary arteries may be affected primarily
    Aortic regurgitation may occur acutely or as a late complication
- Occasional acute revascularization needed for cerebral, cardiac or limb ischemia
- Aggressive atherosclerosis and aneurysmal changes are common in the late or "burned out" phase

COGAN'S SYNDROME
Cogan's syndrome is a rare disease of young adults that presents with keratitis, uveitis, and vestibular symptoms. It often follows an upper respiratory infection. Vertigo, nausea, and hearing changes similar to Meniere's disease may occur. The sedimentation rate is elevated. Fifteen percent of patients have a vasculitis presenting as aortitis or carditis. The most common cardiac manifestation is aortic regurgitation due to aortic cusp involvement. Treatment is high-dose corticosteroids.

MEDIUM VESSEL ARTERITIS

Kawasaki's Disease

Epidemiology
Kawasaki's disease (KD), also known as mucocutaneous lymph node syndrome, affects children under the age of 5, most commonly under age one. Etiology is unclear but it is thought to be infectious. Children of Asian ancestry are affected most commonly, even when living outside of Asia.

Anatomy and Pathology
KD affects medium-sized vessels primarily but not exclusively. The coronary arteries are most commonly affected with aneurysm formation in 25% of untreated children. Myocardial infarction occurs but typically with good functional recovery (Fig. 3). Myocarditis and valvulitis may also be seen.

Symptoms and Findings
Criteria for diagnosis have been set by the American Heart Association reflecting the clinical symptoms. Fever of more than five days despite antibiotics is found in all. Nonsuppurative conjunctivitis; a pleomorphic rash; cervical lymphandenopathy; dry, cracked, red mucous membranes; and brawny edema of the hands and feet with desquamation late are the other findings of the syndrome.

Diagnosis and Treatment
IVIg has been useful in the acute setting for shortening duration of symptoms and reducing coronary artery aneurysm formation. Aspirin alone is not effective in decreasing duration or aneurysm formation. Chronic warfarin therapy is suggested in those with large aneurysms. Long-term survival is good.

- Affects children under age 5
- Cardiac manifestations
    Coronary artery aneurysm common
    Coronary infarction may occur

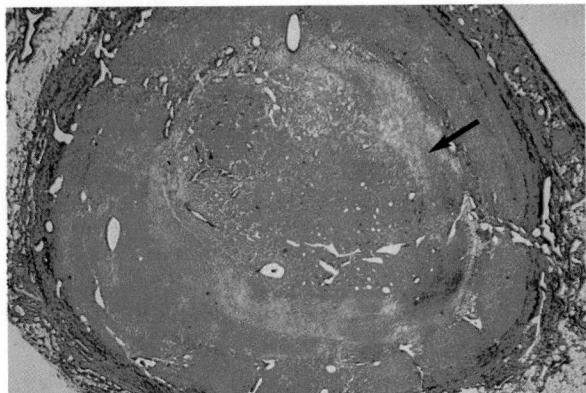

Fig. 3. Left anterior descending artery thrombus in 15-year-old male with Kawasaki's disease and sudden cardiac death. Thrombotic occlusion (*arrow*) of the vessel.

- Treatment with IVIg may decrease duration and complications of disease
- Aspirin alone is not effective therapy

Behcet's Syndrome

Epidemiology
Behcet's syndrome is a rare disorder found most commonly in the Middle East, specifically Turkey, and along the "Silk Road" trading route between East Asia and the Mediterranean.

Anatomy and Pathology
An autoimmune response within the vasovasorum affects large vessels. Aneurysms, stenosis, and occlusion of large and medium-sized arteries and veins may occur. Thrombophlebitis of superficial and deep veins, including cerebral venous thrombosis, occurs. The coronary arteries and valve cusps may be affected.

Symptoms and Findings
Oral aphthous ulcers, genital ulcers, uveitis and skin lesions are the most common presentation.

Treatment
Immunosuppressants are less useful than other vasculitides.

Polyarteritis Nodosa

Epidemiology
PAN may occur in any age group. Hepatitis B is present in 10 to 20% of patients.

Anatomy and Pathology
Muscular arteries of any organ may be involved including the coronaries, although rare. The mesenteric and renal arteries are the most frequently involved vessels. New onset or worsened hypertension is common in patients with renal involvement. Microaneurysm formation is common and occurs due to inflammatory destruction of the media. In the kidney aneurysms are often intra-parenchymal. In contrast, glomerulonephritis is uncommon. The ANCA is negative (Table 6).

Symptoms and Findings
Systemic illness, including fever, malaise, arthralgia, and

myalgia, is common. Localizing symptoms include mental status changes, abdominal pain, flank pain and angina mental status changes, and peripheral neuropathy. Mononeuritis multiplex is present in at least two-thirds of patients. Skin changes are present in up to half with variable manifestation from livedo to vesicular bullae. Orchitis is common. Cardiac involvement is uncommon, but usually presenting as congestive heart failure. Angiography or biopsy is diagnostic.

Treatment

Corticosteroids with cyclophosphamide begun immediately or soon after diagnosis is the usual treatment. Relapse is uncommon.

- Arthralgias, mononeuritis multiplex, skin and gastrointestinal symptoms.
     Cardiac involvement uncommon—congestive heart failure when present.
- No glomerulonephritis or pulmonary involvement.
- ANCA negative. Hepatitis positive in up to 20%.
- Mesenteric angiography best diagnostic test.
- Recurrence uncommon.

SMALL VESSEL ARTERITIS

Microscopic polyangiitis has recently been differentiated

Table 6.   ANCA Antibodies in Vasculitis*

ANCA in vasculitis
  Large vessel
    None
  Medium and small vessel
    Churg-Strauss syndrome
      P-ANCA positive ~70%
    Wegener's granulomatosis
      C-ANCA positive ~90%
    Microscopic polyangitis
      P-ANCA positive ~80%

---

*Antineutrophilic cytoplasmic autoantibodies (ANCA) in a perinuclear (P) or cytoplasmic (C) or atypical pattern. The presence of ANCA autoantibodies is supportive, not diagnostic.

---

from polyarteritis nodosa. Like PAN, micoscopic polyangiitis (MPA) is a necrotizing vasculitis of small vessels with little or no immune complex deposition. Mononeuritis multiplex, arthralgias, and systemic symptoms including fever occur. Unlike PAN, necrotizing glomerulonephritis and pulmonary involvement are common and the P-ANCA is positive in 80%.

Churg-Strauss syndrome is a rare, presenting as fever, asthma, increased eosinophil count, and vasculitis. The histology is a granulomatous inflammation with an eosinophil-rich vasculitis of small to medium-sized vessels most often of the respiratory tract. The P-ANCA is positive in 70%. Involvement of the gastrointestinal tract, kidneys, heart and CNS occur and greatly affect the prognosis (Fig. 4).

Wegener's granulomatosis is a granulomatous vasculitis of small to medium-sized arteries, capillaries and venules of the respiratory tract and kidneys. Necrotizing glomerulonephritis is common, occurring in one-fifth at presentation and up to 80% during the course of the disease. The sinus mucosa and nasal septum are frequently involved and lead to the classic "saddle-nose" deformity. The C-ANCA is positive in 90%. Treatment is usually cyclophosphamide with corticosteroids.

Hypersensitivity vasculitis is a common set of vasculitides with a number of names (allergic vasculitis, leukocytoclastic vasculitis, cutaneous necrotizing vasculitis, etc) all affecting small vessels with cellular debris, primarily on the venular side. The process is immune mediated. Drug hypersensitivity, urticarial vasculitis, mixed cryoglobulinemia, and serum sickness are common clinical syndromes in this class. Skin findings include shallow painful ulceration, purpura, petechiae, urticaria, papules, vesicles, etc. **Henoch-Schönlein purpura** is a small vessel hypersensitivity vasculitis with IgA-dominant immune complexes typically involving the gut, skin, and glomeruli. It affects children under the age of 10 but can be seen in adults.

Small Vessel Vasculitis

- Cardiac involvement in small vessel arteritis is uncommon.
     Occurrs in 10 to 20% of cases.
     When present, myocarditis and coronary artery involvement are the most common pathologies.
- Symptoms of congestive heart failure, angina, dyspnea

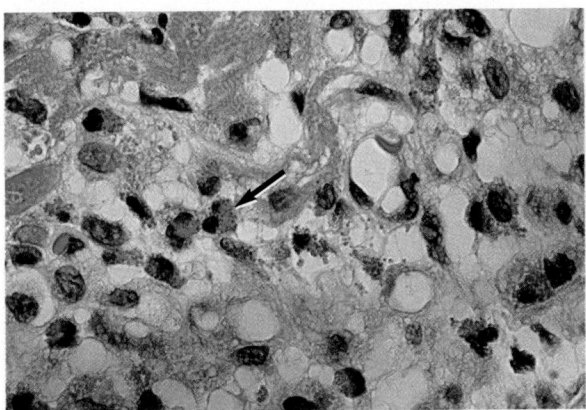

Fig. 4. Eosinophilic myocarditis in Churg-Strauss syndrome; eosinophilic infiltrate (*arrow*).

and arrhythmias in the setting of a suspected or known small vasculitis warrant further investigation.

- The ANCA is positive in microscopic polyangiitis, Churg-Strauss syndrome, and Wegener's granulomatosis.

NONVASCULITIC ARTERITIS

Thromboangiitis Obliterans (Buerger's Disease)

Epidemiology

Thromboangiitis obliterans (TAO) or Buerger's disease is caused by use of or continued exposure to tobacco products. While historically thought to be almost exclusive to men, more recent studies have shown that the male to female ratio reflects smoking patterns in the population. Prevalence of TAO appears to be higher in India and Asia than Europe and North America. Age at presentation must be less than 45 by definition and is frequently much younger.

Anatomy and Pathology

Medium and small vessels are affected, most commonly the distal limb vessels, but coronary, cerebral, and splanchnic arteries may be affected. Involvement of the aorta, iliac, and pulmonary arteries is rare. Histopathology is unique in that the vessel wall is not directly involved. Rather, an intraluminal inflammatory thrombus is present with an intact internal elastic lamina. Three phases of histology have been defined. Acutely,

an inflammatory thrombus, highly cellular, is present with microabscesses and giant cells present. The intermediate phase shows further organization of thombus. Finally the chronic phase demonstrates resolution of inflammation and fibrosis. Superficial thrombophlebitis is common and has the same histology as the arterial findings.

Symptoms and Findings

The presenting complaint is usually a painful ulcer, typically at a single digit or multiple digits in a young smoker. Both the upper and lower extremities may be affected. Claudication may be present. New onset vasospasm (Raynaud's phenomenon) is common. Concurrent or recent symptoms of superficial thrombophlebitis are also common. Examination confirms an ischemic ulcer, decreased or absent pulses, and classically palpable cords consistent with recent phlebitis. Allen's test is frequently positive even if upper extremity symptoms are not present. Embolic cause, hypercoagulable states such as antiphospholipid antibody syndrome, other forms of vasculitis, and arteriopathy due to connective tissue diseases need to be excluded. The sedimentation rate is not elevated in TAO. If elevation is present it could be due to an infected ulcer or another etiology must be considered.

Angiography is confirmatory. The affected limb(s) should be imaged as well as a nonaffected limb. Both upper and lower extremity limb should be imaged on presentation. The classic finding is normal aorta, iliac and proximal femoral arteries with segmental stenosis or occlusion of the distal leg and arm arteries. Corkscrew intra-arterial "collaterals" are frequently seen.

Treatment

Stopping smoking and avoiding second-hand tobacco exposure is a must. Over 90% of those who quit smoking will avoid amputation. The amputation rate in those who continue to smoke is greater than 40%. Thrombolytic therapy or intravenous vasodilators such as iloprost are beneficial in some cases, but not all. Surgical and endovascular revascularization are not indicated in the acute phase except for limb salvage with guarded results. Oral vasodilators and sympathectomy are helpful in the chronic setting.

- Affects tobacco users at an age less than 45.

- Vasculitis, embolism, and connective tissue disease need to be excluded.
- Histopathology shows an inflammatory thrombus, not vessel wall inflammation.
- Medium and small arteries and veins affected.
- Angiography is diagnostic: both upper and lower extremity limbs—clinically affected and non-affected—should be imaged.
- Amputation rate with continued tobacco use is greater than 40%.

Pernio

Chronic pernio or chilblains is a small vessel vasculitis of the toes occurring during the cold weather months and resolving during the warm weather months. The classic teaching is a past history of frostbite but in practice it is more common to have grown up in a cold weather state or have participated in a cold weather sport. The symptoms begin decades after the suspected period of exposure. Debate exists as to the pathophysiology, but many consider it a type of limited vasculitis. Blister over an erythematous base at the toe tips leading to shallow ulcers and pitting is the usual complaint. Mild to moderate pain is common. Symptoms occasionally occur after beta-blockade is started for cardiac disease. Calcium channel blockers or alpha blockers are used to treat symptoms but do not replace good warm footwear during cold-weather months.

Pernio

- Limited vasculitis affecting the toe tips.
- History of cold exposure in past.
- Comes on in cold weather months, resolves in warm months.
- Vasodilators (calcium channel and alpha blockers) helpful.

Connective Tissue Diseases

A number of connective tissue diseases may result in vasculitis, often in the form of an arteriopathy. The vessels affected are very distal in the periphery, such as the digital arteries in the upper and lower extremities. The initial presentation is vasospasm (i.e., Raynaud's phenomenon) and cold intolerance. When new onset vasospasm is present in an adult (third decade or later) and not related to other medical conditions or medications such as beta-blockade, a connective tissue disease should be considered. Scleroderma, CREST syndrome, systemic lupus erythematosis, and mixed connective tissue disease are just some of the possible causes for this. If just one or two digits are affected an embolic event should be considered (Table 3).

Cardiac involvement is uncommon but when present may manifest as either myocarditis or pericarditis. Scleroderma often results in pulmonary hypertension, most commonly with exertional dyspnea as the main complaint. Right-sided heart failure is seen in extreme cases. Myocarditis is the most common presentation in myopathies such as polymyositis.

- Late onset vasospasm (Raynaud's phenomenon) is a common initial presentation of a connective tissue
- Embolism should be considered if sudden ischemia or vasospasm of a single or few digits is present
- Scleroderma is associated with pulmonary hypertension

RESOURCES

Asherson RA, Cervera R, editors. Vascular manifestations of systemic autoimmune diseases. Boca Raton (FL): CRC Press; 2001.

Langford CA. Vasculitis. J Allergy Clin Immunol. 2003;111 Suppl 2:S602-12.

54

MARFAN SYNDROME

Naser M. Ammash, MD

Heidi M. Connolly, MD

INTRODUCTION

Marfan syndrome is the most common inherited multisystem disorder of connective tissue. This autosomal dominant condition has a reported incidence of 2-3 per 10,000 individuals without any particular gender, racial, or ethnic predilection. Early identification and appropriate management improves the outcome of patients with Marfan syndrome who are prone to life-threatening cardiovascular complications.

GENETICS

Marfan syndrome is caused by a mutation of the fibrillin-1 gene located on chromosome 15. Fibrillin-1 protein is an extracellular matrix glycoprotein which is an important component of the connective tissue elastic microfibrils and is essential to normal fibrinogenesis. Fragmentation and disorganization of the elastic fibers in the aortic media is a histological marker on Marfan syndrome, so-called medial degeneration. Those histological changes make the aorta stiffer and less distensible than the normal aorta. More recently, endothelial dysfunction has also been demonstrated in the Marfan aorta.

The penetrance of the fibrillin mutation is high and the phenotypic expression is extremely variable. To date, more than 500 different mutations involving the fibrillin-1 gene have been identified, but no correlation between the specific type of fibrillin-1 mutation and the clinical phenotype has been recognized. In approximately 75% of cases, an individual inherits the disorder from an affected parent. The remaining 25% of cases result from de novo mutation. There is little prognostic information provided by the detection of a mutation beyond the available information provided from the patient's own family history. Therefore, genetic testing is mainly used for adjunctive clinical diagnosis in selected cases.

With current gene testing, approximately 10% of mutations that cause classic Marfan syndrome are missed by conventional screening methods that cost approximately $2,500. Limitations to genetic testing include

1) The mutation in fibrillin-1 gene can cause conditions other than Marfan-like disorder such as MASS syndrome and anuloaortic ectasia.
2) None of the current methods used to find mutations in fibrillin-1 gene identify all mutations that cause Marfan syndrome.
3) Family members of the same mutation causing Marfan syndrome can show wide variation in timing of onset and severity of complications.

CARDIOVASCULAR MANIFESTATIONS

Marfan syndrome is a multisystem disorder involving the cardiovascular and skeletal systems as well as the eyes, lungs, skin, and dura. These clinical features have been codified into the Ghent diagnostic nosology (Table 1). The cardiovascular manifestations of Marfan syndrome include:

1) Dilatation of the ascending aorta and less commonly the descending thoracic aorta, with associated increased risk of aortic valve incompetence, as well as aortic dissection. The latter can involve the coronary artery ostia and as a result myocardial infarction.
2) Mitral valve prolapse with or without mitral valve regurgitation
3) Mitral anular calcification
4) Pulmonary artery dilatation
5) Dilatation or dissection of the descending thoracic aorta.

Aortic root disease leading to aortic root aneurysm is progressive and is the main cause of morbidity and mortality in patients with Marfan syndrome. It is present in 50 to 60% of adults and in 50% of children with Marfan syndrome and can be readily detected by echocardiography (Fig. 1). Both aortic diameter and aortic stiffness are independent predictors of progressive aortic dilatation. The latter predisposes to aortic dissection which involves the ascending aorta in 90% of cases (Fig. 2), and 10% of dissections are distal to left subclavian or type B dissection (Fig. 3).

Marfan syndrome should be suspected in any patient under the age of 40 years with aortic dissection. Recent data suggest that Marfan syndrome is present in 50% of aortic dissection patients presenting under age 40 years and accounts for only 2% of dissections in older patients. Many patients with Marfan syndrome and aortic dissection have a family history of dissection. The two most important determinants of dissection risk are the maximal aortic dimension and family history of aortic dissection.

Mitral valve prolapse with or without mitral valve regurgitation can be seen in 60 to 80% of patients with Marfan syndrome undergoing an echocardiographic examination. However, only an estimated 25% of Marfan patients with mitral valve prolapse have pro-

gressive disease with progressive regurgitation that could be due to worsening degeneration of the valve or spontaneous rupture of the chordae tendineae. Tricuspid valve prolapse with and without regurgitation can occur in presence or absence of mitral valve prolapse.

Ventricular dilatation and/or dysfunction, beyond that explained by aortic or mitral regurgitation, have been reported in patients with Marfan syndrome.

DIAGNOSIS

The diagnosis of Marfan syndrome requires a careful history including information about any family members who may have the disorder or had unexplained early or sudden unexpected death. A thorough physical examination in addition to eye examination by an ophthalmologist, genetics evaluation, x-rays, and echocardiogram are routinely recommended. The goal is to determine whether the diagnosis can be established clinically. The modified Ghent criteria, proposed in 1996, allow a uniform approach to the diagnosis of Marfan syndrome. A comprehensive multidisciplinary approach involving cardiac, orthopedic, ophthalmologic, as well as genetic consultations is warranted in order to confirm or exclude the diagnosis. In the absence of any family history of Marfan syndrome, the diagnosis is made by identifying major criteria in two different organ systems and involvement of a third system or in the presence of fibrillin-1 mutation and major criteria in one system and involvement in a second organ system (Table 1). On the other hand, in the presence of a family history of Marfan syndrome in a first degree relative who meets major criteria independently, the diagnosis of Marfan syndrome can be made in the presence of one major criterion in one organ system and involvement of a second organ system.

Aortic diameter should be measured by transthoracic echocardiogram at multiple levels and related to normal values based on age and body surface area reported by Roman and Devereux (Fig. 4). The maximum aortic dimension is usually located at the sinuses of Valsalva. Other imaging techniques such as transesophageal echocardiogram, computed tomography (CT), angiography, and magnetic resonance imaging (MRI) may also be helpful. Echocardiography however can assess other cardiovascular manifestations of

Table 1.   Summary of the Major and Minor Suggested Ghent Criteria Used to Establish the Diagnosis of Marfan Syndrome

SKELETAL

Major (*at least four of the following constitutes a major criterion*):
- Pectus carinatum
- Pectus excavatum requiring surgery
- Reduced upper to lower segment ratio OR arm span to height ratio >1.05
- Wrist and thumb signs
- Scoliosis of >20° or spondylolisthesis
- Reduced extension at the elbows (<170°)
- Medial displacement of the medial malleolus causing pes planus
- Protrusio acetabuli of any degree (ascertained on radiographs)

Minor
- Pectus excavatum
- Joint hypermobility
- Highly arched palate with crowding of teeth
- Facial appearance: dolichocephaly (long narrow skull)
    - malar hypoplasia (flattening)
    - enophthalmos (sunken eyes)
    - retrognathia (recessed lower mandible)
    - down-slanting palpebral fissures

For involvement of the skeletal system, at least two features contributing to major criteria, or one major and two minor criteria must be present:

OCULAR

Major
- Ectopia lentis

Minor
- Flat cornea
- Increased axial length of globe (<23.5 mm)
- Hypoplastic iris OR hypoplastic ciliary muscle causing decreased miosis

For involvement of the ocular system, at least two of the minor criteria must be present:

CARDIOVASCULAR

Major (*either of the following constitutes a major criteria*)
- Dilatation of the ascending aorta with or without aortic regurgitation and involving at least the sinuses of Valsalva
- Dissection of the ascending aorta

Table 1. (continued)

Minor
  • Mitral valve prolapse with or without mitral valve regurgitation
  • Dilatation of the main pulmonary artery, in the absence of valvular or peripheral pulmonic stenosis, under the age of 40 years
  • Calcification of the mitral anulus under the age of 40 years; or
  • Dilatation or dissection of the descending thoracic or abdominal aorta under the age of 50 years

For involvement of the cardiovascular system, only one of the minor criteria must be present:
PULMONARY SYSTEM

Major
  • None
Minor
  • Spontaneous pneumothorax
  • Apical blebs

For involvement of the pulmonary system, only one of the minor criteria must be present:
SKIN AND INTEGUMENT

Major
  • None
Minor
  • Striae atrophicae (stretch marks) not related to marked weight gain, pregnancy or repetitive stress
  • Recurrent or incisional herniae

For involvement of the skin and integument, only one of the minor criteria must be present:
DURA

Major
  • Lumbosacral dural ectasis by CT or MRI
Minor
  • None

FAMILY/GENETIC HISTORY

Major (one of the following constitute a major criteria):
  • First degree relative who independently meets the diagnostic criterion
  • Presence of mutation in FBN1,
  • Presence of a haplotype around FBN1 inherited by descent and unequivocally associated with diagnosed Marfan syndrome in the family
Minor
  • None

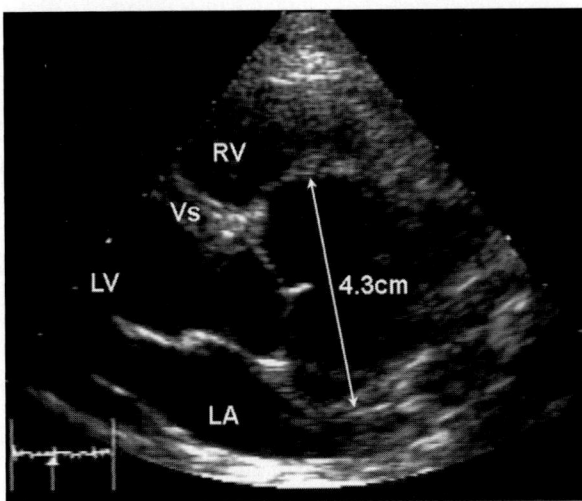

Fig. 1. Parasternal long-axis view of a transthoracic echocardiogram showing aortic root dilation in a patient with Marfan syndrome. LA, left atrium, LV, left ventricle, RV, right ventricle, VS, ventricular septum.

Marfan syndrome and is therefore routinely used in establishing the cardiovascular diagnosis and monitoring patients during follow-up.

The skeletal manifestations of Marfan syndrome require a thorough physical examination. Occasionally pelvic x-ray and lumbosacral MRI or CT may be helpful to document the presence of protrusio acetabula or dural ectasia respectively. However, the latter are only performed for symptoms or occasionally when these findings are required to fulfill the Ghent criteria for the diagnosis of Marfan syndrome. The most common skeletal manifestations can be easily assessed by a full skeletal examination that includes measurements of height, arm span to height ratio, upper to lower segment ratio, and hand and foot examinations, as well as evaluation for scoliosis, pectus deformity (Fig. 5), high arched palate, medial rotation of the medial malleolus causing pes planus (flat feet), joint hypermobility, reduced elbow extension, and arachnodactyly (Fig. 6).

Lens dislocation is the only ocular manifestation that is considered a major criterion and is present in 60% of patient with Marfan syndrome. This is best assessed with a slit-lamp examination with pupillary dilatation performed by an ophthalmologist. Lens dislocation usually occurs early in life but annual ophthalmologic evaluation is recommended due to the recognized risk of early severe myopia, retinal detachment, glaucoma, and cataract formation in Marfan patients. The other manifestations of Marfan syndrome are summarized in Table 1.

Young patients with suspected Marfan syndrome who do not meet the Ghent diagnostic criteria should have repeat evaluation in preschool, before puberty, and at age 18, because some of the clinical manifestations of

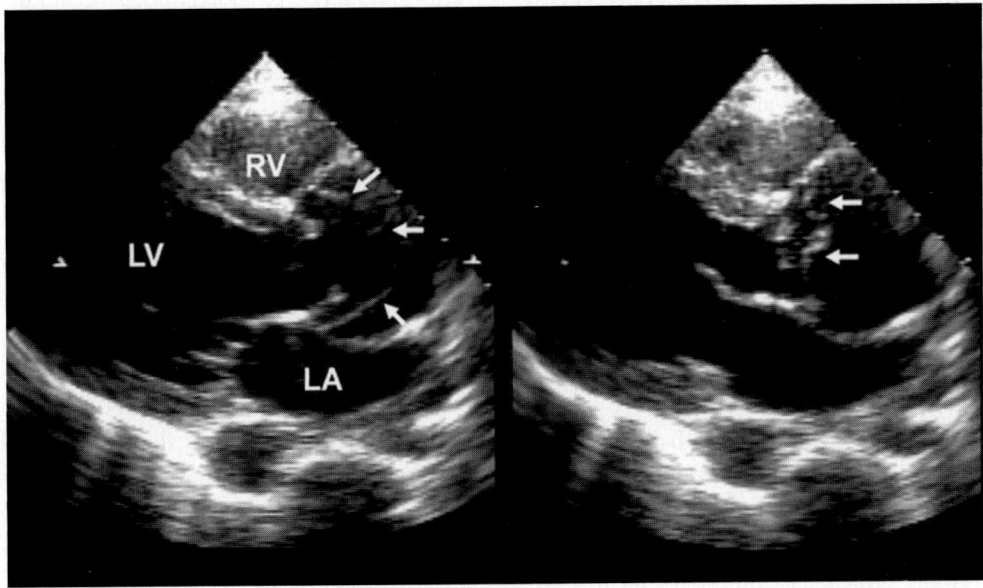

Fig. 2. Long-axis view of a transthoracic echocardiogram showing an ascending aortic dissection with the intimal flap noted in the aortic root (*arrows*). LA, left atrium; LV, left ventricle; RV, right ventricle.

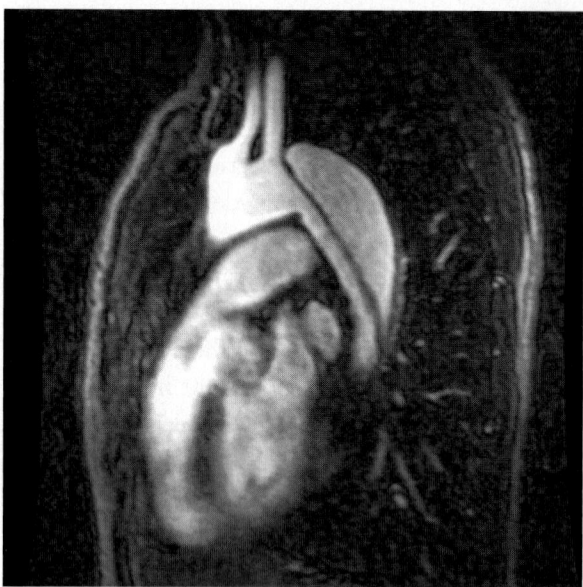

Fig. 3. Magnetic resonance imaging with gadolinium demonstrates a type B aortic dissection, distal to the left subclavian artery.

Marfan syndrome become more evident with age. Serial follow-up is recommended when the aorta is enlarged irrespective of diagnostic criteria.

The differential diagnosis of Marfan syndrome includes

1) *Homocystinuria* which shares several skeletal (tall stature, long bone overgrowth) and ocular features (ectopia lentis) of Marfan syndrome, in addition to mitral valve prolapse. However, by contrast to Marfan syndrome, these affected individuals often have mental retardation and are predisposed to thromboembolism. Homocystinuria is an autosomal recessive disease that is characterized by an elevated urinary homocysteine excretion and can be diagnosed by measuring total homocysteine

2) *MASS phenotype* with myopia, mitral valve prolapse, mild aortic enlargement, and nonspecific skin and skeletal features

3) *Ehlers-Danlos syndrome type IV* where skin laxity, scars, and easy bruising are prominent features in addition to marked joint hypermobility

4) *Stickler syndrome* where retinal detachment and not ectopia lentis is a common feature, in addition to cleft palate and hearing loss

5) *Congenital contractural arachnodactyly or Beals syndrome* is an autosomal-dominant disease manifested also by joint contractures, scoliosis, and crumpled ear malformation in addition to marfanoid appearance

6) *Familial thoracic aortic aneurysm or aortopathy.* These individuals do not show any other systemic manifestation of Marfan syndrome

7) *Congenital bicuspid aortic valve disease with associated aortopathy,* where the dilatation of the ascending aorta is often in its mid section rather then at the aortic root level

8) *Loeys-Dietz syndrome,* which includes unique features of hypertelorism and presence of a broad bifid uvula, in addition to vascular involvement characterized by arterial tortuosity and aneurysms with an increased risk of dissection throughout the arterial tree, often at small arterial sizes

MEDICAL MANAGEMENT

The management of patients with Marfan syndrome should involve a multidisciplinary approach and treatment should be tailored to individual manifestations since different patients have variable degrees of organ involvement. Early diagnosis and treatment are beneficial. Marfan patients of all ages should be encouraged to undergo at least annual evaluation with clinical history, examination, and echocardiogram. Genetic counseling should be provided initially to aid in the diagnosis and should also be provided to potential parents due to the recognized 50% chance of transmission from an affected parent to the child. Phenotypic variability, pregnancy counseling, and the availability of prenatal diagnostic testing should be discussed. Annual ophthalmologic examination, including screening and treatment for myopia, retinal detachment, glaucoma, and cataracts, is also recommended. Those with significant skeletal involvement are best managed by an orthopedic specialist.

The histologic abnormalities noted in the Marfan aorta reduce its distensibility and compliance; as a result, the aorta becomes stiffer and demonstrates excessive dilation with age. Since beta blockade can increase aortic distensibility and reduce aortic stiffness, in addition to lowering the heart rate and left ventricular ejection force, these medications have been the treatment of choice and should be considered in all patients with Marfan syndrome. A randomized trial of propranolol treatment in adolescents and young adults with Marfan syndrome has demonstrated a reduced rate of aortic dilatation and fewer aortic complications in the treatment group. A total of 70 patients with Marfan syndrome were treated with propranolol, mean dose to 112 milligrams a day. At an average follow-up of ten years, the mean slope of regression line for aortic root dimensions was significantly lower in the propranolol group compared to the control group. In another study involving 44 patients with Marfan syndrome followed up for almost four years, those who were taking a beta blocker or calcium channel blocker if intolerant to

beta blocker, showed a slower absolute aortic growth rate of 0.9 vs. 1.8 mm/year after adjustment for age and body size. In addition, prophylactic medical treatment may be most effective in those with an aortic diameter of less than 4.0 centimeters. Those who responded to beta blockade tended to have a smaller aortic diameter (less than 4.0 centimeters) suggesting that a reduction in the rate of aortic dilatation with beta blockade is greatest in young patients with a small aorta. Therefore, beta blockade should be considered in all patients with Marfan syndrome, including children, and those with aortic root diameter of less than 4 cm, unless contraindicated. The beta-blocker dose should be adjusted

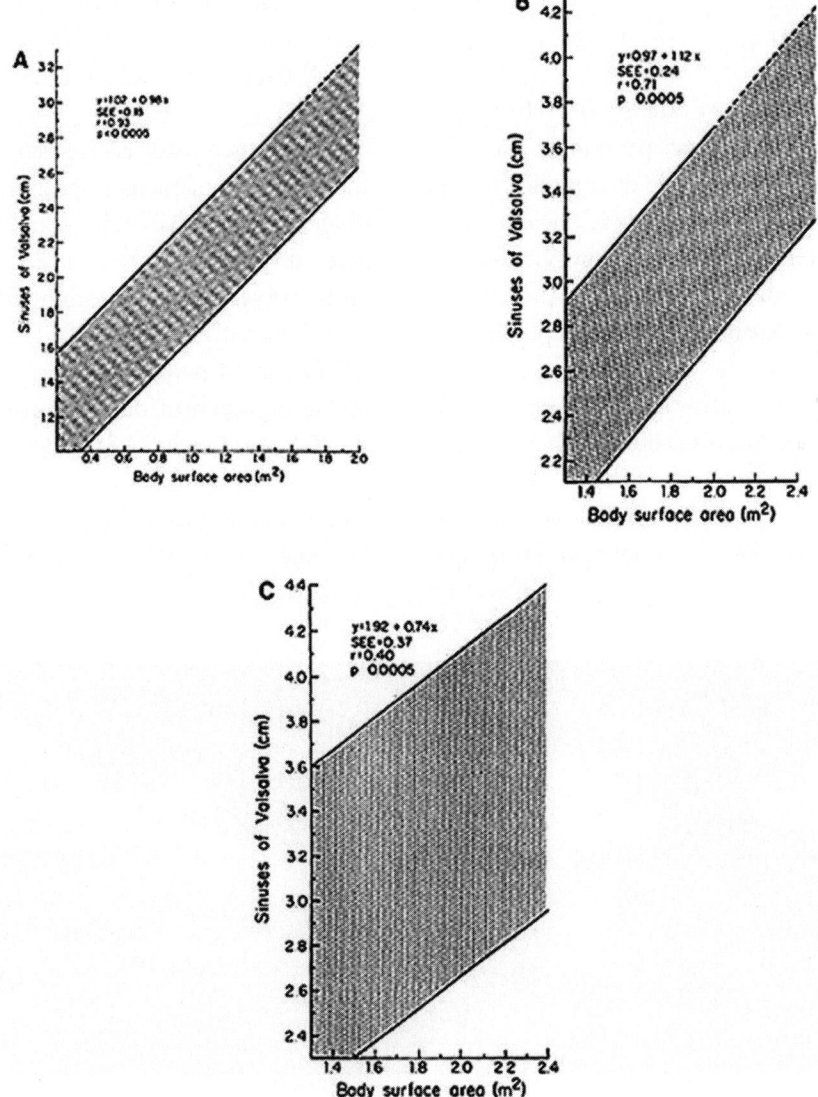

Fig. 4. Normal values of the aortic root diameter at the sinuses of Valsalva level measured by transthoracic echocardiogram in relation to age and body surface area as reported by Roman and Devereux.

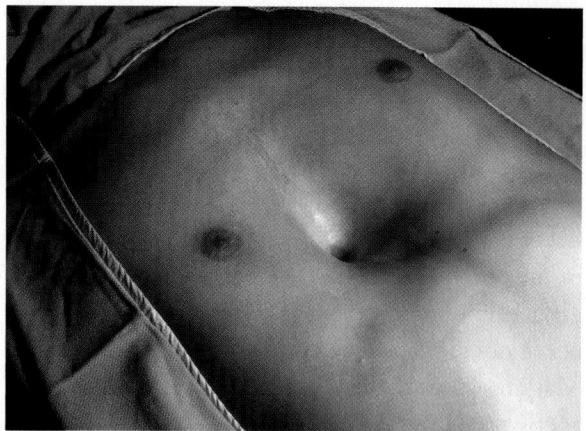

Fig. 5. Severe pectus excavatum in a patient with Marfan syndrome undergoing aortic root replacement.

to maintain a resting heart rate of 60-70 beats per minute or heart rate of 100 beats per minute after submaximal exercise. In patients who do not tolerate beta blockers, alternative treatments include calcium channel blocker, angiotensin-converting enzyme inhibitor, and angiotensin receptor blocker. In the presence of aortic or mitral regurgitation, endocarditis prophylaxis is recommended.

One of the major concerns in Marfan syndrome is the increased risk of aortic dissection which is inherent to the histologic abnormalities of the Marfan aorta. Patients with Marfan syndrome should be counseled to seek urgent medical evaluation for any acute chest pain,

back pain, or abdominal pain, syncope, or sudden change in vision.

Treatment with beta blockers, though beneficial in most Marfan patients, does not protect against aortic dissection. In one study, 20% of patients with Marfan syndrome treated with beta blockers or calcium channel blockers had major cardiovascular complications requiring surgery over a four-year period. The risk factors for aortic dissection in Marfan syndrome include

1) an aortic diameter of more than 5 centimeters,
2) aortic dilatation extending beyond the sinuses of Valsalva,
3) rapid rate of aortic dilatation (more than 5% per year or more than 2 millimeters per year in adults), and
4) family history of aortic dissection.

In adults, a yearly echocardiogram measurement of the aortic root diameter is recommended as long as the diameter is less than 4.5 cm and no major change in aortic dimension has been noted recently. Twice yearly aortic surveillance is recommended when the aortic root diameter is more than 4.5 cm. Alternatively, CT or MRI of the chest could be performed. These imaging techniques do provide a complete assessment of the thoracic aorta including the descending segment that might not be optimally visualized by echocardiography. These imaging modalities complement each other. Periodic CT or MR imaging of the descending tho-

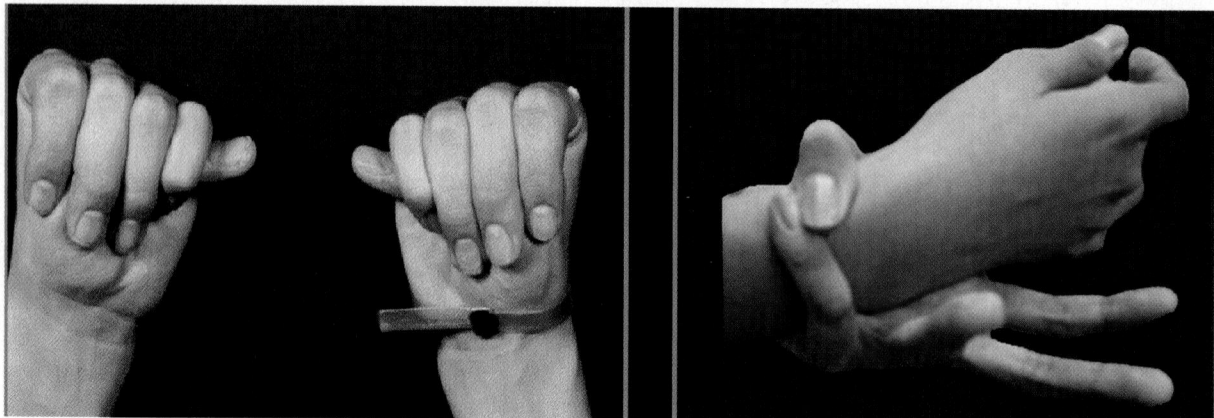

Fig. 6. Arachnodactyly demonstrated using the Steinberg thumb sign where the entire thumbnail projects beyond the ulnar border of the hand and the Walker-Murdoch wrist sign whereby the thumb and the fifth finger overlap around the wrist.

racic and abdominal aorta is recommended in all patients with Marfan syndrome, especially prior to aortic root replacement, due to the recognized risk of aneurysm formation in other parts of the aorta.

Patients should also be educated to avoid smoking and monitor their blood pressure since nicotine use and hypertension are also believed to increase the risk of dilatation of the aorta. The goal blood pressure per JNC-7 is less than 120/80 mm Hg.

Patients with Marfan syndrome should avoid isometric exercise, competitive and contact sports, or exercising to the point of exhaustion. As a general principle, participation in recreational exercise categorized as low to moderate intensity including golf, boating, skating, snorkeling, brisk walking, treadmill or stationary biking, hiking, or doubles tennis are appropriate for patients with Marfan syndrome unless they have had prior aortic root and/or valve replacement. Weight lifting, body building, and competitive sports such as ice hockey, full-court basketball, surfing, and scuba diving should be avoided. Impact sports may also cause ocular complications in patients with Marfan syndrome. For other activities thought to be of intermediate risk such as singles tennis, soccer, touch football, baseball, and skiing, individual assessment is suggested.

SURGICAL MANAGEMENT

There is general agreement based on a number of comparative studies that overall outcome is better in Marfan patients treated with early aortic root surgery, in addition to continuing beta blockade. Prophylactic surgery is recommended when the diameter of the aortic sinuses of Valsalva reaches 5.0 cm. Other factors such as family history of aortic dissection, severe aortic valve regurgitation with associated symptoms or progressive ventricular dilatation or dysfunction, the possibility of a valve-sparing operation, the contemplation of pregnancy, and the rate of aortic dilatation (aortic root growth >2 mm/yr), may indicate the need for surgery at a smaller aortic sinus dimension. It is suggested that the aortic root diameter be plotted serially against body surface area and operation be considered if the diameter begins to increase rapidly from a stable percentile even if the absolute measurement is less than 5.0 centimeters. An increase in aortic dimension of more than 1.0 centimeter per year is regarded as rapid progression in a child,

whereas in the adult an increase of ≥5% per year or an increase of more than 2 mm per year is considered significant, emphasizing the need for regular aortic root and valve surveillance. In the future, assessment of aortic distensibility by carotid artery ultrasound or other methods may become a useful prognostic indicator.

The severity of the aortic valve regurgitation, due to root dilatation, is a major determinant of the kind of surgical intervention offered when aortic root replacement is required. When significant aortic valve regurgitation or valve distortion is present, aortic valve replacement is indicated. The original operation developed for Marfan patients was the Bentall composite graft. This includes aortic root and valve replacement with either a biological or mechanical valve and requires coronary artery reimplantation. The composite aortic graft is a good choice for older children and adults associated with a low operative mortality, especially when done electively, and a 5-, 10-, and 20-year survival of 88, 81, and 75%, respectively.

In absence of important aortic valve regurgitation, a valve-sparing aortic root replacement can be considered. There are two kinds of operations: one is the Yacoub operation (described by Sir Magdi Yacoub) where the aortic conduit is attached to a cuff of a native aorta just beyond the aortic valve and conserving the valve (remodeling); the other was described by Dr. Tirone David. With this operation, the native aortic valve is reimplanted into the aortic graft, which is attached to the left ventricular outflow tract (reimplantation technique). Several modifications of this approach have been described. The mortality risk of the valve-sparing operations is low with a 5-yr survival rate of 96±3%. Mild or no aortic regurgitation may be present in up to 75% of patients as long as 10 years. The risk of requiring aortic valve replacement for severe aortic valve regurgitation is estimated to be 10% at ten years. Aortic valve-sparing operation is an indication for early surgery and therefore an aortic root diameter of <50 millimeters with preserved aortic valve function is an indication to consider surgical repair. In addition, the valve-sparing operation or the use of a biological prosthesis is recommended for a woman who wishes to become pregnant and for other patients with relative contraindication for long-term anticoagulation.

Mitral valve repair for severe mitral regurgitation with associated symptoms or progressive left ventricular dilatation or dysfunction carries a very low operative risk (<1%). In a study of 23 patients with Marfan syndrome having mitral valve repair, the 10-year survival rate was 79% and the 10-year rate of freedom from mitral regurgitation was 87%.

POSTOPERATIVE CARDIOVASCULAR CARE

Marfan patients require long-term medical treatment and lifelong surveillance, even after aortic root surgery, representing a major commitment for patient and doctor. Beta blockers should be resumed postoperatively and continued indefinitely unless contraindicated. Long-term aspirin and endocarditis prophylaxis are recommended in all patients. Long-term anticoagulation with warfarin is recommended for patients with mechanical prostheses or in presence of other indications such as atrial fibrillation. At least annual cardiovascular and ophthalmologic evaluation with a clinical history, examination, and transthoracic echocardiogram is recommended with periodic imaging of the descending thoracic and abdominal aorta. As Marfan patients age, reoperation is often needed if they develop vascular complications elsewhere in the arterial system, reemphasizing the importance of continuing beta-blocker therapy. Mitral valve replacement or repair may be required in up to 10% of those requiring aortic root surgeries. As a group, it is believed that more than 60% of patients with Marfan syndrome require multiple operations during their lifetime and therefore lifelong comprehensive multidisciplinary follow-up is recommended.

Periodic imaging of the entire aorta is recommended indefinitely following initial aortic repair and monitoring can be accomplished with MRI or CT angiography. The rate of change of the aortic diameter should influence follow-up intervals. Indications for replacement of an enlarged segment of the aorta should include

1) a rapid increase in aortic size of more than 5 to 10 millimeters per year,
2) a diameter of more than 50 to 55 millimeters,
3) affected segment diameter twofold greater than the adjacent segment, or
4) symptoms related to aortic dilatation.

An additional late complication of both composite and valve-sparing operation is the development of coronary ostial aneurysms. These aneurysms develop at the site of reimplantation as a result of the perioperative stretch of the weakened wall of the coronary ostium and are not likely to progress.

PREGNANCY IN MARFAN SYNDROME

Pregnancy in Marfan syndrome is possible. There are, however, two major issues that need to be discussed with the patient and family, including the risk of cardiovascular complications in the affected mother and the 50% risk of transmission of Marfan syndrome to the fetus. Due to the autosomal dominant nature of the disorder, each offspring of an affected Marfan parent has a 50% chance of inheriting the genetic mutation. Genetic counseling should be offered to all patients with Marfan syndrome. Mutation detection or linkage can be used for prenatal diagnosis if the parents wish.

The risk of aortic dissection in pregnancy is increased and may be caused by the inhibition of collagen and elastin deposition in the aorta by estrogen and the hyperdynamic hypervolemic circulatory state of pregnancy. Gestational hypertension and preeclampsia may also play a role. Previous reports of pregnancies involving patients with Marfan syndrome have demonstrated a complication rate of approximately 11% mostly related to aortic rupture and endocarditis. The overall risk of death during pregnancy is around 1%. The risk of aortic root complication is increased when the aortic root diameter is more than 4 centimeters at the start of pregnancy and the risk is further increased when the aorta is more than 4.5 cm or if it dilates rapidly during pregnancy. The risk of further dilatation of the aorta during pregnancy is lowest in the first trimester and greatest in the third trimester, as well as during labor and in the first few weeks post partum. In those who become pregnant, beta blocker therapy should be continued throughout pregnancy and patients should have serial follow-up echocardiograms to assess the change in the size of the aorta during pregnancy. Surgery should be considered during pregnancy in patients with progressive aortic dilation or before the aortic root diameter reaches 55 millimeters. A planned cesarean delivery is generally the preferred mode of delivery in patients with the Marfan syndrome and aortic dilatation. Assisted vaginal delivery can be considered when the aortic root diameter is less than 4 centimeters, the aorta has not demonstrated change during pregnancy, and there is no associated severe cardiovascular disease. Antibiotic prophylaxis administered around the time of delivery is appropriate for those patients with significant valvular regurgitation or prior root and valve replacement surgery. Postpartum uterine hemorrhage should be anticipated as a complication of Marfan syndrome and has been reported in nearly 40% of women.

PROGNOSIS

The life expectancy of untreated patients with Marfan syndrome is significantly reduced, with an early study reporting the lifespan to be about 32 years. However, with beta blocker therapy and elective surgical repair, the median cumulative probability of survival has increased gradually to 72 years.

Summary

A marked advance in the understanding of the cause of Marfan syndrome, as well as early recognition of the disorder and subsequent institution of medical and surgical therapy has resulted in dramatic improvement in the prognosis of this patient population over the past few decades. We anticipate that further medical advances, focused primarily on the genetic basis of Marfan syndrome, will allow continued therapeutic improvements with associated prognostic implications in years to come.

KEY POINTS OR PEARLS

1. Marfan syndrome is an autosomal dominant genetic disorder caused by a mutation of the fibrillin-1 gene

2. Marfan syndrome is a multisystem disorder involving the cardiovascular and skeletal systems as well as the eyes, lungs, skin, and dura

3. A comprehensive multidisciplinary approach involving cardiac, orthopedic, ophthalmologic, and genetic consultations is warranted in order to confirm or exclude the diagnosis

4. The cardiovascular manifestations of Marfan syndrome include dilatation of the ascending aorta with associated increased risk of aortic dissection, mitral valve prolapse, mitral anular calcification(age <40 yr), pulmonary artery dilatation, and dilatation or dissection of the descending thoracic aorta

5. Beta blockade should be considered in all patients with Marfan syndrome including children and those with aortic root diameter of less than 4 cm, unless contraindicated

6. The risk factors for aortic dissection in Marfan syndrome include aortic diameter of more than 5 centimeters, aortic dilatation extending beyond the sinuses of Valsalva, rapid rate of aortic dilatation (more than 5% per year or more than 2 millimeters per year in adults), and family history of aortic dissection.

7. Prophylactic surgery is recommended when the diameter of the aortic sinuses of Valsalva reaches 5.0 cm.

8. Patients with Marfan syndrome should also be educated to avoid smoking and monitor their blood pressure with a goal blood pressure less than 120/80 mm Hg.

9. Patients with Marfan syndrome should avoid isometric exercise, competitive and contact sports, or exercising to the point of exhaustion.

10. The risk of aortic root complication during pregnancy is increased when the aortic root diameter is more than 4 centimeters at the start of pregnancy.

SECTION VI

Coronary Artery Disease
Risk Factors

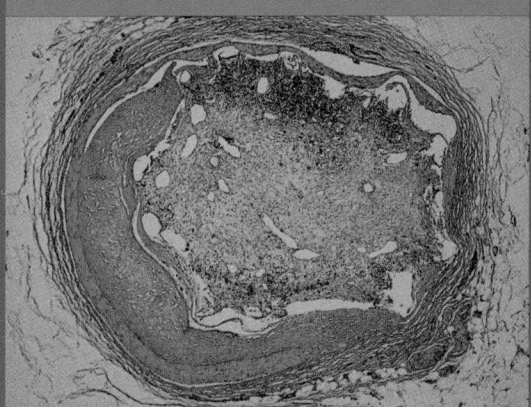

Thrombosed Coronary Stent

Coronary Heart Disease Epidemiology

Thomas G. Allison, PhD

Natural History and Pathophysiology

Coronary heart disease (CHD) develops as a consequence of decreased blood flow to the myocardium due to coronary atherosclerosis (CAD). CAD begins as fatty streaks in the coronaries and other arterial beds quite early in life, with fatty streaks and some raised lesions identified in various autopsy studies in men in their late teens and early 20s and women by late 20s and early 30s. The development of atherosclerosis appears to follow a complex pathway:

1. **Endothelial dysfunction** is caused by a number of factors such as cigarette smoking, hypertension, and hyperlipidemia. This permits entry of various blood components into the arterial intimal layer. These components ordinarily roll along the endothelial layer and do not damage the artery.

2. **Infiltration** of leukocytes, lipids (carried by LDL particles), and macrophages takes places as these blood cells accumulate within the intimal layer of the artery.

3. **Inflammation** occurs, and lipid-rich foam cells form as macrophages ingest LDL particles. These foam cells accumulate and grow into fatty streaks, which eventually bulge out into the arterial lumen. The disease may still be reversible at this stage if LDL cholesterol levels in the blood are decreased, HDL particles increased, and endothelial function restored.

4. **Proliferation** and migration of smooth muscle cells from the medial layer form a fibrous cap over the fatty lesion. *This is now a complex lesion that is not entirely reversible.* Proliferation of the vasovasorum provides the lesion with its own blood supply.

5. Continued **plaque progression** is characterized by growth and eventual necrosis of the lipid core, calcification, hemorrhage within the plaque, and surface erosion with formation of nonobstructive clots. The external elastic lamina may stretch to accommodate this plaque growth without the development of ischemia, but eventually the arterial lumen may narrow to the extent that ischemia may develop during periods of physical or psychological stress. This ischemia may be silent or cause angina.

6. Thinning and weakening of the fibrous cap due to the action of matrix metalloproteinases released from macrophages, coupled with the shear stress of blood flow over the luminal surface of the plaque may cause acute **plaque rupture**. Precipitating factors like nicotine use, excessive physical stress, and psychological stress also appear to play a role in rupture of atherosclerotic plaques. Plaques that are less than 70% obstructive appear to be more likely to undergo rupture, perhaps due to their higher lipid content, thinner fibrous cap, and more irregular configuration with the presence of distinct *shoulders* where shear forces concentrate.

Clinical manifestations of plaque rupture with subtotal or total occlusion of the affected artery, now called *acute coronary syndrome*, include acute myocardial infarction, unstable angina, and sudden death due to ventricular fibrillation. Other manifestations of coronary heart disease include stable or effort angina, which occurs when plaque growth leads to subtotal occlusion of the artery, and ischemic cardiomyopathy. Ischemic cardiomyopathy may be secondary to thinning and dilatation of the myocardium in the first few weeks following a large infarction, or it may develop more gradually as a result of repeated smaller myocardial infarctions and chronic ischemia. Congestive heart failure is a frequent problem in patients with ischemic cardiomyopathy. Heart failure is essentially an end-stage process characterized by exercise intolerance, pulmonary and/or peripheral edema, and high mortality.

Figures 1-6 trace the pathophysiology of coronary disease from fatty streaks to plaque rupture with total occlusion of the artery leading to acute myocardial infarction and sudden death.

PREVALENCE AND INCIDENCE OF CORONARY HEART DISEASE AND TRENDS

The American Heart Association provides an annual statistical report on coronary heart disease. Current data suggest that there are over 13.2 million prevalent cases of CHD in the US. The incidence of CHD death or myocardial infarction is about 1.2 million cases per year with 700,000 being first events and 500,000 being recurrent attacks. The number of cases

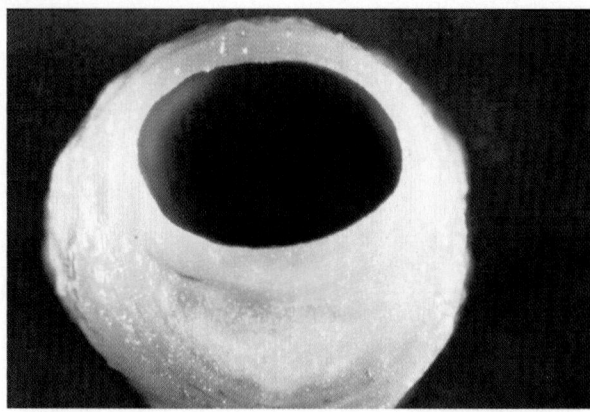

Fig. 2. Advanced lesion with large lipid core. Note lesion is nonocclusive due to remodeling of artery.

of sudden cardiac death is approximately 340,000 per year. Approximately 5 million persons in the US suffer from chronic heart failure. At age 40, an American man has a 49% lifetime risk of developing coronary heart disease versus a 32% risk for a woman at age 40. CHD rates in African Americans are higher than for white Americans, whereas rates for Asian Americans are lower. From an international perspective, coronary heart disease rates in the US are intermediate between the low rates in eastern Asia (1/3 to 1/5 of US rate) and the very high rates in the former socialist countries of Eastern Europe (2-3 times US rate).

Age-adjusted coronary heart disease rates in the US fell by 42% between 1970 and 2000. Rates for whites declined, with the rate of decline greater for

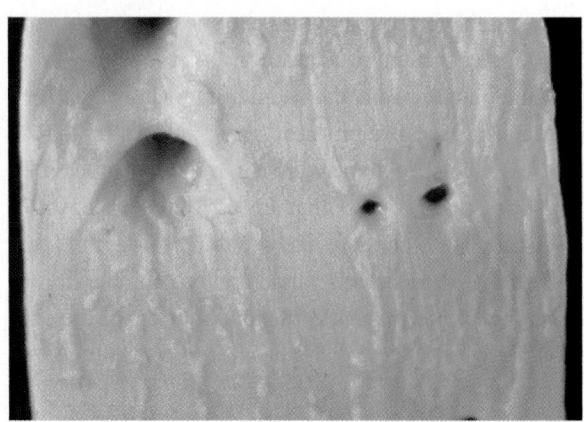

Fig. 1. Fatty streaks in the aorta of a 19-year-old male.

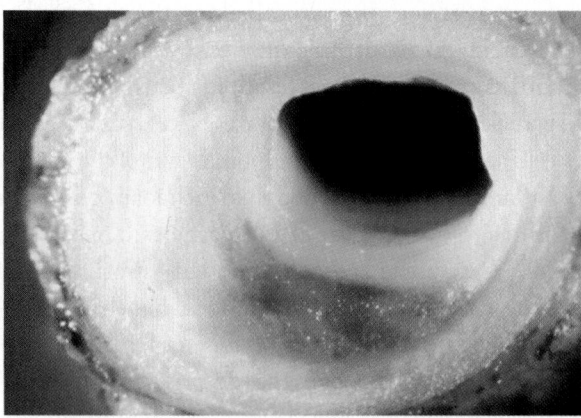

Fig. 3. Advanced lesion with plaque hemorrhage. This lesion is causing relatively severe narrowing of the lumen and may possibly be causing ischemia and effort angina.

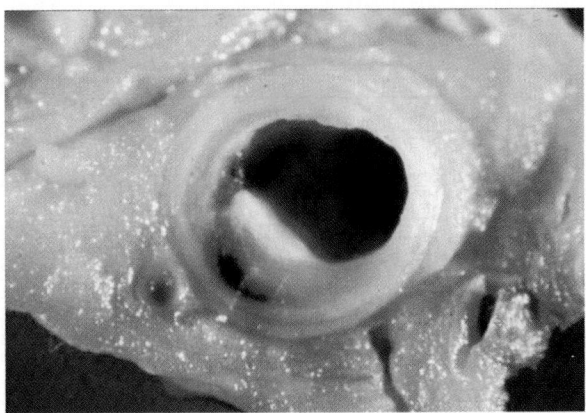

Fig. 4. Intermediate lesion with incorporated thrombus. This appears to be due to plaque erosion rather than frank plaque rupture and may potentially be an asymptomatic event.

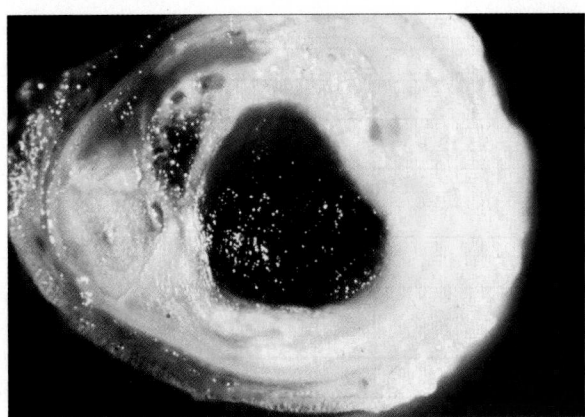

Fig. 6. Advanced lesion occluded with thrombus. This is the end stage of the atherosclerotic process for this patient.

men than women, while rates for African Americans or Mexican Americans actually increased. In the first 15 years of the period 1970-2000, it has been determined that behavior changes—particularly the millions of American men who discontinued cigarette smoking—accounted for most of the decrease in CHD rates, whereas as changes in medical practice (programs teaching cardiopulmonary resuscitation, 911 emergency coverage, coronary care units and defibrillators, emergent coronary angioplasty, and improved medical therapy) accounted for the greatest part of the decrease

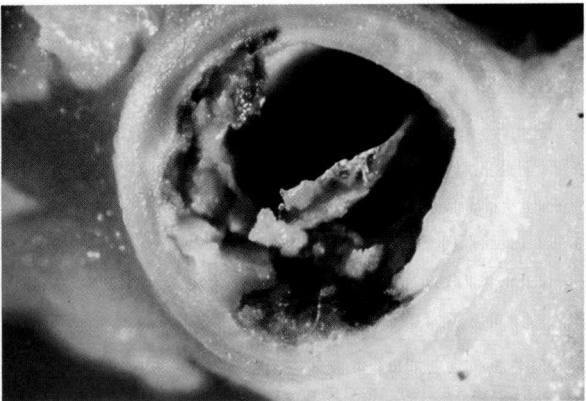

Fig. 5. Plaque rupture with torn fibrous cap. Exposure of collagen to platelets causes increased platelet adhesiveness and aggregation and will likely serve as a platform for thrombus formation in the affected artery. This was likely a symptomatic event.

between 1985 and 2000. Despite the decline in age-adjusted rates, the number of actual cases of CHD have remained stable in men and increased slightly in women over the past 30 years due principally to the aging of the population. Studies from Olmsted County, Minnesota, confirm this shift in the CHD epidemic from middle-aged men towards women and the elderly. Internationally, the coronary heart disease epidemic is gradually moving from countries with established market economies into the developing world (Fig. 7 and 8).

Many epidemiologists are concerned that the decline in CHD rates in the US has already reached or will soon reach a low plateau and then begin to increase again. Cited reasons for the end of the decline and the subsequent resurgence of the CHD epidemic include the failure of smoking rates to decline further below the 22% to 25% level at which they have been stuck for several years and the dramatic increases in obesity, metabolic syndrome, and type 2 diabetes.

RISK FACTORS

Risk factors for CHD were first identified in the Framingham Heart Study which began in 1948 and have been confirmed in numerous subsequent investigations. While the pathophysiology of coronary artery disease, as described above, suggest that it is primarily a lipid disorder, other risk factors play important roles. Risk factors that have long been recognized include

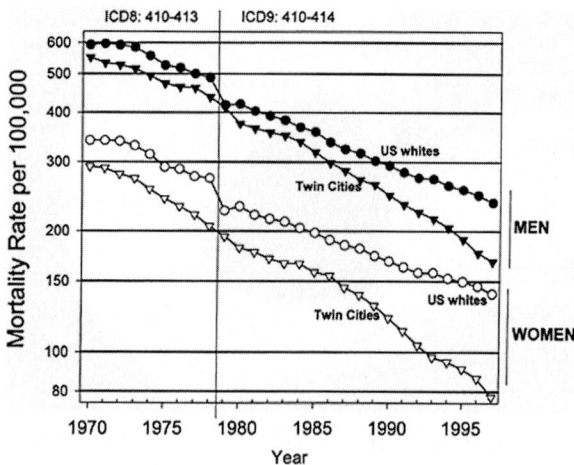

Fig. 7. CHD trends in US and Twin Cities, 1970 to 1997.

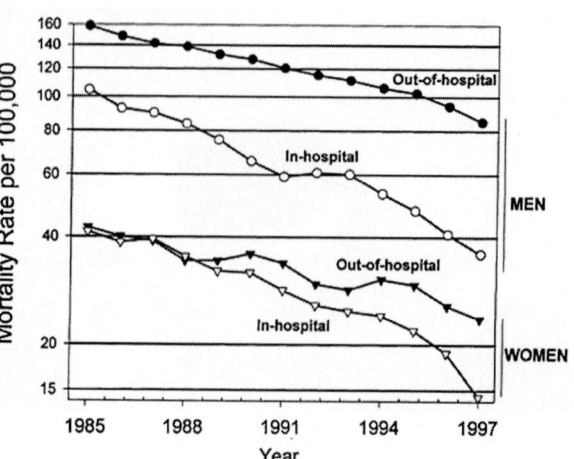

Fig. 8. Comparison of in-hospital and out-of-hospital CHD death trends. The greater rate of decline for in-hospital CHD death suggests that medical care improvements are predominantly responsible for the reduction in CHD death rates after 1985.

non-modifiable factors such as age, male sex, and family history of premature CHD (age of onset <55 years for primary male relative and <65 years for primary female relative). So-called *major* modifiable risk factors include elevated LDL cholesterol, low HDL cholesterol, hypertension, and diabetes. Obesity, lack of regular exercise, and psychological stress are also been recognized as CHD risk factors, but these are frequently termed *minor* risk factors. Reasons for relegating these risk factors to less important status may include weaker or less consistent association with CHD incidence or prevalence in epidemiologic studies, difficulty in accurately defining the level of the factor, and lack of successful interventions by the medical community.

The impact of a risk factor is related to both the strength of its association with CHD, often described in terms of relative risk (RR), and by its prevalence in the population. Table 1 summarizes these aspects of various CHD risk factors applied to the US population.

Though lack of regular exercise has a lower relative risk than the *major* risk factors listed above it, its high prevalence suggests that increasing physical activity levels in the US could have a greater impact than more aggressive treatment of lipid and blood pressure. Indeed, biobehavioral variables—physical activity, diet, and cigarette smoking—appear to predict >75% of CHD deaths worldwide according to multinational INTERHEART study.

The 4 major risk factors for CHD—hyperlipidemia (including both low HDL cholesterol and high LDL cholesterol), hypertension, diabetes, and cigarette smoking—have been shown to consistently and strongly predict CHD incidence and prevalence in a very large number of observational studies, both cross-sectional and longitudinal. Randomized clinical trials to reduce LDL cholesterol and blood pressure have demonstrated conclusively that lowering the level of these risk factors reduces CHD risk. Data for the effect of blood sugar control on CHD risk in diabetes are less extensive to date, and randomized clinical trials of smoking cessation and CHD risk have not nor will likely ever be conducted, but incontrovertible evidence for these latter two risk factors has been established from numerous observational studies.

Optimal levels for each of these CHD risk factors continues to be redefined by new epidemiologic studies and, more importantly, the results of large randomized clinical trials, such as the recent Heart Protection Study of lipid reduction and the ALLHAT study of blood pressure control. For all of the major modifiable risk factors, risk is either linearly or exponentially related to the level of the risk factor (as seen below in Figure 9 for serum cholesterol), but target levels below which risk is acceptable have been developed. For prevention of

CHD, the National Cholesterol Education Program has determined that an LDL cholesterol of less than 100 mg/dL is optimal for CHD prevention, and levels of 70 mg/dL or less are now recommended for individuals with existing CHD plus other risk factors. Ideal blood pressure is now set at 120/80 mm Hg or less by the Joint National Commission on Blood Pressure Awareness and Control. According to the American Heart Association and numerous other groups, smoking and exposure to second hand smoke should be avoided completely. A normal blood sugar is now defined as ≤100 mg/dL by the American Diabetic Association, and the threshold blood sugar used to diagnose diabetes has dropped to 126 mg/dL. For good cardiovascular health, moderately vigorous physical activity should be performed for at least 30 minutes 5 or more days per week, according to the Surgeon General of the US and a number of professional medical groups and agencies. Prevention of obesity is now a national priority, and the nation has been advised to maintain weight within 10% of ideal, generally defined terms of a BMI of 18.5 to 25 kg/m^2.

A meta-analysis of several large epidemiological trials—more than 350,000 patients followed for 21 to 39 years with nearly 40,000 CHD deaths recorded—has shown that fewer than 1 in 10 American adults have an optimal risk profile (i.e., free of any of the major risk factors with LDL cholesterol <130 mg/dL, HDL cholesterol ≥45 mg/dL for men or ≥55 mg/dL

for women, blood pressure ≤120/80 mm Hg, nonsmoker, and no diabetes). However, these ideal individuals have a CHD risk less than 1/5 of all others (with at least 1 risk factor) combined and account for less than 2% of all CHD deaths.

Outcome data from the Framingham Heart Study are used in various equations to predict risk from CHD for a given individual based on the major risk factors listed above (plus age and gender). In turn, targets for LDL cholesterol and, to some extent, blood pressure are indexed to the Framingham Risk Score. A 10-year risk level above 20% is considered high risk, 10-19% intermediate risk, and <10% low risk. Because of the strong relationship of CHD risk to age, however, a Framingham risk score of 12%, for example, is of much greater concern in a 35-year-old than a 65-year-old man. Framingham conveniently provides low and average risk scores for each sex by 5-year age group, so a given individual's risk score can be indexed against those norms.

CHD Epidemiology in Men Versus Women

The age-adjusted risk of CHD in women is approximately 1/3 that for men. Above 75 years of age, the rates of CHD for women eventually catch up to rates for men, but younger men are at significantly greater risk compared to women. Cited reasons for this include a lower-risk lifestyle for women (less smoking, lower fat diet, for example), higher HDL cholesterol levels (mostly secondary to lower testosterone levels), and possible protective effects of endogenous estrogens. Diagnosing CHD in women is somewhat more difficult, however, in that their presentation is more varied both in terms of symptoms and electrocardiographic abnormalities. Once correctly diagnosed, however, women now seem to be receiving appropriate care, at least during the acute hospitalization. Current data suggest that the *gender gap* in appropriate treatment of CHD between men and women has largely or completely disappeared in recent years. Long-term control of CHD risk factors in women may continue to lag behind men, however.

Mortality after myocardial infarction is higher in women versus men, though most of that is due to older age at presentation and more age-associated comor-

Table 1.   CHD Risk Factors

Risk factor	Relative risk	Estimated US prevalence
Hyperlipidemia	2.5	25%
Cigarette smoking	3.0*	23%
Hypertension	2.4	20%
Diabetes	3.0†	7%
Lack of exercise	1.9	59%

*Relative risk higher in men (4.0) versus women (2.0), likely related to number of cigarettes smoked.
†Relative risk higher in women (4.0) versus men (2.0).

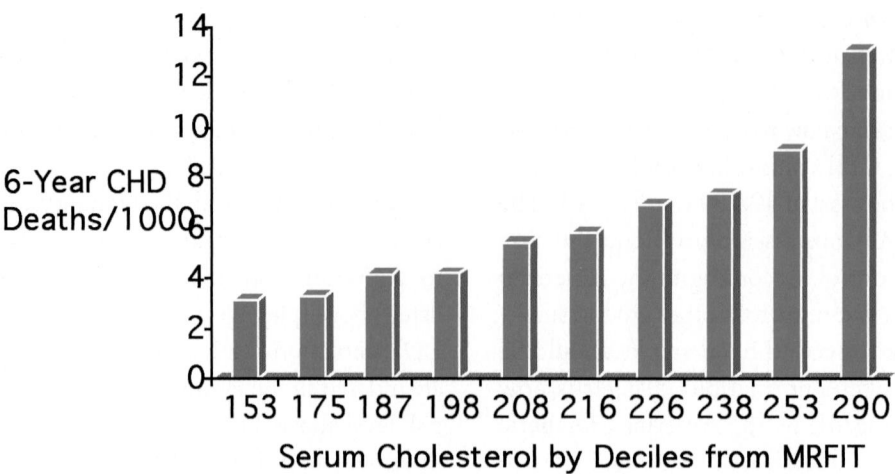

Fig. 9. Relationship of serum cholesterol in mg/dL to 6-year CHD death rate from Multiple Risk Factor Intervention Study.

bidities. Women appear to be more susceptible to development of heart failure than men, however, even after controlling for left ventricular function. Angina, on the other hand, has a more favorable prognosis in women compared to men. Finally, women may not have as favorable an outcome after mechanical interventions for CAD, including angioplasty, stenting, and coronary artery bypass surgery, due to the smaller absolute size of their coronary arteries and a tendency towards more diffuse CAD.

A NEW EPIDEMIOLOGY OF CORONARY HEART DISEASE?

While CHD death in individuals with none of the major risk factors is rare, as discussed above, it is clear that the traditional Framingham risk factors do not fully explain the distribution of CHD in the US population. In the large meta-analysis of >350,000 patients mentioned above, more than 90% of patients dying from CHD in the 21- to 29-year follow-up had at least 1 major modifiable risk factor—but so did nearly 70% of those who did not die from CHD over the same period. As a result of our improved understanding of the biology of atherosclerotic vascular disease, we have developed a number of new markers of CHD risk. Some of these, like lipoprotein (a), appear to be causally related to the development of CAD, though perhaps through mechanisms that are dependent and

synergistic with LDL cholesterol, while others, like C-reactive protein, may more mark the biological steps—in this case inflammation—in the atherosclerotic process than directly causing it. Still other *novel risk factors* serve as anatomical evidence for atherosclerosis presence. Coronary calcium measured by CT and carotid intimal-medial thickness measured by ultrasound represent two such noninvasive markers for atherosclerosis that are now being used clinically to predict CHD risk and identify goals for LDL cholesterol. While it is unlikely that laboratory tests for blood lipids and glucose, measurement of blood pressure, and ascertainment of smoking status and physical activity levels will disappear from CHD risk prediction strategies, the emergence of new markers for CHD risk and/or atherosclerosis presence will likely continue to make inroads into clinical practice and hopefully improve early disease detection and risk prediction, allowing for cost-effective targeting of CHD risk reduction strategies. On the other hand, public health efforts to promote behavioral changes—diet, physical activity, smoking—will always have the greatest potential, if successful, to lower the incidence and prevalence of CHD.

RESOURCES

Behavioral risk factor surveillance system home page. Available from: http://apps.nccd.cdc.gov/brfss/page.asp?cat=EX&yr=1999&state=US#EX.

Department of Health and Human Services, National Institutes of Health. National Heart, Lung, and Blood Institute home page: Available from: http://www.nhlbi.nih.gov/index.htm.

National Heart, Lung, and Blood Institute, National Institutes of Health National Cholesterol Education Program. Available from: http://www.nhlbi.nih.gov/ guidelines/cholesterol/index.htm.

Thom T, Haase N, Rosamond W, et al, American Heart Association Statistics Committee and Stroke Statistics Subcommittee. American Heart Association statistical update: heart disease and stroke statistics—2006 update. January 1, 2006. Available from: http://circ.ahajournals.org/cgi/content/short/113/6/e85.

56

METABOLIC SYNDROME

Thomas G. Allison, PhD

Metabolic syndrome is a novel cardiovascular risk factor that has generated widespread interest—and not a little controversy—since its inclusion in the National Cholesterol Education Program's (NCEP) Adult Treatment Panel III (ATP-III) published in June of 2001. The NCEP lists 5 characteristics for consideration of metabolic syndrome, as shown below. Patients exhibiting at least 3 of these 5 characteristics are said to have metabolic syndrome.

- Waist >40 inches for men or >35 inches for women
- Triglycerides ≥150 mg/dL
- HDL cholesterol <40 mg/dL for men or <50 mg/dL for women
- Blood pressure >130/85 mm Hg
- Fasting blood glucose ≥110 mg/dL

Though metabolic syndrome is dichotomized into absent or present at 3 characteristics, some large studies, such as the West of Scotland primary prevention lipid-lowering trial, have demonstrated that cardiovascular risk increases progressively with each successive characteristic present. Individuals with 4-5 characteristics are at approximately 3 times the cardiovascular risk of those with none. Studies from the US and Finland have identified similar relative risks for cardiovascular events in those with metabolic syndrome.

Alternative definitions of metabolic syndrome have been proposed, most notably by the World Health Organization (WHO). While the NCEP definition could be largely considered a system of counting non-Framingham or "near" risk factors, including impaired fasting glucose, that cluster in overweight and obese individuals, the WHO definition strictly requires diabetes, impaired fasting glucose, glucose intolerance, or demonstration of insulin resistance by the clamp methods—plus 2 or more of 4 additional abnormalities. Though perhaps less mechanistic or physiologically consistent than the WHO definition, the NCEP strategy for identifying metabolic syndrome has the advantage of being somewhat easier to employ clinically, and evidence to date suggests that both definitions are roughly equivalent for predicting future cardiovascular risk. Therefore, this chapter will assume the NCEP definition as metabolic syndrome is discussed further.

There have been well-publicized criticisms of the NCEP definition of the metabolic syndrome, including the abovementioned fact that risk is continuous as the number of characteristics increase rather than dichotomous at 3 characteristics. Concerns have also been raised about vagueness in the definition itself. For example, does blood pressure still count if it is being pharmacologically treated to below 130/85 mm Hg? The cut-points of 40 and 35 inches for waist circumference for men and women may not be fairly applied to extremely short or extremely tall individuals (much as the relationship of body fat percent to body mass index—BMI—is somewhat skewed at the extremes of height), and in fact different criteria for waist circumference have been introduced for Asian populations. Critics also question whether metabolic syndrome adds to the estimate of cardiovascular risk after the effects of individual factors, such as low HDL cholesterol, have been taken into account. Conversely, it has been questioned whether metabolic syndrome is just a more technical way of measuring the impact of obesity on the risk of cardiovascular disease. But in women at least, obesity without metabolic syndrome has been shown to be relatively benign compared to the elevated risk seen in obese women with metabolic syndrome.

The question has also been raised as to whether C-reactive protein, another of the novel risk factors, might explain the excess cardiovascular risk associated with metabolic syndrome. C-reactive protein has been shown to be correlated with all of the metabolic syndrome characteristics. Analysis of the West of Scotland data does show, however, that metabolic syndrome and C-reactive protein each predict cardiovascular risk independently and that the excess cardiovascular risk in subjects with both metabolic syndrome and elevated C-reactive protein was twice that conveyed by either of these two risk factors alone. In other words, C-reactive protein and metabolic syndrome are additive as far as cardiovascular risk is concerned.

Epidemiologic investigations have shown that metabolic syndrome is widely prevalent in the developed countries, especially the US National Health and Nutrition Evaluation Survey (NHANES) data from 1988-1994 suggest a prevalence of 26%, similar to that reported in the West of Scotland study whose subjects were recruited during a similar time frame. Current estimates of metabolic syndrome prevalence in the US range as high as 35%. The increase in metabolic syndrome is thought to be directly related to the increasing prevalence of obesity. While metabolic syndrome prevalence increases with age, the fact that many adolescents in the US may now have metabolic syndrome is generally more concerning to public health officials than its high prevalence in older individuals.

Metabolic syndrome can be readily identified using NCEP criteria by nonphysician health profes-

sionals. Nurses or other allied health personnel working in the clinic setting can be readily trained to measure waist circumference while weight and blood pressure are being checked and recorded, and HDL cholesterol, triglycerides, and fasting blood glucose can be extracted from laboratory record. These data, along with a count of metabolic syndrome characteristics, should be made available to the physician as he or she begins to take a history and examine the patient.

ATP-III includes metabolic syndrome as one of several risk modifiers that can be used to lower LDL cholesterol treatment targets in appropriate patients. The strategy suggested in that document for treating metabolic syndrome itself is to encourage lifestyle modifications—diet, exercise, and weight loss—and then consider focused treatment of those risk factors still not controlled by the lifestyle changes. Use of strategies generally recognized to lower overall cardiovascular risk—including LDL lowering with statin drugs, low-dose aspirin, and fish oil—may be considered depending on the age and estimated cardiovascular risk of individual patients. It is important to recognize that no completed trial to date has specified metabolic syndrome as an entry criterion, but retrospective analyses of some lipid-lowering trials such as 4S (Scandinavian Simvastatin Survival Study) have shown that risk is reduced by statin therapy in the subset of patients with metabolic syndrome—to an equal or slightly greater extent compared to those without metabolic syndrome.

Weight loss registries have shown that individuals who successfully lose more than 10% of body weight and maintain the majority of the lost weight long-term generally exhibit three characteristics:

1) they have developed multiple behavioral strategies for controlling caloric intake;
2) they average more than 60 minutes of physical activity per day; and
3) they weigh themselves regularly.

Patients with metabolic syndrome should be instructed in these principles and advised to make gradual and hopefully permanent modifications in their lifestyles rather than resort to "crash" programs of high-intensity exercise or fad diets. Reducing the intake of both simple carbohydrates and saturated fats has been shown to promote weight loss. Targeting carbohydrate reduction may produce greater weight loss in the short term (first 6 months), but the limited studies that are available suggest that this short-term advantage is largely lost by 1 year. Further, many health professionals—and agencies such as the American Heart Association, have raised concern about the long-term health consequences of high-fat diets (fats being what replaces carbohydrate in some of the low-carbohydrate diet plans). The degree of caloric reduction and the ability to maintain the dietary changes long-term, along with high levels of physical activity, appear to be key factors in sustaining weight loss. Social support and structure provided by various resources, including commercial programs such as Weight Watchers, has also been shown to be useful for long-term maintenance of weight loss. Behavioral strategies, including stress management, should be made available when possible.

Current guidelines from groups such as the American College of Sports Medicine have adopted the concept of 60 minutes or more of daily physical activity of at least moderate intensity (such as brisk walking) for weight loss, going beyond the 30 minutes per day recommended for general cardiovascular health. Patients may be counseled to develop a structured exercise program or use strategies to increase overall daily physical activity. Wearing a digital pedometer is a convenient way of tracking overall physical activity that has been shown to improve compliance with physical activity recommendations and increase weight loss.

Many physicians lack adequate training in nutrition and dietetics or exercise science to actively prescribe dietary therapy, exercise programs, and behavioral weight loss strategies to patients in their office or hospital practice. Even if well-qualified, physicians generally are unable to devote adequate time to patient education and counseling on these topics in the current practice environment. However, the physician can and should promote lifestyle change in the following manner:

1) explain metabolic syndrome and its associated cardiovascular risk to affected patients;
2) underscore the importance of lifestyle modification for treating metabolic syndrome (having presumably identified those who have it);
3) outline general strategies and help patients set realistic weight loss goals;
4) provide materials such as pamphlets, lists of useful books and Web sites, and information on services that might be available through local hospitals and health clubs, along with reputable commercial weight loss programs and psychologists or counselors that might have special interest and expertise in weight loss; and
5) arrange to see patients back at appropriate intervals to recheck labs and weight and to give positive reinforcement as appropriate.

Large group or hospital-based practices may even consider it worthwhile to employ a dietitian or exercise specialist to provide such advice and see patients back at appropriate intervals to review progress. Numerous studies on behavioral change have identified feedback and frequent follow-up as factors that enhance adherence to recommended lifestyle changes and, ultimately, with outcomes such as weight loss, improved cardiovascular fitness, or reduced blood pressure, blood sugar, or lipid levels.

In the absence of satisfactory results of lifestyle modification for weight control, bariatric surgery has been proven effective at resolving over 95% of metabolic syndrome cases. However, at present only the severely obese with BMI >40 or medically complicated obese patients with BMI >35 are generally considered for this procedure. Studies on the effect of waist liposuction on metabolic syndrome characteristics are quite limited and show conflicting results. Weight loss drugs that are currently available, such as Orlistat, have been shown to have some limited benefit in improving metabolic syndrome characteristics, though contemporary pharmacologic strategies for weight loss lag far behind lipid management or blood pressure control drugs in terms of both efficacy and tolerability.

Pharmacologic control of metabolic syndrome lipid parameters (low HDL cholesterol and high triglycerides) is possible using drugs such as niacin or fibrates (or high-dose fish oil in the case of high triglycerides), though data on risk reduction with these agents, particularly in individuals without documented cardiovascular disease, are very limited. In the primary prevention Helsinki Heart Study, gemfibrozil did not reduce mortality or cardiovascular events in the cohort as a whole, though the subgroup with low HDL and high triglycerides (i.e., those most likely to be metabolic syndrome patients) did experience a reduction in nonfatal cardiovascular events. In the VA-HIT (Veterans Affairs High Density Cholesterol Lipoprotein Intervention Trial) secondary prevention trial which contained 25% diabetics and another 25% with impaired fasting glucose, gemfibrozil reduced cardiovascular events and strokes, though no overall mortality benefit was seen. Similar results were reported in the FIELD (Fenofibrate Intervention and Event Lowering in Diabetes) trial, a study of fenofibrate therapy in type 2 diabetics. Large studies using niacin specifically for treatment of low HDL and high triglycerides have not been performed. The NCEP does provide specific guidelines for treatment of non-HDL cholesterol, which incorporates both HDL and triglyceride abnormalities, but recommends control of LDL cholesterol as the primary focus of lipid-lowering therapy, but does not specifically favor one particular lipid-lowering drug over another for treatment of non-HDL cholesterol.

Treatment of impaired fasting glucose or pre-hypertensive blood pressure with drugs is also controversial and generally not included in current guidelines. Unlike lipid treatment, patients may become symptomatic if blood pressure or blood sugar drops below normal levels, so treating borderline levels of these characteristics pharmacologically may result in discomfort to some patients. Drugs such as metformin and the thiazolidine-diones have been shown to delay or prevent conversion of impaired fasting glucose to diabetes, though intensive behavioral programs involving exercise and dietary changes have generally been shown to be more effective.

The Joint National Commission's latest report (JNC-7) continues to utilize a systolic blood pressure of >140 or diastolic blood pressure of >90 mm Hg as an indication to start pharmacologic therapy. Various guidelines advocate lower goals for blood pressure in diabetics and patients with cardiovascular disease. However, there have been no studies addressing the benefits of treating prehypertensive blood pressure in

metabolic syndrome patients. While diuretics and beta blockers represent 2 of the 5 classes of drugs listed by JNC-7 as appropriate first-line therapy for stage I hypertension, some concerns arise over use of these 2 drug classes as initial therapy for metabolic syndrome patients. Specifically, both classes may raise blood sugar and triglyceride levels.

To summarize, metabolic syndrome as defined by the NCEP is highly prevalent in the US and other developed market economies and conveys at least moderate cardiovascular risk. Metabolic syndrome can be easily diagnosed using common laboratory measures and the usual vital signs with the addition of a measurement of waist circumference. The proposed strategy for treating metabolic syndrome is to promote lifestyle change (diet and exercise) and resultant weight loss and then to consider individual treatment of specific characteristics not controlled by lifestyle change. If the overall cardiovascular risk is relatively high—due to age, family history of cardiovascular disease, and smoking, for example—then consideration of general cardiovascular risk reduction with a statin, low-dose aspirin, and fish oil may be appropriate. Studies specifically evaluating various treatments strategies for metabolic syndrome are in progress, but to date there are no completed studies with published results.

RESOURCES

American Heart Association resources on metabolic syndrome [database on the Internet]. Available from: http://www.americanheart.org/presenter.jhtml?identifier=3020263.

Kahn R, Buse J, Ferrannini E, et al, American Diabetes Association: European Association for the Study of Diabetes. The metabolic syndrome: time for a critical appraisal: joint statement from the American Diabetes Association and the European Association for the Study of Diabetes. Diabetes Care. 2005;28:2289-304.

National Cholesterol Education Program [database on the Internet]. Available from: http://www.nhlbi.nih.gov/about/ncep/.

57

PATHOGENESIS OF ATHEROSCLEROSIS

Joseph L. Blackshear, MD

Birgit Kantor, MD, PhD

ARTERIAL ANATOMY, PHYSIOLOGY, AND PATHOLOGY

Cross-section histological examination of arteries reveals 3 concentric regions: the intima, media, and adventitia (Fig. 1 *A*). The boundaries of the intima from the luminal to abluminal sides include the endothelium, a surface monocellular layer with extraordinary biochemical properties, a basement membrane, and the final layer before the media, the internal elastic lamina. The intima is normally extremely thin with endothelial cells in alignment with the direction of flow, except in areas of flow disturbance, such as bifurcations or branches. Normal endothelium is an organ system intimately involved in local vascular regulation. Nitric oxide is produced by endothelial cells and is antithrombogenic, antiproliferative, and vasodilating. Normal endothelial cells also have synthetic capability for endothelin, which is a powerful vasoconstrictor and is promitogenic, and for the vasodilator prostacyclin. Numerous surface receptors are present, including low density lipoprotein receptors.

In addition to the endothelial lining, normal intima may include regions of "cushions" of smooth muscle cells more than one or two layers thick. Cushions tend to occur at sites predisposed to atherosclerosis, including branches, bifurcations, and in the proximal segment of the left anterior descending coronary artery. These appear in infancy and are referred to as *adaptive eccentric intimal thickening* (Fig. 2).

Atherosclerosis is a disease primarily involving pathologic changes in the intima, with reactive changes in media and adventitia. The media is heterogeneous, being thin in conductance vessels such as the aorta and muscular in the coronary arteries. Laminations of smooth muscle cells bounded by elastic membranes form the media, and interstitial spaces, also rich in elastin, are prominent. The abluminal boundary dividing media from adventitia is the external elastic lamina. The arterial wall is normally nourished on the intimal side by oxygen diffusing through the endothelium into the subintima. In large species and in vessels with a wall larger than 250 μm, diffusion of oxygen is insufficient to supply the media and adventitia; to this end vasa vasorum course into the adventitia. Segmental heterogeneity is again present, with variable quantities of networks of nutrient vasa vasorum, lymphatics, and nerves. Aside from vascular, lymphatic or nerve cells, the adventitia is comprised principally of fibroblasts. Coronary artery vasa vasorum originate mostly from side branches of the artery and only in approximately 16% directly from the main lumen. Vasa vasorum may augment delivery of cellular elements to developing atherosclerotic lesions in response to chemical messages originating from the subintima. Although a high density

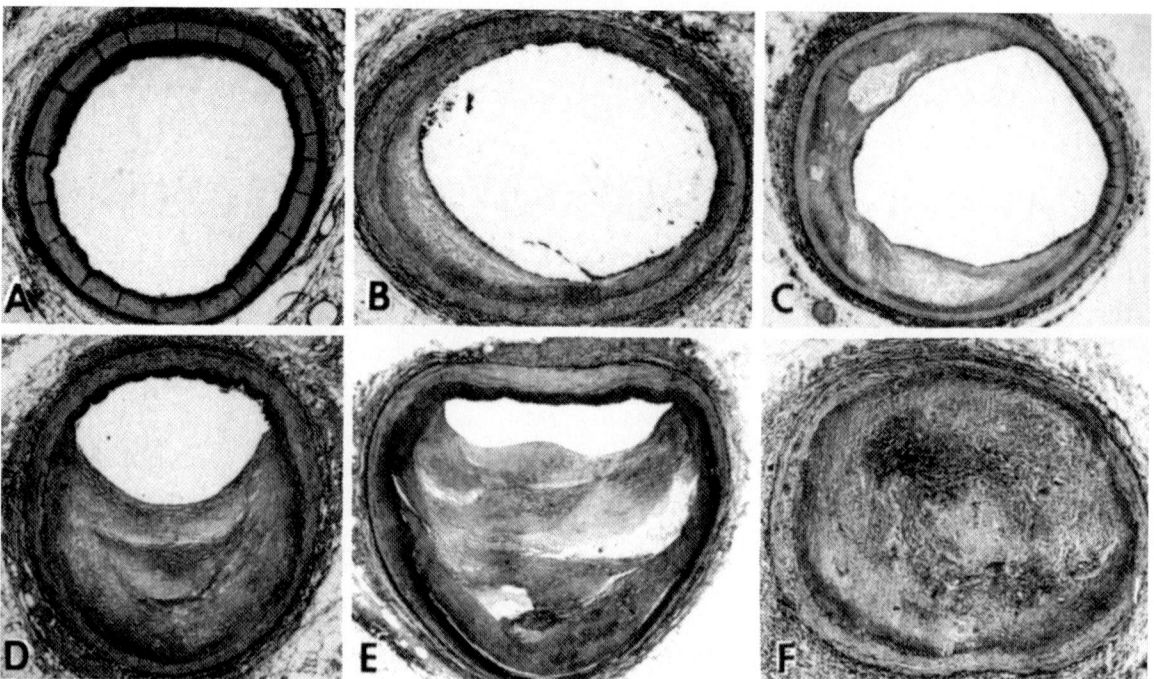

Fig. 1. Elastic-van Gieson stains of coronary artery cross sections. *A*, Normal vessel from 33-year-old woman. *B*, Stage II lesion with subintimal cellular plaque. *C*, Stage III lesion with mostly acellular lipid pool. *D*, Grade IV complex, moderately obstructive plaque with evidence of laminations (74-year-old woman). *E*, Grade V plaque with thin fibrous cap, and greater than 75% luminal compromise in a 69-year-old man. *F*, Total coronary occlusion in a 62-year-old man.

of vasa vasorum may reflect the increased needs for blood supply of the growing plaque, other preclinical data indicate that vasa vasorum actually initiate plaque growth.

Prevalence of atherosclerotic lesions is highest in the abdominal aorta, coronary arteries, femoro-popliteal arteries, internal carotid arteries, and verte-brobasilar arterial regions. Some arteries like the internal mammary artery or radial artery are rarely or never affected by atherosclerosis. Reasons for the regional heterogeneity of pathological response to what is a uni-form systemic exposure to risk factors likely include variation in local response to risk-factor mediated injury. Hemodynamic stresses at branches and bifurca-tions may augment mechanically mediated dysfunction of endothelium, and response to this dysfunction may be different due to differences in vasa vasorum density. Turbulent flow in such areas may also reduce binding of cells that might mediate vascular repair, such as bone marrow-derived endothelial progenitor cells. Local dif-ferences in gene expression and inflammatory reactions may affect the concentrations of growth factors and adhesion molecules.

CARDIAC RISK FACTORS

Major independent risk factors for the development of atherosclerosis include elevated plasma total and low-density lipoprotein cholesterol (LDLc), cigarette smoking, hypertension, diabetes mellitus, advancing age, low plasma high-density lipoprotein cholesterol (HDLc), and a family history of premature coronary artery disease.

The consensus pathogenetic explanation leading to the development of atherosclerosis is that cumulative

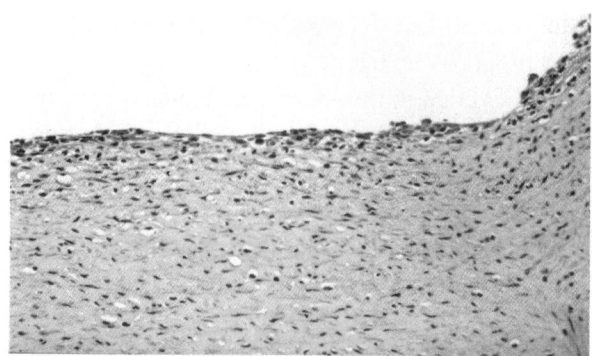

Fig. 2. Intimal smooth muscle cell proliferation.

exposure to risk factors over many years results in a cycle of, or series of cyclical, injury and repair episodes, which culminate in clinical events which include acute coronary thrombotic syndromes, angina, intermittent claudication or acute arterial occlusion, ischemic stroke, and development and rupture of abdominal aortic aneurysm. This explanation is concordant with clinical experience, and strongly implied by coronary artery pathology, in which strata of event and repair cycles may occasionally be seen as laminations within a single arterial segment (Fig. 3).

Acute coronary syndromes and exertional angina are the most important clinical presentations of coronary artery disease. They reflect two main aspects of the disease. Unstable or ruptured plaques are the main reasons for acute myocardial infarction and unstable angina, although plaques responsible for acute clinical syndromes are typically only moderately stenotic. Stable plaques cause exercise-induced chest pain if they occlude more than 75% of the cross-sectional area. Although they become hemodynamically significant, they rarely lead to acute coronary syndromes. Understanding these differences and identifying patients or plaques at risk is currently the focus of intense clinical and basic research.

In the Atherosclerosis Risk in Communities (ARIC) Study, the adjusted rate increases of coronary heart disease and stroke for the well-established, classical risk factors were 67% for smoking, 65% for diabetes, 47% for hypertension, and 59% low-density lipoprotein cholesterol (rate increase due to being in the highest vs lowest quartile). Separate guidelines for management of risk factors are described in detail in other chapters but will be reviewed in brief below because therapeutics addressing these risk factors represents the main activity of daily cardiovascular clinical practice. Several proposed risk factors are under intense study but do not yet affect clinical practice to a significant degree.

Cholesterol

Low density lipoprotein cholesterol can be clearly implicated in the pathogenesis of atherosclerosis. It is instructive to note that while human LDLc concentrations tend to cluster in the 120-200 mg/dL range, and atherosclerotic disease is the largest single cause of death in humans, typical nonhuman mammalian LDLc levels are in the 10-60 mg/dL range, and

atherosclerosis is not seen unless animals are fed high-fat chow. Epidemiologic human data link diets high in saturated fats to the prevalence of atherosclerotic diseases in diverse human populations and also support a direct relationship between cholesterol levels and coronary heart disease death. Relative risk increases in a continuum as total cholesterol increases even from a level as low as 150 mg/dL. Unlike other risk factors, such as diabetes, smoking, and hypertension, cholesterol is present at the scene of the atherosclerotic plaque—mainly in the form of oxidized LDLc or cholesterol esters. In a series of pivotal clinical trials, use of HMG co-A reductase or "statin" drugs were utilized in populations with or without prior coronary disease, and with or without preexisting elevations of LDLc. Statin therapy reduced LDLc by approximately 25%-40%, and lowered coronary artery disease events by approximately 30% (Fig. 4). These

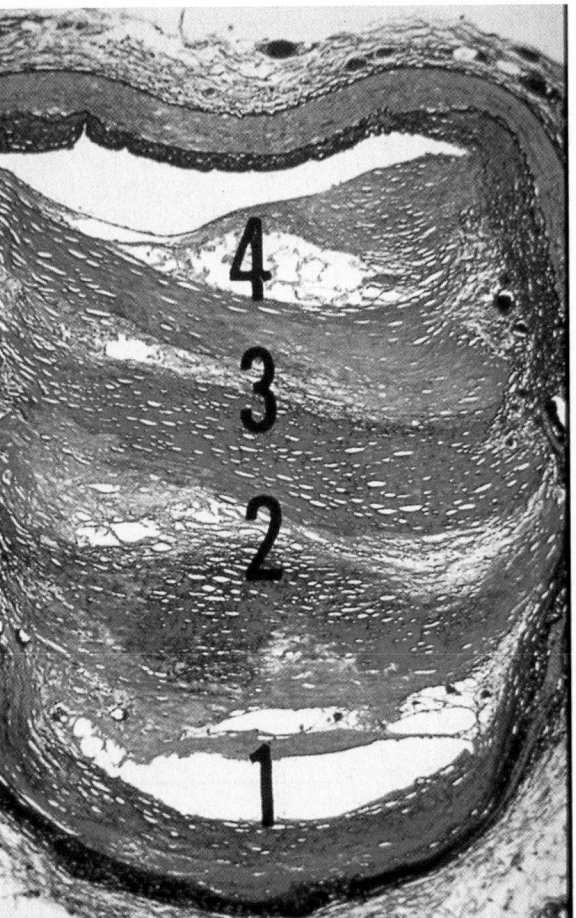

Fig. 3. Complex coronary plaque with distinct laminations, suggesting cycles of progression.

trials have served as final proof of the cholesterol hypothesis of atherogenesis—now widely accepted.

The National Cholesterol Education Project (NCEP) is responsible for digesting new trial data and making therapeutic recommendations regarding treatment targets for practitioners. Its most recent published guidelines support manipulating LDLc to less than 100 mg/dL in patients with known coronary artery disease, and now include an option to manipulate LDLc levels even lower (<70 mg/dL).

Hypertension

Each 20-mm Hg increase in systolic blood pressure or 10-mm Hg increase in diastolic blood pressure doubles coronary heart disease mortality and stroke mortality. Proposed mechanisms by which hypertension promotes atherosclerosis include damage to endothelial cells, promoting activation and incorporation of lipids into subintima, and stimulation of subintimal smooth muscle cell proliferation. The Joint National Committee on Prevention, Detection, Evaluation and Treatment of High Blood Pressure defines normal blood pressure as 120/80 mm Hg or lower, prehypertension as 120-139/80-89 mm Hg, stage I hypertension as 140-159/90-99 mm Hg, and stage II hypertension as >160 mm Hg systolic or >100 mm Hg diastolic. Risk of adverse events from atherosclerosis is seen even in pre-hypertensives. Treatment goal for most patients is <140/90, but more intensive blood pressure lowering is likely desirable, and is already recommended by guidelines for patients with chronic kidney disease or diabetes mellitus (<130/80). Meta-analysis of treatment trials suggests a 16% reduction in coronary artery events and mortality attributable to treatment of mild to moderate high blood pressure. This benefit is twice as strong in elderly vs younger patients.

Diabetes Mellitus

In the National Cholesterol Education Program report, diabetes is considered a coronary artery disease equivalent, thereby elevating it to the highest risk category. This classification is based on the observation that patients with type 2 diabetes without prior history of myocardial infarction are at the same risk for myocardial

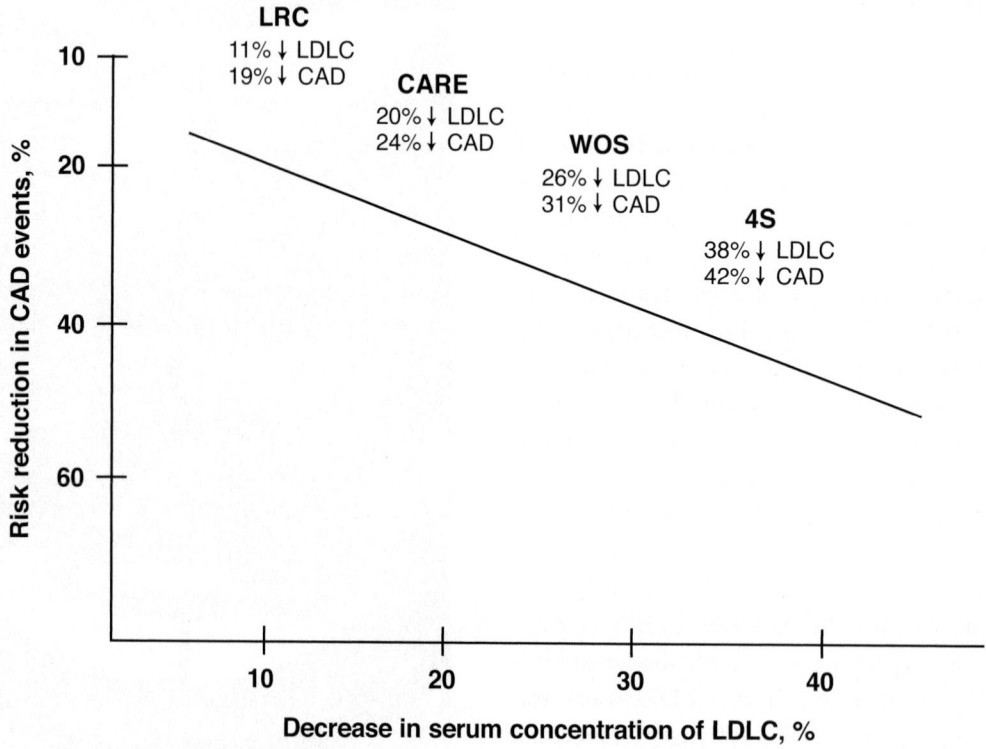

Fig. 4. Coronary heart disease (CHD) risk reduction in placebo-controlled trials of statin drugs. LRC, Lipid Research Clinics Trial; CARE, Cholesterol and Recurrent Events Study; WOS, West of Scotland Study; 4S, Scandanavian Simvastatin Survival Study.

infarction (20%) and coronary mortality (15%) as patients without diabetes who already had an infarction Coronary atherosclerosis is the cause of death in approximately three-fourths of diabetics. Currently, 15 million Americans are known to have diabetes mellitus and this number is projected to double by 2030. Risk for cardiac death and nonfatal myocardial infarction is increased 2-8 times, and the increase in risk appears to occur even in the prediabetic phase. In addition to the increase in mortality, diabetics are also more likely to experience a complication associated with myocardial infarction, including postinfarction angina and heart failure. Possible contributory factors are that diabetic patients are more likely to have multivessel disease and have significantly fewer coronary collateral vessels.

The prevalence of insulin resistance, which usually precedes the onset of overt hyperglycemia is expected to rise significantly as societal obesity continues to increase. The so-called metabolic syndrome (three of five components—fasting hyperglycemia, hypertriglyceridemia, hypertension, waist circumference >88 cm in women, or >102 cm in men, and low HDL cholesterol) is also increasingly prevalent and difficult to manage. The age adjusted prevalence of the metabolic syndrome approximates 25%. The prevalence of coronary artery disease increases in diabetics with vs without the metabolic syndrome from 7.5% to 19.2%.

The exact mechanisms underlying the accelerated progression of atherosclerosis in diabetic patients are unclear. Patients with type 2 diabetes have reduced myocardial flow reserve, a reflection of impaired coronary vasodilator capacity and impaired angiogenesis. Diabetes impairs endothelial function and enhances monocyte adhesion to endothelium, one of the earliest events in the genesis of atherosclerosis. Endothelial dysfunction appears to be an inflammatory result of advanced glycation end product (AGE) formation activating the proinflammatory nuclear transcription factor NF-κ-B, which reduces nitric oxide availability. Although metformin and thiazolidinedione therapy reduce endothelial dysfunction, it is unknown whether such improvement leads to better outcomes.

In the early stages of diabetes, number of vasa vasorum significantly decreases even before atheromas develop. As plaque size, inflammation, and lipid core size increase vasa vasorum rapidly proliferate.

Diabetes has a number of effects on platelet function and the coagulation system which predispose to coronary thrombosis. There is increased platelet aggregation and activation, and enhanced binding of fibrinogen to the glycoprotein IIb/IIIa complex. Diabetic patients also show a plasma increase of the cardiovascular risk factor fibrinogen. Fibrinolytic activity is reduced with increased plasma concentrations and binding of plasminogen activator inhibitor (PAI-1), which is also found locally in atherosclerotic plaques of diabetic patients. Other aspects of plaque composition may differ in diabetics compared to nondiabetics. Coronary artery plaque from diabetic patients contains greater amounts of lipid-rich atheroma, and more macrophage infiltration, both of which are associated with a greater risk of plaque rupture.

There are a number of differences in the lipid profile between diabetics and nondiabetics that may contribute to the increase in atherosclerosis and its complications. In type 1 diabetes, poor glycemic control is characteristically associated with hypertriglyceridemia and low HDL. Among patients with type 2 diabetes, insulin resistance, relative insulin deficiency, and obesity are associated with hypertriglyceridemia, high serum LDL and lipoprotein (a) values. HDLc is decreased, reducing the capacity for reverse cholesterol transport. This pattern can be detected even before the onset of overt hyperglycemia. The LDLc therapeutic target option for diabetic patents is <70 mg/dL with blood pressure target <130/80 mm Hg.

Adiponectin, an adipocyte-derived peptide and its levels correlate with both insulin resistance and atherosclerosis. Low adiponectin concentrations are associated with low HDL concentrations. Both human and animal studies have shown that adiponectin improves insulin sensitivity, lipid profiles, and levels of inflammatory markers including CRP, TNF-α, and IL-6.

Although good glycemic control reduces the risk of *micro*vascular complications and appears to be beneficial during acute MI, protection against macrovascular disease has not been established in type 2 diabetes, suggesting that factors other than hyperglycemia play a significant role.

Cigarette Smoking

In coronary prevention terms, cessation of smoking conveys greater risk reduction than any other modifiable risk factor known. Risk is reduced by slightly more than one-third compared to subjects who continue smoking. At least one pack of cigarettes smoked per day increases risk 2-3 fold, and there is a synergistic increase in risk in women who taking oral contraceptives. Smoking adversely effects endothelial function, promotes platelet aggregation, monocyte adhesion, and reduces endothelial nitric oxide production.

Other Cardiac Risk Factors

C-reactive protein, homocysteine, fibrinogen, D-dimer, lipoprotein(a), plasma creatinine, intimal medial thickness, coronary calcium scores, and systemic markers of infection have all been evaluated as possible potent atherosclerotic risk factors. Thus far, only C-reactive protein (CRP) has found a place in published guidelines.

C-Reactive Protein

High-sensitivity CRP is a systemic marker of inflammation in humans. It is produced in the liver, but also in atherosclerotic plaque and human endothelium, augmented by the presence of macrophages and interleukins-1 and -6. Conditions in which hsCRP is increased include type 2 diabetes, hypertension, sleep apnea, the metabolic syndrome, chronic kidney disease, and all inflammatory diseases. High-sensitivity CRP is an independent marker of risk of coronary events. At present, measurement of hsCRP is recommended in patients judged to be at intermediate risk of coronary events (i.e. 10%-20% risk per 10 years) since an elevated level of hsCRP adds sufficient risk to reclassify such patients as high risk and suggests a need for a more aggressive lipid-lowering therapeutic target. In patients with known coronary artery disease, hsCRP is also an independent prognostic marker for future myocardial infarction, death, or restenosis following percutaneous coronary angioplasty and stenting. Although considerable research has focused on interventions which alter hsCRP, notably aspirin, peroxisome proliferator-activated receptor γ agonists (thiazolidinediones) and statin agents, at the present time primary or secondary prevention therapies should not be based on hsCRP levels, but rather on standard guidelines such as the NCEP Guidelines, the Joint National Committee on Prevention, Detection, Evaluation and Treatment of High Blood Pressure, and use of antiplatelet therapy based on standard guidelines for management of patients with cardiovascular risk factors, stable angina, recent acute coronary syndrome, post-percutaneous coronary intervention or post-coronary artery bypass grafting.

EARLY PROCESSES

The earliest pathological change of atherosclerosis is thickening of the subendothelial intima. Smooth muscle cells in this intima alter their phenotype compared to smooth muscle cells in the medial layer. An early inflammatory reaction of the endothelium, "endothelial activation," is likely mediated through classical risk factors, especially increased LDLc (Fig. 5). Normally, circulating LDLc binds to specific receptors on endothelium and transits through the intima, media, and finally into adventitial vasa-vasorum or lymphatics. Excess LDLc accumulates in the subintima and binds to proteoglycan extracellular matrix in a process likely mediated by apolipoprotein B. Circulating LDLc resists oxidation, but proteoglycan-bound LDLc is exposed to oxidative enzymes. Oxidized LDLc products in the subintima are pro-inflammatory, and inflammatory cascades are initiated in both endothelium and the subintima. Endothelial activation and LDLc receptor binding density may also be enhanced by flow disturbance, smoking, hypertension, and hyperhomocysteinemia.

Endothelial cells injured or "activated" by oxidized LDLc produce adhesion molecules, including vascular cell adhesion molecule-1 (VCAM-1), and chemokines, such as chemoattractant protein-1 (MCP-1), beginning the critical step of binding of circulating blood monocytes to endothelium. Monocytes that are attracted to and bind to endothelial cells are incorporated into the subintima and differentiate into macrophages. Subintimal macrophages scavenge oxidized LDLc, and may accumulate cholesterol to the point where pathological visible cytoplasmic droplets are seen. Oxidized LDLc also promotes further proliferation of macrophages within the subintima. Coalescence of lipid droplets within the macrophage cytoplasm results in the typical "foam cell" of early stage atherosclerotic plaque (Fig. 1 *B* and 6). In this early stage, foam cells are capable of transporting cholesterol back to the endothelial surface to be bound by circulating HDL which binds cholesterol and transports it to the liver, so called "reverse cholesterol transport." However, if the

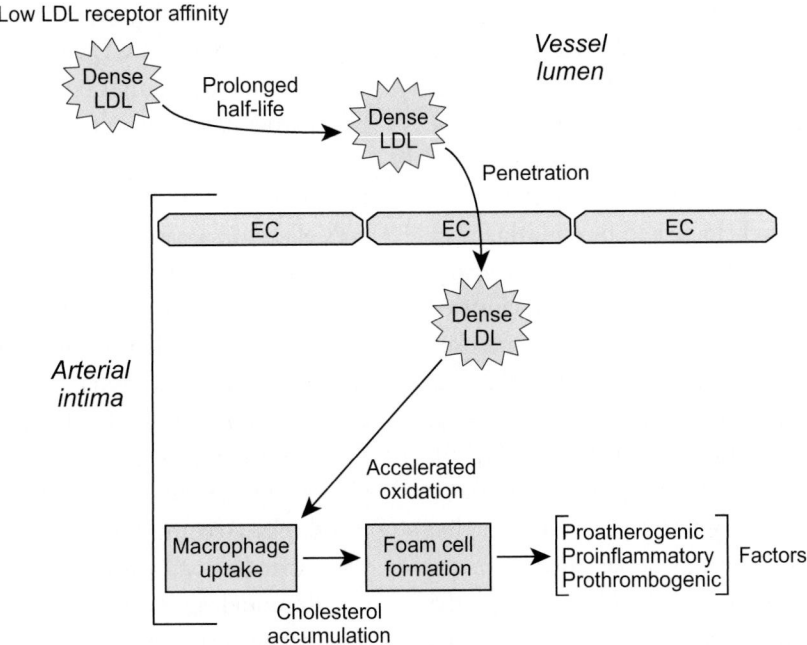

Fig. 5. Pivotal role of LDLc in genesis of early atherosclerosis via subendothelial conversion to oxidized LDLc with macrophage stimulation and activation.

stimulus for atherogenesis remains amplified, foam cells remain in the subintima as repositories of cholesterol (Fig. 1 *C*), until they undergo apoptosis and release lipid into the extracellular subintima forming a mostly acellular subintimal lipid pool (Fig. 1 *D*). Amplification also occurs as macrophage-derived inflammatory cytokines increase the numbers of endothelial cell LDLc receptors, and increase extracellular matrix

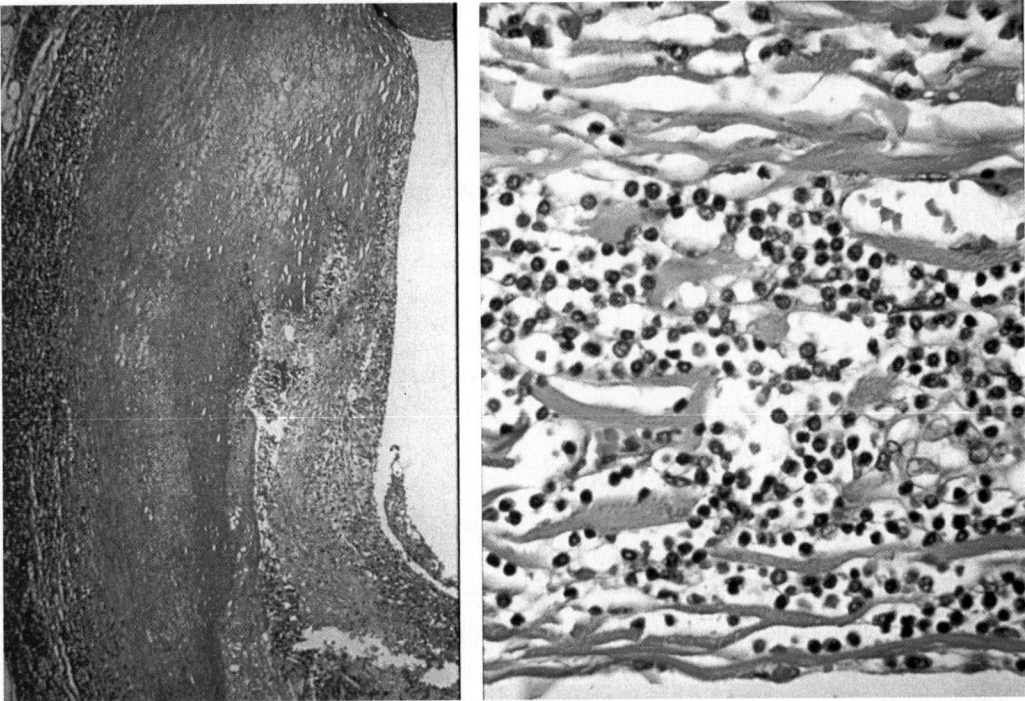

Fig. 6. Foam cells in atherosclerosis.

deposition and fibrosis of adjacent smooth muscle cells. Matrix metalloproteinase enzymes are also promoted, and these digest membranes, including internal and external elastic lamina and also stimulate a proliferative and angiogenic response from the media and adventitia.

Experimental data suggest that adventitial fibroblast activity is strikingly increased by endothelial or adventitial injury, stimulating a migration from adventitia towards media and intima. This migration is fostered by matrix metalloproteinases, which are locally controlled by cytokines and growth factors, including platelet-derived growth factor (PDGF), basic fibroblast growth factor (bFGF), transforming growth factor β (TGF-β), and plasmin. TGF-β importantly influences synthesis or inhibition of other growth factors. In the media, fibroblasts interact further with vascular smooth muscle. Further migration of adventitial fibroblasts through the media to a subendothelial location has been documented experimentally. Apoptosis, cell proliferation, phenotypic alterations in medial vascular smooth muscle cells, and scarring appear all to be controlled by the mixture of matrix growth factors, cytokines, metalloproteinases, tissue inhibitors of metalloproteinases, and oxidized LDLc. The adventitial vascular layer simultaneously undergoes an increase in thickness fostering vasa vasorum growth into the expanding atherosclerotic plaque.

Additional proinflammatory cytokines are numerous in growing plaques. Endotoxin and heat shock protein bind to activated macrophages. T cells of the CD4+ type are recruited and the interaction between macrophages, CD4+ cells and vascular smooth muscle cells results in elaboration of tumor necrosis factor, interleukin-1, and interferon-γ. Activated T cells also stimulate angiogenesis, mediated at least in part by vascular endothelial growth factor (VEGF), and this is one among a number of signals for vasa vasorum proliferation. A number of key observations specifically link CD4+ cells and angiogenesis. First, in mice in which the CD4 system is knocked out, ligation of a hind limb artery is not followed by the usual formation of collateral circulation. Second, when apolipoprotein E knockouts, which phenotypically manifest hypercholesterolemia and accelerated atherosclerosis, are mated with CD4 knockouts, a decrease in atherosclerotic lesion size was seen. Transfusion of the missing CD4+ cells resulted in greater atherosclerotic lesion growth.

Finally, polymorphisms in the genes encoding the expected products of CD4+ activation, such as tumor necrosis factor and interferon-γ, also result in altered phenotypic expression of the atherosclerotic process.

Coronary calcification occurs in vesicles within extracellular matrix. Calcification occurs in collagen and noncollagen-associated organic matrix. Noncollagenous bone-associated proteins that foster calcification, such as osteopontin, are expressed by macrophages in human intima, but expression has also been noted in smooth muscle cells and adventitia. One other mechanism for calcium deposition is intraplaque hemorrhage possibly from immature vasa vasorum with degradation of phosphorous and calcium rich membranes derived from red blood cells. Accumulation of calcium is typical for less vascularized lesions with small or no lipid cores.

Remodeling is a frequently used term. Arterial remodeling occurs in two forms in response to atherosclerotic plaques. Positive remodeling, called the Glagov effect, is a compensatory increase in local vessel size in response to a plaque burden not exceeding 40% of the luminal area. Negative remodeling refers to the local shrinkage of vessel size, which can occur after balloon angioplasty without stenting.

VASA VASORUM, ANGIOGENESIS, NEOVASCULARIZATION

The causes of coronary lesion progression from an asymptomatic fibroatheromatous plaque to a lesion at high risk for rupture with a thin, fibrous cap and necrotic lipid-rich core are not fully understood. Recent research suggests a role of vasa vasorum and neovascularization during this development (Fig. 7 *left*).

At sites of plaque formation there is proliferation of vasa vasorum from the adventitial side into the abluminal side of the plaque. In regions in which new vessels penetrate into the plaque, there are collections of extravascular macrophages, T-lymphocytes, and erythrocytes. Macrophages ingesting erythrocyte membrane are also noted.

Some data indicate that the quantity of vasa vasorum may be associated with symptomatic disease and greater macrophage numbers. There is a clear correlation between increased number of vasa vasorum and plaque size similar to the relationship between vessel wall thickness and vasa vasorum density. Recent data also

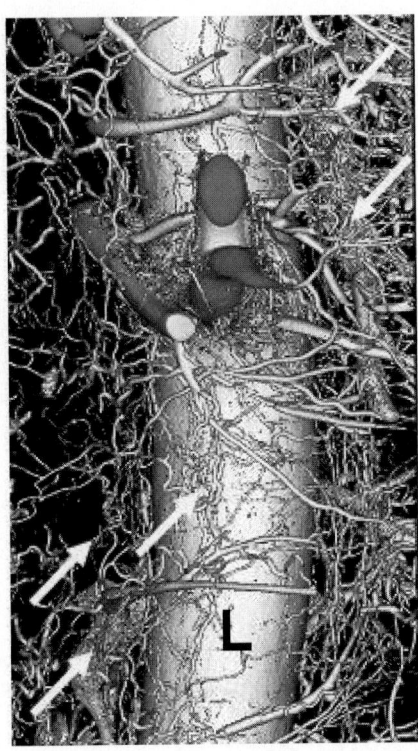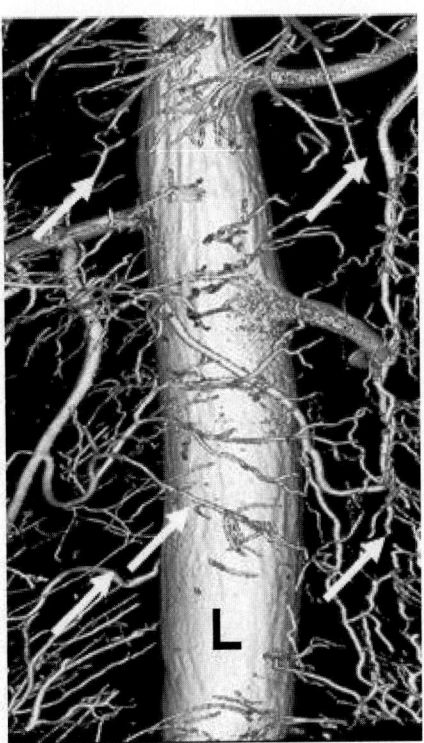

Fig. 7. Microscopic CT images of coronary arteries with vasa vasorum. *Left panel*, Vasa vasorum of a normal coronary artery run longitudinally and across the main artery lumen (L). *Right panel*, Vasa vasorum of a coronary artery during early-stage diabetes before atherosclerotic plaques develop. Number and density of vasa vasorum are markedly diminished in response to hyperglycemia. Artery diameter, 2 mm.

demonstrate a close correlation between vasa vasorum density and size of inflammatory infiltrate. In ruptured or unstable plaques, the necrotic core occupies 30%-50% of the total plaque area, whereas it occupies less than 20% in the majority of stable plaques. This suggests that progressive expansion of the necrotic core precedes plaque rupture.

As the plaque enlarges, subsequent hypoxia and inflammatory cell infiltration promote neovascularization of vasa vasorum which further adds to the total plaque volume. Exposure to this abnormal environment stimulates rapid and abnormal vascular development of the microvessels characterized by disorganized branching and formation of loops with "leaky," imperfect endothelial linings. The entrance of vasa vasorum into plaques occurs at points adjacent to the necrotic plaque core through defects in the medial layer. Intraadventitial and intramedial vasa vasorum are relatively mature, some of which contain cuffs of smooth muscle cells, while proliferating vasa vasorum closest to the arterial lumen are usually thin, immature,

and tortuous. Although endothelialized, they typically lack smooth muscle cells. These immature blood vessels are inherently leaky and permit extravasation of erythrocytes. This hemorrhage into the plaque yields rapid changes in plaque size and composition and may promote the transition from a stable to an unstable lesion. Indeed, autopsy studies indicate that intraplaque hemorrhage is more frequent in patients dying from ruptured plaques compared to patients with stable atherosclerotic lesions (Fig. 8). Erythrocyte membranes are also a potent source of additional cholesterol, particularly in hypercholesterolemic patients. Extravascular erythrocytes in the plaque region further stimulate chemoattraction of macrophages that digest erythrocyte-bound cholesterol which further increases the size of the lipid pool after intraplaque hemorrhage has occurred.

HISTOLOGICAL TYPOLOGY AND CONTENTS
The Committee of Vascular Lesion of the Council on Arteriosclerosis of the American Heart Association has

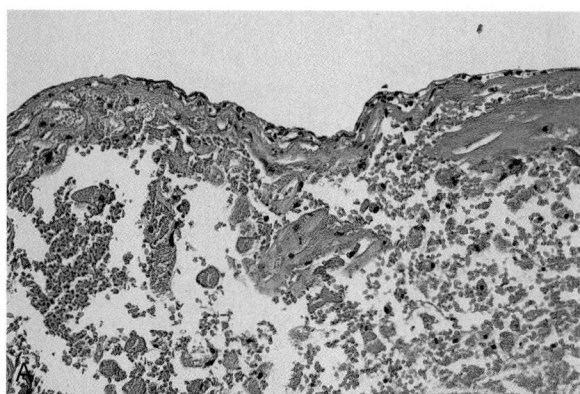 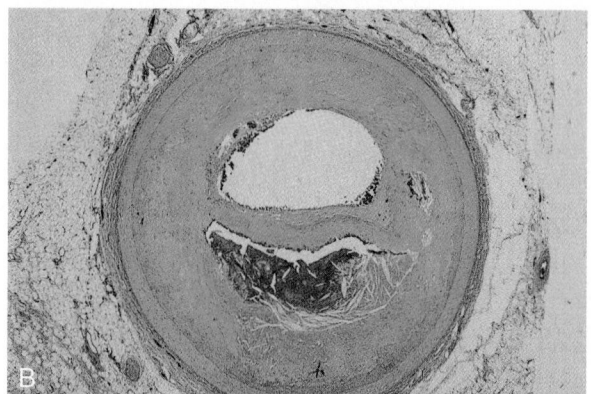

Fig. 8. *A*, High-power (x50) view of severely stenotic plaque with thin fibrous cap and intraplaque hemorrhage. *B*, Lower-power view of intraplaque hemorrhage in a human right coronary artery.

generated a histological classification of atherosclerotic lesions. These build on an earlier classification by Stary (Fig. 9). The early type I lesion is characterized by pathologic intimal thickening and subintimal scattered foam cell macrophages. In addition to foamy macrophages, type II lesions also incorporate lipid-laden smooth muscle cells. These lesions are macroscopically visibly as arterial fatty streaks. Type III lesions are represented by an increase in smooth muscle cells and volumes of surrounding connective tissue matrix, plus collections of extracellular lipid droplets or small lipid pools. The main molecular constituents of type I-III plaques are collagen, proteoglycans in the extracellular matrix, crystalline cholesterol, cholesterol esters and other phospholipids, and cellular components and remnants including macrophages, T-lymphocytes, and smooth muscle cells. In more complex plaque, components of thrombus including platelets, fibrin, and red blood cells may be present, suggesting an important role for repetitive stimuli of either erosion of the plaque surface with hemorrhage, or hemorrhage from vasa vasorum within the plaque in the intermediate term progression of the atherosclerotic process (Fig. 1 *E*, 7 *Right*, and 9).

The type IV lesion is said to be present when extracellular lipid droplets have pooled to create a large confluent extracellular lipid core (Fig. 1 *E*, 9, and 10). When such a core is surrounded by a thick fibrous cap, the lesion is referred as type V (Fig. 11); if heavy calcification is present, Vb, or if calcium is largely absent, Vc. Type VI lesions demonstrate either disruption of the

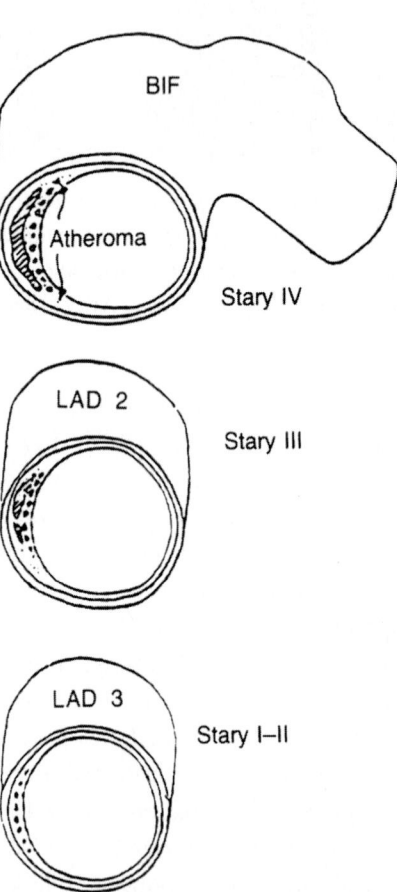

Fig. 9. Stary stages of early atherosclerosis: I, focal intimal thickening due to smooth muscle cell proliferation as seen in human infants; II, fatty streaks composed of subendothelial foam cells with most lipid droplets being intracellular; III, greater space is occupied by a mostly extracellular lipid pool; IV, mixture of cellular and acellular lipid pool with a fibrous cap of variable thickness.

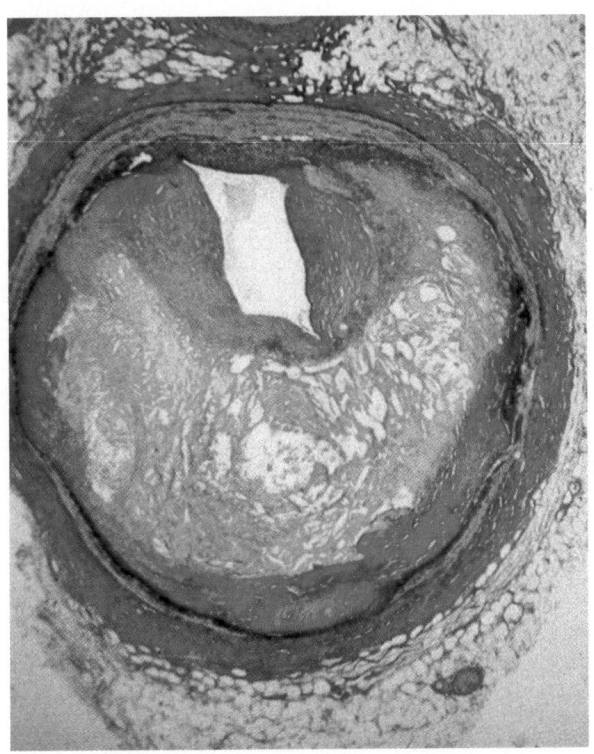

Fig. 10. Highly stenotic coronary plaque. *A*, Vulnerable, relatively thin fibrous cap covering large acellular lipid pool, with some inflammatory cells visible.

fibrous cap with fissure (Fig. 12 and 13), hematoma (Fig. 8 *B*), or thrombus (Fig. 14). Spontaneous disruption of the cap of an unstable plaque is likely the culminating event causing acute myocardial infarction. Intense investigation into the risk factors, mechanisms, and possible therapeutic approaches to this specific occurrence occupies a considerable space in the national effort to combat cardiovascular disease.

VULNERABILITY AND RUPTURE OF PLAQUE

With expansion of the lipid core of type IV plaques and accumulation of macrophages, especially at the luminal edges of the plaque, risk of rupture of the fibrous cap and exposure of the thrombogenic contents of the plaque is increased. Measurements of thickness of the fibrous cap in plaques that have ruptured compared to those which have not indicates that fibrous cap thickness <65 mm thick and the presence of >25 macrophages per high-powered (0.3 mm diameter)

microscopic field increase the risk of plaque rupture. This vulnerability appears to be more likely in moderately stenotic lesions versus severely stenotic lesions, at least as assessed by serial coronary angiography, and theoretically there may be stronger physical forces at play at the edges of a moderately stenotic plaque than anywhere near the surface of a subtotal occlusion (Fig. 15). In subjects dying of acute myocardial infarction, the degree of infiltration of plaque by inflammatory cells is not limited to the lesion causing the fatal infarct— rather greater inflammation is seen in arterial lesions elsewhere in the coronary tree of these subjects, suggesting a diffuse impact of risk factors on the vascular target. In addition to thinness of the cap and degree of inflammatory infiltrate, vasa vasorum are increased approximately 4-fold in ruptured plaques, and twofold in those with vulnerability defined by cap thinness and inflammatory density over plaques that were not associated with acute clinical presentation or were severely stenotic and associated with stable angina.

THROMBOSIS

Rupture of plaque or superficial erosion exposes the bloodstream to thrombogenic stimuli. Superficial erosions or disruptions of fibrous plaque surface attract platelet adhesion and formation of a monolayer of

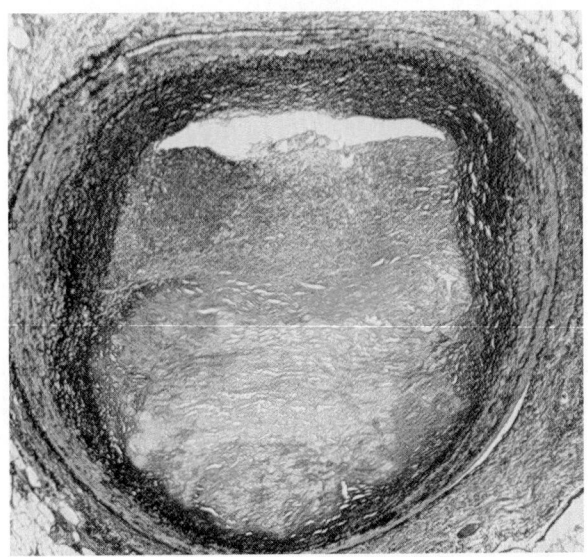

Fig. 11. Highly stenotic plaque in human left anterior descending coronary artery. Although a large lipid pool is present, there is a very thick fibrous cap.

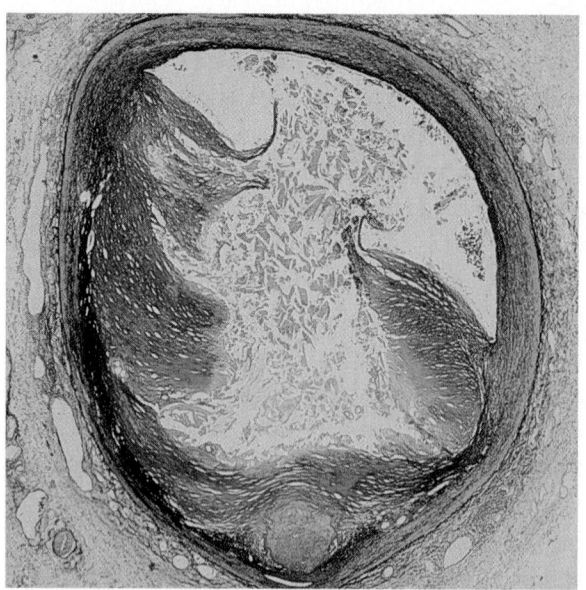

Fig. 12. Acute plaque rupture from center of plaque.

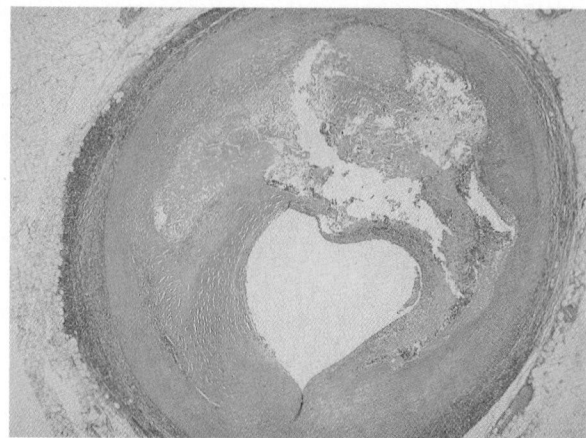

Fig. 13. Acute plaque rupture from "shoulder" of plaque.

platelet thrombus, with platelets binding to collagen and wall-bound von Willebrand's factor. Platelet phospholipids on the newly damaged arterial surface lead to activation of circulating coagulation factors. The activation and amplification of coagulation factors foster binding of additional platelets to the propagating thrombus mass (Fig. 16). This process involves the platelet glycoprotein IIb/IIIa receptor (subject to pharmacological intervention in percutaneous coronary intervention and unstable angina) and fibrinogen. Endogenous inhibitors balancing the propagating thrombus include the fibrinolytic system, antithrombin III, proteins C

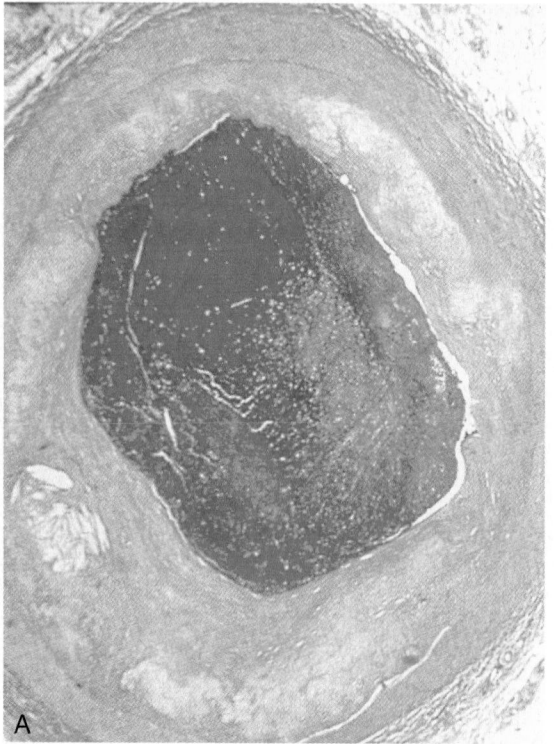

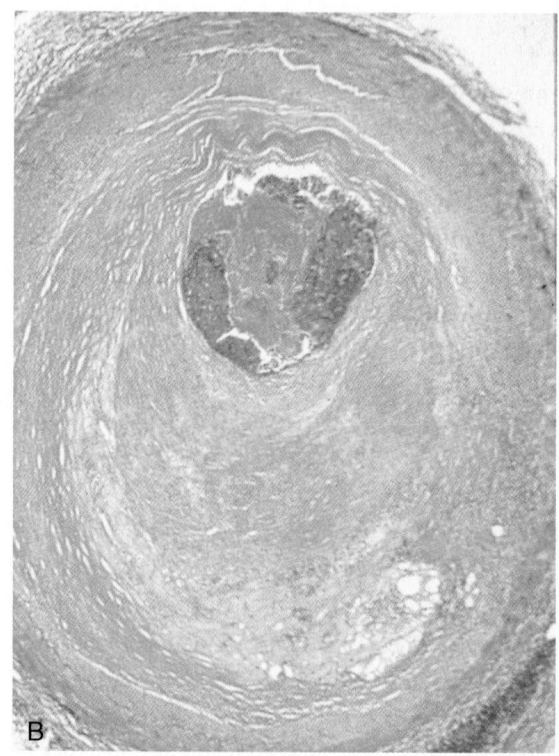

Fig. 14. Occlusive coronary thrombi: *A*, in mildly stenotic underlying plaque; *B*, in severely stenotic plaque.

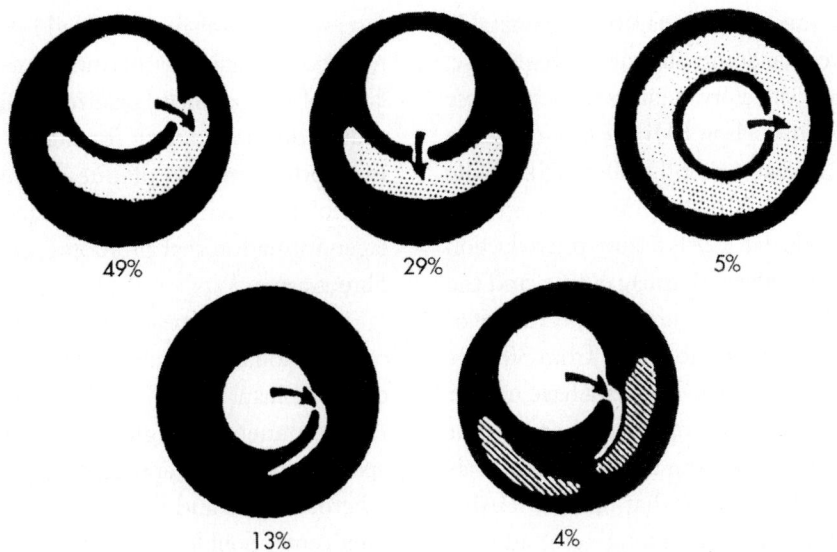

Fig. 15. Frequency of sites of tearing in plaques experiencing plaque rupture. Stippling, lipid pool; Black, fibrous tissue; Cross-hatching, calcification.

and S, and tissue factor inhibitor pathway. In superficial vascular injury, thrombin and erythrocyte incorporation into the thrombus occur only after total occlusion by the platelet plug. The process of occlusion may be dynamic, with stuttering cycles of total or near-total occlusion, distal embolization of platelet plugs by flowing blood, and reformation of thrombus at the site of plaque rupture. As is described elsewhere, the clinical manifestations may vary from sudden death due to ventricular arrhythmias, bradyarrhythmias, acute circulatory failure, or the chest pain and classical ST segment elevation myocardial infarction, non-ST elevation myocardial infarction, or unstable angina. It is also well described that such events may be clinically silent or misinterpreted in as many as 1/4 of patients. If, instead of superficial erosion, a deep arterial fissure or injury occurs, the thrombogenic stimulus is accelerated by the presence of fatty core plaque components such as tissue factor, and an acute occlusive thrombus may develop.

STABILIZATION AND REGRESSION OF ATHEROSCLEROTIC PLAQUE

Therapeutic placebo-controlled and different agent/dose comparative studies, mainly with HMG Co-A reductase or "statin" drugs, have tested differential intensities of lipid-lowering therapy in human subjects both in the setting of acute coronary syndromes and

with manifestations of chronic atherosclerotic disease. Despite therapy, events continue to occur during follow-up which suggest the need for additional therapies and risk factor modification for stabilization or regression of the atherosclerotic process.

In the PROVE-IT trial, patients with acute coronary

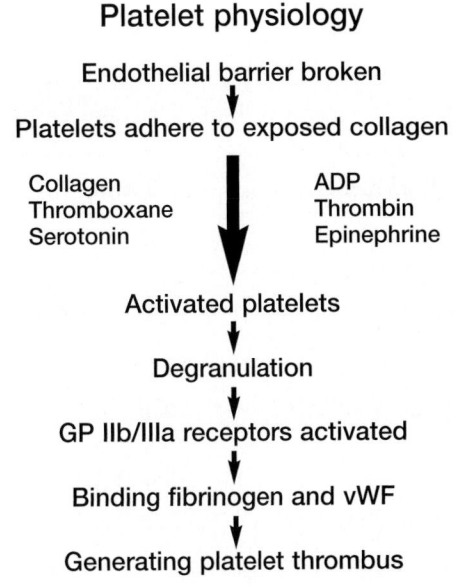

Fig. 16. Physiology of platelet activation and aggregation. ADP, adenosine diphosphate; GP, glycoprotein; vWF, von Willebrand factor.

syndromes (acute myocardial infarction or unstable angina pectoris) were randomly allocated to high-dose, potent statin therapy with atorvastatin vs moderate-dose therapy with pravastatin. Mean LDLc levels at baseline were 106 mg/dL, and at 4 months 60 mg/dL in the atorvastatin group vs 97 in the pravastatin group. Intensive therapy resulted in a 28% relative risk reduction in both early and late adverse cardiac events, and the curves depicting differences in cumulative incidence of subsequent events continued to widen from 30 days through 24 months after entry. Trial data have not yet defined the lower limit of optimal therapy nor described an increase in risk from therapy. Other trials in general support the concept that more intensive statin therapy is likely to reduce long-term adverse events (Table 1).

In a study of different patients but with similar different intensities of statin therapy, intracoronary ultrasound was used to measure changes in coronary plaque volume over time. Intensive therapy (LDLc decreased from 150 mg/dL to 79 mg/dL) with atorvastatin 80 mg per day suggested stabilization of plaque volume over 18 months, while continued increase in plaque volume was seen with pravastatin at a dose of 40 mg per day (LDLc decrease from 150 mg/dL to 110 mg/dL). Thus, most clinicians at present will seek to lower LDLc to below 100 mg/dL for subjects at risk, and below 70-75 mg/dL for those with known disease. Mechanisms proposed for this continuum of reduction of clinical events include reduction in accumulation of subendothelial oxidized LDLc with subsequent reduction in signaling for monocyte adhesion and incorporation into plaque. Reduced macrophage proteolytic activity allows for increased interstitial collagen formation that promotes stability of the plaque fibrous cap.

An additional means of assessing plaque stabilization or regression under active investigation involves the use of recombinant APoA-1 Milano phospholipid complex. A spontaneous single amino acid mutation in apolipoprotein A-1 appears to convey protection from atherosclerosis and is associated with longevity. In a multicenter double-blind randomized trial, exogenous administration of this compound after 5 weekly treatments resulted in a significant regression of atheromatous plaque volume as assessed by intravascular ultrasound. The theoretical basis for regression cited by the authors was enhancement of reverse cholesterol transport from plaque to liver via the apolipoprotein A-1 complex.

The peroxisome proliferator activated receptor (PPAR) is a nuclear receptor present in endothelium, smooth muscle cells, macrophages, and T lymphocytes as well as in liver, skeletal muscle and adipose tissue. Stimulation of PPAR receptors improves insulin-mediated glucose disposal. Agonists of PPAR were initially introduced as therapies in diabetic patients in

Table 1.   Comparative Statin Trials and Frequency of Cardiovascular Events

Trial name	Setting	Therapies	Outcome
A to Z	ACS	Simvastatin 40-80 vs simvastatin 20 mg/d	Nonsignificant trend of ↓CV events
TNT	Stable CAD	Atorvastatin 80 vs atorvastatin 10 mg/d	22% risk reduction in CAD death, nonfatal MI, stroke, or resuscitated cardiac arrest
PROVE-IT—TIMI 22	ACS	Atorvastatin 80 vs pravastatin 40 mg/d	16% risk reduction in death and major cardiac events
IDEAL	Prior MI	Atorvastatin 80 vs simvastatin 20 mg/d	Nonsignificant trend of ↓ CAD death, nonfatal MI, or resuscitated cardiac arrest*

ACS, acute coronary syndromes; CAD, coronary artery disease; CV, cardiovascular; MI, myocardial infarction.
*Significant ↓ in individual events, including nonfatal MI or revascularization.

whom the goal was to improve insulin sensitivity. The thiazolidinediones are PPAR-γ agonists and are in clinical use. In type II diabetics, and even in nondiabetics, however, the agents appear to reduce markers of inflammation and raise HDLc. Pioglitazone, a PPAR-γ agonist, in subjects with hypertension or hypercholesterolemia but without diabetes, reduced blood insulin levels, improved insulin sensitivity, and improved endothelial function, all changes which would be expected to favorably impact risk of complications of atherosclerosis. The sole large clinical trial evaluating outcomes, is the PROactive Study, evaluating pioglitazone in type 2 diabetics with prior evidence of coronary or peripheral atherosclerosis. Over nearly 3 years of follow-up on average, death, myocardial infarction, or stroke was reduced by 16%. Therapy is likely to be most beneficial in patients with type 2 diabetes who have evidence of atherogenic dyslipidemia (small dense LDLc and low total HDLc). PPAR-α agonists are more potent, and dual receptor PPAR agonists are in clinical investigation.

Finally, new research investigates a role for bone marrow-derived circulating endothelial progenitor cells in vascular healing. These cells may bind to injured arterial vessels and promote reestablishment of a healthy nonthrombogenic and antiatherogenic endothelium. Regulatory processes affecting these cells include aging and conventional cardiac risk factors, including diabetes and hyperlipidemia.

ATHEROSCLEROTIC ANEURYSMS

The abdominal aorta is the target for the earliest manifestations of systemic atherosclerosis—the fatty streak—and the site of the most severe bulky plaque formation. The most frequent site of atherosclerotic aneurysmal disease is the infrarenal abdominal aorta (Fig. 17 *A-C*). An association of abdominal aortic aneurysm with diseases such as polycystic kidney disease and chronic obstructive pulmonary disease suggests that matrix degeneration is a common feature. In the coronaries, the laminated structure of the media is preserved despite atherosclerotic plaque development, while in the abdominal aorta there is near complete destruction of the media and loss of the collagen and elastin in the internal elastic lamina. Higher matrix metalloproteinase activity in response to the inflammatory atherosclerotic stimulus is suspected as the cause of media destruction. In the late sixties, Wolinsky and Glagov have observed that the abdominal aorta in humans lacks vasa vasorum in its outermost aspects and have suggested that this may be one of the reasons the abdominal aorta is particularly vulnerable to atherogenesis.

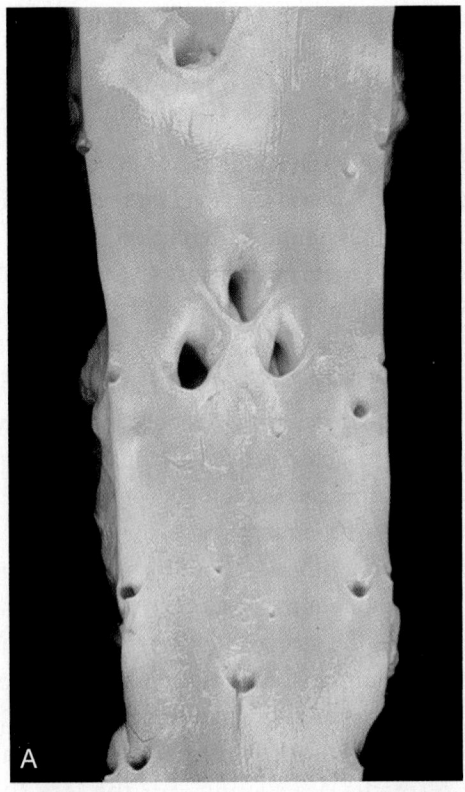

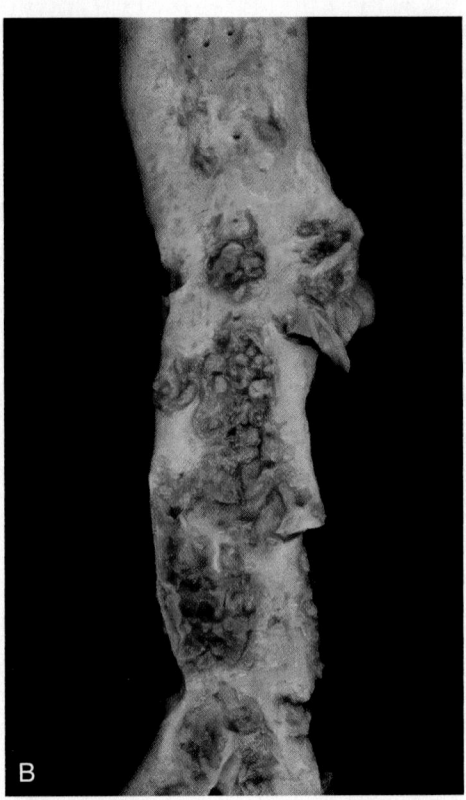

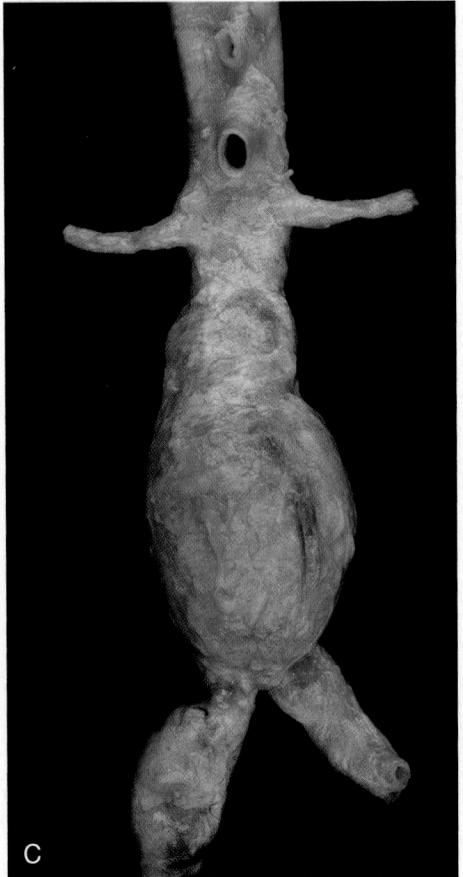

Fig. 17. *A*, Fatty streaks in abdominal aorta. *B*, Severe ulcerocalcific atherosclerosis of the abdominal aorta. *C*, Aneurysmal disease of the aorto-iliac trunk.

58

DYSLIPIDEMIA AND CLASSICAL FACTORS FOR ATHEROSCLEROSIS

Francisco Lopez-Jimenez, MD, MS

Justo Sierra Johnson, MD, MS

Virend K. Somers, MD, PhD

Gerald T. Gau, MD

DYSLIPIDEMIA

Epidemiology

Dyslipidemia, especially hypercholesterolemia, is a major key modifiable risk factor for coronary artery disease (CAD), the leading cause of death in the United States. About one-third of Americans have an elevated total cholesterol, and less than half of patients who would qualify for drug therapy take any prescription drug to reduce cholesterol.

The mere diagnosis of hypercholesterolemia is not straightforward. Mean total cholesterol the US is around 200 mg/dL, while in other parts of the world such as China and Latin America where CAD is less prevalent, the average total cholesterol is much below 200 mg/dL. Therefore, it is probable that our definition of "normal" as a total cholesterol <240 mg/dL is too conservative.

Screening for dyslipidemia is recommended for all men aged 35 or older and women 45 or older. Screening at earlier ages is recommended in patients with family history of CAD at an early age or a history of familial dyslipidemia.

The benefits of lipid-lowering therapy have been demonstrated in persons with and without cardiovascular disease at different levels of hypercholesterolemia. Management strategies for dyslipidemia are discussed at the end of this chapter.

Low-Density Lipoprotein (LDL) Subfractions

An increased LDL concentration is a well-known factor for development and progression of coronary heart disease. LDL is a heterogenous collection of lipoproteins and can be separated into subtypes of different size and density; there are at least 15 distinct subspecies. However, not all LDL particles have the same atherosclerotic potential. LDL can be classified into three classes: large light LDL, intermediate LDL, and small dense LDL. LDL size is inversely related to atherosclerotic risk. The major difference among these classes is the ratio of cholesterol molecules to apolipoprotein B. Large light LDL cholesterol has the greatest cholesterol:apolipoprotein B ratio, and small dense LDL cholesterol has the lowest cholesterol: apolipoprotein B ratio.

Cholesterol Ratios and Apolipoprotein B/AI ratio

There is strong evidence that the risk of atherosclerotic vascular disease is directly related to plasma cholesterol levels. Accordingly, all of the national and international screening and therapeutic guidelines are based on total or LDL cholesterol. However, cardiovascular risk appears to be more directly related to the number of circulating atherogenic particles that contact and enter the arterial wall than to the measured concentration of total cholesterol or LDL and HDL cholesterol fractions alone.

There have been several cholesterol ratios proposed including total cholesterol/HDL-C, LDL-C/HDL-C, and non-HDL-C/LDL-C. Recently, ratios more closely related to apolipoproteins have been investigated. Apolipoproteins are important structural and functional proteins in lipoprotein particles, which transport lipids. Apolipoprotein B100 (apoB) is found in LDL, intermediate-density lipoprotein (IDL), and very low-density lipoprotein (VLDL); thus its quantification presumably accounts for all the potentially atherogenic particles. Measurement of apolipoprotein B plasma concentration is easy, inexpensive, and probably relevant because it is an excellent predictor of cardiovascular disease independent of LDL levels. Non-HDL cholesterol is not a clinically accurate surrogate for apolipoprotein B. These two measurements are correlated but only moderately concordant.

In contrast, apolipoprotein AI is a protein synthesized mainly in the liver and small intestine. It is the primary protein found in HDL. Apolipoprotein AI facilitates reverse cholesterol transport from peripheral tissues to the liver, a physiological pathway thought to be protective against atherosclerosis. Recent reports suggest that measurements of apolipoprotein B and apolipoprotein AI may improve the prediction of risk for cardiovascular disease. Therefore, the apolipoprotein B/apolipoprotein AI ratio may represent the balance between proatherogenic and antiatherogenic lipoproteins. The apolipoprotein B/apolipoprotein AI ratio has been reported to predict cardiovascular risk better than any of the cholesterol indices, and that none of the standard lipid parameters add significant predictive information to the apolipoprotein B/apolipoprotein AI ratio.

Lipoprotein (a)

Lp(a), is composed of low-density lipoprotein (apo B-100) and low-molecular-weight glycoprotein called apolipoprotein (a) which exhibits genetic size polymorphism. Thirty-four isoforms of apolipoprotein (a) have been identified and studies have indicated that the size of apolipoprotein (a) is inversely associated with the lipoprotein (a) levels in plasma. Recent studies indicate that Lp(a) is an independent risk factor for premature coronary artery disease. Serum levels of Lp(a) have been shown to correlate well with the presence, severity and lesion score with coronary angiography as well as with the occurrence and recurrence of myocardial infarction and cardiac death. Also levels of Lp(a) are increased in response to pregnancy, advanced malignancy, and end-stage renal disease. Apolipoprotein (a), has considerable homology with plasminogen and interferes with fibrinolysis and may predispose thrombosis. Serum Lp(a) is largely unaffected by environmental factors and maximum levels are reached early in infancy, which predisposes individuals to CAD at a younger age. Additionally it is important to screen for increased Lp(a) in patients in whom statin treatment does not lower the LDL cholesterol to the desired target level, because Lp(a) can inhibit LDL clearance.

OTHER CV RISK FACTORS

Smoking

Smoking represents the leading modifiable cause of death in the United States, despite the decreased use of tobacco in the last 25 years. People who smoke one pack of cigarettes a day are two times more likely to suffer from a myocardial infarction, die from cardiovascular disease, or to develop other cardiovascular complications when compared to people who do not smoke. The risk seems to be lesser but still significant for people who smoke cigars or for tobacco chewers.

Smoking increases the risk for cardiovascular disease through several mechanisms. Smoking affects both coagulation factors and platelet function. After cigarette smoking, there is a reduced platelet survival time and increased circulating platelet aggregates, factor V, and plasma fibrinogen.

Smoking reduces oxygen delivery because of carbon monoxide. Smokers increase their levels of carboxyhemoglobin at about 5% per pack smoked a day. Exposure to carbon monoxide during exercise increases the risk for complex ventricular arrhythmias. Smoking causes coronary artery constriction as a result of the alpha adrenergic stimulation. There are also several nicotine-mediated hemodynamic effects including increased heart rate and blood pressure.

Smoking also accelerates atherosclerosis through damage to the endothelium. Inhaled carbon monoxide appears to have a direct effect on endothelium, but the development of atherosclerosis in smokers may result as a consequence of different pathophysiologic pathways. Therefore, smoking acts as a trigger for acute coronary syndromes and stroke and also as an atherogenic factor.

Obesity

Obesity is a worldwide epidemic, and its prevalence is steadily increasing. Excess weight is associated with increased mortality and risk of cardiovascular events. The mechanisms whereby excess body fat affects the cardiovascular system include not only an indirect effect on the vascular system through risk factors like dyslipidemia, hypertension, obstructive sleep apnea, or insulin resistance but also by an enhanced inflammatory state, a high turnover of free fatty acids with a lipotoxic effect on myocardial cells, and the potential effects of high levels of leptin. The American Heart Association has declared that obesity is an independent cardiovascular risk factor. Recent data from myocardial infarction surveillance studies suggest that excess weight is the most common cardiovascular risk factor in patients with myocardial infarction and that its prevalence has increased over time. Nevertheless, obesity is underrecognized, underdiagnosed, and undertreated in persons with acute myocardial infarction.

Diabetes Mellitus

A significant component of the risk associated with type 2 diabetes may be related to its characteristic lipid triad profile of raised small dense-LDL levels, lowered HDL, and elevated triglycerides. When patients are diagnosed with type 2 diabetes mellitus, many have already developed early or advanced atherosclerosis. This observation suggests that the atherogenic effect of metabolic dysregulation starts many years before glucose levels become significantly elevated. Type 2 diabetes mellitus represents a higher risk for cardiovascular events in women than in men, and has a multiplicative effect with smoking. The effect of type 2 diabetes mellitus on the development of atherosclerosis is discussed in Chapter 60 "Diabetes Mellitus and Coronary Artery Disease".

Metabolic Syndrome

Metabolic syndrome (MET-Sx) defines a complex metabolic disturbance characterized by a clustering of risk related to increased levels of one or more of the following: insulin, fasting blood glucose, visceral fat,

triglycerides and blood pressure, and decreased HDL cholesterol levels (Table 1). It is estimated that up to 40% of the US adult population has metabolic syndrome. Subjects with this condition are 2-3 times more likely to develop CAD or to die from a cardiovascular cause, risk that is similar to smoking two packs of cigarettes a day and significantly higher than each of the MET-Sx components alone. Thus, there appears to be synergy between components of the MET-Sx in causing cardiac and vascular disease. MET-Sx also precedes type 2 diabetes mellitus. Recent data show that the MET-Sx is highly prevalent and associated with worse prognosis in patients with an acute myocardial infarction.

The mechanisms linking MET-Sx to cardiovascular disease have not been fully elucidated. By definition, patients with MET-Sx are more likely to have an atherogenic lipid profile because elevated triglycerides and low HDL cholesterol are two out of the three diagnostic criteria for MET-Sx. However, some evidence suggests that the cardiovascular disease mechanisms of MET-Sx go beyond the coexistence of hypertension or the atherogenic lipid profile. For example, patients with MET-Sx have impaired fibrinolysis and increased systemic inflammation, which are also characteristics of OSA. MET-Sx is discussed in detail in Chapter 56 "Metabolic Syndrome".

NOVEL CV RISK FACTORS

C-Reactive Protein

Inflammation plays a key role in the pathogenesis of cardiovascular disease, acute atherothrombotic events, and atherosclerosis. Inflammation also regulates the production of the acute phase proteins such as C-reactive protein (CRP). High-sensitivity CRP is an independent predictor of atherosclerosis, cardiovascular events, atherothrombosis, hypertension, and myocardial infarction, even after considering other cardiovascular risk factors such as age, smoking, obesity, diabetes, hypercholesterolemia, and hypertension. CRP may be a causal factor and not just a marker of risk.

The current AHA/ACC recommendations regarding the use of CRP in the prediction of vascular risk state that patients with an intermediate 10-year cardiac risk (between 10-20%) using the Framingham score (Table

Table 1. AHA Criteria for Clinical Diagnosis of Metabolic Syndrome

Measure (any 3 of 5 constitute diagnosis of metabolic syndrome)	Definitions
Increased waist circumference*†	≥102 cm (≥40 inches) in men
	≥88 cm (≥35 inches) in women
Elevated triglycerides	150 mg/dL (1.7 mmol/L) or
	On drug treatment for elevated triglycerides‡
Decreased HDL-C	<40 mg/dL (<1.03 mmol/L) in men
	<50 mg/dL (<1.3 mmol/L) in women or
	On drug treatment for reduced HDL-C‡
Elevated blood pressure	>130 mm Hg systolic blood pressure or
	>85 mm Hg diastolic blood pressure or
	On antihypertensive drug treatment in a patient with a history of hypertension
Increased fasting glucose	>100 mg/dL or
	On drug treatment for elevated glucose

*To measure waist circumference, locate top of right iliac crest. Place a measuring tape in a horizontal plane around abdomen at level of iliac crest. Before reading tape measure, ensure that tape is snug but does not compress the skin and is parallel to floor. Measurement is made at the end of a normal expiration.

†Some US adults of nonAsian origin (eg, white, black, Hispanic) with marginally increased waist circumference (eg, 94-101 cm [37-39 inches] in men and 80-87 cm [31-34 inches] in women) may have strong genetic contribution to insulin resistance and should benefit from changes in lifestyle habits, similar to men with categorical increases in waist circumference. Lower waist circumference cutpoint (eg, ≥90 cm [35 inches] in men and ≥80 cm [31 inches] in women) appears to be appropriate for Asian Americans.

‡Fibrates and nicotinic acid are the most commonly used drugs for elevated TG and reduced HDL-C. Patients taking one of these drugs are presumed to have high TG and low HDL.

2), can be better stratified using CRP. CRP and novel risk factors are discussed in detail in Chapter 59 "Novel Risk Markers for Atherosclerosis".

Homocysteine

Homocysteine is a nonessential sulphur-containing amino acid. Several epidemiologic studies have linked hyperhomocysteinemia with an increased risk for coronary artery disease, although the findings are inconsistent. Levels of homocysteine and cardiovascular disease have also been linked to folate status. Hyperhomocysteinemia may result in direct endothelial injury and a predisposition to a prothrombotic state. Many patients with hyperhomocysteinemia and atherosclerotic vascular disease are also deficient in vitamin B_6 or B_{12}. Despite multiple epidemiologic and basic research

studies in patients with mild to moderate hyperhomocysteinemia, results from recent clinical trials do not support supplementation with vitamin B_6 and folic acid in patients with mild elevation of homocysteine.

Lipoprotein-Associated Phospholipase A2

Lipoprotein-associated phospholipase A_2 (Lp-PLA$_2$) has been proposed as a predictor of CVD event. This enzyme is a member of the phospholipase A_2 superfamily and is produced by monocytes, T-lymphocytes and mast cells. In plasma, ~ 80% of Lp-PLA$_2$ is bound to LDL, and the remaining 20% is linked to HDL and very low-density lipoproteins. Lp-PLA$_2$ has a role in the hydrolysis of oxidized LDL and the resulting formation of lysophosphatidylcholine (LysoPC), a proatherogenic and inflammatory mediator. Lyso PC is

Table 2. Framingham Risk Score*†

Risk factor	Points in men	Points in women
Age group	–9 to 13	–7 to 16
Total cholesterol	0 to 11	0 to 13
Smoking status	0 to 8	0 to 9
HDL levels	–1 to 2	–1 to 2
Systolic blood pressure and treatment status	0 to 3	0 to 6
Diabetes (yes/no)	0 to 2	0 to 2

*This update of the 1991 Framingham coronary prediction algorithm provides estimates of total CAD risk (risk of developing one of the following: angina pectoris, myocardial infarction, or coronary disease death) over the course of 10 years. Separate score sheets are used for men and women and the factors used to estimate risk include age, blood cholesterol (or LDL cholesterol), HDL cholesterol, blood pressure, cigarette smoking, and diabetes mellitus. Relative risk for CAD is estimated by comparison to low risk Framingham participants.

†Estimated 10-year risk by summing points, range from <1% to ≥30%.

an important chemoattractant for macrophage and T-cell, induces migration of vascular smooth muscle cells, affects endothelial function, and increases the expression of adhesion molecules and cytokines. On the other hand, several studies support an antiinflammatory function of Lp-PLA₂. The protein has been shown to play a role in the hydrolysis of the platelet-activating factor (PAF) and manifest a possible antiatherogenic effect when high levels of Lp-PLA₂ are associated with HDL in mice.

Several epidemiological studies have investigated the association between plasma Lp-PLA₂ levels and the risk of subsequent CVD events. Pooled evidence shows that plasma Lp-PLA₂ levels predict CVD beyond traditional risk factors.

Obstructive Sleep Apnea and Ischemic Heart Disease
Obstructive sleep apnea (OSA) activates multiple disease mechanisms associated with myocardial ischemia and infarction. Nocturnal ST segment changes consistent with myocardial ischemia are evident even in patients with OSA who do not have clinically significant coronary artery disease. OSA may contribute to nocturnal angina, and ST depression during sleep appears to be related to the severity of oxygen desaturation. Treatment with CPAP attenuates nocturnal ST depression.

Multiple cohort studies support the notion that OSA is associated with cardiovascular disease. The observational data provide a sound basis for suspecting a causal relationship between OSA and cardiovascular outcomes because the major causality corollaries are met: 1) there is an association between OSA and the *presence* of coronary artery disease; 2) the association is graded based on the severity of OSA; 3) there is a temporal relationship; 4) the risk seems to be attenuated after treatment of OSA. Details of the association between OSA and cardiovascular disease are discussed in Chapter 85 "Sleep Apnea and Cardiac Disease".

TREATMENT STRATEGIES

Treatment Strategies and Goals in Dyslipidemia
The recommendations for treatment of dyslipidemia are based on the Adult Treatment Panel III (ATP III) guidelines published in 2001 and updated in 2004. The management of dyslipidemia is based on the underlying risk for coronary artery disease. The principle target of treatment is LDL cholesterol after secondary causes of hypercholesterolemia have been ruled-out (Table 3). Secondary targets are HDL cholesterol and triglycerides. There is overwhelming evidence that treating hypercholesterolemia in patients with and without CAD improves survival and reduces the incidence of cardiovascular events.

The LDL cholesterol goal depends on the underlying cardiovascular risk. For patients with a clinical history of coronary artery disease, the goal is to achieve an LDL cholesterol of <100 mg/dL. This goal also applies to patients with CAD equivalent such as presence of peripheral vascular disease, abdominal aortic aneurysm, history of stroke, or diabetes mellitus. Patients with CAD or CAD equivalent considered at "very high risk" (those with other modifiable CV risk factors that have not been fully controlled like current

Table 3. Causes of Secondary Hyperlipidemia

Hypertriglyceridemia	Hypercholesterolemia
Excessive alcohol or simple sugars	Excessive dietary cholesterol or saturated fats (or both)
Contraceptives, estrogens, pregnancy	Hypothyroidism
Obesity	Obstructive liver disease
Type 2 diabetes	Nephrotic syndrome
Chronic renal failure	Multiple myeloma or dysglobulinemia
Cushing's disease, corticosteroid therapy	Progestational agents and anabolic steroids

smokers or uncontrolled diabetes mellitus) need to have LDL cholesterol lowered to less than 70 mg/dL.

Among patients without CAD or CAD equivalent, the Framingham risk score can determine if they belong to a moderate or low-risk category for CAD. Further details in LDL cholesterol goals according to the underlying CVD risk are displayed in Table 4.

Epidemiologic research suggests that patients with a high HDL and mild elevation of LDL cholesterol have a CAD risk comparable to patients with normal LDL and subgroup analyses from clinical trials have shown that the clinical benefit of statins is reduced in patients with a low LDL/HDL ratio. However, the current ATP III guidelines do not base any recommendations on LDL/HDL ratios. Patients with elevated LDL would require pharmacologic treatment even if they have a high HDL, as long as they meet criteria based on the Framingham risk score and/or presence of coronary disease or coronary disease equivalent. Conversely, patients with relatively normal LDL cholesterol (between 100-130 mg/dL) with a low HDL may require lipid-lowering therapy if they have other major cardiovascular risk factors resulting in a high Framingham risk score. In both circumstances, patients with high HDL and high LDL or patients with normal LDL with a low HDL should have target LDL values based on the overall Framingham risk score or on the presence of coronary artery disease. A special

challenge are patients who have more than one risk factor for coronary disease that are not accounted in the Framingham score, such as family history of coronary disease in first-degree relatives, central obesity, obstructive sleep apnea, elevated lipoprotein (a), a high ApoB/Apo A1 ratio or chronic renal failure. In those situations, the clinicians should exercise their judgment to determine how low they want the LDL to be. As mentioned in the beginning of this chapter, the current definition of "normal" cholesterol may be too conservative and therefore a more aggressive approach in patients with increased CAD risk—either with traditional risk scores or using novel risk factors—might be of clinical benefit.

Every patient with hypercholesterolemia needs to receive dietary recommendations and to increase his level of physical activity. The optimal dietary recommendations for the management of hypercholesterolemia include a limited fat intake, restricted calories if obesity is present, and increase in the intake of vegetables and fruit. The focus on dietary modification should be on reducing consumption of saturated fat, trans fatty acids, and dietary cholesterol, while allowing "good" fats like mono- and polyunsaturated fatty acids. Patients following these recommendations can achieve a decrease in LDL cholesterol of up to 20%. Some subgroups of patients may have a higher reduction in LDL cholesterol with dietary changes alone, especially those who are fully compliant with the dietary recommendations and those without a genetic trait for dyslipidemia.

Patients at high risk for cardiovascular disease may benefit from receiving lipid-lowering therapy and therapeutic lifestyle changes at the same time. Patients with low-to-moderate risk may start with therapeutic lifestyle changes for three to six months and to start lipid-lowering therapy if the target LDL cholesterol is not achieved. Patients need to be aware that a high intake of saturated fat is a risk factor independent of serum lipids and therefore they should modify their diet even if cholesterol medications achieve LDL cholesterol values.

Patients with isolated low HDL cholesterol represent a special challenge. The priority should be to maintain LDL cholesterol in target values, increase the level of physical activity, and to allow some mono- and polyunsaturated fatty acids in the diet. When patients have a very low HDL cholesterol (less than 25 mg/dL), it would be unrealistic to expect normalization

Table 4.   National Cholesterol Education Program Adult Treatment Panel III for Lipid-Lowering Therapy Recommendations

Risk category	LDL-C goal	Initiate TLC*	Consider drug therapy
High risk: CAD or CAD risk equivalents*(10-year risk >20%)	<100 mg/dL Optional goal: <70 mg/dL	≥100 mg/dL	≥100 mg/dL (≤100 mg/dL optional)‡
Moderately high risk: 2+ risk factors† (10-year risk 10% to 20%)	<130 mg/dL <100 mg/dL		≥130 mg/dL (100-129 mg/dL optional)
Moderate risk: 2+ risk factors (10-year risk <10%)	<130 mg/dL	≥130 mg/dL	≥160 mg/dL
Lower risk: 0-1 risk factor	160 mg/dL	≥160 mg/dL	≥190 mg/dL (160-190 mg/dL optional)

*CAD risk equivalents include history of peripheral vascular disease, abdominal aortic aneurysm, history of stroke or diabetes mellitus.

†Risk factors include cigarette smoking, hypertension, low HDL cholesterol (<40 mg/dl), family history of premature CAD (first degree male relative <55 years; female <65 years), and age (men ≥45 years; women ≥years). If TG 200-499 mg/dL: consider fibrate or niacin after LDL-lowering therapy. If TG ≥500 mg/dL: consider fibrate or niacin before LDL-lowering therapy. Consider omega-3 fatty acids as adjunct for high TG.

‡Patients with recent MI; smoking and previous MI; diabetes mellitus and previous MI or in the setting of an acute coronary syndrome.

of HDL with lifestyle modification alone. In that situation, medications like fibrates or nicotinic acid should be considered, particularly in patients with CAD or CAD equivalent. Factors associated with a high or low level of HDL cholesterol are listed in Table 5.

Patients with isolated hypertriglyceridemia have a good response rate with dietary changes, especially if triglycerides are not higher than 400 mg/dL. Patients on diets with limited refined carbohydrates have shown significant improvement in fasting triglyceride levels. Patients with very high triglyceride levels (more than 500 mg/dL) require immediate treatment to prevent the development of pancreatitis.

Smoking Cessation

Two major meta-analyses assessing the effect of smoking cessation in patients with or without established CAD attributed a 36% reduction of cardiovascular mortality and a 46% reduction in overall mortality to smoking cessation.

Table 5.   Factors Influencing Levels of High Density Lipoprotein

Relatively high levels	Relatively low levels
Females	Males
Blacks in United States	Whites in United States
Exercise	Diabetes
Estrogen	Hypertriglyceridemia
Alcohol	High-carbohydrate diet
Weight reduction	Obesity
Nicotinic acid	Smoking
Fibric acid derivatives	Progesterone
Chlorinated hydro-carbons	Antihypertensive drugs
Familial hyperalphalipo-proteinemia	Sedentary lifestyle
Insulin	

The AHA/ACC recommendation for smoking cessation in primary and secondary prevention is to achieve a complete cessation by providing counseling and pharmacological therapy (which may include nicotine replacement and bupropion). Although most patients who smoke will want to quit after a myocardial infarction, relapse rates can be high. Nicotine replacement therapy, the most frequent pharmacological intervention, has shown minimum benefit when compared to placebo. Because nicotine appears to have cardiotoxic effects during acute ischemic events, nicotine replacement therapy should not be used in a patient experiencing an acute coronary syndrome. For many smokers, however, the question is not whether they will get nicotine, but rather how they will get their nicotine. Because nicotine replacement delivers only about half the dose of nicotine and none of the tar and carbon monoxide delivered by cigarettes, clinicians feel comfortable prescribing nicotine replacement to smokers with stable coronary artery disease. Although bupropion has not been studied in patients with CAD, a panel of experts has concluded that use of bupropion increases the odds of success. If the patient can be entered into a structured program of support, the odds of cessation increase markedly.

Weight Loss

Data from weight loss programs in patients with CAD are limited. Data from small trials have shown that a combination of exercise and diet can effectively induce weight loss in patients with CAD, but attrition is high. When this approach fails, patients can be offered bariatric surgery, which is an effective option for treatment of high-risk obese patients (BMI ≥40). Bariatric surgery, especially gastric bypass, has shown great improvements in many of the major cardiovascular risk factors, such as hypertension, dyslipidemia, diabetes, and obstructive sleep apnea. Mortality for gastric bypass is estimated to be less than 1%, although postoperative complications may occur in up to 20% of patients.

The evidence for long-term efficacy of pharmacologic intervention in weight loss is limited to two medications: sibutramine and orlistat. Treatment with sibutramine produces significantly more maintained weight loss at 2 years than placebo, but the drug is contraindicated in patients with CAD. Orlistat, a medications that blocks the absorption of fat, causes weight loss of about 2.2 kilograms greater than placebo at 4 years, with significantly more patients achieving ≥10% loss of initial body weight (26.2% and 15.6%, respectively).

New drugs like the cannabinoid-1 receptor blocker rimonabant are being studied both for weight loss and smoking cessation. The drug appears to act by decreasing appetite in the brain and stimulating satiety in the gastrointestinal tract. A recent randomized control trial has shown a 6.6 kg greater weight loss with rimonabant (20 mg) when compared to placebo after one year of treatment. Moreover, triglycerides and insulin levels were reduced and HDL-C was increased. Side effects, mild and well tolerated, were mainly limited to dizziness, nausea and diarrhea.

Other medications such as thyroid hormone, amphetamines, phentermine, amfepramone (diethylpropion), phenylpropanolamine, mazindol, and fenfluramines increase risk of angina pectoris, myocardial infarction and death because they increase oxygen demand and vasospasm. Therefore, these medications are contraindicated for weight loss in the secondary prevention of CAD.

The AHA/ACC recommendations for weight control in patients with CAD include calculating BMI and measuring waist circumference during the clinical evaluation and using these measures to monitor response to therapy. The goal of weight management is to achieve a BMI between 18.5 and 24.9 kg/m². When the BMI is 25 kg/m² or greater, the waist circumference goal is <40 inches in men and <35 inches in women.

Diet in Secondary Prevention of Coronary Artery Disease

Many different diets have been advocated for patients with CAD. The diet endorsed by the AHA limits the intake of fat to 30% or less of total calories, from which <10% should come from saturated fat. In recent years, the Mediterranean diet has emerged as a "prudent" diet backed by several clinical trials using hard outcomes in patients with CAD. The Mediterranean diet consists mainly of legumes, cereals, fruits and vegetables with moderate amounts of fish, olive oil, and wine. Consumption of dairy products and meats is limited. The Mediterranean diet is low in saturated fat and high in omega-3 fatty acids.

Dietary recommendations in patients with obesity require caloric restriction and avoid focusing the attention on different types of macronutrients only.

Exercise and Physical Activity

Physical activity can be defined as movements produced by skeletal muscles that result in energy expenditure beyond basal normal energy expenditure. The three major components of exercise and physical fitness are: **dose, intensity and type**. Dose refers to the amount of energy expended in physical activity (kilocalories) and intensity reflects the rate of energy expended during activity. Absolute intensity is usually measured in metabolic equivalents or METs (1 MET = resting metabolic rate @ 3.5 mL O_2/Kg/min), and relative intensity is the percent of aerobic power utilized during exercise and is expressed as the percent of the maximal heart rate or percent of maximum oxygen consumption (VO_2max): moderate-intensity activities are those performed at a relative intensity of 40% to 60% of VO_2max (absolute of 4 to 6 METs), and vigorous intensity >60% of VO_2max (>6 METs). Type of exercise refers to the type of stress on the muscles: isometric (load without movement), isotonic (movement without load), or resistance (movement against a load).

Exercise in patients with CAD in cardiac rehabilitations programs should be increased gradually. Vigorous physical activity increases the risk of myocardial infarction and sudden death, especially in sedentary patients or those with preexisting CAD. Indeed, approximately 5% to 10% of myocardial infarctions are preceded by vigorous physical activity. These facts emphasize the need for well-established physical activity programs that must be gradually increased in time and intensity and with proper supervision.

However, a properly implemented exercise program can decrease mortality rates by up to 27% after myocardial infarction, and a comprehensive rehabilitation program that includes psychosocial and/or educational interventions can decrease mortality rates by up to 31%.

Health professionals should prescribe a well-supervised physical activity program to patients with CAD regardless of age, as elderly patients have similar trainability when compared to younger patients. Therefore, older patients should be encouraged to follow a guided exercise cardiac rehabilitation plan to prevent musculoskeletal injuries. About one-quarter of adults who participate in an exercise program will suffer injuries within a year and, as a result, one-third will stop exercising. An exercise stress test should be used to assess risk and guide prescription.

Exercise Prescription (Table 6)

Exercise should be prescribed in any sedentary patient with moderate or high risk for CAD. The concept "prescription" assumes that the recommendation will be given by a health care provider and that will include at least the following elements:

1) Type of exercise
   The emphasis should be an aerobic exercise like fast walking, jogging, swimming, biking, or other activities that allow a gradual increase in heart rate. Different types of exercise may be needed for patients with special needs (patients with amputations, musculoskeletal conditions, etc.).
2) Intensity
   The two best ways to determine the target intensity of exercise is by achieving between 70-85%

Table 6.   Components of an Exercise Prescription in Primary Prevention of CAD

Type of exercise
- Emphasis on aerobic exercise like fast walking, jogging, swimming, biking, or
- Other activities that allow a gradual increase in heart rate

Intensity
- Achieving between 70-85% of maximum predicted heart rate or
- By the subjective feeling of mildly hard to hard physical effort

Duration
- No more than 10-15 minutes of exercise (sedentary patients)
- Increased gradually five additional minutes every two weeks if tolerated with a goal of 30-45 minutes of aerobic exercise

Frequency
- Five days a week of exercise is recommended in most patients
- Patients also find it easier to develop a daily routine than exercising three to five times a week

of maximum predicted heart rate or by the subjective feeling of mildly hard to hard physical effort. Patients should avoid overexercising to prevent musculoskeletal injuries or even triggering acute coronary syndromes due to atherosclerotic plaque rupture.

3) Duration

For completely sedentary patients, they should start with no more than 10-15 minutes of exercise. This can be increased gradually five additional minutes every two weeks if tolerated, with a goal of 30-45 minutes of aerobic exercise.

4) Frequency

A minimum of five days a week of exercise is recommended in most patients. Patients also find it easier to develop a daily routine than exercising three to five times a week.

Cardiologists should always include practical recommendations for increasing nonexercise physical activity like using stairs and doing small bursts of fast walking during the day to really achieve a meaningful total level of oxygen consumption a day.

Patients with a recent myocardial infarction, a history of congestive heart failure, or ventricular arrhythmias need to be enrolled in a supervised exercise program in a medical setting or cardiac rehabilitation program.

NOVEL RISK MARKERS FOR ATHEROSCLEROSIS

Iftikhar J. Kullo, MD

Cardiovascular risk assessment is a necessary first step prior to implementing preventive and therapeutic interventions. Two algorithms for cardiovascular risk stratification are recommended in the National Cholesterol Education Program (NCEP) Adult Treatment Panel (ATP) III guidelines. The first algorithm involves counting major risk factors and then estimating the 10-year probability of coronary artery disease (CAD) based on an equation derived from the Framingham Study. The second algorithm identifies the presence of the metabolic syndrome. These predictive models have less than desired accuracy in predicting CAD risk in an individual subject, in part because of the widespread prevalence of conventional risk factors in the general population. Thus, although most patients who suffer a cardiovascular event will have one or more of the conventional risk factors, so do many subjects who do not have CAD.

Consequently, there is increasing interest in evaluating circulating biomarkers related to the atherosclerotic process, as well as newer imaging modalities and tests of arterial function that might improve cardiovascular risk stratification (Fig. 1 and Table 1). Risk factors can be classified into several categories (Table 1). NCEP guidelines suggest that 'novel' risk markers… "are associated with increased risk for coronary artery disease although their causative, independent, and

quantitative contributions to coronary artery disease are not well documented." Novel risk markers include C-reactive protein (CRP), fibrinogen, homocysteine, Lp(a), and low-density lipoprotein (LDL) particle size. A fourth category that can be added is that of 'emerging' risk markers (Table 1). The reported association of these factors to CAD will need further confirmatory studies. This chapter provides an update on the "novel" risk markers. The main focus is on the potential utility of these risk markers in the prediction of CAD risk in asymptomatic subjects. The putative mechanisms of

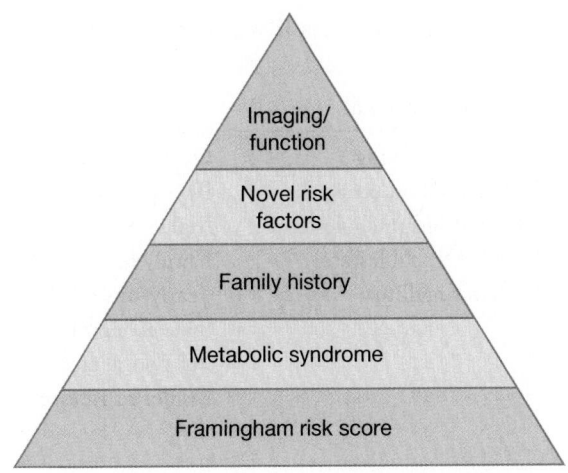

Fig. 1. The cardiovascular risk stratification pyramid.

Table 1.   The Need for Studying Novel Risk
            Markers

Current predictive models have less than desired
    accuracy in predicting CAD risk in an individ-
    ual subject
Conventional risk factors explain <50% of the
    variability in quantitative measures of athero-
    sclerotic vascular disease (assessed by coronary
    angiography or electron-beam computed
    tomography)
The risk of CAD varies among different ethnic
    groups and "novel" risk markers may partly
    explain the variation. An example is the elevated
    CAD risk of South Asians for a given level of
    conventional risk factors. In this ethnic group,
    "novel" risk markers such as insulin resistance,
    lipoprotein(a) (Lp[a]), and homocysteine may
    be important in causation of atherosclerosis
Identifying new risk markers may lead to new
    preventive and therapeutic approaches

risk and the assays available for the measurement of
these risk markers are summarized in Tables 2 and 3.
The evidence for association with atherosclerotic vascular disease and the clinical implications thereof are
discussed below for each novel risk marker.

C-Reactive Protein (CRP)

Although cytokines and cell adhesion molecules are
directly involved in the immune response, assays tend
to have high coefficients of variation. The relatively stable acute-phase reactant CRP is the most widely studied of the inflammatory markers and has been shown
to be a predictor of cardiovascular events in otherwise
asymptomatic patients. In recent years, several prospective studies have related baseline CRP levels to the
future risk of cardiovascular events. In a nested case-
control study of 2,459 patients who had myocardial
infarction or died of CAD derived from a prospective
study of 18,569 participants, CRP in the top tertile
(versus the bottom tertile) was associated with an odds
ratio of 1.45 (Fig. 2). A similar odds ratio was noted in
an accompanying meta-analysis. CRP was a weaker
predictor than increased total cholesterol and smoking
and provided only modest additional risk information
suggesting that the risk due to elevated CRP may have
been overestimated in prior studies.

Clinical Implications

Although several atherogenic properties have been
attributed to CRP (Table 2), CRP does not appear to
be strongly related to extent of coronary atherosclerosis
and may therefore reflect plaque inflammation and
"instability" rather than plaque burden. In a retrospective cohort study, combined assessment of CRP and

Table 2.   Categories of Risk Factors for CAD

Conventional	Predisposing	Novel	Emerging
Cigarette smoking	Overweight and obesity	C-reactive protein	Lipoprotein-associated
Elevated blood pressure	Physical inactivity	Fibrinogen	phospholipase A_2
Elevated serum cholesterol	Male sex	Homocysteine	Pregnancy associated
Low HDL cholesterol	Family history of	Lipoprotein (a)	plasma phosphatase
Diabetes mellitus	early-onset CAD	Small LDL particle	Asymmetric dimethyl-
	Socioeconomic factors	size	arginine
	Behavioral factors		B-type natriuretic
	Insulin resistance		peptide
			Myeloperoxidase
			Measures of oxidative
			stress
			Candidate gene
			polymorphisms

Table 3.   Novel Risk Markers: Mechanisms of Risk

Risk marker	Normal values	Factors influencing marker	Mechanisms mediating risk
CRP	<3 mg/L	Acute phase response, adiposity, metabolic syndrome, poor orodental hygiene, smoking, estrogen use	Increased expression of tissue factor and plasminogen activator inhibitor-1 Activation of complement Decreased nitric oxide production
Fibrinogen	<400 mg/dL	Smoking, increasing age, adiposity, diabetes, and menopause; African Americans tend to have higher levels	Increased plasma viscosity Increased platelet aggregability Vascular smooth muscle proliferation
Homocysteine	<13 μmoL/L	Aging, menopause, hypothyroidism, low plasma levels of vitamin cofactors (B_6, B_{12}, and folate), and chronic renal insufficiency	Increased oxidative stress Vascular smooth muscle proliferation Activation of factor V Inhibition of protein C Enhanced platelet aggregation Activation of NF-κB
Lipoprotein (a)	<30 mg/dL	Renal insufficiency, nephrotic syndrome, diabetes, and menopause. African Americans having higher median levels of Lp(a) than Caucasians	Impaired fibrinolysis Delivery of cholesterol at sites of arterial injury Vascular smooth muscle cell proliferation Endothelial dysfunction
LDL particle size	>265 Å	Obesity, metabolic syndrome, diabetes, and physical activity	Increased ability to cross into the subintimal space Increased binding to intimal proteoglycans Susceptibility to oxidation Reduced affinity for LDL receptor

coronary artery calcium (a surrogate for coronary atherosclerotic plaque burden) had greater predictive value for cardiovascular events than either measure alone. This observation needs confirmation in a prospective study. Guidelines issued jointly by the American Heart Association and the Centers for Disease Control and Prevention suggest optional use of CRP in patients at intermediate risk of CAD based on the Framingham risk equation. A trial is under way that will randomize 15,000 patients with elevated CRP and LDL levels below 100 mg/dL—and who would not therefore qualify for lipid-lowering therapy—to treatment with a statin or to placebo.

FIBRINOGEN

Fibrinogen is an important component of the coagulation pathway, a major determinant of plasma viscosity, and also an acute-phase reactant. Higher plasma fibrinogen concentration has been consistently associated with increased risk of cardiovascular events in multiple studies. Fibrinogen levels are associated with several conventional CAD risk factors, and when these factors are included in multivariate analyses, the association between fibrinogen and cardiovascular disease is attenuated but remains statistically significant. In the largest meta-analysis to date, strong associations of plasma fibrinogen concentration with the risk of CAD, stroke,

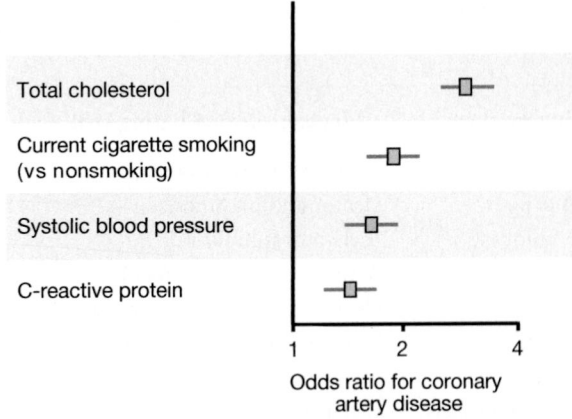

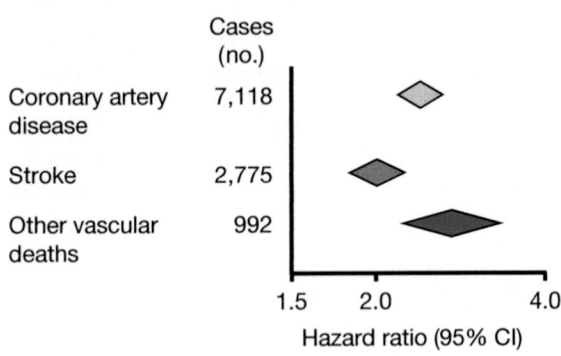

Fig. 2. Odds ratios for coronary artery disease among 2,459 patients with coronary artery disease and 3,969 controls. Comparisons are between patients and controls with values in the top third and those in the bottom third of the distribution of values for controls, except for comparisons involving smoking status. Squares denote odds ratios, and horizontal lines represent 95 percent confidence intervals.

Fig. 3. Hazard ratios for cardiovascular disease per 1-g/L increase in fibrinogen level adjusted for age at screening and stratified by sex, cohort, and trial group. CI indicates confidence interval.

and other vascular mortality were noted in healthy middle-aged adults (Fig. 3). For CAD, the hazard ratio per 1 g/L higher fibrinogen was 2.42 (95% CI 2.24-2.60). After adjustment for established cardiovascular risk factors, the hazard ratio decreased to 1.82 (95% CI, 1.60-2.06).

Clinical Implications

Establishing a standardized assay and uniform cutoffs will increase the utility of fibrinogen as a predictor of CAD risk, particularly since compared to CRP fibrinogen is less likely to be affected by minor inflammatory stimuli and may therefore prove to be a more specific marker. A drug that specifically lowers fibrinogen levels is not yet available; however, availability of such a drug would allow randomized controlled trials to assess the results of fibrinogen lowering on cardiovascular events.

HOMOCYSTEINE

Homocysteine is a sulfur-containing amino acid intermediate formed during the metabolism of methionine, an essential amino acid. McCully demonstrated severe arteriosclerosis in children and young adults with inborn errors of homocysteine metabolism such as cystathionine beta synthase deficiency. Because these dis-

orders are associated with markedly elevated plasma homocysteine levels (>100 μmol/L), McCully postulated that mild to moderate elevations in plasma homocysteine might contribute to atherosclerotic vascular disease.

Despite the demonstrated atherogenic properties of homocysteine (Table 2), it remains to be established whether homocysteine is causal factor for or simply a marker of atherosclerotic vascular disease. Most, but not all, prospective studies of homocysteine and cardiovascular risk show homocysteine to be associated with cardiovascular events. A recent meta-analysis reported that in prospective studies, the increase in risk of cardiovascular events due to elevated homocysteine is modest. After adjustment for the conventional cardiovascular risk factors, a 25% lower homocysteine level was associated with an 11% lower CHD risk and 19% lower stroke risk (Fig. 4).

Clinical Implications

The association of plasma homocysteine concentration with vascular disease is well-established. However, results of several large randomized controlled trials indicate that homocysteine lowering with folic acid and B vitamins does not reduce cardiovascular events. At present, therefore, lowering of homocysteine with folic acid and B vitamins is not recommended for patients with vascular disease, and alternate therapies to reduce homocysteine levels may need to be evaluated.

LIPOPROTEIN (a) (Lp[a])

Lp(a) is a circulating lipoprotein that resembles LDL cholesterol in core lipid composition and in having apoB-100 as a surface apolipoprotein. In addition, it possesses a unique glycoprotein, apo(a), which is bound to apoB-100 by a disulfide bond (Fig. 5). Apo(a) is a glycosylated protein that resembles plasminogen and is comprised of serial "kringle" domains linked to an inactive protease domain. The physiological function of Lp(a) remains obscure, although a role in wound healing has been proposed. Several prospective studies have found Lp(a) levels to be related to future cardiovascular events, with the exception of the Physicians Health Study, Lp(a). A meta-analysis of 27 prospective studies including 5,000 subjects with a mean follow-up of 10 years concluded that an elevated Lp(a) level was an independent risk factor for future CAD events (Fig. 6). Individuals in the top tertile of baseline Lp(a) levels were at a 60% higher risk for a CAD event compared to those in the bottom tertile.

The conflicting data from the prospective studies may be due to variability in the methods used to deter-mine Lp(a) levels and the fact that different isoforms of apo(a) may differ in their atherogenic potential. Elevated Lp(a) levels may be more atherogenic in the presence of small apo(a) size (defined as <22 kringle 4 [K4] repeats) versus larger apo(a) isoforms. In African Americans, high Lp(a) levels are less likely to be associated with the presence of small apo(a) isoforms than in Caucasians. This observation may explain why elevated Lp(a) levels have not been consistently associated with increased CAD risk in African Americans.

Clinical Implications

Measurement of Lp(a) levels may be useful in subjects with early-onset CAD, a family history of early-onset CAD, or those who develop CAD in the absence of conventional risk factors. Levels may need to be measured only once because of little variability within an individual. If elevated levels are detected, testing and counseling of family members may be warranted. The detection of high Lp(a) levels in a patient with CAD or a patient at risk for developing CAD may be an indication for more aggressive therapy and may motivate

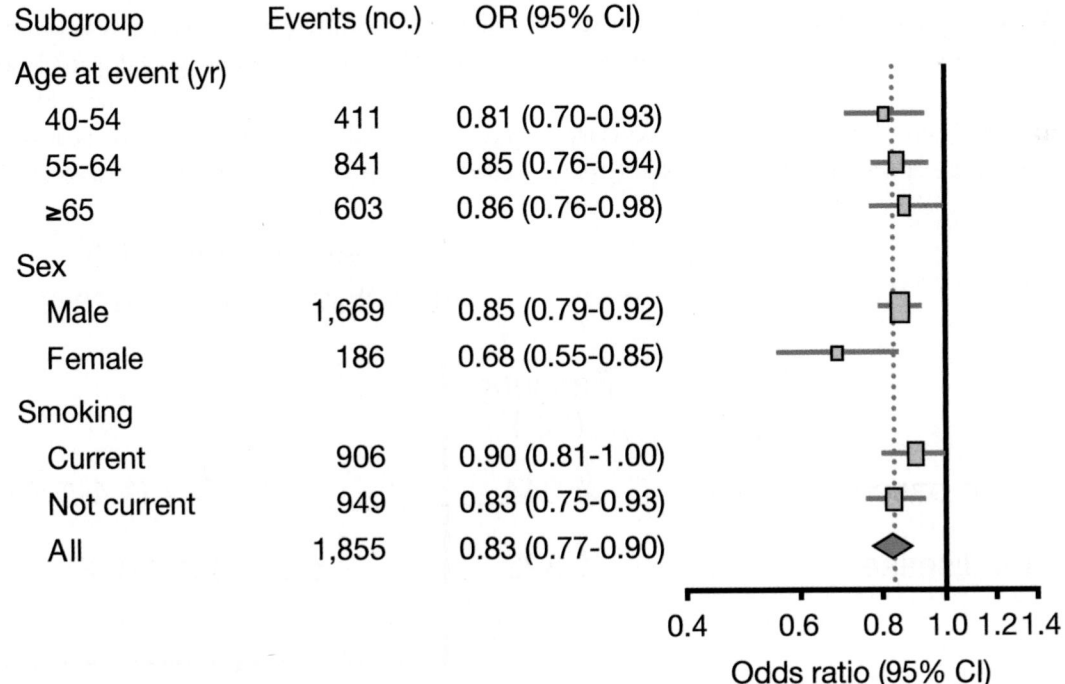

Subgroup	Events (no.)	OR (95% CI)
Age at event (yr)		
40-54	411	0.81 (0.70-0.93)
55-64	841	0.85 (0.76-0.94)
≥65	603	0.86 (0.76-0.98)
Sex		
Male	1,669	0.85 (0.79-0.92)
Female	186	0.68 (0.55-0.85)
Smoking		
Current	906	0.90 (0.81-1.00)
Not current	949	0.83 (0.75-0.93)
All	1,855	0.83 (0.77-0.90)

Fig. 4. Odds ratio of coronary artery disease for a 25% lower than usual homocysteine level among people in prospective studies. Studies are grouped by age at event, sex, and smoking history. The horizontal lines indicate the 95% confidence intervals (CIs). The diamond indicates the total and its 95% CI.

LDL-moiety   **Apolipoprotein (a)**

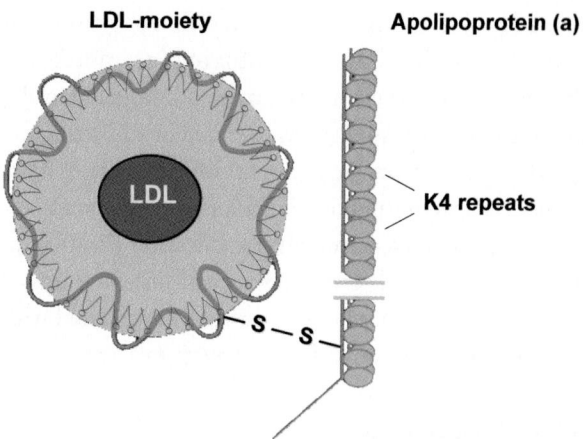

Fig. 5. The structure of the Lp(a) molecule.

patients to make lifestyle changes. A standardized assay for Lp(a) that is insensitive to apo(a) heterogeneity has been recommended. Further refinement of the assays to include information about size of Lp(a) isoforms may improve their predictive value and provide new insights into the role of Lp(a) in atherogenesis. Drugs that specifically lower Lp(a) levels are not yet available.

LDL PARTICLE SIZE

LDL particles differ in size and density. Two distinct phenotypes have been described: pattern B with a predominance of small, dense LDL particles and pattern A with a higher proportion of large, more buoyant LDL particles. Small LDL particles tend to coexist with elevated triglycerides and low HDL cholesterol.

This trait has been called "atherogenic dyslipidemia" and appears to be highly heritable. Small LDL particle size is associated with a number of other cardiovascular risk factors including metabolic syndrome, type II diabetes, and postparandial hypertriglyceridemia. Several retrospective studies show smaller LDL particle size to be associated with an increased risk for CAD. These studies, however, do not clearly establish whether this risk is mediated independent of the coexisting lipoprotein abnormalities. Among prospective studies, the Quebec Heart Study showed LDL particle size to be an independent risk factor, whereas in two other studies, the trait was not independently predictive after adjustment for HDL cholesterol and triglycerides.

Clinical Implications

Although LDL particle size is significantly correlated with plasma triglyceride level, a proportion of subjects with small LDL may not have concomitant elevation of triglycerides. A potential use of measuring LDL particle size may be in aiding decision making regarding the choice of a lipid-lowering agent. Multiple assays, which provide information about LDL particle size and composition, are available for clinical use (Table 3), but large prospective trials that compare the predictive value of these different assays for risk assessment are needed. The utility of measuring LDL particle size will need to be clarified by further clinical and epidemiological studies. Further study is also needed to determine the effects of pharmacologic and nonpharmacologic therapy

Fig. 6. Risk ratios comparing top and bottom thirds of baseline lipoprotein (a) measurements in perspective studies. Diamonds indicate the combined risk ratio and its 95% confidence interval (CI) for each grouping.

on LDL particle size, and whether such therapy influences subsequent outcomes in clinical trials.

CONCLUSION

Some or all of the novel risk markers are now included in a variety of panels that are available to clinicians. The current ATP III guidelines do not have specific recommendations for the use of these risk factors in clinical practice, although the document mentions their potential utility. The European guidelines for cardiovascular disease prevention also acknowledge that the presence of novel risk markers increases the cardiovascular risk due to conventional risk factors. Guidelines for the use of CRP in clinical practice have already appeared, and it is likely that guidelines will also evolve for the use of the remaining novel risk markers. Measurement of novel risk markers should be considered in selected patients such as those with intermediate 10-year CAD risk or those with family history of early-onset CAD (Fig. 7 and Table 4). The resulting information may motivate the patient to make lifestyle changes and help the physician to adjust the threshold for treatment of conventional risk factors. Pharmacologic therapy is available for each novel risk marker but evidence that such an approach would lead to reduction in cardiovascular events is awaited (Table 5).

FUTURE DIRECTIONS

Atherosclerosis is a complex multifactorial disease process involving multiple pathways and both genetic and environmental factors. Conventional risk factors are important determinants of the burden of atherosclerosis in the general population. Efforts need to be intensified to aggressively treat these risk factors or prevent their onset. Further work is needed to elucidate the role of the newer risk markers in refining cardiovascular risk assessment in an individual. Ideally, a new risk marker should add to risk prediction beyond the traditional risk factors, have a standardized and reproducible assay with established cutoff points to guide interpretation of the results, and have available a therapeutic intervention that leads to a reduction in cardiovascular events.

Many risk markers with small to moderate effects are likely to be identified as a result of advances in the genomic and proteomic sciences. Risk prediction could then become personalized, that is, each individual will be assessed with a panel of tests for risk markers, both biochemical and genetic. Preventive and therapeutic interventions could then be implemented based on the composite risk profile. It may also be possible, with a multimarker approach, to identify alterations in specific atherogenic pathways rather than focusing on individual risk markers.

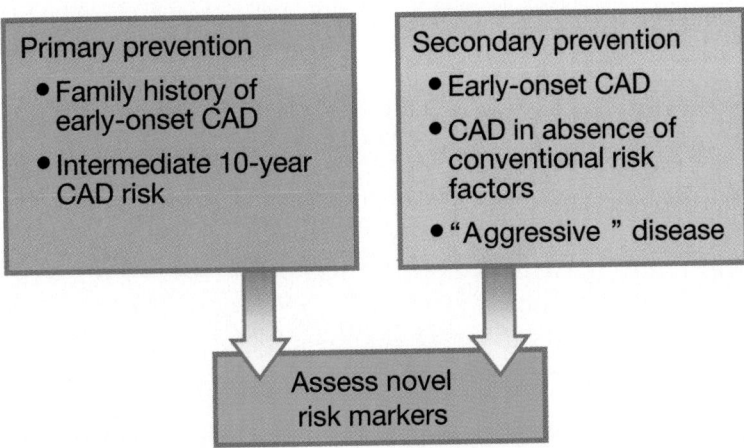

Fig. 7. A potential algorithm for the use of novel risk markers. CHD, coronary heart disease.

Table 4. Assays for Novel Risk Markers

Risk marker	Assays	Comments
CRP	Immunoassays (high sensitivity)	CRP is stable in blood samples and inexpensive, reproducible assays are available.
Fibrinogen	Immunoassay Clotting-time based assay	Levels measured by immunoprecipitation may be more strongly associated with CAD than levels measured by the clotting-time based method.
Homocysteine	High-performance liquid chromatography (HPLC) Enzyme-linked immuno-sorbent assay (ELISA) Mass spectrometry	Nonfasting plasma homocysteine levels have also been shown to be related to future cardiovascular events. Postmethionine load homocysteine levels may classify additional patients as having abnormal methionine metabolism. However at the present time, the clinical utility of the methionine load test is unclear.
Lipoprotein(a)	Gel electrophoresis Immunoassays Lipoprotein electrophoresis	Assay standardization remains a problem. Because apo(a) is variable in size, the antibodies used in immunoassays should react equally well with all apo(a) size isoforms and not cross-react with plasminogen or apoB-100. Information about apo(a) size isoforms may be relevant, as in one study, elevated plasma Lp(a) levels were associated with CAD only among carriers of small apo(a) isoforms.
LDL particle size	Analytic ultracentrifugation Density ultracentrifugation Nondenaturing gradient gel electrophoresis Polyacrylamide gel electrophoresis Nuclear magnetic resonance imaging	Analytic ultracentrifugation is the gold standard, but a difficult and time-consuming method.

Table 5. Lowering Novel Risk Marker Levels

Risk marker	Lifestyle	Drugs	Other
CRP	Weight reduction, smoking cessation, regular exercise, moderate alcohol intake Mediterranean diet, rich in plant sterols, soy protein, viscous fiber, and almonds	Statins Fibrates Fish oil	Drugs that selectively lower CRP are not currently available
Fibrinogen	Smoking cessation, excercise, and moderate alcohol intake Mediterranean diet	Estrogens lower fibrinogen levels in contrast to their effects on raising CRP Fibrates	Drugs that specifically lower fibrinogen are not currently available
Homocysteine	Mediterranean diet	1 mg daily of folic acid alone or supplemented with B_{12} and B_6 In patients with renal failure, much higher doses (up to 20 mg) of folate are often needed to lower homocysteine levels	Based on recent prospective studies, homocysteine lowering with folic acid and B vitamins is not recommended in patients with known vascular disease
Lipoprotein (a)	Diet and exercise have little/no effect	Niacin neomycin Gemfibrozil Omega-3 fatty acids Estrogens	Apheresis is the most effective modality but impractical for most patients. Investigational therapies include selective thyroid hormone receptor stimulation, and inhibitors of disulfide bond formation Statins do not appear to have a significant effect on Lp(a) levels
LDL particle size	Weight reduction, smoking cessation, regular exercise	Fibrates Niacin PPAR (peroxisome-proliferator-activated receptor) agonists	Dual PPAR agonists (α and γ) may have even more favorable effects on LDL particle size Statins have little effect on LDL particle size and primarily reduce the number of LDL particles

60

DIABETES MELLITUS AND CORONARY ARTERY DISEASE

Robert L. Frye, MD

David R. Holmes, Jr, MD

Diabetes mellitus has reached epidemic proportions and continues to increase. Worldwide, the prevalence of diabetes in *all* age groups was estimated to rise from 2.8% in 2000 to a projected 4.4% in 2030. The total number will accordingly increase from 171 million to 366 million diabetic patients in 2030. There is a striking racial interaction (Fig. 1). As can be seen in the age adjusted rates of Americans ≥20 years of age, the prevalence of diabetes is markedly increased in Blacks and Mexican Americans compared to Whites. Mortality rates are also worse in Blacks, Mexican Americans, and Native Americans compared to others. The increase in diabetes has gone hand-in-hand with the marked increase in obesity (Fig. 2).

Type II diabetes has been estimated to account for up to 90-95% of all diagnosed cases of diabetes. In addition to the staggering number of diagnosed cases, a recent United States Department of Health and Human Services study identified that approximately 40% of US adults from 40-71 years of age are "prediabetic." This condition is silent and may not be identified by the patient but results in increasing risk for cardiovascular disease and the development of type II diabetes. The increasing proportion of younger patients with impaired glucose tolerance or type II diabetes represent a critical public health issue with profound future implications for increasing prevalence of cardiovascular

disease in younger age groups after decades that have been spent in hopes of "delaying" cardiovascular disease in the elderly.

Adverse effects of diabetes on short-, intermediate-, and long-term outcome have been the focus of intense investigation. There are societal costs as well as individual adverse outcome measures. It has been estimated that the direct cost of heart disease related to Type II diabetes is $98 billion measured in 2001 dollars. As the prevalence increases, this cost will increase accordingly.

Heart disease is the leading cause of diabetes-related mortality; almost two-thirds of diabetics die of heart or blood vessel disease. In those patients with diabetes, death rates from heart disease are 2-4 times higher than in nondiabetic patients. In addition to heart disease, the presence of diabetes is associated with an increase in the risk of stroke with a relative risk which ranges from 1.6 to almost 6.0. This increased risk is in part related to the increased prevalence of hypertension, which is seen in almost 75% of diabetics and documented in recent National Institutes of Health statistics.

There are substantial gender differences in the outcome of diabetic patients. In women with diabetes, there is a twofold increase in the age-adjusted prevalence of major cardiovascular disease compared with women without diabetes. In addition, there is a signifi-

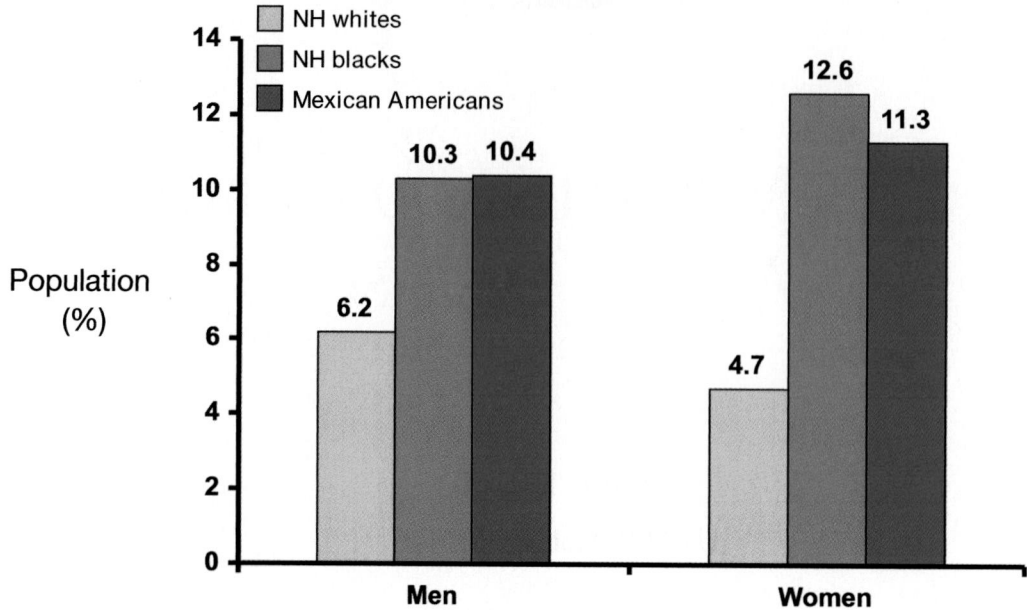

Fig. 1. Age-adjusted prevalence of physician-diagnosed diabetes in Americans age 20 and older by race/ethnicity and sex (NHANES: 1999-2002). NH indicates non-Hispanic.

cantly greater increase in relative risk of stroke compared with men (Table 1). Of particular concern is evidence that the cardiovascular mortality rate among patients with diabetes is increasing, particularly in elderly women. Cardiologists must be aware of these trends and understand the influence of type II diabetes on coronary artery disease.

Most patients with type II diabetes are obese. The link between obesity and type II diabetes is complex. Abdominal or visceral obesity provokes insulin resistance which is the fundamental fault in those with the metabolic syndrome, defined by a cluster of risk factors identifying patients at high risk for progressing to type II diabetes (see Table 2). As insulin resistance worsens,

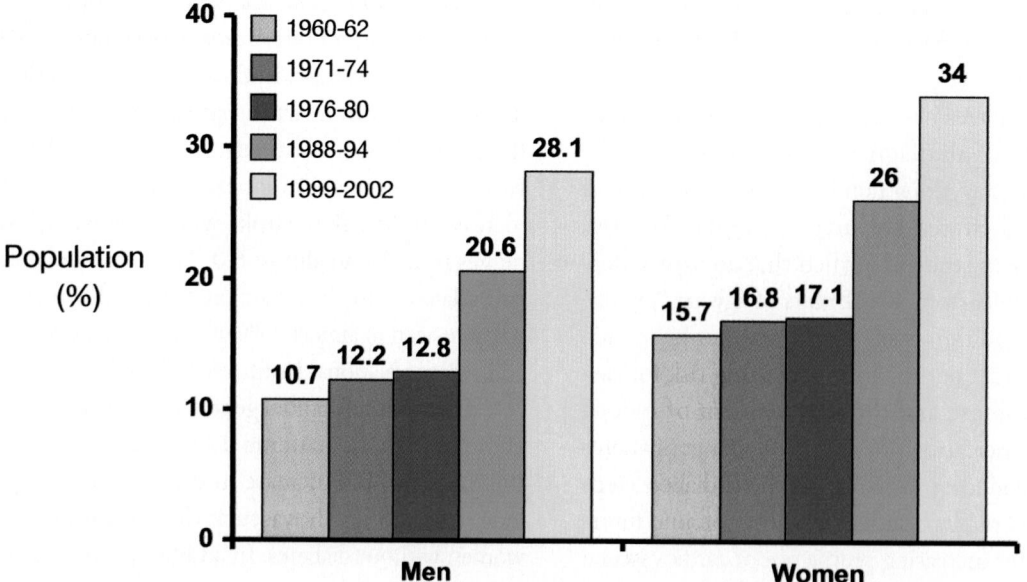

Fig. 2. Age-adjusted prevalence of obesity in Americans ages 20-74 by sex and survey (NHES 1960-62; NHANES: 1971-74, 1976-80, 1988-94 and 1999-2002). Note: Obesity is defined as a BMI of 30.0 or higher.

Table 1. U.S. Demographic Data for Diabetes

Population group	Prevalence of physician-diagnosed diabetes (2003)	Prevalence of undiagnosed diabetes (2003)	Prevalence of pre-diabetes (2003)	Incidence of diagnosed diabetes	Mortality (diabetes) (2003)*	Hospital discharges (2003)	Cost (2002)†
Total	14,100,000 (6.7%)	6,000,000 (2.9%)	14,700,000 (7.0%)	1,500,000	73,965	597,000	$132 billion
Total males	7,000,000 (7.2%)	3,000,000 (3.0%)	8,600,000 (8.9%)	...	35,257	286,000 (47.7%)‡	...
Total females	7,100,000 (6.3%)	3,000,000 (2.7%)	6,100,000 (5.4%)	...	38,748 (52.4%)‡	314,000	...
NH white males	6.2%	3.0%	8.6%	...	28,765	...	...
NH white females	4.7%	2.7%	4.6%	...	30,189	...	...
NH black males	10.3%	1.3%	8.3%	...	5,401	...	...
NH black females	12.6%	6.1%	5.9%	...	7,419	...	...
Mexican-American males	10.4%	3.5%	8.7%	...	...	...	...
Mexican-American females	11.3%	1.8%	7.2%	...	...	...	...
Hispanic or Latino§	8.6%	...	...	...	...	...	...
Asian§	6.5%	...	...	...	...	...	...
American Indians/ Alaska natives§	12.2%	...	...	...	...	...	...

Note: Undiagnosed diabetes is defined here for those whose fasting glucose is 126 mg/dL or higher but who did not report being told they had diabetes by a health care provider. Prediabetes is a fasting blood glucose of 100 to less than 126 mg/dL (impaired fasting glucose). Prediabetes also includes impaired glucose tolerance.

(...) = data not available. NH = non-Hispanic.

*Preliminary.

†CDC/NCHS.

‡These percentages represent the portion of total DM mortality that is males vs. females.

§NHIS (2003), CDC/NCHS; data are estimates for Americans age 18 and older.

Sources: Prevalence: NHANES (1999-2002), CDC/NCHS and NHLBI; percentages for racial/ethnic groups are age-adjusted for Americans age 20 and older. Estimates from NHANES 1999-2002 applied to 2003 population estimates. Incidence: NIDDK estimates. Mortality: CDC/NCHS; these data represent underlying cause of death only; data for white and black males and females include Hispanics. Hospital discharges: National Hospital Discharge Survey, CDC/NCHS; data include people discharged alive and dead.

Table 2. Diagnosis of Metabolic Syndrome

Criteria (any 3 of the 5 below are required for diagnosis):

Increased waist circumference	Greater than 40 inches in males
	Greater than 35 inches in females
Elevated triglycerides	Equal to or greater than 150 mg/dL
Reduced HDL cholesterol	<40 mg/dL
Elevated blood pressure	Equal to or greater than 130/85
	On antihypertensive therapy
Elevated fasting blood glucose	Equal to or greater than 100 mgm/dL

hyperglycemia persists in spite of hyperinsulinemia, leading to the clinical consequences of type II diabetes. Hyperglycemia-induced tissue damage is provoked in part by the glycation of proteins with generation of advanced glycation end products which have toxic effects, including excess oxidative stress, endothelial dysfunction, impaired fibrinolysis, and proinflammatory gene expression among others. While insulin has beneficial effects in glycemic control, it has other complex actions. It exhibits both anti- and proatherosclerosis effects. In addition, hyperinsulinemia has been associated in many studies with a worse clinical outcome.

Cardiologists need to understand that fat cells (adipocytes) are active metabolically and the source of a number of cytokines and other substances that not only influence insulin sensitivity/resistance but have profound effects on the cardiovascular system. An example is leptin, which results in sympathetic stimulation, oxidative stress, and enhancement of platelet aggregation while influencing insulin responsiveness in a tissue-specific manner. Leptin has been demonstrated to be associated with more extensive angiographic evidence of coronary artery disease (CAD). Another fac-

tor is adiponectin which has antiinflammatory and anti-atherosclerosis effects; a low level has been correlated with the presence of CAD, and insulin resistance with type II diabetes as a consequence. There are complex CNS relationships which have been studied. Cerebral pathways may be involved in the susceptibility to obesity. The importance of these has been emphasized with recent reports of inhibitors of cannabinoid receptors which result in significant weight loss and reduction of insulin resistance.

There is general acceptance that the diagnosis of type II diabetes is the "equivalent" of a diagnosis of CAD based upon the work of Hafner, who demonstrated similar survival rates for patients without diabetes and myocardial infarction and those with diabetes but no myocardial infarction. The American Heart Association has thus designated type II diabetes as the equivalent of coronary artery disease, not just a risk factor for the disease. Screening for coronary artery disease is now recommended for asymptomatic patients with type II diabetes with two or more risk factors, though recent studies suggest this may be unduly conservative.

Symptoms typically associated with myocardial ischemia and/or myocardial infarction in patients without type II diabetes may be absent or muted in patients with type II diabetes. Recognizing myocardial ischemia as the cause of an "angina equivalent" of dyspnea or other stress-related symptoms is essential in analyzing clinical symptoms in patients with type II diabetes. Silent infarction is known to be more common in patients with type II diabetes and the size of infarction has been found to be larger among those with diabetes compared to those without diabetes. Congestive heart failure in diabetic patients may be due to ischemia/infarction or a diabetic cardiomyopathy without epicardial coronary flow limiting disease. In these patients the influence of myocardial insulin resistance may play a role along with lipotoxicity in more obese patients. Clinical outcomes are worse among patients with type II diabetes compared to those without diabetes regardless of the clinical event. However, in the setting of acute myocardial infarction (STEMI), diabetic patients benefit acutely from thrombolysis and primary angioplasty, as do patients without diabetes. With longer-term follow-up, those with diabetes have higher event rates. This is true for patients with other acute coronary syndromes. The original Diabetes Mellitus Insulin-Glucose Infusion in Acute

Myocardial Infarction (DIGAMI) trial documented the survival benefit of aggressive control of blood glucose with insulin in the setting of acute myocardial infarction. Other studies in medical intensive care units have confirmed the importance of controlling hyperglycemia in critically ill patients regardless of the presence of diabetes.

Outcomes with revascularization in patients with type II diabetes have been of great interest particularly after the unexpected observation from the original Bypass Angioplasty Revascularization Investigation (BARI) Trial that patients with treated diabetes randomized to PTCA had worse 5-year and 10-year survival than those randomized to coronary artery bypass grafting (CABG). *This was true only if patients having CABG received at least one internal mammary graft.* The difference in survival specifically related to cardiac mortality. In the BARI registry, patients with type II diabetes fared better with PTCA as it appeared the higher-risk patients received CABG. All patients in BARI had multivessel CAD that was selected on the basis of suitability for both procedures; thus patients with the most severe anatomic disease were excluded. As a result of the BARI results, it was recommended that CABG with at least one internal mammary graft was the preferred therapy for patients with characteristics of those in the randomized trial. However, much has changed since the time of the BARI trial with introduction of bare metal and drug-eluting stents, use of clopidogrel, GP IIb/IIIa platelet inhibitors and widespread use of statins. All of the latter interventions have been demonstrated to improve outcomes of patients with type II diabetes undergoing percutaneous interventions (PCI). While the Arterial Revascularization Therapy Study (ARTS I) and the Stent or Surgery (SoS) trials have shown significant reductions in repeat revascularization with bare metal stents, no difference in mortality or a combined end point of mortality, stroke, or myocardial infarction between PCI and CABG have been found. A small cohort of diabetic patients in ARTS I continued to show higher mortality and cardiac events than patients without diabetes, but no difference of significance between PCI and CABG though the trial was not powered to address this point. We await results of the Future Revascularization Evaluation in Patients with Diabetes Mellitus (FREEDOM) trial to provide a comparison of current state-of-the-art PCI and CABG in patients with DM.

New data from a variety of trials clarify issues in medical management of patients with type II diabetes and CAD in relation to:

1. Glycemic control
2. Blood pressure control
3. Effects of thiazolidinediones and metformin
4. Therapy for hyperlipidemia
5. Use of ACE inhibitors and ARBs
6. Antiplatelet therapy

The UKPDS (The United Kingdom Prospective Diabetes Study) tested the following hypothesis: Does intensive glucose control reduce risk of macro/microvascular complications? At 10 years, HbA_{1c} on average was 7.0% on intensive therapy with insulin and sulfonylureas and 7.9% on diet therapy. Patients were free of evidence of CAD at entry. A significant reduction in microvascular complications occurred with intensive glucose control, and there was a trend in favor of a reduction of myocardial infarction rates which did not achieve statistical significance. In addition, blood pressure control, even though it did not achieve current target levels, resulted in a dramatic reduction in rates of congestive heart failure, myocardial infarction, and stroke. A substudy of the UKPDS has also shown that use of metformin in obese patients significantly reduced occurrence of myocardial infarction. A more recent study of the Medicare database of acute myocardial infarction has also shown that in patients with diabetes, a combination of a thiazolidinedione drug (TZD) and metformin is associated with lower mortality with myocardial infarction that either drug alone or only a sulfonylurea. TZD and metformin reduce insulin resistance.

Cardiologists need to be aware of the new TZD drugs, which not only lower blood glucose by their insulin sensitizing action but also have direct effects on atherosclerosis which include improving endothelial function, antiinflamatory effects, reduction in carotid medial thickness, and reducing the proliferative response to injury of balloon angioplasty and implantation of stents. TZDs belong to a fascinating new class of drugs known as peroxisome proliferator antagonist receptor (PPAR) agonists which stimulate nuclear transcription factors influencing genes regulating metabolic processes. Current TZDs in clinical use are primarily PPAR gamma agonists, but others are being developed to explore effects of PPAR alpha receptors. An important complication of TZD drugs is fluid retention based upon enhanced salt and water retention in the distal tubule of the kidney. For these reasons TZDs should not be used in the setting of heart failure or depressed LV function. This is of particular concern in patients taking insulin. The other "insulin sensitizer," metformin, may also be associated with major side effects such as a lactic acidoses and should not be used in patients with congestive heart failure or renal failure.

Sulfonylurea drugs which are used for glycemic control by stimulating beta cells to release insulin are of great interest to cardiologists. These drugs stimulate the KATP channels of the beta cells, but to some degree they also stimulate these channels in the heart. Variation between sulfonylurea drugs in relation to the extent of binding to KATP cardiac channels is important, as those with high cardiac binding may have profound effects on the heart including inhibition of ischemic preconditioning and perhaps cardiac rhythm effects. In observational studies mortality from primary angioplasty in STEMI has been higher among patients with diabetes on sulfonylurea drugs.

Treatment strategies for control of hyperlipidemia should be aggressive in patients with diabetes and CAD. Use of statins has been demonstrated to provide similar benefit among patients with diabetes compared to those without. In addition, patients with diabetes frequently have a pattern of hypertriglyceridemia and low HDL cholesterol (as per discussion of metabolic syndrome). In these patients, use of niacin and/or fibric acid derivative have been shown to improve outcomes (reduce cardiac events) in association with successful elevation of HDL levels. When used in combination with statins, more careful monitoring to screen for early evidence of myositis or liver dysfunction is important as the combination of these drugs with statins result in statin induced complication more frequently than with statins alone.

Diabetic patients need to be screened for microalbuminuria, which is a prognostic marker not only for progression to renal failure but cardiac events. Fortunately, several large trials have documented that probability of progression to renal failure is reduced with ACE inhibitors as well as angiotensin receptor blockers (ARBs). Current guidelines call for all patients with type II diabetes and microalbuminuria to be on an ACE inhibitor or ARB regardless of blood pressure. In most patients with diabetes and hypertension, more than one antihypertensive drug is required and all classes of drugs may be helpful. Diuretics, sometimes feared because of adverse metabolic effects, have been demonstrated to be safe and effective.

Antiplatelet therapy is crucial. Use of aspirin is recommended in all patients with diabetes and CAD, while beneficial effects of clopidogrel prior to or at the time of PCI has been well established, with recommendation for continued use 6-12 months after the procedure. GP IIb/IIIa inhibitors have also been demonstrated to reduce major cardiac events after PCI in patients with type II diabetes.

Cardiologists must also be aware of the profound importance of life style changes in managing CAD in association with type II diabetes. Indeed, type II DM can be prevented by major life style intervention. A major challenge is achieving weight reduction, and some patients may benefit from bariatric surgery. When successful, bariatric surgery may eliminate the presence of or greatly reduce the severity of type II DM. Recent reports of blockade of cannabinoid receptors leading to weight reduction and amelioration of the metabolic syndrome are encouraging.

RESOURCES

Bypass Angioplasty Revascularization Investigation (BARI) [database on the Internet]. Available from: http://www.edc.pitt.edu/bari/.

Future Revascularization Evaluation in Patients With Diabetes Mellitus: Optimal Management of Multivessel Disease (FREEDOM) [database on the Internet]. Available from: http://www.clinicaltrials.gov/ct/show/NCT00086450.

61

HYPERTENSION

Michael J. Hogan, MD, MBA

DEFINITION

It has been customary to define hypertension as a sustained blood pressure in millimeters of mercury above some upper limit of normal. Traditionally, the limits used in the United States have been 139 and 89, for systolic and diastolic blood pressures, respectively. The Joint National Committee on Prevention, Detection, Evaluation and Treatment of Hypertension, in its seventh report, (JNC-7), recognized the continuous and consistent relationship (independent of other risk factors) between blood pressures that exceed 119/79 and cardiovascular events. Hence, blood pressures above this level carry sufficient risk for complications to no longer be considered normal.

BLOOD PRESSURE STAGING

As a consequence of this blood pressure-risk relationship across pressures greater than 119/79, JNC-7 staged blood pressures across four ranges. Table 1 depicts that staging. The blood pressure-cardiovascular risk relationship at systolic blood pressures between 120 and 139 systolic and 80 to 89 diastolic requires health care providers and the public to consider blood pressures within these ranges as greater than desirable. Because the previous designation of "high normal" for these pressure ranges failed to carry sufficient impact to bring about action, with regard to long-term risk, JNC-7

Table 1. JNC-7 Blood Pressure Staging

Normal	<102	and	<80
Prehypertension	120-139	or	80-89
Stage 1 hypertension	140-159	or	90-99
Stage 2 hypertension	≥160	or	≥100

classified blood pressures within this range as *prehypertension*.

The benefit of treatment in reducing cardiovascular and cerebrovascular deaths across the ranges of 140-159 mm Hg for systolic and 90-99 mm Hg for diastolic blood pressures prompted JNC-7 to reiterate this range of pressures as Stage 1. Differing from JNC-6, the current document classifies all pressures greater than 160/100 as stage 2. Reducing the classification numbers from six to four should simplify decision options for health care providers and guides for interventional trials.

PROBLEM MAGNITUDE

With 140/90 mm Hg as the definition point of hypertension, it is estimated that approximately 50 million individuals within the United States meet the criteria for the disease. Twenty times that many worldwide are hypertensive. This can be interpreted as a 90 percent lifetime risk for the 55-year-old normotensive individual of developing hypertension. JNC-7's new definitions will increase the number of individuals at risk to suffer the consequences of abnormal blood pressures—cardiovascular, cerebrovascular, and renal diseases.

The health care community's success in recognizing the disease and informing and treating patients remains less than optimum. Using 140/90 mm Hg as the definition of hypertension, the National Health Awareness and Education Survey (NAHNES) has monitored awareness, treatment, and control over a 25-year span. Improvements in all parameters during the first decade have not persisted during the last half of the study period. The results following the 2000 census suggest a trend toward improvement, but there continues to be a failure on the part of the health care delivery system to optimally treat and control this common and easily diagnosable disease, for which numerous treatments are readily available (Table 2).

BLOOD PRESSURE MEASUREMENT

Accurate blood pressure measurement is the first step in the evaluation and treatment of the hypertensive patient. In the clinic setting, the individual should be seated, comfortably, for five minutes. The back should be fully supported and the brachial artery at heart level. The positive results of interventional trials reflect measurements utilizing a cuff whose bladder encompasses at least 80 percent of the upper arm attached to an accurately calibrated sphygmomanometer.

Stimulants such as caffeine should be avoided for several hours before blood pressure measurement. This is an important caveat for patients doing home blood pressure monitoring.

Employment of ambulatory blood pressure monitoring has increased in the past decade. In the awake state, a normotensive individual's average blood pressure does not exceed 135/85 mm Hg, or 125/75 mm Hg while asleep. Ambulatory blood pressure monitoring provides valuable insight into the management of patients with resistant hypertension, medication-related hypotensive symptoms, stress-related (white coat) increases in blood pressure, and autonomic dysfunction. The circadian rhythm in blood pressure seen in normotensive individuals is maintained in most patients with hypertension (dippers) despite higher pressures throughout the 24-hour cycle. The failure of the blood pressure to fall during sleep (nondippers) correlates with an increased risk of cardiovascular events. However, availability of ambulatory monitoring equipment and reimbursement issues preclude the routine use of ambulatory blood pressure monitoring.

Self-measurement of blood pressure is an alternative means of observing the blood pressure in patients

Table 2.   Hypertension: Awareness, Treatment, and Control of ↑ BP in Adults

	NHANES			
	1988-91	**1991-94**	**1999-2000**	**2001-2002**
Awareness	69%	68%	69%	71%
Treatment	52%	55%	58%	61%
Control*	24%	23%	32%	34%
Control (DM)†	53%	42%	46%	56%
Control (DM)‡	28%	17%	36%	35%

*Adults (18-74) with SBP <140; DBP <90: taking antihypertensive medications.
†<140/90
‡<135/85

under pharmacological treatment. The equipment is readily available, affordable, often covered by insurance, and obviates the need for frequent clinic visits. Symptoms can be correlated better with blood pressure changes and white coat hypertension better identified when patients perform home blood pressure monitoring. The same requirements for cuff size and accuracy of the measuring device apply as for clinic monitoring.

PRIMARY PREVENTION

With the recognition of the major contributors to hypertension—sodium intake, alcohol consumption, excess weight, and lack of exercise—the question that arises is Will correction of these contributors positively impact blood pressure? Even modest reductions in weight have resulted in significant systolic and diastolic blood pressure reductions within groups in whom dietary intervention was initiated. The incidence of hypertension in such a group over almost a decade can be decreased by almost one-third.

Qualitative changes in diet can benefit hypertensive patients. Diets high in fruits and vegetables and low in saturated fats can reduce blood pressure. The addition of sodium restrictions adds to the benefit. As with weight loss, sodium intake reduction has been associated with significantly lower normal blood pressures in meta-analyses of those studies that examined this question. Moderation in alcohol intake and regular exercise also both reduce blood pressure in individuals considered normotensive.

It must be kept in mind that in all the interventional trials the small changes reach statistical significance due to the large numbers of subjects. In addition, subjects classified as normotensive in the earlier studies from which the meta-analyses were created would now fall into the prehypertensive or high-normal classifications of JNC-7. While translation of these data proves difficult in the individual patient, it is difficult to find any detriment to incorporating these healthy lifestyle behaviors.

LIFESTYLE MODIFICATION AS TREATMENT

Just as with primary prevention, lifestyle modification can result in significant blood pressure reduction in the hypertensive population. Correcting each of the contributors, therefore, should be the mainstay of therapy and must be included in any treatment regimen upon which the practitioner decides. Recognition of the importance of lifestyle modification with regard to the contributors to hypertension by JNC-7 can be seen in incorporation in all treatment recommendations.

The correlations between specific behavioral changes and blood pressure reductions are outlined in Table 3. These changes require constant reinforcement with each patient encounter.

PHARMACOLOGICAL INTERVENTION

In an attempt to simplify clinical decision making, JNC-7 created a treatment algorithm incorporating the result of large treatment trials that have been published since JNC-6. The algorithm (Fig. 1) focuses on compelling indications as key decision points in the choice of pharmacological agents. Table 4 presents the compelling indications and the drugs of choice for each.

In each circumstance covered by the compelling indication, the goal of treatment is to prevent progression of the disease or syndrome by reducing the hypertension's contribution. Unfortunately, once the complication has taken place, reversal often is difficult to achieve.

While these recommendations are apropos across populations, treatment must be individualized. Cost,

Table 3.   Lifestyle Modification

Modification	Approximate SBP reduction (range)
Weight reduction	5-20 mm Hg/10 kg weight loss
Adopt DASH eating plan	8-14 mm Hg
Dietary sodium reduction	2-8 mm Hg
Physical activity	4-9 mm Hg
Moderation of alcohol consumption	2-4 mm Hg

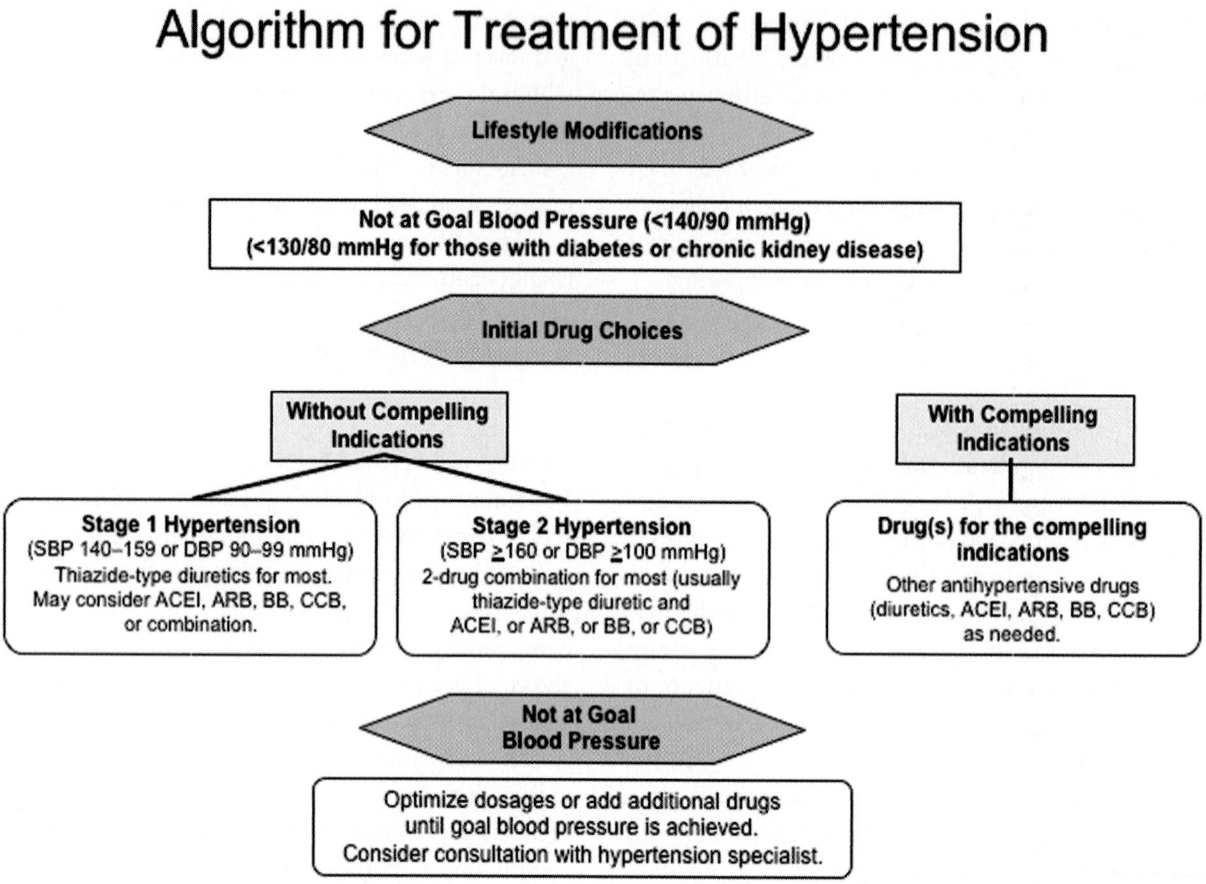

Algorithm for Treatment of Hypertension

Lifestyle Modifications

Not at Goal Blood Pressure (<140/90 mmHg)
(<130/80 mmHg for those with diabetes or chronic kidney disease)

Initial Drug Choices

Without Compelling Indications

With Compelling Indications

Stage 1 Hypertension
(SBP 140–159 or DBP 90–99 mmHg)
Thiazide-type diuretics for most.
May consider ACEI, ARB, BB, CCB,
or combination.

Stage 2 Hypertension
(SBP ≥160 or DBP ≥100 mmHg)
2-drug combination for most (usually
thiazide-type diuretic and
ACEI, or ARB, or BB, or CCB)

Drug(s) for the compelling indications
Other antihypertensive drugs
(diuretics, ACEI, ARB, BB, CCB)
as needed.

Not at Goal Blood Pressure

Optimize dosages or add additional drugs
until goal blood pressure is achieved.
Consider consultation with hypertension specialist.

Fig. 1. Algorithm for treatment decisions.

duration of action, side effects, and drug interactions all bear consideration in the choice of antihypertensive medication. Understanding of the multiple medications patients often take may be limited, and examination of the actual drugs can alleviate much of the misunderstanding and avoid harmful omissions or drug interactions.

The choice of initial drug therapy is open to several options. Low-dose thiazide (thiazide-like) diuretics remain the standard for therapy initiation in most hypertensive patients. 2002 witnessed publication of the results of the Antihypertensive and Lipid-Lowering Treatment to Prevent Heart Attack Trial (ALLHAT). This largest interventional trail for the treatment of hypertension examined the benefits of angiotensin-converting enzyme (ACE) inhibitors, dihydropyridine calcium channel blockers and beta blockers when compared with diuretics in controlling hypertension and positively affecting outcomes of diseases associated with hypertension. Alpha$_2$-adrenergic receptor blockers were dropped from the study prior to

completion because of concerns about this class of drug and a propensity for congestive heart failure in patients receiving it.

As with any interventional trial, the ALLHAT results have been debated in the medical literature since its publication. The results demonstrate equal efficacy in controlling blood pressure among the agents studied for most patients with hypertension. Hyperglycemia and hypokalemia may accompany thiazide administration and limit their applicability. Edema formation would favor avoidance of calcium channel blockers. However, except when compelling indications determine first-line therapy, cost, ease of administration, and efficacy would favor diuretic therapy for the majority of patients with essential hypertension.

A majority of hypertensive patients will require more than one agent to control their blood pressure. Knowledge of appropriate combination therapy then becomes important in the management of these patients. Multiple-drug therapy often affords a level of control without the side effects often encountered

Table 4.   Rx Choice by Compelling Indication

Compelling indication	Diuretic	BB	ACEI	ARB	CCB	Aldo ant
Heart failure	*	*	*			*
Post MI		*	*			*
High risk CAD	*	*	*		*	
Diabetes	*	*	*	*	*	
CRE			*	*		

BB: β-Blocker
ACEI: angiotensin converting enzyme inhibitor
ARB: angiotensin receptor blocker
CCB: dihydropyridine calcium channel blocker
Aldo Ant: aldosterone antagonist

when single-drug therapy requires the agent to be taken to its maximum dose.

Resistant Hypertension

In any hypertensive population there exists a segment whose blood pressure cannot be controlled despite what appears to be adequate therapy. JNC-7 defines such adequate therapy as three drugs, including a diuretic, in recommended doses. Table 5 lists the usual conditions that may contribute to resistant hypertension.

Pseudoresistance refers to the apparent increase in pressure brought about by noncompliant vessels as is often seen in the elderly population. A one-time correlation between an intra-arterial blood pressure and a "cuff" measurement can serve as a guide to efficacy of a treatment program.

Table 5.   Causes of Resistant Hypertension

• Pseudoresistance

• Nonadherence to therapy

• Volume overload

• Drug-related causes

• Sleep apnea

Nonadherence to therapy has several causes. Cost of medications, especially in the elderly population on a fixed income, misunderstanding of directions for use, and insufficient education are some of the reasons why patient fail to comply with instructions.

From a therapeutic standpoint, volume should be considered the prime factor until some other cause is identified. Hence adequate diuretic therapy needs to be achieved before considering other causes.

Proprietary pressor use and caffeine can intermittently elevate blood pressure. There is little data to suggest a relationship with sustained hypertension, but these agents can be of importance when patients are engaged in home monitoring.

Breathing-related sleep disorders are associated with hypertension and may be responsible for failure of drug therapy to successfully control the hypertension. Patients often do not volunteer a history of fatigue or hypersomnolence, necessitating questioning by the clinician regarding daytime fatigue, excessive snoring, or observed interruption of breathing by the patient's sleeping partner.

If these identifiable causes have been eliminated or dealt with and the blood pressure remains uncontrolled attention should then be drawn to the possibility that the patient is in that small group, which has a secondary form of hypertension. In this instance, identifying and treating the primary pathologic process often results in a normalization of the blood pressure.

Secondary Hypertension

More than ninety percent of the hypertensive population suffers from essential or primary hypertension, i.e. hypertension for which a single cause cannot be identified. Hence, an extensive search for a cause of secondary hypertension in all hypertensive patients is not justified. This is particularly true in individuals who present with one or more of the major contributors, easily controlled hypertension, or a strong family history of hypertension.

In the absence of these circumstances the likelihood of secondary hypertension being present increases. Table 6 lists the circumstances which should serve as clues to the existence of secondary hypertension. Table 7 lists the common causes of secondary hypertension. Of these, the conditions which, if treated, often result in improvement in or cure of the hypertension are a) renovascular hypertension, b) mineralocorticoid excess states, e.g. primary aldosteronism, and c) catecholamine-secreting neoplasms.

Renovascular hypertension: Not all renal artery stenotic lesions result in blood pressure elevation. Hence, the presence of renal artery stenosis does not always demand treatment. The criteria for consideration of a secondary form of hypertension apply in the case of renovascular disease. Poor control, evidence of renal dysfunction, or treatment intolerance in the presence of evidence of likely renal artery stenosis (e.g. abdominal bruit, coexistent peripheral vascular disease) are examples of circumstances that warrant a search for renal artery stenosis.

Estimates of renal artery caliber have included excretory urography (IVP), ultrasound, and radionu-

Table 7. Causes of Secondary Hypertension

- Sleep apnea
- Drug-induced or drug-related
- Chronic kidney disease
- Primary aldosteronism
- Renovascular disease
- Chronic steroid therapy and Cushing syndrome
- Pheochromocytoma
- Coarctation of the aorta
- Thyroid or parathyroid disease

cleotide imaging. Varying sensitivity and specificity make these tests less desirable than the "gold standard" of direct renal angiography. The risks of any invasive procedure and the potential nephrotoxicity of standard contrasts have prompted a search for better, less invasive imaging. MRI angiography (Fig. 2) and CT angiography (in individuals for whom nephrotoxicity is not an issue or MRI is not feasible) have filled that need.

For decades surgical correction of renal artery stenosis with vein grafting was the standard treatment. Improvements in angiography techniques, less toxic contrast materials, and stents have all helped angioplasty supplant surgery as the mainstay of therapy.

There exists, however a sizable debate between cardiologists and nephrologists as to whether all instances of renal artery stenosis should be ameliorated angiographically. There exist no trial in which "drive-by" angiography and stenting of stenotic renal arteries is warranted in all patients with renal artery stenosis undergoing coronary angiography.

Primary aldosteronism: Aldosterone is the major mineralocorticoid of the adrenal cortex. Autonomous secretion by the zona glomerulosa, a single neoplasm (adenoma vs. carcinoma), or multiple nodules can result in abnormal aldosterone secretion and blood pressure elevation.

Unprovoked hypokalemia, hypokalemia in the face of minimal diuretic therapy, and "low normal" serum potassium concentrations in conjunction with drug therapy usually associated with elevated potassium concentrations (e.g., ACE inhibitors, angiotensin

Table 6. Clues to Secondary Hypertension

- Recent onset of hypertension
- Loss of blood pressure control
- Resistant hypertension
- Evidence of peripheral vascular disease (↑ creatinine with aniotensin blockade)
- Unprovoked hypokalemia (inappropriately low-normal K^+)

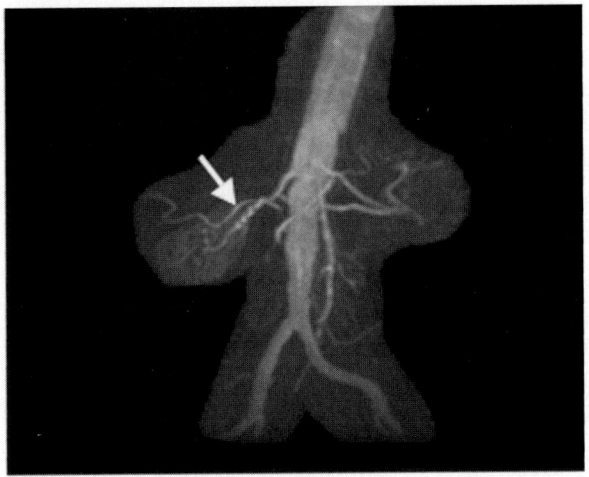

MR Angiogram

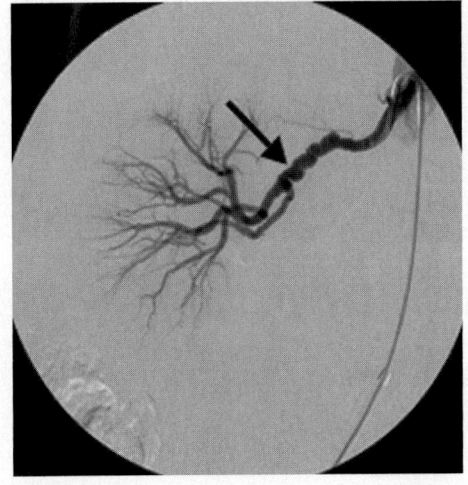

Angiogram

Fig. 2. MRA renal artery stenosis.

receptor blockers, and potassium-sparing diuretics) signal the possibility of primary aldosteronism. The association of hypokalemia, evidence of volume expansion (upper normal to elevated serum sodium concentrations), suppression of the renin-angiotensin axis as reflected by the plasma renin activity (PRA) and aldosterone overproduction (elevated 24 hour aldosterone excretion) are the hallmarks of the syndrome.

To determine which pathologic process is responsible for the syndrome, CT imaging of the adrenal cortex offers the best diagnostic opportunity (Fig. 3). In unusual circumstances, adrenal vein catheterization for measurement of aldosterone may be necessary. In the absence of a single neoplasm, the use of a specific aldosterone antagonist often brings about a normalization of the blood pressure.

Catecholamine-secreting neoplasms: Much less common than either renovascular hypertension or primary aldosteronism are neoplasms of the sympathetic nervous system. The most common of these arise from the adrenal medulla and bear the histologic diagnosis of pheochromocytoma (Fig. 4). Pathologists label those occurring at other sites along the sympathetic chain paraganglioma. Clinically and biochemically there is little to differentiate the different types other than ability of pheochromocytomas to secrete epinephrine. Quantitation of catecholamine production over a 24-hour period (24-hour urine collection) has been the

diagnostic test for the past several decades. Elevations of plasma metanephrine concentrations appear to offer equal, if not greater, predictive value, obviating the need for urine collections.

Once biochemical testing establishes the diagnosis of pheochromocytoma/paraganglioma, localization of the abnormal tissue becomes the goal. Because pheochro-

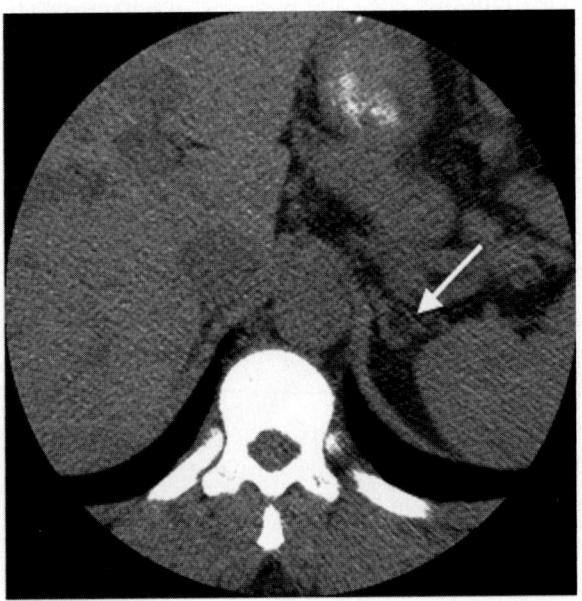

Fig. 3. CT aldosterone producing adenoma (*arrow*).

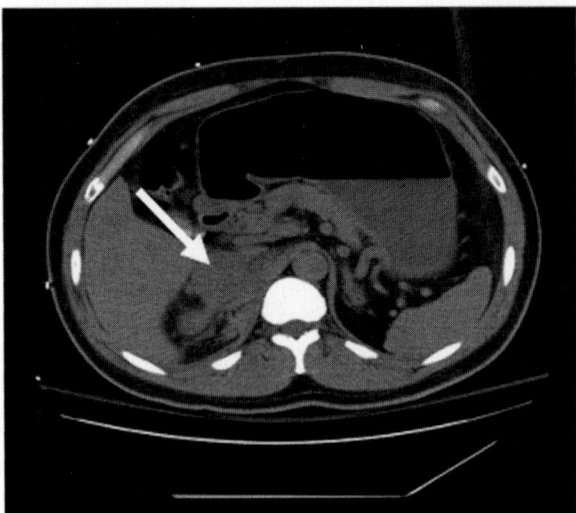

Fig. 4. CT adrenal pheochromocytoma (*arrow*).

mocytomas are more common, computed tomography of the adrenal glands should be the first choice (Fig. 5). In the absence of an unequivocal CT diagnosis, MRI of the abdomen and thorax is the study of choice for examination of the sympathetic chain. Mono-iodo-bis-guanine (MIBG) is a readably radioiodinated compound that can be incorporated into the catecholamine synthetic pathway and will identify overproduction. On occasion, somatostatin receptors on the tumor may make it possible to use the imaging agent octreotide to localize the pathologic tissue. Radionuclide imaging offers little over MRI and is less practical to use except in those individuals in whom CT or MRI is not feasible.

Hypertension in Special Populations

Pregnancy

Hypertension during pregnancy falls into one of four categories according to the NHBPEP working group classification: 1. Preeclampsia-eclampsia; 2. Preeclampsia superimposed on chronic hypertension; 3. Chronic hypertension; 4. Gestational hypertension.

Preeclampsia is a multiorgan disease affecting not only the vasculature but also renal, hepatic, pulmonary, and hematological function as manifest by proteinuria, hepatocellular injury, pulmonary edema, and microangiopathic-hemolytic anemia usually occurring late in pregnancy. This type of hypertension can progress to convulsions (eclampsia) and represents a major risk for maternal and fetal mortality.

Delivery is the definitive treatment for preeclampsia. Pending delivery, magnesium sulfate remains the pharmacologic treatment of choice.

Gestational hypertension refers to mild blood pressure elevations that occur in the second half of pregnancy and are unaccompanied by proteinuria. Blood pressures usually return to normal within 12 weeks of delivery.

Given the limited time course of pregnancy, mild elevations in blood pressure can be tolerated and initiation of pharmacological treatment is reserved for pressures that are consistently in excess of 150 mm Hg. Methydopa remains the drug of choice for women who develop hypertension during pregnancy. Availability has made its use problematic in some

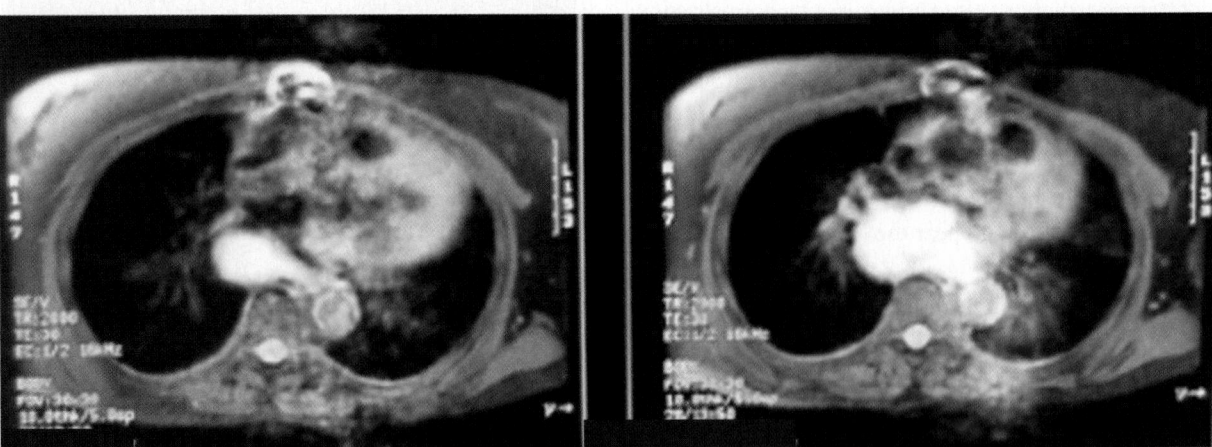

Fig. 5. MRI mediastinal paraganglioma.

locales. Beta blockers are alternatives. Diuretics may be used but with caution to avoid severe volume depletion and resultant uterine underperfusion. ACE-inhibitors and angiotensin receptor blockers are contraindicated due to reported teratongenic effects.

Diabetes
Coincident end-organ damage from diabetes and hypertension has prompted recommendations for more vigorous treatment in diabetic hypertensive patients. Goal blood pressure is <130/80 mm Hg.

In most instances two or more drugs are necessary to achieve goal pressures. Any agent can be selected. The propensity for thiazide diuretics to worsen glycemic control warrants note. However, in small doses this is not a common problem. Beta blockers may mask the cardiovascular symptoms of hypoglycemia in patients prone to this diabetic treatment complication, limiting their use in this population.

Inhibition of angiotensin II generation or its blockade slows the progression of chronic renal disease to dialysis or transplant. This benefit has been applied to patients with diabetes and provides impetus for agents in this category to be used in treating hypertension in the diabetic patient.

Cyclosporine
The growth of organ transplantation has resulted in a moderate population of patients receiving cyclosporine and antirejection therapy. This drug is commonly accompanied by hypertension, often in patients without a history of elevated blood pressure. The mechanism of the blood pressure increase remains a matter of question, but peripheral vasoconstriction has been consistently observed and prompted treatment with dihydropyridine calcium-channel blockers for most.

Hypertensive Urgencies and Emergencies
Because of the often dramatic and potentially lethal effects of extreme blood pressure elevations, attempts at rapid reduction are attractive. However, sudden and rapid declines in blood pressure may offer as great or greater risk as extreme elevations. There is no specific blood pressure that can be defined as presenting either a hypertensive urgency or emergency.

The prompt onset of action of most of the antihypertensive agents in use make oral administration a reasonable approach for any blood pressure level that is unaccompanied by evidence of acute end organ damage. Hypertensive emergencies can best be defined by ongoing end-organ damage and warrant the administration of parenteral agents of rapid onset and offset action. Careful monitoring of organ function and achievement of a safe blood pressure level should be the therapeutic goal. Seldom is it necessary to normalize blood pressure in emergency circumstances. In the face of acute cerebrovascular events, the elevated blood pressure may be a result rather than a cause, and sudden lowering of the blood pressure may worsen the cerebral damage.

RESOURCES
ALLHAT Officers and Coordinators for the ALLHAT Collaborative Research Group, The Antihypertensive and Lipid-Lowering Treatment to Prevent Heart Attack Trial (ALLHAT). Major outcomes in high-risk hypertensive patients randomized to angiotensin-converting enzyme inhibitor or calcium channel blocker vs diuretic. JAMA. 2002;288:2981-16.

Chobanian AV, Bakris GL, Black HR, et al, National Heart, Lung, and Blood Institute Joint National Committee on Prevention, Detection, Evaluation, and Treatment of High Blood Pressure, National High Blood Pressure Education Program Coordinating Committee. The Seventh Report of the Joint National Committee on Prevention, Detection, Evaluation and Treatment of High Blood Pressure: the JNC-7 report. JAMA. 2003;289:2560-72.

Garovic V, Textor SC. Renovascular hypertension: current concepts. Semin Neprhol. 2005;25:261-71.

62

HEART DISEASE IN WOMEN

Patricia J. M. Best, MD

Sharonne N. Hayes, MD

Cardiovascular disease is the number one cause of death in women, outnumbering deaths from all other causes combined. Each year over 500,000 women experience a myocardial infarction and more than 250,000 die from coronary artery disease. Despite the national campaigns to increase the awareness of heart disease in women, including the "Go Red" campaign and the "Red Dress" campaign, only 55% of women in a recent survey are aware that cardiovascular disease is the leading cause of death in women and less than 15% of women surveyed perceive it as a significant risk to themselves. Furthermore, the prevalence of cardiovascular disease in women, including coronary artery disease, congestive heart failure, stroke, and hypertension, exceeds men in the population over 55 years (Fig. 1). Because of the higher proportion of women in the aging population, each year more women die of cardiovascular disease than men. Importantly, increasing prevalence of risk factors for heart disease such as obesity and diabetes, which affect women to a greater extent than men, will likely make heart disease in women more prevalent at an even younger age in the future. The mortality rate from cardiovascular disease in men has declined steadily during the last 20 years. In women, unfortunately, this rate has remained relatively unchanged (Fig. 2).

Despite the magnitude of the problem, women comprise on average only 25% of most cardiovascular trials. Newer studies have demonstrated marked sex differences in response to therapy, outcomes, and preventive strategies which support the need for more information about optimal primary and secondary prevention strategies, diagnostic modalities, and response to medical and surgical therapy in women.

SEX DIFFERENCES VS. GENDER BIAS

Clear sex differences have been identified in the epidemiology and presentation of disease, risk factor prevalence, physiology, and response to diagnostic tests and interventions (Table 1). There are also several factors that solely affect women, including menopausal status, hormone replacement therapy, oral contraceptives, and pregnancy-related heart disease. During the last 2 decades several studies have noted important sex differences in clinical outcomes and in the use of diagnostic and therapeutic interventions during the evaluation and treatment of women with chest pain and myocardial infarction. Despite continued evidence of the importance of heart disease in women, they are still evaluated less intensively, underreferred, and not treated as aggressively as men for comparable presentation and disease. Furthermore, in one study, 10 times as many men with abnormal nuclear stress test results were referred for coronary angiography compared to women with similar

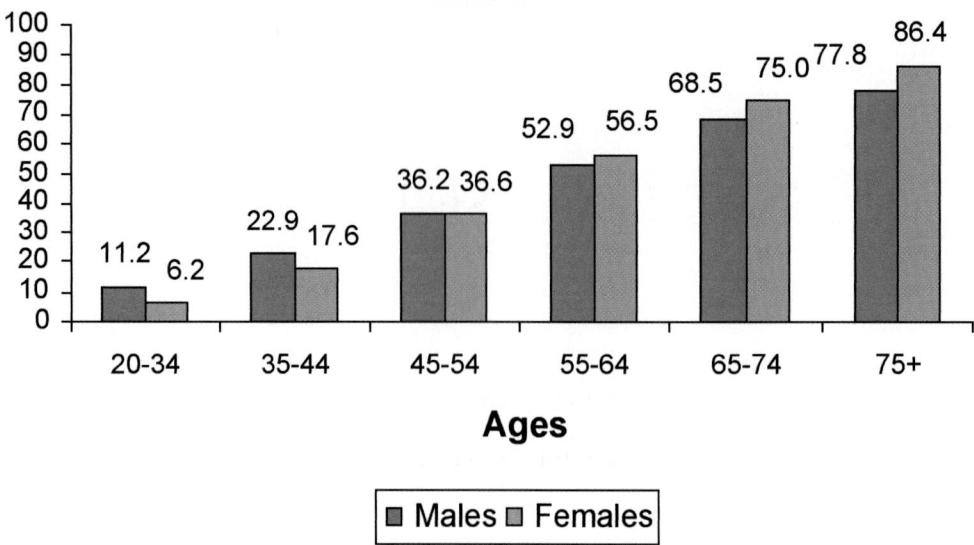

Fig. 1. Prevalence of cardiovascular disease including coronary heart disease, congestive heart failure, stroke, and hypertension in Americans by age and sex.

results, and women with abnormal test results were more than 4 times as likely to have their symptoms attributed to psychiatric causes. Myocardial infarctions are still clinically misdiagnosed at a much greater frequency in women than men. Although most of the differences and apparent bias demonstrated in some studies can be attributed to differences in baseline patient characteristics, some investigators have been concerned that the almost universal worse outcomes of cardiovascular disease in women cannot be explained solely by statistically controlling for older age and comorbid conditions.

CORONARY ARTERY DISEASE

Symptoms
On average women with coronary artery disease present with symptoms, cardiovascular events, or sudden cardiac death approximately 10 years later than men. Although the mechanism for this delay has not been explained completely, it is likely due to the protective effects of endogenous estrogen in premenopausal women. Most men and women present with "typical" symptoms of coronary artery disease. However, disproportionately more women present with atypical symptoms including prominent dyspnea, fatigue, referred pain, indigestion, nausea, syncope, or sweating. For women, advanced age, lower activity level, and increased prevalence of diabetes and other comorbid conditions often contribute to the more frequent occurrence of silent ischemia, dyspnea, and other non-classic symptoms. Furthermore, women typically present later than men to the emergency room with symptoms of an acute myocardial infarction.

Table 1.   Known Sex Differences That May Affect Diagnosis, Treatment, and Outcomes for Heart Disease

Epidemiology and prevalence
Age of onset
Etiology
Presenting symptoms
Risk factor prevalence and strengths
Comorbid conditions including diabetes mellitus, obesity, and chronic kidney disease
Body and coronary artery size
Menopause and hormonal status
Myocardial response to aging, blood pressure, and volume overload
Accuracy of diagnostic tests
Physiologic response to exercise
Response to pharmacologic intervention
Psychosocial/economic factors
Communication style

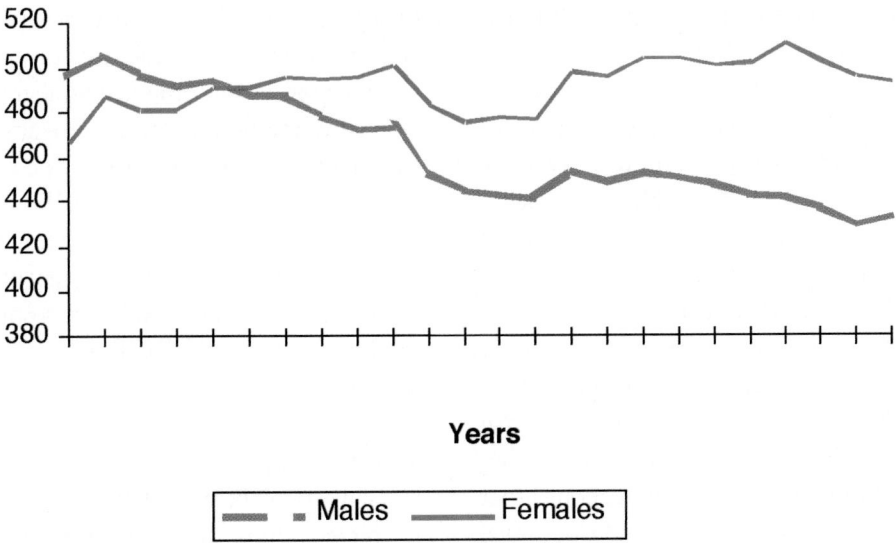

Years

| —— ▪ Males | —— Females |

Fig. 2. Cardiovascular disease mortality trends by sex in the United State.

Because of this later presentation and less typical symptoms, the diagnosis of heart disease in women can be missed and the delays in therapy can result in ineligibility for therapy such as an emergency percutaneous coronary intervention (PCI) or fibrinolysis.

Stress Testing

The noninvasive diagnosis of coronary artery disease in women is challenging. Standard stress electrocardiographic testing is less accurate in women compared to men. This has led some practitioners to adopt a rather negative approach and to treat women empirically without further investigation or use of invasive testing. This attitude is not warranted and could contribute to poor outcomes. Numerous studies have examined the results of exercise electrocardiography in women and found high false-positive rates in women compared with men, perhaps because of the lower prevalence of coronary artery disease in women until the age of 70. Also, there is evidence that the lower specificity is related to gender-specific autonomic and sex hormone effects on the electrocardiogram. In older women, failure to achieve an adequate stress level due to deconditioning or orthopedic limitation may adversely affect the sensitivity of an exercise test. Despite these limitations, normal findings on stress electrocardiography at an adequate workload in a woman are a good indicator that flow-limiting coronary artery disease is unlikely.

Because of these limitations, imaging stress tests have gained popularity for women. However, gender-specific artifacts and physiologic responses have been described in both nuclear and echocardiographic stress test studies. Historically, women have been underrepresented in studies of imaging stress tests, and the reported sensitivities and specificities have varied widely. Therefore, drawing conclusions about the absolute incremental value of stress imaging over standard stress testing is not possible.

Stress thallium scintigraphy improves diagnostic accuracy in women compared to radionucleotide angiography (MUGA), but many of the available clinical trials relied on planar thallium rather than the more commonly used single-photon emission computed tomography. Breast tissue attenuates radioactivity and may produce a false-positive study as a result of artifactual defects in the anterior wall and septum. The use of technetium 99m (Tc99m) sestamibi imaging, a higher energy radiotracer, reduces the breast tissue attenuation artifact, and limited comparison studies have suggested that thallium and sestamibi have similar test sensitivities but test specificity may be enhanced by sestamibi imaging. The use of pharmacologic agents such as adenosine or dobutamine has a similar diagnostic accuracy for both men and women.

Cardiac positron emission tomography (PET) has a similar high sensitivity as conventional stress sestamibi imaging, but PET has a higher specificity. PET imaging is particularly beneficial in the obese patient because of attenuation artifacts that will be present with sestamibi imaging. Even in patients with no significant obstructive coronary disease on angiography, abnormal myocardial blood flow and coronary flow reserve on PET imaging are associated with increased mortality.

Exercise echocardiography improves the accuracy of exercise testing for the diagnosis of heart disease in women and has been proposed as a cost-effective initial approach to the evaluation of chest pain. Also, it has the advantage of providing information about other causes of chest pain, including valvular and myocardial function. Dobutamine echocardiography is safe in women, and studies support a similar diagnostic accuracy for men and women.

As in all stress testing, the pretest probability of disease is likely more important in determining diagnostic accuracy than the specific type of test that is utilized. If the likelihood of coronary artery disease is low, no stress test is very accurate. If the goal is localization of ischemia or the resting electrocardiogram is abnormal, imaging techniques should be used. Additionally, if a woman cannot exercise adequately because of non-cardiac factors, the initial stress test should be pharmacologic. If, however, she can exercise adequately, because of the added benefit of the exercise portion of the test, this type of stress testing should be utilized.

In women with an intermediate probability of coronary artery disease and a normal resting electrocardiogram, standard stress electrocardiography has acceptable sensitivity and specificity. If the results are normal, there is high negative predictive value regarding the absence of coronary artery disease and the prognosis is good. There are not enough data to demonstrate a clearly superior imaging technique in women, so when this approach is chosen, the type of study should depend upon local expertise, patient characteristics, and cost. In women with worrisome symptoms and a high pretest probability of coronary artery disease, an argument can be made to proceed directly to coronary angiography to define the anatomy. Coronary angiography is safe in women, and most studies have demonstrated that despite gender differences in rates of referral to angiography, after the anatomy is defined, women are revascularized at a similar rate to men.

Electron-beam computed tomography (EBCT) is a sensitive method to detect coronary calcium and is similarly predictive of obstructive coronary artery disease in both men and women. Women have significantly lower coronary calcium score compared to men at all ages, even when coronary artery disease is present. However, the specificity and both positive and negative predictive value of EBCT is similar for men and women.

Medical Therapy

Overall aspirin, beta blockers, HMG Co-A-reductase inhibitors (statins), and angiotensin-converting enzyme inhibitors are underutilized in eligible patients especially women and the elderly. This is even true when coronary artery disease is documented or after a myocardial infarction. Women have more commonly been treated with calcium channel blockers, which have no documented survival benefit. Greater utilization of proven effective therapies is needed in our female patients.

Aspirin

In multiple studies, women have been shown to have equal benefit compared to men with the use of aspirin after a myocardial infarction. Recently in a study by Ridker and colleagues of 3,876 healthy women over the age of 45 years, the use of aspirin for primary prevention was studied. Women received 100 mg of aspirin every other day or a placebo and were followed for 10 years. In all women there was a significant benefit in the prevention of strokes (relative risk 0.83). However, there was no impact on the prevention of myocardial infarction in the overall study. However, in the 4,097 women over the age of 65 years there was a significant reduction in the risk of myocardial infarctions (relative risk 0.66) and a reduction in major adverse cardiovascular events (relative risk 0.74). Thus, in women aspirin is effective in secondary prevention and for primary prevention of stroke over the age of 45 and myocardial infarction over the age of 65.

Beta Blockers

The ISIS-I and ISIS-II trials demonstrated improved survival in women receiving beta blockers and aspirin comparable to men, with the greatest benefit in patients at highest risk. Other studies of the use of beta blockers have shown a similar benefit.

HMG Co-A-Reductase Inhibitors (Statins)

The most current studies demonstrate an added benefit for greater LDL reduction to less than 70 mg/dL for secondary prevention. Interestingly, in these studies as well as prior secondary prevention studies, women had generally a greater benefit from LDL reduction with statin therapy. In studies such as the Reversal of Atherosclerosis with an Aggressive Lipid Lowering (REVERSAL) trial the women treated with high-dose statin therapy had a reduction in their atheroma volume on intravascular ultrasound compared to men who just had slowing of disease progression.

Angiotensin-Converting Enzyme Inhibitors (ACE Inhibitors)

ACE inhibitors generally have beneficial effects in women but often less than those in men. This may be reflective of the fact that women typically have less reduction in left ventricular function after a myocardial infarction and less benefit from the treatment of hypertension. Despite these sex differences, ACE inhibitors still should be used in women who meet the appropriate criteria.

Coronary Angiography

Several studies have demonstrated that female gender is an independent predictor of a lower likelihood of receiving coronary angiography, even when baseline factors and severity of disease are considered. When women are referred for angiography they tend to be referred later in the course of their disease. Because coronary angiography is a prerequisite for catheter-based or surgical revascularization, women in these studies had a de facto lower rate of revascularization. Among men and women who undergo coronary angiography, there appears to be little difference in the subsequent use of percutaneous coronary revascularization and coronary artery bypass surgery (CABG), suggesting that once the anatomy is defined, subsequent decisions are based primarily on the severity of disease and not sex. Although the appropriate use of coronary angiography is still debated, these studies showed that appropriate cardiac catheterization was associated with low mortality in both men and women and the relative underuse of coronary angiography in women is associated with adverse long-term outcomes.

Percutaneous Coronary Intervention (PCI)

Early in the interventional era, the procedural success rate for balloon angioplasty in women was lower than in men. In the NHLBI PTCA registry of angioplasty alone, women had an angiographic success rate of 60.3% versus 66.2% in men and lower clinical success rates of 56.6% versus 66.2%. Additionally, women also had higher complications including a higher rate of intimal tears, which in the balloon angioplasty era was associated with an increased need for emergent CABG. Angioplasty was associated with a sixfold increase in short-term mortality in women compared to men. Much of the increased procedural complications and lower success rate in women was attributed to large and nonsteerable catheters and balloons in the generally smaller coronary arteries of women. Subsequent to 1985, sex differences in outcomes after percutaneous coronary revascularization disappeared. With current technology and equipment, no sex difference in procedural success or restenosis rates has been documented. Women undergoing coronary angiography and percutaneous coronary revascularization continue to have increased vascular complications compared to men. Additionally, women have a greater risk of bleeding associated with adjuvant therapies, including glycoprotein IIb/IIIa inhibitors, although with their use generally there is a similar benefit in women. Stenting has decreased the mortality associated with PCI, decreased morbidity, and allowed sicker patients with more complex disease to be treated in both men and women. Women have slightly smaller coronary arteries which contribute to adverse outcomes, but in the stenting era and now drug-eluting stent era, these differences are minimal and sex differences after adjusting for comorbidities are eliminated. Long-term outcomes after PCI are similar for both men and women. There is some suggestion that women may actually have less angiographic restenosis, fewer subsequent myocardial infarctions, repeat PCI, or CABG after the initial procedure. Nearly all reported series show that women have more severe angina and more concomitant illness, including diabetes mellitus, hypertension, and heart failure at the time of their intervention. When these baseline characteristics are considered, there are minimal or no sex differences in short- or long-term survival or rates of myocardial infarction or CABG whether the interventional procedures were performed for unstable angina, acute myocardial infarction, or electively for stable angina.

Women are more likely than men to have residual angina and to take antianginal medications after PCI. This difference is also observed after CABG and has not been explained completely. This may relate to greater microvascular disease and abnormalities in coronary flow reserve associated with left ventricular hypertrophy or diabetes mellitus.

In the current era, PCI should be offered to women who have appropriate indications for revascularization and suitable anatomy without specific concerns over sex. An appropriate referral for coronary angiography is necessary in these women to document their anatomy and lead to subsequent revascularization.

Coronary Artery Bypass Graft Surgery (CABG)

According to the early studies, women who have had CABG experienced greater operative and short-term mortality compared to men. Various explanations for this include technical factors related to smaller body size, more advanced disease at the time of operation, women more often presenting urgently or emergently, and referral bias. However, population studies and long-term results from the Coronary Artery Surgery Study (CASS) registry and Bypass Angioplasty Revascularization Investigation (BARI) trial have reported similar graft patency and long-term survival benefit in men and women following surgical revascularization. The rates of perioperative death and myocardial infarction are greater for women, but this disparity disappears when baseline factors (e.g., age) are considered. Women have a greater risk of heart failure, external wound infections, longer hospital stays, longer postoperative intubation, more blood transfusions, and postoperative congestive heart failure. Women are more likely to have residual angina requiring therapy after CABG. Importantly, in studies such as BARI there was no difference in acute and 5-year outcomes in CABG between men and women and, after adjusting for differences in baseline characteristics, women had a lower mortality at 5 years with an odds ratio for survival of 0.60. Diabetic women also had similar outcomes regardless of whether or not they were treated with PCI or CABG, and the differences in diabetic patients were seen primarily in

men. Thus, women should be referred for CABG when appropriate, and concerns about increased mortality should not influence referral.

MYOCARDIAL INFARCTION

Women consistently have a nearly 50% greater mortality following myocardial infarction compared with men. Much of this increased mortality can be attributed to comorbidities including hypertension, diabetes, heart failure, chronic kidney disease, and advancing age. Debate remains if there is any mortality difference in women and men after adjusting for these factors especially in older patients. However, younger women (<50 years) in the National Registry of Myocardial Infarction-2 had a marked increased in mortality compared with their male counterparts (odds of death 7%, for every 5 years of decreasing age in women). This unusual association of younger patients with increased mortality has been observed in several study populations, but the specific cause of this effect remains unknown.

Women are different in other aspects of their presentation. They have a greater delay to presentation to the emergency room and have a greater delay to treatment after their first electrocardiogram (ECG). Increased public awareness of the risk of heart disease in women will likely improve the delays women have to presentation, but the persistent delays in hospital therapy of women suggest physicians still need to better recognize the risk and symptoms of heart disease in women. Furthermore, in contemporary studies, acute myocardial infarctions are still misdiagnosed more commonly in women. When women present with an acute coronary syndrome, they more commonly present with unstable angina and have a greater increase in B-type natriuretic peptide compared with their male counterparts.

Fibrinolytic Therapy

Fibrinolysis is a highly effective therapy for the reduction of mortality after a myocardial infarction. Women appear to derive similar reduction in mortality with fibrinolytic therapy compared with men, with a risk reduction in most studies of 25-30%. The absolute mortality in women receiving fibrinolytic therapy is still higher than men, given the even higher mortality in women without reperfusion therapy. Women have similar angiographic reperfusion rates compared with men, but have higher bleeding complications including hemorrhagic stroke and major bleeding. The increase in hemorrhagic stroke appears to be particularly higher in women over the age of 70 years. However, the increase in bleeding complications may be at least partially explained by higher activated partial thromboplastin times. Reinfarction also appears to be more than twice that of men after fibrinolytic therapy, which raises the possibility that women may require more aggressive angiography after fibrinolytic therapy. Despite the marked benefit of fibrinolytic therapy in women, there is a lower utilization of this therapy and in those who receive therapy there is a greater time from the initial ECG to treatment.

Percutaneous Coronary Revascularization in Myocardial Infarction

In women, PCI for an acute ST-elevation myocardial infarction reduces mortality and in the Primary Coronary Angioplasty for Acute Myocardial Infarction (PAMI) study, the unadjusted mortality was 3.3 times higher with fibrinolytic therapy compared with PCI. Importantly, PCI is associated with a lower incidence of intracranial hemorrhage compared to fibrinolytic therapy, and given the higher incidence of intracranial hemorrhage in women with fibrinolytic therapy, the overall risk benefit ratio favors PCI for reperfusion therapy more in women than in men. Women still have approximately a 3-fold higher vascular access complication rate with PCI compared to men. In other studies, such as that by Mulller and colleagues, when women are treated as aggressively with primary PCI for acute myocardial infarctions, their mortality after a myocardial infarction is even lower than men. Other studies with a similar goal of aggressive PCI therapy in both women and men have shown that there is no difference in mortality from myocardial infarction when both men and women are treated equally aggressively. However, retrospective data suggests women still have a higher mortality after primary PCI. Exclusion criteria in studies, delays in therapy, and biases in the use of proven strategies to reduce mortality in women with myocardial infarctions may explain some of these differences between the trials and more real world practices.

Adjuvant Medical Therapy

Although no prospective studies have been designed to evaluate the role of adjuvant medical therapy in women, substudies, meta-analyses and retrospective data suggest a similar benefit in women compared to men with aspirin, beta-blockers, and theinopyridines. All efforts should be made to place appropriate women on these therapies according to the current ACC/AHA guidelines.

POSTMENOPAUSAL HORMONE THERAPY

Our current understanding of postmenopausal hormone therapy highlights the importance of prospective studies performed in women at risk for cardiovascular disease or who have established coronary artery disease. Multiple observational studies suggested a 40-50% reduction of cardiovascular events with the use of hormone therapy for both primary and secondary prevention. Furthermore, estrogen is well established to have many mechanisms with potential cardiovascular benefit. These include a 10-20% reduction in LDL cholesterol, a 10-30% increase in HDL cholesterol, and a 25-50% reduction in lipoprotein (a). In the 1990s these findings led to the guidelines for female patients with hyperlipidemia to consider estrogen therapy as the primary therapy for secondary prevention in women with hyperlipidemia. However, in 1998 when the Heart and Estrogen/Progestin Replacement Study (HERS) was presented by Hulley and colleagues, the beneficial effects of estrogen were questioned. In this secondary prevention study of 2,763 women less than 80 years of age treated with continuous combined hormone therapy (conjugated equine estrogen plus medroxyprogesterone) and followed for 4.1 years, they found no reduction in the incidence of cardiovascular events with hormone therapy. Additionally, there were increased thrombotic events including pulmonary emboli with hormone therapy, particularly in the first 2 years of follow-up. Hormone therapy had no significant effect on stroke.

The next important study was the Estrogen Replacement and Atherosclerosis (ERA) Study by Herrington and colleagues which randomized 309 women with a coronary artery stenosis greater than 30% to conjugated equine estrogen, conjugated equine estrogen plus medroxyprogesterone, or placebo. Angiographic follow-up was performed at 3.2 years, and no change in luminal diameter or new lesion development with hormone therapy.

The Women's Health Initiative (WHI) was the largest of these prospective hormone therapy studies.

This study included 16,608 women ages between 50-79 with a mean age of 63.3 years randomized to conjugated equine estrogen plus medroxyprogesterone or placebo with a planned follow-up of 8.5 years. However, this study was terminated at 5.2 years because of no evidence for cardiovascular benefit and excessive risk. This study found a hazard ratio for stroke of 1.4, for pulmonary emboli of 2.1, breast cancer of 1.3, and coronary heart disease of 1.3. In the treated women, there was an excess of stroke of 8 events per 10,000 woman-years. There was, however, a significant reduction in colorectal cancer and hip fractures. In this landmark study of primary prevention in a low-risk population with a wide age range there was no cardiovascular disease benefit to continuous combined hormone therapy. This study led to multiple questions, such as the timing and dose of estrogen replacement therapy as well as the progestin utilized. In the estrogen-alone trial, women who had previously had a hysterectomy were randomized to receive conjugated equine estrogen or placebo. This trial was terminated early after 6.8 years of follow-up (planned 8.5 years). There was no difference in the primary outcome of myocardial infarction or coronary death in those assigned to estrogen therapy compared with placebo (hazard ratio, 0.95; 0.79-1.16). This hazard ratio tended to favor the use of estrogen in women 50 to 59 years (0.63; 0.36-1.08), but did not reach statistical significance. In the 50-59 year-old women, there was less coronary revascularization with estrogen therapy (hazard ratio 0.55; 0.35-0.86). Additionally, the risk of venothromboembolism seen in the conjugated equine estrogen plus medroxyprogesterone study was significantly less with conjugated equine estrogen alone and was associated with a risk of 2.2 women per 1,000 patient years compared with placebo (hazard ratio 1.32; 0.99-1.75).

One criticism of the WHI and HERS has been the fact that participants were postmenopausal for many years before going on hormone therapy. In animal studies, it appears that there is a window of opportunity where estrogen therapy may be beneficial if initiated in the perimenopausal period but not if started later. Prospective studies in women are under way and include the Kronos Early Estrogen Prevention Study (KEEPS). At the current time the FDA has a black box label on estrogen products stating an increased risk for heart disease, myocardial infarction, stroke, and breast cancer. Furthermore the FDA advises that estrogen not be used for heart disease prevention and that it should be used in the lowest effective dose and for the shortest duration possible.

MICROVASCULAR DYSFUNCTION AND ENDOTHELIAL DYSFUNCTION

With the publication of the Coronary Artery Surgery Study (CASS) data it became clear that 50% of women referred for coronary angiography with chest pain did not have significant epicardial coronary artery disease compared to 17% of men. With the NHLBI-sponsored Women's Ischemic Syndrome Evaluation (WISE) study, greater emphasis has been placed on the impact of microvascular dysfunction in women (Table 2). Women presenting with an acute coronary syndrome also have a lower incidence of significant epicardial artery occlusions. Microvascular abnormalities and other markers of age-related arterial stiffness, including increased pulse pressure, can be used to predict ischemic heart disease outcomes in women. These correlations have not consistently been found to exist in men. Microvascular dysfunction is associated with a worse prognosis and may also help to account for abnormal stress tests and anginal symptoms in women without evidence of obstructive disease in the epicardial arteries. In the WISE study, endothelial dysfunction was associated with decreased functional capacity and worse outcomes.

Endothelial dysfunction is also an important component of coronary disease in women. Sex hormones exert effects on vascular reactivity through the endothelium and smooth muscle cells. These hormonal effects

Table 2. Vascular Abnormalities in Women With Heart Disease Compared to Men

Decreased epicardial and microvascular size
Increased arterial stiffness suggesting greater fibrosis and altered remodeling
More diffuse atherosclerotic disease
More endothelial dysfunction

have influenced nitric oxide synthase, L-type voltage-gaited calcium; activated calcium channels; and affect vascular repair. Endothelial dysfunction may also result in coronary artery spasm that can be demonstrated by provocative challenges to the endothelium in the cardiac catheterization laboratory with agents such as acetylcholine or Methergine. Patients with endothelial dysfunction are at increased risk of cardiac mortality and need aggressive management of their cardiovascular disease risk factors and symptoms.

HEART FAILURE

Epidemiology

Heart failure is the most common cause of hospitalization in both men and women. Both the incidence of heart failure and, more dramatically, the prevalence of heart failure are increasing, in part due to the improved survival of patients with risk factors for heart failure such as coronary artery disease. Men have a slightly higher incidence of heart failure at all ages, but because women represent a greater proportion of the elderly population, over half (51%) of the people living with heart failure are women. Women have a 20% risk of developing heart failure in their lifetime. Generally, men have a greater mortality from heart failure. In the Framingham Study, men have a median survival after diagnosis of 1.7 years, while it was 3.2 years in women. Still, 63% of all heart failure deaths in United States are women.

Risk Factors

The most common risk factors for heart failure are coronary artery disease, hypertension, and valvular heart disease in both men and women. Diabetes, obesity, nicotine use, and age are also common risk factors. However, the relative roles of the risk factors differ by sex. Hypertension, diabetes, tobacco use, and left ventricular hypertrophy are more potent risk factors in women than men, and physical inactivity is a risk factor in women, but not in men. Diabetes is associated with an increase in heart failure in women, even when coronary artery disease is not present. Up to 91% of men and women with heart failure have hypertension, and, after the age of 55 years, women are more likely to have heart failure than men. After a myocardial infarction, women are more likely to develop heart failure, even if the overall ejection fraction is preserved.

Systolic vs. Diastolic Heart Failure

Preserved systolic function is present in 40-60% of patients hospitalized for heart failure. In the Framingham Study women represented 65% of the patients with diastolic heart failure but only 25% of those with systolic heart failure. Importantly, most trials which have been conducted in patients with left ventricular systolic dysfunction, and therefore optimal management and outcomes of treatment have not been fully evaluated in this population. The prevalence of diastolic heart failure increases with age, and the mortality in diastolic heart failure is lower than systolic heart failure (annual mortality diastolic heart failure: 8-9%, systolic heart failure: 15-19%).

There may be clear sex differences in the response to pressure overload which may account for the differences in the incidence of diastolic heart failure. In women, there is a 30% increase in the end-diastolic volume in heart failure which is not seen in men, which suggests that women rely on Frank-Starling mechanisms to increase cardiac output, where men rely more on increases in contractility. Sex hormones may contribute to some of these differences. Estrogen decreases renin activity, smooth muscle cell growth, decreases collagen deposition, and inhibits cardiac fibroblasts and monocytes. Testosterone increases renin activity, cardiac hypertrophy, and cardiac fibrosis.

Treatment

Angiotensin-converting enzyme inhibitors (ACE-I) are currently a fundamental part of heart failure regimens. In a meta-analysis of 5 large trials by Flather and colleagues, ACE-I are beneficial in women (odds ratio for death 0.85), but this benefit is less than in men (0.79). Beta blockers are also effective therapy in women and, in a pooled analysis of four of the beta-blocker studies, women had a similar benefit to beta blockers as men (relative risk of mortality women: 0.69, men: 0.66). In studies, aldosterone antagonists also appear to be equally effective regardless of gender. However, special consideration is needed when digoxin is used in women. In the in the Digitalis Investigation Group (DIG) trial, digoxin resulted in a reduction in hospitalizations for heart failure in both men and women, and in the overall trial and in men, this was without an increase in mortality. In women mortality was higher with digoxin therapy (33.1% vs 28.9%, P<0.05), an associated with an increased peak digoxin level in the women. Thus, if digoxin is used in women, careful monitoring of the digoxin level is warranted.

Despite benefit of women to proven heart failure therapy, women are treated with these medications less frequently than men. This may be due to multiple factors, including the increased age in women, and more preserved left ventricular function. Additionally, women are less likely to be referred to a cardiologist for care, which may also impede optimal diagnostic testing and management.

Outcomes

Women with heart failure are generally more symptomatic than men with greater complaints of dyspnea and edema, a greater reduction in exercise capacity, and more overt signs of heart failure (edema, elevated jugular venous distention, rales, and S3). Women also have a lower quality of life with heart failure compared with men, are more likely to be hospitalized with heart failure, and have longer lengths of hospital stay. Despite the increased symptoms in women, the mortality in women is lower (1 year mortality in the Framingham Study 24% for women and 28% for men).

Arrhythmias and Sudden Cardiac Death

Clear sex differences in normal cardiac electrophysiology exist, including a higher resting heart rate in women, even after autonomic blockade, and prolongation of the QT interval. The QT interval is similar in boys and girls, but at puberty the QT interval shortens in boys due to androgens. Boys develop a typical male pattern of ventricular repolarization which is characterized by higher amplitude of the J-point, a shorter and steeper ST segment course, a steeper ascent, and a higher amplitude of the T wave. Further sex differences and potential proarrhythmic effects of medications are caused by the competitive metabolism of estrogen and other agents by the cytochrome P450 enzyme system. Many of these differences are still not well understood.

Paroxysmal Supraventricular Tachycardia (PSVT)

Atrioventricular (AV) nodal reentry tachycardia is twice as common in women compared with men, while AV reentry through an accessory pathway is twice as common in men. Hormonal variations, specifically in the luteal phase of the menstrual cycle, may play a role in triggering these arrhythmias in women with a history of PSVT, but the specific cause has not been elucidated. Possible contributors include estrogen or progesterone level variations, increased catecholamine, increased body temperature or altered calcium channel activity. Despite the sex differences in the frequency of these arrhythmias, radiofrequency ablation is equally efficacious.

Atrial Fibrillation

Atrial fibrillation is the most common arrhythmia in both men and women. Although the incidence is higher in men at all ages, because of the larger number of women over the age of 75 years, the prevalence is higher in women. In the Framingham Heart Study, atrial fibrillation is also associated with a higher mortality in women (adjusted odds ratio for death of 1.9 in women vs. 1.5 in men). Women have faster ventricular rates with atrial fibrillation, a higher incidence of QT prolongation with antiarrhythmic use, and a greater frequency of torsades de pointes. The treatment of atrial fibrillation is similar in men and women, but caution should be used with antiarrhythmic therapy because of QT prolongation.

Sudden Cardiac Death

In the 28-year follow-up of the Framingham study, sudden death was more frequent in men compared with women at all ages. This difference may be partially related to the delayed-onset of coronary artery disease in women. However, even in patients without coronary artery disease, men still have a higher incidence of sudden cardiac death. In recent years, sudden cardiac death has been declining in all age groups except women between the ages of 35 and 44, where there has been a 21% increased incidence. The specific reason for this increase is not known. Prevention of sudden death includes the prevention of coronary artery disease, medical therapy and revascularization for coronary artery disease, and internal cardiac defibrillators (ICD). Although women were underrepresented in most of the ICD trials, women appear to have equal benefit to men when an ICD is indicated.

63

HEART DISEASE IN THE ELDERLY

Imran S. Syed, MD

Joseph G. Murphy, MD

R. Scott Wright, MD

Older patients suffer disproportionately from heart disease compared to younger patients but also benefit more in absolute numbers with aggressive medical therapy, but at the cost of a higher incidence of adverse side effects.

AGE-RELATED CHANGES IN CARDIAC ANATOMY AND PHYSIOLOGY

Ventricle

Heart weight increases about 1 g per year between ages 30 and 90 years, probably due to left ventricular hypertrophy secondary to an age-related increase in systolic blood pressure. This results in an increase in both left ventricular mass and wall thickness. In addition to myocardial cell mass, intercellular collagen also increases with age.

Ventricular hypertrophy leads to significant changes in cardiac function with age, including 1) an increase in left ventricular stiffness; 2) reduced filling during early diastole; and 3) a prolonged diastolic isometric relaxation phase. There is a reduction in the length of the left ventricle from apex to base with the development of an S-, or sigmoid-, shaped septum in some patients.

Conduction System

There are marked changes in the conduction system, including loss of 50% to 75% of the pacemaker cells of the sinoatrial node and fibrosis of the specialized conduction tissue of the bundle of His. Interestingly, some parameters of cardiac function change little with age, including resting cardiac output, stroke volume, and ejection fraction.

■ Systolic function is well preserved in the elderly, but diastolic function is impaired.

ATRIAL FIBRILLATION

The occurrence of atrial fibrillation increases steadily with age and is present in about 5% of subjects older than 65 years. Atrial fibrillation in the elderly is frequently asymptomatic. Atrial fibrillation is associated with an increased long-term mortality primarily due to stroke. In the absence of anticoagulation the stroke risk with nonrheumatic atrial fibrillation is overall approximately 5% percent per year but with a much higher incidence in very elderly patients (>80 years) and in those with rheumatic atrial fibrillation. Independent risk factors for a thromboembolic event in patients with atrial fibrillation include age, diabetes, hypertension, a history of heart failure, a prior transient ischemic attack or stroke, an enlarged left atrium, and poor left ventricular function. Warfarin correctly dosed (INR between 2-3) reduces the risk of stroke by about two-thirds. Age is an independent risk factor for hemorrhagic complications with warfarin therapy, as are poorly controlled hypertension and excessive anticoagulation. Older patients benefit more than younger patients from anticoagulation. Overall, the benefits of warfarin therapy outweigh the bleeding risks in the elderly population, and in general warfarin is indicated for the prophylaxis of thromboembolic events in most elderly patients in atrial fibrillation. Aspirin provides some limited protection from stroke in elderly patients when warfarin anticoagulation is strongly contraindicated. A strategy of rhythm control in which an antiarrhythmic drug is used to lower the risk of recurrent atrial fibrillation does not reduce the stroke risk compared to rate control alone.

The diagnosis of atrial fibrillation may be subtle in the elderly. Atrial fibrillation can worsen or precipitate heart failure and angina in the elderly patient, and the worsening or new onset of these symptoms should merit a search for arrhythmias, including atrial fibrillation. Mental status changes, stroke, or a transient ischemic attack also may be the presenting symptoms for new-onset atrial fibrillation. Occult hyperthyroidism, silent myocardial infarction, hypokalemia due to use of a diuretic, alcoholism, and digoxin toxicity may present with atrial fibrillation. Pulmonary disease, including pneumonia, pulmonary embolism, and chronic obstructive lung disease, may precipitate atrial fibrillation, especially if β-agonists are used.

- Atrial fibrillation occurs in about 5% of subjects older than 65 years.
- Age is an independent risk factor for hemorrhagic complications with warfarin therapy in the elderly.
- Warfarin reduces the stroke risk by about two-thirds.

BRADYCARDIAS

Aging is associated with an increased occurrence of conduction system fibrosis within the sinus node, atrioventricular node, and bundle branches. Sympathetic and parasympathetic neural influence on the conduction system decreases. Maximal heart rate decreases with age, and sinus bradycardia is common in the elderly even in the absence of cardiac disease. The elderly are more dependent than younger patients on atrial systole to complete late ventricular diastolic filling.

- Maximal heart rate decreases with age.

CORONARY ARTERY DISEASE

Dyspnea is a more common presenting symptom of coronary artery disease in the elderly patient than in the younger patient. A fourth heart sound and a soft mitral regurgitation murmur are frequently present in many elderly patients and are poor predictors of the presence of coronary artery disease. The treatment of coronary artery disease in the elderly is similar to that in younger patients. Coronary artery bypass and percutaneous coronary intervention are both very effective in the elderly but are associated with a somewhat higher morbidity and mortality rate.

- A fourth heart sound and a soft mitral regurgitation murmur are poor predictors of the presence of coronary artery disease in the elderly.

MYOCARDIAL INFARCTION

Myocardial infarction is associated with a higher mortality rate, a higher incidence of congestive cardiac failure, and a higher reinfarction rate in the elderly patient than in the younger patient. Fewer elderly patients with myocardial infarction are eligible for thrombolysis because of contraindications (such as stroke, transient ischemic attack, severe hypertension, bleeding), and in those without contraindications, thrombolytics are used less often in part because of the higher occurrence of late and atypical presentations of myocardial infarction. The diagnosis of myocardial infarction is more difficult in the elderly; dyspnea and pulmonary edema are the most common presentation symptoms. Electrocardiography frequently is nondiagnostic because of baseline electrocardiographic abnormalities including left bundle branch block. Non–Q-wave myocardial infarction, cardiogenic shock, cardiac rupture, and death due to electromechanical dissociation are more common. The size of a first infarct does not increase with age, and death from ventricular fibrillation is less common than in the younger patient with infarction. Both primary coronary intervention (PCI) and thrombolysis are beneficial for the treatment of acute ST elevation myocardial infarction (STMI) in the elderly but PCI is associated with a lower rate of stroke compared with thrombolysis in the elderly. PCI is the treatment of choice for elderly patients with STMI but in the absence of a time realistic emergency PCI option, thrombolytic therapy still improves outcomes compared to placebo in older individuals; but at the cost of increasing mortality and bleeding complications and a lowered survival benefit compared to younger patients, particularly in patients older than 75 years. The indications for adjunctive PCI after myocardial infarction in the elderly are similar to those in younger patients and include the occurrence of exercise-induced or spontaneous myocardial ischemia.

- Elderly patients with myocardial infarction are less often candidates for thrombolysis.
- Primary angioplasty is not associated with the excess stroke rate that occurs with use of thrombolytics in the elderly.

STRESS TESTING

Treadmill exercise stress testing is less useful in the elderly population because of the higher occurrence of resting ST-segment changes, higher use of digoxin, and the increased incidence of peripheral vascular, orthopedic, and lung disease that limit exercise capacity. The predictive accuracy of a negative stress test is lower in the elderly patient because of the higher occurrence of occult coronary artery disease. Stress testing with cardiac imaging is the preferred option for noninvasive evaluation of suspect coronary disease in the elderly.

- The predictive accuracy of a negative stress test is lower in the elderly patient.

LIPID MANAGEMENT

Despite their proven benefit, lipid-lowering drugs are markedly underutilized in elderly patients.

Multiple clinical trials of cholesterol lowering medications including the Scandinavian Simvastatin Survival Study (4S trial), the Cholesterol and Recurrent

Events (CARE trial), the LIPID trial, the Heart Protection Study, and the Pravastatin in elderly individuals at risk of vascular disease (PROSPER trial) have included large numbers of elderly patients with hyperlipidemia, both with and without clinical heart disease. These studies have consistently demonstrated significant benefits in the elderly comparable to younger patients in relative terms with an approximate 30%-40% reduction in all cause mortality, major coronary events and number of revascularization procedures. Benefit was present for both patients with established coronary heart disease and those with hypercholesterolemia but without clinically overt heart disease. Older patients benefit more than younger patients in absolute terms because of the higher prevalence of coronary disease in the elderly. Secondary causes of hyperlipidemia, including diabetes and hypothyroidism, are more common in the elderly. Hormone replacement therapy in postmenopausal women is not protective against coronary atherosclerosis, a finding well proven by the Women's Health Initiative and HERS randomized trials.

ISOLATED SYSTOLIC HYPERTENSION IN THE ELDERLY

Hypertension is common in persons older than 65 years with an overall incidence of approximately 50% and a lifetime risk of about 80% in subjects surviving into their 80s. Systolic pressure rises and diastolic pressure falls after age 60 in both untreated hypertensive and nonhypertensive subjects. Isolated systolic hypertension is a common form of hypertension in the elderly and is caused primarily by arterial stiffness and diminished vascular compliance. Pulse pressure increases with age due to an increase in systolic pressure usually with little or no change in diastolic blood pressure. Elevated systolic blood pressure and pulse pressures are strong predictors of cardiovascular events in the elderly.

Isolated systolic hypertension is an elevated systolic blood pressure (above 140-160 mm Hg) with a diastolic pressure below 90 mm Hg. Isolated systolic hypertension is associated with an increased risk of myocardial infarction, left ventricular hypertrophy, renal dysfunction and stroke.

Treating isolated systolic hypertension in the elderly significantly reduces morbidity and mortality as demonstrated by the SHEPS Trial—Systolic Hypertension in the Elderly Program—which used a thiazide diuretic and added a β-blocker if needed. This benefit extends to the primary end point of stroke and the secondary end point of myocardial infarction. An interesting finding in the SHEPS study was that the reduction in cardiovascular events was not seen in patients with with hypokalemia (defined as a serum potassium <3.5 mEq/L). Antihypertensive medication has also been shown to lower the incidence of multi-infarct and vascular dementia in the elderly. Thiazide diuretics should be administered in low doses (equivalent to 12.5 mg to 25 mg of hydrochlorothiazide) to minimize the metabolic complications of high dose thiazide usage which induces depletion of potassium and magnesium, elevation in serum uric acid and mild elevations in plasma glucose and cholesterol. In general systolic pressure should be lowered gradually in the elderly to avoid postural hypotension with a goal systolic pressure 20 mm Hg below the baseline level if the initial value was between 160 and 180 mm Hg or below 160 mm Hg if the initial value was above 180 mm Hg (SHEPS Trial). Excess reduction in diastolic blood pressure may increase cardiovascular events and diastolic blood pressure should not be reduced to less than 65 mm Hg to attain the target systolic pressure.

The Seventh Report of the Joint National Committee on Prevention, Detection, Evaluation, and Treatment of High Blood Pressure (JNC 7) provided the following key recommendations for hypertension management.

1. In middle aged and elderly patients a systolic blood pressure greater than 140 mm Hg was a stronger predictor of future cardiovascular events than diastolic blood pressure.

2. Goal blood pressure is <140/90 mm Hg for most patients but is lower at <130/80 mm Hg for patients with diabetes or chronic kidney disease

3. Pre-hypertension is defined as a systolic blood pressure of 120 to 139 mm Hg or a diastolic blood pressure of 80 to 89 mm Hg and requires aggressive lifestyle modifications to prevent the development of cardiovascular disease.

4. Thiazide-type diuretics should be used in drug treatment for most patients with uncomplicated hypertension, either alone or combined with drugs from other classes.

VALVULAR HEART DISEASE

Calcific aortic stenosis, usually due to degenerative changes in a tricuspid valve, is the most common valvular heart disease in the elderly. The classic physical signs of aortic stenosis seen in younger patients including the parvus and tardus pulse waveform may be absent because of increased arterial stiffness. Benign systolic murmurs due to aortic sclerosis without stenosis are frequent. Aortic valve replacement is superior to balloon aortic valvuloplasty in all but moribund patients with severe aortic stenosis. Mitral regurgitation due to papillary muscle dysfunction resulting from ischemia and myxomatous degeneration of the mitral valve apparatus are both frequent in the elderly. Mitral stenosis is usually the late result of rheumatic fever. The opening snap of mitral stenosis may be absent in the elderly patient because of valve calcification and rigidity. The intensity of the first heart sound also may be reduced for similar reasons. Balloon mitral valvuloplasty is less successful in the elderly patient with mitral stenosis because of the increased occurrence of valvular and subvalvular calcification.

- The physical signs of aortic stenosis may be masked in the elderly.
- The opening snap of mitral stenosis may be absent in the elderly.

CONGESTIVE HEART FAILURE

Heart failure occurs in up to 10% of patients older than 80 years, and in many cases it is due to diastolic ventricular dysfunction with preserved systolic ventricular function. The elderly are relatively more dependent on the Frank-Starling stretch response and less dependent on heart rate to increase cardiac output in response to exercise. The impaired ability of the aged kidney to excrete a fluid challenge contributes to fluid overload. Factors that lead to ventricular diastolic dysfunction and heart failure in the elderly include an impaired ventricular relaxation and increased myocardial stiffness, leading to an increase in left ventricular diastolic filling pressure. Treatment of diastolic ventricular dysfunction is primarily with angiotensin-converting enzyme inhibitors, while diuretics may exacerbate diastolic ventricular dysfunction.

- The elderly are relatively more dependent on the

Frank-Starling stretch response and less dependent on heart rate to increase cardiac output.

Cardiac Drugs

Elderly patients in general have a decreased lean body mass, decreased serum proteins, decreased glomerular filtration rate, and decreased hepatic microsomal oxidation compared with younger patients. Renal clearance of digoxin, quinidine, and procainamide is decreased, and drug toxicity occurs more easily than in younger patients. In the Cardiac Arrhythmia Suppression Trial (CAST study), the incidence of proarrhythmia was higher in elderly patients than in younger patients with the antiarrhythmic agents flecainide, encainide, and moricizine. Adverse drug reactions are at least doubled in the elderly, and patient compliance with drug regimens is poorer. The elderly have blunted baroreceptor reflexes and diminished b-receptor responsiveness.

■ Adverse drug reactions are at least doubled in the elderly.

64

ERECTILE DYSFUNCTION AND HEART DISEASE

Bijoy K. Khandheria, MD

Ajay Nehra, MD

Major advances of significant magnitude have taken place in basic and clinical research pertaining to sexual activity and cardiovascular risk. Sexual dysfunction in men includes decreased libido, anatomical abnormalities such as Peyronie disease, ejaculatory problems, and erectile dysfunction. Erectile dysfunction (ED) is defined as the inability to achieve or maintain an erection that is adequate for intercourse.

Penile erectile function is the result of a complex interplay between vascular, neurologic, hormonal, and psychologic factors. The attainment and maintenance of a firm erection requires good arterial inflow of blood as well as efficient trapping of venous outflow. Disease processes which affect the function of the arterial and venous system would therefore be expected to have a negative impact on the erectile function of a male. Epidemiologic studies have confirmed the high prevalence of ED in middle-aged and older men and the impact of ED on psychologic well-being and quality of life. ED is a physiologic disorder seen among males, which by NIH estimates affects between 10 to 20 million males in the United States. It is generally understood that common risk factors for cardiovascular disease (CVD), such as hypertension, hyperlipidemia, diabetes mellitus, and obesity, are important predictors of ED. In the Rancho Bernardo Study, age, body mass index, and hypercholesterolemia were each significantly associated with an increased risk of ED. In all, 1 in 5 men had >3 risk factors and were at a 2.2-fold increased risk of ED.

It has been proposed and confirmed that ED may be an early marker of endothelial dysfunction preceding the typical symptoms and signs of coronary vascular disease.

SEXUAL ACTIVITY AND THE RISK OF A CARDIAC EVENT

Anecdotal evidence suggests that the risk of MI or death is higher during or immediately after sexual intercourse. The Stockholm Heart Epidemiology Programme (SHEEP) is a study of the magnitude of increased risk with sexual activity. Only 1.3% of patients had sexual activity before the onset of their symptoms. The relative risk (RR) of acute MI was 2.1 during the first hour after sexual activity. The RR among patients with a sedentary lifestyle was 4.4. In another study of 1,774 patients following myocardial infarction, only 1.5% of these events occurred within 2 hours of sexual intercourse, and sex was considered a direct contributing factor in 0.9% of these cases.

Patients with an implanted pacemaker do not appear to be at an increased risk with sexual activity. It is well known that patients with hypertrophic obstructive cardiomyopathy are at increased risk of syncope and sudden death following vigorous exercise. The risk of sexual activity in these patients is currently not known.

Risk of arrhythmias following sexual intercourse

has been evaluated, and most patients with prior known rhythm disturbances did not experience any exacerbation in their arrhythmias with sexual activity. If sexual ventricular ectopic activity did occur during sex, most of it was noted to be similar to that seen with normal daily activity.

Following sexual intercourse, this risk increases around twofold to 2 chances per million per hour, but only for the two hours following intercourse. For low-risk patients without any prior history of cardiovascular disease and an annual myocardial infarction risk of 1% per year, the risk increases to 1.01% with weekly sexual activity. In a high-risk patient with an annual myocardial infarction risk of 10% per year, this risk would only increase to 10.1% per year with weekly sexual activity. Hence, evidence in the literature does not support the anecdotal findings of significantly higher risk of MI or death related to sexual intercourse.

Even though most patients today can be effectively treated for their ED, the question then arises as to whether the resumption of sexual activity is safe in patients after acute coronary syndrome. A study following male patients after coronary artery bypass grafting (CABG) found that 17% of patients and 35% of their partners were afraid of resuming sexual activity. These patients often seek counseling on their relative risk of resuming sexual activity.

The physical activity of sexual intercourse is associated with increased myocardial oxygen demand (MVO_2) and increased sympathetic nervous system activation, both of which can result in myocardial ischemia in the presence of CAD. The effect of sexual activity on total body oxygen consumption (VO_2) and MVO_2 has not been studied extensively. Nonetheless, available research shows that sexual intercourse increases VO_2 modestly to 3 to 5 metabolic equivalents. In one study of men (aged 25 to 43 years) engaged in sexual activity with their wives, foreplay and stimulation had minimal effects on heart rate, VO_2, and rate-pressure product. However, orgasm was associated with maximal increases in all 3 of these parameters. The highest metabolic expenditure at stimulation/orgasm was associated with intercourse, especially the man-on-top position, where 3 to 4 METS were exerted. Furthermore, this increase in VO_2 lasts only for a brief period. It is believed that the small increase in the incidence of myocardial infarction that accompanies

sexual activity within 2 hours of onset is likely related to sympathetic activation and to an increase in MVO_2.

CARDIOVASCULAR RISK ASSESSMENT

The Princeton algorithm for cardiovascular risk assessment places emphasis on the potential risk of sexual activity in patient's cardiovascular risk factors (Table 1) or with comorbid cardiovascular disease (Tables 2, 3, and 4). Patients with ED should be stratified into low, intermediate or indeterminate, or high levels of cardiac risk.

Low-risk patients can safely initiate or resume sexual activity or receive treatment for sexual dysfunction. Patients at intermediate (or indeterminate) levels of risk need further cardiac evaluation, such as stress testing, before being restratified into either the low- or high-risk group. Patients in the high-risk category should be stabilized by specific treatment for their cardiac condition before resumption of sexual activity or initiation of treatment for sexual dysfunction.

Table 1.   Cardiovascular Risk Factors (Princeton Consensus Conference)

Age
Male gender
Hypertension
Diabetes mellitus
Cigarette smoking
Dyslipidemia
Sedentary lifestyle
Family history of premature coronary artery disease

Table 2.   Low-Risk Patients (Princeton Consensus Conference)

Asymptomatic, less than 3 risk factors
Adequately controlled hypertension
Stable angina pectoris
Status after coronary revascularization procedure
Greater than 8 weeks after myocardial infarction
Left ventricular dysfunction (NYHA class I)
Mild valvular heart disease
Atrial fibrillation

Table 3. Indeterminate- or Intermediate-Risk Patient (Princeton Concensus Conference)

Asymptomatic, equal to or greater than 3 risk factors
Moderate, stable angina pectoris (ischemia at reproducible heart rate, blood pressure)
Myocardial infarction greater than 2 weeks but less than 6 weeks previously
Left ventricular dysfunction (NYHA class 2)
Noncardiac sequelae of atherosclerotic disease (e.g., peripheral arterial disease, stroke)

Table 4. High-Risk Patients (Princeton Consensus Conference)

Unstable or refractory angina pectoris
Uncontrolled hypertension
Left ventricular dysfunction (NYHA III, IV)
Recent MI—less than 2 weeks
Hypertrophic obstructive cardiomyopathy
Moderate to severe valve disease
High-risk arrhythmia

TREATMENT OF ERECTILE DYSFUNCTION

A large majority of healthy men remain interested in sex late in life, with studies showing that 83%-90% of men aged 70-90 years old are still interested in sexual activity. The ability to get an erection can now usually be achieved with pharmacotherapy or surgery in patients who suffer from cardiovascular disease. Erectile dysfunction secondary to cardiovascular disease often responds well to the standard ED treatments that have been developed over the last few decades.

Pharmacologic Therapy

Phosphodiesterase type 5 (PDE-5) is found predominantly in the smooth muscle of the corpora cavernosa, but can also be found in smaller quantities on platelets and other vascular smooth muscle throughout the body. PDE-5 is primarily responsible for the breakdown of cGMP in cavernosal tissues. The inhibition of PDE-5 therefore causes continued activation of the NO-cGMP pathway in the cavernosal tissue and improved erectile function. Three PDE-5 inhibitors are currently available: sildenafil, vardenafil, and tadalafil (Table 5).

Sildenafil

Sildenafil revolutionized the treatment of erectile dysfunction when it was released after receiving FDA approval in March of 1998. Sildenafil was the first oral agent that was proven safe and effective for the treatment of ED. Sildenafil is a selective inhibitor of PDE-5 and has a half-life of approximately four hours. Sildenafil enhances the normal response to sexual stimulation but has no effect on erections in the absense of this

stimulation. Recommended doses are 25, 50, or 100 mg taken orally one hour prior to planned sexual activity. It is rapidly absorbed, and peak plasma levels are seen in a fasting state approximately 1 hour after ingestion.

The efficacy of sildenafil in the treatment of male ED has been established in over 21 randomized placebo-controlled trials. Treatment-related improvements in erections with sildenafil range between 70%-90% as opposed to 10%-30% improvement with placebo.

Sildenafil has been noted to have a relatively good safety profile with tolerable side effects. Sildenafil has no effect on bleeding time or prothrombin time when used either alone or in patients taking aspirin or coumadin. Priapism associated with sildenafil use is quite uncommon, and there is a low (<3%) incidence of side effects that lead to discontinuation of the medication. The incidence of the most common side effects include

Table 5. Currently Available Phosphodiesterase Type 5 Inhibitors

Name	Onset of action	Commonly encountered side effects
Sildenafil (Viagra)	30-60 min (if no food 4 hours prior)	Headache, diarrhea, rhinitis, flushing
Vardenafil (Levitra)	30-60 min	Headache, flushing, nausea, rhinitis
Tadalafil (Cialis)	30 min	Headache, dyspepsia, rhinitis

vision changes in 22%, headache in 16%, flushing in 10%, and dyspepsia in 7%.

Conditions in which sildenafil must be used with caution include liver dysfunction and renal impairment, both of which decrease plasma clearance of the medication from the body. In the presence of significant hepatic or renal insufficiency, it is recommended to start sildenafil dosing at 25 mg. Sildenafil is metabolized by the cytochrome p450 3A4 isoenzyme. Medications which inhibit the p450 pathway, such as erythromycin and cimetidine, will decrease metabolic clearance and therefore increase plasma levels of sildenafil. Lower starting dose of sildenafil is recommended in these situations. Elderly patients (>65 years of age) also have decreased clearance of sildenafil, with free plasma concentrations shown to be 40% higher than in younger patients, and therefore lower dosing is recommended. The cardiovascular side effects of sildenafil use have been studied extensively. Overall, it was concluded that sildenafil usage was not associated with an excess of related cardiovascular death.

Vardenafil

The second oral selective PDE-5 inhibitor for ED that was approved is vardenafil. Several double-blind, placebo-controlled studies have shown vardenafil to be more effective than placebo in the treatment of ED. Vardenafil has been shown to be significantly more effective than placebo in the treatment of ED secondary to diabetes mellitus and after radical retropubic prostatectomy. The time to peak serum concentration of vardenafil is 0.75 hour, comparable to that of sildenafil (1.16 hours). Differences that distinguish vardenafil from sildenafil include the fact that unlike sildenafil, vardenafil can be taken after eating a moderately fatty meal and after consumption of alcohol.

Tadalafil

Tadalafil is the third selective PDE-5 inhibitor approved by the US FDA. The efficacy of tadalafil in the treatment of ED has been proved in randomized double-blind, placebo-controlled trials. The time to peak serum concentrations for tadalafil is 2 hours, considerably longer than that of sildenafil. The relative excretion half-life of tadalafil is even longer, at 17.5 hours. This prolonged excretion half-life produces enhanced erections up to 36 hours after oral dosing, thereby potentially allowing for more spontaneous engagement of intercourse. As with vardenafil, food intake does not seem to affect the pharmacokinetics of tadalafil.

Absolute Contraindications to PDE-5 Inhibitors

The use of nitroglycerin or other NO-donor medications represent an absolute contraindication to using sildenafil or other PDE-5 inhibitors for ED.

Other Pharmacologic Therapy

Penile injection therapy is generally offered to patients in whom PDE-5 inhibitors have failed or those who are intolerant or have contraindication to PDE-5 inhibitors. Testosterone replacement therapy is reserved for patients with documented hypogonadism.

Diabetes, the Heart, and ED

Treatment of ED in men with diabetes has undergone revolution with the introduction of PDE-5 inhibitors. However, men with diabetes tend to respond less positively to these agents. This decreased responsiveness may be related to the severity of endothelial function in patients with diabetes. Additional therapeutic strategies may be needed to overcome this problem.

Nonpharmacologic Therapy of ED

These include topical vacuum pump devices and surgically inserted inflatable penile implants.

Conclusions

Cardiovascular disease and male erectile dysfunction represent two common disease processes that are very often intimately associated with one another. A close working relationship between the cardiologist and urologist, as well as a solid understanding of the pathophysiology of these disorders, is essential to providing an effective management strategy for these patients.

Resources

Kostis JB, Jackson G, Rosen R, et al. Sexual dysfunction and cardiac risk (the Second Princeton Consensus Conference). Am J Cardiol. 2005;96:313-21.

Russell ST, Khandheria BK, Nehra A. Erectile dysfunction and cardiovascular disease. Mayo Clin Proc. 2004;79:782-94.

SECTION VII

Myocardial Infarction

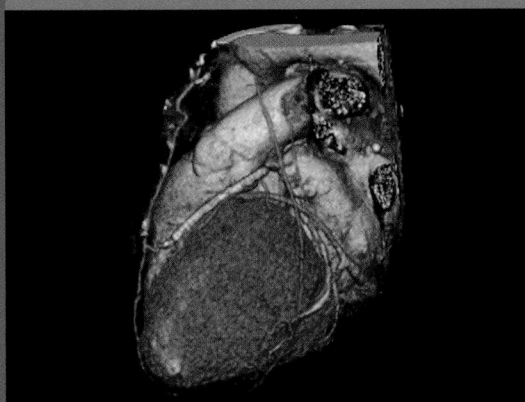

MRI of Internal Mammary Artery Graft

65

CARDIAC BIOMARKERS

Brian P. Shapiro, MD

Luciano Babuin, MD

Allan S. Jaffe, MD

The need for a rapid and reliable diagnosis of myocardial infarction (MI) is crucial. Initially, these efforts focused on clinical assessment and ECG, but, over time, it became clear that they are often non-diagnostic. Therefore, modern day clinicians rely heavily on cardiac biomarkers. Guidelines now call for the routine assessment of cardiac biomarkers for the diagnosis of MI (Table 1).

The interpretation of cardiac biomarkers may be difficult at times. To be successful, clinicians must have an understanding of the kinetics of the biomarkers they use, the mechanisms that can cause elevation, situations in which values can be falsely elevated, and the accuracy of these assays.

CARDIAC TROPONIN

The cardiac troponin (cTn) complex is comprised of 3 subunits (cTnC binds calcium, cTnI inhibits actin-myosin interaction and cTnT binds tropomycin) which are confluent with the actin filament and play a key role in the regulation of calcium-dependent cardiac contraction. While the bulk of cTn exists within the myocardial contractile apparatus, there are traces present in what has been termed the "cytosolic pool" (6% for cTnT and 3% for cTnI). It is thought that the cytosolic pool of unbound cTn are the first molecules

detected in the bloodstream following myocardial injury.

It is likely, though unproven and at times controversial, that the integrity of cell membranes must be compromised to allow cTn to exit the cell. Subsequently, portions of the contractile apparatus are involved and the myofibril-bound portion of cTn enters the intersti-

Table 1. ESC/ACC Criteria for the Diagnosis of MI

Either of the following criteria satisfies the diagnosis of acute, evolving, or recent MI:
  Typical rise and gradual fall (troponin) or more rapid rise and fall (CK-MB) of biochemical markers of myocardial necrosis, with at least one of the following:
    Ischemic symptoms
    Development of pathological Q waves on ECG
    ECG changes indicative of ischemia (ST-segment elevation or depression)
    Coronary artery intervention (e.g., coronary angioplasty)
  Pathological findings of acute MI

tium and eventually the circulation. Newer-generation assays, if used with the sensitive cut-off suggested, document most cTn elevations by 2-3 hours following the onset of MI and nearly 100% by 6 hours. Troponin values typically peak at 24 hours and can remain elevated for 1-2 weeks (Table 2). cTnT stays elevated slightly longer than cTnI.

Due to its enhanced sensitivity and nearly perfect cardiac specificity, cTn is now preferred over CK-MB for the detection of cardiac injury. If one is astute in the use of troponin values, the use of CK-MB should be unnecessary. Newer assays are extremely sensitive and detect even minute traces of myocardial damage. This enhanced sensitivity is due in large part to an increased "release ratio" (the amount of marker depleted from myocardium that arrives in the circulation) compared to CK-MB and the prolonged window during which cTn remains elevated. Multiple studies confirm that in patients with acute coronary syndrome (ACS) that the use of the 99th percentile of a normal population maximizes the ability to determine risk in this group. It is also these low values that have been used to define which treatments will be optimally effective in this group. Higher cut-off values and/or insensitive assays will fail to detect substantial numbers of patients at risk. It should be noted, however, that at very low levels, some values can be increased due to analytic problems alone. An awareness of this problem

by clinicians and the use of a rising pattern of values is often helpful in this situation. With the use of these recommended cut-off values, the use of other testing (e.g., myoglobin and/or CK isoforms) to provide an earlier diagnosis is no longer needed.

The high cardiac specificity of cTn exists because the troponin measured is highly specific for myocardial tissue due to the presence of unique genes which encode cardiac troponin I and T. Although some troponin can exist in skeletal muscle, including some fetal isoforms of cTnT, newer assays employ antibodies that are highly specific and selectively bind to only cardiac forms of troponin. Contemporary assays do not detect the fetal forms of cTnT observed in developing skeletal muscle. While elevated troponin levels indicate damage to the myocardium, they do not necessarily define the mechanism (Table 3). Any stimulus that damages the myoctye will result in release. Thus, clinicians should be aware of the various causes for troponin elevations not related to acute ischemic heart disease.

CREATINE KINASE

Creatine kinase (CK) is a protein located within muscle cells that is essential in ATP generation. Three isoenzymes and a mitochondrial form exist. The cytosolic forms are composed of M and B chains. Thus, there are CK-MB (found predominantly in

Table 2.   Cardiac Biomarkers of Myocardial Injury

Biomarker	Molecular weight, Da	Range of times to initial elevation, h	Mean time to peak elevations (nonreperfused)	Time to return to normal range
Frequently used in clinical practice				
CK-MB	86,000	3-12 h	24 h	48-72 h
cTnI	23,500	3-12 h	24 h	5-10 d
cTnT	33,000	3-12 h	12 h-2 d	5-14 d
Infrequently used in clinical practice				
Myoglobin	17,800	1-4 h	6-7 h	24 h
CK-MB tissue isoform	86,000	2-6 h	18 h	Unknown
CK-MM tissue isoform	86,000	1-6 h	12 h	38 h

Table 3. Nonthrombotic Causes for Elevated Troponin

Diagnosis	Mechanism
Demand ischemia	
Sepsis/systemic inflammatory response syndrome	Myocardial depression/supply-demand mismatch
Hypotension	Decreased perfusion pressure
Hypovolemia	Decreased filling pressure/output
Supraventricular tachycardia/atrial fibrillation	Supply-demand mismatch
Left ventricular hypertrophy	Subendocardial ischemia
Myocardial ischemia	
Coronary vasospasm	Prolonged ischemia with myonecrosis
Intracranial hemorrhage or stroke	Imbalance of autonomic nervous system
Ingestion of sympathomimetic agents	Direct adrenergic effects
Direct myocardial damage	
Cardiac contusion	Traumatic
Direct-current cardioversion	Traumatic
Cardiac infiltrative disorders	Myocyte compression
Chemotherapy	Cardiac toxicity
Myocarditis	Inflammatory
Pericarditis	Inflammatory
Cardiac transplantation	Inflammatory/immune-mediated
Myocardial strain	
Congestive heart failure	Myocardial wall stretch
Pulmonary embolism	Right ventricular stretch
Pulmonary hypertension or emphysema	Right ventricular stretch
Strenuous exercise	Ventricular stretch
Chronic renal insufficiency	Unknown

myocardium, but 1-7% exist in skeletal muscle, and traces in the small intestine, tongue, diaphragm, uterus and prostate), CK-BB (brain and kidney), and CK-MM (skeletal muscle) isoenzymes. Total CK activity and CK-MB (mass and activity) assays are widely available and were considered the biomarkers of choice prior to the development of troponin. Much like cTn, CK may become elevated within 3-6 hours after onset of symptoms and peaks at 24 hours. However, it differs with cTn in that it typically falls to the baseline value by 36-48 hours. Older assays of CK-MB employed gel electrophoresis, which was time-consuming, expensive, and imprecise. Newer assays analyze CK-MB concentration using ELISA assays. This technique is more accurate and rapid and is the preferred method for CK-MB. Most assays for total CK are activity-based assays.

A variety of criteria have been used to define eleva-

tions with total CK and CK-MB. Some have advocated a total CK value greater than 2-fold the normal limit of normal plus a concurrent rise in CK-MB. However, rises in CK-MB despite a normal CK are known to have adverse prognostic significance in patients with ischemic heart disease. Some have suggested the use of a "CK-MB mass index" which takes the ratio of CK-MB to total CK. A value ≥2.5 enhances specificity for cardiac injury but does so at the expense of sensitivity. In addition, it is inaccurate when the total CK is either extremely elevated or if there is concomitant skeletal muscle injury which results in reexpression of the B chain gene as part of the reparative process.

The suboptimal specificity of CK-MB compared to cTn results in an inability of this assay to distinguish between cardiac and skeletal muscle damage. This is in contrast to cTn, which is highly specific to the heart.

Since variable amounts of CK-MB are found in skeletal and smooth muscle and these muscles contain more CK per gram than is found in the heart, muscle damage can cause variable increases in CK and CK-MB. Thus, false positives which are "extracardiac" are common (Table 4).

ADVANTAGES OF TROPONIN VERSUS CREATINE KINASE-MB

Both biomarkers start to rise and peak at similar time intervals. However, cTn has a markedly improved ability to detect myocardial necrosis due to its greater release ratio, which results in a higher concentration of cTn in the bloodstream as compared to CK-MB (Fig. 1). For this reason, there is an enhanced "signal-to-noise" ratio, which enables detection of even minute myocardial damage. Thus, 1/3 of patients with acute MI have an elevated cTn despite a normal CK-MB.

The longer half-life of cTn also gives this biomarker a longer "window" to detect MI. Newer cTn assays detect up to 80% of MIs in 2-3 hours. In addition, cTn levels are highly specific for myocardial damage, as opposed to CK-MB, which is often elevated with injuries involving skeletal muscle.

One potential advantage of CK-MB was thought to be that it did not persist after an ischemic insult. This had the potential benefit of allowing one to estimate the time of onset of MI and diagnose reinfarction

---

Table 4.   Other Causes for CK-MB Elevation

Cardioversion or defibrillation, especially high-dose (>400 J)
Myocardial contusion
Resuscitative chest compressions
Skeletal muscle injury or disorders (e.g., Duchenne's muscular dystrophy)
Reye's syndrome
Hypothyroidism
Postpartum
Heavy binge drinking and delirium tremors
Moderately severe exercise
Severe hypokalemia
Gangrene or severe ischemia of extremities

---

and infarct extension more effectively. However, recent studies suggest that cTn may be just as effective as CK-MB in this regard.

For all of these reasons, the use of CK-MB is diminishing and will continue to do so.

PROGNOSIS AND INFARCT SIZE USING CARDIAC BIOMARKERS

Data support the use of cardiac biomarkers to estimate prognosis and the size of infarction following MI. Numerous studies have confirmed the prognostic importance of elevations of CK-MB as well as troponin. For example, GUSTO-III studied approximately 12,000 patients with ST-segment elevation MI (STEMI). By 30 days, more patients had died who had an elevated cTnT than not (16 vs. 6%). Patients were further stratified into quartiles of cTnT in GUSTO-IV, and those with the highest levels died more frequently if they were in the highest quartile as compared to the lowest. A recent meta-analysis of patients with non-STEMI suggested that patients with an elevated cTn had a greater than 3-fold increase of death as compared to those with a normal value (Fig. 2).

Angiographic data suggest that there is more extensive coronary artery disease, more thrombi and reduced Thrombolysis in Myocardial Infarction (TIMI) flow grades when cTn is elevated. Thus cTn may be helpful in detecting patients who are more in need of aggressive therapeutic measures. Several large trials have shown that a strategy of glycoprotein IIb/IIIa platelet inhibitors, low-molecular-weight heparin, and early revascularization is more efficacious in patients with elevated cTn.

Troponin values correlate well with infarct size as measured by thallium, sestimibi and/or MR imaging. For cTnT, the 72-96-hour value correlates best, but for cTnI, the peak value may be better.

TROPONIN ELEVATION FOLLOWING PERCUTANEOUS CORONARY INTERVENTION (PCI) AND CARDIAC SURGERY

Any elevation of cTn following PCI suggests myocardial injury. However, it is often difficult to know if this rise was related to the MI or to the intervention. Recent data indicate that when one takes into account

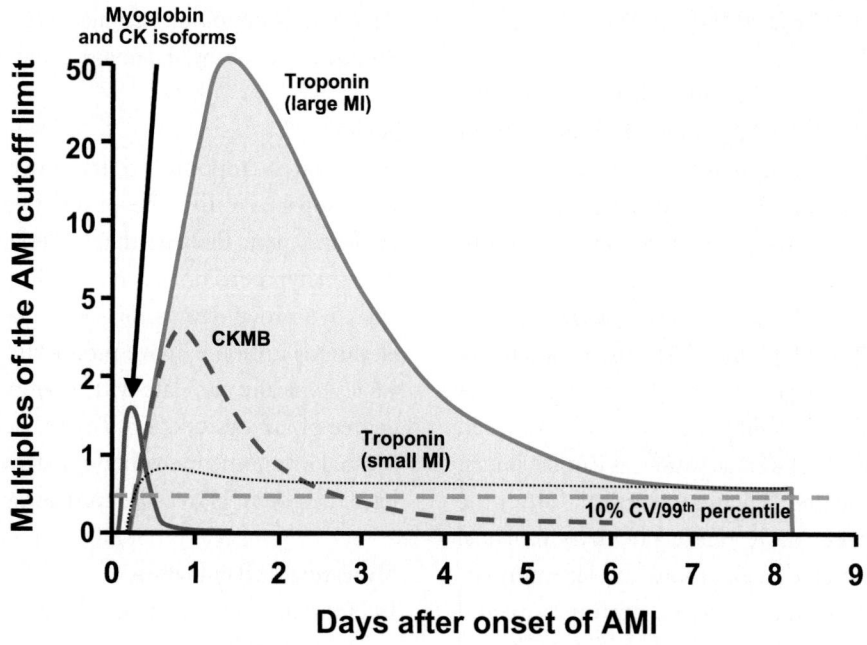

Fig. 1. Time course of the appearance of various markers in the blood after acute myocardial infarction (AMI). Shown are the time concentrations/activity curves for myoglobin and creatine kinase (CK) isoforms, troponin after large and small infarctions, and CK-MB. Note that with cardiac troponin some patients have a second peak in addition. CV, coefficient of variation.

the prognostic significance of baseline elevations, the importance of post-PCI values, both for cTn and CK-MB, vanish. In the absence of baseline elevations, increases are modest and also do not manifest prognostic importance.

Elevations of cTn are ubiquitous following cardiac surgery. Studies suggest that the higher the cTn value following cardiac surgery, the larger the amount of aggregate damage and the worse the prognosis. Only very marked elevations correlate with graft occlusion.

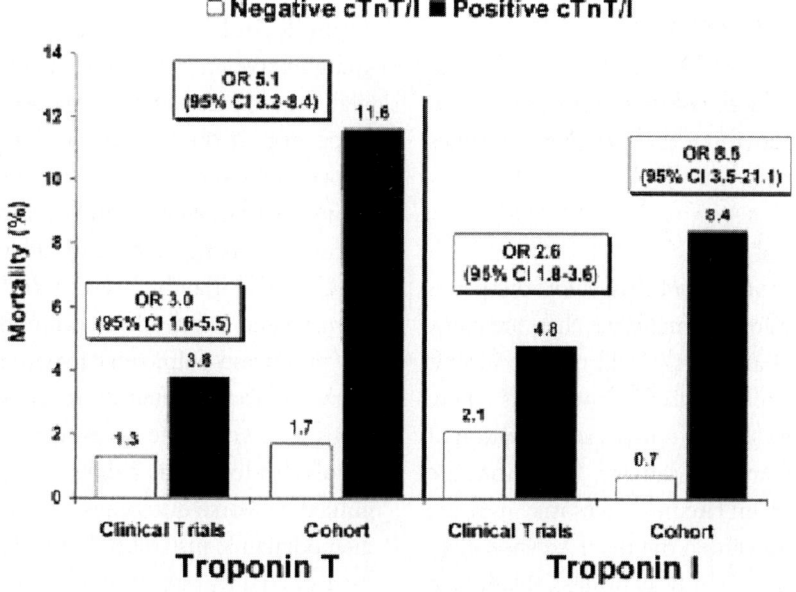

Fig. 2. Meta-analysis depicting the prognostic value of an elevated troponin T/I.

CARDIAC BIOMARKERS AND RENAL DYSFUNCTION

The interpretation of cardiac biomarkers may be difficult in the setting of renal dysfunction. Elevations in cTn and CK-MB are common, but so is the incidence of coronary heart disease in this population. In a study by Apple et al, 733 dialysis patients who were without cardiac symptoms had troponins drawn (cTnI ≥0.1 mg/L and cTnT ≥ 0.01 mg/L represented elevated values). Troponin T was high in 82% of these patients as compared to 6% for cTnI. The reasons for this difference are unclear. Pathological studies have confirmed that the mechanism for cTn elevations is cardiac injury, but it need not be due to acute infarction. Often the abnormalities were more related to myocytolysis. Associations between cTn elevations and left ventricular (LV) hypertrophy, endothelial dysfunction, and acute LV stretch have been reported. Total CK and CK-MB are also highly inaccurate in these patients (>50% false positive rate). In the Apple et al study, there was a significantly worse 2-year survival in dialysis patients with high cTn values (Fig. 3). Even with minor elevations, there was a 2-5-fold decrease in survival.

The following approach is likely to be helpful. If the cTn value is rising, an acute event is likely. If it is elevated but remains unchanged from previous values, an MI is far less likely.

CAUSES OF AN ELEVATED TROPONIN IN THE ABSENCE OF ACUTE ISCHEMIA

While the cTn assay is highly specific for detecting myocardial damage, it does not necessarily point to an exact mechanism, as anything that damages myocytes will result in an elevated value (Table 3).

Mechanical or Electrical Injury

Cardiac trauma from surgery or biopsy and from penetrating or nonpenetrating trauma to the chest are common causes for cardiac and skeletal muscle injury. While CK-MB is often elevated in situations where there is damage to the skeletal muscle, any elevation of cTn suggests cardiac muscle damage. Elevations are often mild, but in certain circumstances may indicate coronary artery or myocardial trauma. Likewise, electrical cardioversion (including ICD firings), ablation, or cardiac arrest may also cause modest elevations in cTn.

Any significant rise should alert the clinician that more significant myocardial damage is present.

Toxins

An elevated troponin occurs in over 50% of patients with sepsis. While the exact mechanism remains unclear, experts theorize that underlying ischemic heart disease, hypotension, microemboli, cytokine activation and myocardial depression likely play a role. Troponin elevations invariably have prognostic significance since values typically correlate with severity of illness and the degree of LV dysfunction. Toxins such as chemotherapy, snake venom, and other vasoactive substances also have the potential to cause cardiac damage.

Myocardial Inflammation

Inflammation of the myocardium and/or pericardium, as occurs in infiltrative cardiomyopathy and in infectious, neoplastic or inflammatory myocardial involvement, can often cause cTn elevations. In symptomatic patients, it may be confused with acute MI. Cardiac biomarker elevation often occurs soon after onset of symptoms, but falls with disease remission. In cases of infiltrative cardiomyopathy such as amyloidosis, cTn elevation often correlates with disease severity and clinical outcome.

Demand Ischemia or Myocardial Strain

While often related to ischemia due to epicardial atherosclerosis, elevation of cardiac biomarkers can result from other causes related to the coronary arteries. For example, in LV or RV hypertrophy, there is a mismatch between supply and demand due to increased wall stress. Therefore, in hypertrophied hearts (e.g., hypertrophic obstructive cardiomyopathy, concentric hypertrophy, pulmonary hypertension, or heart failure) or in situations where significant increases in wall stress occurs (e.g., congestive heart failure), elevations of cTn or CK-MB may be present and reflect myocardial damage and cell death. In pulmonary embolism, acute RV strain and pulmonary hypertension cause troponin elevation that is often more transient than the elevations seen with acute ischemic heart disease and usually resolve in less than 2 days. However, elevations are linked to worse outcomes and are often indicative of hemodynamic instability. Subendocardial ischemia and endothelial dysfunction are also common causes for cTn elevation due to supply/demand mismatch.

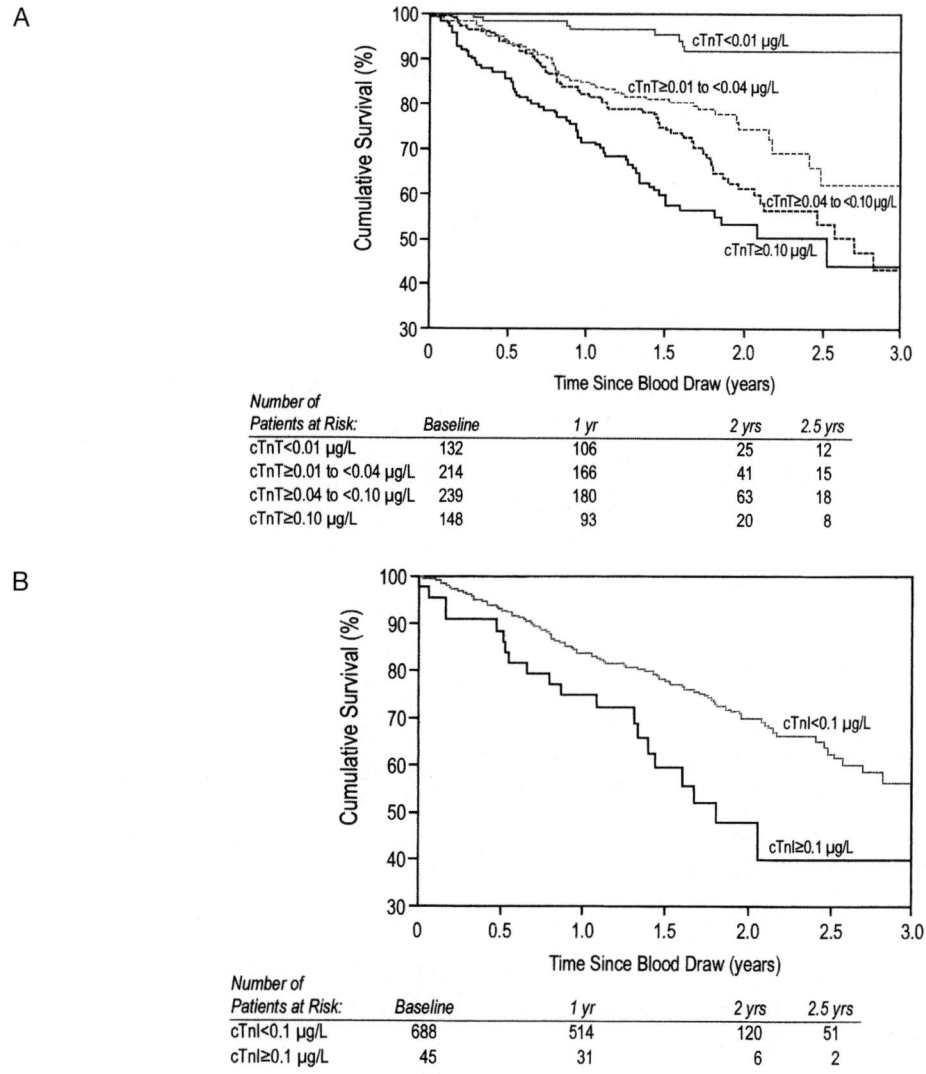

Fig. 3. The top panel represents Kaplan-Meier curves for survival based on quartile of troponin T elevation in patients with renal failure. Patients in the highest quartile survived less than those with a normal troponin. The bottom graph depicts the same analysis using troponin I.

SUMMARY

Cardiac troponin is the preferred biomarker and is highly specific for myocardial damage. It can be helpful in confirming a MI as well as estimating infarct size and prognosis. While the most common cause for an elevated value is acute MI, troponin and CK-MB may be elevated in a number of disease states. Guidelines caution against the use of cardiac biomarkers for routine screening, especially in patients considered to have a low pretest probability of MI, as an elevated value may lead to misdiagnosis and unnecessary clinical evaluation.

66

ACUTE CORONARY SYNDROMES

Anthony A. Hilliard, MD

Stephen L. Kopecky, MD

INTRODUCTION

Unstable angina (UA) and non-ST segment elevation myocardial infarction (NSTEMI) acute coronary syndrome (ACS) are usually caused by atherosclerotic disease. They share a common pathophysiology and may be indistinguishable at initial presentation; the approach to risk stratification and treatment are the same and are differentiated only by the presence or absence of elevated cardiac biomarkers.

PATHOPHYSIOLOGY

NSTE-ACS (non-ST segment elevation acute coronary syndrome) is usually caused by an unstable atherosclerotic plaque rupture with subsequent platelet-rich thrombus overlying the culprit lesion causing severe narrowing (Fig. 1). This abrupt decrease in blood supply often results in chest pain and ECG changes indicative of ischemia, and, if prolonged, results in myocardial necrosis and enzyme elevation. Less commonly, NSTE-ACS is caused by diseases in which myocardial demand exceeds myocardial supply causing a similar clinical presentation. These diseases usually cause a hypermetabolic or high cardiac output state and include hyperthyroidism, anemia, fever, pheochromocytoma, hypertrophic cardiomyopathy, AV fistula and hypertensive urgency/emergency. Rarely NSTE-ACS

is caused by nonocclusive coronary disease in which epicardial or microvascular spasm results in a decrease in myocardial supply.

- NSTE-ACS is usually caused by unstable plaque rupture and thrombus formation.

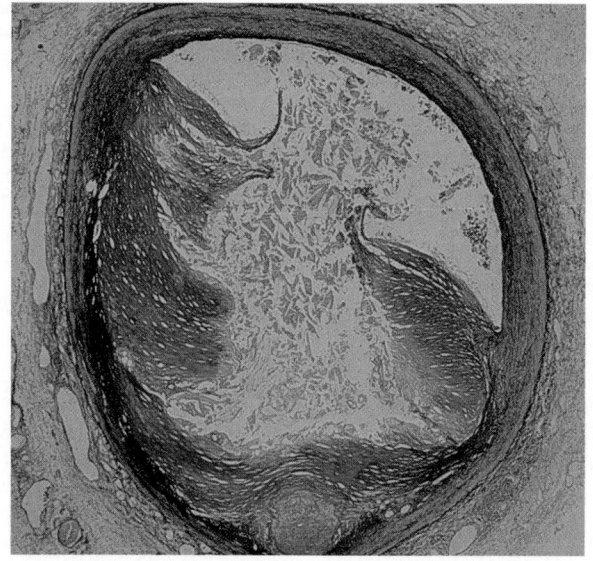

Fig. 1. Acute plaque rupture with apparent atheroembolism.

Rare causes of NSTE-ACS include *h*yperthyroidism, *h*ypertrophic cardiomyopathy, fever (*h*igh temperature), anemia (low *h*emoglobin) and severe *h*ypertension (the "5 *Hs*").

CLASSIFICATION

ACS has evolved to refer to a constellation of clinical symptoms and findings that represent acute myocardial ischemia. It encompasses both ST segment elevation myocardial infarction (STEMI) (historically referred to as the Q-wave MI) and NSTE-ACS. NSTE-ACS is differentiated from STEMI ACS as their clinical characteristics, surface electrocardiogram, approach to treatment and prognosis differ (Fig. 2).

DEFINITION OF UNSTABLE ANGINA

Unstable angina is defined, and differs from stable angina, by the duration and intensity of angina as graded by the Canadian Cardiovascular Society (CCS) classification (Table 1). There are 3 possible presentations of UA: 1) Rest angina (lasting >20 minutes), 2) New-onset angina (at least CCS III intensity), and 3)

Table 1.   Canadian Cardiovascular Society Classification of Unstable Angina

Class	Activity provoking angina	Limits to normal activity
I	Prolonged exertion	None
II	Walking >2 blocks	Slight
III	Walking ≤2 blocks	Marked
IV	Minimal or rest	Severe

Accelerated angina (angina with activity that is occurring earlier, more intense CCS class or with increased duration). Patients initially diagnosed with UA may later be diagnosed with a NSTEMI if initial or serial cardiac biomarkers become elevated.

- UA has 3 presentations: prolonged rest angina, new-onset angina, and accelerated angina.
- NSTEMI typically presents with rest angina and is differentiated from UA simply by elevation of cardiac biomarkers.

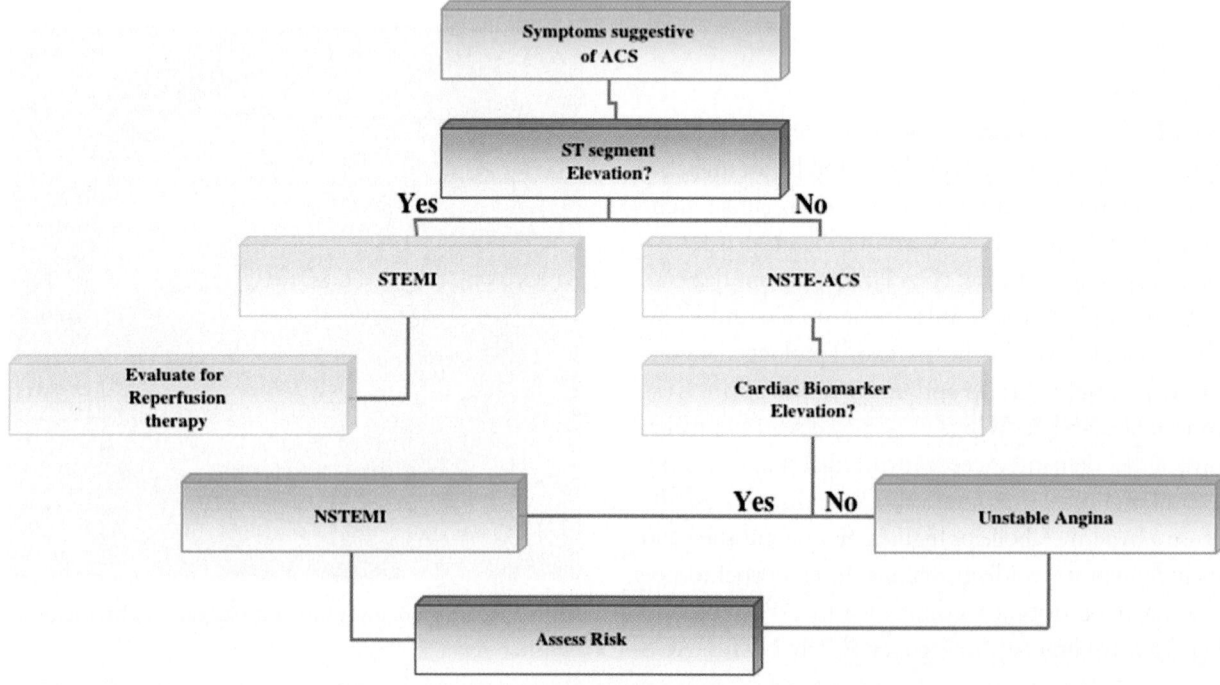

Fig. 2. Acute coronary syndrome (ACS) classification. NSTE-ACS, non-ST-segment elevation-acute coronary syndrome; NSTEMI, non-ST-segment elevation myocardial infarction; STEMI, ST-segment elevation myocardial infarction.

CLINICAL ASSESSMENT

When symptoms raise suspicion for ACS, the goal of the medical evaluation is to answer 2 questions: What is the likelihood (high, intermediate or low) that the patient's presentation is consistent with coronary ischemia (Table 2)? And, if so, what is their risk (see section on risk stratification)?

According to the ACC/AHA (American College of Cardiology/American Heart Association) guidelines for UA/NSTEMI, there are several factors obtained from the initial history, physical exam, ECG, and cardiac biomarkers that are associated with a high likelihood that symptoms reflect acute myocardial ischemia (Table 2). A high likelihood of significant coronary artery disease (CAD) is defined as having >85% chance of having a flow-limiting coronary artery obstruction present, an intermediate risk is a defined as having a 15-85% chance, and a low likelihood is defined as less than a 15% chance.

After estimating the likelihood that the symptoms represent myocardial ischemia, it is important to determine the risk that this portends to the patient as this affects decisions regarding triage. The ACC/AHA risk table (Table 3) provides an estimation of the short-term risk of death or nonfatal MI in patients with NSTE-ACS and assists in the initial triage of these patients. Patients at high or intermediate risk should be hospitalized in a monitored bed for intensive

Table 2. Likelihood of Significant CAD

	High likelihood	Intermediate likelihood	Low likelihood
History	Symptoms same as prior angina History of CAD, MI, sudden death Variant angina (pain with reversible ST-segment elevation) Transient hemodynamic or ECG changes during pain	*Absence of high-likelihood features and any of the following:* Chest or left arm pain as primary symptom Chest pain probably not angina in patients with DM or in non-DM patients ≥2 other risk factors (high cholesterol, hypertension, and smoking) Male age ≥70 Female age ≥60	*Absence of high- or intermediate-likelihood features but may have:* Chest pain not consistent with angina Recent cocaine use One risk factor but not DM
Exam	Hypotension, diaphoresis, pulmonary edema, transient MR	Extracardiac vascular disease	Chest discomfort reproduced with palpation
ECG	ST-segment depression ≥1 mm depression from baseline Marked symmetrical T-wave inversion in multiple leads	Q waves ST segment depression <0.5 mm T-wave inversion >1 mm in leads with dominant R waves	T wave flattening or inversion of ≤1 mm in leads with dominant R waves Normal ECG
Cardiac markers	Elevated TnT, TnI, CK-MB	Normal	Normal

CAD, coronary artery disease; CK-MB, creatine kinase muscle and brain subunits; DM, diabetes mellitus; ECG, electrocardiogram; TnI, Troponin I; TnT, troponin T.

management. However, studies have shown that intermediate and low-risk patients may be observed, when available, in a chest pain observation unit. If the patient does not experience recurrent pain and the follow-up 12-lead ECG and serum cardiac biomarkers are negative after 6-8 hours of observation, the patient may undergo provocative stress testing. This testing may be done prior to discharge from the chest pain unit or can be done within 72 hours of discharge. If the patient has recurrent chest pain consistent with myocardial ischemia or 12-lead ECG is consistent with ischemia or serum cardiac biomarkers become

elevated the patient should be admitted and treated for NSTE-ACS (see below).

History

Factors derived from the clinical history which increase the likelihood that the presenting symptoms are secondary to acute myocardial ischemia include the presence of chest or left arm pain, older age and male sex. The likelihood that chest pain is secondary to acute myocardial ischemia increases with descriptions of chest pain radiation to a shoulder or arm, chest pain that is worse with exertion, chest pain associated with

Table 3.   Factors Increasing Short-Term Risk of Death or Nonfatal MI in NSTE-ACS

	High-risk (at least 1 of the following)	Intermediate-risk (no high-risk features and at least 1 of the following)	Low-risk (no high- or intermediate-risk features and may have 1 of the following)
History	Acceleration of ischemic symptoms over past 2 days	Prior MI, extracardiac vascular disease, CABG, prior aspirin use	
Pain characteristic	Prolonged ongoing (>20 min) rest pain	Prolonged (>20 min) rest pain, now resolved	New-onset or progressive CCS Class III or IV angina the past 2 weeks without prolonged (>20 min) rest pain
Clinical findings	Pulmonary edema, new or worsening MR murmur, S_3 or new/worsening rales, hypo-tension, bradycardia, tachycardia Age >75 years	Age >70 years	
ECG	Angina at rest with transient ST-segment changes >0.05 mV Bundle branch block, new Sustained VT	T-wave inversions >0.2 mV Pathological Q waves	Normal or unchanged ECG during an episode of chest discomfort
Bio-markers	Elevated (e.g., TnT or TnI >0.1 ng/mL)	Slightly elevated (e.g., TNT >0.01 but <0.1 ng/mL)	Normal

CABG, coronary artery bypass grafting; CCS Canadian Cardiovascular Society; min, minutes; mL, milliliter; MR, mitral regurgitation; mV, millivolt; ng, nanogram; TnI, troponin I; TnT, troponin T; VT, ventricular tachycardia.

diaphoresis, nausea or vomiting and chest pain that is worse or similar to symptoms of a prior MI. Chest pain that is pleuritic, positional, sharp, reproducible, inframammary and not associated with exertion decrease the likelihood of being related to acute myocardial ischemia. However, presence of these atypical symptoms alone does not exclude the possibility of ACS. In fact >1/2 of the population over the age of 65 with ACS present with dyspnea rather than chest pain. Women with ACS also tend to present with atypical symptoms and can sometimes delay appropriate medical therapy. It is vital to incorporate this concept into decision making as women with ACS derive similar benefits as men from aggressive medical therapy (per the guidelines) and similar improvement in mortality.

Physical Exam

The physical exam in patients with NSTE-ACS can be very useful in establishing that the patient's presentation is consistent with ACS and their subsequent risk. Prompt review of vital signs can alert the physician to possible cardiogenic shock—systolic hypotension (systolic BP <100), tachycardia (heart rate >100) and tachypnea. The presence of a new mitral regurgitation murmur or increased intensity of a preexisting murmur indicates ischemic dysfunction of a papillary muscle or mitral apparatus. A third or fourth heart sound or an LV lift suggests a significant amount of myocardial ischemia. The presence and extent of pulmonary rales, the Killip classification, in acute myocardial ischemia impacts prognosis (Table 4).

Electrocardiogram

Up to 4% of patients with NSTE-ACS have a completely normal ECG. More commonly, nonspecific ST-segment depression (<0.05 mV) or T-wave inversion (<0.2 mV) are present and provide no significant prognostic information. Transient ST-segment changes of >0.05 mV that develop during a symptomatic episode and resolve with symptom resolution is strongly suggestive of severe CAD. In patients whose history is strongly suggestive of ACS symmetric T-wave inversion of >0.2 mV across the precordial leads strongly suggests acute ischemia of the left anterior descending artery (LAD). The ECG not only adds support to the clinical suspicion of ACS but

also provides prognostic information as patients with NSTE-ACS in whom ST-segment elevation is present in lead aVR are at higher risk for recurrent ischemic events and heart failure during hospitalization and have a higher prevalence of left main coronary artery disease or three-vessel disease.

Laboratory Testing

All patients in whom NSTE-ACS is suspected, creatine kinase muscle and brain subunits (CK-MB) and troponin T or I should be assessed at least twice 6 to 12 hours apart. If clinically indicated, additional laboratory testing including a CBC, comprehensive metabolic panel, and thyroid function should be performed to assess for less common causes of NSTE-ACS and to guide management as anemia and renal failure are associated with adverse outcomes. An ECG should be performed at admission and serially to assess for dynamic ST segment and T wave abnormalities as clinically indicated. A chest radiograph is useful in patients with evidence of hemodynamic instability or pulmonary edema. Serum lipids should be drawn within 24 hours of admission to assess for hypercholesterolemia. Additional laboratory tests when positive in ACS suggest a worse outcome including BNP and CRP. However, more data are required to establish what additional prognostic information these markers provide.

Although troponins are accurate in identifying the presence of myocardial necrosis and portend a worse prognosis when positive, elevation of this enzyme is not always as a result of an acute coronary syndrome. Thus, the diagnosis of NSTEMI, while requiring elevated cardiac biomarkers, should be made in the appropriate

Table 4.   Killip Classification

Class	Exam findings
I	No signs of heart failure
II	S3
	Elevated JVP
	Rales <1/2 of posterior lung fields
III	Overt pulmonary edema
IV	Cardiogenic shock

clinical setting of symptoms and/or ECG changes consistent with myocardial ischemia secondary to plaque rupture.

EARLY RISK STRATIFICATION

Estimation of risk is an integral component of the initial assessment of NSTE-ACS and should be performed simultaneously with initial medical management (see section on initial medical management). Estimation of risk is important as there are population characteristics on initial presentation which are associated with an increased risk of death or complications from myocardial ischemia.

Several tools are used to assess risk and guide the intensity of medical treatment and the need for and timing of coronary angiography. The TIMI (Thrombolysis In Myocardial Infarction) risk score is one commonly used risk stratification tool derived from the TIMI 11B (Thrombolysis In Myocardial Infarction 11B) trial and validated in the ESSENCE (Efficacy and Safety of Subcutaneous Enoxaparin in Non-Q-wave Coronary Events), PRISM-PLUS (Platelet Receptor inhibition for Ischemic Syndrome Management in Patients Limited by unstable Signs and symptoms) and TACTICS-TIMI 18 (Treat Angina with Aggrastat and Determine Cost of Therapy with an Invasive or Conservative Strategy-Thrombolysis In Myocardial Infarction) trials. The risk score predictor variables are 1) age ≥65 years of age, 2)

≥3 risk factors for coronary artery disease (family history of coronary artery disease, hypertension hypercholesterolemia, diabetes, or being a current smoker), 3) prior coronary artery stenosis of ≥50%, 4) ST-segment deviation on presenting electrocardiogram, 5) ≥2 anginal events within the prior 24 hours, 6) use of aspirin within 7 days, and 7) elevated serum cardiac markers. The sum of the 7-point risk score predicts the risk of developing adverse outcomes of death, (re)infarction, or recurrent ischemia requiring revascularization 14 days after randomization. This risk ranged from 5% with a score of 0 or 1 to 41% with a score of 6 or 7 (Fig. 3). Based on this data the ACC/AHA Practice Guidelines have classified patients at low risk (score of 0-2), intermediate risk (score of 3-4) and high risk (score of 5-7).

The Killip classification is an easy bedside assessment of risk (Fig. 4). It was initially used to assess risk in patients with a STEMI but has been validated in patients with NSTE-ACS. Increasing Killip class (class 1 vs class II vs class III/IV) is associated with an increased risk of all-cause mortality at 6 months.

- Early assessment and identification of high risk patients enables the clinician to determine both the intensity of medical therapy and the timing of coronary angiography.
- The TIMI risk score, Killip classification and individual markers of increased age, troponin elevation, ST-segment depression and renal failure all portend a worse outcome in NSTE-ACS.

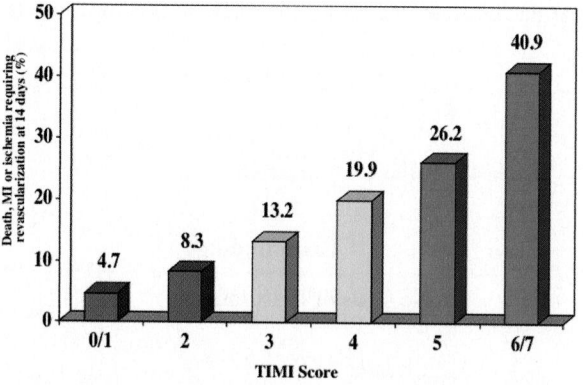

Fig. 3. TIMI risk score bar graph showing colors indicating low (green), intermediate (yellow) or high risk (red). MI, myocardial infarction; TIMI, thrombolysis in myocardial infarction.

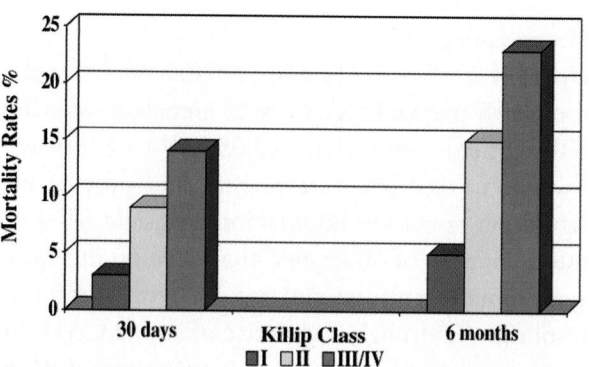

Fig. 4. Mortality rates at 30 days and 6 months in patients with NSTE-ACS based on Killip classification. Killip class I is shown in green; Killip class II is shown in yellow; and Killip class III/IV is shown in red.

PRINCIPLES OF MANAGEMENT OF NSTE-ACS

There are two general strategies to the treatment of patients NSTE-ACS, and these strategies are based largely on the risk of the patient. The early invasive strategy is the recommended approach to treatment in patients at high or intermediate risk. Patients treated with this strategy generally undergo coronary angiography within 48 hours with angiographically directed revascularization. These patients often benefit from administration of clopidogrel (the first dose is often given at the time of angiography) and continuous infusion of a glycoprotein IIb/IIIa inhibitor (GP IIb/IIIa [−]) upstream to coronary angiography in addition to aspirin, β-blockers, heparin and nitrates. Low-risk patients may be assigned to the early invasive strategy or to the early conservative strategy. This latter strategy relies on noninvasive evaluation after a period of observation with catheterization and revascularization reserved for patients with evidence of recurrent ischemia at rest or with provocative testing. Similarly, these patients should be treated with aspirin, β-blockers, heparin, nitrates and clopidogrel. GP IIb/IIIa (−) should be reserved for patients in this strategy who have signs of ongoing ischemia during the period of observation (e.g. crossover into an invasive strategy).

■ Determining whether an early invasive or early conservative strategy for managing patients with NSTE-ACS is largely based on the initial risk assessment.

INITIAL MEDICAL THERAPY

Optimal initial medical management includes the prompt and simultaneous achievement of the following tasks: administration of antiplatelet and antithrombotic agents, relief of ischemic pain and ST deviation, correction of hemodynamic abnormalities, and determination of the timing of diagnostic angiography (early invasive vs. early conservative strategy). Table 5 provides an overview of the mechanism of action, recommended dosages and timing of the commonly used drugs in the treatment of NSTE-ACS.

Antiplatelet Therapy

It is well established that aspirin reduces the risk of vascular death by about one-sixth and the risk of nonfatal myocardial infarction by about one-third in patients with ACS. Thus, in the absence of absolute contraindications, all patients suspected of ACS should receive aspirin 324 mg initially followed by 81-162 mg daily thereafter. The first dose should be chewed as there is measurable platelet inhibition within 60 minutes. Patients with absolute contraindications to aspirin should receive clopidogrel 300 mg initially followed by 75 mg daily.

In addition to those who cannot take aspirin, clopidogrel is recommended in addition to aspirin in NSTE-ACS as the CURE (Clopidogrel in Unstable Angina to Prevent Recurrent Ischemic Events) trial demonstrated that patients receiving dual antiplatelet therapy experienced a 20% relative risk reduction (absolute risk reduction from 11.4 to 9.3%) in the primary combined end point of cardiovascular death, nonfatal MI or stroke at one year. The ACC/AHA recommends continuing clopidogrel for up to 9 months after hospital admission for treatment of NSTE-ACS. Clopidogrel is also efficacious in those undergoing percutaneous intervention. The PCI-CURE (Percutaneous Coronary Intervention-Clopidogrel in Unstable Angina to Prevent Recurrent ischemic Events) subset analysis and the CREDO (Clopidogrel for the Reduction of Events During Observation) trial both demonstrated a reduction in the combined end-point of all-cause mortality, CV death, MI, and/or stroke. Among those who those in whom an early invasive strategy is planned, the benefits of early clopidogrel administration must be weighed against the increased risk of bleeding should the patient require coronary artery bypass grafting (CABG) within 5 days of clopidogrel administration. The ACC/AHA guidelines recommend withholding clopidogrel until the time of diagnostic angiography if it is scheduled with 34-48 hours of admission.

Based on their ability to prevent ischemic complications of percutaneous coronary intervention (PCI), glycoprotein IIb/IIIa inhibitors (GP IIb/IIIa [−]) are recommended in those NSTE-ACS patients treated with an early invasive strategy. Although similar effects have been noted with all three agents (tirofiban, abciximab, and eptifibatide) the timing of angiography should be determined prior to determining which agent to use. Available data favor the use of abciximab if

Table 5.   Drug Therapy in NSTE-ACS

Drug	Action	Dose	Use in NSTE-ACS
Aspirin	Cyclooxygenase 1 inhibitor	324 mg chewed then 81-162 mg daily	Start immediately and continue continue indefinitely
ADP			
inhibitors: Clopidogrel Ticlodipine	ADP receptor blocker	Clopidogrel: 300 mg PO loading dose then 75 mg daily Hold if catheterization within	Start immediately and continue for up to 9 mos in medically and PCI managed patients
		24-48 hrs and/or CABG possible	
GP IIb/IIIa			
inhibitors: Abciximab Eptifibatide Tirofiban	Inhibits interaction of fibrinogen with the GP IIb/IIIa receptor	Example: Eptifibatide: 180 mcg/kg then continuous IV infusion of 2 mcg/kg/min (up to 72 hrs); ↓ infusion to 1 mcg/kg/min if serum Ct >2	Start at admission or at time of PCI in patients at high enough risk to need revascularization
UFH	Binds to, and enhances the activity of, antithrombin III	60 Units/kg bolus then 12 units/kg/hr target to aPTT of 1.5-2.5	Start immediately and continue for 2-7 days as clinically indicated
LMWH Enoxaparin	Factor Xa inhibitor	1 mg/kg every 12 hrs SC with Ct Cl >30 mL/min	Alternative to UFH. Start immediately and continue for 2-7 days as clinically indicated
β-blockers: Cardio- selective	Decrease cardiac workload (↓ HR, ↓ BP, ↓ contrac- tility)	Example: metoprolol 5 mg IV q 5 min x 3 doses then 50 mg po BID, first dose 15-20 min after last IV dose	Start immediately and continue indefinitely
Nitrates	Decrease cardiac workload (↓ preload through veno- dilation)	0.04 mg SL q 5 min x 3 doses. If pain persists 5-100 μg/min IV	Start immediately and continue with IV infusion if pain persists
Morphine sulfate	Venodilation decreases pre- load; opioid analgesic	2-4 mg IV q 5-15 min (should not exceed 25 mg in 24 hour period)	Start after β-blocker and nitrates have been used and pain persists or sooner if anxiety present

ADP, adenosine diphosphate; aPTT, activated partial thromboplastin time; β, beta; BID, twice daily; CABG, coronary artery bypass grafting; Ct, creatinine; Cl, clearance; ↓, decrease; GP, glycoprotein; hrs, hours; IV, intravenous; kg, kilogram; LMWH, low-molecular-weight heparin; μg, micrograms; mg, milligram; min, minutes; mL, milliliters; mos, months; PCI, percutaneous intervention; PO, per os; SC, subcutaneous; SL, sublingual; q, every; UFH, unfractionated heparin.

angiography is planned urgently (<4 hours) with tirofiban and eptifibatide reserved for patients treated medically during the first 48 hours. The role for GP IIb/IIIa (−) in the early conservative strategy is less clear. Currently, the ACC/AHA recommends the use of tirofiban or eptifibatide as a continuous infusion in patients with recurrent ischemia, positive biomarkers or other high-risk features in which there has been a decision to treat conservatively.

Despite these recommendations, the optimal platelet regimen has yet to be established largely due to the lack of clinical trials comparing triple antiplatelet therapy (aspirin, clopidogrel, and GP IIb/IIIa [−]) to dual therapy with aspirin and clopidogrel or aspirin and GP IIb/IIIa (−).

Relief of Ischemic Pain

Rapid relief of ischemia by reducing cardiac workload is a cornerstone of treatment for ACS. This forms the basis for the current recommendation that patients with ongoing chest pain should receive intravenous β-blockade followed by upward titration of oral therapy. β-Blockers relieve ischemia by decreasing contractility, heart rate and ventricular wall tension (preload). Cardioselective agents (atenolol and metoprolol) are preferred in the treatment on NSTE-ACS. The first dose of beta blockade in patients with ongoing pain or high/intermediate risk should be given intravenously. β-Blockers are not recommended in the setting of high-degree AV block, cardiogenic shock, and severe reactive airway disease (in this situation non-dihydropyridine calcium channel blockers should be considered).

Despite little clinical data, nitrates are used extensively in clinical practice due to their success at relieving ischemic pain. Thus, nitrates, in the absence of contraindications, should be given to all patients suspected of ACS. This beneficial effect is thought to occur predominately by decreasing cardiac workload through venodilation. Nitrates should initially be administered sublingually for rapid systemic absorption and if the pain is not well-controlled should be given intravenously, provided the patient is not hypotensive (systolic blood pressure <90). Nitrates are contraindicated in the following patients: those who have taken phosphodiesterase inhibitors in the past 24 hours, those with hypertrophic cardiomyopathy, and those suspected of right ventricular infarction; extreme caution should be taken in patients with severe aortic stenosis.

Narcotics (e.g. morphine sulfate) should be administered only if pain persists despite treatment with β-blockers and nitrates or to help decrease anxiety.

Antithrombin Administration

On the basis of a demonstrated incremental benefit over aspirin alone, UFH or LMWH should be part of the medical regimen of all patients with NSTE-ACS unless the patient is actively bleeding or has a history of heparin-associated thrombocytopenia (HIT) or known hypersensitivity. Heparin in combination with aspirin reduces the incidence of ischemic events in patients with NSTE-ACS by up to one-third compared to patients treated with aspirin alone. Unfractionated heparin (UFH) or low-molecular-weight heparin can be used in the treatment of NSTE-ACS. Comparative trials of LMWH and enoxaparin have demonstrated superiority over UFH in reducing recurrent cardiac events. The ACC/AHA UA/NSTEMI guidelines recommend enoxaparin over UFH (class IIa recommendation). Advantages of LMWH when compared to UFH include ease of administration without the need for monitoring, a lower incidence of heparin-associated thrombocytopenia, and possible improvement in outcomes. LMWH is contraindicated in patients with renal failure (defined as a creatinine clearance of <30 mL/min). UFH should be considered when coronary angiography is expected in <12 hours as there is concern amongst interventional cardiologists about the inability to adequately monitor the level of anticoagulation or to fully reverse its anticoagulant effects. Alternatively, LMWH can be used initially with the last dose administered 12 hours before expected coronary angiography with UFH used thereafter. Data from the SYNERGY (Superior Yield of the New strategy of Enoxaparin, Revascularization and GlYcoprotein IIb/IIIa inhibitors) trial may suggest that enoxaparin may be as safe as UFH in this setting, as the rates of death or nonfatal MI where comparable among these two groups. UFH should be used if CABG is planned within 48 hours because its anticoagulant effect is more easily reversed. Direct thrombin inhibitors are the antithrombin of choice when a patient has a history of HIT. In the absence of HIT, the role for direct thrombin inhibitors as the primary antithrombin is less well-established.

Thrombolytics

Thrombolytic therapy has not been shown to clinically benefit patients with NSTE-ACS. The TIMI-IIIA and IIIB studies showed no benefit of thrombolytic therapy versus standard therapy in this group of patients. In fact, thrombolytic agents increase the risk of myocardial infarction in this group of patients, possibly because of a procoagulant effect due to platelet activation.

- Aspirin, heparin nitrates, β-blockers, clopidogrel and GP IIB/IIIA (–) are the cornerstones of medical treatment of NSTE-ACS.
- Thrombolytic therapy has no documented benefit in NSTE-ACS.

Intra-Aortic Balloon Pump

Intra-aortic balloon pumping should be considered in patients with myocardial ischemia refractory to aggressive medical management outlined above, who have persistent hypotension or who have high-risk obstructions at the time of coronary angiography (significant left main or proximal LAD disease). Contraindications to intra-aortic balloon pumping are 1) severe peripheral vascular disease, 2) significant aortic insufficiency, and 3) severe aortoiliac disease, including aortic aneurysm. Intra-aortic balloon pumping should be used as a bridge to definitive coronary revascularization via percutaneous intervention or CABG.

LATE RISK STRATIFICATION IN THE CONSERVATIVELY TREATED PATIENT

Low- to intermediate-risk patients (by ACC/AHA criteria) treated with an early conservative strategy and have not had recurrent ischemia may undergo stress testing for further risk stratification. In most cases, testing may be done within 72 hours after presentation. The choice of the stress test depends on the patient's resting ECG, the ability of the patient to perform exercise, and the available methods and local expertise.

Exercise treadmill testing is the standard mode of stress testing in patients with a normal ECG who are able to exercise. Conditions precluding accurate interpretation of the stress ECG include digoxin therapy, widespread resting ST-segment depression (≥1 mm), left ventricular hypertrophy, left bundle branch block, significant interventricular conduction delay, and

preexcitation syndrome. In patients with these conditions an imaging modality such as a radionuclide agent (thallium, sestamibi, exercise multiple-gated acquisition [MUGA] scanning, positron emission tomography) or exercise echocardiography should be considered (Table 6). Patients who are unable to exercise because of general debility, chronic obstructive pulmonary disease, peripheral vascular disease, or orthopedic limitations should undergo pharmacologic stress testing with an imaging modality (Table 7). Available agents include adenosine, dobutamine, and dipyridamole, and the agent of choice should be guided by local expertise and patient factors.

Patients who are able to exercise to a high workload (i.e., ≥5 metabolic equivalents [METs]) without ischemia have a good prognosis and may be managed medically. However, patients who have evidence of ischemia, on the basis of symptoms, ECG, or imaging modality at a low workload (i.e., <5 METs) should be considered for angiography.

Patients at low risk on exercise stress testing have a predicted average cardiac mortality of <1% per year, compared with ≥4% per year for those at high risk. It should be remembered that all forms of exercise testing have been shown to be less accurate in women than in men. However, it is still reasonable to use noninvasive testing in women for risk stratification in the early conservative treatment strategy.

- Patients treated with the early conservative strategy should have stress testing done prior to discharge.
- An exercise capacity of ≥5 METs without ischemia indicates a good prognosis.
- Low-risk patients have <1% annual cardiac mortality.
- High-risk patients have ≥4% annual cardiac mortality.

CORONARY ANGIOGRAPHY AND REVASCULARIZATION

Most patients who present with NSTE-ACS undergo coronary angiography. The ACC/AHA recommends patients with new ST-segment depression, troponin elevation, recurrent ischemic pain despite aggressive medical therapy, LV dysfunction and other high risk features undergo coronary angiography (Fig. 5). However, coronary angiography should be performed only in patients who are potential candidates for revascularization.

Table 6. Guidelines for Stress Method in Risk Assessment*

Patient factors	Exercise (treadmill, cycle, arm)	Dipyridamole† (thallium, sestamibi)	Adenosine† (thallium, sestamibi)	Dobutamine (thallium, sestamibi, RNA, echocardiography
Carotid bruits				
Without symptoms	Yes	Yes	Yes	Yes
With recent symptoms	Yes	No‡	Yes§	No‡
Lung disease				
Mild/moderate COPD	Yes	Yes	Yes	Yes
Severe COPD/ asthma	Yes	No	No	Yes
Theophylline	Yes	No	No	Yes
LBBB	No	Yes	Yes	No
β-Blockers	Yes	Yes	Yes	No
Dipyridamole	Yes	Yes	No	Yes
PPM	No	Yes	Yes	No
Poorly controlled HTN	No	Yes	Yes	No
Significant ventricular ectopy	Yes	Yes	Yes	No

β, beta; COPD, chronic obstructive pulmonary disease; ECG, electrocardiogram; HTN, hypertension; LBBB, left bundle branch block; MET, metabolic equivalent; PPM, non-rate-responsive permanent pacemaker; RNA, radionuclide angiography.
*If the patient has normal ECG and can walk, use exercise treadmill. If possible, exercise the patient (to ≥5 METs or to chest discomfort).
†For dipyridamole and adenosine, withhold caffeine for 12 hours.
‡Because of possible high/low blood pressure response.
§Graduated infusion with blood pressure monitoring suggested.

Among patients with NSTE-ACS who undergo coronary angiography, 10-20% have normal or insignificant coronary artery disease, 5-10% have significant left main disease, 20-25% have three-vessel disease, 25-30% have two-vessel disease and 30-35% have single-vessel disease. Patient with significant coronary artery stenosis (i.e. >70% stenosis of the left anterior descending [LAD], circumflex, or right coronary artery or >50% stenosis of the left main coronary artery) are candidates for revascularization. If catheterization shows significant left main coronary artery disease or three-vessel disease with reduced LV function, the patient should be referred for CABG. In general, those patients (particularly those with diabetes mellitus) with two-vessel disease including severe proximal LAD and reduced LV function should be referred for CABG. Currently, in the era of drug-eluting stents, there are several trials comparing CABG with multivessel PCI. Patient enrollment and data collection are still ongoing and it is too early to determine what impact these trials may have in treatment of these groups.

■ The ACC/AHA recommend coronary angiography in NSTE-ACS patients that have new ST-segment depression, troponin elevation, recurrent chest pain, LV dysfunction, and other high-risk features.

Table 7.   Guidelines for Imaging Modality in Risk Assessment*

	Treadmill only	Echo	Thallium	Sestamibi	RNA
Goal of test					
EF	No	Yes	No	Yes	Yes
Screening	Yes	Yes	Yes	Yes	Yes
Low cost	Yes	No	No	No	No
Post MI viability	Yes	Yes	Yes	Yes	Yes
Patient factors					
Large chest	Yes	No	Yes	Yes	Yes
Obese	Yes	Yes	No	Yes	Yes
COPD	Yes	No	Yes	Yes	No
ECG factors					
LBBB	No	Yes	Yes	Yes	Yes
Nonspecific ST-T wave changes due to digoxin, WPW, MVP, LVH, PPM	No	No	Yes	Yes	No
Irregular rhythm (AF, frequent PVCs)	No	Yes	Yes	Yes	No
Cannot exercise	No	Yes	Yes	Yes	No

AF, atrial fibrillation; EF, ejection fraction; COPD, chronic obstructive pulmonary disease; LBBB, let bundle branch block; LVH, left ventricular hypertrophy; MI, myocardial infarction; MVP, mitral valve prolapse; PPM, non-rate-responsive permanent pacemaker; PVC premature ventricular contraction; WPW, Wolff-Parkinson-White syndrome.
*Local expertise/availability is extremely important in choosing imaging modality.

■ Generally, CABG is favored over PCI in patients with LV systolic dysfunction, severe left main coronary artery or three-vessel disease and in two-vessel disease with severe proximal stenosis of the LAD, and in diabetics.

TREATMENT AFTER HOSPITAL DISCHARGE

At the time of hospital discharge the goal of continued pharmacotherapy is to prevent (recurrent) MI and death. Patients hospitalized with NSTE-ACS should be treated indefinitely with aspirin 81-162 mg per day in the absence of contraindications. If aspirin is not tolerated due to hypersensitivity or gastrointestinal intolerance clopidogrel 75 mg per day should used. Additionally, the combination of aspirin and clopidogrel should be used for 9 months after NSTE-ACS, and the dose of aspirin should be 81 mg when clopidogrel is added. β-Blockers should be used indefinitely. Lipid-lowering agents, with preferential use of HMG-CoA reductase inhibitors, and diet should be used in all post NSTE-ACS patients to lower LDL cholesterol to at least <100 mg/dL (and preferentially to <70 mg/dL in high-risk patients). ACE (–) (Angiotensin Converting Enzyme Inhibitors) should be used in all patients with CHF, LV dysfunction (EF <40%), hypertension and diabetes. Special instruction should be given on smoking cessation, optimal weight, diet, exercise, and stress reduction. Additional tailored instruction should be given on the appropriate time to resume routine activities (heavy lifting, climbing stairs, yard work, household activities, sexual activities, and returning to work) and vigorous exercise >200 minutes/week. Patients should have medical follow-up within 6 weeks (sooner if the patient was high-risk). Low-risk patients treated conservatively without coronary angiography that experience recurrent unstable angina or who have severe stable angina (CCS 3 or 4) despite medical therapy and are

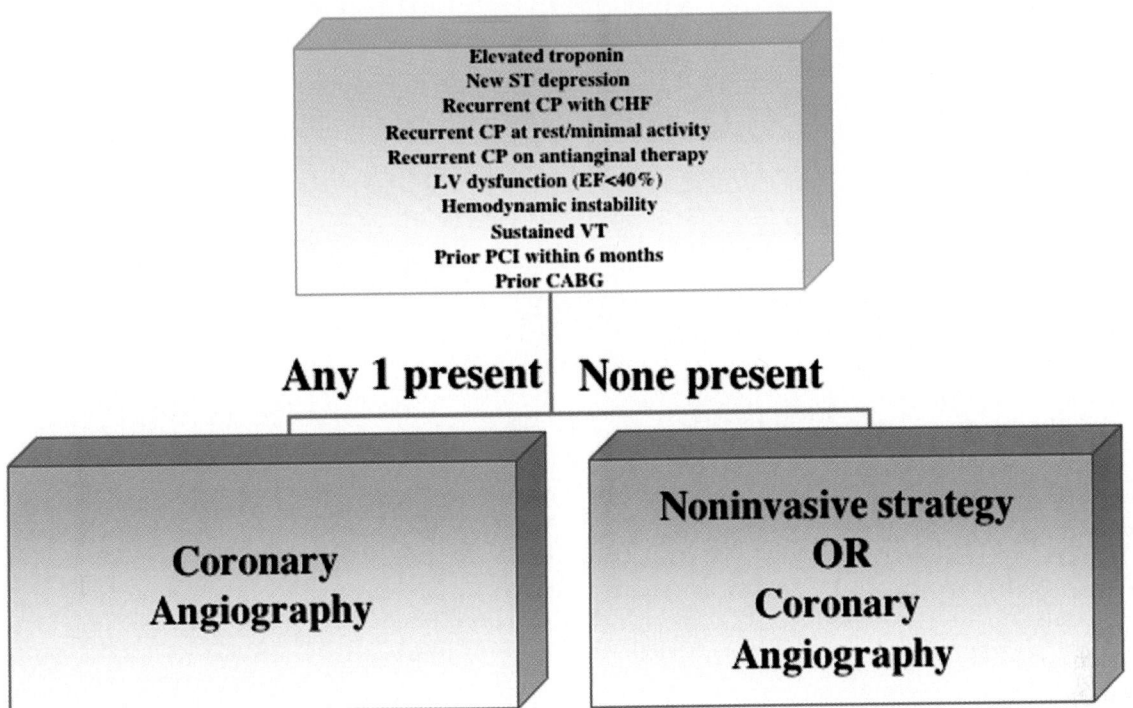

Fig. 5. Clinical factors which determine the ACC/AHA recommendations for an early invasive or early conservative therapy. CABG, coronary artery bypass grafting; CHF, congestive heart failure; CP, chest pain; LV, left ventricular; PCI, percutaneous coronary intervention; VT, ventricular tachycardia.

suitable candidates should undergo coronary angiography. Patients with severe LV dysfunction (EF <30%) at the time of hospitalization for NSTE-ACS who underwent coronary revascularization should have reassessment of LV function >4 weeks from revascularization to determine if they are candidates for ICD (implantable cardioverter-defibrillator) placement (See Chapters 35 and 36 on ICDs).

CHRONIC STABLE ANGINA

Frank C. Chen, MD

Frank V. Brozovich, MD, PhD

SIGNS AND SYMPTOMS

Character

Angina pectoris typically presents as a retrosternal discomfort in the chest and adjacent areas and can vary from being "constricting," "crushing," or "squeezing" in quality to mild and pressure-like with occasional associated numbing or burning sensation. It often radiates down the ulnar surface of the left arm, but radiation can also occur on outer surfaces of both arms. Belching or epigastric discomfort in conjunction with chest pain is not uncommon. Other associated symptoms such as dyspnea, fatigue, and syncope are particularly common in the elderly.

Duration

Typical angina is usually characterized by a crescendo increase in the intensity of pain over minutes, and should neither last hours nor occur in brief spurts of just few seconds. It is often precipitated by exercise, exposure to cold temperature, or carbohydrate-rich meals and relieved within minutes by rest and nitroglycerin. If pain is not relieved within five to ten minutes after rest or nitroglycerin use, it is unlikely to be secondary to myocardial ischemia or alternatively, severe ongoing ischemia is present, such as in the case of unstable angina or acute myocardial infarction. In some patients, exertion interrupted by intermittent periods of rest can lead to greater levels of exertion without symptoms. This is sometimes termed as the "warm-up" phenomenon and is hypothesized to result from either ischemic preconditioning or recruitment of coronary collateral circulation.

Grading of Severity

Grading of angina according to the Canadian Cardiovascular Society (CCS) is a modification of the New York Heart Association (NYHA) functional classification and has since been widely accepted, since the CCS classification allows for more specific categorization of patients according to their activity level (Table 1). Other classification schemes include the Specific Activity Scale developed by Goldman and colleagues and the anginal score by Califf and associates. It should be noted that any functional classification is subject to variability in activity tolerance as perceived by patients and hence its reproducibility is variable. Reproducibility reaches 73% using either the CCS criteria or the Specific Activity Scale, but the latter seems to correlate better with objective measures by treadmill exercise.

PHYSICAL EXAMINATION

Brief episodes of angina can result in transient left ventricular and papillary muscle dysfunction, characterized

Table 1. A Comparison of Three Methods of Assessing Cardiovascular Disability

Class	New York Heart Association functional classification	Canadian Cardiovascular Society functional classification	Specific activity scale
I	Patients with cardiac disease but without resulting limitations of physical activity. Ordinary physical activity does not cause undue fatigue, palpitation, dyspnea, or anginal pain	Ordinary physical activity, such as walking and climbing stairs, does not cause angina. Angina with strenuous, rapid, or prolonged exertion at work or recreation	Patients can perform to completion any activity requiring ≥7 metabolic equivalents (e.g., can carry 24 lb up to 8 steps; carry objects that weight 80 lb; do outdoor work [shovel snow, spade soil]; do recreational activities [skiing, basketball, squash, handball, jog/walk 5 mph])
II	Patients with cardiac disease resulting in slight limitation of physical activity. They are comfortable at rest. Ordinary physical activity results in fatigue, palpitation, dyspnea, or anginal pain	Slight limitation of ordinary activity. Walking or climbing stairs rapidly, walking uphill, walking or stair climbing after meals, in cold, in wind, or when under emotional stress, or only during the few hours after awakening. Walking more than two blocks on the level and climbing more than one flight of ordinary stairs at a normal pace and in normal conditions	Patients can perform to completion any activity requiring ≥5 metabolic equivalents (e.g., have sexual intercourse without stopping, garden, rake, weed, roller skate, dance, fox trot, walk at 4 mph on level ground) but cannot and do not perform to completion activities requiring ≥7 metabolic equivalents
III	Patients with cardiac disease resulting in marked limitation of physical activity. They are comfortable at rest. Less than ordinary physical activity causes fatigue, palpitation, dyspnea, or anginal pain	Marked limitation of ordinary physical activity. Walking one to two blocks on the level and climbing more than one flight in normal conditions	Patients can perform to completion any activity requiring ≥2 metabolic equivalents (e.g., shower without stopping, strip and make bed, clean windows, walk 2-5 mph, bowl, play golf, dress without stopping) but cannot and do not perform to completion any activities requiring ≥5 metabolic equivalents
IV	Patient with cardiac disease resulting in inability to carry on any physical activity without discomfort. Symptoms of cardiac insufficiency or of the anginal syndrome may be present even at rest. If any physical activity is undertaken, discomfort is increased	Inability to carry on any physical activity without discomfort— anginal syndrome *may be* present at rest	Patients cannot or do not perform to completion activities requiring ≥2 metabolic equivalents. *Cannot* carry out activities listed above (Specific Activity Scale, Class III)

by S_3, loud S_4, pulmonary rales, and apical systolic murmurs. Displaced ventricular impulse is a sign of dyskinetic left ventricle, and ischemia can give rise to delayed left ventricular contraction, resulting in the paradoxic split of S_2. A midsystolic click with late systolic murmur seen in mitral valve prolapse can be seen in patients with coronary artery disease (CAD). On peripheral vascular examination, any evidence of peripheral vascular disease such as decreased ankle-brachial index and early carotid disease on ultrasound is strongly associated with the presence of CAD. It should be understood however that patients with angina may have a completely normal physical examination.

OTHER DIFFERENTIAL DIAGNOSES

Acute myocardial infarction; aortic dissection; pulmonary hypertension with right ventricular ischemia; pulmonary embolism; acute pericarditis; gastroesophageal reflux and disorders of esophageal motility, including diffuse spasm, nutcracker esophagus, and achalasia; biliary disorders; cholecystitis; costosternal chondritis or Tietze Syndrome; cervical radiculitis; and shoulder bursitis/tendonitis may all cause pain that mimics the symptoms of chronic angina.

PATHOPHYSIOLOGY

Neuromechanisms of Cardiac Pain

Myocardial ischemia leads to the activation of the chemo- and mechanoreceptors, which in turn causes the release of substances like bradykinin and adenosine. These neurochemicals then stimulate both sympathetic and vagal afferent fibers. Sympathetic afferent impulses converge with somatic sensory fibers from thoracic structures and travels to the thalamus and frontal cortex. Sympathetic activation is responsible for the perception of referred cardiac pain. Failed transmission of afferent impulses from the thalamus to the frontal cortex on PET scan has been postulated to cause silent ischemia in patients with autonomic neuropathy. Vagal afferent fibers synapse in the medulla and innervate the upper cervical spinothalamic tract, which gives rise to the pain in the neck and jaw.

Pathogenesis of Angina Pectoris

Myocardial ischemia can be due to either increased myocardial O_2 requirements or decreased myocardial O_2 supply. Angina precipitated by increased myocardial O_2 requirements is sometimes termed *demand angina* or *fixed-threshold angina*, while angina secondary to a transiently decreased O_2 supply is sometimes termed *supply angina* or *variable-threshold angina*.

Angina Due to Increased Myocardial O_2 Requirement

In demand angina, physiological responses to physical exertion, mental or emotional stresses, and conditions like fever, hypoglycemia, and thyrotoxicosis trigger the release of norepinephrine, which increases myocardial O_2 requirements. Hence, in demand angina with few dynamic (vasoconstrictor) components, the amount of physical activity to precipitate angina is relatively constant.

Angina Due to Decreased Myocardial O_2 Supply

In supply angina, similar to unstable angina, dynamic stenosis can further decrease myocardial O_2 supply in the presence of a fixed organic stenosis; platelets and leukocytes can elaborate vasoconstrictors like thromboxane A_2 and serotonin, which along with the already damaged endothelium and decreased nitric oxide production secondary to coronary atherosclerosis, will lead to vasoconstriction. Other features of supply angina include a circadian variation, in which angina occurs more often in the morning, as well as cold temperature-induced coronary vasoconstriction. High carbohydrate diet can redistribute coronary blood flow away from stenotic vessels and precipitate postprandial angina.

DIAGNOSTIC TESTING

Noninvasive Testing

Biochemical Tests

Initial biochemical evaluation should include a fasting lipid profile and fasting blood glucose to screen for dyslipidemias and insulin resistance. Other markers of increased atherogenicity like lipoprotein Lp(a), small dense LDL, and apolipoprotein B appear to add to traditional tests of total cholesterol/LDL in better predicting future cardiovascular event risk.

Measurement of high-sensitive C-reactive protein (CRP) can be used in secondary prevention to prognosticate patients with established CAD. B-type natriuretic peptide (BNP) and its inactive N-terminal fragment (NT-pro-BNP) have been shown to be strong predictors of morbidity and mortality in patients with heart failure and acute coronary syndromes. Recently, two prospective observational studies from Denmark and Germany showed that in patients with chronic stable angina, higher quartile of NT-pro-BNP level correlated with decreased survival after adjusting for conventional risk factors (e.g., age, sex, history of MI, hypertension, diabetes, LVEF, etc.) (Fig. 1). Another study from Australia and New Zealand demonstrated that in patients with stable CAD (NYHA class II/III), BNP and NT-pro-BNP displayed strong negative predictive value in ruling out severely reduced LVEF and directly correlated with all-cause mortality/worsening heart failure after 1 year follow-up. These data, taken together, suggest that BNP and NT-pro-BNP offer additional prognostic information in patients with stable CAD.

Resting ECG
Approximately half of the patients with chronic stable angina will have normal resting ECG. Most common ECG findings in chronic CAD include nonspecific ST-T wave changes with or without abnormal Q waves. Q waves are relatively specific but not sensitive indicators for previous myocardial infarction. During an anginal episode, ECG becomes abnormal in about 50% of the patients with normal baseline ECG.

Noninvasive Stress Testing
Noninvasive stress testing can be used to diagnose and further assess prognosis in patients with chronic stable angina. However, appropriate stress testing should be directed based on the estimate of the pretest probability (prevalence of disease) of CAD in the particular patient population (Table 2).

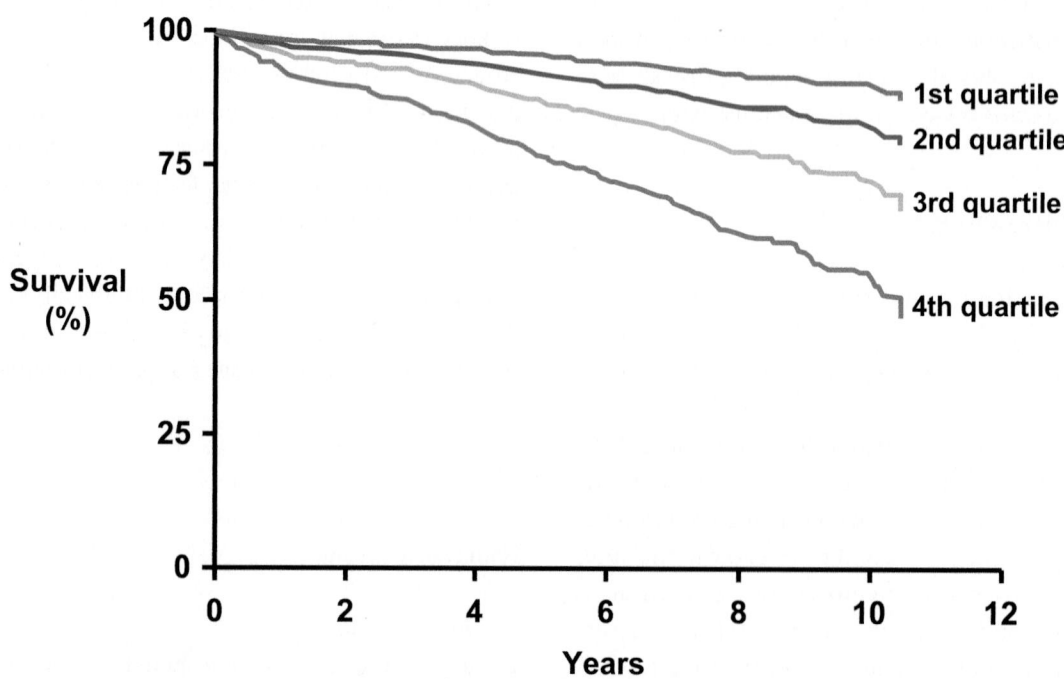

Fig. 1. Adjusted estimates of overall survival among patients with stable coronary disease, according to quartiles of NT-pro-BNP. The survival estimates have been adjusted for age, presence or absence of diabetes, smoking status, left ventricular ejection fraction, presence or absence of suspected heart failure, and severity of angiographic coronary disease. The NT-pro-BNP levels were as follows: first quartile, less than 64 pg/mL, second quartile, 64 to 169 pg/mL, third quartile, 170 to 455 pg/mL, and fourth quartile, more than 455 pg/mL. P<0.001 by the log-rank test for the overall comparison among the groups.

Table 2.   Pretest Likelihood of Coronary Artery Disease in Symptomatic Patients According to Age and Sex*

Age (years)	Nonanginal chest pain		Atypical angina		Typical angina	
	Men	Women	Men	Women	Men	Women
30-39	4	2	34	12	76	26
40-49	13	3	51	22	87	55
50-59	20	7	65	31	93	73
60-69	27	14	72	51	94	86

*Each value represents the precentage with significant coronary artery disease at coronary angiography.

Exercise ECG

In patients with moderate probability of CAD and angina, exercise ECG is particularly helpful provided they have normal resting ECG and achieve an adequate workload. According to the ACC/AHA guidelines on exercise testing, mean sensitivity and specificity are 68% and 77%, respectively. If one corrects for the posttest referral bias, however, sensitivity is further lowered to 45%-50% but specificity increases to 85%-90%. In part the low sensitivity of exercise testing in this population includes the inability of many patients to reach ≥85% of the maximally predicted heart rate, either due to physical inability or the effects of anti-anginal medication.

Stress Myocardial Imaging

In patients with abnormal resting ECGs such as repolarization abnormalities, LVH, LBBB, and digitalis effect, exercise perfusion imaging is superior to exercise ECG alone in localizing diseased vessels, identifying multivessel disease, and detecting areas of ischemia/infarct. Pharmacological vasodilators like adenosine or dipyridamole can be used in elderly patients who are unable to exercise due to comorbid pulmonary or peripheral vascular diseases. The accuracy with exercise echocardiography is similar to that of stress myocardial perfusion imaging. Newer imaging modalities like contrast echocardiography and harmonic imaging have significantly improved endocardial border definition, which enhances the visualization of ischemic myocardium.

Invasive Testing

Coronary Angiography

Among patients with chronic stable angina referred for coronary angiography, ~25% each have single-, double-, or triple-vessel disease (>70% luminal diameter narrowing). 5%-10% of patients have obstruction of the left main coronary artery and 15% do not have detectable critical obstruction. Intravascular ultrasonography (IVUS) allows the assessment of the cross-lumen dimensions and determination of the plaque composition. Angiography also allows the visualization of coronary collateral circulations, coronary artery ectasia/aneurysms, and myocardial bridging and the assessment of LV function using biplane contrast angiography.

PROGNOSIS/RISK STRATIFICATION

Old data from the Framingham Study demonstrated that the annual average mortality in patients with chronic stable angina pectoris was 4%. With the advent of pharmacotherapy like aspirin and beta blockers and aggressive risk factor modifications, more recent data from Britain showed the annual mortality rate in middle-aged men with CAD had decreased down to 1.7%-3%. To predict the presence of severe CAD (triple-vessel or left main CAD), a five-point clinical score is assigned based on the following clinical variables: male sex, typical angina, history and ECG evidence of MI, and diabetes (Fig. 2). The 5-year survival of CAD with medical therapy is based on the number of diseased vessels, the severity of obstruction, and the location (Fig. 3).

THERAPY

Medical Management

Treatment of Associated Diseases
Conditions which can exacerbate previously stable angina include anemia, thyrotoxicosis, fever, infection, tachycardia, and drugs that activate the sympathetic nervous system. Treating these conditions will reduce myocardial O_2 demand and increase O_2 delivery, thus alleviating anginal symptoms.

Reduction of Coronary Risk Factors

Hypertension
The risk of ischemic heart disease doubles for very 20 mm Hg increase (range 115-185 mm Hg) among individuals between the age of 40 to 70. Pharmacological treatment of mild-moderate hypertension demonstrated a statistically significant 16% reduction in CAD events.

Tobacco Smoking
Smoking increases myocardial O_2 demand, causes coronary vasospasm, and decreases the efficacy of antianginal drugs. Among patients with documented CAD, smokers have a higher 5-year risk of sudden death, MI, and all-cause mortality than those who have quit smoking. Hence, smoking cessation is one of the most powerful and cost-effective approach to the prevention of CAD progression.

Dyslipidemia
↑LDL cholesterol. Clinical trials like the Scandinavian Simvastatin Survival Study (4S), Cholesterol and Recurrent Events Trial (CARE), Long-Term Intervention with Pravastatin in Ischemic Disease (LIPID), and Heart Protection Study (HPS) have convincingly demonstrated that, in patients with atherosclerotic vascular disease, 3-hydroxy-3-methylglutaryl coenzyme A (HMG-CoA) reductase

inhibitors (statins) significantly reduce subsequent cardiovascular events (e.g., cardiovascular mortality, rate of MI, need for CABG, etc.). Statins have also been shown to improve endothelial function, lower circulating level of C-reactive protein, reduce thrombogenicity, and stabilize atherosclerotic plaques.

The new ASTEROID (A Study to Evaluate the Effect of Rosuvastatin on Intravascular Ultrasound-Derived Coronary Atheroma Burden) trial showed for first time that high-intensity statin therapy led to the regression of atherosclerotic disease in patients with established CAD. Taken together, these data provide the basis for more aggressive cholesterol-lowering therapy among patients with established CAD.

↓HDL cholesterol. In addition to diet and exercise, pharmacotherapy with gemfibrozil has been shown in the Veterans Affairs High-Density Lipoprotein Cholesterol Intervention Trial (VA-HIT) Study to raise HDL by 6% and reduce death, non-fatal MI, or stroke by 24%.

Exercise
The conditioning effect of exercise lowers the heart rate and increases the cardiac output at any given level of myocardial O_2 consumption. Several small randomized trials have demonstrated improvement in effort tolerance, O_2 consumption, and quality of life in patients with chronic stable CAD undergoing exercise training.

ADDITIONAL PHARMACOTHERAPY FOR SECONDARY PREVENTION OF CAD

Aspirin
Meta-analysis of 140,000 patients from the Antiplatelet Trialists' Collaboration showed that aspirin (75-325 mg/day) reduced the rate of subsequent MI, stroke, and death in patients with history of angina pectoris, MI, CABG, and stroke. In the Swedish Angina Pectoris Aspirin Trial (SAPAT), aspirin (75 mg/day) in conjunction with the beta blocker sotalol conferred an additional 34% reduction in acute MI and sudden death among men and women with chronic stable angina. Aspirin also improves endothelial function and, when used in high dose (300 mg/day), has been shown to reduce circulating levels of C-reactive protein. Dosing in the 75-150 mg/day range appears to have comparable

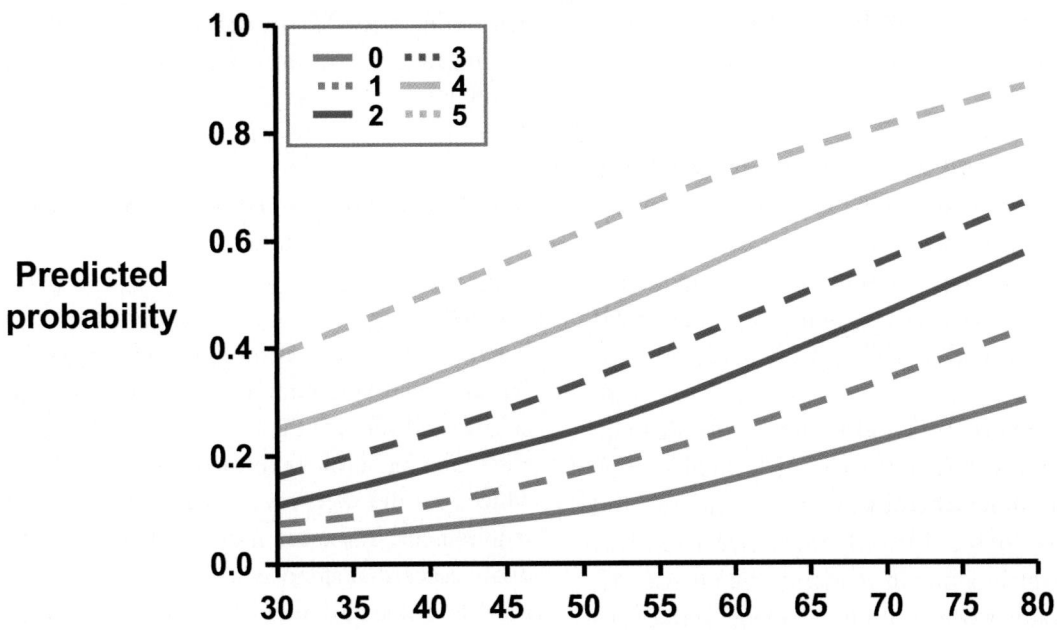

Fig. 2. Nomogram showing the probability of severe (triple-vessel or left main) coronary artery disease based on a five-point clinical score assigned on the basis of the clinical variables: male gender, typical angina, history and electrocardiographic evidence of myocardial infarction, and diabetes.

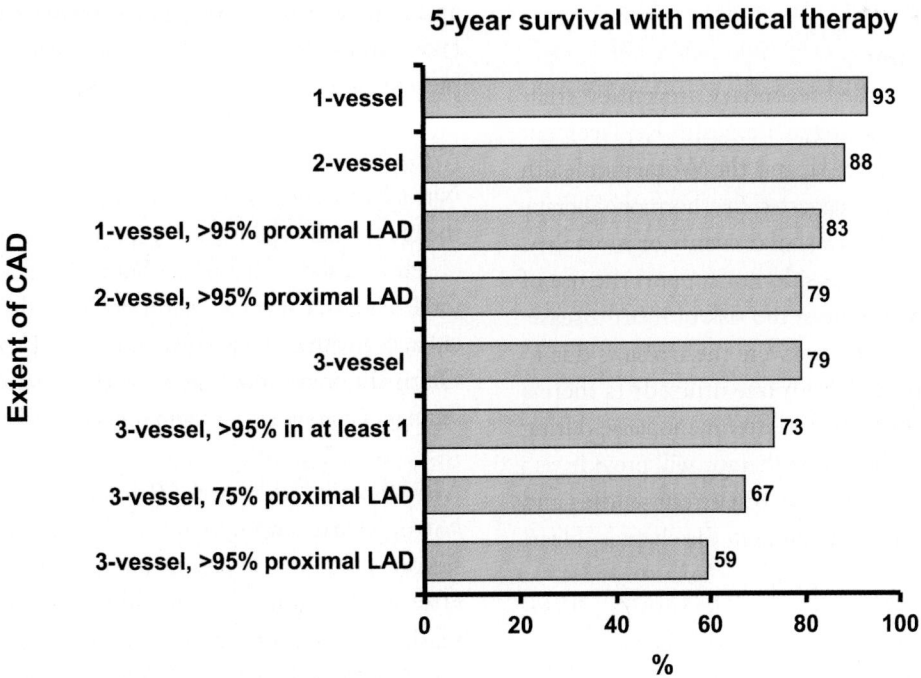

Fig. 3. Angiographic extent of coronary artery disease (CAD) and subsequent survival with medical therapy. A gradient of mortality risk is established based on the number of diseased vessels and the presence and severity of disease of the proximal left anterior descending (LAD) artery.

efficacy for secondary prevention compared to dosing at 160-325 mg/day and also reduces bleeding risk.

Clopidogrel

In the Clopidogrel Versus Aspirin in Patients at Risk of Ischemic Events (CAPRIE) trial, randomized comparison between clopidogrel and aspirin showed that clopidogrel resulted in 8.7% relative reduction in the risk of vascular death, ischemic stroke, or MI among patients with established atherosclerotic vascular disease. In the latest Clopidogrel for High Atherothrombotic Risk and Ischemic Stabilization, Management, and Avoidance (CHARISMA) trial, dual antiplatelet therapy with clopidogrel and aspirin was **not** significantly more effective compared to aspirin alone in reducing the rate of MI, stroke, or cardiovascular death in patients with established vascular disease or at high risk for developing vascular disease. Hence, there is still no data supporting the use of dual antiplatelet therapy in the setting of primary prevention.

THERAPY NO LONGER RECOMMENDED IN THE TREATMENT OF CHRONIC CAD

Estrogen Replacement

Randomized, controlled secondary prevention trials like the Heart and Estrogen/Progestin Replacement Study (HERS), HERS-II, and the Women's Health Initiative (WHI) have suggested that hormone therapy does not reduce cardiovascular events or mortality. Current recommendations do not support the use of hormone therapy to reduce the risk of heart disease. Questions persist, however; were these results due to the dose or regimen of hormone utilized? Is there a small window of opportunity after menopause during which initiation of hormone therapy will provide risk reduction? A full discussion of current studies and recommendations may be found in the chapter "Heart Disease in Women."

Antioxidants

The Heart Protection Study Collaborative Group enrolled more than 20,000 patients with established atherosclerotic vascular disease or diabetes mellitus and conclusively demonstrated no reduction in all-cause mortality, MI, or other vascular events with the regimen of vitamin C, vitamin E, and beta-carotene.

SPECIFIC PHARMACOLOGICAL MANAGEMENT OF ANGINA PECTORIS.

Nitrates

Nitrates induce endothelium-independent vasodilatation. Nitrates relax systemic (including coronary arteries) arteries and veins, but the venodilator effect predominates. The venodilator effect reduces ventricular preload which in turn lowers myocardial wall tension and O_2 requirement. In the coronary circulation, nitrates also dilate epicardial stenosis with eccentric lesions and alleviate endothelial dysfunction, thus improving blood flow across obstructed regions.

Nitroglycerin Tablets

Sublingual nitroglycerin remains to be the treatment of choice for acute anginal episodes. Sublingual administration avoids first-pass hepatic metabolism. The half-life of nitroglycerin is brief, and within 30-60 minutes hepatic breakdown will have abolished the hemodynamic and clinical effects. Sublingual nitroglycerin, when taken prophylactically prior to physical activities, can prevent angina for up to 40 minutes.

Nitroglycerin Ointment

Nitroglycerin ointment (15 mg/inch) can be applied to the chest in 0.5-2.0 inches strips. Its delay in the onset of action is about 30 minutes but the clinical effect lasts for 4-6 hours. Cutaneous permeability of the ointment is enhanced with increased hydration and plastic coverings. Ointment preparations are most commonly used in the settings of chronic severe angina or nocturnal angina.

Nitroglycerin Transdermal Patches

Nitroglycerin impregnated with polymer matrix or silicone gel results in absorption between 24-48 hours after application. The release rate varies from 0.1 mg/hr to 0.8 mg/hr. Administration of nitroglycerin via the transdermal approach has been shown to prolong exercise duration and sustain antianginal effects for 12 hours without significant nitrate tolerance or rebound phenomena.

Isosorbide Dinitrate

Isosorbide dinitrate undergoes rapid hepatic metabolism and thus has low bioavailability after oral administration. One of its subsequent metabolites exerts potent vasodilatory effect and is cleared less rapidly (urinary excretion). Partial or complete nitrate tolerance develops with doses of isosorbide dinitrate at 30 mg three or four times daily. Hence, a dosage schedule which includes a 10 to 12 hour nitrate-free interval should be implemented to prevent tolerance.

Isosorbide 5-Mononitrate

This is the active metabolite of dinitrate which does not undergo first-pass hepatic metabolism. The complete bioavailability of the 5-mononitrate preparation increases the efficacy for treating chronic stable angina. Isosorbide 5-mononitrate reaches peak level between 30 minutes and 2 hours after ingestion and has a plasma half-life of 4-6 hours. The only sustained-release form is given once daily. Nitrate tolerance has not been demonstrated with once-a-day dosing intervals but can be seen with twice-daily dosing at 12-hour intervals.

β-Adrenergic Receptor Blocking Agents (β-Blockers)

β-blockers, via the competitive inhibition of β-adrenoceptors, antagonize the effect of circulating and neuronally released catecholamines. β-blockers slow heart rate and increase diastolic portion of the cardiac cycle, which allows more time for coronary perfusion. By blocking the surges of sympathetic activity during exercise, β-blockers reduce contractility and left ventricular wall tension, resulting in lower myocardial O_2 demand. Many studies have shown that β-blockers decrease the frequency of anginal episodes and raise the anginal threshold. Other salutary properties of β-blockade include reduction in mortality and re-infarction in post-MI patients, as well as reduction in mortality among patients with heart failure. Abrupt withdrawal of β-blockade can precipitate unstable angina and even myocardial infarction in patients with chronic CAD.

ACE Inhibitors

ACE inhibitors reduce LVH, vascular hypertrophy, atherosclerotic progression, plaque rupture and thrombotic risk. ACE inhibition also enhances coronary endothelial vasomotor function and decreases inflammatory changes in animal models of atherosclerosis.

Thus ACE inhibitors promote favorable myocardial O_2 supply/demand relationships and lessen sympathetic activity. The Heart Outcomes Prevention Study (HOPE) Trial showed that ACE inhibitor ramipril (10 mg/day) reduced the relative risk of cardiovascular deaths, MI, and strokes in patients with atherosclerotic vascular disease or diabetes and at least one other CAD risk factor. The European Trial on Reduction of Cardiac Events with Perindopril in Stable CAD (EUROPA) provided further support in the beneficial effect of ACE inhibitors to lower subsequent cardiac events among patients with stable CAD and the absence of heart failure. Therefore, according to 2002 ACC/AHA Guideline Update on the management of chronic stable angina, ACE inhibitors should be recommended for all patients with CAD in conjunction with diabetes and/or impaired left ventricular function.

Calcium Channel Antagonists

Calcium antagonists consist of three subclasses, dihydropyridines (e.g., nifedipine), phenylalkylamines (e.g., verapamil), and the modified benzothiazepines (e.g., diltiazem). The antianginal effect of calcium antagonists primarily derives from their ability to reduce myocardial O_2 demand and enhance myocardial O_2 supply. The latter effect is particularly useful in patients with vasospastic components of angina pectoris, including variable-threshold angina, Prinzmetal (variant) angina, and angina of small coronary arteries with impaired vasodilator reserve. This vasodilatory effect can be seen in both systemic and coronary arterial beds. Inhibition of Ca^{2+} entry into cardiac myocytes can have significant negative inotropic effect on the heart and potentially lead to worsening heart failure in patients with significant LV dysfunction.

Calcium antagonists have also been postulated to have antiatherosclerotic properties. The Prospective Randomized Evaluation of the Vascular Effect of Norvasc Trial (PREVENT) did demonstrate slowing of atherosclerotic progression in carotid but not in the coronary vasculatures. A recent randomized, double-blinded study of 7,665 patients with stable symptomatic CAD showed that long-acting nifedipine had no effect on major cardiovascular event-free survival but did reduce the need for coronary angiography and CABG. Given to patients prior to undergoing PTCA, amlodipine was shown to reduce major cardiovascular end points (death, MI, CABG, repeat PTCA) in the Coronary Angioplasty Amlodipine Restenosis Study (CAPARES).

OTHER ANTIANGINAL AGENTS

Spinal Cord Stimulation

In patients with refractory angina not amenable to coronary revascularization, spinal cord stimulation using specific electrodes inserted into the epidural space uses neuromodulation to reduce painful stimulus. Several observational studies have reported success rates of up to 80% in decreasing anginal frequency and severity. However, more data are still needed and therefore, spinal cord stimulation should be only considered when other treatment options have failed.

Enhanced External Counterpulsation

Enhanced external counterpulsation (EECP) is another alternative therapy for refractory angina. Most data are from observational studies, which have reported improvement in exercise tolerance and reduction in anginal frequency as well as nitroglycerin use among patients treated with EECP. EECP has been postulated to decrease myocardial O_2 demand, enhance myocardial collateral flow via increased transmyocardial pressure, and improve endothelial function. The therapy is usually administered over 7 weeks consisting of 35 one-hour treatments. Possible placebo effect associated with EECP has not been addressed in many studies, which have not included sham controls.

PERCUTANEOUS CORONARY INTERVENTION

Patients with chronic stable angina should be considered for PCI if significant symptoms persist despite intense medical therapy. Technical success rates with PCI are usually high in younger patients (age<70) with single vessel disease (single lesion) and no evidence of CHF (EF >40%). Due to increased operator experience and widespread utilization of stents, PCI can now achieve an overall procedural success rate of 90% with less than 1% expected periprocedural mortality.

In patients with chronic stable angina, no randomized trial to date has demonstrated reduction in death or MI in PCI versus medical therapy. Balloon angioplasty has been shown to reduce angina and improve exercise capacity compared to medical therapy, but in the second Randomized Intervention Treatment of Angina (RITA-2) trial, death and periprocedural MI were higher in the angioplasty group than in the medically treated group. Other data have demonstrated that patients with one- or two-vessel CAD, preserved LV function, and mild symptoms (CCS I-II) have similar rates of cardiac death, MI, revascularization, or hospitalizations for angina when randomized to angioplasty or medical therapy; hence, aggressive medical management should generally be the initial treatment of mildly symptomatic patients with chronic stable angina.

CORONARY ARTERY BYPASS GRAFT (CABG)

CABG is may be an option for patients with refractory angina and surgically approachable vessels. Less invasive CABG has come about with the advent of off-pump coronary artery bypass (OPCAB) and minimally invasive direct CAB (MIDCAB). The avoidance of cardiopulmonary bypass (CPB) reduces the risk of bleeding, systemic thromboembolism, renal insufficiency, myocardial stunning, stroke, and neurological damage. Other advances involve the use of femoral-femoral CPB in totally endoscopic robotically assisted CABG (TECAB). Cardioplegic techniques have also improved substantially with the use of blood and other substrates like glutamate to facilitate myocardial aerobic metabolism and lower lactate production. Retrograde cardioplegia via the coronary sinus provides more uniform distribution of cardioplegic solution and is currently used in conjunction with the more traditional antegrade delivery.

Selection of Patients for CABG

Patients with worse LV function and more reversibly ischemic myocardial involvement will derive the greatest benefit from CABG over medical therapy (Table 3). CABG is highly effective in providing complete relief of angina and other symptoms. Data from a group of patients with saphenous vein grafts demonstrated that 90% of patients were angina-free at 1 year, and in the subsequent 4 years the recurrence rate was approximately 3%/year and 5%/year thereafter. Angina-free rates were 78% at 5 years, 52% at 10 years, and 23% at 15 years.

Table 3.   Effects of Coronary Artery Bypass Grafting on Survival*

Subgroup	Medical treatment mortality rate (%)	P value for CABG surgery vs. medical treatment
Vessel disease		
One vessel	9.9	0.18
Two vessels	11.7	0.45
Three vessels	17.6	<0.001
Left main artery	36.5	0.004
No LAD disease		
One or two vessels	8.3	0.88
Three vessels	14.5	0.02
Left main artery	45.8	0.03
Overall	12.3	0.05
LAD disease present		
One or two vessels	14.6	0.05
Three vessels	19.1	0.009
Left main artery	32.7	0.02
Overall	18.3	0.001
LV function		
Normal	13.3	<0.001
Abnormal	25.2	0.02
Exercise test status		
Missing	17.4	0.10
Normal	11.6	0.38
Abnormal	16.8	<0.001
Severity of angina		
Class 0, I, II	12.5	0.005
Class III, IV	22.4	0.001

LAD, left anterior descending artery; LV, left ventricular.
*Systematic overview of the effect of coronary artery bypass grafting (CABG) vs. medical therapy on survival based on data from the seven randomized trials comparing a strategy of initial CABG surgery with one of initial medical therapy. Subgroup results at 5 years are shown.

PCI vs. CABG

Earlier observational studies comparing PCI to CABG have been limited largely to the use of PTCA. Over a period of 1 to 5 years, the rates of mortality and nonfatal infarction did not differ significantly between patients revascularized with CABG versus PTCA. However, 1 year after PTCA, recurrent symptoms and/or the need for repeat procedures was approximately 40%. In addition, subgroup analysis revealed that patients with certain risk factors derived the highest survival benefit from CABG compared to PTCA: 1) LV dysfunction and 2) proximal LAD stenosis >70%.

OTHER SURGICAL TREATMENT FOR ISCHEMIC HEART DISEASE

Transmyocardial laser revascularization (TMR) is performed by placing a special high-energy, computerized carbon dioxide (CO_2) laser on the epicardial surface of the left ventricle via a lateral thoracotomy incision. The laser beam would then create between 20 to 40 one-millimeter-wide channels from the epicardial to the endocardial surfaces and thereby create a functional network of connections between the left ventricular cavity and the ischemic myocardium. Subsequent observations reveal that these connections close within hours or days after procedure and therefore, other alternative mechanisms must be responsible for the continued relief of angina. Possible explanations include increased perfusion by stimulation of angiogenesis, denervation of the sympathetic pain-sensitive afferent fibers, and a pure placebo effect. Results from two small sham-controlled trials have cast serious doubts on the potential benefit of TMR. Thus the role of TMR in treating refractory angina remains unclear.

68

RIGHT VENTRICULAR INFARCTION

Richard J. Gumina, MD

R. Scott Wright, MD

Joseph G. Murphy, MD

Right ventricular infarction is currently underdiagnosed and its significance with regard to an adverse prognosis is underappreciated. Numerous studies have demonstrated that patients with RV infarction represent an unique subgroup of infarct patients with a distinctive clinical presentation, treatment and prognosis. In patients with an acute inferior myocardial infarct (MI), it is estimated that 10%-50% have evidence of right ventricular (RV) dysfunction or infarction (Fig. 1 and 2).

CULPRIT LESION

RV infarction is commonly associated with acute left ventricular (LV) inferior wall infarction. Postmortem and angiographic data have demonstrated the vast majority of RV infarctions result from occlusion of the proximal right coronary artery (RCA). Inferior RV involvement has also been demonstrated with a "wrap-around" anatomic type distal left anterior descending artery (LAD) occlusion or with left circumflex artery occlusion in a left dominant coronary anatomy. The proximal location of the RCA occlusion is crucial to the development of RV infarction, because it compromises RV branch vessels which supply the RV free wall resulting in the significant RV involvement. Recent studies have demonstrated the importance of RV marginal branches; the magnitude of RV dysfunction was found to correlate with the extent of RV marginal

branch flow impairment and failure to restore marginal branch blood flow is associated with a lack of recovery of RV function, persistent hypotension, low cardiac output and high mortality. RCA occlusions in patients who do not develop RV infarction tend to have more distal RCA lesions or circumflex culprit lesions that spare the RV branch perfusion. However, exceptions in which proximal RCA occlusions that do not result in RV ischemia/dysfunction have also been reported. In necropsy studies of patients deceased from inferior MI, evidence of RV infarction was observed in 14%-60% of cases with evidence of a common triad of infarction involving the LV inferoposterior wall, septal and posterior RV free wall.

- RV infarction is most commonly observed in the setting of inferior LV infarction.
- Occlusion of the proximal RCA is the most common etiology for RV infarction.
- Restoration of RV branch vessel perfusion is key to prevention of RV infarction.

CLINICAL PRESENTATION

In 1930, the classic triad of hypotension, increased jugular venous pressure and clear lung fields was found in a patient with extensive RV necrosis, but minimal LV involvement at postmortem examination was

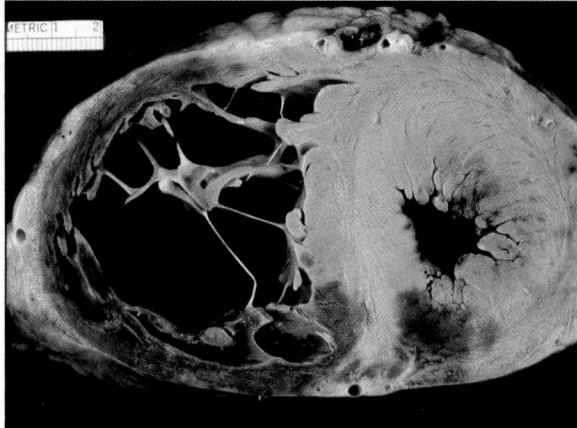

Fig. 1. Acute right ventricular infarct with right ventricular dilatation.

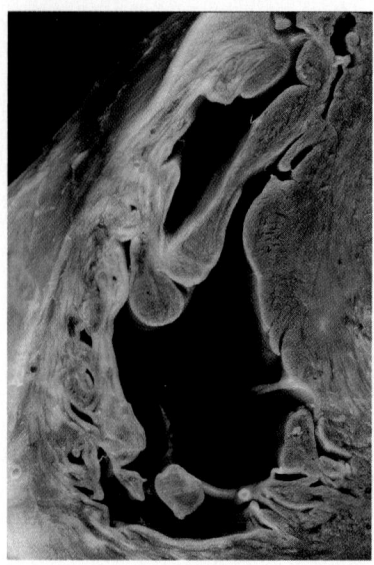

Fig. 2. Healed right ventricular infarct with right ventricular wall fibrosis.

reported. Indeed, the clinical manifestations of RV infarction reveal a distinct hemodynamic syndrome characterized by severe right heart failure, clear lung fields and low cardiac output despite preserved LV systolic function. In addition to this classic triad, Kussmaul's sign (an increase in jugular venous pressure with inspiration), pulsus paradoxus (a fall in systolic blood pressure of greater than 10 mm Hg with inspiration) and a positive hepatojugular reflux test may also be observed in patients with RV infarction. In the setting of an inferior MI, Kussmaul's sign is more predictive of RV involvement. However, in patients with such clinical signs, the differential diagnosis must also include pericardial tamponade, constrictive pericarditis and pulmonary embolus. Despite the RV dilatation that occurs with RV infarction, an RV heave is often not found. Cardiac auscultation may also reveal an RV S3 or S4, due to the RV diastolic dysfunction that occurs with RV infarction. The hepatojugular reflux test is often positive in patients with RV infarction. Additionally, tricuspid regurgitation due to RV dilatation may also result in a holosystolic murmur.

■ The triad of hypotension, increased jugular venous pressure and clear lung fields in patients with acute inferior MI should alert the clinician to the presence of RV infarction.
■ The differential diagnosis should include pulmonary embolus, pericardial tamponade and constrictive pericarditis.

DIAGNOSIS

In the setting of an inferior MI, the potential for RV infarction must always be entertained, especially when accompanied by the clinical findings previously discussed. Additional diagnostic information consistent with RV infarction can solidify the diagnosis.

Electrocardiogram

In the presence of an acute inferior or inferoposterior MI, ST elevation in lead III greater than that observed in lead II is suggestive of acute RV infarction, demonstrating 97% sensitivity but only 56% specificity. First demonstrated in the 1970s, right sided precordial leads, specifically V4R (placed in the 5th intercostal space, right midclavicular line) improve electrocardiographic accuracy, demonstrating 88% sensitivity and 78% specificity for the diagnosis of RV infarction. In fact, the most recent ACC/AHA guidelines for the management of patients with ST-elevation MI list as a class I recommendation that patients with inferior ST elevation MI and hemodynamic compromise should be assessed with a right precordial V4R lead to detect ST-segment elevation.

■ ST elevation in lead III greater than that observed in lead II is suggestive of acute RV infarction.
■ Right-sided precordial lead V4R demonstrates the greatest sensitivity and specificity for the electrocardiographic detection of RV infarction.

Hemodynamic Assessment

As described earlier, the clinical findings of elevated jugular venous pressure, clear lungs fields and hypotension are the manifestation of the hemodynamic compromise resulting from RV infarction. Decreased compliance (diastolic dysfunction) of the RV causes an elevation in right atrial pressure (RAP; ≥10 mm Hg), an increase in the RV filling pressure during inspiration and a severe noncompliant pattern of right atrial pressure. The classic hemodynamic criteria include RAP ≥10 mm Hg and RAP:PCWP ≥0.86. These criteria combined with a noncompliant RAP waveform, demonstrate a sensitivity of 82% and specificity of 97% for RV infarction.

Additionally, right atrial systolic dysfunction may complicate the hemodynamics of RV infarction with studies demonstrating that the magnitude of right atrial a wave relative to the mean RAP provides prognostic information. Patients with small a wave amplitude tend to fare worse clinically.

In the setting of volume depletion, these hemodynamic findings might not be evident; indeed several studies have demonstrated that volume loading may increase the incidence of classic RV infarction hemodynamics.

- The combination of RAP ≥10 mm Hg, RAP/PCWP ≥0.86 and a noncompliant RAP waveform suggest RV infarction.
- In the setting of volume depletion, hemodynamic findings might not be evident; volume loading may increase the incidence of classic RV infarction hemodynamics.

Echocardiography

While echocardiographic views of the RV may be limited (up to 15% in one report) and assessment of RV function obscured by the presence of pulmonary disease, close evaluation can reveal abnormal RV dilatation and free wall motion abnormalities. Additionally, abnormal interventricular septal motion, caused by a reversal of the transseptal pressure gradient due to the increased RV end-diastolic pressure also suggests RV infarction. Echocardiographic criteria have been shown to have sensitivity of 82%, with a specificity ranging from 62% to 93% for hemodynamically important RV infarction. The most recent ACC/AHA guidelines for the management of patients with ST-elevation MI list as a class

I indication that patients with inferior ST elevation MI and hemodynamic compromise should be assessed by echocardiography to screen for RV infarction. Additionally, echocardiography allows differentiation from pericardial tamponade.

- Echocardiographic evidence of RV free wall motion and RV dilatation is suggestive of RV infarction.
- Short axis echocardiographic views have demonstrated a high sensitivity and specificity for detection of hemodynamically significant RV infarction.

Other Imaging Modalities

Radionuclide ventriculography may demonstrate abnormal RV function in patients with inferior MI, using first-pass and gated blood-pool scanning. However, given the wide range of reported normal RV ejection fraction values, interpretation of this value solely is not specific for RV infarction. However, the combination of wall motion abnormalities and low RV ejection fraction demonstrates a 92% sensitivity and an 82% specificity for identifying hemodynamically important RV infarction. Technetium-99m pyrophosphate scintigraphy has also been demonstrated to have a high specificity (94%), but only 25% sensitivity for identifying RV infarction. Dual single photon emission computed tomography (SPECT) using thalium-201 and technetium 99m pyrophosphate has been used to demonstrate RV infarction. Recent studies report the ability of gadolinium-enhanced MRI to identify RV infarction, with a sensitivity and specificity comparable to dual SPECT imaging. However, the inability to conduct these scans emergently has limited applicability of these techniques in the acute diagnosis of RV infarction.

- Radionuclide ventriculography has demonstrated high sensitivity and specificity for identifying hemodynamically significant right ventricular infarction.

COMPLICATIONS

Low Cardiac Output

The hemodynamic complications of RV infarction can be profound right ventricular output is dependent on

RV preload which in turn is very sensitive to patient fluid status. While the RV is now exquisitely preload dependent, LV function in RV infarct has been described as preload deprived, resulting in an overall low cardiac output. However, the overall low-output state in RV infarction is not solely due to a decrease in RV systolic performance. Dilation of the RV also compromises LV filling due to a leftward displacement of the interventricular septum during diastole.

Bradyarrhythmias

Because the ischemic right ventricle has a relatively fixed stroke volume, cardiac output becomes exquisitely heart-rate dependent. Thus, even in the absence of AV dyssynchrony, bradycardia may have profound hemodynamic effects. Bradycardic complications include high-grade atrioventricular block, sinus bradycardia, and secondary hypotension due in part to AV node ischemia and cardioinhibitory (Bezold-Jarisch) reflexes. The development of high-degree atrioventricular block has been reported to occur in as many as 48% of RV infarctions.

Tachyarrhythmias

Several studies have suggested that patients with RV infarction have a greater incidence of ventricular arrhythmias. This incidence is more common in patients with unsuccessful reperfusion. Supraventricular tachyarrhythmias, including atrial fibrillation, appear more common with documented RV dysfunction. Atrial fibrillation has been reported to occur in up to one third of patients with RV infarction, presumably because of concomitant atrial infarction or right atrial dilatation. The loss of atrial contraction can have profound hemodynamic consequences in the setting of RV infarction because the noncompliant RV becomes dependent upon atrial contraction for preload. In view of the importance of atrial contraction in patients with RV infarction, patients requiring ventricular pacing should have atrial or AV sequential pacing.

Mechanical Complications

Severe right heart dilatation and diastolic pressure elevation may result in severe tricuspid regurgitation, which also impairs RV output and exacerbates the overall low cardiac output state. Additionally, the increase in RAP relative to LAP can promote right-to-left shunting across a patent foramen ovale or atrial septal defect, resulting in serious systemic hypoxemia or paradoxical emboli. Clinicians should consider this possible complication in patients with hypoxemia nonresponsive to oxygen therapy.

- The hemodynamic complications of RV infarction can be profound resulting in low cardiac output.
- The development of high-degree atrioventricular block has been reported to occur in as many as 48% of RV infarctions.
- Atrial fibrillation may occur in up to one third of patients with RV infarction, presumably because of concomitant atrial infarction or right atrial dilatation.
- Significant right-to-left shunting across a patent foramen ovale or atrial septal defect, can result from RV infarction in serious systemic hypoxemia or paradoxical emboli.

THERAPY

The treatment of RV infarction involves early reperfusion, maintenance of RV preload, inotropic support of the septum which has a dual blood supply from RCA and LAD coronary arteries and the dysfunctional RV, reduction of RV afterload and maintenance of AV synchrony.

Reperfusion

The goal of reperfusion therapy in all acute ST elevation MIs should be the prompt restoration of epicardial blood flow. In patients with RV infarction, successful reperfusion of the RCA significantly improves RV function and reduces in-hospital mortality. Successful thrombolysis imparts a survival benefit in those with RV involvement and failure to restore infarct artery patency is associated with persistent RV dysfunction and increased mortality. There also appears to be a higher incidence of reocclusion of the RCA following thrombolysis compared to other coronary arteries. Primary angioplasty is more likely to result in successful recanalization of the RCA with resulting benefits on RV performance and clinical outcomes. The presence of preinfarction angina has been shown to predict a lower incidence of RV infarction in patients with acute inferior MI possibly because of ischemic preconditioning of the RV. In addition to early reperfusion, therapy aimed at reversing the diminished filling of the RV (i.e., increasing RV stroke volume) and improving RV function should also be promptly instituted.

Fluid Resuscitation

In RV infarction, the RV becomes preload dependent while the LV is preload deprived. Thus, optimization of ventricular preload is critical to treatment of RV infarction. Expansion of plasma volume to enhance left-sided filling pressures should be promptly instituted in patients with evidence of low cardiac output states. Central venous pressure (CVP) should be raised with administration of isotonic saline. Fluid expansion beyond a capillary wedge pressure >15 mm Hg is unlikely to improve hemodynamic profile. Additionally, in the setting of volume depletion, classic hemodynamic findings might not be evident; indeed several studies have demonstrated that volume loading may increase the incidence of RV infarction hemodynamics. Volume loading may not always produce an increase in cardiac output, therefore it is important to quantitate the effect of volume loading on the stroke volume and cardiac output in order to guide the necessity for additional fluid therapy.

Inotropic Therapy

Dobutamine has been demonstrated to stabilize patients with hemodynamic compromise. When compared to afterload reduction with nitroprusside, dobutamine infusion resulted in a significant increase in cardiac index, stroke volume and RV ejection fraction.

Reduction of RV Afterload With LV Dysfunction

Arterial vasodilators (including sodium nitroprusside and hydralazine) and ACE inhibitors reduce the impedence to LV outflow and in turn LV diastolic, left atrial, and pulmonary pressures, thereby lowering RV outflow impedance and enhancing RV output. When compared to afterload reduction with nitroprusside, dobutamine infusion resulted in a significant increase in cardiac index, stroke volume and RV ejection fraction. Thus, arterial vasodilators should not be considered first line therapy. Additionally mechanical support with intra-aortic balloon counterpulsation, while not directly improving RV performance, may do so via increases in myocardial perfusion pressure. RV assist devices may also provide bridging support in patients with severe hemodynamic deterioration refractory to other therapy.

Therapy to Avoid

Because of the dependency on RV preload, patients with extensive RV infarction demonstrate exquisite sensitivity to nitrates. Profound hypotension with administration of nitrates in patients with inferior MI should alert the clinician to possible extensive RV involvement. Additionally, AV nodal slowing agents such as beta-blockers and calcium channel blockers may potentially increase the risk of bradyarrhythmias and should be used cautiously in RV infarct patients.

Maintenance of Atrioventricular Synchrony

In RV infarction, due to the dependency of the RV on atrial contraction in order to maintain RV output, loss of chronotropy or AV synchrony can have devastating consequences. Therefore, atrial or dual chamber pacing should be considered if ventricular pacing becomes necessary.

- The treatment of RV infarction involves early reperfusion, maintenance of RV preload, inotropic support of the dysfunctional RV, reduction of RV afterload and maintenance of AV synchrony.

PROGNOSIS

RV infarction may result in acute hemodynamic effects, frequent high degree AV block that result in a high in-hospital morbidity and mortality that has been observed in a number of studies as well as a meta-analysis. In patients in whom reperfusion is achieved, there is a significant decrease in in-hospital and short-term morbidity and mortality. While a number of parameters, including ECG and hemodynamic criteria have demonstrated prognostic utility, the application of a simple clinical assessment by TIMI risk score analysis shows predictive value in both in-hospital and 30 day morbidity and mortality in patients with RV infarction. In-hospital mortality was 7, 13 and 26% in patients with TIMI risk scores of 0-1, 2-3, and ≥4 respectively.

In patients surviving RV infarction, both echocardiographic and nuclear studies have demonstrated resolution of RV dysfunction. The clinical implication is that following recovery from RV infarction, there appears to be no additional increased mortality risk in long-term follow-up compared to patients with acute inferior wall myocardial infarct uncomplicated by RV infarction. Chronic right heart failure due to RV infarction is rare. Initial TIMI risk score analysis at presentation has been shown to predict long-term mortality in a small retrospective cohort of RV infarct patients.

- In-hospital and 30 day morbidity and mortality are high with RV infarction.
- Morbidity and mortality is reduced in RV infarct patients with successful prompt revascularization.
- Initial TIMI risk score analysis provides important prognostic data on both short and long-term outcomes in RV infarction.

69

Adjunctive Therapy in Acute Myocardial Infarction

R. Scott Wright, MD

Imran S. Syed, MD

Joseph G. Murphy, MD

Adjunctive therapies in acute myocardial infarction (AMI) target the myocardial infarction "perfect storm" risk triad of high risk atherosclerotic plaque, high risk patient and high risk plasma that are associated with poor clinical outcome (Fig. 1).

Adjunctive Therapy for AMI in the Emergency Department (ED) or Pre-Hospital Setting

Adjunctive therapy for AMI should be initiated as soon as possible in patients with suspected acute myocardial infarction, in many cases before diagnosis confirmation or definitive reperfusion therapy. The adjunctive therapies that should be initiated in the ED or pre-hospital setting, absent contraindication include:

- Aspirin.
- Oxygen.
- Morphine.
- Intravenous unfractionated heparin or subcutaneous low molecular weight heparin.
- Beta blockade, intravenously followed by oral administration.
- Nitroglycerin, except in those with suspected RV infarction.

Early risk stratification of high risk AMI patients (score of 5 or greater) using either the TIMI Risk Score or Mayo Clinic Risk Score is important to facilitate a more aggressive therapeutic approach in those at highest risk. The TIMI score requires knowledge of serum cardiac biomarkers and prior coronary anatomy while the Mayo Clinic risk score is based on earlier available patient data (Tables 1 and 2).

Using either TIMI or Mayo Clinic risk scoring, patients are classified as low mortality risk score of 0 to 2; intermediate risk score of 3 to 4; and high risk with a score of 5 or greater (Fig. 2).

Aspirin

Aspirin inhibits platelet aggregation and activation through its inhibition of the platelet cyclooxygenase pathway. Additionally, aspirin confers antiinflammatory action within the acute atheroinflammatory thrombotic plaque, both acutely and long-term (Fig. 3).

There is substantial evidence documenting the effectiveness of aspirin in all types of AMI and unstable angina. (Americal Heart Association /American College of Cardiology(AHA/ACC) class I evidence of benefit). Aspirin (162 to 325 mg) should be administered immediately in all patients with suspected or established AMI, preferably in the pre-hospital setting.

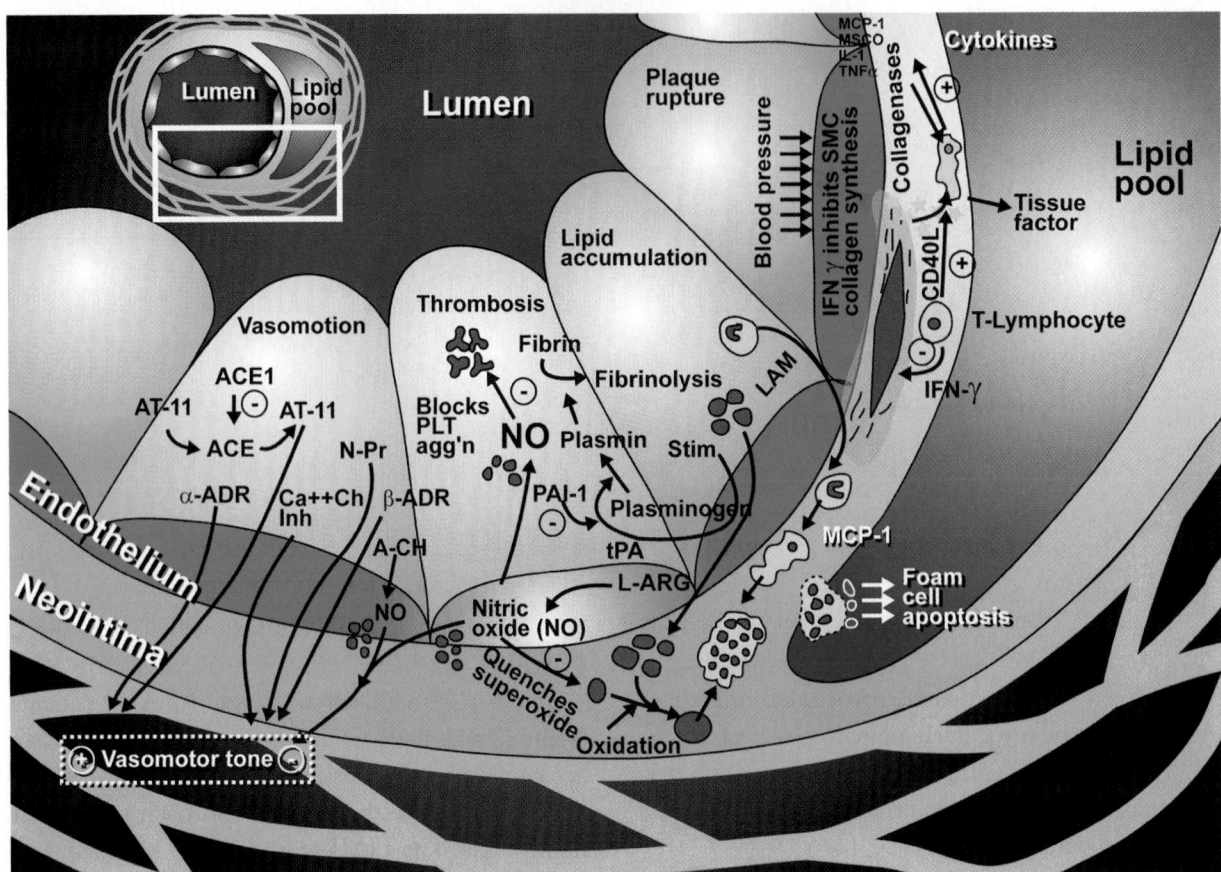

Fig. 1. Atherosclerotic plaque biology.

Aspirin therapy should be withheld only in patients with a documented aspirin allergy or substantive active bleeding. Aspirin should be continued daily at the 162-325 mg dose (reduce dose to 81 mg with concurrent clopidogrel therapy).

- Aspirin should be given initially as a chewed dose of 162-325 mg in the emergency department or pre-hospital setting.
- Aspirin should be continued daily at a dose of 162-325 mg.
- Aspirin should be reduced to 81 mg daily when given in conjunction with clopidogrel.

Oxygen

All patients presenting with AMI require supplemental oxygen preferably in the pre-hospital setting. Patients with documented hypoxemia should have oxygen therapy titrated to increase their arterial oxygen saturation to ≥90%. Oxygen therapy can be discontinued after the initial day of stabilization in patients with a resting saturation >90% on room air and should not be continued in all other AMI patients until they are stabilized.

- Oxygen therapy should be initiated in all AMI patients in the pre-hospital or ED setting.

Table 1.   TIMI Risk Score

Age ≥65 years
Presence of at least three conventional risk factors for CHD
Prior coronary stenosis of ≥50%
Presence of ST segment deviation on initial admission ECG
Two or more anginal episodes in prior 24 hours
Elevated serum cardiac biomarkers
Aspirin use in prior seven days

Table 2.   Mayo Clinic Risk Score

Factor	Points
Age	
>80 years	2
Sex	
Female	3
SBP	
<140 mm Hg	3
Creatinine	
>1.4 mg/dL	1
ST depression	
1-2 μV	1
>2 μV	3
QRS duration	
≥100	1
Killip class	
>I	3
MI location	
Anterior	1

MI, myocardial infarction; SBP, systolic blood pressure.

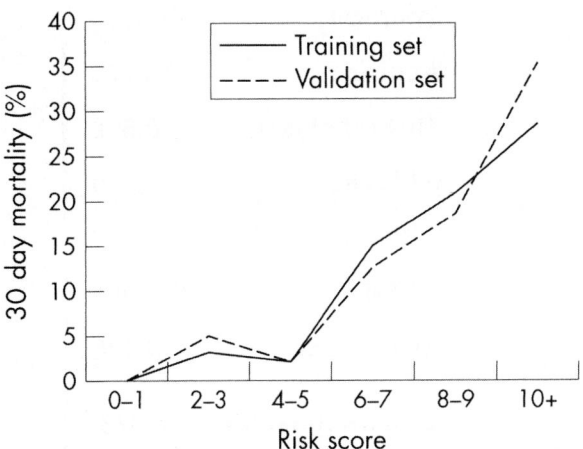

Fig. 2. Thirty day mortality by risk score group in the training and validation sets.

- Oxygen therapy should be titrated to a resting arterial saturation of ≥90%.

Morphine

Intravenous *morphine sulfate* is the drug of choice for relief of chest pain and anxiety in acute myocardial infarction. The initial dose is 2 to 4 mg, with increments of 2 to 8 mg repeated at 5 to 15 minute intervals if needed; watch for respiratory depression.

Heparin

The most commonly used heparin therapy in patients with AMI is unfractionated heparin (UFH). Low molecular weight heparins (LMWH) are increasingly being administered in AMI patients, especially those with non-ST MI. Heparin works by inhibiting thrombin generation and arterial thrombosis. Heparin augments the fibrinolytic action of intravenous fibrinolytic agents and must be given concurrently with the newer fibrin-specific fibrinolytics. Heparin reduces mortality and risk of reinfarction in patients with AMI.

UFH administration should precede or be given concurrently with fibrin specific fibrinolytics in all circumstances. We recommend weight adjusted UFH administration, a bolus of 60 U/kg (maximum of 4,000 U) followed by 12 U/kg/hr infusion (maximum of 1,000 U/hr) adjusted to a partial thromboplastin time at 1.5 to 2.0 times control. There is significant evidence that over anticoagulation with UFH can increase the risk of death in patients with STEMI following fibrinolysis. If using a nonselective fibrinolytic such as streptokinase, UFH can be given selectively to patients with high risk of systemic emboli such as those with a large or anterior wall AMI, those with atrial fibrillation or known LV thrombus and those with severely reduced LV ejection fractions (EF <30%).

For patients treated with primary percutaneous coronary revascularization, we recommend a weight adjusted bolus dose of UFH of 50-70 U/kg accompanied by a 12 U/kg/hr infusion (maximum of 1,000 U/hr).

The use of LMWH is an acceptable alterative to UFH for patients with non-STEMI and should be dose adjusted for those with significant renal dysfunction. The most commonly utilized agents are enoxaparin and dalteparin. Both have been demonstrated to be effective in non-STEMI.

The routine use of LMWH compared to UFH in patients with STEMI has recently been evaluated in the EXTRACT TIMI 25 study. Patients randomized to enoxaparin had lower rates of reinfarction and major adverse cardiovascular events compared to those with UFH. Overall mortality was not significantly different between groups. The FDA has not approved the use of

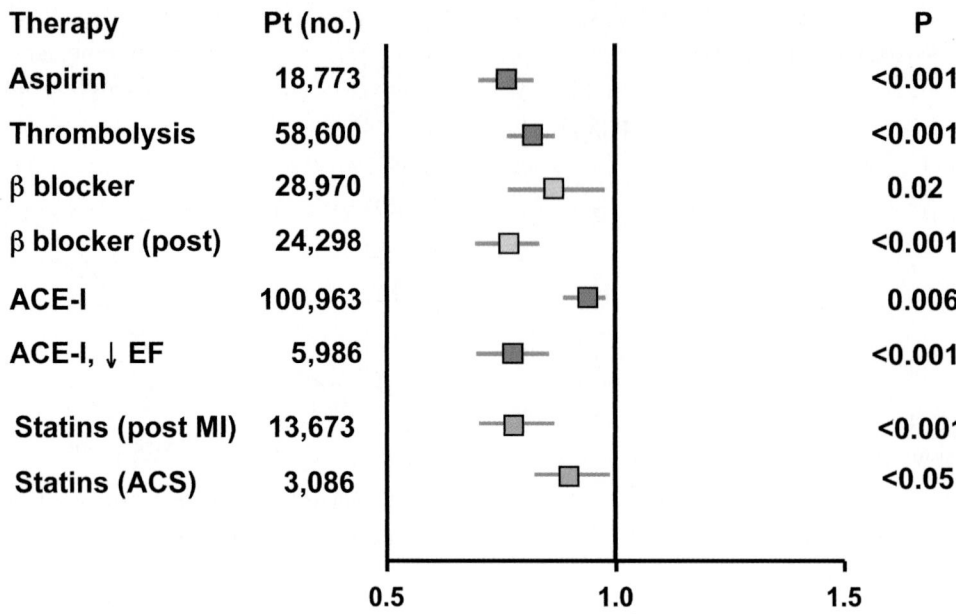

Therapy	Pt (no.)		P
Aspirin	18,773		**<0.001**
Thrombolysis	58,600		**<0.001**
β blocker	28,970		**0.02**
β blocker (post)	24,298		**<0.001**
ACE-I	100,963		**0.006**
ACE-I, ↓ EF	5,986		**<0.001**
Statins (post MI)	13,673		**<0.001**
Statins (ACS)	3,086		**<0.05**

Fig. 3. Therapy for acute MI. Effect on mortality.

enoxaparin in combination with a fibrinolytic as yet, but the data from this study suggest there may soon be an important role for enoxaparin in STEMI.

The duration of heparin therapy during hospitalization for AMI has not been well studied and there is little data from which to extrapolate recommendations. We recommend routine use of heparin therapy following fibrinolytic for ~48 hours or until the time of coronary angiography in patients without another indication for heparin. The routine use of heparin after primary PCI is not indicated unless there is another reason to initiate anticoagulation, such as atrial fibrillation, left ventricular thrombus or a severely reduced LV ejection fraction.

- Heparin therapy should be initiated very early in the initial stabilization of patients with AMI.
- Unfractionated heparin should be administered in a weight adjusted dosing manner in patients receiving IFT: 60 U/kg (maximum of 4,000 U) followed by 12 U/kg/hr infusion (maximum of 1,000 U/hr) and continued for ~48 hours unless coronary angiography is performed earlier.
- The role of LWMH in non-STEMI is well established.
- The use of LMWH in STEMI is supported by early clinical trial data.

- Heparin therapy may be discontinued after coronary angiography and/or PCI unless there is another reason to initiate anticoagulation.

Beta Blocker

Beta blockers play an important role in the initial stabilization of patients with AMI by blocking the beta adrenergic receptors on the myocardium and reducing myocardial oxygen demand enhancing ventricular electrical stability and weakly inhibiting platelet aggregation.

Pooled data from numerous randomized clinical trials including pooled Swedish trial data and GUSTO-1 trial demonstrated that patients given early beta blocker therapy for AMI had lower risks of death, heart failure, electrical instability including ventricular arrhythmias and high grade heart block.

The ACC/AHA AMI guidelines state that oral administration of beta blocker therapy in the initial hours of hospitalization for AMI has class I evidence in nearly all patients, except those with severe heart failure. The use of beta blocker therapy in patients with advanced heart failure can be initiated after initial stabilization and treatment of the heart failure. The guidelines suggest that there is level IIa evidence for the use of intravenous beta blockers in the early hours of hospitalization for AMI: early clinical trials demonstrated the benefit while later trials have been inconclusive.

Beta blockers should not be administered to patients with severe pulmonary edema or to those with bradycardia (HR <50), hypotension, cardiogenic shock, PR interval prolongation ≥0.24 seconds and those with second or third-degree AV block. Additionally, beta blockers should be withheld from those with a history of asthma. Beta blockers can be administered to patients with chronic obstructive pulmonary disease when initiated slowly and uptitrated carefully. It is our practice to administer intravenous beta blocker therapy in the emergency department or pre-hospital setting whenever possible in patients with AMI. Patients are converted to oral beta blocker therapy within a few hours of the initial intravenous dosing and this therapy is continued to hospital discharge and beyond if tolerated.

- Oral beta blocker therapy should be administered in the initial hours of hospitalization for AMI (level I evidence) in all appropriate patients.
- Intravenous beta blocker therapy provides additional benefit when administered very early during the ED or pre-hospital setting.
- Beta blocker therapy should be withheld in those with severe pulmonary edema until they are medically stabilized.
- Beta blocker therapy should not be given to those with severe bradycardia, significant first degree AV block, those with second or third degree AV block and patients with known or suspected asthma.
- Beta blockers can be safely given to those with non-reactive COPD.

Nitroglycerin

Sublingual nitroglycerin at a dose of 0.4 mg every five minutes for a total of three doses is indicated in patients presenting with chest pain thought to be due to myocardial ischemia. Intravenous nitroglycerin is indicated in patients with persistent ischemic chest pain, systemic hypertension or heart failure. *Nitrates* are contraindicated in patients with hypotension (systolic blood pressure less than 90 mm Hg or ≥30 mm Hg below patient baseline), marked bradycardia (<50 beats per minute) or tachycardia (heart rate > than 100 beats per minute) right ventricular infarction, *hypertrophic cardiomyopathy* severe aortic stenosis or in patients who

have taken a phosphodiesterase inhibitor for erectile dysfunction within the previous 36 hours.

While there is no trial data that proves a reduction in mortality with early nitrate use in infarct patients, many patients experience significant symptomatic improvement after nitrate therapy. Nitrates mediate their benefit by reducing both cardiac preload (venous dilatation) and afterload (peripheral arterial dilation) and by vasodilatation of the coronary vasculature which in turn improves coronary blood flow and myocardial oxygen delivery. Nitrates also dilate coronary collateral vessels, potentially creating a favorable subendocardial to epicardial flow ratio.

Nitrates are harmful in patients with hypotension, bradycardia or suspected right ventricular infarction as well as those who have received a phospodiesterase inhibitor-5 for erectile dysfunction within the preceding 36 hours. We recommend an initial nitrate dose of 0.4 mg administered sublingually followed by the initiation of intravenous nitroglycerin or administration of oral isosorbide dinitrate. Nitrates should be continued beyond the initial twenty-four hours of hospitalization only to aid in the symptomatic treatment of ischemia or heart failure.

- Nitrates reduce coronary ischemia by reducing cardiac preload and afterload and by vasodilating the coronary vasculature.
- Nitrates may stabilize AMI by dilating the coronary collateral vasculature.
- Nitrates provide symptomatic relief of angina but have not been demonstrated to reduce mortality in AMI.
- Nitrates should not be continued beyond the initial day of hospitalization except to aid in the symptomatic treatment of angina or heart failure.

Thienopyridine Antiplatelet Therapy

Clopidogrel, a potent antiplatelet agent is a thienopyridine compound that inhibits platelet aggregation through modification of the platelet ADP pathway. The CURE trial randomized patients with unstable angina or non-STEMI to aspirin or aspirin plus clopidogrel with a primary trial end point of cardiovascular death, myocardial infarction, or stroke. CURE demonstrated a significant reduction in the combined primary end point with clopidogrel plus aspirin versus aspirin alone (9.3% versus 11.4 %) due primarily to fewer myocardial infarctions but at the cost of more serious bleeding complications (3.7% versus 2.7%).

The use of clopidogrel in non-STEMI is widespread in the United States, in large part due to the widespread use of coronary angiography and percutaneous coronary revascularization. Clopidogrel is indicated in nearly all patients who are treated with a coronary stent. The routine use of clopidogrel for one month in patients treated with bare metal stents is appropriate and there are data to justify extending therapy for up to one year. The use of clopidogrel following percutaneous coronary revascularization with drug eluting stents (DES) must be tailored to the type of DES used. The FDA has recommended at least three (3) months of therapy for sirolimus eluting DES and at least six (6) months of therapy for paclitaxel eluting DES. Our practice is to routinely use clopidogrel for six months following implantation of any DES; the duration of therapy may be increased if the patient is felt to be at high risk of recurrent thrombosis.

Clopidogrel is also widely used in patients with STEMI following primary percutaneous coronary revascularization. The duration of therapy will follow the general guides as with non-STEMI patients. There is currently no consensus regarding use of clopidogrel routinely following thrombolysis, although some preliminary data have suggested a potential reduction in risk of recurrent reinfarction.

- Clopidogrel is widely utilized following implantation of a bare metal coronary stent for at least one month following PCI and up to one year.
- Clopidogrel should be administered for at least three (3) months following implantation of a sirolimus coated DES.
- Clopidogrel should be administered for at least six (6) months following implantation of a paclitaxel DES.

Renin-Angiotensin-Aldosterone Antagonist Therapy
The use of inhibitors of the renin-angiotensin-aldosterone axis is an important component of managing the AMI patient. These agents reduce mortality, reduce risks of reinfarction and reduce risks of developing heart failure (Fig. 4).

ACE Inhibitors
Angiotensin converting enzyme inhibitors block the conversion of angiotensin I to angiotensin II by inhibiting the angiotensin converting enzyme (ACE).

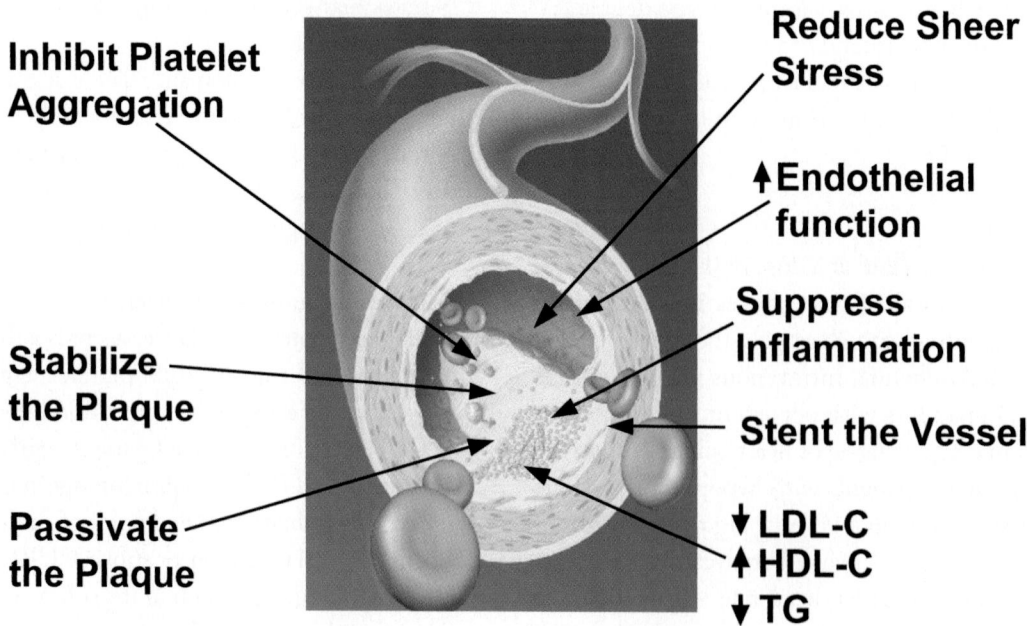

Fig. 4. Medical management of AMI patients.

This results in less sodium retention and arterial vaso-constriction. ACE inhibitors also reduce circulating levels of plasminogen activator inhibitor I (PAI-1), a known prothrombotic substance in the plasma (Fig. 5).

These agents have been widely tested in patients with AMI and overall significantly reduce the risks of death, reinfarction and heart failure. The absolute risk reduction in these end points is most evident in AMI patients with reduced left ventricular ejection fractions (EF <0.40), heart failure, or anterior AMI locations. The benefit of routine ACE inhibitor therapy in all patients with CAD is less robust but likely present. The widespread use of ACE inhibitors in most AMI patients has been recommended by the ACC/AHA guidelines.

The greatest benefit of ACE inhibitor use in AMI patients occurs when the agents are initiated very early during hospitalization, but hypotension should be avoided. There is no proven clinical difference among the available ACE inhibitors with regard to short-term or long-term efficacy following AMI (Table 3).

■ ACE inhibitors should be initiated as early as possible in patients with AMI.
■ Avoid hypotension when up-titrating ACE

inhibitors.
■ Most AMI patients should remain on ACE inhibitors indefinitely.

Angiotensin Receptor Blockers

Much of the endogenous production of angiotensin II in humans occurs through non-ACE pathways. The largest trial of patients with AMI complicated by heart failure and/or left ventricular dysfunction was the VALIANT trial, which enrolled over 16,000 patients and randomized them to captopril, valsartan or the combination of these agents. The results demonstrated that valsartan was equivalent to captopril with regard to all outcomes—survival and freedom from heart failure and/or reinfarction. This trial conclusively established the role for ARB antagonists in patients with AMI and that this class of therapy could be used interchangeably with ACE inhibitors (Fig. 6).

■ ARB agents can be used in AMI patients who are ACE inhibitor intolerant.
■ ARB agents reduce risks of mortality and heart failure equivalent to ACE inhibitors in patients with heart failure or reduced left ventricular function.
■ Valsartan and candesartan are the only currently

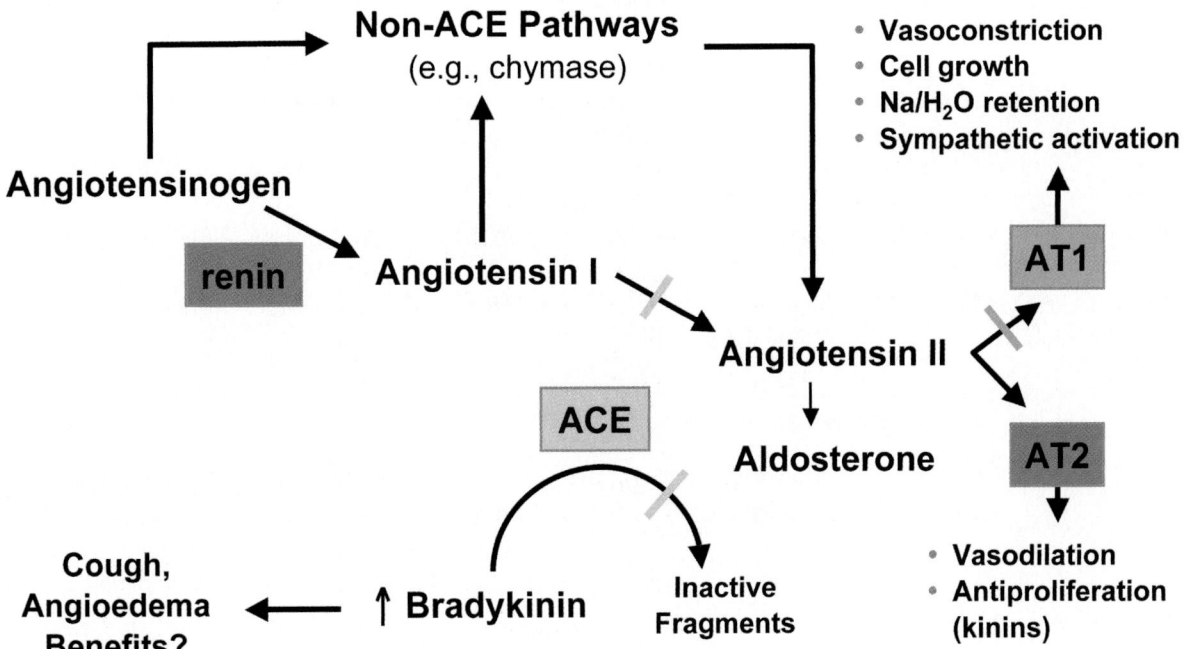

Fig. 5. Renin-angiotensin aldosterone system.

Table 3. Summary of Adjunctive Medical Therapies in Acute Myocardial Infarction

Agent	When to initiate	When to stop	Initial dose	Dose goal	Intended action	Common side effects
Aspirin	Pre-hospital or in ED	Only with aspirin allergy/ intolerance or bleeding	162-325 mg	62-325 mg	Antiplatelet and anti-inflammatory actions	GI bleeding Dyspepsia
Oxygen	Pre-hospital or in ED	After 24 hours and when O_2 saturation >90%	2 L/min	O_2 sat >90%	Improve oxy-genation	Sore or dry nose, epistaxis
Morphine	Pre-hospital or in ED	Pain and anxiety free	Initial 2 to 4 mg, with increment of 2 to 8 mg at 5 to 15 minute intervals	Titrate to response	Pain and anxiety relief	Respiratory depression Hypotension
Nitroglycerin	Pre-hospital or in ED	Hypotension	Sublingual 0.4 mg Repeat every 5 minutes for a maximum of 3 times if needed Intravenous 5 to 10 µg/min and gradually increased	Titrate to response	Dilatation of coronary arteries and arterioles Venous dilatation with decreased preload Relief of coronary spasm	Hypotension Hemodynamic collapse
Heparin	ED arrival	24-48 hours	60 U/kg bolus	12 U/kg/hr	Anti-thrombo-tic action	Bleeding
*Beta blocker (metoprolol) IV	ED arrival	One time administra-tion	5 to 15 mg IV	HR 50-60	Slow heart rate Lower blood pressure Treat ischemia	Bradycardia, Hypotension
Oral	~6 hours after IV	Only with intolerance	25 mg BID	HR 50-55 at rest	Reduce or eliminate ischemia and angina	Low BP, light-headedness Erectile dysfunction

Table 3 (continued)

Agent	When to initiate	When to stop	Initial dose	Dose goal	Intended action	Common side effects
ACE inhibitor (Lisinopril)	First 12 hours	Only with intolerance	2.5 mg	10-20 mg	Lower BP Reduce cardiac remodeling Lower PAI-1 values	Low BP, light-headedness Erectile dysfunction
or ARB (Valsartan)			80 mg bid	160 mg bid	Lower BP Reduce cardiac remodeling	Low BP, light-headedness Erectile dysfunction
Aldosterone antagonist (Aldactone)	Days to weeks	Only with intolerance	12.5 to 25 mg	50 mg	Reduce cardiac remodeling Reduce risk of heart failure	Low BP Hyperkalemia Renal failure
Statin (Atorva-statin)	ED arrival to first day	Only with intolerance	40 mg	LDL <70 CRP <2	Reduce risk of recurrent AMI Lower risk of death Lower LDL Lower CRP Lower PAI-1	Muscle pain LFT elevation Rarely rhabdo-myolysis
Clopidogrel	Following PCI	1 month- bare metal stent 6 months- DES	300-600 mg	75 mg	Reduce risk of stens throm-bosis, re-infarction	Rash Bleeding Bruising

AMI, acute myocardial infarction; BP, blood pressure; CRP, C-reactive protein; DES, drug eluting stent; ED, emergency department; HR, heart rate; PAI-1, plasminogen activatory inhibitor-1; PCI, percutaneous coronary intervention.
*The benefits of ACE inhibition, ARB blockade, aldosterone antagonism, statins and non-ISA beta blockade are class effects with multiple alternative medication available in all classes.

FDA approved ARB agents for use in post-AMI patients with clinical heart failure or reduced left ventricular function.

Aldosterone Antagonists

The use of aldosterone inhibition therapy is also an important adjunctive medical therapy in post-AMI patients. Agents which block aldosterone include aldactone and eplerenone. The EPHESUS trial randomized post-AMI patients to placebo or eplerenone and demonstrated that eplerenone therapy significantly reduced the risk of all cause death, sudden cardiac death and rehospitalization due to a cardiovascular mechanism. The ACC/AHA Guidelines for AMI suggest that long-term aldosterone blockade should be prescribed for post-STEMI patients without significant renal dysfunction (creatinine should be ≤2.5 mg/dL in men and ≤2.0 mg/dL in women) or hyperkalemia (potassium should be ≤5.0 mEq/L) who are already receiving therapeutic doses of an ACE inhibitor,

**Acute Infarction
(hours)**

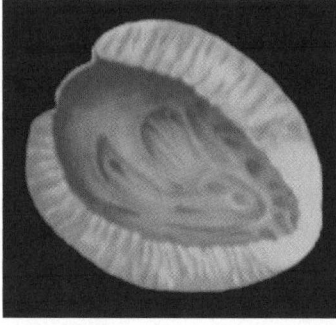

**Infarct Expansion
(hours to days)**

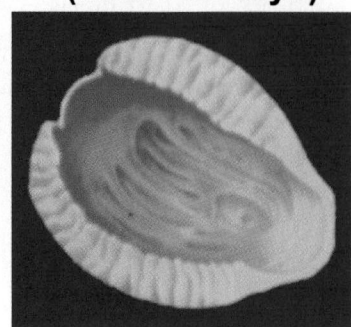

**Global Remodeling
(days to months)**

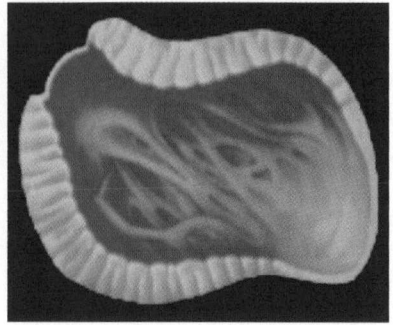

Fig. 6. Left ventricular remodeling following myocardial infarction.

have an LVEF ≤0.40, and have either symptomatic heart failure or diabetes (level of evidence A) (Fig. 7).

■ Long-term aldosterone blockade should be prescribed for post-STEMI patients without significant renal dysfunction (creatinine should be ≤2.5 mg/dL in men and ≤2.0 mg/dL in women) or hyperkalemia (potassium should be ≤5.0 mEq/L) who are already receiving therapeutic doses of an ACE inhibitor, have an LVEF ≤0.40, and have either symptomatic heart failure or diabetes.

STATIN AGENTS AND OTHER LIPID LOWERING THERAPIES

The use of statin agents in AMI is well established and safe. Many patients arrive at hospital on statins which should be continued. Statins primarily lower LDL cholesterol and modestly raise HDL cholesterol but in addition may also secondarily stabilize atherosclerotic plaques, reverse endothelial dysfunction and reduced arterial wall inflammation and the plasma concentrations of inflammatory C-reactive protein (CRP). The cardioprotective benefit of statin therapy following AMI is well proven from the CARE, 4-S and the LIPID trials.

Recent lipid trials including MIRACL (atorvastatin versus pravastatin—Lipitor vs Pravacol) and PROVE-IT (atorvastatin) suggest an early benefit from aggressive high-potency statin therapy (atorvastatin) initiated early (within 24-96 hours) in patients with AMI and unstable angina, long before the established long-term benefits of lipid lowering were likely operative. The **A to Z trial** (Simvastatin-Zocor) did not reproduce this early benefit. It is our practice to initiate in-hospital early potent statin administration in almost all patients with AMI with a treatment goal LDL ≤70 mg/dL and a c-reactive protein (CRP) of ≤2 mg/L.

The use of other lipid lowering therapies in patients with AMI has less clinical evidence of benefit compared to statin therapy. The best studied class of agents are the fibric acid derivatives such as gemfibrozil. All non-statin lipid lowering agents, including niacin, the fibrates, ezetimibe and bile acid binding resins should be utilized to augment statin therapy rather than replace statins (Fig. 8 and 9).

■ Statin therapy should be initiated in all patients with AMI as early as possible during hospitalization and preferably upon admission.

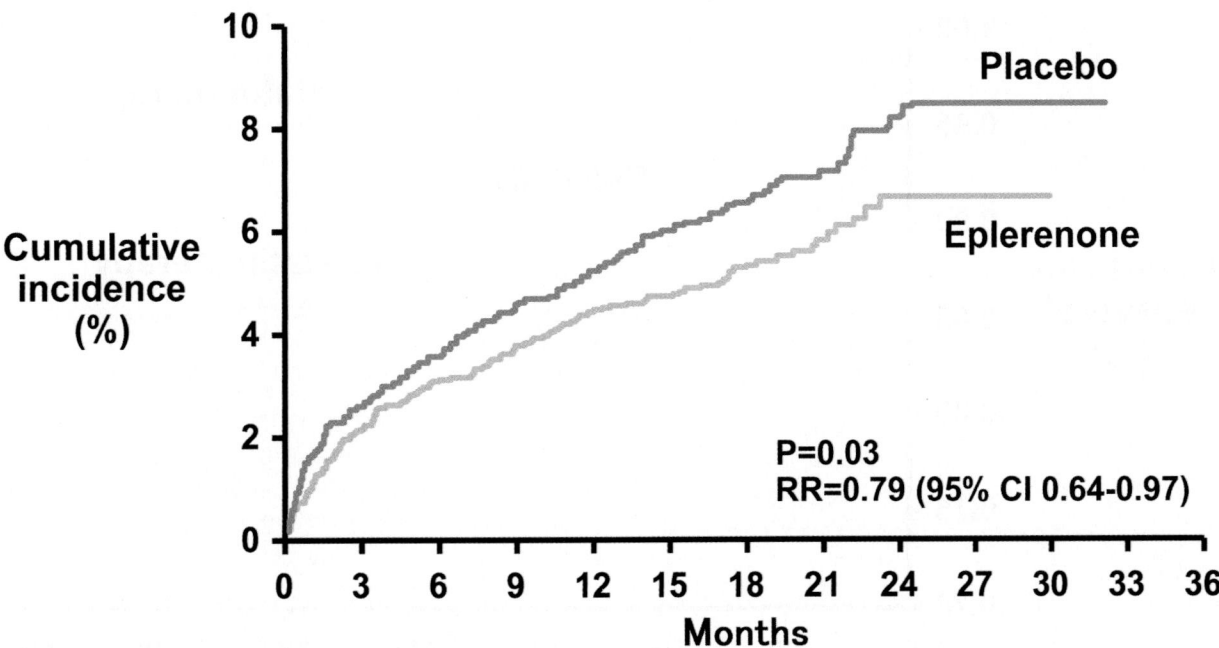

Fig. 7. Rate of sudden death from cardiac causes.

- The goal of statin therapy should be an LDL ≤70 mg/dL and a C-reactive protein of ≤2 mg/L following hospital discharge.
- Other lipid lowering therapy should be utilized only to achieve LDL ≤70 mg/dl, HDL ≥40 mg/dL and a CRP <2 mg/L when statin therapy is insufficient.

MANAGEMENT OF DIABETES MELLITUS

It is imperative to treat the patient with diabetes and AMI very aggressively. We recommend tight glycemic control during the initial period of hospitalization and aggressive diabetic treatment following discharge from hospital. All diabetic patients should receive a potent statin and an added fibrate if necessary to raise the HDL cholesterol.

The choice of which oral agent to use in treatment of Type II diabetes remains somewhat controversial. The data with regard to metformin remain strong and this agent should be utilized if at all possible. There is some evidence that the thiazolidinediones, which are insulin sensitizers, may have a beneficial role in the post-AMI patient especially when given in combination with metformin. On a precautionary note, these agents promote moderate weight gain and also should be used with caution in patients with mild heart failure and not

at all in those with advanced heart failure. Most patients with renal dysfunction and heart failure should probably be managed with insulin therapy.

In addition to glucose modifying therapies, diabetic patients should be encouraged to exercise regularly and maintain ideal body weight. Their LDL cholesterol values should be aggressively lowered to <70 mg/dL.

Hypoglycemic therapy should be inititaed to achieve HbA1c <7% (level of evidence B).

- Thiazolidinediones should not be used in patients recovering from STEMI who have New York Heart Association class III or IV heart failure (level of evidence B).

LONG-TERM ADJUNCTIVE THERAPY

All patients post AMI should be prescribed sublingual nitroglycerin to use at home for recurrent ischemic pain. All AMI patients should receive long-term aspirin and beta blockers unless contraindicated. The dose of aspirin may need to be adjusted if there is concurrent use of clopidogrel.

- Beta blocker therapy should be continued indefinitely in nearly all patients with AMI.

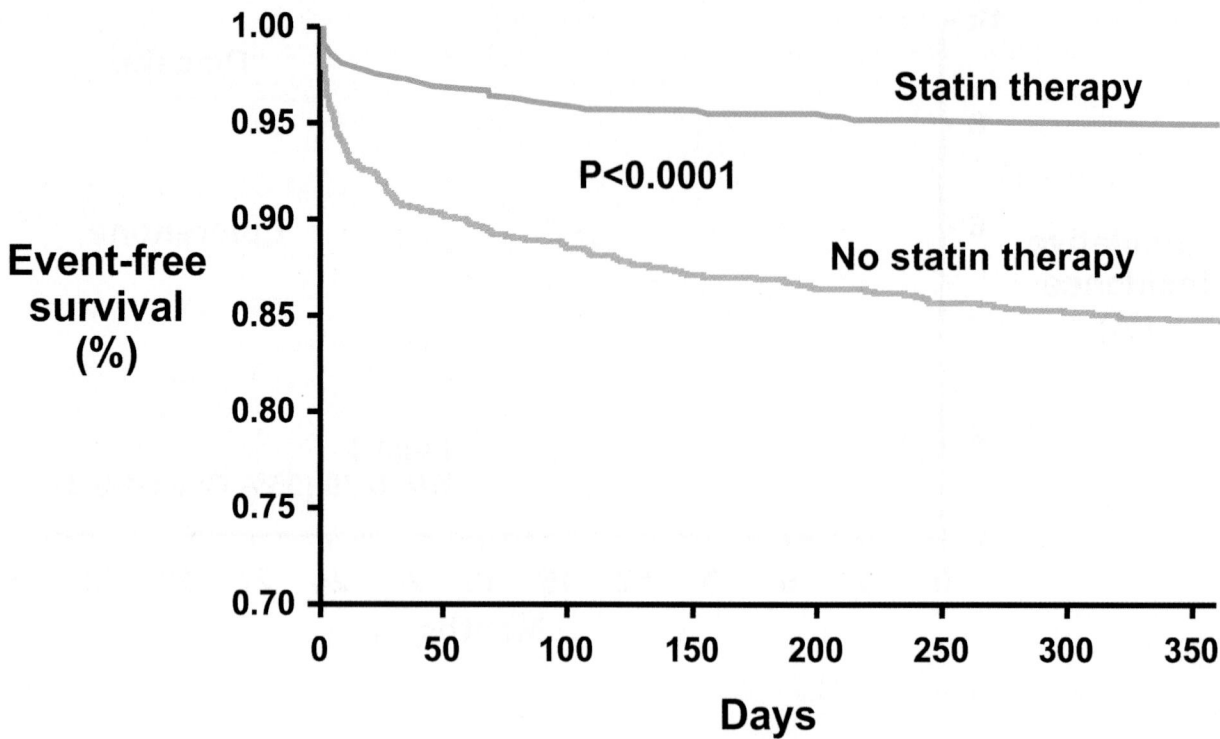

Fig. 8. Survival according to statin therapy initiated within 48 hours of hospitalization vs. no statin therapy.

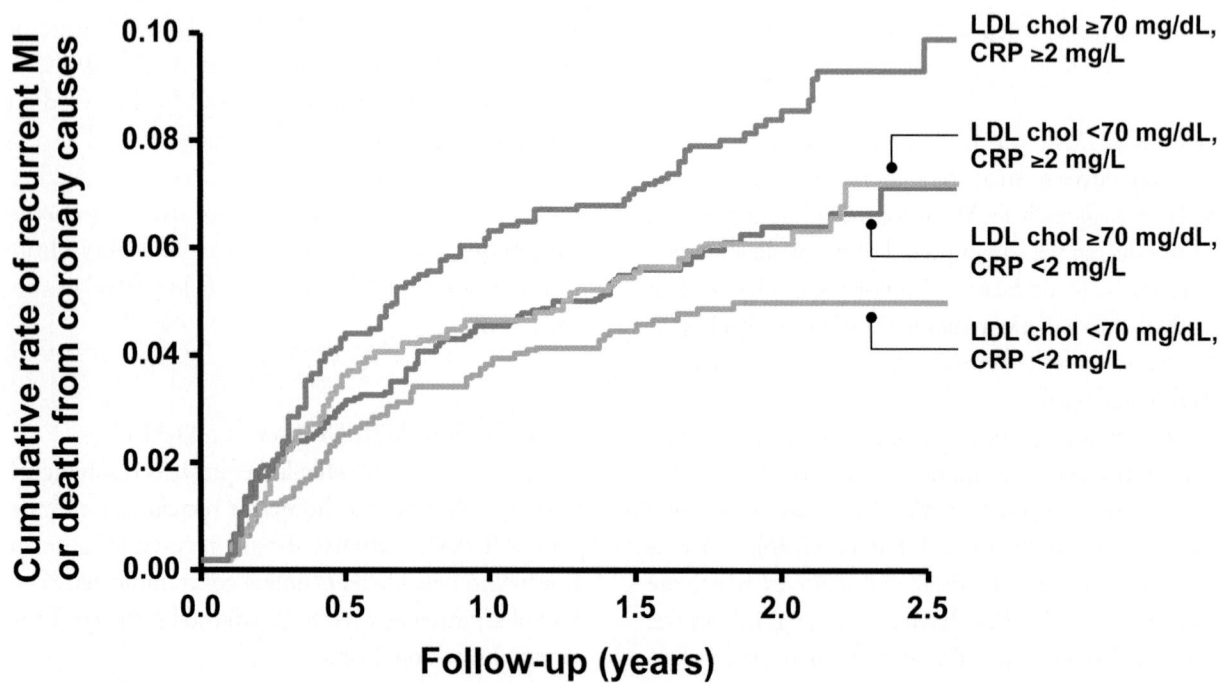

Fig. 9. Cumulative incidence of recurrent MI or death from coronary causes, according to the achieved levels of both LDL cholesterol and CRP.

- Aspirin should be continued indefinitely in all patients with AMI unless contraindicated by aspirin allergy or major bleeding complications.
- Heparin and nitroglycerin therapies can be discontinued during the initial days of hospitalization for AMI.

Lifestyle Risk Factor Management

Lifestyle modification is at least as important in the long-term treatment of AMI as medications. Moderate alcohol intake appears to has a cardioprotective effect on the heart while heavy alcohol usage has an adverse effect. The AHA defines moderate alcohol consumption as an average of one to two drinks per day for men and one drink per day for women. (A drink is one 12 oz. beer, 4 oz. of wine, 1.5 oz. of 80-proof spirits, or 1 oz. of 100-proof spirits.) Alcohol in large doses elevates triglycerides and blood pressure while alcohol in lower doses increases cardioprotective HDL-C. Flavonoids in red wine may also be beneficial. In patients with religious objections to alcohol red grape juice or cranberry juice is indicated.

- Patients with AMI who smoke must be counseled to immediately stop smoking.
- The use of nicotine replacement therapy and bupropion therapy to aid in smoking cessation is safe and effective in AMI patients.
- All AMI patients should receive rehabilitation and exercise counselling.
- Alcohol in moderation is beneficial post AMI.
- Patients who are obese and overweight at the time of AMI should receive intensive lifestyle modification instruction.
- The morbidly obese may be candidates for surgical therapies for obesity management.

70

COMPLICATIONS OF ACUTE MYOCARDIAL INFARCTION

Joseph G. Murphy, MD

John F. Bresnahan, MD

Margaret A. Lloyd, MD

Guy S. Reeder, MD

Complications after myocardial infarction are common and frequently result in patient death.

- Cardiogenic shock and heart failure are the most common causes of death in patients hospitalized with acute myocardial infarction.
- At least 75% of patients with acute myocardial infarction (MI) have an arrhythmia during the peri-infarct period.

SUPRAVENTRICULAR ARRHYTHMIAS AFTER MYOCARDIAL INFARCTION

Sinus Bradycardia

Sinus bradycardia is the most common arrhythmia occurring during the early hours after MI and may occur in up to 40% of inferior and posterior infarctions. Bradycardia may be related to autonomic imbalance or to atrial and sinus node ischemia (or to both). Profound bradycardia may predispose the patient to ventricular ectopy. This arrhythmia usually resolves spontaneously, and treatment is reserved for hemodynamically symptomatic arrhythmias and those accompanied by bradycardia-dependent ventricular arrhythmias. Atropine is often successful in treating symptomatic bradycardia, but it may cause transient rebound tachycardia. Temporary pacing is rarely required (Table 1).

Sinus Tachycardia

Sinus tachycardia may occur in up to one-third of

Table 1. Indications for Temporary Pacing in the Peri-Infarct Period

Sinus bradycardia with hypotension, bradycardia-dependent ventricular arrhythmias, angina, syncope/presyncope, or congestive heart failure and refractory to atropine

Accelerated idioventricular rhythm with symptomatic rate <40 bpm

Prolonged (>3 s) sinus pauses

Atrial fibrillation with inadequate ventricular rate

Asystole

Mobitz II second-degree block

Third-degree (complete heart) block

New or progressive bifascicular block

bpm, beats per minute.

827

patients in the peri-infarct period, especially those with anterior MI. The ischemic left ventricle may have a relatively fixed stroke volume; thus, augmentation of cardiac output is primarily dependent on an increase in heart rate. Sinus tachycardia may also occur as a result of sympathetic stimulation from locally released and circulating catecholamines, concurrent anemia, hypo- or hypervolemia, hypoxia, pericarditis, inotropic drugs, pain, or fear. Treatment includes optimizing hemodynamics and oxygenation, correction of anemia and electrolyte and acid-base abnormalities, pain control, and anxiolytic agents. β-Blockers are indicated for patients without evidence of significant left ventricular dysfunction or hypovolemia. Persistent sinus tachycardia as an early manifestation of heart failure is an indicator of poor prognosis.

Premature Atrial Contractions

Premature atrial contractions may be present in up to one-half of patients with MI. Their occurrence may be due to atrial or sinus node ischemia, atrial infarction, pericarditis, anxiety, or pain. The combination of atrial asystole and a rapid ventricular rate markedly decreases cardiac output and increases myocardial oxygen demands. Attempts should be made to restore sinus rhythm; if not successful, rate control should be pursued aggressively to minimize myocardial oxygen demand. Premature atrial contractions have no prognostic significance after MI.

Atrial Fibrillation

New atrial fibrillation occurs in about 10% to 20% of patients with MI and is usually transient. It may be due to atrial or sinus node ischemia, associated right ventricular infarction, pericarditis, heart failure, or increased atrial pressures. It usually occurs in older patients, more often in those with a history of hypertension, mitral regurgitation, and larger left atria. New atrial fibrillation in the peri-infarct period is associated with a higher infarct mortality.

Atrial systole may contribute up to one-third of the cardiac output in patients with an ischemic left ventricle. Patients with persistent or refractory atrial fibrillation in the peri-infarct period have higher pulmonary capillary wedge pressures and lower ejection fractions and are in a poorer Killip class overall compared with patients who maintain sinus rhythm.

Ventricular Arrhythmias After Myocardial Infarction

Ventricular Fibrillation

Many studies have reported that the incidence of primary ventricular fibrillation (VF) in MI is about 5% in patients in whom a documented rhythm is obtained and occurs without antecedent-warning arrhythmias in over half. The true incidence of primary VF is probably much higher because it has been estimated that one-half of all patients with coronary artery disease die of sudden cardiac death, presumably VF. Factors associated with an increased incidence of VF include current smoking, left BBB, and hypokalemia. Patients with anterior MI and VF have a worse long-term prognosis than those with VF associated with inferior MI. VF may occur with reperfusion after thrombolytic therapy or catheter-based therapy. Treatment consists of prompt defibrillation. β-Blockers appear to decrease the incidence of lethal ventricular arrhythmias, including VF, in the peri-infarct period.

Ventricular Tachycardia

Ventricular tachycardia (VT) occurs in 10% to 40% of cases of MI. Early VT (during the first 24 hours) is usually transient and benign. Late-occurring VT is associated with transmural infarction, left ventricular dysfunction, hemodynamic deterioration, and a markedly higher mortality, both in-hospital and long-term. Treatment of sustained VT consists of cardioversion; if the rate is slow and hemodynamically tolerated, cardioversion may be attempted with drugs. Rapid VT (>150 bpm) or VT associated with hemodynamic deterioration should be treated with prompt DC cardioversion.

Accelerated Idioventricular Rhythm

Accelerated idioventricular rhythm (AIVR) is an ectopic ventricular rhythm consisting of three or more consecutive ventricular beats with a rate faster than the normal ventricular escape rate of 30 to 40 beats per minute, but slower than VT. Onset and offset usually are gradual, and isorhythmic dissociation is often present. AIVR has been reported in 10% to 40% of cases of MI, especially (but not necessarily) with early reperfusion. The incidence is equal in inferior and anterior infarcts and is not related to infarct size. The presence of AIVR during the peri-infarct period is not correlated with increased mortality or incidence of VF. AIVR may also be seen with digitalis toxicity, myocarditis, and cocaine use. Symptoms may be related to loss of atrioventricular (AV) synchrony or slow ventricular rates (or both).

Premature Ventricular Complexes

Premature ventricular complexes (PVCs) occur frequently during MI. Their significance in predicting ventricular tachycardia and fibrillation is unclear. Treatment of PVCs in the peri-infarct period has not been shown conclusively to decrease the incidence of malignant ventricular arrhythmias or to improve mortality; in fact, pooled results of randomized trials in which PVCs were treated prophylactically in the peri-infarct period with lidocaine demonstrated an increased mortality. β-Blockers may be the best option for treating PVCs and preventing malignant ventricular arrhythmias.

MISCELLANEOUS CONSIDERATIONS

Reperfusion Arrhythmias

Typically, AIVR has been credited with being a marker for reperfusion. However, any arrhythmia (or no arrhythmia) may be seen with reperfusion; conversely, AIVR may occur without reperfusion. Other clinical factors should be considered when deciding whether reperfusion has occurred, such as resolution of chest pain, improved hemodynamics, and normalization of electrocardiographic (ECG) changes. The appearance of reperfusion arrhythmias is related to size of infarct, length and severity of ischemia, rate of reperfusion, heart rate, extracellular potassium concentration, and the presence of congestive heart failure or left ventricular hypertrophy (or both).

Asystole and Electromechanical Dissociation

Asystole and electromechanical dissociation occur in a small fraction of patients with MI and are usually associated with large infarcts. The prognosis is extremely poor, even with aggressive therapy. Defibrillation should be attempted in patients with apparent asystole, because the rhythm may actually be fine VF.

T-Wave Alternans

This is a transient ECG finding usually seen with ischemia and most pronounced in leads overlying the affected myocardium.

Other ECG Findings

Regional pericarditis sometimes seen after Q-wave infarctions may present with PR depression, but more commonly with atypical ST-segment and T-wave changes. These changes typically consist of gradual premature reversal of initially inverted T waves or persistent/recurrent ST-segment elevation (or both). Persistent ST-segment elevation after infarct may be due to continuing ischemia or aneurysm formation or may herald free wall rupture.

Left ventricular free wall rupture occurs in approximately 10% of cases of fatal transmural MI. ECG findings include failure of the characteristic evolution of the ST segment, T wave, or both. Persistent, progressive, or recurrent ST-segment elevation in the absence of recurrent ischemia may be seen. Failure of the T wave to invert or initial inversion followed by reversion to the upright may also be seen. Abrupt bradycardia responsive to atropine may occur and is believed to mark the time of rupture.

Other ECG findings may include U waves with hypokalemia and tall peaked T waves with hyperkalemia.

CONDUCTION DISTURBANCES AFTER MYOCARDIAL INFARCTION

Conduction abnormalities after acute myocardial infarction result from autonomic disturbances or interruption of the blood supply to the conduction system.

In most individuals the right coronary artery (RCA) is the most frequent blood supply to the sinusatrial node (SAN) (60% of cases) and the atrioventricular node (AVN) (90% of cases), while the left circumflex artery (LCX) supplies the remaining percentages, SAN (40 %) and AVN (10 %). The bundle of His is supplied from the artrioventricular branch of the RCA with a small contribution from the septal perforator of the left anterior descending coronary artery (LAD). After the His bundle divides into the right and left bundles, the septal perforators of the LAD supply the right bundle with collaterals from the right and left circumflex arteries. The left bundle in turn divides proximally into the left anterior and posterior fascicles. The left anterior fascicle is supplied from the LAD, while the proximal portion of the left posterior fascicle receives a dual blood supply from the nodal artery, generally a branch of the RCA, and from the LAD. The distal portion of posterior fascicle is also supplied from two sources: the anterior and posterior septal perforating arteries.

- Conduction in the left anterior fascicle (blood supply from LAD perforators) is very sensitive to ischemia.
- The overall incidence of high-degree AV block in patients receiving thrombolysis is about 10% with inferior infarcts and 3% with anterior infarcts.
- Heart block complicating inferior infarction increases in-hospital mortality but not long-term mortality in patients discharged from hospital.

First-Degree Block

Approximately 5% to 10% of patients with MI have first-degree block at some point during the peri-infarct period. Almost all have supra-Hisian conduction abnormalities. First-degree block may be associated with drugs that prolong atrioventricular conduction.

Second-Degree, Mobitz Type I Block (Wenckebach)

Wenckebach may be seen in up to 10% of cases of MI, typically inferior infarcts, and is due to increased vagal tone or ischemia. The conduction defect is usually in the AVN and, when seen early in the course of an MI, usually responds to atropine. Resolution usually occurs after 48 to 72 hours. Treatment is initially with atropine and, rarely, temporary pacing for symptomatic bradycardia. Late-occurring Wenckebach is less sensitive to atropine and may be due to recurrent ischemia. Very rarely, Wenckebach will progress to higher grades of block that require permanent pacing. Wenckebach rhythm in the peri-infarct period has no impact on long-term prognosis (Fig. 1).

Second-Degree, Mobitz Type II Block

Mobitz type II block occurs in 1% of cases of MI and is more common after anterior MI. There is a high risk of progression to higher degrees of block, including sudden complete heart block with ventricular asystole. Patients should have a temporary pacing wire placed prophylactically at the first sign of Mobitz type II block in the peri-infarct period. The conduction defect is more likely to be infranodal than in Mobitz type I block, and most patients should be treated with permanent pacing. If it is uncertain whether permanent pacing is indicated,

electrophysiologic evaluation should be performed before hospital dismissal to assess the integrity of the infranodal conduction system. Long-term prognosis is related primarily to the size of the infarct rather than to the conduction abnormality.

Third-Degree (Complete) Block

Complete heart block may occur with either an anterior or inferior MI. With inferior infarcts, the conduction defect is likely to be in the AVN, with escape rhythms exceeding 40 beats per minute and exhibiting a narrow QRS complex. With an anterior MI, the conduction defect is infranodal and the escape rhythm (if present) is usually less than 40 beats per minute with a wide QRS complex. Typically, complete heart block seen with anterior MI is preceded by progressive fascicular, bundle, or Mobitz type II block.

Temporary pacing may be required for complete heart block in association with inferior MI if the patient is hemodynamically unstable. Temporary pacing should always be used in patients with anterior infarcts if progressive or complete heart block is present. Permanent pacing is almost always required for high-grade block in the setting of anterior MI; the prognosis is poor for these patients because of the large amount of myocardium involved. Electrophysiologic evaluation before hospital dismissal should be considered for patients with anterior MI and transient complete heart block to assess the integrity of the infranodal conduction system. Transient complete heart block in the setting of inferior MI rarely requires permanent pacing and usually resolves spontaneously.

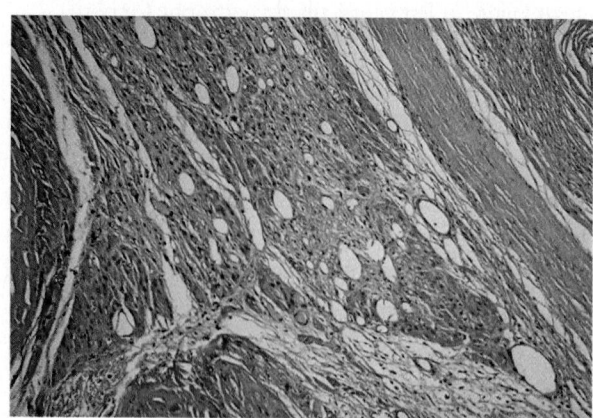

Fig. 1. Edema of the AV node following inferior wall myocardial infarction.

Mechanisms of AV Block

- Anterior infarction: extensive necrosis of infra-His conduction system.
- Multiple mechanisms in inferior MI:
  - Increased parasympathetic tone
  - Ischemic "stunning" of AV node
  - Increased local K^+ due to infarction
  - Increased local release of adenosine
- Autopsy studies show that infarction of the AV node does *not* occur.

Significance of AV Block in MI

- Marker for larger infarction, failure of reperfusion.
- Significant increase in short-term mortality compared to patients without AV block:

	No AV block	AV block
TIMI II	2.2%	9.9%
TAMI	4%	20%
GUSTO-I	6%	21%

The principles of the treatment of heart block complicating myocardial infarction are as follows:

1. Anterior infarctions cause heart block because of septal injury that leads to necrosis of the infra-AV nodal conduction system. Inferior infarctions usually cause heart block because of activation of abnormal cardiovascular reflexes or transient ischemic injury of the AV node. Necrosis of the AV node is rare in inferior infarction because of the presence of collateral vessels from the left anterior descending vessel in addition to the normal blood supply from the AV nodal artery, supplied by the RCA in 85% of cases and the LCX in the remaining 15% of patients (left dominant coronary circulation).

2. Inferior infarcts complicated by high-grade AV block are generally associated with narrow QRS complex escape rhythms with ventricular rates between 40–60 beats per minute. Prognosis for recovery of conduction within a week is good and mortality is low.

3. Symptomatic bradycardia within the first 24 hours of inferior infarction is often due to excess vagal activity (vagotonia) and may respond to IV atropine, administered in 0.5 mg-1 mg increments to a total of 3 mg. Symptomatic bradycardia in anterior infarction is generally atropine resistant.

Atropine does not increase infranodal conduction, may paradoxically slow conduction and the ventricular rate in Mobitz II AV block, is ineffective in transplanted hearts, and rarely can precipitate ventricular fibrillation.

4. First-degree heart block and second-degree heart block type I (Wenckebach) are usually AV nodal in location and frequently are transient, whereas second-degree heart block type II and complete heart block are usually due to injury to the infranodal conduction system and may be permanent.

5. Patients with second degree AV block and anterior infarction can progress to high-grade AV block very rapidly and should be paced at an early stage, whereas inferior infarctions usually progress in a stepwise fashion and can be observed without temporary pacing if clinically stable.

6. Inferior infarctions usually are paced for symptomatic bradycardia and hypoperfusion, whereas anterior infarctions are paced early on the basis of electrocardiographic criteria alone, even if asymptomatic.

Bundle Branch Block

New bundle branch block (BBB) has been reported in about 15% of cases of MI and is associated with an increased risk of complete heart block, congestive heart failure, cardiogenic shock, ventricular arrhythmias, and sudden death. Most commonly seen is right BBB, with left BBB and alternating BBB being less common. This may be related to the discrete anatomical size of the right bundle compared with the broad, fan shape of the left bundle. The correlation between the infarct-related artery and the presence of BBB is strong, with the highest incidence (more than half) of all BBBs occurring in infarcts involving the left anterior descending coronary artery. Progressive infra-Hisian block indicates a significant risk of sudden complete heart block and asystole, and patients demonstrating progression should have temporary pacing wires placed. Persistent BBB confers a significantly higher mortality, because of the large amount of myocardium that must be involved in the infarct to include the bundle branches. Thrombolytic therapy and catheter-based early reperfusion appear to decrease the incidence of BBB in the peri-infarct period.

Mortality With Bundle Branch Blocks

- Mortality rates for patients with BBB are significantly increased:

	BBB	No BBB
TAMI	8.7%	3.5%
GUSTO-I	18%	11%

- Patients who develop BBB in-hospital have higher mortality rates than those who present with BBB.
- Patients whose blocks are transient have similar mortality to patients without block.

Intraventricular Block

New isolated left anterior hemiblock occurs in 3% to 5% of patients with MI; new isolated left posterior hemiblock occurs in 1% to 2% of patients with acute MI. Anatomically, left posterior hemiblock is larger; hence, a larger infarct is required to produce block. Mortality is greater among these patients. Left anterior hemiblock in combination with new right BBB is also indicative of a larger infarct and higher subsequent mortality.

Intraventricular Conduction Defects

- Bundle branch blocks and fascicular blocks are markers for larger infarctions.
- Up to 22% of patients with new BBB will progress to high-grade AV block.
- New bifascicular block ± PR prolongation has highest likelihood of developing complete heart block.
- In approximately 1/4 of patients the conduction abnormalities will be transient.

HEMODYNAMIC CLASSIFICATION OF MYOCARDIAL INFARCTION

Patients with acute myocardial infarction can be divided into four hemodynamic subsets on the basis of the cardiac examination (Killip class I-IV, Table 2) or invasive monitoring (Forrester classification I-IV, Table 3). Although there is overlap between the two classifications, they are not interchangeable in terms of either prognosis or management. Table 4 provides data regarding hemodynamic patterns in cardiovascular disease.

CARDIOGENIC SHOCK

Cardiogenic shock is persistent hypotension conventionally defined as a systolic pressure <80 mm Hg for more than 30 minutes in the absence of hypovolemia. Hypovolemia results in hypotension due to inadequate left ventricular end-diastolic filling pressure (LVEDP) typically measured clinically by its surrogate—a pulmonary capillary wedge pressure (PCWP) <18 mm Hg. Hypotension due to hypovolemia responds to fluid

Table 2.   Killip Class: Clinical Examination

Class	Finding
I	No S3 or rales
II	Rales in less than half of lung field
III	Rales in more than half of lung field
IV	Cardiogenic shock

S3, left ventricular third heart sound.

Table 3.   Forrester Classification: Invasive Monitoring

Class	Finding	PCWP, mm Hg	CI, L/min per m2
I	Normal hemodynamics	≤18	2.2
II	Good cardiac output, pulmonary congestion	>18	≥2.2
III	Low cardiac output, no pulmonary congestion	≤18	<2.2
IV	Low cardiac output, pulmonary congestion	>18	<2.2

CI, cardiac index; PCWP, pulmonary capillary wedge pressure.

Table 4.   Typical Hemodynamic Patterns in Cardiovascular Disease*

| | Pressure | | | | Pulmonary arteriolar resistance index |
	RA	PA	PCW	CI	
Normal	<6	<28/12	<18	>2.4	<2
Tamponade	High	Variable	Low	Low	Normal
Right ventricular infarction	High	Low-normal	Low	Low	Normal
Acute pulmonary embolus	High	Normal-high	Low	Low	Normal-high
Left ventricular failure	Normal	Normal-high	High	Low-normal	Normal
High-output heart failure	High	Normal-high	High	High	Normal
Right ventricular failure	High	Variable	Low-normal	Low-normal	Normal
Cardiogenic shock	High	Normal-high	High	Low	Normal
Septicemia	Low	Low-normal	Low	High	Low
Chronic pulmonary hypertension	High	High	Normal	Low-normal	High
Hypovolemia	Low	Low-normal	Low	Low	Low

*The values and descriptions given reflect typical clinical scenarios, but there is significant patient-to-patient variation. RA, PA, and PCW pressures are in mm Hg. CI is in L/min per m2. Pulmonary arteriolar resistance is in Wood units (multiply by 80 to convert Wood units to dynes · s · cm5).
CI, cardiac index; PA, pulmonary artery; PCW, pulmonary capillary wedge; RA, right atrial.

replacement while cardiogenic shock is associated with an elevated LVEDP and PCWP and is refractory to fluid challenge. Cardiogenic shock is frequently is associated with oliguria or anuria, metabolic acidosis, peripheral hypoperfusion, and cerebral hypoxia. The cardiac index in cardiogenic shock is usually less than 2.0 L/min per m2.

The most common causes of cardiogenic shock include 1) large left ventricular infarct (usually >40% of left ventricle) seen in about 80% of shock patients, 2) right ventricular infarct in 10% of shock patients, and 3) mechanical complications of myocardial infarction (ventricular septal defect, acute mitral regurgitation, tamponade) in 10% of shock patients. Cardiogenic shock also affects the viable perfused myocardium surrounding the infarct zone by rendering it more prone to ischemic necrosis due to hypotension and poor perfusion Cardiogenic shock develops in about 10-20 percent of patients prior to hospitalization but in most patients is delayed several hours after the initial myocardial insult.

Differential Diagnosis of Hypotension Post-Myocardial Infarct

- Cardiogenic shock.
- Right ventricular infarction.
- Papillary muscle rupture.
- Ventricular septal rupture.
- Free wall rupture.
- Conduction abnormalities.
- Hypovolemia.

The incidence of cardiogenic shock is about 8% of all patients with acute myocardial infarction, and mortality is about 80% with conservative management. Thrombolytics are generally ineffective once hypotension has become established. Primary percutaneous coronary intervention (PCI) is generally the treatment of choice for cardiogenic shock while inotropic support from an intra-aortic balloon pump or positive inotropic drugs is also valuable. The clinical management and results of randomized trials in cardiogenic shock are discussed in detail in Chapter 126.

Definition of Cardiogenic Shock

- Decreased cardiac output with evidence of insufficient tissue perfusion in the presence of adequate intravascular volume (Killip class 4).
- Clinical signs: oliguria, cool, cyanotic extremities, altered mental status.
- Hemodynamic criteria: sustained hypotension (SBP <90 mm Hg for >30 min), PAWP >15 mm Hg, CI <2.2 L/min/m^2 (Forrester class 4).

Causes of Noninfarct-Related Cardiogenic Shock

- Myocarditis.
- End-stage cardiomyopathy.
- Myocadial contusion.
- LVOT obstruction (AS or HOCM).
- Ruptured chordae.
- LV inflow tract obstruction, MS or myxoma.
- Septic shock with myocardial depression.
- Pulmonary embolus.
- Aortic dissection with acute AR or tamponade.

HEMODYNAMIC MONITORING IN ACUTE MYOCARDIAL INFARCTION

Generally accepted indications for invasive pulmonary artery pressure monitoring in acute myocardial infarction are as follows:

1. Cardiogenic shock
2. Right ventricular infarction
3. Hypotension unrelated to bradycardia and unresponsive to fluids
4. Combined hypotension and heart failure
5. Suspected or actual mechanical complications of acute myocardial infarction
6. As a guide to the use of inotropic drugs in patients with unfavorable hemodynamics after myocardial infarction

INTRA-AORTIC BALLOON COUNTERPULSATION

Hemodynamic Effects

1. Increased diastolic arterial blood pressure with augmented coronary diastolic blood flow and cardiac output
2. Increased or decreased systolic arterial blood pressure and reduction in left ventricular afterload with lower impedance to left ventricular ejection
3. The above results in a reduction in myocardial oxygen consumption, diminished heart rate, and increased urinary output

Indications

1. Cardiogenic shock
2. Refractory myocardial ischemia
3. To stabilize the patient in association with a myocardial revascularization procedure (coronary artery bypass or PCI)
4. Mechanical complications of infarction

Complications

1. Vascular complications (insertion site, aortic wall, damage from repeated balloon inflations)
2. Hematological problems (hemolysis, systemic emboli)
3. Balloon dependence (unable to wean from support)

Vascular complications are increased in elderly female patients of small stature (smaller caliber vessels) and in patients with diabetes mellitus or peripheral vascular disease

Contraindications

1. Patient not a candidate for aggressive revascularization
2. Aortic incompetence
3. Severe peripheral vascular disease
4. Aortic aneurysm (thoracic or descending aorta)
5. Aortic dissection

RIGHT VENTRICULAR INFARCTION

Suspect right ventricular infarction in any patient with an inferior myocardial infarction complicated by hypotension. Other hemodynamic features of right ventricular infarction include an increased right atrial (RA) pressure (>12 mm Hg) and a normal or decreased right ventricular (RV) systolic and pulmonary artery (PA) systolic pressures. In general, central venous pressure (CVP), RA pressure, and RV diastolic pressure are all increased while RV systolic pressure, PA systolic pressure and cardiac output (CO) are decreased in right ventricular infarction. A hemodynamic pattern that suggests constrictive pericardial physiology (steep right atrial Y descent, square root sign, increased JVP and rarely, a positive Kussmaul sign may occur in RV infarction due to acute RV dilation within a fixed pericardial volume. A clear lung field on chest radiography in a hypotensive patient is a hallmark of right ventricular infarction. Right ventricular infarction is more common in patients with existing right ventricular hypertrophy a finding usually associated with chronic lung disease or congenital heart disease in whom RV infarction can also infrequently occur without flow limiting epicardial coronary artery disease. Right atrial infarction may accompany right ventricular infarction and is usually clinically manifest by atrial arrhythmias. The diagnosis and management of patients with right ventricular infarction is discussed in detail in Chapter 68 (Fig. 2).

- Significant right ventricular infarction is associated with hypotension, an increased jugular venous pressure, and clear lung fields.
- Significant right ventricular infarction rarely occurs in the absence of evidence of an inferior wall infarction.
- Always consider either a pulmonary embolus or a new right-to-left shunt across a patent foramen ovale in a patient with marked arterial desaturation complicating an inferior wall infarction.
- The hemodynamic findings associated with right ventricular infarction are low cardiac output, low pulmonary wedge pressure, and increased right atrial pressure.

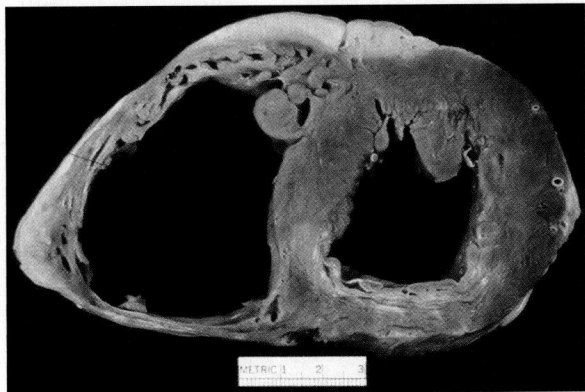

Fig. 2. Old right ventricular infarct with thinning of the inferior and right ventricular wall.

- Right ventricular infarction may be complicated by tricuspid regurgitation due to tricuspid annular dilatation.
- The differential diagnosis of right ventricular infarction is pulmonary embolism, constrictive pericarditis, pericardial tamponade, and cardiogenic shock due to other causes.
- True posterior myocardial infarction often complicated by right ventricular infarction is the only non-ST–elevation myocardial infarction for which thrombolytics should be administered.
- Patients with hypotension or decreased urinary output due to right ventricular infarction should have moderate volume loading with pharmacological inotropic support (dobutamine to augment septal contraction) to achieve a pulmonary wedge pressure of 15-18 mm Hg.
- Avoid "pushing" fluids beyond above parameters. RV overdistention can ↑ RV MVO$_2$ and actually decrease CO by increasing intrapericardial pressure and limiting LV filling.
- Maintenance of AV synchrony is important to maintain RV filling. Temporary pacing should be employed in high-grade AV block. Atrial fibrillation/flutter should be promptly cardioverted.
- Right ventricular infarction complicating inferior infarction increases in hospital mortality but not long–term mortality in patients discharged from hospital.

Failed Reperfusion

Failed thrombolysis is characterized by persistent or worsening chest pain, persistent or worsening ST segment elevation, and/or hemodynamic instability. Absence of these clinical indicators of ongoing myocardial ischemia is not a completely reliable predictor of successful reperfusion for all patients. The success of thrombolytic therapy in patients with an ST elevation myocardial infarction is dependent on complete restoration of normal infarct related artery blood flow (TIMI-3 flow) (Table 5).

Restoration of TIMI-3 blood flow improvement left ventricular function and survival in myocardial patients but restoration of lesser grades of blood flow namely TIMI-2 blood flow or less does not reduce mortality.

Angiographic "no-reflow" or "slow flow" is a special case of non-reperfusion seen at the time of primary

PCI for acute myocardial, in which there is a failure to re-establish normal myocardial perfusion in the absence of a significant residual epicardial coronary stenosis. It is characterized microscopically by swollen endothelial cells which result in capillary plugging by red cells, neutrophils, platelets, and fibrin thrombi which in turn obstructed capillary blood flow. This phenomenon is a predictor of future cardiac events and poorer prognosis including mechanical complications of myocardial infarction.

Infarct Extension and Expansion, Ventricular True and False Aneurysms

Infarct extension or recurrent infarction is an increase in myocardial necrosis remote from the original infarct site and usually occurs between day 2 and 10 following the initial myocardial infarction. It is associated with cardiogenic shock, subendocardial infarct, female gender, and previous infarctions. A secondary elevation in *creatine kinase* (CK-MB) beyond the first 24 hours and a new Q wave on the ECG are suggestive of the diagnosis: serum troponins are less useful diagnostically in this situation as they remain elevated for a longer period after infarction that CK-MB enzyme. Infarct expansion or ventricular remodeling is thinning and dilatation of the infarcted myocardium due the pulsatile hemodynamic pressure without an increase in myocardial necrosis. Infarct expansion stretching the myocyte bundles and

Table 5.   TIMI Angiographic Classification of Coronary Blood Flow

TIMI 0 absence of any antegrade flow beyond a coronary occlusion

TIMI 1 flow is faint antegrade coronary flow beyond the occlusion, although filling of the distal coronary bed is incomplete

TIMI 2 flow is delayed or sluggish antegrade flow with complete filling of the distal territory

TIMI 3 flow is normal flow which fills the distal coronary bed completely

reduces the density of cardiac myocytes in the infarcted wall (Fig. 3). Infarct expansion typically occurs with large anterior wall infarcts and may result in ventricular aneurysm formation, heart failure and refractory ventricular arrhythmias (Fig. 4).

A true left ventricular aneurysm is a discrete thinned segment of the left ventricle that protrudes during both systole and diastole and has a broad neck. In contrast, a false left ventricular aneurysm has a narrow neck, a result of a prior LV free wall rupture and is contained solely by the adherent pericardium. The presence of hypertension and the use of steroids and

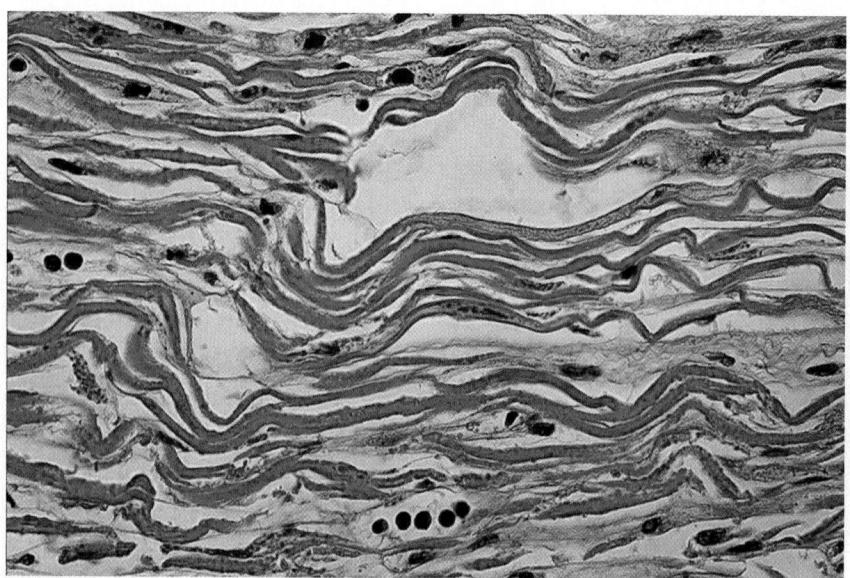

Fig. 3. "Wavy myocytes" following myocardial infarction

nonsteroidal anti-inflammatory drugs may promote aneurysm formation (Fig. 5, 6, and 7).

■ True LV aneurysm rarely rupture, whereas rupture is not uncommon with false LV aneurysms.

Dynamic Left Ventricular Outflow Tract Obstruction

Dynamic left ventricular outflow tract obstruction results from hyperdynamic contraction of the basal portions of the left ventricle in response to catecholamine stimulation usually following an anterior wall infarction. The cross-sectional area of the outflow tract is reduced resulting in a decreased cardiac output, often associated with arterial desaturation and a new systolic ejection murmur. In addition there may be systolic anterior motion (SAM) of the mitral valve leaflets towards the septum due to a Venturi like effect leading to further outflow tract obstruction and mitral regurgitation. The diagnosis is made by echocardiography and treatment is with IV fluids, cessation or reduction in administered inotropic drugs and cautious use of beta blockers.

Myocardial (Cardiac) Rupture

Myocardial rupture after myocardial infarction, encompasses rupture of the interventricular septum and left ventricular free wall rupture, both of which share a similar cellular pathophysiology. Rupture typically occurs

in an area of infarction without myocardial reperfusion with a persistently occluded infarct-related coronary artery. Early thrombolysis or primary PCI decreases the risk of cardiac rupture provided successful reperfusion is achieved. Unsuccessful or late thrombolysis probably does not increase the overall risk of cardiac rupture but may accelerate the process of cell necrosis and lead to earlier ventricular wall rupture usually within 24 hours of administration. Late PCI (>12 hours after presentation) probably reduces the risk of ventricular rupture. Rupture typically occurs at the junction of the normal and infarcted myocardium (Fig. 8 and 9).

RUPTURE OF THE VENTRICULAR FREE WALL

Rupture of the ventricular free wall usually presents catastrophically with either sudden death, usually due to electromechanical dissociation, or tamponade with cardiogenic shock. Rarely, patients present with subacute ventricular rupture manifested by pericardial pain, electrocardiographic evidence of pericarditis, and a pericardial rub. Rupture typically occurs within 4 days after acute infarction. Significant predisposing factors for early ventricular rupture in the TIMI 9B trial were elderly age (>70 years; odds ratio, 5.0) and female sex (odds ratio, 3.6). Other commonly identified risk factors for cardiac rupture include hypertension, absence of ventricular hypertrophy, previous infarction, poor collateral flow, and lateral wall myocardial infarction. Possible additional risk factors also include the use of steroids and anticoagulation.

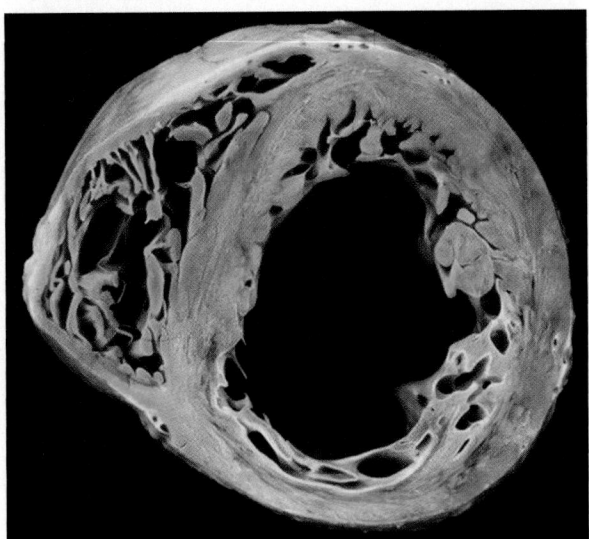

Fig. 4. Thinning and scarring of the inferior wall after a large inferior wall myocardial infarction.

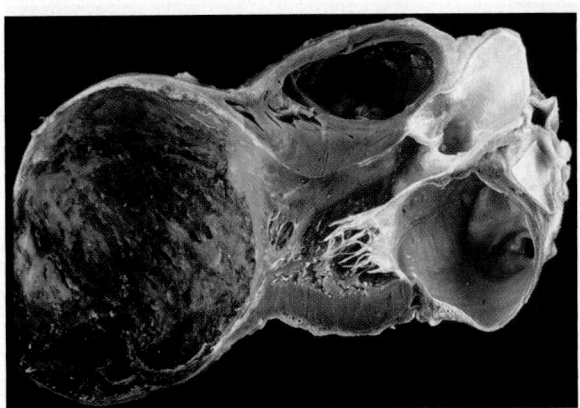

Fig. 5. Very large apical aneurysm with contained thrombus.

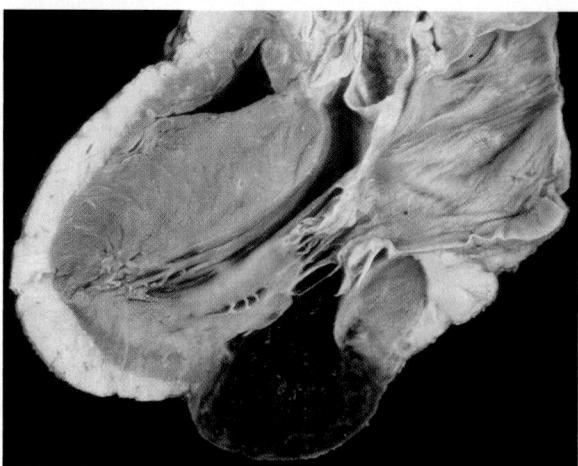

Fig. 6. False aneurysm (contained left ventricle rupture), after myocardial infarction.

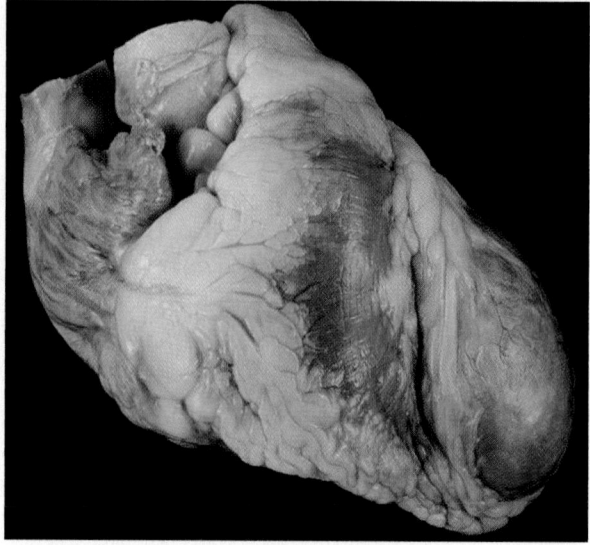

Fig. 7. Apical aneurysm following myocardial infarction.

Myocardial ruptures are of three types:

1. A slit-like tear that occurs early after infarction and is associated with single-vessel coronary disease without any thinning of the left ventricular wall and with good preservation of left ventricular function (most common type of rupture).
2. Rupture that results from a subacute process with localized necrosis of myocardium.
3. Rupture that is preceded by the development of myocardial thinning, with rupture in the center of the thinned area (Fig. 10 and 11).

Late ruptures are associated with multivessel disease and occur days to weeks after infarction. Rupture usually occurs in the left ventricle (8 times more than in the right ventricle), in the terminal distribution of the left anterior descending coronary artery (anterior wall rupture), or in diagonal branches (lateral wall rupture), usually at the junction of normal and infarcted myocardium.

The treatment of rupture of the ventricular free wall is emergency cardiac operation. Rarely, the rupture may be walled off to produce a left ventricular false aneurysm or pseudoaneurysm. Echocardiography is the diagnostic imaging method of choice, and cardiac operation is almost always required pseudoaneurysm because of their to rupture without warning.

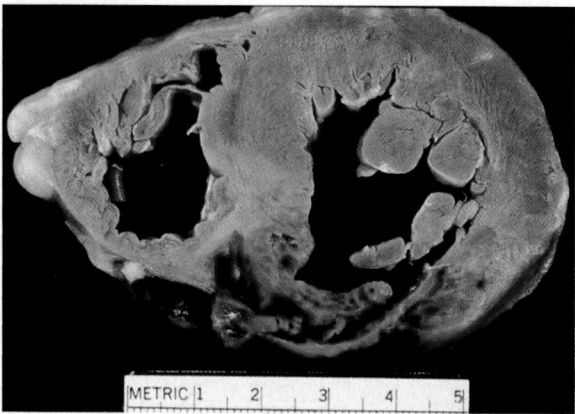

Fig. 8. Myocardial rupture following hemorrhagic infarction and thrombolysis.

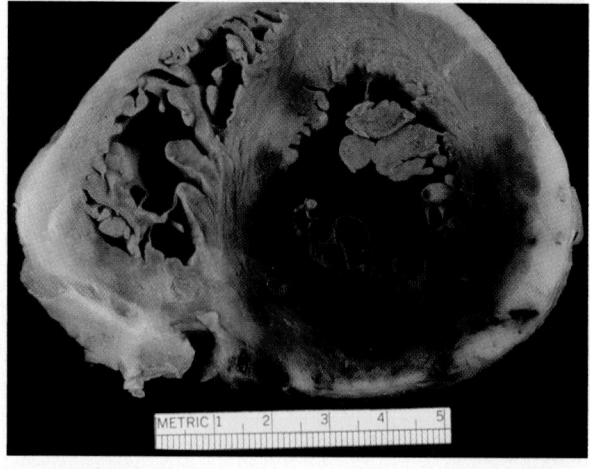

Fig. 9. Hemorrhagic myocardial infarct post thrombolysis.

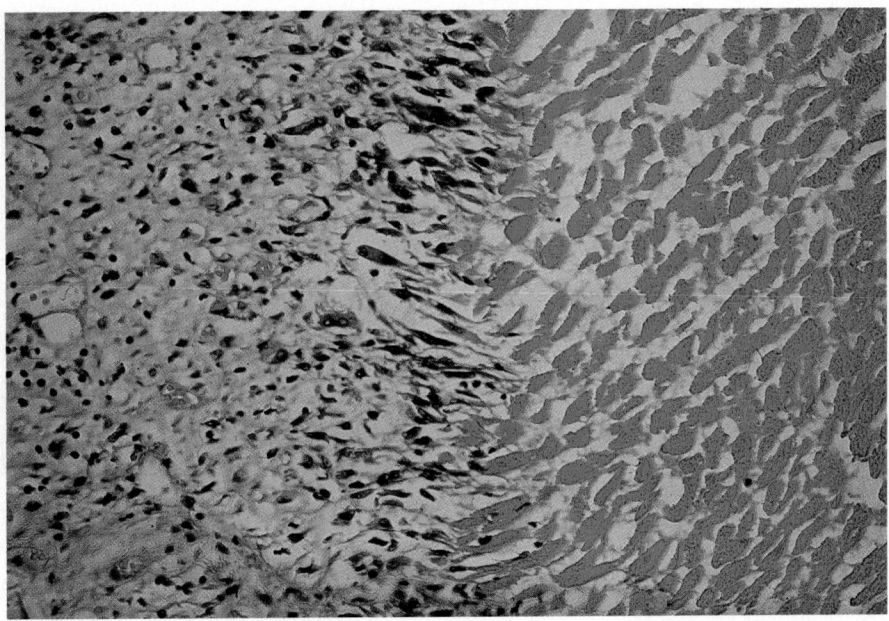

Fig. 10. Junction of infarcted (*left*) and normal myocardium (*right*).

Pseudoaneurysms are also associated with heart failure caused by loss of myocardial power and systemic thromboembolism (Fig. 12 and 13).

- Predisposing factors for ventricular free wall rupture are elderly age (>70 years) and female sex.
- Elderly women are also at higher risk for rupture of the inter ventricular septum.

- A common clinical and examination question is the diagnosis and management of patients with a myocardial infarction complicated by a new systolic murmur. The differential diagnoses include papillary muscle dysfunction or rupture, interventricular septal rupture, dynamic left ventricular outflow tract obstruction, or new tricuspid regurgitation due to right ventricular infarction or massive pulmonary embolus.

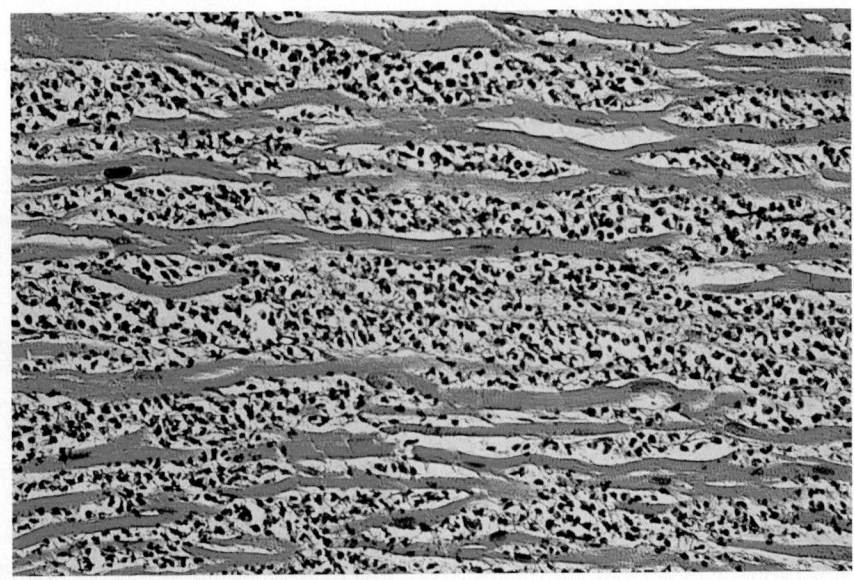

Fig. 11. Inflammatory cell response 72 hours after myocardial infarction.

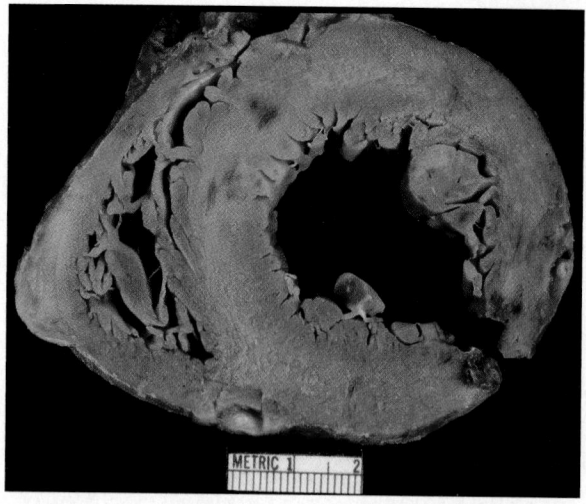

Fig. 12. Cardiac free wall rupture post myocardial infarction.

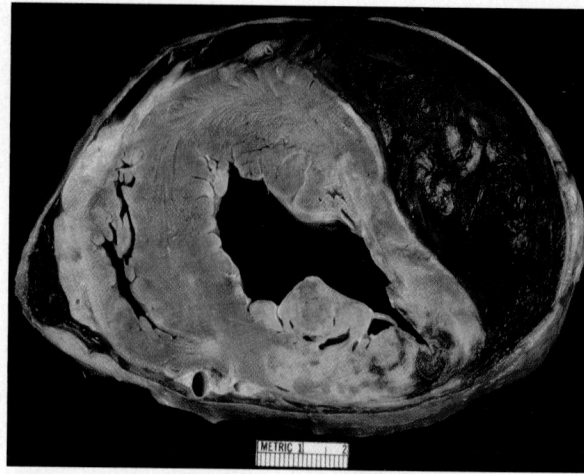

Fig. 13. Pericardial tamponade from left ventricular free wall rupture and hemopericardium.

■ Rarely aortic dissection may present as an inferior wall myocardial infarction due to extension of the dissection into the ostium of the right coronary artery.

RUPTURE OF THE VENTRICULAR SEPTUM

Rupture of the ventricular septum is similar in many ways to rupture of the ventricular free wall in that it almost always occurs within days of acute infarction, is frequently a serpiginous tract rather than a discrete defcet, is associated with transmural infarction, and probably is also associated with hypertension. Ventricular septal rupture usually presents abruptly with hypotension, acute right ventricular failure, and a new pansystolic murmur frequently associated with a systolic thrill. Echocardiography is the diagnostic imaging method of choice. Inferior infarctions cause septal rupture in the basal inferior septum, whereas anterior infarctions cause rupture in the apical septum. Treatment of rupture of the ventricular septum is emergency cardiac surgery or percutaneous defect closure in selected patients (Fig. 14).

■ Ventricular septal rupture presents with hypotension, acute right ventricular failure, and a new pansystolic murmur frequently associated with a systolic thrill.
■ Patients with acute ventricular septal rupture usually lie flat due to systemic hypotension while patients

with acute mitral valve rupture develop pulmonary edema very rapidly and typically cannot lie flat.
■ Septal rupture from inferior wall myocardial infarction has a worse prognosis than that associated with anterior wall infarction.

ACUTE MITRAL REGURGITATION

Acute mitral regurgitation after myocardial infarction can be due to papillary muscle dysfunction caused by fibrosis or ischemia, papillary muscle rupture (either partial or complete), or mitral annular dilatation associated with left ventricular failure. The blood supply to

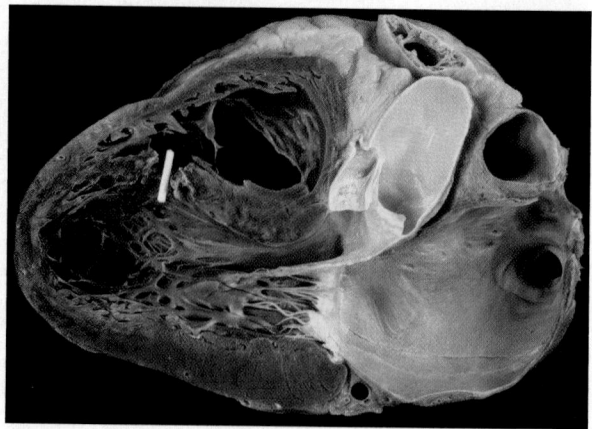

Fig. 14. Septal rupture post myocardial infarction.

the posteromedial papillary muscle (derived only from the posterior descending artery) is more tenuous than that to the anterolateral papillary muscle (derived from both the left anterior descending and the left circumflex arteries). Consequently, 90% of papillary muscle ruptures involve the posteromedial papillary muscle. This is fortuitous because the posteromedial papillary muscle usually has multiple heads (in contrast to the single head of the anterolateral papillary muscle), and rupture of an individual head is frequently survivable, at least in the short term. Complete transection of a left ventricular papillary muscle is usually fatal because of massive sudden mitral regurgitation. Infarctions associated with papillary muscle rupture are usually small, and frequently there is only single-vessel coronary disease. Patients with papillary muscle rupture usually present up to 1 week after myocardial infarction with acute pulmonary edema. The loudness of the mitral regurgitation murmur is variable and may not correlate with the degree of mitral regurgitation. The murmur may be completely absent in some patients with severe mitral regurgitation. A thrill is rarely present in acute mitral regurgitation. Large V waves are present in the pulmonary wedge tracing, and, more rarely, the regurgitant jet may be transmitted through the pulmonary vasculature to lead to increased oxygen saturation in the pulmonary artery; this may suggest an erroneous diagnosis of ventricular septal rupture. Echocardiography is the diagnostic imaging method of choice, and urgent cardiac operation is generally indicated (Fig. 15 and 16).

- In 90% of papillary muscle ruptures, the posteromedial papillary muscle ruptures.
- A thrill is rarely present in acute mitral regurgitation.
- The classical systolic murmur of mitral regurgitation may be absent in acute severe mitral reguritation.

Acute Mitral Regurgitation may be differentiated clinically from ventricular septal rupture by the following features

- A step-up in oxygen saturation between the RA and PA is present in ventricular septal rupture but not in acute mitral regurgitation.
- Large V waves in the pulmonary capillary wedge and pulmonary artery tracings are acute mitral regur-

gitation but not ventricular septal rupture.
- A precordial thrill is common ~50% in ventricular septal rupture but not in acute mitral regurgitation.
- The systolic murmur of ventricular septal rupture is loud and best heard in the lower left sternal area an posteriorly.
- The murmur of acute mitral regurgitation is frequently soft, usually best heard at the apex with radiation to the axilla and may be absent entirely.

Pericardial Effusion and Pericarditis

Early pericarditis and pericardial effusion occur in ~10% of patients with acute myocardial infarction and result from a localized area of pericardial inflammation usually over the site of a transmural infarct. Pericarditis may be associated with non-ischemic type chest pain and a pericardial rub and is more common in patients with anterior infarcts, transmural infarcts, and heart failure. Treatment is with aspirin 650 mg every 4 to 6 hours. Steroids and NSAID's are generally contraindicated due to their effect on fluid retention and the risk of precipitation of heart failure, and their adverse effect on myocardial wound healing and possible association with myocardial rupture.

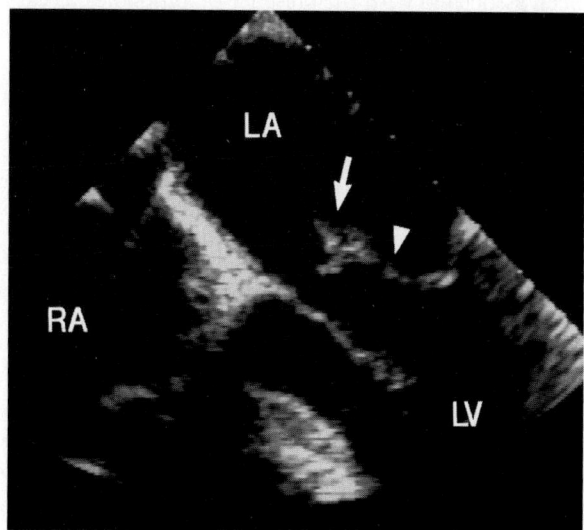

Fig. 15. Papillary muscle rupture complicating acute inferior myocardial infarction; magnified transverse four-chamber view. The ruptured head of the posteromedial papillary muscle (*arrow*) prolapses freely into the left atrium; the posterior mitral valve leaflet (*arrowhead*) is flail.

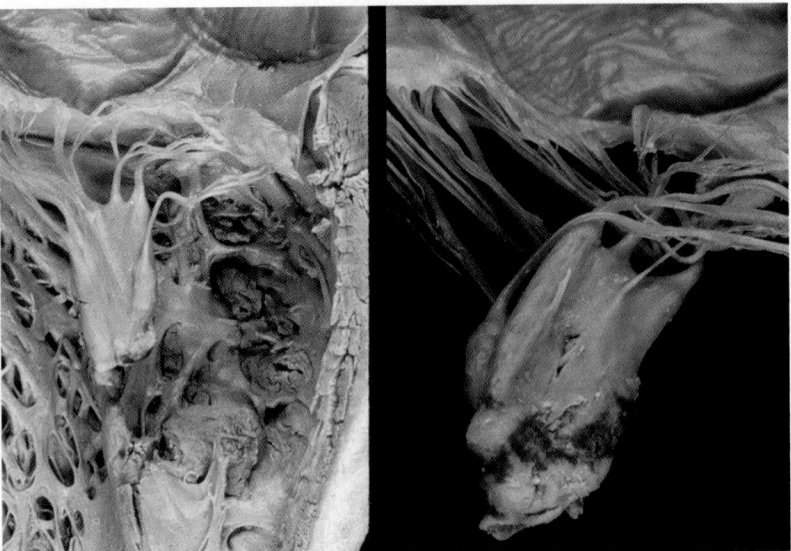

Fig. 16. Ruptured posteromedial mitral papillary muscle in acute myocardial infarction.

Postinfarction Syndrome (Dressler's syndrome)

Dressler's syndrome (~3% of patients) consists of pleu-ro-pericardial chest pain often associated in the early stages with an auscultatory friction rub, fever, arthral-gia, leukocytosis, and pulmonary infiltrates. It typically occurs several weeks after infarction and may be recurrent. Histologically it is characterized by a localized fibrinous pericarditis and neutrophil infiltration and has been associated with the presence of antibodies to cardiac tissue. Treatment is with aspirin 650 mg every 4 to 6 hours or as an alternative NSAID's provided ventricular and renal function are well preserved. Steroids should be avoided.

Left ventricular Mural Thrombus

Mural thrombus formation on the endocardial surface of the left ventricle is common (~50%) in patients with large anterior wall myocardial infarctions. Left ventricular thrombi are associated with reduced global left ventricular function and diminish patient survival. Peripheral embolization may occur in ~10% of patients while coumadin anticoagulation reduces the incidence of left ventricular thrombi and embolization (Fig. 17).

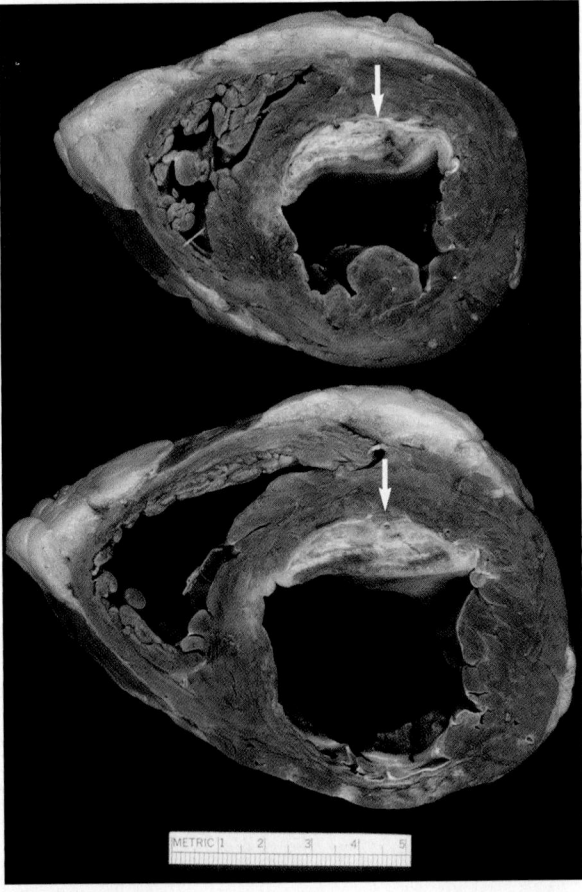

Fig. 17. Left ventricular mural thrombus (*arrows*), after myocardial infarction.

71

REPERFUSION STRATEGY FOR ST-ELEVATION MYOCARDIAL INFARCTION: FIBRINOLYSIS VERSUS PERCUTANEOUS CORONARY INTERVENTION

Henry H. Ting, MD

Coronary artery disease is the leading cause of death in the United States and Europe. More than 500,000 Americans annually suffer an acute myocardial infarction with EKG changes of ST-segment elevation or new left-bundle branch block. ST-elevation myocardial infarction (STEMI) is a medical emergency, analogous to major trauma or aortic dissection, where even "minutes" of delay in initiating appropriate treatment significantly increases mortality. Two important principles guide our approach to myocardial reperfusion:

1. "Time is heart muscle" – Early reperfusion of the infarct related artery as quickly as possible within the first 12 hours of artery occlusion limits infarct size, increases myocardial salvage, preserves left ventricular function, and in turn improves patient survival.

2. "Open artery hypothesis" – Late mechanical opening of the infarct related artery at 12 to 48 hours following artery occlusion may reduce infarct size by salvaging stunned and hibernating myocardium supplied by collaterals vessels and improves left ventricular remodeling.

Based on current trial data and guidelines, there are 2 proven reperfusion strategies for patients with STEMI – namely, full-dose fibrinolysis or primary percutaneous coronary intervention (PCI). Advances in STEMI treatment over the past 2 decades have lowered 30-day mortality to 6% or less among those treated with fibrinolysis and to 4% or less with primary PCI.

Interpretation of the 12 lead electrocardiogram (ECG) makes the diagnosis of STEMI and an EKG should be obtained immediately (within 5 to 10 minutes) in all patients presenting to healthcare providers with chest discomfort.

Definition of STEMI:

1. ECG demonstrates ST-segment elevation greater than 0.1 mV in at least 2 contiguous precordial leads or at least 2 adjacent limb leads.

2. ECG demonstrates new or presumed new left bundle branch block.

DTB is door to PTCA balloon time; DTN is door to needle time.

3. Reperfusion therapy is indicated if the ECG is diagnostic for an acute STEMI even if the patient is free of symptoms.

4. If the initial ECG is not diagnostic but clinical suspicion is high for STEMI, obtain serial ECG at 5 to 10 minute intervals.

THE EVIDENCE FOR FIBRINOLYTICS

Fibrinolysis is most effective for STEMI patients who present within the first 2-3 hours of symptom onset and ideally within the "golden first hour." The Fibrinolytic Therapy Trialists' (FTT) grouped analysis of 9 trials and 58,600 patients randomized to fibrinolysis versus control showed that fibrinolysis saved 39 lives per 1,000 patients treated within 1 hour of symptom onset and 30 lives per 1,000 patients treated within 2-3 hours of symptom onset. There was no significant mortality benefit for fibrinolysis if administered after 12 hours of symptom onset. For every 60 minute delay with fibrinolysis, there was a loss in absolute benefit of 1.6 lives per 1,000 treated. In the CAPTIM trial (Comparison of Angioplasty and Prehospital Thrombolysis in Acute Myocardial Infarction), pre-hospital fibrinolysis for patients within 2 hours of symptom onset showed a trend for improved mortality (2.2% versus 5.7%, P=0.058) and significantly decreased risk for cardiogenic shock compared to primary angioplasty.

Fibrinolysis is indicated for STEMI within the first 12 hours of symptom onset. The main benefits for utilizing fibrinolysis are:

1. Widespread availability in rural and community hospitals.
2. Easily administered with typical door-to-needle time (DTN) <30 minutes.
3. Requires lower personnel and equipment resources than 24 hours access to an onsite cardiac catheterization lab.

The Achilles' heel for fibrinolysis is that TIMI 3 flow is achieved in only 60% to 70% of those treated at 90 minutes; furthermore, up to 30% to 40% of patients have absolute or relative contraindications to fibrinolytic therapy due to bleeding risk (Table 1). Hemorrhagic stroke associated with fibrinolysis occurs in <1% of patients, but remains a catastrophic complication with a mortality >50% in individual patients. In addition,

10%-20% of patients will experience reocclusion of the infarct vessel after successful thrombolytic reperfusion. Patients treated with fibrinolysis should be transferred immediately to a PCI-capable facility because an invasive

Table 1.   Absolute and Relative Contraindications for Fibrinolysis

Absolute contraindications
   Any prior intracranial hemorrhage
   Known structural cerebral vascular lesion
   Known malignant intracranial neoplasm
   Ischemic stroke within the past 3 months (except for acute stroke within 3 hours)
   Suspected aortic dissection
   Active bleeding or bleeding diathesis (excluding menses)
   Significant closed-head or facial trauma within 3 months
Relative contraindications
   History of chronic, severe, poorly controlled hypertension
   Severe uncontrolled hypertension on presentation (systolic pressure >180 mm Hg or diastolic pressure >110 mm Hg)
   History of prior ischemic stroke >3 months previously, dementia, or known intracranial pathology not covered in absolute contraindications
   Traumatic or prolonged CPR (>10 minutes) or major surgery (within last 3 weeks)
   Recent internal bleeding (within last 2-4 weeks)
   Noncompressible vascular punctures
   Pregnancy
   Active peptic ulcer
   Current use of anticoagulants: the higher the INR, the higher the risk of bleeding
   For streptokinase/antistreplase: prior exposure (more than 5 days ago) or prior allergic reaction to these agents

approach is beneficial after successful or failed reperfusion. The GRACIA-1 trial (Routine Invasive Strategy within 24 hours of Thrombolysis versus Ischaemia-Guided Conservative Approach for Acute Myocardial Infarction with ST-Segment Elevation) suggested that STEMI patients treated with fibrinolytic therapy benefit from routine coronary angiography (and percutaneous or surgical revascularization if indicated) within 24 hours of successful reperfusion. Data from the multicenter, randomized REACT trial (Rescue Angioplasty versus Conservative Treatment or Repeat Thrombolysis) showed that among patients who have reperfusion failure with fibrinolysis, an invasive strategy of rescue PCI improved event-free survival compared to those treated with conservative therapy or repeat fibrinolysis. The primary endpoint of death, reinfarction, stroke, or severe heart failure at 6 months occurred in 15.3% treated with rescue PCI, 29.8% treated with conservative therapy, and 31% treated with repeat fibrinolysis ($P<0.01$). Rescue PCI should be considered for patients with reperfusion failure after fibrinolysis (ongoing chest pain or <70% resolution of ST-segment elevation at 90 minutes).

The Evidence for Primary PCI

The benefits from primary PCI can be attributed to improved myocardial salvage (from achieving higher rates of TIMI 3 flow) and to lower risk of reinfarction and reocclusion (from mechanical stabilization of ruptured plaques). Primary PCI is also safer with lower risk of bleeding complications, particularly hemorrhagic stroke and left ventricular rupture due to myocardial hemorrhage. At hospitals with 24 hour PCI-capability, primary PCI has become the preferred reperfusion strategy for all STEMI patients, save for the rare exception where vascular access is not possible or when the patient/family requests conservative management only.

An invasive approach, even when PCI is not performed, has the following advantages:

1. Identification of coronary anatomy more suitable for surgical revascularization (severe left main or 3 vessel disease).
2. Identification of mechanical complications requiring emergency cardiac surgery (acute mitral regurgitation, ventricular septal defect or free wall rupture, aortic dissection associated with STEMI).
3. Shock requiring hemodynamic support with intra-aortic balloon pump or left ventricular assist device.
4. Identification of other causes for ST-segment elevation (pericarditis, myocarditis, ventricular aneurysm, tako-tsubo apical ballooning, coronary bridging or spasm, and old left bundle branch block)

Early trials that demonstrated the benefits of primary angioplasty achieved rapid reperfusion with door-to-balloon time (DTB) of 90 minutes or less. The GUSTO IIb substudy (Global Use of Strategies to Open Occluded Arteries in Acute Coronary Syndromes) demonstrated a direct relationship between time from randomization-to-angioplasty and 30-day mortality as follows: ≤60 minutes (1.0% mortality), 61-75 minutes (3.7% mortality), 76-90 minutes (4.0% mortality), and ≥91 minutes (6.4% mortality) ($P=0.001$). Furthermore, the highest 30-day mortality of 14.1% was observed in the patient subset that did not undergo angioplasty. Cannon and colleagues analyzed a prospective observational registry of 27,080 patients in NRMI 2 (Second National Registry Myocardial Infarction) and showed that the multivariate-adjusted odds of mortality were 40%-60% higher if DTB was longer than 2 hours. In summary, time-to-treatment is an important correlate for mortality for any reperfusion strategy, be it primary PCI or fibrinolysis.

Comparison of Primary PCI versus Fibrinolysis

Keeley and colleagues pooled and analyzed 23 randomized trials in 2003 with 7,739 patients randomized to primary PCI versus fibrinolysis. The authors concluded that primary PCI is preferable to fibrinolysis and demonstrated lower rates of death (7% versus 9%, $P=0.0002$), reinfarction (3% versus 7%, $P=0.0001$), and stroke (1% versus 2%, $P=0.0004$). In a pooled analysis study design, Keeley could not tease out the importance of duration of symptoms and time-to-treatment (i.e., DTB) on the reported clinical outcomes. However, the PRAGUE-2 trial (Primary Angioplasty in Patients Transported From General Community Hospitals to Specialized PTCA Units With or Without Emergency Thrombolysis) demonstrated that primary PCI was beneficial over fibrinolysis only if symptom onset exceeded 3 hours, but 30-day mortality was similar for primary PCI versus fibrinolysis if symptom onset was within 3 hours (7.3% versus 7.4%). Boersma and colleagues have recently updated and confirmed Keeley's findings that primary PCI is the preferred reperfusion strategy if performed rapidly, by experienced operators and institutions, and by facilities with PCI capability and availability. The issue of availability refers to having systems and processes to overcome hospital-dependent delays from first medical contact to balloon inflation during daytime and off-hours.

The largest randomized study comparing primary PCI versus fibrinolysis was the DANAMI-2 trial (Danish Trial in Acute Myocardial Infarction 2) which enrolled 1572 patients. The primary endpoint of death, reinfarction, or stroke at 30 days occurred in 8% of the primary PCI group and 14% of the fibrinolysis group (P=0.0003). The primary PCI group included both patients who presented to PCI-capable hospitals (DTB 93 minutes) and who required transfer to PCI-capable hospitals (DTB 108 minutes). The median time for transport from a regional hospital to PCI capable hospital was only 32 minutes. The benefits for primary PCI in this study hinge on proven systems and networks to achieve these very short DTB.

REVIEW OF RECENT FACILITATED PCI TRIALS

The major limitation with primary PCI arises from the multiple delays between first medical contact and PTCA balloon inflation in the catheterization lab. Hence, there has been intense interest in whether a combination approach of fibrinolysis followed by immediate PCI—so called fibrinolytic facilitated PCI—can restore TIMI 3 flow more rapidly prior to mechanical intervention of the ruptured atherosclerotic plaque, and consequently improve clinical outcomes.

The ASSENT-4 trial (Assessment of the Safety and Efficacy of a New Treatment Strategy with Percutaneous Coronary Intervention) tested the hypothesis that full-dose fibrinolytic (Tenecteplase) facilitated PCI is more effective than standard primary PCI without prior thrombolysis. The trial planned to enroll 4,000 patients, but was terminated early by the data and safety monitoring board after 1,667 patients because of higher in-hospital mortality in the facilitated PCI group compared to the primary PCI group (6%

versus 3%, P=0.0105). TIMI 3 flow *before PCI* was achieved in 43% of the fibrinolytic facilitated PCI group compared to 15% of the primary PCI group (P<0.0001). However, the primary endpoint—namely death, congestive heart failure, or shock within 90 days—was 19% in the facilitated PCI group versus 13% in the primary PCI group (P=0.0045). The higher in-hospital mortality observed in the facilitated PCI group was largely attributable to higher rates of total stroke (1.8% versus 0%, P<0.0001) and hemorrhagic stroke (1.0% versus 0%, P=0.0037). The higher risk of adverse events associated with facilitated PCI may be explained by fibrinolytic-induced platelet activation, intramural coronary hemorrhage, myocardial hemorrhage leading to ventricular free wall rupture, hemorrhagic stroke, and other systemic bleeding exacerbating supply and demand mismatch.

Keeley and colleagues reported a grouped analysis of 17 randomized trials (including ASSENT-4) comparing facilitated and primary PCI among 4504 patients. The pooled trials utilized 3 facilitation strategies—glycoprotein IIb/IIIa inhibitor alone, fibrinolytic alone, and combination therapy. Overall, the facilitated approach achieved higher rates of pre-PTCA TIMI 3 flow compared with primary PCI (37% versus 15%, P=0.0001). However, the facilitated approach demonstrated higher mortality (5% versus 3%, P=0.04), nonfatal reinfarction (3% versus 2%, P=0.006), major bleeding (7% versus 5%, P=0.01), total stroke (1.1% versus 0.3%, P=0.0008), and hemorrhagic stroke (0.7% versus 0.1%, P=0.0014) compared to primary PCI. The higher rates of adverse events were primarily observed among the trials utilizing a fibrinolytic based regimen. Among the trials utilizing glycoprotein IIb/IIIa inhibitor alone, the facilitated approach did not show significant benefit or harm compared to primary PCI. A facilitated PCI strategy with a fibrinolytic based regimen should be avoided.

LATE REPERFUSION (SYMPTOM ONSET FROM 12 TO 48 HOURS)

The BRAVE-2 trial (Beyond 12 hours Reperfusion Alternative Evaluation Trial Investigators) randomized 365 STEMI patients between 12 to 48 hours after symptom onset to an invasive versus conservative strategy. An invasive approach of stenting with

Table 2.   Guidellines for Selecting Fibrinolysis Versus Primary PCI

1. If onset of symptoms is <3 hours and there is no delay to an invasive strategy, then neither fibrinolysis nor primary PCI is preferred
2. Fibrinolysis is generally preferred
   - Early presentation (onset of symptoms <3 hours and anticipated delay to an invasive strategy
   - Cath lab occupied or not available
   - Vascular access difficulties
   - Lack of access to a skilled, high volume PCI facility
   - Prolonged transport delay to primary PCI
   - Door-to-balloon minus door-to-needle >60 minutes
   - Total door-to-balloon >90 minutes
3. Primary PCI is generally preferred
   - Skilled PCI facility with onsite surgical backup
   - Door-to-balloon minus door-to-needle <60 minutes
   - Total door-to-balloon <90 minutes
   - High clinical risk including cardiogenic shock (age <75) or Killip class ≥3
   - Contraindication to fibrinolysis or high bleeding risk
   - Late presentation with onset of symptoms >3 hours
   - Diagnosis is in doubt including pericarditis, myocarditis, aneurysm, tako-tsubo apical ballooning

adjunctive abciximab decreased infarct size compared to a conservative strategy (8% versus 13%, $P<0.001$). Late presenters account for 10% to 30% of STEMI patients and this trial suggested that myocardium may remain viable even after >12 hours of ischemia and salvaged with late PCI. This finding could be explained by ischemic preconditioning, presence of collateral circulation, and stunned or hibernating myocardium in the infarct zone.

GUIDELINES AND RECOMMENDATIONS
The guidelines for selecting reperfusion strategy highlight the importance of 4 critical variables (Table 2):
1. Duration of cardiac symptoms
2. Anticipated delays for primary PCI
3. Patient clinical risk and hemodynamic status
4. Patient bleeding risk

Time of symptom onset, time to reperfusion, and patient risk profile all are important and must be carefully considered for individual patients when selecting the best reperfusion strategy. The relationship between mortality reduction and myocardial salvage as a function of time from symptom onset to reperfusion has been recently described by Gersh and colleagues and is shown in Figure 1.

For patients who present with symptom duration less than 3 hours, time-to-reperfusion is most critical, be it fibrinolysis or primary PCI. Moreover, every 30 minute delay from symptom onset to reperfusion is associated with an 8% increase in relative mortality at 1 year. If DTB of <90 minutes can be reliably achieved, then primary PCI would be the preferred approach. However, if the total delays incurred to diagnose STEMI, to activate the system, and to transport by ground or air ambulance to a PCI-capable facility

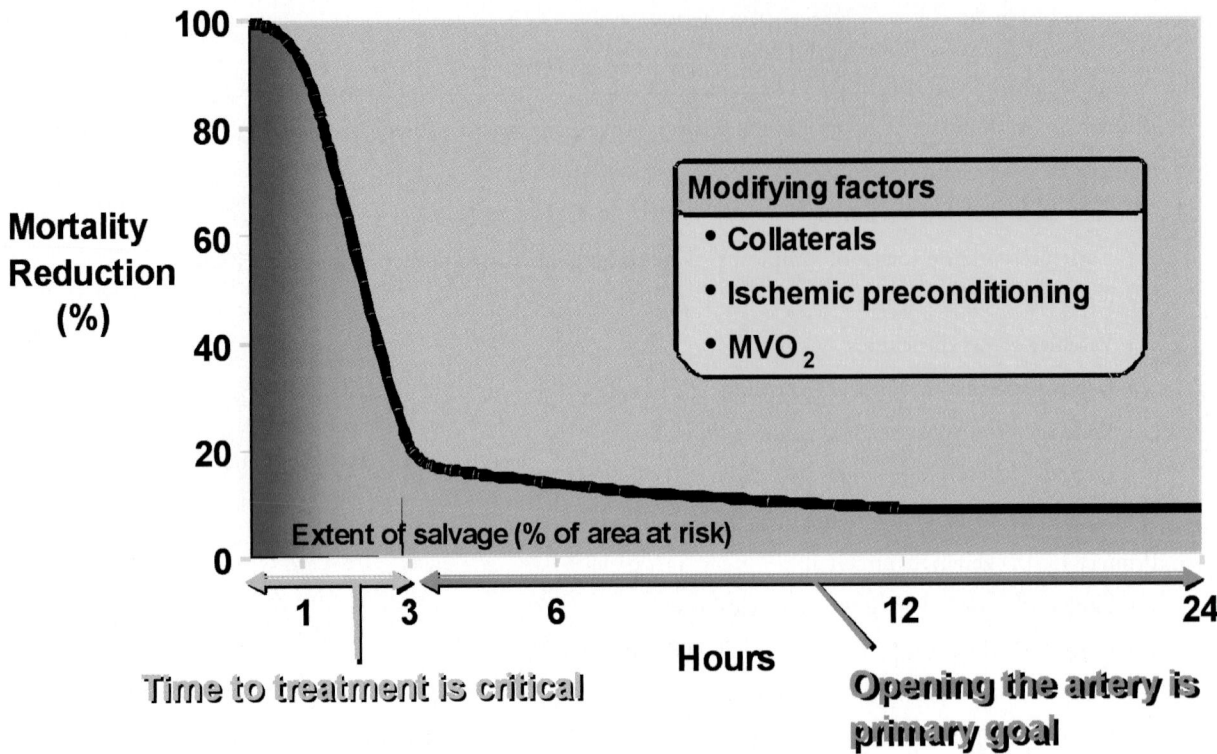

Fig. 1. Relationship between mortality reduction and myocardial salvage

exceed 60 minutes, then consideration should be given to fibrinolysis as the preferred approach.

For patients who present with symptom duration greater than 3 hours, then time-to-reperfusion is less important and opening the artery becomes the primary goal. Primary PCI is the best option and should be pursued as quickly as possible for all patients, except when transfer to a PCI-capable and available facility is not possible, inclement weather prohibits transport, transport distances are extremely long (exceeds 2 hours), or severe peripheral arterial disease precludes vascular access. In these scenarios, fibrinolysis confers some benefit for symptom duration of 3 to 12 hours.

With regard to the observed delays in time to reperfusion, there are two categories for delays. The first delay is patient-dependent—namely, patient awareness of the signs and symptoms of a heart attack and patient activation of the healthcare system. This delay regrettably remains on average 2 to 3 hours and has not changed significantly in recent years. The second delay is hospital-dependent—namely the delays in

processes and systems for delivering reperfusion treatment effectively and efficiently.

Patient risk profiling is the last piece of the puzzle for selecting the best reperfusion strategy. Patients at high clinical risk (including the elderly with age ≥75, in cardiogenic shock, with Killip class ≥3, with pulmonary edema, or with anterior wall infarction) should be immediately transferred for primary PCI. An invasive approach also enables hemodynamic support with assist devices. However, if duration of symptoms <3 hours and there are no bleeding risks, then fibrinolysis may be preferred if transport delay exceeds 60 minutes; conversely, primary PCI may be preferred if transport delay is less than 60 minutes.

MAYO CLINIC FRAMEWORK FOR SELECTING REPERFUSION

In Figure 2 and Table 3, we present an evidence-based and simple framework utilized at Mayo Clinic, Rochester, Minnesota to enable physicians to rapidly select the optimal reperfusion strategy for STEMI. The framework is based upon available clinical trial data integrated with local circumstances by incorporating duration of symptoms ("fixed" ischemia time) and anticipated transport delays to a PCI capable and available facility ("incurred" ischemia time).

FUTURE DIRECTIONS

Primary PCI is preferred if DTB time is <90 minutes or if the difference between DTB and DTN is <60 minutes. These very short DTB times were achieved in the DANAMI-2 trial. Are these DTB times achievable in current clinical practice in the United States? A report from the NRMI 3/4 registry (Third and Fourth National Registry Myocardial Infarction) showed that for patients who required interhospital transfer for primary PCI, the median DTB was 180 minutes and only 4.2% of patients achieved a DTB <90 minutes. A delay on the order of 180 minutes would negate the potential benefits of primary PCI in STEMI patients who present early (duration of symptoms < 3 hours) when "time is heart muscle." Hence, there is still a role for fibrinolysis in STEMI patients who present early and face transfer delays to a PCI-capable and available facility.

Future priorities for investigations should focus on what "total time delay" is acceptable for DTB before fibrinolysis should be recommended and what strategies can effectively shorten symptom onset-to-balloon time and DTB. One potential tactic is "earlier diagnosis of STEMI" including:

1. Pre-hospital electrocardiogram acquisition and ambulance triage directly to catheterization lab and bypassing the emergency room.
2. Earlier patient activation of the system thru increased awareness of signs and symptoms of acute myocardial infarction.

A second tactic is "earlier treatment after diagnosis" including:

1. Systems and networks to expedite transfer to a PCI-capable and available facility.
2. Developing programs for primary PCI at hospitals with a catheterization lab, but without on-site surgical backup.

■ Fixed ischemia time is the time from the onset of ischemic symptoms to clinical presentation (first medical contact)

■ Incurred ischemia time is transport time from clinical presentation to treatment

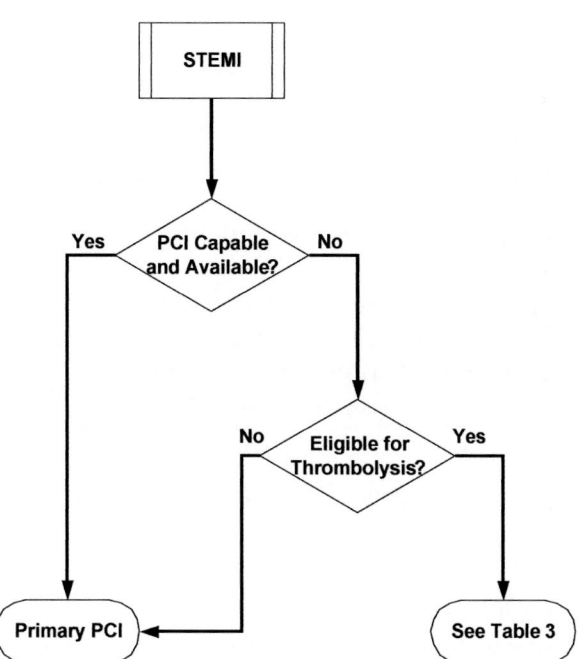

Fig. 2. Selection of reperfusion strategy.

Table 3. Framework for Selecting Reperfusion Strategy

	Duration from onset of symptoms	
Transport time	<3 hours	>3 hours
<30 minutes	Primary PCI	Primary PCI
30-60 minutes	Fibrinolysis	Primary PCI
>60 minutes	Fibrinolysis	Primary PCI
		or
		Fibrinolysis

MAYO FAST TRACK STEMI PROTOCOL FOR REGIONAL HOSPITALS WITHOUT ON-SITE PRIMARY PCI FACILITIES

Patient with New ST Elevation Myocardial Infarction or New LBBB*

Step 1:	**Immediate 12-lead electrocardiogram** and brief history & physical examination
Step 2:	Call Mayo Emergency Department referral nurse who will arrange transport and phone consultation with Mayo Cardiologist
Step 3:	Fax ECG to Mayo Coronary Care Unit

Aspirin 325 mg (four 81 mg non-enteric coated chewable tablets)

Nitroglycerin SL or IV PRN chest pain

Cardiac Monitor

Minimum of (2) peripheral IVs

Choose
one Pathway

   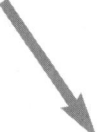

If Onset of Symptoms <3 Hours,	**If Onset of Symptoms >3 Hours,**
Thrombolysis	**Percutaneous Coronary Intervention**
Give full dose **TNK or rPA**	Do <u>not</u> give **TNK or rPA**
Unfractionated Heparin loading dose, 60 Units/kg IV (maximum 4,000 Units) **Heparin infusion**, 12 Units/kg/hour IV (maximum 1,000 Units/hour)	**Unfractionated Heparin loading dose,** 60 Units/kg IV (maximum 4,000 Units) **Heparin infusion**, 12 Units/kg/hour IV (maximum 1,000 Units/hour)
Metoprolol (Lopressor) 5mg IV every 5 minutes, hold if BP<100, HR<60	**Metoprolol (Lopressor)** 5mg IV every 5 minutes, hold if BP<100, HR<60
Give **Clopidogrel (Plavix)** 75mg	†Do <u>not</u> give **Clopidogrel (Plavix)**
Patient transferred to Mayo CCU. Cath Lab is <u>not</u> activated, unless patient arrives at CCU and failed to reperfuse with thrombolytic. Do <u>not</u> give **Eptifibatide (Integrilin)**	Patient will be transferred to Mayo Cardiac Lab directly. Cardiac Lab is activated. Consider giving **Eptifibatide (Integrilin)** on route by Mayo Helicopter Transport Team.

Labs to be drawn and results faxed to Mayo Coronary Care Unit CK-MB, Troponin, CBC, Electrolytes, BUN, Creatinine, Glucose, INR, PTT, Portable chest x-ray.

*New left bundle branch block in the setting of clinical symptoms of myocardial infarction.

†It is clinical practice in many medical centers to give clopidogrel to all patients presenting with acute coronary syndromes. It is our practice to wait until the coronary anatomy is visualized for patients in the PCI pathway. The logic of this approach is to avoid the added bleeding risk associated with clopidogrel in patients that require emergency CABG.

DEFINITION FOR STEMI

1. ECG demonstrates ST elevation greater than 0.1 mV in at least 2 contiguous precordial leads (V1-V6) or at least 2 adjacent limb leads
2. ECG demonstrates new LBBB
3. Reperfusion therapy is indicated if the ECG is diagnostic for STEMI even if the patient is free of symptoms
4. If initial ECG is not diagnostic but clinical suspicion is high for STEMI, obtain serial ECG at 5- to 10-minute intervals

ABSOLUTE CONTRAINDICATIONS FOR THROMBOLYSIS IN STEMI

1. Any prior intracranial hemorrhage
2. Known structural cerebral vascular lesion (e.g., arteriovenous malformation)
3. Known malignant intracranial neoplasm (primary or metastatic)
4. Ischemic stroke within 3 months except acute ischemic stroke within 3 hours
5. Suspected aortic dissection
6. Active bleeding or bleeding diathesis (excluding menses)
7. Significant closed-head or facial trauma within 3 months

RELATIVE CONTRAINDICATIONS FOR THROMBOLYSIS IN STEMI

1. History of chronic, severe, poorly controlled hypertension
2. Severe uncontrolled hypertension on presentation (SBP >180 mm Hg or DBP >110 mm Hg)
3. History of prior ischemic stroke >3 months, dementia, or known intracranial pathology not covered in contraindications
4. Traumatic or prolonged CPR (>10 minutes) or major surgery (within last 3 weeks)
5. Recent internal bleeding (within last 2-4 weeks)
6. Noncompressible vascular punctures
7. For streptokinase/anistreplase: prior exposure (>5 days ago) or prior allergic reaction to these agents
8. Pregnancy
9. Active peptic ulcer
10. Current use of anticoagulants: the higher the INR, the higher the risk of bleeding

CONTRAINDICATIONS FOR EPTIFIBATIDE

1. A history of bleeding diathesis or evidence of active abnormal bleeding within the previous 30 days
2. Severe hypertension (SBP >200 mm Hg or DBP >110 mm Hg) not adequately controlled on antihypertensive therapy
3. Major surgery within the preceding 6 weeks
4. History of stroke within 30 days or any history of hemorrhagic stroke
5. Dependency on renal dialysis

Mayo Acute Coronary Syndrome (Non-ST Elevation MI) Protocol

Step 1:   Patient presents with angina or anginal equivalent symptoms that occurred at rest or are new and/or crescendo.

Immediate 12-lead Electrocardiogram, Troponin and CK-MB—Use STEMI protocol if patients has new ST elevation MI or new LBBB

Brief history and physical examination

Routine labs (electrolytes, BUN, creatinine, glucose, CBC, PT, PTT)

Step 2:   <u>USE</u> **INVASIVE PATHWAY** for patients who are candidates for cardiac catheterization and have any of the following features:

(1) Elevated cardiac biomarker (Troponin and/or CK-MB)

(2) New or transient ST depression

(3) New or transient deep symmetric T wave inversions in V1-V4

<u>CONSIDER</u> **ROUTINE PATHWAY** for patients without above features

Step 3:   • Keep patient **fasting** except for medications

• Cardiac monitoring and supplemental oxygen

• Treat hypertension, heart failure, and ventricular arrhythmias as appropriate

• **Medications** for all patients without contraindications:

(1) **Aspirin** 325 mg (four 81 mg non-enteric coated chewable tablets)

(2) **Nitroglycerin** SL or IV PRN chest pain

(3) **Metoprolol (Lopressor)** 25 mg PO ×1 or 5 mg IV every 5 min ×3 (Hold metoprolol if HR <60, Systolic BP <100, wheezing on exam, CHF, or cardiogenic shock)

(4) **Unfractionated Heparin loading dose**, 60 Units/kg IV (maximum 4,000 Units)
Unfractionated Heparin infusion, 12 Units/kg/hour IV (maximum 1,000 Units/hour)

(5) *Do not give **Clopidogrel (Plavix)** (unless patient is allergic to aspirin, then give clopidogrel 300 mg)

Choose
a Pathway

<u>Invasive Pathway</u>	<u>Routine Pathway</u>
Eptifibatide (Integrilin) loading dose	Do *not* give **Eptifibatide (Integrilin)**
180 mcg/kg bolus ×1	
Eptifibatide (Integrilin) infusion	Obtain serial ECG and cardiac biomarkers every 8 hrs
2 mcg/kg/min if Cr Clearance ≥50 mL/min	Consider other causes of chest discomfort (i.e., dissection,
1 mcg/kg/min if Cr Clearance <50 mL/min	pulmonary embolism, etc. ...)
See contraindications	Stress test if indicated
Urgent transfer for early cardiac catheterization	If patient subsequently has recurrent pain, ECG
and revascularization with PCI or CABG as indicated	changes, elevated biomarkers, or positive stress test,
	then consider invasive pathway

*It is clinical practice in many medical centers to give clopidogrel to all patients presenting with acute coronary syndromes. It is our practice to wait until the coronary anatomy is visualized. The logic of this approach is to avoid the added bleeding risk associated with clopidrogel in patients that require emergency CABG.

TIMI RISK SCORE:

    (1) Age ≥65

    (2) ≥3 cardiac risk factors (Cholesterol, Family History of Premature CAD, Hypertention, Diabetes Mellitus, Active Smoker)

    (3) Known CAD with stenosis >50% on prior cath

    (4) Aspirin use in past 7 days

    (5) >2 episodes of angina in past 24 hours

    (6) Elevated cardiac biomarkers

    (7) New or transient ST segment deviation

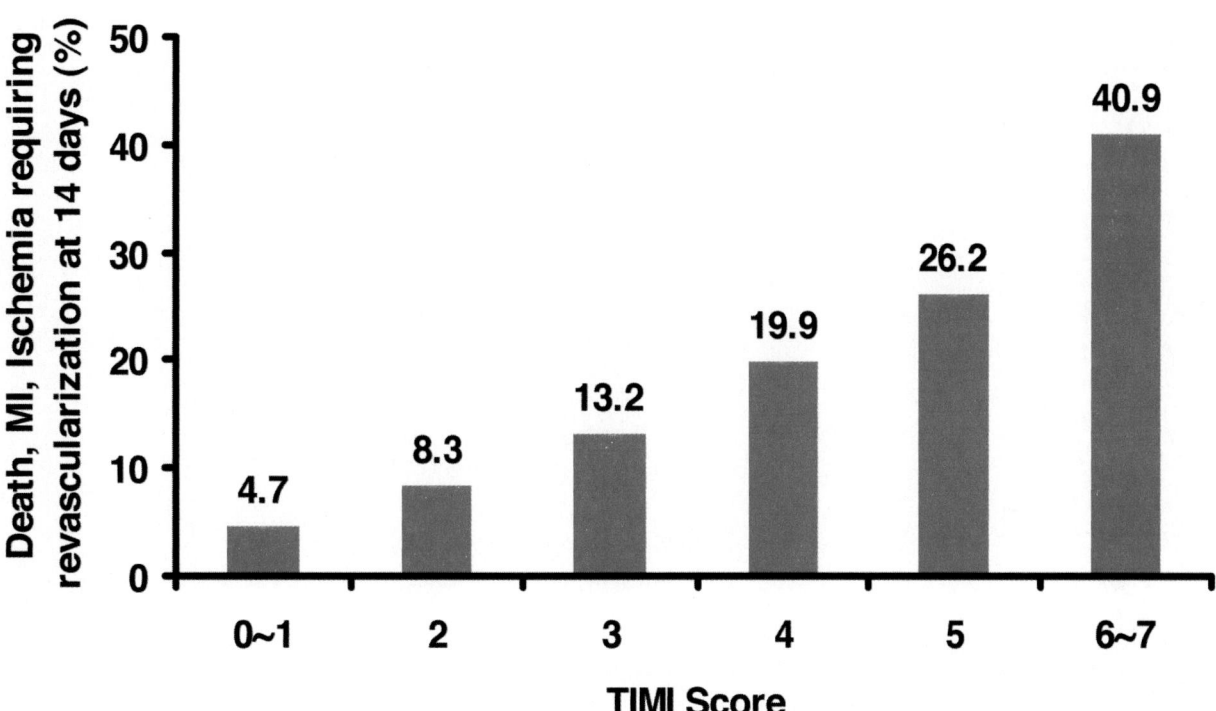

ESTIMATED CREATININE CLEARANCE CALCULATION:

    (1) Male: $\text{Cr Cl} = \dfrac{(140 - \text{age in years}) \times \text{weight in kg}}{(72 \times \text{serum creatinine in mg/dL})}$

    (2) Female: Cr Cl = 0.85 × above formula for males

CONTRAINDICATIONS FOR EPTIFIBATIDE (INTEGRILIN):

    (1) A history of bleeding diathesis or evidence of active abnormal bleeding within the previous 30 days

    (2) Severe hypertension (SBP >200 mm Hg or DBP >110 mm Hg) not adequately controlled on antihypertensive therapy

    (3) Major surgery within the preceding 6 weeks

    (4) History of stroke within 30 days or any history of hemorrhagic stroke

    (5) Dependency on renal dialysis

    (6) Platelet count <100,000

FIBRINOLYTIC TRIALS IN ACUTE MYOCARDIAL INFARCTION

Patricia J. M. Best, MD

Bernard J. Gersh, MB, ChB, DPhil

Joseph G. Murphy, MD

Reperfusion therapy is a critical part of the emergency treatment of acute myocardial infarction, and its use has resulted in a dramatic reduction in both the morbidity and mortality of myocardial infarction over the past 20 years. Nonetheless, reperfusion therapy is markedly underutilized, particularly in subsets of patients at higher risk such as the elderly. A choice now exists between the use of intravenous fibrinolytic therapy or primary percutaneous coronary intervention (PCI) for reperfusion therapy. However, because primary PCI is not available at most hospitals, fibrinolytic therapy remains the mainstay of coronary reperfusion therapy in most countries around the world. Prompt use of fibrinolytic therapy is associated with a marked reduction in mortality and reduces left ventricular failure and subsequent congestive heart failure. Hesitancy with the use of fibrinolytic therapy comes from a lack of a clear understanding of the appropriate guidelines for its utilization and a lack of knowledge of which patients are appropriate, the bleeding risk, and the risk/benefit ratio for patients, particularly those at highest risk.

THROMBOSIS IN THE MECHANISM OF AN ACUTE MYOCARDIAL INFARCTION

The cause of an ST-segment elevation myocardial infarction (STEMI) in most patients is rupture of an atheromatous plaque that leads to occlusive intracoronary thrombus formation. It was not until 1980 that the role of thrombosis as the cause, as opposed to the consequence, of an acute myocardial infarction was unequivocally established despite the initial observations of Herrick in 1912 suggesting thrombus as a putative cause. In animal models of an acute myocardial infarction, ischemic myocardial necrosis proceeds in a "wave front" manner, spreading from the subendocardium to the epicardium. This process begins 20 minutes after acute coronary occlusion and involves most of the myocardial wall within 6 hours. In humans, the time to complete myocardial infarction is variable, affected by the presence or absence of collateral vessels to the ischemic territory, ischemic preconditioning of the myocardium, and the occurrence of intervening periods of spontaneous reperfusion.

PRINCIPLES OF FIBRINOLYSIS

Fibrinolytic agents were first used in the treatment of an acute myocardial infarction in 1958 and gained wide acceptance in the 1980s after several prospective, randomized, controlled trials showed a clear mortality benefit. The single most important predictor of benefit for those treated with fibrinolytic therapy is the time from the vessel occlusion to the restoration of normal

Appendix for clinical trial names is at end of chapter.

coronary blood flow (Fig. 1). Fibrinolytic therapy is equally effective regardless of gender. This therapy is also beneficial for individuals with advanced age, resulting in a significant reduction in the higher mortality attendant in the elderly, but at an increased risk of intracranial hemorrhage. Patients who benefit the most from fibrinolytic therapy are those with an anterior STEMI, diabetes, or the presence of tachycardia. Early administration of fibrinolytic therapy results in the greatest benefit, especially in those who receive therapy within 1 to 3 hours of the onset of symptoms. Intracoronary administration of fibrinolytic therapy was initially thought to be superior to systemic administration, but systemic administration is now considered the clinical delivery method of choice. This is primarily because of the time delay for intracoronary cannulation, and now when cardiac catheterization is performed, primary PCI is the preferred treatment option.

All patients with an acute STEMI presenting within 12 hours of the onset of chest pain should be considered for fibrinolytic therapy or alternatively for primary PCI, if cardiac catheterization facilities and trained interventional staff are available within an expected door-to-balloon time of less than 90 minutes (Table 1). Benefit from fibrinolytic therapy may occur out to 12 hours from the onset of symptoms. However, the greater the time duration from the onset of symptoms, the lower the benefit with reperfusion therapy. The absolute benefit of fibrinolytic therapy is less for

inferior STEMI, except for patients with an inferior STEMI associated with a right ventricular infarction (or anterior ST-segment depression indicative of a greater territory at risk). Therefore, in low-risk patients at increased risk of bleeding complications with fibrinolytic therapy, careful assessment of the risk/benefit ratio needs to be undertaken. Factors associated with a higher risk of intracranial hemorrhage are older age, low body mass index, hypertension, and female gender. Recommendations for treatment with fibrinolytic therapy and contraindications for use have been determined by the American College of Cardiology and American Heart Association (ACC/AHA) (Tables 2 and 3). Fastidious use of these guidelines would result in more patients treated, since currently there is significant under-utilization of fibrinolytic therapy.

MORTALITY TRIALS OF FIBRINOLYTICS IN ACUTE MYOCARDIAL INFARCTION

Several landmark studies (GISSI-1 and ISIS-2) showed convincing beneficial effects of fibrinolytic therapy in patients with an acute myocardial infarction. These beneficial effects were also found in multiple subpopulations at higher risk, including the elderly, diabetics, and patients with a previous myocardial infarction. In spite of the increased fibrinolysis complication risk in these patients, overall they have an equivalent or greater benefit with fibrinolytic therapy. Diabetic patients, because of their increased risks associated with the myocardial infarction, derive greater benefit overall than nondiabetic patients.

The Fibrinolytic Therapy Trialists' Collaborative Group presented the data of nine trials of fibrinolytic therapy, which included 58,600 patients who received therapy. Overall mortality was 10.5%, with a 1% risk of stroke and a 0.7% risk of major noncerebral bleeding. Overall, there was an 18% reduction in mortality with the use of fibrinolytic therapy and an approximately 25% reduction in mortality for patients who presented with a STEMI or left bundle branch block.

Patients with a STEMI or new-onset left bundle branch block benefit the most from fibrinolysis. Patients with a non-STEMI and unstable angina do not benefit from fibrinolysis and there is a trend toward harm. Patients with cardiogenic shock respond poorly to fibrinolysis, probably because of poor penetration of the fibrinolytic

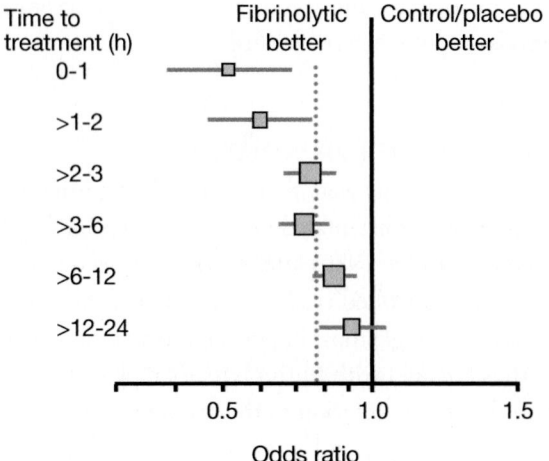

Fig. 1. Proportional effect of fibrinolytic therapy on 35-day mortality according to treatment delay in a meta-analysis of 22 trials (50,246 patients).

agent into the occlusive thrombus and the lack of adequate coronary perfusion pressure, in the setting of severe hypotension, which is needed to prevent recurrent thrombosis and maintain vessel patency. Cardiogenic shock is a strong indication for primary PCI.

Included in this chapter are a select number of the most important clinical fibrinolytic trials that have advanced the treatment of acute myocardial infarction. Fibrinolytic trials are frequently classified by sponsoring organizations (e.g., GISSI, ISIS, TIMI, ECSG, TAMI, GUSTO-1 and MITI).

GISSI

The GISSI trial (or GISSI-1 trial) was the first study that reported the benefit of intravenous streptokinase in 11,816 patients with chest pain accompanied by ST-segment elevation or depression of 1 mm or more in any limb lead or of 2 mm or more in 1 or more of the precordial leads treated within 12 hours of symptom

onset. There was a 17% reduction in mortality at 21 days and at 1 year in patients with STEMI treated within 6 hours of infarction with streptokinase. Early administration resulted in better outcomes, with a mortality reduction at 21 days of 47% if the patient was treated within 1 hour from the onset of chest pain, 23% if within 1 to 3 hours, and 17% if treated within 3 to 6 hours of symptom onset. At 1 year there was still a significant reduction in mortality with earlier treatment (64%, 15%, and 17%, respectively). The overall 21-day mortality was 10.7% in the group treated with streptokinase and 13% in the placebo group. The 1-year mortality was 17.2% in the streptokinase group and 19% in the placebo group (P<0.01). A follow-up to this study demonstrated that the initial mortality benefit was maintained at 10 years. There was no significant

---

Table 1.   Reperfusion Strategy for STEMI

Fibrinolysis usually preferred
- *Early presentation*: ≤3 hours from symptom onset, and primary PCI will have a door-to-balloon time ≥90 min
- *Primary PCI is not an option*: because a catheterization laboratory is not available or is occupied, vascular access difficulties, or lack of access to a skilled PCI laboratory with an operator with >75 PCI cases/y and a team with ≥36 primary PCI cases/y
- *Delay to invasive strategy*: where the transport time is prolonged or there is a >1-hour delay from the door-to-needle time compared with the door-to-balloon time

PCI usually preferred
- *Skilled PCI laboratory is available with surgical backup*: where the door-to-balloon time is expected to be <90 min
- *High risk from STEMI*: Cardiogenic shock or Killip class ≥3
- *Contraindications to fibronolysis*
- *Late presentation*: the symptom onset ≥3 hours
- *Diagnosis of STEMI is in doubt*

PCI, percutaneous coronary intervention; STEMI, ST-segment elevation myocardial infarction.

Table 2.   Indications for Fibrinolytic Therapy

Class I (in the absence of contraindications)
1. Administration to STEMI patients with symptom onset ≤12 hours and ST-elevation >0.1 mV in ≥2 contiguous precordial leads or ≥2 adjacent limb leads
2. STEMI patients with symptom onset ≤12 hours and new or presumably new left bundle branch block

Class IIa (in the absence of contraindications)
1. STEMI patients with symptom onset ≤12 hours and a 12-lead electrocardiogram finding consistent with a true posterior myocardial infarction
2. Symptoms of a STEMI beginning within the prior 12-24 hours with continuing ischemic symptoms and ST-elevation >0.1 mV in ≥2 contiguous precordial leads or ≥2 adjacent limb leads

Class III
1. Fibrinolytic therapy should not be administered to asymptomatic patients whose initial symptoms of STEMI began >24 hours earlier.
2. Fibrinolytic therapy should not be administered to patients whose 12-lead electrocardiogram show only ST-segment depression unless a true posterior myocardial infarction is suspected

STEMI, ST-segment elevation myocardial infarction.

Table 3.   Contraindications to Fibrinolytic
             Therapy

Absolute
- Any prior intracranial hemorrhage
- Structural cerebrovascular abnormality such as an arteriovenous malformation
- Known intracranial malignant lesion
- Ischemic stroke within 3 months (except acute stroke ≤3 hours)
- Aortic dissection
- Active bleeding or bleeding diathesis except menses)
- Significant closed head or facial trauma (≤3 months)

Relative
- History of chronic severely controlled hypertension
- Systolic blood pressure >180 mm Hg or diastolic blood pressure >110 mm Hg on presentation
- Prior ischemic stroke (≥3 months)
- Dementia
- Intracranial pathology
- Traumatic or prolonged (>10 min) cardiopulmonary resuscitation
- Major surgery (<3 weeks)
- Internal bleeding (<2-4 weeks)
- Noncompressible vascular punctures
- For streptokinase/anistreplase: prior exposure or prior allergic reaction to these agents
- Pregnancy
- Active peptic ulcer
- Current use of anticoagulants

mortality benefit in patients with ST-segment depression or in those treated later than 6 hours.

GISSI-2

The GISSI-2 trial was one of the great head-to-head trials of streptokinase and tissue plasminogen activator (t-PA). It compared intravenous streptokinase with t-PA with or without heparin in 12,490 patients admitted within 6 hours after the onset of chest pain. There were no significant differences in the mortality rate, rate of reinfarction, stroke rate, or the incidence of post infarction angina. Subcutaneous heparin had no added benefit on mortality, heart failure, or ventricular function, but it increased bleeding complications.

LATE

In 5,711 patients presenting 6 to 24 hours after the onset of symptoms and electrocardiographic criteria consistent with an acute myocardial infarction randomized to alteplase (t-PA) or placebo, this study demonstrated a trend toward a reduction in death with alteplase (8.86% vs. 10.31%) at 35 days. In patients with symptom onset less than 12 hours, there was a significant reduction in mortality with alteplase (8.90% vs. 11.97%).

ISIS-1

ISIS-1 is a trial of β-adrenergic blockade without fibrinolysis in more than 16,000 patients. Mortality decreased with atenolol in patients with a suspected myocardial infarction who were treated within 12 hours of presentation.

ISIS-2

The ISIS-2 trial compared aspirin and streptokinase and the combination using a 2 × 2 design. It tested four regimens (streptokinase 1.5 million units over 1 hour, aspirin 162.5 mg daily for 1 month, a combination of the two, or placebo) in more than 17,000 patients 24 hours or less after the onset of a myocardial infarction. Aspirin and streptokinase both independently reduced mortality and had a synergistic benefit when used together without increasing the stroke risk, and this benefit was still present at 1 year. The combination of streptokinase and aspirin reduced mortality by 53% when administered within 4 hours of symptom onset and by 38% when administered within 12 to 24 hours of the infarction.

TIMI trials

The TIMI trials were a large series of trials that initially looked at the efficacy of small t-PA (TIMI 1-4), but later hirudin (TIMI 5-9B), tenecteplase (TIMI 10A-10B), enoxaparin (11A to 11B, 23, 25, 28), glycoprotein IIb/IIIa inhibitors (TIMI 12, 14, 15, 16, 18, 20, 24), and prehospital fibrinolysis (TIMI 19). This group also determined the classification of coronary blood flow status by angiography (Table 4).

TIMI-1

Use of recombinant t-PA (rt-PA) resulted in more rapid myocardial infarction reperfusion with streptokinase when assessed angiographically. There was no added benefit in mortality or ejection fraction with rt-PA than with streptokinase. Bleeding complications were similar in both groups. At 90 minutes after thrombolysis, TIMI 2 or 3 coronary flow reperfusion rates were 60% with rt-PA and 35% with streptokinase (*P*<0.001). At 21 days, mortality was 4% with rt-PA and 5% with streptokinase (*P* not significant [NS]).

TIMI-2

In patients who received rt-PA, heparin, and aspirin for an acute myocardial infarction, an invasive strategy of percutaneous coronary angioplasty (PTCA) within 18 to 48 hours of the infarction was of no added benefit over a conservative strategy of only PTCA in patients with spontaneous or exercise-induced myocardial ischemia. There was no difference at 6 weeks or 1 year in mortality or reinfarction rates. Death and nonfatal reinfarction at 1 year were 14.7% and 15.2%, respectively, in the invasive and conservative treatment groups (NS).

TIMI-2A

The TIMI-2A trial differed from the TIMI-2 trial by the addition of an immediate PTCA group (<2 hours after rt-PA administration). This approach was compared with the delayed invasive strategy of PTCA within 18 to 48 hours of rt-PA administration and a conservative arm of PTCA for spontaneous or exercise-induced myocardial ischemia. The conservative strategy was equally effective as the invasive arm when judged according to the predismissal vessel patency, ejection fraction, and 1-year mortality and reinfarction rates.

ECSG Trial

The ECSG trials 1 through 6 analyzed infarct artery patency with t-PA and various conjunctive therapies,

Table 4. TIMI Classification of Coronary Blood Flow

TIMI-0, no antegrade flow
TIMI-1, partial penetration of contrast past the point of occlusion
TIMI-2, opacification but delayed filling of the distal vessel
TIMI-3, normal flow

including PTCA and heparin. The overall conclusion of these studies was that infarct patency with t-PA was superior to that with streptokinase (ECSG-1), heparin improved patency (ECSG-6), and routine PTCA was detrimental (ECSG-4).

TAMI

The TAMI trial consisted of 10 studies (TAMI 1-9 and TAMI-UK) on the efficacy of t-PA, urokinase, and adjunctive therapies (including fluosol, prostacyclin, and glycoprotein IIb/IIIa inhibitors) in acute myocardial infarction. The TAMI-1 trial evaluated the role of immediate PTCA in addition to t-PA in acute infarction and reported no advantage over delayed PTCA.

GUSTO-1

The GUSTO-1 trial randomly assigned 41,021 patients to different thrombolysis regimens to test the hypothesis that early and sustained patency of infarct-related vessel would improve survival in patients with an evolving myocardial infarction. This study reported that rapid restoration of coronary blood flow with t-PA was associated with an improved survival and a 14% reduction in mortality at 30 days when compared with streptokinase and intravenous or subcutaneous heparin. Accelerated t-PA was also associated with a significantly higher incidence of hemorrhagic stroke when compared with streptokinase. For overall benefit, as assessed from the combined end point of total mortality and disabling stroke, t-PA was significantly better than streptokinase with higher risk patients having the greatest benefit. The summary of the GUSTO-1 trial suggested that accelerated t-PA and intravenous heparin resulted in a lower mortality than streptokinase combined with either subcutaneous or intravenous heparin. A secondary finding was that patients with cardiogenic shock benefited from emergency PTCA. The angiographic substudy of GUSTO-1 showed that the 1-year mortality rates favored t-PA (9.1% vs. 10.1% for streptokinase) combined with either intravenous or subcutaneous heparin (*P*≤0.01).

GUSTO-2B Angiographic Substudy Trial

The GUSTO-2B Angiographic Substudy trial was a head-to-head comparison of primary PTCA and fibrinolysis. Primary PTCA was found to be an excellent alternative to thrombolysis in skilled hands and had a small short-term advantage over thrombolysis with t-PA.

GUSTO-3

The GUSTO-3 trial was a head-to-head trial of 2 forms of rt-PA, alteplase, and reteplase (a longer acting mutant variety of alteplase). This study included more than 15,000 patients with STEMI or new left bundle branch block myocardial infarction who presented within 6 hours of symptoms onset. The results with both agents were almost identical. Mortality at 30 days was 7.22% with alteplase and 7.43% with reteplase (NS), and the incidence of hemorrhagic stroke was 0.88% and 0.91%, respectively (NS).

INJECT

In the INJECT trial, 6,010 patients were randomly assigned to receive either 1.5 million units of streptokinase or 2 boluses of 10 units of reteplase (rt-PA) 30 minutes part. Aspirin and intravenous heparin were also given. The 35-day mortality rates were 9% for rt-PA and 9.5% for streptokinase (NS). Mortality at 6 months was 11% and 12.5%, respectively (NS). Hypotension and allergic reactions were more common in the streptokinase group, and there was a small, non-statistically significant excess in nonfatal in-hospital strokes in the rt-PA group.

These studies and others comparing different fibrinolytic agents demonstrated that alteplase, retaplase, and tenecteplase (TNK-t-PA) have fairly similar efficacy in the treatment of acute STEMI. Some differences in the properties of these agents (Table 5), such as the availability of bolus therapy, make retaplase and tenecteplase easier to use and therefore are used more commonly. Streptokinase is slightly less effective than the t-PA agents, but with a lower bleeding risk, and may therefore be an appropriate choice in patients with a lower risk from the STEMI.

ADJUNCTIVE THERAPY WITH FIBRINOLYSIS

Aspirin

The ISIS-2 study provided the strongest evidence that aspirin reduces mortality in STEMI patients. This benefit of aspirin therapy was additive to the benefit of fibrinolytic therapy and did not increase the risk of stroke or intracranial hemorrhage. In an acute STEMI, aspirin reduces mortality by 23% and reocclusion rate by 50%. Therefore, all patients presenting with an STEMI who were not previously receiving aspirin should be given 162 to 325 mg of non–enteric-coated aspirin. Subsequent to this, they should receive 75 to 162 mg of aspirin daily to minimize their bleeding risk.

Oxygen

Because many patients with an uncomplicated myocardial infarction may have mild hypoxemia, possibly because of ventilation perfusion mismatch or pulmonary congestion, oxygen by nasal canula has become part of standard therapy for all patients with a myocardial infarction. Although there is a general recommendation for the use of oxygen, there is little in the way of hard evidence to support its use.

Nitrates

Nitrates are part of standard therapy for patients with an acute myocardial infarction who are experiencing continued pain. Nitrates have multiple effects that may be beneficial, including the reduction of preload and afterload through peripheral arterial venous dilatation, improved coronary blood flow through the vasorelaxation of epicardial coronary arteries, and dilatation of collateral vessels. However, no studies have shown a survival benefit associated with the routine use of nitrates in patients with an acute myocardial infarction (GISSI-3, ISIS-4), and as such they should not be used routinely in all patients. Nevertheless, nitrates are helpful for managing ongoing ischemic pain, congestive heart failure, pulmonary edema, hypertension, and significant mitral regurgitation. However, the use of nitrates must be carefully monitored, especially in the patient who is volume depleted since nitrates may induce hypotension and exacerbate ischemia.

β-Blockers

The effects of β-blockers include a reduction in the cardiac index, heart rate, and blood pressure with an overall reduction in myocardial oxygen consumption. β-Blockers also diminish circulating levels of free fatty acids by blocking the effects of catecholamines on lipolysis, and these free fatty acids augment myocardial oxygen consumption and potentially increase the incidence of arrhythmias.

Table 5. Comparison of Approved Fibrinolytic Agents

	Streptokinase	Alteplase	Reteplase	Tenecteplase-t-PA
Dose	1.5 MU in 30-60 min	Up to 100 mg in 90 min (based on weight)	10 U × 2 each over 2 min	30-50 mg based on weight
Bolus administration	No	No	Yes	Yes
Allergic reactions (especially hypotension)	Yes	No	No	No
Approximate 90-min patency rates, %	50	75	75	75
TIMI grade 3 flow, %	32	54	60	63

TIMI, Thrombolysis in Myocardial Infarction; t-PA, tissue plasminogen activator.

In the prefibrinolytic era, β-blockers resulted in about a 15% reduction in ventricular fibrillation, 15% to 30% reduction in infarct size, and 18% reduction in reinfarction and reoccurrence of myocardial ischemia during hospitalization, and in a summary of over 30 randomized trials involving over 29,000 patients β-blockers were associated with approximately a 13% relative reduction of death. However, the use of β-blockers is not without risk. There is a 3% incidence in the provocation of congestive heart failure or complete heart block and a 2% increase in the incidence of the development of cardiogenic shock.

The effects of β-blockers in conjunction with rt-PA were studied in the 1,431 patients in TIMI-2B. The patients were assigned to immediate metoprolol (intravenous followed by oral) or oral metoprolol starting at day 6 after a myocardial infarction, which did not improve overall mortality or resting ejection fraction at dismissal. There was a lower incidence of reinfarction (2.7% vs. 5.1%, $P = 0.02$) and recurrence of chest pain (18.8% vs. 24.1%, $P<0.02$) within 6 days with immediate metoprolol compared with delayed metoprolol, and there was a trend toward lower intracerebral hemorrhage in the immediate metoprolol group. However, 1-year mortality rates, reinfarction rates, and ventricular function were similar in both groups. The findings from TIMI-2B that immediate β-blocker therapy reduced intracerebral hemorrhage (ICH) was confirmed in the cohort of 60,329 patients from the

National Registry of Myocardial Infarction (NRMI)-2, in which immediate β-blocker therapy was associated with a 31% reduction in the ICH rate (odds ratio [OR] 0.69). The most contemporary study of the use of β-blockers was the COMMIT. In this 2 × 2 study, 45,852 patients suspected of an acute myocardial infarction received either metoprolol or placebo for 28 days or either clopidogrel or placebo for 28 days. In this study 54% of patients received fibrinolysis. Metoprolol therapy did not reduce the composite of death, reinfarction, or cardiac arrest, (9.4% vs. 9.9%). Metoprolol use was associated with lower reinfarction (2.0% vs. 2.5%, $P=0.001$) and ventricular fibrillation (2.5% vs. 3.0%, $P=0.001$) but at increased risk of cardiogenic shock (5.0% vs. 3.9%, $P<0.00001$). Thus, in the current era patients should be hemodynamically stabilized before initiation of β-blocker therapy because of the excessive risk in this population. However, in hemodynamically stable patients, β-blocker therapy is still beneficial.

Heparin

In the GUSTO-1 trial, the patency of the infarct-related artery was significantly higher at 5 to 7 days in patients receiving intravenous heparin (84% vs. 72%, $P=0.04$) after initial t-PA even though there was no difference in the patency rates at 90 minutes and 24 hours. These findings suggest that heparin can prevent reocclusion of the infarct-related artery in an acute STEMI. Currently, unfractionated heparin (UFH) is given routinely to patients receiving fibrinolytic therapy at a dose of 6 U/kg in a bolus (up to 4000 U) followed by 12 Units/kg per hour, up to 1,000 U/h to achieve an aPTT 1.5 to 2 times normal for all patients receiving alteplase, reteplase, or tenecteplase as their fibrinolytic. Patients with a nonselective fibrinolytic agent (such as streptokinase, anistreplase, or urokinase) and who are at high risk for systemic emboli, such as those with a large or anterior myocardial infarction, atrial fibrillation, a previous embolus or known left ventricular thrombus should also receive UFH. The routine use of heparin with streptokinase is less clear but could be considered.

Low-Molecular-Weight Heparin

Low-molecular-weight heparin (LMWH) is a class of depolymerized, fractionated heparinoid compounds that have anti-IIa and anti-Xa activities. The bioavailability is much higher for this class of compounds compared with UFH, with significantly less variability in activity. The incidence of heparin-associated thrombocytopenia and bleeding complications is also much less with these agents.

In the ExTRACT-TIMI 25 trial, 20,506 patients with STEMI receiving fibrinolysis were randomly assigned to enoxaparin throughout the hospitalization or UFH for at least 48 hours. Enoxaparin was associated with a lower incidence of death or nonfatal recurrent myocardial infarction through 30 days than UFH (9.9% vs. 12.0%), and major bleeding occurred in 2.1% receiving enoxaparin compared with 1.4% with UFH.

In the CLARITY—TIMI 28 trial, patients older than 75 years with an STEMI who received fibrinolysis were randomly assigned to low-molecular-weight heparin or UFH and were also randomized to clopidogrel or placebo. Treatment with LMWH was associated with a significantly lower rate of the composite end point of a closed infarct-related artery, death, or myocardial infarction before angiography (13.5% vs. 22.5%, adjusted OR 0.76, $P=0.027$), and a significantly lower rate of cardiovascular death or recurrent myocardial infarction through 30 days (6.9% vs. 11.5%, adjusted OR 0.68, $P=0.030$). Major bleeding rates (1.6% vs. 2.2%, $P=0.27$) and ICH (0.6% vs. 0.8%, $P=0.37$) were similar with both LMWH and UFH use.

In another study of 1,639 patients with STEMI treated with tenecteplase that were randomly assigned to enoxaparin or UFH, enoxaparin was associated with

a trend toward a reduced composite of 30-day mortality, in-hospital reinfarction, or in-hospital refractory ischemia (14.2% vs. 17.4%, $P=0.080$). There was an increased rate of stroke (2.9% vs. 1.3%, $P=0.026$) and ICH (2.20% vs. 0.97%, $P=0.047$) with enoxaparin, particularly in patients older than 75 years.

In the ASSENT-3 trial, 6,095 patients with acute myocardial infarction of less than 6 hours were randomly assigned one of three regimens: full-dose tenecteplase and enoxaparin, half-dose tenecteplase with weight-adjusted low-dose UFH and a 12-hour infusion of abciximab, or full-dose tenecteplase with weight-adjusted UFH for 48 hours. There were significantly fewer efficacy end points in the enoxaparin and abciximab groups than in the UFH group (11.4% vs. 15.4% for enoxaparin and 11.1% vs. 15.4% for abciximab).

Currently, LMWH might be considered as an acceptable alternative to UFH in those patients who are receiving fibrinolytic therapy and are younger than 65 years. LMWH should not be used as an alternative to UFH in patients receiving fibrinolytic therapy if they are older than 75 years or have significant chronic kidney disease (creatinine >2.5 mg/dL in men or >2.0 mg/dL in women). Enoxaparin can be given as a 30-mg intravenously (IV) bolus followed by 1.0 mg/kg subcutaneously every 12 hours until hospital discharge.

The Direct Thrombin Inhibitors (Hirudin and Bivalirudin)

The use of direct thrombin inhibitors decreases the rate of reinfarction by 25% to 30% compared with UFH. However, this benefit was observed primarily while the patient was receiving the thrombin inhibitor, and the magnitude of this difference decreased over time. In the TIMI-5 trial, which evaluated the benefit of hirudin compared with heparin as the adjunct to front-loaded rt-PA treatment of STEMI, hirudin was associated with a higher 18- to 36-hour vessel patency and a lower in-hospital reinfarction rate but at the price of more major hemorrhagic complications. In the TIMI-7 trial, there was no improvement in death, ventricular function, or severe congestive heart failure with hirudin use. The TIMI-9 trial showed that hirudin had no benefit over heparin in patients with an acute myocardial infarction treated with fibrinolysis. Additionally, the GUSTO-2A trial was a hirudin study that was stopped prematurely because of excessive bleeding, although a small benefit for hirudin was found over heparin in patients with a myocardial infarction. In the HERO trial of 412 patients presenting within 12 hours after an STEMI who were randomly assigned to receive streptokinase and heparin or streptokinase and low-dose hirulog (0.125 mg/kg bolus followed by 0.25 mg/kg per hour for 12 hours, then 0.125 mg/kg per hour) or streptokinase and high-dose hirulog (0.25 mg/kg bolus followed by 0.5 mg/kg per hour for 12 hours, then 0.25 mg/kg per hour) with a reduction in the major bleeding complications with hirulog (heparin: 28%; low-dose hirulog: 14%; high-dose hirulog: 19%; $P<0.01$ heparin vs. low-dose hirulog). TIMI-3 flow in the infarct-related artery at 90 to 120 minutes was 35% with heparin, 46% with low-dose hirulog, and 48% with high-dose hirulog (heparin vs. hirulog, $P=0.023$).

Both hirudin and bivalirudin (hirulog) are associated with higher rates of major bleeding when compared with heparin in those patients receiving t-PA fibrinolytic therapy. Currently, the guidelines support that the only patients in whom direct thrombin inhibitors are recommended are patients with heparin-induced thrombocytopenia. In these patients, the use of bivalirudin as an alternative to heparin may be considered. In this case, a bolus of 0.25 mg/kg followed by an IV infusion of 0.5 mg/kg per hour for the first 12 hours and 0.25 mg/kg per hour in the subsequent 36 hours has been used in previous trials with streptokinase. If this regimen is used, a reduction in the bivalirudin is necessary if the partial thromboplastin time is above 75 seconds within the first 12 hours. However, as in the HERO trial, the use of bivalirudin may be a safe and more effective alternative when streptokinase is used for fibrinolysis.

Angiotensin-Converting Enzyme Inhibitors
Angiotensin-converting enyme (ACE) inhibitors are well studied in several large randomized controlled trials involving patients with overt signs of heart failure (SAVE, AIRE, SMILE, and TRACE) and in asymptomatic patients (CONSENSUS-II, GISSI-3, ISIS-4, and Chinese Captopril Trial). In GISSI-3, which evaluated the effect of an ACE inhibitor (lisinopril), transdermal nitrate, or a combination in patients receiving fibrinolysis on left ventricular function in more than 18,000 patients after a myocardial infarction, the use of

lisinopril reduced mortality (6.3% vs. 7.1%) compared with the control group (no ACE inhibitor or nitrate, $P=0.03$) at 6 weeks and reduced the combined end point of death or severe left ventricular function at 6 months (18.1% vs. 19.3%, $P=0.03$). Nitrates were of no statistical benefit for the reduction of death or severe left ventricular dysfunction. In the ISIS-4 trial, in which 70% of 58,058 myocardial infarction patients received fibrinolysis, captopril, oral mononitrate, and IV magnesium, patients presented within 24 hours of symptom onset. Captopril reduced 5-week mortality by 7% ($P = 0.02$), but magnesium and oral nitrates had no mortality benefit. Importantly, in CONSENSUS II, in which 6,090 acute myocardial infarction patients were randomly assigned to receive IV enalapril or placebo within 24 hours of chest pain onset, patients showed no mortality benefit with enalapril at 6 months (10.2% placebo vs. 11.0% with enalapril) and actually trended toward greater risk with enalapril. Early hypotension was four times more likely with enalapril, demonstrating the importance of patients being hemodynamically stable before the initiation of ACE-inhibitor therapy.

Currently, ACE inhibitors should be administered to all STEMI patients in whom there is an anterior infarction, pulmonary congestion, or a left ventricular ejection fraction less than 40% in the absence of hypotension or known contraindications. An angiotensin receptor blocking agent can be administered in those who cannot tolerate ACE inhibitors. In other myocardial infarction and coronary artery disease patients, ACE inhibitors may also be beneficial, but the overall benefit is less.

Thienopyridines
Evidence now supports the use of clopidogrel 75 mg daily in the reduction of adverse events in patients who have received fibrinolytic therapy. (CLARITY-TIMI 28 study and COMMIT trials). In the COMMIT study of 45,852 myocardial infarction patients, 75 mg clopidogrel in addition to 162 mg aspirin continued up to 4 weeks resulted in a decreased incidence of death, reinfarction, or stroke (9.2% vs. 10.1%; $P=0.002$).

Glucose-Insulin-Potassium
The CREATE-ECLA trial included 20,201 STEMI patients who received glucose-insulin-potassium (GIK) IV infusion for 24 hours or usual care for shock; GIK

therapy had no effect on mortality, cardiac arrest, cardiogenic shock, and reinfarction. This definitive trial demonstrated that GIK therapy is not beneficial in STEMI patients and is therefore no longer used.

Glycoprotein IIb/IIIa Receptor Antagonist

These medications bind to platelet glycoprotein IIb/IIIa receptor sites and prevent platelet aggregation. Clinical trials with the combination of fibrinolytic agents with glycoprotein IIb/IIIa receptor antagonists have demonstrated improved patency rates of the infarct-related artery with their use. But virtually all have shown a higher risk of bleeding, and their use with full-dose fibrinolytics is not recommended. In the IMPACT-AMI trial using accelerated t-PA, aspirin, and heparin with eptifibatide, there was a greater incidence of TIMI-3 flow (66% vs. 39%, $P=0.006$) with the use of eptifibatide. PARADIGM was a three-part clinical trial that examined the effects of thrombolysis in combination with the platelet glycoprotein IIb/IIIa inhibitor lamifiban. Patients with an STEMI who were treated with t-PA or streptokinase were enrolled. The mean time to reperfusion, defined electrocardiographically as more than a 50% recovery of the ST-segment elevation, was statistically reduced in the patients receiving lamifiban. At 90 minutes, more patients in the lamifiban group achieved a composite of angiographic, continuous electrocardiographic and clinical markers of reperfusion (80.1% vs. 62.5%, $P=0.001$) but with a higher incidence of bleeding (16.1% vs. 10.3%).

Magnesium

The use of magnesium is no longer part of standard care for an acute myocardial infarction. In the prefibrinolytic era, the LIMIT-2 showed a lower mortality in patients treated with magnesium compared with controls (17.8% vs. 10.3%, $P=0.02$). However, ISIS-4 failed to show a mortality benefit with magnesium in 23,000 patients randomized within 6 hours after the onset of symptoms (7.9% with magnesium vs. 7.6% in controls). ISIS-4 also showed an increase in incidence of hypotension (1.1%) requiring termination of the use of the study drug, bradycardia (0.3%), and cutaneous flushing and burning (0.3%). However, concerns remained after ISIS-4 regarding the dosing regimen of magnesium in this trial and the timing of therapy.

Therefore, the MAGIC study was performed in 6,213 acute STEMI patients using a similar dosing regimen to LIMIT-2 of a 2-g IV bolus of magnesium sulphate administered over 15 minutes, followed by a 17-g infusion of magnesium sulphate over 24 hours. Importantly, only 23% of patients in this study received fibrinolytics and 3% primary PCI, because of the large number of patients included in this study who were ineligible for fibrinolysis. Mortality at 30 days was no different with magnesium therapy or placebo (15.3% vs. 15.2%). Therefore, the current recommendation is to replace magnesium when it is low, but there is no indication for supplemental magnesium therapy for the reduction of mortality in an acute myocardial infarction.

PCI vs. Fibrinolytics

Over the past 15 years, multiple studies compared the safety and efficacy of primary PCI with intravenous thrombolytic therapy for acute myocardial infarctions (PAMI, FAP, and PRAGUE studies). In an analysis of 23 studies, PCI reduced mortality compared with fibrinolytics (7% vs. 9%, $P=0.0002$), reduced nonfatal reinfarctions (3% vs. 7%), and reduced strokes (1% vs. 2%). During long-term follow-up, the benefits of PCI persisted. The relative benefits of primary PCI can be attributed to the more frequent achievement of TIMI 3 coronary blood flow than fibrinolytics, which can increase myocardial salvage and stabilize the disrupted and reocclusion-prone atherosclerotic plaque. Moreover, the significantly lower risk of ICH and other bleeding complications makes PCI a safer reperfusion modality. Thus, if PCI can be performed by an experienced operator in a timely fashion (traditionally within 1 additional hour compared with fibrinolysis), it is the preferred reperfusion modality. However, given that few hospitals have primary PCI capability, fibrinolytics are still a critical therapy for STEMI. Currently, the crucial question is not "if all things are equal, is primary PCI better than fibrinolytics?" but, when a transport delay is entailed, "how much of a delay is acceptable in regard to door-to-balloon time minus door-to-needle time?" Currently the guideline supports up to 60 minutes of added time to perform primary PCI compared with fibrinolytics in patients who are within 3 hours of symptom onset (Table 1).

PREHOSPITAL FIBRINOLYTICS

The attempts to use prehospital fibrinolytics are based on the marked improvement in patients who receive early therapy. Since the greatest mortality benefit is in patients receiving fibrinolytics within 60 to 90 minutes after the onset of symptoms, prehospital fibrinolytics could have a significant advantage. However, trials have not always supported this approach. In particular, with a short transfer time, there was no real advantage. Prehospital fibrinolytics have the best potential mortality impact in patients who have a long transfer time (60-90 minutes). Furthermore, prehospital fibrinolytics require that an electrocardiogram is available and that there are trained personnel in the ambulance for therapeutic decision making and the ability to give this therapy. In a meta-analysis of studies looking at prehospital fibrinolytic therapy, there was a 17% reduction in mortality. Clearly, prehospital fibrinolytic therapy will not be implemented in many communities because of short transport times, but in communities where transport time to hospitals are long, available systems to facilitate prehospital fibrinolytics are needed.

The main studies of prehospital fibrinolysis are the MITI-1 and MITI-2 trials, the GREAT trial, and the European Myocardial Infarct Trial. The MITI trials concluded that there was no demonstrable benefit to prehospital administration of thrombolysis. However, treatment within 70 minutes of symptom onset was extremely beneficial compared with treatment given 70 minutes or later from the onset of symptoms. Mortality was 1.2% in those treated within 70 minutes vs. 8.7% in those treated after 70 minutes with an associated reduction in infarct size and improvement in the ejection fraction. The GREAT trial was conducted in rural Britain and reported a reduction of more than 50% in 1-year mortality (10.5% vs. 21.5%, $P<0.01$) and a time savings of about 2 hours when at-home fibrinolysis was compared with in-hospital fibrinolysis. This trial is particularly relevant in patients with projected long transport time to a hospital. The European Myocardial Infarct Trial was a larger randomized trial of nearly 5,500 patients in which prehospital treatment with anistreplase was compared with in-hospital fibrinolysis. Cardiovascular mortality at 30-days decreased from 9.7% to 8.3% ($P=0.05$) with prehospital fibrinolysis and the time

savings was about 1 hour for drug administration. In a meta-analysis of six trials of prehospital fibrinolysis, prehospital fibrinolysis was associated with a lower all-cause hospital mortality (OR 0.83; confidence interval 0.70-0.98) (Fig. 2). No significant difference was found with 1- or 2-year mortality.

FACILITATED PCI

Facilitated PCI is the use of additional agents with PCI to improve coronary artery patency rates, salvage more myocardium, and decrease mortality in acute myocardial infarctions. This has been attempted with glycoprotein IIb/IIIa inhibitors, fibrinolytics, or both. In a pooled analysis of 17 trials (4,505 patients), facilitated PCI outcomes were compared with primary PCI outcomes. This included 2,957 patients in the fibrinolytic for facilitation studies and 399 patients treated with the combination of fibrinolytics and a glycoprotein IIb/IIIa inhibitor. Facilitated PCI resulted in a far greater initial TIMI 3 flow rate (37% vs. 15%), but the final TIMI 3 flow rates did not differ at the end of the procedure (89% vs. 88%). Mortality was higher with facilitated PCI (5% vs. 3%), as were reinfarction, urgent repeat vessel revascularization, major bleeding (7% vs. 5%), hemorrhagic stroke, and total stroke. These adverse events were seen in studies that used fibrinolytics for facilitation, whereas the glycoprotein IIb/IIIa inhibitors did not have a negative impact. In the ASSENT-4 PCI trial, patients with a STEMI of less than 6 hours' duration and a delay of 1 to 3 hours for primary PCI was anticipated, upfront administration of full-dose tenecteplase before transfer was compared with usual transfer for primary PCI. There was higher in-hospital mortality in the tenecteplase group compared with the standard PCI group (6% vs. 3%, $P=0.0105$), more strokes (1.8% vs. 0, $P<0.0001$), and more reinfarction (6% vs. 4%, $P=0.0279$). Thus, facilitated PCI with fibrinolytic therapy should not be performed as part of routine practice.

Currently, other options for facilitated PCI are being evaluated in the FINESSE study. This study will compare the efficacy and safety of early administration of reduced-dose reteplase and abciximab combination therapy or abciximab alone, with abciximab alone administered just before PCI for acute myocardial infarction patients undergoing primary PCI.

SHOULD THE PATIENT BE TRANSFERRED FOR PCI?

One of the current areas of intense interest is the question of when to transfer patients for primary PCI and when to give patients fibrinolytics. Combined data from five randomized controlled trials demonstrated that primary PCI was associated with a significant reduction in nonfatal reinfarction (1.8% vs. 6.7%), total stroke (1.1% vs. 2.2%), and the combined end point of death, nonfatal reinfarction, and stroke (8.2% vs. 15%). Only three of these five studies individually demonstrated benefit with transfer for primary PCI, although the other two studies had a similar trend. The DANAMI-2 investigators demonstrated that the TIMI risk score clearly identifies those patients most likely to benefit from PCI. Those patients with a TIMI risk score of 0 to 4 had no difference in mortality with either therapy (PCI, 8.0%; fibrinolysis, 5.6%; P=0.11), whereas in those with a TIMI risk score of 5 or more there was a significant reduction in mortality with primary PCI (25.3% vs. 36.2%; P=0.02). Thus, risk stratification is an important method to determine which patients are more likely to benefit from transfer for primary PCI.

The biggest question is "What is an acceptable transport time that still favors PCI?" The largest of the transfer trials, DANAMI-2, had a median transfer time of 67 minutes, with 96% of the patients transferred within 2 hours. Other transfer trials had even better times for transfer, such as a median transfer time of 48 minutes in the PRAGUE-2 study. Since "time is tissue," the time to reperfusion remains a critical question. Importantly, in the United States transfer times to hospitals that can perform primary PCI are significantly longer than those in the countries where these transfer studies were performed. However, in a recent study, in the United States the median time to a PCI hospital is 11.3 minutes and 7.9 miles, with 79.0% of the adult population within 60 minutes of a PCI hospital. Thus, if appropriate transfer mechanisms were in place, the majority of the U.S. population could receive primary PCI if needed.

The current recommendations are to give fibrinolysis unless the time from presentation at the first hospital to balloon therapy is no more than 90 to 120 minutes. In patients who present early (within 2–3 hours of symptom onset) immediate fibrinolytic therapy is warranted. In patients presenting after 3 hours, transfer for PCI is the preferred option depending on the transfer time.

COMPLICATIONS OF FIBRINOLYTIC THERAPY

Bleeding

ICH is the most serious complication that occurs in patients receiving fibrinolytics (0.5% to 1%). There is a slightly higher incidence with t-PA (0.7%) than with streptokinase (0.4%), and it usually occurs within the first two hospital days. The mortality and permanent neurologic damage rate remain high (about two-thirds of patients) after an ICH despite early detection and

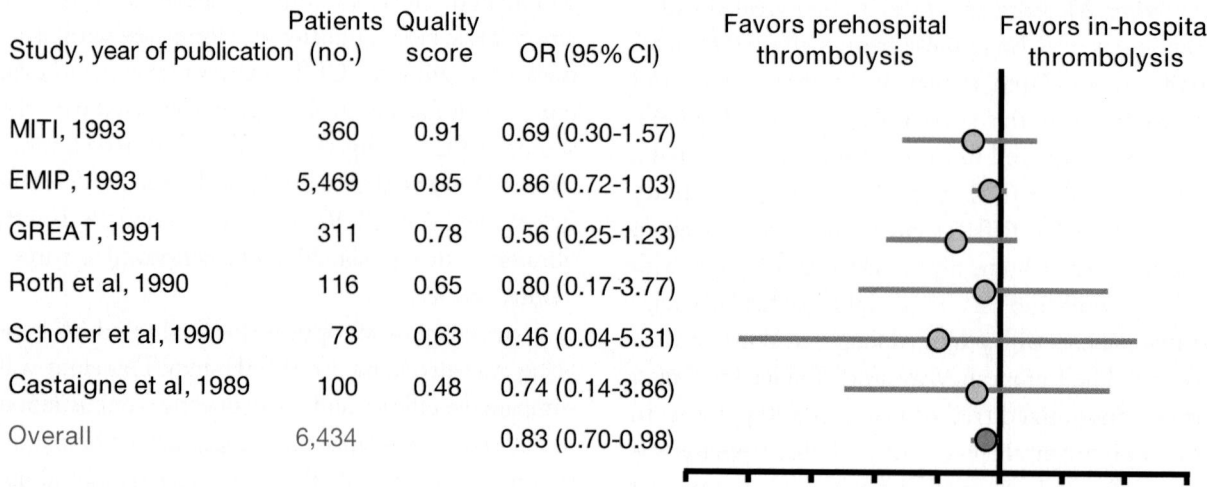

Study, year of publication	Patients (no.)	Quality score	OR (95% CI)
MITI, 1993	360	0.91	0.69 (0.30-1.57)
EMIP, 1993	5,469	0.85	0.86 (0.72-1.03)
GREAT, 1991	311	0.78	0.56 (0.25-1.23)
Roth et al, 1990	116	0.65	0.80 (0.17-3.77)
Schofer et al, 1990	78	0.63	0.46 (0.04-5.31)
Castaigne et al, 1989	100	0.48	0.74 (0.14-3.86)
Overall	6,434		0.83 (0.70-0.98)

Fig. 2. Odds ratios (ORs) and 95% confidence intervals (CIs) for in-hospital mortality with prehospital fibrinolysis compared with in-hospital therapy.

aggressive treatment, and this rate is even higher in patients older than 75 years.

The most common bleeding site is the site of vascular access, which can usually be managed by local pressure for 30 minutes. Other bleeding sites include gastrointestinal, genitourinary, and rarely retroperitoneal sites. In the case of uncontrolled life-threatening bleeding, the fibrinolytic and heparin therapy should be discontinued. In addition to blood transfusion, appropriate antidotes should be administered. For bleeding due to fibrinolytics, cryoprecipitate (10 units) and fresh frozen plasma may be needed to correct hypofibrinogenemic state. ε-Aminocaproic acid is an antifibrinogen agent that competes with plasminogen for lysine binding site on the fibrin. It is used as a last resort because it may cause thrombosis. It is administered at a loading dose of 5 g, followed by a continuous infusion of 0.5 to 1 g per hour until the bleeding stops. Heparin can be neutralized by protamine administration IV (1 mg of protamine uses 100 U of heparin). Platelet transfusions are required for bleeding due to glycoprotein IIb/IIIa inhibitors. Hemorrhage due to hirudin requires administration of prothrombin complex and not fresh frozen plasma because it narrowly corrects the laboratory abnormalities and does not stop the bleeding.

Allergic Reactions

A common nonhemorrhagic complication is allergic reaction. Streptokinase and APSAC (both are derived from group C streptococci) can cause hypotension, flushing, chills, fever, vasculitis, interstitial nephritis, and life-threatening anaphylaxis. Streptokinase and APSAC are not recommended if prior use occurred within 2 years because of the presence of neutralizing antibodies in more than 50% of patients. Urokinase, t-PA, retaplase, and TNK do not usually cause such reactions and can be safely used in patients with prior streptokinase or APSAC exposure.

CLINICAL DETECTION OF REPERFUSION

Clinical detection of reperfusion is even more important than ever, given the option for rescue PCI as part of optimal medical care in patients who do not have improved coronary blood flow with fibrinolytics. Resolution of chest pain, resolution of ST-segment elevation and the presence of a "reperfusion arrhythmia" have limitations as markers of reperfusion. Chest pain may resolve with narcotics or with myocardial denervation as a consequence of myocardial ischemia or necrosis. The ST-segment elevation may return to preinfarct levels as a result of natural postinfarction evolution or the dynamic blood flow pattern so characteristic of the first 12 hours after infarction. Arrhythmias, such as accelerated idioventricular rhythm, are also common with reperfusion. Other techniques such as echocardiography with contrast, continuous vector electrocardiography, and magnetic resonance imaging are used currently only for research purposes. If a patient requires angiography, TIMI frame count can also be a useful tool for perfusion but is not useful in the majority of fibrinolytic patients.

Currently the need to clinically detect reperfusion is important because of the potential for rescue angioplasty. In the REACT trial of 427 patients with an STEMI who did not have reperfusion defined by a resolution of the ST-segment elevation of less than 50% at 90 minutes, patients were randomly assigned to repeat fibrinolysis, conservative therapy, or PCI. Event-free survival was highest in those who were treated with PCI (84.6%), followed by conservative therapy (70.1%) and then repeat fibrinolytics (68.7%). In other studies such as the MERLIN trial, there was no difference in mortality in the rescue angioplasty and conservative groups after thrombolytics, but there was reduction in the composite secondary end point of death, reinfarction, stroke, subsequent revascularization, and heart failure (37.3% vs. 50%, $P=0.02$). Furthermore, a study of 345 patients who received fibrinolytic therapy for a STEMI and underwent 90-minute angiography was performed. Those with TIMI 0-1 flow who underwent rescue PCI had a similar outcome as those patients with initial TIMI 3 flow. Thus, with the possible benefits of rescue angioplasty, a heightened awareness of the potential of reperfusion failure after fibrinolytics will not only help one to risk stratify a patient but may also lead to early percutaneous revascularization.

Appendix
Names of Clinical Trials

AIRE	Acute Infarction Ramipril Efficacy
ASSENT	Assessment of the Safety and Efficacy of New Thrombolytic Regimens
ASSENT-4 PCI	Assessment of the Safety and Efficacy of a New Treatment Strategy With Percutaneous Coronary Intervention
CLARITY-TIMI 28	Clopidogrel as Adjunctive Reperfusion Therapy—TIMI 28
COMMIT	Clopidogrel and Metoprolol in Myocardial Infarction
CONSENSUS	Cooperative New Scandinavian Enalapril Survival Study
CREATE-ECLA	Low-Molecular-Weight Heparin (Reviparin) in Preventing Mortality, Reinfarction, and Strokes in Over 15,500 Patients With ST Elevation Acute Myocardial Infarction
DANAMI	Danish Multicenter Randomized Study on Fibrinolytic Therapy Versus Acute Coronary Angioplasty in Acute Myocardial Infarction
ECSG	European Cooperative Study Group
EMIP	European Myocardial Infarction Project
ExTRACT-TIMI 25	Enoxaparin and Thrombolysis Reperfusion for Acute Myocardial Infarction Treatment—TIMI 25
FAP	Fibrinolytics Versus Primary Angioplasty in Acute Myocardial Infarction
FINESSE	Facilitated Intervention With Enhanced Reperfusion Speed to Stop Events
GISSI	Gruppo Italiano per lo Studio della Streptochinasi nell'Infarto Miocardico
GREAT	Grampian Region Early Anistreplase Trial
GUSTO-1	Global Utilization of Streptokinase and Tissue Plasminogen Activator for Occluded Coronary Artery
HERO	Hirulog Early Reperfusion/Occlusion
IMPACT-AMI	Integrilin to Manage Platelet Aggregation to Combat Thrombus in Acute Myocardial Infarction
INJECT	International Joint Efficacy Comparison of Thrombolytics
ISIS	International Study of Infarct Survival
LATE	Late Assessment of Thrombolytic Efficacy
LIMIT	Leicester Intravenous Magnesium Intervention
MAGIC	Magnesium in Coronaries
MERLIN	Middlesbrough Early Revascularization to Limit Infarction
MITI	Myocardial Infarction Triage and Intervention
PAMI	Primary Angioplasty in Myocardial Infarction
PARADIGM	Platelet Aggregation Receptor Antagonist Dose Investigation and Reperfusion Gain in Myocardial Infarction
PRAGUE	Primary Angioplasty in Patients Transported From General Community Hospitals to Specialized PTCA Units With or Without Emergency Thrombolysis
REACT	Rescue Angioplasty Versus Conservative Treatment or Repeat Thrombolysis
SAVE	Survival and Ventricular Enlargement
SMILE	Survival of Myocardial Infarction Long-term Evaluation
TAMI	Thrombolysis and Angioplasty in Myocardial Infarction
TIMI	Thrombolysis in Myocardial Infarction
TRACE	Trandolapril Cardiac Evaluation

RISK STRATIFICATION AFTER MYOCARDIAL INFARCTION

Randal J. Thomas, MD, MS

BACKGROUND

Risk stratification following myocardial infarction (MI) is the process of estimating the risk of future cardiovascular events in survivors of MI. This process helps health care providers tailor short- and long-term management plans for such patients, with the goal of applying cost-effective treatments that are most appropriate for the risk level of the patient and that are most likely to optimize the patient's quality and quantity of life.

Risk assessment strategies are applicable to patient care at several times during and after MI, including the time of assessment by emergency medical technicians, arrival at the emergency department, admission to the intensive care unit, and before and soon after hospital discharge in the outpatient setting. Although each of these settings is vitally important in risk-stratified treatment approaches to MI care, the focus of this review is on principles that are particularly important in the time frame just before or just after hospital discharge following MI.

Risk-stratified treatment approaches continue to be important today, despite the fact that mortality rates

for cardiovascular diseases (CVDs) have decreased approximately 50% in the United States over the past 4 decades. Evidence suggests that this decline in mortality is due to at least two factors: 1) a reduction in the incidence of CVD events (primary prevention) and 2) a reduction in case fatality following a CVD event (secondary prevention). Incidence of MI has declined in the United States by approximately 20% to 30% during the past 4 decades. In addition, 1-year mortality following MI has also declined, from approximately 20% in 1970 to approximately 5% in 2000.

As improvements in MI-related outcomes have occurred over the past 4 decades, definitions for low-, moderate-, and high-risk subgroups have changed. In the prethrombolytic era, for instance, patients were considered to be at high risk for future CVD events if their estimated 1-year mortality risk was greater than 10%, moderate-risk patients had 5% to 10% risk, and low-risk patients had less than 5% risk of death during the first year after MI. Today, because most patients have a significantly reduced risk following MI compared with patients from previous decades, high-, moderate-,

Clinical trial names are in the Appendix at the end of the chapter.

and low-risk patients are defined as those with 1-year mortality risks of greater than 3%, 1% to 3%, and less than 1%, respectively. With new, more effective, and more costly treatment strategies emerging, the risk-stratified approach to cost-effective and evidence-based risk reduction strategies is as important as ever.

BASIC PRINCIPLES

To incorporate risk stratification into the management of the MI patient, several key principles are important to consider. In MI survivors, future cardiovascular events are generally due to one of the following high-risk conditions:

- Recurrent ischemia
- Left ventricular dysfunction
- High-grade arrhythmias
- Other complications following MI (renal failure, stroke, etc.)

A patient's risk of future CVD events can be estimated by various patient characteristics, including symptoms, physical findings, and test results, to help identify people with recurrent ischemia, left ventricular dysfunction, arrhythmias, and other complications following MI.

A risk-stratified approach to post-MI treatment helps match patients with the most appropriate level of treatment.

- Patients at highest risk for future CVD events generally derive more benefits from aggressive therapies than do patients at lowest risk for future CVD events. (For example, an overweight individual will lose more weight by following an aggressive weight loss program than will an individual at ideal weight.)
- Aggressive therapies, including coronary angiography, percutaneous coronary interventions, surgical revascularization, and antiarrhythmic devices, are treatments with the greatest potential to benefit patients at highest risk, but the associated costs and risks of side effects of these treatments are significant.
- There are several treatments that can be applied to nearly all post-MI patients and can help significantly reduce risk of future CVD events, have a low risk of side effects, and have low-to-moderate costs. These include the "ABCs" of treatment listed in Table 1.

Risk stratification helps guide various parts of post-hospital care, including cardiac rehabilitation and return to work. Patients at highest risk generally have a more gradual and monitored progression of post-MI therapy and recuperation than do post-MI patients at lower risk for future CVD events.

Methods of Risk Estimation

Several published reports and consensus statements have suggested frameworks by which risk stratification can be carried out following MI (Table 2). Published experience from Olmsted County, Minnesota, suggests the following:

- Risk-stratification scoring systems, such as the one from the PREDICT trial, appear to perform equally well for ST-segment elevation MI (STEMI) and non-STEMI, particularly if they include information about comorbid conditions.
- Left ventricular ejection fraction is a powerful predictor of future CVD events in post-MI patients and should be included in risk-stratification strategies.

Guidelines for risk-stratification strategies following STEMI have been published by a joint panel from the American College of Cardiology (ACC) and the American Heart Association (AHA). Highlights from those guidelines are shown in Figures 1 and 2. On the basis of these guidelines, an approach to risk stratification following MI could include the following steps:

Table 1. ABCs of Secondary Prevention Following Myocardial Infarction

A: Antiplatelet agent
    Angiotensin-converting enzyme inhibitor (for those with left ventricular dysfunction)
    Avoid tobacco
B: β-Blockers
    Blood pressure control
C: Cholesterol-lowering drug therapy
D: Dietary control
    Diabetes control
E: Exercise
F: Fish oil (omega-3 fatty acids)

Table 2.   Selected Published Scores for Post-MI Risk Stratification

Feature	TIMI-STEMI	GUSTO-STEMI	TIMI-NSTEMI	PURSUIT-NSTEMI	PREDICT	CCP
Historical data	Age 65-74 y, ≥75 y	Age	Age≥65 y	Age Sex	Age	Older age
	Diabetes mellitus/ hypertension or angina	Prior MI	Pre-MI angina	Pre-MI angina	Prior MI, pre-MI angina, CABG or cardiac arrest, hyper-tension, stroke	
			Prior coronary stenosis ≥50% Aspirin in prior 7 days ≥3 CAD risk factors			
Hemodynamics	Systolic blood pressure <100 mm Hg	In-hospital CHF		Systolic blood pressure (mm Hg)	Shock	CHF/pul-monary edema or cardio-megaly
	HR >100 Killip II-IV	HR LVEF		HR CHF	CHF	LVEF
ECG	Left bundle branch block/ anterior ST elevation		ST-segment deviation	ST depres-sion	ECG severity score	

1. **Assess patient for high-risk symptoms, signs, and comorbid conditions**

   All post-MI patients should be screened for high-risk symptoms and signs, including those that suggest ischemia (angina), left ventricular dysfunction (dyspnea, rales, ventricular gallop), and high-grade arrhythmias (documented ventricular tachycardia/fibrillation, history of cardiac arrest, syncope/presyncope). Comorbid conditions that add prognostic information to risk stratification include age, prior MI, pre-MI angina, hypertension, stroke, coronary artery bypass grafting or cardiac arrest, and renal dysfunction. Individuals with high-risk findings should be considered for more aggressive evaluation (e.g., coronary angiography) and treatment options (e.g., revascularization).

2. **Assess left ventricular function**

   Left ventricular ejection fraction (LVEF) is a powerful predictor of future CVD events after MI. In post-MI patients with an LVEF of less than 30%, 6-month mortality is approximately

Table 2.   (continued)

Feature	TIMI-STEMI	GUSTO-STEMI	TIMI-NSTEMI	PURSUIT-NSTEMI	PREDICT	CCP
Comorbidity	Weight <67 kg				Charlson index Renal function	Body mass index <20 kg/m^2 Renal function Urinary incontinence Assisted mobility Peripheral vascular disease
Other	Time to treatment >4 h		Elevated biomarkers			

CABG, coronary artery bypass grafting; CAD, coronary artery disease; CHF, congestive heart failure; ECG, electrocardiogram; HR, heart rate; LVEF, left ventricular ejection fraction; MI, myocardial infarction.

15%; those with an LVEF of more than 50% have a 1% to 2% 6-month mortality rate. Measurement of LVEF can be performed by echocardiography, nuclear imaging, or at coronary angiography.

3. **Exercise testing**

Exercise testing, with or without echocardiographic or nuclear imaging, has been a long-standing, noninvasive approach to risk stratification of post-MI patients. While exercise testing helps to identify inducible ischemia, an important high-risk condition following MI, it also helps assess exercise capacity, an even more powerful predictor of future CVD events. In addition, exercise testing provides information about heart rate and blood pressure responses to exercise, factors that can add to risk prediction for CVD events. Information about exercise capacity also helps tailor the exercise prescription during cardiac rehabilitation sessions and helps guide return-to-work recommendations for the post-MI patient.

4. **Assess for Arrhythmia Risk**

A small percentage of MI patients have high-grade ventricular arrhythmias during hospitalization and are candidates for further electrophysiologic testing and possible automatic implantable cardioverter-defibrillator (AICD) treatment. For other patients, further tests for significant arrhythmias are of relatively low yield and are generally not recommended.

Recent studies, including the MADIT-II study, suggest, however, that post-MI patients with an LVEF less than 30% derive significant survival benefit from AICD therapy. Patients are considered possible candidates for AICD placement if their LVEF is less than 30% at least 1-month following MI. There is considerable debate regarding the cost-effectiveness of such an approach to risk reduction, given the significant cost of an AICD.

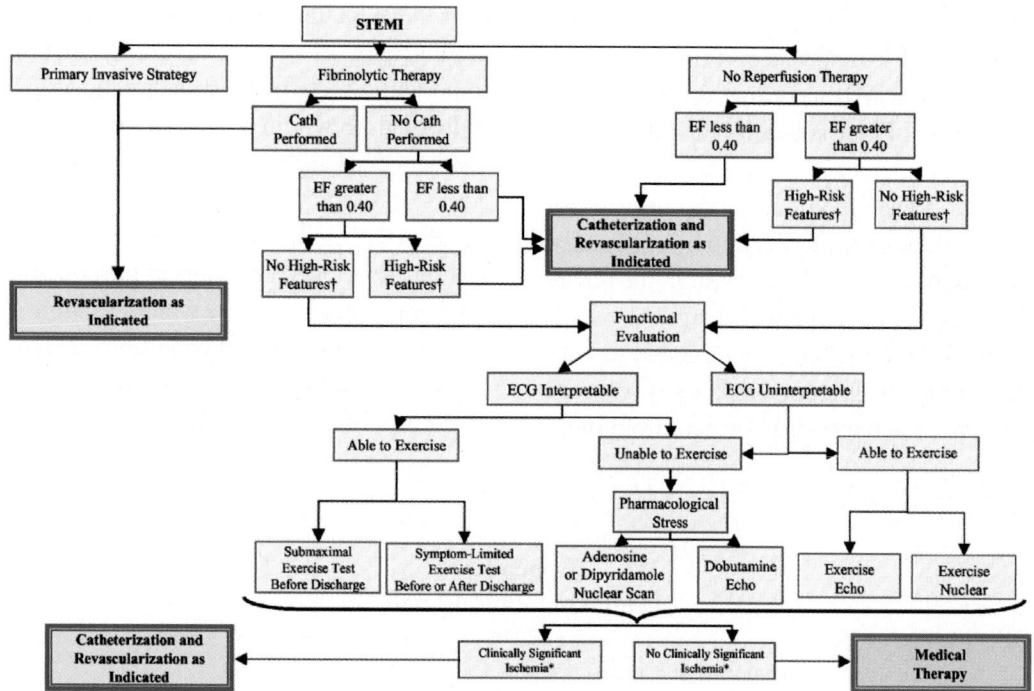

Fig. 1. Approach to risk-stratified management approaches to identify patients with ST-elevation MI (STEMI) who would most likely benefit from more aggressive management strategies, including coronary angiography and revascularization. Cath, catherization; ECG, electrocardiogram; EF, ejection fraction.

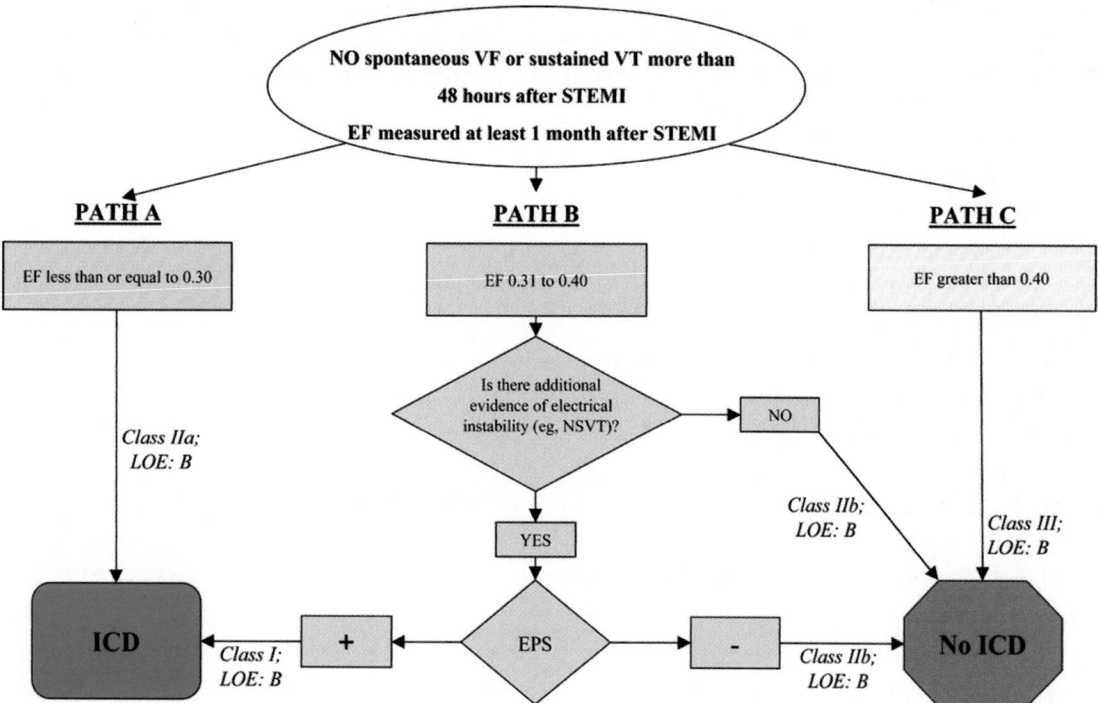

Fig. 2. Algorithm from American College of Cardiology/American Heart Association (ACC/AHA) guidelines for management of ST-elevation myocardial infarction (STEMI) to help select patients with STEMI for implantable cardioverter-defibrillator (ICD) therapy. EF, ejection fraction; EPS, electrophysiologic studies; LOE, level of evidence; LVEF, left ventricular EF; NSVT, nonsustained VT; STEMI, ST-elevation myocardial infarction; VF, ventricular fibrillation; VT, ventricular tachycardia.

SUMMARY

Several strategies and scoring systems exist to help risk stratify patients after MI, according to their risk of future CVD events. These strategies include various patient characteristics and test results that can help risk stratify patients at every point along the health care continuum, from the initial evaluation by emergency medical technicians to the evaluation visit in the physician's office a month after hospital discharge.

Risk-stratification methods are designed to help identify those individuals at increased risk for future CVD events who would most likely benefit from more aggressive management strategies (i.e., coronary angiography or revascularization, or both). More importantly, these methods help to identify lower risk individuals in whom aggressive treatments would be less beneficial and would instead result in additional adverse risks and costs.

A simplified, evidence-based approach to risk stratification for MI patients at or soon after hospital discharge includes: 1) assessment of high-risk symptoms, signs, or comorbid conditions, 2) assessment of left ventricular function, 3) exercise testing, and 4) assessment of arrhythmia risk.

Appendix
Names of Clinical Trials

CCP	Cooperative Cardiovascular Project
GUSTO-STEMI	Global Use of Strategies to Open Occluded Coronary Arteries—ST-Elevation Myocardial Infarction
MADIT-II	Multicenter Automatic Defibrillator Implantation Trial-II
PREDICT	Predilatation vs. Direct Stenting in Coronary Treatment
PURSUIT-NSTEMI	Platelet Glycoprotein IIb/IIIa in Unstable Angina: Receptor Suppression Using Integrilin Therapy—Non–ST-Elevation Myocardial Infarction
TIMI-NSTEMI	Thrombolysis in Myocardial Infarction—Non–ST-Elevation Myocardial Infarction
TIMI-STEMI	Thrombolysis in Myocardial Infarction—ST-Elevation Myocardial Infarction

CARDIAC REHABILITATION

Thomas G. Allison, PhD

DEFINITION

According to the World Health Organization (WHO) definition, cardiac rehabilitation is

the sum of activities required to ensure cardiovascular-diseased patients the best possible physical, mental, and social conditions so that they may by their own efforts regain as normal as possible a place in the community and lead an active life.

The US Public Health Service defines cardiac rehabilitation as follows:

Cardiac rehabilitation services are comprehensive, long-term programs involving medical evaluation, prescribed exercise, cardiac risk factor modification, education, and counseling. These programs are designed to limit the physiologic and psychological effects of cardiac illness, reduce the risk for sudden death or reinfarction, control cardiac symptoms, stabilize or reverse the atherosclerotic process, and enhance the psychosocial and vocational status of selected patients. Cardiac rehabilitation services are prescribed for patients who 1) have had a myocardial infarction, 2) have had coronary bypass surgery, or 3) have chronic stable angina pectoris. The services are in three phases beginning during hospitalization, followed by a supervised ambulatory outpatient program lasting 3-6 months, and continuing in a lifetime maintenance stage in which physical fitness and risk factor reduction are accomplished in a minimally supervised or unsupervised setting (Feigenbaum and Carter, 1988).

More recently, the Agency for Health Care Policy and Research (AHCPR) added in 1991 that

heart transplant patients and patients who have undergone percutaneous transluminal coronary angioplasty or heart valve surgery could benefit from prescribed cardiac rehabilitation programs.

Still others feel that cardiac rehabilitation may be helpful for patients with chronic heart failure, peripheral vascular disease, or a history of stroke. As this chapter is being written, however, only patients in the first 3 classes—post-myocardial infarction, post-bypass surgery, and chronic stable angina pectoris are eligible for reimbursement of cardiac rehabilitation services by Medicare. Coverage of cardiac rehabilitation services for heart transplant, angioplasty, and heart valve surgery have been approved in new guidelines, but implementation of these new guidelines is still pending. Coverage for chronic heart failure and noncoronary vascular patients has not yet been approved.

Cardiac rehabilitation has also been endorsed by the professional medical community. The American Heart Association/American College of Cardiology

Joint Guidelines on Management of Patients With Acute Myocardial Infarction (1999 Update) states:

> The majority of patients need to modify their lifestyle after acute MI. Typical recommendations require a change in previous behavior . . . . Achievement of these goals is often complicated by denial of the significance of the event, physical deconditioning that may reflect a lifelong history of sedentary behavior, and emotional distress . . . (and) may be facilitated through participation in a formal cardiac rehabilitation program.

HISTORICAL PERSPECTIVE

In understanding the history of cardiac rehabilitation, it is important to describe the management of coronary artery disease (CAD) in the 1950s and 1960s, as cardiac rehabilitation developed in large part to deal with the effects of those management practices on exercise capacity, quality of life, and survival of patients with (CAD) treated in that era. In general, CAD patients at that time were younger and more likely male than today, as age-adjusted rates for CAD have been decreasing since 1967—for men especially in part due to the large reduction in smoking. Management of acute myocardial infarction or unstable angina in 1950-1960 largely involved treating symptoms with nitroglycerine and morphine. Procedures to improve or restore blood flow such as PCI, reperfusion therapy, or CABG were unknown. There was not a good understanding of risk factors in the pathogenesis of CAD. Drugs with survival benefit—statins, angiotension converting enzyme inhibitors, beta blockers, and aspirin—were either nonexistent or not yet known to have a protective effect.

It is perhaps instructive to review the treatment schedule devised by Dr. Paul Dudley White for President Dwight Eisenhower's heart attack in 1955 (Table 1). Eisenhower remained in the hospital for 7 weeks and still was not considered capable of climbing the steps into the airplane for his return to Washington from Denver, where he had the heart attack. Interestingly, White was criticized for mobilizing the President too rapidly (Fig. 1).

As a result of the lack of myocardium-sparing therapies and reperfusion strategies to control ischemia,

Table 1. Treatment Schedule

Date (1955)	Event
September 24	Infarct. Bedrest prescribed.
October 11	First allowed to see a cabinet member.
October 22	Sitting up in a chair for a few hours each day, and holding daily conferences about his presidential duties.
November 7	Walking and starting to climb stairs.
November 11	Returned to Washington, the trip delayed a month so that Eisenhower would not be seen being wheeled to the airplane and being lifted on board. After landing in Washington, goes to his farm in Gettysburg, Pennsylvania.
December 26	Eisenhower doubts whether he should run for a second term as president with that "sword of Damocles" over his head. He suggests that Vice President Nixon should run instead.

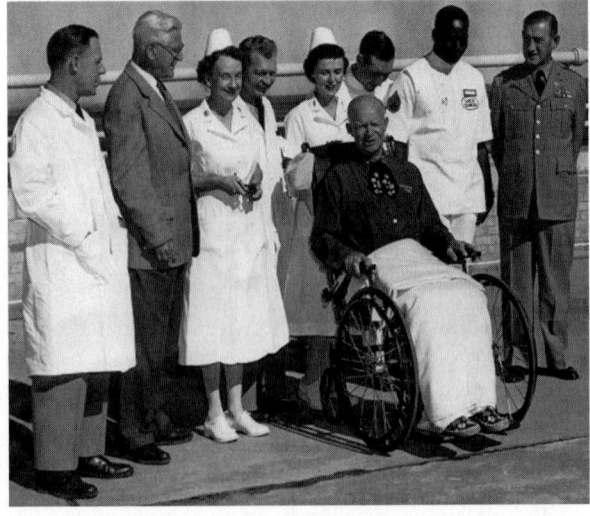

Fig. 1. President Eisenhower following his heart attack in 1955.

transmural infarction, ongoing ischemia, and death were commonly experienced in patients with acute coronary syndromes. Exercise remained one of the few options for control of symptoms and improvement of functional capacity, though exercise also carried greater risk because of uncontrolled ischemia and reduced left ventricular function.

The emphasis in early cardiac rehabilitation programs was largely on aerobic training. Education was a lesser component, and risk factor management was an even smaller part of the effort. Vigorous exercise was pursued not only for its antianginal (and, as later determined) survival benefits but also to some degree for the purpose of educating the cardiology community as to the need to demystify coronary disease free patients from draconian restrictions, social stigma, and inappropriate fear and anxiety over their condition. Exercise physiologists were instrumental in developing cardiac rehabilitation programs at a time when exercise programs were not available in hospitals and the medical community in general considered exercise to be of greater risk than benefit to coronary patients. Currently, appropriate physical activity is recommended for all patients with CAD, including patients with reduced left ventricular function and compensated heart failure.

Constant improvements in the management of CAD and myocardial infarction and attitudes towards physical activity for CAD patients have greatly shaped the nature and content of cardiac rehabilitation programs. Not only is exercise more generally recognized to play an important role in long-term risk reduction in CAD, but exercise is also safer because of better care during the acute event and aggressive use of revascularization and drugs to control ischemia and prevent disease progression. Inpatient programs were gradually reduced in length, as hospital stays decreased markedly and education and counseling gradually became a more important part of these programs since activity was much less restricted—in part due to changing attitudes but also in large part due to myocardial salvage and aggressive management of ischemia. Outpatient programs by and large have moved into hospital settings, where patients exercise on individual ergometers and are continuously monitored by telemetry. Patients begin outpatient (phase 2) cardiac rehabilitation much sooner after their acute event, and program length is limited to 12 weeks in terms of reimbursement for

services, though many patients complete their programs much sooner and return to work—or travel and other normal activities. Recommendations for exercise to be done at home or a community facility on nonclass days are also routinely provided, and weight training, plus nontraditional activities such as tai chi, yoga, and balance training, are frequently included in outpatient cardiac rehabilitation.

CURRENT STRUCTURE OF CARDIAC REHABILITATION

Phase 1
Inpatient cardiac rehabilitation; duration = 3-7 days. Initially a structured activity program conducted by nurses or physical therapists, shortened hospital stays have changed phase 1 programs to be more educational and to refer patients into phase 2 programs.

Phase 2
Early outpatient cardiac rehabilitation; duration = up to 3 months. This is the standard cardiac rehabilitation program now conducted in a hospital setting. Patients exercise 1-3 times per week, generally on ergometers but sometimes around tracks or in swimming pools in those hospitals featuring a comprehensive wellness center. Patients are monitored by telemetry. Dedicated databases are commercially available which interface with telemetry systems to facilitate electronic record-keeping. Exercise not only includes cardiovascular conditioning, such as treadmill walking, but may also include light resistance exercise (weight training) and other activities to improve flexibility and balance. Educational programs are generally offered, and various forms of counseling—dietary, psychological, occupational—may be provided as part of the program. As per Medicare guidelines, each patient's treatment plan is approved and reviewed periodically by a designated physician. Exercise testing—standard exercise electrocardiography, cardiopulmonary exercise testing, and 6-minute walks—is used to evaluate progress and revise the exercise prescription. Phase 2 cardiac rehabilitation programs are also required to track specific patient outcomes, as discussed below under *Current Practices*.

Phase 3
Extended cardiac rehabilitation; duration = up to 3

months. In some cases, patients who progress slowly for various reasons or had initially severely impaired functional status may require an extended course of cardiac rehabilitation before returning to usual activity in the community. These patients may continue in hospital-based programs under close supervision and perhaps further telemetric monitoring.

Phase 4

Lifetime cardiac rehabilitation; duration = months to years. Many hospitals offer a long-term program for patients to continue to exercise in a medically supervised (but generally not continuously monitored) setting on the hospital campus once they have completed phase 2 (and possibly phase 3) cardiac rehabilitation. In some cases, the hospital may contract with a community agency or private health club to provide the facilities while hospital personnel arrive to conduct the actual classes. These programs are generally self-pay on the part of the patient, though an individual employer may in some cases chose to subsidize participation. Patients not qualifying for reimbursement under current Medicare guidelines (such as peripheral vascular disease patients) may participate in cardiac rehabilitation through these phase 4 programs, and some programs may also accept high-risk patients who have not been diagnosed with cardiovascular disease (diabetics are the prime example).

CURRENT PRACTICES

Consistent with the shift in both the epidemiology of coronary heart disease and vastly improved care of the patient presenting with acute coronary syndrome, cardiac rehabilitation today serves a wide range of patients in terms of age, degree of cardiovascular impairment and risk, and number and severity of comorbidities. Young men with recent infarcts likely related to smoking still make up a significant portion of cardiac rehabilitation patients, but their left ventricular function and exercise tolerance is generally well preserved and they are usually free of ongoing ischemia and able to return to work within weeks if not days of their acute event. Thus their cardiac rehabilitation course is considerably accelerated, and ensuring smoking cessation may be the most important task for the cardiac rehabilitation team. At the other end of the spectrum, elderly

patients with recurrent coronary disease—kept alive by medical and technological progress in CHD management—present to cardiac rehabilitation with significant impairments in functional capacity due not only to their extensive cardiac disease but also to the comorbidities associated with aging and obesity. Their progress is obviously much slower, and the burden of care for the cardiac rehabilitation team is much higher. While the ability to actually modify the disease process or prolong survival in these patients is limited, there is great potential to reduce the economic burden of illness by preventing rehospitalization for exacerbation of symptoms that could be adequately managed on an outpatient base.

While participation rates for cardiac rehabilitation are lower for women than for men, increasing numbers of women do now participate in cardiac rehabilitation, and many of them are older and present with multiple comorbidities and poor functional capacity. There is often added challenge due to lack of previous physical activity and attitudes and preferences unfavorable to exercising.

As mentioned above, cardiac rehabilitation programs are organized around the provision of telemetry-monitored cardiovascular conditioning. This is generally provided in a small class format with 4-8 patients exercising at time. Generally, a session lasts 1 hour and is performed 1-3 times per week depending patient availability and the need for close supervision and monitoring. In addition to the cardiovascular conditioning classes, resistance, flexibility, and balance training may be offered. Education and counseling of various forms are also generally provided.

In 1995, the Agency for Health Care Policy and Research published Clinical Practice Guidelines (No. 17) for Cardiac Rehabilitation (link provided below). These guidelines recommended that cardiac rehabilitation programs facilitate and track 8 specific outcomes (Table 2).

In order to carry out these recommendations, a *case management system* has been instituted in many cardiac rehabilitation programs. Each member of the cardiac rehabilitation team is assigned a specific group of patients and is then responsible for evaluating these patients with respect to these recommendations, making appropriate referrals for intervention (such as dietary counseling, smoking cessation counseling, psychological counseling, etc.), and tracking progress.

Table 2.   Recommended Guidelines

1. Smoking
Recommendation: A combined approach of education, counseling, and behavioral interventions in cardiac rehabilitation results in smoking cessation and relapse prevention and is recommended for cardiac risk reduction.

2. Lipids
Recommendation: Intensive nutritional education, counseling, and behavioral interventions improve dietary fat and cholesterol intake. Education, counseling, and behavioral interventions about nutrition—with and without pharmacologic lipid-lowering therapy—result in significant improvement in blood lipid levels and are recommended as components of cardiac rehabilitation.

3. Body weight
Recommendation: Multifactorial rehabilitation that combines dietary education, counseling, and behavioral interventions designed to reduce body weight can help patients lose weight. Education as a sole intervention is unlikely to achieve and maintain weight loss. These multifactorial cardiovascular risk-reduction interventions are recommended as components of comprehensive cardiac rehabilitation.

4. Blood pressure
Recommendation: Expert opinion supports education as an important component of a multifactorial education, counseling, behavioral intervention, and pharmacologic approach to the management of hypertension. This approach is documented to be effective in nonrehabilitation populations and should also be included in cardiac rehabilitation. Education, counseling, and behavioral interventions as sole modalities have not been shown to control elevated blood pressure levels.

5. Exercise tolerance
Recommendation: Cardiac rehabilitation education, counseling, and behavioral interventions without exercise training are unlikely to improve exercise tolerance and are not recommended for that purpose.

6. Symptoms
Recommendation: Cardiac rehabilitation education, counseling, and behavioral interventions are recommended alone or as components of multifactorial cardiac rehabilitation to reduce symptoms of angina.

7. Return to work
Recommendation: Education, counseling, and behavioral interventions have not been shown to improve rates of return to work, which are contingent on many social and policy issues. In selected patients, formal cardiac rehabilitation vocational counseling may improve rates of return to work.

8. Stress and psychological well-being
Recommendation: Education, counseling, and psychosocial interventions—either alone or as components of multifactorial cardiac rehabilitation—result in improved psychological well-being. Education, counseling, and behavioral interventions are recommended to complement the psychosocial benefits of exercise training.

BENEFITS OF CARDIAC REHABILITATION

The 1995 AHCPR Support Clinical Practice Guidelines consider that evidence exists for the following outcomes in cardiac rehabilitation participants versus non-participants:

- Improvement in exercise tolerance.
- Improvement in symptoms.
- Improvement in blood lipid levels.
- Reduction in cigarette smoking.
- Improvement in psychosocial well-being and reduction of stress.
- Reduction in mortality.

Regarding mortality benefit, the Cochrane Library published a meta-analysis of secondary prevention benefits of cardiac rehabilitation programs in 2003. Analyzing outcomes from 8,440 CHD patients in exercise-based rehab programs, they concluded that there was

- 27% reduction in all-cause mortality.
- 31% reduction in CHD mortality.
- No evidence of reduction in nonfatal CHD.

Cardiac rehabilitation programs offering only exercise training seem to show a stronger benefit than comprehensive programs, but that was likely an artifact of the timeframe for the program, in that earlier programs were less comprehensive, likely exercised patients more vigorously, and enrolled patients at higher risk. For a example, an early cardiac rehabilitation program in Finland was able to show significant mortality benefit in a relatively small number of participants due to the exceptionally high risk for cardiac death (10-year risk nearly 50% in control patients) (Fig. 2).

Mayo Clinic published observational data on survival in participants in cardiac rehabilitation after myocardial infarction versus nonparticipants during the years 1982-1998 (Fig. 3). Among eligible men, participation rates were 71% versus 40% for women. Overall, participants had 26% lower mortality compared to nonparticipants. When these figures were adjusted by means of a propensity score for participation in cardiac rehabilitation, the benefit increased to 43%.

FUTURE OF CARDIAC REHABILITATION

Cardiac rehabilitation has a long history of adjustment to improving CHD management strategies, changing CHD epidemiology, and new regulations and guidelines. Challenges for cardiac rehabilitation for the present and near future include

1. Increasing patient referrals and participation rates. In contrast to the Mayo Clinic data cited above, national referral rates have been estimated at only 13-41% for

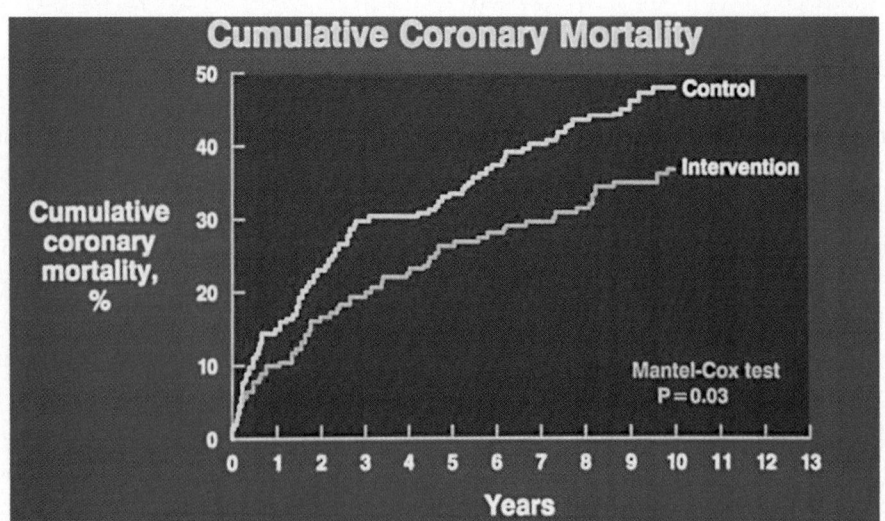

Fig. 2. Finnish cardic rehabilitation study which demonstrated a significant mortality benefit with cardiac rehabilitation in high-risk patients.

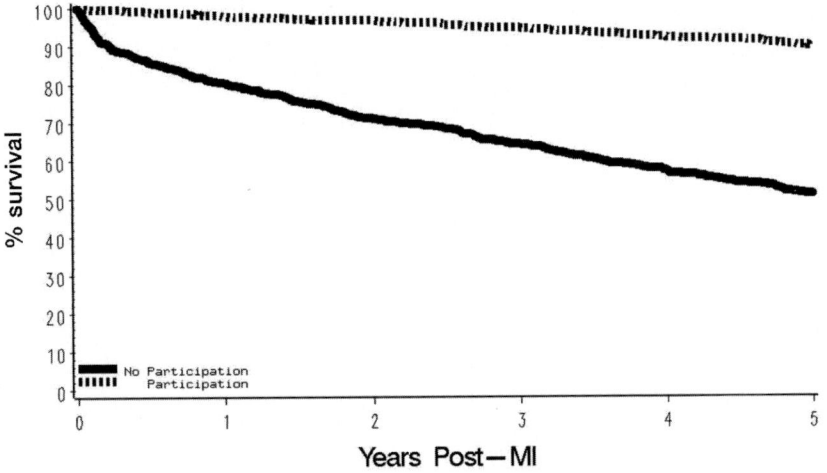

Fig. 3. Observational study of survival post myocardial infarction among participants and non-participants in a cardiac rehabilitation program.

men and 7-22% for women. Many barriers to participation still exist, apart from availability of a program and insurance coverage. Greater distance from cardiac rehabilitation center, more noncardiac comorbidities, older age, living alone, and smoking appear to be significant deterrents to participation. Continuing medical education may play an important role, along with public education and continued research into cardiac rehabilitation benefits.

2. Expanding the range of eligible patients. Recent changes at the federal level may soon allow reimbursement for cardiac rehabilitation services for cardiac transplant, valve replacement or repair, and percutaneous coronary intervention. Adding heart failure, peripheral vascular disease, and stroke as acceptable diagnoses would further expand referral bases. Not only would more patients benefit from cardiac rehabilitation but programs could more readily survive financially with higher patient volumes and not be forced into ever-increasing per session charges to meet expenses.

3. Professional training. As cardiac rehabilitation programs are required to provide more extensive services and administer them to a broader range of patients, public agencies and professional organization will need to upgrade continuing education and certifica-

tion/licensing programs to make sure that cardiac rehabilitation professionals possess the knowledge and skills necessary to provide the level of service required.

RESOURCES

AHA/AACVPR medical director responsibilities for outpatient cardiac rehabilitation/secondary prevention programs. http://circ.ahajournals.org/cgi/content/full/112/21/3354

AHA scientific statement: exercise and physical activity in the prevention and treatment of atherosclerotic cardiovascular disease. Available from: http://circ.ahajournals.org/cgi/content/full/107/24/3109.

AHCPR supported clinical practice guidelines: cardiac rehabilitation. Clinical Guideline No. 17. (AHCPR Publication No. 96-0672, October 1995.) Available from: http://www.ncbi.nlm.nih.gov/books/bv.fcgi?rid=hstat2.chapter.6677.

American Association of Cardiovascular and Pulmonary Rehabilitation. Available from: http://www.aacvpr.org/.

American College of Sports Medicine. ACSM's guidelines for exercise testing and prescription. 6th ed. Philadelphia: Lippincott Williams & Wilkins; 2000.

CORONARY ARTERY BYPASS SURGERY

Thoralf M. Sundt III, MD

BACKGROUND

Surgical coronary revascularization remains a state-of-the-art therapy for cardiac ischemia. Despite scientific and procedural developments that narrow the gap between surgical and percutaneous revascularization strategies, differences in outcome remain, with surgery continuing to demonstrate superior durability and greater long-term cost effectiveness at the expense of greater invasiveness for the patient. Accordingly, it continues to be appropriate for cardiologists to understand the surgical perspective on coronary revascularization with particular attention to the surgeon's view of preoperative assessment, some aspects of intraoperative decision making, and selected aspects of postoperative care.

Preoperative Assessment

Preoperative assessment of the candidate for coronary revascularization includes a determination of the risk/benefit ratio for the individual patient. Several tools are available for the assessment of preoperative risk, the most sophisticated of which is provided by the Society of Thoracic Surgeons Database. This database, which currently includes data on hundreds of thousands of individual cardiac surgical cases, running the gamut from coronary to valvular disease, provides a risk-stratification tool for fee-paying participants. At present, the risk algorithm is proprietary, although this may change in the near future. Nonetheless, the essential elements that help in determining risk are well recognized and have been demonstrated in numerous publications (Table 1).

Unfortunately, there is no statistical tool substituting for the "foot of the bed" test. It is common surgical lore that a successful coronary bypass operation demands three elements: adequate left ventricular function, a suitable conduit, and graftable targets. The optimal results will be obtained when all three are present. Good results can generally be obtained when two of the three are acceptable. One proceeds with extreme caution if only one of these three critical elements is of reasonable quality. Other elements, including general physiologic condition and good function of other organ systems, including, most importantly, renal function, enter into the assessment as well. It should be noted that the perioperative risk of death is dramatically increased among patients who suffer perioperative renal failure. Indeed individuals with marginal renal function who go into renal failure perioperatively fare worse than those who are dialysis dependent preoperatively.

Table 1.   Relative Mortality Risk: Core Coronary Artery Bypass Graft Variables for Operative Mortality

Variable	NNE	VA	STS	NYS	CC	AGH
No. of patients	3,055	12,712	332,064	57,187	4,918	1,567
Year of publication	1992	1992	1997	1994	1997	1996
Years included	1987-1989	1987-1990	1990-1994	1989-1992	1993-1995	1991-1992
Database variables						
Age/year	1.04	1.04	1.1	1.0	1.05	NA
Sex, female	1.2	NA	1.5	1.5	1.63	1.48
Prior heart surgery	3.6	3.2	3.0	3.7	1.72	1.39
Left main disease (70%)	NA	NA	1.3	1.43	NA	NA
No. of diseased coronary vessels						
1	1	NA	1.0	NA	NA	NA
2	1.3	NA	1.0	NA	NA	NA
3	1.6	NA	1.2	NA	NA	NA
Urgency of operation						
Elective	1	1.0	1.0	1.0	1	1
Urgent	2.1	2.4	1.2	1.42	NA	3.5
Emergent	4.4	3.8	2.0	4.0	5.07	7.14
Salvage	NA	NA	6.7	NA	NA	29.9
Ejection fraction						
0.50-0.59		NA	--	--	NA	--
0.40-0.49		NA	--	--	NA	--
0.30-0.39		NA	--	1.6	NA	2.89 (<30%)
0.20-0.29		NA	--	2.2	NA	--
<0.20		NA	--	4.1	NA	--

AGH, Allegheny General Hospital; CC, Cleveland Clinic; NA, not available; NNE, Northern New England Cardiovascular Disease Study Groups; NYS, New York State cardiac surgery reporting systems; STS, Society for Thoracic Surgery national cardiac surgical database; VA, Veterans Affairs cardiac surgical database.

Preoperative Management

Perioperative risk can be modified to some degree by preoperative preparation. Patients fare better if they are not in acute congestive failure at the time of their procedure. The risk of coronary bypass is elevated in the first two weeks after an acute myocardial infarction. While one may argue about the point at which statistical significance is lost, in nearly every study performed, the trend is the same: the closer to the episode of infarction, the higher the perioperative risk. Often an extraordinarily high-risk patient who has had a very large infarct with severely depressed ventricular function will sail through an operation if it can be delayed 2 to 6 weeks as ventricular function recovers. It is important to pay attention to right ventricular performance among patients who have had a recent inferior wall myocardial infarction. A notorious surgical trap is the patient with proximal right coronary artery occlusion and associated right ventricular infarction unrecognized because left ventriculography demonstrates only mildly depressed ventricular function. Echocardiography, if not focused on right ventricular function, may also miss this finding. Such a patient, brought to the operating room, will not be weaned from cardiopulmonary bypass.

Pharmacologic measures, which may be used preoperatively to reduce perioperative risk, include the administration of β-blockers and statins. Data supporting the use of β-blockers are quite solid. β-Blockade should be instituted even if only one dose can be administered preoperatively. Of less certain impact is the preoperative administration of statins. Some evidence suggests that patients receiving statins have a lower operative risk, possibly related to improved endothelial cell function. Although the minimum required duration of treatment with statins is unclear, experimental data suggest that several weeks of therapy are required to achieve this effect. At a minimum, from a practical standpoint, it seems reasonable to initiate statin therapy as soon as a decision has been made to proceed with surgical intervention.

INTRAOPERATIVE MANAGEMENT AND DECISION MAKING

On Pump vs. Off Pump

When a decision has been made to proceed to surgical intervention, several additional decisions must be made about technique. The first is a choice between on-pump and off-pump coronary surgery. Some of the earliest coronary artery bypass procedures performed in the 1950s and 1960s were, in fact, performed without cardiopulmonary bypass, and there has been some ongoing interest in these approaches, particularly in countries with limited economic means. Of late, there has been a resurgence of interest in off-pump

approaches in hopes of reducing neurocognitive deficits following coronary bypass. The term "pump head" was coined to describe alterations in mental status related to cardiopulmonary bypass. Some data have supported the notion that neurocognitive deficits occurring after cardiopulmonary bypass may be persistent. It is logical, therefore, that coronary artery bypass performed without cardiopulmonary bypass may obviate these concerns.

Unfortunately, the data supporting an improvement in neurocognitive outcomes with the use of off-pump techniques has been weak at best. Several nonrandomized studies suggested significant advantages to off-pump surgery. Those studies were followed with several prospectively randomized studies that demonstrated trends toward decreased bleeding and transfusion as well as improved renal function with off-pump surgery but no convincing difference in neurocognitive outcome (Table 2). This paradox can be understood by review of more recent literature concerning neurocognitive outcomes following surgery of all types and patients with coronary artery disease undergoing angioplasty or medical management versus coronary artery bypass graft surgery. These studies indicate that apparent neurocognitive deficits are readily detectable after all manner of surgical procedures in young and old, as well as after general anesthesia or spinal anesthesia. This suggests

Table 2. Results of Randomized Trials of Off-Pump Coronary Artery Bypass Surgery

Study	Year of first publ	Pt, no.		Mortality, %		MI, %		CVA/TIA		Neuropsycho-metric testing	Other findings
		On	Off	On	Off	On	Off	On	Off		
Octupus	2001	139	142	1.4	1.4	6.5	5	1.4	0.4	Decline*	Similar QOL†
BHACAS 1		100	100	2	0	4	1	2	2	No difference	Similar QOL
BHACAS 2	2002	100	100	0	0	1	0	1	1	No difference	Similar QOL
SMART	2003	99	98	2	3	--	--	2	1		Similar QOL‡
PRAGUE	2004	184	204	1.2	1.2	1.7	1.2	1.2	0		

BHACAS, Beating Heart Against Cardioplegic Arrrest Study; CVA, cerebrovascular accident; MI, myocardial infarction; PRAGUE, Primary Angioplasty in Patients Transferred from General Community Hospitals to Specialized PTCA Units With or Without Emergency Thrombolysis; Pt, patients; publ, publication; QOL, quality of life; SMART, Surgical Management of Arterial Revascularization Therapies; TIA, transient ischemic attack.
*At 3 months: on, 29%; off, 21%. At 12 months: on, 34%; off, 31%.
†Similar graft patency (on, 93%; off, 91%).
‡Graft patency early (on, 98%; off, 99%). Graft patency at 1 year (on, 96%; off, 94%).

that some neurocognitive alterations may be related simply to the stress of surgery. Of note, one study tracked perceived neurocognitive deficits to indices of psychologic depression. Additionally, most studies demonstrate a return to baseline neurocognitive function within 3 months of surgery. In short, despite undeniable anecdotal experience with the occasional patient who suffers significant memory loss and occasionally alterations in personality after cardiopulmonary bypass, the vast majority of individuals appear to be no worse for the pump.

Nonetheless, argument can still be made for off-pump surgery. It is an axiom of surgery that the simpler one can make a procedure the better. If the same operation can be performed off-pump as on-pump, why not do so? The issue is completeness of revascularization. Although several studies reported by leaders in the field of off-pump surgery have reported similar indices of revascularization regardless of the modality used, more commonly fewer grafts are performed in the off-pump group vs on-pump registries. Concerns have also been raised about graft patency among off-pump patients. This is hotly debated but remains unresolved. At this time, it is fair to say that off-pump surgery is a reasonable option, provided the patient can be adequately revascularized. There is no clear mandate, however, to perform procedures without bypass and no hard evidence to support the superiority of this approach. It is still reasonable for surgeons and cardiologists to elect either on- or off-pump coronary bypass.

Conduit Choice

A second and likely more critical decision is the choice of conduits to be used in the revascularization strategy. The principle clinical outcome difference between coronary bypass and percutaneous intervention has been and will likely continue to be durability. Although percutaneous coronary intervention is by far the least invasive and the target vessel revascularization failure gap has been narrowed with the use of drug-eluting stents, at this time coronary bypass provides a more durable result. It is also the procedure that has been most solidly associated with an improvement in survival over medical therapy to date. The durability of the procedure, however, depends in large measure on graft patency.

Graft patency depends not only on a technically

perfect anastomosis but also on the characteristics of the conduit used. Saphenous vein is the traditional conduit for coronary revascularization. It is readily harvested and is relatively easy to work with from a technical standpoint. Unfortunately, there are solid data to demonstrate a significant occlusion rate. One can expect 10% of saphenous vein grafts to be occluded at 1 year and 50% of them to be occluded at 10 years. It has been hypothesized, although not proved, that vein graft attrition is largely due to taking a venous structure and subjecting it to arterial hemodynamics. Still, in many settings it has proved to be a satisfactory conduit and is particularly useful in settings of competitive flow.

The internal thoracic artery (ITA) has become the gold standard for a durable conduit. The ITA was used in some of the earliest coronary bypass procedures and its use was held dear by a small group of enthusiasts over the years. In the 1980s it became apparent that use of an ITA graft to the left anterior descending artery actually conferred improved patient survival. This is most likely due in large measure to the demonstrable 10-year patency rate of 90% to 95%. The reason for this patency may relate in part to the unfenestrated internal elastic lamina of the ITA which inhibits migration of smooth muscle cells to the subintimal space, the minimal degree of medial muscularity, or its increased basal excretion of nitric oxide. The downside to the use of the ITA is its fragility and the increased level of difficulty in performing a distal anastomosis between the coronary artery and the ITA. Devascularization of the sternum due to loss of the ITA blood supply to the sternum increases the risks of wound complications. As the population of patients undergoing coronary bypass is enriched for diabetics over time, the concerns for sternal wound infection increase. Good data in the literature suggest that the use of bilateral ITAs significantly increases the risk of sternal wound infection among diabetics. Recent use of skeletonized ITAs may assuage these fears since there appears to be less devascularization of the sternum when the artery is taken in a skeletonized fashion.

A third common conduit is the radial artery. The radial artery was used in the early days of coronary bypass and abandoned because of apparent early failures. Recognition in the past decade that some of the patients with "early string sign" (atresia) of the radial artery had patent radial artery grafts when re-angiogramed many years later suggests that the radial artery is a better conduit than originally thought. Accordingly, there has been an enormous resurgence in interest in the radial artery. It has the advantage of being harvested simultaneously with the ITA and having reduced sternal devascularization. In addition, the radial artery is somewhat longer than the ITA, and this may be advantageous, particularly when performing complex complete arterial revascularization strategies (Fig. 1). The radial artery has been demonstrated in a prospectively randomized trial to have patency superior to that of the saphenous vein but still falling short of the ITA. These patency data, however, need to be viewed in light of the effect of both target vessel stenosis and target vessel identity. As shown in Fig. 2, the radial artery performs particularly poorly in the presence of less than critical stenosis. It is now widely accepted that the radial artery should only be used for targets with a greater than 80% stenosis. It is not uncommon for nicely patent radial artery grafts to undergo involution after angioplasty of stenoses proximal to the target lesion, again attesting to the impact of competitive flow. In addition, target identity is an important factor determining patency regardless of the conduit used. All conduits have the worst patency to the right coronary artery and its branches and intermediate patency to the circumflex artery.

Mitral Regurgitation

Mitral regurgitation (MR) is frequently observed early after myocardial infarction, and delay of surgery until some element of ventricular recovery has occurred may permit resolution of functional MR. Acute MR secondary to papillary muscle rupture, however, is a surgical emergency and requires prompt intervention. In some instances, the mitral valve may be repaired by suture of the ruptured papillary muscle to the left ventricular wall or adjacent papillary muscle. More often the valve is replaced. Either treatment is acceptable. Functional MR due to anular dilatation may be treated with simple anuloplasty. There is controversy among surgeons over the optimal technique for repair—complete versus partial ring and rigid versus flexible ring. Regardless, the rate of recurrent MR is significant. Furthermore, the impact of repair on late outcome is unclear.

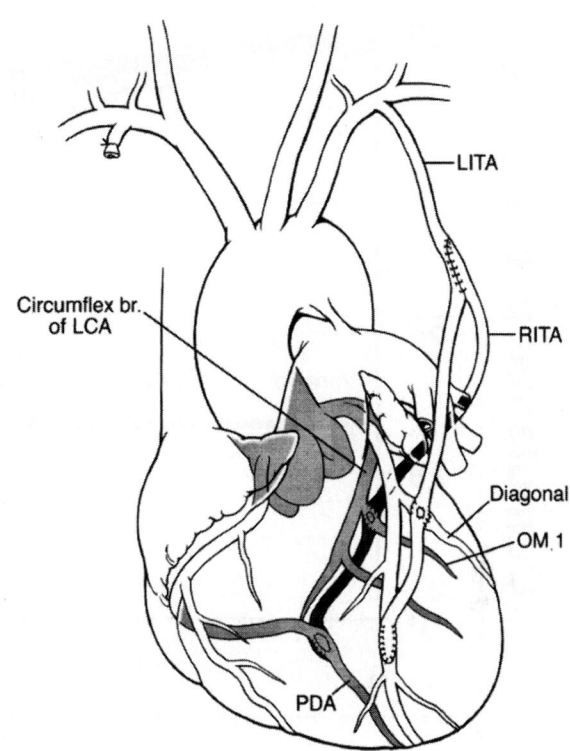

Fig. 1. Use of internal thoracic (mammary) artery grafts for coronary revascularization. br, branch; LCA, left coronary artery; LITA, left internal thoracic artery; OM 1, obtuse marginal branch of circumflex artery; PDA, posterior descending artery; RITA, right internal thoracic artery.

POSTOPERATIVE MANAGEMENT

Hemodynamics

Postoperative management of the coronary bypass patient is like that of any other patient undergoing a cardiac surgical procedure. Of note, patients undergoing off-pump surgery receive much less fluid intraoperatively and require less aggressive diuresis in the postoperative period. Coronary bypass patients should be maintained with a cardiac index (CI) greater than 2.2 L/m2. A CI below this standard should be managed according to a thoughtful algorithm, beginning with assessment of the rate and rhythm. Cardiac surgical patients are particularly sensitive to a loss of sinus rhythm, possibly due to perioperative diastolic dysfunction after the ischemic insult and edema in the myocardium. After ensuring an adequate rate and a sinus rhythm, one should consider the filling pressures. A right atrial pressure of between 8

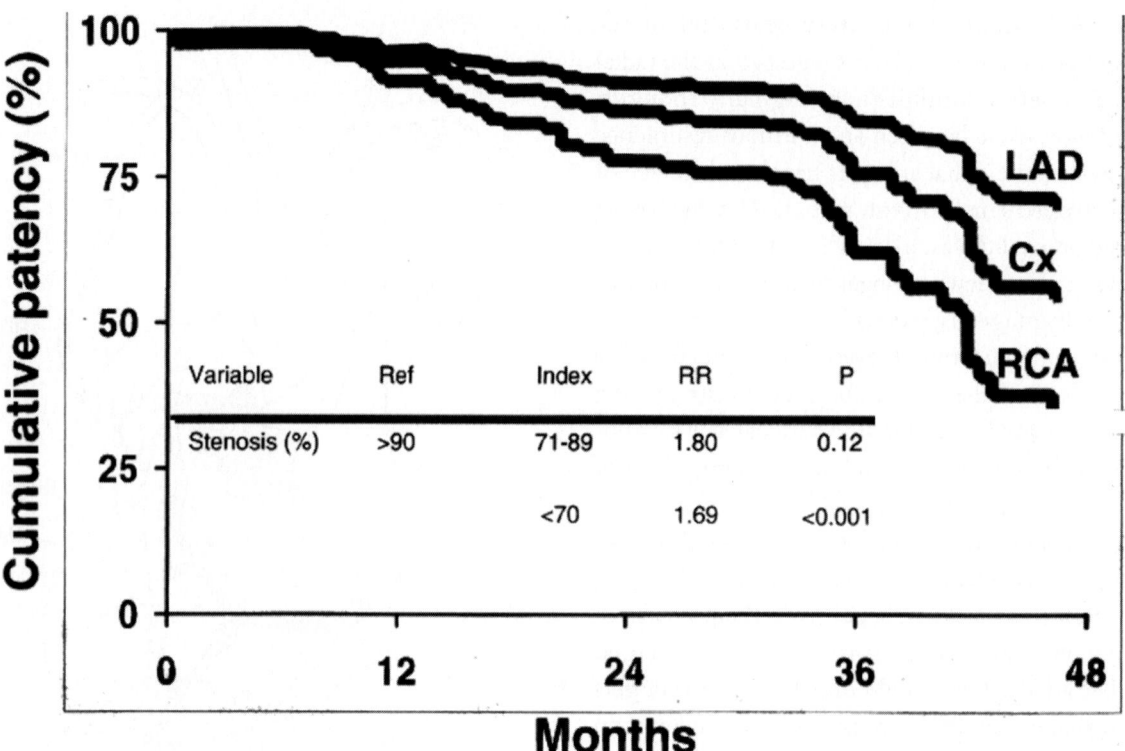

Fig. 2. Radial artery patency in coronary artery revascularization. Cx, circumflex; LAD, left anterior descending; RCA, right coronary artery; Ref, reference; RR, relative risk.

and 12 mm Hg and pulmonary artery diastolic pressure between 16 and 20 mm Hg should be adequate in most instances. Of note, a patient who has adequate hemodynamics but lower filling pressures does not need the administration of fluids. Fluids are required simply for restoring an adequate CI. If filling pressures are adequate or elevated due to left ventricular or right ventricular failure, inotropic support should be initiated. The first-line drugs are often dopamine and dobutamine, with epinephrine an increasingly popular choice among cardiovascular anesthesiologists. Milrinone or other phosphodiesterase inhibitors can also be quite helpful.

An important concept in the postoperative management of patients is their passage through stages of recovery, including the early requirement for additional fluids as the heart recovers, shifting later to a requirement for active diuresis when myocardial function has been restored. This is the rationale behind the seeming paradox that low urine output is treated with volume tonight and furosemide tomorrow.

Pulmonary Function

Coronary artery bypass patients may be extubated early after surgery. In some centers, these patients are extubated in the operating room, provided their core body temperature has returned to normal. During the cardiopulmonary bypass run, some surgeons cool the body temperature and there is some evidence to suggest there are improved neurologic outcomes with this approach, although the data are a bit tenuous. Almost all patients have some core body cooling in the operating room due to ambient temperature loss, but patients having procedures on cardiopulmonary bypass are particularly subject to this. Intubation and mechanical ventilation help to offset the increased oxygen consumption caused by shivering during rewarming. The philosophy of waiting for extubation until the following morning, however, which was popular a decade ago, has given way to "fast-track" protocols that emphasize early extubation. This is accomplished principally through the use of appropriate short-acting anesthetic agents. The vast majority of coronary bypass patients can be extubated within 12 hours of surgery.

Postoperative pulmonary dysfunction can occur secondary to cardiopulmonary bypass, although this is uncommon. Other causes of respiratory insufficiency include pleural effusions, which are relatively common and are in most instances readily manageable with a simple pleural tap. Occasionally postoperative pleural effusions will recur and require several taps. A formal pleurodesis or insertion of a pleural chest tube is seldom required.

Another potential cause of respiratory dysfunction postoperatively is phrenic nerve injury. The phrenic nerve enters the thoracic space adjacent to the internal thoracic artery and it is possible during harvest of the internal thoracic artery to damage the nerve. It is uncommon to transect it; however, use of electrocautery near the nerve can cause a palsy, which is usually transient. The use of intrapericardial ice is becoming less common today; however, in centers where it is still used, phrenic nerve injury can occur simply secondary to the cold.

Sternal Wound

Sternal wound complications are uncommon after coronary bypass but may occur. In most institutions, the rate of deep sternal wound infection is 1% or less. The earliest sign of deep sternal wound infection is often excessive sternal pain. The sternotomy itself should not be particularly painful after the first day or two. Increasing sternal pain, particularly in the first days after surgery, should not be discounted as postpericardiotomy syndrome without a rigorous evaluation for sternal wound infection. This should include physical examination to assess sternal stability as well as a computed tomographic (CT) scan to determine integrity of the sternal bone itself. Occasionally air will be apparent, although often this is secondary simply to the recent presence of a chest tube. It is common to see soft tissue thickening behind the sternum, and the CT scan is often not helpful in that regard. Drainage from the inferiormost portion of the wound is common but can be a harbinger of deep sternal wound problems to come. Drainage from the wound should be taken seriously. There are no clear guidelines for antibiotic use, but most surgeons are liberal given the gravity of sternal wound infections.

The sternum itself should heal in 6 to 12 weeks.

During that time, one should discourage activities that stress the sternum, including swinging a golf club or bowling. If both internal thoracic arteries have been harvested, sternal wound healing is slowed accordingly.

Postoperative Bleeding

Postoperatively, some chest tube output is to be expected. The usual criteria for return to the operating room are 400 mL of chest tube output in a single hour, 300 mL per hour for 2 consecutive hours, or 200 mL per hour for 3 hours. These criteria are not hard and fast and, of course, the decision will be affected by specific surgical factors. Before being returned to the operating room, the patient should have a complete evaluation of coagulation studies, including platelet count, prothrombin time, and partial thromboplastin time. Mild elevation of the prothrombin time is to be expected postoperatively (14-16 seconds); however, if the prothrombin time is significantly prolonged, administration of fresh frozen plasma should be considered. A platelet count should be in excess of 100,000. A prolongation of the partial thromboplastin time early postoperatively may be due to incomplete reversal of heparin. The additional administration of 25-50 mg of protamine may be helpful in this circumstance. Patients with preexisting renal dysfunction are particularly prone to bleeding, and cryoprecipitate can be of benefit in this subgroup for the correction of acquired platelet dysfunction. Administration of clotting factors, however, is not a substitute for a prompt return to the operating room if surgical bleeding is the culprit. Dark blood from the chest tubes is most often venous and can almost always be controlled nonoperatively with increased positive end-expiratory pressure unless the volume of bleeding is excessive. Bright red blood is more problematic and should raise a higher index of suspicion that surgical reexploration will be required. Patients who have experienced excessive chest tube output are at risk of postoperative pericardial tamponade. It is important for the practicing cardiologist to recognize that postoperative tamponade can be due to a localized clot, in contrast to the tamponade more often seen on echocardiogram secondary to pericardial effusion. A localized clot compressing the right atrium but not encasing the ventricles can cause hemodynamic instability (as can a localized thrombus behind the left atrium, etc.).

Echocardiographic criteria for early postoperative tamponade are, therefore, different from those for chronic pericardial effusion. Unexplained hemodynamic deterioration should prompt echocardiographic evaluation.

Weaning Patients From Inotropic Drips

The rate at which patients are weaned from inotropes is as much a matter of style as science. A reasonable approach is to use a rate dictated by the half-life of the drug itself. Therefore, phosphodiestase inhibitors may require a slower wean than β-adrenergic agents. Regardless, weaning should be guided by maintenance of a CI greater than 2.2 L/m^2 in the presence of acceptable filling pressures.

SECTION VIII

Diseases of the Heart, Pericardium, and Pulmonary Circulation

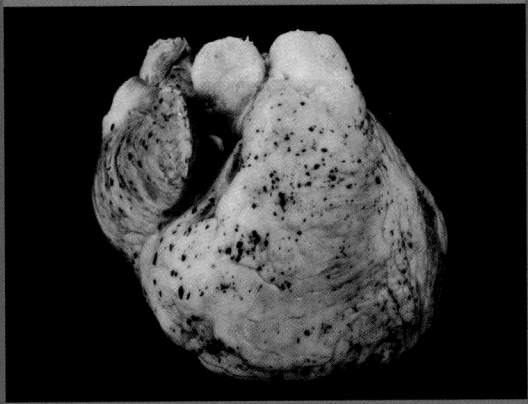

Melanoma Metastases

76

PERICARDIAL DISEASES

Jae K. Oh, MD

ANATOMY AND FUNCTION OF THE PERICARDIUM

Normal pericardium consists of an outer sac, the fibrous pericardium and an inner double-layered sac, the serous pericardium. The visceral layer of the serous pericardium, or epicardium, covers the heart and proximal great vessels. It is reflected to form the parietal pericardium, which lines the fibrous pericardium (Fig. 1). A few centimeters of the proximal portion of the great vessels do reside within the pericardial sac, which explains hemopericardium related to proximal aortic dissection.

The pericardium provides mechanical protection of the heart and lubricates the heart to reduce the friction between the heart and surrounding structures. The pericardium also has a significant hemodynamic impact on the atria and ventricles. Normally, intrapericardial pressure is equal to intrapleural pressure and is transmitted uniformly throughout the fluid-filled intrapericardial space (which usually contains 25-50 mL of clear fluid secreted by the visceral pericardium). The nondistensible pericardium limits acute distention of the heart. Ventricular volume is greater at any given ventricular filling pressure with the pericardium removed than with the pericardium intact. The pericardium also contributes to diastolic coupling between the two ventricles: the distention of one ventricle alters the filling of the other, an effect that is important in the pathophysiology of cardiac tamponade and constrictive pericarditis. Ventricular interdependence becomes more marked at high ventricular filling pressures.

- The pericardium protects and lubricates the heart.
- The pericardium contributes to diastolic coupling of the right and left ventricles, an effect that is important in tamponade and constrictive pericarditis.
- Proximal portions of the great vessels reside in the pericardial sac.

CONGENITAL ABSENCE OF THE PERICARDIUM

Complete absence of the pericardium is very rare and usually asymptomatic. More commonly, a small portion of the pericardium, usually on the left, is absent. Rarely with extreme cardiac shift to the left, the patient may experience left-sided nonexertional chest pain or prominent cardiac pulsation. This condition usually is diagnosed incidentally on chest radiography and displays a marked left-sided shift of the heart without tracheal deviation. Lung tissue is present between the aorta and the main pulmonary artery and between the inferior border of the heart and the left hemidiaphragm. The left ventricular contour is flattened (left upper border) and elongated, giving an appearance of a

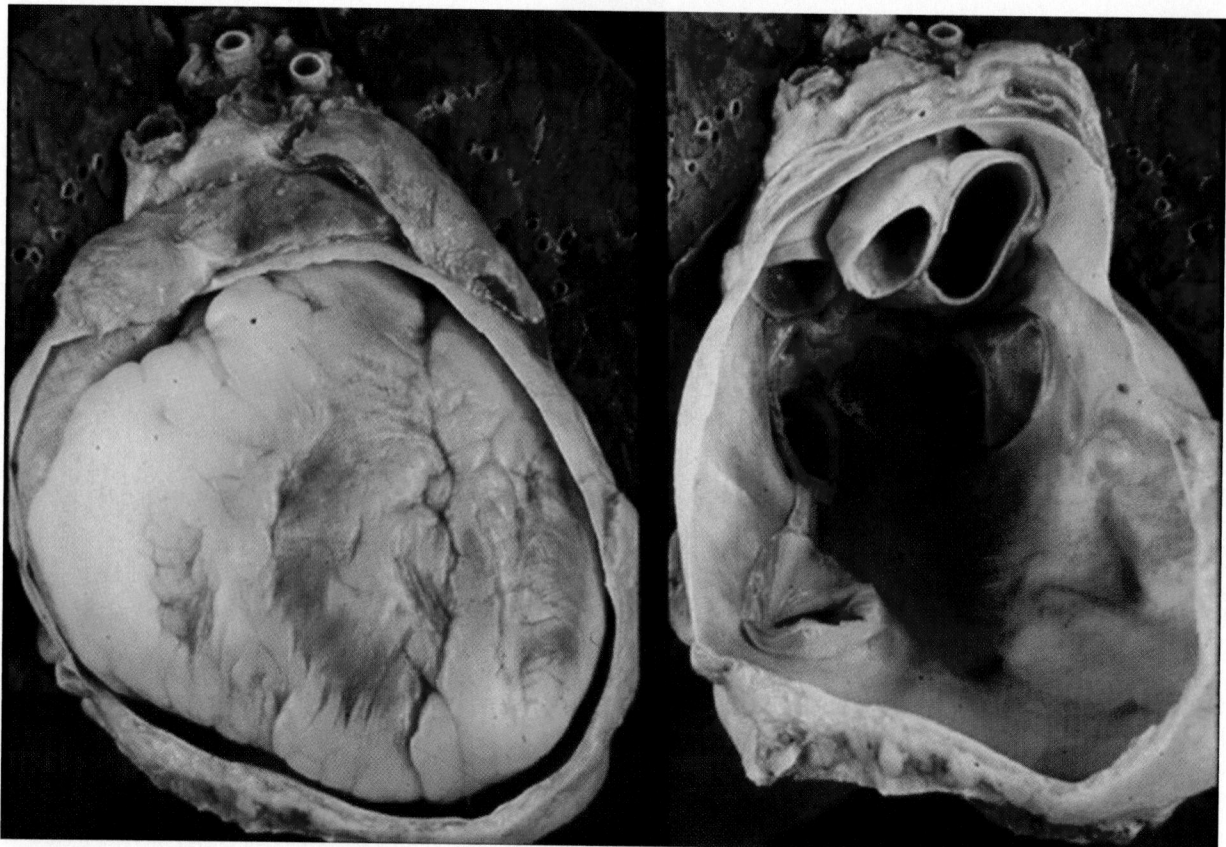

Fig. 1. Gross specimen, normal pericardium.

"Snoopy dog" (Fig. 2 *A* and *B*). The traditional echocardiographic windows demonstrate predominance of the right-sided cardiac chambers and may lead to an erroneous diagnosis of right ventricular volume overload and atrial septal defect. Cardiac motion is exaggerated on echocardiography, especially the posterior wall of the left ventricle. All cardiac structures are shifted to the left, resulting in prominent visualization of the right ventricular cavity and abnormal ventricular septal motion (Fig. 2 *C*). Congenital absence of the pericardium is associated with atrial septal defect, bicuspid aortic valve, and bronchogenic cysts. Rarely, herniation of cardiac chambers through a partial defect of the pericardium may cause sudden death, presumably because of marked ischemia from compression of the coronary artery. Closure of the pericardial defect is necessary in symptomatic patients.

■ Congenital absence of the pericardium gives a "Snoopy dog" cardiac silhouette on a chest radiograph.
■ Congenital absence of the pericardium is associated

with atrial septal defect, bicuspid aortic valve, and bronchogenic cysts.
■ Partial absence of the pericardium has been linked to sudden death.

PERICARDIAL CYST

A pericardial cyst is a benign structural abnormality of the pericardium that usually is detected as an incidental mass lesion on chest radiographs in an asymptomatic person (Fig. 3 *A*). Most frequently, it is located at the right costophrenic angle, but it may also be found at the left costophrenic angle, hilum, or superior mediastinum. The differential diagnoses are malignant tumors, cardiac chamber enlargement, and diaphragmatic hernia. Two-dimensional echocardiography, computed tomography (CT), or magnetic resonance imaging (MRI) may be used to differentiate pericardial cysts from other solid tumors (Fig. 3 *B* and *C*). In asymptomatic patients, no treatment is necessary.

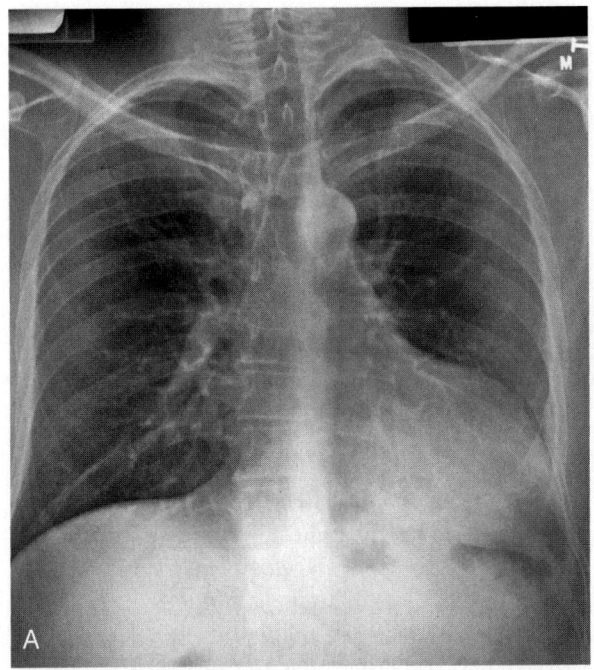

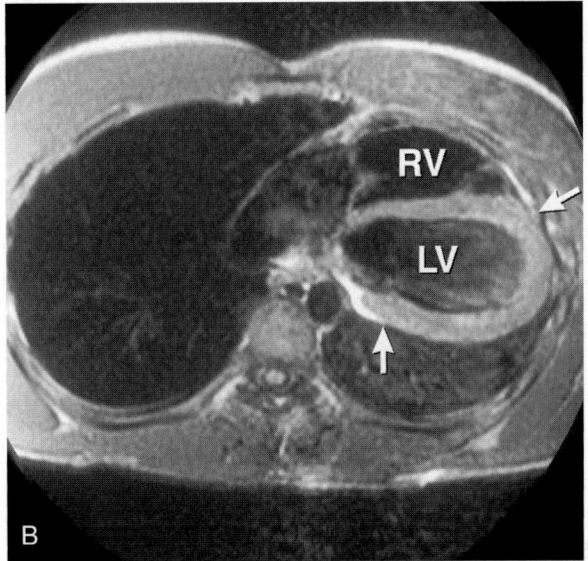

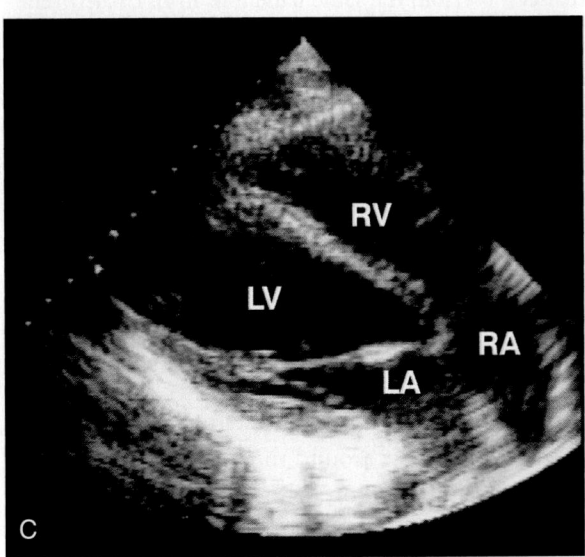

Fig. 2. *A*, Chest radiograph typical of congenital absence of pericardium. *B*, Magnetic resonance scan of chest showing marked cardiac shift to the left due to congenital absence of pericardium. *Arrows*, area of absent pericardium. *C*, Characteristic apical four-chamber view of the heart with congenital absence of pericardium on two-dimensional echocardiography. LA, left atrium; LV, left ventricle; RA, right atrium; RV, right ventricle.

■ Pericardial cyst is usually benign and located at the right costophrenic border.

ACUTE PERICARDITIS

The causes of acute pericarditis are numerous. Acute pericarditis usually is self-limited unless caused by malignancy or other systemic disease. Occasionally, acute pericarditis may undergo a transient constrictive phase. The most prominent symptom of acute pericarditis is pleuropericardial chest pain. Because the visceral pericardium is devoid of pain fibers, the parietal pericardium must be inflamed to cause chest pain. Characteristically, the pain is sharp, stabbing, and pleuritic and radiates to the scapula and back. Pericarditic pain may mimic anginal pain, and clinical differentiation may be difficult on the basis of the medical history alone. It is not uncommon that patients with acute pericarditis undergo urgent coronary angiography because of a concern for its being ST-segment elevation myocardial infarction (STEMI). Patients with acute pericarditis may develop a significant amount of pericardial effusion to the point of hemodynamic compromise, resulting in dyspnea, hypotension, tachycardia, and heart failure. On physical examination, a typical finding is a pericardial friction rub, which is characterized by scratchy high-pitched sounds with three distinct components (coincidental with rapid ventricular filling, ventricular contraction, and atrial contraction). In a subset of patients, however, the pericardial friction

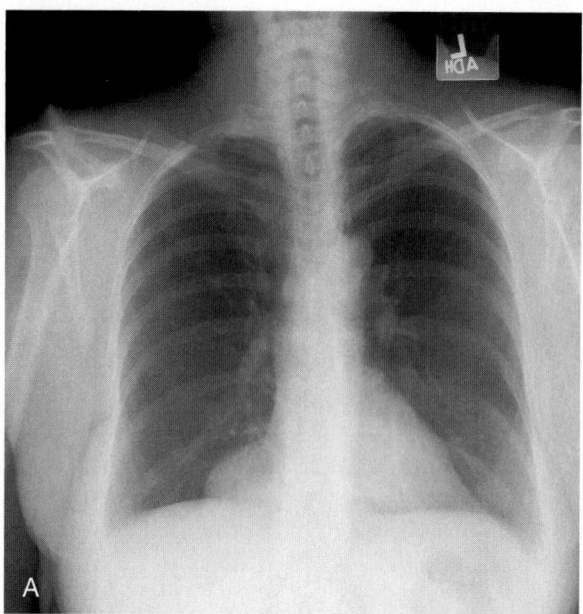

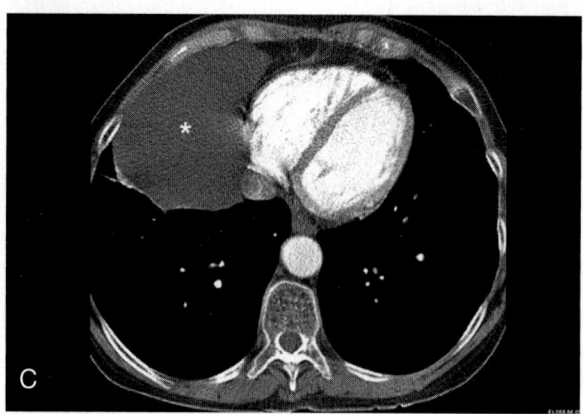

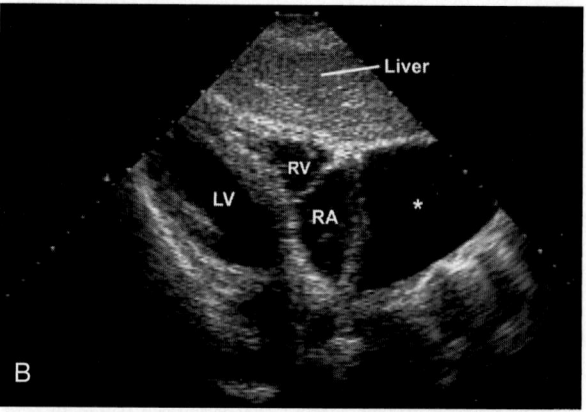

Fig. 3. *A*, Chest x-ray film demonstrating a typical finding in an asymptomatic patient with pericardial cyst. It is usually located in the right side of the heart. *B*, Subcostal echocardiographic view demonstrating a large echo-free cystic structure (*) adjacent to the right atrium (RA) typical of a pericardial cyst. *C*, Computed tomographic scan of the heart demonstrating a pericardial cyst (*) from the same patient as in *B*. LV, left ventricle; RV, right ventricle.

rub may have only one component. A pericardial rub usually is heard best at the left sternal border, with the patient leaning forward during held expiration. It is common for the rub to disappear when a pericardial effusion develops. A pericardial knock does not occur in acute pericarditis.

Electrocardiography in Acute Pericarditis

The ST-segment elevation in acute pericarditis is different from that in acute myocardial infarction (Figs. 4-7). ST-segment elevation in pericarditis is more diffuse, involving both limb and precordial leads. ST-segment elevation is "concave upward" and is associated with upright T waves. After several days of pericarditis, the ST segment returns to baseline and the T wave flattens and, later, becomes inverted. Another electrocardio-

graphic (ECG) characteristic of pericarditis is depression of the PR segment because of atrial involvement (see lead I on Fig. 4). This happens within several days after the onset of pericarditis.

Chest radiographs usually are normal unless the patient has a large amount of pericardial effusion. The most sensitive diagnostic technique for detecting pericardial effusion is echocardiography, which shows an echo-free space around the heart. The absence of pericardial effusion on echocardiography does not exclude the diagnosis of acute pericarditis.

Treatment of Acute Pericarditis

In most patients, acute pericarditis resolves gradually, and treatment is with nonsteroidal anti-inflammatory agents, usually aspirin, 650 mg every 4 hours, or indomethacin, 25 to 75 mg three times daily for 7 to 10 days, with gradual tapering. Rarely, recurrent chest pain may develop, for which more intense nonsteriodal anti-inflammatory agents and/or colchicine (0.6 mg twice daily) should be considered. Treatment of pericarditic pain with a steroid may lead to steroid dependency. Steroid treatment should be considered only when pericarditic pain does not respond to combinations of

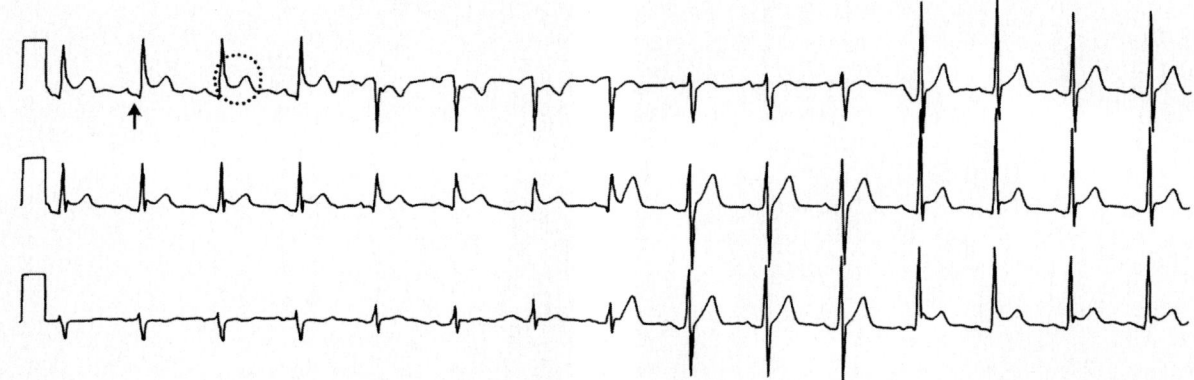

Fig. 4. Electrocardiogram typical of acute pericarditis. *Arrow,* PR depression in lead I. *Circle,* Typical "concave upward" ST-segment elevation.

nonsteroidal anti-inflammatory agents. Colchicine has been used to treat recurrent pericarditic pain, but its benefit is much less if the patient is already receiving steroid treatment. If the pain continues to limit the patient's activity and lifestyle, pericardiectomy may be required, even in the setting of no hemodynamic embarrassment.

Transient Constrictive Phase of Acute Pericarditis
About 7% to 10% of patients with acute pericarditis may have a transient constrictive phase. These patients usually have a moderate amount of pericardial effusion,

and as the pericardial effusion disappears, the pericardium remains inflamed, thickened, and noncompliant, resulting in constrictive hemodynamics. The patient presents with dyspnea, peripheral edema, increased jugular venous pressure, and, sometimes, ascites, as in patients with chronic constrictive pericarditis. This transient constrictive phase may last 2 to 3 months before it gradually resolves either spontaneously or with treatment with anti-inflammatory agents. When hemodynamics and findings typical of constriction develop in patients with acute pericarditis, initial treatment is indomethacin (Indocin) for 2 to 3 weeks and, if

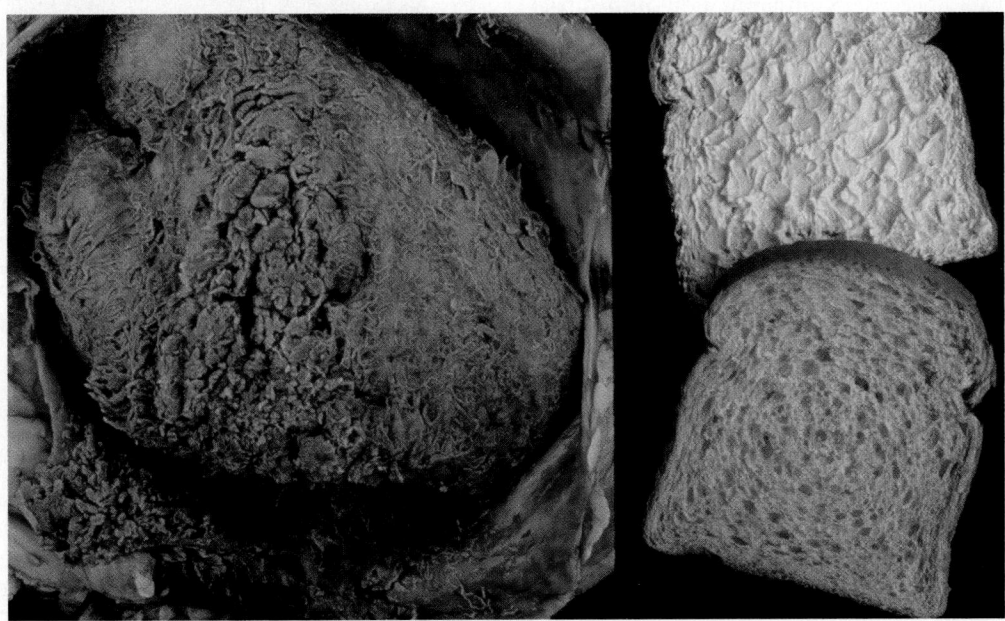

Fig. 5. Fibrinous "bread-and-butter" pericarditis.

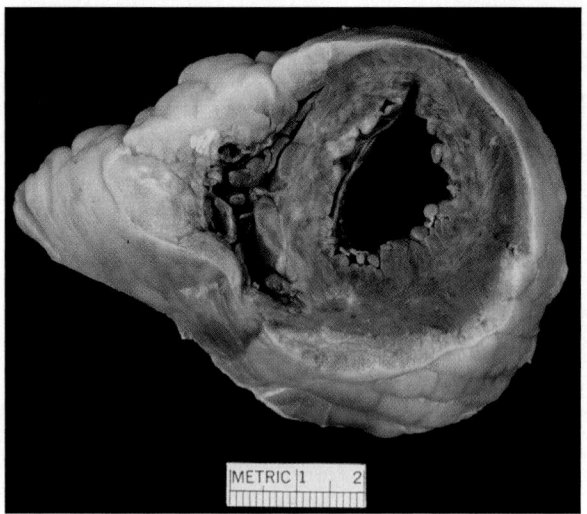

Fig. 6. Epicardial fat necrosis of the heart in pancreatitis.

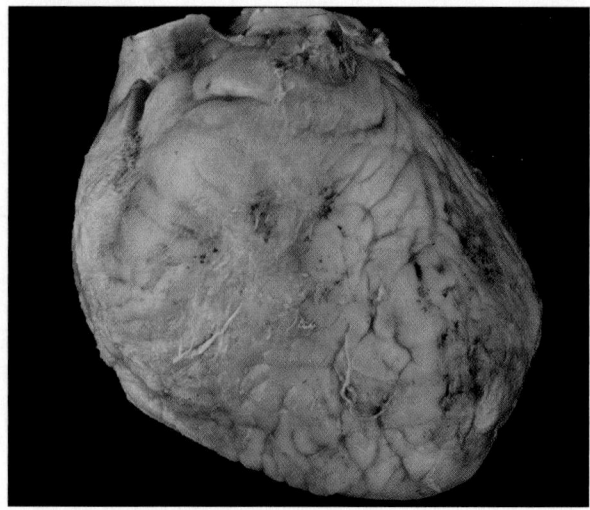

Fig. 7. Healed pericarditis due to systemic lupus erythematosus.

there is no response, steroids for 1 to 2 months after being sure the pericarditis is not caused by bacterial infection, including tuberculosis. Constrictive hemodynamics can be diagnosed readily with Doppler echocardiography (see below); resolution of constrictive physiology can be documented clinically and by follow-up echocardiography (Fig. 8).

■ The classic pericardial rub has three components.
■ Acute pericarditis may cause PR-segment depression on the ECG because of inflammation of the atrial wall.
■ From 7% to 10% of patients with acute pericarditis may have a transient constrictive phase.

PERICARDIAL EFFUSION/TAMPONADE

Pericardial inflammation of any cause may result in a large amount of fluid collecting in the pericardial sac. The pericardium may be filled with blood product (hemopericardium) because of cardiac rupture (injury, iatrogenic, or acute myocardial infarction), aortic dissection, or cardiac bypass surgery. Pericardial effusion may be related to underlying heart failure or abnormality in lymphatic drainage (chylous effusion). When a pericardial effusion develops gradually, so that it does not impair pericardial compliance, the patient may remain asymptomatic, even with a massive amount of pericardial effusion. If the rate of pericardial effusion is

rapid, even a small amount (50-100 mL) of fluid or blood in the pericardium can cause cardiac tamponade. Cardiac tamponade is the result of a critical elevation of intrapericardial pressure produced by accumulation of pericardial fluid.

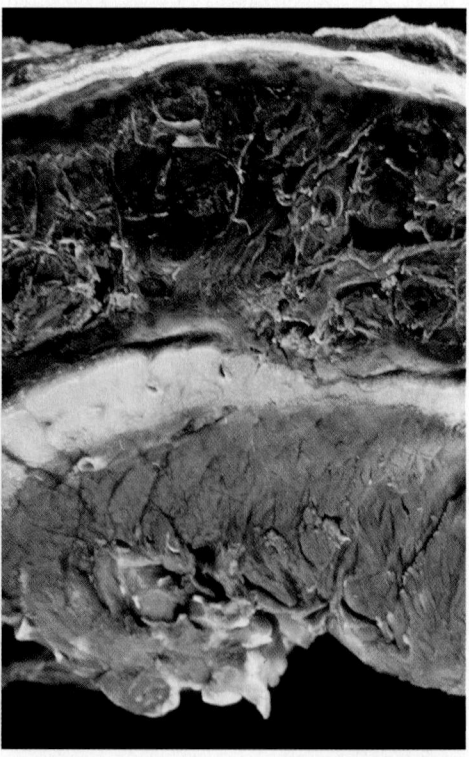

Fig. 8. Postoperative organizing hemopericardium.

Hemodynamics of Pericardial Tamponade

When intrapericardial pressure is increased, atrial pressure is also increased, resulting in impaired venous return. This, in turn, results in systemic venous congestion and reduction in cardiac output (Fig. 9). On physical examination, jugular venous pressure is increased, with prominent systolic x descent and blunted diastolic y descent (Table 1). With pericardial effusion, the precordium is quiet and cardiac sounds are diminished. The Beck triad consists of 1) a decrease in systolic pressure, 2) an increase in systemic venous pressure, and 3) a quiet heart. With reduction in cardiac output, pulse pressure is narrow and systemic venous congestion causes hepatomegaly, peripheral edema, and ascites. In patients with cardiac tamponade, the intrapericardial pressure is increased critically and does not vary with intrapleural pressure. Normally, intrapericardial pres-

sure changes with fluctuations in intrapleural pressure. With inspiration, intrapleural pressure decreases by 5 to 7 mm Hg and similar changes occur in intrapericardial pressure. However, in tamponade, intrapericardial pressure is increased to the level of ventricular diastolic pressures. Both ventricular diastolic pressures equalize with the pericardial pressure. Therefore, left atrial, right atrial, and right ventricular end-diastolic pressure, pulmonary end-diastolic pressure, and pulmonary capillary wedge pressure are equalized within 5 mm Hg of one another.

Intrapericardial and right atrial pressures may not be increased in "low-pressure tamponade," which occurs in the setting of severe hypovolemia. Ventricular filling and stroke volume are affected by relatively normal pressures. Jugular venous distention is absent in this setting.

Pulsus Paradoxus

Pulsus paradoxus is a decrease (>10 mm Hg) in systolic blood pressure during inspiration. This is due to the underlying mechanism of cardiac tamponade. With increased intrapericardial pressure, normal pressure transmission from the intrapleural to the intrapericardial cavity does not occur. Thus, on inspiration, the driving blood pressure across the pulmonary vascular bed decreases as the lungs expand in inspiration. Pulmonary arteriolar pressure decreases, while left atrial and left ventricular pressure remains relatively fixed.

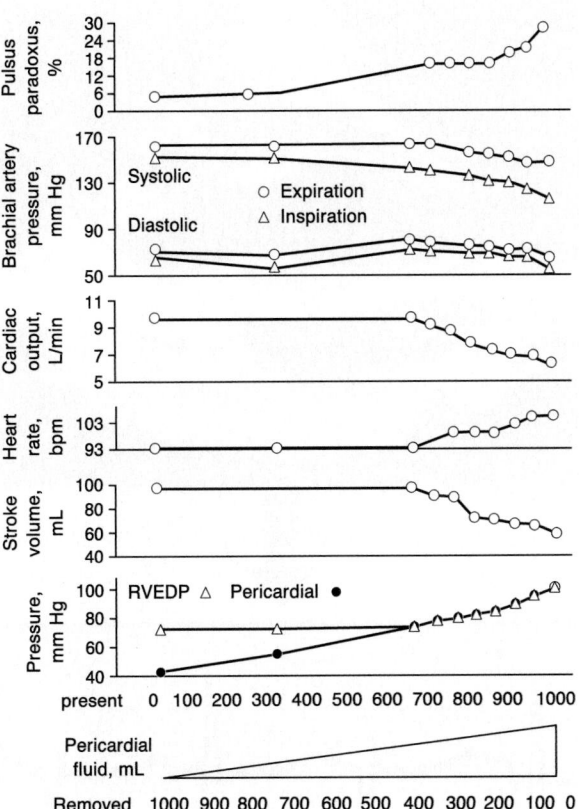

Fig. 9. Hemodynamic changes during pericardial fluid withdrawal in patient with cardiac tamponade. In second frame from top, note the disappearance of pulsus paradoxus. RVEDP, right ventricular end-diastolic pressure.

Table 1.   Comparison of Cardiac Tamponade and Constrictive Pericarditis

	Cardiac tamponade	Constrictive pericarditis
Pulsus paradoxus	Cardiac tamponade	Constrictive pericarditis
Kussmaul sign	Absent	May be present
Pericardial knock	Absent	May be present
Jugular venous pressure	Large x descent	Normal x descent
	Small or absent y descent	Large y descent

Thus, the decrease in pulmonary venous return to the left heart during inspiration translates into a decrease in left ventricular stroke volume, which is detected clinically as pulsus paradoxus. Pulsus paradoxus is characteristic of cardiac tamponade, but it also occurs in other conditions in which there is a significant decrease in forward stroke volume with inspiration, as in patients with acute cor pulmonale (pulmonary embolism), chronic obstructive lung disease, right ventricular infarction, or asthma.

Echocardiographic Diagnosis of Pericardial Effusion/Tamponade

Chest radiography may show cardiomegaly of globular appearance. The best way to detect pericardial effusion and tamponade is with echocardiography. A small amount of pericardial fluid appears as an echo-free space. As pericardial effusion increases, movement of the parietal pericardium decreases. When there is a large volume of pericardial effusion, the heart may have a swinging motion (Fig. 10) in the pericardial cavity, which is responsible for the ECG manifestation of cardiac tamponade, "electrical alternans." However, the swinging motion may be absent in cardiac tamponade. Other M-mode/two-dimensional echocardiographic findings of tamponade include the following:

1. Decreased excursion in the E-A slope of the mitral valve
2. Early diastolic collapse of the right ventricle
3. Late diastolic collapse of the right atrial free wall
4. Plethora of the inferior vena cava with a blunted respiratory change
5. Abnormal ventricular septal motion

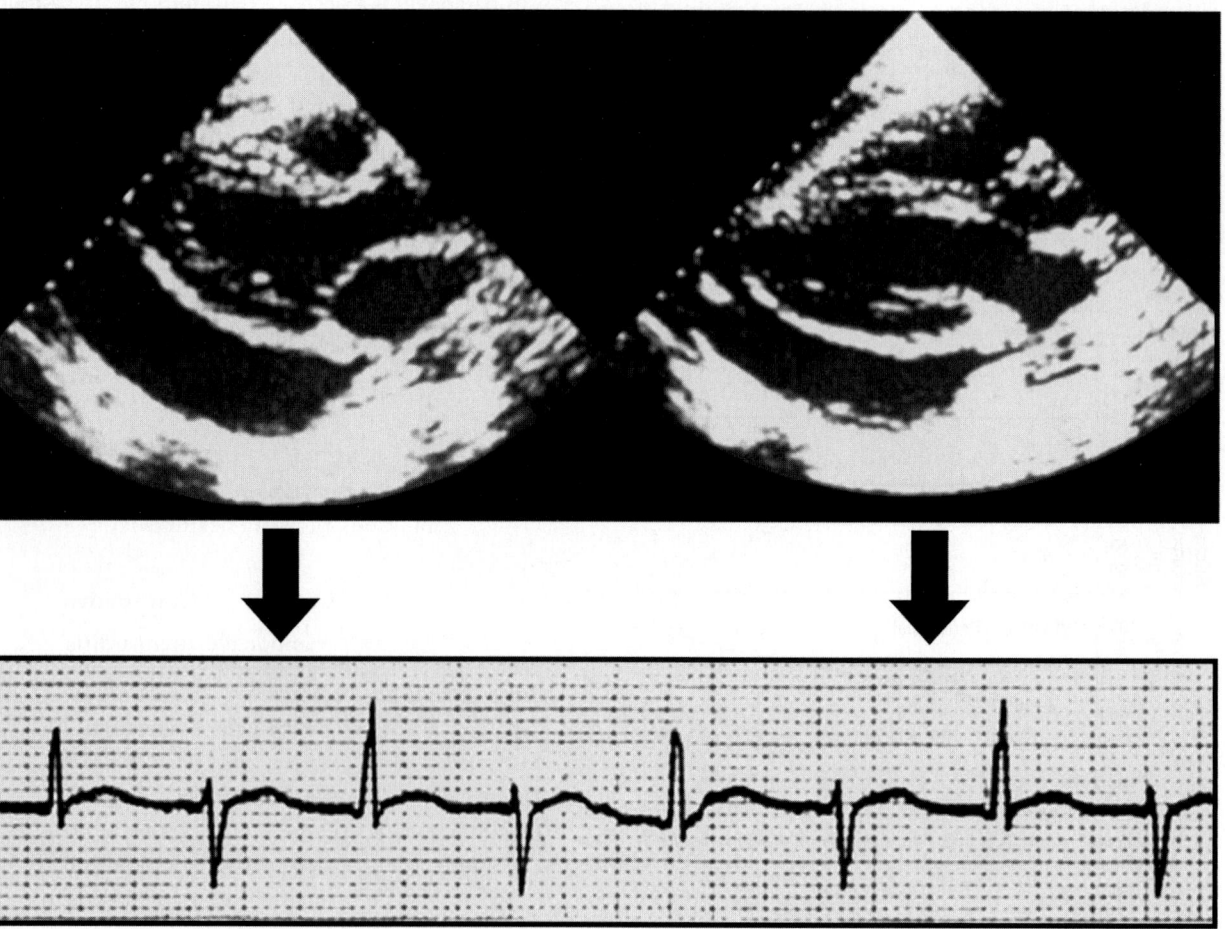

Fig. 10. *Upper*, Parasternal long-axis views demonstrating large pericardial effusion and swinging motion of the heart. *Lower*, With the swinging motion of the heart, the QRS voltage direction alternates, producing "electrical alternans."

In acute myocardial rupture, clotted blood seen in the pericardial sac is highly suggestive of hemopericardium. If there is air in the pericardial sac (pneumopericardium), echocardiographic imaging may be difficult. The Doppler findings in cardiac tamponade are based on the hemodynamic pathophysiology described for pulsus paradoxus. With inspiration, the driving pressure gradient to the left cardiac chamber is decreased so that mitral inflow velocity decreases with inspiration and increases with expiration. Because cardiac volume is relatively fixed with cardiac tamponade, reciprocal changes occur in the right chambers so that increased tricuspid inflow velocity occurs with inspiration and decreased inflow velocity with expiration. With a decrease in filling to the right chambers with expiration, there is significant flow reversal in the hepatic vein, with expiration during diastole (Fig. 11-13).

Treatment of Cardiac Tamponade

The only effective treatment for cardiac tamponade is the removal of pericardial fluid. The best way to perform pericardiocentesis is with echocardiographic guidance, which helps in locating the optimal site for the puncture, in determining the depth of the pericardial effusion, in measuring the distance from the puncture site to the effusion, and in monitoring the results of the pericardiocentesis.

■ Pulsus paradoxus is classically seen in pericardial tamponade.

■ Elective removal of pericardial fluid should always be guided echocardiographically to reduce complications.

Pericardial Effusion Due to Malignancy

Pericardial effusion due to malignancy is a poor prognostic sign. If cytologic examination demonstrates malignant cells in the pericardial effusion, the prognosis is grim regardless of the patient's underlying type of malignancy. Infrequently, pericardial effusion may be the initial presentation of an underlying malignancy. The tumors that spread most frequently to the pericardium are those of the lung and breast, followed by lymphoma and leukemia. Angiosarcoma is a primary cardiac tumor that presents with pericardial effusion and pericarditis. The pericardial fluid in malignancies is usually bloody, but a bloody effusion is not specific

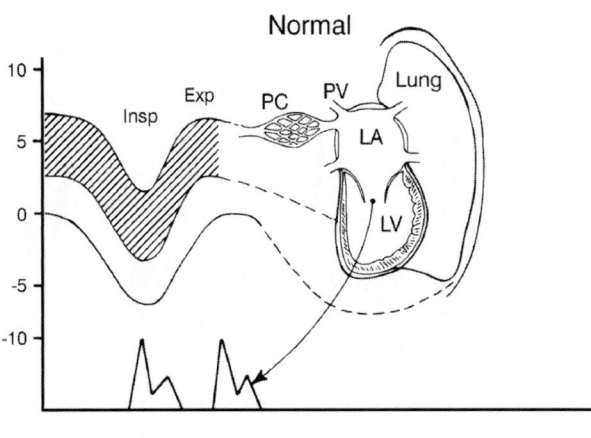

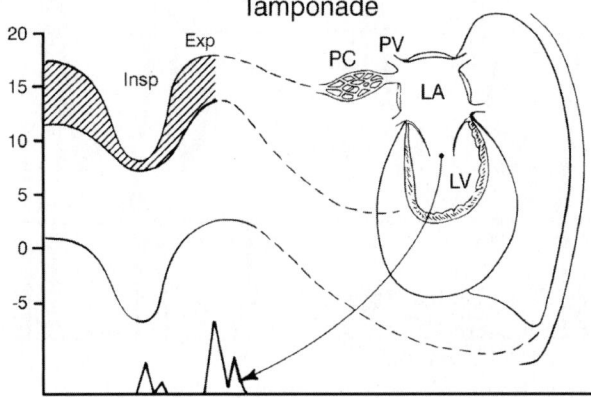

Fig. 11. Diagram of intrathoracic and intracardiac pressure changes with respiration in normal and tamponade physiology. The shaded area indicates left ventricular (LV) filling pressure gradients (difference between pulmonary capillary wedge pressure and LV diastolic pressure). At the bottom of each drawing is a schematic mitral inflow Doppler velocity profile reflecting LV diastolic filling. In tamponade, there is a decrease in LV filling after inspiration (Insp) because the pressure decrease in the pericardium and LV cavity is smaller than that in the pulmonary capillaries (PC). LV filling is restored after expiration (Exp). LA, left atrium; PV, pulmonary vein.

for malignancy. Recurrent pericardial effusion can be treated with repeated pericardiocentesis and sometimes with a pigtail catheter left in place for several days for continuous or intermittent drainage of reaccumulated fluid. Instillation of a sclerosing agent into the pericardium is painful and rarely used in our practice.

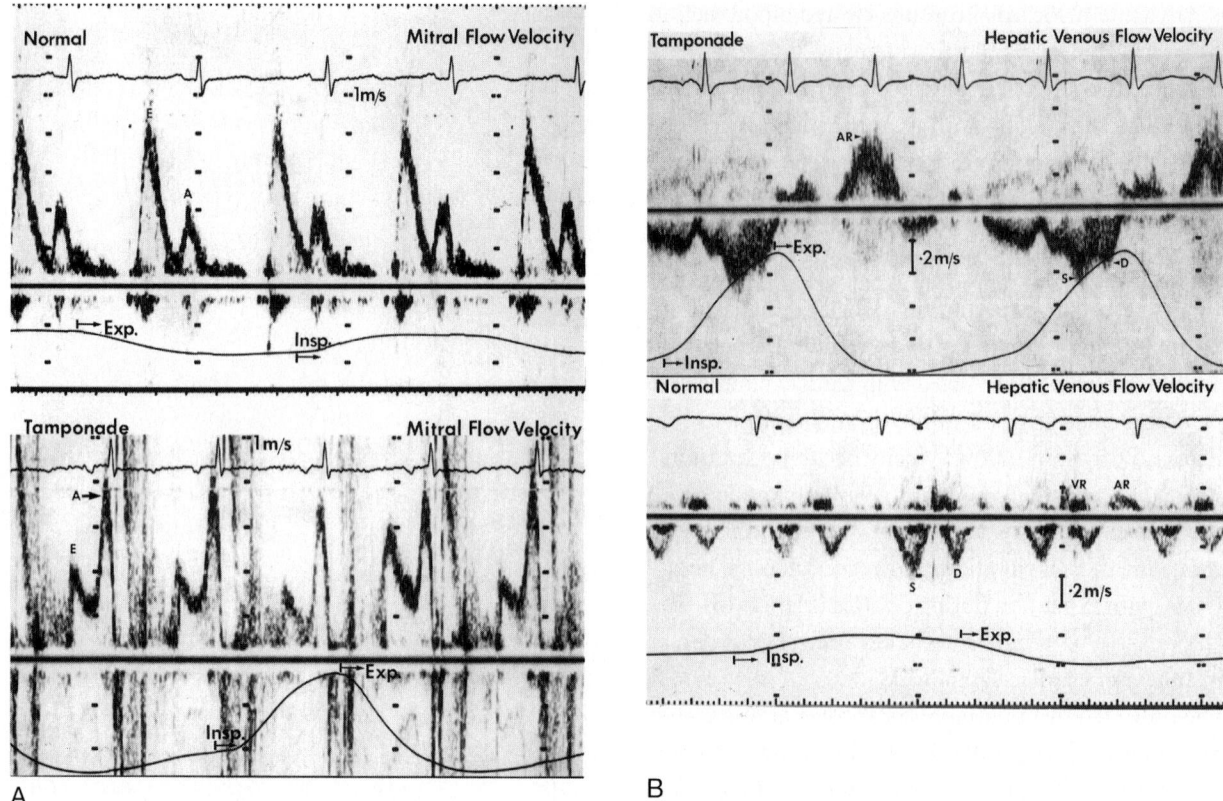

Fig. 12. *A*, Mitral inflow velocity profile typical of a normal subject (*upper*) and a patient with cardiac tamponade (*lower*). *B*, Hepatic venous flow velocity profile in a patient with cardiac tamponade (*upper*, same patient as in *A lower*) and a normal subject (*lower*). Exp, expiration; Insp, inspiration.

PERICARDITIS IN ACUTE MYOCARDIAL INFARCTION

Pericardial effusion occurs in about 20% of patients with acute transmural myocardial infarction, usually associated with a large anterior wall myocardial infarction. The chest pain is different from that of ischemic

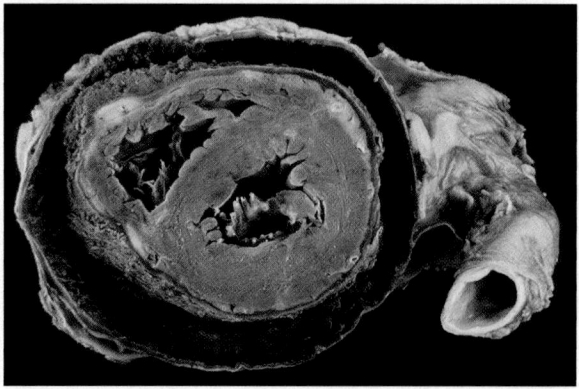

Fig. 13. Pericarditis with pericardial effusion.

chest pain and has a pleuritic component and an associated pericardial rub. The presence of a pericardial effusion with or without pericarditic pain after myocardial infarction is not a contraindication for intravenous treatment with heparin. Hemopericardium can occur after myocardial rupture as a complication of acute myocardial infarction and most frequently is associated with a lateral myocardial infarction (Fig. 14). Most patients with myocardial rupture develop electromechanical dissociation and do not survive. A subgroup of patients may develop subacute cardiac rupture and present with nausea, vomiting, restlessness, and persistent ECG changes. Rarely, the patient may develop a pseudoaneurysm, in which the hemopericardium is contained by the adjacent structures. Although pseudoaneurysm of the left ventricle was considered a surgical emergency, review of the data suggested that rupture of chronic pseudoaneurysm is rare or occurs at a low rate.

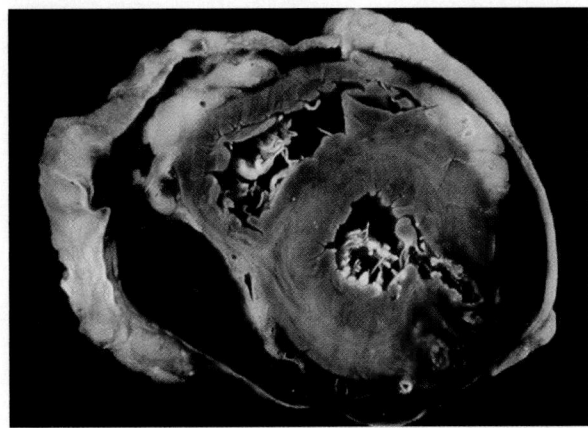

Fig. 14. Pathology specimen of a patient who died of cardiac rupture and hemopericardium.

Dressler Syndrome

Some patients develop pericarditis several weeks after myocardial infarction (Dressler syndrome). It is probably mediated immunologically. Usually it is treated initially with nonsteroidal anti-inflammatory agents, but steroid therapy may be needed for a small number of patients with refractory chest pain.

Postcardiotomy Syndrome

Postcardiotomy syndrome is similar to Dressler syndrome, and an autoimmune response to cardiac antigens has been implicated in this entity. Postcardiotomy syndrome occurs in about 5% of patients who have a cardiac surgical procedure, with symptoms occurring 3 weeks to 6 months postoperatively. It most likely is related to surgical trauma and irritation by blood products in the mediastinum and pericardium. The initial treatment for this syndrome is with nonsteroidal anti-inflammatory agents, and only in the case of refractory symptoms should systemic steroids be used. Pericardiectomy is rarely required.

TAMPONADE RELATED TO AORTIC DISSECTION

Cardiac tamponade or hemopericardium may occur with proximal aortic dissection. After pericardial tamponade is recognized as a result of aortic dissection, urgent surgical repair of the aortic dissection and tamponade is needed. In this clinical setting, pericardiocen-

tesis may increase blood pressure and cause rupture of the dissected aorta. A recent study showed 60% early mortality for patients with an aortic dissection complicated by cardiac tamponade. All patients who underwent pericardiocentesis died shortly thereafter. Hemopericardium due to aortic dissection has a characteristic finding on echocardiogram.

CONSTRICTIVE PERICARDITIS

Constrictive pericarditis is characterized by restrictive ventricular filling due to a thickened and/or calcified pericardium. The pericardium usually contains calcified fibrous scar tissue from an inflammatory process, and in the advanced stage, the scarring may involve the epicardium. The causes of constriction are several, including acute pericarditis, collagen vascular disease, coronary artery bypass surgery, and tuberculosis (Table 2). However, in many patients, the cause may not be identified. In the modern era, the most common cause for constrictive pericarditis is a previous cardiac surgery accounting for one-third of cases at our institution. Where tuberculosis is still common, it is a frequent cause of constriction, but it is rare in our practice.

Table 2. Causes of Constrictive Pericarditis

Unknown (idiopathic)
Post–acute pericarditis of any cause
Post–cardiac surgery
Uremia
Connective tissue disease (systemic lupus erythematosus, scleroderma, rheumatoid arthritis)
Post-trauma
Drugs (procainamide, hydralazine, methysergide)
Radiation-induced
Neoplastic pericardial disease (melanoma, mesothelioma)
Tuberculosis, fungal infections (histoplasmosis, coccidioidomycosis), parasitic infections
Post–myocardial infarct
Post–Dressler syndrome
Post–purulent pericarditis
Pulmonary asbestosis

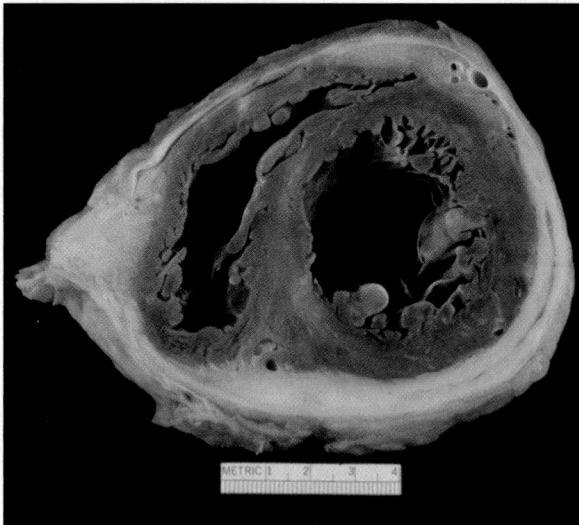

Fig. 15. Noncalcific constrictive pericarditis 4 years after coronary artery bypass grafting.

The main clinical features at presentation are dyspnea, peripheral edema, marked systemic venous congestion with hepatomegaly, and ascites. Frequently, patients are evaluated for primary liver disease and may undergo a liver biopsy before constrictive pericarditis is diagnosed (Fig. 15). The most prominent findings on physical examination are related to systemic venous congestion, such as distention of the jugular vein (Table 3). Venous pressure often increases with inspiration (Kussmaul sign) because of the inability of the right side of the heart to accept the increased cardiac input with inspiration. Unlike the patients with cardiac tamponade with x descent, patients with constrictive pericarditis have rapid y descent, which reflects the early diastolic decrease in right ventricular pressure.

With high atrial pressure, rapid filling of the ventricle is accelerated, and this generates the third heart sound known as "pericardial knock," which usually occurs 80 to 120 ms after aortic valve closure (Fig. 16), corresponding to the nadir of the y descent and the end of the early diastolic filling. Other differential diagnoses of a diastolic gallop occurring 80 to 120 ms after aortic valve closure include opening snap of the mitral valve in mitral stenosis (which is followed by a diastolic rumble), tumor plop from atrial myxoma, and a third heart sound related to left ventricular failure.

The correct diagnosis of constrictive pericarditis is crucial because most of the symptoms can be reversed by pericardiectomy. However, the symptoms and clinical findings mimic those of restrictive cardiomyopathy, which is a progressive disease with no effective treatment (Fig. 17).

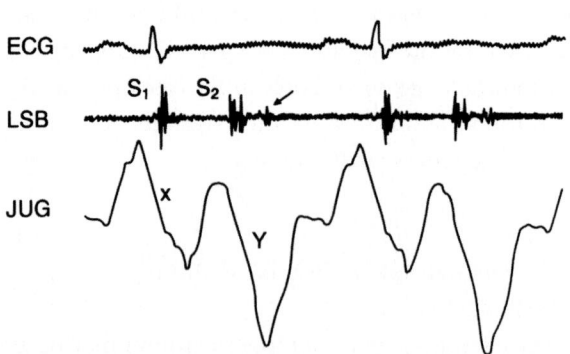

Fig. 16. Simultaneous electrocardiogram (ECG), phonocardiogram (LSB), and jugular venous pressure (JUG) tracing showing the timing of the pericardial knock (*arrow*).

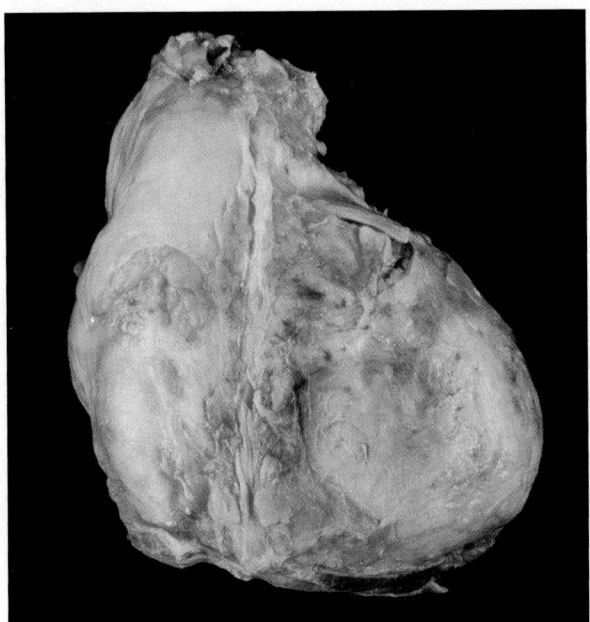

Fig. 17. Constrictive pericarditis after coronary artery bypass grafting.

Pericardial Calcification

When constrictive pericarditis is suspected clinically, a chest radiograph, including a left lateral projection, should be reviewed to look for pericardial calcification (Fig. 18). Pericardial calcification was commonly seen in patients with tuberculous pericarditis, but currently it is seen most commonly in patients with idiopathic constrictive pericarditis. If a patient presents with ascites and other clinical evidence of significant systemic venous congestion and a pericardial knock, chest radiographic findings of pericardial calcification make constrictive pericarditis the leading diagnosis, and in this clinical situation, a patient requires surgical exploration and pericardiectomy. No single ECG abnormality is diagnostic of constrictive pericarditis (Fig. 19).

Echocardiography in Constrictive Pericarditis

Echocardiography is helpful in diagnosing constrictive pericarditis. The characteristic M-mode/two-dimensional echocardiographic findings include abnormal ventricular septal motion (Fig. 20), increased pericardial thickness or calcification, dilated inferior vena cava with no significant changes with inspiration, and flattening of the left ventricular posterior wall during diastole. However, these findings are neither sensitive nor specific.

Although the underlying pathologic mechanism of constriction is different from that of cardiac tamponade, the hemodynamic events of respiratory variation during left and right ventricular filling are similar in the two conditions. The thickened pericardial layer pre-

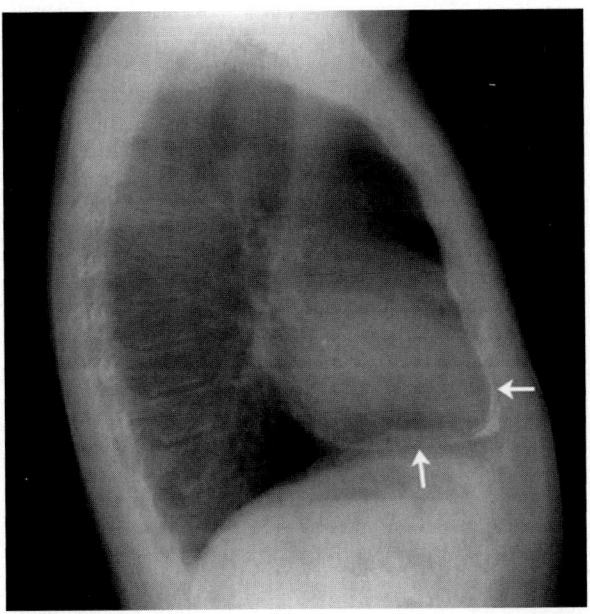
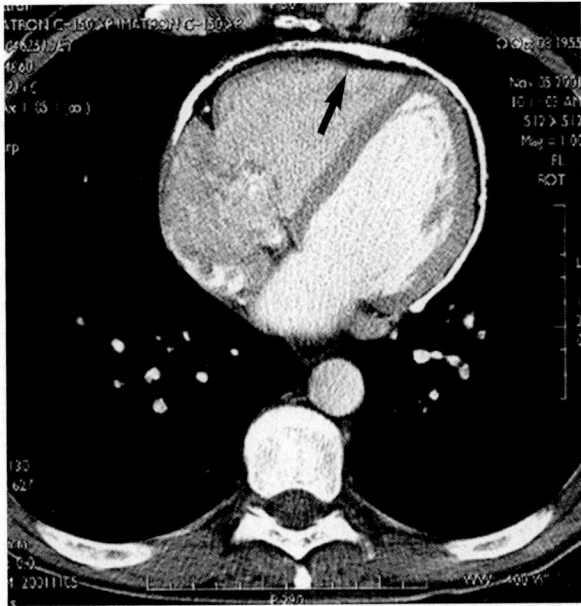

Fig. 18. *A*, Lateral chest radiograph demonstrating calcified pericardium (*arrows*). *B*, Computed tomographic scan of the chest showing egg shell–like calcification of the pericardium (*arrow*).

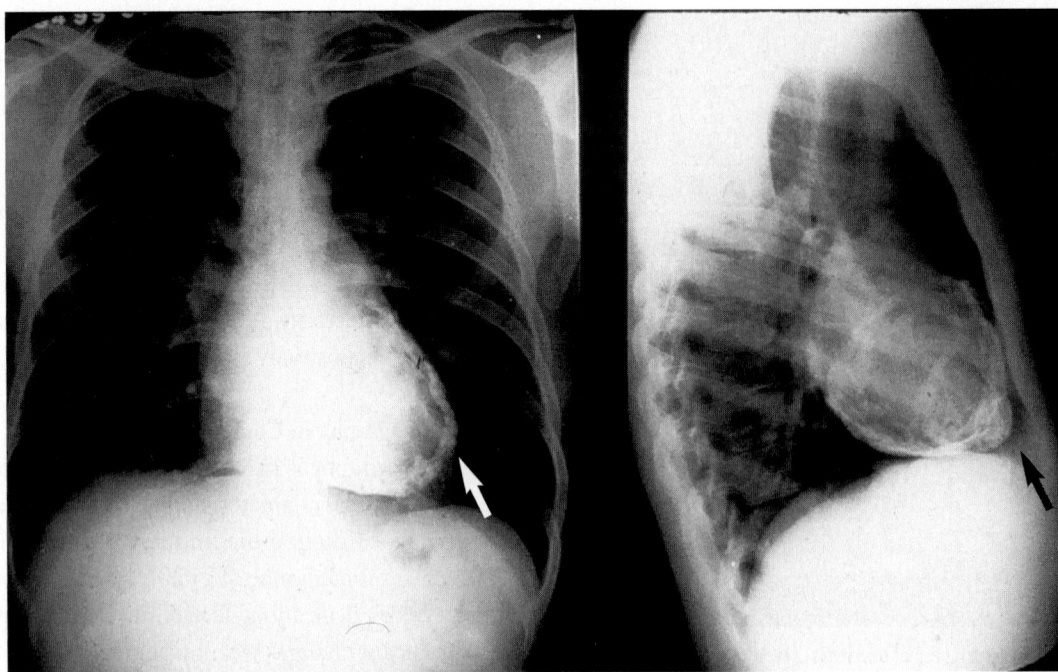

Fig. 19. Chest radiographs showing a calcified pericardium in constrictive pericarditis (*arrows*). *A*, Posteroanterior view. *B*, Lateral view.

vents full transmission of intrapleural pressure changes with respiration to the pericardial and intracardiac cavity, creating respiratory variation in the left-side filling pressure gradient (pressure difference between the pulmonary vein and the left atrium). Therefore, the mitral

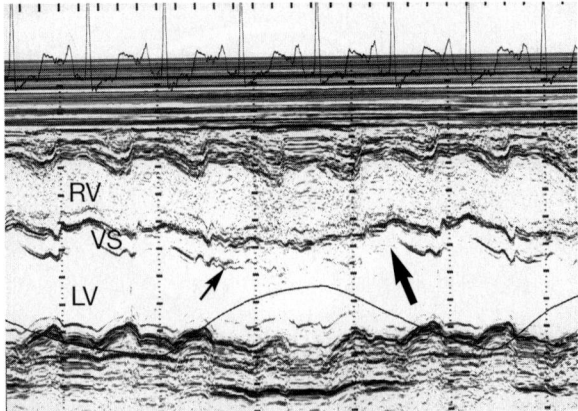

Fig. 20. M-mode echocardiogram with simultaneous respirometer recording. Upward deflection indicates passive inspiration, and downward deflection the onset of expiration. Ventricular septum (VS) moves toward the left ventricle (LV) with inspiration (*small arrow*) and toward the right ventricle (RV) with expiration (*large arrow*). The underlying hemodynamics are explained in the text.

inflow and pulmonary venous diastolic flow velocities decrease immediately after the onset of inspiration and increase with expiration (Fig. 21). Reciprocal changes occur in tricuspid inflow and hepatic venous flow velocity because of the relatively fixed cardiac volume. With decreased filling of the right cardiac chambers on expiration, there are exaggerated diastolic flow reversals and decreased diastolic forward flow in the hepatic vein with the onset of expiration. In contrast, hepatic vein flow reversals are more prominent with inspiration in restrictive cardiomyopathy. However, it is not unusual to see significant diastolic flow reversals in the hepatic vein during both inspiration and expiration in patients with advanced constriction or combined constriction and restriction. A representative Doppler spectrum of constrictive pericarditis is shown in Figure 22. A subgroup of patients with constrictive pericarditis may not have the characteristic respiratory variation of Doppler velocities. Therefore, the absence of respiratory variation in patients with clinical evidence of significant systemic venous congestion does not exclude the diagnosis of constrictive pericarditis, and additional studies should be performed. The typical respiratory variation and Doppler velocities also can occur in other conditions such as chronic obstructive lung disease, right

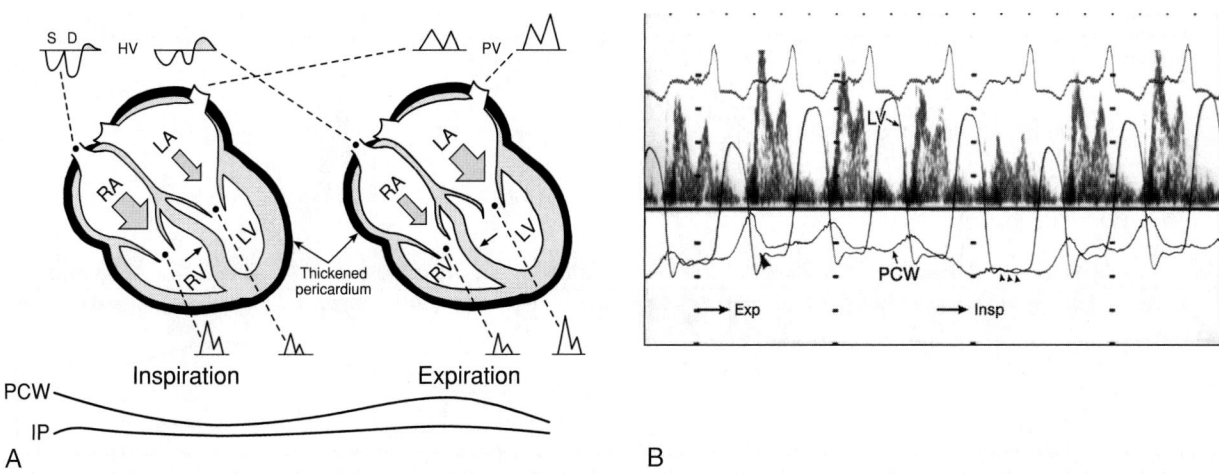

Fig. 21. *A*, Diagram of the heart with a thickened pericardium to illustrate the respiratory variation in ventricular filling and the corresponding Doppler features of the mitral valve, tricuspid valve, pulmonary vein (PV), and hepatic vein (HV). These changes are related to discordant pressure changes in the vessels in the thorax, such as pulmonary capillary wedge (PCW) pressure and intrapericardial (IP) and intracardiac pressures. Hatched area under curve indicates the reversal of flow. *Thicker arrows* indicate greater filling. D, diastolic flow; S, systolic flow. LA, left atrium, LV, left ventricle; RA, right atrium; RV, right ventricle. *B*, Simultaneous pressure recordings from the left ventricle (LV) and pulmonary capillary wedge (PCW) together with mitral inflow velocity on a Doppler echocardiogram. The onset of the respiratory phase is indicated at the bottom. With the onset of expiration, PCW pressure increases much more than LV diastolic pressure, creating a large driving pressure gradient (*large arrowhead*). With inspiration, however, PCW pressure decreases much more than LV diastolic pressure, with a very small driving pressure gradient (*three small arrowheads*). These respiratory changes in the LV filling gradient are well reflected by the changes in the mitral inflow velocities recorded on Doppler echocardiography. Exp, expiration; Insp, inspiration.

ventricular infarct, sleep apnea, asthma, and pulmonary embolism. In these situations, pulsed wave Doppler recording of the superior vena cava demonstrates marked increase in systolic forward flow with inspiration whereas there is less marked increase (less than 20 cm/s) in constrictive pericarditis. A relatively new echocardiographic technique, tissue Doppler imaging, which records the velocity of the myocardium, has considerable diagnostic value in the diagnosis of constriction. Early diastolic velocity (Ea) of the mitral anulus correlates well with the status of myocardial relaxation. Since myocardial relaxation is reduced in myocardial diseases, Ea is reduced in restrictive cardiomyopathy (Ea is normally >10 cm/s, and Ea is <6 cm/s in cardiomyopathy) but is preserved or even increased in patients with constrictive pericarditis. Therefore, if Ea is more than 8 cm/s in a patient with clinical evidence of heart failure, constrictive pericarditis should be considered.

Pericardial Thickness in Constrictive Pericarditis
CT or MRI is best for determining pericardial thickness (Fig. 23). Demonstration of increased pericardial thickness on CT or MRI in patients with significant systemic venous congestion generally indicates constrictive pericarditis. Recently, pericardial thickness has been assessed with transesophageal echocardiography, and the findings correlate well with those of Imatron CT. However, by itself, this finding is not sensitive or specific for constrictive pericarditis.

However, normal pericardial thickness on an imaging test cannot exclude the diagnosis of constriction. In our study, 18% of patients with surgically confirmed constrictive pericarditis had pericardium with a thickness of 2 mm or less. When the pericardial thickness is not increased, the pericardium is usually adhered to the heart, causing constrictive hemodynamics. Therefore, the diagnosis of constriction should be based on hemodynamic abnormalities in addition to anatomical abnormalities.

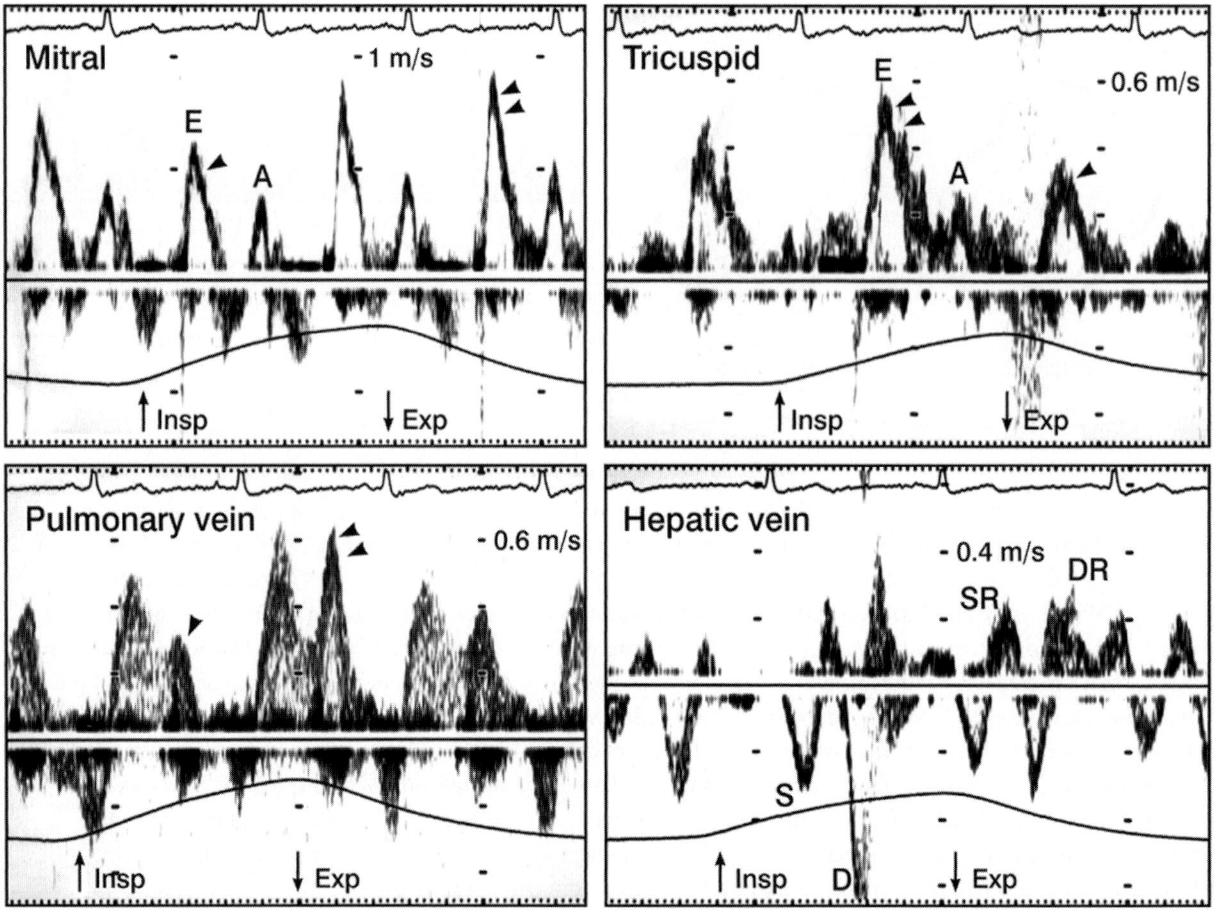

Fig. 22. Composite of mitral valve, tricuspid valve, pulmonary vein, and hepatic venous flow velocities typically seen in constrictive pericarditis. D, diastolic flow; DR, diastolic flow reversal; Exp, expiration; Insp, inspiration; S, systolic flow; SR, systolic flow reversal.

Brain Natriuretic Peptide in Constrictive Pericarditis

Brain natriuretic peptide (BNP) is markedly elevated in patients with heart failure due to systolic dysfunction, and it is less markedly elevated in patients with heart failure due to diastolic dysfunction in the presence of normal ejection fraction. BNP is even less elevated or normal in patients with constrictive pericarditis despite similarly elevated filling pressure.

Hemodynamic Findings in Constrictive Pericarditis

The hemodynamic findings in constrictive pericarditis include an increase in right atrial pressure and a dip-and-plateau configuration of the right and left ventricular diastolic pressure tracings (Fig. 24). Because there is no restriction of early ventricular filling, the y descent is quite prominent, corresponding to a prominent early diastolic dip of the ventricular pressure tracing. Right ventricular

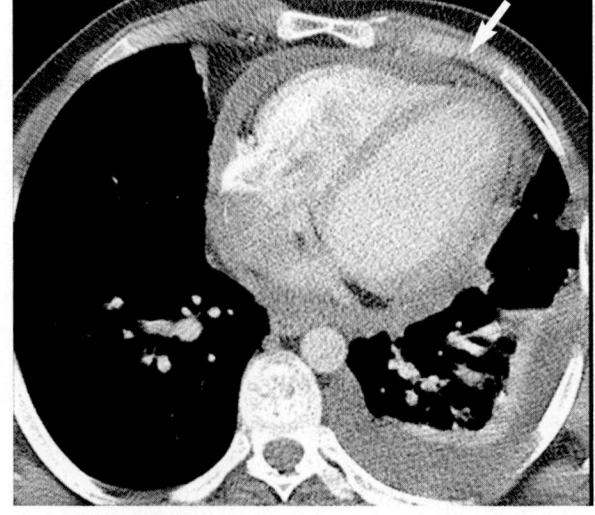

Fig. 23. Computed tomographic scan showing thick pericardium (*arrow*) along with pleural effusion due to constrictive pericarditis.

systolic pressure is usually less than 50 mm Hg, but this finding is not sensitive or specific and cannot be used to differentiate constrictive pericarditis from restrictive cardiomyopathy (Fig. 25). The concept of ventricular interdependence and the reciprocal pressure changes in the right and left ventricles with respiration can be used in hemodynamic assessment. Simultaneous left and right ventricular pressure tracings show a discordant direction of pressure changes with respiration (Fig. 24). Left ventricular pressure decreases with inspiration and right ventricular pressure increases. An opposite change occurs with expiration. Also, simultaneous left ventricular diastolic pressure and pulmonary capillary wedge pressure show significant reduction in the pressure difference between the pulmonary capillary wedge pressure and the left ventricular diastolic pressure with inspiration in comparison with the difference during expiration (Fig. 21).

- There is no characteristic ECG abnormality that is diagnostic of constrictive pericarditis.
- Remember pericardial constriction in a patient who has nonspecific findings on liver biopsy.
- A subset of patients with constrictive pericarditis may not show the typical respiratory changes in Doppler velocities.

- Remember constriction in all patients with heart failure and normal ejection fraction.

RESTRICTION VERSUS CONSTRICTION

The clinical and hemodynamic profiles of restriction and constriction are similar (Fig. 24) despite these conditions having distinctly different pathophysiologic mechanisms. Both are caused primarily by diastolic filling abnormalities, with preserved global systolic function. The diastolic dysfunction in restrictive cardiomyopathy results from a stiff and noncompliant ventricular myocardium, whereas it is due to a thickened noncompliant pericardium in constrictive pericarditis. Both disease processes limit diastolic filling and result in diastolic heart failure (Fig. 26). Pathologically, restriction and constriction may appear similar, with normal-sized ventricles and enlarged atria, but the pericardium is thickened in constriction.

INFILTRATIVE CARDIOMYOPATHY

Infiltrative cardiomyopathy has typical two-dimensional echocardiographic findings and biochemical abnormalities. A prototypical example is cardiac amyloidosis,

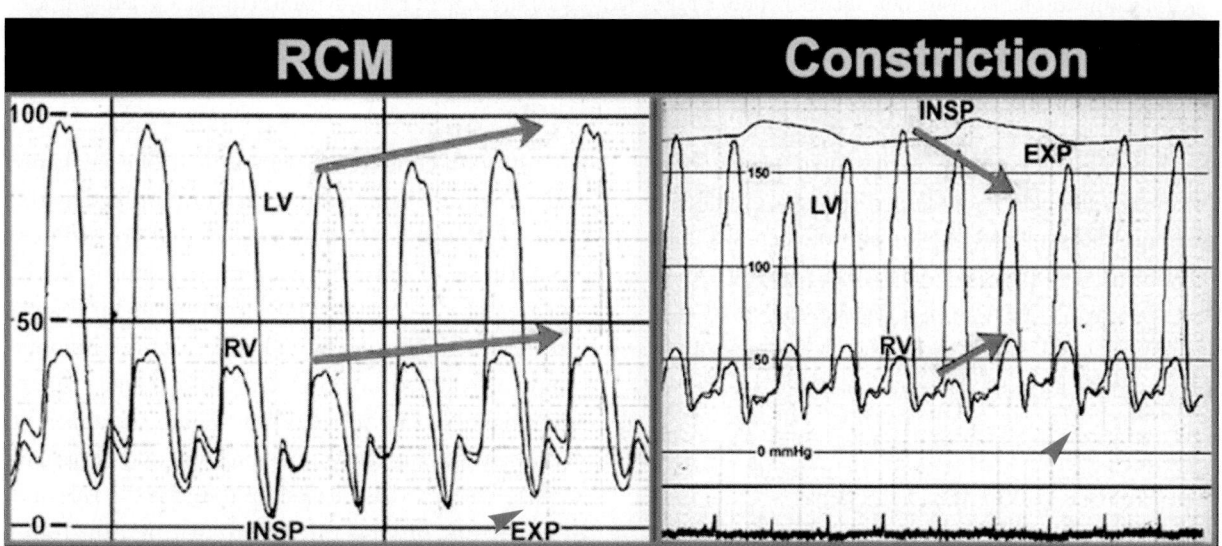

Fig. 24. Simultaneous left ventricular (LV) and right ventricular (RV) pressure tracings in restrictive cardiomyopathy (RCM) and constrictive pericarditis. In both conditions, the tracings show equalization of diastolic pressures and dip-and-plateau (*arrowheads*). There are *concordant* changes in LV and RV systolic pressures with respiration in restrictive cardiomyopathy (both LV and RV pressures increase with inspiration), whereas there are *discordant* pressure changes (LV systolic pressure decreases and RV systolic pressure increases with inspiration) in constrictive pericarditis (slopes of *arrows* show the concordance and discordance).

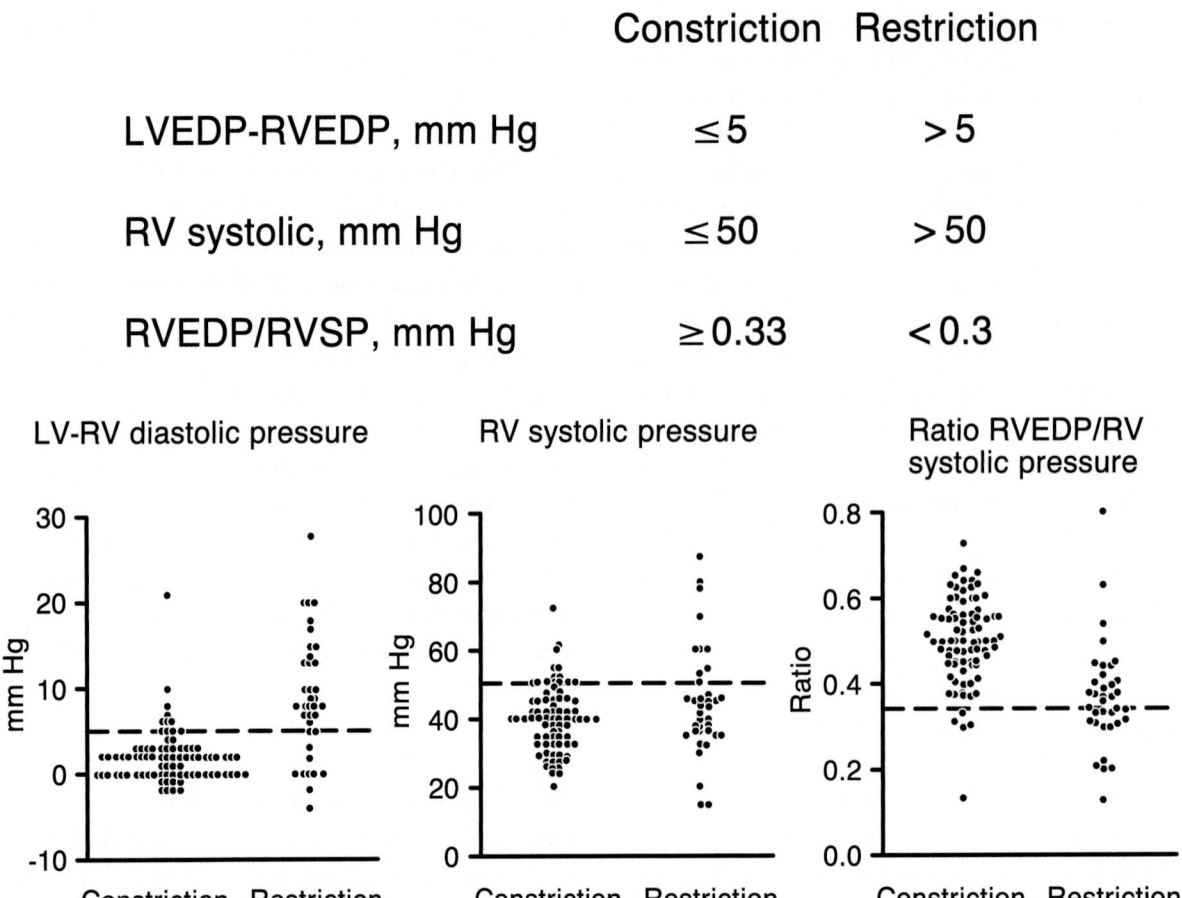

	Constriction	Restriction
LVEDP-RVEDP, mm Hg	≤ 5	> 5
RV systolic, mm Hg	≤ 50	> 50
RVEDP/RVSP, mm Hg	≥ 0.33	< 0.3

Fig. 25. Comparison of constriction and restriction. *Upper*, Hemodynamics. *Lower*, Hemodynamic criteria. LV, left ventricle; LVEDP, LV end-diastolic pressure; RV, right ventricle; RVEDP, RV end-diastolic pressure; RVSP, RV systolic pressure.

which is characterized by increased ventricular wall thickness, a granular or sparkling myocardial appearance on echocardiography, and typical amyloid deposits in fat in myocardial biopsy specimens. Also, patients usually (but not always) have monoclonal gammopathy on serum protein electrophoresis. The ECG shows a low voltage despite increased left ventricular wall thickness.

Noninfiltrative Restrictive Cardiomyopathy

Noninfiltrative restrictive cardiomyopathy is difficult to diagnose. The myocardium becomes noncompliant with fibrosis and scarring, but systolic function is usually maintained. With limited diastolic filling and increased diastolic pressure, the atria become enlarged. In contrast, myocardial compliance usually is not decreased in

patients with constrictive pericarditis. The thickened and sometimes calcified pericardium limits diastolic filling, resulting in hemodynamics that are different from those of restrictive cardiomyopathy. Atrial enlargement in constriction is less prominent than in restrictive cardiomyopathy. When restrictive cardiomyopathy affects both ventricles, clinical signs due to abnormalities of right-sided heart failure are apparent, with increased jugular venous pressure and peripheral edema. An early diastolic gallop sound is the rule and, in restriction, often is difficult to distinguish from a pericardial knock. ECG and chest radiographic findings are nonspecific, except that a calcified pericardium should point to constrictive pericarditis.

Echocardiographically, it is difficult to distinguish between restriction and constriction only on the basis of M-mode and two-dimensional findings. Both con-

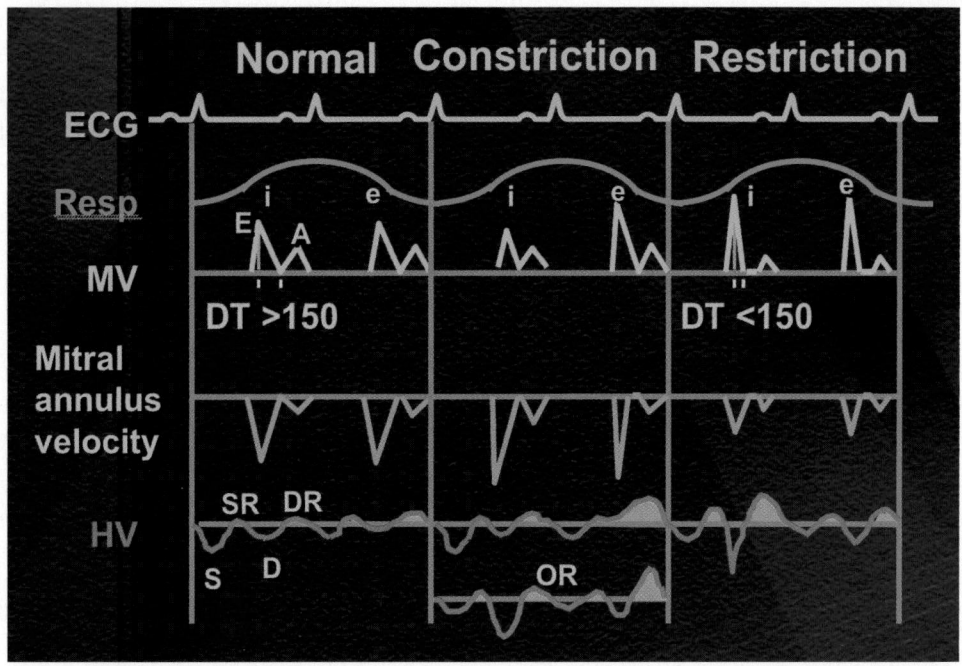

Fig. 26. Summary of mitral valve (MV) inflow, mitral anulus velocity, and hepatic vein (HV) features in normal, constriction, and restriction. DR, diastolic reversal; DT, deceleration time; e, expiration; ECG, electrocardiogram; i, inspiration; Resp, respiration; SR, systolic reversal.

ditions have normal left ventricular systolic function and enlarged atria and inferior vena cava. An increase in ventricular wall thickness, a thickening of the valves, and a small amount of pericardial effusion are typical of cardiac amyloidosis. In constrictive pericarditis, the most striking finding is ventricular septal motion abnormalities, which can be explained on the basis of respiratory variation in ventricular filling. The pericardium usually is thickened, but this may not be obvious on transthoracic echocardiography. Transesophageal echocardiographic measurement of pericardial thickness correlates well with that measured by electron-beam CT. However, constriction cannot be separated from myocardial disease on the basis of pericardial thickness alone.

Diagnostic Strategy to Differentiate Restrictive Cardiomyopathy From Constrictive Pericarditis
The following diagnostic strategy to differentiate restrictive cardiomyopathy from constrictive pericarditis is recommended.

1. The findings of pulsus paradoxus, calcification of the pericardium (seen on chest radiography), and

pericardial knock favor the diagnosis of constrictive pericarditis. Decreased voltage on the ECG may indicate cardiac amyloidosis.
2. Two-dimensional echocardiographic findings of increased left ventricular wall thickness and normal septal motion in conjunction with enlarged atria suggest restrictive cardiomyopathy. A thickened or calcified pericardium and ventricular septal motion favor constrictive pericarditis.
3. In constriction, there is a typical respiratory variation in ventricular filling (decreased filling of the left ventricle with inspiration and increased filling with expiration and significant hepatic venous flow reversal with expiration because of decreased filling on the right side). Restrictive cardiomyopathy is characterized by the restrictive Doppler physiology, with increased E velocity, decreased A velocity, E/A ratio greater than 2, and shortened deceleration time of E velocity. Hepatic vein diastolic flow reversals occur with inspiration instead of expiration. A subgroup of patients with constrictive pericarditis may have similar Doppler findings without respiratory variation. In such cases, the Doppler

examination should be repeated after an attempt has been made to reduce preload (head-up tilt position or diuretic therapy). Respiratory Doppler studies may be difficult to perform in patients with atrial fibrillation, but these patients should have abnormal septal motion and hepatic venous flow velocity changes on Doppler echocardiography. If the diagnosis is still uncer-

tain after a careful clinical examination, review of laboratory data, and two-dimensional Doppler echocardiographic evaluation, additional studies are needed, including CT or MRI, to examine pericardial thickness and cardiac catheterization to look for characteristic discordant respiratory changes in the left and right ventricular pressure tracings.

PULMONARY EMBOLISM

Jason M. Golbin, DO

Udaya B. S. Prakash, MD

EPIDEMIOLOGY OF PULMONARY EMBOLISM

Pulmonary embolism (PE), also called *pulmonary thromboembolism*, is defined as the lodging of blood clot(s) in the pulmonary arterial tree. The thrombus usually originates in the systemic veins of the lower limbs and pelvis and embolizes to the pulmonary arteries, while *pulmonary artery thrombosis* is defined as *in situ* formation of blood clots in the pulmonary arteries.

PE is common in hospitalized patients, with a prevalence rate of about 1%. Although it is the immediate cause of death in about 10% of patients who die in U.S. hospitals, PE is detected in 30% of routine autopsies. The correct antemortem diagnosis is made in less than 30% of cases. Mortality from PE has not diminished in the past 20 years.

PE and deep venous thrombosis (DVT) frequently occur together and are thought to represent two clinical manifestations of the same disease. The annual incidence of PE in the United States is estimated to be 600,000 cases. PE contributes to nearly 200,000 deaths in the United States and is probably the direct cause of death in 60,000 persons. Patients who die of PE die rapidly, usually within 2 hours after the embolism. The majority of deaths are likely due to missed diagnosis rather than failed treatment.

DVT is the cause of PE in more than 90% of patients, and the risk of fatal PE depends on the severity and extent of obstruction of pulmonary arteries and the comorbidities. The risk of PE from untreated proximal DVT is 50% and mortality from untreated PE is 8%. Chronic pulmonary hypertension as a complication of recurrent PE occurs in approximately 2,500 patients/year in the United States (Fig. 1).

- PE is a common problem in hospitalized patients that frequently is not adequately diagnosed.
- Consider PE in *all* patients with respiratory symptoms.
- Prophylaxis against DVT/PE should be considered in all inpatients.
- Risk of PE from untreated DVT is 50%.
- Risk of death from untreated PE is 8%.

ETIOLOGY OF PE

The most important factor responsible for PE is DVT of the lower extremities. DVT results from the triad of Virchow: venous stasis, injury to venous intima, and coagulation disorders. The primary or secondary coagulation disorders are listed in Table 1. The association of factor V Leiden mutation and thromboembolism has gained importance in the last two decades. Factor V Leiden mutation has not been shown to be a significant risk factor for acute DVT in patients undergoing hip or knee replacement surgery. However, it is associated

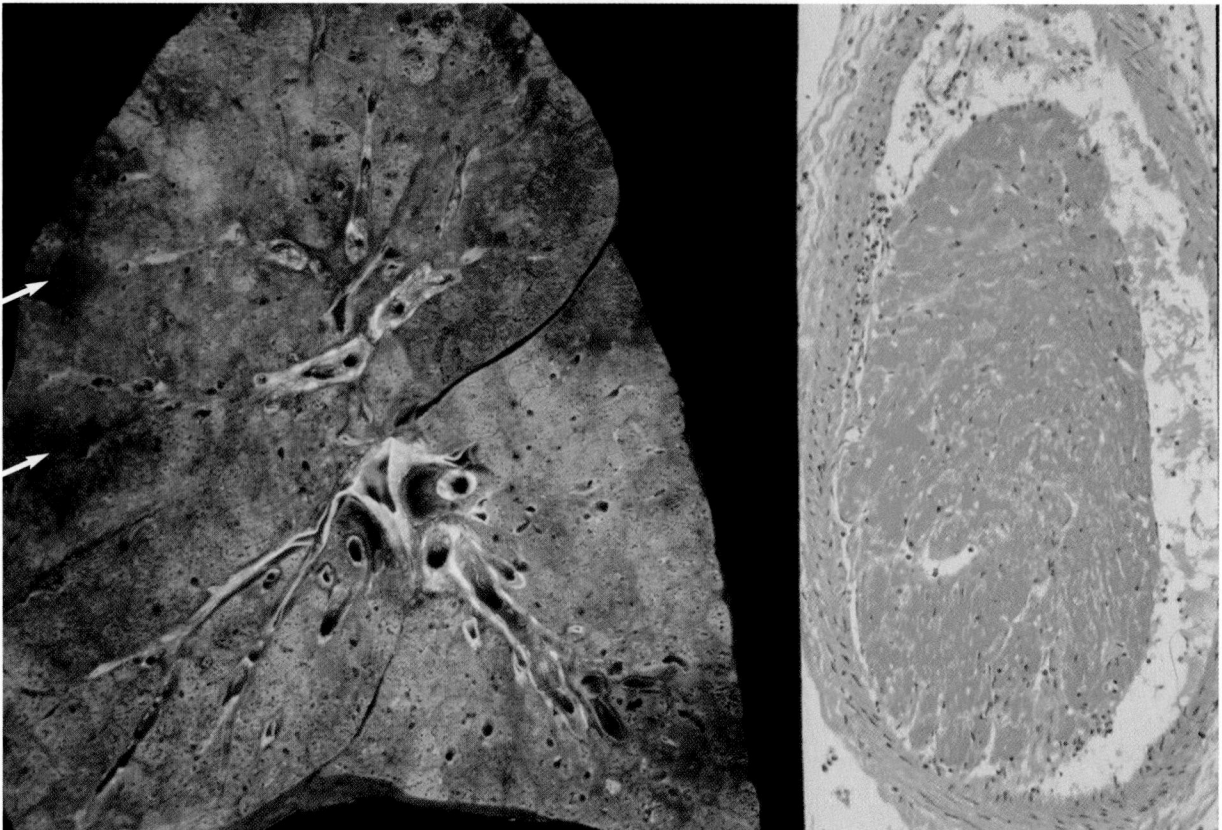

Fig. 1. *A*, Gross lung specimen showing multiple pulmonary emboli with pulmonary infarctions. *B*, Histologic section showing thrombus in a pulmonary vessel.

with increased risk of thromboembolic disease, particularly in men older than 60 years, men with hyperhomocystinemia, and women taking oral contraceptives. A study demonstrated a low annual incidence of spontaneous DVT in asymptomatic carriers of the factor V Leiden mutation. Routine screening for the mutation is not indicated in patients with suspected DVT or PE, nor is it indicated for family members of patients with known factor V Leiden mutation.

Lower Limb DVT

Although most (>90%) PE arise from thrombi of the lower extremities, a recent study demonstrated that compression ultrasonography (CUS) detected DVT in only 60% of patients with symptomatic PE. A large retrospective study found that 82% of patients with angiographically proven PE had venographically proven DVT. Among patients with fatal PE, DVT has been identified clinically in only about 50%. Approximately

45% of femoral and iliac vein DVTs embolize to the lungs. Other sources of PE include clots formed in the veins of the upper extremities, right ventricle, and indwelling venous catheters.

- 20% of calf-only DVTs propagate to the thigh and iliac veins.
- 10% of cases of superficial thrombophlebitis are complicated by DVT.
- Varicose veins do not increase the risk of developing DVT.
- Approximately 45% of femoral and iliac DVTs embolize to the lungs.

Upper Limb DVT

Upper extremity DVT should be considered when the source of PE is not identified. A study of 58 consecutive patients with signs and symptoms suggestive of upper extremity DVT confirmed the diagnosis by venography

Table 1. Coagulation Disorders That Predispose to the Development of Deep Venous Thrombosis (DVT) and Pulmonary Embolism (PE)

Primary hypercoagulable states	Secondary hypercoagulable states
Activated protein C resistance* (factor V Leiden carriers)	Cancer
Antithrombin III deficiency†	Postoperative states (stasis)
Protein-C deficiency†	Lupus anticoagulant syndrome
Protein-S deficiency†	Increased factor VII and fibrinogen
Fibrinolytic abnormalities	Pregnancy
Hypoplasminogenemia	Nephrotic syndrome
Dysplasminogenemia	Myeloproliferative disorders
tPA release deficiency	Disseminated intravascular coagulation
Increased tPA inhibitor	Acute stroke
Dysfibrinogenemia	Hyperlipidemias
Homocystinuria	Diabetes mellitus
Heparin cofactor deficiency	Paroxysmal nocturnal hemoglobinuria
Increased histidine-rich glycoprotein	Behçet disease and vasculitides
	Anticancer drugs (chemotherapy)
	Heparin-induced thrombocytopenia
	Oral contraceptives
	Obesity

tPA, tissue plasminogen activator.

*Prevalence of factor V Leiden in patients with DVT is 16%; presence of V Leiden is associated with a 40% risk of recurrent DVT (N Engl J Med. 1997;336:399-403).

†Prevalence of these protein deficiencies in patients with DVT is 5% to 10%.

in 27 patients (47%). Central venous catheters, thrombophilic states, and a previous lower extremity DVT were statistically significantly associated with upper extremity DVT. PE occurred in 36% of the patients with upper limb DVT. Another study reported that DVT of the upper extremity is associated with higher morbidity and mortality than DVT of the lower extremities.

INCIDENCE OF DVT WITH SPECIFIC CONDITIONS

The incidence of DVT without adequate prophylaxis in various clinical circumstances is as follows: major abdominal surgery, 14% to 33%; thoracic surgery, 25% to 60%; post–myocardial infarction (MI), 20% to 40%; congestive heart failure, 70%; stroke with paralysis, 50% to 70%; postpartum, 3%; and trauma, 20% to 40%. The risks of DVT in other surgical patients who do not receive prophylaxis are listed in Table 2.

Carcinoma and DVT

Idiopathic DVT, particularly when recurrent, may indicate the presence of neoplasm in 10% to 20% of patients. The risk of diagnosis of cancer is significantly elevated only during the first 6 months after the diagnosis of DVT or PE. This risk declines rapidly to a constant low level 1 year after the thrombotic event. The occurrence of thromboembolism in patients with cancer portends a poor prognosis. Among patients with a diagnosis of cancer within 1 year after thromboembolism, 40% will have distant metastases at the time of the diagnosis of cancer.

- About 60% of patients with PE have DVT of the lower extremities.
- Idiopathic DVT, when recurrent, may indicate neoplasm in up to 20% of patients.

Table 2.   Deep Venous Thrombosis (DVT) Risk Without Prophylaxis in Surgical Patients

Type of surgery	Specific factors	Risk of DVT, %
General	Age >40 y	16-42
	Age >60 y	46-61
	Cancer resection	40-59
Gynecologic	Procedure duration <30 min, age <40 y, benign disease	<3
	Minor procedure, age 40-70 y	10
	Major procedure, age 4-70 y	0-40
	Cancer resection	35
Urologic	Open prostatectomy	28-42
	TURP	10
	Other procedures	31-58
Neurologic	Craniotomy	18-40
	Laminectomy	4-25
Orthopedic	Total hip arthroplasty	40-78
	Hip fracture	48-75
	Tibial fracture	45
	Knee procedure	57

TURP, transurethral resection of the prostate.

■ Risk of DVT: thoracic surgery, 25%-60%; hip surgery, 50%-75%; post-MI, 20%-40%; congestive heart failure, 70%; and stroke with paralysis, 50%-70%.

DIAGNOSIS OF DVT

DVT is diagnosed in only 50% of clinical cases. A diagnosis based on physical examination alone is unreliable.

Homans sign (pain and tenderness on dorsiflexion of the ankle) is a poor physical sign for the diagnosis of DVT and is elicited in less than 40% of patients with proven DVT. A false-positive Homans sign occurs in 30% of high-risk patients.

Impedance plethysmography (IPG) and CUS together are the most commonly used noninvasive tests and have a diagnostic accuracy of 90% to 95% in detecting iliac and femoral deep venous thromboses, but their accuracy in the diagnosis of calf vein thrombosis is low. Repeated CUS examinations are not needed in patients with clinically suspected DVT who have had a negative initial CUS and a negative sensitive D-dimer test. D-Dimer is a degradation product released into the circulation when cross-linked fibrin undergoes endogenous fibrinolysis. In patients with low to moderate clinical probability of suspected DVT, a normal-range sensitive D-dimer level effectively rules out DVT and eliminates the need for further testing.

Contrast venography remains the gold standard for the diagnosis of DVT if noninvasive testing is equivocal. In patients in whom recurrent DVT is suspected, venography may help differentiate a new thrombosis from an old one. Reliable signs of DVT on venography include a reproducible intraluminal filling defect evident in two or more views or an abrupt cutoff of a deep vein.

■ DVT is diagnosed in only 50% of clinical cases.
■ Impedance plethysmography plus ultrasound are up to 95% accurate for detection of iliac and femoral DVT.
■ Serial CUS studies are important in high-risk patients hospitalized long-term.

CLINICAL FEATURES

PE has no pathognomonic clinical symptoms and signs. Tachypnea and tachycardia are observed in nearly all patients with PE. Other common (>75% of patients) symptoms include dyspnea and pleuritic pain. Less common symptoms (<25% of patients) are hemoptysis, pleural friction rub, wheezing, and fever. The differential diagnosis of PE includes MI, pneumonia, congestive heart failure, pericarditis, esophageal spasm, asthma, exacerbation of chronic obstructive lung disease, intrathoracic malignancy, rib fracture, pneumothorax, pleurisy from any cause, pleurodynia, anxiety, and nonspecific skeletal pains. Acute cor pulmonale occurs if more than 65% of the pulmonary circulation is obstructed by emboli.

- PE has no pathognomonic signs or symptoms.
- Acute cor pulmonale occurs when >65% of vasculature is obstructed by PE.

DIAGNOSTIC TESTS

Clinical examination, electrocardiography (ECG), chest radiography, blood gas abnormalities, and elevated plasma D-dimer level, although helpful, have low specificity and sensitivity for the diagnosis of PE. Clinical suspicion remains the most important single factor in steering the clinician toward appropriate diagnostic tests for PE.

Chest Radiography in PE

The most common chest radiographic abnormality in PE is diaphragmatic elevation (about 60% of patients), followed by pulmonary infiltrates in 30%, focal oligemia in 10% to 50%, pleural effusion in 20%, and an enlarged pulmonary artery in 20%. Chest radiographs are normal in 30% of patients with PE.

- Chest radiographs are normal in 30% of patients with PE.

Electrocardiography

The most common ECG abnormalities in PE are nonspecific changes (noted in 80% of patients), ST and T changes in 65%, the pattern of S wave in lead I and Q wave in lead III (S_1Q_3) in 15%, right bundle branch block in 12%, and left-axis deviation in 12%. Nonspecific T-wave inversion in the precordial leads is commonly seen and is the ECG sign best correlated with the severity of PE.

- The classic pattern of S wave in lead I and Q wave in lead III (S_1Q_3) is seen in only 15% of patients with PE.
- T-wave inversion in the precordial leads is the ECG sign best correlated with the severity of PE.

Arterial Blood Gases

Both the PaO_2 and $P(A-a)O_2$ gradient may be normal in up to 20% of patients. The $(A-a)O_2$ gradient shows a linear correlation with the severity of the PE, but a normal $(A-a)O_2$ does not exclude PE. Indeed, in the Prospective Investigation of PE Diagnosis (PIOPED) study, about 20% of patients with angiographically documented PE had a normal $P(A-a)O_2$ gradient (≤20 mm Hg). Most patients with acute PE demonstrate hypocapnia secondary to hyperventilation.

- The $P(A-a)O_2$ gradient linearly correlates with the severity of PE.
- Of patients with PE, 20% have a normal $P(A-a)O_2$ gradient (≤20 mm Hg).

Serum Markers in Pulmonary Embolism—Troponin and D-Dimer

Both Troponin T (cTnT) and Troponin I (cTnI) are highly sensitive and specific markers for myocardial cell injury, and patients with increased troponin levels presenting with PE have significantly higher in-hospital mortality than PE patients with normal troponin levels.

D-dimer, a specific fibrin degradation product, is typically increased in patients with DVT and PE. A high level of D-dimer is a nonspecific finding and on its own has a very low positive predictive value for PE. Equally, normal levels of D-dimer alone do not exclude DVT or PE. It is important to combine clinical probability of PE, concomitant imaging studies, and serum markers into a diagnostic algorithm of PE. Advancing age, pregnancy, trauma, cancer, critical illness, and prior DVT/PE are all associated with increased D-dimer levels.

- Normal levels of D-dimer do not exclude DVT or PE without concomitant use of a diagnostic algorithm or imaging study.
- Elevated D-dimer levels have very low positive predictive value for PE.
- Various D-dimer assays are available—verify your hospital's test.

Echocardiography

Echocardiography identifies thrombi in the right side of the heart in up to 15% of patients with PE. Occasionally, the presence of rare cardiac abnormalities, such as intracardiac tumors, poses difficulty in distinguishing these lesions. Patients with a mobile right heart thrombus-in-transit have a 98% risk of acute PE and a 1-week mortality of 50%. In patients with massive or submassive PE, abnormalities are often apparent on the transthoracic echocardiogram (TTE), including right ventricular dilatation and hypokinesis, abnormal interventricular septal movement, and tricuspid regurgitation.

In these patients, echocardiographic detection of a patent foramen ovale signifies a high risk of death, stroke, and other arterial thromboembolic complications. Transesophageal echocardiography (TEE) has a sensitivity of 97% and a specificity of 86% for the diagnosis of centrally located pulmonary arterial thrombi. Echocardiography is very helpful in the assessment of secondary pulmonary hypertension caused by recurrent PE.

Ventilation-Perfusion Lung Scan

The ventilation-perfusion (V/Q) lung scan is commonly used in the diagnosis of PE. It is designed to detect areas of the lung that are ventilated but not perfused, a mismatch that suggests PE. A high probability lung scan has a sensitivity of 41% and a specificity of 97%. The likelihood of PE in a scan that shows high-probability is 90% (Fig. 2). A normal lung scan excludes PE in nearly 100% of patients. A low-probability lung scan excludes the diagnosis of PE in approximately 85% of patients. An intermediate-probability scan is associated with PE in 20% to 30% of patients. Therefore, patients with an intermediate probability V/Q scan usually require pulmonary angiography or other imaging modalities. Intermediate scans are encountered in 60% of patients with chronic obstructive lung disease and in 43% of those with prior cardiac or pulmonary disease. In the PIOPED study, only 41% of patients with angiographically proven PE had a high-probability V/Q scan; the remaining 59% of patients with acute PE had either a low-probability or intermediate-probability scan. Both ventilation and perfusion scans are not necessary in all patients with suspected PE. If the initial perfusion scan is normal, no ventilation scan is needed. A V/Q scan is useful in patients with contraindications to contrast imaging studies, such as renal failure and contrast hypersensitivity.

- High-probability V/Q scan = 90% probability of PE.
- Normal scan excludes PE in nearly 100%.
- The majority of patients require further testing.

Computed Tomographic Angiography

Multidetector-row computed tomography (CT) permits ultrafast scanning (in a single breath hold) of pulmonary arteries during injection of contrast material

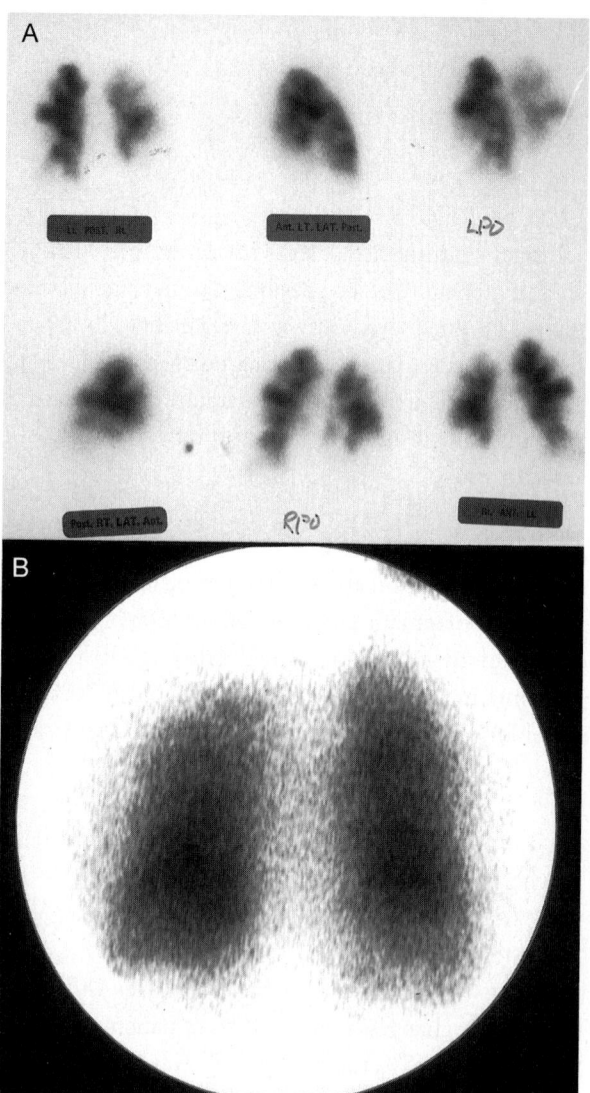

Fig. 2. Ventilation-perfusion scan showing multiple bilateral perfusion defects (*A*) even though the ventilation scan is normal (*B*). This was interpreted as showing a high probability of pulmonary embolism.

into peripheral veins, providing a major advance in the diagnosis of PE. Overall, the sensitivity for CT varies from 57% to 100% and the specificity varies from 78% to 100%. PE located in the main or lobar arteries are more easily identified than those in segmental or subsegmental arteries. A recent study demonstrated that a negative multidetector-row CT scan, in conjunction with a clinical diagnostic algorithm and a negative D-dimer test, can effectively rule out PE without the use of CUS (Fig. 3 and 4).

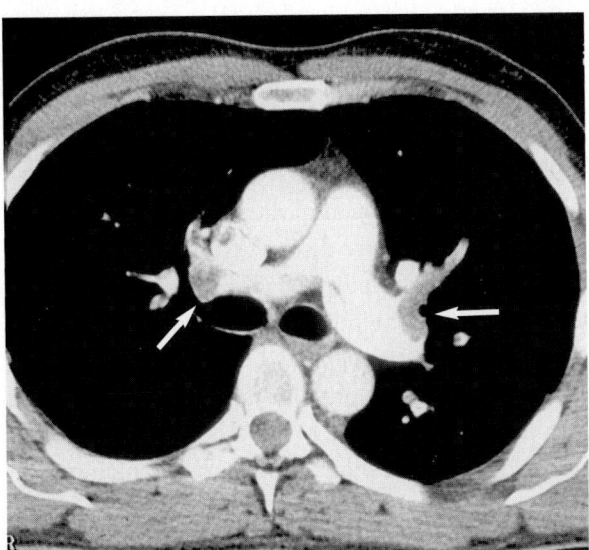

Fig. 3. Ultrafast computed tomography showing large pulmonary emboli occluding major pulmonary arteries bilaterally (*arrows*).

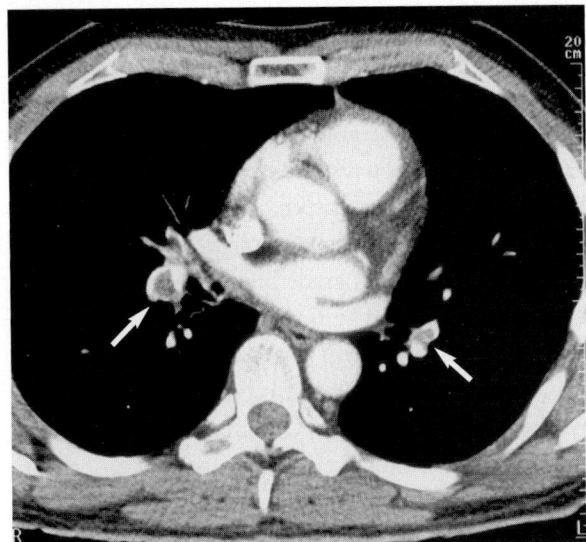

Fig. 4. Ultrafast computed tomography showing occlusion of the lobar and segmental pulmonary arteries bilaterally (*arrows*).

- Traditional single-detector-row CT cannot reliably exclude PE, particularly in subsegmental arteries.
- New generation multidetector-row CT, in conjunction with a clinical diagnostic algorithm and D-dimer testing, can effectively rule out PE.

Magnetic Resonance Imaging
The role of magnetic resonance imaging (MRI) in the diagnosis of DVT and PE is still undergoing validation. MRI has shown a sensitivity of 100% and a specificity of 95% for detecting DVT in pelvic and thigh veins. The sensitivity and specificity for DVT of calf veins are 85% and 98%, respectively. The role of MRI in the diagnosis of PE continues to evolve.

Pulmonary Angiography
Pulmonary angiography remains the gold standard for the diagnosis of pulmonary embolism (Fig. 5). Ideally it should be performed within 24 to 48 hours of symptom onset if the diagnosis of PE is of at least moderate clinical probability and noninvasive testing has been equivocal. Pulmonary angiography represents the last stop on most diagnostic algorithms when the diagnosis cannot be obtained through other methods. False-negative results are observed in 1% to 2% of pulmonary angiograms. In the PIOPED study, experts disagreed

on the presence of PE in 8% of patients and on PE absence in 17%; 3% of the angiograms were rated as nondiagnostic.

- Major complications of pulmonary angiography = 1%.

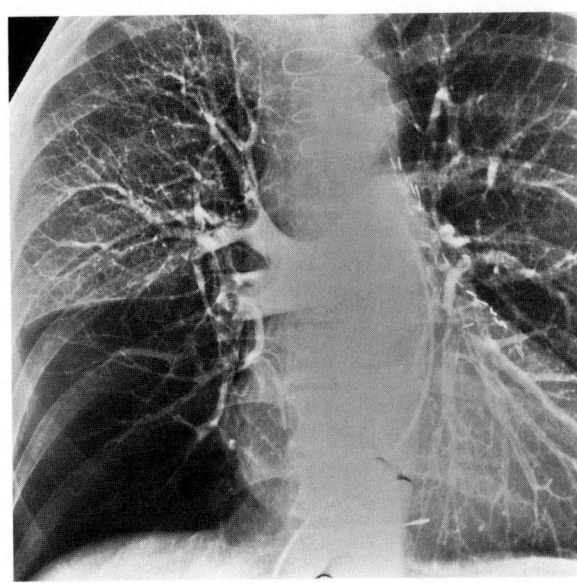

Fig. 5. Pulmonary angiogram showing almost total occlusion of the pulmonary arteries to the right middle and lower lobes.

- Minor complications of pulmonary angiography = 2%.
- Mortality = 0.5%.

Clinical Scoring Systems

Assessing clinical pretest probability of venous thromboembolism is a crucial aspect of the current diagnostic algorithm for pulmonary embolism. The original PE algorithm by Wells is graded in 3 levels: low, moderate/intermediate, and high probability, based on clinical signs, symptoms, and risk factors (Table 3 and Fig. 6).

This score then guides the need for further diagnostic work-up, including CUS, CT imaging, or ultimately pulmonary angiography. The low–clinical probability group has a PE prevalence of approximately 10% or less; the intermediate, approximately 30%; and the high-probability group, greater than 70%.

Many algorithms have been proposed to best identify and exclude DVT safely. The most crucial point is to consistently follow an algorithm. A recent study demonstrated that inappropriate follow-through of diagnostic criteria was independently associated with a thromboembolic event. See sample algorithms in Figures 7 and 8.

TREATMENT OF PULMONARY EMBOLUS

The treatment of uncomplicated DVT is the same as that of PE. For acute disease, treatment with both heparin and warfarin can be initiated simultaneously, unless warfarin is contraindicated. An overlap period of 4 to 5 days is recommended. Unfractionated heparin (UFH), 80 U/kg, is administered as a bolus, followed by a maintenance dose of 18 U/kg per hour intravenously. The dose should be adjusted to maintain an activated partial thromboplastin time (APTT) greater than 1.5 times the control value. Fixed-dose subcutaneous low-molecular-weight heparin (LMWH) was shown to be as effective and safe as dose-adjusted intravenous heparin for the treatment of PE in a large meta-analysis. Caution should be used with LMWH in certain clinical situations, such as pregnancy, severe obesity (body mass index>50 kg/m^2), and severe renal failure; plasma anti-Xa levels should be monitored in these situations 4 hours after administration.

- In acute DVT and PE, treatment with heparin and warfarin can be initiated simultaneously.
- Heparin dose: bolus = 80 U/kg; maintenance = 18 U/kg per hour.
- LMWH is now preferred over UFH in the treatment of nonmassive PE.

Long-term anticoagulation can be maintained with either heparin or warfarin. Heparin (either UFH or LMWH) is indicated when warfarin is contraindicated or not tolerated. The usual dose of heparin is 5,000 to 10,000 U subcutaneously twice daily. However, the dose should be adjusted on the basis of APTT. Weight-based heparin dosage is not reliable for maintenance therapy by the subcutaneous route. LMWH, 30 mg twice daily subcutaneously, has been used in patients with difficulty in monitoring APTT. LMWH has been shown to be at least as effective and safe as unfractionated heparin in the treatment of both DVT and acute PE without increasing the risk of major bleeding.

Warfarin is recommended at the dose needed to achieve an international normalized ratio (INR) of 2 to 3. The starting dose of warfarin is either 5 or 10 mg/d

Table 3. Rules for Predicting the Probability of Embolism

Variable	No. of points
Risk factors	
Clinical signs and symptoms of deep venous thrombosis	3.0
An alternative diagnosis deemed less likely than pulmonary embolism	3.0
Heart rate >100 beats/min	1.5
Immobilization or sugery in the previous 4 wk	1.5
Previous deep venous thrombosis or pulmonary embolism	1.5
Hemoptysis	1.0
Cancer (receiving treatment, treated in the past 6 mo, or palliative care)	1.0
Clinical probability	
Low	<2.0
Intermediate	2.0-6.0
High	>6.0

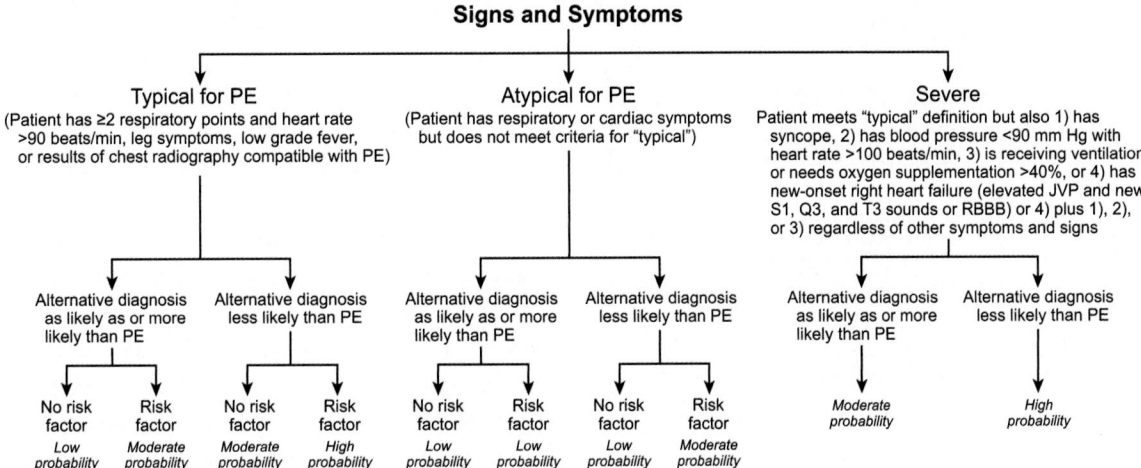

Fig. 6. Algorithm for the clinical model to determine the pretest probability of pulmonary embolism (PE). Respiratory points consist of dyspnea or worsening of chronic dyspnea, pleuritic chest pain, chest pain that is nonretrosternal and nonpleuritic, an arterial oxygen saturation less than 92% while breathing room air that corrects with oxygen supplementation less than 40%, hemoptysis, and pleural rub. Risk factors are surgery within 12 weeks, immobilization (complete bedrest) for 3 or more days in the 4 weeks before presentation, previous deep venous thrombosis or objectively diagnosed pulmonary embolism, fracture of a lower extremity and immobilization of the fracture within 12 weeks, strong family history of deep venous thrombosis or pulmonary embolism (two or more family members with objectively proven events or a first-degree relative with hereditary thrombophilia), cancer (treatment ongoing, within the past 6 months, or in the palliative stages), the postpartum period, and lower-extremity paralysis. JVP, jugular venous pressure; RBBB, right bundle branch block.

for 1 to 3 days, followed by adjustment of dosage to maintain an INR of 2.0 to 3.0. Some trials have shown that the 5-mg starting dose is associated with fewer episodes of excessive anticoagulation than starting with 10 mg, but other studies have validated an advantage of the higher dose. The frequency of APTT and prothrombin time testing may vary from patient to patient and often in the same patient, depending on the metabolism of anticoagulants, use of interfering drugs, and new medical problems.

Current American College of Chest Physicians tratment recommendations include the following:

- Patients with first episode of DVT secondary to a transient risk factor: 3 months.
- Patients with first episode of idiopathic DVT: at least 6 to 12 months.
- Patients with DVT and cancer: LMWH for at least 3 to 6 months.
- Patients with first episode and antiphospholipid antibodies or 2 or more thrombophilic conditions: at

least 12 months.
- Patients with first DVT or one thrombophilic condition (other than antiphospholipid antibodies): 6 to 12 months.
- Patients with 2 or more DVTs: indefinite treatment.

Bleeding Complications

Among patients receiving chronic warfarin therapy, the cumulative incidence of fatal bleeding is 1% at 1 year and 2% at 3 years. Presence of malignant disease at initiation of warfarin therapy is significantly associated with major hemorrhage. Among patients with PE treated with thrombolytic agents, the risk of intracranial bleeding is about 1%.

Drugs that prolong the effect of warfarin include salicylates, amiodarone, heparin, estrogen, antibiotics, clofibrate, quinidine, and cimetidine. Drugs that decrease the effect of warfarin include rifampin and barbiturates. This is only a partial list of drugs that interfere with warfarin metabolism, and it is wise to review possible interactions when a new drug is administered to a warfarin patient.

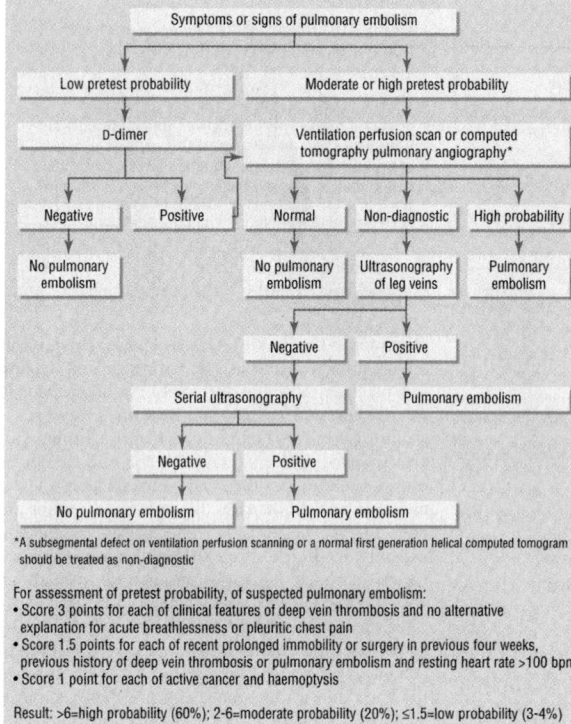

Fig. 7. Clinical approach to the diagnosis of pulmonary embolism.

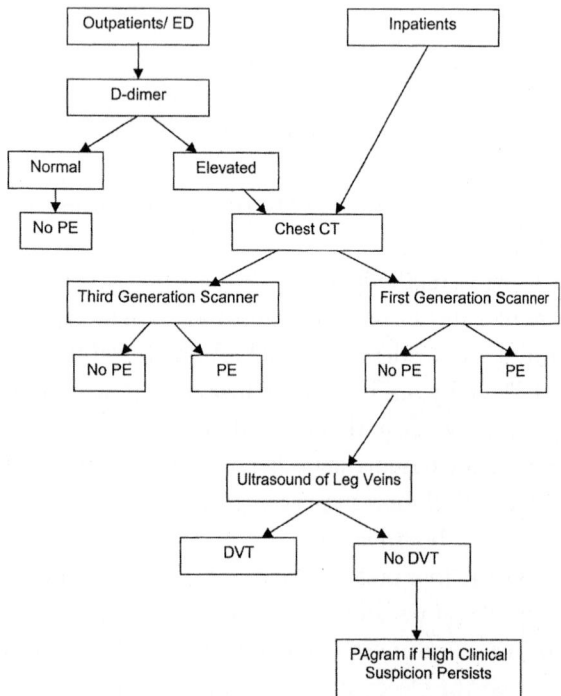

Fig. 8. Proposed diagnostic strategy. CT, computed tomography; DVT, deep venous thrombosis; ED, emergency department; PE, pulmonary embolism.

Inferior Vena Caval Interruption

Inferior vena caval (IVC) interruption is aimed at preventing PE while maintaining blood flow through the IVC. IVC plication or insertion of a filter into the inferior vena cava is indicated in recurrent DVT in a patient who recently had a massive PE, presence of bleeding disorder or other contraindication to anticoagulation therapy, or failure of anticoagulation therapy. The routine use of an IVC filter in patients with cancer and DVT or PE is not recommended. IVC plication or IVC filter insertion does not replace anticoagulant therapy; many patients require both. Anticoagulation therapy after filter insertion is aimed at preventing DVT at the insertion site, IVC thrombosis, cephalad propagation of clot from an occluded filter, and propagation or recurrent DVTs of the lower extremities. Most IVC filters are inserted through the internal jugular vein. Multiple types of filters are available in the United States. Probably the most well known is the Greenfield filter (Fig. 9 and 10).

PE occurs in 2.5% of patients even after insertion of an IVC filter. The complications of filter insertion include DVT at the insertion site (2%), change in position after insertion (migration, tilting in up to 50%), perforation of the IVC (15% to 24%, but most are radiologically diagnosed and have no clinical problems), obstruction of the IVC below the filter (6%), and edema of the

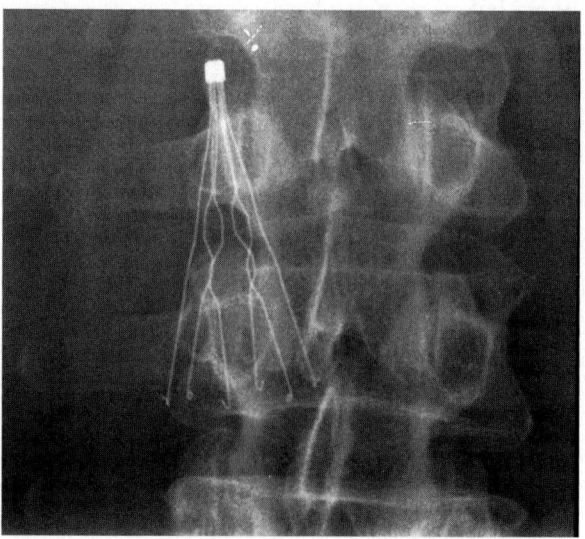

Fig. 9. A properly placed inferior vena caval filter in a patient with recurrent pulmonary emboli and secondary pulmonary hypertension.

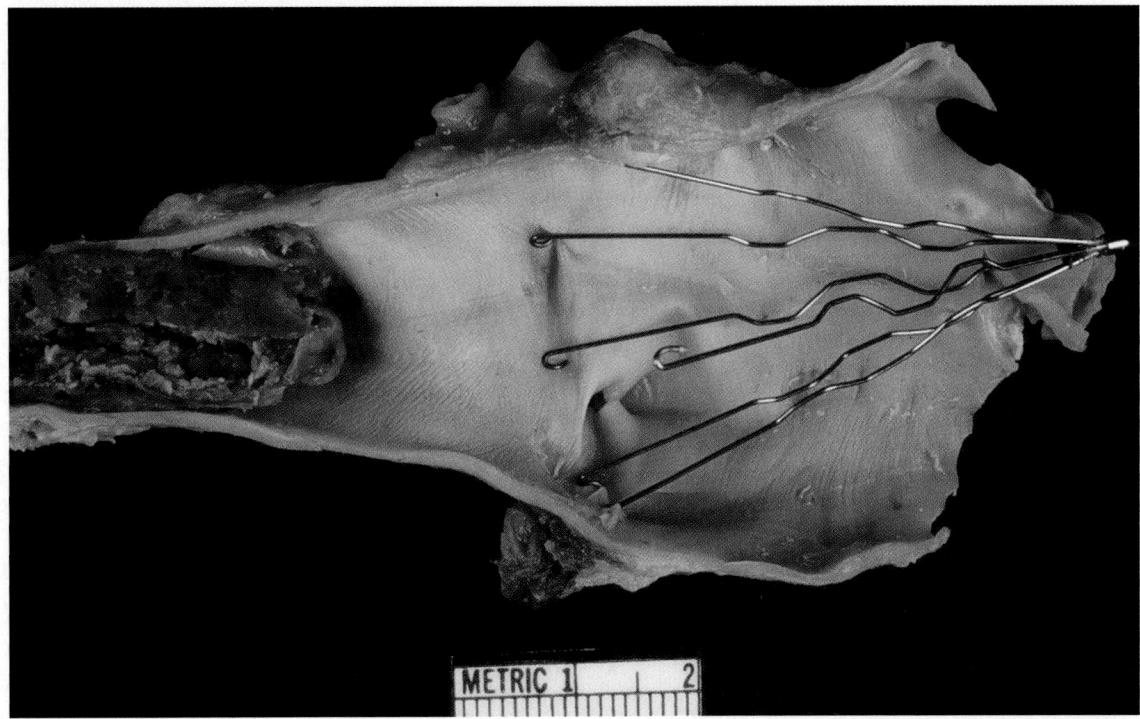

Fig. 10. Greenfield inferior vena cava filter with occluding thrombus after pelvic irradiation for uterine cancer.

lower extremities (5%). Infections from filter insertion are extremely rare. Most complications are clinically insignificant, and the mortality rate from IVC filters is 0.12%.

- IVC plication does not replace chronic anticoagulation therapy.
- Recurrent PE occurs in 2.5% patients after filter insertion.
- IVC plication does not affect mortality from PE.
- The role of the IVC in PE has not yet been full determined.
- Complications: DVT (2%), migration (50%), perforation of IVC (24%), and edema of legs (5%).

Prophylaxis of DVT and PE
Less than 50% of hospitalized patients in the United States received adequate prophylaxis against DVT or PE. Prophylaxis includes early ambulation after surgery or immobilization, intermittent pneumatic compression of the lower extremities, active and passive leg exercises, and low-dose unfractionated heparin (LDUH) or LMWH subcutaneously.

Current American College of Chest Physicians recommendations include the following:

- Aspirin should not be used alone as thromboprophylaxis.
- For moderate-risk general surgery patients, use LDUH (5,000 U twice daily) or LMWH (>3,400 U daily).
- For higher risk general surgery patients, use LDUH (5,000 U three times daily) or LMWH (>3,400 U daily).
- For high-risk general surgery with risk factors, combine pharmacologic methods with compression stockings/pneumatic compression devices.
- Use prophylaxis in major gynecologic and urologic operations with LDUH (5,000 U three times daily).
- For elective total hip/knee arthroplasty, use either LMWH, fondaparinux, or warfarin (INR, 2-3).
- For hip fracture surgery, use fondaparinux, LMWH, warfarin, or LDUH.
- For hip/knee arthroplasty and for hip fracture surgery, use thromboprophylaxis for at least 10 days.
- For acutely ill medical patients who have heart failure

or respiratory disease, or who are confined to bed, and have at least one risk factor, use LDUH or LMWH.

■ All patients admitted to an intensive care unit should be assessed for their risk of thromboembolism, and most should receive prophylaxis.

CHRONIC THROMBOEMBOLIC PULMONARY HYPERTENSION

Chronic thromboembolic pulmonary hypertension (CTPH) is likely more common than previously thought and occurs in about 3% of patients after a pulmonary embolus. Many patients with the initial diagnosis of idiopathic pulmonary hypertension are subsequently found to have CTPH. Risk factors for increased risk of CTPH after PE include younger age, a larger perfusion defect, and idiopathic PE at presentation. A subset of patients can develop CTPH even though the occurrence of recurrent PE cannot be documented. In some patients, multiple emboli may not be the cause of CTPH, but rather recurrent in situ

thrombosis following an initial PE may be the culprit.

Less than 50% of patients with CTPH have a history compatible with a previous episode of DVT or PE. Lupus anticoagulant is present in about 10% of patients with CTPH, and 1% have deficiencies of either antithrombin III, protein C, or protein S. CTPH develops in many patients without an underlying coagulopathy because of a delayed or missed diagnosis of PE or inadequate anticoagulation for previously documented DVT or PE. Lung biopsy specimens from patients with CTPH show plexiform lesions, suggesting that factors other than obstructive PE may have a role in the onset of CTPH. Indeed, the degree of angiographic obstruction correlates poorly with the degree of pulmonary hypertension (Fig. 11 and 12).

■ Recurrent PE leads to development of CTPH in about 3% of patients.
■ Chronic recurrent in situ thrombosis initiated by the first PE may be responsible for many cases of CTPH.
■ Plexiform histologic lesions are found at lung biopsy in CTPH.

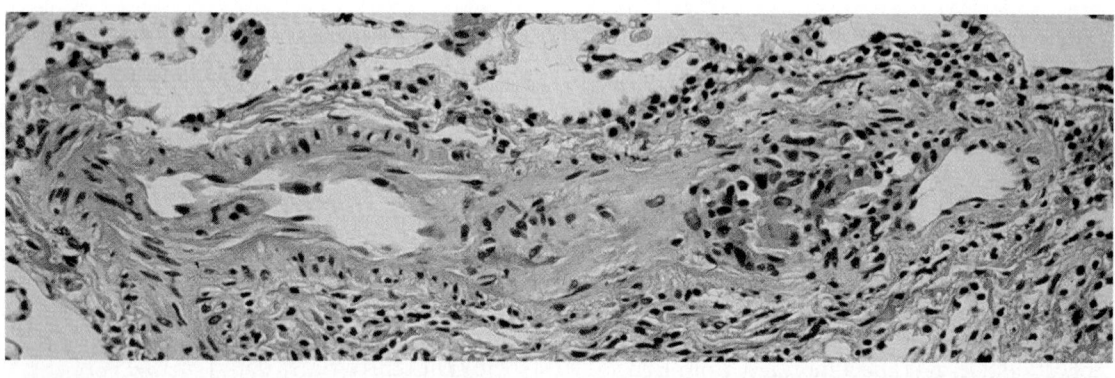

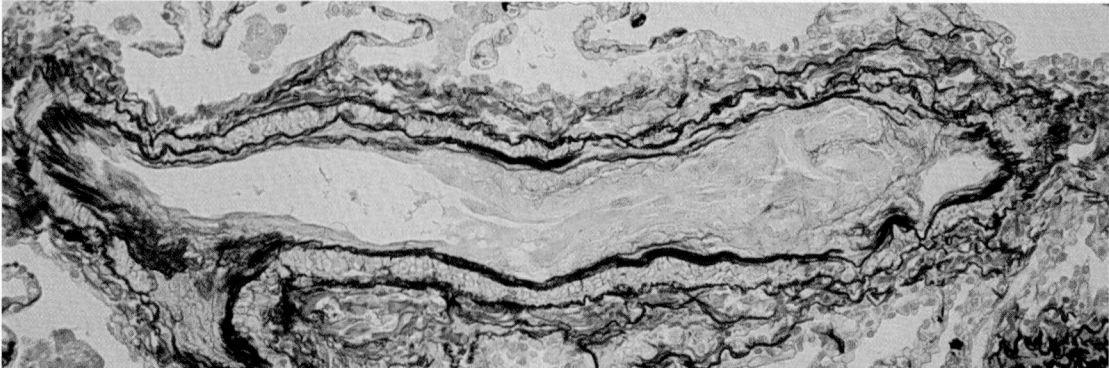

Fig. 11. Lung biopsy specimens of thromboembolic pulmonary hypertension with organized arterial thrombus formation. Plexiform lesions are not present. (x50.)

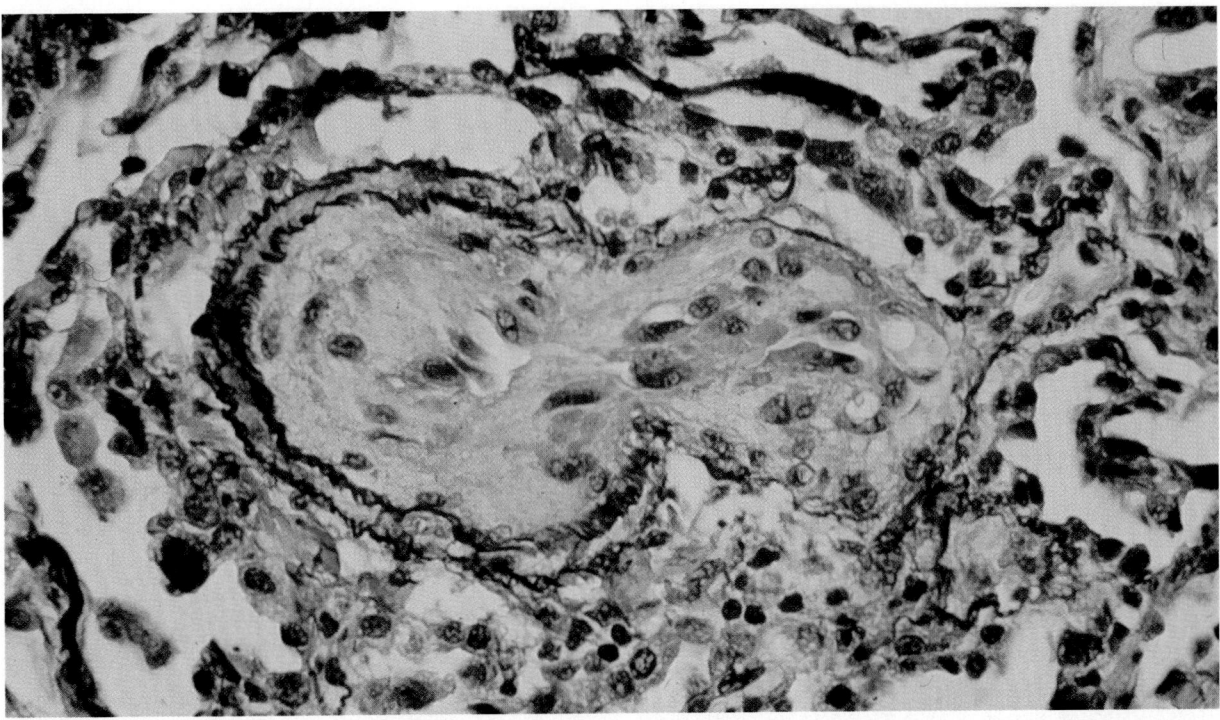

Fig. 12. Lung tissue with pulmonary arteriolar obstruction in thromboembolic pulmonary hypertension. (x100.)

Many patients remain asymptomatic—in a "honeymoon period"—despite extensive PE. When symptoms develop, they are similar to those of idiopathic pulmonary hypertension. An uncommon clinical finding is the presence of low-pitched flow murmurs or bruits, systolic or diastolic, in areas of partial branch pulmonary artery stenosis caused by intra-arterial clots and fibrotic bands, present in up to 20% of patients. Chest radiographic findings are usually unremarkable. The diffusing capacity of the lung for carbon monoxide (DLCO) is either normal (in many patients) or reduced (in a minority); a normal value does not exclude CTPH. A mild to moderate restrictive defect is noted in 20% of patients. P(A-a)O$_2$ is usually widened and PaO$_2$ decreases with exercise in most patients. In almost all patients with CTPH who undergo V/Q scanning, at least one segmental or larger perfusion defect (with corresponding ventilation mismatch) is observed. However, the V/Q often underestimates the extent of central pulmonary vascular obstruction (Fig. 13).

■ "A honeymoon" (asymptomatic) period occurs despite extensive PE in many patients.

■ Low-pitched flow murmurs or bruit, systolic or diastolic, are heard over lung fields in up to 20% of patients.
■ Diffusing capacity of the lung for carbon monoxide: either normal or reduced (in a minority); a normal value does not exclude CTPH.
■ Mild-to-moderate restrictive pulmonary dysfunction in 20% of patients.

Pulmonary thromboendarterectomy (PTEA) is the treatment of choice in symptomatic patients, whether symptomatic at rest or during exercise. The mean pulmonary vascular resistance in patients undergoing surgery is 800 to 1,000 dynes/s/cm^{-5}. Selection criteria for PTEA include thrombi accessible to a surgical approach, acceptance of surgical risk by patient, acceptable patient age and comorbidity, and the absence of severe underlying lung disease, either obstructive or restrictive. However, none of these criteria is absolute. Complications of PTEA include reperfusion pulmonary edema, right ventricular failure secondary to residual pulmonary hypertension, aortic dissection, cerebrovascular accident, mediastinal hemorrhage, and intraoperative cardiac arrest. Overall mortality is

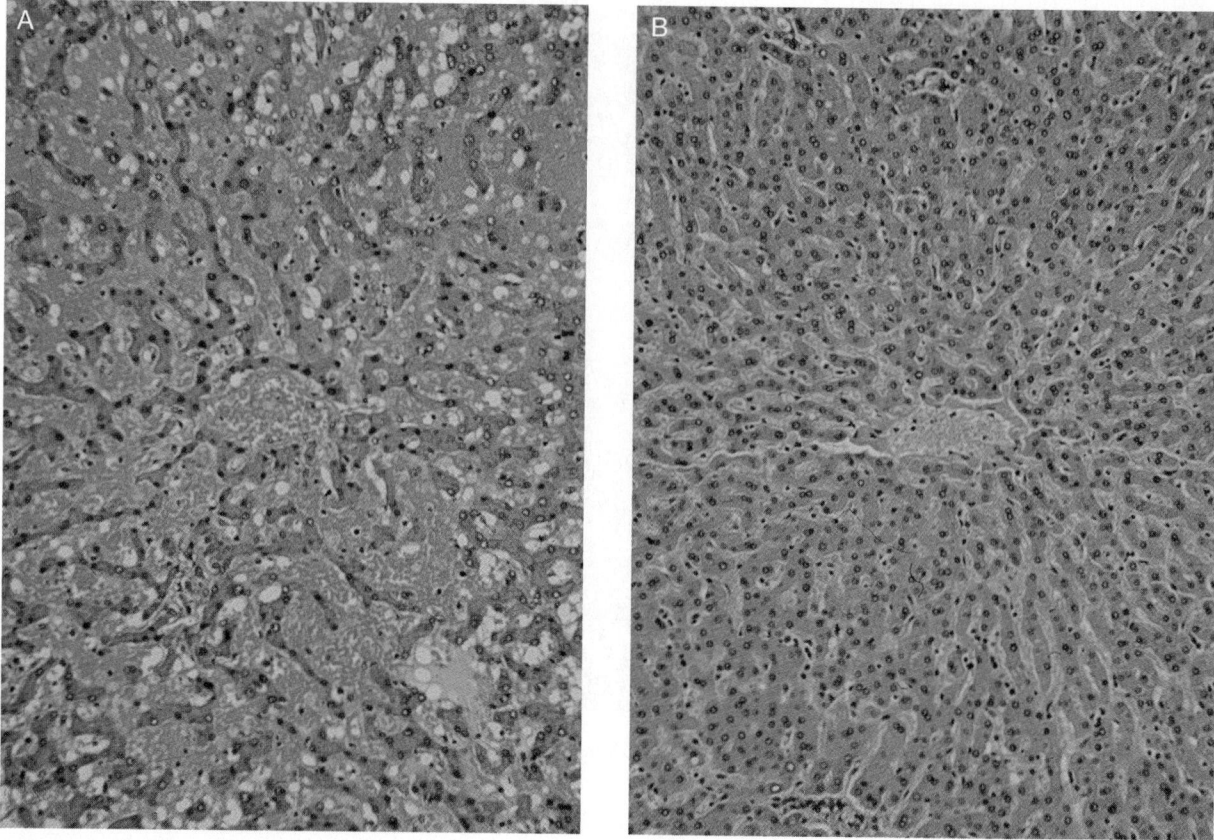

Fig. 13. *A*, Congested liver in thromboembolic pulmonary hypertension. *B*, Normal liver.

approximately 10%, with a perioperative mortality of approximately 5%. Although small numbers of patients do not show an immediate positive response to PTEA, symptomatic improvement may occur over a prolonged period of up to 12 months. Long-term anticoagulation and IVC filter placement is indicated in all patients who undergo PTEA. Lung transplantation may be considered for patients who are not candidates for PTEA or for those who have inadequate results.

- PTEA: overall mortality: 10%; perioperative mortality: 5%.
- PTEA selection criteria: thrombi accessible to PTEA, acceptance of surgical risk by patient, age, and comorbidities, including coexisting lung disease.
- Lifelong anticoagulation is indicated after PTEA.

Massive PE

Massive PE is defined as a PE causing hemodynamic shock. In most patients, the degree of hypoxia and its acuteness and effect on hemodynamics, as well as the underlying cardiopulmonary disease, determine the "massive" nature, rather than the volume of emboli that occlude the pulmonary vasculature (Fig. 14). The incidence of massive PE is about 4% to 5%. Massive PE is associated with mortality rates estimated at 10% within 1 hour after the occurrence of PE and up to 85% in the first 6 hours. The sudden onset of severe dyspnea, syncope, and hemodynamic collapse and clinical detection of acute right ventricular failure (elevated jugular venous pressure, right-sided S_3, and parasternal lift or heave) and hypoxia in a high-risk patient should suggest the possibility. Massive PE may acutely increase the right atrial pressure and open a patent foramen ovale, with a resultant right-to-left shunt and worsening hypoxia. A more serious complication is paradoxical embolization into the systemic circulation. Chest radiography may demonstrate acute oligemia. An ECG is more likely to exhibit S_1Q_3 and new incomplete right bundle branch block in massive PE than in nonmassive

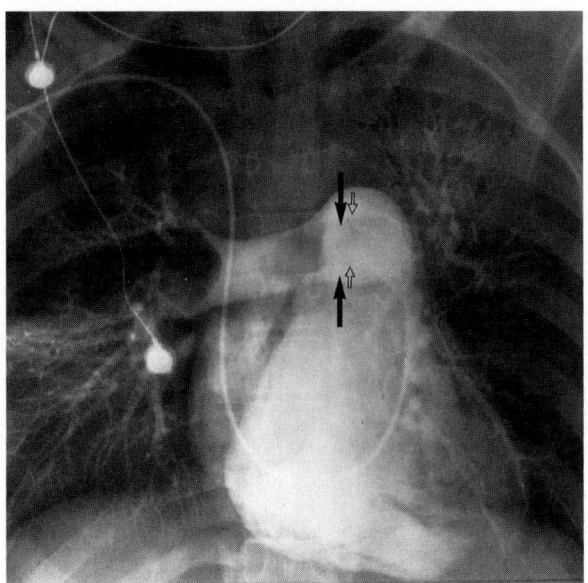

Fig. 14. Massive pulmonary embolism involving the main pulmonary artery (*arrows*). Reduced perfusion of contrast agent into the right upper lobe arteries is evident.

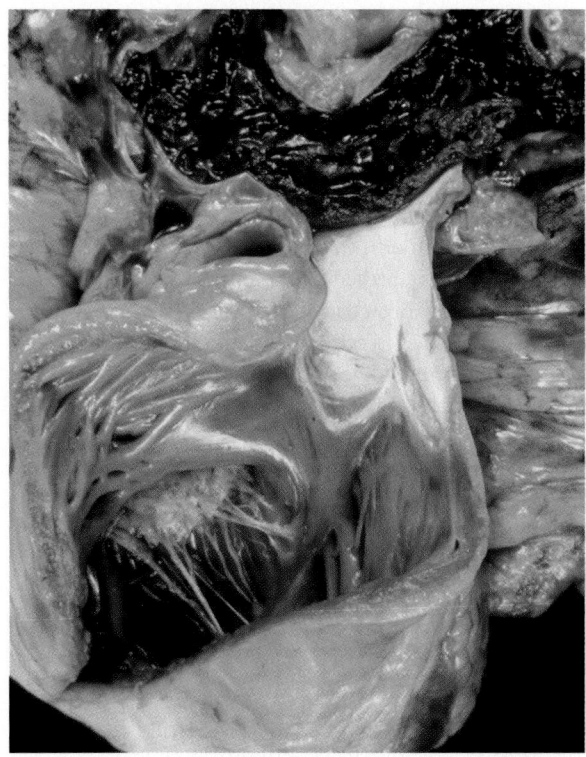

Fig. 15. Massive fatal pulmonary embolus occupying the right and left pulmonary trunks. The pulmonary valve and pulmonary outflow tract are seen inferiorly.

PE (Fig. 15). If available, bedside echocardiography should be obtained as soon as the diagnosis is suspected. This is useful for substantiating the diagnosis by visualizing right ventricular dilatation and dysfunction and for exclusion of other diseases that may mimic PE, such as tamponade or myocardial infarction.

Treatment recommendations include hemodynamic resuscitation and stabilization, oxygenation, and close follow-up in the intensive care unit. Heparinization should be commenced as quickly as possible.

Thrombolytic agents (streptokinase, urokinase, and tissue plasminogen activator [tPA]) are used to treat massive PE and massive iliofemoral thrombosis. The role of thrombolytics remains controversial and several meta-analyses have not provided definitive guidance. Individual thrombolysis trials have not proven that thrombolysis decreases mortality in massive PE, but most surrogate markers, including improvement in right ventricular function, suggest a benefit. The risk/benefit ratio with thrombolysis in PE appears to be most favorable in the sickest patients with massive PE. In the absence of contraindications, thrombolysis is indicated for massive PE with hypotension or severe hypoxemia.

Ideally, thrombolytic agents are administered within

24 hours after PE. Dosages for different agents are as follows: streptokinase, loading dose of 250,000 IU infused over 30 minutes, followed by maintenance dose of 100,000 U/hour for up to 24 hours; urokinase, loading dose of 4,400 IU/kg, infused over 10 minutes followed by continuous infusion of 4,400 IU/kg per hour, for 12 to 24 hours; and tPA, a total dose of 100 mg intravenously over a 2-hour period. Heparin infusion is begun or resumed if APTT is less than 80 seconds after thrombolytic therapy. The contraindications to thrombolytic therapy are listed in Table 4.

- Thrombolytic agents should be given within 24 hours of massive PE.
- Heparin therapy is necessary following thrombolytic therapy.
- Mortality in massive PE: 10% within 1 hour; up to 85% in 6 hours.
- Important signs of massive PE: sudden dyspnea, syncope, shock, and acute right ventricular failure.
- Bedside echocardiography should be obtained as soon as the diagnosis is suspected.

Table 4. Contraindications to Thrombolytic
Therapy in Venous Thromboembolism

Absolute
  Intracranial disorders (neoplasms, vascular
    accidents, hemorrhagic stroke, aneurysm)
  Intracranial or intraspinal surgery or trauma
    within the preceding 2 months
  Operation, obstetric delivery, or organ biopsy
    within the preceding 10 days
  Active internal bleeding within the preceding
    6 months
  Bleeding diathesis
  Severe hypertension (systolic blood pressure
    >200 mm Hg or diastolic blood pressure
    >110 mm Hg)
  Recent trauma (including cardiopulmonary
    resuscitation)
Relative
  Pregnancy
  Infective endocarditis
  Pericarditis
  Diabetic hemorrhagic retinopathy or other
    hemorrhagic ophthalmic conditions

PULMONARY HYPERTENSION

Michael D. McGoon, MD

DEFINITION

The pulmonary vascular bed is normally a low-pressure, low-resistance circulation with compliant thin-walled vessels. Pulmonary hypertension (PH) is considered to be present when the pulmonary artery (PA) systolic pressure exceeds 35 mm Hg or the PA mean pressure (mPAP) is over 25 mm Hg at rest. Clinically significant PH is usually associated with substantially higher PA pressures. Although PH can be suspected based on echocardiographic estimates, the diagnosis cannot be established in the absence of invasive measurements.

The above figures are based on a general consensus that this degree of PA pressure elevation over the average population is clinically significant. Unlike systemic hypertension, the prognostic significance of minimally abnormal pulmonary pressures has not been determined. Similarly, a mPAP >30 mm Hg with exercise while considered abnormal, is currently without rigorous assessment of its clinical implications. In determining whether PH is present, it should be noted that a PA systolic pressure >40 mm Hg (when measured by echocardiography) is present in 6% of otherwise normal individuals older than 50 years and 5% of people with a body mass index (BMI) >30 kg/m2. Athletic men also have a higher resting PA systolic pressure.

PA pressure is related to PV pressure, PA blood flow (Qp), and pulmonary vascular resistance (Rp) by the following equation:

$$Qp(L/min\ per\ m2) = \frac{PA - PV\ (mm\ Hg)}{Rp\ (U \cdot m2)}$$

DIAGNOSTIC CLASSIFICATION

The current World Health Organization (WHO) taxonomy of diseases causing or associated with PH incorporates pathology, etiology, clinical presentation, and functional data. The term *primary pulmonary hypertension* has been replaced by idiopathic pulmonary arterial hypertension (IPAH) or, when specific genetic findings or a heritable pattern are present, familial PAH (FPAH) (Table 1).

PULMONARY ARTERIAL HYPERTENSION

Pulmonary arterial hypertension comprises pulmonary hypertensive diseases of various substrates which have similar pathologic lesions, clinical presentations and responses to treatment. These include, in addition to

Table 1.   WHO Classification of Pulmonary Hypertension

1. **Pulmonary arterial hypertension (PAH)**
    1.1.   Idiopathic (IPAH)
    1.2.   Familial (FPAH)
    1.3.   Associated with (APAH):
        1.3.1. Collagen vascular disease
        1.3.2. Congenital systemic-to-pulmonary shunts
        1.3.3. Portal hypertension
        1.3.4. HIV infection
        1.3.5. Drugs and toxins
        1.3.6. Other (thyroid disorders, glycogen storage disease, Gaucher's disease, hereditary hemorrhagic
                 telangiectasia, hemoglobinopathies, chronic myeloproliferative disorders, splenectomy)
    1.4.   Associated with significant venous or
             capillary involvement
    1.4.1. Pulmonary veno-occlusive disease (PVOD)
    1.4.2. Pulmonary capillary hemangiomatosis (PCH)
    1.5.   Persistent pulmonary hypertension of the newborn
2. **Pulmonary hypertension with left heart disease**
    2.1.   Left-sided atrial or ventricular heart disease
    2.2.   Left-sided valvular heart disease
3. **Pulmonary hypertension associated with lung diseases and/or hypoxemia**
    3.1.   Chronic obstructive pulmonary disease
    3.2.   Interstitial lung disease
    3.3.   Sleep-disordered breathing
    3.4.   Alveolar hypoventilation disorders
    3.5.   Chronic exposure to high alititute
    3.6.   Developmental abnormalities
4. **Pulmonary hypertension due to chronic thrombotic and/or embolic disease (CTEPH)**
    4.1.   Thromboembolic obstruction of proximal pulmonary arteries
    4.2.   Thromboembolic obstruction of distal pulmonary arteries
    4.3.   Non-thrombotic pulmonary embolism (tumor, parasites, foreign material)
5. **Miscellaneous**
    Sarcoidosis, histiocytosis X, lymphangiomatosis, compression of pulmonary vessels (adenopathy, tumor, fibros-
      ing mediastinitis)

IPAH and FPAH, pulmonary hypertension related to left-to-right shunts, connective tissue diseases, portal hypertension, human immunodeficiency virus (HIV) infection, exposure to certain drugs or dietary products, and persistent pulmonary hypertension of the newborn. In addition, *pulmonary venopathy* (previously called pulmonary veno-occlusive disease) and *pulmonary microvasculopathy* (previously called pulmonary capillary hemangiomatosis) are included in the catego-

ry of PAH because they also demonstrate arteriopathy, similar risk factors and possibly genetic substrates.

Idiopathic

Idiopathic PAH is pulmonary hypertension of undetermined cause. It is a rare disease, with a prevalence of less than 0.2%. It is more common in women than men; the female preponderance is greater among black patients, and the mean age at onset is 35 years.

The clinical course of untreated idiopathic pulmonary hypertension is generally one of inexorable progression toward death. Among patients who do not undergo heart-lung transplantation or treatment with an effective vasodilator, actuarial survival is 68% to 77% at 1 year, and 22% to 38% at 5 years. The most frequent cause of death is right ventricular failure. Survival has a direct relation with cardiac index and an inverse relationship to right atrial mean pressure, mean pulmonary arterial pressure, exercise capacity (particularly 6-minute walk distance), BNP level, pulmonary arterial oxygen saturation and presence of a pericardial effusion.

Familial (Genetic)

A pattern of autosomal dominant inheritance has been observed in families with two or more members having PAH and no other underlying or associated condition. The specific gene is on chromosome 2q31-32 and codes for bone morphogenetic protein receptor 2 (*BMPR2*), a member of the TGF-β superfamily of signaling molecules. Mutant *BMPR2* leads to increased proliferation and decreased apoptosis of vascular smooth muscle cells, thereby promoting constrictive lesions.

The phenotypic expression of the genetic abnormality is very variable and incomplete. The penetrance of disease for all known *BMPR2* mutations is 15% to 20% in most families. Individuals known to have the genetic mutation may not develop pulmonary hypertension, though they may still transmit the disease to their offspring. Thus, the siblings or children of FPAH patients have an overall risk of 50% of inheriting the gene, so with a 20% penetrance their risk of acquiring the clinical disease is 10%. There is a female preponderance and a tendency for FPAH to develop at earlier ages in subsequent generations within a family (genetic anticipation). The natural history of FPAH is indistinguishable from IPAH, including response to treatment. Between 10 and 25% of patients with apparently sporadic IPAH, have the genetic mutation associated with FPAH.

It is generally felt that although the genetic substrate sets the stage for the development of PAH, a second environmental or coexisting genetic condition triggers the clinical expression of the disease. Mutations of the *BMPR2* gene have been reported in PAH associated with fenfluramine derivatives, but not in patients with PAH in the scleroderma spectrum of disease or HIV-associated PAH. Mutation of the ALK1 receptor gene confers susceptibility to pulmonary hypertension in some patients with hereditary hemorrhagic telangiectasia. This appears to be a less common cause of heritable PAH. ALK1 is also a member of the TGF-beta family.

- Genetic testing and professional genetic counseling should be offered to relatives of patients with FPAH.
- Patients with IPAH should be advised about the availability of genetic testing and counseling for their relatives.

Associated With Connective Tissue Disease

PAH has been observed in all of the connective tissue diseases, but occurs most frequently (mean from several studies, 16%) in systemic sclerosis. In limited scleroderma (CREST syndrome), PAH is the cause of death in up to 50% of patients who die of scleroderma-related complications. Isolated PAH is relatively uncommon in diffuse scleroderma; when seen it most often occurs in association with the antinucleolar antibody, anti-U3-RNP. Pulmonary artery hypertension is especially associated with the presence of autoantibodies (including anticentromere antibodies and antinucleolar antibodies) in those with long-standing limited scleroderma.

In mixed connective tissue disease (an overlap syndrome of features of scleroderma, systemic lupus erythematosus and polymyositis associated with the anti-U1-RNP antibody), PAH is the most common cause of death. PAH is less frequent in SLE, rheumatoid arthritis, or polymyositis. Anticardiolipin antibodies are associated with PAH in up to 68% of patients with SLE.

- In patients with unexplained PAH, testing for connective tissue disease and HIV infection should be performed.

Bulleted items in blue are key recommendations based on the consensus statement from the American College of Chest Physicians (2004). Strength of recommendation and level of evidence not given.

Associated With Toxic Exposure

PAH has been associated with the ingestion of appetite suppressants which have a molecular similarity to amphetamine, including aminorex, fenfluramine and dexfenfluramine. Dexfenfluramine increases the likelihood of developing PAH by a factor of over 20 times in patients who took the drug longer than 3 months. PAH has been observed in users of illicit methamphetamine, and may become an increasing health problem with widening abuse of the drug. Other toxic associations include contaminated rapeseed oil (an epidemic of 20,000 cases of toxicity occurred in Spain in 1981, of which 2.5% developed clinically significant PAH and 20% died). Contaminated tryptophan caused the eosinophilic myalgia syndrome, and PAH was a severe complication in some patients.

Associated With Right-to-Left Shunting

The term "Eisenmenger syndrome" refers to systemic-to-pulmonary (left-to-right) arterial shunts leading to PAH and ultimately resulting in a right-to-left or bidirectional shunt. The pulmonary vasculopathy is preceded by a period of low pulmonary resistance and high pulmonary blood flow. The likely cause of the development of PAH is endothelial damage related to elevated shear stress caused by high blood flow.

The likelihood of developing PAH usually depends on the site and the severity of the defect. Ventricular septal defects (VSD) cause PAH more commonly than atrial septal defects (ASD), followed by patent ductus arteriosus (PDA). VSD or PDA patients tend to develop earlier Eisenmenger syndrome compared to ASD, and complex anomalies, such as atrioventricular septal defects or truncus arteriosus, tend to develop PAH early. Rarely, PAH may develop even after the defect is corrected.

Compared to a patient with IPAH, a patient with Eisenmenger syndrome and a comparable degree of pulmonary hypertension has a probability of survival that is significantly longer. Their degree of disability due to hypoxemia may be considerable, however (Table 2).

Associated With Portal Hypertension

Among patients with portal hypertension who undergo evaluation for orthotopic liver transplantation 10-20% have a PASP of 30-50 mm Hg. These patients are often asymptomatic, but the possibility of PAH should be considered and investigated since the mortality of liver transplantation is demonstrably increased if mPAP exceeds 35 mm Hg. Patients with portopulmonary hypertension often have a hyperdynamic circulation with high cardiac output.

Associated With HIV Infection

HIV infection has a 0.5% prevalence of PH, significantly above the general population.

Associated With Other Diseases

Patients who have had a *splenectomy* have been reported to exhibit an 11.5% prevalence of clinically significant PAH after an interval of 4 to 32 years. Some *hemoglobinopathies* appear to be at higher risk for developing PAH, including sickle-cell disease, in which it is the cause of death in 3%. The cause of PAH has been postulated to be related to increased shear stress from abnormal erythrocytes passing through the pulmonary microvasculature and/or reduced nitric oxide bioavailability. Beta-thalassemia may also be related to PAH.

Chronic myeloproliferative disorders, including polycythemia vera, essential thrombocytosis, and myelofibrosis with myeloid metaplasia accompanying chronic myeloid leukemia or the myelodysplastic syndrome have been associated with PAH.

Certain *rare genetic diseases* have been reported to exhibit findings of PAH in some patients. These include type Ia glycogen storage disease (Von Gierke disease), Gaucher disease, hereditary hemorrhagic telangiectasia (Osler-Weber-Rendu disease).

Table 2. Causes of Pulmonary Hypertension Due to Left-to-Right Shunts

Extracardiac shunts
    Patent ductus arteriosus
    Aortopulmonary window
    Rupture of aortic sinus
    Peripheral arteriovenous fistula
    Hemodialysis shunts
Intracardiac shunts
    Ventricular septal defect
    Atrial septal defect

Some metabolic *conditions* appear to have a higher-than-expected association with PAH. These include both hypothyroidism and hyperthyroidism, and hyperuricemia.

Pulmonary Venopathy and Pulmonary Microvasculopathy

Both pulmonary venopathy and pulmonary microvasculopathy are rare entities, but overlap in terms of pathology, clinical presentation and response to therapy. They are classified within the category of PAH because of similar histological changes in the small pulmonary arteries (including intimal fibrosis, medial hypertrophy, and plexiform lesions), and similar clinical presentation. The gene associated with familial and IPAH has been identified in a patient with pulmonary venopathy. Pulmonary occlusive venopathy and pulmonary microvasculopathy are rare, with less than 200 reported cases, but substantially more unreported cases. Patients with pulmonary venopathy or pulmonary microvasculopathy may develop severe pulmonary edema after administration of vasodilators.

Persistent Pulmonary Hypertension of the Newborn

This form of PAH, occurring in almost 2 per 1000 live births, is present when pulmonary vascular resistance remains high after birth and results in arterial hypoxemia due to right-to-left shunt through fetal circulatory pathways.

PULMONARY VENOUS HYPERTENSION WITH LEFT HEART DISEASE

Disorders of the left heart that raise pulmonary venous pressures lead to increases in pulmonary arterial pressure, initially due to passive reflection of venous pressures into the arterial bed. The transpulmonary pressure gradient and pulmonary vascular resistance are within a normal range while direct measures of left atrial pressure and left ventricular end-diastolic pressure are elevated. With time, pulmonary arterial remodeling can occur, and is associated with an increase in the transpulmonary gradient due to high pulmonary vascular resistance.

Diagnosis of this type of PH is based on features of the examination, cardiac imaging and functional assessment, and hemodynamic measurements reflecting the underlying left heart problem (Table 3).

PULMONARY HYPERTENSION ASSOCIATED WITH LUNG DISEASE AND/OR HYPOXEMIA

The predominant cause of this type of PH is inadequate oxygenation of arterial blood as a result of lung disease, ventilatory disorders, or prolonged exposure to high altitude (Table 4). The elevation of mPAP is usually rather modest (25-35 mm Hg). However, a subset of patients with chronic obstructive pulmonary disease have severe PH despite relatively minimal reduction of FEV_1/FVC. The diagnostic strategy of PH in this setting should include evaluation of possible obstructive or restrictive pulmonary disease, pulmonary fibrosis, hypoxic sleep disorders or other neurologic hypoventilation syndromes.

CHRONIC THROMBOEMBOLIC DISEASE (CTEPH)

Up to 3.8% of patients who survive an acute pulmonary embolism develop evidence of PH within 2 years. In addition, patients with documented chronic thromboembolic pulmonary hypertension (CTEPH) often do not have a recognized history of an acute embolic event. Since many cases of proximal CTEPH are amenable to surgical intervention, investigation directed to this entity is important (Table 5).

Table 3. Left Heart Causes of Pulmonary Hypertension

Location	Condition
Aorta	Coarctation
	Supraventricular aortic stenosis
Left ventricle	Aortic stenosis
	Aortic regurgitation
	Congenital subaortic stenosis
	Hypertrophic cardiomyopathy
	Constrictive pericarditis
	Restrictive cardiomyopathy
	Dilated cardiomyopathy
	Mitral stenosis
	Mitral regurgitation
Left atrium	Ball-valve thrombus
	Myxoma
	Cor triatriatum

- Ventilation-perfusion scanning should be performed to rule out CTEPH; a normal scan effectively excludes a diagnosis of CTEPH.
- A normal contrast-enhanced CT or MRI does not exclude the diagnosis of CTEPH and should not be used to screen for CTEPH.
- In patients with PAH, when a ventilation-perfusion scan is suggestive of CTEPH, pulmonary angiography is required for accurate diagnosis and best anatomic definition to assess operability for surgical pulmonary thrombectomy.

PH Caused by Diseases Affecting the Pulmonary Vasculature

This category of PH includes miscellaneous disorders causing inflammatory processes or mechanical obstruction. Specific disorders include schistosomiasis, sarcoidosis, histiocytosis X, and lymphangiomatosis. Extrinsic compression of pulmonary vessels (arterial or venous) by adenopathy, malignancy or mediastinal fibrosis may also lead to significant PH.

PATHOLOGY

Medial hypertrophy of muscular and elastic arteries, dilation and intimal atheromas of elastic pulmonary arteries, and right ventricular hypertrophy due to pressure overload are noted in all forms of PH. Pulmonary artery hypertension specifically is characterized by constrictive and complex arterial lesions.

The *plexiform lesion* is a focal proliferation, often located at branches of pre- and intra-acinar pulmonary vessels of endothelial channels lined by myofibroblasts, smooth muscle cells, and connective tissue matrix. It is typically associated with idiopathic or familial PAH (though the prevalence is unclear), or with Eisenmenger syndrome, but is virtually never observed in PAH associated with connective tissue diseases. The endothelial cells in plexiform lesions of IPAH have been reported to be monoclonal in origin and express vascular endothelial growth factor (VEGF) and are thought to perhaps represent a neoplastic-like disordered angiogenesis. Dilation lesions are venous-like vessels sometimes observed downstream from plexiform lesions.

Other pathological findings include intimal hyperplasia, adventitial thickening, and arteritis (Fig. 1). Enlargement and hypertrophy of the right ventricle (Fig. 2 *A*) and right atrium (Fig. 2 *B*) are often prominent in severe pulmonary hypertension.

Table 4.   Causes of Respiratory or Hypoxic Pulmonary Hypertension

Long-term dwelling in a high altitude
Restrictive respiratory dysfunction
   Obesity
   Kyphoscoliosis
   Neuromuscular disorders
   Severe pleural fibrosis
   Lung resection
Chronic upper airway obstruction
   Congenital webs
   Enlarged tonsils
   Obstructive sleep apnea
Chronic lower airway obstruction
   Chronic bronchitis
   Asthmatic bronchitis
   Bronchiectasis
   Cystic fibrosis
   Emphysema
Chronic diffuse parenchymal disease
   Interstitial fibrosis
   Pneumoconioses
   Granulomatous disease
   Alveolar filling disorders
   Connective tissue disorders (scleroderma, rheumatoid lung)

Table 5.   Causes of Arterial Obstructive Pulmonary Hypertension

Thrombotic disease
   Sickle cell disease
   Coagulation disorders
Embolic disease
   Chronic thromboemboli
   Tumor emboli
   Schistosomiasis
   Connective tissue disorders
   Lupus
   Systemic sclerosis

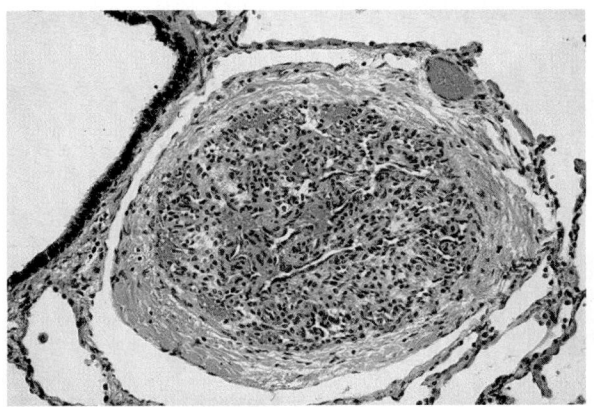

Fig. 1. Plexiform lesion in pulmonary arteriole in pulmonary hypertension.

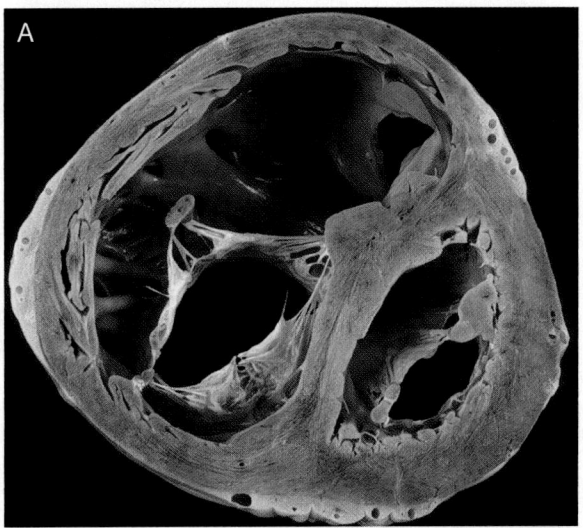

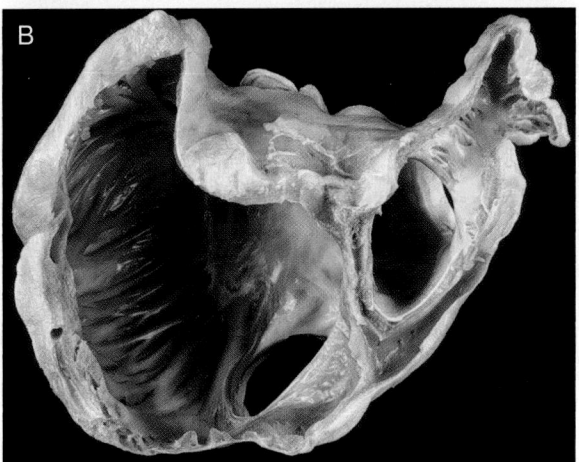

Fig. 2. *A*, Right ventricular hypertrophy and dilatation in pulmonary hypertension. *B*, Right atrial dilatation and normal left atrium.

MECHANISMS

A number of mechanisms and genetic factors appear to contribute to the initiation and progression of pulmonary hypertensive states (Fig. 3). Pulmonary vasoconstriction is believed to be an early component of the process. Mechanisms promoting vasoconstriction in PH include abnormal function or expression of potassium channels, reduced production of vasodilators such as nitric oxide (NO) and prostacyclin, and overexpression of vasoconstrictors such as endothelin (ET)-1. All of these factors also have a role in stimulating vascular remodeling. The endothelial production of prostacyclin, an endogenous pulmonary vasodilator and platelet inhibitor, is decreased in PH patients. In clinically apparent PH, vascular remodeling appears to be the major abnormal process contributing to PH.

The level of lung and circulating endothelin-1 (ET-1) is increased in patients with various types of PH and likely contributes to both abnormal vasoconstrictive and proliferative abnormalities. Reduced expression of nitric oxide synthase in endothelial cells decreases production of nitric oxide from the substrate amino acid arginine. This decreases the conversion of GTP to guanosine 3'-5' monophosphate (cGMP), facilitating entry of calcium ions into vascular smooth muscle cells and promotion of vasoconstriction and cellular proliferation.

Circulating serotonin levels are elevated and platelet stores are depressed in patients with PAH, and may have a direct role in causing the increased pulmonary vascular resistance due to vasoconstriction and cellular proliferation. Increased serotonin levels may be

one mechanism by which appetite suppressants such as fenfluramine increase the risk of developing PAH. The appetite suppressants also block K$^+$ channels in pulmonary vascular smooth muscle cells, resulting in increased entry of calcium ions into the cell and consequent vasoconstriction. Inflammatory mechanisms may participate in some forms of PAH, such as that related to connective tissue diseases and human immunodeficiency virus infection. Elevated circulating levels of pro-inflammatory cytokines IL-1 and IL-6 have also been observed. Thrombotic processes and platelet dysfunction are involved in PAH, both by promoting intravascular thrombus formation and by

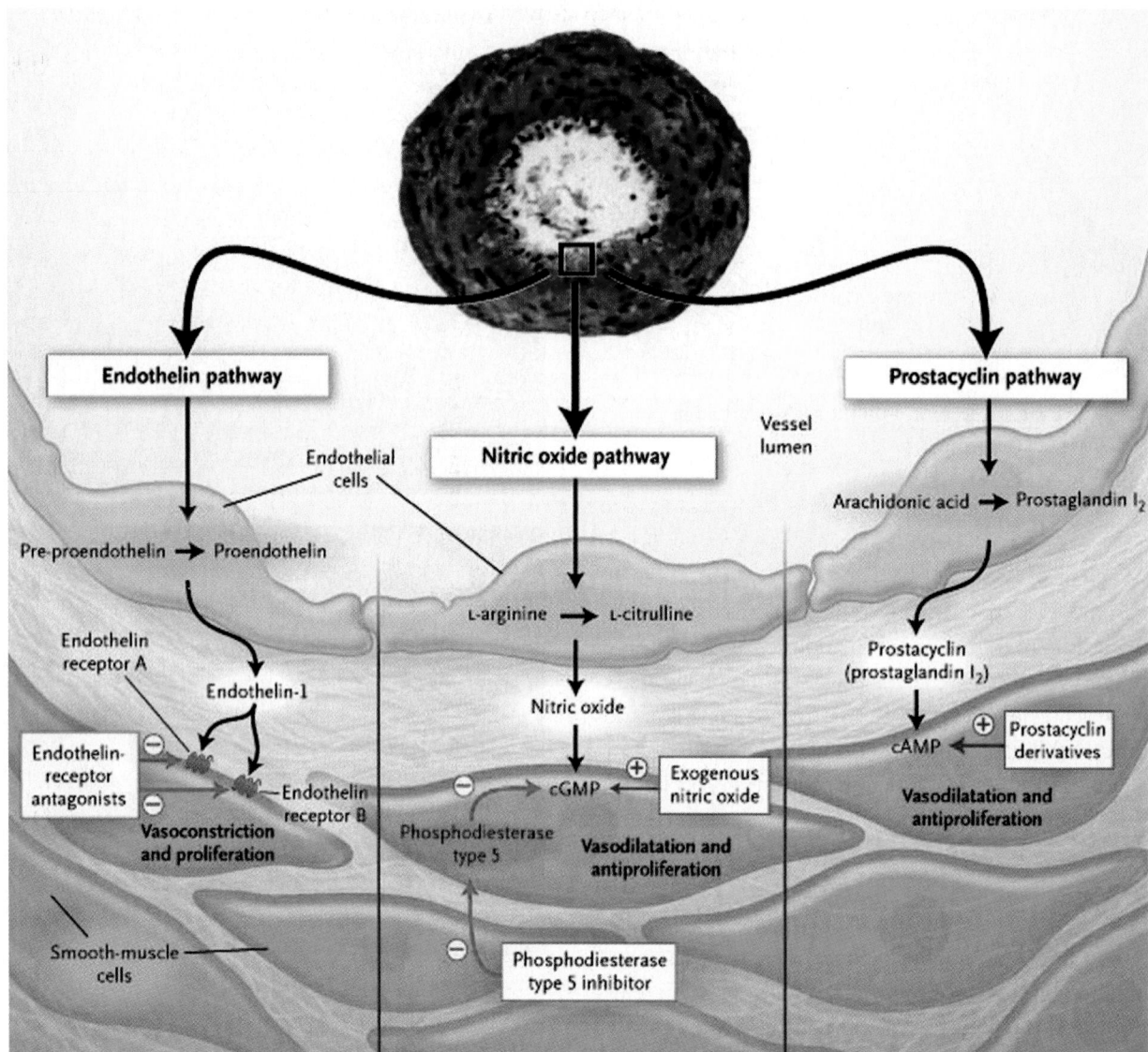

Fig. 3. Targets for current or emerging therapies in pulmonary arterial hypertension. Three major pathways involved in abnormal proliferation and contraction of the smooth-muscle cells of the pulmonary artery in patients with pulmonary arterial hypertension are shown. These pathways correspond to important therapeutic targets in this condition and play a role in determining which of four classes of drugs—endothelin-receptor antagonists, nitric oxide, phosphodiesterase type 5 inhibitors, and prostacyclin derivatives—will be used. At the top of the figure, a transverse section of a small pulmonary artery (<500 μm in diameter) from a patient with severe pulmonary arterial hypertension shows intimal proliferation and marked medial hypertrophy. Dysfunctional pulmonary-artery endothelial cells (blue) have decreased production of prostacyclin and endogenous nitric oxide, with an increased production of endothelin-1—a condition promoting vasoconstriction and proliferation of smooth-muscle cells in the pulmonary arteries (red). Current or emerging therapies interfere with specific targets in smooth-muscle cells in the pulmonary arteries. In addition to their actions on smooth-muscle cells, prostacyclin derivatives and nitric oxide have several other properties, including antiplatelet effects. Plus signs denote an increase in intracellular concentration; minus signs blockage of a receptor, inhibition of an enzyme, or a decrease in the intracellular concentration; and cGMP cyclic guanosine monophophosphate.

contributing to structural remodeling of the blood vessel itself. In situ pulmonary artery thrombosis is present in a significant number of patients.

DIAGNOSIS: ESSENTIAL TESTS

A general algorithm for the assessment of patients with PH is shown in Figure 4.

Exertional dyspnea is present in 60% of patients at the time of initial diagnosis and ultimately develops in all patients as the disease progresses. Angina or syncope are each reported by approximately 40% of patients during the course of the disease. Elevated right ventricular pressure overload leads to right ventricular failure and tricuspid regurgitation in later stages of PAH. The symptomatic manifestations are leg edema, abdominal bloating and distension due to ascites, anorexia, plethora, and more profound fatigue. Additional signs are outlined in Tables 6, 7, 8, and 9.

Electrocardiography

Electrocardiography characteristically shows evidence of right ventricular hypertrophy and right atrial enlargement. Up to 13% of patients with severe PAH have an unremarkable ECG. P-wave amplitude in lead II of ≥0.25 mV is associated with a greater risk of death (Fig. 5).

- In patients with a suspicion of PAH, ECG should be performed to screen for a spectrum of cardiac anatomic and arrhythmic abnormalities.
- ECG lacks sufficient sensitivity to serve as an effective screening tool for PAH, but contributes prognostic information in patients with known PAH.

Chest X-Ray

The chest x-ray in PAH reflects central pulmonary artery and right ventricular enlargement. Findings specific to advanced PAH include a prominent pulmonary trunk and hilar pulmonary arteries with "pruning" of the peripheral pulmonary arteries, and obliteration of the retrosternal clear space by the enlarged, anteriorly situated right ventricle (Fig. 6).

- In patients with a suspicion of PAH, a chest x-ray should be obtained to reveal features supportive of a

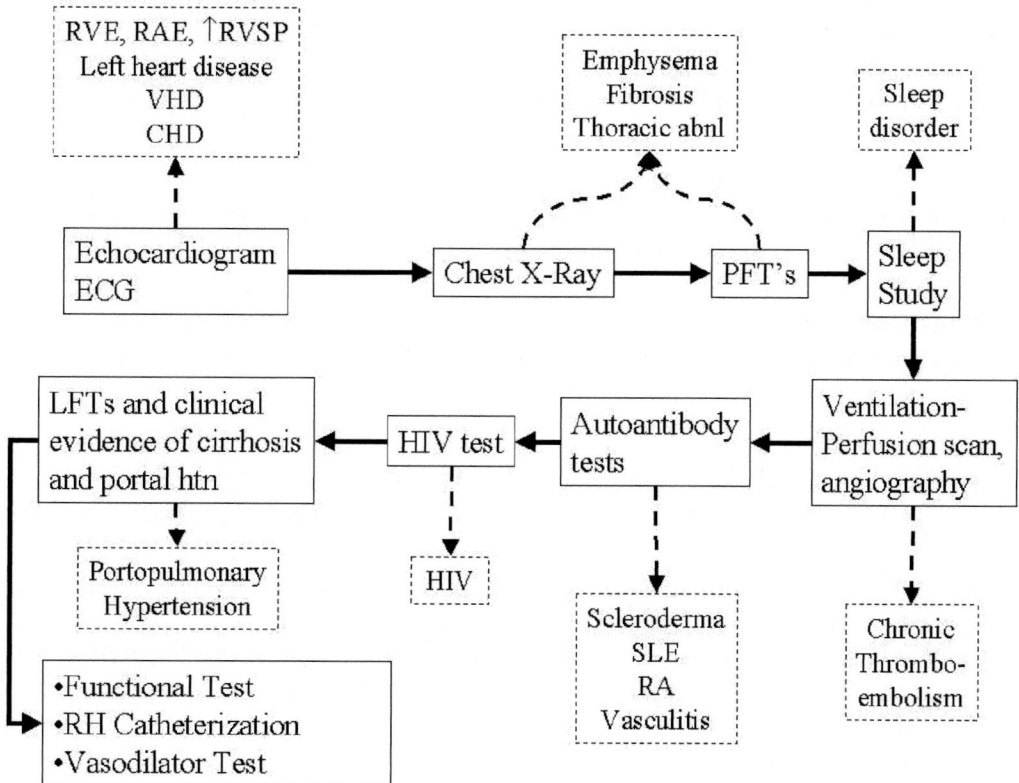

Fig. 4. Algorithm for the assessment of patients with pulmonary hypertension.

Table 6.   Physical Signs That Indicate Significant Pulmonary Hypertension

Sign	Implication
Accentuated pulmonary component of S2 (audible at apex in over 90%)	High pulmonary pressure increases force of pulmonary valve closure
Early systolic click	Sudden interruption of opening of pulmonary valve into high-pressure artery
Midsystolic ejection murmur	Turbulent transvalvular pulmonary outflow
Left parasternal lift	High right ventricular pressure and hypertrophy present
Right ventricular S4 (in 38%)	
Increased jugular "a" wave	High right ventricular filling pressure

Table 7.   Physical Signs That Indicate Severity of Pulmonary Hypertension

Sign	Implication
Moderate to severe pulmonary hypertension	
Holosystolic murmur that increases with inspiration	Tricuspid regurgitation
Increased jugular v waves	
Pulsatile liver	
Diastolic murmur	Pulmonary regurgitation
Hepatojugular reflux	High central venous pressure
Advanced pulmonary hypertension with right ventricular failure	
Right ventricular S3 (in 23%)	Right ventricular dysfunction
Marked distention of jugular veins	
Hepatomegaly	Right ventricular dysfunction or tricuspid regurgitation or both
Peripheral edema (in 32%)	
Ascites	
Low blood pressure, diminished pulse pressure, cool extremities	Reduced cardiac output, peripheral vasoconstriction

Table 8.   Physical Signs That Detect Possible Underlying Cause or Associations of Pulmonary Hypertension

Sign	Implication
Central cyanosis	Hypoxemia, right-to-left shunt
Clubbing	Congenital heart disease, pulmonary venopathy
Cardiac auscultatory findings, including systolic murmurs, diastolic murmurs, opening snap, and gallop	Congenital or acquired heart or valvular disease
Rales, dullness, or decreased breath sounds	Pulmonary congestion or effusion or both
Fine rales, accessory muscle use, wheezing, protracted expiration, productive cough	Pulmonary parenchymal disease
Obesity, kyphoscoliosis, enlarged tonsils	Substrate for disordered ventilation
Sclerodactyly, arthritis, rash	Connective tissue disorder
Peripheral venous insufficiency or obstruction	Possible venous thrombosis

Table 9. Parameters of Severity With Prognostic Significance

Category	Observation
Pulmonary vascular resistance and mean pulmonary arterial pressure (mPAP)	mPAP <55 mm Hg: median survival, 48 mo mPAP ≥85 mm Hg: median survival, 12 mo
Response to vasodilator therapy	Patients in whom pulmonary arteriolar resistance decreases with test administration of pulmonary vasodilators NO or epoprostenol tend to survive longer, and this benefit may be independent of subsequent treatment status Treatment with vasodilators may also enhance survival
New York Heart Association (NYHA) functional classification	NYHA I-II: median survival, 58.6 mo NYHA III: median survival, 31.5 mo NYHA IV: median survival, 6 mo
6-Minute walk distance (6MWD)	6MWD <332 m: 4-year survival <20% 6MWD >332 m: 4-year survival ~90%
Right atrial pressure (RAP)	RAP <10 mm Hg: median survival, 46 mo RAP >20 mm Hg: median survival, 1 mo
Cardiac index (CI)	CI ≥4.0 L · m2/min: median survival, 43 mo CI <2.0 L · m2/min: median survival, 17 mo
Pulmonary arterial (mixed venous) oxygen saturation (SvO2)	SvO2 ≥63%: mean 3-year survival, 55% SvO2 <63%: mean 3-year survivval, 17%
Pulmonary stroke volume/pulmonary pressue (capacitance)	Inversely related to mortality over 4 years
Brain natriuretic peptide (BNP)	>180 pg/mL after 3 months of treatment with epoprostenol: mean 3-year survival, ~20% <180 pg/mL after 3 months of treatment with epoprostenol: mean 3-year survival, ~90%

diagnosis of PAH and to screen for other cardiopulmonary diseases.

Transthoracic Doppler Echocardiography (TTE)
Doppler echocardiographic criteria can estimate pulmonary arterial systolic, diastolic, and mean pressures. Systolic pressure can be extrapolated from right ventricular pressure in the absence of pulmonary stenosis. Right ventricular pressure is determined with continuous-wave Doppler echocardiography to measure the retrograde velocity across the tricuspid valve (Fig. 7). Careful Doppler examination by experienced sonographers yields quantifiable tricuspid regurgitant signals in 74% of patients. The tricuspid pressure gradient is derived from the modified Bernoulli equation: $\Delta P_{TV} = 4V^2_{TR}$, in which ΔP_{TV} = maximal systolic pressure gradient across the tricuspid valve and V_{TR} = peak Doppler signal velocity across the tricuspid valve. The

addition of estimated right atrial pressure (RAP) yields right ventricular systolic pressure (RVSP): ΔP_{TV} + RAP = RVSP. The RAP can either be a standardized value or an estimated value from characteristics of the inferior vena cava ultrasound or from degree of jugular venous distension.

End-diastolic pulmonary regurgitant velocity can be measured with continuous-wave Doppler echocardiography (Fig. 8). Pulmonary artery diastolic pressure (PADP) corresponds to the regurgitant pressure gradient plus the right atrial (that is, right ventricular end-diastolic) pressure (RAP): $\Delta P_{PV} = 4V^2_{PR}$ and ΔP_{PV} + RAP = PADP, in which ΔP_{PV} = end-diastolic pressure gradient across the pulmonary valve and V_{PR} = regurgitant Doppler signal velocity across the pulmonary valve.

Echocardiographic imaging also can provide information about right ventricular size and function, right atrial size, pericardial effusion and disclose underlying

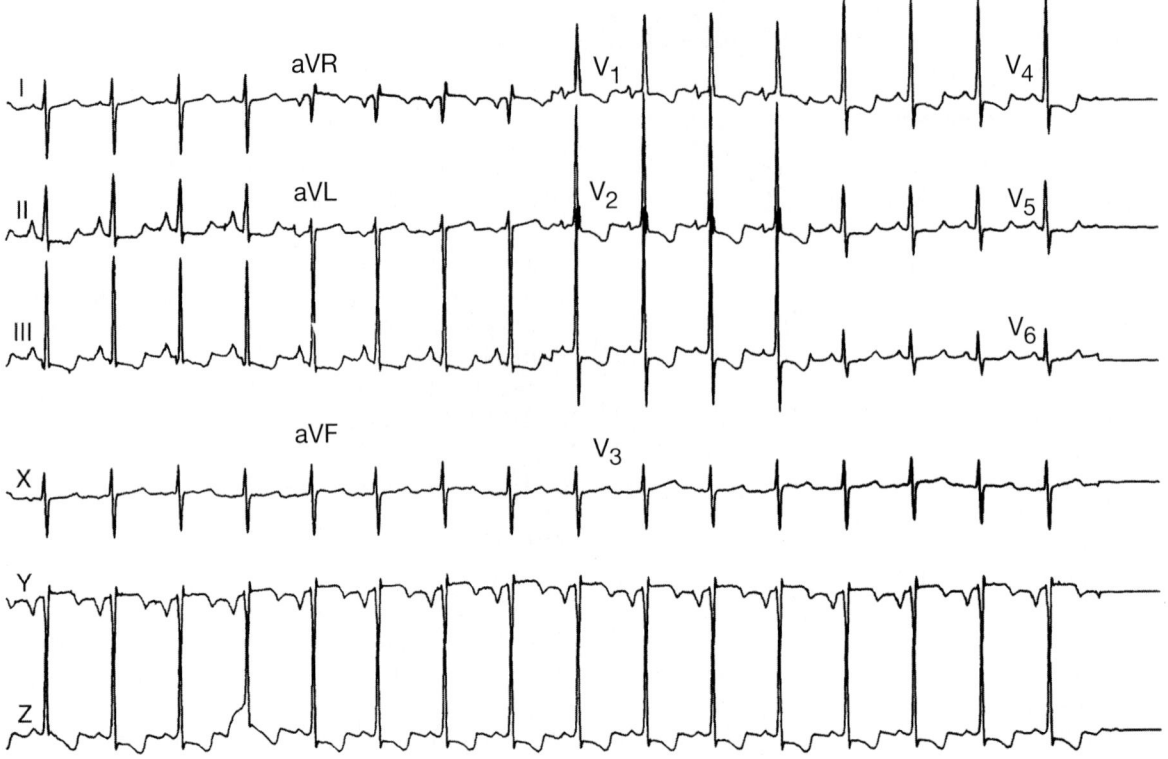

Fig. 5. Electrocardiogram from 28-year-old woman with primary pulmonary hypertension, showing right atrial enlargement, right ventricular hypertrophy, and right ventricular strain pattern.

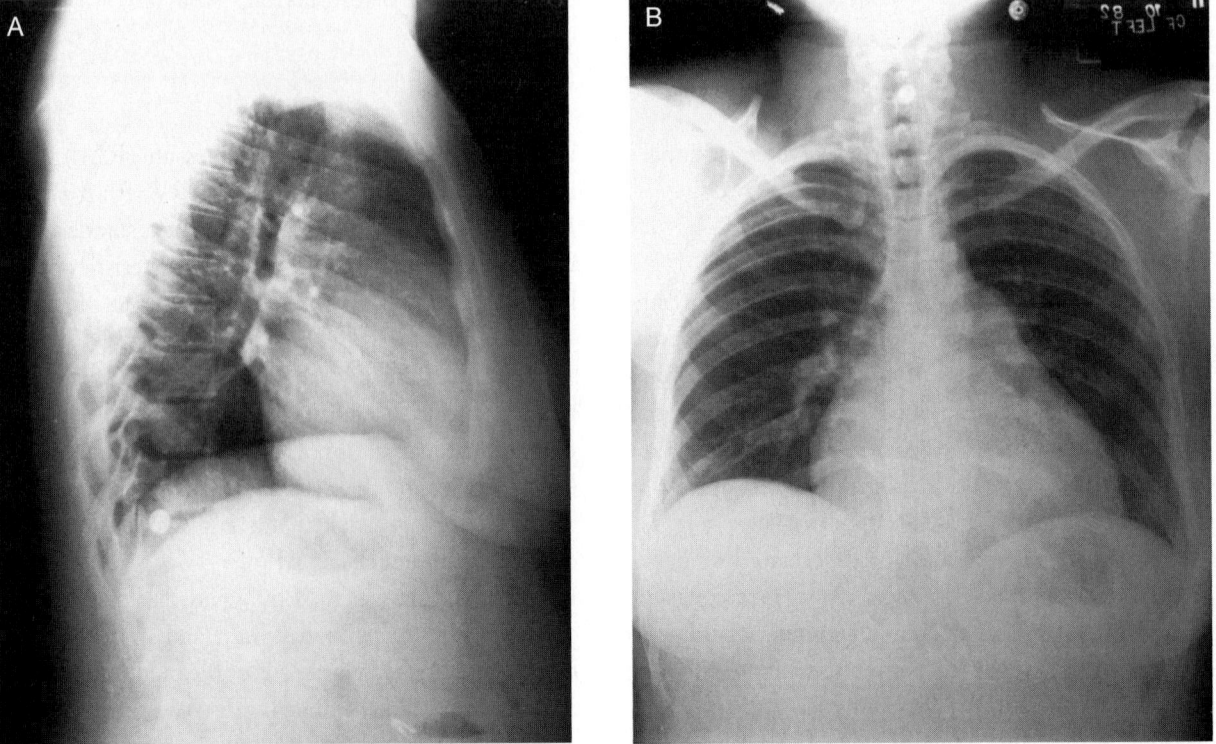

Fig. 6. Chest radiographs from patient with primary pulmonary hypertension. *A*, Lateral view. *B*, Posteroanterior view.

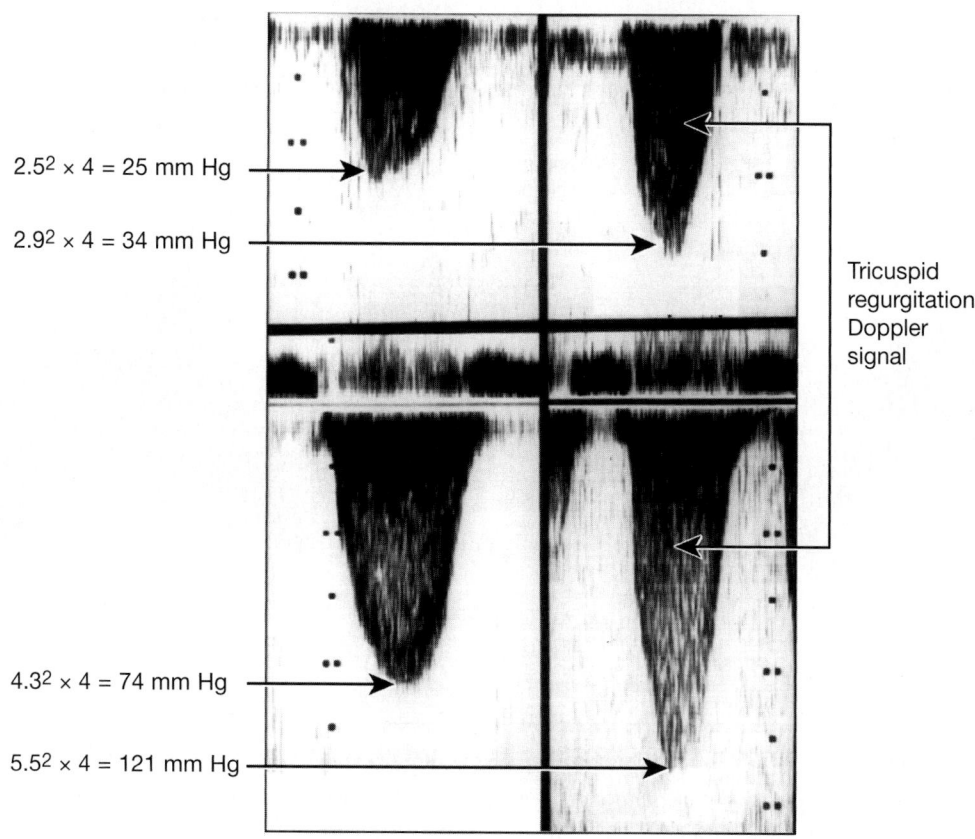

$2.5^2 \times 4 = 25$ mm Hg

$2.9^2 \times 4 = 34$ mm Hg

Tricuspid
regurgitation
Doppler
signal

$4.3^2 \times 4 = 74$ mm Hg

$5.5^2 \times 4 = 121$ mm Hg

Fig. 7. Continuous-wave Doppler echocardiography signals of varying degrees of tricuspid regurgitant velocity which are used to estimate right ventricular systolic pressure.

causes of PH such as left-sided valvular lesions, ventricular dysfunction or intracardiac shunt. A D-shaped septum with normally contractile left ventricle on two-dimensional echocardiography supports the diagnosis of a pressure overloaded an enlarged right ventricle (Fig. 9).

Left atrial enlargement in the absence of mitral valve disease suggests that an elevated left-sided filling pressure that may be contributing to pulmonary pressure elevation even if left ventricular systolic function is normal.

Echocardiography provides one of the best evaluations of congenital heart disease. Although the diagnosis of congenital heart disease often precedes the discovery of PH, if PH is discovered in a patient without a specific causal diagnosis, an echocardiographic contrast ("bubble") study using agitated saline solution is warranted to detect evidence of intracardiac shunting. This procedure is best suited for detecting right-to-left shunting (i.e., shunt reversal). Anomalous pulmonary venous return or pure left-to-right shunts may be missed by transthoracic echocardiogram and transesophageal echocardiography may be warranted for best anatomic definition.

- In patients with a clinical suspicion of PAH, Doppler echocardiography should be performed as a noninvasive screening test to detect PH.
- Doppler echocardiography should be performed to evaluate both the level of RVSP, and to assess the presence of associated anatomic abnormalities such as right atrial enlargement, right ventricular enlargement, and pericardial effusion.
- In asymptomatic patients at high risk of PAH, Doppler echocardiography should be performed to detect elevated pulmonary arterial pressure.
- Doppler echocardiography is less accurate in

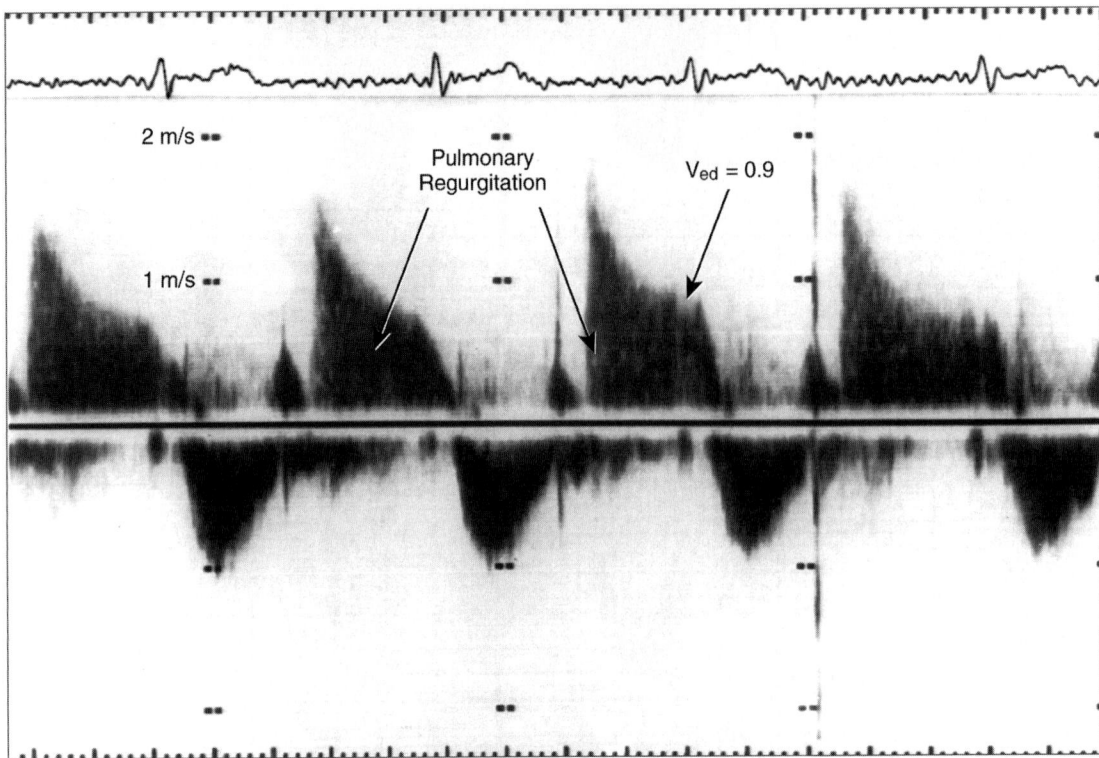

Fig. 8. Continuous-wave Doppler signal of pulmonary regurgitation. The regurgitant velocity at end-diastole (V_{ed}) is used to estimate pulmonary artery diastolic pressure. An end-diastolic velocity of 0.9 m/s corresponds to an estimated pressure gradient of 4 (.9²) = 3.24. If the right atrial pressure is 14 mm Hg, then the pulmonary artery diastolic pressure is 3 + 14 = 17 mm Hg.

determining actual pulmonary artery pressure than invasive pressure measurement in many patients.

- In patients with suspected or documented PH, Doppler echocardiography should be obtained to look for left ventricular systolic and diastolic dysfunction, left-sided chamber enlargement, or valvular heart disease.

- Doppler echocardiography with contrast should be obtained to look for evidence of intracardiac shunting in patients with suspected or documented PH.

Radionuclide Studies

Ventilation-perfusion lung scanning is recommended for screening for CTEPH. The high sensitivity of the test (90-100%) in this setting means that while a negative or very low probability result essentially rules out CTEPH. Segmental perfusion defect visualized on V/Q scanning should be pursued for definitive assessment using pulmonary angiography. The V/Q scan correlates poorly with severity of obstruction. False-positive scans may occur with pulmonary artery sarcoma, large-vessel pulmonary vasculitis, extrinsic vascular compression, pulmonary venopathy or pulmonary microvasculopathy (Fig. 10).

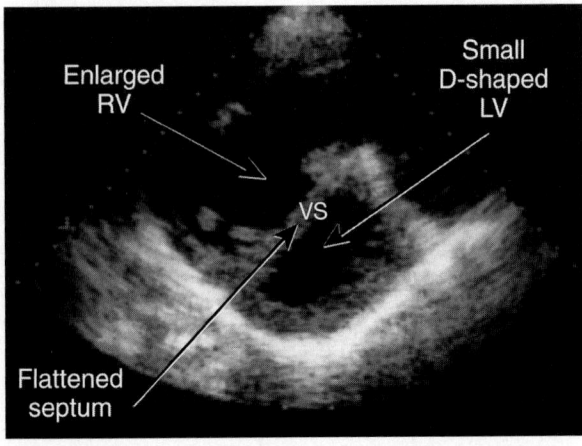

Fig. 9. Still frame of two-dimensional echocardiogram of a patient with severe primary pulmonary hypertension. LV, left ventricle; RV, right ventricle; VS, ventricular septum.

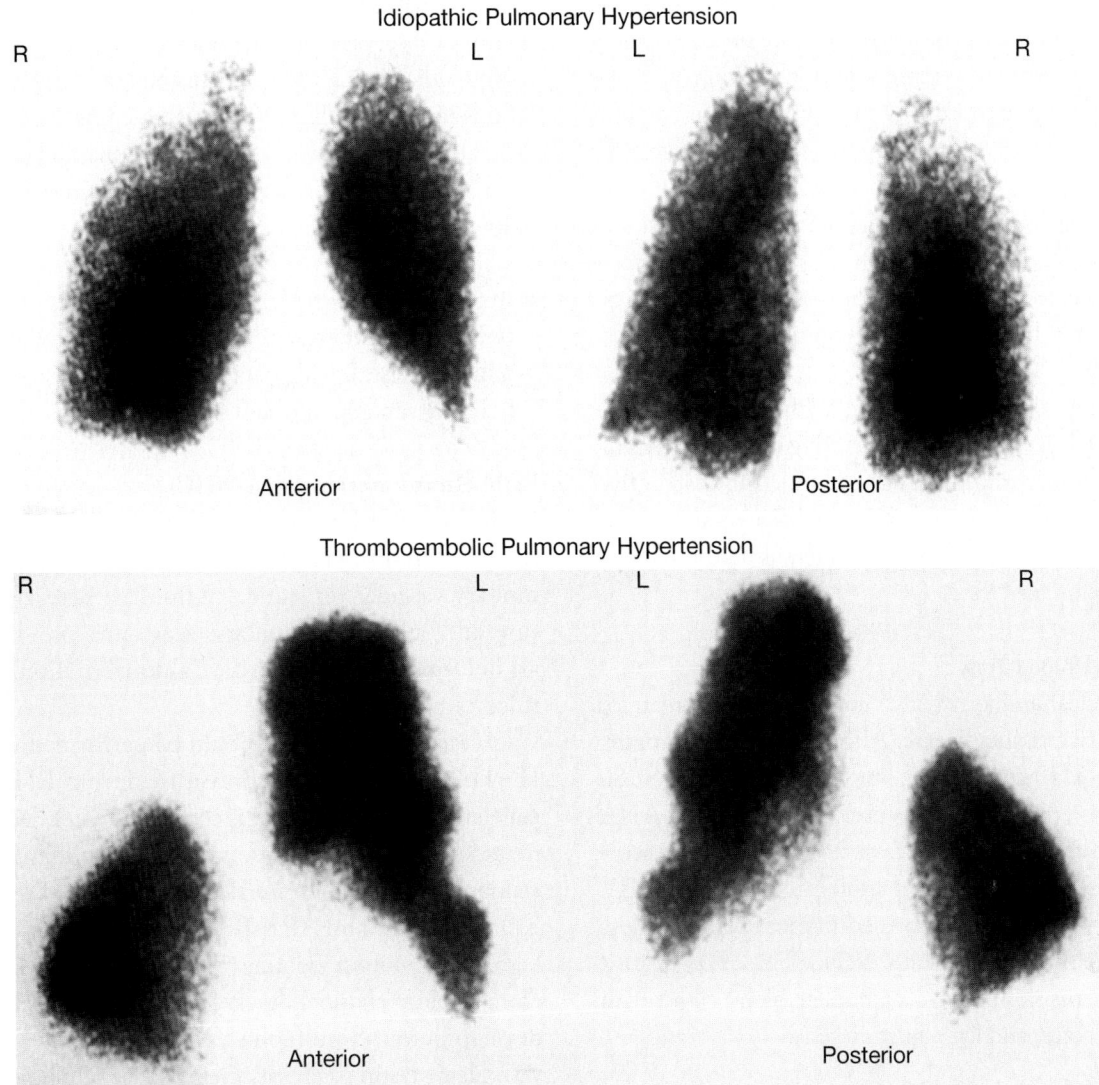

Fig. 10. Perfusion lung scans, showing diffuse inhomogeneity of perfusion, especially apically, suggestive of idiopathic pulmonary hypertension (*Top*) and segmental and subsegmental defects consistent with chronic major vessel thromboembolic pulmonary hypertension (*Bottom*). Ant, anterior; L, left; Post, posterior; R, right.

Pulmonary Function Testing (PFT)

Pulmonary function testing is used to diagnose underlying airway or parenchymal lung disease. Obstructive pulmonary disease with hypoxemia may be confirmed by PFT testing. Abnormalities also are present in other types of PH. About 20% of patients with CTEPH have restrictive lung parameters (i.e., lung volumes <80% predicted) yet may have near normal DLCO. A DLCO of <55% of predicted in patients with systemic sclerosis in the presence of normal rest pulmonary artery pressures may be predictive for an increased risk for the future development of PAH.

The DLCO is mildly reduced, to approximately 60 to 80% of predicted, in both IPAH.

In all forms of PAH, desaturation during exercise is primarily related to the inability of the right ventricle to augment cardiac output, resulting in further depression of mixed venous oxygen saturation.

Screening Overnight Oximetry

Overnight oximetry can screen for significant obstructive sleep apnea or hypopnea during sleep.

■ In patients with PAH, pulmonary function testing and

arterial blood oxygenation determination should be performed to evaluate for the presence of lung disease.

- In patients with systemic sclerosis, pulmonary function testing with DLCO should be performed periodically (every 6 to 12 months) to improve detection of pulmonary vascular or interstitial disease.
- In patients with PAH, lung biopsy is not routinely recommended because of the risks, except under circumstances in which a specific question can only be answered by pulmonary tissue histologic examination.
- In the evaluation of patients with PAH, an assessment of sleep disordered breathing is recommended.
- Polysomnography is recommended if obstructive sleep apnea is suspected on the basis of a positive-screening test for OSA or if there is a high clinical suspicion for OSA.

Essential Blood Tests

Antinuclear antibody (ANA) titer is used to screen for connective tissue disease. Although 40% of patients with IPAH have positive but low ANA titers (≥1:80 dilutions), patients with a substantially elevated ANA and/or suspicious clinical features require further serologic assessment and rheumatology consultation. HIV serology should be performed in most people unless exposure can be confidently excluded based on history. All patients should have a complete blood count with platelet count and liver function tests.

Assessment of Exercise Capacity

An objective assessment of exercise capacity is important for several reasons:

1) eliminate alternative reasons for dyspnea;
2) determine maximal exercise tolerance;
3) characterize a patient's comfortable activity level;
4) provide prognostic information;
5) establish exercise capacity at baseline and during therapy;
6) in some cases, to assess the hemodynamic response to exercise as a possible cause of symptoms in patients with unremarkable resting hemodynamics.

The 6-minute walk test (6MWT) distance is predictive of survival in PH and also correlates inversely with WHO functional status severity. Arterial oxygen desaturation >10% during the 6MWT increases

mortality risk 2.9 times over a median follow-up of 26 months. Observations from cardiopulmonary exercise testing indicate that the mechanism(s) of exercise limitations in PAH include V/Q mismatching, lactic acidosis at a low work rate, arterial hypoxemia, and inability to adequately increase stroke volume and cardiac output.

- In patients with PAH, serial determinations of functional class and exercise capacity assessed by the 6-min walk test provide benchmarks for disease severity, response to therapy, and progression.

Right Heart Catheterization (RHC)

Right heart catheterization is mandatory to confirm the diagnosis of PH. Cardiac output, pulmonary vascular resistance, pulmonary artery pressure, and pulmonary capillary wedge pressure should all be obtained. Intracardiac shunting should be ruled out.

A vasodilator study should be performed when IPAH is discovered or confirmed during RHC in patients in whom treatment is contemplated. A decrease in response to short acting vasodilators (typically intravenous epoprostenol or inhaled nitric oxide) of mPAP ≥10 mm Hg to a mPAP ≤40 mm Hg with a normal or high cardiac output identifies patients who may benefit from calcium channel blocker treatment. The abrupt development of pulmonary edema during acute vasodilator testing suggests the presence of pulmonary venopathy or pulmonary microvasculopathy and is a contraindication to chronic vasodilator treatment.

- In patients with suspected PH, right-heart catheterization is required to confirm the presence of PH, establish the specific diagnosis, and determine the severity of PH.
- In patients with suspected PH, right-heart catheterization is required to guide therapy.
- Patients with IPAH should undergo acute vasoreactivity testing using a short-acting agent such as IV epoprostenol or adenosine, or inhaled NO.
- Patients with PAH associated with underlying processes, such as scleroderma or congenital heart disease, should undergo acute vasoreactivity testing.
- Patients with PAH should undergo vasoreactivity testing by a physician experienced in the management of pulmonary vascular disease.

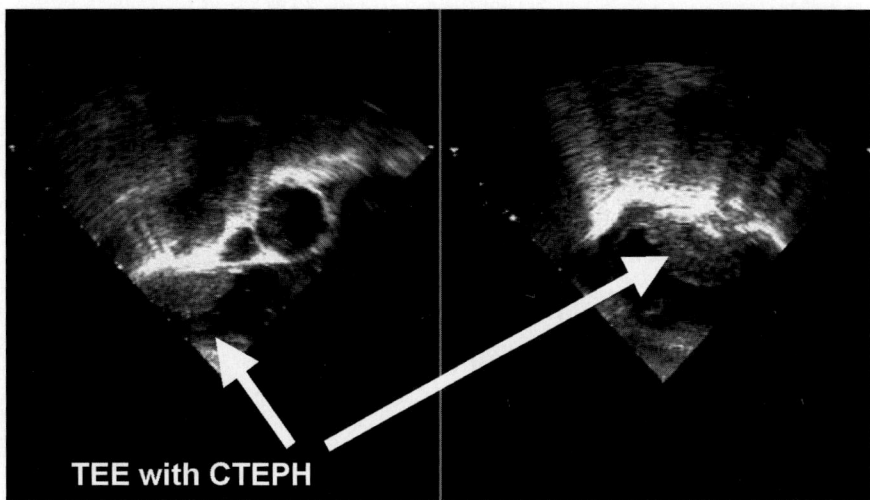

Fig. 11. TEE showing chronic thrombus in main pulmonary artery.

DIAGNOSIS: CONTINGENT TESTS

Presymptomatic Screening

Screening for PH using Doppler echocardiography is warranted when risk of PH is sufficiently high: 1) a patient with a known genetic mutation associated with PAH or a first-degree relative in a family with FPAH; 2) a patient with scleroderma spectrum of disease; 3) patients with congenital heart disease and systemic-to-pulmonary shunts; or 4) patients with portal hypertension undergoing evaluation for orthotopic liver transplantation. Patients with other potential PAH risk factors do not warrant routine screening in the absence of symptoms because of the infrequency of diagnosis and/or low likelihood of instituting treatment at a presymptomatic stage.

Transesophageal Echocardiography (TEE)

TEE provides important data that may alter treatment in up to 25% of patients. It is valuable in the detection of intracardiac shunts, especially atrial septal defects. TEE can also detect chronic central pulmonary emboli (Fig. 11) with a reported sensitivity of 80% to 96%, and a specificity of 88%.

TEE may be required to visualize anomalous pulmonary venous connections.

Chest Computed Tomography (CT)

CT may provide further supportive evidence of CTEPH if the screening ventilation/perfusion scan is suggestive. However, a negative CT scan in the setting of high suspicion of PH should not defer pulmonary angiography. A mosaic pattern of lung attenuation in a noncontrast CT scan raises the possibility of chronic thromboembolism.

Contrast-enhanced *spiral (or helical) CT* or *electron-beam CT* (EBCT) can visualize central chronic pulmonary thromboemboli (Fig. 12). The CT features of chronic thromboembolic disease are complete occlusion of pulmonary arteries, eccentric filling defects consistent with thrombi, recanalization, and stenoses or webs. Sensitivity of spiral CT for detecting central pulmonary embolism is >85% to 90%. Diagnostic accuracy for both proximal and distal pulmonary emboli will likely improve markedly with new generation scanners.

Signs of pulmonary venopathy on EBCT or high resolution CT are smooth thickening of interlobular septa, peribronchovascular cuffing, and alveolar ground-glass opacification. In addition, high resolution CT assists in the diagnosis of pulmonary fibrosis.

A ground-glass, mosaic attenuation pattern in the lower lobes on CT scan is suggestive of pulmonary venopathy.

Pulmonary Angiography

A pulmonary angiogram is required to confirm CTEPH and assess candidacy for surgical pulmonary thrombectomy in patients with a positive ventilation-perfusion scan or images suggestive by contrast-enhanced CT scan. Chronic thrombi appear different

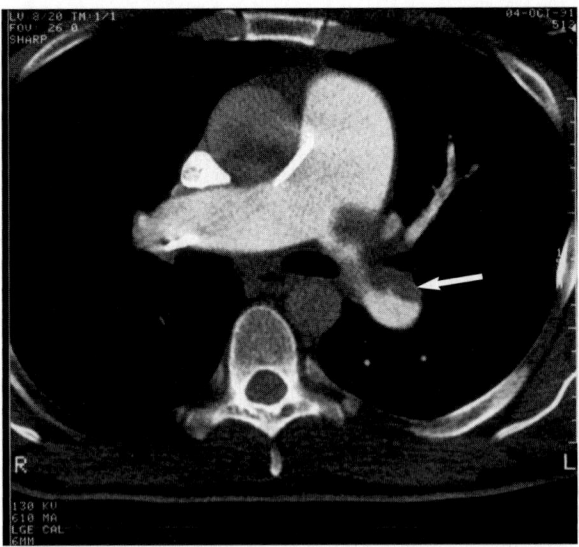

Fig. 12. Cardiac computed tomography scan, showing thrombus in the left main pulmonary artery (*arrow*).

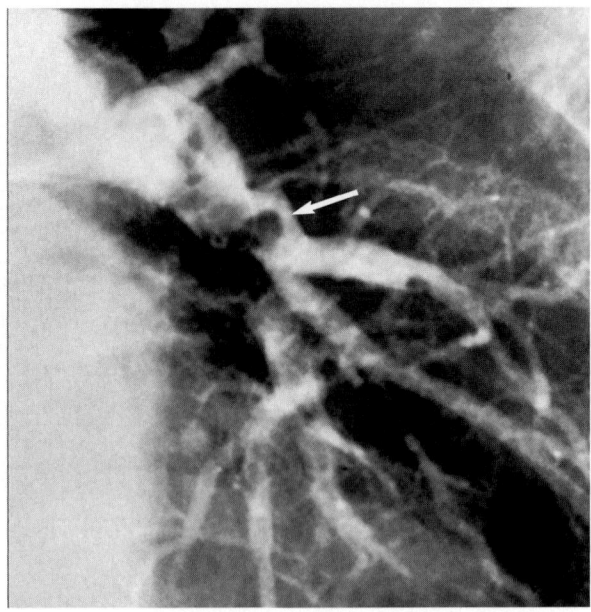

Fig. 13. Pulmonary angiogram showing features of chronic pulmonary embolism. *Arrow* shows thrombus.

from acute thrombi on the angiogram and occur in highly variable locations, often incorporated into and retracting the vessel wall. Obstructions can take the form of bands or webs, sometimes with post-stenotic dilation. Irregular intimal surface, rounded or pouch-like termination of segmental branches, luminal narrowing of the central vessel, and odd-shaped pulmonary arteries all may indicate the presence of chronic pulmonary embolism (Fig. 13).

Contingent Blood Tests

For patients with known or suspected CTEPH, further evaluation of a potential *clotting diathesis* is warranted (bleeding time; coagulation Factors VIII, VII, II, and V; von Willebrand factors; Protein C and S; lupus anticoagulant and anticardiolipin antibodies). Factor V Leiden mutation (the most common cause of activated protein C resistance) has been implicated as a risk for idiopathic venous thromboembolism, though not specifically in pulmonary embolism or CTEPH. Serum viscosity, serum protein electrophoresis, and Hgb electrophoresis may be helpful under certain circumstances.

Arterial blood gas or *oximetry* measurements showing desaturation may suggest abnormal gas exchange, right-to-left shunting, ventilation/perfusion mismatching, interstitial fibrosis, other parenchymal lung disease, or hypoventilation. The degree of rest arterial hypoxemia in IPAH is usually mild to moderate; when

hypoxemia is severe, it should suggest another contributing problem. Failure of blood gases to normalize with high inhaled FiO_2 oxygen suggests a component of direct pulmonary-to-systemic circulation, either due to intra- or extracardiac shunts or intrapulmonary shunting.

Exercise desaturation suggests that supplemental oxygen may be useful to improve exercise capacity. Right-to-left shunting through a patent foramen ovale during exercise may contribute to desaturation in PAH.

Overnight oximetry may disclose nocturnal desaturation associated with sleep apnea. Nocturnal hypoxemia occurs in >75% of IPAH patients.

Hyperuricemia occurs with high frequency in patients with PH and correlates with hemodynamic abnormalities (e.g., right atrial pressure) and mortality in IPAH.

Brain natriuretic peptide (BNP) is elevated in right ventricular pressure overload and correlates with severity of right ventricular dysfunction and mortality in PAH.

Polysomnography

If the history and/or screening overnight oximetry is suggestive, a sleep study should be considered to assess a possible contributory role for OSA in PH. Up to 27%

of patients with sleep apnea syndromes have a degree of PH which is usually mild and correctable by treatment with continuous positive airway pressure.

Lung Biopsy

Lung biopsy is risky in patients with PH, and should be limited to circumstances in which histopathologic findings are required to direct treatment, such as excluding or establishing a diagnosis of active vasculitis, granulomatous pulmonary disease, pulmonary venopathy, pulmonary microvasculopathy, interstitial lung disease, or bronchiolitis. In general, routine performance of a lung biopsy to establish a diagnosis of PAH or to determine its cause is discouraged.

TREATMENT

Calcium-Channel Blockers (CCBs)

Patients who demonstrate a significant response to the acute administration of a short-acting vasodilator may be treated cautiously with oral CCBs and monitored closely to determine both the efficacy and safety of such therapy. CCBs with a significant negative inotropic effect, such as verapamil, should be avoided; nifedipine, diltiazem, or amlodipine are used most frequently and are titrated to the highest tolerated dose. Clinical improvement with CCBs is rarely marked and replacement or combination with additional medications should be considered in symptomatic patients.

Prostanoids

Three prostacyclin analogs have been FDA approved for use in symptomatic patients with PAH.

Epoprostenol Sodium

Epoprostenol is a synthetic prostacyclin. Its use is intended to replace the deficiency of prostacyclin in patients with PH in order to provide vasodilation, platelet inhibition and antiproliferative effects. The mechanism is via the cyclic AMP pathway. Treatment with epoprostenol is complex since it must be administered by continuous IV infusion through a portable pump and indwelling central venous catheter due to its half-life of several minutes. The short half-life also accounts for its most feared adverse effect: the risk of rebound exacerbation of PH with interruption of the

infusion. The dose must be carefully titrated and adjusted.

Epoprostenol treatment produces improved exercise capacity, reduces symptoms of dyspnea, enhances survival (Fig. 14) and improves pulmonary hemodynamics. The hemodynamic improvement is relatively modest, but may become more notable with increasing duration of treatment. Early effects are likely due to vasodilation, whereas later benefits may result from reversal of vascular remodeling due to antiproliferative mechanisms.

Common side effects of epoprostenol therapy include headache, flushing, jaw pain with initial mastication, diarrhea, nausea, a blotchy erythematous rash, and musculoskeletal aches and pain (predominantly involving the legs and feet). Long-term high dosage can lead to the development of a hyperdynamic state. Other complications of long-term IV therapy with epoprostenol include infusion catheter line-related infections, catheter-associated venous thrombosis, thrombocytopenia, and ascites.

Treprostinil

Treprostinil is a prostacyclin analog with a serum half-life of 4 1/2 hours and, unlike epoprostenol, is stable at room temperature. It can be administered either by

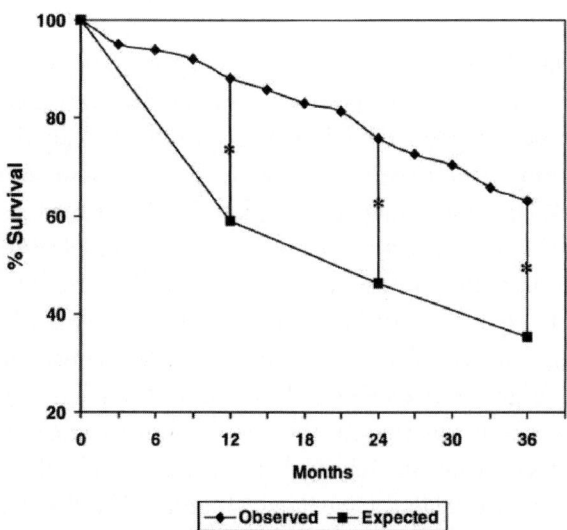

Fig. 14. Probability of survival of patients treated with epoprostenol versus expected survival based on prediction by baseline hemodynamic parameters.

continuous subcutaneous or intravenous infusion. Like epoprostenol, it improves symptoms and modestly improves hemodynamics, but a definite survival benefit has not been convincingly demonstrated. In addition, adverse events including headache, diarrhea, flushing, jaw pain, and foot pain are common, as they are with epoprostenol. An additional side effect of frequent pain and erythema at the infusion site occurs with subcutaneous infusion. Because of the longer half-life of treprostinil, interruptions of the drug due to dislodgment of the catheter or pump malfunction tend to be less serious.

Inhaled Iloprost

Iloprost is a prostacyclin analog with a serum half-life of 20 to 25 minutes. It is approved in the U.S. for administration as an aerosolized inhalant. An advantage of an inhaled agent is that it is selectively distributed to ventilated areas of the lungs, so that its local vasodilatory effect results in optimal ventilation-perfusion matching. The clinical benefits and adverse effects are similar to those of the other prostanoids. A unique disadvantage, however, is that because of the relatively short duration of action it must be inhaled six to nine times a day for about 8-10 minutes at a time. The hemodynamic effects disappear within 30 to 90 min after inhalation, but may be extended by coadministration of other medications, such as sildenafil.

Endothelin Receptor Antagonists (ETRAs)

Endothelin antagonists address the excess effect of endothelin that has been observed in patients with PH.

Bosentan: Bosentan is an orally administered nonselective endothelin receptor antagonist, blocking the action of endothelin-1, a potent vasoconstrictor and smooth muscle mitogen, at endothelin A and B receptors. Its therapeutic effect is due to reduction of vasoconstriction and pulmonary vascular hypertrophy caused by increased plasma levels of endothelin-1 in patients with PAH, and mediated predominantly via endothelin A receptors. The demonstrable clinical vasodilatory effect of the drug is quite modest in patients with established PAH, but clinical studies have demonstrated an augmented 6 minute walk distance compared to placebo and improved functional classification over 16 weeks. Some of its benefit may be related to antiproliferative and antifibrotic effects which stabilize the disease process and promote remodeling. The

medication is administered orally in pill form twice daily and liver function tests are monitored monthly.

Adverse effects associated with bosentan include dose-dependent elevation of transaminases reflecting hepatic toxicity. Bosentan is also associated with a reduction of hemoglobin, which seems typically to be mild. Syncope and flushing may occur in some patients. Drug interactions with glyburide cyclosporine, ketoconazole, statins, and coumadin are recognized; bosentan may interfere with the action of hormonal contraceptives. The drug has potential teratogenic effects.

Phosphodiesterase-5 Inhibition

Phosphodiesterases are enzymes that hydrolyze the cyclic nucleotides, including cGMP, to inactive monophosphates (5′-guanosine monophosphate). Drugs that inhibit cGMP-specific phosphodiesterases increase the pulmonary vascular effect of the NO pathway.

Sildenafil

Sildenafil is a potent and specific orally administered phosphodiesterase type-5 inhibitor, which is a safe and effective for treatment of erectile dysfunction. The drug is approved by the FDA for use in PAH at a dose of 20 mg three times daily. There are relatively few minor side effects, such as headache, nasal congestion, and visual disturbances. Whether other phosphodiesterase type-5 inhibitors have similar beneficial effects has not been determined.

Warfarin, Supplemental Oxygen, Diuretics, Digoxin

In situ microscopic thrombosis has been documented in some patients with IPAH, and numerous prothrombotic abnormalities have been identified. Patients with right ventricular failure and venous stasis are at increased risk for pulmonary thromboembolism. Improved survival has been reported with oral anticoagulation in patients with IPAH. The target international normalized ratio (INR) in patients with IPAH treated with warfarin is approximately 1.5 to 2.5.

Hypoxemia is a potent pulmonary vasoconstrictor, and can contribute to the development and/or progression of PAH. Supplemental oxygen should be used to maintain oxygen saturations >90% if possible at all times, though significant shunting may preclude achieving this goal.

Diuretics are required in patients with right ventricular failure causing peripheral edema and/or ascites. Digitalis is warranted for right ventricular inotropic support and treatment of atrial arrhythmias in patients with refractory right ventricular failure.

- Patients with IPAH, in the absence of right-heart failure, demonstrating a favorable acute response to a vasodilator (defined as a fall in mPAP of at least 10 mm Hg to <40 mm Hg, with an increased or unchanged cardiac output), should be considered candidates for a trial of therapy with an oral calcium-channel antagonist.
- Patients with PAH associated with underlying disease processes such as scleroderma or congenital heart disease, in the absence of right-heart failure, demonstrating a favorable acute response to vasodilator (defined as a fall in mPAP of at least 10 mm Hg to <40 mm Hg, with an increased or unchanged cardiac output), should be considered candidates for a trial of therapy with an oral calcium-channel antagonist.
- In patients with PAH, CCBs should not be used empirically to treat PH in the absence of demonstrated acute vasoreactivity.
- Patients with IPAH should receive anticoagulation with warfarin. In patients with PAH occurring in association with other underlying processes, such as scleroderma or congenital heart disease, anticoagulation should also be considered.
- In patients with PAH, supplemental oxygen should be used as necessary to maintain oxygen saturations >90% at all times.
- Patients with PAH in functional class II who are not candidates for, or who have failed, CCB therapy may benefit from further treatment. However, limited data are available, and no specific drug can be recommended. Enrollment in clinical trials is encouraged.
- Patients with PAH in functional class III who are not candidates for, or who have failed, CCB therapy are candidates for long-term therapy with:
  - Endothelin-receptor antagonists (bosentan).
  - IV epoprostenol.
  - Subcutaneous treprostinil.
  - Inhaled iloprost.
- Patients with PAH in functional class IV who are not candidates for, or who have failed, CCB therapy

are candidates for long-term therapy with IV epoprostenol (treatment of choice).
- Other treatments available for patients with PAH in functional class IV include, in no hierarchical order:
  - Endothelin-receptor antagonists (bosentan).
  - Subcutaneous treprostinil.
  - Inhaled iloprost.
- In patients with PAH who have failed or are not candidates for other available therapy, treatment with sildenafil should be considered.
- In patients with OSA and PAH, treatment of OSA with positive airway pressure therapy should be provided with the expectation that pulmonary pressures will decrease, although they may not normalize, particularly when PAH is more severe.

Procedures and Surgery for Treatment of Pulmonary Arterial Hypertension

Atrial Septostomy
Creation of an interatrial right-to-left shunt by graded balloon pullback techniques (atrial septostomy) appears to decompress the failing right ventricle and increase left ventricular preload.

Pulmonary Endarterectomy
Surgical excision of fibrotic obstructive tissue following failure of pulmonary embolism to resolve medically may yield a cure or marked improvement in PH in patients with central (main, lobar, or segmental) CTEPH. This intervention improves cardiac output, pulmonary arterial pressure, right ventricular function, symptomatic status and survival in appropriately selected patients.

Lung and Heart-Lung Transplantation
Heart-lung, single lung and bilateral lung transplant have been employed in the treatment of patients with PAH, who compose about 24%, 2% and 8% of recipients, respectively. Each approach has advantages and disadvantages. Heart-lung transplant is hampered by a shortage of available organs, though it has advantages of requiring only one airway anastomosis, has a very low rate of vascular complications, and generally yields the best hemodynamic outcomes. Single lung transplantation is easier to perform, requires less operative, ischemic and cardiopulmonary bypass time, but there is

potential for ventilation-perfusion mismatch and reperfusion injury. Bilateral lung transplantation may produce better hemodynamics, less ventilation-perfusion mismatch, fewer early complications, better immediate overall lung function, and possibly improved long-term survival, but the operation is longer and more difficult to perform.

Survival of patients with IPAH following heart-lung transplantation or lung transplant is approximately 70% at 1 year, 40% at 5 years, and 25% at 10 years. Among operative survivors, most patients had an early improvement from a preoperative mPAP of 60 to 70 mm Hg to 20 to 25 mm Hg, and concomitant improvements in cardiac index and pulmonary vascular resistance. Among long-term survivors of lung or heart-lung transplant, over 80% have no limitation in activity at 1 year and 5 years following transplantation, and 40 to 50% work at least part-time.

■ In select patients with PAH unresponsive to medical management, atrial septostomy should be considered.

■ In patients with PAH, atrial septostomy should be performed only at institutions with significant procedural and clinical experience.

■ Patients with suspected CTEPH should be referred to centers experienced in the procedure for consideration of pulmonary endarterectomy.

■ In patients with operable CTEPH, pulmonary endarterectomy is the treatment of choice to improve hemodynamics, functional status, and survival.

■ In patients with CTEPH deemed inoperable or with significant residual postoperative PH, balloon dilation, PAH medical therapy, or lung transplant may be considered.

■ PAH patients with NYHA functional class III and IV symptoms should be referred to a transplant center for evaluation and listing for lung transplant or heart-lung transplant.

■ Listed patients with PAH whose prognosis remains poor despite medical therapy should undergo lung transplant or heart-lung transplant.

■ In patients with PAH who are undergoing transplantation, the procedure of choice is bilateral lung transplant.

■ In children with PAH who are undergoing transplantation, the procedure of choice is bilateral lung transplant.

■ In adult patients with PAH and simple congenital heart lesions, bilateral lung transplant with repair of the cardiac defect is the procedure of choice.

■ In adult patients with PAH and complex congenital heart disease who are undergoing transplantation, heart-lung transplant is the procedure of choice.

RESOURCE

Advances in Pulmonary Hypertension. Available from: http://www.phassociation.org/Medical/Advances_in_PH/.

PREGNANCY AND THE HEART

Heidi M. Connolly, MD

Approximately 2% of pregnancies occur in women with heart disease. Congenital heart disease is the predominant form of heart disease among pregnant women in developed countries, whereas rheumatic heart disease predominates in developing countries. Heart disease does not preclude successful pregnancy but increases the risk to both mother and baby and requires special management.

Knowledge of the normal hemodynamic changes that occur during pregnancy and the resultant effect on common cardiovascular diseases is required for cardiology examinations.

PHYSIOLOGY

Hemodynamic Changes During Normal Pregnancy

Substantial hemodynamic changes occur during normal pregnancy, including a 20% to 30% increase in red blood cell mass and a 30% to 50% increase in plasma volume. As a result, there is an increase in total blood volume, with a relative anemia (Fig. 1). Heart rate increases about 10 beats/min, and there is a reduction in systemic and pulmonary vascular resistance. Blood pressure decreases slightly during pregnancy. These hemodynamic changes result in a steady increase in cardiac output during pregnancy until the 32nd week,

at which time cardiac output plateaus at 30% to 50% above the prepregnancy level (Fig. 2). The pregnant uterus can require up to 18% of cardiac output. Oxygen consumption increases steadily throughout pregnancy and reaches a level of approximately 30% above the prepregnant level by the time of delivery. This increase is due to the metabolic needs of both mother and fetus. During the last half of pregnancy, cardiac output is significantly affected by body position, because the enlarging uterus decreases venous return from the lower extremities. The left lateral position minimizes this reduction in venous return. Normally, the hemodynamic

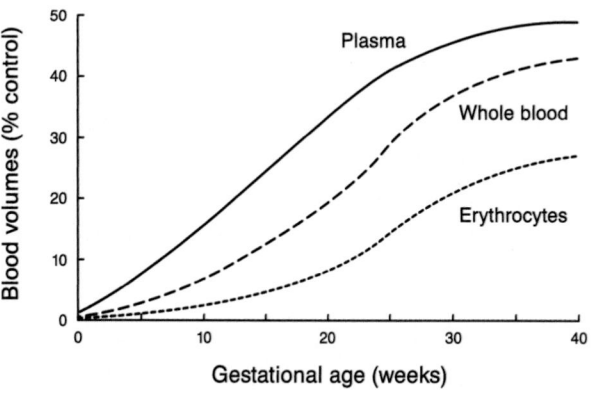

Fig. 1. Hemodynamic changes during normal pregnancy.

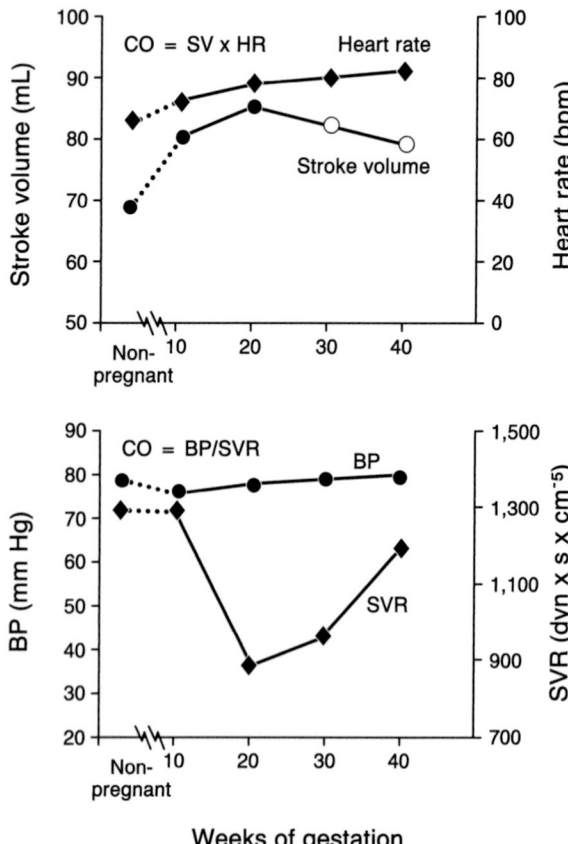

Fig. 2. Cardiac output (CO) can be determined from other variables in at least 3 ways: CO = heart rate (HR) x stroke volume (SV), CO = mean arterial pressure (BP) minus right atrial pressure/systemic vascular resistance (SVR); CO = oxygen (O_2) consumption/arteriovenous (A - V)O_2 difference. The expected values for these variables measured in the supine position during pregnancy are based on information acquired from many studies.

changes that occur during pregnancy are well tolerated by the mother. Heart disease may be manifested initially during pregnancy because of increased cardiac output or because minor preexisting symptoms may be exacerbated.

Cardiac Examination in Normal Pregnancy

During normal pregnancy, there is a brisk and full carotid upstroke, and jugular venous pressure is normal or mildly increased, with prominent "a" and "v" waves. The left ventricular impulse is displaced laterally and is enlarged. The first heart sound is louder than normal.

The pulmonic second sound may be prominent, and there often is persistent splitting of the second heart sound. A third heart sound is audible in more than 80% of normal pregnant women (Fig. 3). An early peaking ejection systolic murmur is audible in more than 90% of normal pregnant women and is caused by a pulmonary outflow murmur. Venous hums and mammary continuous murmurs are common but without significance. Peripheral edema and venous varicosities are common. Abnormal physical findings include a fourth heart sound, a loud (≥3/6) systolic murmur, and a diastolic murmur or fixed splitting of the second heart sound. These do not occur during normal pregnancy in the absence of heart disease.

■ Normal physical findings during pregnancy may be misinterpreted as abnormal.

Cardiac Studies in Pregnancy

On chest radiographs, the cardiac silhouette is enlarged, with increased vascular markings. On echocardiography, there is a small increase in right and left ventricular volumes. The electrocardiogram shows an increase in heart rate, with a leftward shift of the QRS and T-wave axes because of the upward and horizontal displacement of the heart by the pregnant uterus.

Hemodynamic Changes During Labor and Delivery

With uterine contractions, an additional 300 to 500 mL of blood enters the circulation. This increase in blood volume in conjunction with increased blood pressure and heart rate during labor increases cardiac output. At the time of delivery, cardiac output increases as much as 80% above the prepregnancy level (and may be as great as 9 L/min). Administration of epidural anesthesia decreases cardiac output to about 8 L/min, and the use of general anesthesia decreases it further. Approximately 500 mL of blood is lost at the time of vaginal delivery, and approximately 1,000 mL is lost during a normal cesarean delivery.

Hemodynamic Changes Post Partum

After delivery, venous return increases because of relief from fetal compression on the inferior vena cava. Spontaneous diuresis occurs during the first 24 to 48 hours after delivery; however, it takes about 2 to 4

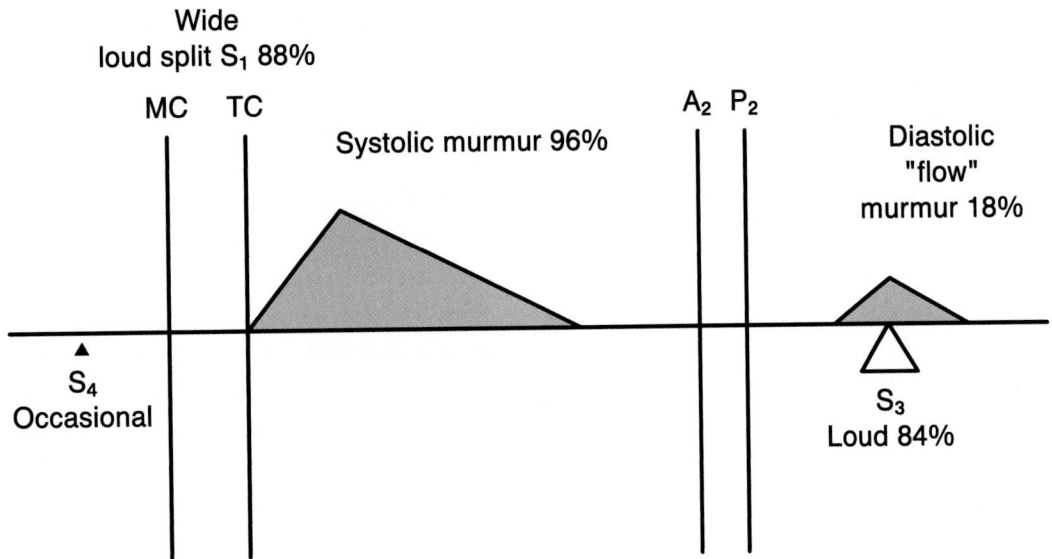

Fig. 3. Normal auscultatory findings during pregnancy. A₂, aortic second sound; MC, mitral valve closure; P₂, pulmonic second sound; TC, tricuspid valve closure.

weeks for hemodynamic values to return to baseline after vaginal delivery and longer after cesarean delivery.

- Cardiac output increases by 30% to 50% during normal pregnancy.
- Cardiac output increases to about 80% above baseline during labor and delivery.
- Hemodynamics return to baseline 2 to 4 weeks after vaginal delivery and may take up to 6 weeks to return to normal after cesarean delivery.

CARDIAC DISEASE IN PREGNANCY

Principles of Management

Antepartum management of women with heart disease should include an anatomical and hemodynamic assessment of any cardiac abnormality to determine the maternal and fetal risks of pregnancy. Doppler echocardiography is ideal for the evaluation of pregnant women with heart disease. When evaluating women with cardiovascular disease, the safety of the mother is always the highest priority. Specific cardiovascular conditions pose an unacceptable risk of death to both mother and baby, and in these situations, pregnancy should be avoided

Fetal growth and development are monitored with ultrasonography. Fetal heart ultrasonography is also recommended in women with congenital heart disease. Special attention to the woman's hemodynamic response to pregnancy is required.

The time and route of delivery should be planned before spontaneous labor to facilitate the delivery and to intervene as appropriate. With few exceptions, vaginal delivery with a facilitated second stage (forceps delivery or vacuum extraction) is preferred for women with heart disease. Cesarean delivery is indicated for obstetrical reasons and when delivery is required in a patient who is fully anticoagulated with warfarin due to the risk of fetal intracranial hemorrhage (Table 1). In addition, cesarean delivery should be considered for patients with fixed cardiac obstructive lesions and pulmonary hypertension. The optimal anesthesia and analgesia as well as administration of prophylactic treatment for endocarditis should be considered before pregnancy. Invasive hemodynamic monitoring is occasionally recommended for severe maternal heart disease. Maternal postpartum care should include early ambulation, attention to neonatal concerns, and consideration of contraception if appropriate.

- Anatomical and hemodynamic assessment of cardiac

Table 1. Indications for Cesarean Section in Women With Cardiovascular Disease

Obstetrical reasons
Anticoagulation with warfarin
Fixed obstructive cardiac lesions
Pulmonary hypertension
Dilated/unstable aorta

status ante partum is imperative to determine the maternal and fetal risk of pregnancy.

■ Vaginal delivery is the preferred mode of delivery in most women with heart disease.

Prognosis of Heart Disease in Pregnancy

Maternal prognosis during pregnancy is strongly related to functional class. Siu and colleagues reported New York Heart Association (NYHA) Functional Class greater than 2 is the strongest predictor of cardiovascular complication during pregnancy. Additional factors which contribute to the risk of cardiovascular complications during pregnancy include a prior history of heart failure, transient ischemic attack, stroke or arrhythmia, the presence of cyanosis, left heart obstruction with either mitral stenosis with a mitral valve area <2 cm^2, or aortic stenosis with a peak left ventricular outflow tract gradient >30 mm Hg and AVA <1.5 cm^2 by echocardiographic Doppler examination.

The management of pregnant women in NYHA class I or II should include limiting strenuous exercise, having adequate sleep and rest, maintaining a low-salt diet, avoiding anemia (keep hemoglobin >11 g), having frequent prenatal examinations (both obstetrical and cardiovascular), and monitoring for arrhythmias. In symptomatic women (NYHA functional class > II) and those with systemic ventricular dysfunction (ejection fraction less than 40%), pregnancy should be avoided because of the risk of pregnancy-related complications. The option to continue or interrupt the pregnancy should be discussed with the patient. If the patient opts to continue her pregnancy, bed rest is often required during part of the pregnancy, and close cardiac and obstetric monitoring are mandatory. Treatment of congestive heart failure is more challenging in pregnant

than in nonpregnant women. Conservative measures are very important; however, pharmacologic therapy may be required, and safe medical options are limited due to adverse effects on the fetus.

Because of the hemodynamic changes that occur during pregnancy, fixed obstructive cardiac lesions or those associated with pulmonary hypertension generally are poorly tolerated, primarily due to the inability to increase cardiac output. In contrast, regurgitant lesions are relatively well tolerated because of the pregnancy-related decrease in systemic vascular resistance.

High-risk pregnancy includes women with 1) prosthetic valves; 2) obstructive lesions, including uncorrected coarctation of the aorta; 3) Marfan syndrome; 4) hypertrophic obstructive cardiomyopathy; 5) cyanotic congenital heart disease; 6) pulmonary hypertension; 7) systemic ventricular dysfunction (ejection fraction <40%), or 8) significant uncorrected congenital heart disease (Table 2).

CARDIAC CONTRAINDICATIONS TO PREGNANCY

There are certain cardiac conditions in which pregnancy should be avoided, and if pregnancy occurs, termination should be considered (Table 3). These include severe pulmonary hypertension (pulmonary artery pressure ≥3/4 systemic pressure) and Eisenmenger syndrome. Cardiomyopathy with class III or IV congestive heart failure or left ventricular dysfunction (ejection fraction <40%) with significant symptoms is another situation in which pregnancy is contraindicated. Any form of severe obstructive cardiac lesion such as aortic stenosis, mitral stenosis, pulmonary stenosis, coarctation, or hypertrophic obstructive cardiomyopathy may result in important limitations during pregnancy. Intervention before pregnancy is the preferred management option. Women with Marfan syndrome with an aortic root of 40 mm or more should be strongly counseled to avoid pregnancy, because of the unpredictable risk of aortic dissection and rupture. Severe cyanosis is a relative contraindication to pregnancy, primarily because of adverse fetal outcome. A patient with a history of peripartum cardiomyopathy should be counseled to avoid additional pregnancies. The risk of recurrence is approximately 50%, and recurrence carries a risk of progressive heart failure and death.

Table 2.   High-Risk Pregnancy

Prosthetic valves
Obstructive lesions, including uncorrected coarctation of the aorta
Marfan syndrome
Hypertrophic obstructive cardiomyopathy
Cyanotic congenital heart disease
Pulmonary hypertension
Systemic ventricular dysfunction (ejection fraction ≤40)
Significant uncorrected congenital heart disease

Table 3.   Cardiac Contraindications to Pregnancy

Severe pulmonary hypertension
Eisenmenger syndrome
Cardiomyopathy, with class III or IV congestive heart failure
Systemic ejection fraction <40%
Severe obstructive cardiac lesions
Marfan syndrome, with aortic root ≥40 mm
Severe cyanosis
A history of peripartum cardiomyopathy

Congenital Heart Disease in Pregnancy

In patients with repaired complex congenital heart disease, some uncertainties still remain about the ability to conceive, the effects of pregnancy on maternal heart disease, and the effects of heart disease on the fetus.

Currently, an increasing number of women with congenital heart disease are reaching childbearing age and are considering pregnancy. This is primarily because congenital heart disease is being diagnosed and managed earlier and women are surviving to childbearing age.

Patients should be counseled about pregnancy and the increased risk of congenital heart disease in the fetus. The incidence of congenital heart disease in the general population is about 1%. The offspring of women with congenital heart disease have a 5% to 6% incidence of congenital heart disease. Usually, the lesion in the offspring is not the same as in the mother, except for syndromes in which the incidence of recurrence with each pregnancy may be up to 50% (e.g., autosomal dominant disorders such as Marfan syndrome or hypertrophic cardiomyopathy). Occasionally familial left-sided obstructive lesions and atrial septal defects may occur. Bicuspid aortic valve is now also recognized to be inherited and family screening is recommended.

Fetal cardiac ultrasonography is used routinely in women with congenital heart disease to detect congenital heart disease in the fetus.

Endocarditis prophylaxis is generally recommended around the time of delivery in high risk patients (for specific recommendations, see chapter "Infections of the Heart").

Cyanosis inhibits fetal growth and development

(Fig. 4). Pregnancy is generally contraindicated in women with severe cyanosis. Surgical repair of the underlying cardiac anomaly should be considered before pregnancy, if possible (e.g., an Ebstein's anomaly with cyanosis from a right-to-left shunt related to an atrial septal defect).

- Pregnant cyanotic women have a high risk of fetal loss. Also, cyanosis is a recognized handicap to fetal growth, resulting in low birth weight infants.
- Congenital heart disease is the most common form of structural heart disease that affects women of childbearing age in the U.S.
- Congenital heart disease has important implications for both the mother and the fetus.
- The incidence of congenital heart disease in the offspring of women with congenital heart disease is increased.

Rarely, device intervention such as atrial septal defect or patent foramen ovale closure is indicated during pregnancy. However, the procedure can usually be postponed until after delivery.

Marfan Syndrome and Other Aortopathies in Pregnancy

The pregnancy risk in patients with Marfan syndrome relates to the underlying medial changes affecting the aorta. The hormonal and physiologic changes that occur during pregnancy may adversely affect an abnormal aorta. This results in an unpredictable maternal risk of aortic dissection and rupture. Patients with Marfan syndrome who have an aortic dimension over 40 mm

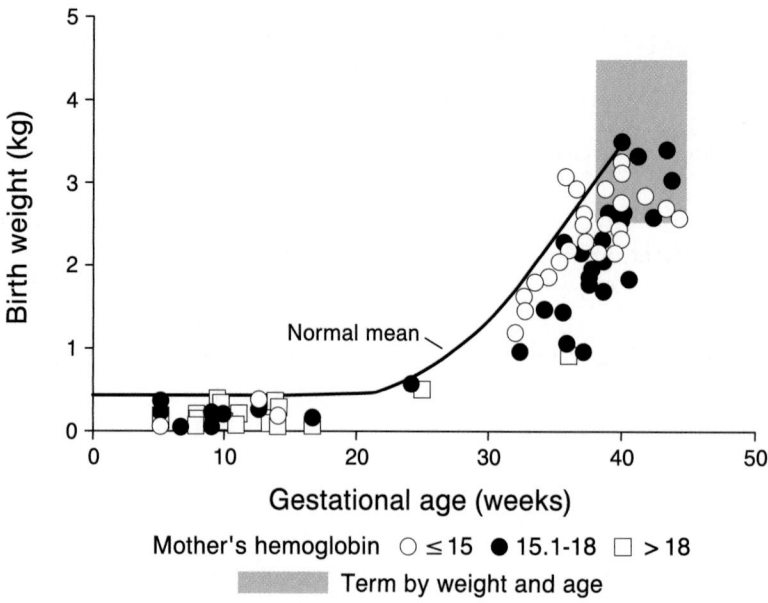

Fig. 4. Severity of maternal cyanosis, as indicated by the hemoglobin level, is related directly to fetal loss (gestational age <20), prematurity, and infant birth weight.

should be counseled against pregnancy due to the unpredictable risk of a cardiovascular event.

If pregnancy is being considered in a patient with Marfan syndrome, careful prepregnancy cardiovascular evaluation and counseling is recommended. Genetic counseling is also vital prior to pregnancy and should include a discussion about the inheritance of Marfan syndrome, the variability of the disorder and the possibility of prenatal diagnosis. Once pregnant, patients with the Marfan syndrome should be followed closely with regular aortic imaging by echocardiography. Treatment with a β-blocker during pregnancy is recommended. Fetal heart ultrasonography is often performed to assess the aorta and cardiac status of the fetus. Rare cases of severe Marfan syndrome may be diagnosed in the fetus. The risk of inheriting the Marfan syndrome is 50% per pregnancy. Near term, a facilitated delivery should be planned to avoid excessive strain on the aorta. If the aorta is over 40 mm, or has enlarged during pregnancy, cesarean delivery should be considered. Endocarditis prophylaxis should be administered around the time of delivery as indicated. The postpartum period requires special monitoring. The risk of aortic dissection persists during this time and there is also an increased risk of postpartum hemorrhage.

Patients with bicuspid aortic valves, coarctation of the aorta and other aortopathies have a predisposition for aortic dissection and aneurysm formation, and this risk may be increased during pregnancy. Prepregnancy aortic assessment is imperative in these patients. Once pregnancy occurs β-blockers may decrease the rate of dilatation of the aortic root and should be considered in all pregnant patients with aortopathy. Regular aortic follow-up using echocardiography when feasible is recommended during pregnancy in patients with aortopathy.

Peripartum Cardiomyopathy

Peripartum cardiomyopathy is defined as congestive heart failure that occurs late in pregnancy or during the early postpartum period (the last trimester or up to 6 months post partum) in the absence of congenital, coronary, or valvular heart disease or another recognized cause of heart failure. Most commonly, it is diagnosed during the first month post partum. The incidence in the United States ranges from 1:1,300 to 1:15,000 pregnancies and is higher in certain parts of the world such as Africa and Haiti. Peripartum cardiomyopathy occurs more frequently in multifetal pregnancies, multiparous women, women older than 30 years, in black women, in women with gestational hypertension or preeclampsia, and those treated with tocolytic therapy. The cause is unknown, and the prognosis varies. Peripartum cardiomyopathy is a major cause of pregnancy-related deaths in the United States, with a maternal mortality of 10-15%. Mortality is increased in patients with persistent left ventricular dysfunction >6 months after delivery. Maternal death is related to profound left ventricular dysfunction with heart failure, thromboembolic events, or arrhythmias.

Improvement in left ventricular function within 6 months after delivery is expected in 50% of women. The recommended management is supportive and includes delivery of the baby when cardiomyopathy is identified before parturition and standard medical treatment for congestive heart failure. Intravenous immune globulin and pentoxifylline should be considered. Anticoagulation should also be considered when the ventricular ejection fraction is less than 35% due to the risk of thromboembolism. Referral to transplantation should be considered in select patients.

Recurrence with subsequent pregnancies is common, and further pregnancy should be avoided in patients with a history of peripartum cardiomyopathy. Subsequent pregnancy is often associated with a decrease in ventricular function, clinical heart failure and death; the risk of these complications is significantly greater in women with persistent left ventricular dysfunction at the time of subsequent pregnancy.

- Fifty percent of women with peripartum cardiomyopathy have improvement in left ventricular function within 6 months after delivery.
- Because recurrence of peripartum cardiomyopathy is common, repeated pregnancy is contraindicated.
- Administration of angiotensin-converting enzyme inhibitors and angiotensin II inhibitors is contraindicated during pregnancy. These agents can be used during breast feeding. Digoxin and hydralazine are considered safe during pregnancy and breast feeding.
- Pregnancy should be avoided if the systemic ventricular ejection fraction is less than 40% or the NYHA functional class is higher than II.

CARDIOVASCULAR DRUGS IN PREGNANCY

The U.S. Food and Drug Administration categorize drugs according to their potential to cause birth defects.

The categories depend on the reliability of documentation of fetal risk and the potential risk-to-benefit ratio. The classifications are as follows:

Class A—No documented fetal risks.

Class B—Animal studies suggest risk, but unconfirmed in controlled human studies (e.g., methyldopa, thiazides, and dipyridamole).

Class C—Animal studies have demonstrated adverse fetal effects, but no controlled human studies (e.g., propranolol, digoxin, hydralazine, heparin, furosemide [Lasix], quinidine, procainamide, and verapamil). These drugs should be given only if the potential benefits justify the risk.

Class D—Evidence of human fetal risk. These drugs should be given only in a life-threatening situation or for a serious disease for which safer drugs either cannot be used or are ineffective. Informed consent is advised when administering these agents during pregnancy (e.g., phenytoin and captopril).

Class X—Documented fetal abnormalities; the drug is contraindicated during part or all of pregnancy (e.g., warfarin).

Pharmacologic Management of Congestive Heart Failure During Pregnancy

The treatment of congestive heart failure is more difficult in pregnant than in nonpregnant women due to the hemodynamic changes associated with pregnancy and limited safe treatment options available. Conservative measures such as salt restriction and limitation of activity are extremely important. Pharmacologic therapy may be required.

Digoxin and Diuretics

Digoxin can be safely administered during pregnancy.

No teratogenic effects of diuretics have been described; however, cases of neonatal thrombocytopenia, jaundice, hyponatremia, and bradycardia have been reported with the use of thiazides. No single diuretic is clearly contraindicated. Experience is greatest with thiazide diuretics and furosemide. Diuretics impair uterine blood flow and placental perfusion. Continuation of diuretic therapy initiated before conception does not seem unfavorable. However, routine initiation of diuretic medications during pregnancy is not recommended. Use of diuretics should be limited to the treatment of symptomatic congestive heart failure with clear evidence of elevated central venous pressure.

Maternal use of furosemide during pregnancy has not been associated with toxic or teratogenic effects, although metabolic complications have been observed. Neonatal hyponatremia and fetal hyperuricemia have been reported.

ACE Inhibitors and Angiotensin II Blockers

The use of angiotensin converting enzyme (ACE) inhibitors and angiotensin II receptor blockers is contraindicated during pregnancy. Maternal-fetal transfer of captopril has been documented, and, in animals, exposure to ACE inhibitors during pregnancy has produced prolonged fetal hypotension and death. In addition, use of ACE inhibitors during pregnancy increases the risk of early delivery, low birth weight, oligohydramnios, or neonatal anuria and renal failure (or some combination of these). These agents can be safely used during lactation.

Nitrates

The use of organic nitrates during pregnancy has been reported in the treatment of hypertension; however, in one case, the decrease in blood pressure with nitroglycerin was associated with fetal heart rate decelerations. Therefore, treatment with nitrates requires further evaluation for the management of pregnancy-related hypertension and congestive heart failure. Nitrates are excreted in breast milk and may cause methemoglobinemia in infants.

■ The administration of ACE inhibitors and angiotensin II blockers are contraindicated during pregnancy.

Management of Arrhythmias During Pregnancy

Most cardiovascular drugs cross the placenta and are secreted in breast milk. The risk-to-benefit ratio must be considered when administering any medications during pregnancy. Cardiac arrhythmias during pregnancy should be evaluated the same as in a nonpregnant patient and the underlying disease or precipitating factors treated if possible.

Direct Current Cardioversion

Direct current cardioversion may be used safely during pregnancy. This is the treatment of choice for arrhyth-

mias causing hemodynamic compromise during pregnancy. For less urgent situations, pharmacologic management of arrhythmias may be required.

Pharmacologic Management of Arrhythmias During Pregnancy

Digoxin and Quinidine

Digoxin is thought to be safe for treating arrhythmias except for an increased risk of prematurity and intrauterine growth retardation. Quinidine is an alternate antiarrhythmic medication. Adverse fetal effects have not been reported when quinidine is given at a therapeutic dose, but toxic doses may induce premature labor. Limited information is available on the use of procainamide and disopyramide during pregnancy, but to date, no adverse fetal effects have been reported.

Amiodarone and Verapamil

The use of amiodarone during pregnancy has been reported in several cases and may result in fetal hypothyroidism. The manufacturer recommends against using amiodarone during pregnancy. Amiodarone use should be limited to patients with refractory life-threatening arrhythmias, and serum amiodarone levels should be kept as low as possible. Fetal electrocardiographic monitoring should be performed before, during, and after birth, and neonatal thyroid function should be monitored at birth and continued for as long as exposure to amiodarone lasts. Amiodarone and its active metabolite have been found in human breast milk in significant concentrations, therefore the use of amiodarone is not recommended in breastfeeding women.

Verapamil has been used in pregnancy for the management of supraventricular arrhythmias, and no adverse effects have been reported. However, it has been recommended that verapamil therapy be discontinued at the onset of labor to prevent dysfunctional labor or postpartum hemorrhage.

β-Blockers

The use of β-blockers during pregnancy has been reported to cause intrauterine growth retardation, apnea at birth, fetal bradycardia, hypoglycemia, and hyperbilirubinemia. Large studies have not confirmed these concerns, and β-blocking agents have been used in a large number of pregnant women without adverse effects. β₂-Blockers now are thought to be relatively safe and may be used in the treatment of arrhythmias, hypertrophic cardiomyopathy, and hyperthyroidism during pregnancy if clinically indicated. All available β-blockers cross the placenta and are present in human breast milk. These agents can reach significant levels in the fetus or newborn. Therefore, if used during pregnancy, it is appropriate to monitor fetal and newborn heart rate as well as blood glucose and respiratory status after delivery.

Adverse fetal effects have been associated with the use of atenolol during pregnancy especially when atenolol was initiated early in the pregnancy, according to a retrospective analysis of pregnancies complicated by hypertension. Babies born to mothers in the atenolol group weighed significantly less than babies of mothers who used other antihypertensive monotherapy. There was also a trend, among mothers using atenolol, for early delivery and small for gestational age infants, especially when atenolol was administered early in pregnancy.

The World Health Organization considers atenolol unsafe during breastfeeding as it concentrates in breast milk, resulting in pharmacologically significant dose to the breastfed infant with an associated risk for hypoglycemia and bradycardia. Metoprolol should be considered as an alternative.

Adenosine

Adenosine has been used successfully to treat supraventricular tachycardia during pregnancy. To date, no adverse fetal or maternal effects related to adenosine have been reported.

- Adenosine has been used safely to treat acute supraventricular tachycardia in pregnancy.
- β-Blockers and calcium channel blockers can be used for supraventricular tachycardia prophylaxis in pregnancy, but discontinuation of these agents is advised near the time of delivery.
- Atenolol should be avoided during pregnancy and lactation.

Management of Coronary Artery Disease During Pregnancy

Coronary artery disease is occasionally encountered in the pregnant population, and carries a high risk. Careful evaluation must be carried out to exclude other causes of chest pain or acute coronary syndromes such as aortic or coronary artery dissection. Treatment depends on the presentation and the resources available. Acute myocardial infarction has a high risk of death during pregnancy and should be treated aggressively with acute percutaneous intervention when feasible. Abdominal shielding will limit the radiation exposure to the fetus.

Pharmacologic Management of Coronary Artery Disease During Pregnancy

Heparin, low dose aspirin, nitrates and β-blockers are all routinely and safely used during pregnancy. The role and safety of thrombolytic agents, glycoprotein IIb/IIIa inhibitors, and clopidogrel have not been established. These agents should be reserved for emergency management.

Valvular Heart Disease in Pregnancy

Because of the blood volume expansion and resultant increase in stroke volume and cardiac output during pregnancy, fixed obstructive cardiac valve lesions, particularly left-sided obstructive lesions (such as mitral and aortic valve stenosis), generally are poorly tolerated during pregnancy. In contrast, regurgitant valve lesions are relatively well tolerated because of the decrease in systemic vascular resistance. The effect of pregnancy on a patient with valve disease depends on the specific valve lesion, ventricular function, pulmonary artery pressures and on the New York Heart Association (NYHA) functional class. A careful cardiovascular evaluation should be performed prior to pregnancy in patients with valvular heart disease.

Percutaneous Valve Intervention

Interventional procedures are effective alternatives to surgery in several cardiac disorders that occur during pregnancy. Preliminary reports are optimistic; however, no large series have reported on the safety of cardiac interventions during pregnancy.

Percutaneous mitral commissurotomy is the strategy of choice in pregnant women with severe mitral stenosis whose symptoms cannot be controlled with medication. Marked relief of symptoms and excellent maternal and fetal outcomes have been reported. This procedure should only be attempted in centers that have extensive experience with percutaneous mitral procedures and also have surgical backup. Special considerations for balloon valvuloplasty in the gravid state include radiation exposure and pregnancy outcome. No increase in the incidence of reported congenital malformations or abortions has been reported with fetal radiation exposure of less than five rads, which can be achieved by shielding the gravid uterus and keeping fluoroscopy time to a minimum. Transesophageal or intracardiac echocardiographic guidance has also been used during the procedure to reduce radiation exposure. Percutaneous balloon aortic valvuloplasty has been reported as a safe and effective palliative procedure during pregnancy. Pulmonary balloon valvuloplasty is rarely required during pregnancy but has been reported. These procedures should be considered alternatives to surgery in patients with severe symptomatic native-valve stenosis identified during pregnancy.

Cardiac Surgery During Pregnancy

Cardiac surgery should be reserved for patients refractory to medical management in whom further delay would prove detrimental to maternal and fetal health. Cardiopulmonary bypass can adversely affect both the mother and fetus. High-flow, high-pressure, normothermic perfusion appears safest from a fetal standpoint. Fetal heart rate monitoring is recommended during cardiopulmonary bypass. When cardiac surgery is necessary during pregnancy, the optimal time is between weeks 24 and 28 of pregnancy and the duration of cardiopulmonary bypass should be kept as short as possible. A multidisciplinary team approach is required to optimize maternal and fetal outcomes.

Prosthetic Heart Valves

The best type of heart valve prosthesis to use in women of childbearing age who have critical valvular heart disease is debated. Some data have suggested that premature valve deterioration occurs in bioprosthetic valves during pregnancy, but this has not been documented conclusively or demonstrated experimentally. One report has suggested that reoperation (required for most patients with bioprosthetic valves) carries a higher risk of morbidity and mortality than the risk of anticoagulation during pregnancy. Recent surgical data would substantially higher than the risk of the initial operation,

depending on patient characteristics. Pregnant women with a mechanical heart valve have an increased risk for developing prosthetic valve thrombosis or other life-threatening complication during pregnancy. The complication rate depends on the anticoagulation regimen used during pregnancy. The best management for a pregnant woman who requires anticoagulation is controversial.

Anticoagulants

Hematologic changes that occur during normal pregnancy include an increase in clotting factor concentrations, an increase in platelet adhesiveness, and a decrease in fibrinolysis and protein S activity. These changes result in an overall increased risk of thrombosis or embolism.

Heparin

Unfractionated heparin does not cross the placenta. The primary concern with heparin use is the increased risk of thromboembolic complications, including fatal valve thrombosis, in high-risk pregnant women given subcutaneous unfractionated heparin. The efficacy of adjusted-dose subcutaneous heparin has not been established, and for high-risk patients (those with caged-ball or the Bjork-Shiley tilting-disk mitral prostheses), this form of anticoagulation should be used only between the 6th and 12th weeks of pregnancy and around delivery. The heparin dose should be adjusted so that the activated partial thromboplastin time is at least 2.5-3.5 times the control value 6 hours after the dose is administered for high-risk patients. Lower level anticoagulation may be appropriate for patients with other prostheses.

Prolonged heparin therapy (intravenous or subcutaneous) can result in thrombocytopenia, osteoporosis, and alopecia. Erratic absorption of subcutaneously delivered heparin may occur, and frequent monitoring of the activated partial thromboplastin time to ensure therapeutic anticoagulation is mandatory.

Warfarin

Because warfarin has a low molecular weight, it crosses the placenta and results in fetal anticoagulation. The effect of warfarin on the fetus is greater than that on the mother because of reduced vitamin K–dependent factors in the fetal liver. Fetal anticoagulation increases the risk for spontaneous abortion, prematurity, fetal deformity, and stillbirth. Retroplacental hemorrhage and fetal intracranial hemorrhage are additional risks to the fetus. Warfarin use throughout pregnancy, until near term, provides the lowest risk for maternal thromboembolic events complications and death.

Warfarin Embryopathy

Historic reports describe a 30% risk of embryopathy with administration of warfarin during the first trimester (6th to 12th week of gestation). More recent data suggest the incidence of warfarin embryopathy to be less than 10%. The maternal dose of warfarin during the first trimester appears to be important. The risk of warfarin embryopathy appears to be low with a warfarin dose less than 5 mg daily. Warfarin embryopathy results in bone and cartilaginous abnormalities with chondrodysplasia, nasal hypoplasia, optic atrophy, microphthalmia, blindness, minor neurologic dysfunction, reduced intelligence quotient, and seizures. Warfarin does not enter breast milk and, thus, can be administered safely to women who breastfeed their infants.

Low-Molecular-Weight Heparin

Data are currently insufficient to support use of low-molecular-weight heparin (LMWH) for anticoagulation of patients with mechanical heart valves during pregnancy. No teratogenic effects have been reported with LMWH, and they do not cross the placenta. They are used regularly in patients requiring anticoagulation during pregnancy for causes other than mechanical valves.

Concern regarding the safety of LMWH is based in part on an unpublished South African study that was stopped early due to two maternal deaths in the LMWH group. Although anti-Xa levels were measured, and were low in both deceased patients, the dose of LMWH was not adjusted when the levels were low. Subsequently, Oran et al reviewed the literature and reported on 81 pregnancies in 75 women with mechanical prostheses, treated with LMWH. Valve thrombosis occurred in 8.6% of these pregnancies. However, when 51 pregnancies were reviewed in which anti-Xa levels were monitored and LMWH dose adjusted, only one thromboembolic event occurred. Barbour et al have demonstrated that LMWH requirements increase during pregnancy and that the dose should be adjusted according to anti-Xa levels.

Anticoagulation Management During Pregnancy

The American Heart Association and American College of Cardiology provided recommendations regarding anticoagulation during pregnancy. For patients with high-risk prostheses or prior thromboembolic events, continuous intravenous heparin during the first trimester and continuation of warfarin and aspirin are considered the treatment options of choice. Subcutaneous dose-adjusted heparin with a partial thromboplastin time 2.5 to 3.5 times the control value is considered a less safe regimen. In the United States, owing to the risk of embryopathy, informed consent should be obtained if warfarin is used during the first trimester of pregnancy (Fig. 5). The warfarin package insert states that warfarin is contraindicated during pregnancy.

Warfarin is the anticoagulation agent of choice for patients with mechanical valves during the second trimester of pregnancy. The warfarin dose should be adjusted to the prosthesis appropriate international normalized ratio.

During the third trimester, warfarin therapy should be continued until 36 weeks of pregnancy. In anticipation of delivery, patients should be hospitalized and treatment with intravenous heparin should be started. The activated partial thromboplastin time should be over 2.5 times the control value.

Labor and delivery is a particularly high-risk time for patients who require anticoagulation during pregnancy. Delivery should be planned, and intravenous heparin treatment should be stopped peripartum. Cesarean delivery should be performed if labor occurs during warfarin anticoagulation because of the risk of fetal intracranial hemorrhage with vaginal delivery. Heparin should be resumed four to six hours after Cesarean or vaginal delivery in the absence of bleeding. The European Society of Cardiology suggests continuation of warfarin anticoagulation during pregnancy and the American College of Chest Physicians recommend avoiding warfarin and using aggressive dose adjusted LMWH or unfractionated heparin during pregnancy. Addition of low-dose aspirin for the high-risk patient was also suggested.

Thus, there is no consensus on the best anticoagulation regimen during pregnancy for patients with mechanical valve prostheses. An informed discussion with the patient and her partner, and meticulous

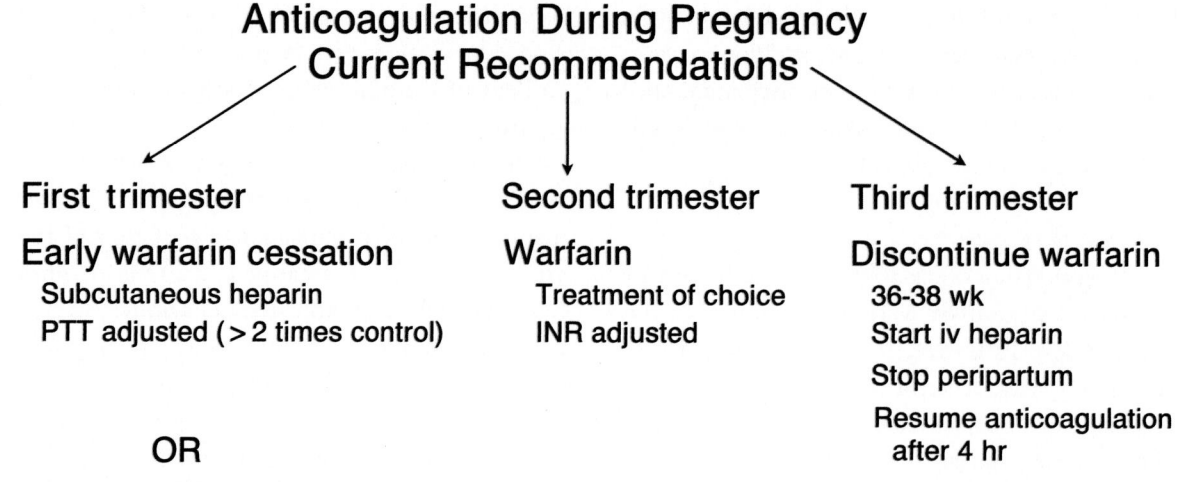

Fig. 5. Anticoagulation options during the 3 trimesters of pregnancy. Treatment must be individualized for each patient. INR, international normalized ratio; PTT, partial thromboplastin time.

monitoring of the chosen anticoagulation regimen is mandatory. An updated regimen incorporating the recommendations by the American Heart Association and American College of Cardiology recommendations with those from the American College of Chest Physicians has been suggested by Elkayam (Fig. 6).

Antiplatelet Agents

Low-dose aspirin (81 mg) is safe to use during pregnancy. It is recommended for patients with intracardiac shunts (e.g., those with atrial septal defect), cyanosis, or a valve prostheses. However, the antiplatelet effect has not been proved.

Dipyridamole should not be used during pregnancy. No data are available on the effects of ticlopidine or clopidogrel during pregnancy. Information is limited on administration of glycoprotein IIb/IIIa inhibitors during pregnancy. Thrombolytic therapy has been used in pregnancy, and is the recommended treatment of choice for patients with mechanical valve thrombosis during pregnancy. Operation is recommended when patients have contraindications for thrombolytic therapy. Thrombolytic therapy should be considered in the critically ill patient with acute coronary syndrome

when urgent percutaneous intervention is not available or feasible.

- Use of warfarin during the first trimester of pregnancy is associated with an increased risk of miscarriage and warfarin embryopathy, but is the safest method of anticoagulation for the mother, especially with older mechanical mitral prostheses.
- Adjusted dose, unfractionated heparin administered between weeks 6 and 12 of pregnancy, decreases the risk of fetal complications but doubles the risk of maternal thromboembolism and death compared to warfarin.
- Data regarding the safety of LMWH for anticoagulation of pregnant women with mechanical prostheses remain insufficient to recommend this form of anticoagulation routinely.
- Considerable controversy exists about the best method of anticoagulation during pregnancy.

Endocarditis Prophylaxis

The American Heart Association does not recommend endocarditis prophylaxis for patients expected to have an uncomplicated cesarean or vaginal delivery. However,

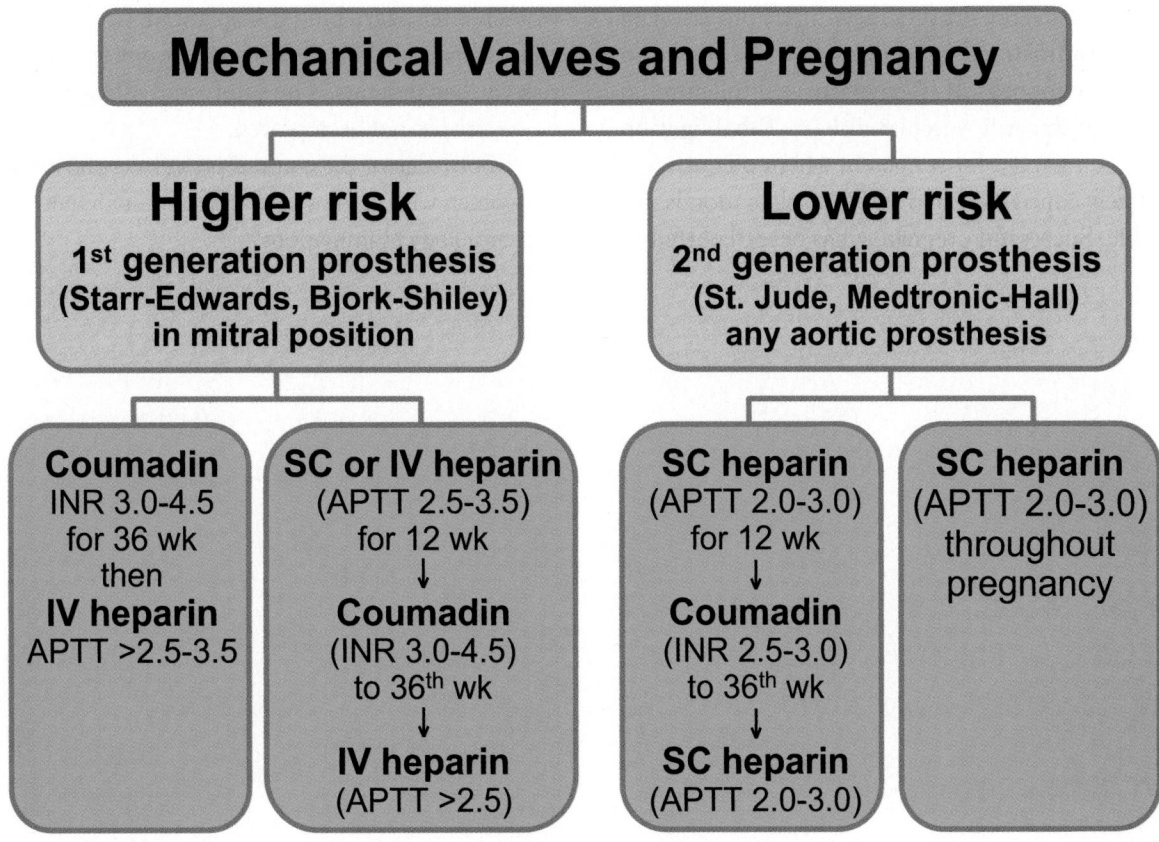

Fig. 6. Anticoagulation strategies in pregnant patients with mechanical heart valves.

standard prophylactic treatment with antibiotics given intravenously or intramuscularly is recommended for the placement of a urinary catheter in the presence of urinary tract infection and for vaginal delivery in the presence of vaginal infection.

Our recommendations are more conservative. We recommend the intravenous administration of antibiotics for endocarditis prophylaxis using the gastrointestinal or genitourinary regimen in all high-risk cardiac patients because of the risk of undiagnosed infections and the significant patient morbidity and mortality should infective endocarditis occur. Antibiotic therapy should be administered 30 to 60 minutes before delivery is expected and repeated 8 hours later.

CONTRACEPTION IN PATIENTS WITH HEART DISEASE

More than 50% of teenagers are sexually active and 10% of the women in the U.S. who are 15 to 19 years old have unplanned pregnancies.

The estrogen-containing oral contraceptive pill, or "combination pill," has an increased risk of thromboembolic events, pulmonary embolism, and fluid retention; therefore, it should be prescribed with caution for women with severe structural heart disease. Alternative methods include the progesterone-only pill, or "mini pill," which is an option for patients with pulmonary hypertension, right-to-left shunts, or a prosthetic valve. The failure rate of the progesterone-only pill is higher than that of the combination pill and is similar to the failure rate of barrier methods. Also, the progesterone-only pill must be taken at the same time each day. Breakthrough bleeding is common and, when this occurs, contraceptive coverage is not reliable. Barrier methods also have a high failure rate (18% per year) and should be used with caution in patients in whom pregnancy is absolutely contraindicated. An intrauterine device is not suggested for women with heart disease, because of the potential risk of infection. Depo-Provera is synthetic progestogen that is administered as an intramuscular injection every three months. It is generally well tolerated in patients with cardiovascular disease. Tubal ligation should be reserved for women in whom pregnancy is absolutely contraindicated and transplantation is not possible. Successful pregnancy has been reported in women after heart-lung transplantation. The Essure endovaginal tubal ligation is another option for high-risk cardiac patients. The safety and efficacy of this procedure has not been proven.

Knowledge of the contraception risks and options for women with cardiovascular disease are required for the cardiology examinations.

ADULT CONGENITAL HEART DISEASE

Carole A. Warnes, MD

ATRIAL SEPTAL DEFECT (ASD)

Secundum ASD

The secundum type of ASD is the most common adult congenital heart defect after bicuspid aortic valve. The defect is in the central portion of the atrial septum and is associated with left-to-right shunting and right ventricular volume overload. Adults are often asymptomatic, and the murmur may be found incidentally on physical examination. The natural history of unrepaired ASD is that atrial fibrillation develops in patients in their 40s or 50s in association with tricuspid regurgitation and often right ventricular failure. Death is usually from heart failure or thromboembolic stroke, although survival into old age occurs in some patients.

Physical Examination

The jugular venous pressure is often normal and the "a" and "v" waves may be equal in amplitude. Other findings are a right ventricular lift, an ejection systolic murmur from the pulmonary area (always less than grade 3/6), fixed splitting of the second heart sound, and a tricuspid diastolic flow rumble if the shunt is large (Qp/Qs more than 2.5 to 1).

Electrocardiography

Typical electrocardiographic findings include an RSR pattern and partial right bundle branch block, often with right-axis deviation.

Chest Radiography (Fig. 1 and 2)

A prominent pulmonary artery, right ventricular enlargement, and pulmonary plethora are found on chest radiographs. Left atrial enlargement does not typically occur unless the patient is older than 40 years or has atrial fibrillation. If left atrial enlargement is present in a young person with an ASD in sinus rhythm, consider a primum ASD in the differential diagnosis or coincidental mitral valve disease.

Diagnosis and Management

The diagnosis of ASD can usually be made with echocardiography, but if the image is suboptimal, transesophageal echocardiography should be performed. Cardiac catheterization is usually unnecessary to confirm an ASD unless coexistent coronary artery disease is suspected. If there is evidence of right ventricular volume overload, the ASD should be closed to prevent right heart failure, paradoxical embolus, and atrial arrhythmia. (Closing an ASD later in life, although still beneficial, is associated with an increased risk of atrial arrhythmias during late follow-up.) Percutaneous device closure of the ASD is successful in experienced hands, as long as the defect has an adequate rim. Surgical closure is an

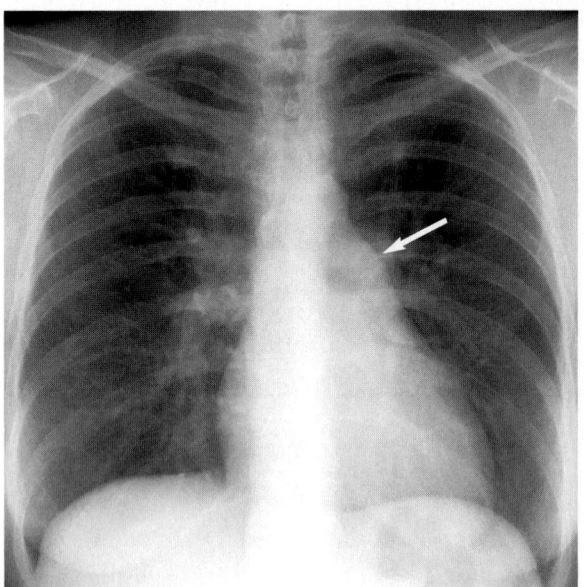

Fig. 1. Chest radiograph showing mild cardiomegaly with prominence of the pulmonary artery (*arrow*). There are increased pulmonary vascular markings from a left to right shunt consistent with a significant atrial septal defect.

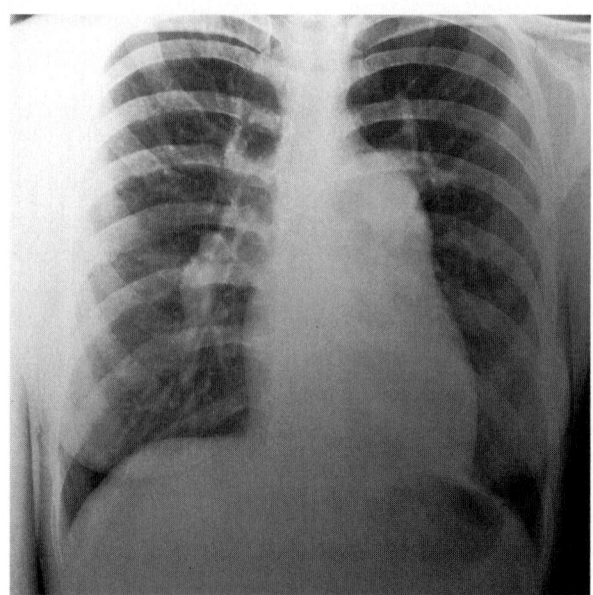

Fig. 2. Chest radiograph of 35-year-old woman with atrial septal defect. There is severe pulmonary vascular obstructive disease with prominence of the main pulmonary artery and decreased peripheral pulmonary vascularity.

alternative. Symptomatic patients usually improve after closure.

- The secundum type of ASD is the most common adult congenital heart defect after bicuspid aortic valve.
- Cardiac catheterization is usually unnecessary to confirm an ASD unless coexistent coronary artery disease is suspected.

Primum ASD

The primum type of ASD is in the lower portion of the atrial septum and is a defect in the atrioventricular septum. Both atrioventricular valves are on the same anatomical level and are congenitally abnormal. Classically, the mitral valve is cleft, but 4% of defects may be associated with double-orifice mitral valve. The mitral valve, therefore, has various degrees of regurgitation and may occasionally be stenotic. The septal leaflet of the tricuspid valve often is deficient, with varying degrees of tricuspid regurgitation. The findings on physical examination in primum ASD are the same as those for secundum ASD, with the addition of variable signs of mitral regurgitation.

Electrocardiography

Electrocardiography shows left-axis deviation with right bundle branch block. First-degree atrioventricular block occurs in approximately 75% of cases.

Diagnosis

The condition is diagnosed with echocardiography, and cardiac catheterization is usually unnecessary. Because of the elongated ventricular outflow tract, the so-called gooseneck deformity is produced on angiography. Subaortic stenosis is a recognized association.

Management

Patch closure is used for the ASD, and the mitral cleft is repaired if the valve is regurgitant.

- The findings on physical examination in primum ASD are the same as those for secundum ASD, with the addition of variable signs of mitral regurgitation.

Sinus Venosus ASD

Sinus venosus ASD is a defect in the superior portion of the septum usually associated with anomalous pulmonary vein (classically, the right upper pulmonary vein).

Diagnosis
The diagnosis usually can be made with echocardiography (this may require transesophageal echocardiography), and the pulmonary vein also should be diverted at the time of surgical repair.

■ Eisenmenger syndrome develops in approximately 5% of patients with ASD.

VENTRICULAR SEPTAL DEFECT
Small defects (so-called *maladie de Roger*) often produce a loud murmur but are of little or no clinical significance apart from the need for endocarditis prophylaxis. Defects can occur at many different areas in the septum, the most common being in the membranous and muscular parts of the septum. These defects have the possibility of closing spontaneously up to about age 20 years. Defects in other positions never close spontaneously (such as subaortic defects, subpulmonary defects, and canal-type defects) (Fig. 3).

Small defects may be associated with a thrill at the left sternal edge, usually in the fourth interspace. The murmur is usually holosystolic, but it may be shorter if it is in the muscular septum because the defect may be occluded during late systole. Large defects also may produce a mitral diastolic flow rumble at the apex, particularly when the shunt has a Qp/Qs more than 2.5 to 1.

■ Ventricular septal defect is the most common congenital heart defect to produce the Eisenmenger syndrome.

PATENT DUCTUS ARTERIOSUS
This classically is associated with maternal rubella. A small ductus may be of little or no hemodynamic consequence and is consistent with a normal life span. A patent ductus arteriosus commonly calcifies in adult life.

Physical Examination
Because it produces an "arteriovenous fistula," the pulse pressure is usually wide with a prominent left ventricular impulse and a continuous "machinery murmur" enveloping the second heart sound. This usually is audible beneath the left clavicle in the second intercostal space.

Therapy
Percutaneous device closure of the ductus is the most common therapy; surgical ligation is an alternative if it is not amenable to device therapy. After successful closure antibiotic prophylaxis is no longer necessary.

Differential Diagnosis
The differential diagnosis of a patent ductus arteriosus includes pulmonary atresia with systemic collateral vessels in a patient with cyanosis, aortopulmonary window, and ventricular septal defect with concomitant aortic regurgitation. Other fistulae such as coronary and pulmonary fistulae may also produce continuous murmurs, and rarely, coarctation.

PULMONARY STENOSIS
Pulmonary stenosis may be associated with Noonan syndrome, in which case the valve is frequently dysplastic. The condition usually produces few or no symptoms unless the pulmonary stenosis is very severe. Usually the

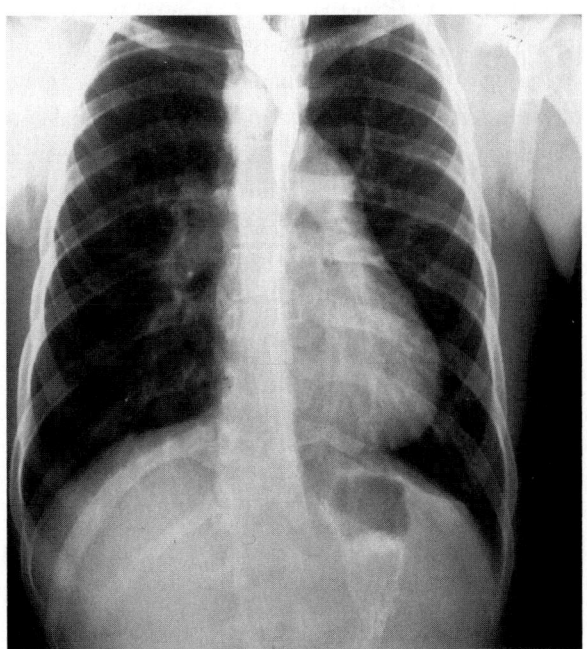

Fig. 3. Chest radiograph of 22-year-old man with ventricular septal defect complicated by pulmonary vascular obstructive disease. Note nearly normal cardiac size with apex tilted upward, marked dilatation of central pulmonary arteries, and decreased peripheral pulmonary vascularity.

valve remains pliable until well into middle age; thus, an ejection click is common until later life.

Physical Examination

The following features suggest pulmonary stenosis: a prominent "a" wave in the jugular venous pressure, right ventricular lift, ejection click (the earlier the click, the more severe the stenosis), systolic murmur, and delayed pulmonary component of second heart sound (P_2) (absent in severe pulmonary stenosis).

Electrocardiography

Right ventricular hypertrophy is seen on the electrocardiogram.

Chest Radiography

When stenosis is at valve level, there is poststenotic dilatation of the main and left pulmonary arteries, which is a typical radiographic appearance (Fig. 4). Lung fields are oligemic *only* in severe pulmonary stenosis.

Diagnosis and Management

The diagnosis is made from the findings on clinical examination and echocardiography. Severe stenosis is usually a gradient of more than 50 mm Hg (right ventricular pressure more than two-thirds of systemic pressure). Most patients have good results from balloon valvotomy. Often, coexistent subpulmonary stenosis is due to hypertrophy of the infundibulum. This usually regresses with time after pulmonary valvotomy. Midterm results appear to be comparable to those with surgical commissurotomy; hence, balloon valvotomy is now the procedure of choice for treatment of pulmonary stenosis.

- Pulmonary stenosis may be associated with Noonan syndrome, in which case the valve is frequently dysplastic.
- Severe stenosis is usually a gradient of more than 50 mm Hg.
- Balloon valvotomy is now the procedure of choice for treatment of pulmonary stenosis.

COARCTATION OF THE AORTA

Coarctation of the aorta most often is diagnosed in childhood and is usually a discrete narrowing of the

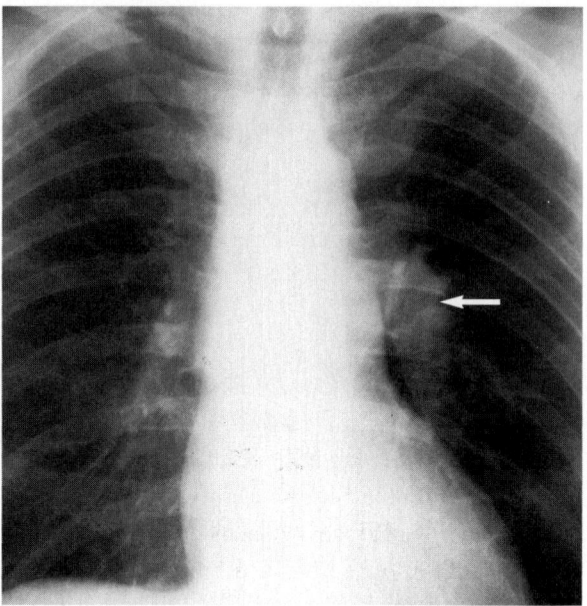

Fig. 4. Chest radiograph showing severe pulmonary stenosis. Note the poststenotic dilatation of the main and left pulmonary arteries (*arrow*), indicating that this is valvular pulmonary stenosis.

aorta just distal to the left subclavian artery. Occasionally there may be an elongated, narrowed thoracic aorta. Coarctation is much more common in males than females and often is associated with a bicuspid aortic valve. It is the most common anomaly associated with Turner syndrome. It also is associated with ventricular septal defect, Shone syndrome, and cerebral aneurysms in the circle of Willis.

It may be noted as an incidental murmur, but if it is not detected in childhood it may present with systemic hypertension in adulthood. The narrowing in the aorta produces systemic hypertension above the coarctation and reduced blood pressure below the coarctation in the legs. Sometimes patients present because of signs of hypertension on retinal examination.

As a result of the coarctation, systemic collateral vessels frequently develop from the subclavian, axillary, internal mammary, scapular, and intercostal arteries. It is the intercostal artery collateral vessels that produce the classic rib notching.

Physical Examination

Findings on physical examination include radiofemoral delay and a decrease in blood pressure between the upper and lower extremities. An ejection systolic murmur is present in the second space at the left sternal edge. This occasionally extends into diastole, producing a continuous murmur when the coarctation is severe. Collateral murmurs may be audible and palpable over the thorax and particularly the back over the scapulae. An ejection click may be heard when there is an associated bicuspid aortic valve. The aortic component of the second heart sound (A_2) may be loud, and a fourth heart sound may be present if there is systemic hypertension.

Electrocardiography
Electrocardiography shows varying degrees of left ventricular hypertrophy.

Chest Radiography
Chest radiographs may show the classic "figure-3" sign beneath the aortic knob, which represents dilatation of the aorta above the coarctation and then dilatation below. This is uncommon however. Rib notching is a variable feature (Fig. 5 *A* and *B*).

Complications
The major complications of coarctation include aortic rupture or dissection, coexistent aortic valve disease, left ventricular failure, stroke (due to either systemic hypertension or rupture of a cerebral aneurysm), endocarditis, and endarteritis.

Pregnancy in patients with coarctation is associated with an increased risk of aortic dissection and rupture. The risk of aortic dissection and rupture also is increased in Turner syndrome, even in the absence of coarctation.

Diagnosis
Coarctation of the aorta is diagnosed from findings on physical examination and Doppler echocardiography (Fig. 6). Doppler echocardiography at rest may demonstrate a systolic and diastolic gradient, and exercise Doppler echocardiography may improve the diagnostic accuracy. If the coarctation is not well visualized, be cautious with the gradient interpretation because collateral vessels may reduce the gradient even when significant coarctation is present. If Doppler echocardiographic imaging is not satisfactory, consider magnetic resonance or CT or aortography.

Treatment
Percutaneous balloon angioplasty and stent placement is successful in appropriately selected cases in experienced

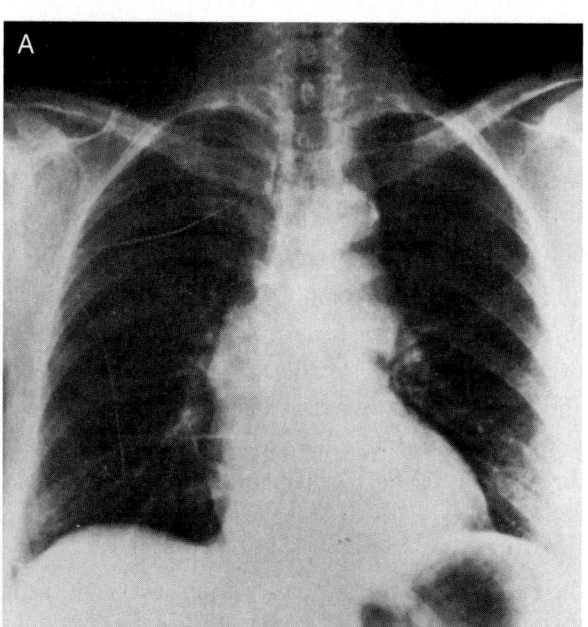
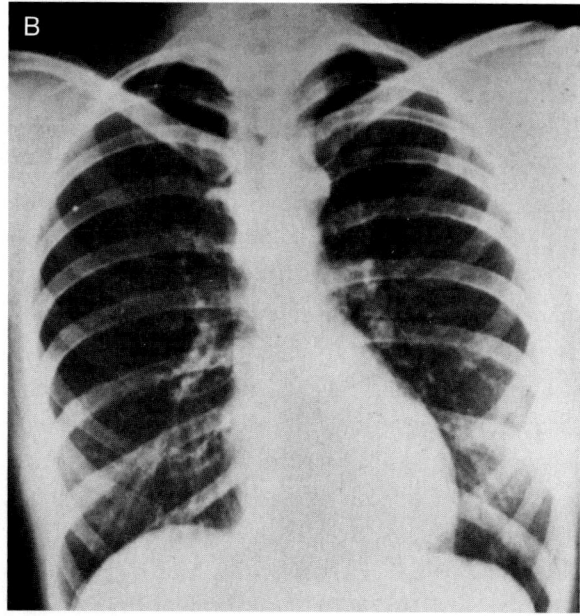

Fig. 5. *A*, Coarctation of aorta with "figure-3" sign seen along upper aspect of left cardiac silhouette; indentation just below aortic arch represents coarcted segment with poststenotic dilatation below this. *B*, No other characteristics of aortic coarctation are present except notching beneath the undersurface of the ribs, evident on the left side.

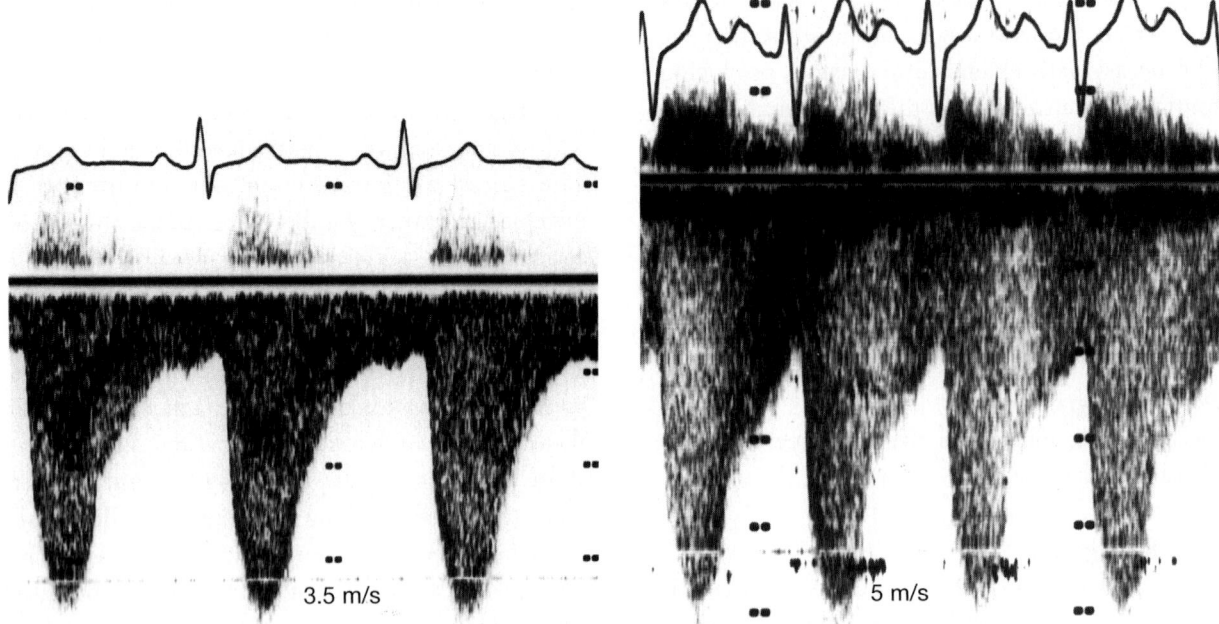

Fig. 6. Continuous-wave Doppler recordings down the descending aorta in a patient with coarctation of the aorta. *Left*, Resting recording with a peak systolic velocity of 3.5 m/s indicates a maximal instantaneous gradient of approximately 49 mm Hg. Note the persistence of high velocity (approximately 1 m/s) in diastole. *Right*, With exercise, the peak velocity increases to 5 m/s (100 mm Hg maximal instantaneous gradient) and the diastolic flow also is increased, to 2 m/s. These measurements are consistent with severe coarctation.

hands, but it is less successful in patients with higher gradients and may be complicated by dissection and rupture.

Surgical repair by left lateral thoracotomy is the accepted treatment. Recoarctation, however, is possible, and there is still a significant incidence of systemic hypertension (75% at 30 years) after coarctation repair. Even after successful repair of coarctation, the aorta is still abnormal and patients are still at increased risk of dying of dissection and rupture. They also die of premature coronary artery disease, heart failure, and stroke. The earlier the age of repair, the less chance of systemic hypertension and its complications. In one Mayo Clinic series, patients who had operation at younger than 14 years had a 20-year survival rate of 91%, and patients who had operation at age 14 years or older had a reduced 20-year survival rate of 79%.

■ Coarctation is much more common in males than females and commonly is associated with a bicuspid aortic valve.

■ The major complications of coarctation include aortic rupture or dissection, coexistent aortic valve disease, left ventricular failure, stroke (due to either systemic hypertension or rupture of a cerebral aneurysm), endocarditis, and endarteritis.

EBSTEIN ANOMALY

The major abnormality in Ebstein anomaly is inferior displacement of the tricuspid valve into the right ventricle, producing an "atrialized" right ventricle above and a small right ventricle below, which often has impaired contraction. The degree of displacement is variable, as is the degree of abnormality of the tricuspid valve. The septal leaflet is variably deficient or even absent. The posterior leaflet also often is deficient, and there is a large "sail-like" anterior leaflet that is the hallmark of the condition. Among patients with Ebstein anomaly, 50% have either a patent foramen ovale or a secundum ASD, and 25% have one or more accessory atrioventricular conduction (Wolff-Parkinson-White syndrome) pathways. The anomaly is thought to be associated with maternal lithium ingestion.

Physical Examination

Findings include a low-volume pulse with cool extremities and sometimes peripheral cyanosis reflecting low cardiac output. Central cyanosis may be present if there is an atrial communication. A "v" wave may be present in the jugular venous pressure, although this is uncommon even in the presence of significant tricuspid regurgitation because the large right atrium absorbs the tricuspid regurgitant volume. There is a subtle right ventricular lift. The loud tricuspid component of the first heart sound (T_1) is produced by the sail-like anterior leaflet of the tricuspid valve. The holosystolic murmur of tricuspid regurgitation is often associated with one or more systolic clicks in Ebstein anomaly.

Chest Radiography

Varying degrees of cardiomegaly with marked right atrial enlargement are seen on chest radiographs (Fig. 7). In contrast to cardiomyopathy, the pedicle is very narrow (small pulmonary artery). Usually, the lung fields are normal or oligemic.

Electrocardiography

Right atrial enlargement produces tall P waves, which may be the largest of any anomaly (Himalayan P waves) (Fig. 8). Right bundle branch block often is present, or there may be evidence of preexcitation.

Diagnosis and Management

The diagnosis is made with echocardiography. Cardiac catheterization is unnecessary unless coexistent coronary artery disease is suspected. Surgical repair is indicated when 1) patients have functional limitation or deteriorating exercise capacity on stress testing, 2) progressive right ventricular enlargement is demonstrated on echocardiography, 3) an atrial communication is present and the patient is cyanotic (risk of stroke), 4) a bypass tract is present, and 5) there is severe tricuspid regurgitation (especially if the valve is reparable).

Surgical Repair

Surgery consists of closure of the atrial communication, repair of the tricuspid valve if there is sufficient mobility to the anterior leaflet, and plication of the atrialized right ventricle. If the valve is tethered and immobile, tricuspid valve replacement may be necessary.

■ Among patients with Ebstein anomaly, 50% have either a patent foramen ovale or a secundum atrial septal defect, and 25% have one or more accessory atrioventricular conduction (Wolff-Parkinson-White syndrome) pathways.

CYANOTIC HEART DISEASE

There are many "natural survivors" with cyanotic heart disease who reach adulthood without having had surgery. These include patients with tetralogy of Fallot, anatomical variants with a very large interventricular shunt (single ventricle), pulmonary stenosis with atrial septal defect, Ebstein anomaly with ASD, and Eisenmenger syndrome.

Tetralogy of Fallot

One of the so-called conotruncal abnormalities, tetralogy of Fallot consists of a large subaortic ventricular septal defect and obstruction to the pulmonary outflow, usually at the infundibular level and often at the pulmonary valve level also. This produces right ventricular hyper-

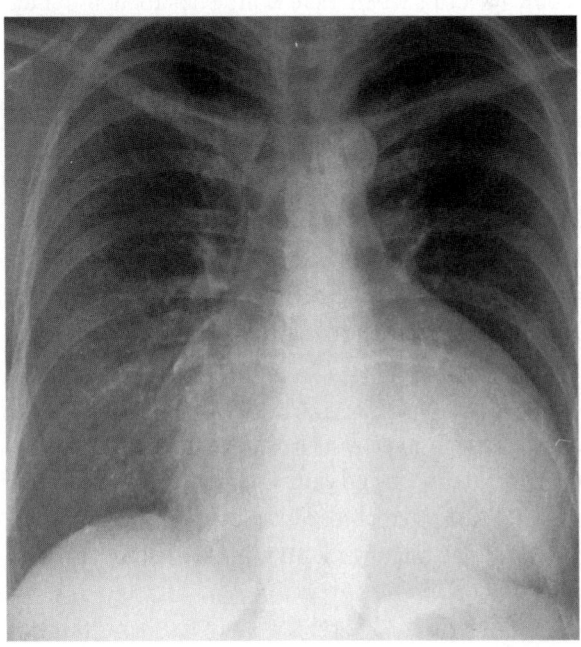

Fig. 7. Patient with severe Ebstein anomaly, severe right atrial enlargement, and huge cardiomegaly with a very narrow pedicle.

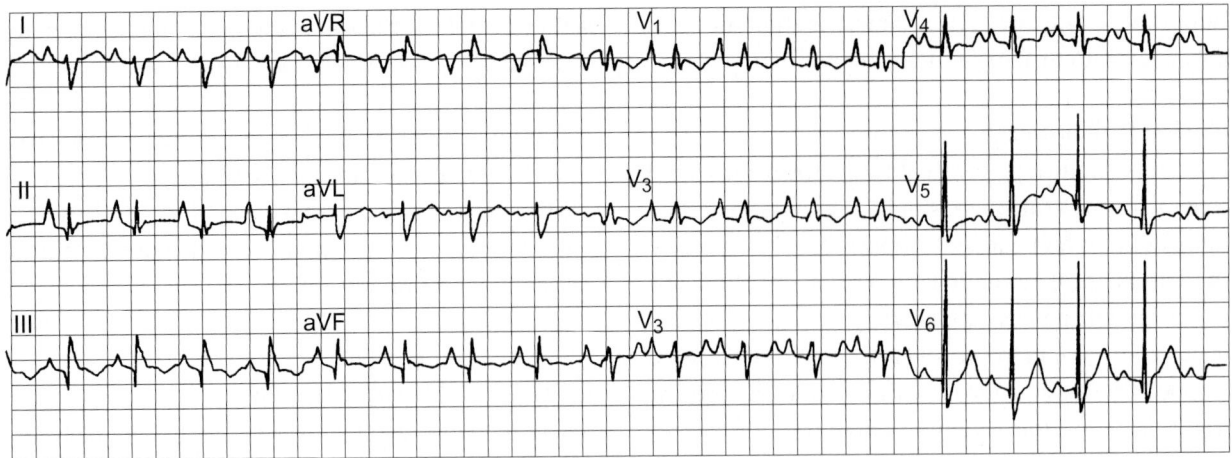

Fig. 8. Electrocardiogram from 15-year-old boy with Ebstein anomaly. Note prominent P wave, prolonged atrioventricular conduction, and delay in right ventricular conduction.

trophy. In addition, the aorta overrides the ventricular septal defect.

The pressure in the right ventricle is the same as that in the left because of the large ventricular septal defect. The obstruction to pulmonary blood flow causes desaturated blood to be diverted into the aorta, which is often large; thus, the degree of right ventricular obstruction determines the degree of cyanosis. Hence, in childhood, the so-called acyanotic Fallot or the pink tetralogy occurs when there is little obstruction to pulmonary blood flow and patients do not have cyanosis. The infundibular hypertrophy, however, tends to be progressive; thus, the cyanosis increases with advancing age.

Most patients have repair in childhood, but occasionally they reach adulthood without surgical intervention. These adult patients do not have right ventricular failure until they are at least 40 years of age, unless they have a superimposed arrhythmia.

Physical Examination

Findings on physical examination include varying degrees of cyanosis and clubbing, right ventricular lift, a thrill at the left sternal edge if the pulmonary obstruction is severe, long systolic murmur in the pulmonary area, and absent P_2.

Adult patients who have not had operation may have aortic regurgitation, because the aorta is large and the cusps prolapse into the defect. Aortic regurgitation may be of varying degree. The aortic regurgitant jet

may enter the right ventricle, and this may ultimately produce right ventricular failure.

Chest Radiography

Tetralogy of Fallot is associated with right aortic arch (approximately 25% of cases), right ventricular enlargement, concave pulmonary bay, and possibly pulmonary oligemia.

Electrocardiography

Tetralogy of Fallot is associated with right ventricular hypertrophy, usually right-axis deviation, and tall, peaked P waves.

Diagnosis and Management

The diagnosis can usually be made with echocardiography. The coronary anatomy should also be determined because of the increased incidence of anomalous coronary anatomy if surgical correction is being contemplated. If the pulmonary arteries are of adequate size, surgical repair involves closure of the ventricular septal defect and relief of the outflow obstruction. In simple cases, this involves resection of the infundibular muscle, but if the pulmonary anulus is small, it may involve pulmonary valvotomy, right ventricular outflow patch, transanular patch, excision of the pulmonary valve, or placement of a conduit from the right ventricle to the pulmonary artery.

The most common long-term problem after surgical repair of tetralogy is pulmonary regurgitation, which occurs when the pulmonary anulus has been patched. This may cause exercise limitation or arrhythmias. The presence of atrial or ventricular arrhythmias should always prompt a search for an underlying hemodynamic abnormality. Pulmonary valve replacement should be performed before there is irreversible right ventricular dysfunction. Other problems include residual pulmonary stenosis, right ventricular aneurysm formation at the site of the surgical patch, residual ventricular septal defect, and aortic dilatation and aortic regurgitation. Sudden death may occur due to ventricular arrhythmias and is more common in patients with residual hemodynamic abnormalities and ventricular dysfunction and those who had late surgical repair.

Other patients with tetralogy of Fallot may survive because of earlier palliative shunts that improve pulmonary blood flow and help pulmonary arteries to grow. Types of shunt include Blalock-Taussig (a subclavian artery-to-pulmonary artery anastomosis—can be used on either the right or the left side); Waterston shunt between the ascending aorta and the right pulmonary artery; Potts shunt (descending aorta-to-left pulmonary artery shunt); and a central shunt constructed with a polytetrafluoroethylene (PTFE, Gore-Tex) graft.

Problems with palliative shunts include distortion of the pulmonary arteries, which may kink, thrombose, or occlude, and pulmonary vascular disease when the shunt is too large. Patients with large shunts are at risk of volume overload on the ventricle and ultimately ventricular failure with pulmonary vascular disease. These patients are not accepted for heart-lung transplantation because of the lateral thoracotomy scar and the profound risk of bleeding.

- Tetralogy of Fallot consists of a large subaortic ventricular septal defect and obstruction to the pulmonary outflow.
- Problems with palliative shunts include distortion of the pulmonary arteries, which may kink, thrombose, or occlude, and pulmonary vascular disease when the shunt is too large.

Other Causes of Cyanosis

Pulmonary Atresia With Ventricular Septal Defect
This is also a conotruncal abnormality and has the same intracardiac anatomy as tetralogy of Fallot, except that the right ventricular outflow tract is blind or atretic. Pulmonary blood flow arises from collateral vessels from the descending aorta which are congenital, patent ductus arteriosus, bronchial collateral vessels, and coronary collateral vessels.

Collateral vessels may be end arteries feeding into the lung tissue directly, or one or more collateral vessels may enter into central pulmonary arteries.

Forty percent of patients with pulmonary atresia have a right aortic arch.

Transposition of the Great Arteries
Patients with transposition of the great arteries have virtually all had surgery by the time they reach adulthood, either in the form of an atrial baffle procedure (Mustard or Senning) or an arterial switch procedure. Long-term complications of atrial baffle procedure are significant because the right ventricle still supports the systemic circulation; hence, right ventricular failure and tricuspid regurgitation are common. Atrial arrhythmias, particularly junctional rhythm and atrial flutter, are also common late in follow-up.

Tricuspid Atresia
Patients with tricuspid atresia have almost always had operation by the time they reach adulthood. The tricuspid valve is absent, so systemic blood flows from the right atrium to the left atrium. It then enters the left ventricle and reaches the pulmonary artery through a ventricular septal defect into a hypoplastic right ventricle. This pattern occurs when the great arteries are normally related. Most patients have reduced pulmonary blood flow because of a small ventricular septal defect with or without pulmonary stenosis. If the ventricular septal defect is large, there may be pulmonary hypertension.

Single Ventricle
There are many forms and combinations of abnormalities; the most common type in adulthood is a double-inlet left ventricle with pulmonary stenosis. Patients therefore will have cyanosis with *left* ventricular hypertrophy and signs of pulmonary stenosis.

Truncus Arteriosus
In this condition, the pulmonary arteries arise from the aorta, and the intracardiac anatomy is the same as that for pulmonary atresia. The pulmonary arteries are usually

not stenosed, and so the clinical features are those of Eisenmenger syndrome. Truncal regurgitation is common.

Total Anomalous Pulmonary Venous Drainage

In this condition, all the pulmonary veins drain to the right atrium or a major systemic vein, producing right-sided volume overload. An atrial communication is obligatory. When the venous confluence connects to the left innominate vein, it produces the "snowman" sign on chest radiography. Total anomalous pulmonary venous drainage is very rare in adulthood.

Corrected Transposition With Ventricular Septal Defect and Pulmonary Stenosis

Corrected transposition (levo [L]-transposition) is an anomaly in which there is atrioventricular discordance and ventriculoarterial discordance. Thus, the right atrium enters into the left ventricle, which ejects into the pulmonary artery. The left atrium enters into the morphologic right ventricle, which ejects into the aorta. Thus, the circulation flows correctly (hence the term "corrected" transposition) but flows through the wrong chambers. Atrioventricular valves enter the appropriate ventricle; thus, the flimsy tricuspid valve sits at the mouth of the right ventricle in the systemic circulation. The coronary artery pattern is also reversed. The common associated anomalies are ventricular septal defect; abnormalities of the left atrioventricular valve (tricuspid valve), which is usually regurgitant; and pulmonary stenosis.

Complete heart block is also a common association. Patients may survive to their 50s or 60s if they have corrected transposition and no associated anomalies, but problems often occur because of the morphologic right ventricle supporting the systemic circulation. The presence of an associated defect, particularly left atrioventricular valve regurgitation, usually causes presentation earlier in life. The presence of pulmonary stenosis and ventricular septal defect will produce varying degrees of cyanosis (depending on the severity of the pulmonary stenosis), and the clinical features may resemble those of tetralogy of Fallot.

Electrocardiography

Findings on electrocardiography include absent Q waves in the left precordial leads and Q waves present in the right precordial leads (QR pattern in leads II, III, and V_1).

Chest Radiography

A straight left aortic border (because the aorta does not ascend on the right and the pulmonary trunk is not border-forming on the left) is seen on chest radiographs. The ventricle may show a hump-shaped contour in the region of the left atrial appendage.

Surgical Treatment

The ventricular septal defect, if present, is closed. Relief of pulmonary stenosis may be difficult because of access problems and the danger of producing heart block or damage to the right coronary artery. A conduit is often, therefore, necessary. The left atrioventricular valve cannot be repaired and always needs replacement if regurgitant. This should be performed before there is significant deterioration of the vulnerable right ventricle which is the systemic ventricle.

Eisenmenger Syndrome

Babies born with either a large ventricular septal defect or a large patent ductus arteriosus have a large left-to-right shunt in early childhood with increased blood volume and pressure transmitted to the right side of the heart. The result is pulmonary hypertension and subsequent pulmonary vascular disease, which may become established within the first 2 years of life. Rarely, other intracardiac shunts may also result in Eisenmenger physiology. This reversal of the left-to-right shunt causes cyanosis, and the original congenital heart defect then becomes inoperable. Some infants with large shunts never have any decrease in their pulmonary vascular resistance and have pulmonary vascular disease from an early age. The right-to-left shunting associated with pulmonary hypertension is called Eisenmenger syndrome. It may rarely occur with secundum ASD (<5% of cases), usually later in life.

Physical Examination

Physical examination reveals the following findings: cyanosis and clubbing, jugular venous pressure that may be normal or with a slightly prominent "a" wave, right ventricular lift, ejection click from the dilated pulmonary artery, *little or no* murmur (pressure in both ventricles is equal), loud P_2 (may be palpable), and variable murmur of pulmonary regurgitation. There may be differential cyanosis between the limbs if the patient has a patent ductus arteriosus.

Electrocardiography

Right ventricular hypertrophy is found on electrocardiography.

Chest Radiography

On chest radiography, the following are findings: prominent central pulmonary arteries (may be calcified; these are sometimes mistaken for lymphadenopathy), right ventricular contour, and peripheral pulmonary artery pruning.

Diagnosis

The diagnosis can be made from the findings on physical examination and echocardiography. Rarely, the shunt is missed because the pressure is equal in both chambers and the ventricular septal defect is overlooked. A patent ductus arteriosus may be difficult to see because there is little blood flow through the ductus. The differential diagnosis of Eisenmenger syndrome is primary pulmonary hypertension, but, in comparison patients with Eisenmenger syndrome have a much better long-term survival. Death may occur from acute hypoxia, sudden ventricular arrhythmia, or massive hemoptysis. Patients frequently experience symptomatic deterioration in their 40s but may survive to their 60s. Vasodilatation should be avoided (such as hot tubs and vasodilator therapy). Patients should be followed for progressive right ventricular dilatation and tricuspid regurgitation, which may herald right ventricular failure. They may become extremely symptomatic with the onset of atrial arrhythmias, and sinus rhythm should be maintained whenever possible. Treatment options for primary pulmonary hypertension have been applied to patients with Eisenmenger syndrome and may improve symptoms. These include prostacyclin analogs, endothelin receptor antagonists and phosphodiesterase inhibitors. Other options, rarely performed, are heart-lung transplantation or single-lung transplantation with closure of the defect.

■ Patients with Eisenmenger syndrome have a much better long-term survival than patients with primary pulmonary hypertension.

Hematologic Abnormalities

Patients with cyanosis have increased erythrocytes (it is *not* polycythemia), and management of erythrocytosis may be difficult. Patients with high degrees of erythrocytosis (hemoglobin >20 g/dL, hematocrit >65%) may experience symptoms of hyperviscosity (poor concentration, headache, and fatigue). This condition is uncommon with lower hemoglobin levels (unless the patient is dehydrated). Patients therefore should *not* have therapeutic phlebotomy unless the hemoglobin value is more than 20 g/dL. Frequent phlebotomies, in particular, should be avoided, because they destabilize the erythropoiesis and produce a rebound response from the bone marrow and, ultimately, iron deficiency anemia. When iron-deficient microcytes are produced, this condition not only causes a deterioration in exercise capacity but also, because iron-deficient red cells are less deformable than normal red cells, paradoxically increases the risk of stroke.

Phlebotomy should *never* be performed in patients without concomitant fluid replacement, particularly in patients with Eisenmenger syndrome, who may experience hypotension and even sudden death.

In contrast, although patients with cyanotic heart disease have a slightly increased risk of stroke, they also have hemostatic problems and are at increased risk of bleeding. These hemostatic problems include prolonged prothrombin time, prolonged activated partial thromboplastin time, decreased coagulation factors, decreased platelet count, and abnormal platelet function.

Thus, patients with cyanotic heart disease should never receive anticoagulation therapy unless there is a very strong indication to do so, and, ideally, the international normalized ratio (INR) should be kept on the low side of the therapeutic range.

If a patient with cyanosis is to undergo surgery and the hemoglobin value is more than 20 g/dL, therapeutic phlebotomy with fluid exchange will tend to normalize the hemostatic problems.

Renal Abnormalities

Adults with cyanotic congenital heart disease frequently have abnormal renal function with a reduced glomerular filtration rate, proteinuria, and hyperuricemia. The high uric acid levels are due to a low fractional uric acid excretion and the overproduction of urate from red cell turnover. Hyperuricemia is particularly important when cyanotic patients have cardiac catheterization, and they should *not* be dehydrated around the time of the procedure, particularly because they may require a large amount of imaging contrast, which may induce acute renal failure. Intravenous fluid hydration is indicated in very cyanotic patients, with meticulous attention to fluid balance and good urine output.

Orthopedic Abnormalities

Scoliosis is also much more common in patients with cyanotic heart disease (even in the absence of a lateral thoracotomy). In addition, patients may have a painful arthropathy due to hypertrophic changes in the long bones.

Pulmonary Abnormalities

Patients with Eisenmenger syndrome are at particular risk of hemoptysis (which can be life-threatening and may be due to pulmonary hemorrhage, pulmonary embolus, or in situ pulmonary infarction). In addition, they are vulnerable to vasodilatation, which may prove fatal. Any decrease in blood pressure (such as that produced by vasodilators) may cause increased right-to-left shunting, cerebral hypoxia, and sudden death; thus, patients should not be given injudicious vasodilator therapy. Extreme caution must be used when patients with Eisenmenger syndrome are undergoing noncardiac surgery, and even relatively minor procedures such as appendectomy may prove fatal.

- Adults with cyanotic congenital heart disease frequently have abnormal renal function with a reduced glomerular filtration rate, proteinuria, and hyperuricemia.
- Patients with Eisenmenger syndrome are at particular risk of hemoptysis.

SYNDROMES ASSOCIATED WITH CONGENITAL HEART DISEASE

- Syndromes associated with congenital heart disease include the following:
- Down syndrome: atrioventricular septal defects (atrioventricular canal, primum ASD), ventricular septal defect
- Turner syndrome: coarctation of the aorta, bicuspid aortic valve
- Holt-Oram syndrome: secundum ASD
- Marfan syndrome: aortic dilatation, dissection, and rupture; mitral valve prolapse
- Noonan syndrome: pulmonary stenosis

Right aortic arch is associated with the following:

- Pulmonary atresia
- Truncus arteriosus
- Tetralogy of Fallot

With cardiac apex on one side and gastric bubble on the other, consider the following:

- Corrected transposition
- Single ventricle

If both the cardiac apex *and* the gastric bubble are on the right, the heart may be normal (situs inversus totalis)

THE ELECTROCARDIOGRAM IN ASD

- Right bundle branch block and right-axis deviation: secundum ASD
- Right bundle branch block and left-axis deviation (with or without first-degree atrioventricular block): primum ASD

AMERICAN HEART ASSOCIATION RECOMMENDATIONS FOR ENDOCARDITIS PROPHYLAXIS

Endocarditis prophylaxis is recommended for all patients with congenital heart disease, with the following exceptions:

- For isolated secundum ASD
- More than 6 months after surgical repair of secundum ASD, ventricular septal defect, patent ductus arteriosus (with no residual defect)

HIV INFECTION AND THE HEART

Joseph G. Murphy, MD

Zelalem Temesgen, MD

Cardiac involvement in human immunodeficiency virus (HIV) infection has been described by several autopsy and echocardiography-based studies and is much more prevalent than is clinically apparent. Additionally, as HIV-infected patients live longer as a result of highly active antiretroviral therapy (HAART), cardiovascular problems are becoming more prominent. This is due to the direct effects of HIV infection and indirectly due to its treatment as well as the contribution of other established causes of cardiac disease in other populations.

PERICARDITIS

Pericarditis, often associated with pericardial effusion, is the most common finding in patients with HIV infection. Autopsy series have reported up to 37% prevalence of pericardial disease in HIV-infected patients. The prevalence observed in echocardiographic series is as high as 59%. A 1998 review of the literature on HIV-associated pericardial disease estimated a 21% average incidence of pericardial disease based on analysis of 15 autopsy and echocardiographic series involving 1139 patients with HIV infection. The spectrum of pericardial disease in HIV-infected patients ranges from asymptomatic effusions incidentally detected by echocardiography to potentially fatal tamponade. Most asymptomatic pericardial effusions in HIV patients do not have a specific identifiable etiology. On the other hand, a specific etiology can be established in two-thirds of symptomatic pericardial effusions. The etiologic spectrum of HIV-related pericardial disease is wide and includes infectious organisms and malignancy. Among the infectious causes of pericarditis, mycobacterial organisms, including *M. tuberculosis* and atypical mycobacteria, are often isolated from pericardial effusions in HIV patients—in 34% of 66 published cases of cardiac tamponade. Other infectious causes of pericardial disease in HIV-infected patients include *Staphylococcus aureus*, *Streptococcus pneumoniae*, *Nocardia asteroides*, *Listeria monocytogenes*, *Chlamydia* species, *Histoplasma capsulatum*, *Cryptococcus neoformans*, herpes simplex virus, CMV, and Coxsackie virus. The neoplastic causes of pericardial effusions in AIDS patients are commonly Kaposi's sarcoma and lymphoma.

HIV-infected patients with small nonsymptomatic pericardial effusions should be managed conservatively with follow-up echocardiography at regular intervals but without specific diagnostic or therapeutic interventions. Symptomatic patients and those with large effusions require pericardiocentesis and fluid analysis for cytology, culture and biochemical studies. Pericardial biopsy will increase the diagnostic yield, particularly for the diagnosis of tuberculosis.

Cardiac tamponade may occur with large, or moderately sized but rapidly accumulating pericardial effusions and may be the presenting feature of pericarditis. Cardiac tamponade requires urgent catheter drainage and in many cases a surgically performed pericardial window via a subxiphoid pericardiotomy for refractory effusions. Percutaneous balloon pericardiotomy is generally ineffective and rapidly obstructs. Bacterial or fungal pericarditis should be treated with appropriate drugs. Patients with large refractory pericardial effusions in whom no specific etiology has been established may require empiric antituberculous chemotherapy. Steroids used as an adjunct to antituberculous therapy in patients with HIV infection and tuberculous pericarditis are probably beneficial. Pericarditis due to lymphoma may respond in the short term to radiation therapy and chemotherapy.

- Approximately two-thirds of AIDS patients with symptomatic pericarditis have an identifiable and potentially treatable etiology.
- Mycobacterial infections are a common infectious cause of tamponade in AIDS patients
- Surgical pericardial biopsy is the diagnostic test of choice if pericardial fluid microscopy is negative in patients with suspected tuberculous pericarditis.

MYOCARDITIS AND CARDIOMYOPATHY

The spectrum of myocardial involvement in HIV infection is wide and includes inflammatory myocarditis, dilated cardiomyopathy, and infiltrative neoplastic disease (Fig. 1).

The prevalence of myocarditis in HIV infection is variable depending on the population selected and the methods used. Autopsy studies of HIV-infected adults have reported myocarditis in up to 52% of patients. Echocardiographic series have identified cardiomyopathy in 30 - 40% of HIV-infected patients. A prospective long-term clinical and echocardiographic follow-up study of 952 asymptomatic HIV-positive patients identified dilated cardiomyopathy in 76 patients (8%), with a mean annual incidence rate of 15.9 cases per 1000 patients. A histologic diagnosis of myocarditis was made in 63 of the patients with dilated cardiomyopathy (83%). Association of higher rates of left ventricular dysfunction with lower CD4 counts has

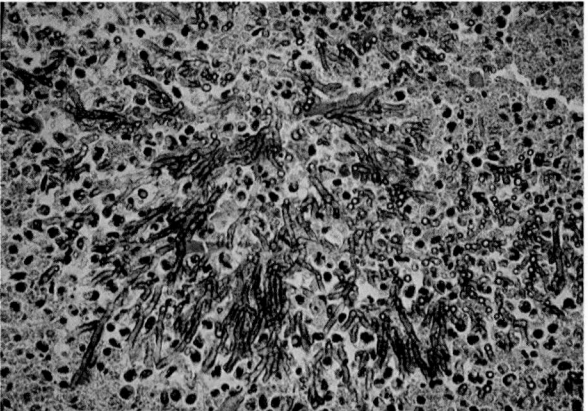

Fig. 1. Aspergillus myocarditis.

also been reported. However, cardiomyopathy has been known to occur before the development of advanced HIV disease. Recent reports have suggested a decline in the prevalence of HIV-associated cardiac disease with the introduction of HAART.

The etiologic spectrum of myocarditis in HIV-infected individuals is wide. HIV has been detected in cardiac tissue by culture, immunohistochemistry, and molecular techniques. However, a direct causal link between the presence of HIV in the myocardium and the induction of myocarditis has not been established. The lack of CD4 cell receptor on myocardial cells further argues against the direct role of HIV in causing myocarditis. A number of mechanisms through which HIV may indirectly cause myocardial disease have been proposed. These include release of various cytokines (interleukin 1-β, interleukin 6, interleukin 9, endothelin-1, tumor necrosis factor α), hypersensitivity from uncontrolled hypergammaglobulinemia, and autoimmunity. Several infectious agents have been implicated in HIV-associated myocardial disease. These include toxoplasmosis, tuberculosis, atypical mycobacterial infections, cryptococcosis, histoplasmosis, CMV, Coxsackie virus, and Chagas disease (Fig. 2). A number of nutritional deficiencies, including selenium, L-carnitine, and vitamin B deficiencies have also been associated with myocardial dysfunction and cardiomyopathy. Several drugs, used either for the treatment of HIV infection itself or its complications, have been associated with cardiac related toxicities. These are listed in Table 1. Finally, cocaine, methamphetamine, and alcohol have been reported to cause cardiac toxicity.

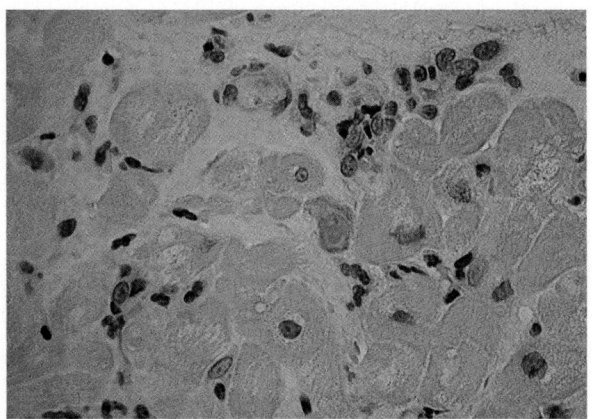

Fig. 2. Cytomegalovirus (CMV) myocarditis.

been identified. The routine use of immunosuppressive therapy to treat myocarditis is not indicated. Treatment of congestive heart failure is the same as for HIV-negative patients. Digoxin should be used in patients with heart failure but myocarditis may increase sensitivity to the drug arrhythmias.

Mortality in HIV-infected patients with cardiomyopathy is increased when compared to HIV-infected patients without cardiomyopathy or non HIV-infected patients with idiopathic dilated cardiomyopathy.

Diagnostic modalities and findings are in general similar to those reported for non HIV-infected patients. Chest radiographs may show cardiomegaly; ECG findings are nonspecific. Echocardiography is the main diagnostic tool in documenting cardiac dysfunction. Myocardial biopsy may be useful but suffers from a lack of sensitivity. A specific etiology is found on biopsy only in a small minority (20%) of cases. Histology generally shows only small focal collections of mononuclear cells, usually without evidence of myocardial necrosis.

The treatment of HIV-associated myocardial disease is directed towards a treatable etiologic agent if one has

PULMONARY VASCULAR DISEASE AND PULMONARY HYPERTENSION

Right ventricular dysfunction is a well documented cardiac complication of HIV infection and occurs in about 10% of AIDS patients with cardiovascular disease. The etiology is probably multifactorial and is seen more frequently in intravenous drug users and patients with a history of chronic pulmonary infections including *Pneumocystis carinii* infection.

Many cases of HIV-related pulmonary hypertension have no additional risk factors for pulmonary hypertension other than the HIV infection itself. The estimated incidence of this entity is 0.5%, 2,500 times greater than the incidence of primary pulmonary hypertension in the general population. No correlation between CD4 cell counts or the presence of opportunistic infection

Table 1.   Select Drugs Used for the Treatment of HIV and/or Its Complications That Have Potential to Cause Cardiac-Related Toxicity

Drug	Effect
Nucleoside analogue reverse transcriptase inhibitors	Mitochondrial toxicity, cardiomyopathy
Non-nucleoside reverse transcriptase inhibitors	Dyslipidemia
Protease inhibitors	Dyslipidemia, increased risk of coronary artery disease, insulin resistance
Trimethoprim-sulfamethoxazole	Torsades de pointets
Pentamidine	Ventricular arrhythmia, torsades de pointes
Anabolic steroids	Increased risk of coronary artery disease
Interferon	Hypertension, hypotension, tachycardia, cardiomyopathy
Doxorubicin	Cardiomyopathy
Vinblastine	Increased risk of coronary artery disease

and the development and progression of pulmonary hypertension has been observed. The pathophysiology of this condition is unclear and there is no evidence that HIV directly infects pulmonary artery endothelial cells. Attempts to detect HIV or its proteins in lung tissue by electron microscopy, immunohistochemical or molecular techniques have not been successful. An indirect role for HIV virus through the release of cytokines (IL-1, IL-6, TNF, endothelin-1) has been proposed. Some studies have suggested a genetic basis for individual susceptibility. Recently, the viral cyclin gene and the latency-associated nuclear antigen (LANA-1) of HHV-8 were detected in 10 out of 16 patients with primary pulmonary hypertension. Only three of these patients were HIV positive and only one of these three patients had the viral cyclin gene detected in lung tissue. An etiologic role for HHV-8 has not yet been established. The histopathology of HIV-associated pulmonary hypertension is similar to that noted in primary pulmonary hypertension in the general population and includes plexogenic pulmonary arteriolar lesions, in-situ thrombotic pulmonary arteriopathy, and pulmonary venoocclusive disease. Symptoms, clinical features, and findings from diagnostic studies are not different from those reported for non HIV-infected patients with primary pulmonary hypertension. Progressive dyspnea is the most common presenting symptom. Chest radiographs show cardiomegaly and pulmonary artery prominence, while right ventricular hypertrophy, right atrial abnormality, and right axis deviation are commonly noted on ECG tracings. Echocardiographic findings usually consist of right heart enlargement, tricuspid regurgitation, and paradoxical septal motion. Doppler echocardiography shows pulmonary arterial systolic pressure >30 mm Hg. Cardiac catheterization confirms increased pulmonary artery and right atrial pressures. Pulmonary capillary pressure is normal.

The treatment of HIV-associated pulmonary hypertension is similar to that of patients with primary pulmonary arterial hypertension: options include pulmonary vasodilators (epoprostenol), calcium channel blockers, oral anticoagulation therapy, diuretics, and sildenafil. Responses have been variable. The effect of antiretroviral therapy on the course of HIV-related pulmonary hypertension is controversial. Some studies have shown a benefit, others have failed to do so.

Worsening of the clinical course with antiretroviral therapy has also been reported.

The prognosis of HIV-related pulmonary hypertension is poor with a median interval from the diagnosis of pulmonary hypertension to death of 6 months.

Endocardial Disease

A common incidental finding at autopsy in patients dying of AIDS is thrombotic nonbacterial marantic endocarditis, a condition in which sterile valvular vegetations occur without an infectious cause. Systemic embolization is an uncommon clinical presentation of marantic endocarditis: valve destruction or clinical valve dysfunction is rare.

Infective endocarditis in HIV-infected patients is uncommon and occurs almost exclusively in intravenous drug users. In a retrospective review of infective endocarditis in HIV-infected patients between 1979 and 1999 at a tertiary care hospital, only 8 out of 599 cases of infective endocarditis were diagnosed in non intravenous drug users. In another review, infective endocarditis was responsible for 5-20% of hospital admissions and for 5-10% of total deaths in intravenous drug using patients with HIV infection. The clinical presentation was similar to what has been observed in HIV-negative patients. The clinical outcome of the patients appeared to depend more on the affected valve and the causative organism rather than the HIV serostatus of the patient. In intravenous drug users, the most common valve involved is the tricuspid valve and the most common causative organism, *Staphylococcus aureus*. The microbiologic spectrum in non-intravenous drug use-related infective endocarditis in HIV-infected patients is wide and includes unusual organisms such as *Salmonella, Aspergillus, Cryptococcus,* and *Candida* species in addition to the usual bacteria causing endocarditis in the general population.

Cardiac Tumors

Kaposi's sarcoma as seen in patients with AIDS, can involve the myocardium and pericardium and classically presents with pericardial effusion or less commonly cardiac tamponade. Primary cardiac lymphoma is a rare malignancy associated with AIDS that presents with heart failure or ventricular arrhythmias secondary to diffuse infiltration of the ventricular wall or less commonly mechanical obstruction to valve function due to localized nodules or intracavitary masses. Surgery, chemotherapy and radiation are generally palliative (Figs. 3 and 4).

CORONARY ARTERY DISEASE

With continued use of HAART and longer survival of HIV-infected patients, a number of metabolic complications of HIV infection and its treatment have been observed. These include dyslipidemias, insulin resistance, hyperglycemia, and body composition changes (lipodystrophy, lipoatrophy). The appreciation of these metabolic disorders associated with antiretroviral therapy has led to a growing concern about a possible increased risk for cardiovascular disease. Results from studies that have attempted to analyze this risk have not always been consistent but the weight of evidence suggests that there is a link between antiretroviral therapy, particularly the use of protease inhibitors, and an increased risk for coronary artery disease. In an analysis of data from a cohort of 5,672 outpatients with HIV-1 at nine US HIV clinics, the use of protease inhibitors (PI) was associated with an increased risk of myocardial infarction. In a study of 19,795 HIV-infected French men receiving a PI-based regimen, morbidity ratios were greater with longer exposure to PIs. Similarly, receipt of a PI-based regimen was associated with myocardial infarction after adjustment for age in the Frankfurt HIV Cohort. The D/A/D study, a large international collaborative observational study, evaluated the incidence of myocardial infarction (MI) in 23,400 HIV-infected

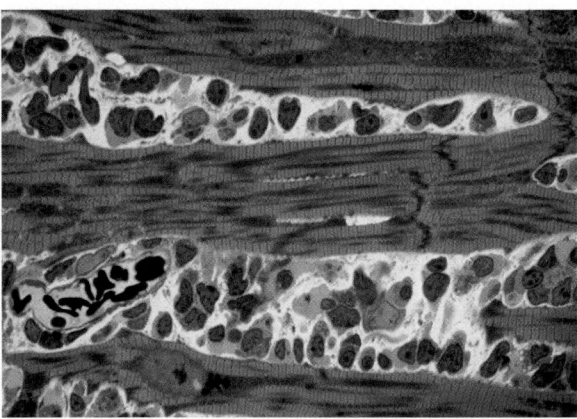
Fig. 4. Lymphoma cells in the myocardium.

patients from 11 cohorts in Europe, Australia, and the United States. The risk for MI rose progressively with the number of years on combination antiretroviral therapy (adjusted relative risk [RR] 1.16/year of exposure [95% CI 1.09 to 1.23]). Increased PI exposure was associated with an increased risk of MI, which is partly explained by dyslipidemia. Age, male sex, a past history of cardiovascular disease, smoking, elevated total cholesterol level at baseline and the presence of diabetes mellitus at baseline were also independent predictors for MI. Contrary to these results, data from a large cohort of HIV-infected patients (n = 36,766) in the Veterans Affairs Health System did not indicate increases in myocardial infarction related hospitalizations, despite the substantial use of PIs.

The risk of HAART-related cardiovascular disease is outweighed by the benefits of antiretroviral therapy and should not be a reason to withhold therapy. While consideration of dyslipidemia and cardiovascular risk is appropriate in the construction of an antiretroviral regimen, virologic suppression remains the overriding goal of antiretroviral therapy. Current guidelines recommend that HIV-infected adults undergo evaluation and treatment on the basis of the National Cholesterol Education Program Adult Treatment Panel (NCEP ATP) guidelines for dyslipidemia. Nonpharmacologic interventions such as dietary counseling, exercise, and modification of other risk factors (e.g. smoking) should generally be attempted first before instituting drug therapies. Pharmacologic therapy of dyslipidemias usually includes treatment with statins with or without fenofibrates. Protease inhibitors are in general sub-

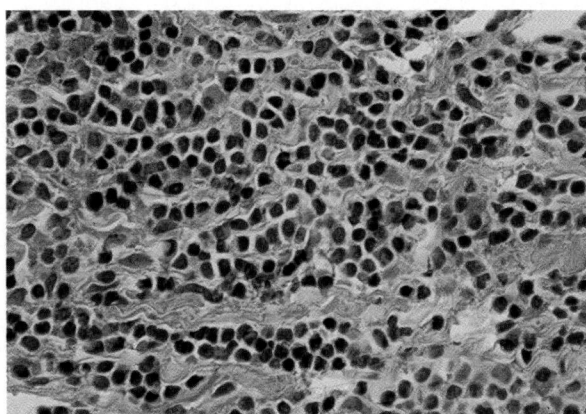
Fig. 3. Primary cardiac lymphoma.

strates as well as inhibitors of cytochrome P450. The primary route of metabolism for most statins is also cytochrome P450. Thus a significant potential for drug interaction exists. Simvastatin and lovastatin should not be used in patients taking PIs or the nonnucleoside reverse transcription inhibitor (NNRTI) delavirdine. Atorvastatin, fluvastatin, pravastatin, and rosuvastatin appear to be safe for use with PIs. Fibrates are metabolized by glucuronidation and thus do not present a significant potential for drug interaction.

INFECTIVE ENDOCARDITIS

Robin Patel, MD

Joseph G. Murphy, MD

James M. Steckelberg, MD

NATIVE VALVE INFECTIVE ENDOCARDITIS

Epidemiology

There are about 15,000 new cases of infective endocarditis annually in the U.S. The annual number of cases of endocarditis has remained relatively constant, but the spectrum of underlying cardiac conditions and the etiologic organisms have changed over time. The median age of patients with infective endocarditis has increased, and currently, about one-half of all patients are older than 60 years, with the median age of those with enterococcal endocarditis even higher.

Infective endocarditis is rare in children and is usually associated with underlying structural congenital heart disease, surgical repair of congenital heart disease, or nosocomial catheter-related bacteremia, especially in infants. Complex congenital heart disease and unrepaired ventricular septal defect are the most common underlying structural cardiac lesions in children.

■ Complex congenital heart disease and unrepaired ventricular septal defect are the most common underlying cardiac lesions predisposing to infective endocarditis in children.

Men are affected 2.5 times more commonly than women by infective endocarditis. Chronic rheumatic valvular disease has been supplanted by mitral valve prolapse with mitral regurgitation and degenerative aortic valve disease as the leading cardiac conditions predisposing to bacterial endocarditis in adults. Nosocomial endocarditis associated with therapeutic interventions (intravenous catheters, hyperalimentation lines, pacemakers, dialysis shunts, etc.) is increasing in frequency. A high proportion of cases of right-sided endocarditis occur in intravenous drug users.

Predisposing Heart Lesions for Endocarditis

The heart valve most commonly involved in infective endocarditis is the mitral valve (Fig. 1), followed by the aortic valve. Isolated aortic valve endocarditis is more common in men than women and often is associated with congenitally bicuspid aortic valve. The mitral valve is infected in more than 85% of cases of infective endocarditis that follow damage by rheumatic fever. The tricuspid valve is typically involved in intravenous drug users, while the pulmonary valve is rarely infected. Both right- and left-sided endocarditis may occur simultaneously (Fig. 1).

We would like to acknowledge Walter R. Wilson, MD, for the generous provision of patient photographs in Figure 1 and Figures 3-14.

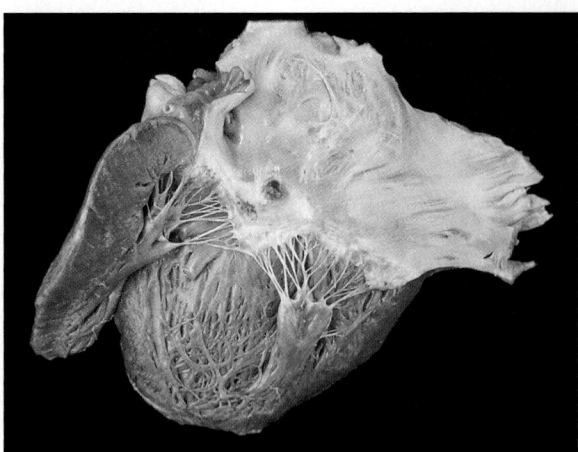

Fig. 1. Infective endocarditis involving the mitral valve.

■ The heart valve most commonly affected by endocarditis is the mitral valve, followed by the aortic, tricuspid, and pulmonary valves.

High Risk

Congenital heart lesions include patent ductus arteriosus, ventricular septal defect, coarctation of the aorta, bicuspid aortic valve, tetralogy of Fallot, and, rarely, pulmonic stenosis. Surgical closure of ventricular septal defect decreases the risk of infective endocarditis provided no residual shunt is present. Endocarditis is extremely rare in secundum atrial septal defects. Patients with hypertrophic cardiomyopathy (HCM) are at increased risk for infective endocarditis, especially those with hemodynamically severe forms of the disease (high peak systolic pressure gradient and markedly symptomatic patients). Either the mitral or aortic valve, or both valves, may be infected.

■ Endocarditis is extremely rare in secundum atrial septal defects.
■ Patients with HOCM and high gradients are at increased risk for endocarditis.

Infective endocarditis is associated with mitral valve prolapse, especially in patients with marked valvular redundancy, valve leaflet thickening, or significant mitral regurgitation.

Unusual organisms may cause endocarditis after immunosuppressed patients following in solid organ transplantation, including *Corynebacterium*, *Candida* species, and *Aspergillus flavus* endocarditis in liver transplant recipients, cytomegalovirus and *Staphylococcus epidermidis* endocarditis in heart transplant recipients, and *Staphylococcus aureus* and *Candida albicans* endocarditis in heart-lung transplant recipients.

Other conditions associated with an increased incidence of infective endocarditis include poor dental hygiene, long-term hemodialysis, diabetes mellitus, and infection with the human immunodeficiency virus (HIV).

■ Mitral valve prolapse with regurgitation and degenerative aortic valve disease are the most common predisposing lesions for infective endocarditis in adults.

Pathogenesis

The development of infective endocarditis (Fig. 2) requires that the valve surface must first be damaged to uncover a suitable site for bacterial attachment and colonization. Typically, this damage is caused by blood flow turbulence, which leads to the deposition of platelets and fibrin and the formation of "nonbacterial thrombotic endocarditis." Hemodynamic factors contribute to the localization of these lesions downstream from a regurgitant flow, characteristically on the atrial surface of the mitral valve and on the ventricular surface of the aortic valve. Lesions with high degrees of turbulence (small ventricular septal defects with jet lesions, valvular stenoses) valve regurgitation readily create conditions that lead to bacterial colonization, whereas defects with large surface areas (large ventricular septal defects), low flow (ostium secundum atrial septal defects), or attenuation of turbulence (congestive heart failure) are rarely implicated in infective endocarditis.

■ Infective endocarditis characteristically occurs on the atrial surface of the mitral valve and on the ventricular surface of the aortic valve.

After the formation of the nonbacterial thrombotic media, bacteria colonize the lesion. Transient bacteremia typically occurs when a mucosal surface heavily colonized with bacteria is traumatized, as with dental procedures and with gastrointestinal, urologic, and gynecologic procedures. The degree of bacteremia is proportional to the trauma produced by the procedure

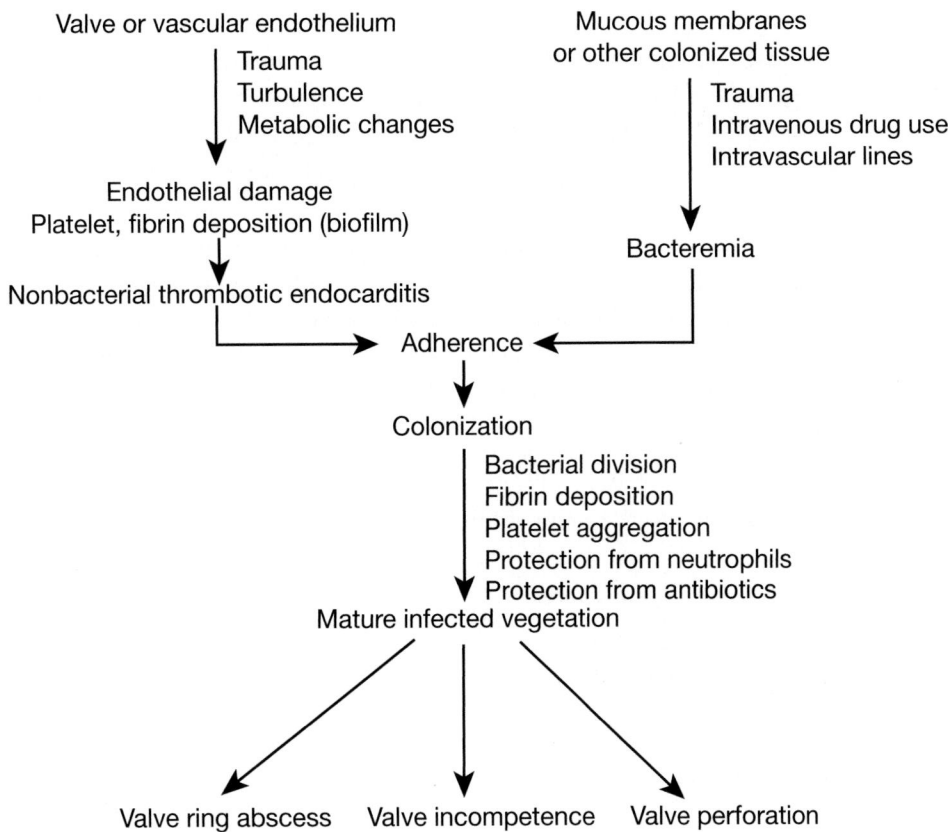

Fig. 2. Pathogenesis of infective endocarditis.

and the number of organisms inhabiting the area. Most of the cases of bacterial endocarditis cannot be attributed to an identifiable invasive procedure.

Certain species and strains of bacteria appear to have a selective advantage in adhering to platelets, fibrin, or valvular endothelium and/or formation of biofilm. Biofilm is particularly important in the context of foreign bodies (e.g., prosthetic heart valves, cardiovascular devices).

After colonization of the valve occurs and a critical mass of adherent bacteria develops, the vegetation enlarges by additional deposition of platelets and fibrin and continued proliferation of bacteria.

■ Less than one-half of the cases of bacterial endocarditis can be attributed to an identifiable invasive procedure.

Infective endocarditis stimulates both humoral and cellular immunity. Rheumatoid factor develops in about one-half of the patients with infective endocarditis of more than 6 weeks' duration. Antinuclear

antibodies may also occur in infective endocarditis and contribute to musculoskeletal manifestations, low-grade fever, and pleuritic pain. Circulating immune complexes are found with increased frequency in connection with a long duration of illness, extravalvular manifestations, hypocomplementemia, and right-sided infective endocarditis. Concentrations decrease with successful therapy. Patients with infective endocarditis and circulating immune complexes may develop a diffuse glomerulonephritis. Immune complexes and complement are deposited subepithelially along the glomerular basement membrane to form a "lumpy-bumpy" pattern. Some of the peripheral manifestations of infective endocarditis, such as Osler nodes, may also result from the deposition of circulating immune complexes.

■ The vascular endothelium is damaged most often by turbulent blood flow; platelets and fibrin are deposited; the nonbacterial thrombotic endocarditis lesion is seeded during a bacteremic episode, and a mature vegetation develops.

Pathologic Changes

Pathologic changes of infective endocarditis are shown in Table 1. The classic vegetation is located along the line of closure of the valve leaflet. Vegetations may be single or multiple, vary from a few millimeters to several centimeters in size. With treatment, healing occurs by fibrosis and, occasionally, calcification. In acute endocarditis, the vegetation is larger, softer, and more friable. Infection may lead to perforation of the valve leaflet or rupture of the chordae tendineae, interventricular septum, or papillary muscle. Endocarditis, especially *S.* *aureus* endocarditis, may produce valve-ring abscesses, with fistula formation into the myocardium or pericardial sac. Aneurysms of the valve leaflet or sinus of Valsalva are also seen. Myocardial abscesses are associated with *S. aureus* endocarditis, high fever, rapid onset of congestive heart failure, and conduction disturbances. Embolic phenomena are common in infective endocarditis; major embolic episodes occur in at least one-third of patients. Most emboli occur before diagnosis, the incidence of emboli falls once effective antimicrobial therapy begins. Embolic phenomena most frequently involve

Table 1. Pathologic Findings in Infective Endocarditis

Location	Manifestation	Comment
Central nervous system	Cerebral emboli	
	Cerebral infarction	
	Arteritis	
	Abscess	
	Mycotic aneurysm	
	Intracerebral or subarachnoid hemorrhage	
	Cerebritis	
	Meningitis	
Spleen	Splenic infarct	
	Splenic abscess	
	Splenic enlargement	Pathologic findings include hyperplasia of lymphoid follicles, proliferation of reticuloendothelial cells, scattered focal necrosis
Lung	Pulmonary emboli	Associated with right-sided infective endocarditis
	Pleural effusion	
	Empyema	
Skin	Petechiae	
	Osler nodes	Consist of arteriolar intimal proliferation with extension to venules and capillaries, which may be accompanied by thrombosis and necrosis; diffuse perivascular infiltrate consisting of neutrophils and monocytes surrounds dermal vessels; immune complexes may be seen in dermal vessels
	Janeway lesions	Consist of bacteria, neutrophilic infiltration, necrosis, and subcutaneous hemorrhage; secondary to septic emboli; subcutaneous abscesses on histologic examination
Eye	Roth spots	Consist of lymphocytes surrounded by edema and hemorrhage in nerve fiber layer of retina

the cerebral, renal, splenic, or coronary circulation. When large emboli occlude major vessels, consider fungal endocarditis, marantic endocarditis, or an intracardiac myxoma.

- Circulating immune complexes have been found in high titer in virtually all patients with infective endocarditis.
- *S. aureus* is frequently associated with valve-ring abscesses and myocardial abscess.

Renal Complications of Infective Endocarditis

Abscess, infarction, or glomerulonephritis may be found in the kidney in infective endocarditis (Fig. 3 and 4). Glomerulonephritis may be a focal, local, or segmental process characterized by endothelial and mesangial proliferation, hemorrhage, neutrophilic infiltration, fibrinoid necrosis, crescent formation, and healing by fibrosis. Diffuse glomerulonephritis, consisting of generalized cellular hyperplasia in all glomerular tufts, may also be seen. Less commonly, membranoproliferative glomerulonephritis, characterized by marked mesangial proliferation and by splitting of the glomerular basement membrane, may be found.

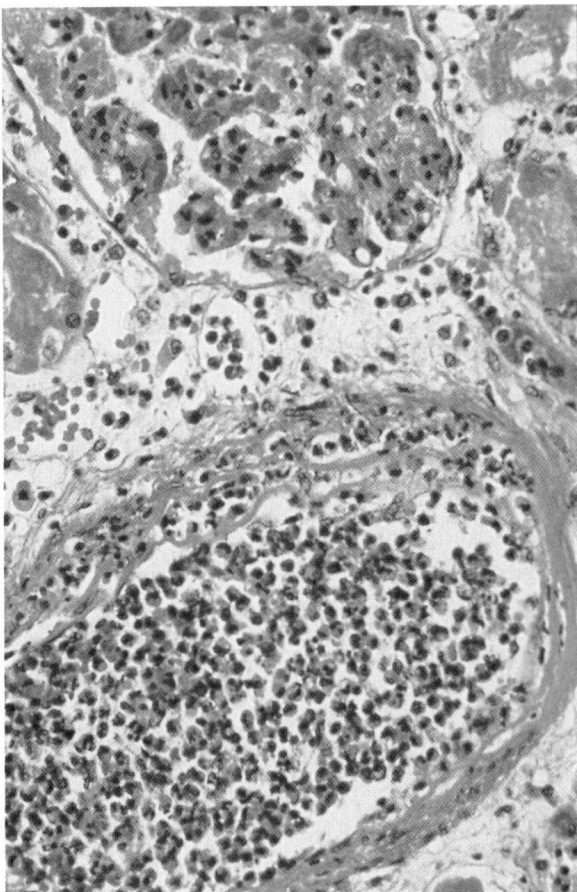

Fig. 4. Microscopic appearance of kidney in *S. aureus* endocarditis.

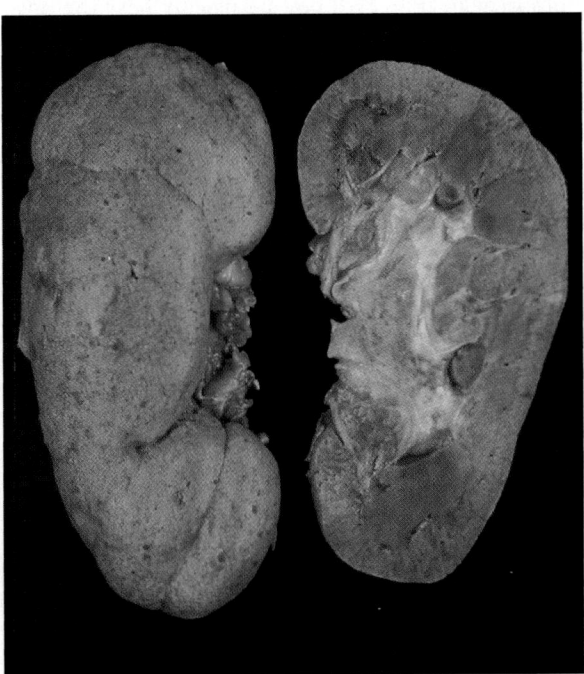

Fig. 3. Gross appearance of kidney in *S. aureus* endocarditis.

- Glomerulonephritis may be a focal, local, or segmental process.

Mycotic Aneurysms

Mycotic aneurysms may develop during active infective endocarditis, rarely months to years after successful therapy. They may arise by 1) direct bacterial invasion of the arterial wall, with subsequent abscess formation or rupture; 2) septic or bland embolic occlusion of the vasa vasorum; or 3) immune complex deposition, with resultant injury to the arterial wall. Mycotic aneurysms tend to occur at bifurcation points and are found in the cerebral vessels (especially the peripheral branches of the middle cerebral artery), but they also occur in the abdominal aorta, sinus of Valsalva, ligated patent ductus arteriosus, and in splenic, coronary, pulmonary, and superior mesenteric arteries. Importantly, mycotic aneurysms often are silent clinically until rupture occurs.

■ Central nervous system mycotic aneurysms are usually silent clinically until rupture occurs.

Clinical Manifestations

Clinical manifestations of infective endocarditis are listed in Table 2. Fever is the most common manifestation but is not present in elderly patients who have blunted febrile responses. Prolonged fever is associated with *S. aureus*, gram-negative bacilli, fungi, culture-negative endocarditis, embolization of major vessels, myocardial abscess, tissue infarction, pulmonary emboli, drug fever, and nosocomial infection. In patients with prolonged fever, abdominal computed tomography (CT) may be helpful to rule out splenic abscess, and transesophageal echocardiography, to exclude valve-ring abscess.

Table 2.   Clinical Manifestations of Infective Endocarditis

Symptom	Physical finding
Fever	Fever
Chills	Heart murmur
Weakness	Changing murmur
Dyspnea	New murmur
Sweats	Embolic phenomena
Anorexia	Skin manifestations--Osler
Weight loss	nodes, petechiae, Janeway
Malaise	lesions
Cough	Splenomegaly
Skin lesions	Septic complications--
Stroke	pneumonia, meningitis, etc.
Nausea	Mycotic aneurysms
Vomiting	Clubbing
Headache	Retinal lesions
Myalgia	Signs of renal failure
Arthralgia	Arthritis--reactive or infectious
Edema	Mucosal petechiae (e.g., palate,
Chest pain	conjunctiva)
Abdominal pain	Splinter hemorrhages
Delirium	
Coma	
Hemoptysis	
Back pain	

Heart murmurs occur in most patients but may be absent with right-sided endocarditis. The classic changing murmur or new murmur is uncommon but may be seen with acute staphylococcal disease. More than 90% of patients who demonstrate a new regurgitant murmur will develop congestive heart failure (the leading cause of death in infective endocarditis). Pericarditis is rare, and when present, it is usually accompanied by myocardial abscess formation as a complication of *S. aureus* infection.

■ Prolonged fever is associated with *S. aureus*.
■ More than 90% of patients who demonstrate a new regurgitant murmur will develop congestive heart failure.

Peripheral Lesions in Endocarditis

Osler nodes are small, painful nodular lesions usually found on the pads of the fingers or toes and occasionally on the thenar eminence (Fig. 5). They range in size from 2 to 15 mm and are frequently multiple. They disappear in a matter of hours to days. Janeway lesions are hemorrhagic, macular, painless plaques with a predilection for the palms or soles (Fig. 6). They persist for several days and are thought to be embolic in origin. Roth spots are oval pale retinal lesions surrounded by hemorrhage (Fig. 7). They are usually near the optic disk. They are not specific for infective endocarditis. Musculoskeletal manifestations of infective endocarditis include proximal arthralgias, lower extremity mono- or oligoarticular arthritis, low back pain, and diffuse myalgias. Splinter hemorrhages and palatal or conjunc-

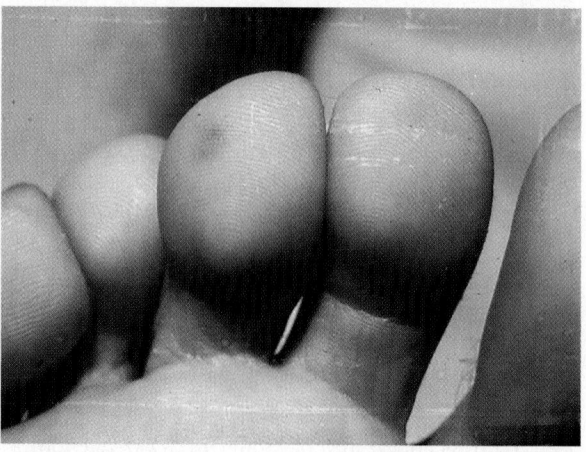

Fig. 5. Osler node.

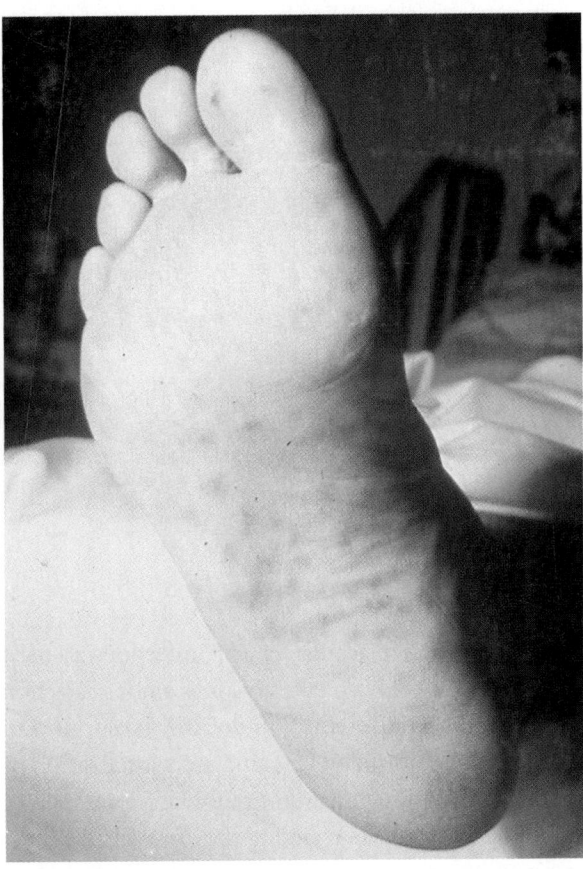

Fig. 6. Janeway lesions.

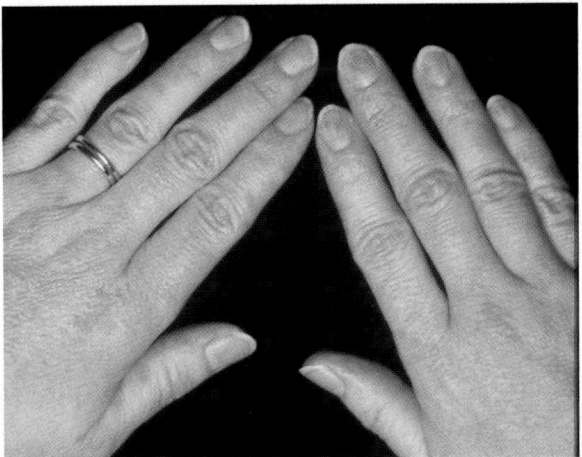

Fig. 8. Splinter hemorrhage.

tival petechiae may occur but are not specific for infective endocarditis (Fig. 7-10).

- Osler nodes are small, painful nodular lesions usually found on the pads of the fingers or toes.
- Janeway lesions are hemorrhagic, macular, painless plaques with a predilection for the palms or soles.

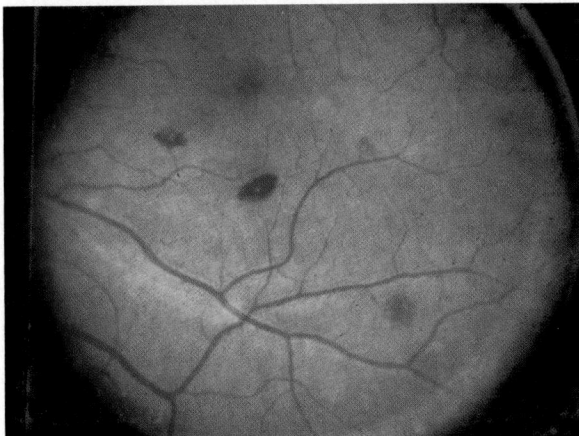

Fig. 7. Roth spots.

Embolic Events

Major embolic episodes are an important complication of infective endocarditis. Splenic artery emboli with infarction may result in left upper quadrant abdominal pain (with radiation to the left shoulder), splenic or pleural rubs, or left pleural effusion. Renal infarctions may be associated with microscopic or gross hematuria. Retinal artery emboli are rare and may be manifested by a complete, sudden loss of vision. Pulmonary emboli arising from right-sided endocarditis are a common feature in intravenous drug users. Coronary artery emboli usually arise from the aortic valve and may result in septic myocarditis with arrhythmias or myocardial infarction. Major vessel emboli (femoral, brachial, popliteal, or radial arteries) are more frequent in fungal endocarditis. Major cerebral emboli may result in hemiplegia, sensory loss, ataxia, aphasia, or alteration in mental status.

- Splenic artery emboli with infarction may result in left upper quadrant abdominal pain (with radiation to the left shoulder).
- Renal infarctions may be associated with microscopic or gross hematuria.

Neurologic Complications

Neurologic manifestations occur in one-third of patients with infective endocarditis. Up to 50% of these patients present with neurologic signs and symptoms as heralding features of their illness. Mycotic aneurysms

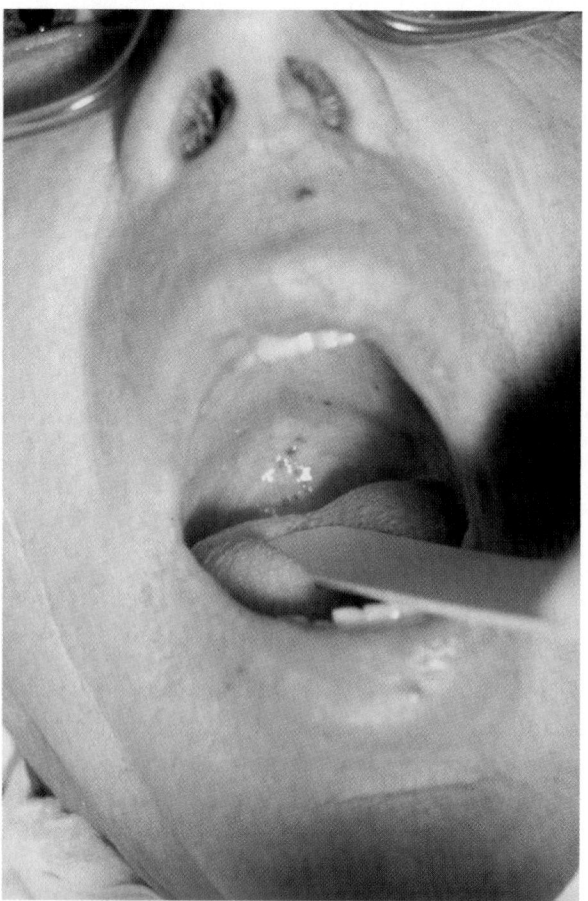

Fig. 9. Palatal petechiae.

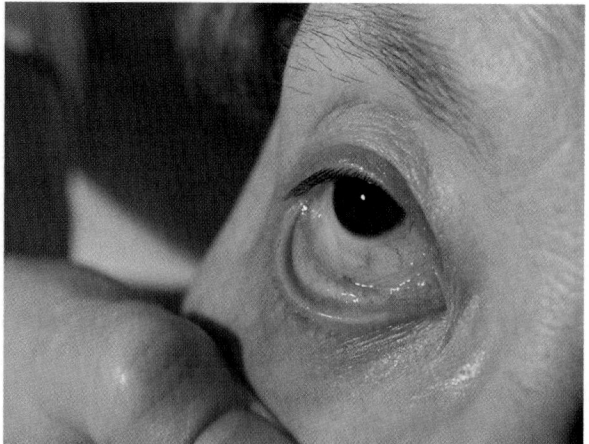

Fig. 10. Conjuctival petechiae.

of the cerebral circulation occur in 2% to 10% of patients (Fig. 11). Typically, these aneurysms are single, small, and peripheral and may lead to devastating subarachnoid hemorrhage. Other neurologic features include seizures, severe headache, visual changes, choreoathetoid movements, mononeuropathy, cranial nerve palsies, and toxic encephalopathy. Most central nervous system complications of infective endocarditis precede the diagnosis of infective endocarditis and initiation of effective therapy (Fig. 12).

■ Neurologic manifestations occur in one-third of patients with infective endocarditis.

Infective Endocarditis in Injection Drug Addicts
The risk for the development of endocarditis among injection drug addicts is as high as 5% per patient per year and may be higher in patients who previously had

prosthetic valve replacement. Acute infections account for the majority of hospital admissions among injection drug addicts, and infective endocarditis is found in ~10% of these episodes. Cocaine use, visualization of vegetations with echocardiography, and presence of embolic phenomena are among the most reliable indicators of infective endocarditis in febrile injection drug users. In this group of patients, two-thirds have no clinical evidence of preexisting underlying heart disease, and there is a predilection for infection of the tricuspid valve. The predominance of right-sided endocarditis in injection drug addicts is presumed to be due to the injection of both drug and adjunctive compounds used

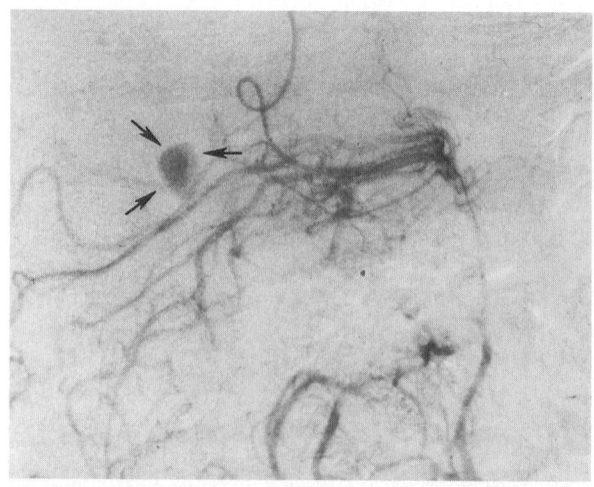

Fig. 11. Mycotic aneurysm (*arrows*).

to dilute the active agent, resulting in endocardial damage of the tricuspid (and pulmonic) valves. Tricuspid valve infection may result in pleuritic chest pain, cough, and hemoptysis, with chest radiographic findings of infiltrates and effusions. Signs of tricuspid insufficiency are present in a small proportion of these cases. The microbiology of endocarditis associated with injection drug addicts differs from that of nonaddicts, with a higher prevalence of gram-negative, fungal, and staphylococcal organisms identified. The course of acute *S. aureus* endocarditis in injection drug addicts tends to be less severe than in nonaddicts.

- Changing murmurs or new murmurs are important findings in endocarditis but are uncommon.
- Cutaneous manifestations of endocarditis include petechiae, Osler nodes, and Janeway lesions.

Laboratory Findings in Infective Endocarditis

Anemia is seen in ~75% of patients and typically is a mild normochromic normocytic anemia. Leukocytosis is seen in about one-third of patients and typically is mild; leukopenia is occasionally noted, especially in conjunction with splenomegaly. Large mononuclear cells (histiocytes) may be noted in peripheral blood. Positive rheumatoid factor, hypocomplementemia, a false-positive VDRL test, and a false-positive Lyme serologic test may occur in endocarditis. Circulating immune complexes as well as mixed-type cryoglobulins may also be detected. The results of urinalysis may reveal proteinuria, microscopic hematuria, red blood cell casts, gross hematuria, pyuria, white blood cell casts, or bacteriuria.

- A false-positive VDRL test and a false-positive Lyme serologic test may occur in endocarditis.

Blood Culture

Blood culture is the most important laboratory test for diagnosing infective endocarditis. The bacteremia of infective endocarditis is typically continuous and low grade. When bacteremia is present, the first two blood cultures will yield the etiologic agent in more than 90% of cases. At least three blood culture sets should be obtained during the first 24 hours. More cultures may be necessary if the patient has received an antimicrobial agent in the preceding 2 weeks. Nutritionally variant streptococci require supplementation of the culture media. Some unusual organisms, such as *Brucella* species, *Nocardia* species, and members of the HACEK group (see below), are slow-growing, sometimes requiring that cultures be held for extended incubation (4 weeks). Special culture techniques or media may be required for some organisms (e.g., *Legionella* species, mycobacteria). Tissue cell culture may be useful for isolating obligate intracellular bacteria (e.g., *Coxiella burnetii*, *Chlamydia* species) from blood, vegetations, or valvular tissues. Blood culture results are negative in more than 50% of cases of fungal endocarditis.

When embolization to major vessels occurs, embolectomy should be performed and the material examined with stains and culture for fungi.

Serologic studies are useful for the diagnosis of Q fever, murine typhus, bartonellosis, brucellosis, legionellosis, and psittacosis. Gram stain of resected valve specimens may be helpful in the diagnosis of infective endocarditis.

- Blood culture is the most important test for diagnosing infective endocarditis.
- Blood cultures are negative in more than 50% of cases of fungal endocarditis.
- Endocarditis is often associated with anemia and an increased erythrocyte sedimentation rate.
- At least three blood culture sets should be obtained during the first 24 hours.

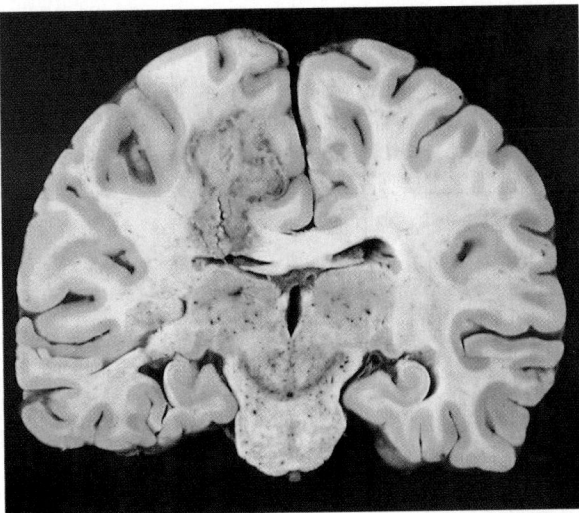

Fig. 12. Brain abscess caused by *Aspergillus* species in a patient with *Aspergillus* infective endocarditis. (From same patient as in Fig. 14.)

Polymerase Chain Reaction

The polymerase chain reaction (PCR) can be used to detect organisms which grow poorly (or not at all) using conventional culture techniques. It can be applied to blood, excised vegetations, or systemic emboli. There are two basic approaches to PCR for the diagnosis of infective endocarditis. The first detects a genetic target unique to a specific genus or species of microorganism. The second broadly detects nucleic acid common to a large group of organisms based on a conserved genetic target. A common target used for broad range detection of bacteria using PCR is 16S ribosomal DNA which is present in all bacteria (but not in humans). Broad range amplification of 16S ribosomal DNA can be followed by sequencing of amplified DNA to identify the source bacterium. Several caveats about PCR should be noted. PCR is a very sensitive technique and can be associated with false-positive results. A positive PCR result must always be interpreted within the clinical context. Even several months after therapy for infective endocarditis, PCR results may still be positive. Since PCR does not provide information about antimicrobial susceptibility, routine culture and susceptibility testing remain important in the microbiologic diagnosis of infective endocarditis.

Echocardiography

Echocardiography is central in both the diagnosis and management of infective endocarditis. Specific echocardiographic findings are part of the Duke major diagnostic criteria. The objectives of the echocardiographic evaluation in a patient with suspected infective endocarditis are summarized in Table 3.

There may be one or more vegetations involving one or more valves. Infrequent locations for vegetations (e.g., left atrial or ventricular wall in the path of a regurgitant jet) should also be assessed. When a vegetation is detected, size, location, and connections with other structures and associated local complications should be assessed. The characteristic finding noted in patients with endocarditis is shaggy dense irregular echoes distributed uniformly on one or more leaflets. The average size of vegetations is similar on the aortic and mitral valves. Tricuspid valve vegetations are typically significantly larger and pulmonic valve vegetations usually smaller.

Large vegetations on the mitral valve, especially on the anterior leaflet, are associated with a higher risk of embolism than vegetations of similar size elsewhere. Overall, the presence or absence of a vegetation and its size does not accurately predict future embolic events. Also, vegetation size has no definite relationship to the incidence of heart failure, the risk of death during the acute phase of infective endocarditis, or the final outcome. There is no size or location threshold that accurately predicts increased mortality associated with embolization in such a way as to justify surgery for the prevention of embolization. An increase in the size of vegetations detected by echocardiography during the course of therapy may identify a subgroup of patients with a higher rate of complications. Persistence of vegetations, as determined by echocardiography, is common after successful medical treatment of infective endocarditis and is not closely associated with late complications. Conversely, sudden disappearance of a vegetation may imply fragmentation and embolization (Fig. 13).

Transthoracic echocardiography has excellent specificity (98%) but low sensitivity (30%-40%) for detection of small vegetations. Transthoracic echocardiography is inadequate in up to 20% of adult patients because of obesity, chronic obstructive pulmonary disease, endotracheal intubation, or chest-wall deformities. Transthoracic echocardiography may be used in the initial evaluation of patients with suspected infective endocarditis involving native valves but is generally much less useful in prosthetic valve endocarditis

---

Table 3.   Objectives of Echocardiography in a Patient With Suspected Infective Endocarditis

Detection of presence, location, and size of vegetations

Evaluation of functional deficiencies of involved valves (e.g., valvular regurgitation)

Identification of anatomy of infected valves and other possible companion diseases

Assessment of consequences of valvular dysfunction (e.g., left ventricular function, pulmonary hypertension)

Detection of other intracardiac complications (e.g., myocardial abscess)

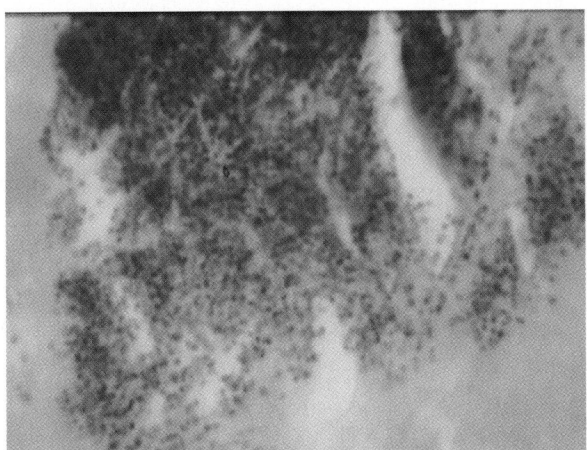

Fig. 13. Gram stain of *S. aureus* vegetation from a patient with infective endocarditis.

because of acoustic shadowing of the valve. If the clinical probability of native valve infective endocarditis is less than 4%, a negative transthoracic echocardiography is cost effective and clinically satisfactory in excluding infective endocarditis. In patients in whom the clinical probability of infective endocarditis is 4% or greater, negative transthoracic echocardiography should be followed by transesophageal echocardiography. Patients who should undergo urgent transesophageal echocardiography include those with gram-positive coccal bacteremia, those with catheter-associated *S. aureus* bacteremia, and those admitted with fever or bacteremia in the setting of injection drug use. Transesophageal echocardiography does not significantly improve the diagnostic accuracy of transthoracic echocardiography in the detection of vegetations associated with right-sided endocarditis in injection drug abusers, but is useful for detecting paravalvar abscess formation and for diagnosing unusual forms of right-sided endocarditis such as pulmonary valve involvement or infection of the eustachian valve. Transesophageal echocardiography is more sensitive than transthoracic echocardiography in detecting intracardiac vegetations, perivalvular abscesses, vegetations associated with prosthetic valves and vegetations smaller than 5 mm. Transesophageal echocardiography with color-flow Doppler techniques can be used to demonstrate the distinctive flow patterns of a fistula, pseudoaneurysm, or unruptured abscess cavity and is more sensitive than transthoracic echocardiography for identifying valvular perforation.

Negative findings on transesophageal echocardiography decrease the likelihood of endocarditis but do not exclude the diagnosis. Causes of such negative findings include an incomplete study, vegetation size less than 2 mm, prosthetic valve endocarditis, calcified valves, and vegetation fragmentation and embolization prior to the study. For patients with suspected right-sided infective endocarditis who are injection drug abusers, a transthoracic echocardiogram should first be performed. If there is a moderate or high suspicion of infective endocarditis, and initial transthoracic echocardiography is negative, this study should be repeated after an interval of about one week. Transesophageal echocardiography is recommended for patients in whom quality images are not obtained with transthoracic echocardiography.

The development of a new high-grade atrioventricular block or bundle branch block seen on electrocardiography is highly specific as a predictor of perivalvular abscess. The degree of mitral valve preclosure in patients with aortic insufficiency, as determined by echocardiography, correlates with increased left ventricular end-diastolic pressure and the severity of hemodynamic compromise.

CT and/or MRI of the head is indicated in all patients with endocarditis and neurologic symptoms. Infarction, hemorrhage, or abscess usually can be differentiated by these techniques. Cerebral angiography should be considered for selected patients with neurologic symptoms not readily explained with other imaging to exclude intracranial mycotic aneurysm.

■ Transesophageal echocardiography is more sensitive than transthoracic echocardiography in the detection of intracardiac vegetations and perivalvular abscess.

Diagnostic Criteria

The Duke diagnostic criteria for infective endocarditis are listed in Table 4*A*, and definitions of the diagnostic terms are given in Table 4*B*.

Microbiology

Streptococcal Endocarditis

Streptococci are the most common causative agents of native valve infective endocarditis in nonintravenous drug users (Table 5). Of these, viridans group streptococci are the most common subgroup and frequently

Table 4A. Duke Criteria for Diagnosis of Infective Endocarditis

Definite infective endocarditis
    Pathologic criteria
        1. Microorganism demonstrated by culture or histologic examination* of a vegetation, a vegetation that has embolized, or an intracardiac abscess specimen; or
        2. Pathologic lesions; vegetation or intracardiac abscess confirmed by histologic examination showing active endocarditis
    Clinical criteria
        1. 2 major criteria; or
        2. 1 major criteria and 3 minor criteria; or
        3. 5 minor criteria
Possible infective endocarditis
        1. 1 major criterion and 1 minor criterion; or
        2. 3 minor criteria
Rejected
        1. Firm alternate diagnosis explaining evidence of infective endocarditis; or
        2. Resolution of infective endocarditis syndrome with antimicrobial therapy for ≤4 days; or
        3. No pathologic evidence of infective endocarditis at surgery or autopsy, with antimicrobial therapy for ≤4 days; or
        4. Does not meet criteria for possible infective endocarditis, as above

*Some authors suggest that a microorganism detected by molecular-based techniques or by Gram stain, may fulfill a pathologic criterion.

are of oral origin. The cure rate of streptococcal endocarditis exceeds 90%, although complications occur in more than 30% of cases. An association of *Streptococcus gallolyticus* (formerly *Streptococcus bovis*) bacteremia with carcinoma of the colon and other lesions of the gastrointestinal tract has been shown; colonoscopy and/or barium enema should be performed when this organism is isolated from blood cultures.

Streptococcus pneumoniae is a rare cause of infective endocarditis; however, when present, it typically has a fulminant course and often is associated with perivalvular abscess formation and pericarditis. In *S. pneumoniae* infective endocarditis, the aortic valve is typically involved and many such patients have a history of alcohol abuse. Concurrent meningitis is present in ~70% of patients. Infective endocarditis due to *Abiotrophia defectiva* and *Granulicatella adiacens* (formerly nutritionally variant streptococci) is typically indolent in onset and associated with previous heart disease. Therapy is difficult because of systemic embolization and frequent relapse.

Group B streptococcus (*Streptococcus agalactiae*) may cause infective endocarditis. Risk factors for group B streptococcal infective endocarditis in adults include diabetes mellitus, carcinoma, alcoholism, liver failure, elective abortion, and injection drug abuse. Group B streptococcal endocarditis has been associated with villous adenomas of the colon. The mortality of this type of infection approaches 50%. A similar clinical picture with a destructive process, left-sided predominance, frequent complications, and high mortality has been observed with group A or G streptococcus. *Streptococcus anginosus* is a rare cause of infective endocarditis, but it is notable because it has a predilection for suppurative complications involving the brain and liver; perinephric, myocardial, and other abscesses; cholangitis; peritonitis; pericarditis; and empyema more characteristic of *S. aureus* infections.

■ Viridans group streptococci are the most common causative agents of native valve infective endocarditis in noninjection drug abusers.

Table 4B. Definition of Terms Used in the Diagnostic Criteria

Major criteria

Blood culture positive for infective endocarditis

1. Typical microorganisms consistent with infective endocarditis from 2 separate blood cultures:
   Viridans group *Streptococcus* species; *Streptococcus gallolyticus* (formerly *Streptococcus bovis*),
   HACEK group, *Staphylococcus aureus*; or community-acquired *Enterococcus* species, in the
   absence of a primary focus or

2. Microorganism consistent with infective endocarditis from persistently positive cultures, defined as
   follows:
   At least 2 positive cultures of blood samples drawn >12 h apart; or
   All of 3 or a majority of ≥4 separate cultures of blood (with first and last sample drawn at least
   1 h apart)

3. Single positive blood culture for *Coxiella burnetii* or antiphase I IgG antibody titer >1:800

Evidence of endocardial involvement

Echocardiogram positive for infective endocarditis (transesophageal echocardiography recommended in
   patients with prosthetic valves, rated at least "possible infective endocarditis" by clinical criteria, or
   complicated infective endocarditis (paravalvular abscess); transthoracic echocardiography as first test in
   other patients), defined as follows:

1. Oscillating intracardiac mass on valve or supporting structures, in the path of regurgitant jets, or on
   implanted material in the absence of an alternative anatomic explanation; or

2. Abscess; or

3. New partial dehiscence of prosthetic valve

New valvular regurgitation (worsening or changing of pre-existing murmur not sufficient)

Minor criteria

Predisposition, predisposing heart condition or injection drug use

Fever, temperature >38°C

Vascular phenomena, major arterial emboli, septic pulmonary infarct, mycotic aneurysm, intracranial
   hemorrhage, conjunctival hemorrhage, and Janeway's lesions

Immunologic phenomena: glomerulonephritis, Osler nodes, Roth spots, and rheumatoid factor

Microbiological evidence: positive blood culture but does not meet a major criterion as noted above[†] or
   serological evidence of active infection consistent with infective endocarditis[‡]

---

*Including *Abiotrophia defectiva, Granulicatella adiacens*.
[†]Excludes single positive cultures for coagulase negative staphylococci and organisms that do not cause endocarditis.
[‡]Serologic test result positive for *Brucella* species, *Chlamydia* species, *Legionella* species, *Bartonella* species.

- The cure rate of nonenterococcal streptococcal endocarditis is more than 90%.
- Viridans group streptococci are often of oral origin.
- *S. gallolyticus* (formerly *S. bovis*) may be associated with colon lesions.

Enterococcal Endocarditis

Enterococcal endocarditis typically affects older men after genitourinary tract manipulation or younger women after an obstetric procedure. More than 40% of patients with enterococcal endocarditis have no previously recognized underlying heart disease, although more than 95% develop a heart murmur during the course of the illness. Classic peripheral manifestations are uncommon. Factors that suggest that a patient with enterococcal bacteremia may have infective endocarditis include no identifiable extracardiac focus of infection and preexistent valvular heart disease or heart murmur.

Staphylococcal Endocarditis

Staphylococci are the second most common cause of infective endocarditis. Of the staphylococci, *S. aureus* is the most common cause of native valve infective endocarditis (Fig. 13) and may attack normal heart valves in addition to diseased ones. The course of *S. aureus* infective endocarditis is typically fulminant when it involves the mitral or aortic valve, with widespread metastatic infection and a 40% chance of death. Myocardial abscesses, purulent pericarditis, valve-ring abscesses, and peripheral foci of suppuration (lung, brain, spleen, kidney, etc.) are common with *S. aureus* infective endocarditis. Approximately one-third of patients with *S. aureus* endocarditis experience neurologic manifestations, with two-thirds or more of this group presenting with neurologic symptoms before initiation of antimicrobial therapy. The most frequent neurologic presentation is hemiparesis. In injection drug addicts, *S. aureus* is the most frequent cause of infective endocarditis, but the disease tends to be less severe than that in nonaddicted patients. Children with endocarditis due to *S. aureus* are more likely than those with infections due to viridans group streptococci to have prolonged fever, complications and to require surgery. Infective endocarditis caused by methicillin-resistant *S. aureus* is increasingly common, especially in injection drug addicts. Coagulase-negative staphylococci are an important cause of prosthetic valve endocarditis.

- Staphylococci are an important cause of infective endocarditis.
- In injection drug addicts, *S. aureus* is the most frequent cause of infective endocarditis.
- *S. aureus* endocarditis has frequent intra- and extra-cardiac complications.

Gram-Negative Endocarditis

Gram-negative bacilli may also cause infective endocarditis. Typically, the gram-negative bacilli involved are fastidious organisms such as those belonging to the HACEK group (see below), although occasionally the *Enterobacteriaciae* may be involved. Persons addicted to narcotics, prosthetic valve recipients, elderly individuals, and patients with cirrhosis appear to be at increased risk for gram-negative bacillary endocarditis. Congestive heart failure is common in this group of patients, and the prognosis is poor, with the mortality

rate approaching 80%. *Salmonella* species are associated with valvular perforation or destruction (or both), atrial thrombi, myocarditis, and pericarditis. Several cases of infective endocarditis due to *Serratia marcescens* have been noted in injection drug abusers. Typically, this infection has involved the aortic and mitral valves, with large vegetations and near-total occlusion of the valve orifice in the absence of significant underlying valvular destruction.

Pseudomonas species infective endocarditis occurs in injection drug addicts and usually affects normal valves. Major embolic phenomena, inability to sterilize valves, neurologic complications, ring and anular abscesses, splenic abscesses, bacteremic relapses, and rapidly progressive congestive heart failure are common. *Pseudomonas aeruginosa* endocarditis has been associated with the use of pentazocine and tripelennamine.

Neisseria gonorrhoeae occasionally causes infective endocarditis and typically follows an indolent course, with aortic valve involvement, large vegetations, associated valve-ring abscesses, congestive heart failure, and nephritis. A high frequency of complement component deficiencies has been noted in patients with gonococcal endocarditis.

- Persons addicted to narcotics, prosthetic valve recipients, and patients with cirrhosis appear to be at increased risk for gram-negative bacillary endocarditis.
- *P. aeruginosa* endocarditis has been associated with the use of pentazocine and tripelennamine.

HACEK Endocarditis

Members of the HACEK group of organisms include *Haemophilus* species, *Actinobacillusactinomycetemcomitans*, *Cardiobacterium hominis*, *E. corrodens*, and *Kingella* species. Infective endocarditis due to the HACEK group of organisms (normal inhabitants of the human oropharynx) has been reported in patients who have dental infections and a history of dental procedures and in injection drug abusers who have "cleaned" the injection site with saliva. HACEK endocarditis characterized by a lengthy (i.e., 2 weeks to 6 months) course before diagnosis, large friable vegetations, frequent emboli, and the development of congestive heart failure, with eventual valve replacement. The HACEK group of organisms are fastidious and may require weeks for primary isolation.

Other Agents

The microbiology of infective endocarditis in injection drug abusers is distinct from that in noninjection drug abusers (Table 5).

Fungal Endocarditis

Fungal endocarditis his increasing in occurance because of the increased number of immunocompromised patients and drug users, the extensive use of broad spectrum antimicrobial agents, and the use of indwelling central venous catheters or hyperalimentation. *Candida parapsilosis* and *Candida tropicalis* predominate in injection drug addicts, and *C. albicans* and *Aspergillus* species cause most cases of fungal infective endocarditis in noninjection drug addicts. Fungal endocarditis carries a poor prognosis because of large bulky vegetations, tendency for fungal invasion of the myocardium, widespread systemic septic emboli, and poor penetration of antifungal agents into vegetations (Fig. 14-16). Surgical intervention is almost always required. In patients with *Aspergillus* endocarditis, most blood cultures will be negative, in contrast to the continuous bacteremia in bacterial endocarditis. Other peripheral lesions (e.g., emboli, cutaneous lesions, oropharyngeal lesions, sputum, and bronchoalveolar lavage fluid) should be examined and cultured for fungi in suspected settings. Valvular vegetations are not always seen on echocardiography, and clinical manifestations of endocarditis are not always present in *Aspergillus* endocarditis. The case fatality rate associated with fungal endocarditis is more than 80% for molds and more than 40% for yeasts.

■ In patients with *Aspergillus* infective endocarditis, most blood cultures will be negative.

Culture-Negative Endocarditis

Culture-negative endocarditis accounts for a small proportion of cases (<5%). It may occur because of several factors: 1) recent administration of antimicrobial agents masking growth of conventional microbes; 2) slow growth of fastidious organisms such as members of the HACEK group of organisms; 3) fungal endocarditis; 4) endocarditis caused by nonculturable intracellular organisms such as *Bartonella* species, *Chlamydia* species, *T. whipplei*, or 5) noninfectious (marantic) endocarditis (Table 6). *Bartonella* species are slow-growing gram-negative bacteria that may require a month or longer for culture isolation.

C. burnetii, the agent of Q fever, may also cause endocarditis. It occurs most commonly in males, and

Table 5.   Etiologic Agents of Native Valve Infective Endocarditis

Agent	Cases, %	
	Noninjection drug abusers	Injection drug addicts
Streptococci	60-80	27
Viridans streptococci	30-40	15
Enterococci	5-18	2
Other streptococci	15-25	10
Staphylococci	20-35	66
S. aureus	10-27	66
Coagulase-negative staphylococci	1-3	0
Gram-negative aerobic bacilli	1.5-13	2
Fungi	2-4	1-20
Miscellaneous bacteria	< 5	1
Mixed infections	1-2	1
"Culture negative"	<5-24	2

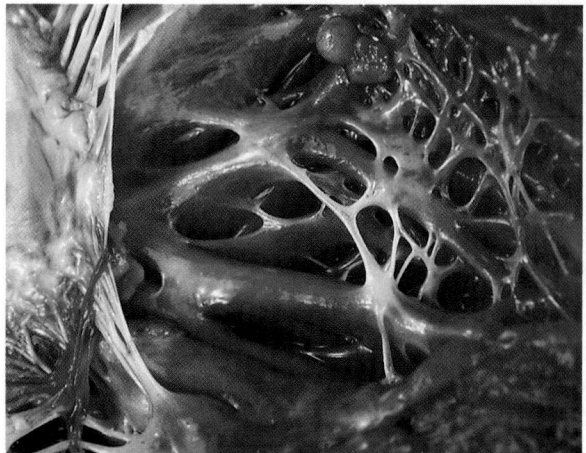

Fig. 14. Gross appearance of the heart from a patient with Aspergillus infective endocarditis.

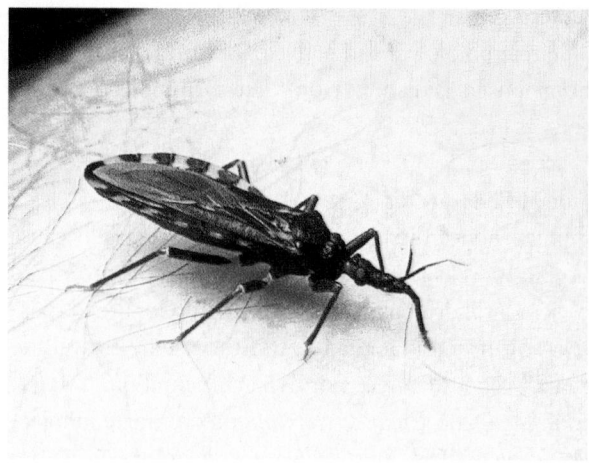

Fig. 16. Reduviid bug.

most patients have underlying heart disease. Typically, the presentation of Q fever endocarditis is chronic, with a history of an influenzalike illness 6 to 12 months previously. More than half of *C. burnetii* endocarditis occurs in patients with prosthetic valves. Risk factors include exposure to sheep, cattle, rabbits, or parturient cats. Most commonly, the aortic valve is involved, and there may be associated hepatosplenomegaly, hepatitis, thrombocytopenia, hypergammaglobulinemia, and immune complex glomerulonephritis. Underlying immunocompromising conditions, including HIV infection and cancer, may be present.

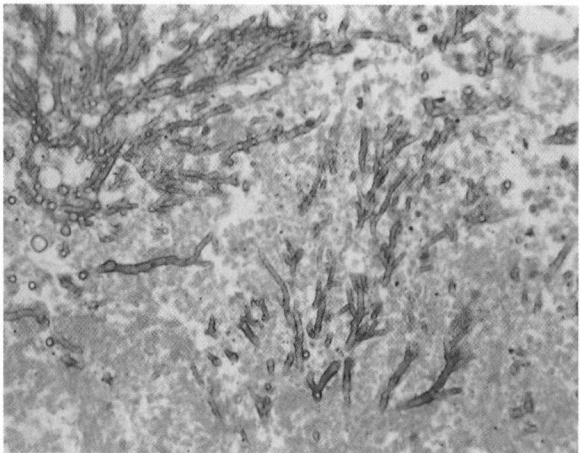

Fig. 15. Microscopic appearance of the brain abscess shown in Figure 12.

- *C. burnetii*, the agent of Q fever, may cause endocarditis.
- Premature antimicrobial therapy may render blood cultures falsely negative and complicate therapy.

Antimicrobial Therapy of Infective Endocarditis
Several principles govern the therapy of infective endocarditis. 1) The selection of antimicrobial agents to be used must be based on microbial susceptibility testing after isolation of the causative microbe. 2) Generally, parenteral antimicrobial agents are preferred because of the erratic absorption of oral agents, although some highly orally bioavailable agents (e.g., fluoroquinolones) may be suitable for treatment of compliant patients in selected cases. 3) Generally, treatment requires prolonged administration of antimicrobial agents. 4) Bactericidal agents or antimicrobial combinations that produce synergistic, rapidly bactericidal effects are required. 5) When aminoglycosides are used for treatment, the concentration of antibiotic in the serum should be measured periodically because these agents have a low toxic-therapeutic ratio, especially in elderly patients and in those with renal dysfunction. Peak and trough concentrations should be measured and the dose adjusted accordingly. Regimens for treatment of infective endocarditis are shown in Table 7.

- Penicillin-susceptible viridans group streptococcal endocarditis may be treated with a 2-week course of penicillin G and gentamicin.

Table 6.   Clues to the Diagnosis of Culture-Negative Endocarditis

Epidemiologic clues
    Travel to endemic areas—*Coxiella burnetii*, *Brucella* spp.
    Exposure to animals or their products—*C. burnetii*, *Chlamydia psittaci*, *Brucella* spp., *Bartonella henselae*
    Risk factors for fungal endocarditis
    Travel to areas endemic for demographic fungi
    Injection drug abuse—fungi, *Corynebacterium* spp.
    Homeless persons, chronic alcoholism, human immunodeficiency virus—*Bartonella* spp.
    Underlying immunocompromised host—*Listeria* spp., *Corynebacterium* spp., *Legionella* spp.
    Poor dental hygiene—HACEK group, *Granulicatella adiacens*, *Abiotrophia defectiva*
Echocardiographic clues
    Large vegetations—HACEK group, fungi
    Vegetations with "fingerlike projections"—*Chlamydia* spp.
Clinical clues
    Periodontal disease, emboli—HACEK group, *Granulicatella adiacens*, *Abiotrophia defectiva*
    Underlying neoplasm (atrial myxoma, adenocarcinoma, lymphoma, rhabdomyosarcoma, carcinoid tumor)—
        noninfective endocarditis
    Underlying autoimmune disease (rheumatic heart disease, systemic lupus erythematosus)—Libman-Sacks
        endocarditis, antiphospholipid syndrome, polyarteritis nodosa, Behçet disease, noninfective endocarditis
    Postvalvular operation—noninfectious process (e.g., thrombus, suture[s], other postvalvular surgical change)
    Miscellaneous conditions associated with noninfective endocarditis (e.g., eosinophilic heart disease, ruptured
        mitral chordae, myxomatous degeneration)

HACEK, *Haemophilus* spp, *Actinobacillus actinomycetemcomitans*, *Cardiobacterium hominis*, *Eikenella corroden*s, and *Kingella* species.

Anticoagulation does not prevent embolization related to infective endocarditis. In patients with infective endocarditis in whom anticoagulation is needed for an underlying condition (e.g., prosthetic heart valves, mitral stenosis with atrial fibrillation), anticoagulation treatment should be given. Persistent or recurrent fever despite appropriate antimicrobial therapy may be due to pulmonary or systemic emboli or drug hypersensitivity; however, the most common cause is extensive infection of the valve ring or adjacent structures.

■ Anticoagulation does not prevent embolization related to infective endocarditis.

Antibiotic Treatment of Enterococcal Endocarditis

Enterococci deserve special mention because of their relative or absolute resistance to certain antimicrobial agents. Most enterococci are only inhibited—but not killed—by clinically relevant concentrations of all effec-tive antimicrobials used singly. However, penicillin, ampicillin, or vancomycin in combination with certain aminoglycosides exert a synergistic bactericidal effect on these organisms. The degree of resistance of enterococci to aminoglycosides is highly variable. A minimal inhibitory concentration greater than or equal to 2,000 µg streptomycin/mL or 500 µg gentamicin/mL is considered the dividing point between low-level and high-level resistance of enterococci to these agents. Enterococci that are highly resistant to an aminoglycoside are not synergistically killed when that aminoglycoside is combined with either penicillin or vancomycin. For enterococci that do not exhibit high-level resistance to streptomycin or gentamicin, either aminoglycoside provides synergistic killing when combined with penicillin or vancomycin.

Because high-level resistance to gentamicin and streptomycin is encoded by different genes, isolates of enterococci that cause endocarditis should be screened with both compounds, and an aminoglycoside to which the strain is not highly resistant should be used for treatment. If endocarditis is caused by an enterococcal isolate that exhibits high-level resistance to both gentamicin and streptomycin, the addition of an aminoglycoside to a cell-wall active agent will not be beneficial. Instead, prolonged (i.e., 8 to 12 weeks) treatment with high doses of penicillin or ampicillin may cure ~50% of these patients. Surgical intervention should be considered for those in whom medical therapy fails. Along with the increasing incidence of aminoglycoside resistance, both penicillin and vancomycin resistance are increasingly present in enterococci.

- Most enterococci are inhibited—but not killed—by clinically relevant concentrations of all effective antimicrobials used singly.
- Enterococcal endocarditis must be treated with a cell-wall active agent to which the organism is susceptible and an aminoglycoside when high-level resistance is not present.

Antibiotic Treatment of Staphylococcal Endocarditis

Methicillin-susceptible staphylococcal endocarditis is treated with nafcillin or, alternatively, cefazolin or vancomycin for 4 to 6 weeks, with aminoglycosides optional for the first 3 to 5 days of treatment. The combination of nafcillin plus gentamicin, in comparison with nafcillin alone, results in a more rapid rate of eradication of *S. aureus* bacteremia but it does not improve mortality and is associated with increased nephrotoxicity. In methicillin-susceptible staphylococcal endocarditis, a β-lactam agent is more rapidly effective than vancomycin. Importantly, in HIV negative (or HIV positive and CD4 counts ≥ 200/mm3) injection drug addicts with right-sided *S. aureus* endocarditis without complications, 2 weeks of treatment with an antistaphylococcal penicillin plus an aminoglycoside may be effective. For selected injection drug abusers with uncomplicated right-sided *S. aureus* endocarditis, oral therapy with a 28-day course of ciprofloxacin and rifampin may be effective. In patients with infective endocarditis caused by methicillin-resistant *S. aureus* or methicillin-resistant coagulase-negative *Staphylococcus* species, vancomycin is the therapy of choice.

Regimens for treating endocarditis caused by HACEK microorganisms are listed in Table 7.

Antibiotic Treatment of Fungal Endocarditis

Fungal endocarditis is commonly treated with a combination of medical and surgical approaches. The mainstay of antifungal drug therapy is amphotericin B, ideally administered as a lipid preparation to optimize continued uninterrupted therapy and reduce toxicity. After 1 to 2 weeks of antifungal therapy, surgery may be considered. Caspofungin alone or fluconazole with or without oral flucytosine may also bear consideration for treatment of *Candida* endocarditis. Likewise, caspofungin, itraconazole or voricanazole may bear consideration for treatment of *Aspergillus* endocarditis. Relapse may occur in as many as 30% to 40% of patients who have received short-term antifungal therapy; long-term suppression may be beneficial. If isolated tricuspid endocarditis is present (as in an injection drug abuser), total tricuspid valvulectomy may be sufficient. Valve replacement is necessary for left-sided mold endocarditis. It is less clear if *Candida* endocarditis itself is an indication for surgery; reported data suggest that there may be a survival advantage to valve replacement.

Q fever endocarditis is usually treated with a prolonged course (at least 18 months) of doxycycline and hydroxychloroquine. Valve replacement is often required. The long-term prognosis is guarded. Relapses can occur after years of therapy.

Therapy for culture-negative endocarditis is controversial. Recommended empiric antimicrobial therapy for patients with apparent culture-negative endocarditis is outlined in Table 8.

Cardiac Surgery in Infective Endocarditis

Congestive heart failure and hemodynamic compromise are the strongest indication for surgery in infective endocarditis (Table 9). The hemodynamic status of the patient at the time of valve replacement surgery is the main determinant of operative mortality and early surgical intervention should be balanced against the advantage of "valve sterilization." If metastatic infection of other organs is present, surgery should be delayed if possible to avoid relapse of infection of the prosthetic valve, seeded from these sites of metastatic infection.

Embolic neurologic complications during infective endocarditis are associated with a two- to fourfold increase in mortality. Recurrent emboli after appropriate antimicrobial therapy can be considered an indication for surgery. Delay of valve replacement, however, is

Table 7. Antimicrobial Treatment in Adults With Infective Endocarditis

Causative agent	Antibiotic	Dosage and route	Duration of treatment, wk	Comments
I. Native valve endocarditis				
Viridans group streptococci and *Streptococcus gallolyticus* (formerly *Streptococcus bovis*) penicillin-susceptible (MIC, <0.1 µg/mL)	1) Aqueous crystalline penicillin G *or* Ceftriaxone	12-18 million U/24 hr IV continuously or 6 equally divided doses 2 g once daily IV or IM*	4 4	Preferred in most patients older than 65 yr and in those with impaired CN VIII or renal function
	2) Aqueous crystalline penicillin G *with* Gentamicin†	12-18 million U/24 hr IV continuously or 6 equally divided doses 1 mg/kg IM or IV every 8 hr	2 2	When obtained 1 hr after 20-30 min IV infusion or IM injection, serum concentration of gentamicin of ~3 µg/mL is desirable; trough concentration should be <1 µg/mL
	3) Vancomycin‡	30 mg/kg per 24 hr IV in two equally divided doses, not to exceed 2 g/24 hr unless serum levels are monitored	4	Vancomycin is recommended for patients allergic to β-lactams
Viridans group streptococci and *S. gallolyticus* (formerly *S. bovis*) relatively resistant to penicillin (MIC, 0.1-0.5 µg/mL)	1) Aqueous crystalline penicillin G *with* Gentamicin†	18 million U/24 hr IV continuously or 6 equally divided doses 1 mg/kg IM or IV every 8 hr	4 2	Cefazolin or other first-generation cephalosporins may be substituted for penicillin in patients with penicillin hypersensitivity not of the immediate type
	2) Vancomycin‡	30 mg/kg per 24 hr IV in 2 equally divided doses, not to exceed 2 g/24 hr unless serum levels are monitored	4	Vancomycin is recommended for patients allergic to β-lactams
Enterococci (and viridans group streptococci with penicillin MIC >0.5 µg/mL, *Granulicatella adiacens*, *Abiotrophia defectiva*)	1) Aqueous crystalline penicillin G *with* Gentamicin	18-30 million U/24 hr IV either continuously or 6 equally divided 1 mg/kg IM or IV every 8 hr	4-6 4-6	4-wk therapy recommended for patients with symptoms <3 mo duration; 6-wk therapy for patients with symptoms >3 mo duration
	2) Ampicillin *with* Gentamicin	12 g/24 hr IV either continuously or 6 equally divided doses 1 mg/kg IM or IV every 8 hr	4-6 4-6	

Table 7.   (continued)

Causative agent	Antibiotic	Dosage and route	Duration of treatment, wk	Comments
	3) Vancomycin	30 mg/kg per 24 hr IV in 2 equally divided doses, not exceeding 2 g/24 hr unless serum levels are monitored	4-6	Vancomycin is recommended for patients allergic to β-lactams; cephalosporins are not acceptable alternatives for patients allergic to penicillin
	with Gentamicin	1 mg/kg IM or IV every 8 hr	4-6	
Staphylococci—penicillin-susceptible	Aqueous crystalline penicillin G	10 million U/24 hr IV either continuously or 6 equally divided doses	4-6	
Staphylococci—methicillin-susceptible	1) Nafcillin or oxacillin *with*	2 g IV every 4 hr	4-6	Benefit of additional aminoglycosides has not been established
	Optional addition of gentamicin*	1 mg/kg IM or IV every 8 hr	3-5 days	
	2) Cefazolin (or other first-generation cephalosporin in equivalent dosages) *with*	2 g IV every 8 hr	4-6	For β-lactam-allergic patients, cephalosporins should be avoided in those with immediate-type hypersensitivity to penicillin
	Optional addition of gentamicin†	1 mg/kg IM or IV every 8 hr	3-5 days	
Staphylococci—methicillin-resistant	Vancomycin‡	30 mg/kg per 24 hr IV in 2 equally divided doses, not exceeding 2 g/24 hr unless serum levels are monitored	4-6	
II. Prosthetic valve endocarditis				
Staphylococci—methicillin-resistant	Vancomycin‡	30 mg/kg per 24 hr IV in 2 or 4 equally divided doses, not exceeding 2 5/24 hr unless serum levels are monitored	≥6	
	with Rifampin and	300 mg orally every 8 hr	≥6	Rifampin increases amount of warfarin sodium required for antithrombotic therapy
	Gentamicin	1.0 mg/kg IM or IV every 8 hr		

Table 7. (continued)

Causative agent	Antibiotic	Dosage and route	Duration of treatment, wk	Comments
Staphylococci— methicillin-sensitive	Nafcillin or oxacillin *with*	2 g IV every 4 hr	≥6	First-generation cephalosporins or vancomycin should be used in patients allergic to β-lactams
	Rifampin and	300 mg orally every 8 hr	≥6	
	Gentamicin	1.0 mg/kg IM or IV every 8 hr	2	Cephalosporins should be avoided in patients with immediate-type hypersensitivity to penicillin or with methicillin-resistant staphylococci
Streptococci— coccal-penicillin-susceptible (MIC, ≤0.1 μg/mL)	1) Aqueous crystalline penicillin G *with*	20 million U/day IV in divided doses every 4 hr	6	
	Gentamicin	1 mg/kg body weight (not exceeding 80 mg) IV or IM q8h	2	
	2) Cephalothin	2.0 g IV every 4 hr	6	
	3) Cefazolin	2.0 g IV every 8 hr	6	
Diphtheroids— gentamicine-susceptible (MIC, ≤4 μg/mL)	1) Aqueous crystalline penicillin G *with*	20 million U/day in divided doses every 4 hr	6	
	Gentamicin	1 mg/kg body weight (not exceeding 80 mg) IV or IM every 8 hr	6	
	2) Vancomycin	30 mg/kg body weight IV in divided doses every 12 hr or 6 hr	6	
Diphtheroids— gentamicin-resistant (MIC, >4 μg/mL)	1) Vancomycin	30 mg/kg body weight IV in divided doses every 12 hr or 6 hr	6	
	2) Ampicillin§	2 g IV every 4 hr	6	
HACEK micro-oganisms	1) Ceftriaxone	2 g once daily IV or IM*	4-6	Cefotaxime or other third-generation cephalosporins may be substituted

Table 7.   (continued)

CN, cranial nerve; HACEK, *Haemophilus* spp, *Actinobacillus actinomycetemcomitans, Cardiobacterium hominis, Eikenella corrodens*, and *Kingella* species; IV, intravenous; IM, intramuscular; MIC, minimal inhibitory concentration.

*Patients should be informed that IM injection of ceftriaxone is painful.

†Dosing of gentamicin on an mg/kg basis will produce higher serum concentrations in obese than in lean patients. Thus, in obese patients, dosing should be based on ideal body weight. (Ideal body weight for men is 50 kg + 2.3 kg/in. over 5 ft and for women, 45.5 kg + 2.3 kg/in. over 5 ft.) Relative contraindications to use of gentamicin are age > 65 yr and renal or CN VIII impairment. Other potentially nephrotoxic agents (e.g., nonsteroidal anti-inflammatory drugs) should be used cautiously in patients receiving gentamicin.

‡Vancomycin dosage should be decreased in patients with impaired renal function. Vancomycin given on an mg/kg basis will produce higher serum concentrations in obese than in lean patients. Thus, in obese patients, dosing should be based on ideal body weight. Each dose of vancomycin should be infused over at least 1 hr to reduce risk of histamine-release "red man" syndrome.

§Ampicillin should not be used if laboratory tests show β-lactamase production.

recommended for two or three weeks in embolic infarcts, and for at least one month in intracerebral hemorrhages, if possible.

Infective endocarditis caused by an organism which is unlikely to respond to antimicrobial therapy (e.g., fungi-resistant enterococci for which there is no synergistic bactericidal regimen) is another indication for early surgery because of the aggressive course of these infections and the poor response to medical therapy alone.

In right-sided infective endocarditis, persistent infection is the usual indication for surgery. Most of these patients are injection drug abusers with endo-carditis caused by organisms that are difficult to eradicate with antimicrobial therapy alone. Currently, tricuspid valvulectomy or resection of the vegetation with valvuloplasty is the procedure of choice for refractory right-sided endocarditis. A recently described alternative is transplantation of a cryopreserved mitral homograft into the tricuspid position.

PROSTHETIC VALVE ENDOCARDITIS

Prosthetic valve endocarditis occurs in up to 10% of patients during the lifetime of their prosthesis. For mechanical prostheses, the incidence peaks in the first

Table 8.   Empiric Antimicrobial Therapy for Patients With Apparent Culture-Negative Endocarditis

Clinical setting	Antimicrobial therapy	Alternative regimen
Acute onset		
Native valve	Nafcillin plus an aminoglycoside	Vancomycin hydrochloride plus an aminoglycoside
Subacute onset		
Native valve	Ampicillin-sulbactam plus an aminoglycoside	Vancomycin-ceftriaxone sodium and an aminoglycoside
Prosthetic valve	Vancomycin plus an aminoglycoside plus rifampin (consider broader coverage for gram-negative bacilli)	
Intravenous drug use	Nafcillin plus an aminoglycoside (consider broader coverage for gram-negative bacilli)	Vancomycin plus an aminoglycoside

Table 9.   Indications for Cardiac Surgery in Patients With Native Valve Infective Endocarditis[*]

Left-sided endocarditis
    Accepted indications
        Acute aortic regurgitation or mitral regurgitation with medically uncontrolled heart failure
        Acute aortic regurgitation with tachycardia and early closure of the mitral valve
        Fungal endocarditis
        Evidence of valve dysfunction and persistent infection after a prolonged period (7 to 10 days) of
            appropriate antimicrobial therapy, as indicated by presence of fever, leukocytosis, and
            bacteremia, provided there are no noncardiac causes of infection
    Relative indications
        Evidence of anular or aortic abscess, sinus or aortic true or false aneurysm
        Recurrent emboli after appropriate antibiotic therapy
        Infection with gram-negative organisms or organisms with a poor response to antimicrobials in
            patients with evidence of valve dysfunction
Right-sided endocarditis
    Uncontrolled sepsis despite adequate antimicrobial treatment
    Intractable right heart failure despite appropriate medical treatment
    Paravalvular abscess or fungal endocarditis
    Very large (>20 mm) vegetations (some authors also identify large vegetation size >10 mm in the context
        of persisting fever as an indication for surgery)

[*]Criteria also apply to repair mitral and aortic allograft or autograft valves.

few weeks after valve replacement which then decreases to a stable low incidence rate during subsequent months to years. The risk of infection for mechanical and bioprosthetic valves is similar and there is no difference in the risk of endocarditis between mitral or aortic prostheses. Prosthetic valve endocarditis has been classified arbitrarily as "early" the first 60 days after implantation and "late" after 60 days. Classically, it was thought that "early" cases were acquired at the time of implantation and "late" cases thereafter. Subsequently, it was shown that many cases of prosthetic valve endocarditis that occur during the first year after surgery are acquired at the time of implantation. Some investigators have recommended that the time limit for "early" disease be extended to 6 months or even 1 year.

The mortality associated with prosthetic valve endocarditis is 30% to 80% in the "early" form and 20% to 40% in "late" postsurgical endocarditis, with a worse prognosis associated with a new or changing murmur, new or worsening heart failure, persistent fever despite appropriate antimicrobics, new conduction myocardial

abscess, renal insufficiency, *S. aureus* as the causative agent, and neurologic complications.

- Prosthetic valve endocarditis has been reported to occur in up to 10% of patients during the lifetime of the prosthesis.
- Prosthetic valve endocarditis has been classified arbitrarily as "early" when it occurs within the first 60 days after implantation and "late" when it occurs after 60 days.

Pathogenesis of Prosthetic Valve Endocarditis

Early *S. epidermidis* prosthetic valve endocarditis is thought to result from valve contamination during the perioperative period. This may occur at the time of surgery or in the immediate postoperative period when the prosthetic valve and sewing ring are not yet endothelialized and are susceptible to microbial adherence. Nosocomial bacteremia is an important risk factor for prosthetic valve endocarditis. Another potential (but uncommon) source of infection is contamination of the prosthesis before implantation (e.g., contamination of glutaraldehyde-fixed porcine prosthetic valves with *Mycobacterium chelonei*).

The pathogenesis of late prosthetic valve endocarditis is similar to that of native valve endocarditis, with microorganisms from a transient bacteremia localizing on a prosthesis or area of damaged endothelium.

Valve-Ring Abscess

Valve-ring abscess is a serious complication of prosthetic valve endocarditis and is seen with both mechanical and bioprosthetic valves. Valve-ring abscesses occur where infection involves the sutures used to secure the sewing ring to the perianular tissue; this may result in dehiscence of the valve. The clinical finding of a new perivalvular leak in a patient with prosthetic valve endocarditis is presumptive evidence of a valve-ring abscess. Extension of the abscess beyond the valve ring may result in myocardial abscess formation, septal perforation, or purulent pericarditis. In addition to sewing-ring abscesses, prosthetic valve endocarditis of the bioprosthesis may cause leaflet destruction, with resulting valvular incompetence. Large vegetations occasionally obstruct blood flow and lead to functional valvular stenosis or a combination of stenosis and insufficiency. This complication appears to be more common in mitral prosthetic valve endocarditis than in aortic disease. Bioprosthetic valve endocarditis may involve only the valve cusps, the sewing ring, or both.

- Early prosthetic valve endocarditis results from valve contamination during the perioperative period.
- Late prosthetic valve endocarditis results more often from transient bacteremia.

Echocardiography in Prosthetic Valve Endocarditis

Transthoracic echocardiography is less accurate in the diagnosis of prosthetic valve endocarditis than in native valve endocarditis, because the echoes generated by the prosthesis may mask subtle abnormalities such as small vegetations. Transesophageal echocardiography is more sensitive than transthoracic echocardiography for the detection of vegetations, periprosthetic tissue destruction with prosthetic dehiscence, myocardial abscesses, fistulas, pseudoaneurysms, and perivalvular abscesses.

Since infective endocarditis involving mechanical prostheses usually starts at the prosthetic ring, the search of vegetations in such patients must focus on the prosthetic ring. In contrast, infective endocarditis of biological prostheses involves both the ring and the valvular leaflets. For patients with negative transesophageal echocardiography and an intermediate probability of infective endocarditis, repeat transesophageal echocardiography is recommended after a week, especially if an aortic prosthesis could be involved.

- Transesophageal echocardiography is recommended for diagnosis of prosthetic valve endocarditis.
- CT and/or MRI of the head is indicated in patients with prosthetic valve endocarditis and neurologic symptoms.

Diagnostic Criteria

The currently accepted diagnostic criteria for infective endocarditis are outlined in Table 4.

Microbiology

Among cases of prosthetic valve endocarditis, coagulase-negative staphylococci are the dominant cause of endocarditis occurring in the first postoperative year. The organisms causing prosthetic valve endocarditis more than 12 months after valve implantation are similar to those associated with native valve endocarditis (except for nosocomial and drug abuse-associated infective endocarditis). During this late postoperative period, the predominant causes of infection are streptococci, coagulase-negative staphylococci, enterococci, *S. aureus*, and members of the HACEK group of organisms. A broad range of bacteria have also caused sporadic cases of prosthetic valve endocarditis. *Corynebacterium* species cause prosthetic valve endocarditis that occurs within the first 6 postoperative months and are notable because of their relative resistance to many antimicrobial agents (other than vancomycin) and their fastidious growth requirements.

Fungi not only account for a number of cases of prosthetic valve endocarditis but are associated with high case fatality rates. *Candida* species followed by *Aspergillus* species are the two most common fungi that cause prosthetic valve endocarditis. Fungal vegetations formed on prosthetic valves are bulky and may partially occlude the orifice or embolize and occlude medium-sized arteries. Notably, patients with prosthetic heart valves who develop nosocomial candidemia are at risk for either having or developing candidal prosthetic valve endocarditis months or years later. Late-onset candidemia and lack of an identifiable portal of entry should heighten concern about candidal prosthetic valve endocarditis in such patients.

■ Coagulase-negative staphylococci are the most common cause of prosthetic valve endocarditis in the first postoperative year.

Treatment

Antimicrobial therapy is based on laboratory identification of the etiologic microorganism and in vitro susceptibility testing. Bactericidal antimicrobials are necessary. Recommended antimicrobial regimens are listed in Table 7. Many isolates of coagulase-negative staphylococci isolated from patients with prosthetic valve endocarditis are resistant to oxacillin. For methicillin-resistant staphylococcal infection on prosthetic valves, treatment with a combination of vancomycin, rifampin, and gentamicin is recommended. Fungal prosthetic valve endocarditis usually requires combined medical and surgical therapy. For *Candida* endocarditis, high doses of amphotericin B given intravenously in combination with oral flucytosine are often used. Alternative considerations include caspofungin or combined fluconazole and oral flucytosine. For culture-negative prosthetic valve endocarditis, treatment must be individualized. When prosthetic valve endocarditis is considered but the level of clinical suspicion is low, 3 or 4 blood specimens should be obtained by separate venipunctures for culture and the patient observed. If valve replacement surgery is imminent, it is reasonable to initiate empiric antimicrobial therapy with vancomycin and gentamicin. The diagnosis of prosthetic valve endocarditis can usually be confirmed or excluded at the time of valve replacement.

■ For methicillin-resistant staphylococcal infection on prosthetic valves, treatment with a combination of vancomycin, rifampin, and gentamicin is recommended.

After initiation of antimicrobial therapy, blood should be cultured daily for the first few days and weekly thereafter until the completion of therapy. Usually, blood cultures will be sterile within 3 to 5 days after appropriate antimicrobial therapy is initiated. After completion of therapy, blood should be cultured weekly for 1 month. A relapse necessitates reinstitution of antimicrobial therapy, retesting of the microorganism for antimicrobial susceptibility, and consideration of valve replacement.

Indications for cardiac surgery in patients with prosthetic valve endocarditis are listed in Table 10. Moderate to severe congestive heart failure associated with prosthesis dysfunction is a common indication for surgery. Few patients with prosthetic valve endocarditis-induced heart failure are alive 6 months after medical treatment, whereas combined surgical and medical treatment has resulted in survival rates of up to 64%. Patients with culture-negative endocarditis who continue to experience fever during empiric antibiotic therapy are candidates for surgical intervention. Surgery may allow a definitive microbiologic diagnosis and development of specific, effective antimicrobial therapy. Also, some of these patients will be found to have fungal endocarditis or unrecognized invasive infection that warrants surgery.

■ Medical therapy alone is appropriate for some patients with prosthetic valve endocarditis.

The timing of cardiac surgery in patients with prosthetic valve endocarditis must be individualized. The hemodynamic status of the patient is the most important consideration in determining the timing of operation. As in patients with native valve endocarditis, the likelihood of those with prosthetic valve endocarditis surviving valve replacement is inversely related to the severity of the patient's heart failure at the time of operation. Thus, although in theory it may be desirable to control infection with antimicrobial therapy preoperatively, this must not be attempted at the expense of progressive destruction of perivalvular tissue and further deterioration in the patient's hemodynamic status. Longer periods of antimicrobial therapy preoperatively do not correlate with inability to recover bacteria from intraoperative cultures or with a more favorable outcome. Renal dysfunction preoperatively is one of the most important predictors of both increased operative mortality and overall long-term poor prognosis. Renal failure is often associated with advanced decompensated heart failure and low cardiac output.

Table 10. Recommendations for Surgery for
Prosthetic Valve Endocarditis*

Indication
>   Early prosthetic valve endocarditis (first 2
>   months or less after surgery)
>   Heart failure with prosthetic valve dysfunc-
>   tion
>   Fungal endocarditis
>   Staphylococcal endocarditis not responding
>   to antimicrobial therapy
>   Evidence of paravalvular leak, anular or
>   aortic abscess, sinus or aortic true or false
>   aneurysm, fistula formation, or new-onset
>   conduction disturbances
>   Infection with gram-negative organisms
>   with a poor response to antimicrobials
>   Persistent bacteremia after prolonged
>   course (7 to 10 days) of appropriate
>   antimicrobial therapy without noncardiac
>   causes for bacteremia
>   Recurrent peripheral embolus despite
>   therapy

*Criteria exclude repaired mitral valves or aortic allograft
or autograft valves.

■ The hemodynamic status of the patient is the most
important consideration in determining the timing
of operation.

In selected patients with prosthetic valve endocarditis, the results of treatment with antimicrobial
agents alone are comparable to the results of combined
surgical and medical therapy; for these patients, medical
therapy is recommended. Included in this subgroup are
patients with late-onset prosthetic valve endocarditis
(12 months or more postoperatively) who are infected
with less virulent organisms (viridans group streptococci,
enterococci, and fastidious gram-negative coccobacilli)
and who do not develop complicated endocarditis.

Careful anticoagulation therapy is recommended
for patients with mechanical prosthetic valve endocarditis involving prostheses that usually would warrant
maintenance of anticoagulation. Anticoagulation
should be reversed temporarily, however, if a patient

experiences a hemorrhagic central nervous system
event. Anticoagulation is not recommended for
bioprosthetic valve endocarditis that under usual circumstances do not require anticoagulation therapy.

PROPHYLAXIS OF INFECTIVE ENDOCARDITIS

Prophylaxis for infective endocarditis is advised for
patients who have an underlying cardiac condition that
places them at increased risk for endocarditis and who
are undergoing a procedure that carries a risk of transient bacteremia due to an organism that causes endocarditis. Endocarditis prophylaxis is recommended in
high-risk and, in most cases, moderate-risk patients; it
is not required in low-risk patients (Table 11).

Mitral valve prolapse is common and represents a
spectrum of abnormalities. A clinical approach to
determine the need for prophylaxis in persons with
suspected mitral valve prolapse, as recommended by the
American Heart Association, is shown in Figure 17.
When normal valves prolapse without leaking, as in
patients with one or more systolic clicks but no murmurs and no Doppler-demonstrated mitral regurgitation,
the risk of endocarditis is not increased above that of
the normal population. Therefore, antimicrobial prophylaxis against endocarditis is not necessary. This is
because it is not the abnormal valve motion but the jet
of mitral insufficiency that creates the shear force and
flow abnormalities that increase the likelihood of bacterial
adherence on the valve during bacteremia. However,
patients with prolapsing and leaking mitral valves,
evidenced by audible clicks and murmurs of mitral
regurgitation or by Doppler-demonstrated mitral
insufficiency, should receive prophylactic treatment
with antimicrobials. Similarly, patients with myxomatous mitral valve degeneration with regurgitation valve
leaflet thickening should receive endocarditis prophylaxis. Because older age and male sex have been shown
to be risk factors for the development of endocarditis,
men older than 45 years with mitral valve prolapse,
even without a consistent systolic murmur, may warrant
prophylaxis even in the absence of resting regurgitation.

The American Heart Association has identified
common procedures for which prophylaxis is recommended or not recommended according to the perceived degree of risk (Table 12). The recommended
antimicrobial regimens for infective endocarditis

Table 11. Cardiac Conditions Associated With Endocarditis*

Endocarditis Prophylaxis Recommended

High-risk category
> Prosthetic cardiac valves, including bioprosthetic and homograft valves
> Previous bacterial endocarditis
> Complex cyanotic congenital heart disease (e.g., single ventricle states, transposition of the great arteries, tetralogy of Fallot)
> Surgically constructed systemic pulmonary shunts or conduits

Moderate-risk category
> Most other congenital cardiac malformations (other than above and below)
> Acquired valvar dysfunction (e.g., rheumatic heart disease)
> Hypertrophic cardiomyopathy
> Mitral valve prolapse with valvar regurgitation and/or thickened leaflets

Endocarditis Prophylaxis Not Recommended

Negligible-risk category (no greater risk than the general population)
> Isolated secundum atrial septal defect
> Surgical repair of atrial septal defect, ventricular septal defect, or patent ductus arteriosus (without residua beyond 6 mo)
> Previous coronary artery bypass graft surgery
> Mitral valve prolapse without valvar regurgitation
> Physiologic, functional, or innocent heart murmurs
> Previous Kawasaki disease without valvar dysfunction
> Previous rheumatic fever without valvar dysfunction
> Cardiac pacemakers (intravascular and epicardial) and implanted defibrillators

*Please consult the original table for references to the sources of the data.

prophylaxis are outlined in Tables 13 and 14.

Before elective valve replacement, the dental health of every patient should be evaluated and any necessary dental work completed under close observation and with appropriate antibiotic coverage.

The number of organisms in the mouth and gingival crevices can be decreased temporarily by local irrigation with an antiseptic solution such as iodinated glycerol. Some dental experts recommend routine use of this measure before dental extractions.

Occasionally, a patient may be taking an antimicrobial agent when going to see a physician or dentist. If the patient is taking an antimicrobial agent normally used for endocarditis prophylaxis, it is prudent to select a drug from a different class rather than to increase the dose of the current antibiotic. In particular, antimicrobial regimens used to prevent the recurrence of acute rheumatic fever are inadequate for the prevention of bacterial endocarditis. Persons who take an oral penicillin for secondary prevention of rheumatic fever or for other purposes may have viridans group streptococci in their oral cavities that are relatively resistant to penicillin, amoxicillin, or ampicillin. In such cases, clindamycin, azithromycin, or clarithromycin should be selected for endocarditis prophylaxis. Because of possible cross-resistance with cephalosporins, this class of antibiotic should be avoided. If possible, one should delay the procedure until at least 9 to 14 days after completion of the antimicrobial agent to allow the usual oral flora to be reestablished.

■ Patients receiving a low dose of penicillin for rheumatic fever prophylaxis should not receive penicillin for endocarditis prophylaxis.

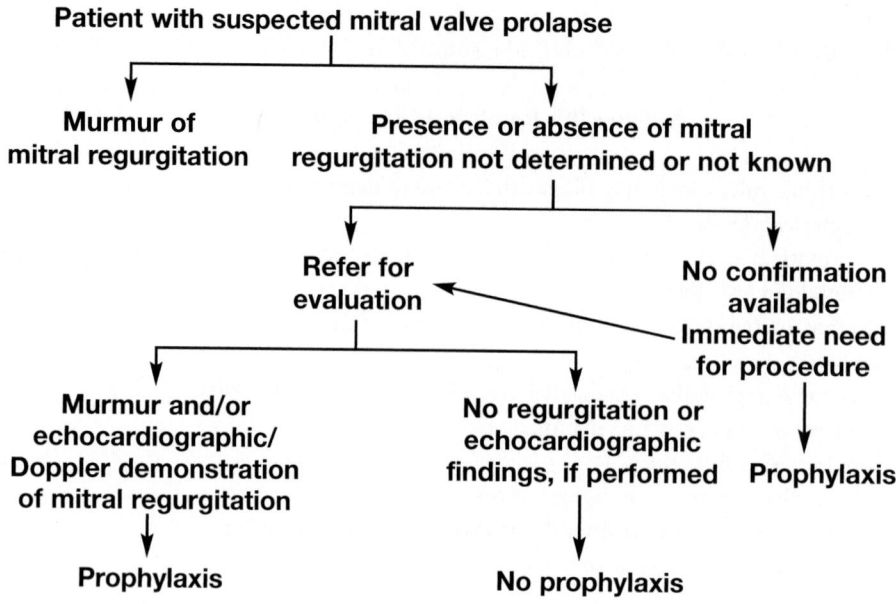

Fig. 17. Clinical approach to determination of need for prophylaxis in patients with suspected mitral valve prolapse.

INFECTIONS OF CARDIOVASCULAR DEVICES

Symptoms and signs of cardiovascular device-related infections depend on the location of the infected part(s) of the device. When infected intravascular or endovascular portions of a device are present, clinical manifestations resemble those of infective endocarditis or endarteritis. Fever is often present, as are embolic events, which involve either the pulmonary or systemic vasculature (depending on the site of the infected device). Virulent pathogens, such as *P. aeruginosa* and *S. aureus* may be associated with sepsis. Subacute and chronic presentations are found in association with less virulent organisms. As with endocarditis, immune-mediated events (e.g., immune complex-mediated nephritis, vasculitis) may be present. Cardiovascular device-related infections may present as bacteremia with fever in the absence of other clinical findings. Alternatively, findings may include local pain, erythema, induration, warmth and/or purulent drainage at the exit site of the device (e.g., percutaneous drivelines). Cellulitis or abscess formation may be present in association with subcutaneously implanted devices. Pseudoaneurysms may develop in cases of infections of vascular graft anastomoses; occlusion of a graft may lead to ischemia or necrosis.

The microbiology of cardiovascular device-related infections involves predominantly *S. aureus* and coagulase-negative staphylococci. The incidence of cardiovascular device-related infections depends on the device; details are provided in Table 15. Endothelialization is viewed as a healing response following device implantation in humans, and is considered important in the prevention of subsequent infection. The exact length of time required for endothelialization of implanted cardiovascular devices is not known, but is likely in the range of 1 to 3 months.

Pacemaker and Implantable Cardioverter-Defibrillator Infections

Pacemaker infections most commonly occur in the pocket in which the generator is placed. Involvement of the electrode leads occurs less frequently.

In pacemaker or implantable cardioverter-defibrillator infective endocarditis, vegetations may form on the tricuspid valve and/or anywhere along the course of the electrode, including in the endocardium of the right ventricle or atrium. Pulmonary emboli or empyema may be present. The pathogenesis of generator box infections is thought to relate to contamination of the device by skin flora at the time of implantation. Most

Table 12. Recommendations for Prophylaxis During Various Procedures That May Cause Bacteremia*

Endocarditis Prophylaxis Recommended

Dental Procedures†
  Dental extractions
  Periodontal procedures including surgery, scaling
    and root planing, probing, and recall maintenance
  Dental implant placement and reimplantation of
    avulsed teeth
  Endodontic (root canal) instrumentation or surgery
    only beyond the apex
  Subgingival placement of antibiotic fibers or strips
  Initial placement of orthodontic bands but not
    brackets
  Intraligamentary local anesthetic injections
  Prophylactic cleaning of teeth or implants where
    bleeding is anticipated

Other Procedures
  Respiratory tract
    Tonsilectomy and/or adenoidectomy
    Surgical operations that involve respiratory
      mucosa
    Bronchoscopy with a rigid bronchoscope
  Gastrointestinal tract‡
    Sclerotherapy for esophageal varices
    Esophageal stricture dilation
    Endoscopic retrograde cholangiography with
      biliary obstruction
    Biliary tract surgery
    Surgical operations that involve intestinal mucosa
  Genitourinary tract
    Prostatic surgery
    Cystoscopy
    Urethral dilation

Endocarditis Prophylaxis Not Recommended

Dental Procedures
  Restorative dentistry§ (operative and prosthodontic)
    with or without retraction cord//
  Local anesthetic injections (nonintraligamentary)
  Intracanal endodontic treatment; post placement
    and buildup
  Placement of rubber dams
  Postoperative suture removal
  Placement of removable prosthodontic or ortho-
    dontic appliances
  Taking of oral impressions
  Fluoride treatments
  Taking of oral radiographs
  Orthodontic appliance adjustment
  Shedding of primary teeth
Other Procedures
  Respiratory tract
    Endotracheal intubation
    Bronchoscopy with a flexible bronchosope,
      with or without biopsy¶
    Tympanostomy tube insertion

Gastrointestinal tract
  Transesophageal echocardiography¶
  Endoscopy with or without gastrointestinal
    biopsy//
Genitourinary tract
  Vaginal hysterectomy¶
  Vaginal delivery¶
  Cesarean section¶
  In uninfected tissue:
    Urethral catheterization
    Uterine dilatation and curettage
    Therapeutic abortion
    Sterilization procedures
    Insertion or removal of intrauterine devices
Other
  Cardiac catheterization, including balloon angio-
    plasty
  Implanted cardiac pacemakers, implanted de-
    fibrillators, and coronary stents
  Incision or biopsy of surgically scrubbed skin
  Circumcision

*Please consult the original table for references to the sources of the data.
†Prophylaxis is recommended for patients with high- and moderate-risk cardiac conditions.
‡Prophylaxis is recommended for high-risk patients; optional for medium-risk patients.
§This includes restoration of decayed teeth (filling cavities) and replacement of missing teeth.
//Clinical judgment may indicate antibiotic use in selected circumstances that may create significant bleeding.
¶Prophylaxis is optional for high-risk patients.

Table 13. Prophylactic Regimens for Dental, Oral, Respiratory Tract, or Esophageal Procedures*

Situation	Agent	Regimen†
Standard general prophylaxis	Amoxicillin	Adults: 2.0 g; children: 50 mg/kg orally 1 hr before procedure
Unable to take oral medications	Ampicillin	Adults: 2.0 g intramuscularly (IM) or intravenously (IV); children: 50 mg/kg IM or IV within 30 min before procedure
Allergic to penicillin	Clindamycin	Adults: 600 mg; children: 20 mg/kg orally 1 hr before procedure
	or	
	Cefalexin‡ or cefadroxil‡	Adults: 2.0 g; children: 50 mg/kg orally 1 hr before procedure
	or	
	Azithromycin or clarithromycin	Adults: 500 mg; children: 15 mg/kg orally 1 hr before procedure
Allergic to penicillin and unable to take oral medications	Clindamycin	Adults: 600 mg; children: 20 mg/kg IV within 30 min before procedure
	or	
	Cefazolin‡	Adults: 1.0 g; children: 25 mg/kg IM or IV within 30 min before procedure

*Please consult the original table for references to the sources of the data.
†Total children's dose should not exceed adult dose.
‡Cephalosporins should not be used in persons with immediate-type hypersensitivity reaction (urticaria, angioedema, or anaphylaxis) to penicillins.

such infections are present soon after pacemaker implantation but may not become clinically evident for two years or longer. Wound infection or erosion of the box through the overlying skin may also lead to microbial contamination and subsequent infection. Microorganisms from the pocket can spread along the electrode to the endocardium and electrode tip. Hematogenous seeding of the endovascular electrode during transient bacteremia may also occur. Pacemaker or implantable cardioverter-defibrillator endocarditis most commonly occurs as a result of pocket infection; the most common pathogens of pacemaker and implantable cardioverter-defibrillator endocarditis are skin flora, including staphylococci and corynebacteria. Hematogenous seeding from a distant source of infection may account for late-onset infection due to *S. aureus* or other organisms (e.g., viridans group streptococci, enterococci, gram-negative bacilli, anaerobes, fungi, nontuberculous mycobacteria).

Risk factors for infection include the presence of diabetes mellitus, steroid use, underlying malignancy, overlying dermatologic disorders (especially pustular disorders), hematoma formation within the pocket, urgent placement or frequent replacement of the generator, and inexperience of the implantation team.

The diagnosis should be entertained in patients with pacemakers or implantable cardioverter-defibrillators and unexplained fever. The diagnosis is typically confirmed by positive blood cultures and an echocardiogram that demonstrates vegetations on a pacemaker or implantable cardioverter-defibrillator lead. Transesophageal echocardiography is more sensitive than transthoracic echocardiography. The blood, the pacemaker pocket, and any other wound site should be cultured. A definitive diagnosis of pacemaker infection depends on isolation of the etiologic microorganism from the pacemaker pocket or the blood.

Ideally, all of the hardware should be removed in

Table 14. Prophylactic Regimens for Genitourinary and Gastrointestinal (Excluding Esophageal) Procedures*

Situation	Agent†	Regimen‡
High-risk patients	Ampicillin plus gentamicin	Adults: ampicillin 2.0 g intramuscularly (IM) or intravenously (IV) plus gentamicin 1.5 mg/kg (not to exceed 120 mg) within 30 min of starting the procedure; 6 hr later, ampicillin 1 g IM/IV or amoxicillin 1 g orally Children: ampicillin 50 mg/kg IM or IV (not to exceed 2.0 g) plus gentamicin 1.5 mg/kg within 30 min of starting the procedure; 6 hr later, ampicillin 25 mg/kg IM/IV or amoxicillin 25 mg/kg orally
High-risk patients allergic to ampicillin/amoxicillin	Vancomycin plus gentamicin	Adults: vancomycin 1.0 g IV over 1-2 hr plus gentamicin 1.5 mg/kg IV/IM (not to exceed 120 mg); complete injection/infusion within 30 min of starting the procedure Children: vancomycin 20 mg/kg IV over 1-2 hr plus gentamicin 1.5 mg/kg IV/IM; complete injection/infusion within 30 min of starting the procedure
Moderate-risk patients	Amoxicillin or ampicillin	Adults: amoxicillin 2.0 g orally 1 hr before procedure, or ampicillin 2.0 g IM/IV within 30 min of starting the procedure Children: amoxicillin 50 mg/kg orally 1 hr before procedure, or ampicillin 50 mg/kg IM/IV within 30 min of starting the procedure
Moderate-risk patients allergic to ampicillin/amoxicillin	Vancomycin	Adults: vancomycin 1.0 g IV over 1-2 hr; complete infusion within 30 min of starting the procedure Children: vancomycin 20 mg/kg IV over 1-2 hr; complete infusion within 30 min of starting the procedure

*Please consult the original table for references to the sources of the data.
†Total children's dose should not exceed adult dose.
‡No second dose of vancomycin or gentamicin is recommended.

both generator box and electrode infections. Infection relapse has been strongly associated with failure to remove all of the hardware. The mortality of patients with pacemaker or implantable cardioverter-defibrillator endocarditis treated with antimicrobial agents alone is significantly higher than the mortality of such patients treated with a combination of antimicrobial agents and electrode removal. In patients with *S. aureus* bacteremia and a pacemaker or implantable cardioverter-defibrillator, removal of the device is recommended in the following situations: 1) if there is clinical or echocardiographic evidence of device infection; 2) if there is no other source of *S. aureus* bacteremia identified; 3) if there is relapsing *S. aureus* bacteremia after a course of appropriate antimicrobial therapy. Removal of pacemaker wires may be challenging because of neoendothelialization and fibrocollagenous sheath formation along the electrode. Options for removal of such leads include the use of a locking stylet introduced onto the lead and affixed close to the distal end of the electrode to apply traction directly to the tip, the use of a telescoping sheath that can be advanced over the lead to disrupt fibrous attachments of the lead to vein or cardiac tissue and to free the lead by countertraction, the use of a laser sheath to photoablate the fibrous attachments, or the use of minimally invasive video-assisted pacemaker removal under thoracoscopic guidance. The need for reimplantation should be reassessed, as 13% to 52% of patients may no longer require pacemaker support following pace-

maker removal. Device reimplantation should be at a new site when the patient is no longer bacteremic.

■ Staphylococci are the most common cause of pacemaker infections.
■ When possible, all the hardware should be removed in pacemaker infections.

Left Ventricular Assist Device Infections
Infection is a frequent complication of left ventricular assist device use; the risk increases with the duration of use, and most commonly occurs in patients in whom the device has been in place for at least two weeks. Infection has been reported to complicate 25% to 70% of left ventricular assist device placements.

Table 15. Nonvalvular Cardiovascular Device-Related Infections

Type of device	Incidence of infection, %
Intracardiac	
Pacemakers (temporary and permanent)	0.13-19.9
Defibrillators	0.00-3.2
Left ventricular assist devices	25-70
Total artificial hearts	
Ventriculoatrial shunts	2.4-9.4
Pledgets	Rare
Patent ductus arteriosus occlusion devices (investigational in the United States: plugs, double umbrellas, buttons, discs, embolization coils)	Rare
Atrial septal defect and ventricular septal defect closure devices (Bard clamshell occluders, discs, buttons, double umbrellas)	Rare
Conduits	Rare
Patches	Pare
Arterial	
Peripheral vascular stents	Rare
Vascular grafts, including hemodialysis	1.0-6
Intra-aortic balloon pumps	≤5-26
Angioplasty/angiography-related bacteremias	<1*
Coronary artery stents	Rare
Patches	1.8
Venous	
Vena caval filters	Rare

*Closure device use ≤1.9%.

Ventricular assist device infections can be divided into three different syndromes. Drive-line infection is the most common type of left ventricular device infection, and typically presents with local inflammatory changes and drainage at the cutaneous exit site. The second syndrome is infection of the left ventricular assist device pocket; this causes local inflammatory changes. The third and most rare syndrome is endocarditis due to infection involving either or both the valve or the internal lining (i.e., parts in contact with the blood) of the device. Patients can have more than one different type of infection at the same time.

Interestingly, the left ventricular assist device may induce an immunodeficiency state that may predispose to infection. Left ventricular assist devices have been shown to induce aberrant T-cell activation leading to programmed cell death of CD4-positive T-cells.

Pathogens associated with ventricular assist device infections depend on the infection syndrome and whether or not the infection involves the blood. Staphylococci are the main bacteria isolated followed by gram-negative bacilli (*P. aeruginosa*, *E. coli*), *Enterococcus* species, *Corynebacterium* species, and *Candida* species.

Risk factors for infection of left ventricular assist devices are related to patient comorbidities (e.g., diabetes, obesity, chronic obstructive airway disease) and perioperative events (e.g., postoperative bleeding, blood product transfusion, surgical reexploration, thrombosis). Common clinical findings in left ventricular assist device infection are fever, leukocytosis, and local signs of infection. Antimicrobial therapy should be directed towards the causative organism and administered for 3 to 4 weeks; for unresolved infection, removal of the device may be needed. Importantly, left ventricular assist device infection, including persistent bacteremia or fungemia, is not a contraindication to cardiac transplantation.

Peripheral Vascular Stent Infections

Peripheral vascular stent infection is rare, but when it does occur can cause severe complications, including pseudo- and mycotic aneurysms, abscesses, arterial necrosis, septic emboli, refractory sepsis, need for amputation, and death. Most such infections occur in the first month after stent placement. *S. aureus* is the most common pathogen. Risk factors for endovascular stent infection include prolonged use of a catheter sheath or reuse of the same sheath after 24 hours, local hematoma formation, multiple interventions on the same origination sites, prolonged procedural time, and use of the same femoral artery for vascular access within one week of a prior catheterization. Excision with extra-anatomic revascularization in combination with antimicrobial therapy is the treatment of choice. For patients in whom surgical intervention is not feasible, long-term suppressive antimicrobial therapy has been used.

Prosthetic Vascular Graft Infections

The long-term incidence of prosthetic vascular graft infection is 1% to 6%. The risk of infection for aortic grafts is less than that for aortofemoral grafts which in turn is less than that of inguinal grafts. Infection is thought to occur in the intra- or perioperative setting, and most commonly presents within two months of prosthetic graft placement. Less virulent organisms, such as coagulase-negative staphylococci, may result in delay of symptom onset for 6 months or longer after graft placement. Risk factors for vascular graft infection include groin incisions, emergent surgery, history of multiple invasive interventions before or after graft placement, contiguous infection of the graft area, diabetes mellitus, chronic renal disease, obesity, and immunocompromising conditions.

Infections involving an extremity may present with focal inflammatory changes; infections involving an intracavitary graft location may be challenging to diagnose. Gastrointestinal bleeding due to aortoenteric fistula formation or erosion is seen in a minority of patients with aortic graft infection. The management of prosthetic graft infections includes excision of the graft, wide incomplete debridement of devitalized, infected tissue, maintenance of vascular flow to the distal bed, and administration of prolonged antimicrobial therapy.

Hemodialysis Prosthetic Vascular Graft Infections

Infections of hemodialysis prosthetic vascular grafts are unique because hemodialysis patients are immunocompromised, have increased carriage rate of *S. aureus,* and undergo repetitive needle puncture of the graft for access. *S. aureus* is the most common cause of infection followed by coagulase-negative staphylococci. Antimicrobial-resistant bacteria are not infrequently involved because of the repetitive exposure of hemodialysis patients to antimicrobial agents and clinical environments conducive to the transmission of multi-drug-resistant bacteria.

Coronary Artery Stent Infections

Infections of intracoronary stents are rare but often fatal and occur secondary to contamination of a stent at the time of delivery or subsequent transient bacteremia. The incubation period has been reported to range from four days to four weeks. *S. aureus* and *P. aeruginosa* have been reported as pathogens. Associated findings consist of local abscess formation, suppurative pancarditis, and pericardial empyema.

Intra-Aortic Balloon Pump Infections

Infections of intra-aortic balloon pumps are rare. Local wound infections are most common, and most cases of bacteremia are due to spread from a colonized or infected insertion site. Risk factors for such infections include contamination of the femoral area, especially in obese patients, and insertions performed in the coronary care unit or surgical intensive care unit, especially on an emergent basis (as compared to in an operating room or cardiac catheterization suite). Treatment consists of appropriate antimicrobial therapy and local wound care in addition to removal of the intra-aortic balloon pump, if possible.

83

SYSTEMIC DISEASE AND THE HEART

Marian T. McEvoy, MD

Joseph G. Murphy, MD

Many systemic diseases affect the heart either directly or indirectly. This chapter, while not exhaustive, provides a summary of the most frequently encountered systemic diseases in clinical practice that affect the heart. An important issue is how the systemic disease modifies either the diagnosis or the management of the cardiac problem and how the cardiac disease, in turn, modifies the approach to the systemic disease.

NEUROLOGIC DISEASE
Cardiac involvement in neurologic disease is unusual; the most important examples are summarized below.

Friedreich Ataxia
Friedreich ataxia is an autosomal recessive neurologic disorder that has been associated with variant hypertrophic type cardiomyopathy and, less commonly, dilated cardiomyopathy. The hypertrophic cardiomyopathy seen in Friedreich ataxia differs from the classical type in that septal myofibrillary disarray is absent, malignant ventricular arrhythmias are rare, and left ventricular systolic and diastolic function remain relatively normal. Concentric left ventricular hypertrophy is more common than asymmetric septal hypertrophy. A dilated cardiomyopathy may also be seen in Friedreich ataxia and has a poor prognosis.

■ The hypertrophic cardiomyopathy seen with Friedreich ataxia is more benign than the more classical form.

Duchenne Muscular Dystrophy
Duchenne muscular dystrophy is an X-linked recessive disorder that affects all muscle types. It is characterized by the absence of the protein dystrophin normally found on the sarcolemma of muscle cells. This disease may selectively involve the posterior wall of the left ventricular wall including the posterolateral papillary muscle. Atrial and ventricular arrhythmias are common, especially inappropriate sinus tachycardia or atrial flutter, a malignant arrhythmia when encountered in childhood, because of 1:1 atrioventricular node conduction.

■ Duchenne muscular dystrophy preferentially involves the posterobasal and posterolateral left ventricular wall and is associated with inappropriate sinus tachycardia and atrial flutter.

Myotonic Muscular Dystrophy
Myotonic muscular dystrophy is an autosomal dominant genetic muscle disorder characterized by delayed relaxation of skeletal muscles after contraction. Cardiac involvement is usually limited to conduction system disturbances, but heart failure rarely occurs. All degrees

of heart block are seen. Deep abnormal Q waves may be seen in the ECG in the absence of myocardial infarction.

Other Neurologic Diseases
Kearns-Sayre syndrome is a genetic disease transmitted through mitochondrial DNA and characterized by progressive external ophthalmoplegia, pigmentary retinopathy, and heart block that frequently requires permanent pacemaker implantation.

Guillain-Barré syndrome is a nonhereditary demyelinating neuropathy associated with autonomic dysfunction and, rarely, sudden death that is probably due to cardiac arrhythmias.

Head injuries and cerebral hemorrhage may be associated with marked ECG changes, including QT prolongation, prominent U waves, ST-segment elevation or depression, and deep symmetrical T-wave inversion in the precordial leads.

ENDOCRINE AND METABOLIC DISEASE

Acromegaly
Acromegaly, a growth hormone disorder, is associated with cardiomegaly, hypertension, focal myocardial fibrosis, lymphocytic myocarditis, premature atherosclerosis, and a specific acromegalic cardiomyopathy characterized by myocardial fibrosis and degeneration of myofibrils. Acromegalic cardiomyopathy complicated by heart failure is poorly responsive to conventional heart failure treatment but may respond to octreotide. The hypertension of acromegaly is a low renin-type hypertension due to plasma volume expansion, which responds well to diuretics and sodium restriction.

Hyperthyroidism
Thyroid hormone has effects on the heart similar to those of α-adrenergic receptor stimulation. In hyperthyroidism, the heart is hyperdynamic, with an increase in heart rate, systolic blood pressure, cardiac output, and stroke volume and a decrease in systemic vascular resistance. Atrial fibrillation occurs in 25% of patients and is is problematic because of increased atrioventricular node conduction and relative refractoriness to digoxin. β-Blockers in large doses are the drug of choice pending definitive treatment. About 40% of patients have

spontaneous reversion from atrial fibrillation to sinus rhythm when they become euthyroid. It is important to check for occult hyperthyroidism in patients with unexplained new-onset atrial fibrillation. Ventricular tachycardia can occur in uncontrolled hyperthyroidism—"thyroid storm."

Hypothyroidism
Hypothyroidism is associated with a decrease in heart rate, ventricular contractility, and cardiac output but an increase in systemic vascular resistance and systemic blood pressure. It may also be associated with pericardial effusion and an abnormal lipid profile (increase in low-density lipoprotein cholesterol and triglycerides) (Fig. 1).

Cushing Syndrome
Cushing syndrome results from glucocorticoid excess due to ACTH-producing adenomas of the pituitary. Other causes include ectopic ACTH-producing tumors and primary adrenal tumors. Iatrogenic Cushing disease may be caused by the therapeutic use of steroids. Cushing syndrome is associated with hyperkalemia, systemic hypertension, and left ventricular hypertrophy. The hypertension of Cushing syndrome is relatively resistant to conventional antihypertensive medications but may respond to ketoconazole because of its inhibitory effect on adrenal enzymes (Fig. 2).

Addison Disease
Addison disease, or other causes of adrenal insufficiency including abrupt withdrawal of steroid medication, is associated with arterial hypotension, postural hypotension, and syncope. Specific electrocardiographic (ECG) changes, low-voltage ECG, prolonged QT interval, and sinus bradycardia may occur.

Hyperaldosteronism
This is the result of excess secretion of aldosterone. It is associated with hypokalemia and hypertension.

Fabry Disease
This is an X-linked recessive lysosomal storage disorder that results in glycosphingolipid infiltration of the heart, skin, brain, and kidneys. Infiltration of cardiac myocytes results in ventricular hypertrophy and dysfunction, myocardial ischemia and infarction, endothelial

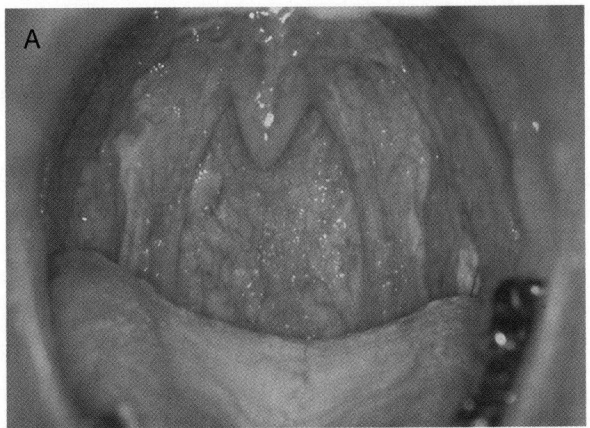

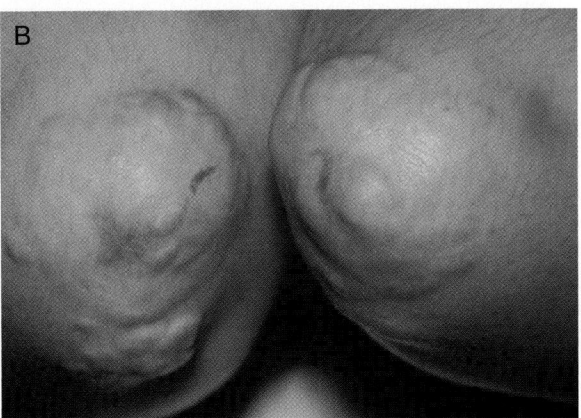

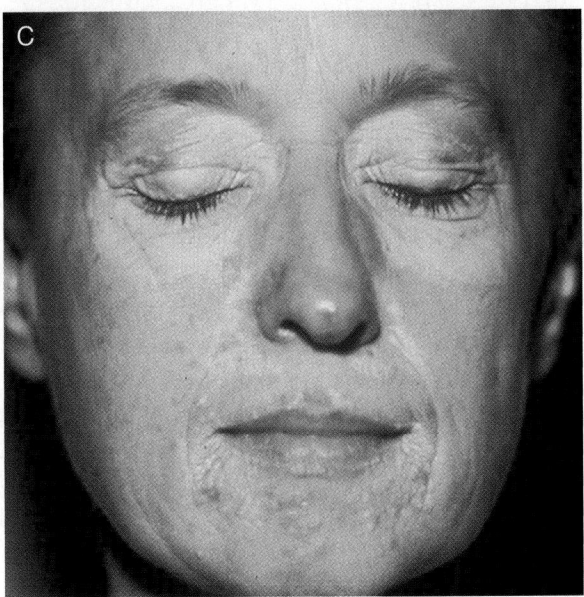

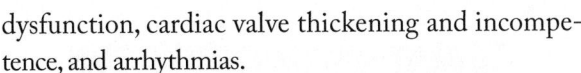

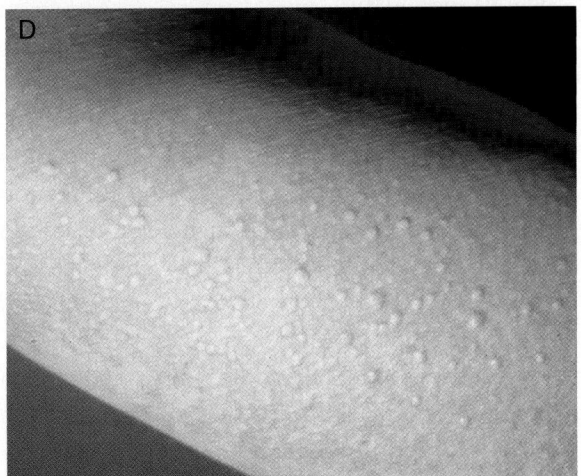

Fig. 1. *A*, Diffuse-plane nomolipemic xanthomatosis. *B*, Xanthoma tuberosum. *C, D*, Biliary hypercholesterolemic xanthomatosis.

dysfunction, cardiac valve thickening and incompetence, and arrhythmias.

Refsum Disease

This is an autosomal recessive neurodegenerative disorder due to accumulation of phytanic acid that these patients cannot metabolize. Cardiac involvement includes conduction disorders (atrioventricular node and bundle branch), arrhythmias, and an increased occurrence of sudden death.

GLYCOGEN STORAGE DISEASES

In type II glycogen storage disease (Pompe disease) and type III disease, cardiomyopathy due to myocardial deposition of abnormal glycogen occurs, leading to cardiomyopathy.

Amyloidosis

Amyloid infiltration of the heart may occur in many of the inherited amyloidoses and lead to cardiomyopathy with features of restrictive, dilated, and hypertrophic variants. The prognosis is poor without cardiac transplantation. Cardiac amyloidosis may also occur with minimal or no systemic involvement (Fig. 3).

CONNECTIVE TISSUE DISEASE

Rheumatoid Arthritis

Rheumatoid arthritis may be associated with involvement of all cardiac structures, including the pericardium, valves, myocardium, conduction system, coronary arteries, aorta, and pulmonary circulation. Rheumatoid arthritis can cause both granulomatous and nongranulomatous inflammation of the leaflets of cardiac valves, rarely leading to severe mitral or aortic valve incompetence. The myocardium may be involved by an inflammatory myocarditis or by the deposition of amyloid. The pericarditis of rheumatoid arthritis is characterized by a low glucose value and complement depletion in the pericardial fluid. Constrictive pericarditis rarely occurs. Rheumatoid nodules may be deposited in the conduction system, leading to all degrees of heart block. Aortitis and pulmonary hypertension due to pulmonary vasculitis are rare complications.

■ The pericarditis of rheumatoid arthritis is characterized by a low glucose value and complement depletion.

Systemic Lupus Erythematosus

Systemic lupus erythematosus can involve all cardiac structures. Special features of cardiac involvement in systemic lupus erythematosus include nonbacterial endocarditis, antiphospholipid antibody syndrome, and congenital heart block in the offspring of mothers with subacute cutaneous lupus erythematosus.

The offspring of mothers with anti-Ro and anti-La antibodies are at risk for the development of both myocarditis and inflammation and fibrosis of the conduction system, leading to congenital heart block. Treating the mother with corticosteroids may be beneficial if fetal complete heart block is detected ultrasonographically.

■ The offspring of mothers with anti-Ro and anti-La antibodies are at risk for the development of congenital heart block.

Polymyositis and Dermatomyositis

Polymyositis is associated with myocarditis, pericarditis, and conduction system disease (Fig. 4). Myocarditis is rare in the absence of systemic myositis but may respond to systemically administered corticosteroids, hence the importance of endomyocardial biopsy if myocarditis is suspected in polymyositis. All degrees of conduction system disease may be seen with polymyositis. Pericarditis, rarely leading to constrictive pericarditis, may occur (Fig. 5).

Ankylosing Spondylitis

Ankylosing spondylitis is associated with aortic incompetence in up to 10% of patients and, more rarely, mitral valve prolapse and mitral regurgitation. Histologically there is an infiltrate of lymphocytes and plasma cells in the aortic wall and around the vasa vasorum, with resultant shortening and thickening of the aortic valve leaflets and aortic root dilatation. Conduction system disease due to both fibrosis and acute inflammation may occur.

Scleroderma

Pericardial disease (pericarditis, pericardial effusions, tamponade, constrictive pericarditis) and pulmonary

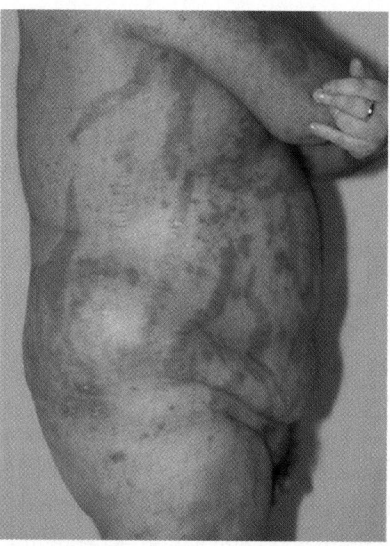

Fig. 2. Exogenous Cushing disease.

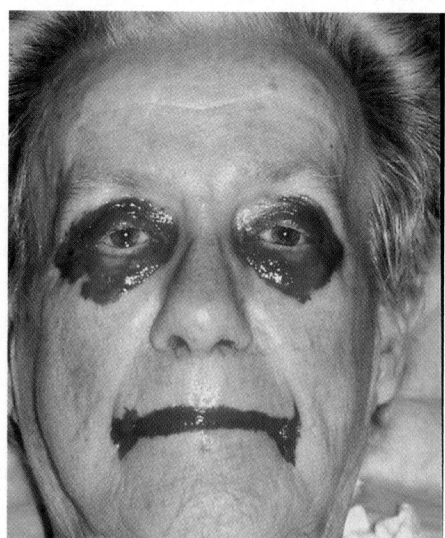

Fig. 3. Amyloidosis.

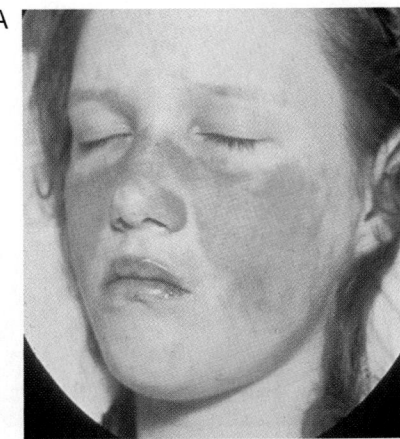
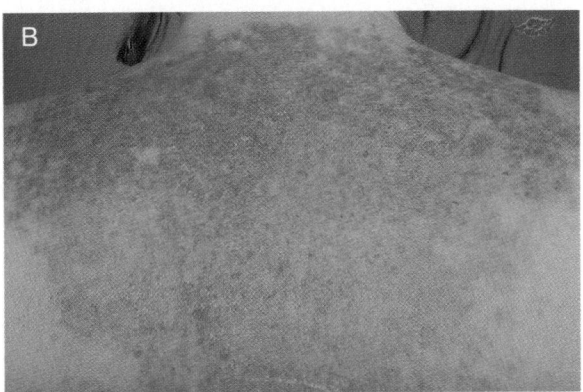
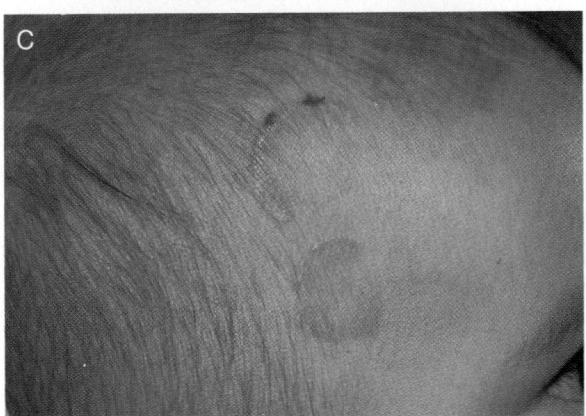
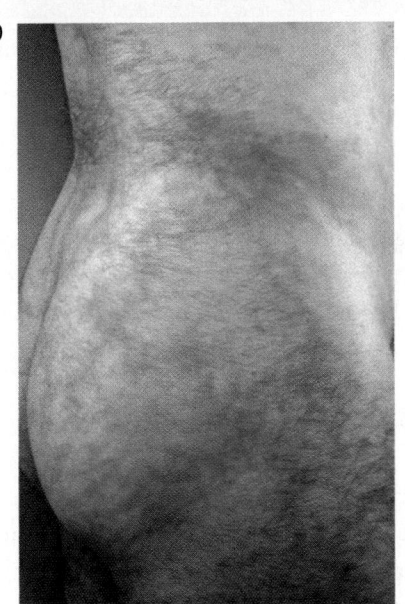

Fig. 4. *A* and *B*, Lupus erythematosus, systemic. *C*, Neonatal lupus. *D*, Livedo reticularis.

hypertension are the classic cardiac complications associated with diffuse scleroderma, although conduction system disease and myocardial fibrosis also occur. Patients with CREST syndrome (calcinosis cutis, Raynaud phenomenon, esophageal dysfunction, sclerodactyly, and telangiectasia) are at higher risk for cardiac complications, particularly pericarditis, than patients with uncomplicated scleroderma (Fig. 6).

Relapsing Polychondritis
Relapsing polychondritis is associated with aneurysms of the ascending aorta and with aortic incompetence due to inflammation of cartilaginous supporting tissues. Vasculitis of large- and medium-sized arteries, including the coronary vessels, may also occur.

Reiter Syndrome
Reiter syndrome is associated with aortitis, aortic incompetence, heart block, and pericarditis.

Behçet Disease
Behçet disease is associated with aneurysms of the arch vessels and abdominal aorta, aortitis, and aortic incompetence.

Churg-Strauss Syndrome
Classically, Churg-Strauss syndrome is associated with eosinophilic myocarditis and restrictive cardiomyopathy; however, acute pericarditis, constrictive pericarditis, myocardial infarction, arrhythmias, and heart failure may also occur (Fig. 7).

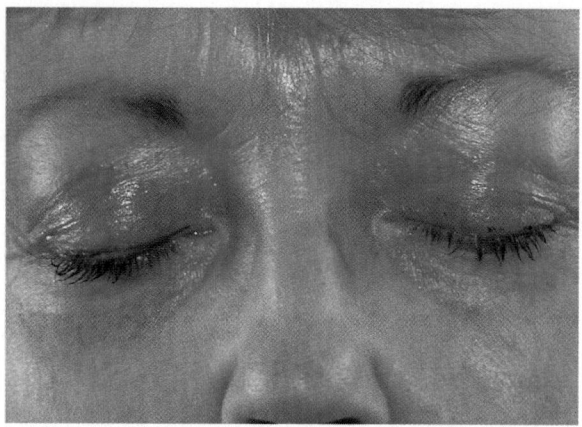

Fig. 5. Heliotrope periorbital rash seen in dermato-myositis.

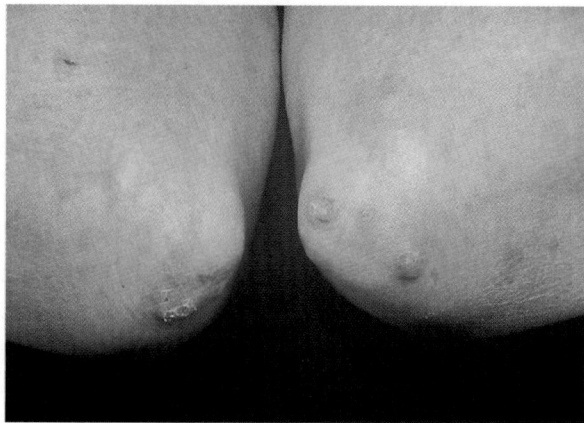

Fig. 7. Churg-Strauss granuloma.

Polyarteritis Nodosa

Polyarteritis nodosa is associated with arteritis and aneurysm formation of the epicardial coronary arteries. Myocarditis and pericarditis may also occur (Fig. 8).

HEMATOLOGY/ONCOLOGY DISEASES

Anemia

Chronic anemia leads to a compensatory increase in cardiac output due to increased venous preload and decreased systemic vascular resistance. Venous return and systemic catecholamines increase, and, rarely, high-output cardiac failure occurs. Left ventricular dilatation and hypertrophy are common. Anemia lowers the threshold for angina and may cause nonspecific ST changes even in the absence of cardiac disease. The rapidity of the development of anemia is a major determinant of symptoms. Severe anemia may cause abnormal findings on a cardiac examination, including a hyperdynamic apex, systolic flow murmurs across the aortic and pulmonary valves, diastolic flow murmurs across the mitral and tricuspid valves, and third and fourth heart sounds.

Thalassemia

Thalassemia frequently is associated with systemic iron overload and myocardial iron deposition due to extravascular hemolysis and multiple blood transfusions. This leads to systolic and diastolic ventricular dysfunction, with eventual heart failure. Recurrent pericarditis, pericardial effusions, and, rarely, pericardial tamponade

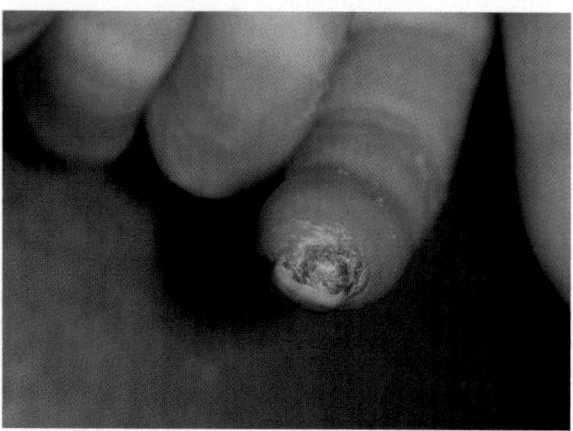

Fig. 6. Scleroderma, systematic.

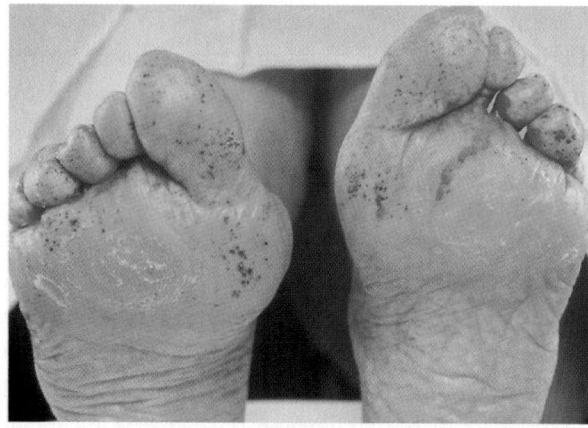

Fig. 8. Vasculitis

may occur. Heart block may occur because of iron deposition in the atrioventricular node. Chronic anemia is common in thalassemia, and transfusions are frequently required. Chelation agents significantly reduce the occurrence of transfusion-associated cardiac dysfunction.

Sickle Cell Disease

Sickle cell disease is associated with chronic anemia, heart failure, myocardial infarction, and pulmonary infarction. Myocardial infarction in the absence of coronary atherosclerosis occurs because of in situ thrombosis of sickled cells. Sickling is aggravated by high oxygen extraction by the myocardium. Papillary muscle infarction is a well-recognized complication of sickle cell disease. Pulmonary infarction can result from thrombosis in situ as well as from pulmonary emboli and can predispose to recurrent pulmonary infections. Cardiac complications due to iron overload are less common in sickle cell disease than in thalassemia.

Primary Hemochromatosis

Primary hemochromatosis is a genetic disorder of increased iron absorption that results in an increase in the serum level of iron and ferritin and a decrease in total iron binding capacity. Cardiac manifestations include atrial and ventricular arrhythmias, heart block, biventricular enlargement, restrictive cardiomyopathy, and heart failure. Repeated phlebotomy is protective against the cardiac complications of hemochromatosis if started before organ damage has occurred. When phlebotomy is initiated later in the course of the disease, it may partially reverse end organ dysfunction.

Cardiac Radiation Damage

Cardiac radiation damage occurs after irradiation of the mediastinum, usually for Hodgkin or non-Hodgkin lymphoma. All cardiac structures can be damaged, and initial cardiac symptoms may not develop for years to decades after irradiation. All forms of pericarditis may occur, including acute pericarditis with or without effusion, chronic pericarditis, effusive-constrictive pericarditis, and constrictive pericarditis. Asymptomatic pericardial thickening without signs of constriction is a common late finding in patients who had mediastinal (mantle) irradiation in the past.

Cardiac irradiation may cause an acute or, more likely, a chronic valvulitis that results in valve stenosis or incompetence. Dilated cardiomyopathy due to myocardial microvasculature damage is a late consequence of cardiac irradiation. Cardiac irradiation can cause significant endothelial damage of the coronary arteries, leading to nonatherosclerotic coronary artery disease. Irradiation in childhood increases fourfold the relative risk of myocardial infarction in adulthood. Irradiation during childhood and the concomitant use of anthracycline chemotherapy agents increase the risk of myocardial damage.

Cancer Chemotherapy

The anthracyclines, including daunorubicin and doxorubicin, are the major causes of chemotherapy-induced cardiomyopathy. The probability of developing cardiomyopathy is dependent on the cumulative dose of medication administered. The risk of cardiomyopathy is less than 1% up to 400 mg/m^2 but increases to 7% at 550 mg/m^2 and to more than 15% at 700 mg/m^2. Preexisting cardiac disease, concomitant use of cyclophosphamide, previous chest irradiation, or age older than 70 years all increase the risk of cardiomyopathy. All patients requiring anthracycline chemotherapy should have a baseline evaluation of ventricular function. If the ejection fraction is 50% or greater, the risk of cardiomyopathy is small, but the ejection fraction should be determined again after dose levels of 300 mg/m^2 and 400 mg/m^2 and after each subsequent dose of doxorubicin. Chemotherapy should be stopped if the ejection fraction decreases by 10% or more or to less than 50%.

In patients with a baseline ventricular dysfunction, chemotherapy should not be initiated if the ejection fraction is 30% or less. If EF is between 30% and 50%, chemotherapy may be administered in patients with high-risk malignancies provided the ejection fraction remains greater than 30% and does not decrease by more than 10% from baseline. The risk to benefit ratio needs to be assessed for individual patients. Children are more sensitive than adults to the adverse effects of chemotherapy, even with a surface area-adjusted dose, and for unknown reasons, females are more sensitive than males.

Cyclophosphamide administered in a high dose is associated with hemorrhagic myocarditis, cardiomyopathy, and pericardial effusion. Paclitaxel (Taxol) may cause atrioventricular block and bundle branch block, and 5-fluorouracil is associated with coronary vasospasm, angina pectoris, and, rarely, myocardial infarction or myocarditis. Interleukin-2 is associated with capillary leak syndrome and, rarely, myocarditis. Cardiomyopathy is a rare reported association of interferon-α therapy.

DRUGS

Cocaine has numerous adverse cardiovascular effects. Many of these effects are related to the sympathomimetic effect of cocaine, which is due to blockage of reuptake of catecholamines in sympathetic nerve terminals. Cocaine has been associated with acute myocardial infarction, sudden cardiac death, noninfarction chest pain, myocarditis, and cardiomyopathy. Hypertension is often a prominent feature because of systemic vasoconstriction. Other effects include accelerated atherosclerosis, subarachnoid hemorrhage, and aortic dissection. Supraventricular and ventricular arrhythmias are common. β-Blockers should be avoided because of the risk of further vasoconstriction due to unopposed vasoconstrictor effects. Labetalol (combined α- and β-blockers) may be used, as may nitrates and calcium channel blockers. Lidocaine used to treat ventricular arrhythmias may precipitate seizures (Fig. 9 and 10).

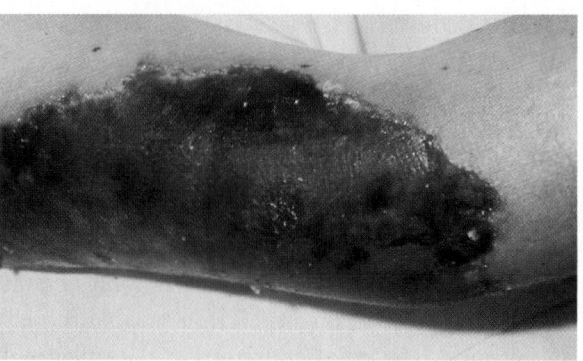

Fig. 10. Coumadin skin necrosis.

SPECIFIC SYNDROMES WITH CARDIAC INVOLVEMENT

Kartagener Syndrome

This syndrome is caused by an autosomal recessive genetic disorder that affects microtubule function. Clinically, it is characterized by situs inversus, including dextrocardia, bronchiectasis, sinusitis, and sterility due to abnormal sperm and cilia.

Marfan Syndrome

Marfan syndrome is an autosomal dominant disorder characterized by musculoskeletal, cardiovascular, and ocular abnormalities. Cardiac involvement includes mitral valve prolapse leading to mitral regurgitation, aortic root dilatation leading to aortic regurgitation, aortic aneurysm, aortic dissection, and rupture. This syndrome is caused by a genetic mutation in the fibrillin gene. The risk of aortic dissection and rupture increases significantly during pregnancy, especially in women with moderate or greater aortic root dilatation before pregnancy. All patients with Marfan syndrome should receive β-blockers, which decrease the rate of aortic root expansion and the risk of aortic rupture. Aortic replacement should be considered in asymptomatic patients with aortic root diameters of 6 cm or greater (Fig. 11).

Ehlers-Danlos Syndrome

This is an autosomal dominant disorder associated with hyperextensile joints, spontaneous pneumothoraces, scoliosis, arthritis, and cardiovascular abnormalities that include mitral and tricuspid valve prolapse, aortic root dilatation and rupture, and dissection and rupture of

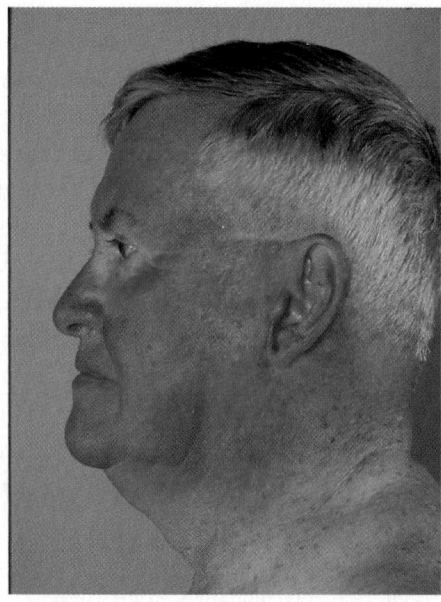

Fig. 9. Amiodarone skin pigmentation.

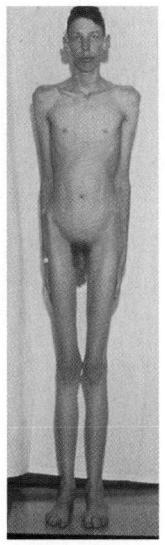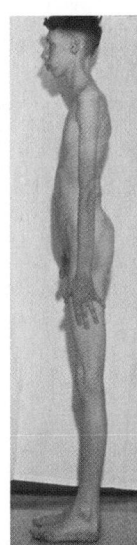

Fig. 11. Marfan syndrome.

other major arteries. Marked variation in the risk of cardiovascular abnormalities is found among the different forms of this syndrome, of which at least 15 are known (Fig. 12).

Pseudoxanthoma Elasticum
This condition is associated with yellow skin papules, angioid streaks in the retina, and cardiovascular disease. Coronary arteries, peripheral arteries, cardiac valves,

and the cardiac conduction system may all be affected in this disease. There is a high risk of atherosclerosis even in the absence of traditional risk factors (Fig. 13).

Osteogenesis Imperfecta
Osteogenesis imperfecta is characterized by blue sclera, increased bony fragility, and hearing loss and is associated with mitral valve prolapse and aortic incompetence.

Noonan Syndrome
This syndrome is characterized by impaired mental abilities, a characteristic facies, variant hypertrophic cardiomyopathy, pulmonary valve stenosis or infundibular stenosis, peripheral pulmonary artery stenosis, patent ductus arteriosus, atrial septal defect, and tetralogy of Fallot.

Williams Syndrome
This syndrome is characterized by mental impairment, a characteristic facies, supravalvular aortic stenosis, peripheral pulmonary artery stenosis, ventricular septal defect, atrial septal defect, major artery stenoses, and hypercalcemia in infancy.

Osler-Weber-Rendu Syndrome
This syndrome is associated with diffuse hemangiomas throughout the body (Fig. 14).

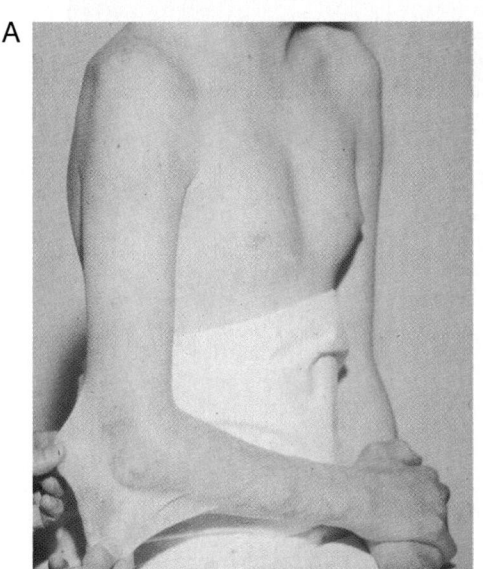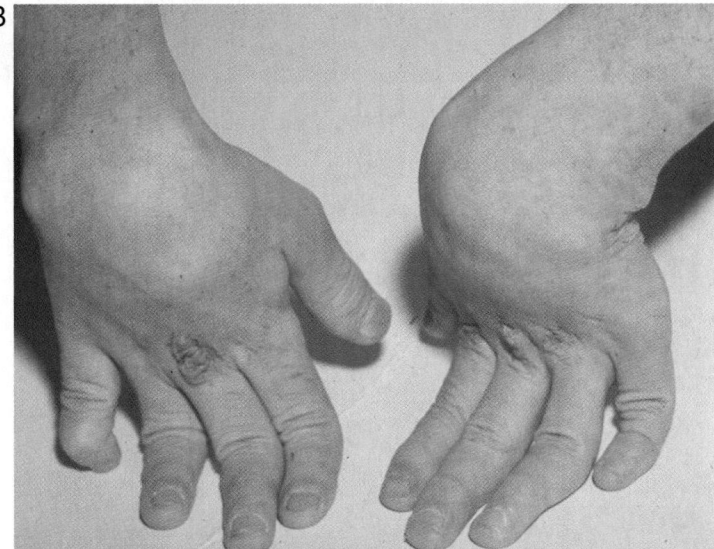

Fig. 12. *A* and *B*, Cutis hyperelastica (Ehlers-Danlos syndrome).

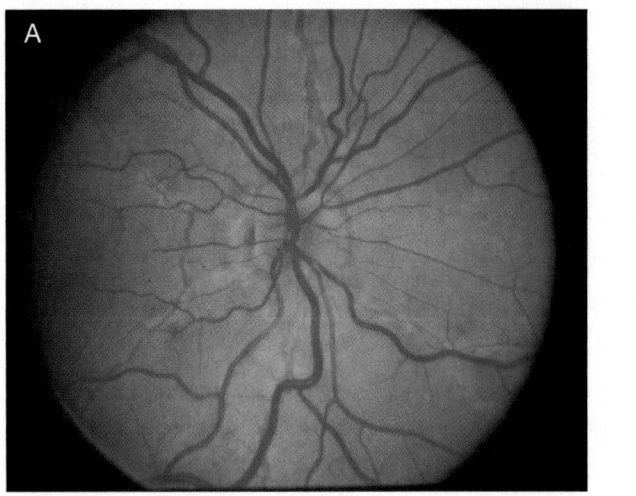
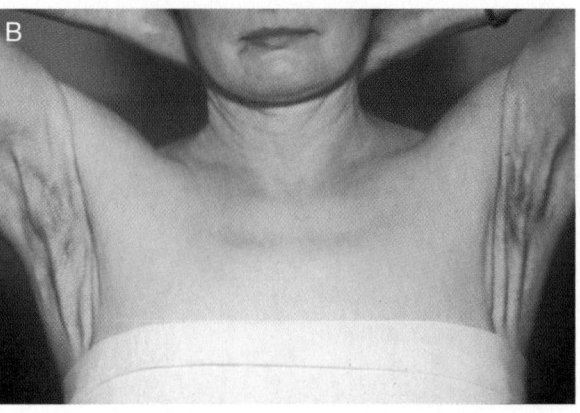

Fig. 13. *A*, Angioid streak in pseudoxanthoma elasticum. *B*, Pseudoxanthoma elasticum.

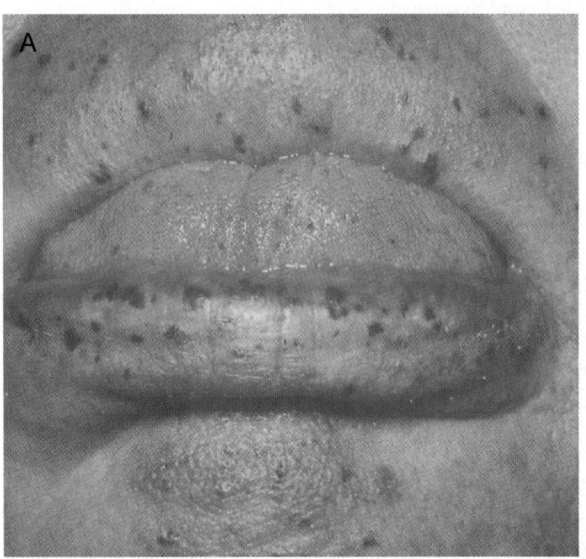
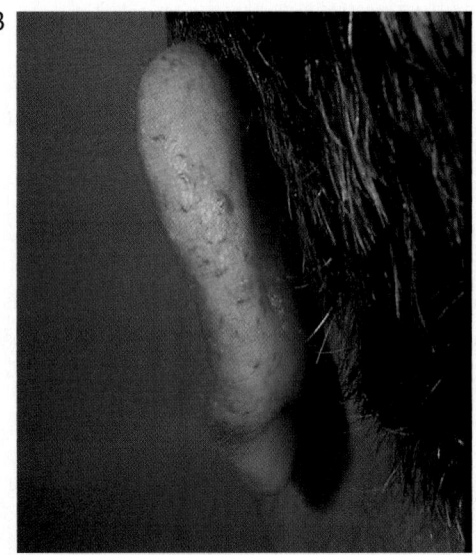

Fig. 14. *A* and *B*, Osler-Weber-Rendu disease.

84

CARDIAC TUMORS

Joseph G. Murphy, MD

R. Scott Wright, MD

Primary tumors of the heart are exceedingly rare, accounting for less than 5% of all cardiac tumors; the remaining 95% of tumors are metastatic tumors to the heart. The most common primary cardiac tumors in adults are myxomas (usually occurring in the left atrium, Fig. 1), followed by lipomas and fibroelastomas (Table 1). The most common cardiac tumor in children is rhabdomyoma.

- Primary cardiac tumors are 5% of all cardiac tumors.
- Metastatic cardiac tumors are 95% of all cardiac tumors.
- The most common primary cardiac tumors in adults are myxomas.
- 20% of patients dying from cancer have pericardial metastases.

Table 1. Common Types of Primary Tumors of the Heart

Benign (75%)
  Myxoma
  Rhabdomyoma
  Fibroma
  Lipoma and lipomatous hypertrophy of the atrial septum
  Atrioventricular node tumor
  Papillary fibroelastoma
  Hemangioma
Malignant (25%)
  Angiosarcoma
  Rhabdomyosarcoma
  Fibrosarcoma

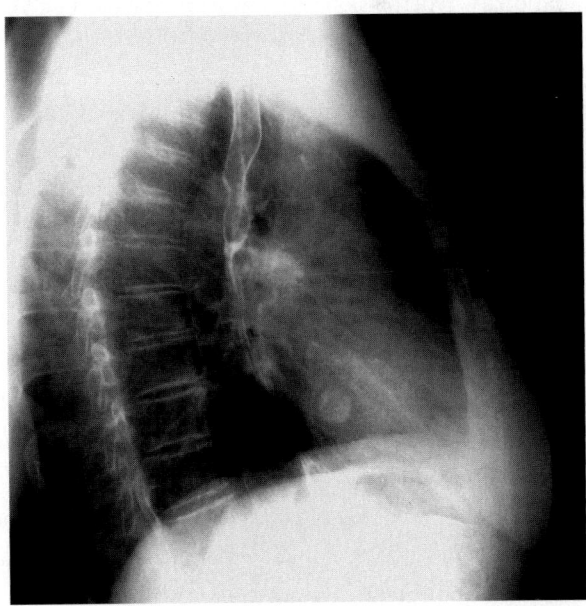

Fig. 1. Lateral chest radiograph demonstrating calcified left atrial myxoma.

CLINICAL FEATURES OF CARDIAC MYXOMA

Cardiac myxoma may result in systemic symptoms, largely due to embolic phenomenon or its secretion of interleukin-6 (IL-6). Constitutional symptoms include fever and weight loss. Embolic phenomena are due to tumor fragmentation and thromboembolism from the tumor surface. These embolic episodes may mimic systemic vasculitis or infective endocarditis. Right-sided cardiac tumors may result in recurrent pulmonary emboli. The most common presenting symptoms of left-sided cardiac myxomas are dyspnea on exertion, paroxysmal nocturnal dyspnea, and fever, but sudden death and hemoptysis also may occur. The most common physical finding with a left atrial myxoma is a mitral diastolic murmur (similar to mitral stenosis but without the opening snap) (Table 2) or a mitral systolic murmur due to mitral incompetence. Other features include an added heart sound or tumor plop, atrial fibrillation, clubbing, and Raynaud phenomenon. Left atrial tumors may mimic mitral stenosis or incompetence, endocarditis, or vasculitis. Right atrial tumors may mimic Ebstein anomaly, atrial septal defect, or constrictive pericarditis (Fig. 2). Left ventricular tumors may mimic aortic stenosis or hypertrophic obstructive cardiomyopathy, and right ventricular tumors may mimic pulmonary stenosis, pulmonary hypertension, or pulmonary emboli (Fig. 3).

PRESENTATION OF CARDIAC TUMORS

- Asymptomatic—incidental discovery on Echo, CT or MRI of chest.
- Pericardial effusion with or without cardiac tamponade (usually due to pericardial metastases)
- Obstruction to myocardial filling or emptying
- Obstruction to valve opening or closing
- Atrial or ventricular arrhythmias including heart block.
- Thromboembolism to systemic or pulmonary circulations.
- Systemic symptoms (fever, weight loss).

The most common malignant cardiac tumor in adults is angiosarcoma. In children, rhabdomyosarcoma is the most common malignant tumor. A malignant lymphoma may occasionally develop in the adult heart.

The locations of cardiac myxomas are listed in Table 3.

- Cardiac myxoma results in systemic symptoms, largely due to its secretion of interleukin-6 (IL-6).
- Right atrial tumors may mimic Ebstein anomaly, atrial septal defect, or constrictive pericarditis.

Table 2. Features Differentiating Left Atrial Myxoma From Mitral Valve Disease

Parameter	Myxoma	Mitral valve disease
History	Short duration	Chronic
	Associated constitutional symptoms	No associated constitutional symptoms
	Syncope occasionally noted	Syncope rare
Symptoms	Occasionally episodic	Progressive
Physical examination	Tumor "plop"	Opening snap
	Murmurs varying with position	Murmurs constant
	Associated valve disease unusual	Associated valve disease common
Electrocardiogram	Sinus rhythm	Atrial fibrillation
Chest radiograph	Tumor calcification	Valve calcification
	Left atrium small	Left atrium enlarged
Echocardiogram	Characteristic findings	Characteristic findings

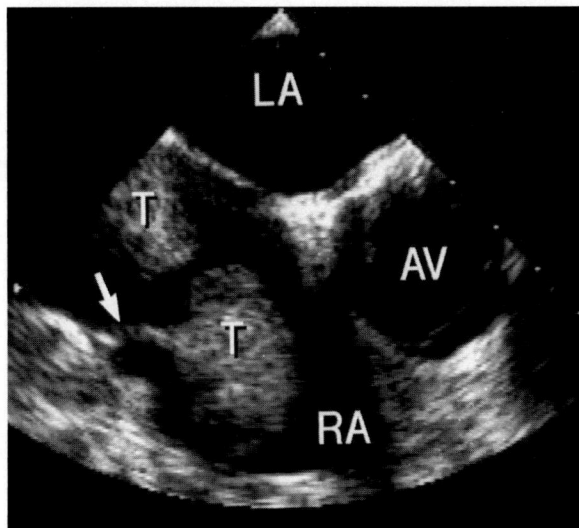

Fig. 2. Multicentric right atrial myxomas; modified basal transverse transesophageal echocardiography plane. Two of three right atrial myxomas (T) are visible in this plane. The larger has a well-defined slender stalk (*arrow*) attaching the tumor to the lateral wall of the right atrium (RA). The smaller myxoma has a broad-based attachment to the posterior atrial septum. AV, aortic valve; LA, left atrium.

FAMILIAL CARDIAC TUMORS

The familial cardiac myxoma syndromes constitute approximately 10% of myxomas and have an autosomal dominant transmission.

In Carney syndrome, myxomas arise in noncardiac locations (usually breast or skin), pigmentation of the skin occurs (usually lentigines or pigmented nevi), and there may be endocrine tumors, including pituitary

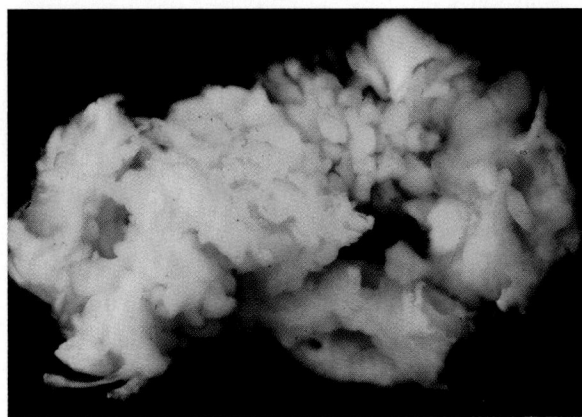

Fig. 3. Left atrial myxoma.

adenomas, adrenocortical disease, or testicular tumors. Other syndromes include the NAME syndrome (nevi, atrial myxoma, myxoid neurofibroma, and ephelides) and the LAMB syndrome (lentigines, atrial myxoma, and blue nevi). Familial cardiac myxoma syndromes differ from nonfamilial (sporadic) myxomas in that they occur in younger patients, have less of a female preponderance, are frequently multiple, are more frequently recurrent postoperatively, and occur more often in a ventricular site. Familial myxomas are associated with freckling and noncardiac tumors in approximately two-thirds of cases and with endocrine tumors in one-third of cases. Cardiac rhabdomyomas are associated with the tuberous sclerosis syndrome, which is characterized by hematomas in multiple organs, epilepsy, mental deficiency, and adenoma sebaceum. Cardiac fibromas are benign connective tissue tumors that occur predominantly in children. Imaging of cardiac tumors is usually with echocardiography, Imatron computed tomography, or magnetic resonance imaging. Atrial myxomas may recur in approximately 5% of patients. Malignant cardiac tumors have a uniformly poor prognosis.

- NAME syndrome (nevi, atrial myxoma, myxoid neurofibroma, and ephelides).
- LAMB syndrome (lentigines, atrial myxoma, and blue nevi).

LIPOMATOUS HYPERTROPHY OF THE ATRIAL SEPTUM (FIG. 4)

Lipomatous hypertrophy of the atrial septum, although not a true tumor, is the accumulation of nonencapsulated adipose tissue (both fetal and adult type) within the atrial septum (Fig. 5). This can lead to massive atrial septal hypertrophy that may protrude into the right atrium. It is more common in elderly, obese women.

Table 3. Locations of Cardiac Myxomas

Location	%
Left atrium	75
Right atrium	15
Right ventricle	5
Left ventricle	5

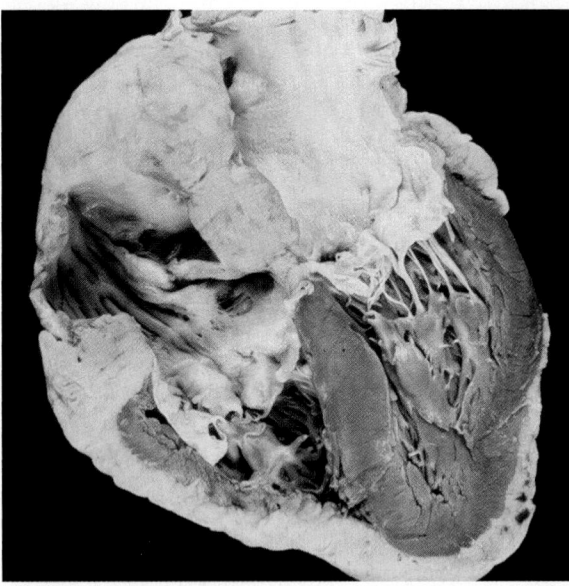

Fig. 4. Lipomatous hypertrophy of atrial septum.

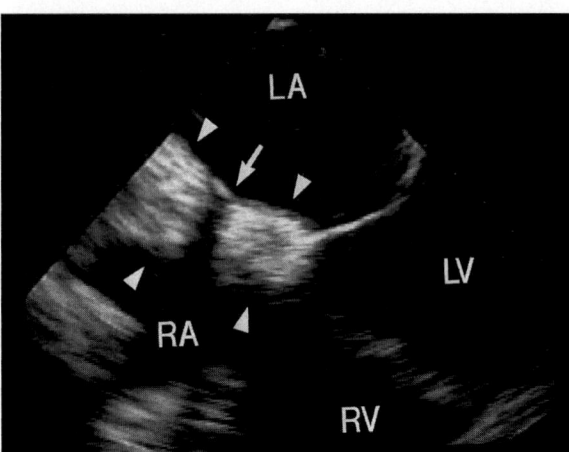

Fig. 5. Lipomatous hypertrophy of the atrial septum; transverse transesophageal echocardiography plane, four-chamber view. Extensive fatty tissue accumulation within the atrial septum (*arrowheads*) spares the fossa ovalis membrane (*arrow*), imparting the typical dumb-bell appearance of lipomatous atrial septal hypertrophy. LA, left atrium; LV, left ventricle, RA, right atrium; RV, right ventricle.

Lipomatous hypertrophy of the atrial septum has been variably associated with supraventricular arrhythmias. The diagnosis is usually made with echocardiography.

Cardiac sarcomas are the commonest primary malignant tumor of the heart and include severe histologies including angiosarcomas derived from malignant vascular forming cells, and rhabdomyosarcomas usually arising from the ventricular walls. Prognosis is poor with median survival of less than one year. Rare patients have been successfully treated with surgery. Cardiac transplantation is of unproven benefit when combined with complete heart removal for cardiac tumor.

MESOTHELIOMA OF THE ATRIOVENTRICULAR NODE (FIG. 6)

The mesothelioma of the atrioventricular node is a cystic tumor usually diagnosed at autopsy. It is a rare cause of sudden death due to complete heart block, ventricular fibrillation, or cardiac tamponade.

Malignant mesothelioma of the pericardium usually presents acutely with features of cardiac tamponade or chronically with features of pericardial constriction. Its relationship to asbestos exposure is unproven unlike pleural mesothelioma where asbestos is a proven etiologic agent. Treatment is largely palliative and prognosis for cure is very poor (Fig. 7).

PAPILLARY FIBROELASTOMA

Papillary fibroelastomas are benign tumors that arise from the cardiac valves (Fig. 8). They may cause valvular incompetence, coronary obstruction if located on the arterial side of the aortic valve, and thromboembolic complications. Surgical excision is curative (Fig. 9).

■ Cardiac tumors associated with AIDS infection include Kaposi sarcoma and primary lymphoma of the heart.

METASTATIC CARDIAC TUMORS

Metastatic tumors of the heart, predominantly from carcinoma of lung and breast, malignant melanoma, and the leukemias and lymphomas, constitute the majority of cardiac tumors, outnumbering primary cardiac tumors approximately 20 to 1.

Pericardial metastasis presenting with pericarditis is the most common symptom of metastatic heart disease. Less commonly the patient may have an asymptomatic pericardial effusion detected on chest radiography or echocardiography. If the pericardial fluid collects

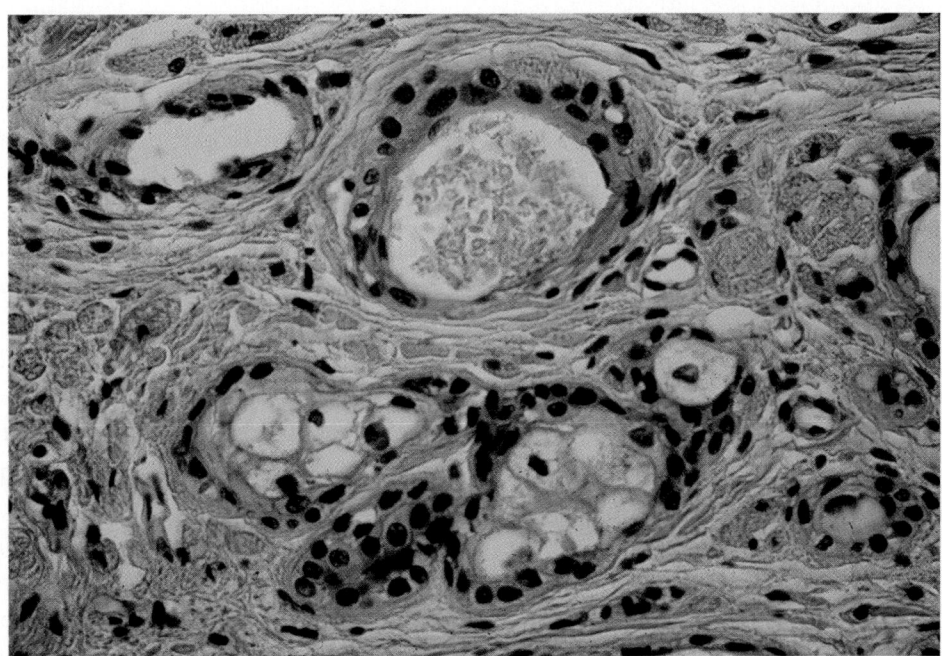

Fig. 6. Mesothelioma of atrioventricular node associated with sudden death.

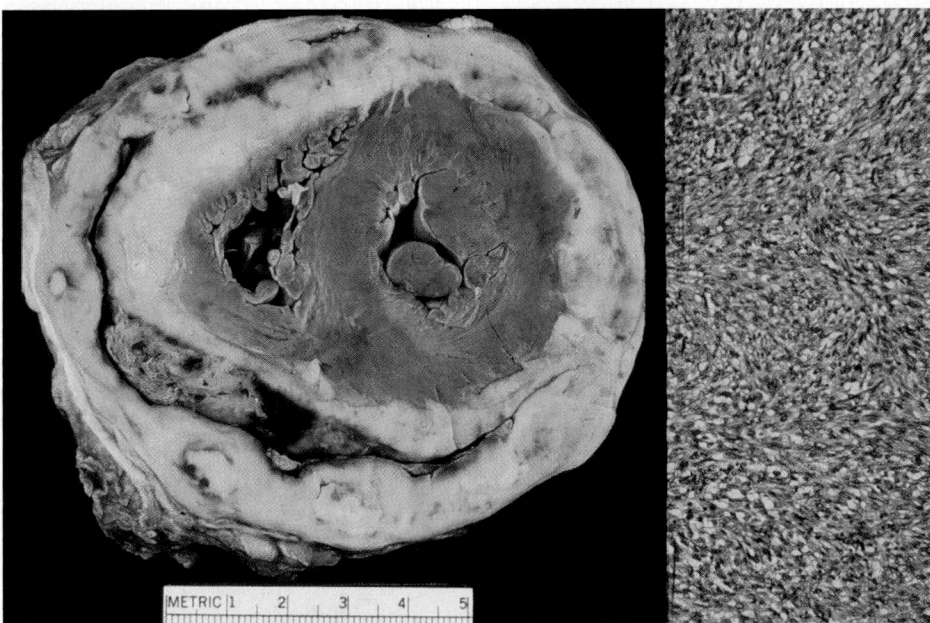

Fig. 7. Mesothelioma with pericardial constriction.

rapidly, the patient may present with pericardial tamponade. Myocardial metastasis is frequent in patients dying of widespread carcinomatosis, but it is rarely diagnosed before death. Endomyocardial and valve metastases may mimic primary cardiac tumors, but they are rare.

Neoplastic Pericarditis

At autopsy, approximately 10% of patients dying of malignancy have pericardial involvement, 5% of which have myocardial metastases. Table 4 lists tumors that can cause neoplastic pericarditis.

Nephroblastoma (Wilms tumor) and neuroblastoma

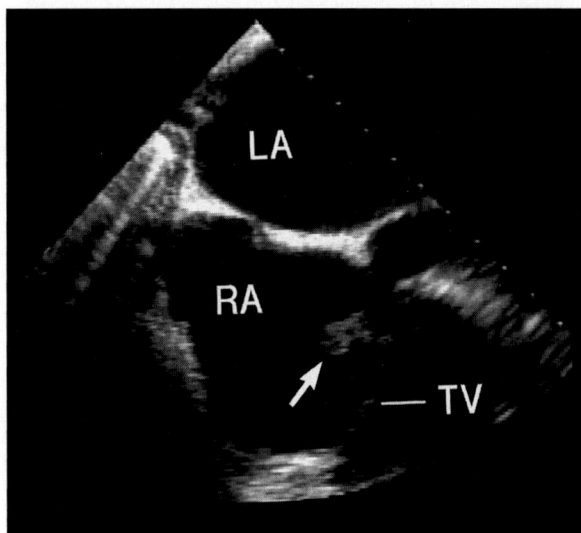

Fig. 8. Papillary fibroelastoma of the tricuspid valve; transverse transesophageal echocardiography plane. A broad-based mass (*arrow*) is attached to the atrial surface of the septal leaflet of the tricuspid valve. The "shimmering" mobility of its fronds on real-time examination was typical of papillary fibroelastoma. LA, left atrium; RA, right atrium; TV, tricuspid valve.

are additional causes of neoplastic pericarditis in children.

Primary pericardial tumors are very rare. They include mesothelioma (possibly associated with asbestos exposure), pheochromocytoma, and sarcomas (fibrosarcoma, liposarcoma, angiosarcoma) (Fig. 10).

A hemorrhagic pericardial effusion may be due to extramedullary intrapericardial hematopoiesis in chronic myeloid leukemia and myelomonocytic leukemic blast crisis.

Small nonprogressive, asymptomatic pericardial effusions may occur in 50% of patients with breast cancer, probably as a result of lymphatic obstruction.

Carcinoma of the bronchus and breast spreads to the heart primarily via lymphatics but also by direct extension and, more rarely, via the pulmonary veins (bronchogenic carcinoma). Carcinoma of the testis and kidney may spread via the venous system and lead to intracardiac metastasis.

Myocardial metastasis may be clinically asymptomatic or may present with nonspecific ST-T wave changes, cardiac arrhythmias, heart block, or myocardial dysfunction. Echocardiography is the most commonly used imaging method in suspected cardiac metastatic disease, but magnetic resonance imaging and computed Imatron tomography imaging are also valuable. Pericardiocentesis under echocardiographic guidance allows diagnosis of pericardial metastases in 70% to 80% of patients.

Treatment of pericardial metastasis is usually palliative, but radiation therapy and chemotherapy are valuable. Malignant pericardial effusion can be treated in the short term by an indwelling drainage catheter and more long term by a pericardial window. Surgical pericardiectomy may be required if the pericardial

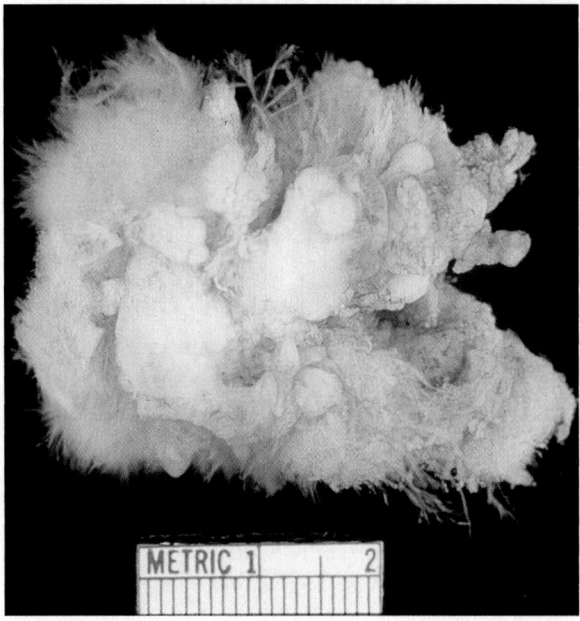

Fig. 9. Papillary fibroelastoma of mitral papillary muscle.

Table 4. Tumors That Cause Neoplastic Pericarditis

Tumor	%
Lung carcinoma	40
Breast carcinoma	20
Hodgkin disease, leukemia, lymphomas	15
Other carcinoma	10
Melanoma	5
Sarcoma	5
Others	5

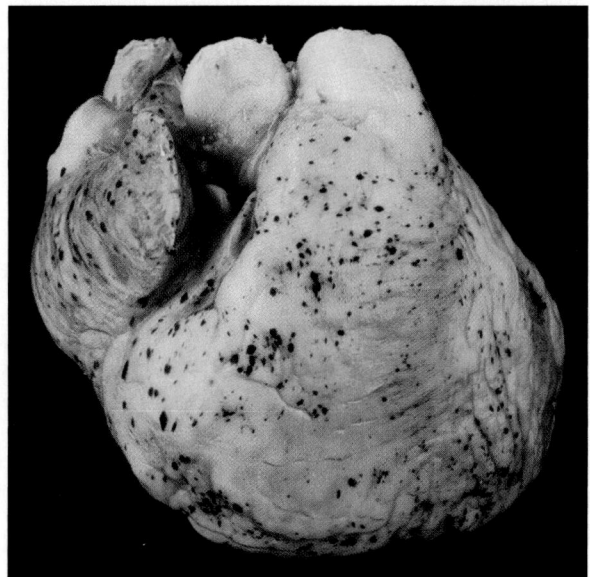

Fig. 10. Metastatic melanoma affecting the epicardial surface of the heart.

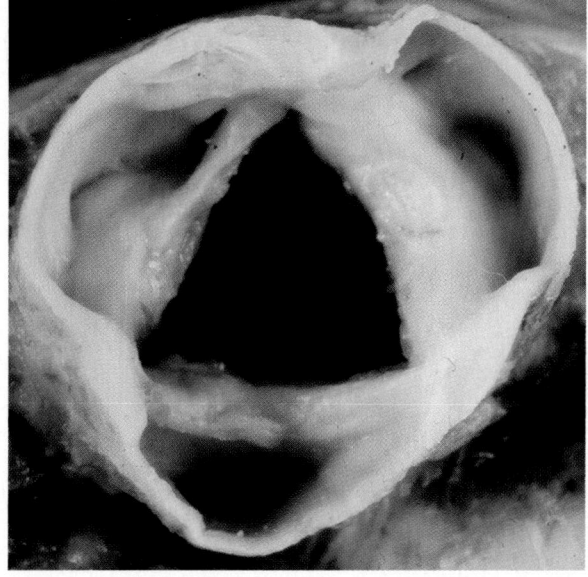

Fig. 11. Carcinoid heart disease causing a combination of pulmonary valve stenosis and incompetence.

window obstructs. In patients with acquired immuno-deficiency syndrome (AIDS), cardiac tumors may be due to non-Hodgkin lymphoma or metastatic Kaposi sarcoma (Fig. 11 and 12).

Carcinoid heart disease is characterized by plaque-like deposits of fibrous tissue on the endocardial surface of valve cusps and leafelets usually on the right heart valves (90% of time) but less commonly on the left heart valves (10% of time) if there is a patent foramen ovale or the carcinoid tumor is a bronchial carcinoid. Carcinoid tumor cells are not found in the heart but seratonin secreted remotely is considered the mechanism of carcinoid heart disease.

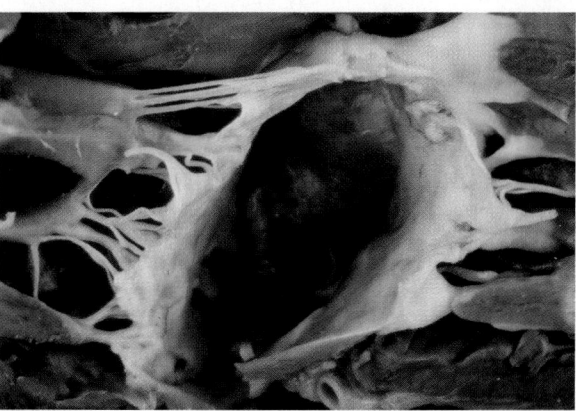

Fig. 12. Carcinoid heart disease causing a combination of tricuspid valve stenosis and incompetence.

SLEEP APNEA AND CARDIAC DISEASE

Tomas Kara, MD, PhD

Robert Wolk, MD, PhD

Virend K. Somers, MD, PhD

Sleep represents about one-third of our lives and disordered sleep may contribute significantly to the initiation, long-term prognosis, and treatment of cardiovascular disease.

NORMAL SLEEP

Normal sleep is divided into REM (associated with rapid eye movements) and non-REM (NREM) stages: NREM sleep is further divided into stages I, II, III and IV, representing progressively deeper stages of sleep, with gradual reductions in sympathetic activity and consequently in heart rate, stroke volume, cardiac output, systemic vascular resistance and blood pressure. Simultaneously, ventilation and metabolic rate also decline. During stage IV of sleep sympathetic activity, heart rate, blood pressure and ventilation are usually at their nadir. Conversely, parasympathetic or vagal activity increases in NREM sleep, particularly in stage IV.

REM sleep, by contrast, is a state of neural activation. It is characterized by sporadic rapid eye movements and is the time of sleep when dreams are most likely to occur. During REM there is a marked sympathetic activation with intermittent surges in blood pressure and heart rate. Surprisingly, sympathetic activity is about twofold the levels recorded during quiet wakefulness, and blood pressure and heart rate are similar to

wakefulness measures. Occasional bursts of parasympathetic activity, manifest as bradyarrhythmias, may also occur during REM.

Normal adults spend approximately 85% of their total sleep time in NREM sleep—generally a time of cardiovascular relaxation. Sleep apnea can seriously disrupt the structured autonomic and hemodynamic profile of normal NREM and REM sleep.

DEFINITION OF SLEEP APNEA

Sleep apnea is defined as repetitive episodes of attenuated or absent respiratory airflow during sleep, leading to a fall in oxygen saturation and to repetitive arousals with sleep fragmentation. Sleep apnea can be central or obstructive. **Central sleep apnea (CSA)** is characterized by apneas secondary to diminution or cessation of thoracoabdominal respiratory movement due to decreased central respiratory drive. CSA is primarily seen in patients with congestive heart failure (CHF), although it occasionally may occur in healthy normal subjects, in people at high altitude, and in association with central neural lesions. By contrast, **obstructive sleep apnea (OSA)** is caused by upper airway collapse during inspiration and is accompanied by strenuous breathing efforts (i.e. increased respiratory drive) (Fig. 1). When defined as >5 episodes of apnea or hypopnea per hour

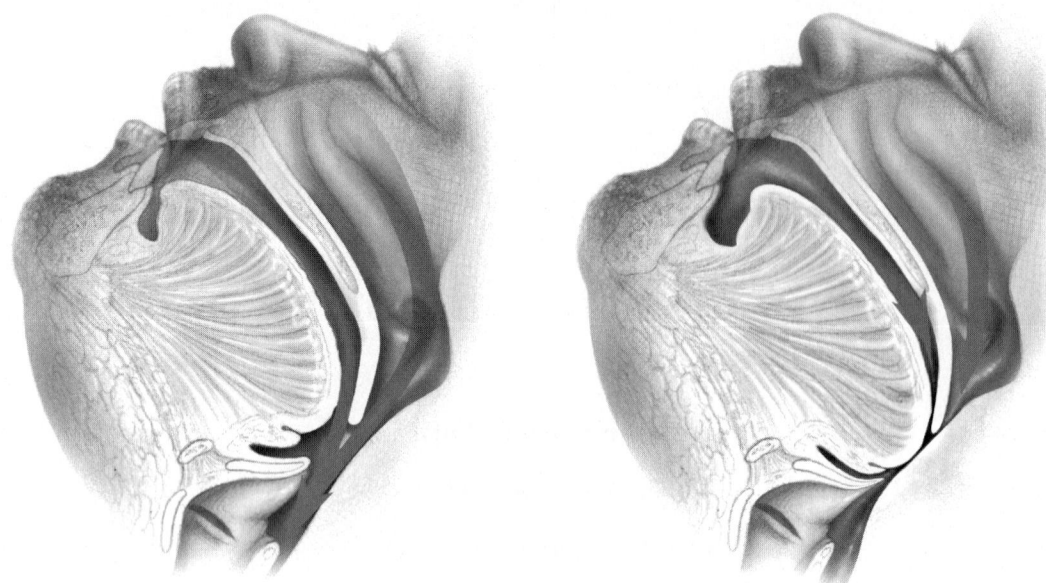

Fig. 1. Schematic of patent upper airways during sleep (*left*) and collapsed upper airways (*right*) causing obstructive sleep apnea.

of sleep, OSA is relatively common, affecting 24% and 9% of middle-aged men and women, respectively.

Sleep apnea, particularly OSA, constitutes a major public health problem and is closely associated with obesity. Emerging evidence strongly links OSA to cardiovascular morbidity.

OBSTRUCTIVE SLEEP APNEA

Acute Responses

Repetitive apneas can induce nocturnal oxygen desaturation to levels as low as 40-50%. This hypoxemia, together with CO_2 retention, activates the peripheral and central chemoreflexes, resulting in sympathetic activation with vasoconstriction and surges in blood pressure. Blood pressure can reach levels as high as 240/130 mm Hg (Fig. 2), at a time when there is severe simultaneous hypoxic and neurohumoral stress on homeostatic mechanisms.

Also implicated in the acute effects of OSA are the hemodynamic and cardiac structural consequences of inspiration against a closed airway, also known as the Mueller maneuver. The intrathoracic negative pressure generated during obstructive apneas, which can reach up to −60 mm Hg, may elicit consequences such as

increased ventricular load and elevated left ventricular transmural pressure, thereby increasing cardiac wall stress. These hemodynamic effects may be particularly important in OSA patients with coexisting heart disease.

Hypoxemia may also activate the diving reflex, which is able to simultaneously elicit both sympathetic vasoconstriction to multiple vascular beds (with the exception of the heart and the brain) and vagal activation to the heart. Thus, in perhaps ~10% of sleep apnea patients, the nocturnal apneas may be associated with severe bradyarrhythmias including AV block and occasionally sinus arrest.

Severe sleep apnea may also acutely trigger the release of several vasoactive substances, including catecholamines, atrial natriuretic peptide, and endothelin (Fig. 3).

Sustained Effects of OSA Persisting Into Daytime Wakefulness

There is considerable evidence that the acute pathophysiologic mechanisms activated by repetitive apneas may carry over into daytime disease processes. Even during normoxic wakefulness, patients with OSA have higher sympathetic activity, faster heart rates, diminished heart rate variability and increased blood pressure variability. High sympathetic drive may in part be due to

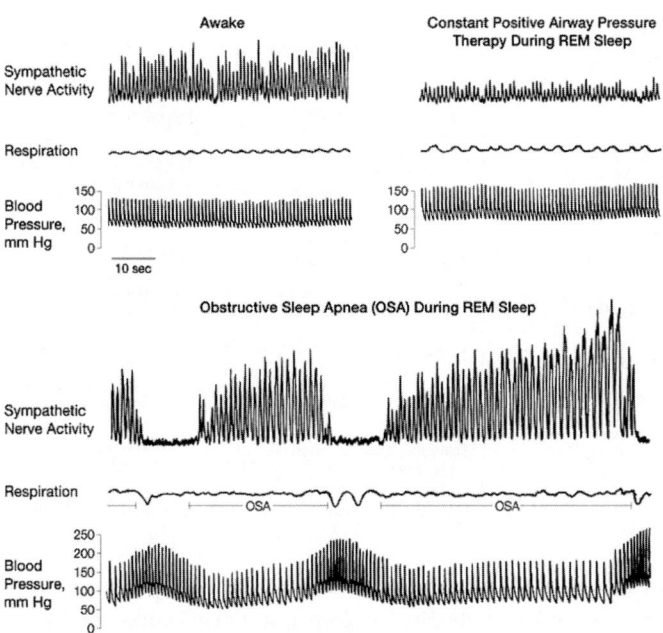

Fig. 2. Neural and circulatory changes in obstructive sleep apnea. Recordings of sympathetic nerve activity, breathing, and intra-arterial blood pressure in the same individual when awake, with OSA during rapid eye movement (REM) sleep, and with elimination of OSA episodes by continuous positive airway pressure (CPAP) therapy during REM sleep. Sympathetic nerve activity is very high during wakefulness, but increases even further secondary to obstructive apnea during REM sleep. Blood pressure increases from 130/65 mm Hg when the patient is awake to 256/110 mm Hg at the end of the apneic episode. Elimination of apneic episodes by CPAP therapy results in decreased sympathetic activity and prevents blood pressure surges during REM sleep.

tonic chemoreflex activation, since chemoreflex deactivation by 100% O_2 lowers sympathetic drive, slows heart rate, and lowers blood pressure in OSA patients.

There is also evidence for a chronic systemic inflammatory state, as indicated by higher levels of C-reactive protein and of serum amyloid A (Fig. 4). In addition, there is evidence of increased leukocyte activation and binding to endothelial cells.

Inflammatory and other mechanisms that may damage the endothelium can contribute to resistance vessel endothelial dysfunction in OSA.

OSA and Cardiovascular Disease Conditions

Hypertension

While many reports have shown an association between both pulmonary and systemic hypertension with OSA, studies from the Wisconsin Sleep Cohort have provided the first prospective evidence of a dose response association between the severity of OSA and the likelihood for development of systemic hypertension

4 years later in subjects who were normotensive at baseline (Fig. 5). This association was independent of other known risk factors such as baseline blood pressure, body mass and habitus, age, gender and alcohol and cigarette use. No single causal factor responsible for the occurrence of incident hypertension in OSA has been identified. The mechanisms are probably multifactorial and include activation of the sympathetic nervous system, endothelial dysfunction (including that caused by systemic inflammation), and increased endothelin, all of which would potentiate vasoconstriction.

Treatment of obstructive sleep apnea may induce decreases in blood pressure not only at night but also during the daytime. Sleep apnea should be especially considered in patients with resistant hypertension, particularly if they are also obese. Sleep apnea should also be suspected in patients who are "nondippers," i.e. in those in whom blood pressure does not fall appropriately during the night.

The most recent JNC Guidelines have listed sleep apnea as an important identifiable cause of hypertension.

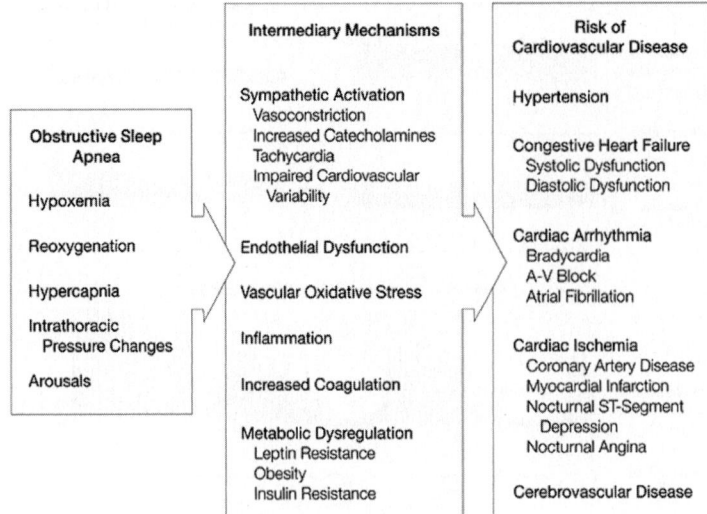

Fig. 3. Intermediary mechanisms associated with obstructive sleep apnea that potentially contribute to risk of cardiovascular disease. Abnormalities associated with obstructive sleep apnea may be intermediary mechanisms that contribute to the initiation and progression of cardiac and vascular pathology. These mechanisms may interact with each other, thus potentiating their pathophysiological implications.

Atherosclerosis and Coronary Artery Disease

In the presence of coexisting coronary artery disease, OSA may trigger acute nocturnal cardiac ischemia with ST-segment depression. Such nocturnal exacerbation of ischemic heart disease by OSA may be a result of oxygen desaturation, high sympathetic activity, increased cardiac oxygen demand (due to tachycardia and increased systemic vascular resistance), as well as a prothrombotic state. Whether these mechanisms may also lead to coronary plaque rupture and an acute coronary event is not known. Nevertheless, from the clinical perspective, OSA should be considered in the differential diagnosis of patients with evidence of cardiac ischemic events triggered at nighttime. Indeed, it has been

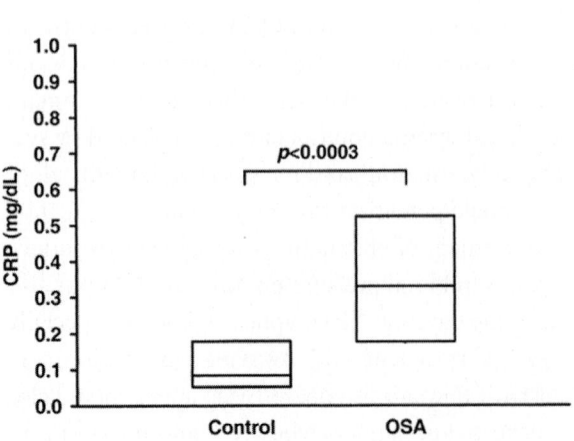

Fig. 4. Box plot showing plasma CRP in OSA patients (n=22) and controls (n=20). Middle horizontal line inside box indicates median. Bottom and top of the box are 25th and 75th percentiles, respectively.

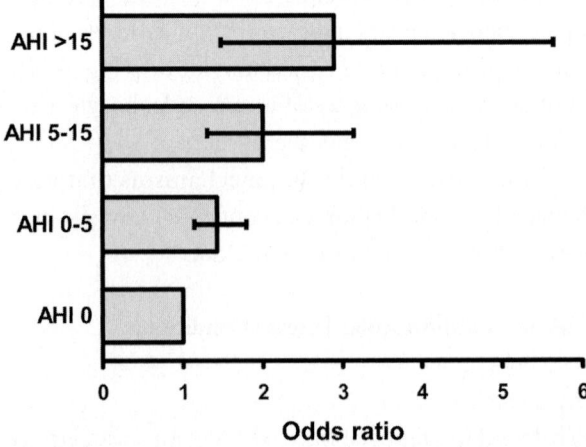

Fig. 5. Adjusted odds ratios for the presence of incident hypertension at 4-year follow-up according to the apnea-hypopnea index (AHI) at baseline. Data are shown as odds ratio (line bars indicate lower and upper 95% confidence intervals). P for trend=0.002.

proposed that OSA may be a poor prognostic factor in patients with coronary artery disease. 5-Year mortality in those with OSA was 38% compared to 9% mortality in patients without OSA.

There is epidemiological evidence that OSA may be etiologically linked to the development of atherosclerosis. There is a high prevalence of OSA in patients with coronary artery disease, and several case-control or prospective studies implicate OSA as an independent predictor of coronary artery disease. Observational studies suggest that treatment of OSA in patients with stable coronary artery disease by continuous positive airway pressure may decrease the incidence of new cardiovascular events.

The exact mechanisms of any atherogenic effects of OSA have not been established. However, recent reports linking OSA to inflammation lend support to the possibility that systemic or local inflammation may play a direct role in atherogenesis in OSA subjects. The role of oxidative stress in the vascular pathophysiology of OSA remains controversial. Finally, OSA-induced hypertension may contribute to endothelial damage and thereby to atherosclerosis.

Atrial Fibrillation and Bradyarrhythmias

In an unselected population of atrial fibrillation patients presenting for cardioversion, the risk for OSA (assessed using the Berlin questionnaire) is approximately 50%, as compared to a 30% risk in a general cardiology clinic population. Patients with OSA undergoing coronary artery bypass grafting have an increased likelihood of post-op atrial fibrillation. Furthermore, in atrial fibrillation patients undergoing cardioversion, the presence of untreated OSA was associated with a twofold greater risk of one year recurrence of atrial fibrillation (82%) as compared to the recurrence risk in those OSA patients receiving appropriate therapy (42%) (Fig. 6). Several pathophysiological mechanisms may contribute to the association between OSA and atrial fibrillation. OSA-related hypoxia, atrial stretch, sympathetic activation, acute blood pressure surges, and increased C-reactive protein may all reasonably be expected to predispose to increased risk for atrial fibrillation.

Other arrhythmias frequently associated with OSA are sinus arrest, sinoatrial block, and atrioventricular block, all of which may lead to ventricular asystole. The mechanism of these bradyarrhythmias is usually a reflex

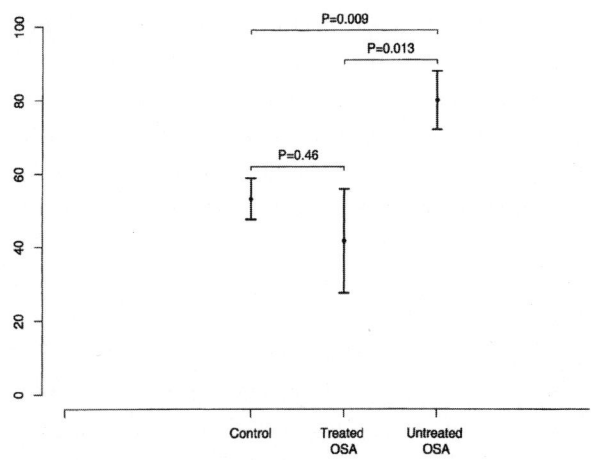

Fig. 6. Recurrence of atrial fibrillation at 12 months comparing patients who did not have sleep studies (controls) with treated OSA patients and with untreated (including noncompliant) OSA patients (mean±SD).

increase in cardiac vagal tone triggered by a combination of apnea and hypoxemia. It occurs in the presence of peripheral vasoconstriction (due to increased sympathetic outflow to resistance vessels), and represents the response to activation of the diving reflex by simultaneous hypoxemia and apnea.

Arryhthmias and/or cardiac ischemia may contribute to the increased likelihood of sudden cardiac death during the nighttime hours in patients with OSA. In contrast to patients without OSA, who are more likely to experience sudden cardiac death in the morning hours between 6 am and noon, about 50% of sudden cardiac deaths in OSA patients occur at night, between 10 pm and 6 am.

Stroke

The association between OSA and atrial fibrillation may in part explain the increased stroke risk in OSA. Atherosclerosis, vascular inflammation, hypertension, and procoagulant effects of OSA are also important risk factors for stroke. Furthermore, the decreased cardiac output and increased intracranial pressure during acute OSA episodes, with a consequent reduction in cerebral blood flow, may also play an important role. However, the nature of the association between stroke and OSA remains unclear. It is known that patients with stroke have a high prevalence of OSA, exceeding 40%. What is uncertain is whether OSA is a causal factor in the occurrence of stroke, or whether sleep apnea is a consequence of stroke and results from stroke-induced impairment of respiratory and muscle tone control. Also, whether patients with transient ischemic attacks who also have OSA have an increased risk for stroke compared to those without OSA remains controversial. Nevertheless, recent prospective observational data show the presence of severe OSA to be an important predictor of risk for new stroke. What is also clinically important is that OSA in stroke survivors could further compromise physical and cognitive functions, and have detrimental effects on prognosis. The diagnosis of sleep apnea in stroke patients should be pursued and, if indicated, appropriate therapy should be instituted.

Heart Failure

The acute hemodynamic and cardiac structural effects of OSA, together with adrenergic activation, systemic inflammation, increased endothelin, endothelial dysfunction, hypertension, and ischemic heart disease, are some of several mechanisms that may underlie the association between OSA and chronic heart failure, as well as between OSA and acute exacerbations of heart failure. Heart failure, by virtue of soft tissue edema, may predispose to OSA. While it is not clear whether the prevalence of OSA in heart failure is greater than the prevalence of OSA in the general population, OSA should be suspected in heart failure patients who are obese. Treatment of OSA may significantly improve clinical status. The very high risk for development of heart failure over 20-year follow-up noted in the Framingham population may in part be explained by occult sleep apnea in obese subjects.

Diagnosis and Treatment of OSA

OSA should always be considered in patients with risk factors for OSA (especially obesity, age, and male gender) as well as in those with symptoms suggestive of a sleep disorder, including daytime sleepiness, fatigue, snoring and witnessed cessation of breathing during sleep. It should also be suspected in patients with specific clinical features, such as resistant hypertension (especially the "non-dipping pattern"), resistant heart failure with frequent nocturnal exacerbations, sleep-time cardiac ischemia, recurrent atrial fibrillation, stroke, etc. The risk for OSA can be further assessed by overnight oximetry (severe and repetitive oxygen desaturations

being suggestive of OSA) and by using questionnaires (e.g. the Berlin questionnaire), which contain scoring systems indicating the probability of OSA. However, the definitive diagnosis can be made only by polysomnography, which is usually performed in a specialized sleep center.

The severity of OSA will often be attenuated by behavioral and lifestyle modifications, such as weight loss, avoidance of sedatives and alcohol, and avoidance of sleeping on the back. In selected patients surgical procedures designed to increase the diameter of the upper airway (such as uvulopalatopharyngoplasty and laser assisted uvuloplasty) can be used, but beneficial effects on OSA may be transient and unpredictable. Other treatment options include dental applicances which serve to minimize posterior displacement of the mandible during sleep, and may be helpful in less severe OSA.

The treatment of choice in OSA remains continuous positive airway pressure (CPAP), which should be used in patients with moderate to severe OSA, and perhaps also in those with mild OSA. CPAP therapy is associated not only with a decrease in OSA severity and OSA-related symptoms (leading to a marked improvement in the quality of life) but it can also favorably affect the risk and the course of OSA-related cardiovascular disease. Specifically, in OSA patients with hypertension, effective CPAP treatment has been shown to significantly reduce daytime and nocturnal blood pressure (Fig. 7). Nocturnal ST-segment depression and nocturnal angina might be significantly reduced after CPAP therapy. Observational data suggest that CPAP treatment of patients with severe OSA is accompanied by a reduction in acute cardiovascular events. CPAP has also been shown to reduce the recurrence of atrial fibrillation in patients undergoing cardioversion. Treatment of OSA in heart failure has been associated with improvements in ejection fraction, lower blood pressure and slower heart rate. However, whether treatment of OSA results in any mortality benefit in heart failure or in any other OSA-related cardiovascular conditions remains unknown.

An important and as yet unresolved question is how to treat those OSA patients who are not compliant with CPAP therapy or in whom CPAP is not effective in alleviating OSA severity. In patients with life threatening OSA, who cannot tolerate CPAP, tracheostomy

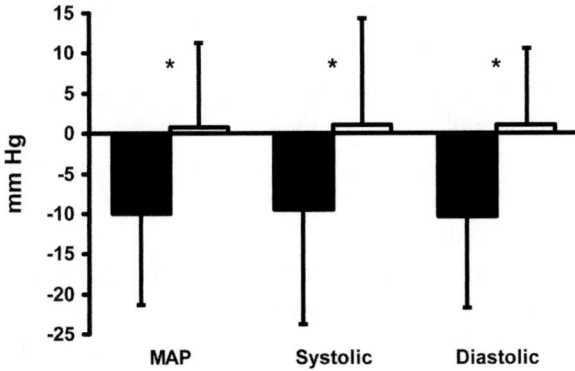

Fig. 7. Changes in mean (MAP), systolic, and diastolic blood pressure with effective (*closed bars*) and subtherapeutic (*open bars*) continuous positive airway pressure (CPAP). *Significant difference.

should be considered. Better understanding of the biology of OSA may help in developing new pharmacologic and nonpharmacologic therapies acting on specific pathophysiological pathways involved in the development of OSA and/or OSA-associated cardiovascular disease.

CENTRAL SLEEP APNEA

Acute and Chronic Effects

Many acute and sustained effects of CSA are similar to those of OSA as described earlier. These effects are related primarily to chemoreceptor activation by hypoxia, and lead to elevated sympathetic drive and an increase in circulating catecholamines. Similarly, frequent arousals and sleep fragmentation due to apneas can result in sleep deprivation and daytime fatigue and somnolence.

However, in contrast to OSA, CSA is not accompanied by airway occlusion and strenuous respiratory efforts, and thus hemodynamic effects related to changes in intrathoracic and cardiac transmural pressures are modest, and hypoxemia is usually less marked.

The Association Between CSA and Cardiovascular Disease

The main clinical association of CSA is with chronic heart failure (CHF), although it can also occur in healthy individuals during exposure to hypobaric

hypoxia at altitudes. In the setting of CHF, CSA occurs in the form of Cheyne-Stokes respiration, characterized by repetitive episodes of apnea/hypopnea and hyperpnea (i.e. hyperventilation) manifested as crescendo-decrescendo (a waxing-waning pattern) changes in tidal volume (periodic breathing).

Although the pathophysiology of CSA in CHF is not fully understood, its etiology is probably multifactorial and includes instability in the respiratory rhythm control (such as heightened chemoreceptor drive and fluctuating arterial CO_2 levels), upper airway narrowing, pulmonary venous congestion (resulting in reflex afferent stimulation of pulmonary mechanoreceptors), and prolonged circulation time, which leads to a delay in sensing changes in arterial blood gases by chemoreceptors. It occurs predominantly during stage I and II of non-REM sleep, when ventilation is regulated by the levels of arterial CO_2.

The prevalence of CSA in CHF has been estimated to be between 33 to 70 percent of patients with stable systolic heart failure, although it depends on various factors including heart failure etiology, gender (being more common in men), age, ejection fraction and hemodynamic status. What is important is that CSA is frequent not only in patients with advanced CHF but also in those with asymptomatic left ventricular dysfunction.

The clinical significance of CSA in CHF is twofold. First, CSA is associated with the severity of CHF. The nature of this reciprocal association between CSA and CHF severity is complex and not fully understood. On the one hand, CHF patients with CSA are characterized by lower exercise capacity and ejection fraction, increased left ventricular volumes, elevated pulmonary capillary wedge pressure, and a higher prevalence of cardiac arrhythmias, indicating that the presence of CSA may be merely an index of CHF severity. On the other hand, it is conceivable that CSA may lead to the progression of CHF through several mechanisms, such as neuroendocrine effects (elevated catecholamines), hypoxia, blood pressure and heart rate fluctuations, cardiac arrhythmias etc. In fact, even in patients with asymptomatic left ventricular dysfunction, CSA is accompanied by impaired cardiac autonomic control and increased cardiac arrhythmias, suggesting that perhaps CSA may precede the development of overt heart failure.

Secondly, irrespective of the mechanisms involved,

the presence of CSA is an important risk factor and impairs prognosis in CHF—an effect that is independent of other known risk factors, such as left ventricular ejection fraction, hemodynamic parameters, or peak oxygen consumption. For example, in clinically stable patients with CHF, CSA has been shown to be an independent predictor of cardiac death and transplantation during 2 year follow-up.

Treatment

The primary goal of treating CHF patients with CSA is optimization of pharmacological heart failure therapy. Decreased CHF severity and hemodynamic improvement of CHF is often associated with a significant decrease in CSA. More aggressive treatment of CSA may be indicated in case of persistent CSA and refractory CHF. Theophylline or nocturnal oxygen supplementation or acetazolamide have been suggested to decrease the severity of CSA, but their long-term effects on outcome are not known. Pilot studies suggest that CPAP therapy may improve transplant-free survival, but the recent CANPAP trial showed no mortality benefit from CPAP treatment of CSA in CHF patients. However, the efficacy of CPAP in reducing CSA was limited, with suboptimal patient compliance, which may help explain the absence of benefit.

A new potentially promising therapeutic strategy is cardiac resynchronization therapy, which has been suggested to have beneficial hemodynamic effects in CHF as well as decrease the severity of CSA.

CONCLUSIONS

Both OSA and CSA are associated with cardiovascular disease. While a causal relationship between sleep apnea and cardiovascular disease is not definitively proven, the coexistence of sleep apnea with cardiovascular disease exacerbates symptoms and may accelerate progression. The diagnosis of sleep apnea should always be considered in cases of refractory heart failure, resistant hypertension, transient ischemic attacks, and nighttime cardiac ischemia or arrhythmias, especially in persons with risk factors for sleep apnea. Treating sleep apnea may improve CV disease management. The diagnosis and treatment of sleep apnea is important even in the absence of any clinically overt cardiovascular disease, because sleep apnea might be conducive to their development. Randomized trials examining the cardiovascular effects of treatment of sleep apnea are lacking. Whether treatment of sleep apnea truly prevents cardiovascular events and has a mortality benefit remains unknown.

CARDIOVASCULAR TRAUMA

Joseph G. Murphy, MD

R. Scott Wright, MD

Cardiovascular trauma is a significant cause of death particularly in young men in our society. Cardiovascular trauma is classified into penetrating injuries, blunt, nonpenetrating trauma, and medical injuries to the heart sustained at the time of an invasive cardiovascular procedure, medical device implantation, or cardiopulmonary resuscitation.

Penetrating cardiac injury is due primarily to knife or gunshot injuries, whereas blunt cardiac injury is usually due to automobile or motorcycle accidents or industrial incidents. Iatrogenic cardiac trauma also may occur as a result of cardiopulmonary resuscitation, endomyocardial biopsy, or the use of intravascular catheters, including Swan-Ganz catheters (Table 1).

- Males between the ages of 15 and 35 are the most common victims of cardiac trauma.
- Nonpenetrating cardiac trauma usually results from automobile or industrial injuries, whereas penetrating cardiac injuries usually result from knife or gunshot wounds.
- 50% of patients with traumatic penetrating cardiac injury die rapidly, usually before hospitalization.

PENETRATING CARDIAC INJURY

Penetrating cardiac trauma most commonly affects the right ventricle, followed in order by the left ventricle, right atrium, and left atrium. Cardiac injury may occur from direct injury or indirectly from rib fractures that puncture the cardiac chambers. The principal consequences of perforating cardiac injury are cardiac tamponade and exsanguinating hemorrhage, both of which lead to death rapidly if not treated on an emergency basis. Whether cardiac tamponade develops will depend on the chamber penetrated, the size of the penetration, and whether the pericardium is also lacerated. The left ventricle is usually capable of sealing a small hole because of the thickness of the surrounding muscle, whereas a perforation of the right atrium or right ventricle usually leads to rapid hemopericardium. If the pericardium also is opened by the initial injury, tamponade usually will be prevented and the bleeding will present as a hemothorax. Occasionally, the pericardial tear also may act as a flap valve and prevent blood drainage into the pleural space and lead to tamponade. The signs and treatment of pericardial tamponade are discussed in the chapter on pericardial disease (Fig. 1).

Table 1. Traumatic Cardiac Lesions

I. Pericardial
   A. Hemorrhagic pericarditis
   B. Pericardial laceration
   C. Tamponade
   D. Purulent pericarditis, due to associated
      rupture of esophagus
   G. Constrictive pericarditis
   H. Intrapericardial diaphragmatic hernia
II. Myocardial
   A. Contusion
   B. Ischemic infarction, secondary to trau-
      matic occlusion of coronary artery
   C. Myocardial hematoma
   D. Myocardial laceration
   E. Myocardial rupture
   F. Aneurysm
   G. Pseudoaneurysm
   H. Diffuse calcification ("myocarditis ossifi-
      cans")
III. Endocardial
   A. Thrombus
IV. Valvular
   A. Atrioventricular valves (chordal rupture,
      papillary muscle rupture, torn leaflet)
   B. Semilunar valves (avulsion of cusp, avul-
      sion of commissure, torn cusp, intimal
      tear in adjacent aorta with cusp displace-
      ment, sinus of Valsalva aneurysm with
      cusp displacement)
V. Coronary artery (laceration, arteriovenous
   fistula)
VI. Aorta and pulmonary artery
   A. Rupture
   B. Aneurysm

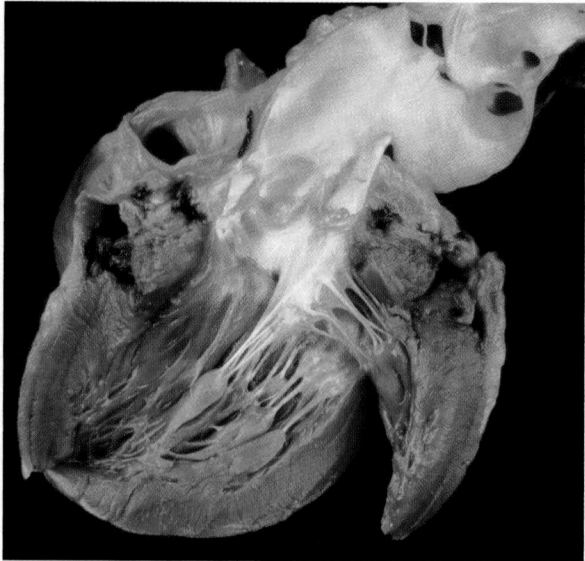

Fig. 1. Motor vehicle accident resulting in cardiac trauma and fatal hemopericardium.

frequent in automobile accidents. Nonpenetrating cardiac trauma may result in myocardial contusions; chamber or vessel lacerations; rupture of chordae tendineae, papillary muscles, or cardiac valves; pericarditis; pericardial lacerations; and, rarely, the late development of constrictive pericarditis.

PERICARDIAL INJURY

Pericardial injury may result from blunt or pentrating chest injuries and may lead to rapid death due to cardiac tamponade or slowly progressive pericardial inflammation and fibrosis leading to late pericardial constriction. Delayed pericardial tamponade and localized pericardial tamponade are variants of pericardial injury that are often difficult to diagnose.

MYOCARDIAL CONTUSION

Myocardial contusion is primarily a pathologic diagnosis, and there are no definitive clinical methods to establish this diagnosis. Although late complications from blunt cardiac trauma may occur in a small number of patients, in the majority of patients with cardiac trauma who present with stable vital signs, a short period of electrocardiographic monitoring (about 24 hours) is usually sufficient to determine whether arrhythmia or heart failure will develop. Sudden cardiac death due to

■ Cardiac injury may occur from direct injury or indirectly from rib fractures that puncture the cardiac chambers.

BLUNT CARDIAC INJURY

Nonpenetrating cardiac trauma may result from a direct force on the chest wall or indirectly from pressure on the abdomen displacing a large volume of blood suddenly into the heart. Both forms of injury are

ventricular fibrillation may occur with low-energy impact to the chest wall (such as from a baseball impact) if the blow coincides with a narrow window of time during cardiac repolarization. Damage to the coronary artery may result in occlusion, laceration, or, more rarely, fistula formation. Rupture of the intraventricular septum, myocardial aneurysm, and pseudo-aneurysm formation also have been reported.

■ Damage to the coronary artery may result in occlusion, laceration, or, more rarely, fistula formation.

MEDICAL CARDIAC INJURY

CPR frequently results in nondisplaced rib fractures and may also lead to rupture of the left ventricle or right ventricle if performed too vigorously, especially in the setting of a recent myocardial infarction when softening of the myocardium has occurred. Other complications include rupture of the papillary muscles that support the tricuspid valve, resulting in severe tricuspid regurgitation, and, more rarely, rupture of the aorta. Penetrating cardiac injuries caused by medical trauma occur during endomyocardial biopsy of the right ventricle or after perforation with a temporary pacemaker wire. Dissection of the aorta or coronary ostia may occur during coronary angiography. In rare cases, coronary angioplasty has resulted in coronary artery rupture and tamponade. Intra-aortic balloon counterpulsation also may cause aortic dissection, but it is more likely to cause thromboembolic complications as a result of pulsation against the atheromatous plaques in the aorta. Indwelling venous catheters may migrate and perforate the pulmonary arteries, and improper use of balloon-tipped pulmonary artery catheters may lead to branch pulmonary artery rupture and intrapulmonary hemorrhage (Fig. 2).

DIAGNOSIS OF CARDIAC INJURY

Cardiac trauma must always be suspected in the setting of blunt or penetrating trauma to the chest or abdomen. A rapid assessment of the patient (airways, breathing, circulation [ABC]), neck veins, and extremities, looking for clues to tamponade or hemorrhagic shock, is mandatory. Cardiac contusion is frequently unrecognized. Myocardial contusion may lead to regional wall

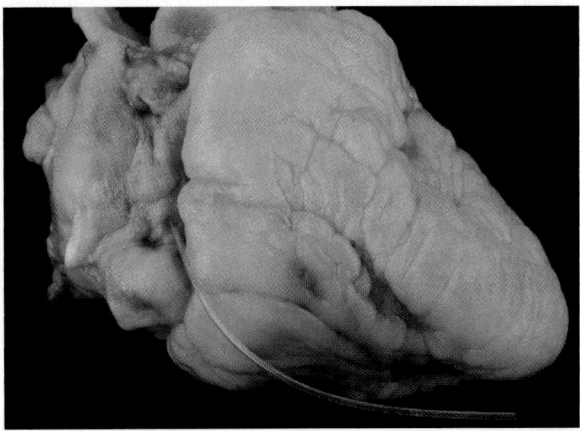

Fig. 2. Catheter perforation of right atrium with tamponade.

motion abnormalities and associated hemorrhagic infiltrate and myocyte necrosis on histologic examination. Acute heart failure and ventricular arrhythmias may occur, but they usually resolve within hours or days. Cardiac injury can occur in the absence of sternal or rib fractures or other significant chest injuries. In cases of blunt cardiac injury, the electrocardiogram may show 1) nonspecific ST-T wave changes, 2) electrocardiographic changes of acute pericarditis, or 3) pathologic Q waves. An increase in the troponin level confirms the presence of cardiac injury.

Echocardiography is the imaging method of choice for identification of cardiac injury. The findings include pericardial contusion, pericardial tamponade, regional wall motion abnormalities, chamber enlargement, valvular incompetence, and the presence of intracardiac shunts. An adequate transthoracic echocardiographic examination is not possible in up to 30% of trauma victims, and transesophageal echocardiography may be needed. Transesophageal echocardiography may not be possible in patients with cervical, maxillary, or mandibular injuries (Fig. 3).

■ Cardiac injury can occur in the absence of sternal or rib fractures or other significant chest injuries.
■ Echocardiography is the imaging method of choice for identification of cardiac injury.

TREATMENT OF CARDIAC INJURY

Emergency pericardiocentesis for cardiac tamponade

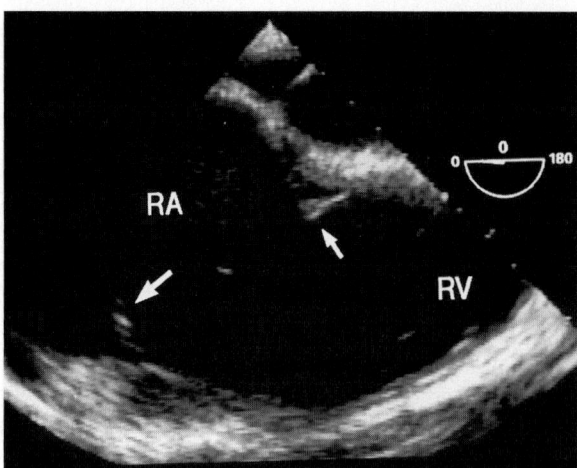

Fig. 3. Traumatic right ventricular contusion and tricuspic valve disruption; modified right ventricular inflow view at 0°multiplane imaging. The right ventricle (RV) is markedly enlarged and was nearly akinetic on real-time examination. The anterior tricuspid leaflet (*large arrow*) is unsupported and flail; both the anterior and the septal (*small arrow*) leaflets are dwarfed by profound tricuspid annular dilatation, which is responsible for an expansive gap between the noncoapting leaflets. RA, right atrium.

may be life-saving if the patient is hemodynamically unstable. Echocardiography-guided pericardiocentesis is preferred if immediately available. Emergency thoracotomy is the treatment of choice for severe hemorrhage due to cardiac trauma. Lesser degrees of cardiac contusion may be managed conservatively. For hypotensive patients who have multiple-injury trauma and do not respond to fluids, consider cardiac tamponade or ventricular hypokinesia—both conditions are easily diagnosed with echocardiography. Inotropic agents and intra-aortic balloon counterpulsation (provided there is no aortic injury) may be beneficial in patients with ventricular hypokinesia due to myocardial contusion. Traumatic rupture of the atrial or ventricular septum or major valve injury generally requires surgical repair. Traumatic cardiac rupture due to blunt trauma occurs most commonly in the right or left ventricle. Late cardiac rupture may occur from contusion complicated by intramyocardial hemorrhage, necrosis, and softening. Emergency operation is the treatment of choice for patients with cardiac rupture. Patients who present with pseudoaneurysm formation should have surgical repair because future rupture is unpredictable.

DAMAGE TO INTRACARDIAC STRUCTURES

The aortic valve is the most frequently damaged valve in nonpenetrating chest injuries. Patients with underlying valvular heart disease are considered to be at a higher risk than those without preexisting disease. Aortic or mitral incompetence due to valve leaflet tears usually presents early and worsens with time. Tricuspid valve injury is unique in that it may be recognized only years after the original injury. Aortic incompetence may result from a combination of damage to the aortic wall and damage to the valve leaflets, and it may improve when perivalvular edema and hemorrhage subside. Sudden traumatic obstruction to left ventricular outflow during systole may result in papillary muscle or mitral valve rupture. The risk of cardiac valve injury is dependent on the time at which the injury occurs during the cardiac cycle. Injury during systole damages the mitral valve, whereas injury during diastole damages the aortic valve. Severe abdominal injury, even in the absence of chest trauma, may result in tricuspid valve or right ventricular papillary muscle rupture. Definitive treatment for significant valve injury is valve replacement or repair. Injury to the coronary arteries from blunt or penetrating trauma may lead to coronary occlusion and myocardial infarction. Left ventricular pseudoaneurysm or aneurysm formation may result from coronary trauma. Atrioventricular fistula formation is a rare complication of penetrating trauma and most commonly affects the right coronary artery. The fistula may extend from the right coronary artery into the coronary sinus, the great cardiac vein, the right ventricle, or the right atrium (Fig. 4).

- The risk of cardiac valve injury is dependent on the time at which the injury occurs during the cardiac cycle.
- Atrioventricular fistula formation is a rare complication of penetrating trauma and most commonly affects the right coronary artery.

INJURY TO THE AORTA AND GREAT VESSELS

Rupture of the aorta is the most frequent nonpenetrating injury to the great vessels and occurs in about 8,000 cases annually in the United States. Traumatic rupture of the aorta occurs after rapid deceleration injuries such as high falls or automobile accidents. Traumatic aortic

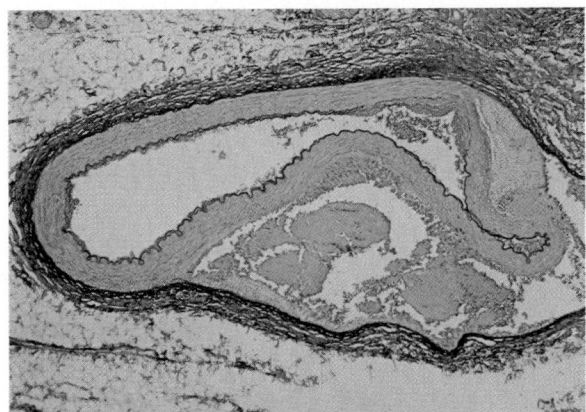

Fig. 4. Traumatic rupture of right coronary artery. (x5.)

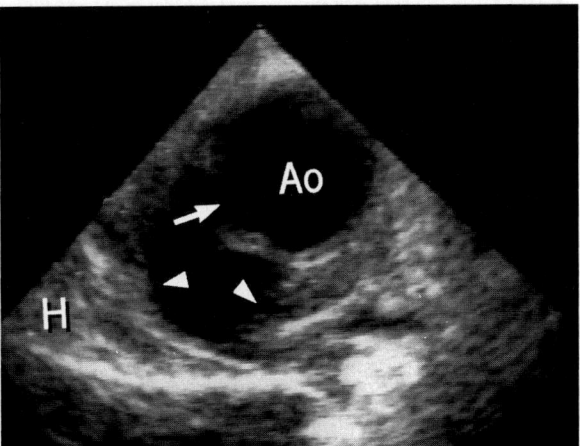

Fig. 5. Traumatic rupture of the descending thoracic aorta after a motor vehicle accident; transverse transesophageal echocardiographic plane. A large rent in the aorta (Ao) is clearly visualized (*arrow*) communicating with an adjacent para-aortic space (*arrowheads*); there is also hematoma formation (H).

rupture is present in about 20% of patients who die of injuries from motor vehicle accidents. The site of the aortic tear is usually the junction of the aortic arch and the descending aorta at a point where the descending aorta is fixed to the spine by the intercostal arteries just distal to the origin of the left subclavian artery. This injury is usually fatal in 80% to 90% of patients, but survival has been reported with emergency cardiac operation. Partial rupture of the aorta is associated with increased arterial pressure in the upper extremities, decreased arterial pressure in the lower extremities, and evidence of widening of the superior mediastinum on chest radiography or computed tomography. Pseudoaneurysm of the aorta tends to expand and rupture, but it also may contain thrombus that embolizes to distant sites. Fistulas may form to adjoining structures. Transesophageal echocardiography, computed tomography, and aortic angiography are the imaging methods of choice in cases of suspected aortic injuries (Fig. 5). The commonest angiographic findings are an intimal flap and a pseudoaneurysm. With aggressive surgical intervention, about 80% of patients who reach a hospital will survive; without surgery, 2% to 5% of patients will develop a chronic pseudoaneurysm (Figs. 6 and 7).

■ The site of the aortic tear is usually the junction of the aortic arch and the descending aorta.

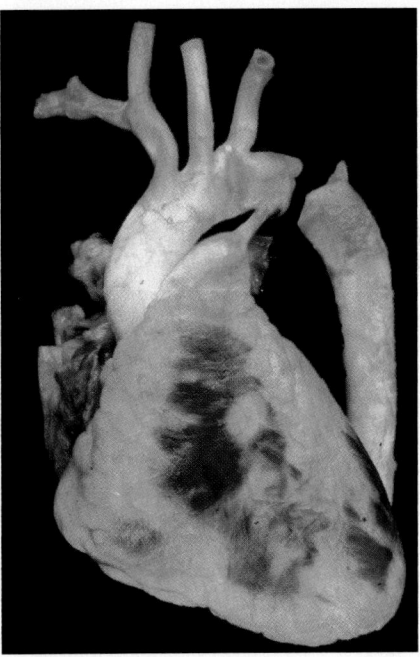

Fig. 6. Motor vehicle accident with aortic transection just distal to the ligamentum arteriosum.

ELECTRICAL INJURY TO THE HEART

Electrical injury to the heart may occur from a lightning strike (about 100 deaths annually in the United States), industrial, home electrical accident, or from an electronic stun gun (Taser). Ventricular fibrillation is the usual cause of death. Drug intoxication with cocaine or phencyclidine (PEP) may increase the lethality of an electrical injury by increasing catecholamines and predisposing to fibrillation.

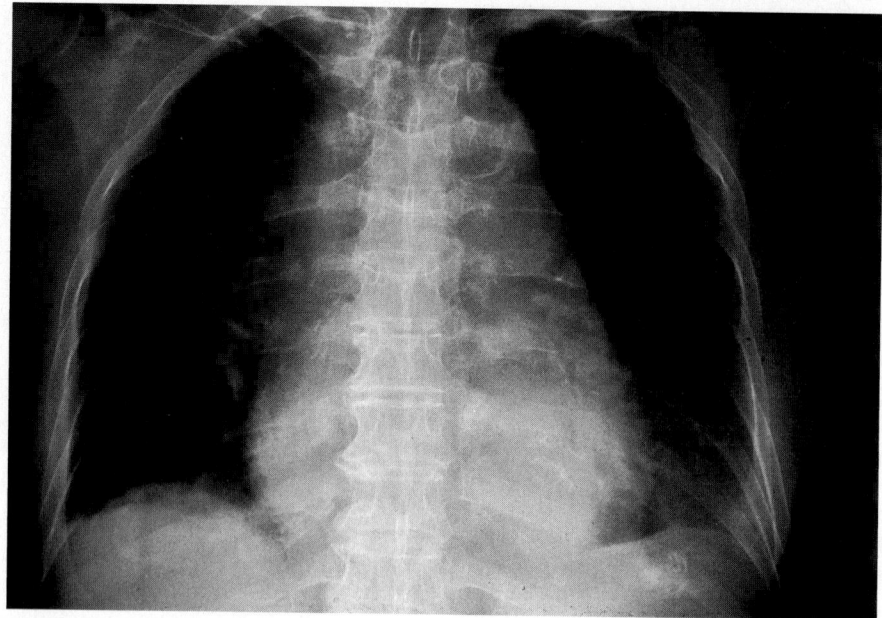

Fig. 7. Wide mediastinum (on chest radiograph) in acute aortic dissection with rupture and hemopericardium.

87

ACUTE BRAIN INJURY AND THE HEART

Nandan S. Anavekar, MB, BCh

Sarinya Puwanant, MD

Krishnaswamy Chandrasekaran, MD

Neurological and cardiovascular functions are closely intertwined: cerebral perfusion is dependent on cardiac performance while much of cardiac function is regulated by higher brain centers. Dysfunction in either organ system can precipitate dysfunction in the other.

Acute brain injury may result from vascular injury (stroke, subarachnoid or parenchyma hemorrhage), trauma (closed head injury), and inflammation (encephalitis, meningitis). Cardiac sequelae may manifest as fluctuations in blood pressure and hemodynamics, electrocardiographic changes, arrhythmias, and elevations in cardiac biomarkers.

CARDIAC INNERVATION

The autonomic nervous system (Fig. 1) strongly influences the electrical and mechanical activities of the heart; it is composed of two broad categories of efferent pathways, namely the parasympathetic and sympathetic nervous system. These efferent pathways are modulated by higher brain centers which constitute a functional unit referred to as the central autonomic network. Neurons in the cerebral cortex, basal forebrain hypothalamus, midbrain, pons, and medulla participate in autonomic control. The central autonomic network integrates visceral, humoral, and environmental information to produce coordinated autonomic, neuroendocrine, and behavioral responses to external or internal stimuli.

Parasympathetic Innervation of the Heart

The heart is innervated by both arms of the autonomic nervous system. The parasympathetic preganglionic neurons originate in the nucleus ambiguus of the medulla and synapse with intracardiac ganglia, via the vagus nerve. From these ganglia, short postganglionic parasympathetic neurons innervate the myocardial tissue. The parasympathetic innervation of the heart is particularly abundant in the sinus node and atrioventricular conduction system. Parasympathetic innervation of the heart is mediated entirely via the vagus nerve. The right vagus nerve innervates the sinoatrial node and when stimulated excessively predisposes to sinus node bradyarrhythmias. The left vagus nerve innervates the atrioventricular node and when hyperstimulated predisposes the heart to atrioventricular (AV) blocks. The parasympathetic postganglionic neurons release acetylcholine which activates M2 muscarinic receptors in the heart, the effects of which result in slowing of the heart rate, reduced contractile forces of the atrial cardiac muscle, and slowing of conduction velocity through the atrioventricular node (AV node). Vagal stimulation has no effect on ventricular muscle function. Excessive

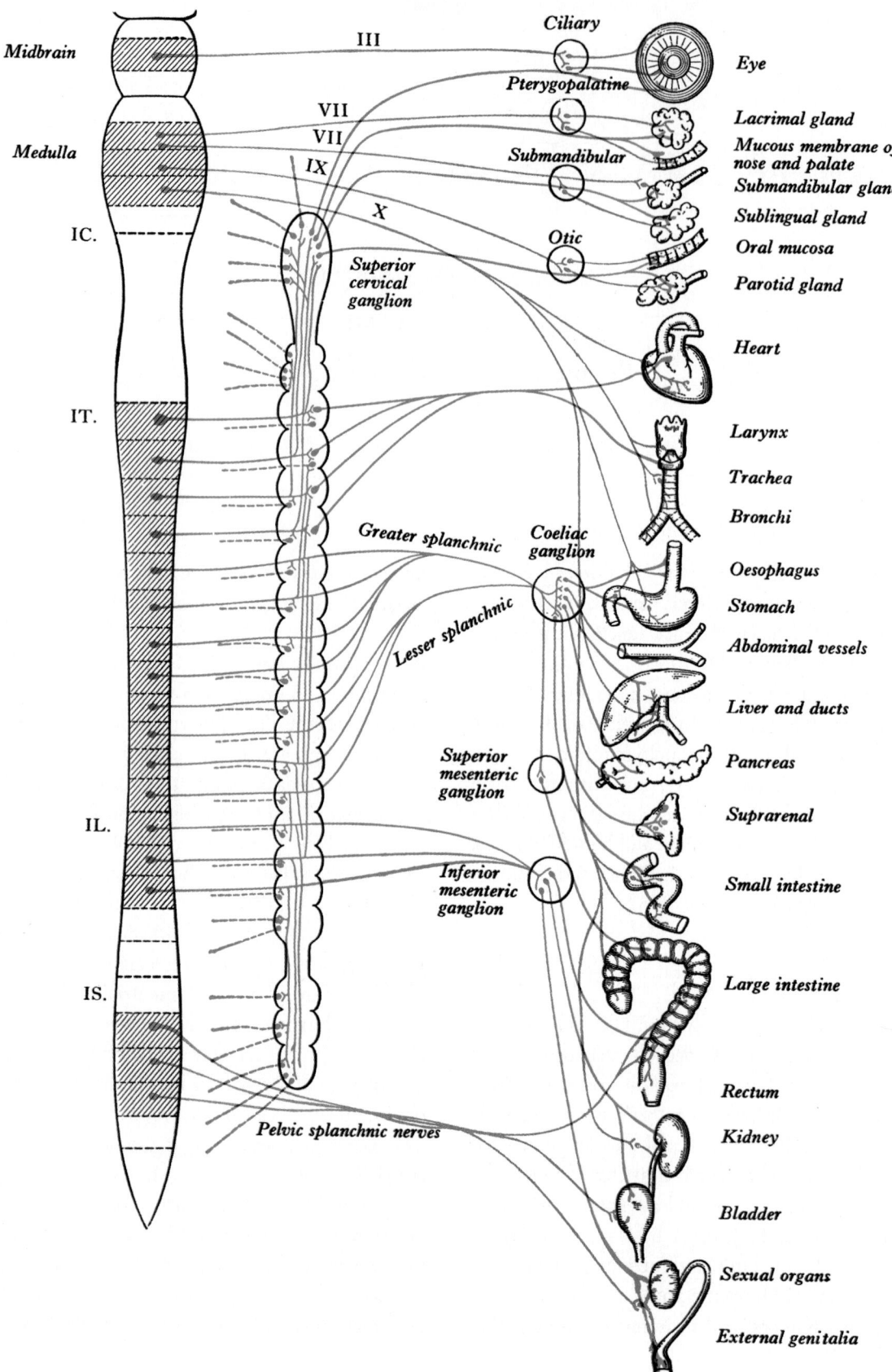

Fig. 1. Demonstrates the innervation of the heart.

vagal tone during emotional stress, which is usually a parasympathetic overcompensation to strong sympathetic activation during stress, can cause syncope because of a sudden drop in blood pressure and heart rate. Patients with bulimia and anorexia or spinal cord injury may have high vagal activity which is associated with the cardiac arrythmias often seen in these patients.

Sympathetic Innervation of the Heart
The sympathetic innervation of the heart originates from the intermediolateral column of the thoracic spinal cord and synapses with the sympathetic postganglionic neurons in the superior, middle and inferior cervical ganglia. The postganglionic sympathetic neurons innervate the sinoatrial and atrioventricular nodes, the conduction system and myocardial fibers, most prominently in the ventricles. The postganglionic sympathetic nerves release norepinephrine, which primarily through β-adrenergic receptor stimulation increases heart rate, conduction velocity through the atrioventricular node (AV node) and contractility of the heart. The sympathetic outflow to the peripheral circulation can produce vasoconstriction via activation of alpha adrenergic receptors. Such activation can increase the metabolic requirements of the heart which can manifest clinically as myocardial ischemia.

The autonomic outflow to the heart and peripheral vasculature fluctuates on a moment to moment basis. It is regulated by a variety of reflexes, which are initiated by arterial baroreceptors and chemoreceptors as well as a variety of intracardiac receptors. The autonomic innervation of the heart can also be influenced by pathologic events occurring in the central nervous system which alter the balance between parasympathetic and sympathetic outflow. These alterations can ultimately lead to disturbances in cardiac function and hemodynamics. Thus cardiac innervation serves as the common link between acute brain injury and its cardiac complications.

CARDIOVASCULAR COMPLICATIONS OF CEREBROVASCULAR ACCIDENT

Stroke
Patients who suffer a stroke are predisposed to cardiac disturbances. It is often difficult to ascertain in an individual patient whether the cerebrovascular event was initiated by a primary cardiac disturbance or the converse namely that the stroke caused a cardiac disturbance since the prevalence of cardiac morbidity in stroke patients is high.

ECG Abnormalities in Stroke
ECG abnormalities are present in up to 90% of patients presenting with acute stroke. Typical ECG demonstrates large upright T-waves and prolonged QT intervals (Fig. 2). Such ECG changes are also seen in the setting of subarachnoid hemorrhage, transient ischemic attacks, and nonvascular cerebral lesions. The ECG changes have been postulated to arise from subendocardial ischemia as a result of increased centrally mediated catecholamine release in the setting of hypothalamic hypoperfusion.

Repolarization Abnormality
ECG repolarization abnormality manifesting as QT prolongation is seen in about 38% of stroke patients. QT prolongation increases the vulnerable period of the cardiac cycle for arrhythmias and sudden death. QT prolongation in the absence of hypokalemia in stroke patients identifies high risk patients vulnerable to arrhythmia related sudden death. QT prolongation is more common after right middle cerebral artery stroke.

ST Segment Abnormality
Nonspecific ST segment changes are seen in over 20% of patients presenting with acute stroke and commonly include ST segment depression, a feature more frequently seen with left middle cerebral artery strokes. Dynamic ST segment changes may also be indicative of true myocardial ischemia: ST segment changes secondary to stroke are generally transient and paradoxically improve with brain death.

Q waves
New Q waves occur in up to 10% of patients with acute stroke. The Q waves may be a transient feature of the ECG, or may proceed through the typical evolutionary changes seen in myocardial infarction. Q waves seen in this setting do not reflect myocardial ischemic damage.

U Waves
The presence of U waves is a common finding in the

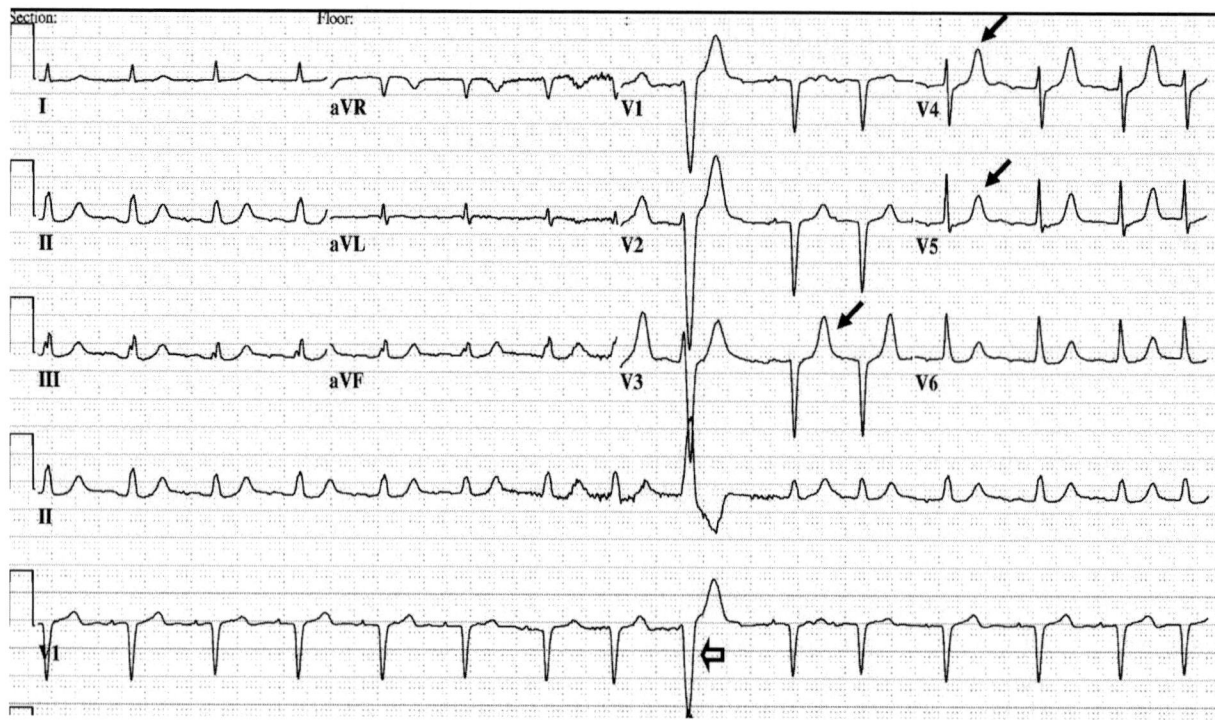

Fig. 2. Electrocardiography in a patient with acute ischemic stroke demonstrates classic tall upright T wave (*arrows*) in leads V3-5 and prolonged corrected QT interval of 471 msec. Note occasional ventricular extrasystole (*open arrow*) is also seen.

setting of acute stroke. These are usually unrelated to any electrolyte abnormality and may be found alone or in concert with T wave changes or prolonged QT intervals.

Arrhythmias

Cardiac arrhythmias frequently follow an acute stroke, even when not present on the admission ECG. All types of dysrhythmia can be seen including ventricular extrasystoles, atrial extrasystoles, supraventricular tachycardia, and ventricular tachycardia. Only ventricular arrhythmia is associated with increased mortality in stroke patients. Many cardiac arrhythmias occur in patients with normal cardiac function, suggesting a neurogenic etiology. Furthermore, the type and location of a stroke predicts the type of arrhythmia seen. The pathophysiologic mechanism of these dysrhythmias is postulated to be alterations in the central autonomic outflow to the heart. Bradycardia and vasodepressor effects are more common with injury to the right insular region whereas tachycardia and hypertension are more common with injury to the left insular region.

Restoration of normal autonomic tone can take up to 6 months after the acute cerebrovascular event: during this period, there is an increased risk of sudden cardiac death.

Cardiac Biomarkers

Elevation in cardiac biomarkers including troponin T, creatine kinase, and myoglobin may be seen in acute stroke. The magnitude of rise is usually small. Often troponin will only become elevated in stroke patients when there is existing coronary artery disease, and then it is associated with left ventricular dysfunction and poor prognosis. Increased autonomic sympathetic discharge increases myocardial oxygen demand and may result in both myocardial stunning and elevation in cardiac biomarkers. Classical myocardial infarction occurs in up to 6% of patients with acute stroke and is a therapeutic dilemma as many myocardial infarct therapies increase the risk of intracerebral bleeding.

Neurogenic LV Dysfunction

"Neurogenic stunned myocardium" is a clinical term

that describes neurologically mediated cardiac injury that is reversible in nature and clinically manifest by ventricular dysfunction with or with out hemodynamic instability. Commonly it is accompanied by ECG changes, arrhythmias, and cardiac biomarker release. This phenomenon is unrelated to any underlying coronary artery disease and is frequently seen in stroke patients, more commonly with left insular stroke. Pathologic findings include a characteristic pattern of petechial subendocardial hemorrhage and "contraction band necrosis." Excessive autonomic sympathetic discharge and catecholamine release is thought to be the pathogenic mechanism. Catecholamine blockade is protective against neurogenic cardiac injury. Tako-tsubo syndrome (apical balloon cardiomyopathy), a condition generally seen in elderly women that closely mimics the clinical presentation of acute anterior wall myocardial infarction is postulated to result from stress associated catecholamine released. It is associated with a characteristic pattern of abnormal ventricular wall motion, with hypokinesis of the cardiac apex and mid ventricle

with relative sparing of the cardiac base (Fig. 3). Prognosis for recovery is excellent.

Subarachnoid Hemorrhage

Subarachnoid hemorrhage is associated with significant patient morbidity and mortality and accounts for 10% of all strokes. It usually results from rupture of a saccular intracerebral aneurysm, but other causes include trauma, arteriovenous malformation and illicit drug use including cocaine and amphetamine use. Almost all the changes observed in the ECG, cardiac biomarkers and LV dysfunction can be seen in SAH, however, there are certain characteristics typically seen in SAH.

Acute ECG changes are noted in greater than 50% of patients with subarachnoid hemorrhage classically described as deep T wave inversions or "cerebral T waves" (Fig. 4 and 5). ECG changes may be seen up to 2 weeks after the acute bleed. Prolongation of the QT interval and QT dispersion are seen in >70% of patients presenting with subarachnoid hemorrhage, a finding that predisposes to ventricular arrhythmia and sudden

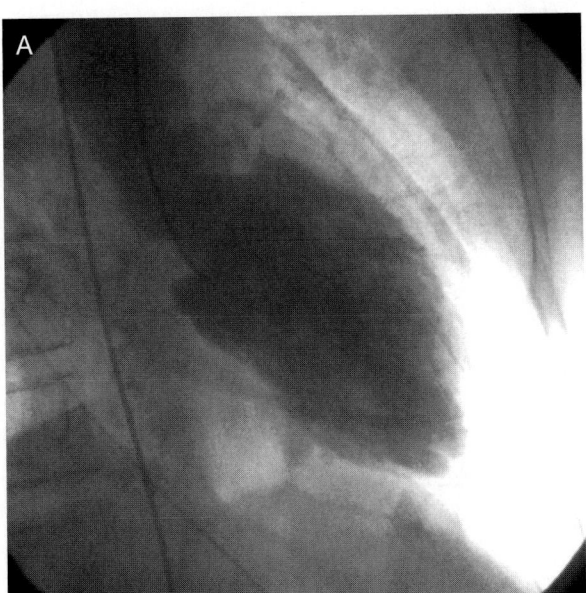 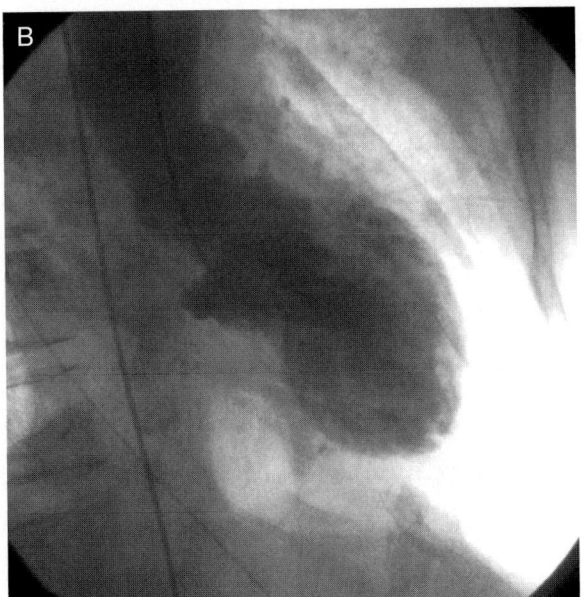

Fig. 3. Left ventriculography in a patient with apical ballooning syndrome. End diastolic (*A*) and end systolic (*B*) frames demonstrate akinesis of mid, and dyskinesis of apical regions of the left ventricle with hyperdynamic contraction of basal left ventricle. The appearance is similar to "ampulla" or "tako-tsubo"—a vessel used for catching octopus in Japan. This phenomenon can be seen in all acute brain injury situations including inflammation. However, it is more common in SAH and any ischemic stroke involving thalamus, and brainstem. In SAH the apex and base are spared and only mid ventricle demonstrates systolic ballooning (dyskinesis).

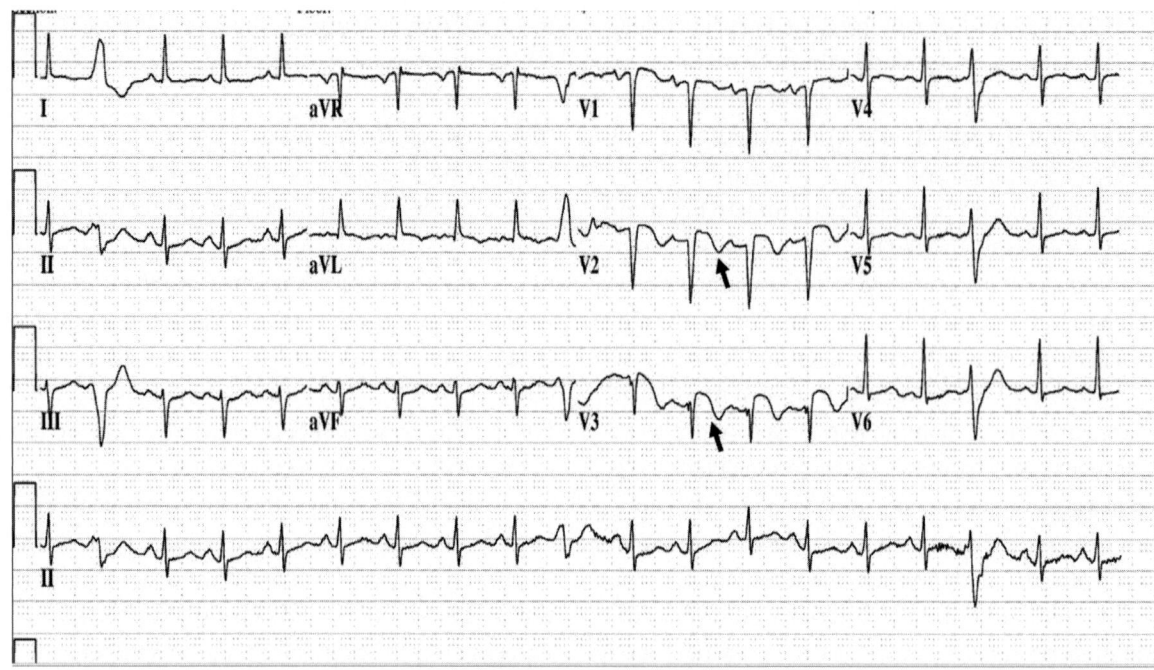

Fig. 4. Electrocardiography in a patient with a subarachnoid hemorrhage demonstrates ST elevation and T wave inversion (*arrows*) in leads V2-V3 suspicious for ST-elevation anteroseptal infarction. However, absence of reciprocal changes and marked prolongation of QT interval are common in SAH and help diffferentiate from ST elevation myocardial infarction (STEMI).

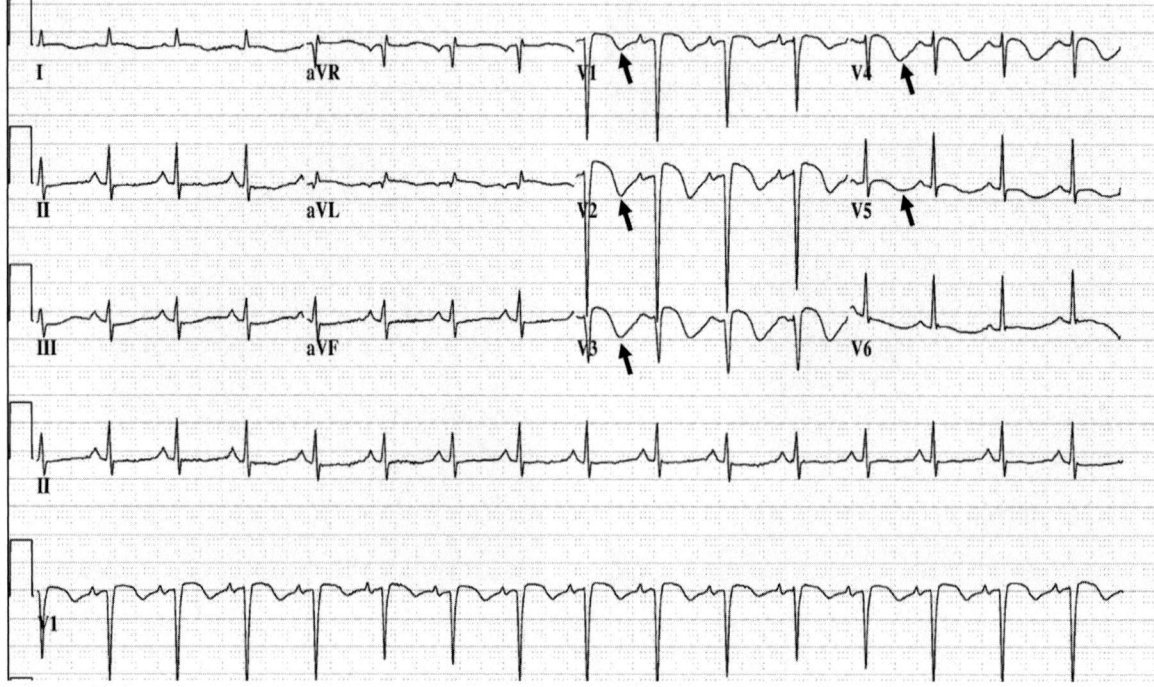

Fig. 5. Follow-up electrocardiography from the same patient shown in Figure 2, with subarachnoid hemorrhage, demonstrates persistence of ST elevation and changes in the T waves. Note the T waves are large and are symmetrically inverted (*arrows*) in leads V1-V5 with markedly prolonged corrected QT interval.

death. A prolonged QTc interval of >440 msec identifies severe head trauma patients at risk for ventricular arrhythmias and sudden death.

Elevations in cardiac enzymes are common after subarachnoid hemorrhage, the putative mechanism being excessive sympathetic discharge. The greater the troponin rise, the worse the clinical outcome.

Neurogenic left ventricular dysfunction is much more common in subarachnoid hemorrhage than in ischemic stroke with an incidence of about 10%. The pathophysiology of left ventricular dysfunction is similar to that seen in stroke, namely cardiac myocyte injury from catecholamine surge due to increased sympathetic discharge. In some patients with subarachnoid hemorrhage the apex and the base of the left ventricle contract normally while the mid ventricle demonstrates akinesis, a condition Japanese authors have coined "panic myocardium."

CARDIAC COMPLICATIONS OF HEAD TRAUMA

Closed head trauma leads to 175,000 deaths and 500,000 hospitalizations per year with a peak incidence in men 15 to 24 years of age. Head trauma is associated with significant cardiac complications that can negatively impact clinical outcomes including cardiac rhythm and conduction disturbances. EKG findings include diffuse tall upright or deep inverted T waves, prolonged QT intervals, ST segment depression or elevation, and U waves. Dysrhythmias in head-injured patients often resolve when intracranial pressure is reduced. QT prolongation and associated fatal arrhythmias are more commonly associated with intracerebral hemorrhage with raised intracranial pressure. Reduction of ischemic cerebral injury is dependent on preservation of adequate cardiac output, and in the setting of concomitant cardiac dysfunction, neurologic outcome is also worsened.

Brain Death and the Heart

Patients with brain death following head injury, ischemic stroke or subarachnoid hemorrhage are potential organ donors for cardiac transplantation. Cardiac dysfunction from neurogenic mechanisms generally will recover with time as excess autonomic sympathetic activity subsides which may take from 72

hours to 1 week. Myocardial recovery is dependent upon the maintenance of adequate mean arterial pressure to ensure coronary perfusion. β-Blockers can protect the myocardium from the toxic effects of catecholamines and the use of glucocorticoids has also been shown to reduce cardiac dysfunction after brain death.

Head Injury and Anticoagulation

Head injury in patients who are on anticoagulation adversely effects survival by increasing the incidence of intracranial hemorrhage. An international normalized ratio (INR) greater than 3.3 has been shown to be associated with an increased incidence of intracerebral hemorrhage following a head trauma and an adverse outcome.

CARDIAC MANIFESTATION IN EPILEPSY

Cardiovascular manifestations of epileptic seizures are common and symptoms and signs can occur in the pre-ictal, ictal or post-ictal period. The typical cardiovascular effects of alterations in autonomic function include changes in heart rate, blood pressure and ECG changes. ECG manifestations of epilepsy include ST-depression, ST elevation, and T-wave inversion. ECG changes can occur in the absence of changes in cardiac rhythm, in the setting of a seizure. Sinus tachycardia is seen in greater than 60% of patients. Sinus tachycardia accompanied with peripheral vasoconstriction and an increase in blood pressure is associated with hypothalamic lesions. Bradyarrhythmias occur in less than 5% of seizures and include sinus bradycardia, sinus arrest, AV block and prolonged asystole. Other cardiac arrhythmias seen in the setting of seizures include acceleration and deceleration of heart rate, enhanced sinus arrhythmia, atrial premature beats, sinus pauses, AV block, nodal escape, paroxysmal supraventricular tachycardia and ventricular ectopy.

Electroconvulsive Therapy

Electroconvulsive therapy (ECT) is an artificially induced seizure often associated with a significant catecholamine elevation and autonomic discharge particularly parasympathetic discharge. ECG changes occur fairly commonly during treatment with ECT and are similar to those changes seen in primary seizure disorders. There has been one prospective study analyzing the effects of

ECT on left ventricular systolic function which showed that ECT associated left ventricular systolic dysfunction is a common but transient early phenomenon. Multiple ECT treatments do not have a cumulative effect on ventricular function, and tolerance to shocks appears to develop after multiple treatments.

CARDIAC COMPLICATIONS OF ENCEPHALOMYELITIS

Encephalomyelitis is an inflammatory disorder of the central nervous system, dorsal root ganglia, and autonomic nerves due to an infectious or noninfectious etiology, the latter often associated with vasculitis or paraneoplastic syndromes.

Encephalomyelitis may be associated with cardiac manifestations owing to profound disturbances in autonomic function that are common in this condition. These findings include hypertension, tachycardia and high plasma catecholamine levels, consistent with a hypersympathetic state. The plethora of cardiac manifestations in brainstem encephalitis is explicable by the density of autonomic fibers that traverse the brainstem and the location of the primary vasomotor area.

88

NONCARDIAC ANESTHESIA IN PATIENTS WITH CARDIOVASCULAR DISEASE

Laurence C. Torsher, MD

The perioperative period stresses the cardiovascular system due to hemodynamic and neuroendocrine physiologic changes induced by the trauma attendant to the surgical interventions, fluid compartment shifts, blood loss, as well as anesthetic medications.

Preoperative evaluation, in addition to giving information about operative risk, should also provide information that will affect perioperative management decisions, e.g. decision to forgo or modify proposed surgical procedure, delay a procedure to optimize the

PREOPERATIVE PREPARATION

Screening and Mitigation of Perioperative Cardiovascular Risk

Preoperative patient assessment has the role of stratifying patients into risk groups such that physicians and patients can make informed decisions about the risks and benefits of proposed surgery. Preoperative assessment should also provide information to the perioperative caregivers that will allow them to optimize care of the patient. Risk scoring systems like the Goldman and Detsky systems allow caregivers to identify patients at high or low operative risk but do not provide information to optimize patients care. The American Society of Anesthesiologists' classification (Table 1) is an extremely simple global risk stratification scheme that is based solely on functional status. In spite of its simplicity it has proven to be as sensitive as many more sophisticated schemes.

Table 1. ASA Physical Status Classification System*

ASA-I: Healthy patient with no systemic disease

ASA-II: Mild systemic disease, no functional limitations

ASA-III: Moderate to severe systemic disease, some functional limitations

ASA-IV: Severe systemic disease, incapacitating, and a constant threat to life

ASA-V: Moribund patient, not expected to survive >24 hours without surgery

ASA-VI: Brain-dead patient undergoing organ harvest

E: Added when the case is emergent

---

*The American Society of Anesthesiologists physical status classification, developed in 1941, is used for risk stratification in outcome studies.

patient's medical conditions, choice of intra- and postoperative monitoring methods, modification of perioperative medical therapy, disposition of patient postoperatively (floor, ICU, outpatient) and even location of care (outpatient surgicenter, small community hospital, tertiary care center).

With respect to coronary artery disease, emphasis should be placed on identifying the extent of the disease and left ventricular performance. The impact of the disease and its impact on outcome have been formalized in the 2002 ACC/AHA guideline entitled "Perioperative Cardiovascular Evaluation for Noncardiac Surgery." By identifying clinical predictors, patients are classified as major, intermediate, or minor risk (Table 2). The surgical procedure being proposed is classified as high, intermediate, or low risk (Table 3). Then a stepwise approach as outlined in Figure 1 is utilized to determine whether to

immediately proceed to surgery, or proceed with further physiologic testing. The recurring theme throughout the guidelines is an assessment of functional status (as a clinical reflection of left ventricular performance) as reflected by exercise tolerance. Patients with minor or no clinical predictors with moderate or excellent exercise capability (>5METs) may proceed directly to the operating room without further work-up.

Aortic stenosis is the most important valvular heart lesion that needs identification before surgery because of the associated incidence of sudden death as well as the well documented ineffectiveness of cardiac massage should cardiac arrest occur. Surgical aortic valve replacement may be appropriate for some patients with severe aortic stenosis while patients with moderate aortic stenosis can generally be managed medically with avoidance of tachycardia, maintaining of vascular

Table 2. Clinical Predictors of Increased Perioperative Cardiovascular Risk (Myocardial Infarction, Heart Failure, Death)*

Major	**Intermediate**
Unstable coronary syndromes	Mild angina pectoris (Canadian Cardiovascular Society class I or II)
Acute or recent myocardial infarction†	Prior myocardial infarction by history of pathological Q-waves
with evidence of important ischemic risk by clinical symptoms or noninvasive study	Compensated or prior heart failure
Unstable or severe‡ angina (Canadian Cardiovascular Society class III or IV)§	Diabetes mellitus (particularly insulin-dependent)
Decompensated heart failure	Renal insufficiency
Significant arrhythmias such as	
High-grade atrioventricular block	**Minor**
Symptomatic ventricular arrhythmias in the presence of underlying heart disease	Advanced age
Supraventricular arrhythmias with uncontrolled ventricular rate	Abnormal electrocardiogram (left ventricular hypertrophy, left bundle branch block, ST-T abnormalities)
Severe valvular disease	Rhythm other than sinus (e.g., atrial fibrillation)
	Low functional capacity (e.g., inability to climb one flight of stairs with a bag of groceries)
	History of stroke
	Uncontrolled systemic hypertension

*In conjunction with exercise tolerance and surgical risk factors, will determine degree of preoperative cardiac investigations as well as need for β-blockade.
†The American College of Cardiology National Database Library defines recent myocardial infarction as greater than 7 days but less than or equal to 1 month (30 days); acute MI is within 7 days.
‡May include "stable" angina in patients who are unusually sedentary.
§Campeau L. Grading of angina pectoris. Circulation. 1976;54:522-3.

Table 3.   Cardiac Event Risk* Stratification for Noncardiac Surgical Procedures†

High
(Reported cardiac risk often >5%)
    Emergent major operations, particularly in the elderly
    Aortic and other major vascular surgery
    Peripheral vascular surgery
    Anticipated prolonged surgical procedures associated
      with large fluid shifts and/or blood loss

Intermediate
(Reported cardiac risk generally <5%)
    Intraperitoneal and intrathoracic surgery
    Carotid endarterectomy surgery
    Head and neck surgery
    Orthopedic surgery
    Prostate surgery

Low‡
(Reported cardiac risk generally <1%)
    Endoscopic procedures
    Superficial procedures
    Cataract surgery
    Breast surgery

*Combined incidence of cardiac death and nonfatal myocardial infarction.
†Classifies common surgical types into a risk classification.
‡Further preoperative cardiac testing is not generally required.

preload and preservation of ventricular contractility.

Patients with mitral stenosis are at increased risk for pulmonary edema and perioperative management goals include control of heart rate, maintenance of sinus rhythm (with a low threshold to move to DC cardioversion if atrial fibrillation occurs) and maintenance of preload and afterload.

- Regurgitant valve lesions pose a much lower perioperative risk than stenotic valve lesions .
- Congenital heart patients with Eisenmenger type physiology (pulmonary hypertension and right to left shunting) are at significant perioperative risk with major noncardiac surgery
- Pulmonary hypertension due to any cause increases perioperative risk

Hypertrophic obstructive cardiomyopathy (HOCM) may become hemodynamically more significant in the perioperative period because of large fluid shifts that lead to ventricular underfilling and surgical stress and pain that lead to increased ventricular contractility and tachycardia that shortens diastole more than systole and thus reduces ventricular filling. All of these factors increase the intraventricular gradient of HOCM and

may exacerbate symptoms including dyspnea and angina.

Systemic hypertension, unless severe and uncontrolled, has not been shown to be an independent risk factor for perioperative cardiac events. Antihypertensive medications should be continued throughout the perioperative period.

Medications
Perioperative fasting guidelines have changed dramatically over the last 10 years. Clear fluids are now allowed up to 2 hours before surgery, so this should not be used as an excuse for withholding medications. Diuretics should be held on the day of surgery to avoid exacerbation of hypovolemia in a fasting patient. Anticoagulation, including aspirin, should be evaluated on a case by case basis taking into account the surgery proposed and the initial indication for anticoagulation. All of the patient's other usual medications should be given on the day of surgery with a sip of water.

β-Blockers should be continued throughout the perioperative period in any patient who normally takes them. In the postoperative period the beta blockers should be given intravenously if the patient is not able to take them by mouth. If the patient is not already on a beta blocker and there is no contraindication, current

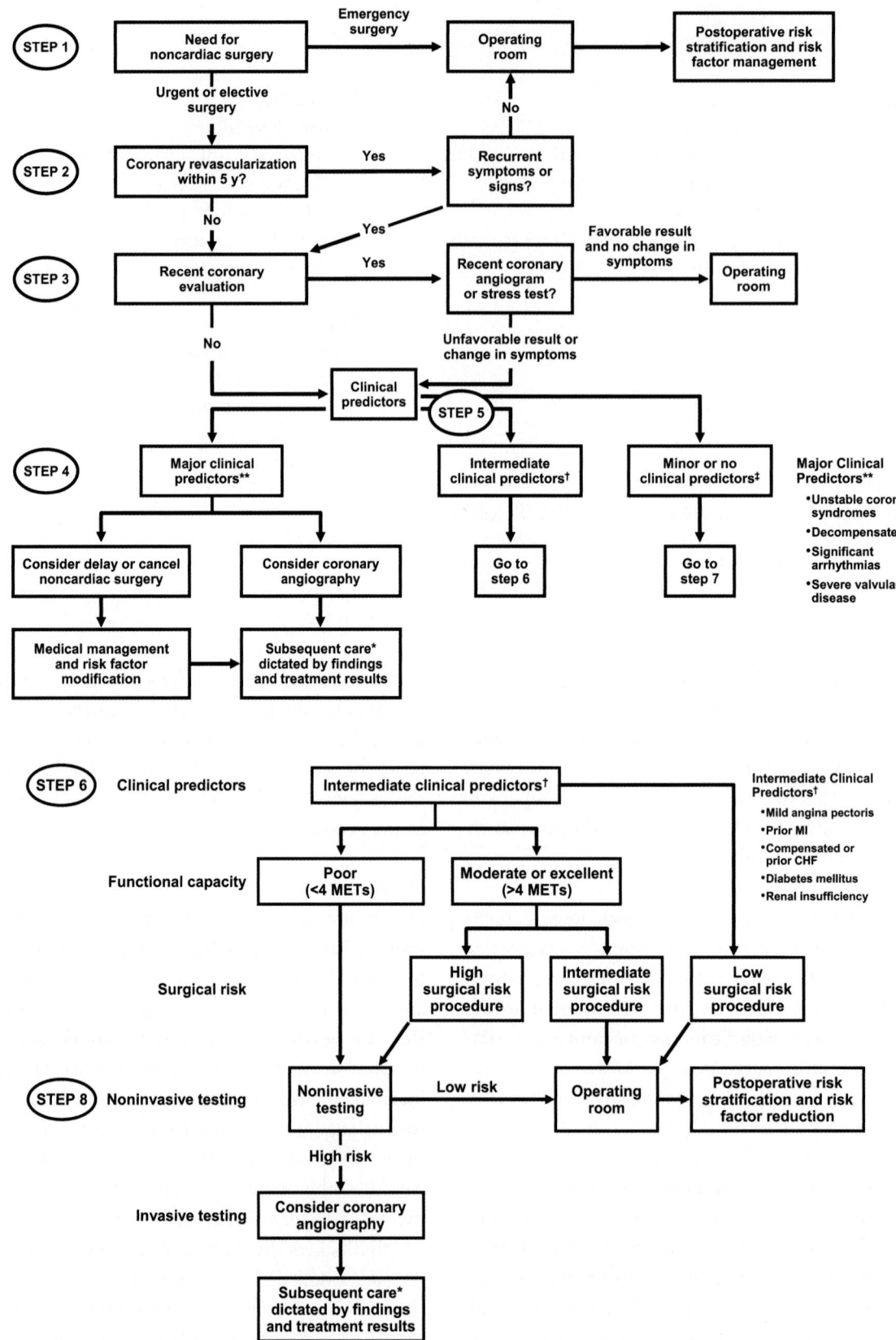

Fig. 1. Continued on next page.

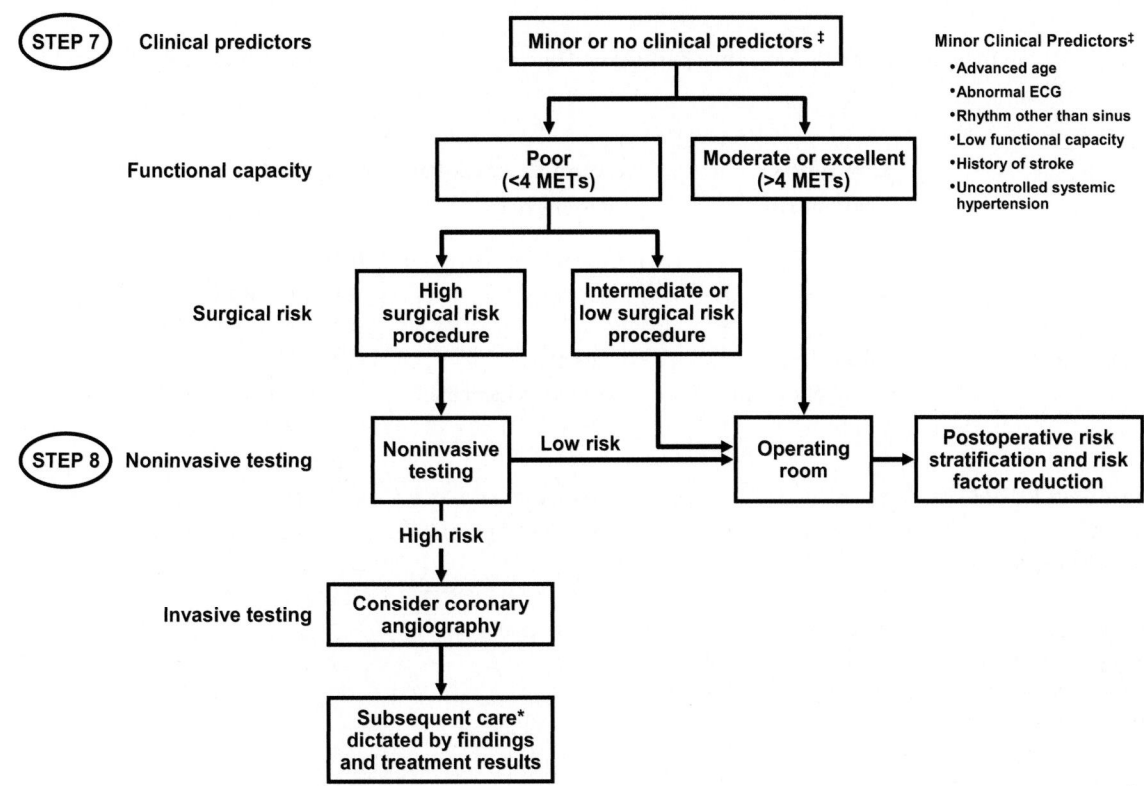

Fig. 1. A stepwise approach to preoperative cardiac assessment. Progressing through steps 1 through 5 for major clinical predictors, 6 through 8 for intermediate predictors, and an alternative steps 7 and 8 for minor clinical predictors. *Subsequent care may include cancellation or delay of surgery, coronary revascularization followed by noncardiac surgery, or intensified care. CHF indicates congestive heart failure; ECG, electrocardiogram; MET, metabolic equivalent; MI, myocardial infarction.

ACC/AHA guidelines suggest that the high risk patient should receive β-blockers for all surgical procedures. The intermediate risk patient will benefit from receiving beta blockers for vascular, high and intermediate risk procedures and the low risk patient for vascular procedures (Table 4). β-Blockade should be started prior to surgery and continue postoperatively. Target heart rate should be less than 80 beats/minute in the operating room and immediate postoperative period and less than 60 beats/minute otherwise. There is evidence to suggest that beta blockade without adequate heart rate control does not provide the optimal degree of protection from perioperative cardiovascular events. There is insufficient evidence to state definitively which beta blocker to use, or how long to continue therapy postoperatively although it should probably be continued for at least 7 postoperatively and possibly as long as 30 days following surgery.

Clonidine has been shown to decrease the risk of perioperative cardiac events in intermediate and high risk patients undergoing surgery when started preoperatively and continued throughout the perioperative period in both β-blocked and non-β-blocked patients. It may be an alternative for those patients in whom beta blockade is contraindicated. If the patient is taking clonidine already it must be continued in the perioperative period either orally, by transcutaneous patch or intravenously to avoid a catastrophic hypertensive rebound effect.

HMG-CoA reductase inhibitors (statins) appear to decrease the rate of cardiac events in high risk cardiac patients. Patients for whom long term statin therapy would normally be indicated appear to benefit from them in the perioperative period; however the data is not robust enough to suggest starting statins in all patients. Statins, like β-blockers, should be continued through the postoperative period.

Table 4. Recommendations for Perioperative β-Blocker Therapy Based on Published Randomized Clinical Trials

	Low cardiac patient risk	Intermediate cardiac patient risk	CHD or high cardiac patient risk
			Patients found to have myocardial ischemia on preoperative testing
Vascular surgery	Class IIb	Class IIb	Class I*
	Level of evidence: C	Level of evidence: C	Level of evidence: B
			Class IIa†
			Level of evidence: B
High-/intermediate-risk surgery	‡	Class IIb	Class IIa
		Level of evidence: C	Level of evidence: B
Low-risk surgery	‡	‡	‡

*Applies to patients found to have coronary ischemia on preoperative testing.
†Applies to patients found to have coronary heart disease.
‡Indicates insufficient data. See text for further discussion.
CHD, coronary heart disease.

Devices

Indications for pacemaker and AICD placement perioperatively are no different than if the patient were not going to the operating room.

Pacemakers should be interrogated for proper function prior to surgery and rate responsive features and any rate enhancement functions should be turned off, since electrical interference "noise" from the electrosurgical units (Bovie) may interfere with them. The patient's underlying rate and rhythm should be documented and the effect of a magnet on the particular device should be communicated to the anesthesia team. Implantable cardioverter-defibrillator units (ICDs) should be disabled prior to going to the operating room. Pacemaker functions deactivated prior to surgery and ICDs should be reactivated as soon as the patient returns to the recovery room.

Not every implanted generator palpated in the chest wall is a pacemaker or ICD. Pain stimulators, thalamic stimulators for Parkinson's disease, phrenic nerve stimulators for diaphragmatic drive or vagus stimulators for seizure control may also be placed in the upper chest.

INTRAOPERATIVE MANAGEMENT

Anesthetic Choice

There is no definitive evidence to show that a well conducted general anesthetic is any more or less successful than a regional anesthetic in minimizing cardiac complications with noncardiac surgery. There are inconclusive reports of a lower incidence of thromboembolism in patients undergoing regional anesthesia with lower extremity surgery and a slightly lower incidence of graft failure in vascular patients presumably by decreasing the degree of surgical neuroendocrine stress that triggers the perioperative hypercoagulable state.

General Anesthesia

General anesthesia results not only in unconsciousness but also amnesia, analgesia and muscle relaxation. The patient may breathe spontaneously or may require positive pressure ventilation. The patient's airway may be secured with an endotracheal tube, laryngeal mask, or the patient may be breathing simply through a face mask.

Commonly used anesthetic drugs and their effects on cardiovascular physiology are outlined in Table 5.

Table 5. Hemodynamic Effects of Common Drugs Used in General Anesthesia

	Heart rate	Preload	Afterload	Contractility	Notes
Sedatives					
Benzodiazepines	↓	--	Slight ↓	--	
Clonidine	↓	--	↓	--	
Scopolamine	Slight ↑	--	--	--	
Induction drugs					
Propofol	↓	↓	↓	↓	Dose dependent effect
Thiopental	↓	↓	↓	↓	
Etomidate	--	--	Slight ↓	--	
Dexmedetomidine	↓	--	↓	--	
Ketamine	↑	--	↑	--	Increases myocardial O_2 consumption
Narcotics					
Fentanyl	↓	--	--	--	
Sufentanil	↓	--	--	--	
Morphine	↓	↓	↓	--	Histamine release mediated vasodilation
Methadone	↓	--	--	--	Torsades de pointes associated with high doses
Meperidine	↑	--	--	↓	
Muscle relaxants					
Succinylcholine	↓	--	--	--	Transient hyperkalemia may lead to dysrhythmias
Pancuronium	↑	--	--	--	
Vecuronium	--	--	--	--	
Rocuronium	--	--	--	--	
Atracurium	--	↓	↓	--	Vasodilation due to histamine release
Cisatracurium	--	--	--	--	
Inhaled agents					
Halothane	--	--	↓	↓↓	Sensitizes myocardium to proarrhythmic effects of epinephrine
Isoflurane	↑	↓	↓	↓	
Sevoflurane	↓	↓	↓	↓	
Desflurane	↑	↓	↓	↓	
Nitrous oxide	--	↑	↑	↑	Increases sympathetic tone
Xenon	--	--	--	--	
Antiemetics					
Droperidol	--	↑	↓	--	Prolongs QT
Ondansetron	--	--	--	--	

Systemic hypotension may arise from blood loss, fluid shifts between the vascular and extravascular space or decreases in preload, afterload or ventricular contractility secondary to anesthetic agents. Increased intrathoracic pressure associated with positive pressure ventilation may also contribute to decreased preload and resultant hypotension.

Regional Anesthesia

Regional anesthesia may consist of a peripheral or a central neuraxial block. Peripheral techniques include blockade of a single extremity, e.g. axillary plexus block for hand or forearm surgery, or block of a single peripheral nerve, e.g. femoral nerve block for analgesia of the anterior thigh. Central neuraxial techniques refer to those in which a needle is placed within the spinal canal, e.g. spinal or epidural injections.

Contraindications to regional anesthesia include preexisting neurological abnormality, coagulopathy, allergy to local anesthetic agents, systemic infection, local infection at needle insertion site and lack of patient cooperation. Regional anesthesia carries the risk of a failed or patchy block which will then require either conversion to a general anesthetic or heavy sedation. Patients are also at risk for local anesthetic toxicity usually manifesting as short, self limited seizure or cardiac dysrhythmias.

The neuraxial techniques, e.g., single-dose spinal or continuous epidural, provide nerve blockade in a dermatomal distribution. In addition to the sensory and motor blockade, sympathetic blockade leads to venodilation, decreased preload and arterial vasodilation with subsequent hypotension. If the height of the nerve block extends above the fourth thoracic level (T4), it will impinge upon the cardiac accelerator fibers of the sympathetic nervous system and can result in unopposed parasympathetic tone to the heart with profound bradycardia (Fig. 2). The hypotension seen with central neuraxial techniques is usually treated with IV fluids to supplement preload as well as alpha agonists, usually phenylephrine, to reverse the vasodilation. Anticholinergics like atropine or glycopyrrolate will reverse the bradycardia associated with the high spinal block.

Bleeding from needle trauma within the spinal canal is potentially catastrophic because pressure from a spinal hematoma may impinge on the spinal cord and roots and result in irreversible neurological deficit. Therefore the anesthesiologist should be especially cognizant of coagulation abnormalities in these patients both at the time of surgery and postoperatively. Patients are at risk for bleeding with initial needle placement, subsequent placement of the indwelling epidural catheter and also with catheter removal. The American Society of Regional Anesthesia and Pain Medicine (ASRA) drafted a consensus statement with recommendations regarding the use of neuraxial techniques in the face of anticoagulation:

1. Avoid antifibrinolytics for 10 days after spinal or epidural anasthesia. In the event that a patient requires antifibrinolytic therapy within that window, the patient should have frequent assessment of neurological function on a 2 hourly basis.

2. There are no contraindication to using mini-dose subcutaneous unfractionated prophylactic heparin while therapeutic levels of anticoagulation with heparin infusion are a contraindication to spinal/epidural anesthesia. Heparin infusions should be stopped 4 hours before starting spinal/epidural anesthesia. If a neuraxial technique is anticipated and intraoperative anticoagulation is planned, then this is acceptable provided no other concomitant coagulopathies are present and heparin is given more than one hour after spinal/epidural occurred. If there is a postoperative indwelling epidural or spinal catheter, heparin should be discontinued for 2-4 hours before it is removed and should not be restarted for at least an hour after its removal. An indwelling spinal catheter should be used with minimal dose of local anesthetics to avoid masking new neurological deficits. Antiplatelet or oral anticoagulants in addition to the heparin will increase the risk of bleeding.

3. In patients receiving prophylactic dosing of low molecular weight heparin (LMWH) preoperatively, the last dose should be at least 12 hours prior to needle placement. Patients receiving therapeutic doses of LMWH preoperatively should have a 24 hour window prior to needle placement. Patients starting on postoperative LMWH for thromboprophylaxis on a twice daily regimen should have the first dose started at least 24 hours

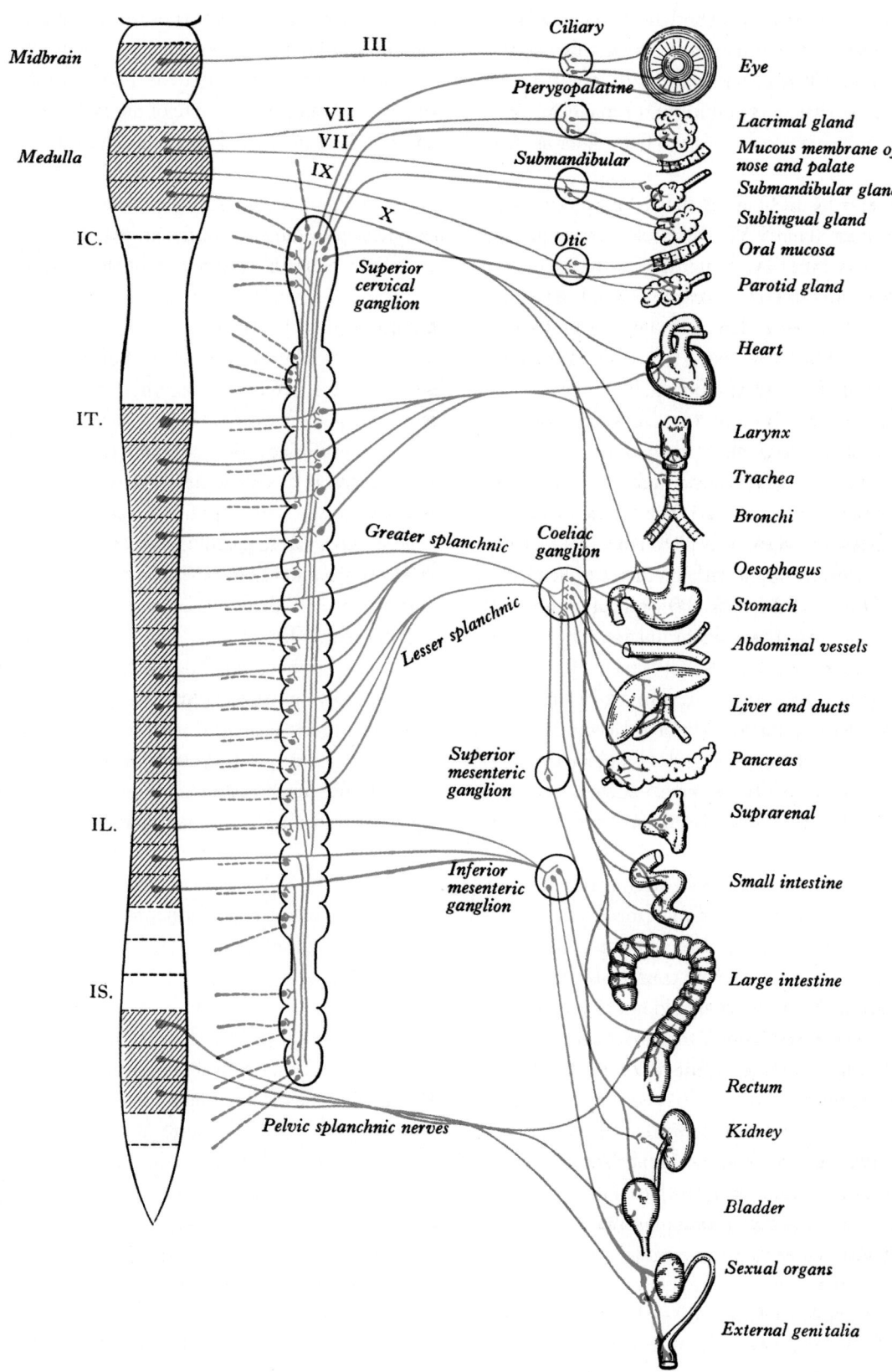

Fig. 2. Sympathetic pathways are shown in red. Cardiac accelerator fibers from T1-T4. Vascular tone mediated by T5-T12.

after needle placement and the epidural catheter should be removed at least 2 hours prior to the first dose. With once a day dosing, the first dose may be given 6-8 hours after needle placement with the next dose at least 24 hours after the first dose. An indwelling catheter should be removed at least 10-12 hours after LMWH dosing and the next dose of LMWH should be given at least 2 hours after the catheter was discontinued.

4. Warfarin should be discontinued at least 4 days prior to the procedure and a normal INR documented. If warfarin is being started for perioperative thromboprophylaxis and the first preoperative dose was taken more than 24 hours prior or a second dose was taken preoperatively, a normal INR should be documented prior to needle placement. If warfarin is being taken while an indwelling catheter is in place, daily INRs should be checked and the catheter discontinued if the INR >1.5. If the INR>3.0 while an indwelling catheter is in place, warfarin should be held to facilitate removal of the catheter.

5. Nonsteroidal anti-inflammatory drugs by themselves pose no additional bleeding risk for neuraxial placement. Patients should stop taking ticlopidine for 14 days and clopidogrel for 7 days prior to spinal needle placement. Normal platelet function returns 24-48 hours after abciximab cessation and 4-8 hours after eptifibatide or tirofiban discontinuation. One should avoid spinal/epidural needle placement within that time. Product inserts are more conservative and suggest that these agents should not be used within 4 weeks after surgery. Other anticoagulants used in addition to these agents will increase the risk of bleeding.

When indwelling catheters are used as part of a postoperative analgesia regimen, a mechanism should be in place to flag and bring to special attention any new orders for anticoagulation or antiplatelet therapy in patients with indwelling catheters.

Sedation or Monitored Anesthesia Care

Intuitively one would expect that patients having only moderate sedation or sedation with local anesthesia would be at very low risk of cardiac events: confidential reporting of anesthetic complications in Australia have shown that overall there is a similar risk of patient death with sedation compared with other anesthesia techniques. This may be a result of decreased vigilance by caregivers because of the misperception that sedation is very low risk, inadequate local anesthesia blockade of procedural site resulting in escalating dosing of sedation, different staffing models with less skilled caregivers providing care or the proceduralist attempting to simultaneously take responsibility for sedation care.

Monitoring

The role of pulmonary artery catheter placement for perioperative patient management during and after major surgery is now less clear than once thought. Numerous clinical trials conducted both within the operating room as well as the intensive care environment have shown no patient survival benefit. Transesophageal echocardiographic (TEE) monitoring during surgery and close clinical observation after surgery seems to be as successful as invasive pulmonary artery catheter monitoring.

Transesophageal echocardiography (TEE) has been used by anesthesiologists for many years during cardiac surgery cases and its role is now expanding beyond the cardiac surgery to monitoring cardiac anatomy and function during major noncardiac surgery, e.g., liver transplantation to evaluate both RV and LV function and filling and to screen for patent foramen ovale and air emboli in patients with unusual anesthesia positioning, e.g., sitting for neurosurgical patients or some orthopedic cases.

Other

Maintaining perioperative normothermia decreases surgical infections, as well as cardiac complications. Presumably the detrimental physiologic mechanism is shivering and increased systemic vascular resistance (SVR) noted in the hypothermic patient.

Transfusion thresholds for the surgical patient continue to be debated. Transfusing patients with heart failure to a hemoglobin >12.5 g/dL improves outcomes. Patients with preexisting cardiovascular disease have an increased incidence of complications with hemoglobin levels below 10 g/dL. It is reasonable to extrapolate from these data that a hemoglobin level >10 g/dL is optimal for surgical patients with cardiac disease.

POSTOPERATIVE CARE

Disposition

Postoperatively patients at significant risk of myocardial ischemia, cardiac rhythm disturbances, or major bleeding should be monitored in an intensive care setting (ICU). Achievement of optimal pain control and monitoring of marginal respiratory status with a propensity for secondary cardiac stress may also be indications for ICU admission.

Postoperative Analgesia

Poor postoperative pain control can lead to increased cardiac and pulmonary events. Aggressive pain control can decrease these complications. Pain control may be achieved with careful titration of narcotics, often with a patient controlled analgesia (PCA) pump, although this still requires careful choice and alteration of dosing by caregivers. Indwelling epidural catheters, running narcotic with or without dilute local anesthetic, can be very effective for lower extremity, abdominal or thoracic pain. Anticoagulant considerations as outlined earlier in this chapter as well as increased sensitivity to respiratory depression from concomitant use of additional narcotics or sedatives require thoughtful analgesia management. Peripheral nerve catheters infusing local anesthetic, in which an indwelling catheter is laid next to a peripheral nerve covering the surgical site, e.g. femoral nerve for knee surgery, allow analgesia with few systemic side effects.

Early data suggested that epidural analgesia decreased the rate of cardiac complications with noncardiac surgery but later, carefully designed studies now suggest that aggressive pain control, whether epidural or narcotic, is the key rather than anesthesia type.

RESOURCES

Auerbach A, Goldman L. Assessing and reducing the cardiac risk of noncardiac surgery. Circulation. 2006;113:1361-76.

Eagle KA, Berger PB, Calkins H, et al, American College of Cardiology; American Heart Association. ACC/AHA guideline update for perioperative cardiovascular evaluation for noncardiac surgery: executive summary: a report of the American College of Cardiology/American Heart Association Task Force on Practice Guidelines (Committee to Update the 1996 Guidelines on Perioperative Cardiovascular Evaluation for Noncardiac Surgery). J Am Coll Cardiol. 2002;39:542-53. Erratum in: J Am Coll Cardiol. 2006;47:2356.

Fleisher LA, Beckman JA, Brown KA, et al. ACC/AHA 2006 guideline update on perioperative cardiovascular evaluation for noncardiac surgery: focused update on perioperative beta-blocker therapy. A report of the American College of Cardiology/American Heart Association Task Force on Practice Guidelines (Writing Committee to Update the 2002 Guidelines on Perioperative Cardiovascular Evaluation for Noncardiac Surgery). J Am Coll Cardiol. 2006;47:2343-55.

SECTION IX

Cardiomyopathy and Heart Failure

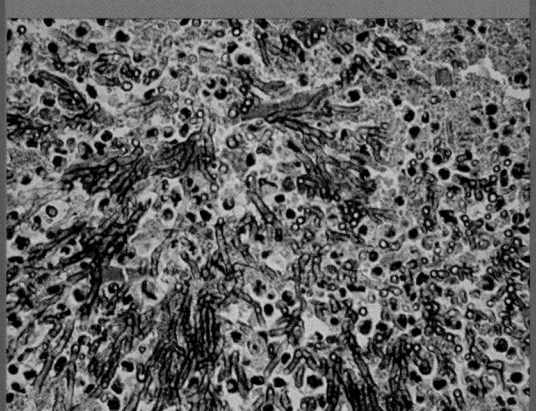

Aspergillus Myocarditis

CARDIOVASCULAR REFLEXES AND HORMONES

Alfredo L. Clavell, MD

John C. Burnett, Jr, MD

Optimal regulation of the circulation is dependent on an integration of cardiovascular reflexes with local and circulating humoral factors that regulate myocardial contractility, vascular tone, and intravascular volume (intravascular volume is regulated primarily through renal sodium excretion). Under physiologic conditions, cardiovascular reflexes function in short-term cardiovascular control, whereas humoral mechanisms function as more long-term modulators of cardiovascular homeostasis.

CARDIOVASCULAR REFLEXES

Two principal cardiovascular reflex arcs are involved in the regulation of blood pressure:

1. Arterial baroreceptors are located in the carotid sinus and aortic arch and respond with increasing neural discharge in response to stretch caused by increases in arterial blood pressure.
2. Cardiopulmonary baroreceptors are located in the ventricular myocardia and also in the atria and venoatrial junctions.

Normal Cardiac Function

The arterial and cardiopulmonary reflexes discharge during cardiac systole; their rate of discharge is directly related to the force of myocardial contraction and to cardiac filling pressure. Afferent signals from both arterial and cardiopulmonary receptors go to the nucleus solitarius in the brain stem. The principal functions of these receptors are twofold:

1. To inhibit efferent sympathetic neural outflow to the heart and circulation, resulting in decreases in arterial blood pressure and systemic vascular resistance.
2. To augment efferent parasympathetic neural outflow to the heart, resulting in sinus node slowing and prolongation of atrioventricular conduction.

During reductions in arterial pressure and cardiac filling pressures under physiologic conditions, the inhibitory discharge of these receptors declines. Efferent sympathetic neural outflow increases, resulting in an increase in systemic vascular resistance, and efferent parasympathetic outflow decreases, resulting in tachycardia. Conversely, during increases in arterial blood pressure and cardiac filling pressures, the inhibitory discharge of these receptors is enhanced.

Efferent sympathetic neural outflow decreases, resulting in a decrease in systemic vascular resistance, and parasympathetic outflow increases, resulting in bradycardia.

Congestive Heart Failure

In chronic congestive heart failure (CHF), a chronic reduction in arterial filling results in a decrease in inhibitory signaling to the cardiovascular reflex center, causing a significant increase in systemic vascular resistance. Despite high cardiac filling pressures due to ventricular dysfunction, an attenuation in the inhibitory action of the cardiopulmonary baroreceptors occurs. The dysfunction of cardiovascular reflexes in CHF results in enhanced adrenergic activity with systemic vasoconstriction. Additionally, sympathetic activation may have secondary actions and lead to activation of local and neurohumoral systems (such as the renin-angiotensin system) and to avid sodium retention due to increased sodium resorption by the kidney.

■ Arterial baroreflexes are located in the carotid sinus and aortic arch and respond to increases in arterial blood pressure.

■ Dysfunction of cardiovascular reflexes in congestive heart failure results in enhanced adrenergic activity with systemic vasoconstriction.

LOCAL AND CIRCULATING HUMORAL SYSTEMS

Vasodilatory, Natriuretic, and Antimitogenic Systems

Natriuretic Peptides

The natriuretic peptide system encompasses a family of cardiovascular peptides: atrial (ANP) and brain (BNP) natriuretic peptides are of cardiac myocyte origin, whereas C-type natriuretic peptide (CNP) is of endothelial cell origin. These peptides are released in response to both acute and chronic atrial stretch (ANP and BNP) and in response to numerous other humoral stimuli (CNP). They have important actions on the heart, functioning through autocrine and paracrine mechanisms, and on other organ systems such as the kidney, adrenal gland, and the vascular wall (Fig. 1).

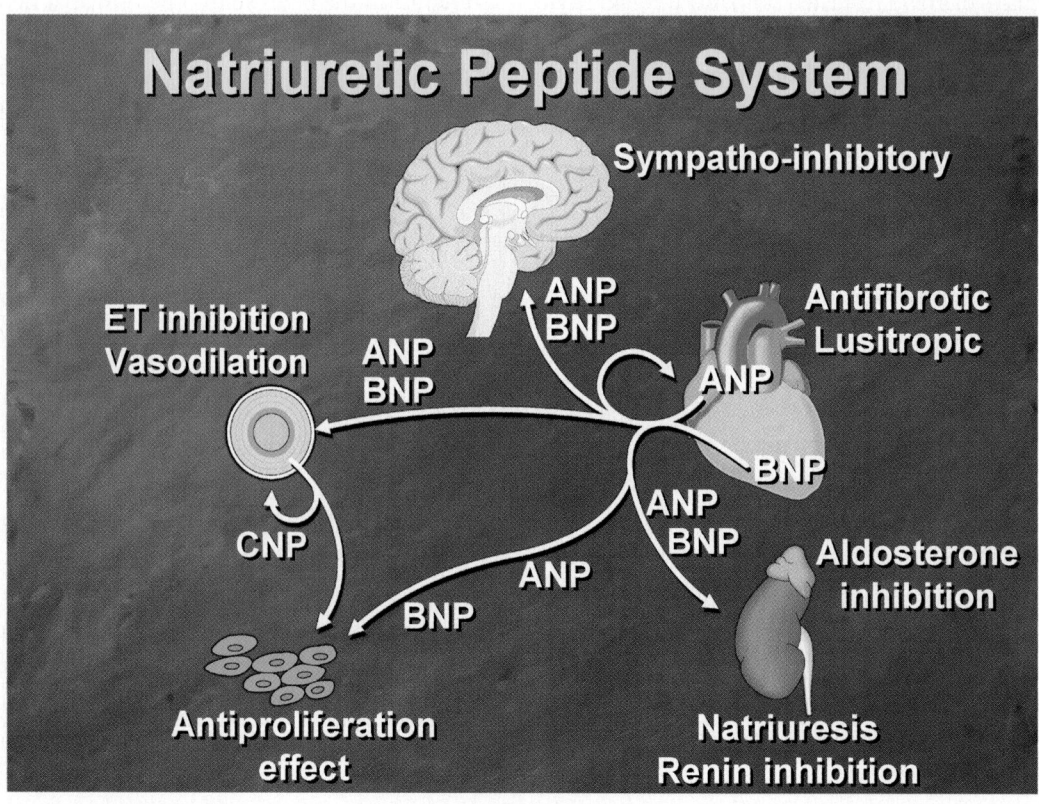

Fig. 1. Natriuretic peptide system.

Important biologic actions include modulation of myocardial function and structure, natriuresis, inhibition of the renin-angiotensin-aldosterone system, vasodilatation, and an antimitogenic effect on vascular smooth muscle cells. CNP is devoid of natriuretic actions but is a powerful vasodilatory and antimitogenic peptide. The biologic actions of this important cardiovascular humoral system are via activation of specific particulate guanylate cyclase receptors, which function via the second messenger cyclic guanosine monophosphate. Importantly, the activity of this system is modulated by two pathways responsible for clearance and degradation of the natriuretic peptides, including neutral endopeptidase and a unique receptor-based clearance mechanism (Fig. 2).

In chronic CHF, ANP and BNP circulating levels are increased. They have functional significance in the overall regulation of the cardiovascular system in CHF because their inhibition with unique receptor antagonists results in a rapid deterioration in experimental animal models of heart failure, as manifested by rapid activation of the renin-angiotensin-aldosterone system together with vasoconstriction and sodium retention (Table 1).

The increase of the levels of the natriuretic peptides in heart failure has significance for both prognosis and diagnosis of early asymptomatic left ventricular dysfunction. In particular, BNP has been recognized as a marker for left ventricular dysfunction and hypertrophy. Because of this functional importance, therapeutic strategies have emerged to potentiate the endogenous natriuretic peptides through inhibition of their degradation by neutral endopeptidase and by exogenous administration of natriuretic peptides via the intravenous and subcutaneous routes. However, the use of a peptidase inhibitor in a recent clinical trial had disappointing results.

■ In chronic CHF, ANP and BNP levels are increased.

Other causes of elevated BNP are listed in Table 2.

Endothelium-Derived Relaxing Factor (Nitric Oxide)
In addition to the natriuretic peptides, an endothelial

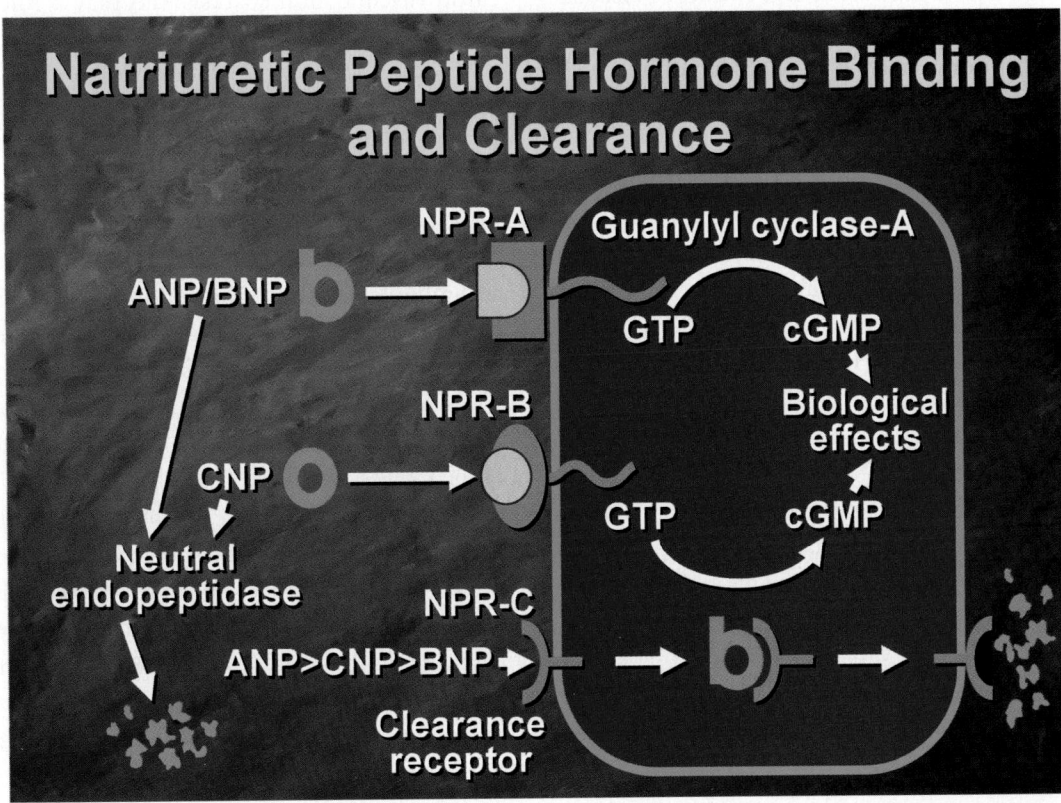

Fig. 2. Natriuretic peptide hormone binding and clearance.

Table 1. Neurohumoral Mechanisms in Congestive Heart Failure

Vasodilatory, natriuretic, and antimitogenic factors	Vasoconstrictive, antinatriuretic, and mitogenic factors
Natriuretic peptides	Renin-angiotensin-aldosterone system
Kallikrein, kinins	
Prostaglandin	Sympathetic nervous system
Dopamine	
Endothelium-derived relaxing factor—nitric oxide	Vasopressin
	Thromboxane
	Endothelin
Adrenomedullin	Cytokines

Table 2. Other Causes of Elevated BNP

LVH
Myocarditis
Cardiac allograft rejection
Kawasaki disease
Primary pulmonary hypertension
Renal failure
Ascitic cirrhosis
Cushing's disease
Primary hyperaldosteronism
Advanced age

cell-derived relaxing factor, nitric oxide (NO), also functions via activation of cyclic guanosine monophosphate through stimulation of soluble guanylate cyclase. The functional role of this endogenous factor is to cause vasodilatation and natriuresis and to inhibit vascular proliferation. Indeed, inhibition of endogenous NO by unique inhibitors results in systemic, renal, and pulmonary vasoconstriction and sodium retention. Long-term inhibition of the endogenous NO system results in hypertension and ventricular and vascular remodeling.

Nitric oxide synthetases (NOS) are responsible for NO production; several isoenzymes have been identified. At the level of the endothelium the production and function of NO appears to be impaired in CHF. Other factors such as cytokines, free radicals and changes in cellular calcium handling contribute to the apparent dysfunction of the NO system in CHF. However, studies conflict with regard to NO activity in CHF. Some studies suggest that NO activity is enhanced in human and experimental animal heart failure, because inhibition of its generation in heart failure results in further ventricular dysfunction and systemic vasoconstriction.

■ Nitric oxide (NO) functions via activation of cyclic guanosine monophosphate through stimulation of soluble guanylate cyclase.
■ The clinical significance of NO activity in CHF is unclear.

Vasoconstrictor, Antinatriuretic, and Mitogenic Systems
Endocrine mechanisms exist to modulate vascular tone, growth of cardiac myocytes and vascular smooth muscle, and sodium excretion by the kidney. The sympathetic, renin-angiotensin-aldosterone, and endothelin systems emerge as three important vasoconstrictor, antinatriuretic, and mitogenic systems that control cardiovascular homeostasis and play a role in the pathophysiology of CHF.

Sympathetic Nervous System
Plasma catecholamines (norepinephrine and epinephrine) are the circulating humoral counterparts of the sympathetic nervous system. Norepinephrine is released locally from sympathetic nerve endings adjacent to myocardium and modulates myocardial contractility. The adrenal medulla also releases both catecholamines in response to diverse stimuli and amplifies the cardiovascular response to sympathetic nervous system activation. The myocardium is rich in β receptors, which are the target of these cardiovascular hormones.

In chronic CHF there is activation of the sympathetic nervous system as a response to the reduction in myocardial contractility and cardiac output. Although the resultant vasoconstriction and increase in myocardial contractility are essential for maintaining blood pressure, eventually this response becomes deleterious and contributes to a further decline in myocardial function. In the presence of chronically increased serum norepinephrine levels, there is down-regulation of myocardial β receptors, perhaps as a protective mechanism.

Circulating levels of norepinephrine correlate with patient mortality in CHF.

β-Adrenergic blockade is an important strategy in the therapeutic neurohumoral modulation of CHF. Recent studies demonstrate a paradoxic increase in left ventricular function with β-blockers, improved clinical symptoms, and better prognosis in heart failure, regardless of the cause of the CHF and in addition to angiotensin-converting enzyme inhibition. Additionally, studies suggest that non-selective β-blockade is superior to selective β–1 blockade in the management of CHF. In fact, the mortality benefit of β-blockade appears to be superior to the benefit observed with angiotensin converting enzyme inhibition.

■ In CHF there is chronic activation of norepinephrine and down-regulation of myocardial β receptors.
■ Treatment with β-blockade results in improved left ventricular function, clinical symptoms, and prognosis in patients with CHF.

Renin-Angiotensin-Aldosterone System
Angiotensin II is one of the most potent vasoconstrictor and mitogenic peptides that is produced both systemically and locally in the heart, lung, kidney, and vascular endothelium as a result of the abundant presence of angiotensin-converting enzyme (Table 3). Angiotensin II, which functions via specific receptor subtypes, also is responsible for stimulation of norepinephrine release and sympathetic activation. Metabolism and growth in myocyte and non-myocyte cells also are altered by circulating and locally generated angiotensin II, which increases cellular proliferation and impairs myocyte contractile activity. Additionally, aldosterone produced by the adrenal gland is activated by angiotensin II and has effects on non-myocytes in addition to its sodium-retaining action in the kidney.

Most recently, studies have suggested that aldosterone may be responsible for cardiac fibrosis via specific receptors within the heart. These two important hormones, angiotensin II and aldosterone, have emerged as the targets for pharmacologic inhibition in the treatment of CHF; in severe human CHF, inhibition of angiotensin II generation has resulted in improvement in mortality and morbidity. However, escape from angiotensin-converting enzyme inhibition is noted chronically, and newer strategies relying on angiotensin

II receptor and aldosterone antagonists have proved useful in the management of refractory heart failure.

■ Angiotensin II, which functions via specific receptor subtypes, is responsible for stimulation of norepinephrine release and sympathetic activation.

Endothelin System
Endothelin is a 21-amino acid peptide that is produced by the endothelium. Much like angiotensin II, an endothelin-converting enzyme cleaves large endothelin into its biologically active form. Its biological actions are mediated through several ET-receptors. Although its role in physiology continues to be elucidated, most likely, as with angiotensin II, it serves to maintain vascular tone and arterial blood pressure. In CHF, it functions as a compensatory mechanism to mediate vasoconstriction and possibly augment inotropic function. Myocardial responsiveness to endothelin also may be preserved in late heart failure when the myocardium has become refractory to other endogenous agonists.

As with angiotensin II, endothelin has growth-promoting and mitogenic potential and, therefore, may contribute to cardiac and vascular remodeling. Endothelin stimulates renin and aldosterone release and augments activation of cardiac fibroblasts.

Table 3.   Angiotensin II: Sites and Actions

Targets	Actions
Heart	Positive inotropism, hypertrophy
Kidney	Renin release, mesangial contraction, sodium resorption
Adrenal body	Aldosterone release
Brain	Vasopressin release, thirst, increased sympathetic outflow
Sympathetic nervous system	Norepinephrine release
Vascular smooth muscle	Vasoconstriction, hypertrophy

Endothelin also has potent renal vasoconstricting and sodium-retaining actions in CHF. Studies also have suggested that an increase in plasma endothelin may have adverse prognostic implications in CHF. However, chronic endothelin receptor blockade resulted in no benefit in a recent randomized study in CHF patients. Selective ET-A receptor blockade has proven efficacious in the management of pulmonary hypertension.

- An increase of plasma endothelin may have prognostic implications in CHF.
- Endothelin receptor blockade is emerging as a new strategy in the management of pulmonary hypertension.

90

SYSTOLIC HEART FUNCTION

Wayne L. Miller, MD, PhD

Lyle J. Olson, MD

CELLULAR ASPECTS OF LV CONTRACTION

Microanatomy

The myocardium is composed of cardiac myocytes enveloped in a dense extracellular matrix of collagen, the main structural protein of the heart. Cardiac myocytes account for 70-75% of the myocardium by cell volume but only 25-30% by cell number. Cardiac myocytes contain myofibrils that are composed of longitudinally repeating sarcomeres separated by Z bands (thickened and invaginated portions of the surface membrane called the sarcolemma). The sarcomeres occupy about 50% of the mass of cardiac myocytes. Thin filaments composed of actin are attached to each Z line and interdigitate with the thick filaments composed of myosin molecules. The thick and thin myofilaments slide past one another in a "ratchet-type" mechanism to generate force and shorten the myocyte. The myofilaments maintain a fixed length throughout contraction. Mitochondria compose about 20% of the cell volume and are the organelles in which adenosine triphosphate (ATP) is generated and located in close proximity to the myofibrils, as well as just beneath the sarcolemma. Platelike folds, or cristae, project inward from the surface membrane of the mitochondria and contain the respiratory enzymes necessary for energy production (Fig. 1).

- Contractile sarcomeres occupy about 50% of the mass of cardiac myocytes.

Excitation and Contraction Coupling

The coupling of cardiac excitation (electrical event) and contraction (mechanical event) are fundamentally molecular in character. The sarcolemma is a thin phospholipid membrane which functions to maintain electrical polarization. The phospholipid bilayer acts as an ionic barrier and maintains relative high intracellular potassium $[K^+]$, and low intracellular sodium $[Na^+]$ and calcium $[Ca^+]$ concentrations (Fig. 2).

Near the Z lines are wide invaginations of the sarcolemma, the T (tubule) system, which branch through the cell. Closely coupled to but not continuous with the T system is the sarcoplasmic reticulum, a complex network of anastomosing membrane-limited intracellular tubules that surround each myofibril and play a critical role in the excitation-contraction coupling of the heart muscle.

Troponin (which is composed of troponin C, I, and T) and tropomyosin are regulatory proteins found in the thin filaments. In the absence of troponin and tropomyosin, the contractile proteins actin and myosin are activated, requiring only the presence of Mg^{2+} and ATP. The regulatory proteins, when present prevent cross-bridge formation between myosin and actin.

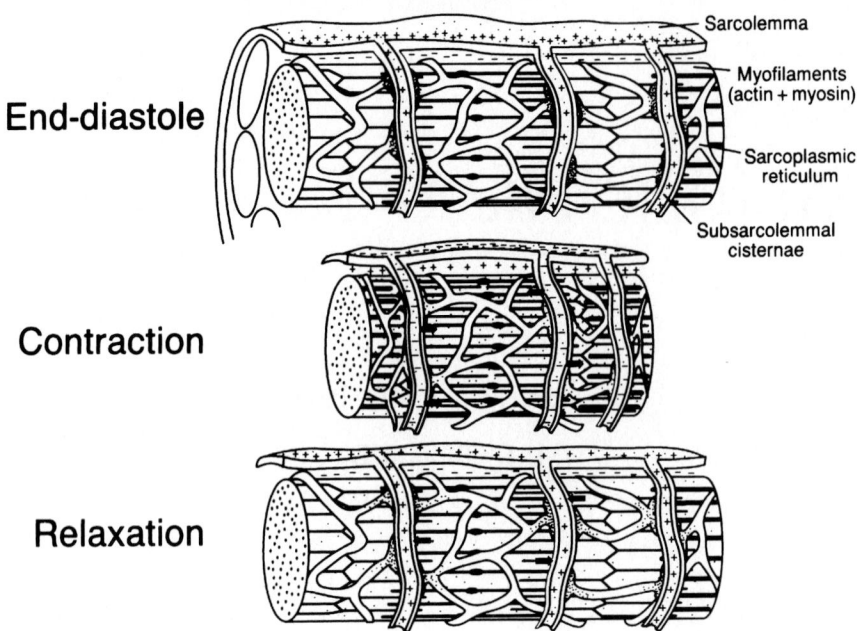

Fig. 1. The major shifts of calcium ions during myocyte excitation-contraction coupling and relaxation. The dots represent calcium ions, and the positive and negative signs indicate electrical charge across membrane partitions.

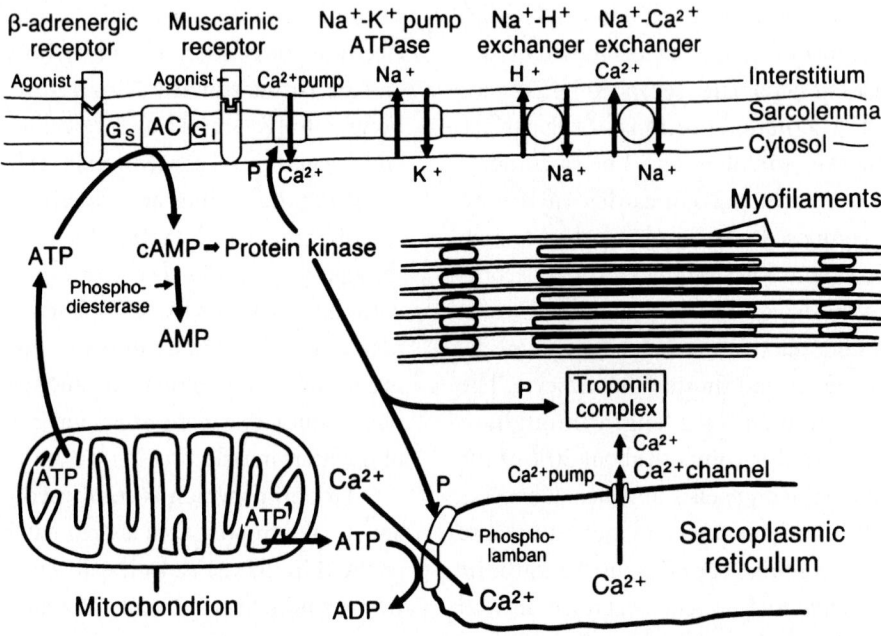

Fig. 2. The regulation of excitation-contraction coupling. The sarcolemma and sarcoplasmic reticulum modulate cytoplasmic calcium availability, and the troponin-tropomyosin complex regulates responsiveness to cytoplasmic calcium. AC, adenylate cyclase; ADP, adenosine phosphate; AMP, adenosine monophosphate; ATP, adenosine triphosphate; ATPase, adenosine triphosphatase; cAMP, cyclic adenosine monophosphate; G_I, guanine nucleotide-binding regulatory protein that inhibits adenylate cyclase; G_S, guanine nucleotide-binding regulatory protein that stimulates adenylate cyclase.

When Ca2+ binds to troponin C, the binding of troponin I to actin is inhibited, which in turn causes a conformational change in tropomyosin, such that tropomyosin instead of inhibiting, now enhances cross-bridge formation. Thus, Ca2+ blocks an inhibitor of the interaction between actin and myosin. The key element in the initiation of contraction is the release of sarcoplasmic [Ca2+]. Depolarization of the sarcolemma caused by the upstroke of the action potential opens the ion channels that carry the inward Ca2+ current, which in turn triggers a release of the large stores of calcium in the sarcoplasmic reticulum. With cellular depolarization, the myoplasmic [Ca2+] rises and is bound to troponin. Once each cross-bridge sliding action is completed, the myosin head releases its ATP breakdown products, binds another ATP molecule, and detaches from the actin site. The myosin head then returns to its original configuration and the cycle is repeated.

Relaxation is brought about by the active (ATP-requiring) reuptake of the calcium into the sarcoplasmic reticulum. Thus, calcium is essential to the excitation-contraction coupling, and when the calcium concentration decreases to a critical point, contraction ceases.

- Troponin and tropomyosin are regulatory proteins found in the thin filaments.
- The key element in the initiation of cardiac contraction is the release of sarcoplasmic [Ca2+].
- The transmembrane calcium current does not directly cause cardiac contraction but promotes release of sarcoplasmic Ca2+.

Mechanics of Contraction

The motion of the LV during contraction can be summarized in the mnemonic TARTT. During systole, the LV *T*ranslates (moves from side-to-side), *A*ccordions (moves with the base and apex attempting to approximate each other), *R*otates (about the LV "long axis"), *T*ilts (perpendicular to the long axis), and *T*hickens (Fig. 3).

Myocardial fibers are arranged in a spiral fashion around the central LV cavity. The subendocardial and subepicardial fibers run largely parallel to the long axis of the cavity, and the mid-wall fibers are mostly perpendicular to the long axis (i.e. circumferential). During ventricular ejection, these fibers shorten and thicken,

and as the LV cavity decreases circumferentially and longitudinally, the inner surface decreases more than the external surface (as dictated by geometry). Because muscle mass remains constant, an increase in wall thickness must occur.

During isovolumic LV contraction, the chordae tendineae become tense, the mitral valve closes, and the ellipsoid LV becomes more spherical. During LV ejection with the opening of the aortic valve, the longitudinal axis shortens by only about 10%, whereas the short-axis diameter shortens by about 25%, thus accounting for 80% to 90% of the normal stroke volume.

Isovolumic contraction refers to the interval (about 50 ms) between the onset of ventricular systole and the opening of the semilunar (aortic and pulmonic) valves. The LV pressure must exceed that in the aorta during diastole for the valves to open. There is a small increase of pressure in the aorta just before the semilunar valves

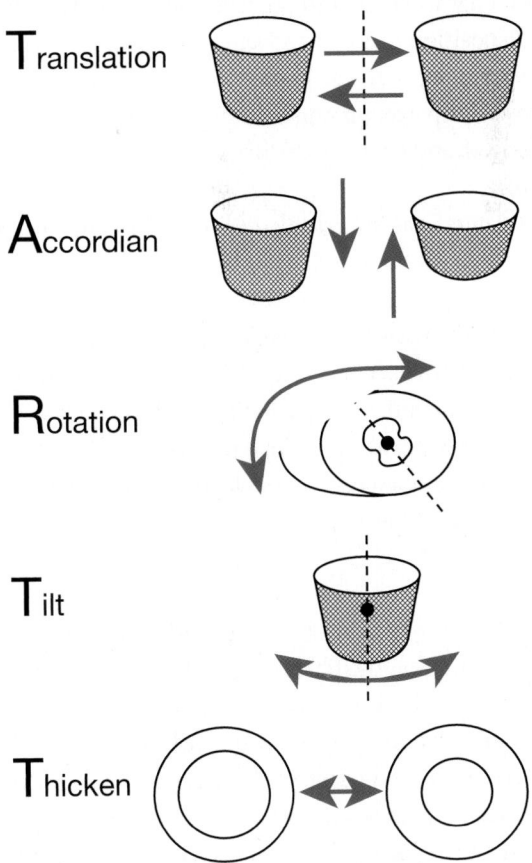

Translation

Accordian

Rotation

Tilt

Thicken

Fig. 3. Mechanisms of contraction and motion of the heart.

open causing the incisura or dicrotic notch. Ventricular ejection is that phase of ventricular systole (about 350 to 400 ms in duration at a normal heart rate) in which blood is ejected through the aortic valve. The first phase (about 100 ms) is rapid, and then ejection slows toward the end of ventricular systole. The increase in ventricular pressure is more marked in the rapid phase.

■ Myocardial fibers are arranged in a spiral fashion around the central LV cavity.

DETERMINANTS OF CONTRACTION OF THE INTACT LV

The mechanical determinants of cardiac function are preload, afterload, contractility and heart rate. When the intact heart is compared with isolated muscle, heart volume and pressure are analogous to muscle length and tension. *Starling's Law of the Heart* is a fundamental property of heart muscle in which the force of contraction at any given tension depends on the initial muscle fiber length. This, in turn, depends on the ultrastructural disposition of thick and thin myofilaments within the sarcomeres. It was in the classic isolated heart and muscle strip experiments that the concepts of preload, afterload, and contractility first became clinically useful terms.

Alterations in preload, operating through changes in end-diastolic fiber length, are important determinants of the performance of the intact ventricle and provide the basis for the length-function curves of the intact ventricle. The ability to augment preload provides a functional reserve to the heart in situations of acute stress or exercise. Preload is thus an important factor in maintaining LV systolic performance in many disease states (Fig. 4).

Afterload

Afterload in the intact LV is the tension (force or wall stress) acting on the fibers of the LV after the onset of shortening. This is primarily the arterial pressure and is a major determinant of stroke volume. An abrupt increase in the impedance to LV ejection, when preload is constant, causes a decrease in fiber shortening and LV stroke volume. The LV becomes smaller during normal ejection and its walls thicken. Thus, despite an increase in aortic pressure during LV ejection, the

afterload or wall stress decreases during ejection. In this situation, there is an inverse relationship between afterload (systolic pressure or wall stress) and stroke volume, extent of wall shortening, and velocity of shortening. In the normal individual, stroke volume can be maintained despite a modest increase in arterial pressure by augmenting LV end-diastolic pressure and volume; that is, the increment in afterload is met by an increase in preload. However, in the diseased heart with little preload reserve (such as heart failure), the LV stroke volume would decrease. Also, even in the normal heart, when there is relative hypovolemia (such as with sepsis or hemorrhage), the preload cannot increase sufficiently and an increase in afterload will reduce the stroke volume (Fig. 5). Table 1 shows LV loading in disease states.

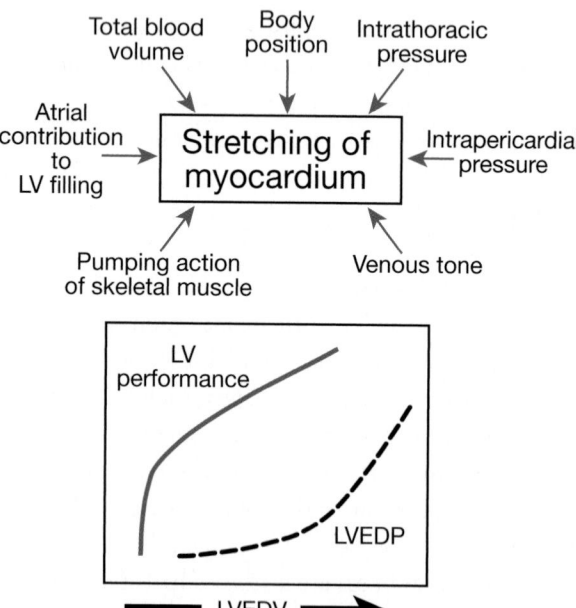

Left Ventricular Preload:
- "Stretch" in isolated muscle preparations
- End-diastolic wall stress in intact heart
- Common to use LVEDV with substitution of LVEDP frequently in clinical situations

Contributing factors:

Fig. 4. Factors affecting myocardial stretch and left ventricular (LV) preload. LVEDP, left ventricular end-diastolic pressure; LVEDV, left ventricular end-diastolic volume.

Contractility

The term "contractility" has been used synonymously with "inotropic state." It is difficult to define in a quantitative sense because there is no clear-cut single measurement of contractility that provides a numeric value that can be assigned to a given heart. However, when loading (preload and afterload) conditions remain constant, an improvement in contractility augments cardiac performance, whereas a depression in contractility lowers cardiac performance. Inotropic influences generally act through altered Ca^{2+} availability to the myofilaments or through an alteration of myofilament Ca^{2+} sensitivity. Additional factors that directly or indirectly affect contractility are sympathetic neural activity and circulating catecholamines (Fig. 6).

The LV pressure-volume relationship is a convenient assessment framework used to understand the responses of LV contraction to alterations in preload, afterload, and contractility.

In its simplest sense, the average circumferential wall stress (σ, force per unit of cross-sectional area of wall) in the intact heart is the product of intraventricular pressure (P) and the internal radius of curvature of the chamber (a) divided by the thickness of the muscle walls (h x 2). Laplace's law for a spherical chamber is

$$\sigma = Pa/2h$$

Preload

Defining preload for the intact LV as the ventricular end-diastolic wall stress provides a direct analogy to the preload of the isolated muscle strip, which in turn determines the resting length of the sarcomeres. Increases in preload augment the stroke volume, as well as the extent and velocity of wall shortening. At a constant preload, there is an inverse relation between systolic wall stress and stroke volume.

■ The ability to augment preload provides a functional reserve to the heart in situations of acute stress or exercise.

Heart Rate

Increasing the frequency of contraction does not produce a shift of the ventricular performance curve relating LV end-diastolic pressure and stroke work, but it does increase stroke power at any given level of filling pressure. Thus, increasing the heart rate will improve myocardial contractility, because the systolic fraction of the cardiac cycle is increased. The positive inotropic effect resulting from an increase in heart rate is more prominent in the depressed heart than in the normal heart. In the normal heart, an artificial increase in heart rate (such as via a pacemaker) will not increase cardiac output, because venous return to the heart is reflexly

Table 1.   Left Ventricular Loading in Disease States

Condition	Preload	Afterload	Contractility	Therapy
Sepsis	↓	→↓	→↓	Fluids and antibiotics
Dehydration	↓	→	→	Fluids
Heart failure	↑	→	↓	Diuretics
Cardiogenic shock	↑	→	↓	Inotropes Intra-aortic balloon pump
RV infarct	↓	→	→	Increase intravenous fluids to maintain high RV filling pressure
Acute mitral regurgitation	↑	→	→	Intra-aortic balloon pump Surgery, if severe
Aortic stenosis	→	↑	→	Surgery, if severe
Systemic hypertension	→	↑	→	Antihypertensive medications

RV, right ventricle.

Left Ventricular Afterload:
- Tension, force, or wall stress acting on the fibers of the LV after the onset of shortening
- Although LV systolic pressure and systemic vascular resistance can affect afterload, and thus cardiac output, neither is its equivalent

Contributing factors:

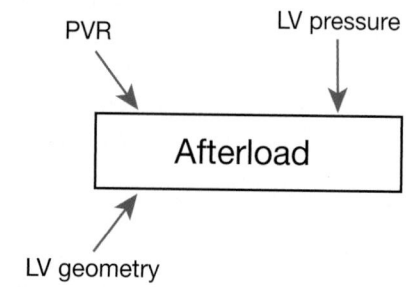

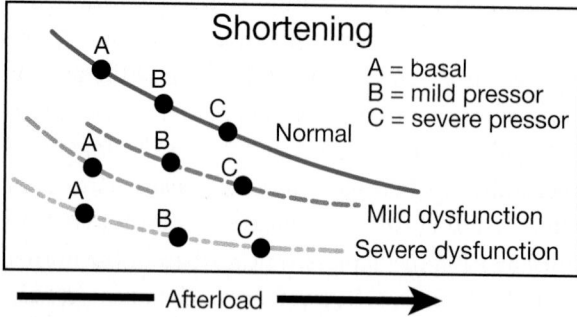

Fig. 5. Factors affecting left ventricular (LV) afterload. PVR, peripheral vascular resistance.

Left Ventricular Contractility:
- Synonymous with "inotropic state," but there is no single measurement of its value
- Generally mediated through altered Ca^{2+} availability or via alteration of myofilament Ca^{2+} sensitivity
- Contractility by definition is independent of loading conditions

Contributing factors:

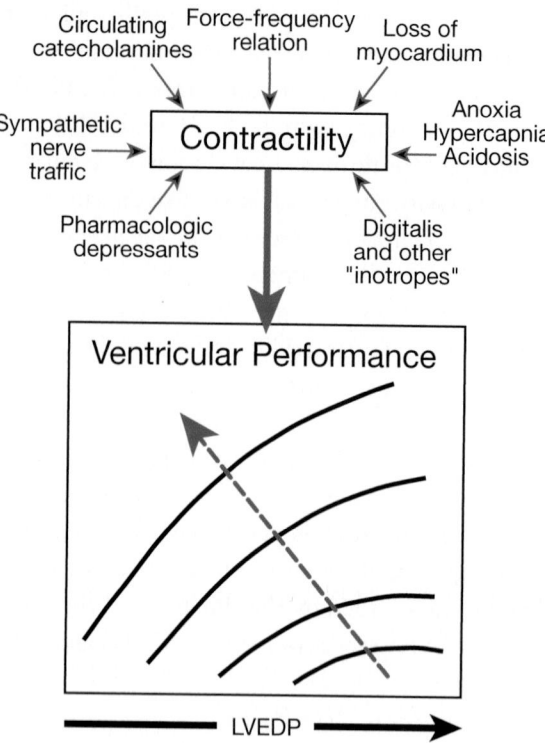

Fig. 6. Determinants of left ventricular contractility. LVEDP, left ventricular end-diastolic pressure.

and metabolically stabilized. However, if the diastolic volume of the LV is increased by increasing venous return, as during exercise, then tachycardia plays a major role in increasing cardiac output. This assumes, however, that not only the speed of contraction but also the speed of relaxation is increased. This effect requires preservation of both systolic and diastolic function. Of course, when the heart rate is too fast, the short duration of diastole can impede ventricular filling, and a decrease in cardiac output can be observed, generally with rates greater than 180 beats/min (Table 2).

Myocardial Infarction
Infarction of 30% or more of the LV mass results in a decrease in LV ejection fraction. Initially, the cardiac output will be depressed and, in circumstances of considerable damage to the LV, function may deteriorate

further, leading to hemodynamic compromise and death. However, in most circumstances, when adequate reserve is present, the cardiac stroke volume is augmented by increases in ventricular preload within hours of the infarction. This change is generally accomplished by an increase in LV end-diastolic pressure and reflects a direct consequence to Starling's law of the heart. Increases in afterload may also accompany these changes and thus may offset the increases in stroke volume brought about by increased preload. There are limits to preload reserve, and further increases in cardiac output must then be brought about by increased heart rate. This situation is also observed in patients with dilated cardiomyopathy and congestive heart failure. In such circumstances, use of agents to reduce afterload

**Table 2.   Effect of Heart Rate on Left
Ventricular Systolic Function**

Heart rate:

  Positive inotropic effect. Note there is little
  effect by ventricular pacing on stroke volume
  in normal patients because of reflex stabilization of venous return

  In the overloaded LV (e.g., CHF), increases in
  heart rate augment stroke volume (to a point)

  In exercise, with increased venous return,
  increases in heart rate are the major contributors to increased cardiac output; in normals,
  the speeds of LV contraction and relaxation
  are increased, facilitating accommodation of
  the increased venous return (up to 180-220
  beats/min, but much lower rates in CHF)

CHF, congestive heart failure; LV, left ventricle.

may be beneficial in augmenting LV stroke volume
(Table 3).

■ Myocardial infarction of 30% or more of the LV
mass results in depression of the LV ejection fraction.

Left Ventricular Hypertrophy
Left ventricular hypertrophy may occur in conditions

**Table 3.   Effect of Loss of Myocardium on Left
Ventricular Systolic Function**

Loss of myocardium:

  Infarction (> 30% of LV mass), fibrosis, infiltration, "myopathies" all reduce LV systolic
  performance

  Generally, preload reserve (Starling's law) can
  assist in augmentation of stroke volume

  However, in some circumstances, reflex and
  intrinsic regulatory humoral factors may
  "pathologically" increase SVR (increase
  afterload); when preload reserve is exhaust-
  ed, there is an afterload-preload "mismatch"

LV, left ventricle; SVR, systemic vascular resistance.

of pressure and volume overload. Acquired disorders
associated with a pathologic increase in LV preload
include chronic aortic and mitral valvular regurgitation,
dilated cardiomyopathy, and, often, myocardial infarction. Disorders associated with a pathologic increase in
LV afterload include severe aortic stenosis and chronic
systemic hypertension. Although the changes in the
sarcomeres are different for these two overload states,
in both situations the overall mass of the LV is
increased. Nevertheless, the hypertrophic response,
which is an important adaptive process that enables the
heart to compensate for overloading, is a complex
process that is both beneficial and detrimental to LV
performance. The hypertrophied cells are not necessarily normal, and abnormalities in inotropic response and
vascular reactivity have been shown. LV hypertrophy
increases myocardial oxygen demand and, along with
changes in ventricular loading (primarily afterload) and
heart rate, is a major contributor to increased myocardial oxygen consumption (Table 4).

PHYSIOLOGIC MEASURES OF LV SYSTOLIC FUNCTION

Ejection Fraction
The most commonly available measure of LV systolic
performance or contraction is the ejection fraction
(EF). This is simply a ratio of the LV stroke volume

**Table 4.   Effect of Left Ventricular Hypertrophy
on Left Ventricular Systolic Function**

Left ventricular hypertrophy:

  Common in both chronic "pressure" and "volume" overloading; also common in dilated
  cardiomyopathy and after myocardial infarction (if > 20% of LV)

  May assist in "normalizing" LV wall stress, but
  is a major component of myocardial oxygen
  demand and can be associated with reduced
  myocardial flow reserve (?mechanism of
  "angina" in aortic stenosis) and altered
  inotropic responsiveness

LV, left ventricle; SVR, systemic vascular resistance.

(SV) to the LV end-diastolic volume. It can be determined with various imaging methods (Table 5). Many of these methods rely on an assumption that the LV shape can be approximated by an ellipsoid. However, the geometry of the LV can be distorted by various diseases, and thus the accuracy of any measure of EF is dependent on the completeness of the measurements. For instance, use of simple formulas derived from two-dimensional echocardiographic measures of end-systolic and end-diastolic dimensions and estimates of LV long-axis length can be erroneous if there are regional LV wall abnormalities of contraction, such as after infarction. In such instances, accurate measures of EF can be derived with radionuclide ventriculography (which does not require assumptions of ventricular shape) or directly via quantitation of LV end-diastolic volume (EDV) and end-systolic volume (ESV) with magnetic resonance imaging or electron beam computed tomography. Thus:

$$\text{Ejection Fraction (EF)} = \frac{\text{EDV} - \text{ESV}}{\text{EDV}} = \frac{\text{SV}}{\text{EDV}}$$

- The most commonly applied and clinically available measure of systolic performance or contraction is the ejection fraction.

Table 5. Clinical Methods of Measuring Left Ventricular Systolic Function

1. Ejection fraction (EF) can be determined with available imaging tools; be cautious of methods that rely on assumptions of LV geometry; acute increase in preload or decrease in after-load will increase EF, and vice versa
2. The velocity of circumferential fractional shortening (VCF) is a better index of contractility than the actual amount of shortening; is relatively insensitive to acute changes in preload; difficult to calculate clinically
3. PER: peak LV systolic emptying rate; load-dependent index of systolic function; use angio, RNA, cine-CT

---

angio, angiography; cine-CT, cine-computed tomography; RNA, radionuclide angiography.

Maximal Elastance

Another method for measurement of left ventricular contractility is the concept of Emax (maximal elastance). This is based on the observation that there is a linear relationship between pressure and volume at end-systole. Stated another way, all end-systolic pressure-volume intercepts form a straight line on the pressure-volume curve for a given degree of contractility. The slope of this line is called the Emax. With an increase in contractility, there is an increase in the slope of the Emax; with a decrease in contractility, there is a decrease in the slope of the Emax. Calculation of Emax requires construction of pressure-volume curves and manipulation of either preload or afterload (Fig. 7).

MYOCARDIAL RELAXATION

Myocardial relaxation is the process by which the myocardium returns to its initial length and tension relationship. Cardiac relaxation is an energy-dependent process that consumes high-energy phosphates. At the cellular level, abnormalities of calcium reuptake may account for LV diastolic abnormalities and impaired relaxation. Relaxation also depends on systolic and diastolic loads and the passive elastic characteristics of the ventricle.

Relaxation may be simplistically regarded as occurring during the isovolumic relaxation period and part of the rapid filling period. If the ventricle is able to fully and quickly complete relaxation, the ventricle will rapidly expand and a large portion of blood flows in from the left atrium to the LV after mitral valve opening. However, if there is a delay in the rate and duration of relaxation, the ventricle will continue to expand slowly even after mitral valve opening. Thus, there will be a decrease in the rate of early rapid filling.

Ventricular Compliance

In mid and late diastole, pressure and volume increase, and the passive diastolic properties of the ventricle, namely, chamber stiffness (or its inverse, chamber compliance), can be assessed. LV compliance is the change in volume per unit pressure as the LV fills with blood from the left atrium. Thus, a decrease in compliance will result in less blood entering the LV for a given increase in pressure. Myocardial fibrosis from any cause can be

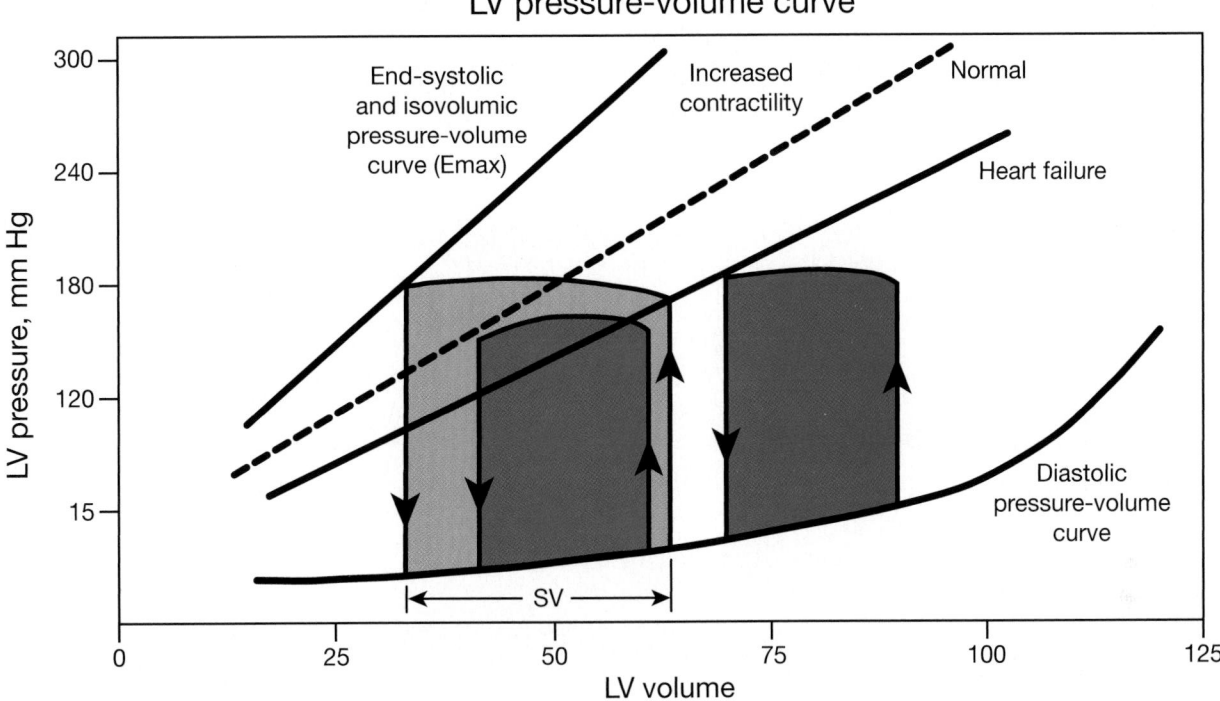

Fig. 7. Maximal elastance (Emax) is a sensitive measure of left ventricular (LV) function and is derived from LV pressure-volume loops.

expected to in-crease ventricular stiffness because collagen fibers are very rigid and virtually nondistensible at normal pressures.

The term "myocardial stiffness" is used to differentiate changes in the stiffness properties of each unit of muscle as opposed to overall chamber stiffness. Thickening of ventricular walls from any cause (for example, LV hypertrophy) tends to increase both myocardial and chamber stiffness. An increased volume/mass ratio is often associated with increased chamber stiffness, whereas in other cases increased chamber stiffness may occur in the presence of a normal volume/mass ratio, implying increased myocardial stiffness.

91

DIASTOLIC HEART FUNCTION

Christopher P. Appleton, MD

Normal left ventricular (LV) diastolic function can be defined as the ability of the ventricle to fill to a normal end-diastolic volume, during both rest and exercise, with a mean left atrial (LA) pressure that does not exceed 12 mm Hg. Because the process of LV relaxation is more energy dependent than contraction, abnormalities of LV diastolic function occur earlier than systolic dysfunction in virtually all cardiac diseases. They increase in frequency with aging, so that about 50% of patients over 70 years old with symptoms of heart failure (HF) have a normal LV ejection fraction, or "diastolic heart failure" (DHF) as their primary cardiac problem. Studies show the symptoms of diastolic and systolic heart failure (SHF) are clinically indistinguishable. Patients with DHF are either unable to adequately distend their slowly relaxing and stiffened left ventricles, or can do so only with elevated filling pressures. This results in symptoms due to pulmonary congestion, atrial arrhythmias or reduced exercise capacity due to a inability to increase LV stroke volume at faster heart rates. Recognition of patients with DHF is important because they have a prognosis nearly as poor as SHF, and even asymptomatic patients with diastolic dysfunction are at increased risk for adverse cardiovascular events. In addition, in patients with

SHF, the degree of diastolic dysfunction is a powerful predictor of mortality. Reliable, noninvasive ways to diagnose diastolic function at its earliest stages continue to be pursued and potential therapies for LV diastolic function are being studied.

- The symptoms of HF from LV systolic and diastolic dysfunction are indistinguishable.
- Recognition of patients with a normal LVEF who have asymptomatic LV diastolic dysfunction is important because of their increased risk for future adverse cardiovascular events.
- Once symptomatic DHF is present, the prognosis is nearly as poor as that of symptomatic SHF.
- In patients with SHF the degree of diastolic abnormality is a powerful predictor of survival.

EPIDEMIOLOGY

In the United States over 500,000 new cases of HF are diagnosed yearly. Epidemiological studies show risk factors for new onset HF to be advancing age, coronary artery disease, hypertension, LV hypertrophy and diabetes mellitus. In patients <65 years old new onset HF is most often associated with male gender, ischemic heart disease and a reduced LV ejection fraction, or "systolic heart failure" (SHF). The increasing importance of genetic familial forms of non-ischemic dilated cardiomyopathy is increasingly recognized. In contrast, almost half the patients over 70 years old with new HF have normal LV ejection fractions (>50%) or "diastolic heart failure" (DHF) as their primary cardiac abnormality (Fig. 1). In this more elderly group female gender and hypertension predominate. These patients complain of dyspnea on exertion and reduced exercise capacity. They may present acutely with marked hypertension and pulmonary edema. They are also at increased risk for new onset atrial fibrillation or stroke. Although the mortality associated with symptomatic LV DHF had previously been thought to be about one third of that seen in SHF, many studies now indicate that cardiovascular (CV) events and mortality are nearly equal for the two types of HF (Fig. 2). It has also been shown that the burden of unrecognized and asymptomatic LV diastolic dysfunction is common in the general community, and increases the risk for cardiovascular events. With our aging population increasing numbers of patients with DHF will be seen, and yet compared to SHF there are few clinical studies on therapy to guide clinical practice.

- In patients >70 years old who have HF symptoms, new onset atrial fibrillation or stroke, DHF should

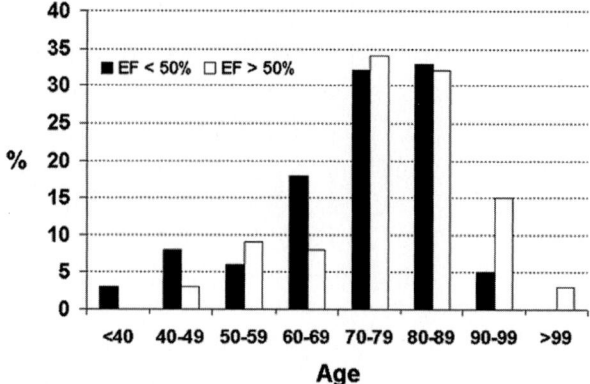

Fig. 1. Age distribution of new onset HF in 216 patients from Olmsted County, Minnesota in 1991. Patients with diastolic HF tend to be older (>70 years) than those with a reduced LVEF.

always be suspected, especially if the LV ejection fraction is normal.

- In the elderly the CV event rate associated with DHF appears to be higher than previously thought, and approaches that of patients with SHF.
- Since asymptomatic LV diastolic dysfunction is common and associated with increased future cardiovascular risk, reliable cost effective methods for identifying these patients are needed.
- The best therapies for DHF are unknown at the present time.

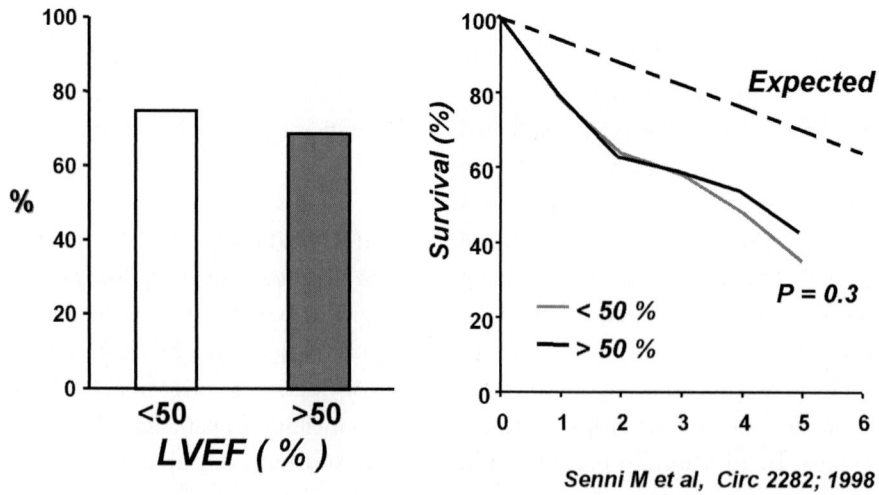

Fig. 2. Survival of patients with new onset HF in Olmsted County, Minnesota in 1991. Survival is markedly reduced regardless of LV ejection fraction (LVEF) compared to that expected for an age matched group.

HEMODYNAMIC PHASES OF DIASTOLE

Diastole is divided into four phases: 1) isovolumic relaxation, 2) early LV filling, 3) diastasis, and 4) filling at atrial contraction. As shown in Figure 3, the determinants of LV diastolic performance vary in their importance and interaction during these different phases. Isovolumic relaxation begins with aortic valve closure, and continues until LV pressure falls below left atrial (LA) pressure. Early diastolic LV filling begins with mitral valve opening and ends when the rising ventricular pressure equals or exceeds the LA pressure. If the diastolic filling period is relatively long, a period of diastasis follows where LA and LV pressures are nearly equal and little additional LV filling is occurring. Finally, atrial contraction reestablishes a transmitral pressure gradient and a variable amount of blood is transferred from atrium to ventricle in late diastole.

■ Diastole is divided into four phases: 1) isovolumic relaxation, 2) early LV filling, 3) diastasis, and 4) filling at atrial contraction.

Although dividing diastole into phases aides description and quantitation of LV diastolic properties, in reality such a separation is artificial in that the factors that influence each phase usually influence all others, especially in disease states. This interaction of diastolic properties, the multiple other factors which influence these properties (systolic function, pericardial restraint, coronary artery turgor, etc.) and the overlap of their effects on the different phases of diastole, has contributed to the difficulty and understanding in studying LV diastolic function.

LV DIASTOLIC PROPERTIES

LV Relaxation

The process of LV contraction and relaxation is dependent upon two biologic systems, cellular Ca^{2+} extruding pumps and exchangers, and myofilament (actin-myosin) interaction (Fig. 4). In mammalian hearts contraction occurs after cellular depolarization results in the passive release of large stores of Ca^{2+} from the sarcoplasmic reticulum (SR), and subsequent activation of the Ca^{2+}/troponin/actin/myosin cascade. In contrast to the process of Ca^{2+} release, the reuptake of cytosolic Ca^{2+} back into the SR is an active, energy (ATP) and load-dependent process accomplished by a powerful SR Ca^{2+} (SERCA) pump. The energy dependence of Ca^{2+} resequestration explains why diastolic properties are altered before contraction becomes abnormal.

Under normal circumstances the rate of Ca^{2+} reuptake is rapid so that LV relaxation occurs largely by "elastic recoil" from energy stored in compressible interstitial elements during systolic compression. Delay in deactivation of the contractile proteins interferes with this process, occurs by several different mechanisms, and is a consistent finding early in the course of all cardiac diseases. Electrical dyssynchrony, increased

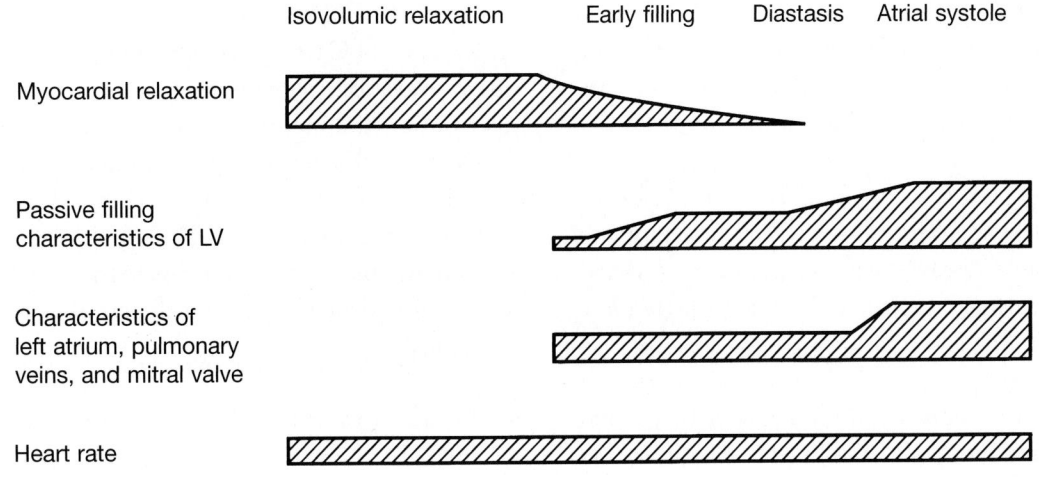

Fig. 3. Determinants of LV diastolic performance and their relation to phases of diastole.

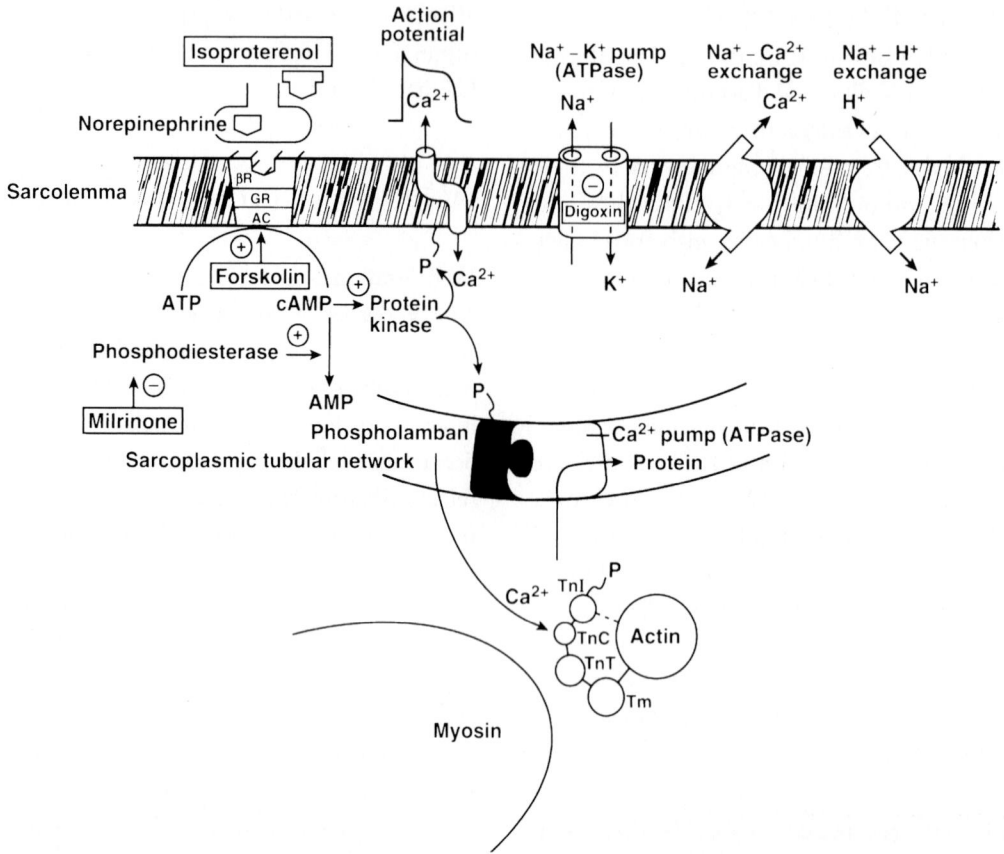

Fig. 4. Schematic diagram of calcium dependent excitation-contraction coupling and relaxation in the heart (see text for discussion). AMP, adenosine monophosphate; ATP, adenosine triphosphate; cAMP, cyclic AMP; BR, β-adrenergic; P, degree of phosphorylation; Tm, tropomyosin; TnC, troponin C; TnI, troponin I; TnT, troponin T.

mechanical loading (hypertension, aortic stenosis), arterial endothelial dysfunction, ischemia, and negative inotropic drugs are some of the ways LV relaxation can be slowed or "impaired," decreasing the rate of elastic recoil and time available for ventricular filling. Genetic alterations in the SERCA handling of Ca2+ are induced by LV hypertrophy and thyroid hormone.

■ In contrast to LV contraction, LV relaxation is an energy dependent process and more susceptible to disruption by disease states such as electrical dyssynchrony, increased mechanical loading (hypertension, aortic stenosis), and coronary artery disease.

The cellular processes and molecular biology that influence myocyte Ca2+ handling, LV relaxation, and their alteration in cardiac diseases is becoming clearer (Fig. 4). The SERCA pump has an endogenous regulator

phospholamban (PLB), which is stimulated by phosphorylation with a cAMP dependent protein kinase. β1-adrenergic phosphorylation of PLB by drugs speeds relaxation. SERCA pump dysfunction can result in a reduced rate of Ca2+ uptake, which may limit the rate of LV relaxation, or result in incomplete crossbridge dissociation and increased chamber stiffness. Other factors that influence LV relaxation include shifts in myofilament Ca2+ sensitivity, mechanical stretch or load on the ventricle and displacement and load dependence of the myofilaments themselves, whose effects differ depending on which part of systole they are applied.

■ The sarcoplasmic reticulum Ca2+ (SERCA) pump, helps control the rate of LV relaxation, and has an endogenous regulator, phospholamban.

■ LV contraction and relaxation is also be affected by

mechanisms which alter the availability of Ca^{2+} to the contractile proteins, the sensitivity of the proteins to Ca^{2+}, or the mechanical stretch and load on the ventricle.

In the intact mammalian heart both experimental and clinical studies suggest the normal left ventricle contracts to a volume below its equilibrium volume, compressing elastic cardiac elements. This creates early diastole restoring forces that produce elastic recoil, a "suction" effect that lowers LV minimum pressure and increases early LV diastolic filling. In the normal canine heart approximately 20% of filling occurs while LV pressure is falling. Rapid LV relaxation helps maximize the beneficial effect of these restoring forces and together they result in a normal pattern of LV filling that occurs predominantly in early diastole, rather than at atrial contraction. Slower LV relaxation antagonizes the "suction" effect of normal restoring forces on LV filling and results in a delayed mitral valve opening, lower early transmitral gradient and a shift to an LV filling pattern which has a greater proportion of filling at atrial contraction. This filling pattern is less favorable, especially during faster heart rates, because a shorter diastolic filling time may not allow the ventricle to relax and fill to an optimal end-diastolic volume without elevating mean LA pressure and causing pulmonary congestion and dyspnea.

■ Normal ventricular contraction compresses elastic elements whose recoil in early diastole helps augment early diastolic myocardial filling.

LV PASSIVE DIASTOLIC PROPERTIES

After LV relaxation is complete, the remainder of LV filling is influenced by more "passive" LV characteristics. These are composed of inherent cardiac elements such as collagen fibers and sarcomeric proteins that affect myocyte and *myocardial* compliance, and external elements such as the pericardium and pulmonary airway pressure that affect LV *chamber* compliance. Together the sum effect of all components is described by the exponential diastolic LV pressure-volume (P-V) relationship. This describes the ability of a relaxed or "passive" left ventricle to distend with increasing volume. A decrease in LV chamber compliance means that

increased filling pressures will be required to maintain a normal LV end-diastolic volume, stroke volume and cardiac output.

Left ventricular myocardial compliance is related to the cardiac interstitial elements; the collagen-elastic struts and network that help connect and provide support for the cardiac myocytes. Normally these supporting structural interstitial elements compose less than 5% of cardiac mass. With increase in heart size due to aerobic athletic training, collagen increases in proportion to myocardial mass. However, in the presence of pressure overload induced LV hypertrophy, LV ischemia, or dilated cardiomyopathy, release of angiotensin II and aldosterone occurs and stimulates a disproportionate increase in interstitial elements. An increase in diastolic myocardial stiffness occurs when the collagen concentration increases two to threefold without a similar increase in myocyte volume. Increased resting passive stiffness in DHF may also be due to abnormal phosphorylation of sarcomeric proteins. Viscoelastic properties, or loss of potential energy due to frictional forces associated with LV elastic recoil, are small enough to be ignored except when marked cardiac fibrosis is present.

■ Myocardial compliance is affected by inherent cardiac elements such as sarcomeric proteins and cardiac interstitial elements, especially collagen fibers.
■ LV chamber compliance is determined by both myocardial compliance and external elements that affect LV compliance such as the pericardium.

Under normal circumstances about 40% of resting diastolic pressure is due to extrinsic cardiac forces, mostly from the pericardium. However, the effect of pericardial restraint in limiting cardiac filling becomes clinical significant only during maximal exercise, or when there is acute cardiac dilatation or pericardial disease present. Left ventricular chamber compliance decreases with increasing LV volume, in part due to the increased stretch on the elastic interstitial elements. Similarly, only with a marked increase in pulmonary airway pressures, as seen in asthmatics or with positive pressure ventilation, are intracardiac pressures affected sufficiently to inhibit LV filling or decrease cardiac output.

■ The effect of pericardial restraint in limiting cardiac

filling becomes clinically significant only during maximal exercise or when acute cardiac dilatation or pericardial disease is present.

MEASURING LV DIASTOLIC PROPERTIES

LV Relaxation

The rate of LV relaxation can be measured from high-fidelity (micromanometer) pressure recordings taken during LV isovolumic relaxation (Fig. 5). LV pressure change is usually exponential between maximal -dP/dt (occurring approximately at aortic valve closure) and the time of mitral valve opening. The pressure decrease can be described by the relationship:

$$P(t) = P_o \cdot e^{-t/T}$$

where P_o is LV pressure at maximal -dP/dt (the point at which the rate of LV pressure decline is maximal), t is the time after onset of relaxation, and T is the time constant of isovolumic relaxation (τ). This time constant represents the time for the LV pressure to decrease to $1/e$ of its initial value, τ typically being 30-40 milliseconds in humans, with lower values representing faster relaxation. Relaxation is believed to be "complete" after three to four time constants (120-150 ms in humans), which corresponds in time to shortly after peak early diastolic filling in normals. In mammalian hearts, τ appears proportional to heart rate, being as short as 10 milliseconds in rats, in which the normal resting heart rate is 350 beats/min.

- LV relaxation is quantitated by analyzing the exponential decrease in LV pressure during isovolumic relaxation.
- Tau (τ) is a quantitative measure of LV relaxation. Lower values represent faster relaxation.

Despite its usefulness, several limitations of quantitating LV relaxation with a simple exponential model are recognized. In patients with hypertrophic cardiomyopathy or markedly asynchronous relaxation, LV pressure decline may significantly deviate from an exponential relation. The simple model also assumes that LV pressure decays to zero pressure, which does not take into account the effect of either LV elastic recoil or external

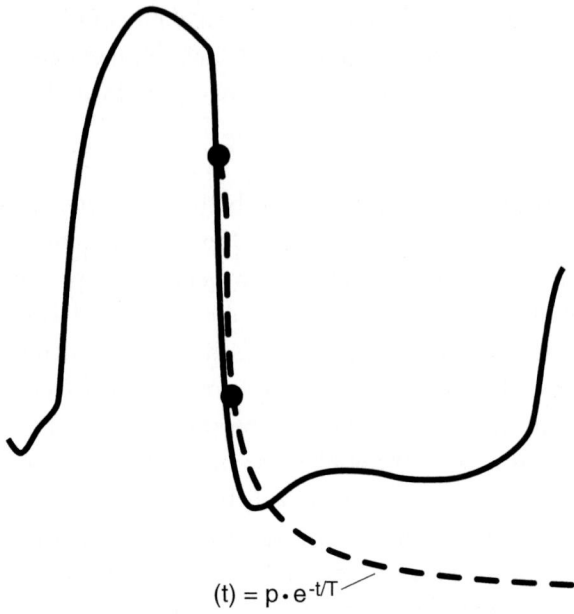

$$(t) = p \cdot e^{-t/T}$$

Fig. 5. Calculation of time constant of myocardial relaxation (tau, τ). LV pressure is plotted on y-axis, and time is plotted on x-axis. Pressure is measured by high-fidelity, manometer-tipped catheters. Pressure from time of aortic valve closure (upper dot) to mitral valve opening (lower dot) is fited to a monoexpoential equation. Time constant of relaxation (T) is obtained from equation, as shown. E, natural logarithm; p, pressure; t, time; T, τ.

forces. Studies in normal animals suggest that if LV filling did not occur, LV minimum pressure would be negative. Although the addition of an intercept term to the original equation provides for a "floating" or non-zero LV asymptote pressure, the method to best quantify LV relaxation under different circumstances remains uncertain.

LV PASSIVE PROPERTIES

Developing a stress-strain relationship quantitates LV myocardial compliance, or the ability of the muscle to distend. This requires applying a force to a known mass of myocardium while simultaneously measuring its deformation. Because of the many assumptions about LV geometry, and the inability to exclude the effects of external and "active" (relaxation, viscoelastic properties) LV forces, it has been impractical to measure in vivo. Therefore, the sum effect of myocardial compliance, chamber compliance, and external forces is studied by constructing LV pressure-volume (P-V) relationships obtained during diastasis (Fig. 6). Operating chamber compliance, or its reciprocal term "chamber stiffness," is defined as the slope of a tangent to the P-V relationship at a specified point. The steeper the slope of the tangent, the less compliant or "stiffer" the LV chamber (Fig. 6 *A*). Because chamber stiffness depends on which point of the P-V curve is used for assessment, several methods have been proposed to normalize this value so that it can be compared after interventions, in serial studies, or between ventricles of different sizes. Although no consensus exists on this point, operating chamber compliance is most commonly measured at LV end-diastolic pressure.

■ LV chamber compliance is evaluated by analyzing the diastolic portion of pressure-volume (P-V) relationships.

Shifts and shape changes in the LV P-V relationship have different implications. Because the P-V relationship is exponential, the same incremental increase in volume results in a greater pressure increase as the ventricle progressively distends (Fig. 6 *B*). If the shape of the P-V curve does not change, a shift leftward indicates decreased chamber compliance (same slope tangent at smaller LV volume), and a shift rightward indicates increased compliance (Fig. 6 *C*). In reality, when measured in sequential studies, curve shifts to the right and left are usually accompanied by alterations in the shape of the P-V curve, and so the incremental change in pressure for a given volume is also changing.

The requirements for accurate construction of LV P-V relationships are formidable. The points should be taken after LV relaxation is complete (during diastasis), so that only passive properties are in effect. High-fidelity LV pressure recordings should be used and transmural LV pressure (LV pressure-intrapleural pressure) should be calculated to avoid inaccuracies caused by respiratory-induced changes in intrapleural pressure. To characterize the P-V relationship over its entire clinical range, LV volume must be varied by rapid changes in preload and afterload without markedly affecting heart rate or LV contraction and relaxation. Accurate calculation of LV volume itself is difficult by current angiographic and echocardiographic methods. These requirements have proved impractical for most clinical studies. As a result, most research involving chamber compliance, or sequential changes in LV chamber compliance has been performed in experimental studies.

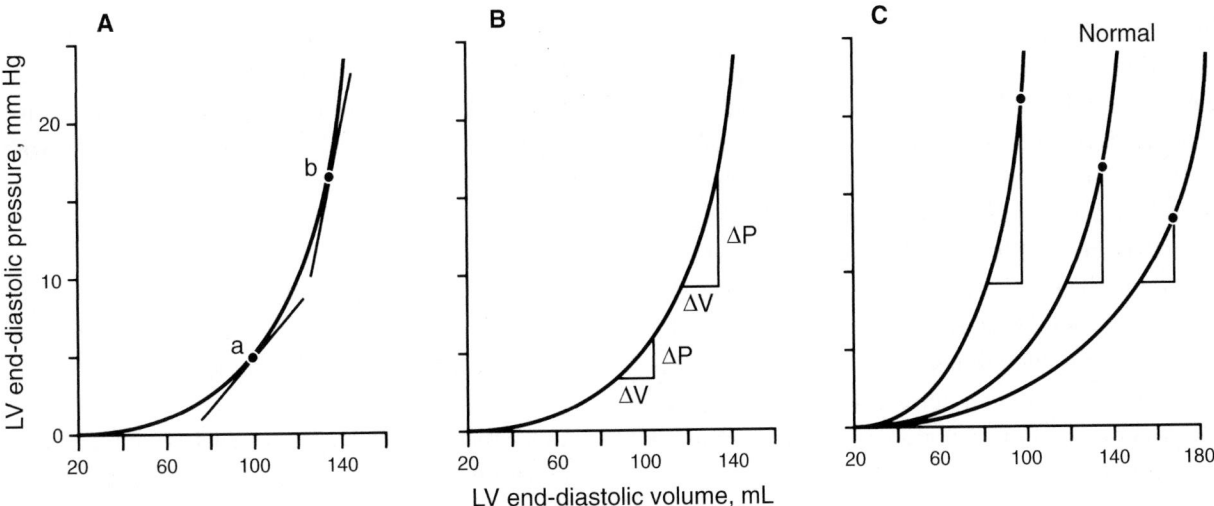

Fig. 6. Left ventricular (LV) pressure-volume relationships. Slope of tangent at different pressures (a and b, panel *A*) represents chamber compliance at different end-diastolic volumes and pressures in the same ventricle. The steeper the slopes the greater the incremental pressure change for the same amount of volume increase (panel *B*). A leftward shift of the PV relation represents a stiffer chamber, while a rightward shift, a more compliant chamber compared to normal (panel *C*). P, pressure; V, volume.

LV Diastolic Properties in Cardiac Disease States

It is estimated that as many as 30 million Americans have high blood pressure (>140/80 mm Hg), with only 30% being adequately treated. Therefore, the most common cardiac abnormality encountered in clinical practice is impaired LV relaxation due to hypertension with or without LV hypertrophy. A minority of these patients shows clinical evidence of reduced LV chamber compliance and increased LA pressures. Patients with ischemic heart disease are similar, with the majority showing mostly LV relaxation abnormalities, and only about 10% having altered compliance that raises mean LA pressure to abnormal values. Patients with hypertrophic cardiomyopathy also have abnormal LV relaxation (sometimes severe), but a higher proportion of individuals also demonstrate a decrease in chamber compliance.

■ The most common cause of LV diastolic dysfunction when the ejection fraction is normal is ventricular hypertrophy due to hypertension.

Patients with dilated cardiomyopathies typically have both impaired LV relaxation and reduced chamber compliance. Interestingly, the LV pressure-volume relation is shifted right (more compliant) in most cases, but this is offset by the increase in LV volume so that filling pressures are often elevated. More rarely (<10%) operating chamber compliance and filling pressures will remain normal. In restrictive cardiomyopathies LV relaxation is also usually impaired. However, the hallmark of this disorder is a severe decrease in LV chamber compliance at normal, or near normal, LV volumes. This indicates a shift of the diastolic pressure-volume relation to the left. A similar leftward shift of the P-V relation is seen in patients with constrictive pericarditis due to the thickened, noncompliant pericardium. Constrictive pericarditis is unusual in that LV relaxation can be normal in the presence of severely altered chamber compliance.

■ Shifting of the normal LV P-V relationship to the right indicates a more compliant ventricle and is a compensatory mechanism in patients with dilated cardiomyopathies, even though filling pressures are often elevated due to the increased end-diastolic volume.

■ A leftward shift of the P-V relationship occurs in patients with DHF due to increased myocardial stiffness. A similar leftward shift is seen in restrictive cardiomyopathies and constrictive pericarditis due to a thickened, noncompliant pericardium.

Patients with isolated mitral or aortic regurgitation most often show little change in LV relaxation or chamber compliance. When the left ventricle is enlarged this indicates a remodeling of the ventricle to an eccentric type hypertrophy whose P-V relation has shifted to the right keeping filling pressures normal despite the increase in cardiac volume. A marked decrease in cardiac compliance in MR or AR indicates severe acute regurgitation or additional ventricular disease.

■ Patients with isolated chronic mitral or aortic regurgitation have increased LV volume, but a shift of the P-V curve to the right helps keep filling pressures normal.

Relationship of LV Systolic and Diastolic Function

LV systolic and diastolic function is a continuum, intimately related on a beat-to-beat basis. Through its effect on compression of elastic elements LV end-systolic volume affects the rate of LV relaxation, while end-diastolic volume through sarcomere stretch affects LV stroke volume and contractility. Loading conditions, inotropic stimulation and neurohumoral factors likewise generally affect both systolic and diastolic function in parallel fashion.

■ Loading conditions, inotropic stimulation, and neurohumoral factors generally affect both systolic and diastolic function in parallel fashion.

Despite this close interaction, a hysteresis of LV systolic and diastolic function can occur. This is common with LV hypertrophy, where LV end-systolic volume and ejection fraction remain normal yet LV relaxation is impaired because of slowing of the rate in Ca^{2+} reuptake. Hypertrophic and restrictive cardiomyopathies are diseases where reduced chamber compliance, as well as prolonged relaxation, can be seen with a normal LV ejection fraction. The reverse situation, abnormal LV systolic function with normal diastolic properties is not observed, although shifts of the LV P-V relation to the right help minimizes the decrease in LV chamber compliance expected when ventricular volume is increased.

LV DIASTOLIC FILLING PRESSURES

Familiarity with different LV filling pressures and their pathophysiologic correlates aids understanding of LV diastolic function. The relation between LA and LV pressures in diastole, or the transmitral pressure gradient, determines whether there is forward mitral blood flow and LV filling (Fig. 7). LV end-diastolic pressure, or the pressure immediately preceding systole, distends the myocardium to its optimal volume and helps maintain normal stroke volume via the Frank-Starling mechanism. When an elevated LV end-diastolic pressure is needed to fill a noncompliant ventricle, two different situations may be present. In early disease a contraction from a hypertrophied left atrium confines the abnormal pressure increase to the short period in late diastole, so that mean LA pressure remains normal. In these patients the loss of atrial contraction due to atrial fibrillation results in an immediate drop in cardiac output and higher filling pressures, which may precipitate pulmonary edema. In more advanced disease LV compliance is reduced throughout diastole and mean LA pressure is elevated. Pulmonary congestion is often present and there is an early and abnormally rapid increase in early diastolic pressure. The atrium may already demonstrate systolic failure and contribute relatively little to ventricular filling and maintaining a normal end-diastolic pressure. Paradoxically, developing A-fib in this group may result in less hemodynamic deterioration and fewer symptoms.

LV FILLING PATTERNS

At Rest and With Exercise and Aging

Although many factors influence diastolic function, LV relaxation and LV chamber compliance (through its affect on left atrial pressure) are the chief determinants of the transmitral pressure gradient and LV filling. For a given left atrial pressure, slower LV relaxation results in a later mitral valve opening, reduced early diastolic

transmitral gradient, and a compensatory increase in the proportion of filling at atrial contraction. Conversely, for the same rate of LV relaxation a higher left atrial pressure will result in opposite effects.

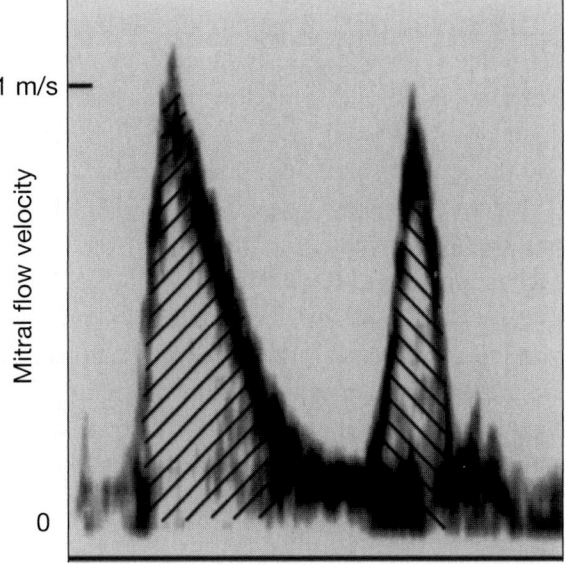

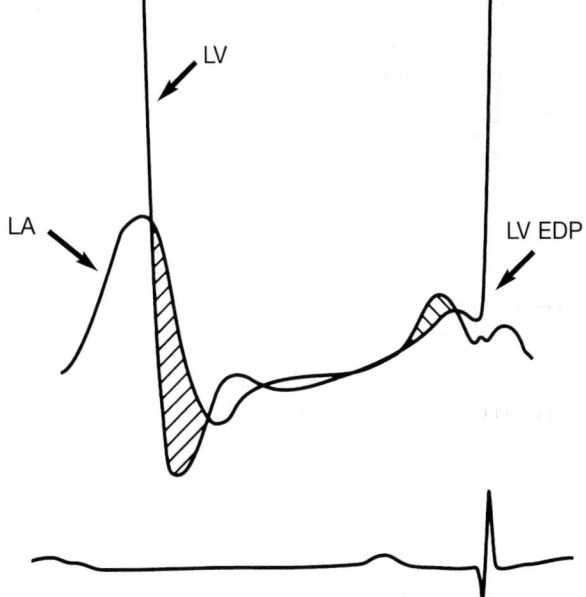

Fig. 7. *Upper panel*, diastonic LV filling pattern obtained with PW Doppler technique. *Lower panel*, transmitral pressure gradient (hatched areas) that causes this filling. A slower rate of LV relaxation will decrease the early diastolic pressure gradient, while a higher LA pressure will increase it. LA, left atrium; LV, left ventricle; LV EDP, left ventricular end-diastolic pressure.

■ At normal heart rates and PR intervals atrial contraction occurs after LV relaxation and early diastolic filling are complete. This separation of early and late diastolic filling optimizes mechanical efficiency and helps maintain normal left atrial filling pressures.

In young individuals LV relaxation is rapid, LV restoring forces are prominent, and the majority of LV filling (70%-90%) occurs during early diastole. With aging, LV relaxation slows in association with an increase in systolic blood pressure and LV mass, and the proportion of filling that occurs with atrial contraction increases, typically to 30%-40% by age 65. During exercise, the rate of LV relaxation becomes faster and the PR interval shortens. These changes partially offset the reduction in diastolic filling time at faster heart rates and help maintain the separation between early and late diastolic filling. Despite increases in cardiac output of three to four times that present at rest, LA pressure does not appreciably rise in the normal heart.

■ In normal subjects the LV filling pattern changes with age, with the proportion of filling in early diastole decreasing and that at atrial contraction increasing.

■ In normals with sinus tachycardia or exercise, LV relaxation becomes faster and the PR interval shortens to help maintain the normal separation between early and late diastolic filling, and normal filling pressures.

LV FILLING PATTERNS IN DISEASE STATES

Three basic abnormalities of LV filling patterns are recognized and are associated with changes in LV diastolic properties, filling pressures and prognosis. The most common and least abnormal pattern is reduced filling in early diastole, due to impaired LV relaxation in the presence of normal LA pressure. Patients who have this "impaired LV relaxation" filling pattern generally have minimal symptoms at rest, but may show a functional limitation with exercise. In many instances this is due to premature "fusion" of early and late diastolic filling at faster heart rates that result in a reduced end-diastolic volume and elevation in LA pressure.

A second abnormal LV filling pattern has been termed "pseudonormal," to indicate that although the LV filling pattern appears normal, moderate diastolic abnormalities are present. This seemingly paradoxical situation occurs when the effect of impaired LV relaxation on early diastolic filling is offset by a moderate decrease in LV compliance and increase in LA pressure. In contrast to a truly normal LV filling pattern, blood is partially forced, rather than sucked, into the left ventricle in early diastole due to the elevated LA pressure. Patients with pseudonormal LV filling have a moderate functional limitation that is between those with impaired LV relaxation and restrictive type physiology. New onset A-fib is common in this group.

A third, and the most abnormal LV filling pattern is termed "restrictive." Patients with this filling pattern also have impaired LV relaxation. However, a severe decrease in LV compliance results in a markedly elevated LA pressure and rapid ventricular filling in early diastole. The stiff ventricle causes pressure to increase rapidly with an abrupt, premature termination. Only minimal filling occurs at atrial contraction. A reduced atrial contribution indicates LA systolic failure is present due to pressure overload. Patients with this pattern are severely symptomatic, demonstrate marked functional impairment and have a guarded prognosis.

■ Three abnormal LV filling patterns are recognized. In order of increasing severity they are: "impaired" relaxation, "pseudonormal" filling and "restrictive" filling.

Gradations in LV filling patterns between the three described above are common. Unusual patterns can also been seen in the presence of a prolonged PR interval, or intraventricular conduction defects. However, the abnormal LV filling patterns remain specific to the alterations in LV relaxation and compliance rather than the type of cardiac disease, with all three patterns (depending on disease stage) being seen in disorders as diverse as restrictive and dilated cardiomyopathies. The progression of abnormalities in LV filling patterns with disease states (from impaired relaxation to pseudonormal to restrictive), together with changes in LV relaxation and compliance, has been documented in experimental models of HF and clinically observed in patients with restrictive cardiomyopathies. When added to the normal changes observed with aging a "natural history" of LV filling patterns in health and disease can be constructed (Fig. 8).

NONINVASIVE EVALUATION OF LV DIASTOLIC FUNCTION

Because of the impracticality of invasively measuring diastolic properties in most patients, noninvasive methods for indirectly evaluating LV diastolic function have been developed. These methods have focused on evaluating the LV filling pattern. The techniques have included digitized M-mode echocardiograms, radionuclide ventriculograms, pulsed wave (PW) Doppler mitral flow velocities and more recently Doppler tissue imaging (DTI) and cardiac cine-CT or MRI.

Because of ease of performance, lack of ionizing radiation, and associated information about cardiac anatomy, systolic function, valvular disease, and filling pressures, echo-Doppler technique is currently the method used to assess LV filling and indirectly diastolic function. The basic analysis includes PW Doppler recording of mitral, pulmonary venous and when appropriate right heart inflow velocities. Nomograms for normal, age related mitral and pulmonary venous flow velocities and related variables are established. The relation of mitral and pulmonary venous A-wave duration is currently the best way to identify the earliest stages of LV diastolic dysfunction, when mean LA pressure is normal but A-wave pressure rise and LV end-diastolic pressure is elevated. With disease progression a decrease in LV and LA compliance increases the mean LA pressure, so the proportion of LA filling that occurs during the LA reservoir phase (ventricular systole) decreases. A systolic fraction of forward flow of <40% indicates increased mean LA pressure, and that a pseudonormal LV filling pattern is likely present. The sensitivity of this finding is low because of compensatory LA hypertrophy, so other ancillary data to help identify pseudonormal LV filling have been developed. These include increased maximal LA volume, LV filling changes in response to preload reduction (the Valsalva maneuver), and the mitral anular motion as assessed by Doppler DTI .

In the absence of mitral valve disease or atrial arrhythmias, LA pressure and volume increase as LV compliance decreases. The technique for LA maximum volume measurement has been standardized and normal values published. When indexed for body surface area these do not change with age. Increased maximal LA volume is an independent risk factor for new onset DHF and A-fib, so that it is now done as part of a diastolic function assessment. The diastolic mitral anular velocity pattern in normals obtained with TDI is similar to mitral flow velocity, with longitudinal movement in early diastole toward the pulmonary veins (the E' wave) being larger than that at atrial contraction (the A' wave). LV hypertrophy reduces longitudinal mitral annular displacement so the E'/A' ratio becomes <1. If this is

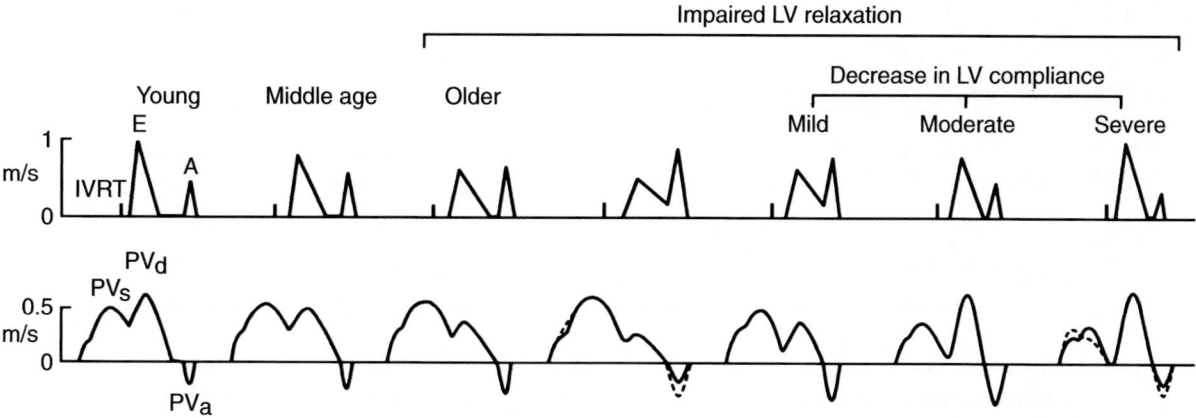

Fig. 8. Natural history of left ventricular (LV) filling patterns as reflected in PW Doppler mitral (top) and pulmonary venous (bottom) flow velocity patterns. The first three patterns are normal. The fourth, sixth, and seventh represent impaired LV relaxation, pseudonormal and restrictive filling respectively. A, mitral flow velocity at atrial contraction; E, mitral flow velocity in early diastole; IVRT, LV isovolumic relaxation time; PV$_a$, reverse pulmonary venous flow at atrial contraction; PV$_d$, pulmonary venous flow velocity in diastole; PV$_s$, pulmonary venous flow velocity in systole.

seen when the mitral E/A wave velocity ratio appears normal, a pseudonormal mitral flow velocity pattern is present. Performing a Valsalva maneuver decreases preload, and if the mitral flow velocity pattern reverts to one that shows impaired LV relaxation (E/A ratio <1), mean LA pressure was elevated at baseline. Studies show that mitral flow velocity, TVI of the mitral anulus and LA volume measurements are easier to perform and more reproducible than pulmonary venous flow recordings or the Valsalva maneuver, so these are done most frequently. Since all the variables discussed above have situations which decrease their positive predictive value they are used in aggregate when assessing LV diastolic abnormalities. A composite diagram of the different Doppler variables for normal and the three abnormal filling patterns is shown in Figure 9.

■ A 2-D echocardiogram and PW Doppler mitral and pulmonary venous flow velocity recordings remain the basic variables for assessing LV diastolic function
■ Ancillary data such as maximal LA volume, response

of LV filling pattern to the Valsalva maneuver and mitral anulus motion as assessed by Doppler TDI also help assess LV filling patterns and grade diastolic abnormalities and normal and abnormal LA pressures.
■ Mitral flow velocity, maximal LA volume and mitral anular motion by TDI are the most easily performed and reproducible echo-Doppler measurements in most labs.

ESTIMATING LV DIASTOLIC FILLING PRESSURES

The three abnormal LV filling patterns demonstrate different combinations of diastolic abnormalities and have a general qualitative relation to LV filling pressures, with impaired relaxation the most normal and restrictive the most elevated. Individual echo-Doppler variables, such as mitral deceleration time, systolic fraction of pulmonary venous flow, LA minimum volume and peak pulmonary venous A-wave flow velocity reversal in the pulmonary veins can sometimes be related to LV

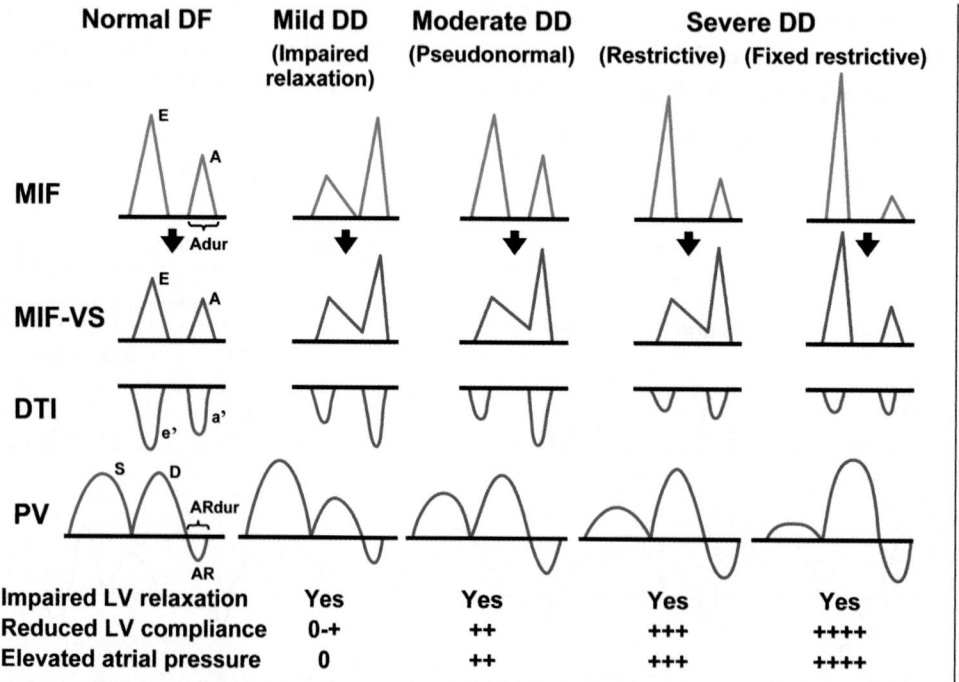

Fig. 9. Summary of LV filling patterns relating PW Doppler mitral (MIF) and pulmonary venous (PV) flow velocity patterns to response to Valsalva maneuver (MIF-VS) and mitral anular Doppler tissue imaging findings (DTI). The difference in mitral flow velocity response to VS and differences in DTI help distinguish normal from "pseudonormal" filling and moderate diastolic HF.

filling pressures. However, age, valvular regurgitation, LV ejection fraction, and heart rate, influence these variables so they cannot be used in all individuals. An exception is the relation of mitral to pulmonary venous A-wave duration. Regardless of age, when retrograde pulmonary venous flow at atrial contraction exceeds that of forward mitral flow by 35 ms LV A-wave pressure and LV end-diastolic pressure are increased. TDI of mitral anular velocity has allowed for a rapid screening of mean LV diastolic pressure (Fig. 10). When the ration of peak mitral E wave velocity to TDI E' velocity (E/E') is <8 mean filling pressures are normal. When this ratio is >15 they are increased. Ratios of 8-15 are indeterminate and in these cases LA size, pulmonary venous recordings and the Valsalva manuever are used in an attempt to estimate filling pressures. Differences in published results between studies and a preponderance of older patients with CAD in reported data suggest that further study is necessary to determine the applicability of these methods to all types of cardiac disease.

The prognostic value of mitral flow velocity patterns for predicting survival has been demonstrated in patients with dilated (Fig. 11) and restrictive cardiomyopathies. In some studies the deceleration time of early mitral flow velocity was the strongest predictor of reduced survival, and was independent of LV systolic function. The response of LV filling patterns to altered loading conditions has also been shown to relate to future cardiac events. In other studies of dilated cardiomyopathy LV systolic function was a more powerful predictor. Prospective studies to compare the prognostic significance of LV systolic and diastolic indices in heart failure patients are now underway.

- The prognostic value of LV filling and mitral flow velocity patterns for predicting survival has been demonstrated in patients with dilated and restrictive cardiomyopathies.
- An impaired LV relaxation pattern has the best prognosis, while a restrictive LV filling pattern indicates a poor prognosis regardless of disease type or LV ejection fraction.
- If reducing preload by a Valsalva maneuver changes a pseudonormal or restrictive pattern to one that is less abnormal the prognosis is better than if their filling pattern remains unchanged.

THERAPY FOR LV DIASTOLIC DYSFUNCTION

Optimal therapy for LV diastolic dysfunction is unknown because few studies on therapy for symptomatic patients have been published. Randomized trials are currently underway. Awaiting further data it seems reasonable that once identified, the immediate goals of therapy are to favorably improve cardiac loading conditions, heart rate or atrioventricular coupling intervals while simultaneously treating the underlying cause of

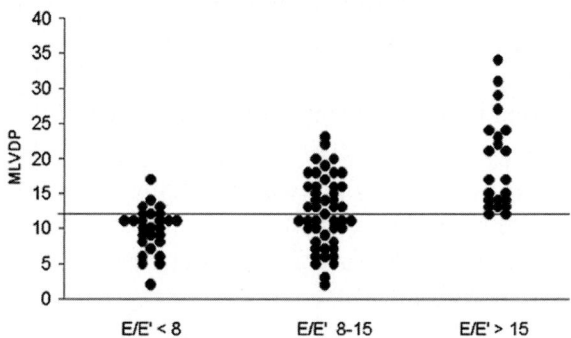

Fig. 10. Mean LV diastolic pressure (MLVDP) versus patient groups defined by the ratio of peak mitral E' wave flow velocity and mitral anular septal E' velocity (E/E').

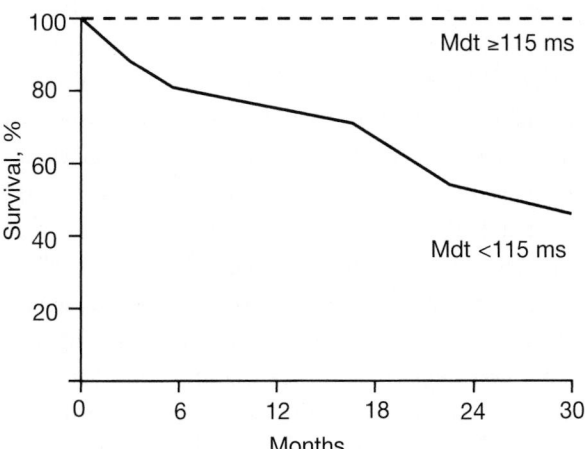

Fig. 11. Actuarial survival curves of patients with dilated cardiomyopathy and SHF by PW Doppler mitral deceleration time (Mdt). An Mdt <115 ms indicates severe diastolic dysfunction (restrictive physiology) and a markedly reduced survival.

the diastolic dysfunction.

■ The immediate goals of therapy for DHF are to normalize cardiac loading conditions, and optimize the resting heart rate to provide a normal separation of early and late diastolic LV filling.

Patients with DHF may present acutely with pulmonary edema due to severe hypertension. In these cases therapy with intravenous diuretics and lowering blood is beneficial. Interestingly, during the acute episode the LV ejection fraction remains normal showing that diastolic abnormalities are truly the cause of their acute HF symptoms. In patients with dyspnea on exertion and moderate DHF treatment with diuretics and afterload reduction to normalize these is also appropriate. Angiotensin converting enzyme (ACE) inhibitors have been shown to improve exercise tolerance in patients with a hypertensive blood pressure response to exercise. Loop diuretics may be less useful if there is no evidence of increased filling pressures at rest (impaired relaxation LV filling pattern) and should be used carefully in patients with thick-walled, "restrictive" like cardiomyopathies where decreasing preload may result in a fall in cardiac output.

In patients whose predominant abnormality is impaired LV relaxation therapy focuses on reversing the underlying disease process. This is most typically hypertension, diabetes, coronary artery disease, obesity or sleep apnea. Non-dihydropyridine calcium channel or beta-blockers may be beneficial by slowing the heart rate, and allowing the ventricle to relax more completely and fill before atrial contraction. The potential beneficial effects of slowing the heart rate are most easily appreciated by examining a PW Doppler mitral flow velocity pattern. Patients likely to have the most benefit from lowering their heart rates are those with continued filling into the diastasis period, or fusion of early and late LV diastolic filling with normal PR intervals. Patients with first degree AV block may respond less well to these medicines, as the increase in PR interval with Ca^{2+} and β-blockers may actually result in an

unphysiologic (>280 ms) first degree AV block, with more fusion of early and late diastolic filling, diastolic MR and a reduced exercise tolerance. In patients with a pacemaker atrial or dual chamber cardiac pacing can normalize the PR interval and help improve the LV filling profile if the QRS duration does not markedly increase and cause dyssynchronous LV contraction.

Over a longer treatment period, lowering blood pressure in hypertensive patients and regression of LV hypertrophy often improves symptoms. Thiazide diuretics and ACE inhibitors reduce LV hypertrophy and lisinopril and aldosterone antagonists may decrease cardiac fibrosis even without LVH regression. In the future, more specific agents that accelerate collagen degradation, or reduce phosphorylated sarcomeric proteins may be developed.

■ Long-term therapy for diastolic dysfunction involves treating the underlying abnormality that is causing the diastolic abnormality.
■ Although optimal therapy for many patients with diastolic dysfunction is unknown, ACE inhibitors and aldosterone antagonists have been shown to reduce blood pressure, LV hypertrophy and fibrosis.

Of course the best therapy for LV diastolic dysfunction and DHF would be prevention. Approximately 40 million Americans are hypertensive with only 30% adequately treated. Most cases of poorly controlled hypertension involve isolated systolic hypertension and are in the elderly, the exact group with a high incidence of DHF. Treatment in this group reduces the incidence of CHF, myocardial infarction and stroke. More aggressive and effective therapy of risk factors for coronary artery disease, adult onset diabetes mellitus and obesity would also be expected to help prevent the development of LV diastolic dysfunction.

■ The best primary prevention therapy for diastolic CHF would be increased identification and adequate treatment of hypertension, diabetes and coronary artery disease.

HEART FAILURE: DIAGNOSIS AND EVALUATION

Richard J. Rodeheffer, MD

Margaret M. Redfield, MD

HEART FAILURE

Classically, heart failure has been defined as the pathophysiologic state in which an abnormality of cardiac function is responsible for failure of the heart to pump blood at a rate commensurate with the requirements of the metabolizing tissues, or to do so only when filling pressures are excessively increased. Not all patients with ventricular dysfunction have the clinical syndrome of heart failure. In recognition of the continuous and progressive nature of ventricular dysfunction, heart failure is now divided into four stages: stage A patients have risk factors for heart failure (hypertension, coronary heart disease, diabetes, obesity) but normal ventricular function and no heart failure symptoms; stage B patients have structural abnormality but no heart failure symptoms; stage C patients have ventricular dysfunction and symptoms of inadequate cardiac output (exercise intolerance) and/or fluid overload (congestion); stage D patients have advanced symptoms and severe disability. The stages are associated with increasing morbidity and mortality (Fig. 1).

SYSTOLIC AND DIASTOLIC HEART FAILURE

Systolic heart failure refers to the pathophysiologic state in which systolic ventricular contraction is impaired. Diastolic heart failure is a condition in which there is resistance to filling of one or both ventricles, leading to increased ventricular filling pressures and congestive symptoms in the presence of normal or near-normal systolic function.

EPIDEMIOLOGY OF HEART FAILURE

Heart failure has been termed the "new epidemic of cardiovascular disease" for the 21st century. Mortality rates from acute coronary syndromes have decreased with improved coronary disease management (coronary care units, reperfusion therapy, aspirin, β-adrenergic blockers, angiotensin-converting enzyme inhibitors, and revascularization), resulting in an increase in the prevalence of patients surviving with chronic coronary disease and ventricular dysfunction. In combination with the aging of the population, the effect of decreasing acute mortality from myocardial infarction has led to an increase the prevalence of heart failure. This trend is expected to continue. Mortality from hypertension-related cerebrovascular accidents has also declined and thus more patients are surviving with chronic hypertensive heart disease who are at risk for heart failure. Unfortunately, increases in awareness and control of hypertension have plateaued, and hypertensive heart disease continues to play a major role in the development of heart failure.

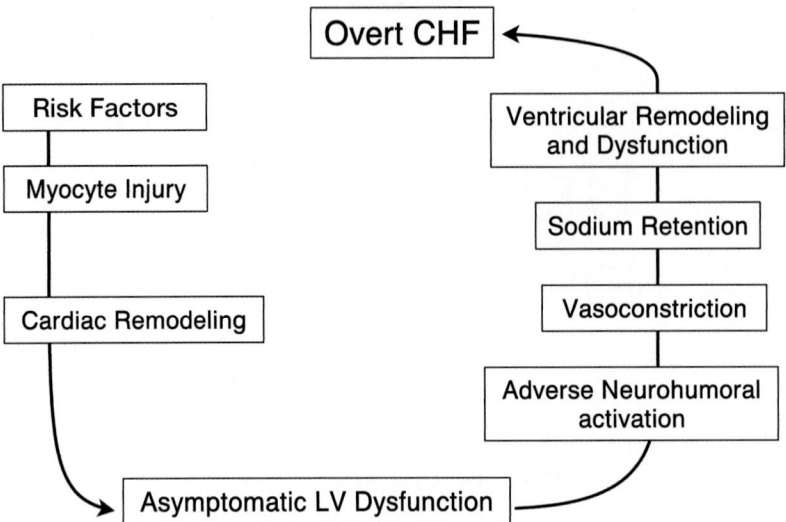

Fig. 1. Progression to heart failure. Myocardial damage leads to ventricular dilatation and hypertrophy (cardiac remodeling), but in the early stages a patient may be well compensated hemodynamically without fluid retention or symptoms or signs of congestive heart failure. Ultimately, adverse neurohumoral activation and progressive ventricular dysfunction lead to excessive vasoconstriction, sodium retention, and clinical congestive heart failure (CHF). LV, left ventricular.

More than 400,000 new cases of heart failure are diagnosed each year in the United States, and 2 to 3 million persons have stage C (symptomatic) heart failure. The population with stage B (asymptomatic ventricular dysfunction) is estimated to be 3-5 million persons. The annual number of deaths approaches 200,000, and heart failure is the leading diagnosis at hospital dismissal for patients older than 65 years.

The incidence and prevalence of heart failure in the general population increase greatly with age. Approximately half of new onset heart failure cases occur after age 80 years, making heart failure a major disease of the very elderly.

Community data in persons over age 45 years show that about one-quarter have stage A (risk factors) heart failure, one-third have stage B (asymptomatic ventricular systolic and/or diastolic dysfunction) heart failure, 2-3% have stage C (overt symptoms and signs) heart failure, and <1% have stage D (end stage) heart failure. From the perspective of objectively measured ventricular function approximately 6% of such a community cohort have mild systolic dysfunction (ejection fraction <50%), 2% have moderate to severe systolic dysfunction (ejection fraction <40%), and 6-7% have moderate to severe diastolic dysfunction. Among those

with stage C symptomatic heart failure about half have predominantly systolic dysfunction and half have predominantly diastolic dysfunction.

■ Heart failure is a progressive disorder that begins with risk factors and evolves from asymptomatic to symptomatic ventricular dysfunction.
■ In the community about half of heart failure patients have predominantly diastolic dysfunction.

Natural History of Heart Failure

Accurate estimation of prognosis in patients with congestive heart failure is difficult because of the multiple causes that produce the syndrome, the large number of factors that influence prognosis, the different modes of death (ischemic events, progressive heart failure, and sudden death), and the variable and evolving treatment strategies. Observed mortality in asymptomatic and symptomatic patients enrolled in representative recent randomized trials is shown in Fig. 2 and 3 and Table 1.

Poor prognostic factors in ventricular dysfunction are listed in Table 2. When ejection fraction and symptom class are similar, most studies have documented a poorer survival in patients with ventricular dysfunction

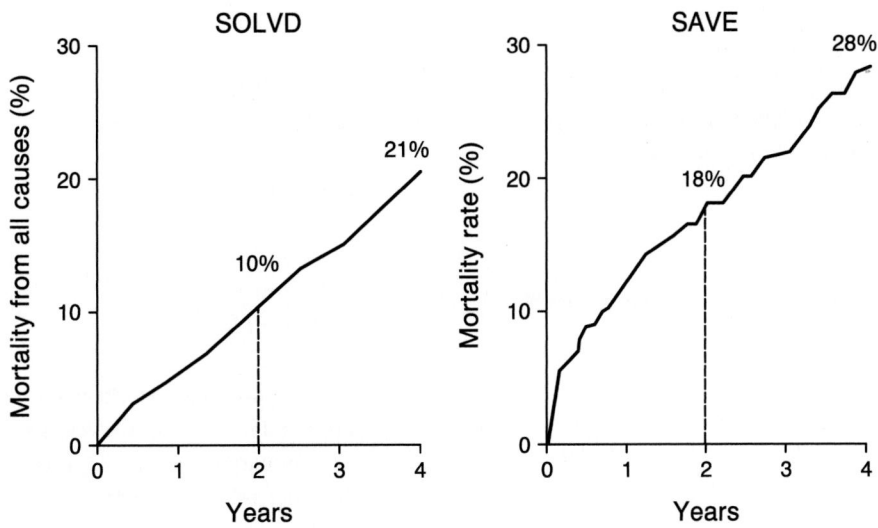

Fig. 2. Mortality among untreated patients with asymptomatic ventricular dysfunction in the SAVE and SOLVD trials.

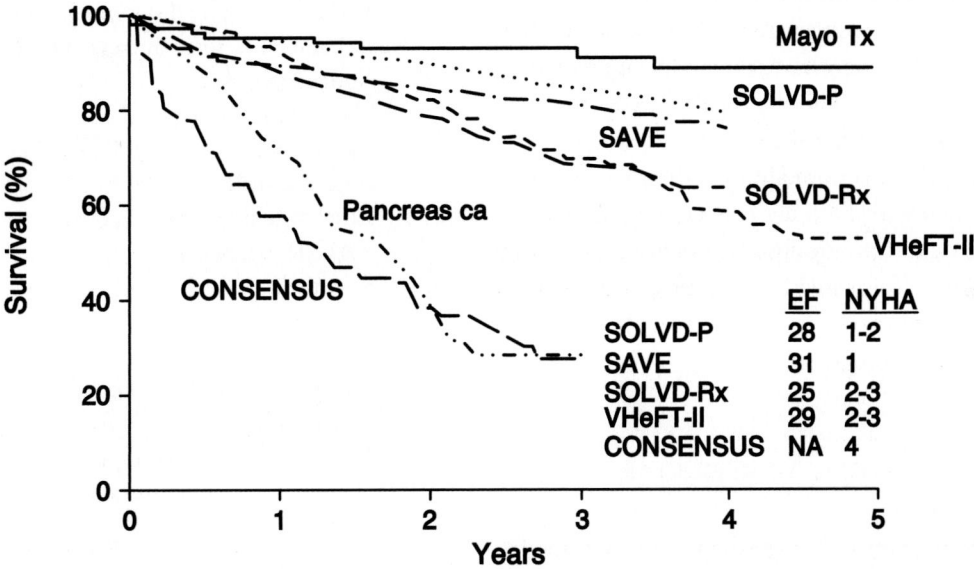

Fig. 3. Observed mortality in patients with systolic dysfunction and heart failure treated with angiotensin-converting enzyme inhibitors in recent clinical heart failure trials. EF, ejection fraction; NYHA, New York Heart Association.

due to coronary artery disease than in "nonischemic" ventricular dysfunction. Most studies have reported that in congestive heart failure, advanced age is a poor prognostic factor. Patients with recent onset of symptoms probably have a better chance of having improvement in systolic function (especially in myocarditis, peripartum cardiomyopathy, or alcoholic cardiomyopathy) and, thus, have a better prognosis. Left ventricular ejection fraction is a powerful independent prognostic factor in

heart failure. Most patients with advanced heart failure have an ejection fraction less than 20%, and further decrements do not add significant prognostic value. Thus, in patients referred for cardiac transplantation, ejection fraction is not helpful in determining short-term prognosis and priority for early transplantation. Furthermore, among patients with an ejection fraction less than 20%, symptoms and prognosis vary widely. Several studies have suggested that symptoms and

Table 1. Approximate 2-Year Mortality of Patients With Left Ventricular Dysfunction Treated With Angiotensin-Converting Enzyme Inhibitors

New York Heart Association class	Mortality, %
I	10
II	20
III	30-40
IV	40-50

prognosis worsen markedly when *right* ventricular function deteriorates and that this may represent a useful prognostic factor in patients with very poor left ventricular function. Hemodynamic values measured after optimization of therapy have some value in predicting prognosis, especially pulmonary capillary wedge pressure and stroke work index. Likewise, several studies have demonstrated that abnormalities in diastolic function as determined with Doppler echocardiography have prognostic value. Specifically, a "restrictive" transmitral Doppler pattern (increased E/A, decreased deceleration time of E, short isovolumic relaxation time) was associated with a worse prognosis.

CAUSES OF SYSTOLIC VENTRICULAR DYSFUNCTION

Systolic dysfunction and congestive heart failure are the common end points of a wide range of cardiovascular disease processes (Tables 3 and 4). In the Framingham Heart Study, hypertension was the most common precursor of the development of heart failure. Of patients with a clinical diagnosis of heart failure, 75% had hypertension. Hypertension was the sole cause of heart failure in 25% of these patients. Hypertension or coronary artery disease (or both) remain the major risk factors for heart failure in the United States.

Global ventricular dilatation and systolic dysfunction are often referred to as cardiomyopathy even when the underlying cause is known (eg, ischemic cardiomyopathy, alcoholic cardiomyopathy, hypertensive cardiomyopathy).

Table 2. Poor Prognostic Factors in Ventricular Dysfunction

Ischemic cause*
Advanced age
Duration of symptoms
Ejection fraction
    Left ventricular <25%*
    Right ventricular <35%
Hemodynamics
    Low cardiac index, stroke work index
    High pulmonary capillary wedge pressure, pulmonary artery systolic pressure
    "Restrictive" filling pattern on Doppler echocardiography
Functional
    NYHA functional class III or IV*
    Decreased exercise duration
    Peak oxygen consumption <14 mL/kg per min*
    6-Minute walking distance <350 m
Neurohumoral factors—increased levels of:
    Norepinephrine
    Plasma renin activity
    Aldosterone
    Angiotensin II
    Atrial or brain natriuretic factor
    Arginine vasopressin
    Endothelin
    Tumor necrosis factor
Arrhythmias
    Sudden death and symptomatic ventricular tachycardia*
    Asymptomatic premature ventricular contraction and nonsustained ventricular tachycardia

NYHA, New York Heart Association.
*Most useful clinically.

A list of disease processes that produce cardiac dilatation and systolic dysfunction is provided in Table 4. Two well-conducted studies have demonstrated that idiopathic dilated cardiomyopathy is familial in at least 20% to 25% of cases. The diagnosis of idiopathic dilated cardiomyopathy is increasing, and this may reflect a true increase in the incidence of this disease or an increased awareness of the entity and the increasing use

Table 3.   Causes of Ventricular Dysfunction in Recent Studies of Congestive Heart Failure

Study	History of hypertension, %	Ischemic, %	Nonischemic, %
CONSENSUS*	19	74	26
VHEFT†	40	44	56
VHEFT II	50	54	46
SOLVD treament	42	72	28
SOLVD prevention	37	83	17

*Cooperative North Scandinavian Enalpril Survival Study.
†Veterans Administration Cooperative Vasodilator-Heart Failure Trial.

of noninvasive assessment of systolic function, such as echocardiography.

Acute inflammatory myocarditis may be associated with viral infection or systemic inflammatory conditions, and occasionally can evolve into dilated cardiomyopathy. Cardiac manifestations of human immunodeficiency virus (HIV) infection have been described, including pericarditis, lymphocytic myocarditis, and dilated cardiomyopathy.

It now is well recognized that in patients with excessive tachycardia (eg, atrial fibrillation with poorly controlled ventricular rates) can result in a reversible dilated cardiomyopathy. Since these patients are often unaware of their tachycardia and may have reasonable resting heart rates, exercise testing or Holter monitoring is needed to detect the poor rate control. Patients who do not respond to, or are intolerant of, negative chronotropic medications may require atrioventricular node ablation and pacemaker implantation or ablation of an accessory pathway.

Cocaine use is associated with a myocarditis with persistent ventricular dysfunction as well as microvascular disease, coronary artery spasm, and myocardial infarction.

Reversible left ventricular dysfunction associated with severe sleep apnea has been described recently.

- Hypertension and coronary disease are the most important heart failure risk factors in the U.S.
- Idiopathic dilated cardiomyopathy is familial in 20% to 25% of cases.

Table 4.   Causes of Dilated Cardiomyopathy*

Idiopathic

Familial

Infectious agents: bacterial, viral (including human immunodeficiency virus), fungal, *Borrelia burgdorferi* (Lyme disease)

Acute rheumatic fever

Infiltrative disorders: amyloid, hemochromatosis, sarcoid

Toxic: heroin, cocaine, alcohol, amphetamines, doxorubicin (Adriamycin), cyclophosphamide, sulfonamides, lead, arsenic, cobalt, phosphorus, ethylene glycol, some antiviral agents

Nutritional deficiencies: protein, thiamine, selenium

Electrolyte disorders: hypocalcemia, hypophosphatemia, hyponatremia, hypokalemia

Collagen vascular disorders: lupus, rheumatoid arthritis, systemic sclerosis, polyarteritis nodosa, hypersensitivity vasculitis, Takayasu's syndrome, polymyositis, Reiter's syndrome

Endocrine and metabolic diseases: diabetes mellitus, thyroid disease, hypoparathyroidism with hypocalcemia, pheochromocytoma, acromegaly

Tachycardia-induced cardiomyopathy

Miscellaneous: peripartum cardiomyopathy, sleep apnea syndrome, Whipple's disease, L-carnitine deficiency

■ In patients with atrial fibrillation, poorly controlled ventricular rates can result in a reversible dilated cardiomyopathy.

Causes of Diastolic Ventricular Dysfunction

Diastolic dysfunction is discussed in more detail in Chapter 91. The principal conditions associated with diastolic heart failure are hypertension and coronary artery disease. Infiltrative cardiomyopathies account for a very small number of diastolic dysfunction patients.

CLINICAL PRESENTATION OF HEART FAILURE

The symptoms of heart failure are listed in Table 5. Symptoms are similar for systolic and diastolic ventricular dysfunction. Dyspnea on exertion and fatigue are early but very nonspecific symptoms of heart failure. Pulmonary disease, obesity, deconditioning, and advanced age can also produce these symptoms. Edema is also nonspecific. Paroxysmal nocturnal dyspnea and true orthopnea are more specific for heart failure but are relatively insensitive indicators. The physical findings in heart failure, listed in Table 6, also lack sensitivity and specificity for heart failure. Patients with advanced ventricular symptoms may have few of the typical symptoms and signs of heart failure.

Diagnostic criteria for heart failure were established before the widespread use of noninvasive assessments of systolic and diastolic function. The Framingham clinical criteria are listed in Table 7; while they have been important for identifying heart failure in epidemiologic studies, these criteria are more specific than sensitive, and probably miss mild cases of heart failure.

When heart failure is suspected, the physician should provide an estimation of the functional class of the patient based on an assessment of the patient's daily activity and the limitations imposed by the patient's symptoms of heart failure. Although imperfect, the New York Heart Association classification has long been used to categorize patients with heart failure, and this classification provides important prognostic information (Table 8).

EVALUATION OF HEART FAILURE

The goals of the evaluation in patients with chronic heart failure are 1) to determine the type of cardiac

Table 5.   Symptoms of Congestive Heart Failure

None
    Truly asymptomatic
    Asymptomatic because of sedentary lifestyle
Dyspnea on exertion
Decreased exercise tolerance
Orthopnea
Paroxysmal nocturnal dyspnea
Fatigue
Edema
Abdominal pain and distention
Palpitations
Syncope or presyncope
Embolic events (central nervous system, peripheral)

Table 6.   Physical Findings in Congestive Heart Failure

Carotid	Normal or ↓ volume
Jugular venous pressure	Normal or ↑
Hepatojugular refllux	+ or -
Parasternal lift	+ or -
Apical impulse	Normal or diffuse in character, normal in position or laterally displaced
S_3, S_4	+ or -
MR or TR murmur	+ or -
Rales	+ or -
Pulsus alternans	+ or -
Edema	+ or -
Ascites	+ or -
Hepatomegaly	+ or -
Muscle wasting	+ or -
Blood pressure	Normal, ↑, orthostatic, or ↓

+ or -, Present or absent; MR, mitral regurgitation; TR, tricuspid regurgitation.

Table 7.   Framingham Criteria for the Diagnosis of Congestive Heart Failure

Major criteria
   Paroxysmal nocturnal dyspnea or orthopnea
   Neck vein distention
   Rales
   Cardomegaly
   Acute pulmonary edema
   S_3 gallop
   Increased jugular venous pressure >16 cm H_2O
   Circulation time >25 s
   Hepatojugulr reflux
Minor criteria
   Ankle edema
   Night cough
   Dyspnea on exertion
   Hepatomegaly
   Pleural effusion
   Vital capacity decresed 1/3 from maximum
   Tachycardia (heart rate >120 beats/min)
Major or minor criterion
   Weight loss >4.5 kg in 5 days in response to treatment

Definite congestive heart failure = 2 major criteria or 1 major and 2 minor criteria

Table 8.   New York Heart Association Functional Classificaton for Congestive Heart Failure

Class I — Patients with cardiac disease but without resulting limitations of physical activity. Ordinary physical activity does not use undue fatigue, palpitation, dyspnea, or anginal pain

Class II — Patients with cardiac disease resulting in slight limitation of physical activity. They are comfortable at rest. Ordinary physical activity results in fatigue, palpitation, dyspnea, or anginal pain

Class III — Patients with cardiac disease resulting in marked limitation of physical activity. They are comfortable at rest. Less than ordinary physical activity causes fatigue, palpitation, dyspnea, or anginal pain

Class IV — Patients with cardiac disease resulting in inability to carry on any physical activity without discomfort. Symptoms of cardiac insufficiency or of anginal syndrome may be present even at rest. If any physical activity is undertaken, discomfort is increased

dysfunction (systolic vs. diastolic, right ventricular vs. left ventricular failure, valvular vs. myocardial), 2) to uncover correctable etiologic factors, 3) to determine prognosis, and 4) to guide therapy.

In addition to the history and physical examination, the routine laboratory evaluation for suspected heart failure or ventricular dysfunction and the pertinent findings are listed in Table 9.

Coronary Angiography

Because many patients with systolic dysfunction have coronary artery disease, it is important to assess the presence and extent of coronary disease. Revascularization should be considered to prevent further ischemic injury and to restore function to "hibernating" myocardium, but the role of CABG in patients without angina is unclear. All major trials of coronary artery bypass grafting (CABG) versus medical therapy excluded patients with congestive heart failure or ejection fraction less than 35%. Several small uncontrolled cohort studies in patients with systolic dysfunction have demonstrated significant benefit of CABG over medical therapy. In patients with severe systolic dysfunction who are candidates for revascularization, some assessment of viability with thallium imaging, PET scanning, or dobutamine echocardiography to document the extent of salvageable myocardium is reasonable.

■ Evaluation of ventricular dysfunction includes assessment for coronary artery disease.

Endomyocardial Biopsy

Endomyocardial biopsy for the detection of lymphocytic myocarditis is no longer routinely recommended; there is significant sampling error leading to a high false negative rate, and immunosuppression was not found to

Table 9.   Routine Laboratory Evaluation for Suspected Heart Failure or Systolic Dysfunction*

Class I—usually indicated, always acceptable
Chest radiography
Electrocardiogram
    Rhythm, Q waves, ST-T changes, left ventricuar hypertrophy
Complete blood cell count
Urinalysis
Sodium, phosphorus, magnesium, calcium, BUN, creatinine, glucose
Serum albumin
T_4 and TSH or sensitive TSH
Transthoracic echocardiography
Cardiac catheterization/coronary angiography—in patients:
    With angina
    With significant area of ischemia on noninvasive stress test
    At risk for coronary artery disease who are to undergo a corrective noncoronary cardiac surgical procedure
    With diastolic heart failure and angina or risk factors for coronary artery disease
Noninvasive stress testing—to detect ischemia in patients who are candidates for revascularization:
    Without angina but with a high probability of coronary artery disease
    Without angina but with previous myocardial infarction to detect viability and residual ischemia (thallium
        or dobutamine echocardiography probably is preferable to sestamibi to provide optimal information on
        viability)
Screening for other rare causes
    Only as suggested by history and physical examination findings
Exercise testing with respiratory gas analysis
    As needed for prognosis/timing of transplantation in transplantation candidates
Class II—acceptable but of uncertain efficacy and may be controversial
Serum iron and ferritin
    For patients without features to suggest hemochromatosis
Sensitive TSH
    In nonelderly patients in normal sinus rhythm with unexplained congestive heart failure
Noninvasive stress testing
    To detect ischemia in all patients with unexplained congestive heart failure who are candidates for
        revascularization
Coronary angiography
    In all patients with unexplained congestive heart failure who are candidates for revascularization
Endomyocardial biopsy—in patients:
    With recent onset of rapidly deteriorating cardiac function
    Receiving chemotherapy with doxorubicin
    With systemic disease and possible cardiac involvement (hemochromatosis, sarcoidosis, amyloidosis,
        Löffler's endocarditis, endomyocardial fibroelastosis); some argue that currently there is little to support
        its use to detect lymphocytic myocarditis because there is no proven benefit to standard immunosup-
        pressive therapy and it has no prognostic value; exception for transplantation candidates
Exercise testing
    To determine functional limitation in patients for whom history is unclear
    To address specific clinical questions (rate control in patients with atrial fibrillation, chronotropic
        competence, exercise-induced arrhythmias, blood pressure control in those with congestive heart failure
        and hypertension, response to therapy)

Table 9 (continued)

Class III—generally not indicated
  Endomyocardial biopsy
    Routine evaluation of patients with unexplained congestive heart failure
  Screening for asymptomatic arrhythmias
    Patients who have symptoms suggestive of sustained arrhythmia or syncope should undergo electro-
      physiologic evaluation
  Multiple echocardiographic or radionuclide studies
    For patients responding to therapy unless normalization of systolic function is suspected
  Coronary angiography
    In patients who are not candidates for revascularization, valve surgery, or heart transplantation

BUN, blood urea nitrogen; T_4, thyroxine; TSH, thyroid-stimulating hormone.
*Based on guidelines of the American College of Cardiology and the American Heart Association.

have an impact on survival in a multicenter trial. Endomyocardial biopsy is recommended if a systemic disease (amyloidosis or hemochromatosis) is suggested by the clinical presentation. If giant cell myocarditis is suspected (acute onset, young patient, ventricular arrhythmias), a biopsy should be considered because of the poor prognosis and the potential for improvement with immunosuppression.

Exercise Testing in Heart Failure
Increasingly, more objective quantification of functional capacity is obtained with exercise testing with respiratory gas analysis for calculating oxygen consumption. The maximal oxygen consumption indexed to body surface area $\dot{V}O_2$max has prognostic value even in patients with severe systolic dysfunction and heart disease who are being considered for transplantation. According to a study in patients with severe systolic dysfunction and advanced symptoms of congestive heart failure who were referred for cardiac transplantation, $\dot{V}O_2$max less than 14 mL/kg per m^2 was predictive of a poorer 1-year survival with medical therapy than with cardiac transplantation, and $\dot{V}O_2$max more than 14 mL/kg per m^2 was predictive of a 1-year survival at least equivalent to that afforded by transplantation. Thus, patients with preserved exercise tolerance can be followed closely on medical therapy until exercise capacity deteriorates. The prognostic value of $\dot{V}O_2$max must be interpreted in view of the age, sex, and conditioning status of the person

and should not be viewed as an inflexible guideline. A functional classification scheme based on respiratory gas exchange and $\dot{V}O_2$max is presented in Table 10. Because $\dot{V}O_2$max reflects the cardiac output during peak exercise, the corresponding levels of cardiac index are also presented.

- $\dot{V}O_2$max less than 14 mL/kg per m^2 is suggestive of a poorer 1-year survival.

ACUTE DECOMPENSATION OF CHRONIC HEART FAILURE
The initial evaluation of patients with acute decompensation of chronic heart failure includes clinical and hemodynamic stabilization. Always look for potential precipitating factors that may cause deterioration in a previously stable heart failure patient (Table 11).

ACUTE HEART FAILURE
Acute heart failure may present as pulmonary edema ("backward failure") or cardiogenic shock ("forward failure"). Common causes of acute heart failure include the following:
1. Coronary artery disease with ischemia or infarct
2. Mechanical complications of myocardial infarction (ventricular septal defect, acute mitral regurgitation, left ventricular rupture)

3. Arrhythmia (high-grade atrioventricular block or tachyarrhythmia)

4. Tamponade

5. Pulmonary embolus

6. Myocarditis

7. Valvular lesion (acute mitral regurgitation due to papillary muscle dysfunction, chordal rupture or endocarditis; acute aortic regurgitation due to dissection or endocarditis; prosthetic valve dysfunction due to endocarditis, thrombosis or dehiscence)

8. Hypertensive or ischemic heart disease, with an acute increase in hypertension or plasma volume

9. Acute renal failure or insufficiency leading to increased plasma volume, in association with underlying cardiac disease

Initial Evaluation of Acute Pulmonary Edema

The initial evaluation of a patient presenting with pulmonary edema or cardiogenic shock includes the following:

1. A directed history and physical examination

2. 12-Lead electrocardiography (ECG) and continuous ECG monitoring

3. Complete blood cell count, electrolytes, urea, creatinine, cardiac enzymes, and arterial blood gases

4. Chest radiography

5. Transthoracic echocardiography

6. Consider cardiac catheterization, transesophageal echocardiography, or pulmonary artery balloon catheterization

If there is no specific cause that requires emergency intervention such as percutaneous transluminal coronary angioplasty or cardiac surgery, stabilize the patient with oxygen, diuretic agents, afterload reduction, inotropic agents, and morphine sulfate. Perform further evaluation and treatment as needed.

Initial Evaluation of Cardiogenic Shock

Cardiogenic shock is associated with a high mortality rate if untreated (approximately 85%). Remember that 10% to 15% of patients presenting with cardiogenic shock have inadequate left ventricular filling pressures and need fluid. Consider right ventricular infarction, usually in the setting of an inferior infarct. The initial evaluation also should include determination of prothrombin time, activated partial thromboplastin time, serum glucose level, liver transaminases, and lactate concentration. Focus on the following key steps:

1. Assess volume status—consider fluid challenge unless the signs of left-sided fluid overload are clear-cut (pulmonary artery catheter may be of value in uncertain cases)

2. Assess left ventricular systolic function (transthoracic echocardiography)

Table 10. Functional Classification for Congestive Heart Failure Based on $\dot{V}O_2max$

Class	Severity	$\dot{V}O_2max$, mL/kg per m²	Maximal cardiac index, L/min per m²
A	None	>20	>8
B	Mild	16-20	6-8
C	Moderate	10-15	4-6
D	Severe	6-9	2-4
E	Very severe	<6	<2

$\dot{V}O_2max$, maximal oxygen consumption.

Table 11. Precipitating Factors for Acute Decompensation of Chronic Congestive Heart Failure

Noncompliance with diet or therapy
Arrhythmia
Systemic infection
Pulmonary embolism
High-output states—anemia, pregnancy, hyperthyroidism
Unrelated illness—renal, pulmonary, hypothyroidism, gastrointestinal
Ischemia
Hypertension
Toxins—alcohol, street drugs
Inappropriate drug therapy—negative inotrope, salt-retaining

3. Rule out infarct or ischemia

4. Rule out correctable mechanical lesion (transthoracic echocardiography and perhaps transesophageal echocardiography)

If infarct or ischemia is suspected, catheterization with percutaneous transluminal coronary angioplasty, if immediately available, is preferable to treatment with thrombolytic agents. Stabilize the patient with volume-expanding or diuretic agents, inotropic agents, and afterload reduction. Consider an intra-aortic balloon pump if the initial measures are inadequate, especially after revascularization. Intra-aortic balloon pump is most appropriate as a bridge to surgery (mitral regurgitation or ventricular septal defect) or transplantation. Exclude aortic regurgitation or dissection before pump placement. Continue evaluation for underlying cause.

■ Acute heart failure requires urgent hemodynamic stabilization and diagnosis of a cause of the sudden deterioration in clinical status.

93

PHARMACOLOGIC THERAPY OF SYSTOLIC VENTRICULAR DYSFUNCTION AND HEART FAILURE

Richard J. Rodeheffer, MD

Margaret M. Redfield, MD

PRINCIPLES OF TREATMENT

Aggressive treatment of the underlying cardiovascular disease, especially coronary artery disease, valvular heart disease, or hypertension, should be pursued in all cases of systolic ventricular dysfunction. Concurrent with the evaluation of the underlying cause of systolic ventricular dysfunction, specific medical therapy should be commenced to reduce both morbidity and mortality. Treatment strategies common to all patients with systolic dysfunction regardless of the underlying myocardial disorder are discussed below according to the severity of symptoms of heart failure (Table 1). Therapies proven to reduce morbidity and mortality (angiotensin-converting enzyme [ACE] inhibitors and beta-blockers) should be used in all patients with reduced systolic function. Therapies that control symptoms (digoxin, diuretics) but have not been proved to reduce mortality should be guided by symptoms. Nonpharmacologic measures appropriate for all patients with systolic dysfunction are also outlined in Table 1. Revised ACC/AHA practice guidelines for the evaluation and management of chronic heart failure in the adult suggest a new approach to the classification of heart failure that emphasizes both the evolution and progression of the disease. Accordingly, four stages of heart failure have been identified: 1) stage A have heart failure risk factors but have no structural heart disease; 2) stage B refers to patients with a structural disorder of the heart, but no history of symptoms; 3) stage C are patients with past or present symptoms of heart failure with associated structural disease of the heart; and 4) stage D are patients with end-stage disease who may require specialized treatment strategies (Table 2).

■ Medical therapy should be initiated early in the course of heart failure to reduce or delay progression of ventricular dysfunction.

ACE INHIBITORS

Angiotensin II is an important regulator of blood pressure and has a large number of biologic actions (Fig. 1). It is produced from the precursor angiotensin I peptide by an angiotensin-converting enzyme, and angiotensin I, in turn, is formed from cleavage of angiotensinogen by renin. This system is referred to as the "renin-angiotensin system" (RAS) or, because angiotensin II stimulates production of aldosterone, as the "renin-angiotensin-aldosterone system" (RAAS). Angiotensin may be produced by several tissues (including the heart and vasculature), and tissue RAS may be upregulated independently from circulating or systemic RAS. Circulating RAS is activated primarily in decompensated heart failure or in patients taking

Table 1. General Approach to Medical Therapy for a Patient With Systolic Dysfunction

In all patients
    Assess and aggressively treat ischemia and cardiac risk factors
    Control hypertension
    Dietary counseling as needed
    Exercise program
    Maintain sinus rhythm if posible
    Monitor electrolytes
    Instruct in daily weights and adjustment of diuretics
    Referral to appropriate center if candidate for transplantation
NYHA class I before therapy (asymptomatic left ventricular dysfunction)
    ACE inhibitor*
    β-blocker
    Consider warfarin
NYHA class II
    ACE inhibitor*
    β-blocker
    Consider warfarin
    Loop diuretic if symptoms persist while taking ACE inhibitor
    Digoxin if symptoms persist
NYHA class III
    Consider hospitalization for initiation of therapy
    ACE inhibitor*
    Loop diuretic
    Digoxin
    β-blocker
    Consider warfarin
NYHA class IV
    Hospitalization
        Hemodynamic monitoring, intravenous inotropic support, and intravenous vasodilators to stabilize
        condition may be necessary, with gradual weaning and up-titration of oral regimen
    ACE inhibitor*
    Loop diuretic
    Digoxin
    β-blocker for euvolemic, stable patients
    Consider warfarin
    Consider additional vasodilator (hydralazine and isosorbide dinitrate or amlodipine)
    Consider combination diuretic therapy for diuretic resistance

ACE, angiotensin-converting enzyme; NYHA, New York Heart Association.
*Titrate to maximal recommended dose as tolerated; use hydralazine and isosorbide dinitrate or angiotensin II receptor block-
er if patient cannot tolerate drug because of cough; use hydralazine and isosorbide dinitrate if patient cannot tolerate drug
because of renal insufficiency.

diuretics. Some studies have suggested that tissue RAS is activated in patients with systolic dysfunction without overt heart failure. On this basis, antagonism of the deleterious actions of angiotensin II should be beneficial in all patients with systolic dysfunction, regardless of the level of symptoms. This hypothesis is supported by the results of several large multicenter trials evaluating the impact of therapy with ACE inhibitors in patients with systolic dysfunction with or without overt heart failure (Table 3). As summarized in Table 3, ACE inhibitor therapy reduces symptoms, retards progression of heart failure (including need for hospitalization), and

Table 2. Stages of HF

Stage	Description	Examples
A	Patients at high risk of developing HF because of the presence of conditions that are strongly associated with the development of HF. Such patients have no identified structural or functional abnormalities of the pericadium, myocardium, or cardiac valves and have never shown signs or symptoms of HF	Systemic hypertension; coronary artery disease; diabetes mellitus; history of cardiotoxic drug therapy or alcohol abuse; personal history of rheumatic fever; family history of cardio-myopathy
B	Patients who have developed structural heart disease that is strongly associated with the development of HF but who have never shown signs or symptoms of HF	Left ventricular hypertrophy or fibrosis; left ventricular dilatation or hypercontractility; asymptomatic valvular heart disease; previous myocardial infarction
C	Patients who have current or prior symptoms of HF associated with underlying structural heart disease	Dyspnea or fatigue due to left ventricular systolic dysfunction; asymptomatic patients who are undergoing treatment for prior symptoms of HF
D	Patients with advanced structural heart disease and marked symptoms of HF at rest despite maximal medical therapy and who require specialized interventions	Patients who are frequently hospitalized for HF or cannot be safely discharged from the hospital; patients in the hospital awaiting heart transplantation; patients at home receiving continuous intravenous support for symptom relief or being supported with a mechanical circulatory assist device; patients in a hospice setting for the management of HF

reduces mortality among patients with systolic dysfunction regardless of functional class. Mortality reduction is most striking in the most symptomatic patients and in those with severe systolic dysfunction, especially post myocardial infarction.

Effects of ACE Inhibitors in Systolic Dysfunction

As combined arterial and venous vasodilators, ACE inhibitors have favorable hemodynamic effects in patients with systolic dysfunction. Reduction in afterload, preload, and wall stress are observed without an increase in heart rate.

ACE inhibitors augment renal blood flow and reduce production of aldosterone and antidiuretic hormone. Thus, they promote excretion of sodium and water.

ACE inhibitors have effects on cellular metabolism independent of their hemodynamic effects. Their potent antihypertrophic effects on ventricular and vascular cells are at least partially independent of blood pressure reduction and contribute to their role in the prevention of ventricular remodeling. ACE inhibitors have been demonstrated to blunt progressive dilatation of the ventricle in patients with systolic dysfunction and are among the most potent agents for reducing ventricular hypertrophy in patients with hypertension.

ACE inhibitors also have been demonstrated to reduce ischemic events in patients with systolic dysfunction due to myocardial ischemia. This has led to studies that have examined an expanded role for the use of ACE inhibitors in patients with acute myocardial

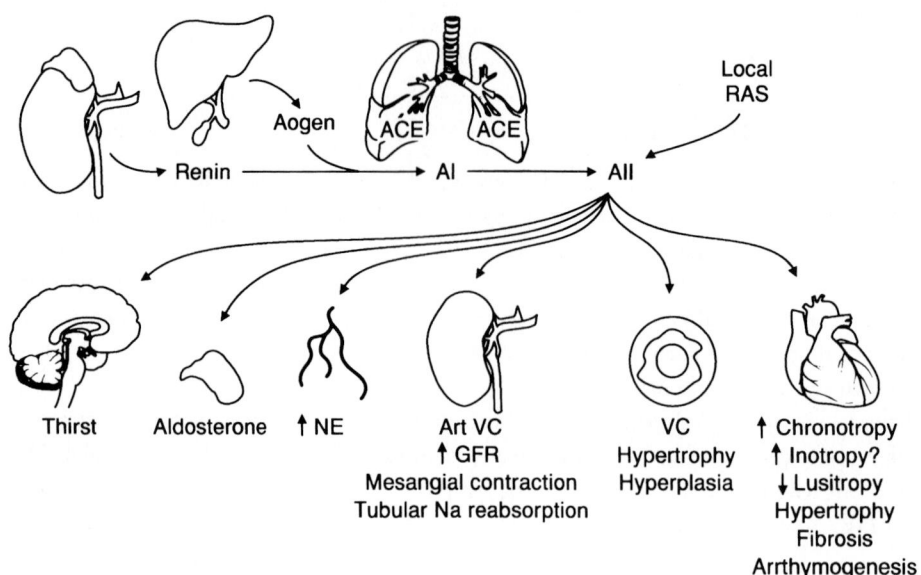

Fig. 1. Circulating and local renin-angiotensin system (RAS). Renin from kidney converts angiotensinogen (Aogen) to angiotensin I (AI), which is converted to angiotensin II (AII) by angiotensin-converting enzyme (ACE) in lungs. AII, either from this pathway or produced independently in tissues, exerts effects on brain, adrenals, sympathetic nervous system, kidney, vasculature, and heart. NE, norepinephrine; GFR, glomerular filtration rate; NA, sodium; VC, arterial vasoconstriction.

infarction without definite systolic dysfunction (Table 2). Completed trials support the use of ACE inhibitors in stable patients with large myocardial infarctions regardless of ejection fraction.

Specific ACE Inhibitors

Specific ACE inhibitors differ in chemical structure, which imparts differences in potency, half-life, bioavailability, route of elimination, and affinity for tissue-bound ACE. The clinical relevance of these differences is unproven. The most widely prescribed ACE inhibitors (captopril, enalapril, lisinopril) are those used in the large clinical trials. ACE inhibitors with a sulfhydryl group (captopril) are more likely to produce rash, neutropenia, and nephrotic syndrome. These side effects are dose-related, and neutropenia is more likely to occur in patients with collagen vascular disease.

Special Considerations With ACE Inhibitors

Correct Dosage of ACE Inhibitors

Use of the optimal dose of ACE inhibitors is an important clinical issue. In clinical practice, ACE inhibitors commonly are prescribed at doses well below those demonstrated to be efficacious in clinical trials. Up-titration to target doses established to be efficacious in clinical trials should be attempted in all patients (Table 4). Careful monitoring of renal function, potassium, and blood pressure is required during the titration phase. Diuretic dosage may need to be decreased in the face of systemic hypotension. Over-diuresis should be avoided before initiation and titration of ACE inhibitor dose. In the Evaluation of Losartan in the Elderly (ELITE) trial, more than 70% of elderly patients in the ACE inhibitor arm tolerated full doses of the drug and only about 10% of all patients developed a significant increase in creatinine levels.

ACE Inhibitors in Renal Dysfunction

Mild renal impairment and a mild increase in the serum level of creatinine during the up-titration of ACE inhibitors are not contraindications to initiation of goal doses of ACE inhibitors, although meticulous monitoring of electrolytes during up-titration is required. ACE inhibitors are contraindicated in the presence of significant renal artery stenosis.

Table 3. Clinical Trials of ACE Inhibitors in Systolic Dysfunction

Study	Patient population	ACE inhibitor	Time of administration after MI	Treatment duration	Outcome
Studies in systolic dysfunction with heart failure					
CONSENSUS	NYHA IV (n=253)	Enalapril vs. placebo		1 day-20 mo	Decreased mortality; decreased CHF
SOLVD-Treatment	NYHA II and III (n=2,569)	Enalapril vs. placebo		22-55 mo	Decreased mortality; decreased CHF
V-HeFT II	NYHA II and III (n=804)	Enalapril vs. hydralazine isosorbide		0.5-5.7 y	Enalapril decreased mortality compared with hydralazine and isosorbide
Studies in asymptomatic systolic dysfunction					
SOLVD-Prevention	Asymptomatic LV dysfunction (n=4,228)	Enalapril vs. placebo		14.6-62 mo	Decreased combined end point of mortality and CHF hospitalizations
SAVE	MI, decreased LV function (n=2,231)	Captopril vs. placebo	3-16 days	24-60 mo	Decreased mortality, progression to CHF and recurrent MI
Studies in systolic dysfunction/acute MI					
AIRE*	MI and CHF (n=2,006)	Ramipril vs. placebo	3-10 days	Minimum of 6 mo	Decreased mortality
TRACE*	MI, decreased LV function (n=1,749)	Trandolapril vs. placebo	3-7 days	24-50 mo	Decreased mortality
Studies in patients with acute MI					
CONSENSUS II	MI (n=6,090)	Enalaprilat/ enalapril vs. placebo	24 h	41-180 days	No change in survival; hypotension with enalaprilat
ISIS-4	MI (n>50,000)	Captopril vs. placebo	24 h	28 days	Decreased mortality
GISSI-3	MI (n=19,394)	Lisinopril vs. control	24 h	6 wk	Decreased mortality
SMILE	MI (n=1,556)	Zofenopril vs. placebo	24 h	6 wk	Decreased mortality

ACE, angiotensin-converting enzyme; CHF, congestive heart failure; LV, left ventricular; MI, myocardial infarction; NYHA, New York Heart Association.
*Study involved patients with MI.

Table 4.   Recommended Dosage of Commonly
           Used Angiotensin-Converting
           Enzyme Inhibitors for Treatment of
           Systolic Dysfunction

Agent	Dose
Captopril	50 mg tid
Enalapril	10 mg bid
Lisinopril	20-40 mg qd

Side Effects of ACE Inhibitors

In addition to renal insufficiency, hyperkalemia, and
hypotension, other class-related side effects of ACE
inhibitors include cough, angioedema, and dysgeusia
(metallic taste). Cough is related to an increase in
bradykinin and occurs in 5% to 10% of white persons
but may be more common among Asians. Because
ACE inhibitors prevent the breakdown of bradykinin,
the potentiation of bradykinin may mediate some of
the beneficial effects of ACE inhibitors as well as some
of the side effects. ACE inhibitors may be teratogenic
and should not be used in the treatment of females of
childbearing age who are not using effective birth control.

■ ACE inhibitors are indicated for all patients with
   systolic ventricular dysfunction regardless of symptoms.

Angiotensin II Receptor Blockers (ARB)

These agents were developed as antagonists of the
RAS that do not cause potentiation of bradykinin. The
findings of the ELITE and ELITE-II trial suggest
that angiotensin II antagonists and ACE inhibitors
have similar beneficial effects on symptoms and survival.
In the Val-HeFT trial, the benefit of the *addition* of the
angiotensin II receptor blocker valsartan to standard
therapy (including ACE-inhibition) for congestive
heart failure was evaluated. Overall, patients did benefit
from this strategy with reduction of the combined end
point of mortality and morbidity. However, the benefit
was observed primarily in patients intolerant of ACE-
inhibition. Furthermore, there appeared to be increased
mortality in patients in whom valsartan was added to

ACE-inhibitors and beta-blockers. In the CHARM
trial, candesartan was evaluated in three separate
substudies: CHARM-added (ARB added to ACE-
inhibitor), CHARM-alternative (ARB instead of ACE-
inhibitor) and CHARM-preserved (ARB in patients
with probable diastolic heart failure). In the overall
composite CHARM program analysis candesartan led
to a 1.6% reduction in overall mortality. The magnitude
of benefit was greatest in patients not already taking an
ACE-inhibitor. In current practice angiotensin II
receptor blockers are recommended primarily for
patients who are intolerant of ACE-inhibitors.

■ Angiotensin II receptor antagonists have benefits
   comparable to ACE-inhibitors and should be used
   in ACE-inhibitor intolerant patients.
■ Angiotensin II receptor antagonists do not have a
   lower incidence of renal insufficiency or hyperkalemia and thus are not an alternative to ACE-
   inhibitors for patients intolerant of ACE-inhibitors
   because of renal effects.
■ Angiotensin II receptor antagonists do not cause
   cough.

Hydralazine and Isosorbide Dinitrate in Heart Failure

The combination of hydralazine and isosorbide dinitrate
was shown in the VHeFT-I trial to reduce mortality
and improve symptoms in patients with heart failure.
In the VHeFT-II trial, ACE inhibitors reduced mortality more than hydralazine and isosorbide dinitrate.
This combination is particularly efficacious in African-
American patients.

Calcium Channel Blockers in Heart Failure

First-generation calcium channel blockers (verapamil,
diltiazem, nifedipine) are contraindicated in the presence
of heart failure because they reduce survival and exacerbate symptoms of heart failure.

   Newer generation dihydropyridines have been
tested for the treatment of heart failure. These agents
have higher vascular-to-myocardial specificity and
fewer negative inotropic effects. The PRAISE trial
tested amlodipine versus placebo (in addition to standard therapy including ACE inhibitors) in patients
with heart failure, and amlodipine had no effect on survival or hospitalization for major cardiovascular events.
There was a suggestion of improved survival for

patients with nonischemic cardiomyopathy. PRAISE II evaluated whether the addition of amlodipine (vs. placebo) to standard therapy improved survival in patients with nonischemic dilated cardiomyopathy; no benefit was observed. The VHeFT-III trial examined felodipine, another dihydropyridine, in patients with heart failure. No beneficial (or detrimental) effect on survival or symptoms was demonstrated.

■ Amlodipine may be an option for treating heart failure in patients who are still hypertensive while receiving maximal doses of standard therapy, as it does not appear to increase mortality.

DIGITALIS GLYCOSIDES IN HEART FAILURE

Although the consensus is that digitalis is of modest value in controlling ventricular rate in atrial fibrillation when this rhythm complicates heart failure, its efficacy in ventricular dysfunction for patients in sinus rhythm has been questioned.

In the RADIANCE trial, patients receiving digoxin treatment who were in sinus rhythm and had an ejection fraction of 35% or less and New York Heart Association class II or III symptoms were randomized to continuation of digoxin or substitution of digoxin by a placebo. All patients continued to take ACE inhibitors and diuretics. Those in whom digoxin treatment was discontinued had a 25% probability of clinical deterioration, in comparison with 5% of those who continued receiving digoxin (Fig. 2). The RADIANCE trial documented the benefit of digoxin in ventricular systolic dysfunction with sinus rhythm.

The Digoxin Study enrolled 6,800 patients with symptomatic congestive heart failure and sinus rhythm, with or without evidence of systolic dysfunction. There were few patients with class IV heart failure in this trial. Digoxin treatment did not alter overall mortality during an average follow-up of 3 years. However, digoxin-treated patients did have reduced risk of hospitalization for worsening heart failure. In a subsequent post-hoc analysis of this same data, women randomized to therapy were found to have increased risk for mortality, associated with increased digoxin level.

The dose of digoxin should be adjusted downward in patients with renal insufficiency and in those taking verapamil, amiodarone, quinidine, or propafenone.

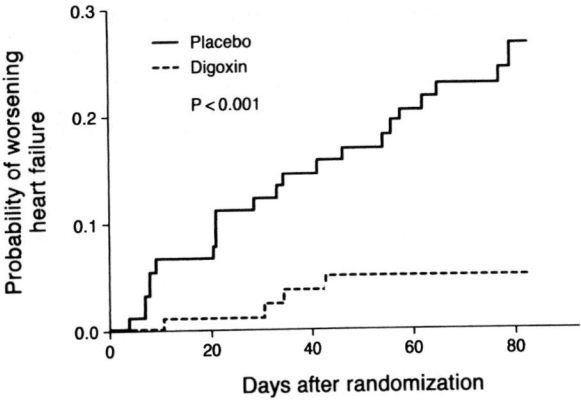

Fig. 2. RADIANCE study. Kaplan-Meier analysis of cumulative probability of worsening heart failure in patients continuing to receive digoxin (*n*=85) and those with treatment switched to placebo (*n*=93). Patients in the placebo group had a higher risk of worsening heart failure throughout the 12-week study (relative risk, 5.9; 95% confidence interval, 2.1 to 17.2; *P*<0.001).

Plasma levels should not exceed 1.0 mg/mL.

■ Digitalis provides symptomatic benefit but no mortality benefit in heart failure.

ALDOSTERONE ANTAGONISTS

The RALES Trial was a randomized trial of aldactone in 1,663 patients with severe heart failure and an ejection fraction less than 35% who were being treated with an ACE inhibitor, a loop diuretic, and, in some cases, digoxin. Spironolactone decreased mortality (46% in the placebo group to 35% in the spironolactone group, P<0.001). This 30% reduction in mortality among patients in the spironolactone group was due to a lower risk of both death from progressive heart failure and sudden death. The frequency of hospitalization for worsening heart failure was 35% lower in the spironolactone group. In addition, patients who received spironolactone had a significant improvement in the symptoms of heart failure, as assessed on the basis of the New York Heart Association functional class (P<0.001). A controlled trial of 6,632 patients with systolic heart failure using eplerenone also showed reduced mortality. Blockade of aldosterone receptors, in addition to standard therapy, further reduces the risk of both morbidity and death among patients with severe heart failure. Addition of aldosterone antagonists can cause serious hyperkalemia and serum K+ levels should be carefully monitored during initiation of treatment.

■ Spironolactone and eplerenone further reduce mortality in patients with advanced heart failure who are on ACE-inhibition and beta blockers.

β-Blockers in Heart Failure

The rationale for use of β-blockers in heart failure stems from the sympathetic nervous system being activated in asymptomatic left ventricular dysfunction, and this activation increases with the severity of heart failure. Experimental data suggest that chronic heightened sympathetic nervous system activation and increased plasma norepinephrine may exacerbate myocyte dysfunction and cell death.

Although acute administration of β-adrenergic blockade decreases contractility and heart rate in systolic heart failure, chronic administration improves contractility. This effect becomes apparent in 3 to 6 months. The increase in ejection fraction is positively related to β-blocker dose.

Controlled trials have demonstrated that beta-blockers prolong survival and improve functional class,

cardiac hemodynamics, left ventricular ejection fraction and quality of life in patients with class II, III and IV CHF (Table 5). These benefits are incremental to ACE-inhibition and have been proved for carvedilol, bisoprolol and metoprolol. Carvedilol demonstrated significant mortality benefit in patients with class II and III CHF. Two other trials, CIBIS II (bisoprolol) and MERIT-HF (metoprolol succinate), demonstrated significant improvement in survival primarily in patients with class II-III CHF with these cardioselective beta-blockers. The COPERNICUS trial demonstrated that carvedilol is safe and lowers mortality in class IV CHF. The COMET trial compared the efficacy of short-acting metoprolol tartrate to carvedilol in CHF patients; carvedilol therapy resulted in lower mortality than metoprolol tartrate therapy.

Once initiated, beta blocker therapy should be continued indefinitely; discontinuation may result in deterioration of cardiac function.

■ Beta-blocker therapy is usually well tolerated and is a foundation in the treatment of systolic heart failure.
■ Beta-blocker therapy may result in improved systolic function.

Oral Inotropic Agents in Heart Failure

Phosphodiesterase inhibitors were developed as

Table 5. Selected Clinical Trials of β-Blockers in Systolic Dysfunction

Agent	Patient population	β-blocker	Follow-up, y	Outcome
U.S. Carvedilol	NYHA class II, III, IV (n=1,094)	Carvedilol vs. placebo	0.7	All cause mortality ↓ 65% (P=0.001)
CIBIS-II	NYHA class II, III, IV (n=641)	Bisoprolol vs. placebo	1.3	All cause mortality ↓ 34% (P=0.001)
MERIT-HF	NYHA class II, III, IV (n=3,991)	Metoprolol vs.	1	All cause mortality ↓ 34% (P=0.0001)
COPERNICUS	NYHA class IV (n=2,289)	Carvedilol vs. placebo	0.94	All cause mortality ↓ 35% (P=0.00013)
COMET	NYHA class II-IV (n=3,029)	Carvedilol vs. metoprolol tartrate	5.8	All cause mortality ↓ 18% (P=0.0017)

NYHA, New York Heart Association.

inotropic agents for the treatment of heart failure. The first of these, amrinone, was shown to have effective inotropic and vasodilator properties when used for short-term, intravenous support of critically ill patients. A similar compound, milrinone, was developed for both short-term intravenous use and long-term oral administration.

These agents are hemodynamically effective and increase cardiac output, decrease pulmonary capillary wedge pressure, and improve exercise capacity. However, in a controlled clinical trial, when these agents were administered orally for long periods, their short-term efficacy was overshadowed by an increase in long-term mortality. The PROMISE trial, which compared oral milrinone with placebo, showed increased mortality in the milrinone group, with detrimental effects most prominent in patients in New York Heart Association class IV heart failure. Because of the poor results of long-term oral administration, phosphodiesterase inhibitors currently are restricted to short-term use as intravenous inotropic support agents. They can be of value in the intensive care setting in stabilizing the condition of patients with heart failure who have hemodynamic decompensation.

Two important lessons can be learned from "failed drug" experiences with inotropes:

■ Short-term improvements in hemodynamic variables and exercise capacity do not necessarily imply a long-term mortality benefit in heart failure.
■ Only adequately designed clinical trials with sufficient statistical power can assess the long-term safety and efficacy of drugs for heart failure.

Intermittent and Continuous Intravenous Inotropic Therapy

During the 1980s, a few small clinical studies suggested that the periodic use of short-term intravenous inotropic support provided long-lasting symptomatic benefit. It was hypothesized that short-term exposure to intravenous inotropic drugs resulted in "conditioning" of the myocardium, with subsequent sustained clinical improvement. Larger, more definitive clinical trials have not been performed, and the theoretical basis for this form of therapy is unproven.

Although continuous low-dose intravenous inotropic therapy is administered on an outpatient basis

in selected end-stage patients, adequately controlled clinical trials have not been performed to demonstrate the safety and efficacy of this therapy. The potential for toxicity with home use of powerful inotropic drugs should be considered.

DIURETICS IN HEART FAILURE

Recent data from the Systolic Hypertension in the Elderly Program (SHEP) showed that diuretic-based therapy of hypertension reduced new onset of heart failure, especially in patients with a history of myocardial infarction (80% decrease in initial episodes of heart failure). Diuretics may be required for patients with established heart failure who remain symptomatic despite treatment with ACE inhibitors, beta blockers and digoxin. Patients who present with pulmonary edema need diuretics immediately.

The minimal dose of diuretics needed to control congestion should be used. Over-diuresis exacerbates the activation of the RAS and may result in hypotension, prerenal azotemia, hyponatremia, hypokalemia, and hypomagnesemia. Over-diuresis also results in excessive thirst and may result in excessive fluid intake and apparent "diuretic refractoriness." Education of patients about the use of higher doses of diuretics for transient increases in fluid retention can eliminate the need for hospitalization or office visits and is an important part of heart failure management programs.

If congestive symptoms persist despite treatment with maximal doses of ACE inhibitors, digoxin, and beta-blockers, an increased dose of diuretics may be needed. It is important to determine whether the current dose of diuretics is effective (produces a diuretic response). If not, the morning dose should be increased. In advanced heart failure, twice-daily dosing may be required. In the absence of renal failure, if there is need for doses greater than 120 mg furosemide twice daily, consideration should be given to combination therapy with a thiazide diuretic such as metolazone (Zaroxolyn). Metolazone may be given daily, every other or every third day, or only if weight increases substantially. Metolazone potentiates the action of loop diuretics, because it blocks sodium reuptake in the distal nephron. With chronic use of loop diuretics, there is hypertrophy and enhanced sodium retention by the distal nephron, blunting the response to loop diuretics.

Blockade of the distal nephron by a thiazide prevents this augmented sodium reuptake. Such combination diuretic therapy can result in profound hypokalemia and volume depletion. Thus, careful monitoring of electrolytes and blood pressure is required. Patients with refractory hypokalemia may benefit from a small dose of a potassium-sparing diuretic such as spirono-lactone (Aldactone). Careful monitoring of potassium levels is required, especially in patients taking ACE inhibitors.

- Diuretics are required for patients with heart failure who remain symptomatic despite treatment with ACE inhibitors, digoxin, and beta-blockers.
- The minimal dose of diuretics needed to control congestion should be used.
- Metolazone potentiates the action of loop diuretics but should be used cautiously because it may result in profound hypokalemia and volume depletion.

ANTICOAGULATION IN HEART FAILURE

The Stroke Prevention in Atrial Fibrillation (SPAF) trial and other atrial fibrillation trials have demonstrated that patients with decreased ejection fraction or clinical heart failure and atrial fibrillation are at high risk for cardioembolic events. The efficacy of warfarin (Coumadin) in reducing embolic events in these patients has also been well documented. Similarly, patients with a recent anterior or large myocardial infarction are at markedly increased risk for cardioembolic events, and anticoagulation is recommended for at least the first 3 to 6 months after infarction. Patients with systolic dysfunction who have had a cardioembolic event are also at increased risk regardless of rhythm, and anticoagulation is recommended for them.

The value of chronic anticoagulation in patients with sinus rhythm and chronic ischemic or nonischemic dilated cardiomyopathy without a recent large myocardial infarction or previous cardioembolic event is a matter of controversy. The clinical practice guidelines of the National Health Care Policy and Research Agency for Heart Failure do not recommend anticoagulation for these patients. However, the American Heart Association/American College of Cardiology guidelines indicate that use of anticoagulation in patients with a very low ejection fraction (<25%) or an intracardiac thrombus is a "class II" therapeutic intervention, that is, "acceptable but of uncertain efficacy."

In an analysis of major heart failure studies, the incidence of arterial thromboembolism in the largest studies was 2-3% per 100 patient-years. A post hoc analysis of anticoagulation use in 6,513 patients enrolled in the SOLVD trials demonstrated that, after adjustment for baseline differences in other predictors of outcome in warfarin treatment was associated with lower all-cause mortality and lower mortality due to cardiovascular disease. There was no decrease in deaths due to stroke, pulmonary embolism, or other vascular cause. After adjustment for baseline differences in other predictors of outcome in patients receiving warfarin and those not receiving it, warfarin treatment was also associated with lower rates of hospital admission for nonfatal myocardial infarction. The mortality benefit was evident in patients with ischemic or nonischemic cause of heart failure as well as in patients with or without atrial fibrillation and was independent of the treatment arm or symptom status of the patient. Because this was a post hoc analysis, the mortality benefit may reflect other management factors not assessed in this observational study. Until randomized trials are conducted, this issue remains a matter of debate.

- Chronic anticoagulation is indicated in patients with decreased ejection fraction and atrial fibrillation, previous cardioembolic event, or recent large myocardial infarction.
- Use of chronic anticoagulation in sinus rhythm patients with low ejection fraction remains a matter of controversy.

Other Therapeutic Issues

Atrial Fibrillation in Heart Failure

Atrial arrhythmias such as atrial fibrillation can aggravate heart failure and increase the risk of stroke. Restoration of sinus rhythm may improve symptoms as well as left ventricular function itself. For most patients, an attempt to restore and maintain sinus rhythm is warranted. If sinus rhythm cannot be restored, good rate control remains an important therapeutic goal.

The most appropriate antiarrhythmic agent for maintenance of sinus rhythm in patients with heart failure and atrial fibrillation is amiodarone. Other antiarrhythmic agents such as propafenone and sotalol may exacerbate heart failure and increase mortality in patients with ischemic heart disease. Amiodarone does not increase mortality or symptoms in patients with heart failure and, in some patients with heart failure, may improve symptoms.

■ Excessive ventricular response rate in atrial fibrillation can in itself cause deterioration of left ventricular function. Restoration of normal sinus rhythm or at least good control of ventricular rate is an essential aspect of management.

Sudden Death and Sustained Ventricular Tachycardia in Heart Failure

Sudden death is common in heart failure and accounts for approximately one-third of the deaths among these patients. Although sudden death was widely assumed to be a consequence of ventricular tachycardia or fibrillation, recent data suggest that bradyarrhythmias and electromechanical dissociation may account for a significant proportion of these cases of sudden death. Patients who survive an episode of cardiac arrest or who present with sustained ventricular tachycardia should be referred to an electrophysiologist for consideration of a defibrillator and antiarrhythmic therapy. For patients with ischemic LV dysfunction with LVEF <35%, with or without nonsustained ventricular arrhythmia, prophylactic insertion of an implantable cardioverter defibrillator is indicated based on outcomes of controlled trials. Further discussion of the indications for defibrillator therapy in heart failure patients is provided in "Implantable Cardioverter-Defibrillator Trials and Prevention of Sudden Cardiac Death."

Cardiac Resynchronization Therapy

Recent trials have documented that biventricular pacing can improve symptoms and survival in patients with significant dyssynchrony of left ventricular contraction. The indications for biventricular pacing are still evolving and are discussed in greater depth in "Cardiac Resynchronization Therapy." Biventricular pacing should only be undertaken after a comprehensive pharmacologic heart failure treatment program has been instituted.

Nesiritide in Heart Failure

Nesiritide is synthetic brain natriuretic peptide (BNP), identical to the endogenous circulating peptide. This agent has been extensively evaluated in clinical trials and is labeled for the treatment of acute CHF. It is available for parenteral administration and is intended for short-term infusion for management of decompensated CHF. Nesiritide has no inotropic action, and hence, is significantly different from pressor agents such as dopamine or dobutamine. It is not indicated for the treatment of acute cardiogenic shock.

Nesiritide has vasodilatory effects and has compared favorably to intravenous nitroglycerin in head to head trials. Favorable actions include reduction of cardiac filling pressures with relief of dyspnea, as well as diuresis and natriuresis. The agent is unique in that it reduces concentrations of circulating catecholamines and endothelin. However, it has the potential to significantly aggravate renal dysfunction. The role of nesiritide therapy in routine clinical practice is still being defined.

Exercise

Although exercise programs do not alter mortality in patients with congestive heart failure, physical conditioning improves exercise capacity and the sense of well-being. It is recommended that patients with chronic heart failure engage in regular exercise to maintain peripheral muscle tone. For many patients, a monitored exercise program is an important adjunctive therapy.

MYOCARDITIS

Leslie T. Cooper, Jr, MD

Oyere K. Onuma, SB

INTRODUCTION

Myocarditis is defined histologically as an inflammation of the myocardium associated with injury to cardiac myocytes (Fig. 1). Although many if not most cases of myocarditis remain idiopathic, a variety of treatable specific causes should be considered and excluded during the initial evaluation. These include infectious, autoimmune, toxic, and hypersensitivity reactions (Table 1). Myocarditis usually presents as an acute or fulminant illness, with new onset congestive heart failure and dilated cardiomyopathy. However, it may present as sudden death, acute myocardial infarction-like syndrome, new atrial or ventricular arrhythmias, or complete heart block. Occasionally, the physiologic presentation of acute myocarditis is more suggestive of a hypertrophic or restrictive than a pure dilated cardiomyopathy. Important clinicopathologic variants also include the endocardial eosinophilic and fibrotic diseases and pericarditis associated with focal of diffuse epicarditis (also called myopericarditis). In most acute cases of lymphocytic myocarditis, left ventricular function improves over one to six months with standard heart failure care. However a substantial minority will fail to clear a cardiotropic virus or develop persistent

Table 1. Common Causes of Myocarditis

Associated disorder or agent	Clinical clues	Diagnostic method
Viral/Coxsackie B	Flu-like prodrome	Endomyocardial biopsy
Acute rheumatic fever	Jones criteria	Throat culture, antistreptolysin O titer
Lyme disease	History of tick bite	
Doxorubicin/anthracycline	Previous cancer treatment	Serology
Chagas disease	Travel to Central or South America	Clinical, endomyocardial biopsy
Peripartum cardiomyopathy*	Last trimester or first 6 mo postpartum	Serology
		Clinical

*Reviewed in Heart Disease in Pregnancy chapter.

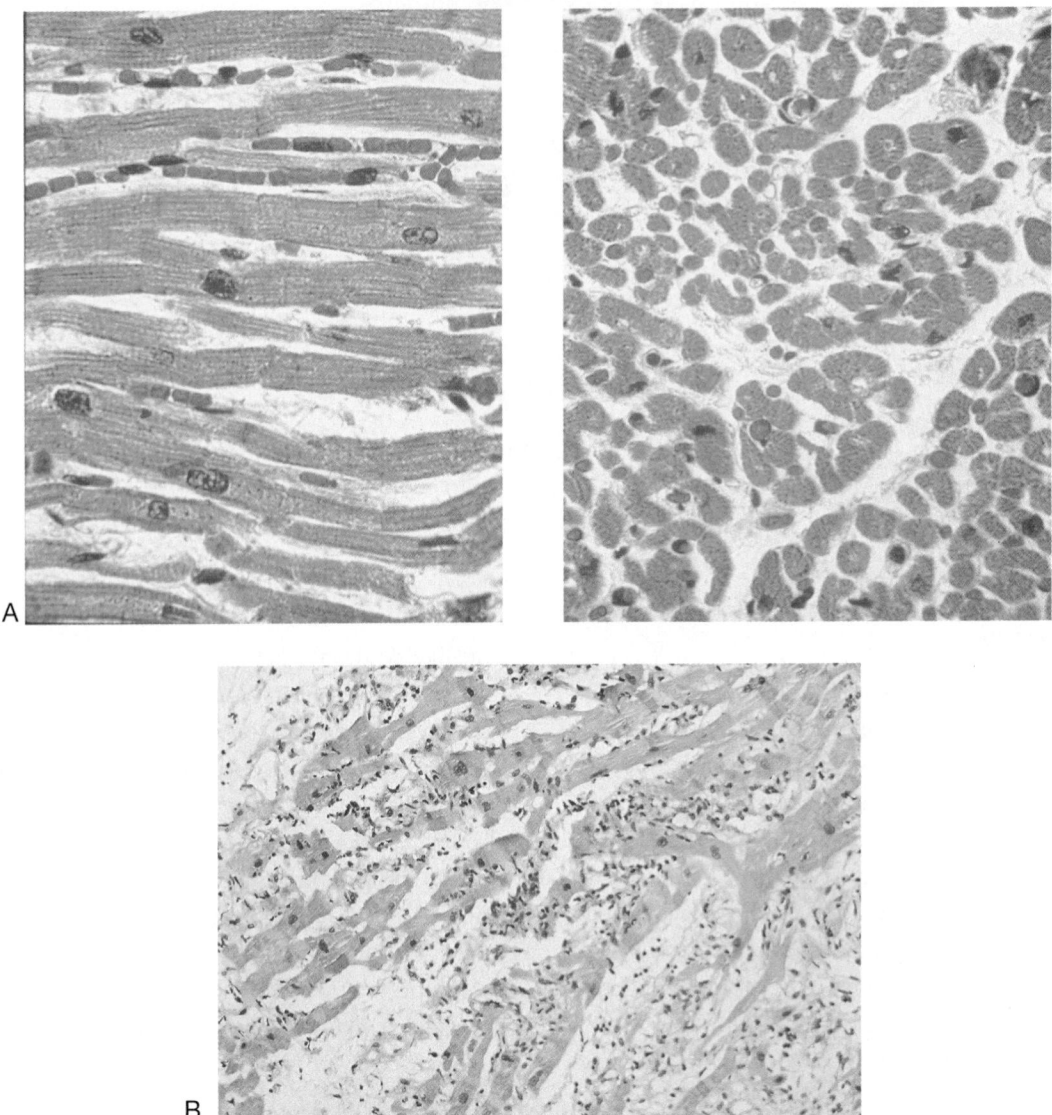

Fig. 1. *A*, Normal myocardium in longitudinal (*left*) and cross (*right*) sections. *B*, Lymphocytic myocarditis with a mixed inflammatory infiltrate and associated myocyte necrosis.

inflammation that leads to chronic cardiomyopathy. In the patients who develop chronic cardiomyopathy, the risk of heart transplantation and death is high.

ETIOLOGY OF ACUTE MYOCARDITIS

For over 40 years, seroepidemiologic studies have linked enteroviral infections with acute cardiomyopathy. The most common enterovirus identified in these studies is usually Coxsackie B. As our ability to diagnose viral infection has improved with the advent of molecular biologic techniques, about 20 viruses have been associated in case reports and case series with acute and chronic dilated cardiomyopathy. In the past decade, adenovirus, parvovirus B19, hepatitis C (in Japan), influenza virus, cytomegalovirus and Epstein-Barr virus (Table 2) have been identified with increasing frequency in pediatric and adult populations. Acute cardiomyopathy associated with viral infection is often also associated with a lymphocytic infiltrate or altered expression of immunologic markers on cardiac myocytes suggesting acute myocarditis.

Table 2. Viral Myocarditis

Cause	Clinical features	Pathologic findings	Comments
Coxsackievirus	See text	Lymphocytic infiltrate with myocyte necrosis	Sensitivity of endomyo-cardial biopsy is about 35%
Influenza	Tachycardia, ECG abnor-malities, dyspnea, anginal chest pain, congestive failure, complete heart block, and death	Myocarditis present in one-third of fatal cases; biventricular dilatation, subendocardial and subepi-cardial hemorrhage, and mononuclear perivascular inflammation	Treat type A with amanta-dine
Cytomegalovirus	Symptomatic disease rare; pericardial effusion occasionally present	Focal lymphocytic infiltra-tion and fibrosis	
Poliomyelitis	Often found in fatal cases; cardiovascular collapse, heart failure, and pulmo-nary edema		Immunization effective, maintain proper oxygena-tion and pulmonary function
Infectious mono-nucleosis	ECG changes common, cardiac symptoms unusual, congestive heart failure or death rare	Myocardial infiltrates of atypical lymphocytes and necrosis	Consider treatment with corticosteroids
Human immuno-deficiency virus	Pericarditis, arrhythmias, ECG abnormalities, and dilated cardiomyopathy	Lymphocytic myocarditis, opportunistic myocardial infections, and ventricular dilatation	Consider adverse drug effects, opportunistic infections, and malignancy
Viral hepatitis	Usually transient; ECG abnormalities of brady-cardia, ventricular premature complexes, ST-T change; congestive failure and sudden death in severe cases	Focal necrosis and inflam-mation; petechial hemorrhage, including hemorrhage into con-duction system	
Mumps	Clinical and cardiac involvement uncommon, ST- and T-wave abnor-malities more frequent	Cardiac dilatation and hypertrophy, mural thrombi, interstitial fibrosis and infil-tration of mononuclear cells and focal necrosis, possible relationship of maternal mumps and fetal endocardial fibroelastosis	
Rubeola	Transient ECG abnor-malities, rare congestive heart failure	Perivascular lymphocyte infiltrate	

Table 2. (continued)

Cause	Clinical features	Pathologic findings	Comments
Varicella	Rare bundle-branch block, conduction defects, heart failure, and sudden death; nonsustained ventricular tachycardia and fibrillation	Intranuclear inclusion bodies within myocardial cells, interstitial edema, cellular infiltrates, and myonecrosis	
Variola and vaccinia	Myocarditis rare but may be fatal, myocarditis may follow vaccination by 2 weeks	Mononuclear infiltrate, interstitial edema, and necrosis	Variola now eradicated and immunization no longer recommended; severe myocarditis after vaccination has responded to short course of steroids
Arbovirus (chikungunya, dengue)	Myocarditis frequent; chest pain, dyspnea, palpitations, murmurs, gallops, and cardiomegaly; ST-T abnormalities, supraventricular and ventricular arrhythmias, and sudden death; chronicity	Embolization	
Respiratory syncytial viruses	Rare congestive failure, complete heart block, and arrhythmias		
Herpes simplex virus		Chronic interstitial inflammation and fibrosis	Treat with adenine arabinoside or acyclovir, but effectiveness not proved
Adenovirus	Myocarditis rare	Dilated right and left ventricles, mononuclear infiltrate	
Yellow fever virus	Hepatitis, gastrointestinal bleeding, cardiovascular collapse, and bradycardia inappropriate to the fever	Pericardial petechial hemorrhages and myocyte degeneration	
Rabies	Rare tachycardia, gallop rhythm, and hypotension	Diffuse interstitial infiltrate, myocardial necrosis	

ECG, electrocardiographic.

■ Coxsackie B virus, an enterovirus, and adenoviruses are associated with lymphocytic myocarditis.

Although the possible causes of acute myocarditis are many, viral cardiomyopathy remains the most common form of acute myocarditis in North American adults. The diagnosis of a viral cardiomyopathy may be suggested by an antecedent upper respiratory tract illness or by acute changes in serologic titers of antiviral immunonoglobulins. However, the specificity of acute changes in viral serologic titers is low, because similar serologic changes have been observed in unaffected family members of patients with myocarditis. Indeed, during outbreaks of Coxsackie B infection only 3.5 to 5 percent of patients develop symptoms of myocarditis. The diagnosis may be confirmed by polymerase chain reaction (PCR) from a sample of fresh frozen myocardium obtained by biopsy, but this is not routinely performed at most medical centers (see diagnosis and treatment of myocarditis below).

Although much clinical research in the 1980s and 1990s focused on the effects of the immune response to viral infection as a cause for cardiomyopathy, recent research has focused on the role of direct viral injury. Viral infection can lead acutely to myocyte death, release of sequestered intracellular antigens, and an innate and adaptive immune response in the myocardium. Cytokines, such as tumor necrosis factor-alpha (TNF-α), and autoantibodies associated with this inflammatory reaction can impair cardiac myocyte contractility, and released cellular products, such as major basic protein (MBP), can lead directly to myocyte cell death. Alternately, protein products of the enteroviral genome, including viral protease 2a, can cleave host proteins, including dystrophin, and lead to cardiomyopathy independently of any immune response. Thus, therapeutic strategies that try to eliminate viral infection are currently being investigated in patients with dilated cardiomyopathy and evidence of persistent viral infection.

A three-phase model has been proposed that characterizes the progression of acute viral infection to dilated cardiomyopathy. In the first phase, acute infection of cardiac myocytes results in myocyte cell death, activation of the innate immune response, including, interferon gamma, natural killer (NK) cells, and nitric oxide. Antigen presenting cells phagocytize released viral particles and cardiac proteins and migrate out of the heart to regional lymph nodes. The second phase consists of an adaptive immune response in a subset of patients. Antibodies to viral proteins, and to some cardiac proteins (often including cardiac myosin and receptors such as the β_1 receptor) are produced along with a proliferation of T helper cells. In the third phase, the immune response is down regulated with fibrosis replacing a cellular infiltrate in the myocardium. Under neurohumoral stimulation and hemodynamic stress, the ventricles dilate leading to chronic cardiomyopathy. Late into the third phase, viral genome may persist in the heart and inflammatory mechanisms may contribute to ventricular dysfunction.

In acute myocarditis, the inflammation may have the beneficial result of complete viral clearance. This may be one explanation for the largely negative results of treatment trials aimed at altering this acute immune response. Most patients with acute myocarditis have a mild illness with partial or complete recovery of ventricular function (see treatment of myocarditis below). Patients who fail to respond to usual heart failure care, or who develop progressive heart block or ventricular arrhythmias in the context of acute cardiomyopathy may have a distinct pathologic disorder such as granulomatous or giant cell myocarditis, and should be considered for heart biopsy. In contrast, patients who have evidence of persistent inflammation in the myocardium or persistent viral infection in the context of chronic, symptomatic congestive heart failure usually do not improve if they are already on optimal standard treatment for heart failure. In these patients with chronic viral or inflammatory cardiomyopathy, therapy aimed at eliminating virus or altering the immune response may have therapeutic benefits. The management of chronic myocardits is an area of active clinical research.

CLINICAL PRESENTATION AND DIAGNOSIS

The clinical presentation of myocarditis is highly variable, ranging from subclinical disease to fulminant heart failure. There is a slight male predominance in most case series. Of the 111 patients enrolled in the Myocarditis Treatment Trial 62% were male. Patients may report fatigue, decrease in exercise tolerance, palpitations and precordial chest pain. Chest pain may be anginal in quality and associated with ST-segment elevation in EKG. Chest pain typical of pericarditis is not unusual and suggests epicardial inflammation. Patients with myocarditis who present with syncope have a particularly high risk of death or transplant. However, the clinical symptoms rarely identify an etiologic cause and are not specific enough to establish the diagnosis with certainty.

- Myocarditis often presents as subacute congestive heart failure in an otherwise healthy person.
- One should suspect myocarditis in a previously healthy young adult male who presents with new onset heart failure and dilated cardiomyopathy.
- Median age of affected persons is about 42 years.

- Most patients report a flu-like prodrome.
- Left ventricular function usually improves over several months with standard heart failure management.
- Myocarditis is an important cause of chronic dilated cardiomyopathy.

Physical Examination

The physical examination findings in patients with acute myocarditis are those of acute decompensated heart failure. Patients may shows signs of fluid overload with rales, elevated jugular venous pressure, hepatomegaly and lower extremity edema. They are usually tachycardic and the apex may be diffuse and laterally displaced suggesting cardiomegaly. S_1 may be soft and there may be an S_3, S_4 or both.

Certain physical exam findings imply a specific cause of myocarditis. Enlarged lymph nodes might suggest systemic sarcoidosis. A pruritic, macopapular rash may suggest a hypersensitivity reaction, often to a drug or toxin. Sustained ventricular tachycardia or new heart block in the setting of rapidly progressive congestive heart failure suggests giant cell myocarditis. Acute rheumatic fever can present with the modified Jones criteria.

Biomarkers of Cardiac Injury

Cardiac enzyme elevations are seen in a minority of patients with acute myocarditis and can help confirm the diagnosis. Standard markers of myocardial damage including troponin-I and CK-MB have a high specificity but limited sensitivity in the diagnosis of myocarditis. Clinical and experimental data suggest that cardiac troponin-I is increased more frequently than creatnine kinase MB subunits (CK-MB) in patients with myocarditis. Other serum immunologic biomarkers including cytokines, complement and anti-heart antibodies have not been prospectively validated for sensitivity and specificity in the diagnosis of myocarditis. Certain serum biomarkers, including sFAS, sFAS ligand and IL-10 have been associated with poor prognosis in single case series of patients with severe, acute myocarditis.

A mild to moderate leukocytosis with fever, elevated erythrocyte sedimentation rates (ESR), C-reactive proteins (CRP), and moderate elevations in AST, ALT and lactase dehydrogenase (LDH) are sometimes present in acute myocarditis but these are nonspecific signs of inflammation.

Electrocardiogram

The electrocardiogram (ECG) in acute myocarditis often shows sinus tachycardia with non-specific ST-segment and T-wave abnormalities. Occasionally, the ECG changes are suggestive of an acute myocardial infarction; intraventricular conduction delay is common. In a small proportion of patients, various degrees of heart block may occur. In the Myocarditis Treatment Trial, pacemaker implantation occurred in approximately 1% of subjects, secondary to high-grade heart block. Sustained and nonsustained ventricular arrhythmias may also be present, but occur more commonly in cardiac sarcoidosis and giant cell myocarditis.

Echocardiography

The most common echocardiographic features of acute myocarditis are unfortunately not specific. Echocardiographic patterns of dilated, hypertrophic, restrictive, and ischemic cardiomyopathy have been described in histologically proven myocarditis. Segmental wall motion abnormalities (hypokinesia, akinesia and even dyskinesia) can simulate myocardial infarction in myocarditis. Acute myocarditis can show a restrictive hemodynamic pattern out of proportion to the degree of systolic dysfunction. In addition, diastolic relaxation abnormalities are common. In the Myocarditis Treatment Trial, increased sphericity and left ventricular volume occured in acute, active myocarditis.

- Echocardiographic findings are not specific for acute myocarditis, but are useful to exclude other known causes of heart failure.

Left ventricular cavity size may be normal in very early myocarditis and increase over time due to remodeling. Felker et al suggested that fulminant myocarditis can be distinguished from acute myocarditis by echocardiographic criteria. They performed echocardiography on 11 fulminant and 43 acute myocarditis patients at presentation and after six months. Patients with fulminant myocarditis had near normal LV diastolic dimensions (5.3 ± 0.9 cm) with increased septal thickness (1.2 ± 0.2 cm) at presentation, while those with acute myocarditis had increased diastolic dimensions (6.1 ± 0.8 cm, *P*<0.01 vs. fulminant) but normal septal thickness (1.0 ± 0.1 cm, *P* = 0.01 vs. fulminant). The prognosis in the patients with fulminant myocarditis was better than those with acute disease.

Certain echocardiographic variables may predict prognosis in acute myocarditis. Right ventricular function (RVF) may be an independent predictor of death or cardiac transplantation. In a study of 23 patients with biopsy confirmed myocarditis by Mendes et al, the likelihood of death or heart transplantation was greater in patients with abnormal RVF (RV descent ≤1.7cm) than in patients with normal RVF(>1.7). Sixty percent of patients with RV descent <1.7 died or required transplantation, compared to none of the patients with RV descent >1.7 cm (*P*=0.03) after 2 years. In this study, multivariate analysis revealed that right ventricular dysfunction as quantitated by right ventricular descent was the most powerful predictor of death or cardiac transplantation. In a separate study, Naqvi et al demonstrated that contractile reserve assessed by dobutamine echocardiography predicted left ventricular functional recovery in 22 patients with new onset DCM, some of which may be due to myocarditis. Baseline variables that were significantly predictive of follow-up LVEF were deceleration time (r=0.69, *P*=0.0006), wall motion score index (WMSI) (r=–0.63, *P*=0.002), LV mass (r=0.56, *P*=0.008) and LVEF after dobutamine (r=0.84, *P*=0.0001).

Cardiac Magnetic Resonance

Cardiac Magnetic Resonance (CMR) is increasingly becoming an important tool for the diagnosis of myocarditis. Serial CMR using T1-weighted images with gadolinium have been used to visualize the myocardial injury in myocarditis and track its progression. The Myocardial Delay Enhancement (MDE) technique provides additional diagnostic value with improved sensitivity and utility for guided endomyocardial biopsies. Histopathologic evaluation of biopsies directed by cardiac magnetic resonance with delay enhancement (DE) demonstrated active myocarditis in 19 of 21 patients. In contrast, only 1 in 7 patients showed active myocarditis in biopsies guided by non-MDE cardiac magnetic resonance. Thus CMR may provide diagnostic value both in the diagnosis of myocarditis and for the targeted use of endomyocardial biopsy.

CMR may differentiate ischemic from non-ischemic cardiomyopathy. McCrohon et al performed gadolinium enhanced CMR in 90 patients with heart failure and LV systolic dysfunction of whom 63 patients had idiopathic DCM. All patients (100%) with ischemic cardiomyopathy had either subendocardial or transmural enhancement. In contrast, the DCM group had three patterns of enhancement: no enhancement, myocardial enhancement indistinguishable from the patients with CAD and patchy or longitudinal striae of mid wall enhancement. This and other similar studies suggest that diffuse and/or heterogeneous involvement in the lateral wall, subepicardial, mid-myocardial or combined enhancement is highly suggestive of myocarditis.

Because of its availability and low risk, CMR is being used with increasing frequency as a diagnostic test in suspected acute myocarditis. Current limitations of CMR include the inability to differentiate types of myocarditis that may require specific therapy such as granulomatous or giant cell myocarditis and myocarditis due to specific diseases, such as idiopathic hypereosinophic syndrome. Not all patients are candidates for CMR due to claustrophobia, implantable devices, tachyarrhythmias and hemodynamic instability. The prognostic value of CMR beyond clinical and hemodynamic variables has not been established.

Endomyocardial Biopsy

The current gold standard for the diagnosis of acute myocarditis is by transvenous right ventricular endomyocardial biopsy (EMB) (Fig. 2). Although the specificity of EMB for lymphocytic myocarditis is high at 79%, the sensitivity is only 35% when compared with the clinical standard of improved left ventricular function over time. A positive EMB unequivocally establishes the diagnosis of myocarditis. However, due to widespread sampling error, the absence of histologic evidence should not preclude the diagnosis of myocarditis in the appropriate clinical settings.

The incidence of positive right ventricular biopsy findings on specimens from patients with suspected myocarditis averages 10%. In the Myocarditis Treatment Trial, only 214 of 2,233 patients with heart failure and suspected myocarditis had diagnostic biopsy findings. The low incidence of diagnostic findings on EMB is due the sampling error from small biopsy

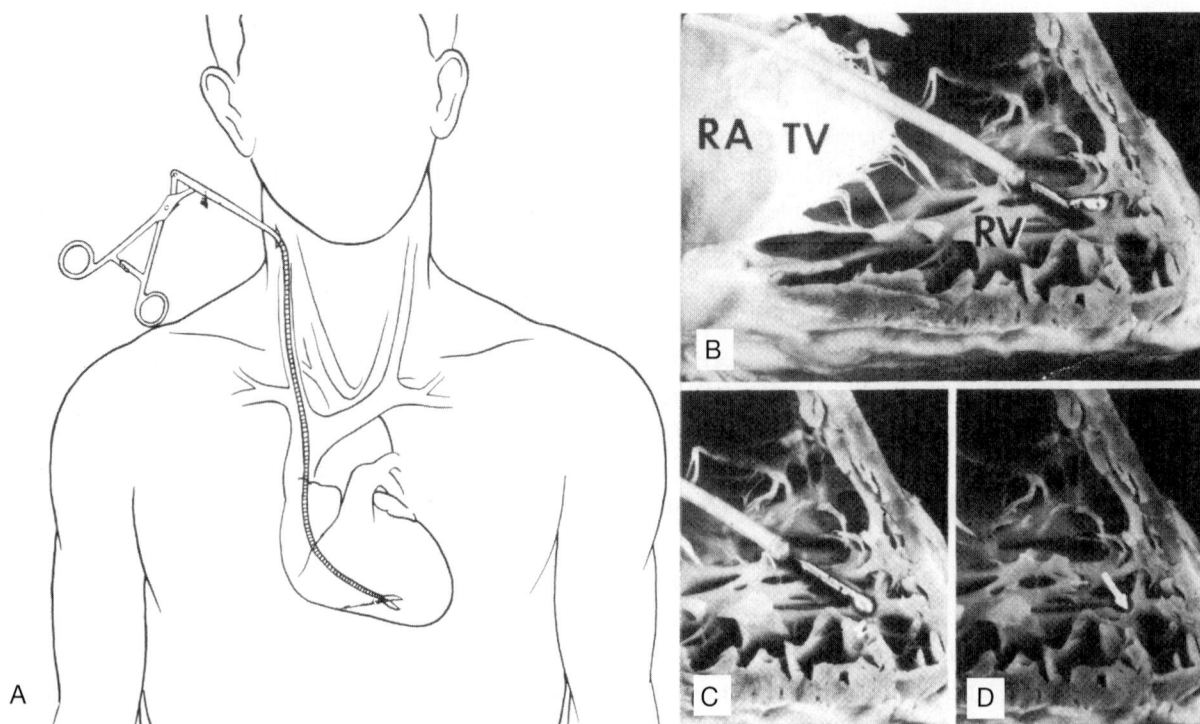

Fig. 2. Right ventricular endomyocardial biopsy. *A*, Diagram showing ease of access to right ventricular apex via right internal jugular vein. *B* to *D*, Autopsy specimen used to simulate biopsy procurement, with bioptome jaws opened around a trabecula carnea (*B*), jaws closed (*C*), and appearance of biopsy site (*arrow*) (*D*). RA, right atrium; RV, right ventricle; TV, tricuspid valve.

specimens, the insensitivity of routine histologic techniques (Dallas Criteria, Table 3) for detecting inflammation, and considerable intraobserver variability in the identification of inflammatory infiltrates.

Routine use of EMB is also limited by the complications of this invasive technique which include a 1 in 1,000 risk of death, 1 in 250 risk of perforation in experienced hands, and a risk of arrhythmias. Because of relatively high risk, many clinicians have questioned the role of routine EMB in the diagnosis of lymphocytic myocarditis. EMB is currently listed as a class IIb recommendation in current American College of Cardiology/American Heart Association (ACC/AHA) guidelines; i.e. it is not recommended for routine evaluation of suspected myocarditis. This is based in part on the evidence from the Myocarditis Treatment Trial which failed to demonstrate a benefit for EMB-guided treatment in acute myocarditis. In most cases of acute DCM, EMB does not affect treatment, and therefore there is no need to obtain a specific histologic diagnosis. However, in patients with a rapidly deteriorating course

particularly if complicated by heart block or ventricular arrhythmias, an EMB remains the only way to diagnosis giant cell myocarditis, a disorder with poor prognosis that usually responds to heart transplantation or multidrug immunosuppression.

The role of EMB in the evaluation of patients with chronic DCM is more controversial than its role in acute DCM. PCR of viral RNA and DNA from EMB specimens can be used to diagnose viral myocarditis. Expression of major histocompatability antigens (MHC) is a more sensitive marker than the Dallas criteria for myocardial inflammation, and can be detected using immunoperoxidase-based stains for HLA-ABC and HLA-DR antigens. Indeed, the sensitivity and specificity of MHC expression for detecting biopsy-proven myocarditis was 80% and 85% respectively from a recent study. Because of the potential to influence outcome with antiviral or immunomodulatory treatment in chronic DCM, there is a renewed interest in the use of EMB combined with these novel methods of tissue analysis in the management of chronic

Table 3.   Dallas Criteria for the Diagnosis of Lymphocytic Myocarditis*

First biopsy
    Active myocarditis (with or without fibrosis)
    Borderline myocarditis (not diagnostic and requiring further biopsy)
    No evidence of myocarditis
Subsequent biopsies
    Ongoing (persistent) myocarditis
    Resolving (healing) myocarditis
    Resolved (healed) myocarditis

*The histologic diagnosis of active myocarditis requires an inflammatory infiltrate with necrosis and/or degeneration of adjacent myocytes without evidence of Chagas disease or features of ischemic heart disease.

DCM. At this time, the role of EMB to diagnose and treat viral infection and inflammation in chronic DCM is under active investigation. No firm recommendations regarding the use of EMB in the setting outside of research protocols can be made at this time.

TREATMENT OF MYOCARDITIS

The **Myocarditis Treatment Trial** was a prospective, randomized, double-blinded, placebo-controlled trial of prednisolone plus cyclosporine or azathioprine for the treatment of biopsy-proven lymphocytic myocarditis in persons with acute congestive heart failure. There was no benefit to immunosuppression over placebo in survival or improvement of left ventricular function. The mean left ventricular ejection fraction increased from 24% to 35% in both groups and the mortality (death or heart transplantation) was approximately 56% by 4.5 years in both groups.

The **IMAC (Immune Modulation for Acute Cardiomyopathy)** trial evaluated the role of intravenous immunoglobulin treatment and enrolled patients with left ventricular ejection fraction less than 40% and heart failure symptoms for less than 6 months. The trial showed an average increase in left ventricular function of 14% regardless of treatment.

These results were in agreement with the findings from the Myocarditis Treatment Trial that immune modulation in most cases of acute DCM does not provide additional benefit beyond usual care.

Most patients with acute cardiomyopathy will improve with treatment that includes the standard heart failure regimen of ACE inhibitors or angiotensin receptor blocking agents, beta-blockers such as carvedilol or metoprolol, and diuretics if needed. Heart block and tachyarrhythmia may be treated with standard agents, including a pacemaker if needed.

■ Current recommendations do not indicate routine treatment with immunosuppressive agents for acute post-viral or lymphocytic myocarditis.

Prognosis for Lymphocytic Myocarditis
In a multivariate analysis, predictors of death or heart transplantation after acute myocarditis included syncope, low ejection fraction (<40%), and bundle branch block. Increased pulmonary pressures are consistently associated with poor prognosis. The prognosis in myocarditis depends on the etiology of myocardial inflammation (Fig. 3).

SPECIFIC FORMS OF MYOCARDITIS

Giant Cell Myocarditis
Idiopathic giant cell myocarditis is a rare and usually fulminant form of myocarditis diagnosed by the pres-

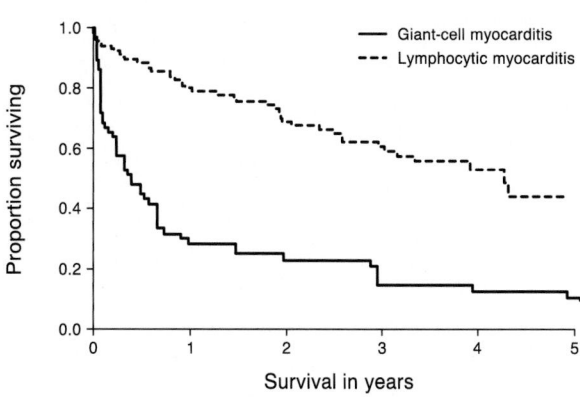

Fig. 3. Kaplan-Meier survival curve for patients with giant-cell myocarditis.

ence of multinucleated giant cells associated with eosinophils and myocyte destruction in the absence of granulomas (Fig. 4). Unlike lymphocytic myocarditis, giant cell myocarditis generally causes progressive left ventricular failure complicated by arrhythmias. Of the 63 patients enrolled in the multicenter Giant Cell Myocarditis Treatment Trial, 75% presented with congestive heart failure and 14% with ventricular arrhythmia.

Giant cell myocarditis is also associated with worse prognosis than lymphocytic myocarditis; the median survival from the onset of symptoms is only 5.5 months and has an 89% rate of death or transplantation (Fig. 3). Given this poor prognosis, a biopsy-proven diagnosis of giant cell myocarditis prompts consideration of immunosuppression and early evaluation for cardiac transplantation. Timely institution of combination immunosuppressive therapy including cyclosporine and prednisone prolongs time to survival or transplantation. Despite a 25% incidence of post-transplantation recurrence of giant cell myocarditis detected by biopsy, the 5-year survival after transplantation is about 71% which is comparable to survival after transplantation for cardiomyopathy.

Cardiac Sarcoidosis

Cardiac sarcoidosis occurs clinically in about 5% of patients with clinical sarcoidosis although autopsy series have reported higher rates of about 25%. Isolated cardiac sarcoidosis can present clinically with ventricular tachycardia, heart block, or congestive heart failure.

Definite diagnosis is by EMB which shows characteristic noncaseating granulomas (Fig. 5). However, the diagnosis can also be inferred if there is a tissue diagnosis of sarcoidosis from an extracardiac source in the presence of a cardiomyopathy of unknown origin. Transplant-free survival in cardiac sarcoidosis is similar to that of lymphocytic myocarditis, but the rates of syncope, pacemaker, and AICD placement are higher.

Acute Rheumatic Fever

Acute rheumatic fever may present as a pancarditis that affects the endocardium, myocardium and pericardium. Although the incidence of acute rheumatic fever is low in the United States at about 2 cases per 100,000 persons, there is a much higher incidence in Asia, Africa and South America with an incidence of 100 cases per 100,000 persons. It remains one of the most important cardiovascular diseases in developing countries. It is thought to result from an immunologic response to a pharyngeal infection with certain strains of group A streptococci and occurs in about 3% of persons with untreated streptococcal pharyngitis.

The risk of rheumatic fever is related to the presence of certain virulent types of streptococci that induce a strong immune response to M-type mucoid proteins that encapsulate the organism in genetically susceptible individuals. Patients with HLA-DR 1, 2, 3 and 4 haplotypes may be at increased risk for rheumatic fever. A more detailed discussion of rheumatic fever is presented in the Rheumatic Heart Disease chapter.

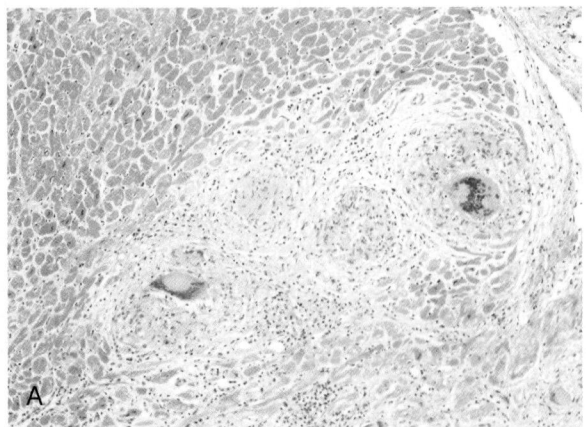
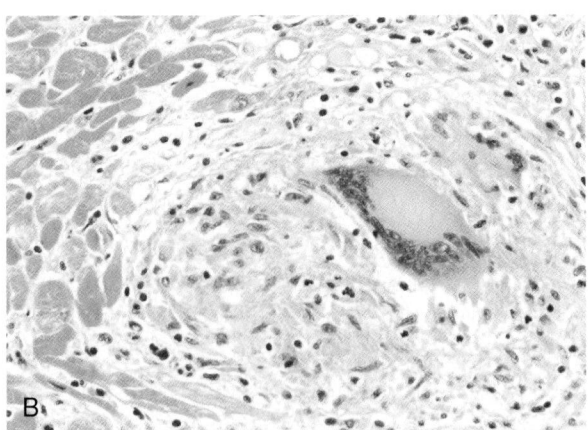

Fig. 4. *A*, Cardiac sarcoidosis. Well-formed granuloma with giant cells may be seen without myocyte necrosis. (Original magnification, x125.) *B*, Follicular granuloma in cardiac sarcoidosis. (Original magnification, x400.)

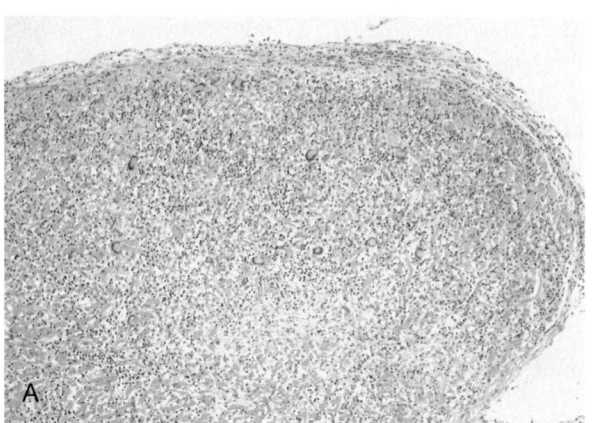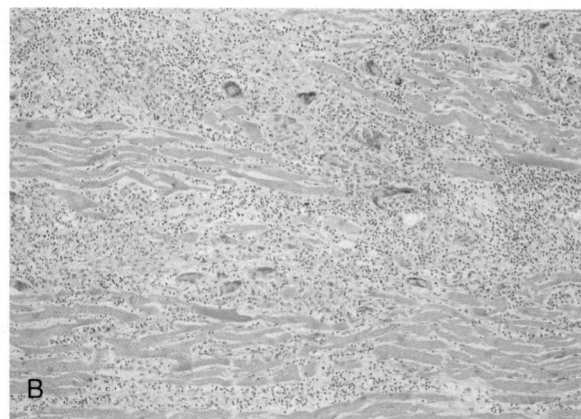

Fig. 5. *A*, Idiopathic giant cell myocarditis. Diffuse endomyocardial inflammatory infiltrate with multinucleated giant cells in the absence of granuloma. (Original magnification, x25.) *B*, Widespread mixed inflammatory infiltrate with multinucleated giant cells and myocyte necrosis. (Original magnification, x100.)

Hypersensitivity and Eosinophilic Myocarditis

Drug induced hypersensitivity reactions can sometimes affect the myocardium. Numerous medications including antidepressants (tricyclics), antibiotics (penicillins, cephalosporins, sulfonamides) and antipsychotics (clozapine) have been implicated in hypersensitivity myocarditis (Tables 4 and 5). Clinically, the presentation is different from lymphocytic myocarditis, in that the patients are generally older (mean age, 58 years) and are often taking several medications. Patients often present acutely with rash and fever; liver function test abnormalities are commonly, but not always, present. ECG changes are similar to lymphocytic myocarditis with sinus tachycardia and nonspecific T-wave abnormalities and ST-elevations may be seen.

Eosinophilic myocarditis may occur in association with systemic diseases such as hypereosinophilic syndrome (HES), Churg-Strauss syndrome and Löffler's endomyocardial fibrosis (Table 6). These syndromes are commonly marked by peripheral eosinophilia and an infiltration of mature eosinophils in many organ systems including the heart. Clinical manifestation of eosinophilic myocarditis include endocardial fibrosis, fibrosis of the cardiac valves leading to regurgitation, right and left congestive heart failure and formation of thrombi on the endocardial surface. Eosinophilic myocarditis may also occur in association with parasitic helminthic or protozoal infections such as Chagas disease, toxoplasmosis, schistosomiasis, trichinosis, hyatid cysts and visceral larval migrans. Acute necrotizing eosinophilic myocarditis is

an aggressive form of eosinophilic myocarditis with acute onset and high mortality rates.

In general, the treatment for eosinophilic myocarditis depends on the underlying cause. High-dose corticosteroids might be beneficial in the setting of systemic disease, while surgical treatment might aid in endomyocardial fibrosis.

Lyme Myocarditis

Myocarditis occurs in association with the infection by the spirochete *Borrelia burgdorferi* (Lyme disease). Lyme myocarditis should be suspected in patients who have a history of travel to the endemic regions or in patients who give a history of a tick bite. Clinical presentation may include transient or permanent heart block or cardiac arrhythmia. The diagnosis of Lyme disease is confirmed by serologic testing, however, this does not establish the diagnosis of myocarditis.

Endomyocardial biopsy may show a lymphocytic myocarditis with a prominent plasmacytic component. The organism may be visualized in the section with special stains. In a patient with suspected Lyme disease after a tick bite, the possibility of coinfection with *Ehrlichia* (ehrilichiosis) and *Babesia* (babesiosis) should be considered as both can also cause myocarditis. Serologic tests are available for both disorders.

Chagas Cardiomyopathy

Chagas cardiomyopathy is an acute myocarditis that may present secondary to an infection with *Trypanosoma*

Table 4.   Possible Effects of Various Drugs on the Heart

Hypersensitivity myocarditis	Toxic myocarditis	Dilated cardiomyopathy
Acetazolamide	Amphetamines	Amphetamines
p-Aminosalicylic acid	Antihypertensives	Anthracyclines
Amitriptyline	Antimony	Chloroquine
Amphotericin B	Arsenicals	Cobalt
Carbamazepine	Barbiturates	Cocaine
Chloramphenicol	Caffeine	Ephedrine
Diphenylhydantoin	Catecholamines	Ethanol
Diphtheria toxin	Cocaine	Lithium
Horse serum	Cyclophosphamide	
Hydrochlorothiazide	Emetine	**Endocardial fibrosis**
Indomethacin	5-Fluorouracil	Anthracyclines
Isoniazid	Immunosuppressives	Busulfan
Methyldopa	Lithium	Ergotamine
Penicillins	Paraquat	Mercury
Phenindione	Phenothiazines	Methysergide
Phenylbutazone	Plasmocid	Serotonin
Smallpox vaccine	Quinidine	
Spironolactone	Rapeseed oil	**Myocardial fibrosis**
Streptomycin	Theophylline	Cyclosporine*
Sulfonamides		
Sulfonylureas		
Tetanus toxoid		
Tetracycline		

*In transplanted hearts only.

cruzi or as a chronic cardiomyopathy. It is a major cause of cardiomyopathy worldwide and may be seen in immigrants from rural Central or South America. In these endemic areas, Chagas cardiomyopathy is a leading cause of dilated cardiomyopathy and congestive heart failure.

Clinically, Chagas cardiomyopathy may present with symptoms of cardiac arrhythmia, or heart block in 10 to 20% of infected persons (Table 7). These symptoms may be related to congestive heart failure due to left ventricular dysfunction or ventricular arrhythmia resulting from progressive damage to the myocardium, extracellular matrix, autonomic innervation and coronary microvessels. An additional 20% to 30% of affected persons have asymptomatic cardiac involvement. The disease is clinically suspected if the patient has a strong history of environmental exposure, and the diagnosis is confirmed by serologic testing or poly-merase chain reaction. Electrocardiography may show evidence of conduction system disease including right bundle branch block or left anterior fasicular block. Echocardiography or contrast ventriculography may reveal a left ventricular apical aneurysm, regional wall motion abnormalities, or diffuse cardiomyopathy.

There is no specific treatment for Chagas cardiomyopathy, the best treatment is the institution of preventive measures. Improvements in housing and the use of pesticides may eradicate the reduviid bugs that transmit the disease, thus reducing infection and disease rates. Antiparisitic treatments directed against T. cruzi may eradicate the disease in acute or subacute infection. Congestive heart failure can be managed symptomatically with ACE inhibitors at high doses, diuretics and digoxin. Ventricular arrhythmias may respond to electrophysiology guided treatments. Although heart transplantation for Chagas cardiomy-

Table 5.   Hypersensitivity Myocarditis

Drug	Symptoms	Mode of death	Pathology
Methyldopa	Shortness of breath, malaise, headache, fever, cerebro-vascular accident	Sudden	Myocarditis, vasculitis, hepatitis
Sulfonamides (sulfadiazine, sulfisoxazole, sulfamethoxypyrid-azine, carbutamide)	Fever, shortness of breath	Sudden	Myocarditis, petechial hemor-rhages, vasculitis, granulomas
Penicillin, ampicillin	Rash, congestive heart failure	Sudden	Myocarditis, granulomas, pericarditis, myocardial infarction
Phenylbutazone	Shortness of breath, fever, rash, chest pain, hypo-tension	Sudden	Myocarditis, hepatitis, myo-cardial giant cells, perivascular granulomas, fibrinoid degenera-tion, pericarditis
Oxyphenbutazone	Congestive heart failure	Sudden	Myocarditis
Chlortetracycline	Fever, tachycardia		Interstitial and perivascular infiltrates
Chloramphenicol		Sudden	Myocarditis, hepatitis
Streptomycin	Chest pain, fever, rash	Sudden	Myocarditis, petechial hemor-rhage, pericardial effusion
p-Aminosalicylic acid	Heart failure, hypotension, ventricular irritability		
Phenytoin	Epistaxis	Sudden	Myocarditis
Carbamazepine	Jaundice, fever, rash	Sudden	Myocarditis
Indomethacin	Cardiac arrest, fever	Brain damage	Myocarditis
Spironolactone with hydrochlorothiazide	Low back pain, fever	Sudden	Myocarditis
Acetazolamide	Fever, rash	Uremia	Myocarditis, hepatitis
Amitriptyline		Sudden	Myocarditis
Phenindione			Myocarditis
Interleukin-2	Congestive heart failure; may occur within days after therapy initiated		Myocarditis

opathy has been successfully performed, reactivation of *Trypanosoma cruzi* is common.

HIV Myocarditis

Myocarditis is the most common cardiac pathologic finding at autopsy of HIV-infected patients with a prevalence as high as 70%. HIV-associated myocarditis is often characterized by a focal nonspecific myocardial infiltrate in the presence of left ventricular dysfunction. HIV1-RNA has also been detected in the myocardial tissue of patients with acquired immunodeficiency syndrome (AIDS). A prospective study of asymptomatic HIV-positive patients showed a mean annual incidence of progression to dilated cardiomyopathy of 15.9 cases per 1,000 patients. However, the pathogenesis of myocarditis and left ventricular dysfunction in immunocompromised patients is unclear, as the myocardial inflammation could be secondary to HIV itself, other opportunistic viruses and coinfections, or even due to the medications used in treatment. The prognosis for HIV-associated myocarditis is significantly poorer than that of lymphocytic myocarditis, and in a large cardiomyopathy cohort, HIV-related myocarditis was the strongest predictor of death.

Table 6.   Causes of Various Histopathologic Forms of Myocarditis in Biopsy Tissues

Lymphocytic	Eosinophilic
Idiopathic	Idiopathic
Viral syndrome	Hypereosino-
Polymyositis	philia
Sarcoidosis	Restrictive car-
Lyme disease	diomyopathy
Mucocutaneous	Churg-Strauss
lymph node	syndrome
syndrome	Parasitic infesta-
(Kawasaki disease)	tions
Acquired immuno-	Drug hypersen-
deficiency syndrome	sitivity
Mycoplasma pneumoniae	
Drug toxicity	
Neutrophilic or mixed	**Giant cell or granu-**
Bacterial infection	**lomatous**
Acute drug toxicity	Idiopathic
Infarction	Sarcoidosis
	Infective
	Rheumatoid
	Rheumatic
	Drug hypersensi-
	tivity
	Foreign body
	reaction

Table 7.   Clinical Presentation of North American Patients With Chagas Heart Disease

Feature	Patients No.	%
Atrioventricular block	9	21
Congestive heart failure	8	19
Chest pain	6	14
Conduction abnormality on ECG	8	19
Aborted sudden death	3	7
Sustained ventricular tachy-cardia	3	7
Embolic event	3	7
Other	2	5
Total	42	

ECG, electrocardiography.

95

DILATED CARDIOMYOPATHY

Horng H. Chen, MD

Cardiomyopathy is an important topic to review for cardiology examinations; special attention should be paid to the physical signs and possible causes of dilated cardiomyopathy. The diagnosis and management of heart failure, myocarditis, and systolic and diastolic ventricular function are reviewed elsewhere in this book.

The American Heart Association (AHA) published a scientific statement in April 2006, "Contemporary definitions and classification of the cardiomyopathies." Prior to this AHA scientific statement, the most widely accepted definition and classification of cardiomyopathies was developed by the World Health Organization [WHO]/International Society and Federation of Cardiology in 1995.

DEFINITION OF CARDIOMYOPATHIES

<u>WHO definition</u>: Cardiomyopathies are diseases of heart muscle associated with cardiac dysfunction

<u>AHA definition</u>: Cardiomyopathies are a heterogeneous group of diseases of the myocardium associated with mechanical and/or electrical dysfunction that usually (but not invariably) exhibit inappropriate ventricular hypertrophy or dilatation and are due to a variety of causes that frequently are genetic. Cardiomyopathies either are confined to the heart or are part of generalized systemic disorders, often leading to cardiovascular death or progressive heart failure–related disability.

CLASSIFICATION OF CARDIOMYOPATHIES

<u>WHO classification</u>: Cardiomyopathies are classified as either dilated cardiomyopathy (DCM) or hypertrophic cardiomyopathy (HCM) on the basis of ventricular morphology; or as restrictive cardiomyopathy (RCM) primarily on the basis of a characteristic hemodynamic pathophysiology; arrhythmogenic right ventricular dysplasia (a rare type of cardiomyopathy associated with sudden death in young patients); and unclassified cardiomyopathies. Specific cardiomyopathies refer to heart muscle diseases that are associated with specific cardiac or systemic diseases.

<u>AHA classification</u>: Cardiomyopathies are divided into 2 major groups based on predominant organ involvement. <u>Primary cardiomyopathies</u>: genetic, nongenetic or acquired, and solely or predominantly confined to heart muscle (Fig. 1). <u>Secondary cardiomyopathies</u> show pathological myocardial involvement as part of a large number and variety of generalized systemic (multiorgan) disorders (Table 1). These systemic diseases associated with secondary forms of cardiomyopathy have previously been referred to as "specific cardiomyopathies" or "specific heart muscle diseases" in the WHO classifications.

PREVALENCE OF CARDIOMYOPATHY

DCM is the most common type of cardiomyopathy,

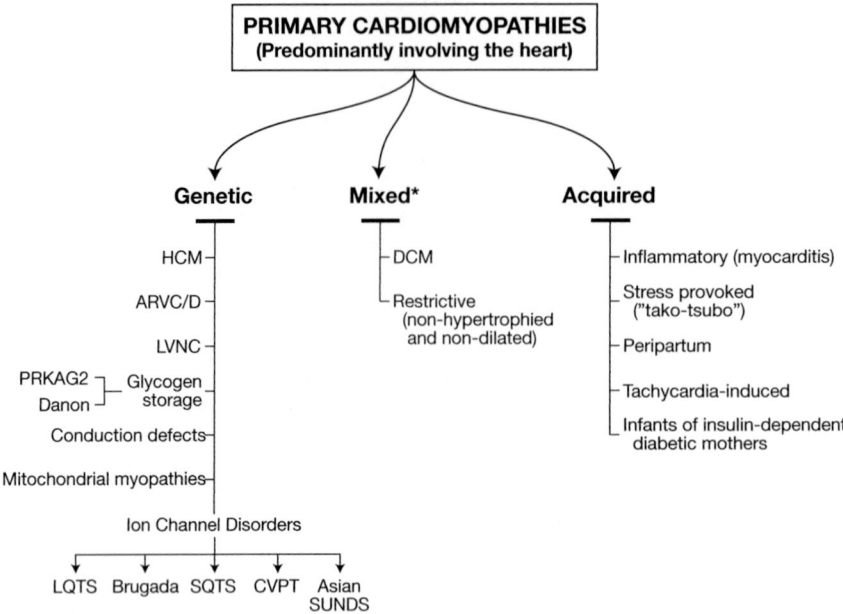

Fig. 1. Classification of primary cardiomyopathies.

with an estimated prevalence in the general population of 40 to 50 cases per 100,000. HCM is about one-fifth as common, and RCM and arrhythmogenic right ventricular dysplasia are extremely rare.

CHARACTERISTIC FEATURES OF CARDIOMYOPATHIES

The characteristic features of each of the main types of cardiomyopathy can readily be identified with two-dimensional and Doppler echocardiography on the basis of chamber size, wall thickness, and systolic and diastolic function of the left ventricle (Table 2).

DCM consists of an enlarged left ventricular cavity with depressed systolic function. HCM is characterized by a small-to-normal size left ventricular cavity, massive hypertrophy of the myocardium, and hyperdynamic systolic function. The major abnormality in RCM is diastolic dysfunction.

It is important to remember that there is some overlap among the types of cardiomyopathies. End-stage HCM may exhibit ventricular dilatation and have features of both HCM and DCM. Some cases of HCM in which the ventricular walls are only mildly thickened may mimic the restrictive hemodynamic profile of RCM. RCM may also exhibit some degree

of ventricular dilatation; this is referred to as "minimally dilated restrictive cardiomyopathy." Although each type of cardiomyopathy has a pure form, some degree of clinical overlap can exist among these entities.

DILATED CARDIOMYOPATHY

Definition

The WHO defined dilated cardiomyopathy as myocardial disease "characterized by dilatation and impaired contraction of the left ventricle or both left and right ventricles. It may be idiopathic, familial/genetic, viral and/or immune, alcoholic/toxic, or associated with recognized cardiovascular disease in which the degree of myocardial dysfunction is not explained by the abnormal loading conditions or the extent of ischemic damage. The histologic findings are frequently nonspecific. Presentation is usually with heart failure, which is often progressive. Arrhythmias, thromboembolism, and sudden death are common and may occur at any stage."

Features

The macroscopic pathologic features of DCM are distinct and almost identical in all patients: four-chamber dilatation is usual and thrombi are frequent in the

Table 1.   Secondary Cardiomyopathies

Infiltrative*
  Amyloidosis (primary, familial autosomal
    dominant,† senile, secondary forms)
  Gaucher disease†
  Hurler's disease†
  Hunter's disease†
Storage‡
  Hemochromatosis
  Fabry's disease†
  Glycogen storage disease† (type II, Pompe)
  Niemann-Pick disease†
Toxicity
  Drugs, heavy metals, chemical agents
Endomyocardial
  Endomyocardial fibrosis
  Hypereosinophilic syndrome (Löffler's
    endocarditis)
Inflammatory (granulomatous)
  Sarcoidosis
Endocrine
  Diabetes mellitus†
  Hyperthyroidism
  Hypothyroidism
  Hyperparathyroidism
  Pheochromocytoma
  Acromegaly
Cardiofacial
  Noonan syndrome†
  Lentiginosis†
Neuromuscular/neurological
  Friedreich's ataxia†
  Duchenne-Becker muscular dystrophy†
  Emery-Dreifuss muscular dystrophy†
  Myotonic dystrophy†
  Neurofibromatosis†
  Tuberous sclerosis†
Nutritional deficiencies
  Beriberi (thiamine), pallagra, scurvy, selenium,
    carnitine, kwashiorkor
Autoimmune/collagen
  Systemic lupus erythematosis
  Dermatomyositis
  Rheumatoid arthritis
  Scleroderma
  Polyarteritis nodosa
Electrolyte imbalance

Table 1 (continued)

Consequence of cancer therapy
  Anthracyclines: doxorubicin (Adriamycin),
    daunorubicin
  Cyclophosphamide
  Radiation

---

*Accumulation of abnormal substances between
  myocytes (ie, extracellular).
†Genetic (familial) origin.
‡Accumulation of abnormal substances within
  myocytes (ie, intracellular).

apices of both ventricular chambers. Left ventricular wall thickness is entirely normal, but left ventricular mass is markedly increased in tandem with the increased ventricular diastolic dimension. There also is a concomitant increase in right ventricular size. In clinical practice, patients may present in the early stage of the disease with only left ventricular dilatation, followed later by left atrial dilatation, and finally with dilatation of all four cardiac chambers. Right ventricular dilatation in DCM carries a poor prognosis. DCM occurs more frequently in males than females (about 3:1) and is more common in African Americans than in whites (the ratio is about 2.5:1). Patients with DCM frequently have a history of an increase in alcohol intake and systemic hypertension. Echocardiographically, DCM has similar features in all patients: marked dilatation of the left ventricular cavity, normal wall thickness, and globally reduced systolic function. Regional wall motion abnormalities can be superimposed on DCM even if no flow-limiting coronary disease is present. Regional wall motion abnormalities do not exclude a diagnosis of idiopathic DCM. Anginal pain does not occur in DCM, and its presence should lead to a search for coronary artery disease.

■ Regional wall motion abnormalities do not exclude a diagnosis of idiopathic DCM.

Etiology of Dilated Cardiomyopathy

The most important causes of DCM are listed in Table 3. It is important to remember the reversible forms of heart disease that may mimic idiopathic DCM. One of

Table 2. Comparison of Dilated, Hypertrophic, and Restrictive Cardiomyopathies

Feature	Dilated	Hyper- trophic	Restrictive
Cavity size	Enlarged	Small	Normal
Wall thick- ness	Normal	Marked	Normal
Systolic function	Severely depressed	Hyper- dynamic	Normal/ reduced
Diastolic function	Abnormal	Abnormal	Abnormal
Other		Outflow tract obstruction	

Table 3. Important Causes of Dilated Cardiomyopathy

Post-chemotherapy (doxorubicin)
Acquired immunodeficiency syndrome
Infiltrative disease (hemochromatosis)
Peripartum cardiomyopathy
Associated with muscular dystrophy
Tachycardia-induced
Alcohol-induced

these is tachycardia-induced cardiomyopathy, which may be seen in patients with recurrent supraventricular tachycardia or atrial fibrillation of long duration. By treating the arrhythmia, left ventricular dysfunction can be reversed. Patients with very frequent premature ventricular contractions may also develop left ventricular dysfunction. Successful suppression of the premature ventricular contractions may allow ventricular function to normalize. Hibernating myocardium is another cause of cardiac dysfunction.

Infiltrative diseases, in particular hemochromatosis, may cause a DCM that improves with reduction in iron overload. In spite of being an infiltrative cardiomyopathy, hemochromatosis does not produce thickened ventricular walls as amyloidosis does. Phlebotomy performed weekly in patients with hemochromatosis-induced cardiomyopathy results in marked improvement of ventricular function and decrease in left ventricular size. In contrast, amyloid heart disease, another infiltrative disease, is not reversible.

■ In patients with a dilated, poorly functioning left ventricle, always check the serum levels of iron and ferritin, a fat aspirate for amyloid, and protein electrophoresis.

The incidence of a familial form of DCM is up to 20% of all cases of DCM. Family members of patients

with DCM should have echocardiographic screening even if asymptomatic.

The prognostic factors in DCM predictive of poor survival are listed in Table 4.

OTHER CARDIOMYOPATHIES*

Ischemic cardiomyopathy presents as dilated cardiomyopathy with impaired contractile performance not explained by the extent of coronary artery disease or ischemic damage.

Valvular cardiomyopathy presents with ventricular dysfunction that is out of proportion to the abnormal loading conditions.

Hypertensive cardiomyopathy often presents with left ventricular hypertrophy in association with features of dilated or restrictive cardiomyopathy with cardiac failure.

Inflammatory cardiomyopathy is defined by myocarditis in association with cardiac dysfunction. Myocarditis is an inflammatory disease of the myocardium and is diagnosed by established histologic, immunologic, and immunohistochemical criteria. Idiopathic, autoimmune, and infectious forms of inflammatory cardiomyopathy are recognized. Inflammatory myocardial disease is involved in the pathogenesis of dilated cardiomyopathy and other cardiomyopathies (e.g., Chagas disease, human immunodeficiency virus, enterovirus, adenovirus, and cytomegalovirus).

Metabolic cardiomyopathy includes the following categories: endocrine (e.g., thyrotoxicosis, hypothyroidism, adrenal cortical insufficiency, pheochromocytoma, acromegaly, and diabetes mellitus), familial storage

Table 4. Prognostic Factors in Dilated
Cardiomyopathy That Predict Poor
Survival

Abnormal ventricular function
  Decreased ejection fraction is the most power-
    ful prognostic indicator in dilated cardiomy-
    opathy
  Increased left ventricular size (assessed by the
    cardiothoracic ratio on chest radiography or,
    more accurately, by left ventricular end-
    diastolic dimension on echocardiography)
  Right ventricular dilatation is an independent
    predictor of poor survival in cardiomyopathy
Functional class
  Poor New York Heart Association functional
    class
  Maximal oxygen uptake <12 mL/kg per
    minute on cardiopulmonary exercise testing
Electrocardiography
  Left bundle branch block
  Asymptomatic nonsustained ventricular
    tachycardia
Clinical features
  Clinical left or right heart failure
  Syncope
Endocrine activation and electrolyte levels
  Hyponatremia (serum sodium concentration
    <135 mmol/L)
  Increased plasma concentrations of
    norepinephrine, atrial natriuretic factor, and
    renin
Hemodynamic
  High (>18 to 20 mm Hg) left ventricular end-
    diastolic pressure or pulmonary capillary
    wedge pressure used as a surrogate for left
    ventricular end-diastolic pressure
  Low cardiac output (cardiac index <2.5 L/min
    per m^2)
  Pulmonary hypertension (pulmonary artery
    systolic pressure >35 mm Hg)
Cardiac biopsy
  Loss of intracellular cardiac myofilaments
  Persistence of enteroviral RNA

disease and infiltrations (e.g., hemochromatosis, glycogen storage disease, Hurler syndrome, Refsum syndrome, Niemann-Pick disease, Hand-Schüller-Christian disease, Fabry-Anderson disease, and Morquio-Ullrich disease), deficiency (e.g., disturbances of potassium metabolism, magnesium deficiency, and nutritional disorders such as kwashiorkor, anemia, beri-beri, and selenium deficiency), amyloid (e.g., primary, secondary, familial, and hereditary cardiac amyloidoses), familial Mediterranean fever, and senile amyloidosis.

General systemic diseases include connective tissue disorders (e.g., systemic lupus erythematosus, polyarteritis nodosa, rheumatoid arthritis, scleroderma, and dermatomyositis). Infiltrations and granulomas include sarcoidosis and leukemia.

Muscular dystrophies include Duchenne, Becker-type, and myotonic dystrophies.

Neuromuscular disorders include Friedreich ataxia, Noonan syndrome, and lentiginosis.

Sensitivity and toxic reactions include reactions to alcohol, catecholamines, anthracyclines, irradiation, and miscellaneous. Alcoholic cardiomyopathy is associated with heavy alcohol intake. Currently, we cannot define a causal versus a conditioning role of alcohol or apply precise diagnostic criteria.

Peripartal cardiomyopathy may first manifest in the peripartum period. This is probably a heterogeneous group.

Arrhythmogenic Right Ventricular Dysplasia: cardiomyopathy characterized by progressive fibrofatty replacement of the right ventricle, ventricular arrhythmias, and sudden death at a relatively young age. Autosomal dominance with incomplete penetrance is common

Stress ("Tako-Tsubo") Cardiomyopathy: stress cardiomyopathy, first reported in Japan, is a recently described clinical entity characterized by acute but rapidly reversible LV systolic dysfunction in the absence of atherosclerotic coronary artery disease, preferentially involves the distal portion of the left ventricle ("apical ballooning") and triggered by profound psychological stress.

(*This section is from Richardson P, McKenna W, Bristow M, et al. Report of the 1995 World Health Organization/International Society and Federation of Cardiology Task Force on the Definition and Classification of cardiomyopathies. Circulation. 1996;93:841-2. Used with permission.)

RESTRICTIVE CARDIOMYOPATHY

Sudhir S. Kushwaha, MD

DEFINITION AND ETIOLOGY

Restrictive cardiomyopathy (RCM) is defined as myocardial disease that results in impaired ventricular filling with normal or reduced diastolic volume of either or both ventricles with normal or near-normal systolic function and wall thickness. The condition usually results from increased stiffness of the myocardium that causes pressure within the ventricles to rise precipitously with only small increases in volume. RCM can affect either or both ventricles and so may cause symptoms or signs of right or left ventricular failure. Often, right sided findings may predominate, with elevated jugular venous pressure, peripheral edema, and ascites. When the left ventricle is affected, there are symptoms of breathlessness and evidence of pulmonary edema, usually with normal cardiac dimensions. The diagnosis should therefore be considered in a patient with heart failure but no evidence of cardiomegaly or systolic dysfunction. The importance of an accurate diagnosis lies in distinguishing RCM from constrictive pericarditis, which can also present with "restrictive physiology" but which is often possible to cure surgically.

RCM is the least common of the cardiomyopathies. Outside the tropics, cardiac amyloidosis is the most thoroughly studied. Endomyocardial fibrosis is endemic in parts of Africa, Central America and Asia and occurs sporadically throughout the world. There are a variety of local and systemic disorders which may cause the condition (Table 1), many of which may not be encountered in clinical practice. Conditions such as amyloidosis are more common and may present with congestive heart failure. In idiopathic RCM, the hemodynamic abnormalities occur in the absence of specific histopathological changes.

PATHOGENESIS AND NATURAL HISTORY

Idiopathic RCM

Idiopathic RCM may be familial and associated with a distal skeletal myopathy and atrioventricular block. There may be a genetic predisposition although some cases are sporadic and the result of spontaneous mutation. In childhood, idiopathic RCM may be more common in girls and have a worse prognosis, with a median survival of only one year. The clinical course is more variable in adults and most small series suggest a protracted clinical course. The condition is characterized by a mild to moderate increase in cardiac weight. Biatrial enlargement is common with thrombi often present in the atrial appendages. Systolic function tends to be preserved or may be mildly reduced and ventricular size tends to be normal. Depending on the degree of pulmonary hypertension, the right ventricle may become

Table 1.   Causes of Restrictive Cardiomyopathy

Primary (idiopathic) restrictive cardiomyopathy
Eosinophilic endomyocardial disease and endomy-
     ocardial fibrosis
Infiltrative cardiomyopathies
     Amyloid heart disease
     Hemochromatosis
     Glycogen storage disease
     Fabry disease
     Mucopolysaccharidoses
     Sarcoidosis
Scleroderma
Post-heart transplantation
Post-mediastinal irradiation
Pseudoxanthoma elasticum
Doxorubicin and daunorubicin chemotherapy
Carcinoid heart disease
Malignant disease with encasement of the heart
     from pericardial metastases
Associated with the eosinophilia-myalgia
     syndrome due to toxic contamination of
     L-tryptophan dietary supplements

enlarged. On microscopy, the pericardium is normal and patchy interstitial fibrosis may be present. If fibrosis affects the conducting system, complete heart block may occur which requires permanent pacing.

Amyloidosis

Cardiac involvement with amyloid is more common in primary amyloidosis, caused by the production of immunoglobulin light chains by plasma cells, often due to multiple myeloma. It can also occur with familial amyloidosis. RCM results from injury to tissue due to replacement of normal myocardium with infiltrative interstitial deposits (Fig. 1). Abnormalities of diastolic filling can occur even in the absence of clinical evidence of RCM. Patients with cardiac amyloid may also present with angina. The presence of RCM in amyloid is strongly predictive of a poor prognosis, with 55% of patients dying of arrhythmia or cardiac failure. Amyloid infiltration of the heart is common in the elderly, as well as in patients with chronic heart diseases, such as rheumatic or congenital disease. Cardiac amyloid can be

characterized by analyzing endomyocardial biopsy tissue and immunohistochemical staining may help in distinguishing the various types.

The myocardium of patients with cardiac amyloidosis is firm and noncompliant, with small or dilated ventricular cavities and thrombi in the atrial appendages. Typically there is interstitial deposition of insoluble amyloid fibrils in all four cardiac chambers which can result in increased wall thickness without cavity dilatation. The pericardium, cardiac valves, and the coronary arteries may also be involved. The left-ventricular wall thickness is one of the prognostic variables. In patients with normal wall thickness, the survival may be up to 2.4 years but only a few months in those with markedly increased wall thickness. Increased wall thickness is also correlated with the characteristic granular sparkling appearance seen on 2-D echocardiography (Fig. 2). Abnormalities of diastolic filling can also occur and may also be predictive of decreased survival.

Amyloid deposits can be found in the conducting system, and as a result a variety of cardiac arrhythmias can occur, including complex ventricular arrhythmias. Frequently a combination of atrial fibrillation with low voltage on ECG and a slow ventricular response is seen. A classic scenario typical for cardiac amyloidosis involves a patient with atrial fibrillation and low voltage on the ECG undergoing pacemaker placement, and difficulty finding a spot in the right ventricle with adequate pacing thresholds. The severity of arrhythmias tends to be correlated with the severity of heart failure and abnormalities seen on echocardiography. Depending on the stage of the disease, the patient can present with some combination of asymmetric septal thickening, angina, heart failure, abnormal diastolic function, and a reduced ejection fraction.

Other Infiltrative and Storage Diseases

A number of infiltrative conditions can result in RCM. Gaucher's disease and related syndromes can result in the accumulation of cerebroside in a number of organs including the heart (Fig. 3). Hurler's syndrome leads to a RCM due to the deposition of mucopolysaccharide in the myocardium as well as the cardiac valves and coronary arteries. Patients with Fabry's disease can also present with RCM.

Cardiac sarcoidosis may initially present with impaired diastolic function with normal systolic function.

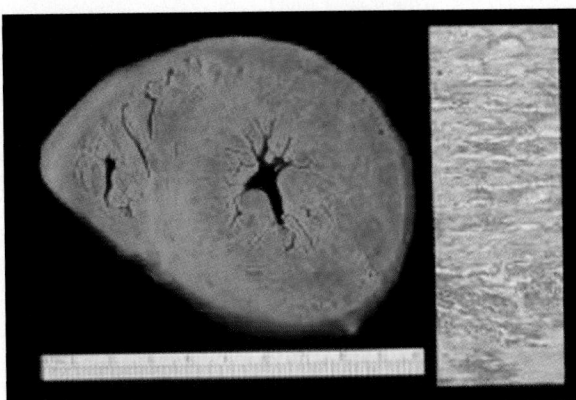

Fig. 1. Amyloid simulating hypertrophic cardiomyopathy (HCM) (675 g heart).

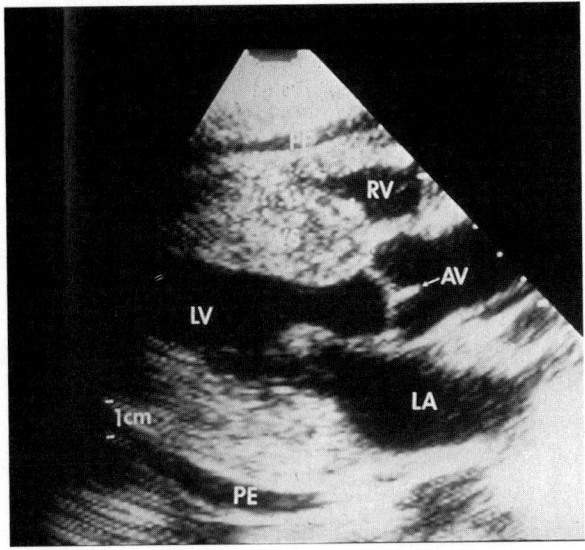

Fig. 2. Echocardiogram of amyloid heart disease with abnormal myocardial texture ("scintillating granular myocardium") and wall thickening. AV, aortic valve; LV, left ventricle; LA, left atrium; PE, pericardial effusion; RA, right atrium; RV, right ventricle

Subsequent injury and fibrosis can result in systolic dysfunction resulting in diffuse hypokinesis as well as regional wall motion abnormalities. In patients with systemic sarcoidosis the myocardium may be involved resulting in subclinical cardiac dysfunction. Cardiac sarcoidosis may present with sudden death or high degree atrioventricular block due to involvement of the conducting system. Endomyocardial biopsy may be useful in the diagnosis of cardiac sarcoidosis (Fig. 4), although a negative biopsy does not rule out the diagnosis.

Endomyocardial Fibrosis and Eosinophilic Endomyocardial Disease

Endomyocardial fibrosis and Löffler's endocarditis (eosinophilic cardiomyopathy) are different manifestations of restrictive obliterative cardiomyopathy, both associated with eosinophilia (Fig. 5). Severe prolonged eosinophilia of any cause (allergic, autoimmune, parasitic, leukemic, or idiopathic) can lead to eosinophilic infiltration of the myocardium which can lead to decreased myocardial compliance. Eosinophilic degranulation results in myocardial damage through the action of major basic and cationic proteins. This disease, also called Löffler syndrome, in its late stages is associated with dense endomyocardial fibrosis, intraventricular thrombus formation, and obliteration of the ventricular cavity. Occasionally the fibrosis may be localized and produces valvular regurgitation or stenosis which can be treated with valve replacement. The eosinophilia-myalgia syndrome associated with the use of tryptophan containing a contaminant resulted in RCM, suggesting

that eosinophilia may have been responsible for the RCM. End-stage cardiac structure is similar to that of a condition called "endomyocardial fibrosis" found almost exclusively in equatorial Africa and, less frequently, in Asia and South America.

Tropical endomyocardial fibrosis is a common form of RCM that occurs in equatorial Africa, Asia, and South America. Because most patients with this condition also have heavy parasite loads, it was thought for many years that endomyocardial fibrosis represented an end stage of eosinophilic endomyocardial disease in response to an allergic/immune reaction to parasitosis. This is now considered incorrect because patients with the tropical form of endomyocardial fibrosis do not exhibit eosinophilia. The prognosis for endomyocardial fibrosis is poor, but surgical removal of fibrotic disease and valve repair or replacement may be helpful. The disease may have an insidious onset with development of right or left sided cardiac failure. Sudden death and syncopal episodes are not common in endomyocardial fibrosis compared with other causes of RCM. Atrial fibrillation does occur. Other ECG abnormalities include low QRS voltage, first degree AV block and left atrial enlargement. Echocardiographically, endocardial

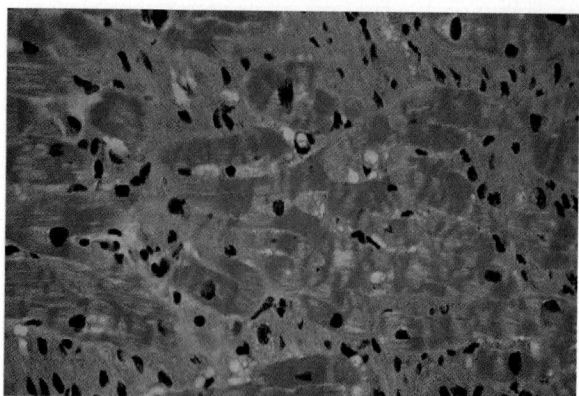

Fig. 3. Gaucher's disease (right ventricle (RV bx.).

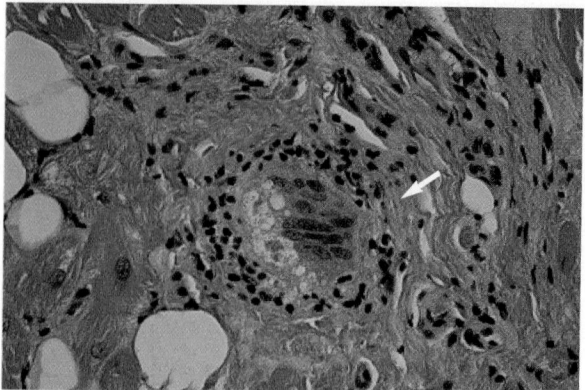

Fig. 4. Cardiac sarcoidosis with solitary granuloma (right ventricle RV bx.).

deposition of thrombus with apical obliteration and mitral regurgitation may be observed. Systemic or pulmonary emboli are uncommon.

Clinical Presentation of Restrictive Cardiomyopathy

The underlying cause of RCM may not be obvious on presentation. Symptoms include dyspnea, paroxysmal dyspnea, orthopnea, peripheral edema, and ascites, as well as general fatigue and weakness. Angina does not occur except in amyloidosis, in which it may be the presenting symptom. In advanced cases, all the signs of heart failure may be present except cardiomegaly. The findings may resemble those of severe constrictive pericarditis. Up to one third of patients with idiopathic

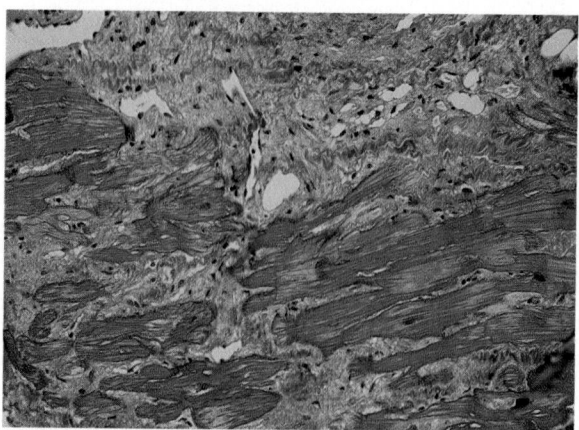

Fig. 5. Right ventricular endomyocardial biopsy specimen showing eosinophilic restrictive cardiomyopathy (16% eosinophils).

RCM may present with thromboembolic complications. In amyloidosis and sarcoidosis, cardiac conduction disturbances are particularly common. Atrial fibrillation is common in idiopathic RCM and cardiac amyloidosis. In the elderly, RCM remains a diagnosis of exclusion, but it should be differentiated from age-related changes in diastolic compliance.

Diagnostic Evaluation

The initial diagnostic approach should attempt to rule out constrictive pericarditis, which results in clinical signs and symptoms similar to those of RCM, as described below.

The physical examination is remarkable for increased venous pressure with rapid x and y descents if sinus rhythm is present, but the most prominent wave is the y descent. The jugular venous pulse fails to fall during inspiration and may actually rise (Kussmaul's sign). Peripheral edema and ascites are present in advanced cases, and the liver may be enlarged and pulsatile. The carotid upstroke may be low volume and sinus tachycardia may be present, consistent with a low output state. The left ventricular systolic impulse is usually normal. The first and second heart sounds are usually normal with normal splitting of the second heart sound. The pulmonary component of the second heart sound is not accentuated. There may be a third heart sound that is right or left ventricular in origin and less commonly a fourth heart sound. The precordium is usually normal. Murmurs of mitral and/or tricuspid valve regurgitation may be present.

The chest radiograph shows that heart size is usually normal. Atrial enlargement may be present, particularly if there is atrioventricular valvular regurgitation. Pulmonary congestion may be seen, as well as interstitial edema, with Kerly B lines. Pleural effusions may also occur. The ECG shows nonspecific ST and T wave abnormalities. Depolarization abnormalities may also be present as well as bundle branch block, atrioventricular block or findings of ventricular hypertrophy.

One should consider serum protein electrophoresis, iron studies, ACE levels, and appropriate parasitic screening if the history and clinical findings are suggestive.

Echocardiography in Restrictive Cardiomyopathy

The imaging modality of choice for diagnosing RCM is echocardiography. In most instances, a two-dimensional echocardiogram shows normal left ventricular size and function and marked dilatation of both atria (Fig. 6). The wall thickness in idiopathic RCM is usually normal, while cases of infiltrative disease causing RCM (amyloidosis) may have increased wall thickness. Doppler echocardiography shows features of a restrictive filling pattern, indicating a marked decrease in chamber compliance. There is an increased early diastolic filling velocity (≥1.0 m per second), decreased atrial filling velocity (≤0.5 m per second), an increased ratio of early diastolic filling to atrial filling (≥2), a decreased deceleration time (≤150 msec), and a decreased isovolumic relaxation time (≤70 ms). There is a high E/A ratio, with a short deceleration time on the mitral inflow velocities, indicating an abrupt cessation of ventricular filling, and as a low systolic-to-diastolic flow ratio of the pulmonary venous flow velocities. Evidence of moderate pulmonary hypertension is usually present.

Cardiac Catheterization in Restrictive Cardiomyopathy (Fig. 7)

The characteristic hemodynamic feature is a deep and rapid early decline in ventricular pressure at the onset of diastole, with a rapid rise to a plateau in early diastole. This is the dip and plateau square-root sign, manifested in the atrial-pressure tracing as a prominent y descent followed by a rapid rise to a plateau. The right atrial pressure is elevated, as in constrictive pericarditis, and the y descent may become deeper during inspiration. Although the right ventricular pressure may be elevated, the diastolic hypertension is usually more prominent

with mean right atrial pressures of 15 to 20 mm Hg. The left ventricular diastolic pressure has the same wave form as the right ventricular diastolic pressure, and although it may be 5 mm Hg higher than the right ventricular pressure, the value may be the same. This difference may be accentuated by exercise.

Distinction Between RCM and Constrictive Pericarditis

Constrictive pericarditis (CP) is more likely with a clinical history of pericarditis. A history of tuberculosis may suggest CP, particularly in non-industrialized nations. CP may also follow trauma, cardiac surgical procedures, radiation therapy as well as acute pericarditis, with CP appearing years later. Although rare, some causes of RCM may also lead to CP, including sarcoidosis and amyloidosis. Table 2 summarizes the important differences between the two conditions. No technique is completely reliable and sometimes the only way to make the diagnosis may be to perform pericardectomy.

TREATMENT OF RESTRICTIVE CARDIOMYOPATHY

Symptomatic Therapy

Diuretics are used to treat pulmonary and systemic venous congestion, but they have to be used with caution because their excessive use may result in the reduction of ventricular filling pressures and a consequent decrease in cardiac output with symptoms and signs of hypotension and hypoperfusion. Digoxin is usually not recommended because it is potentially arrhythmogenic, particularly in patients with amyloidosis. It is important to try and maintain sinus rhythm. The development of atrial fibrillation with removal of the atrial contribution to ventricular filling may worsen existing diastolic dysfunction and this may be further compromised by a rapid ventricular response. Advanced conduction system disease may need to be treated with implantation of a pacemaker. In RCM, stroke volume tends to be fixed so the development of bradyarrhythmias can precipitate cardiac failure, so the heart rate will need to be supported. For this reason, calcium channel blockers and beta-blockers are also not helpful. Malignant ventricular arrhythmias which are a frequent mode of presentation in cardiac sarcoidosis may need to be treated with an implantable defibrillator system with a pacemaker.

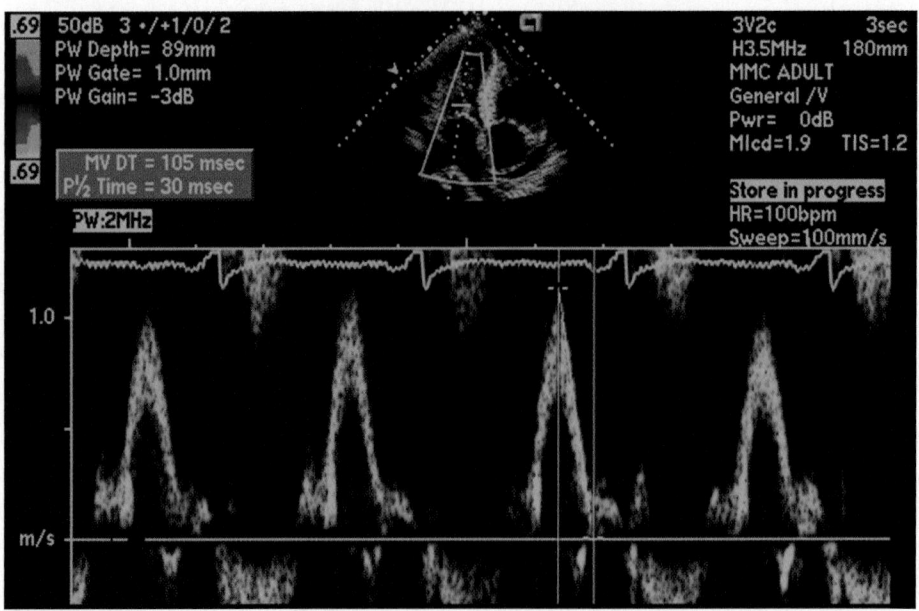

Fig. 6. Characteristic restrictive inflow profile by Doppler echocardiography in patient with restrictive cardiomyopathy. The inflow profile demonstrates increased peak E velocity with rapid deceleration time and diminutive peak A velocity.

Because of the propensity for thrombus formation in the atrial appendage with risk of embolic complications, anticoagulation with warfarin is recommended in most patients.

SPECIFIC THERAPY

Cardiac Amyloidosis
Overall the prognosis tends to be poor, although chemotherapy may have benefits in terms of cardiac as

well as systemic manifestations in specific cases. In specialized centers cardiac transplantation has been performed with success. Without subsequent stem-cell transplant in primary amyloidosis or liver transplant in familial amyloidosis, recurrence will occur in the transplanted heart.

Endomyocardial Fibrosis and Eosinophilic Cardiomyopathy
Treatment with steroids and cytotoxic drugs may be helpful in the early stages of Löffler's endocarditis and

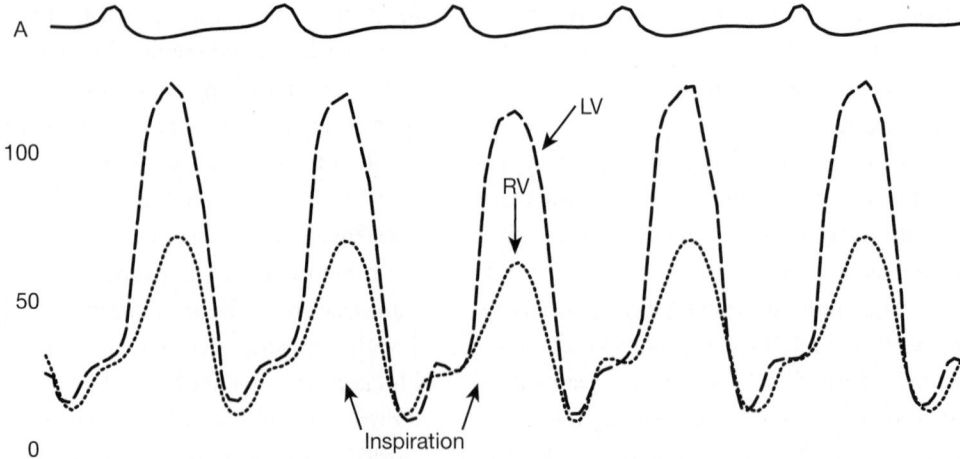

Fig. 7. Hemodynamic tracing of restrictive cardiomyopathy. LV, left ventricle; RV, right ventricle.

improves symptoms and survival. Surgical excision of the fibrotic endocardium and replacement of the mitral and tricuspid valves may also provide symptomatic relief in the fibrotic stage of the disease.

Other Conditions

The prognosis and complications of hemochromatosis depend on the degree of iron overload. This condition may respond to early treatment with venesection or iron-chelation therapy, with reversal of many of the hemodynamic abnormalities associated with heart failure in this condition. Combined heart and liver transplantation has been successful.

In idiopathic or familial RCM, cardiac transplantation has been successful and should be considered. Although transplantation may be an option for cardiac sarcoidosis, there tends to be recurrence in the transplanted heart.

Table 2.   The Differential Diagnosis of Restrictive Cardiomyopathy and Constrictive Pericarditis

Type of evaluation	Restrictive cardiomyopathy	Constrictive pericarditis
Physical examination	Kussmaul's sign may be present Apical impulse may be prominent S3 may be present, rarely S4 Regurgitant murmurs common	Kussmaul's sign usually present Apical impuse usually not palpable Pericardial knock may be present Regurgitant murmurs uncommon
Electrocardiography	Low voltage (especially in amyloidosis), pseudoinfarction, left-axis deviation, atrial fibrillation, conduction distrubances common	Low voltage (<50 percent)
Echocardiography	Increased wall thickness (especially thickened interatrial septum in amyloidosis) Thickened cardiac valves (amyloidosis) Granular sparkling texture (amyloid)	Normal wall thickness Pericardial thickening may be seen Prominent early diastolic filling with abrupt displacement of interventricular septum
Doppler studies	Decreased RV and LV velocities with inspiration Inspiratory augmentation of hepatic vein diastolic flow reversal Mitral and tricuspid regurgitation common	Increased RV systolic velocity and decreased LV systolic velocity with inspiration Expiratory augmentation of hepatic vein diastolic flow reversal
Cardiac catheterization	LVEDP often >5 mm Hg greater than RVEDP, but may be identical	RVEDP and LVEDP usually equal RV systolic pressure <50 mm Hg RVEDP >one third of RV systolic pressure
Endomyocardial biopsy	May reveal specific cause of restrictive cardiomyopathy	May be normal or show nonspecific myocyte hypertrophy or myocardial fibrosis
CT/MRI	Pericardium usually normal	Pericardium may be thickened

LV, left ventricular; RV, right ventricular; LVEDP, left ventricular end-diastolic pressure; RVEDP, right ventricular end-diastolic pressure; CT, computed tomography; MRI, magnetic resonance imaging.

97

HYPERTROPHIC CARDIOMYOPATHY

Steve Ommen, MD

DEFINITION

The World Health Organization (WHO) defined hypertrophic cardiomyopathy (HCM) as "left and/or right ventricular hypertrophy, which is usually asymmetric and involves the interventricular septum. Typically, the left ventricular volume is normal or reduced (Fig. 1). Intraventricular systolic gradients are common. Familial disease with autosomal dominant inheritance predominates, which in turn leads to mutations in sarcomeric contractile proteins. Typical morphological changes include myocyte hypertrophy and myocardial disarray. Arrhythmias and premature sudden death, while still infrequent, are more common than in the general population. HCM is also defined as inappropriate ventricular hypertrophy without a cardiac or systemic cause."

GENETIC ETIOLOGY

HCM is present in approximately 1:500 individuals; a rate that appears constant across many ethnic backgrounds. Mutations in the gene encoding for cardiac β-myosin heavy chain were the first to be associated definitively with HCM. To date, hundreds of mutations encoding for defects in at least 21 genes were recognized as responsible for HCM. The vast majority of these mutations involve the proteins of the cardiac sarcomere:

β-myosin heavy chain, myosin binding protein C, cardiac troponin T, cardiac troponin I, alpha tropomyosin, essential myosin light chain, regulatory myosin light chain, cardiac alpha actin, and titin (Table 1). These mutations are inherited in an autosomal dominant pattern. Mutations in other cellular structures (Z-disc, mitochondrial, etc) have also been described.

Evidence suggests that gene mutations alter sarcomeric function and secondarily lead to hypertrophy and fibrosis. Putative abnormalities include alteration of the protein structure, change in sensitivity to regulators such as calcium or adenosine triphosphate, impaired energy metabolism, and/or decrease in the force or velocity of myocyte contraction. Hypertrophy may thus be a compensatory mechanism for sarcomeric dysfunction. There may be other determinants or disease-modifying genetic polymorphisms that play a role in the extent and distribution of hypertrophy.

PATHOLOGY AND MORPHOLOGY OF HCM

The histologic hallmark of HCM is myocardial disarray consisting of short runs of severely hypertrophied fibers interrupted by connective tissue (Fig. 2). Disarray is noted not only in the ventricular septum but in all myocardial segments (Fig 3). Additional findings

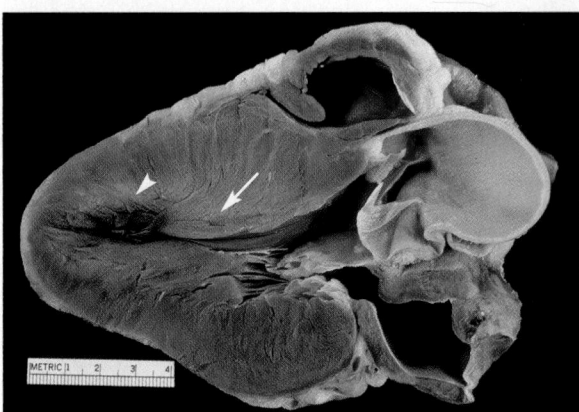

Fig. 1. Autopsy specimen of hypertrophic cardiomyopathy showing marked septal hypertrophy (*long arrow*), a small left ventricular cavity, and a moderately dilated left atrium. Subendocardial myocardial infarct (*arrowhead*).

include large and bizarre myocyte nuclei, fibrosis, and degenerating muscle fibers (Fig. 4). Another microscopic feature is intramyocardial fibrosis, an integral determinant of arrhythmogenesis and diastolic dysfunction. Finally, thrombosis and obliteration of the small vessels within the myocardium is observed, which can predispose to subendocardial ischemia.

While asymmetric hypertrophy of the basal to mid-ventricular septum is common, any pattern of left ventricular hypertrophy can be seen in HCM (Figs. 5-7). In addition to subaortic obstruction, there may be diffuse hypertrophy of the septum and papillary muscles at the midventricular level, resulting in combined midventricular obstruction. Endocardial plaque formation or thickening of the subaortic portion of the ventricular septum is frequently seen in the obstructive variant of the disease where the anterior mitral leaflet contacts the ventricular septum. The severity of hypertrophy is also highly variable (Fig. 8). The maximal left ventricular wall thickness is frequently measured between 20-30 mm, but can be in excess of 35-40 mm. Finally, abnormalities of mitral valve and its support structures are common in HCM. Elongation of the mitral leaflets and anterior displacement of the papillary muscles are common. Additionally, very short chordae tendineae, or direct insertion of the papillary muscle onto the mitral leaflets has been observed. The precise HCM variant present will determine the pathophysiologic findings.

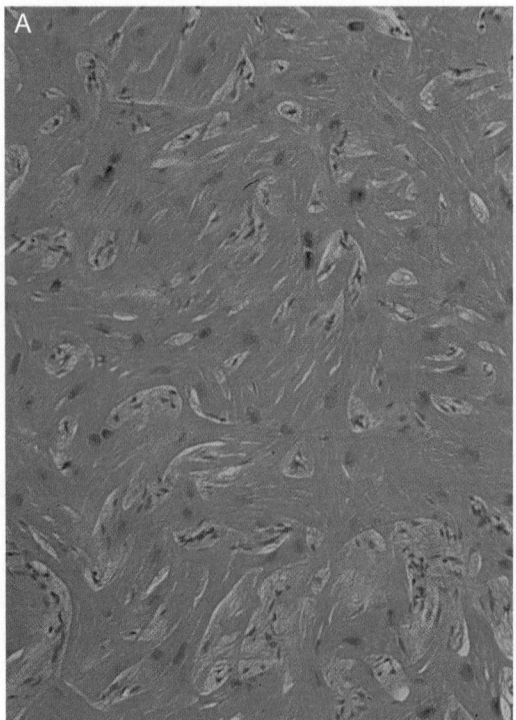
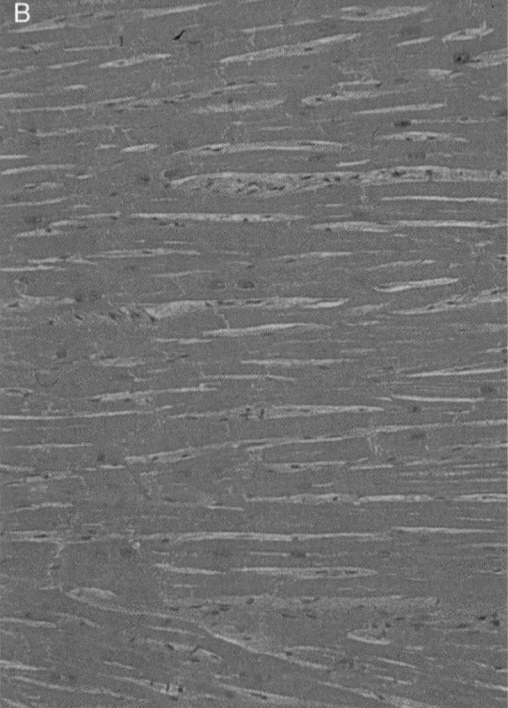

Fig. 2. *A*, myocardial disarray in hypertrophic cardiomyopathy compared with, *B*, normal myocardium.

Table 1. Frequency of Identified Chromosome and Protein Abnormalities in Hypertrophic Cardiomyopathy

Protein	Chromosome	Distribution
Cardiac myosin binding protein C (MYBPC3)	11	15-25
β-myosin heavy chain (MYH7)	14	15-25
α-myosin heavy chain (MYH6)	14	<1
Regulatory myosin light chain (MYL2)	12	<2
Essential myosin light chain (MYL3)	3	<1
Cardiac troponin T (TNNT2)	1	<5
Cardiac troponin I (TNNI3)	19	<5
α-tropomyosin (TPM1)	15	<5
Cardiac α-actin	15	<1
Titin (TTN)	2	<1
Muscle LIM protein (CSRP3)	11	<1
Telethonin (TCAP)	17	<1
Vinculin/metavinculin (VCL)	10	<1
Z-band alternatively spliced PDZ protein (ZASP/LBD3)	10	<5
α-actinin (ACTN2)	1	<1
Cardiac ryanodine receptor (RyR2)	1	<1
Junctophilin-2 (JPH2)	20	<1
AMP-activated protein kinase (PRKAG2)	7	<1
Lysosome-associated membrane protein 2 (LAMP2)	X	<1
Frataxin (FRDA)	9	<1

GENOTYPE-PHENOTYPE CORRELATIONS

The potential that the clinical features of HCM could be determined by the individual mutations or gene defects has led to intense investigation. Studies of large families affected by HCM have suggested that mutations in β-myosin heavy chain are associated with severe hypertrophy, while mutations in cardiac troponin have only mild hypertrophy. Some family-based studies have suggested that certain mutations higher or lower risks for sudden cardiac death. However, subsequent investigations of unrelated patients with HCM suggest that the neither the phenotypic expression nor the natural history of HCM can be distinguished on the basis of the specific mutation. Notably, mutations in myosin heavy chain, cardiac actin, troponin T, alpha-tropomyosin, and titin can result in either hypertrophic or dilated cardiomyopathy. Several reports have shown that delayed penetrance (late onset hypertrophy in the 5th or 6th decade) can occur, particularly if the underlying mutation involves myosin binding protein C.

Contrary to the previous belief that phenotypic expression would be complete in early adulthood, this finding has led to a significant change in the recommendations for family screening. It is now recommended that adult family members of HCM patients undergo surveillance echocardiography every 5 years, while adolescents should be screened every 12-18 months (more often if they wish to participate in competitive athletics). Among patients with clear clinical HCM, the yield of currently available genetic testing is only about 50%. Undoubtedly, there are many mutations that have yet to be discovered.

■ Among patients with clear clinical HCM, the yield of currently available (2006) genetic testing is only about 50%.

PATHOPHYSIOLOGY OF HCM

The complex pathophysiology of HCM results from a

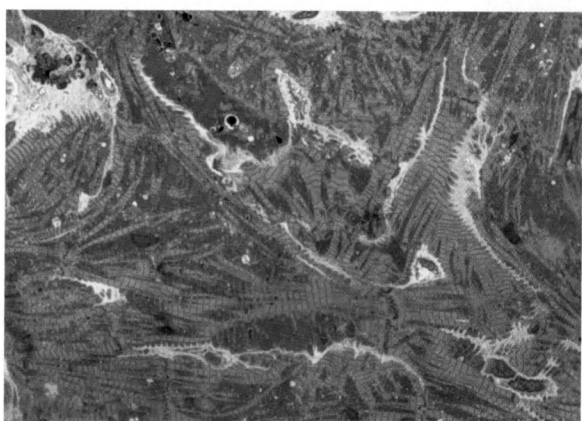

Fig. 3. Right ventricular biopsy specimen showing myofiber disarray in familial hypertrophic cardiomyopathy.

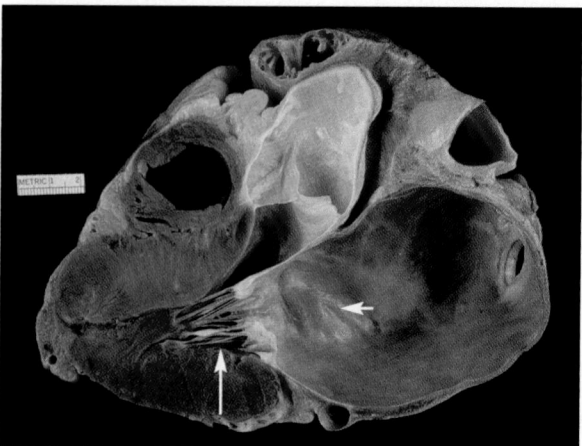

Fig. 5. Autopsy specimen of hypertrophic cardiomyopathy with predominant apical involvement of the left ventricle and massive left atrial enlargement (*short arrow*). Also, the papillary muscles are malpositioned and misoriented (*long arrow*).

mix of left ventricular diastolic dysfunction, myocardial ischemia, arrhythmias, left ventricular outflow obstruction, mitral regurgitation, and autonomic dysfunction.

Diastolic Dysfunction in HCM

Diastolic dysfunction is thought to be one of the major pathophysiologic mechanisms present in all patients with HCM, frequently leading to diastolic heart failure. Marked abnormalities of both ventricular relaxation and chamber stiffness may be present. Multiple abnormal loads are imposed on the left ventricle, including contraction loads (from outflow obstruction) and relaxation loads as well as nonuniformity of relaxation. The thick, hypertrophied ventricular muscle causes abnormalities of passive filling because of the increased stiffness of the left ventricle. Abnormalities of relaxation have

been observed using tissue Doppler echocardiography prior to the development of hypertrophy in animals and humans.

Left Ventricular Outflow Obstruction and Mitral Regurgitation

Left ventricular outflow tract obstruction is present in 25-40% of HCM patients under resting conditions and with physiologic provocation may be observed in the majority of patients. It can be severe in the resting state, labile (mild in the resting state but significant with provocation) or latent (not present in the resting state but produced with provocation). Outflow obstruction is exacerbated in the presence of a decreased ventricular preload, decreased ventricular afterload, or increased ventricular contractility. The mechanism of outflow obstruction involves basal septal hypertrophy and flow-mediated displacement of the mitral valve anteriorly into the left ventricular outflow tract such that the mitral leaflet can come into contact with the ventricular septum (Fig. 9 and 10). The temporal sequence has been described as "eject-obstruct-leak." The accelerated flow around the hypertrophied basal septum pushes the mitral leaflet at the same time there may be "suction" forces which both contribute to the systolic anterior motion of the mitral valve. Other anatomic features may contribute to the obstruction

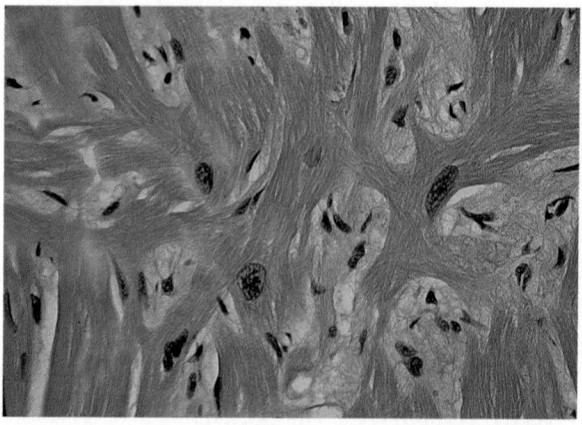

Fig. 4. Myofiber disarray in hypertrophic cardiomyopathy.

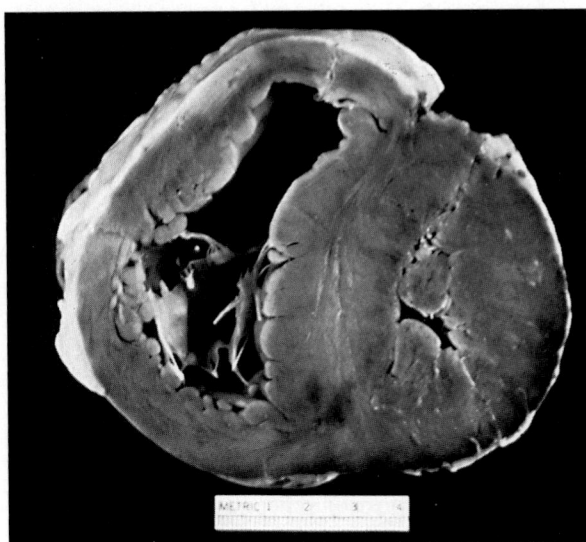

Fig. 6. Autopsy specimen of hypertrophic cardiomyopathy showing hypertrophy of the inferior wall and right ventricle in addition to that of the septum and antero-lateral wall.

including anterior displacement of papillary muscles, hypertrophied papillary muscles and direct insertion of the papillary muscles onto the mitral valve.

The outflow tract obstruction can produce symptoms by several mechanisms. The obstruction itself can limit the cardiac output and result in effort related symptoms such as dyspnea or pre-syncope. Obstruction also increases left ventricular pressures, which can induce ischemia through increased demand and

decreased perfusion pressure. The high contraction load on the left ventricle will impair diastolic filling of the left ventricle. The mitral regurgitation that is associated with the obstruction can cause further elevation of left atrial pressure.

Arrhythmias in HCM

Arrhythmias contribute to the pathophysiology of HCM. Atrial arrhythmias are common (up to 25% of patients in some series) and may cause severe hemodynamic deterioration from loss of atrial contraction as well as from rapid heart rates. Ventricular ectopy is a common finding on Holter monitoring. Sustained ventricular tachycardia and fibrillation are the most likely mechanisms of syncope and sudden death in these patients. Patients with HCM are very dependent on normal atrial function for filling of the stiff hypertrophied left ventricle. Cardiac output may decrease as much as 40% if atrial fibrillation occurs, leading to rapid deterioration of the patient's symptoms. For a more comprehensive review of the impact of arrhythmias in HCM (see Chapter 31, Heritable Cardiomyopathies).

Autonomic Dysfunction in HCM

Approximately 25 percent of HCM patients will have an abnormal blood pressure response to exercise as defined by either a failure of systolic blood pressure to rise greater than 20 mm Hg or a fall in systolic blood pressure. The inability to augment and sustain systolic blood pressure occurs despite an appropriate rise in cardiac output and is due to inappropriate systemic vasodilatation during exercise. It is speculated that there is a high degree of abnormal autonomic tone in patients with HCM and is associated with a poorer prognosis.

CLINICAL MANAGEMENT OF HCM

Successful treatment of HCM requires careful appreciation of the pathophysiology as it applies to each individual patient.

Clinical Presentation and Diagnosis of HCM

HCM may be newly diagnosed at any age from early childhood to advanced age. The clinical presentation of HCM varies widely. Patients may be completely asymptomatic, with the diagnosis made on the basis of

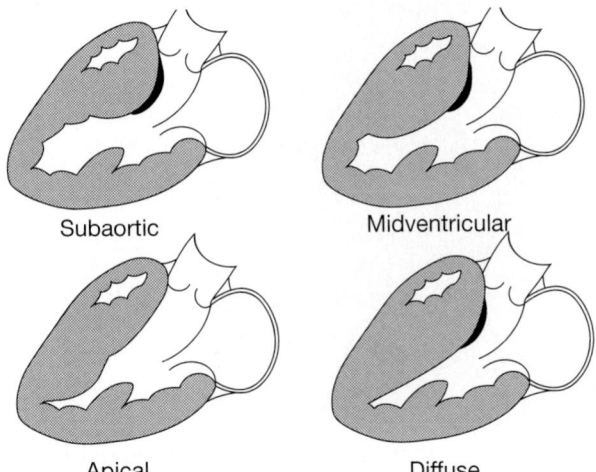

| Subaortic | Midventricular |
| Apical | Diffuse |

Fig. 7. Diagram of hypertrophic cardiomyopathy variants.

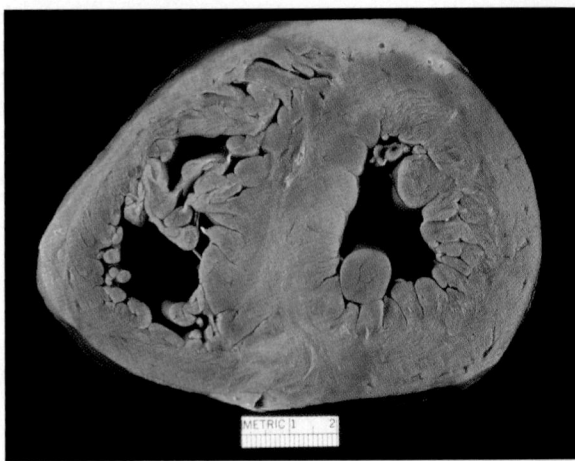

Fig. 8. Hypertrophic cardiomyopathy (short-axis-view).

a heart murmur, abnormal ECG (Fig. 11), or during screening prior to participation in competitive athletics. Even patients with massive hypertrophy of the heart can be completely asymptomatic and some patients are not diagnosed until they present with sudden cardiac death.

The typical triad of symptoms in HCM includes dyspnea on exertion, angina, and presyncope or syncope (Fig. 12). Patients with atrial fibrillation may also present with systemic embolism. The dyspnea in HCM is due to increased left atrial pressure, which can result from abnormal left ventricular diastolic function, outflow tract obstruction, or significant mitral regurgitation. Angina pectoris is common even in the absence of epicardial coronary artery disease and is related to an abnormal myocardial oxygen supply/demand mismatch due to the hypertrophied left ventricular walls, increased arteriolar compressive wall tension caused by diastolic relaxation abnormalities, and endothelial dysfunction. Syncope may be due to arrhythmias or a sudden increase in outflow tract obstruction. Patients with HCM frequently have abnormal autonomic function, and vasodepressor syncope may be part of the mechanism of syncope.

HCM is a clinical disease that is defined by the finding of left ventricular hypertrophy in the absence of identifiable provocative etiology. The primary diagnostic test is two-dimensional echocardiography. Cardiac magnetic resonance imaging and computed tomography can also confirm the presence of left ventricular hypertrophy. It is crucial that other stimuli for hypertrophy (hypertension, valvular/subvalvular aortic stenosis) or wall thickness (cardiac amyloidosis, Fabry's cardiomyopathy, Freidrich's ataxia) are considered before the label of HCM is applied to an individual patient.

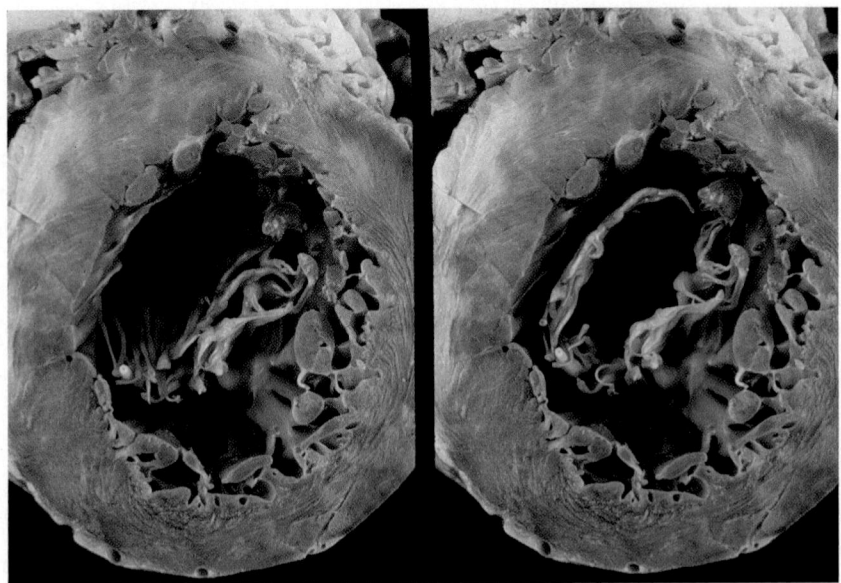

Fig. 9. Hypertrophic cardiomyopathy with simulated systolic anterior motion of the anterior leaflet of the mitral valve. *Left*, Mitral valve closed in systole. *Right*, Mitral valve open in diastole, with systolic anterior motion of the anterior leaflet.

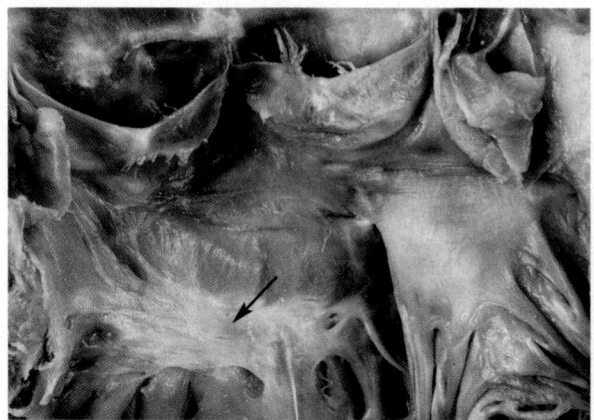

Fig. 10. Subaortic septal patch (mitral contact lesion) in hypertrophic cardiomyopathy (*arrow*).

HCM may be distinguished from the "athletic heart" by careful evaluation that includes echocardiography and potentially other imaging modalities such as cardiac magnetic resonance imaging. In HCM, left ventricular septal wall thickness is typically unusual or asymmetric and greater than 15 mm, the left atrium is dilated (>4 cm), and the left ventricular end-diastolic diameter is less than 45 mm. In the athletic heart, the hypertrophy is more commonly concentric in distribution and less than 15 mm for the septum, less than 4 cm for the left

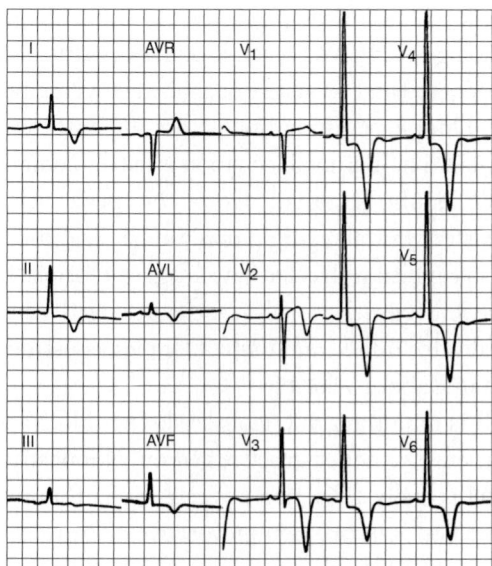

Fig. 11. ECG of patient with apical hypertrophic cardiomyopathy variant with deeply inverted T waves in chest leads V_2-V_6 and limb leads II, III, and AVL.

atrium, and greater than 45 mm for left ventricular end-diastolic diameter. In the athletic heart, the left ventricular hypertrophy will regress after training stops, usually within 3 months. Diastolic function is normal in the athletic heart in contradistinction to HCM where diastolic function is abnormal.

Physical Examination in HCM

Physical examination findings are always abnormal when there is obstruction of the outflow tract, but in non-obstructive HCM the physical examination may be less obvious. The hallmark of the physical examination in HCM is the finding of severe myocardial hypertrophy. This is detected by palpation of the left ventricular apex, which is localized but markedly sustained. There frequently is a palpable presystolic impulse of the augmented atrial contraction present (palpable S4). In the presence of outflow obstruction, there is a "triple ripple," though this classic finding is rarely observed. A bifid apex or double apical impulse is more common. The first impulse is the large atrial kick (atrial boost, presystolic boost), and the next impulse is a sustained left ventricular apical impulse. The atrial kick is due to a forceful atrial systole secondary to atrial hypertrophy in response to the chronically elevated left ventricular diastolic pressure and mitral regurgitation. The jugular venous pressure may be slightly increased, with a prominent "a" wave indicating abnormal diastolic function of the right side of the heart.

The carotid pulse has a rapid upstroke due to the hyperdynamic systolic function and rapid ventricular emptying. In the presence of ventricular outflow tract obstruction, the carotid upstroke has a distinctive "jerky" bifid quality (spike-and-dome pulse). The spike is the initial rapid ventricular emptying phase, whereas the dome corresponds to the onset of ventricular obstruction, followed by the more gradual increase in ventricular pressure to overcome the gradient.

A harsh systolic ejection murmur is heard across the entire precordium and radiates to the apex and base of the heart but not the neck. In many instances, a separate mitral regurgitation murmur may be auscultated. Both murmurs respond in a similar manner to examination maneuvers that change the loading conditions of the left ventricle.

The murmur of HCM is increased by maneuvers that decrease left ventricular end-diastolic volume

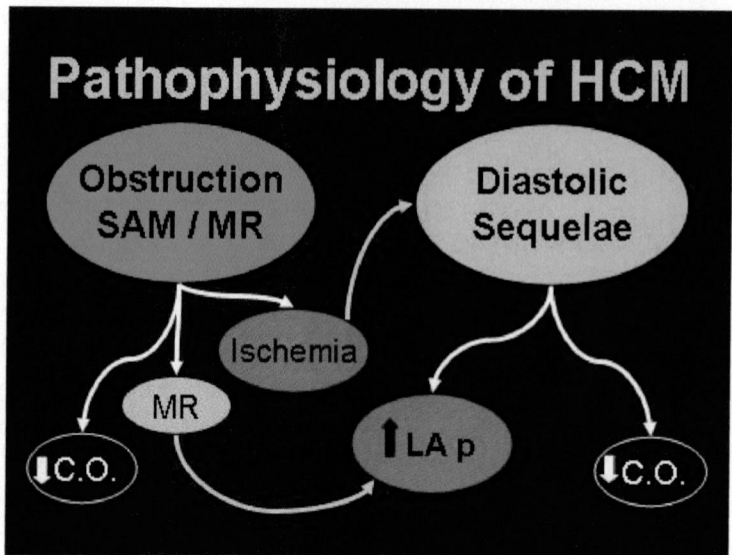

Fig. 12. Pathophysiologic mechanisms in hypertrophic cardiomyopathy. C.O., cardiac output; LAp, left atrial pressure; MR, mitral regurgitation; SAM, systolic anterior motion of the mitral valve.

(decreased venous return, decreased afterload, increased contractility, pure vasodilators, inotropes, dehydration, and the Valsalva maneuver). The murmur decreases with squatting, passive leg raising, negative inotropes such as β-blockers, verapamil, disopyramide, and any maneuver that increases left ventricular end-diastolic volume. Examination of the patient after a brisk walk or stair climb also reveals an intensification of the murmur.

In addition to an S4 gallop, there may be an S3 gallop. Previously, it was thought that a dilated chamber was necessary for an S3 gallop, but both S3 and S4 gallops are frequent in HCM, even in the absence of left ventricular dilatation.

ECHOCARDIOGRAPHY IN HYPERTROPHIC CARDIOMYOPATHY

Two-Dimensional Echocardiography

Two-dimensional and Doppler echocardiography are the standard tests for the diagnosis and evaluation of HCM. Two-dimensional echocardiography is able to visualize and characterize the site and extent of the hypertrophy of the myocardium. Although in the majority of cases the hypertrophy is classically asymmetric septal hypertrophy with anterolateral extensions, it can also be diffuse concentric hypertrophy or localized to specific areas such as the apex or free wall of the left ventricle. Echocardiographic contrast enhancement can aid in the detection of some variants such as apical HCM. Systolic anterior motion of the mitral valve is frequently present when there is outflow tract obstruction.

Doppler Echocardiography

Doppler echocardiography is used to study the pathophysiology of HCM. Dynamic outflow obstruction can be diagnosed and accurately quantified by a continuous-wave Doppler examination across the outflow tract (Fig. 13). The Bernoulli equation is used to obtain the peak systolic gradient from the peak velocity. Coexistent mitral regurgitation can be diagnosed and semi-quantified with color-flow imaging. Diastolic filling of the left ventricle can also be characterized using the mitral valve inflow and tissue Doppler assessment of the mitral anular velocity.

It is important to establish whether HCM is the obstructive or nonobstructive variant. Nonobstructive HCM is really a diagnosis of exclusion, if no resting obstruction is noted, then provocative maneuvers must be used. The Valsalva maneuver and inhalation of amyl nitrite are used to exclude the presence of latent obstruction; occasionally, isoproterenol is infused. When obstruction is present, the site and severity should be quantified and defined, the associated mitral regurgitant severity should be defined, and the diastolic ventricular dysfunction should be assessed.

Doppler is used to quantify and localize the level and severity of obstruction. It is important to distinguish between the mitral regurgitant signal and the signal due to the intracavitary obstruction. The typical appearance of the HCM Doppler signal is late-peaking and frequently referred to as "dagger-shaped" (Fig. 13). To distinguish the HCM signal from mitral regurgitation, look for the aortic closure signal. The mitral regurgitant signal in HCM may be late-peaking, but it continues until mitral valve forward flow begins in diastole, while the left ventricular outflow obstruction signal ends with aortic valve closure. Doppler-derived gradients in patients with HCM correlate well with catheter-derived gradients during simultaneous examinations.

Cardiac catheterization is not necessary to diagnose HCM or to evaluate the severity of left ventricular outflow tract obstruction or mitral regurgitation, however, it may be useful in select patients with challenging echocardiographic studies.

- The typical appearance of the HCM Doppler signal is a late-peaking signal frequently referred to as "dagger-shaped."
- The Brockenbrough response is a classic hemodynamic function in HCM (Fig. 14).

MANAGEMENT OF OBSTRUCTIVE HCM

General Principles
There are several general guidelines for management of HCM:

- All first-degree relatives should undergo screening with echocardiography, and younger affected members of the family should have genetic counseling if they plan to have a family.
- For adults, screening should be repeated every 5 years, while children and those participating in competitive athletics should be screened every 12-18 months.
- HCM patients should avoid competitive athletics or other types of strenuous activity, but may participate

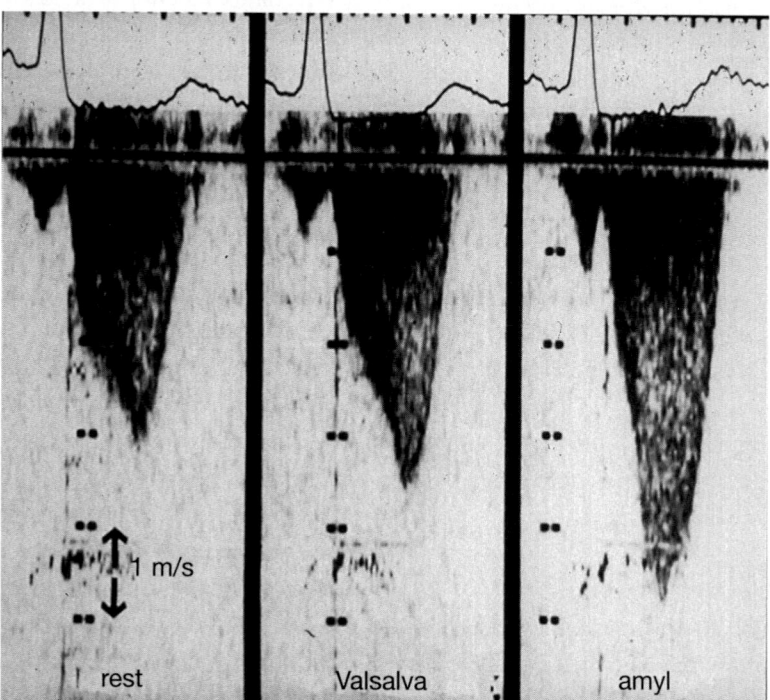

Fig. 13. Doppler "dagger-shaped" late-peaking signal of intracavitary gradient in hypertrophic cardiomyopathy accentuated by Valsalva response and by inhaled amyl nitrite. At rest, the velocity is 3.0 m/s (gradient, 36 mm Hg) and increases to 3.5 m/s (gradient, 50 mm Hg) during Valsalva and to 4.7 m/s (gradient, 88 mm Hg) after inhalation of amyl nitrite.

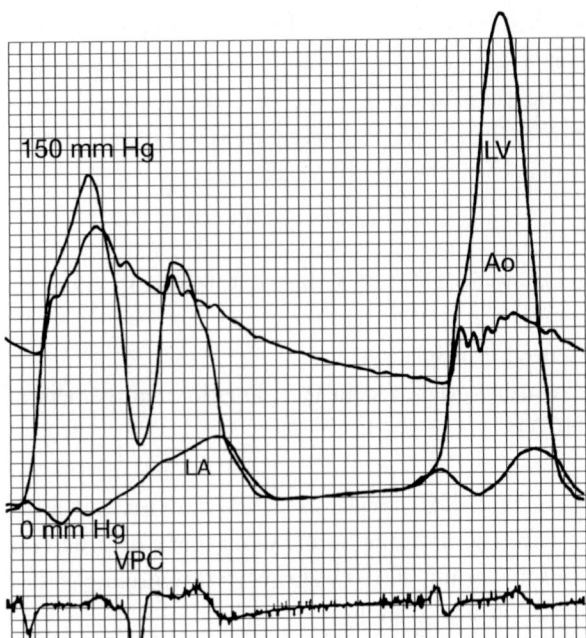

Fig. 14. Brockenbrough response shows an increase in left ventricular (LV) systolic pressure, a decrease in ascending aortic (Ao) systolic pressure, and an increase in the gradient between the LV and ascending aorta. Note that there is also a decrease in the height of pulse pressure in the ascending aorta (systolic-diastolic blood pressure).

in low-level aerobic exercise to promote general cardiovascular health.

- Antibiotics should be given prophylactically according to the AHA guidelines before medical and dental procedures to prevent infective endocarditis.
- Dehydration should be avoided.
- Holter monitoring should be performed for 24-48 hours to detect ventricular arrhythmias and for risk stratification.
- Pure vasodilators, high-dose diuretics and positive inotropes should be avoided as they may exacerbate left ventricular outflow obstruction.

β-Blockers, Calcium Blockers, Disopyramide

For patients with obstructive cardiomyopathy and symptoms, first-line pharmacologic therapy should be negative inotropic agents. β-Blockade with large dosages in the range of 200 to 400 mg propranolol or equivalent per day is a good first choice. Selective β-blockers lose their selectivity at high doses so there is little to be gained by using a β_1 selective β-blocker.

β-Blockers relieve symptoms in about 50% of patients by slowing the heart rate, which allows a longer diastolic filling time and decreases myocardial oxygen consumption, thus reducing myocardial ischemia and left ventricular outflow tract obstruction through a direct negative inotropic effect. If this does not adequately decrease the intraventricular gradient and control symptoms, calcium channel blockers may be added, usually verapamil in dosages of 240 to 320 mg per day. Care must be taken when prescribing calcium channel blockers for patients with large outflow tract obstruction, because acute hemodynamic deterioration may occur because of peripheral vasodilatation. Dihydropyridine class calcium channel blockers are contraindicated in obstructive HCM as these agents are pure vasodilators. Disopyramide, a class I antiarrhythmic agent with strong negative inotropic properties, may also be used to treat HCM, especially in patients with outflow tract obstruction, however, anticholinergic effects can causes urinary retention in men and dry mouth.

Surgery for HCM

If patients with obstructive HCM continue to have severe, disabling effort related symptoms, then surgical septal myectomy is the primary treatment strategy (Tables 2 and 3). Septal myectomy is a well-proven therapy that can abolish the outflow tract gradient and provide excellent long-term relief. The resected muscle does not regrow. Procedural complications are infrequent (<5%) and mortality associated with the operation is rare (<1%), across all age-ranges, in reports from high-volume centers. With surgery, the outflow tract is effectively widened; thereby abolishing the gradient and eliminating systolic anterior motion mediated mitral regurgitation. In non-randomized comparison, it appears that septal myectomy improves survival compared to patients managed without surgery.

Alcohol Septal Ablation for HCM

Alcohol septal ablation has emerged as a potential alternative to surgical myectomy for selected patients with drug-refractory symptoms with obstructive HCM. In this percutaneous, catheter-based procedure, pure ethanol is injected into the septal perforator coronary artery that supplies the hypertrophied myocardium adjacent to the point of outflow obstruction (SAM-septal contact point). This renders this portion of the

Table 2. Comparison of Surgical Septal
Myectomy and Percutaneous Septal
Ablation

	Myectomy	Ablation
Procedural mortality	≤1%	1-2%
Residual gradient (immediate)	<10 mm Hg	<25 mm Hg
Success rates	≥95%	≥85%
Need for permanent pacemaker	1-2%	≥5-10%
Subsequent sudden death or ICD discharge risk	Very low	Uncertain
Intramyocardial scarring	None	Present

septum akinetic, and eventually leads to scarring (thinning) in this area which dramatically reduces the outflow obstruction. There is a relatively high rate of complete heart block necessitating permanent pacing; 5-10% in experienced centers. The procedural mortality rate has

been ~2% in pooled data. As this procedure induces a non-reperfused septal infarction there are concerns about proarrhythmia. Septal ablation cannot offer relief from coexistent structural valve abnormalities, and the ability to treat the precise site is dependent on appropriate coronary anatomy. Given these limitations and complication profile, septal ablation has a more limited patient eligibility and should only be performed after careful discussion with the patient.

Dual-Chamber Pacing in HCM
Dual-chamber pacing was advocated as another means of relieving outflow obstruction. The proposed mechanism for the beneficial effects of pacing include optimization of atrioventricular synchrony, alteration of ventricular activation sequence (i.e. apex to base), and potentially long-term remodeling to widen the outflow tract (Fig. 15). While initial observational series were encouraging, randomized controlled trials did not demonstrate significant objective improvements. It now appears that only ~30% of patients treated with pacemakers to relieve obstruction have lasting benefit. Unfortunately, no preprocedural variables can identify which patients will respond favorably to pacing therapy.

Table 3. Selection Criteria for Invasive Therapy in Obstructive HCM

	Good candidates	Poor candidates
Surgical septal myectomy	LVOTO with class III-IV symptoms Any age Coexistent mitral valve or other structural cardiac abnormalities	Severe comorbidity that markedly increases risks
Percutaneous septal ablation	LVOTO with class III-IV symptoms Isolated basal septal hypertrophy Moderate gradient (40-60 mm Hg) Older age Pre-existing PPM Contraindication to surgical septal myectomy	More diffuse hypertrophy Extreme gradients (>80 mm Hg) Left bundle branch block Abnormal mitral valve or mitral support structures Pre-existing risk factors for SCD in the absence of ICD
Dual-chamber pacing	LVOTO with class III-IV symptoms Coexistent chronotropic incompetence Contraindication to surgical septal myectomy and percutaneous septal ablation	Rapid native atrioventricular conduction Abnormal mitral valve or mitral support structures

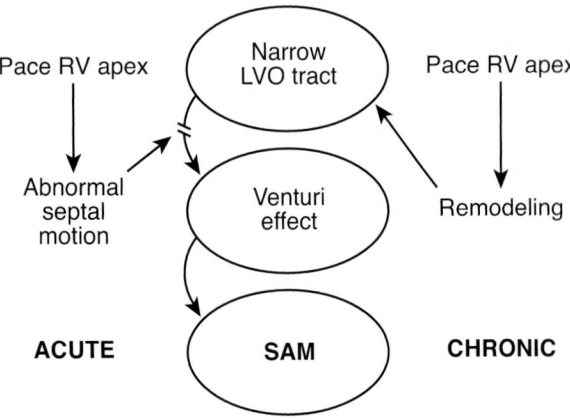

Fig. 15. Possible mechanisms of the benefit of dual-chamber pacing in hypertrophic cardiomopahty. LVO, left ventricular outflow; RV, right ventricle; SAM, systolic anterior motion of the mitral valve.

Based on these findings, pacemaker therapy to relieve symptomatic outflow obstruction is reserved for patients with contraindication to myectomy and septal ablation.

MANAGEMENT OF NONOBSTRUCTIVE HCM

The majority of patients with HCM do not have outflow obstruction. If these patients become symptomatic it is usually heart failure symptoms due to the inherent diastolic dysfunction and/or atrial arrhythmias. The treatment options for these patients are limited. Diuretics are often useful in the early stages of management. There are emerging data that suggest that inhibition of the renin-angiotensin-aldosterone cascade may favorably alter the diastolic properties of the left ventricle. If symptoms continue to progress, cardiac transplantation becomes an option.

Risk Assessment for Sudden Cardiac Death in HCM

The natural history of HCM is highly variable, but population-based studies suggest that most HCM patients have near-normal longevity. Unfortunately, there remains an approximately 1%/year rate of sudden cardiac death. HCM is the leading cause of sudden death in competitive and school-age athletes. The challenge for the clinician is to identify those patients who are at increased risk so that preventive strategies (implantable defibrillators) may be appropriately utilized. A personal history of resuscitated cardiac arrest or sustained ventricular tachycardia is a clear indication for implantation of a defibrillator. Several other clinical features also portend a poorer prognosis including positive family history of sudden death, history of syncope in the young, repetitive non-sustained ventricular tachycardia, massive (>30 mm) left ventricular hypertrophy, and failure to augment systolic blood pressure by 20 mm Hg with exercise. If two or more of these factors is present, a defibrillator is indicated (Fig. 16). The finding of only one of these factors requires individualized discussion with the patient. There is little to suggest that electrophysiologic testing is of benefit in the risk assessment.

Summary

Hypertrophic cardiomyopathy is disease marked by heterogeneity. It is generally thought to be an autosomal dominant disease with mutations often localized to the proteins comprising the cardiac sarcomere. While sudden cardiac death is more common than in the general population, it remains rare in HCM. Risk stratification remains a challenging art. Left ventricular outflow tract obstruction is a common feature that predisposes to effort-related dyspnea, angina, and presyncope. Pharmacologic treatment is usually successful in controlling symptoms. Surgical septal myectomy remains the primary treatment strategy for symptomatic patients who are refractory to medications, while alcohol septal ablation can be offered to select patients (i.e. those with considerable comorbidity) as an alternative to an operative approach.

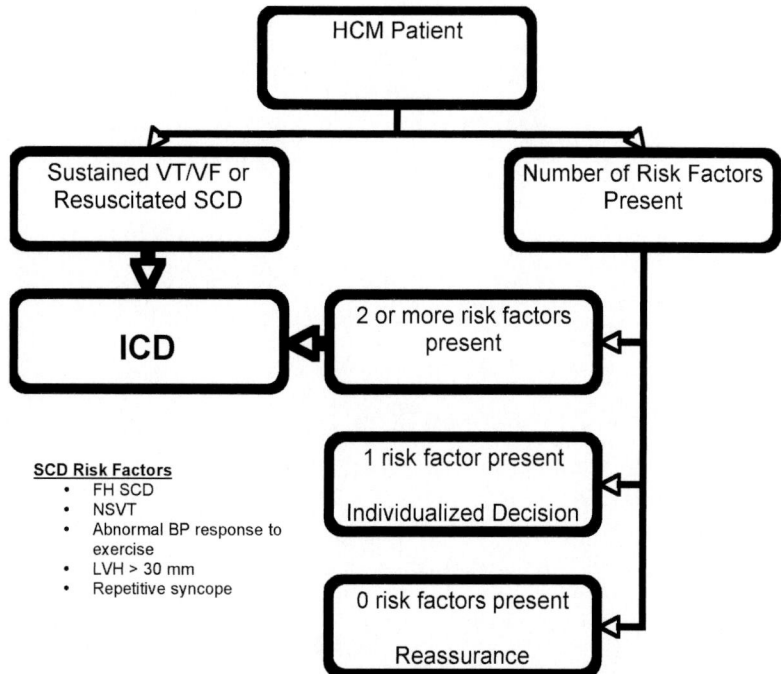

Fig. 16. Sudden cardiac risk stratification in hypertrophic cardiomyopathy. FH, family history; HCM, hypertrophic cardiomyopathy; ICD, implantable cardioverter defibrillator; LVH, left ventricular hypertrophy; NSVT, nonsustained ventricular tachycardia; SCD, sudden cardiac death; VF, ventricular fibrillation; VT, ventricular tachycardia

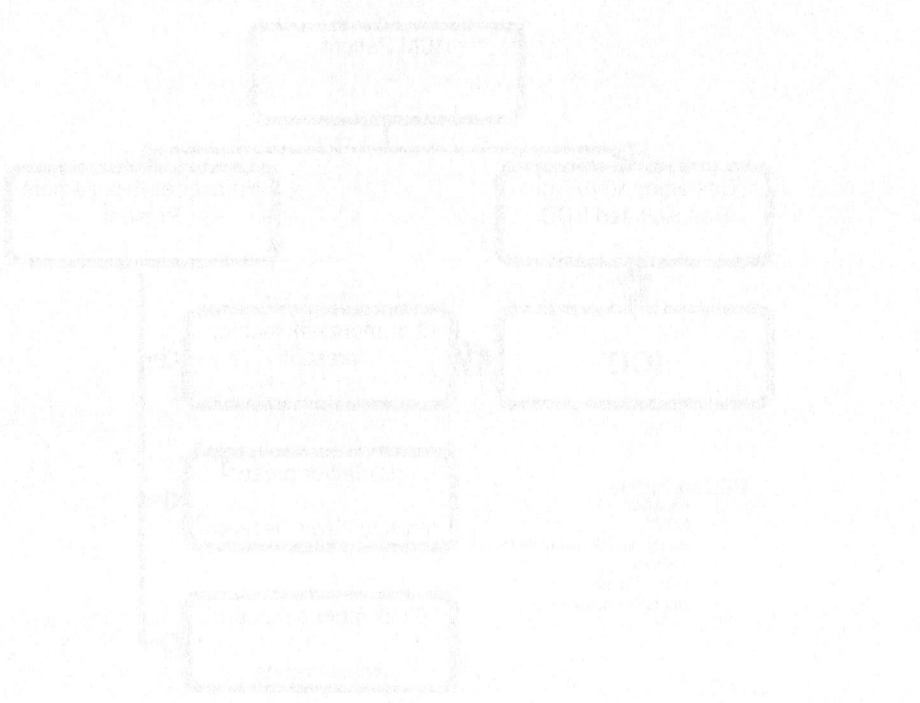

98

RIGHT VENTRICULAR FAILURE

Robert P. Frantz, MD

INTRODUCTION

Right ventricular failure is a clinical syndrome that often represents a difficult diagnostic and therapeutic challenge. It should not be considered a freestanding diagnosis, but should lead the clinician to search for clues to the underlying disease substrate. Most often occurring in the context of left heart failure, it is a harbinger of adverse prognosis. Signs and symptoms of right heart failure are listed in Table 1.

Suspicion of right heart failure requires the clinician to ponder the considerable list of associated conditions and differential diagnosis. Edema often does not represent right heart failure. Consider also the possibility of simple stasis, venous insufficiency, venous thrombosis, lymphedema, lymphatic obstruction, intraabdominal processes impeding lower extremity venous or lymphatic return, intrinsic liver disease, side effects of medication such as dihyropyridine calcium channel antagonists and nonsteroidal antiinflammatory agents, and nephrotic syndrome. The medical history can provide important clues in this regard. The medical history should include a thorough review of systems including questions targeting symptoms of obstructive sleep apnea, prior exposure to diet drugs, tobacco and alcohol, illicit drug use, risk factors for pulmonary embolus including recent prolonged travel or bedrest and use of birth control pills or estrogen replacement therapy, and risk factors for

HIV. Obstructive sleep apnea is increasingly prevalent in the context of the obesity epidemic. The associated nocturnal hypoxemia results in pulmonary vasoconstriction that may aggravate right ventricular failure. The past medical history and family history are also critical in providing context for the presenting symptoms and guiding the differential diagnosis.

The physical examination requires particular attention to study of the neck veins, since presence or

Table 1. Manifestations of Right Heart Failure

Symptoms	Signs
Diminished appetite	Jugular venous distention
Abdominal distention/ pain	Hepatomegaly
	Ascites
Peripheral swelling	Peripheral edema
Nasal congestion	Right ventricular lift
Dyspnea on exertion	Right sided S3
Exertional chest discomfort	Accentuated pulmonic closure sound
Weight gain	Murmur of tricuspid insufficiency
	Murmur of pulmonic insufficiency

absence of abnormal jugular venous waveforms and pressure can be extremely helpful in defining whether right heart failure is in fact present. Abdominal compression to elicit the abdomino-jugular reflex should routinely be performed.

ADDITIONAL DIAGNOSTIC EVALUATION

Following a thorough history and physical examination, a chest x-ray and ECG should be obtained. These tests should be studied to search for clues of underlying left heart disease that commonly accompanies right heart failure. The chest x-ray should also be examined for signs of right heart enlargement. This includes enlargement of the cardiac border to the right of the spine, and loss of the anterior mediastinal clear space on lateral film due to right ventricular enlargement. Other features of disease that may accompany right heart failure, such as enlargement of the central pulmonary arteries in pulmonary arterial hypertension, hyperinflation in COPD, or interstitial changes that may accompany a variety of inflammatory/fibrotic lung diseases, should also be sought. A CXR from a patient with pulmonary arterial hypertension is shown in Figure 1.

The electrocardiogram may show signs of right atrial enlargement, right axis deviation, and/or right ventricular hypertrophy. A typical ECG from a patient with idiopathic pulmonary arterial hypertension resulting in right ventricular hypertrophy is shown in Figure 2.

Echocardiography is an essential tool in further assessment of suspected RV failure. Defining whether left heart disease accompanies the right heart failure is essential. This should include complete Doppler analyses in order to assess LV diastolic function. Estimation of right ventricular systolic pressure by interrogation of the tricuspid regurgitant signal and application of the modified Bernoulli equation (RV pressure = 4(triscuspid regurgitant velocity)^2 + estimated right atrial pressure) is important in assessing presence and estimating severity of pulmonary hypertension. Definitive diagnosis of pulmonary hypertension requires right sided heart catheterization.

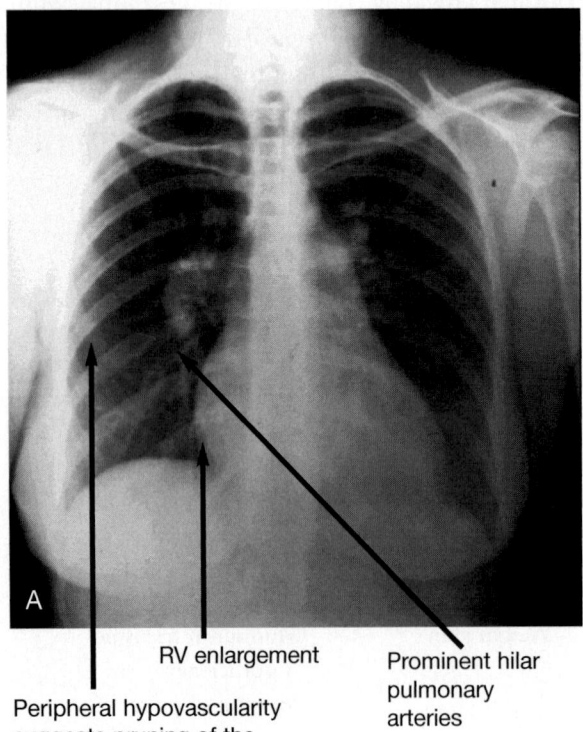
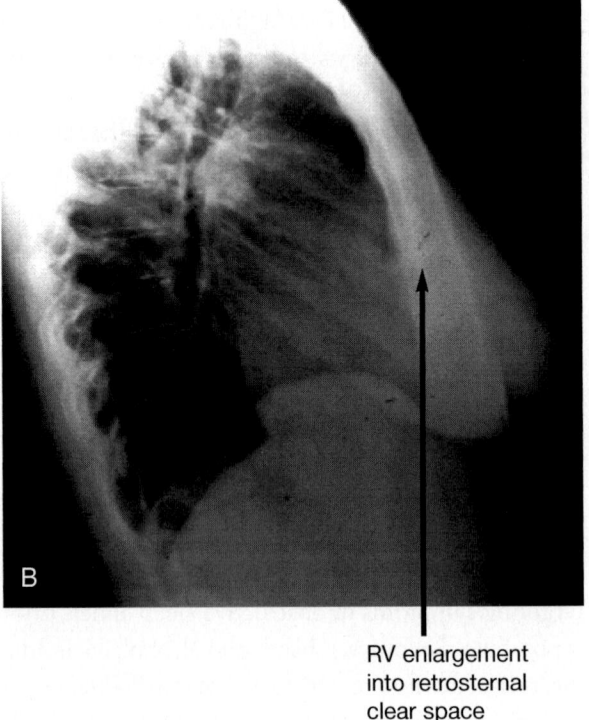

RV enlargement

Prominent hilar pulmonary arteries

Peripheral hypovascularity suggests pruning of the vascular tree consistent with pulmonary arterial hypertension

RV enlargement into retrosternal clear space

Fig. 1. Chest x-ray from a patient with pulmonary arterial hypertension.

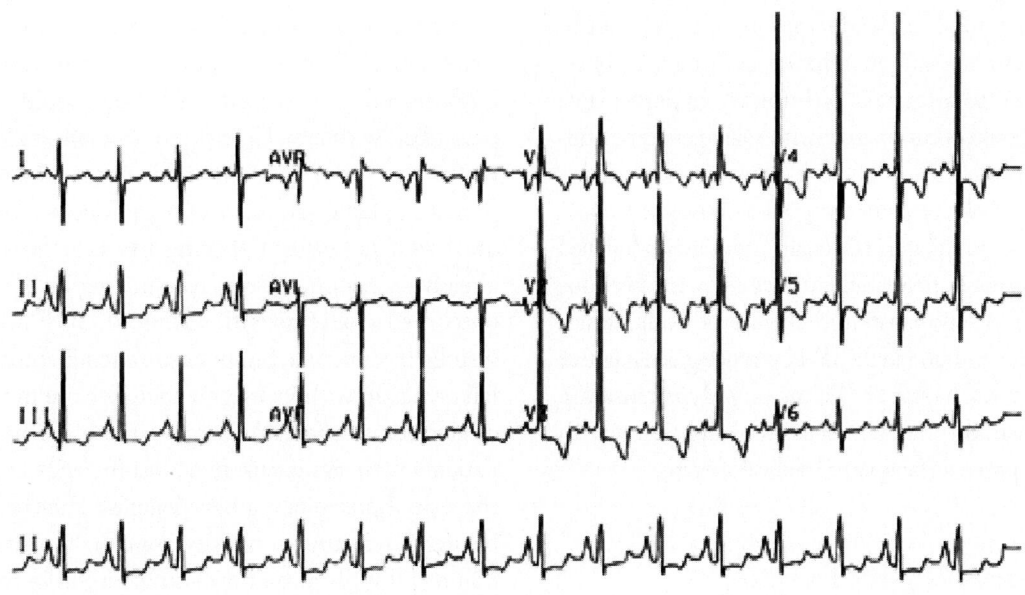

Fig. 2. Electrocardiogram from a patient with pulmonary arterial hypertension, reflecting right atrial enlargement, right axis deviation and right ventricular hypertrophy.

CLASSIFICATION OF PULMONARY HYPERTENSION

Pulmonary hypertension often accompanies RV failure. When present, pulmonary hypertension should be classified based upon the Venice classification system (Tables 2 and 3). This system divides patients into those with pulmonary arterial hypertension (PAH) and those with non-PAH. Diagnosis of PAH requires that the following criteria be met:

1. Mean pulmonary artery pressure that is greater than 25 mm Hg
2. Normal pulmonary capillary wedge or left ventricular end-diastolic pressure (15 mm Hg or less)
3. Absence of left heart disease or other diseases that fall into the non-PAH category

This distinction is useful because patients with PAH may respond to selective pulmonary vasodilators. Patients with non-PAH who have elevated PCW pressure may deteriorate with administration of selective pulmonary vasodilators due to the increase in pulmonary blood flow that may further congest the pulmonary bed. Patients with non-PAH but normal PCW pressure have generally been excluded from randomized trials of selective pulmonary vasodilators, so no confident recommendations can be made regarding the role of selective pulmonary vasodilators in such patients.

MANAGEMENT OF RV FAILURE ASSOCIATED WITH PAH

Treatment of RV failure associated with PAH includes use of diuretics, digoxin, warfarin (in effort to reduce risk of associated venous thrombosis or in situ pulmonary

Table 2.   Non-PAH

Pulmonary hypertension (PH) with left heart disease
LV systolic or diastolic dysfunction
Valvular heart disease
Pulmonary hypertension with lung disease/hypoxemia
Chronic obstructive pulmonary disease
Interstitial lung disease
Sleep-disordered breathing (obstructive sleep apnea, hypoventilation syndromes)
Developmental abnormalities
PH due to chronic thrombotic and/or embolic disease
Thromboembolic obstruction of proximal PA
Thromboembolic obstruction of distal PA
Non-thrombotic pulmonary embolism (PE)

vascular thrombosis), and supplemental oxygen to maintain systemic saturation in normal range.

Referral to a tertiary pulmonary hypertension program should occur to assist with management of this complex problem. Use of selective pulmonary vasodilators such as endothelin receptor antagonists (bosentan), phosphodiesterase-5 inhibitors (sildenafil), prostanoids (inhaled or intravenous iloprost, subcutaneous or intravenous treprostinil or epoprostenol) should be considered; guidance can be found in the PAH practice guidelines (see Resources and Chapter 78 "Pulmonary Hypertension"). Lung transplant may be necessary in patients with PAH who prove refractory to medical therapy.

Management of RV Failure Complicating LV Systolic Dysfunction

Efforts in this situation should focus on optimizing left ventricular performance, lowering left ventricular end-diastolic pressure, and lessening mitral regurgitation by effective afterload reduction. This includes optimization of doses of angiotensin converting enzyme inhibitors and/or angiotensin II receptor antagonists. In some situations tenuous renal function may greatly complicate management of biventricular failure; if there is a need to withdraw or reduce these drugs, substitution of nitrates and hydralazine should be considered in order to maintain proper preload and afterload reduction. Avoiding hypotension may be important in preserving renal perfusion.

Patients with biventricular failure may present with rapidly progressive ascites and peripheral edema. This leads to edema in the intestinal wall, impeding absorption of oral diuretics and preventing effective diuresis with oral agents. Patients should be questioned carefully regarding recent fluid or salt indiscretion or use of nonsteroidals, since these are common precipitants of progressive fluid retention. In this situation, intravenous loop diuretics either as a bolus or drip can be extremely helpful in achieving diuresis. Use of oral metolazone can also help to achieve diuresis in resistant patients. By blocking reuptake in the distal tubule, metolazone works synergistically with loop diuretics. Metolazone must be used with extreme caution due to potential for precipitation of electrolyte disturbances (hypokalemia, hyponatremia) and renal failure. Patients should weigh daily and have electrolytes checked at least twice weekly during periods

of augmented diuresis. Use of metolazone once or twice a week 30 minutes prior to administration of a loop diuretic is often effective, but should never be prescribed without a clear commitment to follow electrolytes in serial fashion, and is not a substitute for proper fluid and salt restriction. Spironolactone can be used as a potassium sparing diuretic for patients already on a loop diuretic, recognizing its benefits on outcome in patients with advanced CHF due to LV systolic dysfunction, but potassium requirements often fall or vanish with its use, mandating close monitoring of electrolytes. Spironolactone should be avoided in patients with significant renal insufficiency because of the risk of precipitating hyperkalemia. Paracentesis can be useful in setting of massive ascites complicating RV failure. Ultrafiltration may also be useful in removing large volumes, but may aggravate renal dysfunction. Inotropes such as dopamine, dobutamine or milrinone may be useful for treatment of the hospitalized patient with refractory right ventricular failure, but do increase risk of arrhythmia.

Patients being considered for placement of left ventricular assist devices should undergo efforts to optimize volume status and lower right sided pressures prior to device placement; this reduces risk of development of intractable RV failure following LVAD placement, which may necessitate biventricular support.

Summary

Right ventricular failure is a serious complication of a wide variety of medical conditions. Careful definition of the underlying disease is essential. A thorough understanding of the hemodynamics is also important. Optimal outcomes can be achieved only with a commitment to vigilant longitudinal assessment and management.

Resources

Badesch DB, Abman SH, Ahearn GS, et al. Medical therapy for pulmonary arterial hypetension: ACCP evidence-based clinical practice guidelines. Chest. 2004;126 Suppl 1:S35-S62.

McGoon M, Gutterman D, Steen V, et al. Screening, early detection, and diagnosis of pulmonary arterial hypertension: ACCP evidence-based clinical practice guidelines. Chest. 2004;126:S14-S34.

Table 3.   Pulmonary Arterial Hypertension

Idiopathic PAH
Familial PAH (documented bone morpho-
  genetic protein receptor II mutation)
PAH related to:
      Connective tissue disease (CTD)
      Human immunodeficiency virus (HIV)
      Portal hypertension
      Anorexigens
      Congenital heart disease (CHD)
      Persistent pulmonary hypertension of the
        newborn (PPHN)
      PAH with venule/capillary involvement

99

Congestive Heart Failure: Surgical Therapy and Permanent Mechanical Support

Richard C. Daly, MD

Brooks S. Edwards, MD

Surgery for Heart Failure

The decision to offer conventional surgical procedures to patients with severe cardiac dysfunction is difficult due to the significantly increased risk and the fact that outcomes are not well studied even for those who survive the surgical procedure. For patients who are potential transplant candidates, surgical outcomes need to be viewed relative to late outcomes that can be obtained with transplantation (the Mayo Clinic experience is detailed in another chapter). On the other hand, heart transplantation is only available to a limited number of patients because donor numbers are limited and many heart failure patients are not candidates for transplantation. As heart failure continues to increase in incidence and prevalence, other therapeutic options are being evaluated including higher risk surgery for ischemic disease or valvular lesions, ventricular remodeling procedures, and – what may eventually have the greatest impact – permanent implanted pumps.

Conventional Surgical Procedures

Ischemic Disease: Coronary Artery Bypass Grafting

Large trials such as the Coronary Artery Surgery Study (CASS) established that patients with extensive coronary artery disease and systolic ventricular dysfunction have better survival after revascularization. Unfortunately, these large, prospective, randomized trials which established the importance of coronary revascularization excluded patients with symptoms of heart failure and with left ventricular ejection fractions less than 35% (among seven randomized trials only 7% had an EF<40%, and only 4% had symptoms of heart failure). The STICH trial is an ongoing multi-institutional, international, prospective, randomized trial comparing surgical revascularization with medical therapy for patients with heart failure or low left ventricular ejection fraction. The trial will finish enrollment in late 2006 and will be able to report medium term outcomes in the next few years. Awaiting the results of this trial and potential identification of subgroups of patients that will benefit from surgery, current decisions are based on smaller reports and retrospective reviews. A manuscript published in the *Journal of the American Medical Association* in 1994 reviewed 7 publications which reported on outcomes after CABG in patients with an EF between 25% and 40%. Six of the seven papers found that survival was best in the patients who had CABG. Since that time, in might be argued, medical therapy has improved for patients with heart failure, but surgical care including myocardial protection has also improved.

Identification of patients with heart failure who

might be candidates for surgical revascularization includes evaluation of suitability of target vessels, presence of myocardial viability and presence of comorbid conditions.

The presence of suitable target vessels for surgical coronary artery bypass grafting is important for patients with heart failure. Most cohort reports ignore this because patients in these reports have been selected for surgery. One trial, however, found that poor target vessels in patients with an EF ≤25% was 100% predictive of operative mortality. Suitable target vessels should be at least >1 mm in diameter, and probably >1.5 mm.

The importance of identifying significant myocardial viability in patients being considered for CABG is probably important, but it has not been well clarified. Thallium scanning has a positive predictive value for identifying myocardial viability of only 60%, but this increases to 85-90% with 24 hour delayed views. PET scanning has a positive predictive value of 83%, but a negative predictive value of 94% so is highly sensitive. Dobutamine stress echo has been reported to have lower positive and negative predictive values but is the only test that can identify recruitable myocardium which may help predict perioperative response to inotropic support as well as providing additional important information discussed below.

Identifying viability and potential "hibernating" myocardium (flow-metabolism mismatches in PET, delayed redistribution on thallium or recruitable myocardium by stress echo) does not necessarily predict improved ejection fraction. Other measures of clinical outcome, however, may be more important. Certainly, anecdotal experience of dramatic improvement in EF after CABG exists. Average improvement in EF has only been 7% in an informal meta-analysis of 9 surgical reviews by this author. More importantly, flow-metabolism mismatch on PET has been shown to predict improvement in heart failure symptoms, and viability identified by thallium scanning has been shown to predict improved late survival after CABG, while an increase in EF did not predict such improvement.

Comorbid conditions that are associated with poorer outcome after cardiac surgery in heart failure patients are different from those conditions in patients without heart failure. Suitable target vessel and viability were discussed above. The conditions that predict poor surgical outcome in patients with heart failure undergoing CABG are severe LV dilatation, high cardiac filling pressures and poor RV function. These factors are so important that they probably outweigh the usual conditions that are related to poor outcome in patients who undergo CABG without heart failure (although these conditions certainly are important and cannot be ignored (e.g., age, cerebral or peripheral vascular disease, renal dysfunction, diabetes, etc.). LV end-diastolic diameter of >7 cm and LV end systolic volume index of >100 mL/m^2 have each been shown to be associated with high operative mortalities. Dilated ventricles are probably also much less likely to have improved EF after revascularization even if they seem to have a large amount of "hibernating" myocardium on viability testing.

Performing CABG in patients with heart failure and high filling pressures (two studies identified a PCWP >24 mm Hg and mean pulmonary artery pressure >40 mm Hg on statistical analysis) is clearly a very high risk undertaking. Fortunately, this will often respond to aggressive preoperative treatment. The authors have used several days of preoperative hospitalization for aggressive diuresis, often including intravenous inotropes, to improve the condition of heart failure patients having CABG. Dramatic changes in filling pressures, and even RV function, can frequently be achieved.

The combination of poor RV function and poor LV function is a difficult situation in patients having surgery. Indeed, several authors have strongly cautioned that biventricular failure is an absolute contraindication to CABG. Fortunately, most patients with ischemic heart disease have well preserved RV function. When RV failure is present, it may indicate previous RV infarct or, ominously, long-standing high left sided filling pressures. We have found that some patients can become operable with aggressive preoperative therapy attempting to rduce the right atrial pressure to <12 to 15 mm Hg.

Occasional patients with severe LV dilatation will have anatomy suitable for surgical ventricular remodeling (SVR). Direct surgical remodeling has been most successful for selected patients with ischemic disease.

Surgical Ventricular Remodeling
The concept of reducing the volume of a dilated LV is appealing as a surgical approach to treating heart failure. Reduction in LV volume will also reduce LV radius

and, by the law of LaPlace, result in decreased wall tension. At the level of the myocyte, wall tension is similar to LV afterload. The concept that reducing LV volume will have a benefit on physiology of the LV as a whole and on the myocytes themselves is crucial to understanding the potential benefits of surgical intervention for heart failure patients. Surgical volume reduction can be accomplished by direct intervention on the LV or by reducing volume overload related to valvular regurgitation.

In the mid 1990s, Randas Batista, a surgeon from a remote aspect of Brazil, championed a procedure directed at reducing the volume of the LV in patients with dilated cardiomyopathy. This procedure involved resection of that portion of the lateral wall of the LV between the papillary muscles. It was hoped that this would reduce LV volume, short axis radius, sphericity and wall tension, and that improvement in these parameters would translate to improved LV function and patient outcome. Some patients clearly had considerable benefit; we had a few patients that improved from NYHA class IV to class II. However, the procedure proved to be very unpredictable. The largest experience was reported by McCarthy in 2001; among 62 patients, 3 year survival was 60% but 3 year survival free of death, need for LVAD support or return to class IV symptoms was only 26%. Thus, the Batista procedure has very limited, if any, application today.

Surgical ventricular remodeling (SVR), or the Dor procedure, is another direct surgical approach to reduce LV volume. This is a procedure applicable to patients with ischemic cardiomyopathy who have suffered an anterior infarct with subsequent remodeling. The SVR procedure involves exclusion of dyskinetic or akinetic apical and (importantly) septal components of a dilated LV when (also importantly) other walls have reasonable preservation of contractility. A small patch is used to exclude the affected LV walls. Care is taken to avoid creating an LV volume that is too small (the procedure is not applicable to the acute infarct), targeting the LV end diastolic volume to be about 60 mL/m². Experience in over 1000 patients has been reported from Dor (in Monaco) and Menicanti (in Italy). Survival at 5 years is 70% for anterior dyskinetic LV and 50% for akinetic LV. Operative mortality is increased substantially for patients in NYHA class IV, those with an EF <25%, and those with significant mitral insufficiency. Most patients improved from class III to IV (89%) to class I

or II (76%). A prospective, randomized trial evaluating the SVR procedure in patients undergoing CABG is one of the arms of the STICH trial; enrollment in this arm is completed and reporting of results in anticipated in 2 to 3 years as follow-up is completed.

Interestingly, LV filling pressures did not decrease with either the Batista or the SVR procedure in the few patients in whom this was evaluated after the procedures.

Valvular Heart Disease
Indications for surgical treatment of valvular heart disease are generally well established. However, when LV function is severely reduced, surgical risk is greatly increased and it is not clear when it is futile to offer surgery. This is particularly the case for mitral regurgitation (MR) which, when severe, may cause a false elevation in LVEF. Further, when encountering the combination of severe MR and poor LV function, it is generally not possible to distinguish between the etiologies of primary MR with subsequent LV failure versus primary dilated cardiomopathy with subsequent mitral anular dilatation and MR. Whether the underlying etiology is important in outcome after surgical correction of the MR is unknown, but this uncertainty clouds interpretation of reports of surgery in this patient population.

Early surgical correction of severe MR, even for asymptomatic patients with normal LV function, is known to be very important to maintain a normal long term prognosis. This has been well studied by Sarano and others at Mayo Clinic. Among patients with heart failure, presence of even mild MR is associated with poor outcome. In a study by Blondheim, 3-year survival was 60% with no MR, 26% with mild MR and 17% with moderate to severe MR. Whether the MR is a marker for more severe myocardial disease, more advanced heart failure or actually contributes to progression of the heart failure is unclear.

Severe MR results in volume overload of the left ventricle and, conceptually, correction of the MR will reduce LV volume, diameter, and wall tension. There has been an opinion that MR results in a "pop-off" effect for the LV and correction in the presence of severe LV dysfunction will be poorly tolerated. However, as noted above, correction of MR may result in reduced LV volume and wall tension, and—paradoxically—a reduction in afterload at the myocyte level.

Bolling, at the University of Michigan has pioneered surgical repair of mitral regurgitation in patients with severely reduced LV function (LVEF <25%). Operative mortality has been reported as low as 2%. A good understanding of patient selection, indications and contraindications has been elusive. Indeed, careful reading of serial papers published by Bolling imply an increase in operative mortality after the initial clinical experience, probably related to relaxing the criteria for inclusion in surgical care. Repair of MR in these patients with heart failure selected for surgery did reduce LV end-diastolic volume, improve EF and improve functional class. In 2005, Bolling reported late outcome for patients having surgical repair of severe MR and it was not possible to show that surgical intervention in this high risk group improved late survival.

Surgical therapy for other valvular lesions when LV function is severely reduced is high risk. Patient selection and surgical benefit remain unclarified. Patients with many comorbid conditions require very careful consideration and may not be surgical candidates.

Other Surgical Treatment
A number of techniques and devices have been developed to provide external support to the failing left ventricle. Dynamic cardiomyoplasty involved pacing the latissimus dorsi muscle after wrapping it around the heart so that it contracted with the heart. The procedure improved functional class in heart failure patients, but was not applicable to those in class IV due to the time it took to condition the muscle. Advances in medical therapy limited the application of cardiomyoplasty to such an extent that the manufacturer of the pacing device stopped making the device.

The Acorn Corcap (Acorn Cardiovascular, Inc.) passive restraint device is a polyester yarn that can be placed around the heart with minimally invasive techniques and provides compliant, uniform stress distribution. Report of the initial 300 patients was presented at the American Heart Association in 2004. Functional capacity improved in 38% of Acorn patients compared with 27% of controls, but two-thirds of all patients also received mitral valve repair, which clearly confounds interpretation of the results.

The Myosplint (Myocor, Inc.) is another passive restraint device in which cables are passed through the LV and secured from the outside with button-like devices. This results in a bilobular LV with each chamber having a lower radius compared to baseline and potentially reduced wall stress. The devices can be placed off-pump. Evaluation is pending.

MECHANICAL CIRCULATORY SUPPORT

Destination Therapy with Left Ventricular Assist Devices
Fifteen years ago, the Institute of Medicine estimated that by the year 2010 approximately 50,000 patients in the U.S. per year would benefit from cardiac replacement or support with transplant or a mechanical device. Heart transplant volume in the U.S. has been limited to about 2500 per year for the last decade. This estimate has fueled industry attempts to develop a mechanical device to provide cardiac support. Total artificial heart (TAH) development has been pursued to a limited extent (the CardioWest manufactured by SynCardia Systems, Inc. and the Abiocor manufactured by Abiomed, Inc.). Most efforts have centered on developing left ventricular assist devices (LVAD) that can provide flows that will replace the entire cardiac output of the LV or are true assist devices that pump only a portion of the cardiac output. The development of a suitable TAH or LVAD for long term support has been challenging and elusive; the National Heart, Lung and Blood Insititute set a priority for providing support to develop such a device more than 40 years ago—landing men on the moon proved to be a less formidable challenge. In 2003 the FDA approved the first mechanical LVAD as a permanent device ("Destination Therapy").

LVADs (and TAHs) have undergone development and evaluation as a bridge to transplant (BTT) in more than 3500 patients. Over half of recent recipients of implantable LVADs have been able to be discharged from the hospital and about 70% survive to transplant. This experience has led to expanding these pumps to use as destination therapy (DT).

The landmark REMATCH trial (Randomized Evaluation of Mechanical Assistance for the Treatment of Congestive Heart Failure) was reported in the *New England Journal of Medicine* in 2001. This trial established DT as superior to medical management in an exceptionally ill group of heart failure patients and led to FDA approval of the Heartmate I device (Thoratec, Inc.) for DT. To date, it is the only approved device for

DT, and represents the first generation of LVADs: large, implantable, pulsatile devices that require air venting and are capable of pumping up to 10-12 liters per minute of blood.

REMATCH randomized heart failure patients to LVAD or optimal medical management (OMM), and inclusion criteria approximated criteria for transplantation: class IV heart failure, LVEF <25%, and either peak oxygen consumption <12 to 14 mL/kg/min or dependence on intravenous inotropic support. The enrolled population was the sickest entered in a randomized heart failure trial. Indeed, most patients randomized were already beyond current medical therapy: 32% were intolerant to ACE inhibitors. Survival at 1 year was 52% and 25%, and at 2 years was 28% and 11% (intention to treat analysis: OMM survival at 2 years was 8% excluding those crossing over to LVAD) for LVAD and OMM patients, respectively (p = 0.0015). The cause of death for the OMM group was primarily heart failure. Cause of death among patients with LVAD was primarily sepsis (37% of deaths) and mechanical device failure (19% of deaths).

Quality of life was superior in the LVAD group as analyzed by the Minnesota Living with Heart Failure Score, and LVAD patients reported improvement in NYHA class from IV to either II or III.

Following REMATCH, improvement in survival after LVAD placement for DT has been demonstrated using the same LVAD device (Heartmate I, Thoratec, Inc.). Among experienced centers, one year survival of 61% has been achieved with the same population group as the REMATCH trial indicating improvements in patient management including an eightfold decrease in death rate due to sepsis. Patients entered into the later part of the REMATCH trial were not evaluated separately in the initial publication, but these patients had a 2 year survival of 43%. These improved results indicate that better outcomes can be achieved as experience accumulates.

One of the limitations of the REMATCH trial involved the relatively high device failure rate of the Heartmate I device: 0.15 failures per patient-year. Another first generation LVAD, the Novacor (Worldheart, Inc.) has been reported to have a device failure rate of 0.033 per patient-year. Device failure of second generation, rotary style pumps is reported to be uncommon.

The patients entered in the REMATCH trial were extremely sick, as indicated by the survival in the OMM group. Improved patient selection would clearly help improve outcome. The process of patient selection will be facilitated with better understanding of predictors of survival in these patients with advanced heart failure. The patients selected using the Seattle Heart Failure Model, non-responders to resynchronization therapy, and specific clinical factors such as hematocrit, serum sodium level, and other factors may contribute to a better patient selection process. Outcomes are also improving with the understanding that some patients can become "too sick." Evaluation of the Thoratec Registry database has identified predictors of in-hospital death after DT LVAD placement which include (followed by the risk ratio for each): platelets <150x10^9/liter (10), body surface area <1.8 m^2 (8.8), creatinine clearance <30 mL/min (7.7), white blood cell count >12 x10^9/liter (6.5), mean pulmonary artery pressure <25 mm Hg (5.9), INR >1.1 seconds (4.6), albumin <3.3 g/dL (3.6). Multiple risk factors predicted mortality to a much greater degree than would be expected from a simple additive effect.

Interestingly, LVAD use for DT has been very uncommon given the earlier prediction of the Institute of Medicine. From FDA approval in 2002 to May 2006 only 420 patients have been entered in the mandatory Thoratec Registry with an average of 6.7 implants per center. The reasons for the slow adaptation of the technology are many. Certainly, implants will increase as outcomes improve and patient selection is better understood. However, improvements in the technology itself will also contribute. The current first generation devices (Heartmate I and Novacor) are very large, pulsatile devices that require large diameter, relatively rigid drivelines to vent air with each cycle and have relatively high power requirements. The size of these devices, alone, limits their application. The large, rigid drivelines contribute to driveline infections and the exit sites require vigilant care.

Second generation LVADs are small, rotary pumps that are quieter, easier to implant, more comfortable for the patient and have smaller, more pliable drivelines. The consequences of the non-pulsatile, continuous flow that they provide are still being studied. Current devices in clinical trials include the Heartmate II (Thoratec, Inc.), the Jarvik 2000 (Jarvik, Inc.) and the Debakey-Micromed

(Micromed, Inc.). While all these devices have bearings, mechanical failure has been very rare. All require systemic anticoagulation, have thromboembolic rates equal to or less than the first generation pumps, and are less prone to infection (probably related to the smaller size and driveline exit sites that are easier to manage). Third generation pumps currently in laboratory and very early clinical trials are magnetically suspended centrifugal pumps that eliminate potential for bearing wear.

One of the exciting aspects of long term LVAD support has been the recognition that occasional patients will have recovery of their LV function. This has been an anecdotal experience at this point, though it is common enough that most experienced centers have had patients recover enough LV function to allow explantation of their LVADs. Yacoub and Khaghani at Harefield Hospital in London, U.K. have reported LV recovery in 10 of 16 patients entered into a clinical protocol of aggressive medical heart failure therapy. The potential to provide mechanical support with the LVAD while new technology such as stem cell therapy is provided will be an exciting area of future research.

CONCLUSION

Heart failure continues to increase in incidence and prevalence, and now is the most common reason for hospitalization of patients over the age of 65 in the U.S. Medical therapy has dramatically improved survival for many patients. However, many patients with potential hibernating myocardium or valvular disease may benefit from surgery. Left ventricular remodeling may benefit some patients with antero-apico-septal LV dyskinesia. Ultimately, long term or permanent therapy with LVADs may provide improved prognosis with an acceptable quality of life for a large number of patients with advanced or end-stage heart failure.

100

CARDIAC TRANSPLANTATION

Brooks S. Edwards, MD

Richard C. Daly, MD

Cardiac transplantation is now considered a well established treatment for patients with intractable end-stage cardiac failure with about 2000 heart transplants performed annually in the United States at 130 transplant centers.

CARDIAC TRANSPLANTATION CURRENT STATUS

Indications for Cardiac Transplantation

Cardiac transplantation is indicated for patients with end-stage congestive heart failure (ACC/AHA Stage D) whether due to primary systolic dysfunction or diastolic dysfunction (Table 1). In general, candidates with severe ventricular dysfunction resulting in NYHA class IV congestive heart failure should be considered for cardiac transplantation. The limited number of donor hearts limits recipient patients to those most in need of transplantation and those who will derive the greatest benefits from the procedure. Various studies have demonstrated the utility of maximal exercise testing in identifying patients who are at high risk for poor outcome with medical therapy. These studies have shown a peak $\dot{V}O_2$ of 14 mL/kg/min or a peak $\dot{V}O_2$ less than 50% of predicted age adjusted maximum peak $\dot{V}O_2$ will identify patients at particularly high risk

Table 1. Common Selection Criteria for Cardiac Transplantation

End stage CHF (ACC/AHA stage D) despite optimal medical management

Impaired functional capacity ([oxygen consumption $\dot{V}O_2$] usually less than 14 mL/kg/min or 50% predicted)

Intractable Arrhythmias not amenable to usual therapy

Severe CAD not suitable for revascularization

Congenital heart disease not amenable to conventional surgery

Ability to follow a complex medical regimen

Adequate psychosocial support

for poor outcomes with medical therapy alone. Many third-party payers have established a peak $\dot{V}O_2$ of less than 14 mL/kg/min as a firm cut point for cardiac transplantation. It is our opinion that no one single test or cutoff value should be used alone to determine transplant candidacy. Rather the patient's entire clinical picture needs to be assessed to determine suitability for heart transplantation. In addition to the patient with severe heart failure, transplantation may be utilized in patients with intractable coronary artery disease even when left ventricular function is preserved if prognosis from the coronary artery disease is so poor as to justify transplantation and there are no other acceptable options for adequate revascularization. Patients with intractable arrhythmias not adequately treated by other modalities may also be considered for cardiac transplantation.

Transplantation may be utilized for individuals with severe congenital heart disease who cannot be adequately treated with conventional heart surgery. This includes neonates with hypoplastic left heart syndrome as well as older children and adults who frequently have had previous surgery for congenital heart disease and now have severe ventricular dysfunction. Patients post Fontan procedure who develope late congestive heart failure may be suitable candidates although those who have developed protein losing enteropathy with associated cachexia have not historically done well. Among patients with a history of left to right shunting, special attention needs to be directed to the state of the pulmonary vasculature and pre-transplant assessment of pulmonary vascular resistance is important.

Patients with infiltrative disorders such as primary amyloidosis or familial amyloidosis are considered for transplantation in some centers. In general, for patients with primary systemic amyloidosis the strategy is to treat the infiltrative disorder with bone marrow/stem cell transplantation. In patients with reasonably well preserved cardiac function stem cell transplant can be performed with careful cardiac monitoring. In patients with advanced cardiac involvement and symptomatic heart failure cardiac transplantation followed by stem cell transplantation as a staged procedure may be appropriate in a highly selected individuals. Extensive extracardiac amyloid deposition may make cardiac transplantation impractical. Individuals with familial amyloid, in which the transthyretin protein is produced by the liver, may benefit from combined heart-liver transplantation. Many of these patients experience peripheral and autonomic neuropathy which may not improve with transplantation.

Contraindications to Transplantation (Table 2)
Patients with coexistent systemic diseases which are not likely to be improved by transplantation or could

Table 2. Contraindications for Cardiac Transplantation

Severe irreversible pulmonary hypertension PVR >6 Wood units

Pulmonary parenchymal disease resulting in an inability to adequately rehabilitate

Recent acute pulmonary emboli with unresolved pulmonary infarction

Coexistent systemic disease which will severely impact on life expectancy

History of neoplastic disease with substantial chance for recurrent disease

Ongoing systemic infectious process

Severe cerebral or peripheral vascular disease

History of unresolved or untreated substance abuse

High titer of multiple preformed anti-HLA antibodies

Inability to follow a complex medical program

actually be aggravated by transplantation need careful evaluation. Patients with history of noncutaneous malignancies or melanoma when there has not been adequate time to assess whether the patient has been cured are not are considered good candidates for transplantation. If, however, there has been an adequate period of time since the treatment of the malignancy to the development of congestive heart failure these individuals may be reasonable transplant candidates. The required duration of the tumor free interval varies with different neoplasms. Transplantation for primary cardiac tumors has had disappointing results.

Patients with severe fixed (not responsive to vasodilator agents) pulmonary hypertension are not candidates for transplantation because the donor heart is not used to generating high right-sided pressure and will likely fail in this setting. If the pulmonary hypertension can be reduced by vasodilator therapy then candidacy may be considered. In general, one should be careful when considering heart transplantation alone for patients with a transpulmonary gradient (mean pulmonary artery pressure minus mean wedge pressure) greater than 15 mm Hg in the presence of vasodilator therapy such as nitroprusside. Pulmonary vascular resistance (PA mean – PCWP/Cardiac Output) measured in Wood units greater than 6 Wood units in spite of vasodilator therapy should be considered as a contraindication to transplantation.

Patients with unresolved chemical addiction including nicotine should not undergo transplantation until they have been adequately treated and followed. A strong social network with adequate psychosocial support is important for successful transplantation and the absence of such a support system raises considerable concern regarding the long-term outcome for patients undergoing cardiac transplantation.

Patients with diabetes mellitus may be considered candidates for transplantation depending upon the extent of diabetic complications. The presence of severe diffuse microvascular disease is a particular concern. Many patients with mild diabetes mellitus without severe vascular disease have been successfully transplanted.

Renal insufficiency is common among patients with severe cardiac dysfunction. In some cases the renal function improves with improved cardiac output but often this improvement is limited. Various factors post transplant (prolonged period of cardiac pulmonary bypass time and cyclosporine or tacrolimis treatment) may result in further renal damage. In heart failure patients with pretransplant GFR less then 30 mL/min consideration should be given to simultaneous heart/kidney transplantation. In some situations a renal biopsy can help distinguish intrinsic renal disease from prerenal hypoperfusion.

Waiting List

The annual number of patients listed for cardiac transplantation exceeded those transplanted by the late 1990s: since then the divergence has continued and presently there are about twice as many patients waiting for organs than transplants done in any given year.

Transplant organs are allocated through an agency licensed by the federal government—United Network for Organ Sharing (UNOS) based on a combination of severity of recipient's disease and waiting time. Candidates for cardiac transplantation wait in one of four categories. These are as follows: Status 1A, the patient is waiting in an ICU or on a mechanical assist device (for 30 days or less) or those patients requiring multiple inotropes for support or mechanical ventilation. Status 1B are patients requiring a single inotrope or multiple inotropes but the patient does not have indwelling hemodynamic monitoring and is not required to be in an ICU. Long-term (greater than 30 days after the inplant) ventricular assist device (VAD) patients are also considered status 1B. Status 2 are patients treated with oral therapy either in hospital or as outpatients and status 7 are inactive patients for transplantation because of medical or social issues.

Organs are matched for ABO blood type and then allocated to the patient with the longest waiting time in the region with the highest status. Rh antigen is not carried on the myocyte and therefore Rh incompatibility poses no barrier to heart transplantation.

Perioperative Management

Induction of anesthesia and initiation of cardiopulmonary bypass for planned heart transplant recipients can be challenging because of the underlying severe cardiac dysfunction that these patients typically exhibit. Patients with multiple previous operations represent increased surgery challenge because of the development of adhesions, substantial bleeding risk and the potential for disruption of patent cardiac grafts during the dissection and cannulation.

The donor heart can withstand a maximum period of cold ischemia of about four hours after which the function of the heart declines and the outcome from transplantation is less favorable. Close communication between the donor surgical team and the recipient surgical team is mandatory.

The donor heart is anastomosed either to the posterior wall of the recipients right and left atrium (Figure 1) or the right-sided structures may be anastomosed with a bicaval approach. The bicaval approach has been favored recently because of the reported lower incidence of postoperative heart block and possibly lower incidence of postoperative tricuspid valve insufficiency.

The transplanted heart often exhibits some degree of sinus node dysfunction in the early postoperative period and frequently requires support with isoproterenol or cardiac pacing for several days. About 15% of donor hearts may exhibit long-term sinus node dysfunction or AV node dysfunction requiring implantation of a permanent pacemaker. The incidence of pacing appears to rise with the use of older donor hearts.

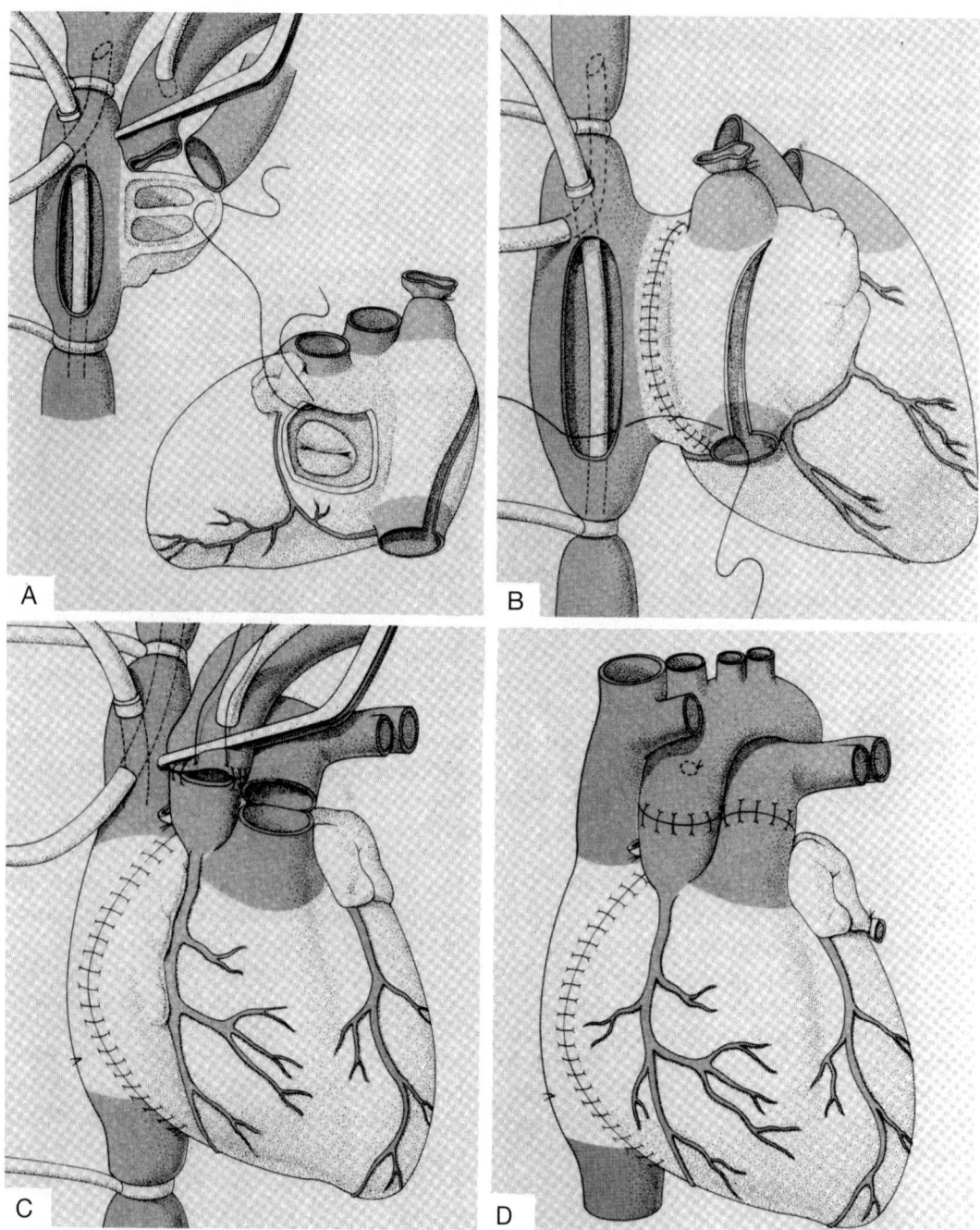

Fig. 1. *A* to *D*, Surgical techniques of orthotopic cardiac transplantation.

Chronic Immunosuppression

Since the 1980s the standard immunosuppression for cardiac transplantation has consisted of "triple" therapy. The triple therapy has included a calcineurin inhibitor (cyclosporine or tacrolimus), an antimetabolite (azathioprine or mycophenolic acid), and corticosteroids. In approximately 50% of patients weaning of long-term corticosteroids is possible after the first year post transplantation.

Recent advances in immunosuppression include the development of a new class of drugs including rapamycin and everolimus both of which inhibit a proliferative step in the cell cycle and in doing so provide significant immuno-suppression. This anti-proliferative effect may also inhibit wound healing and hence their use in the early postoperative period has been complicated by delayed and diminished wound healing. The advantages of these drugs include less nephrotoxicity than calcineurin inhibitors and in preliminary studies they appear to have a favorable effect on the prevention of graft related coronary vasculopathy. Studies are ongoing to assess whether rapamycin should be given as an alternative to calcineurin inhibitors or as an alternative to antimetabolite therapy.

All immunosuppressive drugs share the complication of increasing the risk of opportunistic infections. These infections can be bacterial, viral, or fungal. Most patients treated with immunosuppressive therapy should receive prophylaxis for *Pneumocystis* either in the form of trimethoprim/sulfamethoxazole or with monthly inhaled pentamidine.

There are specific complications associated with the specific immunosuppressive drugs. Cyclosporine is associated with renal insufficiency, tremor, hirsutism and some element of hyperlipidemia. Gingival hyperplasia also can occur with cyclosporine. Tacrolimus shares the nephrotoxic potential of cyclosporine but does not cause hirsutism or gingival hyperplasia and therefore may be a more acceptable choice in individuals who are particularly concerned about their appearance. Tacrolimus does appear to increase the incidence of post-transplant glucose intolerance and diabetes.

The antimetabolite drugs include mycophenolic acid (CellCept) and azathioprine have been associated with cytopenias and increased risk of viral infections. Azathioprine can result in hepatic dysfunction and CellCept at higher doses is associated with a GI intolerance. Azathioprine and allopurinol share a common metabolic pathway and, great care is needed if used together as allopurinol will markedly increase azathioprine levels and if unchecked can result in profound bone marrow suppression.

The complications of corticosteroids are well-known and the transplant population is particularly prone to diabetic complications and osteopenic bone disease. All of the manifestations of Cushing's syndrome with exogenous corticosteroids can be observed.

Rapamycin has been associated with hyperlipidemia and bone marrow suppression and oral lesions including aphthous ulcers. Wound healing is delayed and great caution should be exercised in patients having major surgery while on rapamycin.

LONG-TERM OUTCOMES OF CARDIAC TRANSPLANTATION

Since the introduction of cyclosporine in the 1980s the outcomes for transplantation have improved dramatically. Based on data from UNOS the overall one-year survival after cardiac transplantation ranges between 80-85%. The five-year survival ranges between 50-60%. In individual centers outcomes can be considerably better. At Mayo Clinic the one-year survival after cardiac transplantation is in excess of 90% and the five-year survival is approximately 80%.

Most patients after transplantation can return to a relatively normal lifestyle although it does require a regimented approach to medical care with attention to daily medication administration and monitoring for signs of rejection or infection. Most patients can return to full-time employment with little or no restrictions.

Numerous studies have evaluated the cost effectiveness of cardiac transplantation and it appears to be favorable in terms of dollars spent for prolongation of active life. Compared to other medical procedures including dialysis, and routine screening mammography, transplantation compares favorably.

COMPLICATIONS

While the overall results from cardiac transplantation are excellent with most patients returning to an active lifestyle with a good quality of life, recipients should recognize that they are at risk for multiple long-term complications.

Coronary Artery Vasculopathy

Regardless of the initial indication for cardiac transplantation, recipients commonly develop some degree of obstructive coronary arterial disease in the donor heart. There are several distinct morphologic types of disease recognized. Classical post transplant coronary arterial disease develops in small distal vessels and results in obstruction with "drop out "of branch vessels. Over time the disease may involve the entire length of the artery (Fig. 2). Histologically, this process appears to resemble post coronary stent restenosis and is charac-

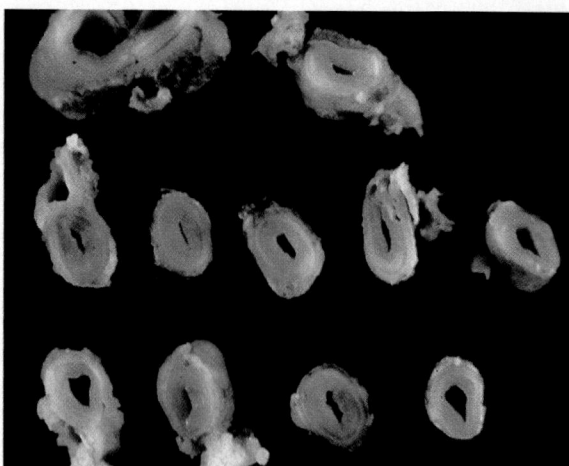

Fig. 2. Posttransplant coronary vasculopathy. The entire epicardial coronary artery has been removed and cut in cross-section. Diffuse severe intimal proliferation is seen in the length of the artery.

terized by a marked proliferative fibrotic appearance without typical lipid laden atheromas. Coronary angiography detects some degree of coronary vascular disease in approximately 40% of recipients 5 years following heart transplantation. Utilizing intravascular ultrasound the incidence is even higher. This process may develop rapidly in some cases and be detected at angiography one year following the transplant. Among long term recipients (greater then >5 years post transplant) some will exhibit more classical coronary arterial atherosclerosis with proximal arterial stenosis. The results of percutaneous coronary intervention or coronary artery bypass surgery are less favorable than in non-transplanted hearts.

The mechanism of posttransplant vasculopathy appears to be multifactorial in nature and includes both chronic forms of immune rejection as well as more traditional causes for atherosclerosis including hyperlipidemia which probably plays a role in the development of coronary artery disease in long term transplant recipients. Smoking post heart transplant has not been systematically studied but in our experience the few patients who resume smoking post transplant often develop a very malignant form of vascular disease.

Transplanted hearts are denervated at surgery and typically don't exhibit angina with myocardial ischemia: the presenting manifestation of coronary artery vasculopathy is often sudden death. Most post transplant surveillance programs perform annual coronary angiography (with our without intravascular ultrasound) to detect coronary vasculopathy early. Preliminary studies suggest that the antiproliferative immunosuppressive agents sirolimus and everolimus may be effective in preventing or retarding the development of post transplant coronary vasculopathy.

Infectious Complications

Patients following cardiac transplantation are increasingly susceptible to a variety of infectious agents. These can be broken down based on the origin of the infection. Certain infections are donor acquired. These include viral infections (CMV, Epstein-Barr virus, HIV, West Nile virus) and toxoplasmosis. Viral hepatitis (B and C) can also be transmitted via a donor organ. Community acquired infections include influenza and *Legionella* as well as other bacterial and viral infections.

Infections associated specifically with the immunosuppressed state include fungal infections. In patients exposed to a significant inoculum of *Aspergillus* this is a major concern. Most transplant patients should be treated with prophylactic therapy to prevent *Pneumocystis* lung infections.

Hypertension

Post-transplant hypertension is a common phenomenon with estimates of its prevalence ranging from 65-90% of patients posttransplant. While it has been generally associated with cyclosporine use, the phenomenon of posttransplant hypertension was identified before the introduction of cyclosporine and occurs with other immunosuppressive regimens as well. The mechanism of hypertension has been rather illusive but preglomerular vasoconstriction in the kidney is probably important. Some of the hypertension appears to be volume dependent phenomenon. Treatment of posttransplant hypertension may require multiple agents. There is often a loss of normal diurnal variation of blood pressure.

Rejection

Cardiac rejection represents an ongoing risk for patients following cardiac transplantation. The highest risk of rejection occurs in the first year following transplantation. While the risk of rejection never goes to zero it does diminish over time as organ immune tolerance develops. Patients need to understand that they will need chronic immunosuppressive therapy for life.

Because there are currently no noninvasive tests to accurately detect graft rejection patients undergo routine right ventricular endomyocardial biopsy. The biopsy is usually done from the right internal jugular approach but can be accomplished via a femoral venous approach. Typically 4-6 pieces of myocardium are collected for light microscopy and if necessary immunostaining. There are several noninvasive tests for rejection in development and early clinical application which may reduce the need for cardiac biopsy. These noninvasive techniques include an analysis of gene activation or measurement of immune mediators.

The predominant mechanism for cardiac rejection is based on a T cell mediated phenomenon. This can be identified by cardiac biopsy and graded as noted below. There is also an additional phenomenon of humeral or antibody mediated rejection which is more difficult to identify but sometimes correlates with a fall in ventricular function and the development of thickened ventricular walls on echo imaging a finding consistent with myocardial edema. Immunostaining for antibodies and complement can sometimes identify humeral rejection.

The International Society for Heart and Lung Transplantation published a new grading system for cardiac rejection in 2005. It is based on a scheme that looks for both T cell mediated rejection and humeral (antibody mediated) rejection. Grade 1R represents mild cell mediated rejection, grade 2R represents moderate cell mediated rejection, and grade 3R represents severe cell mediated rejection (Fig. 3). In general, most physicians would not treat a grade 1R rejection but would treat grade 2R and beyond. The higher levels of rejection are associated with myocyte damage and heavy cellular infiltrate. Humeral rejection is graded 1H, 2H, and 3H, similarly.

On cardiac biopsy there is a phenomenon known as the "Quilty phenomenon." This represents a prominent endocardial collection of lymphocytes. This may be associated with EBV activation but does not in itself represent rejection or post-transplant lymphoproliferative disease.

Most cases of allograft rejection are identified by cardiac biopsy before the occurrence of ventricular dysfunction. Advanced forms of rejection may present with low-grade fever and evidence of congestive heart failure. Any patient presenting with hemodynamic

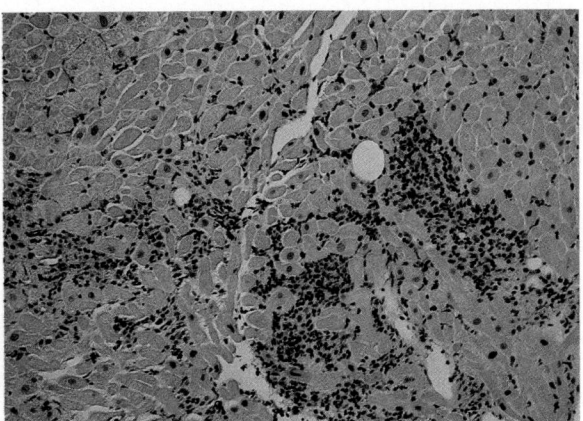

Fig. 3. Photomicrograph of acute cell medicated rejection. This is a moderate grade 2R cell mediated rejection. The lymphocytic infiltrate is seen in blue.

compromise suggestive of rejection should be treated aggressively even before biopsy confirmation can be confirmed.

Standard treatment for cell mediated rejection includes augmented corticosteroids. Humeral rejection may require plasmapheresis and targeted anti B-cell therapy. Severe forms of cell mediated rejection may require antilymphocyte antibody therapy.

Posttransplant Neoplastic Disease

Chronic immunosuppression can lead to the development of post transplant malignancies the most common of which include non-melanotic cutaneous malignancies. This includes both localized basal cell carcinoma as well as cutaneous squamous cell cancers. Occasionally the squamous tumors may present with regional or distant metastatic disease. Patients with fair skin type and a history of extensive sun exposure are a particular risk of post transplant tumors.

Posttransplant lymphomas may develop with chronic immunosuppression. These disorders are often times related to Epstein-Barr virus (EBV) activation especially in the patients who have not previously been exposed to EBV and receive an organ from an EBV positive donor. The so called posttransplant lymphoproliferative disorder (PTLD) may sometimes respond to a reduction in immunosuppression while at other times systemic chemotherapy may be required (Fig. 4).

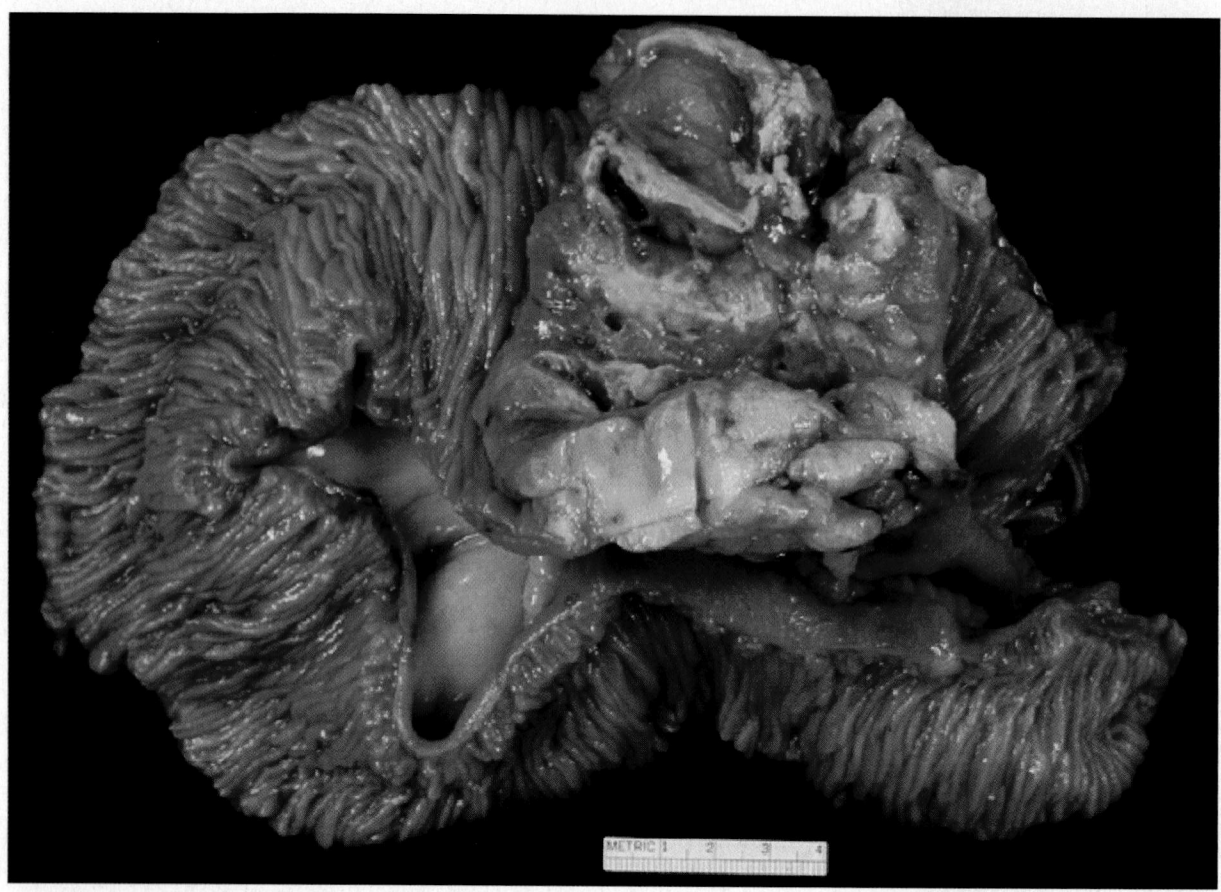

Fig. 4. Posttransplant lymphoproliferative disorder (PTLD). Lymphoma present in the mesentery of the small intestine. This PTLD responded to a surgical resection with a reduction in overall immunosuppession.

Cardiac Pharmacology

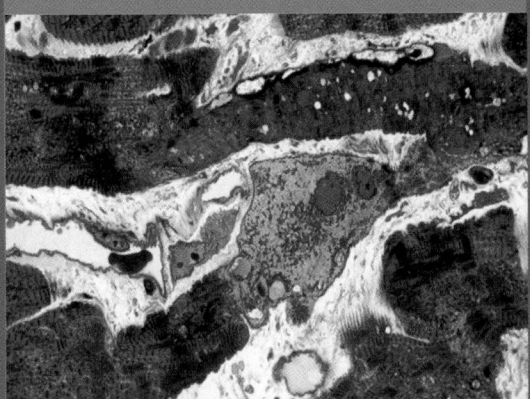

Doxorubicin Cardiac Toxicity

—

101

Principles of Pharmacokinetics and Pharmacodynamics

Arshad Jahangir, MD

Leonid V. Zingman, MD

Andre Terzic, MD, PhD

Pharmacology defines the pharmacokinetics and pharmacodynamics of drugs.

- *Pharmacokinetics* (PK) describes the fate of a drug following administration.
- *Pharmacodynamics* (PD) defines the mechanism(s) of a drug including interaction with targets and induced response.

Understanding the pharmacokinetics and pharmacodynamics of drugs is essential in individualizing the therapeutic plan to secure optimum clinical benefit while avoiding adverse effects.

PHARMACOKINETIC PRINCIPLES

Pharmacokinetics comprises the processes of drug **a**bsorption, **d**istribution, **m**etabolism, and **e**limination (ADME) (Fig. 1). Pharmacokinetic principles help determine the dosage of the drug taking into account the patient's age, sex, weight, liver and renal function and specifying routes of administration and dosage regimen to achieve appropriate concentration at target/receptor sites.

Absorption

Absorption refers to the transfer of a drug from its site of delivery into the circulation. This commonly occurs by diffusion across plasma membranes with carrier-mediated transfer or active transport recognized for certain drugs. P-glycoprotein encoded by the multidrug resistance-1 (*MDR1*) gene is an important drug transporter that acts as an efflux pump and limits drug absorption in enterocytes by causing transport of the drug back into the intestinal lumen subsequent to its absorption by passive diffusion.

Drug absorption into systemic circulation is dependent on many factors including those related to formulation and physicochemical properties of the drug, patient's pathophysiology, genetic make up (P-glycoprotein polymorphism) or use of concomitant drugs that alter drug absorption by changing gut motility, bacterial flora or P-glycoprotein function (Table 1). Absorption is more efficient for small, lipid soluble and electrically neutral molecules. However, many drugs behave as weak acids or bases and have different absorption rates depending on their ionic charge. The ratio between the charged and uncharged form is determined by the pH at the site of absorption and the

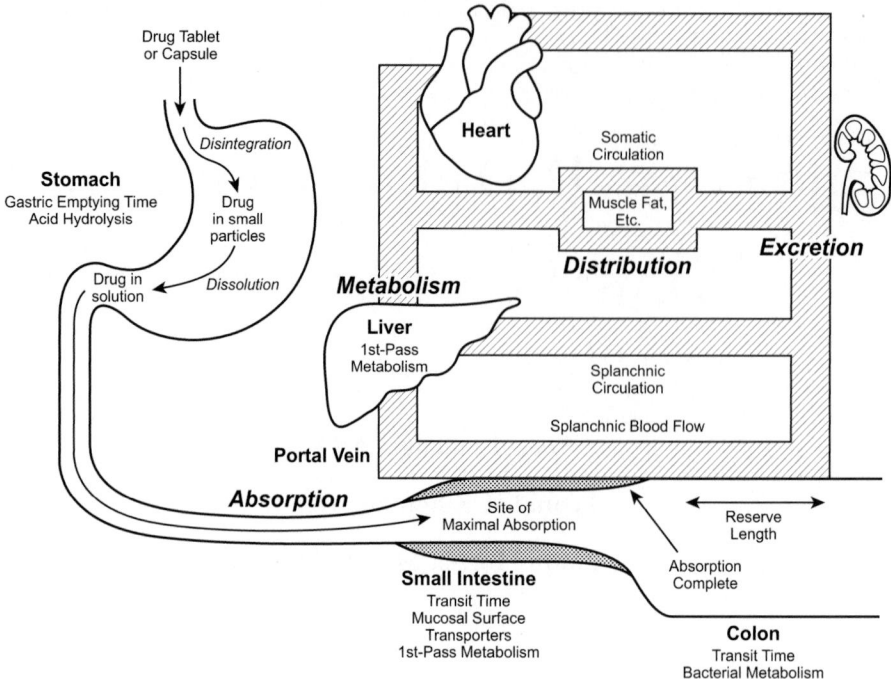

Fig. 1. Pharmacokinetic steps from absorption to elimination of drugs. Physiologic processes that affect the rate and extent of absorption of a drug are highlighted.

strength of the weak acid or base, which is represented by the pK_a value. Acidic or neutral drugs remain unionized and get absorbed well from the stomach with its acidic pH, while basic drugs are poorly absorbed until they pass into the duodenum (Fig. 1).

The sustained release formulations produce a lower peak concentration and prolong the duration of drug effects. This allows less frequent dosage regimens compared to rapid release forms. It is important to avoid crushing or splitting the extended release formulation as the drug's physical and chemical properties will be altered and could result in loss of drug action or excessive systemic delivery causing toxicity.

Bioavailability describes the fraction of the unchanged drug that is absorbed into the systemic circulation. Bioavailability is 100% following intravenous administration but is variable with other routes as only a fraction of the administered dose is absorbed. Orally administrated drugs may also undergo metabolism in the gut wall or liver (first-pass effect) contributing to further reduction in bioavailability. After oral administration the bioavailability of a drug can be determined by comparison of the area under the plasma concentration-time curve following oral and intravenous drug administration (Fig. 2). These curves also provide information about peak plasma levels and time necessary to attain peak levels.

Drug metabolism that occurs en route from the gut lumen to the systemic circulation is referred to as *"first-pass metabolism."* The first-pass effect of some drugs (such as lidocaine and ibutilide) is so extensive that only a minute fraction of the orally administered drug reaches its target and therefore these drugs have to be given intravenously. Individual variation in first-pass metabolism is present in a population due to genetic heterogeneity and could be further affected by disease conditions resulting in higher bioavailability and potential for toxicity, especially for drugs with a narrow therapeutic index. Table 2 lists some of the drugs used in cardiovascular medicine that undergo high first-pass metabolism.

Points to Remember for the Cardiology Examinations

- The most important factors governing rate and extent of absorption of a drug are solubility and intestinal permeability.
- Crushing or splitting the extended release formulation affects physical and chemical properties of a drug

Table 1. Determinants of Drug Absorption and Bioavailability

Absorption
Drug/dosage form
Formulation (drug + vehicle)
Liquid form (solution, elixirs, and suspension)
Solids (tablets, capsules, soluble, sustained-released)
Creams and ointments
Physical/chemical properties of drug
Particle size of the molecule
Solubility (nature of diluent, lipophilic vs. hydrophilic)
Ionization or charge (salt or ester form)
pH
Patient related
Local conditions at the site of administration
Blood flow
Temperature of the tissue
Adiposity
Surface area (integrity of gastrointestinal tract)
Contact time (gastrointestinal motility)
Concomitant drugs
Food
Presystemic metabolism
First-pass effect
Transport (P-glycoprotein polymorphism)
Comorbidities
Diarrhea, malabsorption
Liver disease
Heart failure

Table 2. Common Cardiovascular Drugs Undergoing First-Pass Metabolism

Labetalol, metoprolol, propranolol
Lidocaine
Verapamil, nifedipine
Aspirin
Ibutilide
Isosorbide dinitrate
Morphine
Prazosin

Distribution

After absorption, a drug enters the blood stream and distributes into interstitial and intracellular fluids. Volume of distribution is a hypothetical volume of fluid into which the drug is disseminated. Distribution depends on several factors, including cardiac output, regional blood flow, capillary permeability, tissue volume, plasma concentration of the drug, its solubility and binding to plasma proteins. In conditions where cardiac output is diminished such as during cardiac arrest and asystole, even an intravenously administered drug may not be effective unless circulation is maintained by cardiopulmonary resuscitation. A well-perfused tissue may become saturated with the drug earlier than less perfused areas. Lipophilic drugs can diffuse rapidly across lipid membranes, whereas water-soluble drugs that diffuse through gap junctions between endothelial cells may not diffuse so readily in tissues lacking these specialized intercellular junctions, such as the brain (blood-brain barrier).

The "*volume of distribution*" (V_d) is the volume of body fluid in which a drug is distributed. It can be calculated using the amount of drug in the body and the plasma concentration of the drug after a given time following administration.

$$V_d = \frac{\text{Amount of drug in body}}{\text{Concentration of drug in plasma}}$$

Hydrophilic drugs have a low volume of distribution and are mainly confined to the vascular space, whereas,

and may result in loss of efficacy or excessive drug delivery causing toxicity.

■ A decrease in first-pass metabolism, such as with severe liver dysfunction, can lead to an unexpectedly high bioavailability and risk for toxicity, especially for drugs with a narrow therapeutic index.

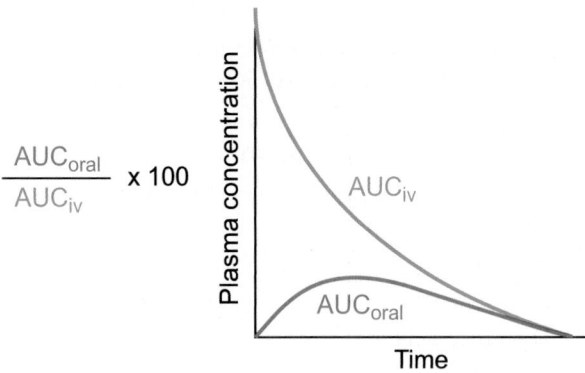

$$\frac{AUC_{oral}}{AUC_{iv}} \times 100$$

AUC = Area Under the Curve

Fig. 2. Bioavailability is determined by comparison of the area under the plasma concentration-time curve (AUC) following oral and intravenous drug.

lipophilic drugs have a high volume of distribution and are distributed in both vascular and extravascular tissue (Fig. 3). If the plasma concentration is low, the volume of distribution will be high. The volume of distribution varies among individual patients and with disease conditions, nutritional status, age and sex and is influenced by total body water, the quantity and binding capacity of plasma proteins, body fat and lean muscle mass composition.

Binding to Plasma Proteins

Many drugs circulate in the bloodstream bound to plasma proteins. Acidic drugs predominantly bind to albumin and basic drugs to α1-glycoprotein (Table 3). To a lesser extent drugs also bind to lipoproteins and globulins. Since the protein-bound complex is too large to cross membranes, only the unbound (free) drug fraction distributes to the target tissue and determines clinical effects. Access of drugs to their extravascular tissue receptors, as well as metabolism, storage and excretion are affected to some extent by plasma protein binding. Increasing the dose of a drug beyond the binding capacity of plasma proteins may increase the unbound fraction. Similarly, drugs may compete with one another for binding on plasma proteins and, by displacement interaction, result in a transient increase in free drug concentration (Fig. 4) that may lead to undesired effects, especially by drugs with a small volume of distribution, long elimination half-life and a narrow therapeutic index. Therefore, a drug that is 98% bound to plasma protein (such as the anticoagulant warfarin) has only 2% of the free drug available for action at the target receptor. If another 2% of the drug is displaced from plasma proteins by addition of a second drug, the unbound level may double, at least transiently and result in adverse effects. In addition, disease conditions in which serum albumin levels decrease (such as malnutrition, burns, nephrotic syndrome or liver disease)

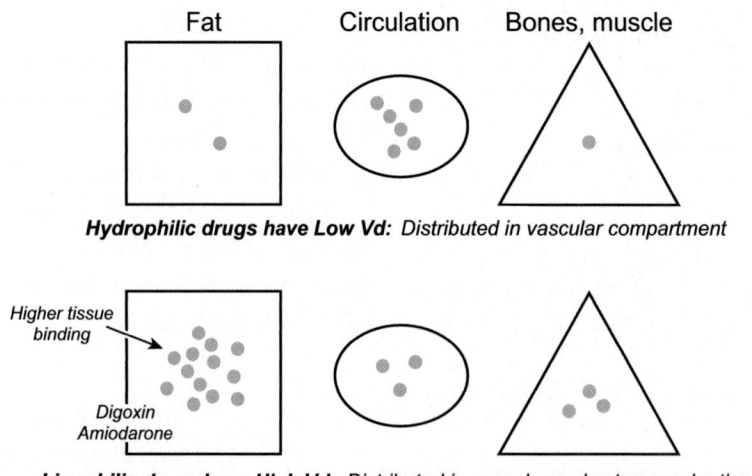

Fig. 3. Hydrophilic drugs have a low volume of distribution and are mainly confined to the vascular space, whereas lipophilic drugs have a high volume of distribution and are distributed in both vascular and extravascular tissue.

Table 3.   Drug Binding to Plasma Proteins

Bind primarily to albumin	Bind primiarly to α1-glycoprotein	Bind primarily to lipoproteins
Barbiturates	Alprenolol	Amitriptyline
Benzodiazepines	Dipyridamole	Nortriptyline
Bilirubin	Disopyramide	
Penicillins	Imipramine	
Phenytoin	Lidocaine	
Sulfonamides	Methadone	
Tetracycline	Prazosin	
Valproic acid	Propranolol	
Warfarin	Quinidine	
	Verapamil	

may require dosage reduction to avoid toxicity with increased amount of the free drug. Dosage of drugs that are bound to α1-glycoprotein (Table 3) need to be increased in conditions, such as acute myocardial infarction, inflammation or postoperatively when this acute phase reactant protein is increased.

Many drugs accumulate within tissues (muscle or fat) at higher concentrations than the extracellular fluids or blood. The tissue may then serve as a reservoir for drugs, prolonging their duration of action.

Points to Remember for the Cardiology Examination

■ Hydrophilic drugs are mainly confined to the vascular space and have a low volume of distribution, whereas, lipophilic drugs are distributed in both vascular and extravascular tissue and have a high volume of distribution.

■ Drugs may compete with one another for binding on plasma proteins and, by displacement interactions, result in a transient increase in free drug concentration that may lead to undesired effects.

■ Drug dosage may need to be adjusted for some drugs in conditions that cause hypoalbuminemia or increase in α1-glycoprotein levels.

Drug Metabolism and Elimination

Drugs are eliminated from the body mainly by two mechanisms, liver metabolism and renal excretion. Non-renal, non-hepatic pathways play only a minor role. Small water soluble drugs are eliminated unchanged by simple renal excretion, whereas larger or lipid soluble drugs first undergo biotransformation in the liver to hydrophilic polar metabolites, which are then excreted through the kidneys or in the bile.

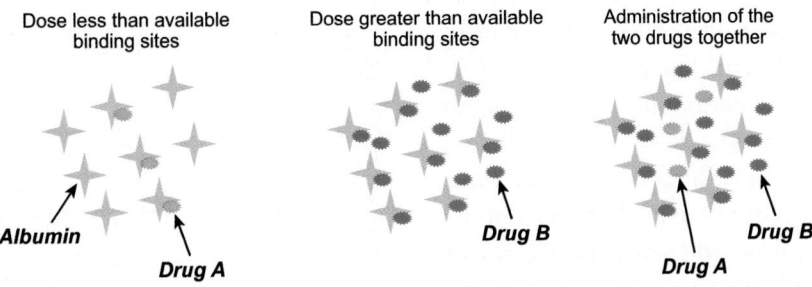

Fig. 4. Drug and plasma protein interaction. Increasing the dose of a drug beyond the binding capacity of plasma proteins or the addition of a drug with higher binding capacity may displace a drug with lower binding affinity and increase the unbound drug fraction.

Drug clearance is defined as the volume of blood cleared of the drug per unit time (mL/min). Total clearance (CL) of a drug can be calculated by:

$$CL = \frac{0.69 \cdot V_d}{t_{1/2}}$$

where, V_d = volume of drug distribution, and
$t_{1/2}$ = half life of the drug

Clearance can be used to determine dosage when the desired plasma concentration has been predetermined.

$$Dosage = CL \cdot C_{SS}$$

where, CL = clearance
C_{SS} = steady state plasma drug concentration

In situations where a rapid therapeutic response is required, the desired plasma concentration can be achieved with a quick loading dose to fill the entire volume of distribution to the desired concentration calculated by:

$$LD = \frac{V_d \cdot C}{F}$$

where V_d = apparent volume of distribution
C = desired plasma concentration, and
F = fraction of oral dose reaching the systemic circulation (bioavailability)

Half-Life of a Drug

The half-life ($t_{1/2}$) of a drug is defined as the time required for the plasma concentration to be decreased by one-half and is usually independent of the route of administration and dosage. The concentration of a drug in the blood most commonly decreases in an exponential manner, through *first-order kinetics*, that is, a *constant percent* of drug is eliminated per unit time. The half-life for each drug can be derived from the first-order reaction calculated from a semilog plot of the plasma concentration versus time (Fig. 5) during the elimination phase that reflects the sum of renal and hepatic metabolism and excretion. For some drugs, such as alcohol, phenytoin or high-dose aspirin, the

rate-limiting step can be saturated and elimination occurs by *zero-order kinetics*, that is, a *constant amount* of drug is eliminated per unit time. Thus even a small increase in drug dose can increase plasma concentration markedly, resulting in toxicity (Fig. 6).

The plasma steady state level of a drug, where the rate of entry is equal to the rate of elimination, is attained after approximately five half-lives (Fig. 7) and is independent of dosage, rate of administration or concentration. After withdrawal, the converse is seen and the plasma levels are reduced by 50% in one half-life, 75% in two, 87.5% and 93.75% in three and four half-lives.

Hepatic Drug Metabolism

The rate and extent of hepatic drug metabolism depends on blood flow to the liver and the type, number, affinity, and activity of hepatic enzymes. Drugs that are extensively extracted by the liver are mainly affected by the hepatic blood flow, whereas those with lower extraction rates are affected by the activity of liver enzymes (Fig. 8). Diminished hepatic extraction capacity, as seen in patients with liver disease or heart failure, may decrease clearance of these drugs.

Metabolism of drugs in the liver occurs in two phases (Fig. 9):

Phase one reactions involves oxidation, reduction or hydrolysis of the drug to generate a more polar, water soluble compound.

Phase two metabolism involves conjugation of the

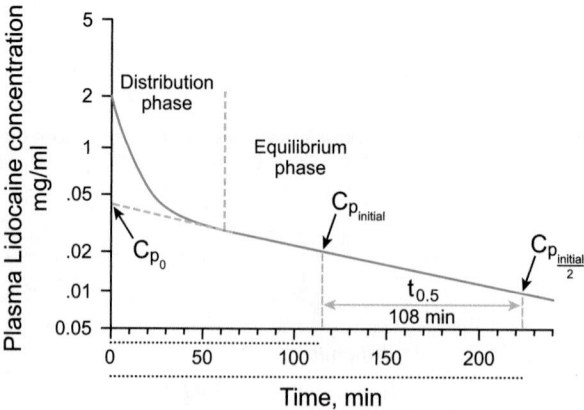

Fig. 5. Half-life ($t_{1/2}$) is the time for the plasma concentration of the drug during equilibrium to decrease by half.

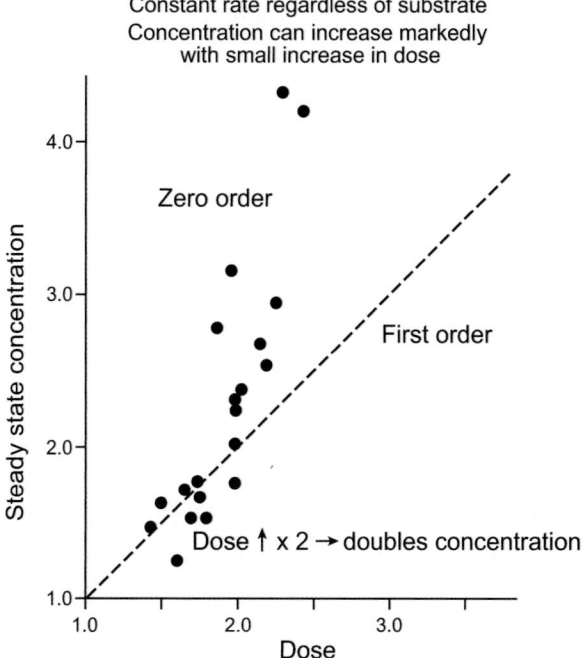

Fig. 6. Zero and first order elimination kinetics. The concentration of many drugs decrease in an exponential manner through first-order kinetics, with a constant percent removed per unit time. Other drugs, such as alcohol, phenytoin and aspirin are removed by zero order kinetics, in which a constant amount of drug is removed per unit time such that even a small increase in drug dose can increase plasma concentration markedly, resulting in toxicity.

phase one metabolite with glucuronic acid, sulfates or glutathione that can then be eliminated by the kidneys or in the bile.

The oxidation reactions in the liver are catalyzed by microsomal mixed function mono-oxygenate system, also known as the cytochrome P450 (CYP450) system. CYP450 is a large family of isozymes coded by 14 CYP genes, however most of the drugs are metabolized by enzymes belonging to only three CYP families (CYP 3, 2 and 1). They have broad substrate specificity and may catalyze the metabolism of different drugs. About 50% of drugs undergo metabolism by the CYP3A family, 25% by CYP2D6, 20% by CYP2C9 and 5% by CYP1A2. Table 4 lists the CYP isoforms and common drugs used in cardiovascular practice that are metabolized by these enzymes.

Many factors can affect the clearance of drug from the circulation (Table 5). Drug metabolizing isoenzymes are determined by genetic factors and are also modulated by disease or concomitant drug therapy. About 5-10% of Caucasians are deficient in CYP2D6, the isozyme that converts codeine to morphine, its active analgesic metabolite. Thus, individuals lacking CYP2D6 do not obtain much pain relief from codeine and may also experience more side effects related to β-adrenergic blockade with β-blockers or the antiarrhythmic drug propafenone, which possesses both sodium channel blocking (class I antiarrhythmic) and β-adrenergic receptor blocking (class II antiarrhythmic) effects.

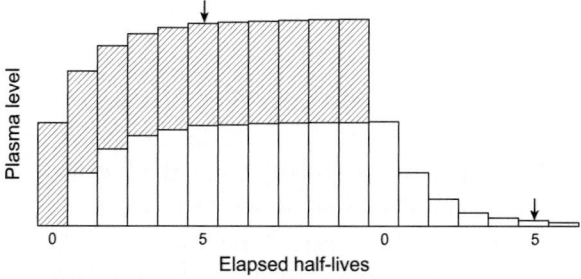

(↓) Steady state = rate of entry equals rate of elimination

Fig. 7. Steady state plasma levels are attained after ~5 half-lives. With the first-order kinetics, 50% of steady state is attained after one half-life; 75% after two; 87.5% and 93.75% after three and four half-lives.

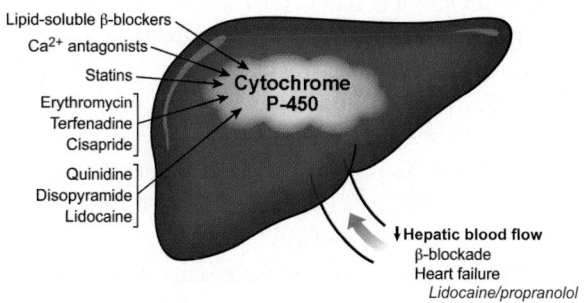

Fig. 8. Hepatic metabolism. Drugs that are extensively extracted by the liver are mainly affected by the hepatic blood flow, whereas those with lower extraction are affected by the activity of liver enzymes and not blood flow.

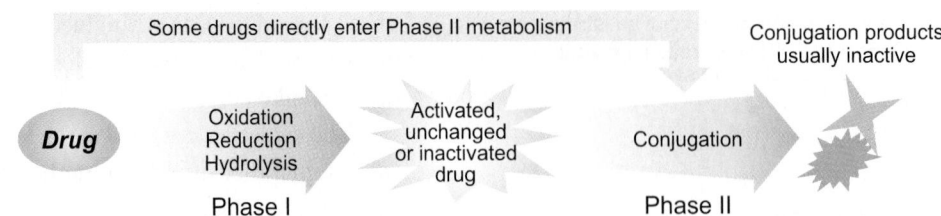

Fig. 9. Drug metabolism. Metabolism of drugs in the liver occurs in two phases. A phase I reaction involves oxidation, reduction, or hydrolysis of the drug to generate a more polar, water soluble compound. Phase II involves conjugation of the phase one metabolite with glucuronic acid, sulfates or glutathione that can be then eliminated by kidneys or in the bile.

CYPP450 enzyme activity is inhibited or induced by different drugs (Table 6) and dietary or other environmental factors. Such interactions can be of clinical relevance as inhibition of metabolism of an active drug can raise its serum levels and cause toxic effects. Cimetidine, a commonly used drug can profoundly decrease drug clearance by both reduction in hepatic blood flow and inhibition of CYP450 system activity, including CYP1A2, CYP2C, and CYP3A resulting in elevations of drugs such as lidocaine, propranolol or statins normally metabolized by these enzymes. CYP3A4 isozymes are also inhibited by macrolide antibiotics and ketoconazole and life-threatening arrhythmias were reported when these drugs were used with the long-acting antihistamine terfenadine, a prodrug that is metabolized by CYP3A4. An interesting interaction also occurs with consumption of grapefruit juice that inhibits CYP3A enzymes in the bowel that can increase the bioavailability and clinical effects of coadministered drugs (Table 7 and Fig. 10) normally metabolized by this enzyme.

Induction of CYP450 isozymes by drugs (Table 6) can accelerate clearance of other concomitantly used drugs normally metabolized by these enzymes, thus reducing their plasma level that may result in therapeutic failure. On the other hand, discontinuation of the enzyme inducer may result in increased drug levels and risk for toxicity.

Renal Drug Clearance

The clearance of drugs by the kidneys depends on the

Table 4.   Cytochrome P-450 Families and Common Drugs Metabolized by the Specific Isozymes

CYP3A4: amiodarone, dihydropyridine calcium channel blockers, diltiazem, verapamil, lidocaine, quinidine, HMG CoA reductase inhibitors, warfarin (partially), benzodiazepines, cisapride, clarithromycin, cyclosporine, cortisol, estrogens, erythromycin, fentanyl, indinavir, methadone, sildenafil, terfendine, troglitazone

CYP2E1: ethanol, isoflurane

CYP2D6: β-blockers, codeine, fluoxetine, mexiletine, propafenone, tricyclic antidepressants

CYP2C9: celecoxib, ibuprofen, irbesartan, losartan, tolbutamide, warfarin

CYP2C19: indomethacin, diazepam, omeprazole, phenytoin

CYP2B6: cycloposphamide, diazepam, lidocaine, procainamide, temazepam

CYP1A2: acetaminophen, caffeine, cimetidine, theophylline, nicotine

---

Table 5.   Factors Affecting Drug Clearance

Genotype (enzyme isoforms or transport protein)
Functional integrity of the organ responsible for clearance (renal or hepatic disease)
Concurrent illnesses (affecting perfusion, volume of distribution, protein or tissue binding)
Concomitant drugs
    Inducers of metabolic enzymes
    Inhibitors of metabolic enzymes

Table 6. Drugs Affecting Hepatic Metabolism

CYP3A inhibitors
    Allopurinol
    Amiodarone
    Ciprofloxacin
    Clarithromycin, erythromycin
    Cimetidine
    Diltiazem, verapamil
    Isoniazid
    Fluconazole, itraconazole, ketoconazole
    Fluoxetine
    Protease inhibitors (HIV)
    Terfenadine
    Grapefruit juice (intestinal CYP3A)
CYP450 inducers
    Barbiturates (CYP3A4)
    Carbamazepine (CYP3A4)
    Dexamethasone (CYP2B6)
    Ethanol (CYP2E1)
    Glucocorticoids (CYP3A4)
    Omeprazole (CYP1A)
    Phenobarbital (CYP3A4, CYP1A)
    Phenytoin (CYP2C, CYP3A4)
    Prednisone (CYP2C19)
    Rifampin (CYP3A4, CYP2B6, CYP2C19,
      CYP2C9)
    St. John's wort (CYP3A4)
    Troglitazone (CYP3A4)

Table 7. Examples of Drugs Whose Oral
         Bioavailability Is Increased by
         Grapefruit Juice

Benzodiazepines
Calcium channel blockers (felodipine, nifedipine,
  verapamil)
Cyclosporine
Estradiol
HMG CoA reductase inhibitors
Saquinavir
Sildenafil
Terfenadine

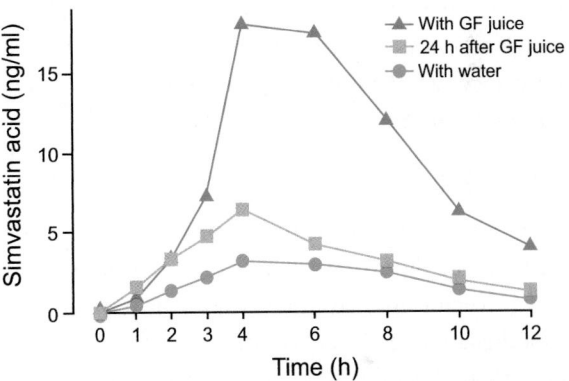

Fig. 10. Effect of grapefruit juice on simvastatin plasma concentration when given concomitantly with grapefruit juice (pink line) or 24 hour after grapefruit juice (yellow line) compared to levels when given with water.

rate of renal blood flow, glomerular filtration, tubular secretion and reabsorption. The glomerular filtration rate can be estimated from creatinine clearance taking into account the age, body weight, serum creatinine level and sex:

$$\text{Creatinine clearance (CrCl)} = \frac{(140\text{-age}) \times \text{weight in kg}}{[72 \times \text{serum creatinine (mg/dL)}]}$$

For women, multiply CrCl by 0.85

The estimation of creatinine clearance is useful for dosing renally eliminated drugs, such as digoxin, dofetilide, sotalol, aminoglycosides or lithium with narrow therapeutic indices. In the elderly, especially women, it is important to remember that serum creati-

nine concentrations alone may not accurately reflect the extent of renal impairment and marked renal dysfunction may be present despite near-normal or only mildly elevated serum creatinine levels.

Points to Remember for the Cardiology Examinations
- Small water soluble drugs are eliminated unchanged by simple renal excretion, whereas larger or lipid soluble drugs are first metabolized in the liver to hydrophilic polar metabolites, which are then excreted through the kidneys or in the bile.
- About 5-10% of Caucasians are deficient in CYP2D and may not obtain pain relief from codeine or expe-

rience side effects related to β-adrenergic blockade with use of β-blockers or propafenone.

■ Remember drug interactions between drugs metabolized and drugs that inhibit or induce CYP 450 enzyme.

■ Serum creatinine concentrations alone may not accurately reflect the extent of renal impairment in patients with reduced muscle mass, such as elderly women.

PHARMACODYNAMICS

Pharmacodynamics addresses the mechanism of action and the effect of a drug at the subcellular, cellular, tissue, organ, and organism levels. Understanding the interaction of drugs with their receptors in the targeted and nontargeted organs helps to explain their efficacy and predict side effects. By increasing the selectivity of a drug's action for a particular receptor in a tissue, the efficacy could be enhanced and unwanted adverse effect minimized.

Targets of Drug Action

To produce pharmacologic response, a drug interacts with one or more constituents on or within the cell. Drug receptors may be located within the plasmalemma, subcellular compartments or nucleus. Most drugs produce their effects by binding to proteins serving as ion channels, receptors, enzymes, transporters or structural proteins (Table 8). Some of these receptors are coupled to signal transduction cascades directly or through intermediate molecules, such as guanosine triphosphate (GTP)-binding proteins through which they regulate distant cellular functions. Thus, a drug may modulate cellular function by activation or inhibition of enzyme activity, translocation of molecules by carriers or ion permeance through ion channels. General anesthetics and some antiproliferative and antimicrobial agents modulate cellular function by interacting with nonprotein targets such as lipids or nucleic acids modifying gene expression.

Affinity denotes the ability of a drug to bind to a receptor, and can be described by the disassociation constant (K_A) of the drug-receptor complex as:

$$\text{Affinity} = 1/\,K_A$$

Thus, a higher K_A reflects a lower affinity of a drug for a receptor, whereas a lower K_A reflects a higher affinity.

Selectivity denotes the drug's ability to elicit a specific effect and is determined by the drug's affinity for a single versus multiple targets.

The ability of a drug to activate a receptor reflects the *intrinsic activity* of the drug (Fig. 11). A *full agonist* is defined as a drug with intrinsic activity (=1). A *partial agonist* is a drug with partial intrinsic activity (<1). An *antagonist* is a drug lacking intrinsic activity (=0) but exhibiting an affinity for the receptor blocking interaction of the agonist to its receptor and therefore antagonizing its effect.

The Dose-Response Relationship

Almost all drugs demonstrate a characteristic relationship between the dose administered and the magnitude of the elicited response which can be plotted as a graph with the drug effect on the ordinate and the drug dose or concentration (log scale) on the abscissa (Fig. 11). At a lower dose, a drug produces smaller effect, which increases as the dose increases until a maximal effect is reached (Fig. 12). Drug dose-response relationship typically exhibits a sigmoid-shaped curve from which the concentration (EC_{50}) or dose (EC_{50}) at which 50% of the maximal effect (E_{max}) is achieved can be calculated.

The *potency* of a drug is described as the concentration required to achieve the half-maximal effect, whereas *efficacy* refers to the maximum response achieved (Fig. 12). Therapeutic effect of a drug relates to the percentage of maximal response elicited when

---

Table 8.   Major Classes of Drug Receptors

Ion channels
  Na^+, Ca^{2+}, K^+
Receptors activating signaling pathways
  β-adrenergic, α-adrenergic, muscarinic,
    purinergic, AT II
Enzymes
  Na^+-K^+ ATPase, ACE
Transporter/carrier proteins
  Na^+-Ca^{2+} exchanger
Nucleic acids
  Thyroxine

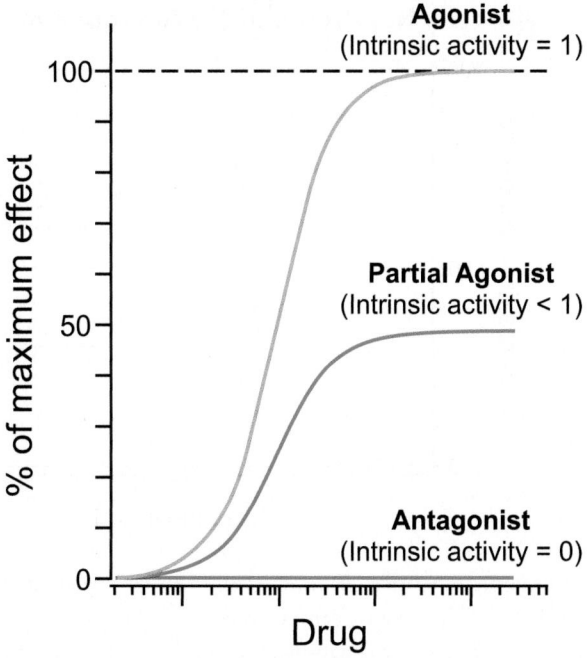

Fig. 11. Drugs' intrinsic activity. Full agonists (yellow) produce maximum stimulatory effects similar to endogenous ligand. Antagonists (red) produce no direct effects, but inhibit action of an endogenous compound or a drug. Partial agonists (green) produce less than maximum stimulatory effect; possess both agonist and antagonist properties.

the drug binds to its receptor. Drug A in Figure 12 is more potent than drug B but has a similar efficacy to drug B, because the EC_{50} of drug A is less than the drug B but the two drugs can achieve similar maximal response (E_{max}). Potency largely determines the dose that needs to be administered to achieve the desired effect and is not as important in selection between drugs with the same maximal response (efficacy), as similar effects can be obtained with less potent drugs by giving a larger dose. The efficacy of a drug largely determines the magnitude of the achievable therapeutic affect. The effect of a drug with a lower efficacy cannot be increased to one with a higher efficacy by increasing the drug concentration (Fig. 12).

The dose-response curves are also useful to differentiate between *competitive* vs. *non-competitive antagonism* of an agonist by a drug (Fig. 13). The *margin of safety* of a drug can also be determined by determining the dose at which 50% of the toxic effect, also called the "median toxic dose" (TD_{50}) is observed. The ratio between the therapeutic dose of drug (ED_{50}) and the toxic dose (TD_{50}) is known as the *therapeutic index* (Fig. 14). The narrower is the therapeutic index (ratio closer to 1), the greater is the chances of toxicity, as observed with digoxin or warfarin. Caution should be

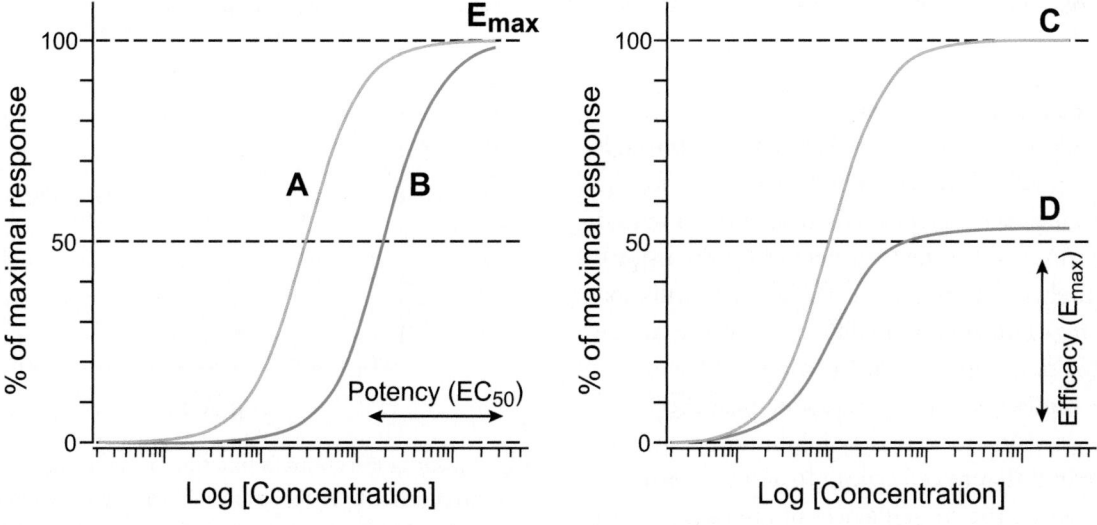

Fig. 12. Dose-response curves illustrating a drug's potency and efficacy. Potency of a drug is describd as the concentration (EC_{50}) required to achieve the half-maximal effect, whereas efficacy refers to the maximum response (E_{max}) achieved. Drug A has the same effect (efficacy) as drug B but at lower concentration (lower potency). Drug C and D have similar potencies but C is more efficacious with higher maximum response than D. Increasing the dose of drug D does not increase the response.

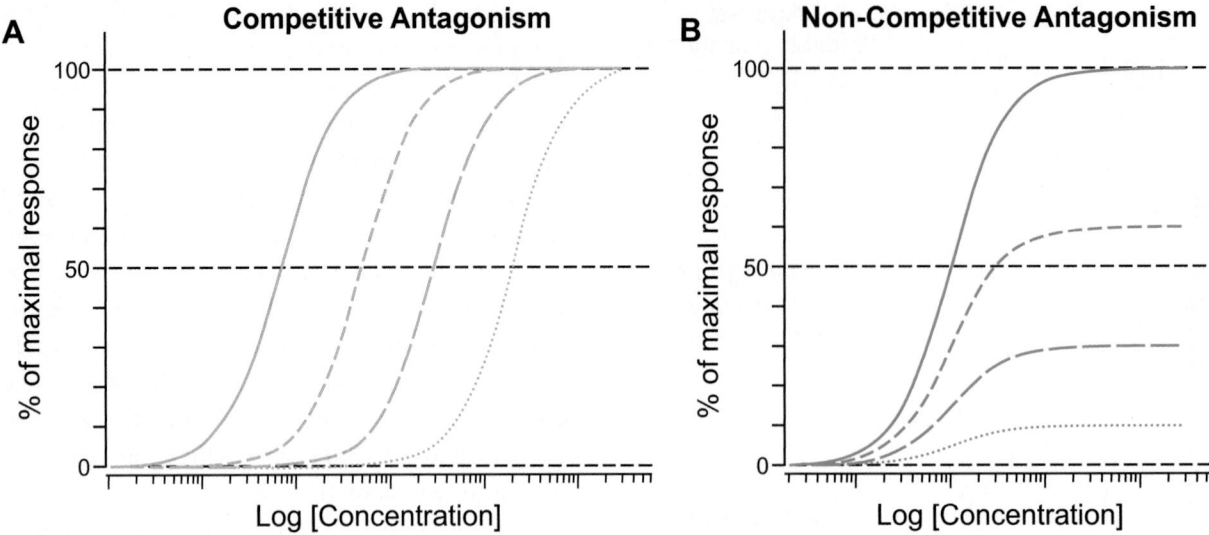

Fig. 13. Log dose-response curves illustrating competitive (*A*) and noncompetitive (*B*) inhibition. Competitive antagonist—competes with the agonist for receptor sites. Giving larger doses of the agonist can overcome the antagonist effects. Noncompetitive antagonist—binds to receptors and blocks the effects of the agonist. Giving larger doses of the agonist does not increase the maximal response and cannot reverse its action. Solid lines are dose-response curves in the presence of an agonist alone. Broken lines are dose-responses in the presence of increasing concentration of a competitive (*A*) and noncompetitive inhibitor (*B*).

used in using these drugs (especially in the elderly) and the drug level or its effect monitored to adjust the dosage to maintain optimum concentration without loss of therapeutic efficacy or increased risk of toxicity. The clinically acceptable risk of toxicity strongly depends on the severity of the disease being treated.

Adverse Effects and Drug Toxicity

A toxic effect of a drug may be mediated through interaction with the same receptors responsible for the therapeutic effect (e.g., postural hypotension induced by prazosin used for the treatment of hypertension). Alternatively, an adverse effect could be due to activation of the drug's receptors but in different tissues (e.g., digitalis glycosides augment cardiac contractility but also produce cardiac arrhythmia, gastrointestinal effect, and changes in vision mediated by inhibition of Na^+/K^+ ATPase in different cell types). In addition, adverse effects may be the consequences of interaction with different types of receptors (antipsychotic drugs exhibit therapeutic affect through action on dopamine receptors, but they may decrease blood pressure through action on adrenergic receptors).

Adverse drug events (ADE) are common with over

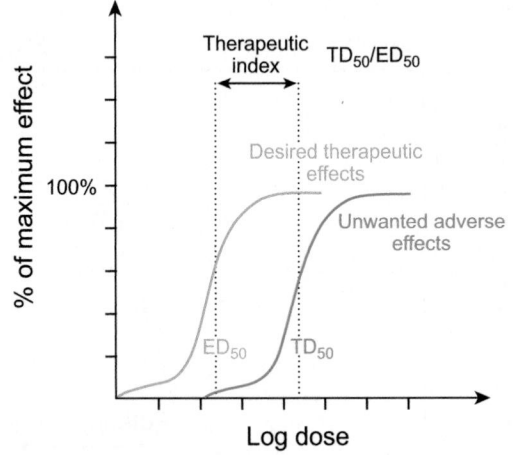

Fig. 14. Drug effects are a function of the drug concentration. Increasing concentration beyond what's required for maximum effect can only increase side effects. Therapeutic index of a drug is given by the ratio of a drug's dosage causing 50% of maximal toxic effect (TD_{50}) to 50% of maximal therapeutic effects (ED_{50}). The lower the index, the higher chance of toxicity and the greater need to monitor plasma levels.

2 million incidents per year that add significantly to morbidity and the length and cost of hospitalization. It is estimated that adverse drug reactions are the 4th leading cause of death ahead of diabetes, AIDS, pulmonary disease, accidents and automobile deaths accounting for more than 100,000 deaths per year in the USA. In more than one-fourth of cases adverse drug events are preventable. Common causes for errors in drug prescriptions by physicians and adverse drug events in the elderly are summarized in the Tables 9 and 10, respectively.

Rational Dosage Regimen

After a drug class has been selected for treating a clinical condition, a rational dosage regimen is required to individualize pharmacotherapy. A rational dosage regimen is based on achieving a target concentration at the site of drug action that will produce the desired therapeutic effect.

Pharmacokinetic Considerations

In most clinical situations, drugs are administered in such a way as to maintain a steady-state concentration of the drug in the body; that is, each dose is given to replace the amount of drug that has been eliminated since the preceding dose. At steady-state, the dosing rate ("rate-in") should equal the rate of elimination ("rate-out"). Therefore,

$$\text{Maintenance Dosing Rate} = CL \cdot C_{ss}$$

where CL = clearance and C_{ss} = target concentration.

If the bioavailability of the drug is less than 1, then the dosing rate (DR) needs to be divided by F, the drug bioavailability. The maintenance dose is calculated as follows:

$$MD = DR \cdot DI$$

where MD = maintenance dose, DR = dosing rate, and DI = dosing interval that equals the time elapsed between 2 doses.

The pharmacokinetic variables that may affect dosage regimens include absorption, clearance, volume of distribution, and drug half-life. The most frequent cause of underdosage or overdosage is inadequate patient compliance. This can be determined by measuring the concentration of the drug in the blood. If compliance is adequate, other causes of absorption alteration should be considered. Kidney, liver, or heart failure would decrease the clearance of a drug. In the elderly, the relative decrease in skeletal muscle mass tends to produce a smaller volume of distribution of a drug. The volume of distribution can be overestimated in obese patients if dosage is based on body weight but the drug used does not distribute into fatty tissue. Also, abnormal

---

Table 9.   Common Causes for Errors in Drug Prescriptions by Physicians

Failure to compensate for renal or hepatic impairment
Failure to recognize drug allergies
Writing the wrong drug name or dosage
Use of abbreviation causing confusion

Table 10.   Common Causes for Adverse Drug Events in the Elderly

Prescription of higher doses
Lack of adjustment to reduced hepatic and/or renal clearance, volume of distribution, plasma protein concentration
Use of drugs likely to produce side effect (such as anticholinergics causing urinary retention)
Polypharmacy, unnecessary prescriptions
Combinations with drugs with additional adverse effect
Comorbidities increasing side effects (orthostatic hypotension, stroke, dementia, frequent falls, constipation, reduced appetite, malnutrition)
Miscommunication regarding dosage and timing of different drugs
Noncompliance
Over- and underuse of medications
Financial concerns
Cognitive decline
Poor vision or hearing
Complicated drug regimen

accumulation of fluid (edema, ascites, pleural effusion) can markedly increase the volume of distribution of certain drugs. Changes in drug clearance and volume of distribution alter the half-life of a drug.

Clinical Monitoring of Dosage

In many cases, the action of a drug can be monitored by clinical observation and dosage regimens modified accordingly. Measurement of drug concentration in the blood can be performed to help optimize therapy. In this regard, the physician should address the following questions:

1. Is the patient responding to therapy or showing symptoms/signs of toxicity?
2. Does the concentration measured in the blood reflect the administered dose?
   Is the concentration within the therapeutic or target range?
3. If the patient is not responding or manifests adverse effects, how should the therapy be modified? Should the drug be discontinued?

Pharmacodynamic Considerations

If increasing the dose of a drug in a particular patient does not lead to further changes in the clinical response, it is possible that a maximal effect of a drug has been reached. Recognition of a maximal drug effect is important in avoiding further increase in dosage that could increase the risk of toxicity. Failure of therapy can be due to changes in the sensitivity of a target organ to a drug. This can be detected by measuring therapeutic drug concentrations in a patient whose response is not adequate to the administered therapy. This may result from drug-drug interactions, downregulation of target receptors, an abnormal condition or a disease state. Some important drug-drug interactions and drug-disease interactions important for cardiology board examination are summarized in Tables 11-13.

Pregnant Patient

No drugs should be prescribed for pregnant women unless careful consideration for potential benefits to the mother or fetus outweighs the potential risks to both. Points to remember for the Cardiology Board Examination for drug prescription in pregnant patients are summarized in Tables 14 to 16.

Table 11. Digoxin-Drug Interactions

Increased serum level
  Increased absorption
    Atropine
    Propantheline
  Decreased clearance
    Amiodarone
    Quinidine
    Flecainide
    Propafenone
    Verapamil
    Cimetidine
    Spironolactone
    Macrolides
    Benzodiazepines
    Indomethacin
Decreased serum level
  Decreased absorption
    Antacids
    Cholestyramine
    Colestipol
    Metoclopramide
    Neomycin
    Phenytoin
    Sulfasalazine
  Increased clearance
    Thyroxine

Table 12. Warfarin-Drug Interactions

Potentiation
  Amiodarone
  Aspirin and salicylates
  Cimetidine
  Clofibrate
  Erythromycin
  Propafenone
  Quinidine
  Sulfonamides
Antagonism
  Barbiturates
  Rifampin
  Vitamin K

Table 13. Examples of Drugs That Can Prolong QT Interval and Increase the Risk of Torsades des Pointes

Antiarrhythmics
    IA: quinidine, procainamide, disopyramide
    III: sotalol, NAPA, ibutilde, dofetilide, amiodarone, azimilide
Antimicrobials
    Antibiotics: erythromycin, TMP/SMX
    Antifungals: itraconzaole, ketoconazole
    Antimalarials: chloroquine
    Antiparasitic: pentamidine
    Antivirals: amantadine
Antihistamine
    Terfenadine, astemizole
Antidepressants
    Tricyclics, tetracyclics
Psychotropics
    Haloperidol, droperidol
    Phenothiazines
Miscellaneous
    Cisapride
    Probucol
    Ketanserin
    Vasopressin
    Organophosphate poisoning
    Chloral hydrate overdose

Table 14. Drug Categories Classified by Fetal Toxicity Rating

Category	Data from human	Data from animals	Fetal risk
A	+++		± (safest)
B	±	+++	±
C	--	++	+
D	+++		++
X	++	++	+++ (high risk)

Drug Development

Before a new drug is released, extensive testing and clinical trials are conducted to assess the safety and effectiveness of the drug for its indicated use. The drug evaluation and development proceed in specified phases of preclinical and clinical assessment (Fig. 15).

Preclinical Assessment

This is mainly performed in tissues or experimental animals to determine safety of the compound.

Table 15. Teratogenic Effects of Commonly Used Drugs

Drug	Teratogenic effects
ACE inhibitors	Oligohydramnios, postnatal renal failure, lung hypoplasia
Alcohol	Facial dysmorphogenesis, growth and mental retardation
Beta blockers	Growth retardation, fetal hypoglycemia
Carbamazepine	Cranial, facial dysmorphogenesis and neural tube defect
Diethylstilbestrol	Vaginal adenosis and carcinogenesis, uterine anomalies
Lithium	Cardiac effects (Ebstein's anomaly)
Narcotics	CNS depression, apnea, and low APGAR score
Phenytoin	Cranial, facial and limb anomalies; growth and mental retardation
Retinoic acid	Cranial, facial, cardiac and CNS anomalies
Valproate	Lumbosacral spina bifida, facial dysmorphogenesis
Warfarin	Facial anomalies (nasal hypoplasia), chondrodysplasia punctata, optic atrophy, anomalies of the central nervous system

Clinical Assessment

Phase I determines the safety of the drug and involves an initial trial in a few healthy volunteers. Characterization of the pharmacokinetics and pharmacodynamics is performed mainly to assess the safety profile.

Phase II determines the safety in a small number of patients and involves drug characterization in the patient population it is intended for. Phase II trial determines the drug efficacy, adverse effects, and safety.

Phase III trial is conducted in a larger number of patients to assess drug safety and therapeutic efficacy. Marketing authorization is requested after phase III clinical trial.

Phase IV is a postmarketing pharmacovigilance phase where monitoring for adverse events is continued.

Table 16. Drugs Preferred and Contraindicated for Pregnant Women

Disease condition	Recommended	Not recommended
Hypertension	Methyldopa	Hydralazine, diuretics, ACE inhibitors calcium channel blockers
Diabetes	Insulin	Sulfonylureas
Infection	Ampicillin, cephalosporin	Sulfonamides, floxacillin
Hyperthyroidism	PTU	Radioactive iodine
Thrombophlebitis	Low-molecular-weight heparin	Warfarin in first and third trimester

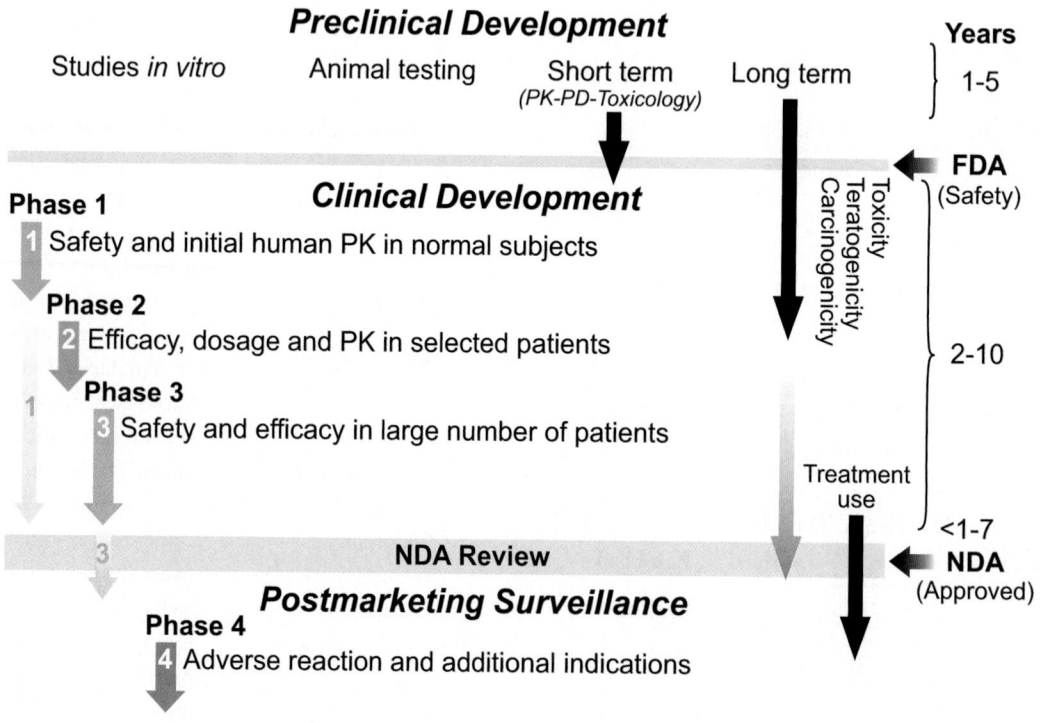

Fig. 15. Phases of drug development. PK, pharmacokinetics; PD, pharmacodynamics; FDA, Food and Drug Administration application; NDA, new drug application.

ANTIARRHYTHMIC DRUGS

Peter A. Brady, MD

GENERAL CONCEPTS

Clinical practice and cardiology examinations emphasize appropriate use of antiarrhythmic drug therapy in patients with heart rhythm disorders. Although some knowledge of the basic pharmacology of these agents is required, the most commonly tested areas include:

- Recognition of specific patients and circumstances in which antiarrhythmic drug therapy is contraindicated.
- Drug-drug interactions.
- Mode of elimination of specific agents.

CLASSIFICATION

It is important to know the Vaughan Williams classification of antiarrhythmic drug therapy which is the most clinically useful and commonly used. This classification denotes sodium channel blocking agents as class I, beta blocking agents class II, potassium channel blocking agents as class III, and calcium channel blocking agents as class IV. Adenosine and digoxin are unclassified within this scheme. The "Sicilian Gambit" scheme is more complex and classifies drugs based upon their cellular mechanism of action. Specifics will likely not be tested on cardiology examinations other than in very broad terms (Fig. 1).

EFFECT OF ANTIARRHYTHMIC DRUGS ON REENTRANT CIRCUITS

A common model for understanding the action of antiarrhythmic drug therapy is that of the propagating wave front, the refractory tail, and the excitable gap. This is shown in Figure 2. Reentrant arrhythmias require a functional circuit around which a activating wave front of depolarization can travel. Nondepolarized areas of myocardium within the circuit that are available for depolarization constitute the excitable gap. To sustain reentry, the advancing wave front must encounter readily excitable tissue. Reentry can be terminated by slowing of conduction or reducing or elimination of the excitable gap.

In general, drugs that block sodium channels (class I) slow the velocity of the propagating wave front (i.e. conduction velocity is decreased) whereas drugs that block outward potassium channels (most commonly I_{ks}) increase tissue refractoriness and thereby decrease the excitable gap (Fig. 3).

a) Slowed conduction promotes abolition of the propagating wave front.

b) Increased refractoriness reduces the excitable gap decreasing the available myocardium for re-excitation by the advancing wave front.

c) Marked slowing of conduction or large increase

Class I

Na⁺ channel block

1a: Depress phase 0
- Slow conduction
- Prolong repolarization

1b: Little effect on phase 0 in normal tissue
- Depress phase 0 in abnormal fibers
- Shorten repolarization

1c: Markedly depress phase 0
- Markedly slow conduction
- Slight effect on repolarization

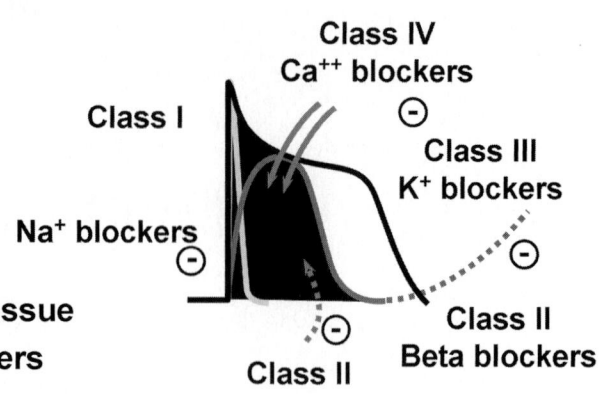

Class II

Sympatholytic drugs

Class III (K⁺ channel block)

Drugs that prolong repolarization

Class IV

Calcium channel-blocking drugs

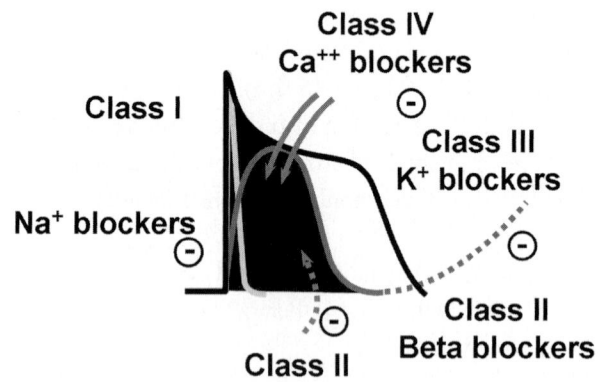

Fig. 1. Vaughan Williams classification of antiarrhythmic drugs.

in the excitable gap can lead to a proarrhythmic effect (Fig. 4).

This model for understanding both the antiarrhythmic and proarrhythmic action of antiarrhythmic drugs is useful when deciding upon a specific drug and/or combination of drugs to maximize efficacy and minimize proarrhythmic potential.

The cellular action of antiarrhythmic drugs can be viewed in light of major ion shifts responsible for both atrial and ventricular action potential.

A ventricular action potential is shown in Figure 5.

Differences in ion channel components, of myocardial and nodal cells are summarized in Figure 6.

Important components of the cardiac cell AP include rapid inward sodium current (I_{Na}) responsible for the rapid upstroke of this action potential and calcium and outward potassium currents that are responsible for the repolarization phase of the action potential. Sodium channel blocking drugs act at phase 0 of the ventricular action potential whereas class III agents act during repolarization. Block of sodium channels by class I agents decreases available sodium channels for cellular activation resulting in slowing of conduction manifest as prolongation of the QRS width on the

Effect of Drugs on Reentrant Circuits

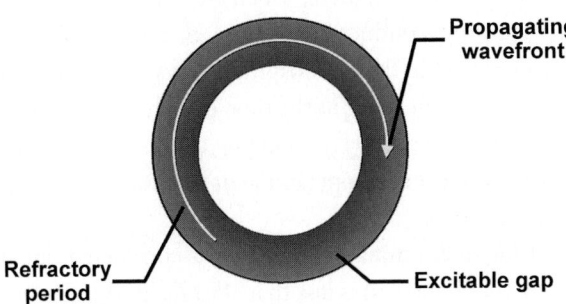

Fig. 2. Model of myocardial depolarization.

surface ECG (Fig. 7). Block of outward potassium current (class III agent) results in prolongation of the action potential duration manifest as QT prolongation on the surface ECG (Fig. 7).

USE DEPENDENCY

The concept of use dependency is important. In broad terms, drugs that bind to open or inactivated channels show greater drug effect at faster heart rates, a phenomenon termed "use dependent" channel block. In resting contrast, drugs binding predominantly during the rested state of the channel show greatest effect at slower heart rates, termed "reverse use dependent" channel block. The importance of this concept is that agents that show use dependent channel block (especially flecainide and propafenone) have the greatest activity at faster heart rates whereas drugs that demonstrate reverse use dependent block (commonly sotalol and dofetilide) have the greatest effect at slower (resting) heart rates. Drugs that show use dependent block are therefore most commonly monitored by increasing heart rate (for example with treadmill exercise testing) to maximize drug-channel block and assess for QRS widening when maximal channel block would be occurring. Agents that show reverse use dependency are most likely to have the greatest effect during rest or with bradycardia and therefore QT interval prolongation caused by agents such as sotalol and dofetilide is best observed at rest, and treadmill exercise testing is not indicated or useful when using these drugs. Theoretically, agents that show use dependence block may be more effective at chemical cardioversion of

Effect of Drugs on Reentrant Circuits

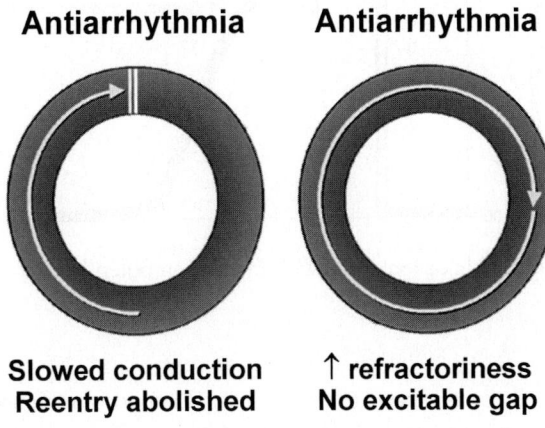

Fig. 3. Slowed conduction abolishes the propagating wave front.

tachyarrhythmias due to the drug having greatest effect at elevated heart rates whereas agents that show reverse use dependence may be more efficacious at *preventing* arrhythmias and maintaining sinus rhythm.

HOSPITAL VERSUS OUTPATIENT INITIATION OF AAD

The decision to initiate antiarrhythmic drug therapy in hospital versus the outpatient setting is determined

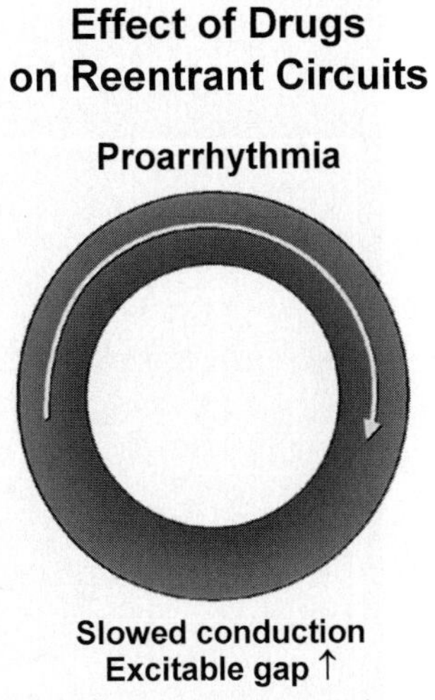

Effect of Drugs on Reentrant Circuits

Proarrhythmia

Slowed conduction
Excitable gap ↑

Fig. 4. Marked slowing of conduction or large increase in the excitable gap can lead to a proarrhythmic effect.

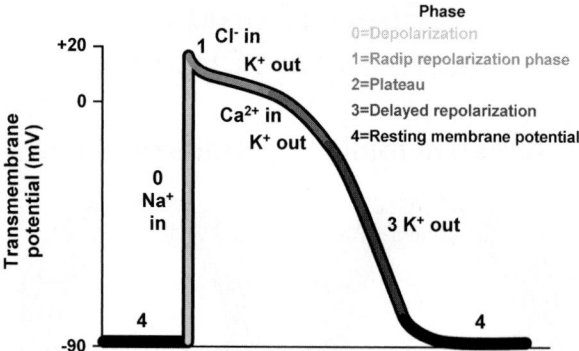

Fig. 5. Major ion shifts with fact action potential

recovery sufficient to cause syncope and injury on termination of AF. If outpatient loading of propafenone or flecainide, which worsen AV node and His-Purkinje conduction is planned, cardioversion to restore sinus rhythm in hospital allows assessment of the impact of the drug at the time of arrhythmia termination. Due to the QT prolonging effects of quinidine, procainamide and disopyramide in hospital initiation is recommended.

Outpatient initiation of sotalol is considered safe if baseline QT interval is less than 450 ms in the absence of renal dysfunction and risk factors for TdP (Table 1).

Despite causing prolongation of the QT interval, amiodarone is only rarely associated with Tdp and is commonly initiated in the ambulatory setting, even in patients with persistent AF, provided significant sinus node dysfunction has been excluded and AV nodal blocking agents have been discontinued or dosage reduced to avoid significant AV block.

largely by likelihood of risk versus cost and inconvenience of inpatient drug loading. In the case of ventricular arrhythmias, and use of dofetilide, in-hospital initiation is necessary or mandated.

For atrial arrhythmias, outpatient loading and arrhythmia termination should generally be avoided in patients with evidence of sinus node dysfunction, AV conduction disturbance, bundle branch block, structural heart disease and QT prolongation. Unsuspected sinus node dysfunction, aggravated by use of AADs, especially class IC agents may cause prolongation of sinus node

■ In general, in patients who are in sinus rhythm without evidence of sinus node disease, ventricular systolic dysfunction, myocardial ischemia or baseline QT prolongation, outpatient initiation of AAD is safe.

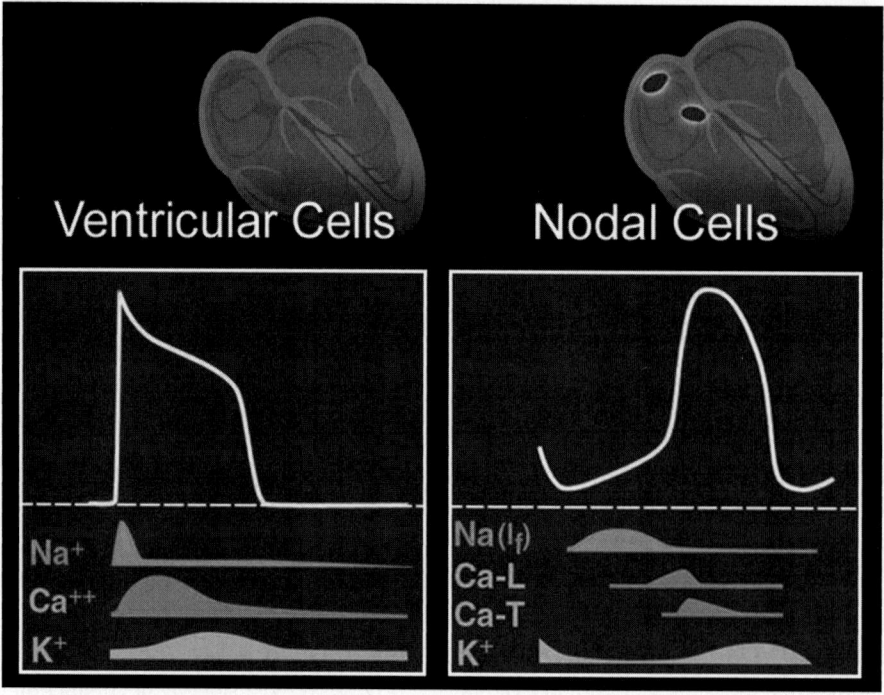

Fig. 6. Differences in ion channel components between ventricular and nodal cells.

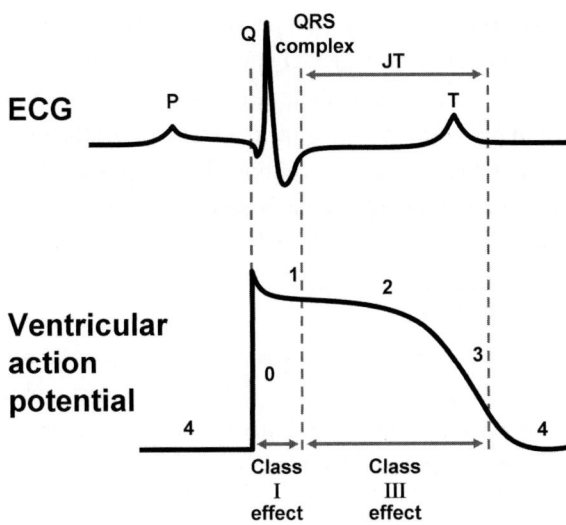

Fig. 7. Effects of class I and class III agents on ventricular action potential correlated with surface ECG.

Table 1.   Risk Factors for Torsades de Pointes

Patient factors
  Female gender
  Sinus node dysfunction leading to pauses after
    arrhythmia termination
  $\downarrow K^+/Mg^{2+}$
  Baseline QT $\uparrow$
  Use of a class III agent
Pharmacologic factors
  Concomitant use of drugs that interfere with
    metabolism of QT prolonging agent
  Renal impairment of renally excreted agents
    that prolong QT (sotalol, procainamide,
    dofetilide)

MONITORING OF ANTIARRHYTHMIC DRUGS

Class I

Since sodium channel blocking agents slow conduction velocity, drug tissue effect is best monitored with reference to the PR and QRS interval and duration. Class I drugs, especially class IC agents, flecainide and propafenone, exhibit "use-dependence" in that the degree of sodium channel blocking increases as heart rate increases. Thus, increasing heart rate using a pre-dismissal treadmill exercise test is a useful screening tool for proarrhythmic effect. In general, widening of the QRS should not exceed 150% of pretreatment interval.

Class III

Increased cardiac repolarization manifests as QT prolongation on the surface ECG. In most cases, corrected QT interval should not exceed 520 ms during therapy with class III agents. The incidence of torsades de pointes with use of class III agents is around 1-3%. Unlike class I agents, the efficacy with which class III drugs block potassium channels increases with slower heart rates (reverse use dependence) increasing the likelihood of TdP at slower heart rates.

In most cases, risk of TdP increases with drug dosage but in the case of quinidine, TdP is unrelated to serum drug levels may occur even after the first dose.

VAUGHAN WILLIAMS CLASS I ANTIARRHYTHMIC DRUGS

The characteristic of drugs in Vaughan Williams class I is that they block the cardiac sodium channel. The magnitude of sodium channel block depends upon heart rate, membrane potential, and specific drug characteristics. Class I agents are subclassified as class IA, class IB, and class IC according to the efficacy of sodium channel blockade.

Class IC > Class IA > Class IB (Fig. 8).

Class IA drugs with intermediate sodium channel block generally only cause significant prolongation of conduction at higher heart rates. Class IB drugs (lidocaine and mexilitine) have minimal effect on the sodium channel in normal tissue but cause significant conduction slowing in depolarized tissue. Hence, these agents are preferable for use in ischemic tissue where partial depolarization is present. Class IC drugs (flecainide and propafenone) cause significant prolongation of conduction in cardiac tissue (manifest as increase in the QRS complex duration of the ECG at normal heart rates). Lidocaine (and mexilitine) is used frequently in patients with ventricular arrhythmias due to myocardial ischemia whereas drugs in class IA and class IC are used predominantly in patients with supraventricular arrhythmias, most commonly atrial fibrillation.

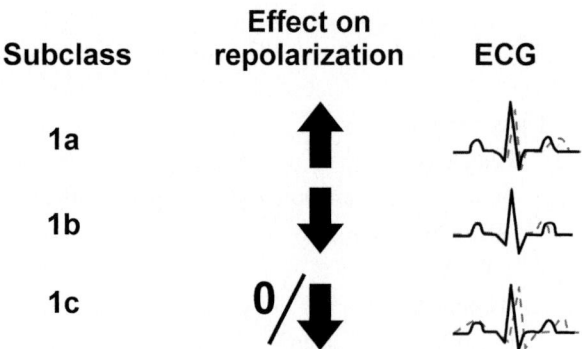

Subclass	Effect on repolarization	ECG
1a		
1b		
1c	0/	

Fig. 8. Effects of class I drugs on surface ECG.

CLASS IA DRUGS (QUINIDINE, PROCAINAMIDE, DISOPYRAMIDE)

General Properties

In addition to sodium channel block, class IA agents also block outward potassium currents leading to prolongation of the action potential duration manifest as increased QT interval (Fig. 8). In addition, quinidine blocks alpha adrenergic receptors and both quinidine and disopyramide inhibit muscarinic receptors. These latter effects may enhance the efficacy of these agents in "vagal" mediated arrhythmias.

Quinidine

Quinidine metabolism is via the cytochrome P450 3A4 system. Drugs that increase metabolism via this pathway (e.g. **phenytoin and phenobarbital**) may increase quinidine dose requirements while drugs decreasing metabolism via this pathway (**cimetidine, verapamil**) may increase quinidine plasma concentrations. Quinidine is a potent inhibitor of cytochrome P450 2D6 which forms the basis for a number of drug interactions with quinidine (increase in **propafenone** or increase in beta blockade). Quinidine reduces **digoxin** clearance leading to significant increases in digoxin concentrations.

■ Be aware of cytochrome P450 3A4 metabolism and the interaction with **phenytoin** and **phenobarbital**, **cimetidine** and **verapamil**. Also note the interaction between **digoxin** and **quinidine**.

Procainamide

Procainamide is conjugated by *N*-acetyltransferase to *N*-acetyl procainamide. This compound (NAPA) is an electrophysiologically active class III drug with a half life of 6-10 hours. The rate of metabolism varies in the population with more than half being rapid acetylators. In the presence of renal impairment, continued use of procainamide may lead to accumulation of *N*-acetylprocainamide with consequent effects on QT prolongation predisposing to torsades de pointes ventricular tachycardia.

■ Be aware of the use of procainamide in patients with renal impairment as accumulation of the metabolite NAPA may lead to TdP despite apparent normal parent compound blood level (Tables 2 and 3).

Disopyramide

Disopyramide is a rarely used antiarrhythmic medication with strong negatively inotropic properties (sometimes used for this reason in HOCM) and anticholinergic side effects—blurred vision, urinary retention, constipation, and dry mouth.

Proarrhythmia With Class IA Drugs

Proarrhythmia with class IA agents is most likely due to the QT prolonging effects leading to TdP that occur in 0.5-8% of cases. In addition, quinidine effect is idiosyncratic in that TdP may occur after the first or second dose when plasma concentrations are still low (Fig. 9). Thus, quinidine therapy should be initiated in the hospital with continuous electrocardiographic monitoring. Perhaps based on risk of TdP, meta-analysis of randomized clinical trials have suggested that quinidine when used to treat atrial fibrillation is associated with increased mortality.

Efficacy

Quinidine, procainamide, and disopyramide all have documented efficacy for the treatment of atrial arrhythmias. However, the vagolytic effect of quinidine may enhance conduction through the atrioventricular node and sufficiently slow atrial rates allowing 1:1 AV response during atrial flutter with ventricular rates >250, which may be fatal. Thus, coadministration of an AV nodal blocking drug should be considered when quinidine is used for treatment of atrial rhythm disorders.

Adverse Effects of Quinidine

Gastrointestinal side effects (most commonly abdominal

Table 2.   Summary Table of Antiarrhythmic Drugs

Drug	Dose (mg/24 hr)	Ion channel block	Cardiac toxicity	Noncardiac toxicity
			Class I	
Quinidine	600–1,500	Na+, K+	↑ QT, TdP, vagolytic effects and enhanced AV node conduction	Nausea, vomiting, diarrhea
Procainamide	1,000–4,000	Na+, K+	↑ QT, TdP, ↑ cimetidine and trimethoprim	Lupus-like syndrome GI upset Agranulocytosis
Disopyramide	400–750	Na+, K+	TdP, exacerbation of CHF	Urinary retention Dry mouth Avoid with history of glaucoma
Flecainide	200–300	Na+	Atrial flutter with 1:1 conduction Ventricular tachycardia	CNS effects, dizziness and blurred vision
Propafenone	450–900	Na+	Atrial flutter with 1:1 conduction Ventricular tachycardia ↑ digoxin/warfarin	Metallic taste Wheezing Dizziness
			Class III	
Sotalol	160–320	K+	↑ QT, TdP Bradycardia Exclusive renal elimination	COPD or asthma exacerbation
Dofetilide	500–1,000	K+	↑ QT, TdP	-
Amiodarone	200–400 g	K+, Ca2+, Na+	Bradycardia, TdP (rare) ↑ warfarin/digoxin	Thyroid, liver, lung, optic neuritis (rare)

Table 3.   Summary of Antiarrhythmic Drug Therapy of AF

Drug	Lone AFib	CHF, CAD	CAD (normal EF)	Renal failure
First line	Flecainide Propafenone	Dofetilide Amiodarone	Sotalol	Amiodarone
Second line	Sotalol Procainamide Disopyramide Amiodarone			Propafenone
Avoid		Flecainide Propafenone	Flecainide Propafenone	Sotalol Procainamide Dofetilide

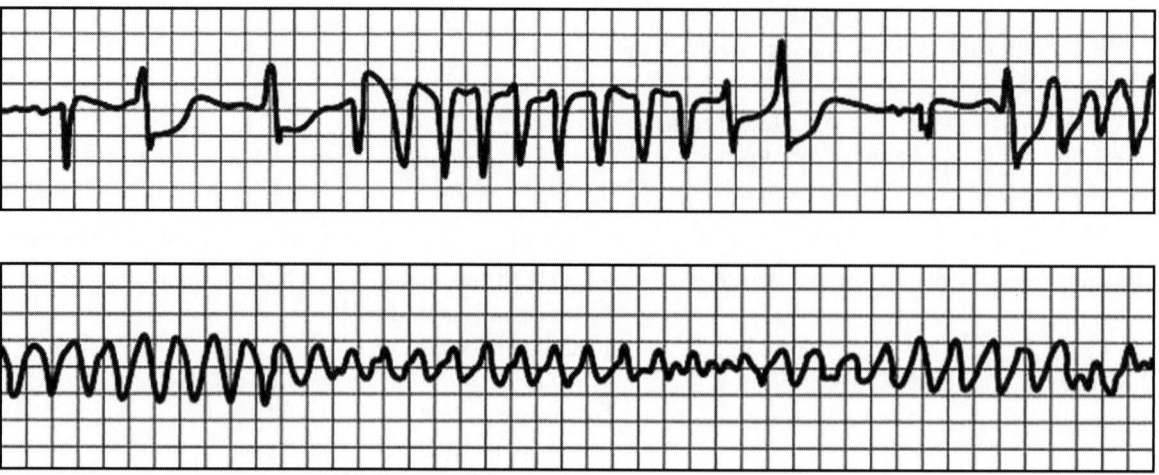

Fig. 9. A 46-year-old woman after 3 doses of quinidine.

cramping and diarrhea) occur in one third. Granulomatous hepatitis is rare but well described. **Rash** is common. "Cinchonism" consists of decreased hearing, tinnitus, and blurred vision. Delirium may also occur. **Thrombocytopenia** and **Coombs-positive hemolytic anemia** along with **Lupus syndrome** with development of antihistone antibodies has been reported.

Quinidine toxicity is characterized by marked QRS widening and ventricular arrhythmias which may be reversed with infusion of sodium lactate or bicarbonate.

An approximate 30% concordance rate for drug-induced ventricular arrhythmias in patients with class IA drugs is described. Thus, if ventricular fibrillation or polymorphic VT occurs with one class IA drug then the likelihood of similar findings with other class IA drugs is high.

The idiosyncratic nature of TdP and polymorphic VT in patients taking class IA drugs mandates initiation of these drugs in hospital. In general, if the QTC is prolonged >500 msec, the antiarrhythmic drug should be stopped to prevent proarrhythmia. However, polymorphic VT may occur with quinidine at normal QT intervals. Plasma levels of quinidine or its metabolites do not predict proarrhythmia.

Class IB Drugs (Lidocaine, Mexiletine)

General Properties

The efficacy of Class IB drugs are increased at very rapid heart rates and in depolarized tissue, hence, the usefulness of these drugs in patients with ventricular arrhythmias in the setting of myocardial ischemia.

Lidocaine

Pharmacokinetics

Lidocaine undergoes extensive first pass hepatic metabolism and therefore must be administered parenterally. Lidocaine is highly bound to an alpha-1 acid glycoprotein which may increase in myocardial infarction and heart failure causing a reduction in available drug. In addition, the volume of distribution and clearance of lidocaine are decreased in heart failure leading to increased plasma levels.

■ Lidocaine and mexilitine toxicity are increased in patients with myocardial infarction and heart failure.

Mexiletine is metabolized to inactive metabolites via the cytochrome P450 system and genetic variation leads to individuals who are slow and fast metabolizers of mexiletine which affects both efficacy and risk of toxic effects.

Proarrhythmia

Lidocaine proarrhythmia is uncommon. Prophylactic lidocaine in acute myocardial infarction may reduce ventricular fibrillation but increases overall mortality and should not be used. Intravenous amiodarone has replaced both procainamide and lidocaine as the initial drug of choice for hemodynamically stable wide complex tachycardia. Lidocaine remains acceptable for treatment of shock refractory ventricular fibrillation and pulseless VT. Mexiletine is most commonly used as an oral equivalent of lidocaine especially with inappropriate ICD shocks refractory to amiodarone. Recently mexiletine has been advocated to correct the QT interval prolongation associated with type 3 long QT syndrome.

Although lidocaine has minimal effect on hemodynamics, transient hypotension may be seen with intravenous administration of a bolus of lidocaine in patients with severely depressed left ventricular function.

Drug Interactions
Propranolol, metoprolol, and cimetidine decrease hepatic blood flow resulting in reduced metabolism of lidocaine with up to 80% increase in plasma levels of the drug. Lidocaine levels are decreased by phenobarbital.

Adverse Effects
Central nervous system side effects predominate including perioral numbness, paresthesias, diplopia, hyperacusis, slurred speech, altered consciousness, seizures, respiratory arrest, and coma. Nystagmus is a common early sign of lidocaine toxicity.

Mexiletine

Mexiletine has minimal hemodynamic effects although in patients with markedly impaired left ventricular function an approximate 2% exacerbation of congestive heart failure may be seen.

Drug Interactions
Metabolism of mexiletine is increased by **phenytoin**, **phenobarbital**, and **rifampicin**. Reduced hepatic metabolism (**cimetidine, chloramphenicol,** and **isoniazid**) increases mexilitine levels. **Theophylline levels** are increased a mean of 65% with mexiletine, **digoxin**, and **warfarin** levels are unaffected by mexilitine.

Adverse Effects
Gastrointestinal and central nervous system side effects predominate. Most commonly, tremor is the first sign of CNS toxicity but blurred vision, dysarthria, ataxia and confusion may occur. Tremor caused by mexiletine may respond to a beta adrenergic blocker. Thrombocytopenia has been reported rarely. Increased liver function tests and other blood dyscrasias are rare.

Class IC Antiarrhythmic Drugs (Flecainide, Propafenone)

Pharmacodynamics
Flecainide and propafenone cause profound slowing of conduction which is exaggerated in depolarized tissue and at increased heart rate (use dependency). Because of the use dependence properties of flecainide and propafenone, evaluation of drug efficacy is best at higher heart rates. Thus, interval or predismissal exercise stress testing looking for a QRS widening less than 20% is useful.

Pharmacokinetics
Both flecainide and propafenone undergo hepatic metabolism via the cytochrome P450 2D6 system. Metabolites of flecainide are electrophysiologically inactive. However, 5 hydroxy propafenone is equipotent to propafenone as a sodium channel blocker but is much less potent as a beta blocker. Because hepatic metabolism of propafenone is saturable resulting in nonlinear relationship between dose and steady state mean concentration, individuals lacking cytochrome P450 2D6 (i.e. poor metabolizers) demonstrate less first pass hepatic metabolism. Because of this, plasma propafenone concentrations increase which is associated with greater beta blocker effect from the parent compound. Metabolic rate is also correlated with drug efficacy with slow metabolizers experiencing greater suppression of atrial fibrillation than rapid metabolizers. In individuals who experience marked beta-blocker side effect or who fail to respond to propafenone, this mechanism should be considered.

Flecainide and propafenone exert marked negative inotropic effect similar to that of disopyramide which may exacerbate congestive heart failure in patients with left ventricular dysfunction. In patients with normal left ventricular function, flecainide has no effect on ejection fraction.

Flecainide

Drug Interactions
Flecainide causes increased **digoxin** levels (mean of 25%) via decreased drug clearance. **Amiodarone** and **cimetidine** increase flecainide levels. When given concomitantly, **propanolol** and flecainide levels are mildly

increased. **Quinidine** inhibits hepatic metabolism of flecainide increasing elimination half life by 20% (Table 4).

Adverse Effects

Most common side effects are central nervous system reactions with blurred vision, headaches, and ataxia. Congestive heart failure may be provoked in patients with underlying reduced ventricular function.

Proarrhythmia With Class IC Drugs

Both the Cardiac Arrhythmia Suppression Trials (CAST I and II) (Fig. 10 *A* and *B*), the Cardiac Arrhythmia Suppression Trial Hamburg (CASH) and the Multicenter Unsustained Tachycardia Trial (MUSTT) demonstrated increased risk of sudden cardiovascular events in patients with coronary artery disease treated with flecainide. Thus class IC drugs are contraindicated in patients with a prior history of myocardial infarction or history of sustained ventricular arrhythmias.

The incidence of ventricular proarrhythmia with flecainide or propafenone in the absence of structural heart disease is low. Both flecainide and propafenone may cause acceleration of the ventricular rate in patients with atrial flutter or atrial fibrillation presenting as a wide QRS complex tachycardia. Thus, co-administration of an AV nodal blocking agent is recommended.

Propafenone

In addition to class IC effect, propafenone also has negative inotropic effect due to beta adrenergic and calcium channel blocking action which may cause exacerbation of heart failure in patients with impaired left ventricular function. However, the negative inotropic effects of propafenone are somewhat less than those of disopyramide and flecainide. Note that approximately 7% of the U.S. population lack cytochrome P450 2D6 enzyme activity responsible for metabolism of propafenone to 5 hydroxy propafenone. This leads to increased levels of the parent compound and lower levels of 5 hydroxy propafenone which result in greater beta blocker symptoms.

Drug Interactions

Propafenone markedly increases **digoxin** levels due to a decrease in nonrenal clearance and volume of distribution. **Warfarin** clearance is also decreased leading to an increased anticoagulant effect. Both **propranolol** and **metoprolol** are metabolized via the cytochrome P450 system and therefore levels of these drugs are increased in the presence of propafenone. **Theophylline** and **cyclosporin** levels are also increased by propafenone. **Phenytoin**, **phenobarbital**, and **rifampicin** increase metabolism of propafenone. **Quinidine** blocks the cytochrome P450 system inhibiting the conversion of propafenone to 5 hydroxy propafenone in extensive metabolizers. **Cimetidine** causes an increase in propafenone levels resulting in a small but significant lengthening of the QRS complex.

Adverse Effects

Most common are metallic taste (especially with dairy products), nausea, and dizziness. Occasionally, blurred vision, paresthesias, constipation, and increased liver function tests. Exacerbation of asthma may occur (most likely due to the beta adrenergic blocking effects). CNS side effects appear to be related to propafenone plasma concentrations and are more frequent in poor metabolizers.

Both polymorphic VT and ventricular fibrillation have been reported shortly after initiation of propafenone therapy. However, the incidence of serious proarrhythmia with propafenone is low. In patients with atrial fibrillation, propafenone may cause organization of AF to atrial flutter with potential for 1:1 AV conduction in the absence of AV nodal blocking agents.

■ Note that approximately 7% of the U.S. population lack cytochrome P450 2D6 enzyme activity responsible for metabolism of propafenone to 5 hydroxy propafenone. This leads to increased levels of the parent compound and lower levels of 5 hydroxy propafenone which results in greater beta blocker symptoms.

Table 4.   Selected Drug Interactions: Quinidine

Interacts with	Effects
Digoxin	↑ digoxin
Phenytoin, rifampicin, phenobarbital	↓ quinidine
Ketoconazole, azole antifungals	↑ quinidine

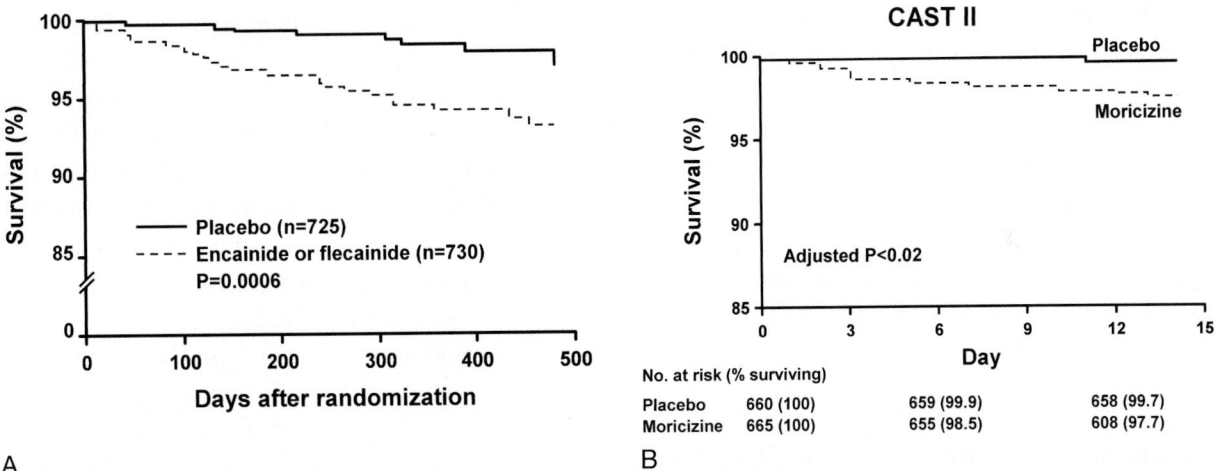

Fig. 10. *A*, Cardiac arrhythmia suppression trial (CAST). *B*, Survival in the CAST II cardiac arrhythmia suppression trial.

VAUGHAN WILLIAMS CLASS III ANTIARRHYTHMIC DRUGS

General Properties of Class III Antiarrhythmic Drugs

The defining property of all class III antiarrhythmic drugs is block of outward potassium channels (Fig. 1). This action prolongs cellular repolarization increasing the cardiac action potential duration and consequent lengthening of the refractory period (Fig. 5).

Increased duration of the cardiac action potential increases the QT interval on the surface ECG (Fig. 7). An important property of class III drugs is reverse use-dependence. This property means that maximal drug action is at SLOWER heart rates. Therefore, QT interval is best measured at rest. All clinically available class III agents block the IKr channel.

Action of Class III Drugs on the Reentry Circuit

Prolongation of the action potential increases the wave length of the reentrant circuit thereby reducing the excitable gap. Reduction of the excitable gap reduces the amount of potentially excitable tissue ahead of the leading edge of activation and increases the likelihood that the advancing wave front will be extinguished (Fig. 3).

Amiodarone

Amiodarone is a complex drug with electrophysiological characteristics of all four Vaughan Williams classes. In addition, the electrophysiological effects of Amiodarone are different when given intravenously to those of chronic use. Acutely, amiodarone inhibits both sodium and calcium currents giving it a class I and class IV effect which is both use dependent (i.e. works better at faster heart rates) and voltage dependent with inhibition being greatest in tissue that is relatively depolarized (i.e. in the presence of myocardial ischemia). The acute effects make amiodarone an effective drug for ventricular arrhythmias in the setting of acute myocardial ischemia. Acutely, amiodarone also has an antagonistic effect on outward potassium currents but this is less potent than its effects on sodium and calcium currents. Specific ion channel currents affected include IK_1 IK_r and Ito (the transient outward current associated with early repolarization during phase 1 of the action potential) and IK_S. Amiodarone has other effects on sodium dependent potassium channels and acetylcholine dependent potassium channels.

Pharmacokinetics

Amiodarone is highly lipid soluble with a large volume of distribution (approximately 5000 liters). Therefore several weeks of drug therapy are required to reach steady state. Typically, a dose of 15 grams or more is required to saturate body fat stores. Elimination half life is greater than 30 days and plasma levels can be detected for more than 9 months after discontinuation of the drug. Metabolism occurs primarily in the liver to *N*-desethylamiodarone (DEA) which has effects similar to those of the parent compound. The kidney does not significantly metabolize or eliminate amiodarone.

Therefore dosage adjustment for renal dysfunction is unnecessary. Neither hemodialysis nor parenteral dialysis removes amiodarone.

Adverse Effects

Most side effects of amiodarone relate to other organ systems. With the exception of the kidney, nearly every organ system is affected with amiodarone use. In general, risk of adverse effect is associated with both daily dosage and duration of therapy.

Cardiac Effects

Torsades de pointes (TdP) is rare, most likely due to the multiple ion channel effects that balance out the potential for QT prolongation to cause TdP.

Bradycardia

Bradycardia is not uncommon especially in patients with sinus or AV nodal dysfunction or with concomitant use of beta-adrenergic blockers due to the effects of amiodarone on both the sinus and AV node. Therefore, dosage of beta-adrenergic blockers should be reduced or discontinued.

Extracardiac Adverse Effects

1. Pulmonary Toxicity

    Pulmonary toxicity is a potentially serious adverse effect of amiodarone. Most commonly this manifests as **chronic interstitial pneumonitis**. Organizing pneumonia with bronchiolitis obliterans and acute respiratory distress syndrome may also occur. Although pulmonary toxicity may develop acutely, it is more commonly associated with chronic use. Symptoms and signs of amiodarone pulmonary toxicity are nonspecific leading to diagnostic difficulties and chest radiographic findings often may mimic those of congestive heart failure. The role of high resolution CT to detect pleural based high attenuation lesions is uncertain. Although commonly used, decreased DLCO from baseline is nonspecific as are findings on bronchoalveolar lavage.

    Treatment includes discontinuation of amiodarone and pulmonary support. Systemic steroids have been used with some efficacy.

2. Thyroid Dysfunction

    Clinical *hypothyroidism is* most common, occurring in close to one-third of patients taking amiodarone depending upon duration of use and is due to inhibition of peripheral de-iodination of T_4 by amiodarone with resultant increasing T_4 and reverse T_3 levels and decreasing T_3 levels. Treatment usually involves thyroid supplementation if continued amiodarone use is required. In occasional cases hypothyroidism persists despite discontinuation of the drug.

    Amiodarone induced *hyperthyroidism* is less common (incidence ~2-10%) typically occurring between three and five years after initiation but is more challenging to manage than hypothyroidism. Treatment with antithyroid agents such as propylthiouracil, methimazole, or in refractory cases, thyroidectomy, is frequently required. Assessment of iodine uptake with a thyroid scan is often helpful in distinguishing amiodarone induced thyrotoxicosis from other causes of thyroid gland overactivity. Note, thyroid ablation using radioactive iodine (I^{131}) is usually ineffective since this agent is not concentrated in the thyroid gland due to the high concentration of iodine already present secondary to amiodarone use.

3. Skin Photosensitivity

    Amiodarone induces sunlight photosensitivity and therefore use of a sun screen is recommended. Long term use is associated with blue-gray discoloration of the skin. These changes are reversible after discontinuation of the drug.

4. Gastrointestinal

    GI symptoms are common and include liver enzyme abnormalities which are usually reversible.

5. CNS

    Peripheral neuropathy, headache, ataxia and (rarely) blindness have all been described. Corneal deposits due to secretion of lacrimal fluid are common and can be visualized on ophthalmologic evaluation. These changes are harmless and are reversible with discontinuation of the drug.

Drug Interactions

Amiodarone reacts with a variety of drugs particularly those that are highly protein bound. Two important effects include amiodarone augmentation of **warfarin** and **digoxin**. Thus, dosages of warfarin and digoxin should be reduced (or discontinued) prior to starting amiodarone.

All drugs that prolong the QT interval may increase the likelihood of torsades de pointes with amiodarone use.

Monitoring Amiodarone Use

Recommended monitoring includes baseline liver function tests, thyroid function tests, electrolytes and creatinine, chest x-ray, pulmonary function test, and ECG. Liver function tests and thyroid function test are generally performed semiannually. A chest x-ray and ECG should be repeated yearly. Ophthalmologic and followup pulmonary function tests are recommended if symptoms or changes occur.

Amiodarone Device Interactions

Chronic amiodarone therapy increases the energy requirement for conversion of ventricular fibrillation to normal sinus rhythm (increase in defibrillation threshold). Therefore in patients who have an ICD, strong consideration should be given for defibrillation threshold testing after initiation of amiodarone.

Clinical Efficacy

The efficacy and safety (in terms of proarrhythmia) of amiodarone has been evaluated in several clinical trials of patients after myocardial infarction including European Myocardial Infarction Amiodarone Trial – EMIAT, and the Canadian Amiodarone Myocardial Infarction Trial-CAMIAT and in patients with congestive heart failure (GESICA and STAT-CHF). Based on pooled data from these trials, and others, amiodarone use is associated with a small (13%) reduction in mortality in high risk patients. However, data from the SCD-Heft Trial that compared amiodarone to ICD and placebo, suggests greater benefit with ICD in high risk patients when compared with amiodarone. Thus, the important message for CV boards from these trials is that amiodarone is safer than other antiarrhythmic agents in terms of proarrhythmia even in post MI and CHF patients but not as good as an ICD.

Sotalol

Sotalol is another class III drug (potassium channel blocking effect) which also has beta adrenergic antagonist properties.

Pharmacokinetics

Bioavailability of sotalol is near 100% and it is eliminated almost entirely unchanged by the kidney. Liver dysfunction has no appreciable effect upon sotalol metabolism. Elimination half life ranges from 12 to 16 hours. Drug accumulation occurs in the setting of renal insufficiency increasing the risk of TdP. Therefore drug dosages should be tailored to patient's creatinine clearance. Doses less than 120 mg twice daily appear to have primarily a beta adrenergic effect and little class III action.

Adverse Effects

Adverse effects of sotalol relate mostly to the beta adrenergic blockade and class III effects. These include bradycardia, fatigue, bronchospasm, and dyspnea. The incidence of TdP due to QT prolongation is estimated at around 2-2.5%. Most events occur early after initiation of the drug or after a change in drug dosage.

Clinical Efficacy

Sotalol is superior to placebo, beta blocker, and class I antiarrhythmic agents for the treatment of supraventricular tachycardia and ventricular arrhythmias. Currently sotalol is most frequently used for the treatment of atrial arrhythmias and to prevent both appropriate and inappropriate ICD shocks in patients with implanted ICD. When compared to placebo, sotalol reduces the number of both appropriate and inappropriate ICD shocks. Unlike amiodarone sotalol decreases the defibrillation threshold. The efficacy of sotalol for maintaining sinus rhythm in patients with atrial fibrillation is not as good.

■ Like other agents in class III Sotalol DECREASES defibrillation threshold (the minimum amount of energy needed to be discharged from an ICD and restore normal rhythm after induction of VF)

Ibutilide

Although technically a class III agent, ibutilide does not exhibit reverse use dependence like other class III agents and has no apparent effect on sinus node function or the cardiac conduction system. Ibutilide exerts antiarrhythmic action via block of potassium channels (IK and IK_r) causing increase in the action potential duration and QT interval prolongation which increases the risk of TdP.

Clinical Efficacy

Ibutilide is superior to placebo in terminating atrial fibrillation or atrial flutter when used alone. In addition,

Ibutilide is useful to facilitate electrical cardioversion of both atrial fibrillation and flutter and overdrive pacing of atrial flutter.

Pharmacokinetics

Ibutilide is only available as an intravenous preparation. Initial dose is 1 mg given over 10 minutes with a second 1 mg dose being given after this period if atrial arrhythmias persist.

Adverse Effects

The most important adverse effect of ibutilide is TdP which is observed in around 3.5-8% of patients. Thus, after administration of ibutilide rhythm should be closely monitored for at least four hours. Importantly, occurrence of TdP may be delayed and risk is increased in patients with decreased left ventricular function. Ibutilide is contraindicated in patients with baseline QTc interval >440.

Clinical Use

The most frequent clinical use of ibutilide is facilitation of direct current cardioversion after initial failure in patients without significant left ventricular dysfunction. Ibutilide is indicated for acute rhythm conversion of atrial fibrillation or atrial flutter in patients with WPW syndrome and preserved ventricular function when duration of arrhythmia is <48 hours.

Dofetilide

Dofetilide, unlike sotalol that also exhibits β-adrenergic blocking effect or amiodarone with complex class I, II, III and IV antiarrhythmic effects, is a pure potassium channel blocker that prolongs the action potential duration and effective refractory periods in both the atria and ventricles.

Pharmacokinetics

The bioavailability of dofetilide following oral administration is >90% and maximal plasma concentrations occur at about 2 to 3 hours. Renal elimination is the main route of excretion and dosage needs to be adjusted based on creatinine clearance.

Indications

Dofetilide is indicated for the treatment of atrial fibrillation and flutter and has greater efficacy when compared with placebo (Fig. 11). It is rarely useful in ventricular arrhythmias.

Adverse Effects

The most serious concern is QT interval prolongation and risk of TdP. This is directly related to its plasma concentration and caution should be used with factors that can increase plasma concentrations, such as reduced creatinine clearance and drug interactions. Dofetilide is contraindicated in patients with severe renal impairment (creatinine clearance <20 mL/minute), a baseline QT_c interval >440 msec or congenital or acquired long QT syndrome. Concurrent use with drugs that inhibit renal cationic secretion (such as cimetidine, ketoconazole and verapamil) is contraindicated and use with agents that are known to cause QT prolongation should be avoided.

Digoxin

Although an older drug, digoxin is still commonly used (>70% patients in rate control arm of AFFIRM trial were taking digoxin) and remains a favorite for CV board questions.

Antiarrhythmic action of digoxin is mediated via its central and peripheral actions to augment vagal tone. Direct action of digoxin on the AV node and atria is seen only at high concentrations (above that used clinically). At toxic concentrations, digoxin increases sympathetic tone and intercellular calcium loading leading to enhanced automaticity and increase in delayed after depolarizations. Direct inhibition of the sodium potassium adenosine triphosphate pump mechanism caused by digoxin increases intracellular calcium concentration via modulation of slow calcium channels and inhibition of the sodium calcium channel and enhances excitation contraction coupling, which is believed to be the mechanism for the positive inotropic effects of cardiac glycosides.

Electrophysiology

Digoxin shortens the refractory period of some accessory pathway fibers and should be avoided in patients with manifest preexcitation (WPW pattern). The reason for this is that the combination of digoxin induced increase in vagal tone (which slows conduction in the AV node) and increased conduction within the atria and accessory pathways increases the likelihood of preexcited atrial fibrillation leading to ventricular fibrillation.

At therapeutic plasma concentrations, digoxin has only minor electrocardiographic effects (PR and QRS intervals usually unchanged).

Clinical Pharmacology

Digoxin is absorbed in the stomach and small intestine with bioavailability of around 80%. Absorption is increased by cholestyramine, colestipol, antacids, calan and sucralfate which bind digoxin in the gut lumen. Absorbed digoxin is excreted back into the gut via the P glycoprotein system. Inhibition of this system can result in decreased levels of digoxin. In the kidney, P glycoprotein is also involved in renal elimination. In patients with normal renal function, elimination half life is approximately 36 hours.

Drug Interactions

Drug-drug interactions with digoxin are common and important.

Quinidine displaces digoxin from tissue binding sites and inhibits the P glycoprotein system increasing the availability of digoxin. **Amiodarone, propafenone,** and **verapamil** decrease both renal and nonrenal clearance also increasing digoxin levels. **Cyclosporin, antiviral** and **antifungal agents,** and **benzodiazepines** also significantly increase serum digoxin concentrations by interfering with the P glycoprotein system.

Adverse Effects

Digoxin toxicity may be precipitated by deterioration in renal function, hypoxia and electrolyte imbalances (particularly changes in serum potassium concentration).

Noncardiac Manifestations

Common noncardiac side effects of digoxin include anorexia, nausea, vomiting, headache, malaise, and changes in vision including scotoma, halo-vision, and altered color perception. Cardiac toxicity is most commonly due to exaggerated effects on the AV node causing bradycardia along with intracellular calcium overloading leading to delayed after depolarizations and increased automaticity leading to development of arrhythmias.

Most common arrhythmias associated with digoxin toxicity include **high grade AV block, accelerated junctional rhythm and bidirectional ventricular tachycardia and atrial tachycardia with block** (Fig. 12 *A* and *B*).

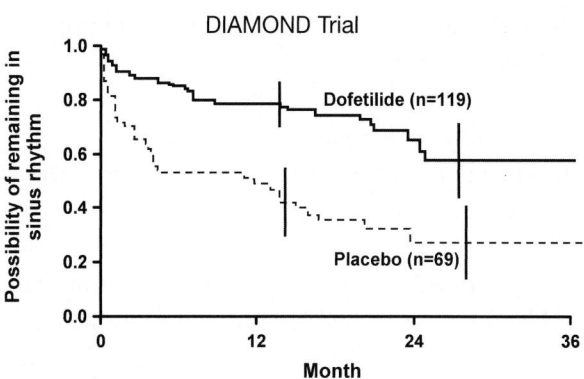

Fig. 11. Efficacy of dofetilide in AF.

Massive digoxin ingestion results in marked inhibition of the sodium potassium exchange leading to severe hyperkalemia and ventricular arrhythmias.

Treatment of Known or Suspected Digoxin Toxicity

Rhythm abnormalities without hemodynamic consequences are best managed with cessation of therapy and observation. Hyperkalemia and hypermagnesemia should corrected. Direct current cardioversion should be avoided wherever possible due to an increased likelihood of precipitating ventricular fibrillation. If hyperkalemia is present, calcium administration should be avoided because it may potentiate arrhythmias caused by intracellular calcium overloading. Digoxin immune FAB antibody therapy may be used to reverse severe digoxin toxicity as evidenced by high serum digoxin levels or the occurrence of malignant ventricular arrhythmias or heart block when it may be life saving. Plasma exchange is of limited value because of the large volume of distribution of digoxin.

Adenosine

Adenosine has a complex mode of action but in cardiac cells acts via the adenosine A1 receptor. Direct effects of adenosine occur via activation of an outward potassium current (IK_{ADO} and IK_{ACH}) present in the atrium, sinoatrial and atrioventricular nodes. These ion channels are not present in ventricular cardiomyocytes and therefore adenosine has no effect in ventricular myocardium. Activation of the IK_{ADO} channel results in shortening of the atrial action potential and hyperpolarization of the membrane which results in depression of sinus node rate and transient AV block. Adenosine also has indirect actions via inhibition of intracellular C_{AMP} generation.

Clinical Electrophysiology

Rapid intravenous bolus of adenosine results in transient (less than 10 seconds) sinus slowing, AV nodal Wenckebach and conduction block. Because of this action adenosine is most frequently used for termination of PSVT due to AV nodal reentry and AV reentry.

Use of Adenosine in Patients With Idiopathic Ventricular Outflow Tract Tachycardia (Right Ventricular Outflow Tract VT)

Although adenosine has no direct effects in ventricular myocardium, it does inhibit catecholamine stimulated calcium currents. A group of adenosine sensitive ventricular tachycardias have been described. Typically, these arise from the right ventricular outflow tract and have a left bundle branch block inferior axis morphology.

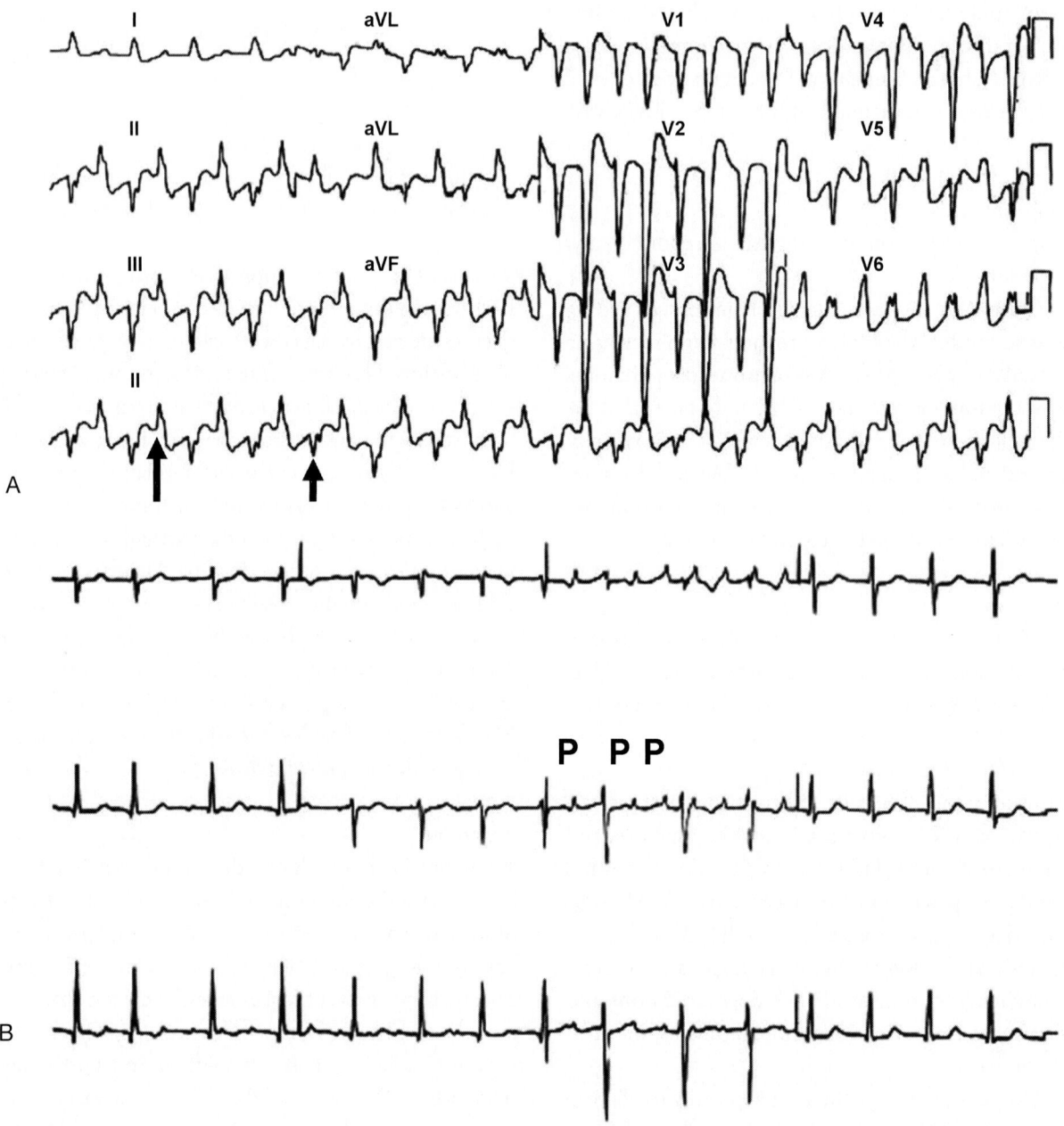

Fig. 12. *A,* Bidirection ventricular tachycardia due to digoxin toxicity. *B,* Atrial tachycardia with AV block due to digoxin toxicity.

Clinically, this form of VT is usually exercise-induced and in the EP lab is facilitated by isoproterenol.

Effects of Adenosine on Other Atrial Arrhythmias
Other than development of AV block, the effect of adenosine on atrial arrhythmias is inconsistent. Use of adenosine for diagnostic purposes in patients with atrial tachycardia is limited.

Drug Interactions and Adverse Effects of Adenosine
Most common reported side effects include facial flushing, chest pain or pressure and dyspnea. These effects are dose related and typically brief.

Proarrhythmia
Shortening of the atrial refractory period by adenosine allows micro-reentry within the atrium and may precipitate atrial fibrillation. The incidence of atrial fibrillation with use of adenosine is 10-15%. Bradycardia due to sinus bradycardia, sinus arrest, or AV block is observed commonly especially upon termination of PSVT. A bradycardia-dependent polymorphic VT has been reported in patients with use of adenosine.

Transplanted Heart
Transplanted hearts are highly sensitive to the effects of adenosine. Therefore, adenosine dosage should be reduced.

Dipyridamole
Dipyridamole decreases reuptake of adenosine which significantly prolongs the effect of adenosine.

Theophylline
Theophylline along with other methylxanthines block adenosine A1 and A2 receptors and prevent the action of adenosine (Table 5).

Table 5.   Choice of Agent in PSVT

Adenosine preferred	Calcium channel blocker preferred (verapamil/diltiazem)
Uncertain diagnosis (especially wide complex tachycardia)	PSVT recurs
	Dipyridamole (adenosine effect prolonged)
Hypotension	Theophylline (adenosine no effect)
Heart failure	Bronchospasm or intolerance of adenosine
	Transplanted heart

ANTIARRHYTHMIC DRUG-DEVICE INTERACTIONS

Effect of Antiarrhythmic Drugs on Pacing Thresholds
The effect of antiarrhythmic drugs on pacing threshold is summarized in Table 6.

■ Drugs that block sodium channels increase the energy required to "reach threshold" ie they increase pacing thresholds whereas drugs that block potassium channels decrease the energy required to reach threshold.

Effect of Antiarrhythmic Drugs on Defibrillation Thresholds
The defibrillation threshold (DFT) is the minimum energy required to restore normal rhythm during ventricular fibrillation (spontaneous or induced). Antiarrhythmic drugs can increase or decrease defibrillation thresholds (Table 7).

Table 6.   Effect of Antiarrhythmic Drugs on
           Pacing Thresholds

Increase	No effect	Decrease
Class IA and C directly proportional to degree of sodium channel block)	Class IB Class III	Digitalis

Table 7.   Effect of Antiarrhythmic Drugs on
           Defibrillation Thresholds

Increased DFT	Decreased DFT
All drugs that block sodium channels Amiodarone	All drugs that block potassium channels (i.e., class III agents EXCEPT amiodarone

103

MODULATORS OF THE RENIN-ANGIOTENSIN SYSTEM

Garvan C. Kane, MD

Peter A. Brady, MD

RENIN-ANGIOTENSIN SYSTEM

The angiotensin-converting enzyme (ACE) regulates the balance between two opposing systems that modulate blood pressure: the renin-angiotensin system (RAS) and the kallikrein-kinin system (Fig. 1). ACE exists in the blood, body fluids, and tissues such as the lung. Increased activity of the RAS leads to salt and water retention and increased vascular tone, which increases blood pressure. Activation of the kallikrein-kinin system leads to the formation of bradykinin, which promotes vasodilatation and natriuresis.

RAS activation occurs under three main conditions: 1) decreased delivery of sodium to the renal macula densa, 2) a decrease in renal perfusion, and 3) sympathetic stimulation leading to release of renin by renal juxtaglomerular cells. Renin acts on angiotensinogen, a prohormone, which leads to the formation of angiotensin I. Angiotensin I is acted upon by ACE to produce angiotensin II. Angiotensin II acts mainly on type 1 angiotensin receptors (AT_1) in vascular smooth muscle cells to induce intense vasoconstriction. It also causes vasoconstriction indirectly through stimulation of the sympathetic nervous system, both centrally and peripherally. Angiotensin II increases circulating plasma volume by stimulating the release of aldosterone from the adrenal cortex, which promotes retention of salt and water, and the release of antidiuretic hormone (ADH),

or vasopressin, from the posterior pituitary, which promotes fluid retention. In tissues, angiotensin II promotes cell migration, proliferation, and growth, pathogenic mechanisms that are likely important in many disease states including myocardial hypertrophy. ACE also increases degradation of bradykinin. In the cardiovascular system, bradykinin promotes vasodilatation through the production of arachidonic acid, its metabolites, and nitric oxide by vascular endothelium. In the kidney, bradykinin promotes natriuresis through direct action on the renal tubules. Thus, bradykinin acts to oppose many of the actions of angiotensin II. The inhibition of ACE alters the balance between RAS and the kallikrein-kinin system in favor of vasodilatation and natriuresis and may have beneficial antiproliferative and anti-hypertrophic effects.

PHARMACOLOGY OF ANGIOTENSIN-CONVERTING ENZYME INHIBITORS

ACE inhibitors differ in potency, bioavailability, plasma half-life, and route of elimination. Most clinically useful ACE inhibitors are prodrugs that require esterification in the liver before they become active, a property that increases bioavailability. ACE inhibitors can be divided into three groups on the basis of their chemical structure: sulfhydryl-containing (captopril), phosphinyl-containing

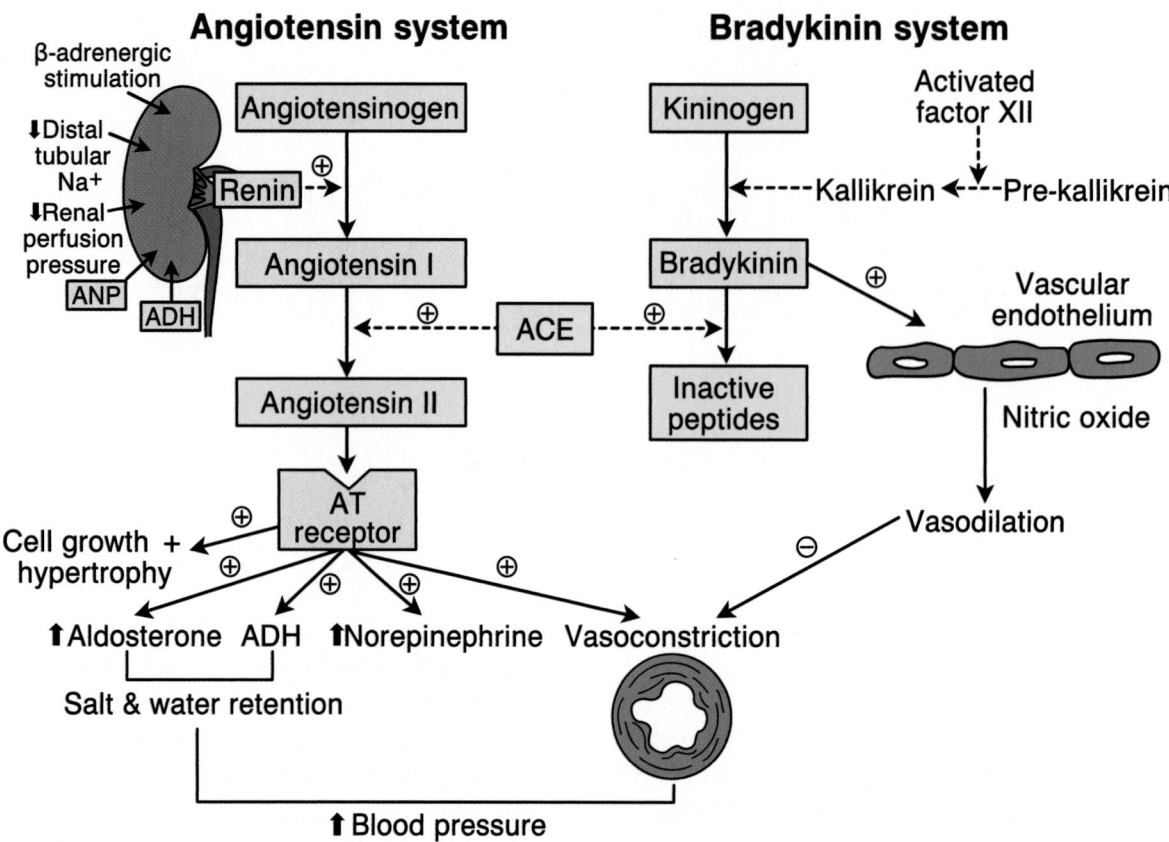

Fig. 1. Regulation of blood pressure by the renin-angiotensin and kallikrein-kinen (bradykinin) systems. ACE, angiotensin-converting enzyme; ADH, antidiuretic hormone; ANP, atrial natriuretic peptide; AT, angiotensin.

(fosinopril), and carboxyl-containing (enalapril, lisinopril, trandolapril, benazepril, and ramipril). Captopril, the first clinically available ACE inhibitor, differs from the others by having the shortest plasma half-life. Evidence suggests that the sulfhydryl-containing moiety may confer additional properties such as free-radical scavenging and effects on prostaglandins. Because most ACE inhibitors are excreted by the kidneys, dosages need to be reduced in patients with renal dysfunction. Exceptions are fosinopril and trandolapril, which are also excreted by the liver.

PHARMACOLOGY OF ANGIOTENSIN RECEPTOR BLOCKERS

The overwhelming effect of ACE inhibitors is on the formation of angiotensin II. Hence, angiotensin (AT1) receptor blocking agents (ARBs) that block the final common pathway of angiotensin II action, share many

of their actions. ARBs also block the action of angiotensin II produced by pathways independently of the RAS system (e.g., chymase and cathepsin) or produced locally in different tissues. They have no effect on bradykinin metabolism. Due to these differences, ARBs have a lower incidence of the kinin-mediated side-effects of cough or angioedema. Available clinical data suggest that ARBs are safe, well tolerated, and at least as effective as ACE inhibitors.

HEMODYNAMIC EFFECTS OF ACE INHIBITORS AND ANGIOTENSIN RECEPTOR BLOCKERS

ACE inhibitors and ARBs decrease systemic vascular resistance, with little change in heart rate. In normotensive and hypertensive persons with normal left ventricular function, ACE inhibitors and ARBs have minimal effect on cardiac output or pulmonary capillary wedge pressure. In systolic dysfunction, both ACE inhibitors and ARBs reduce afterload, preload, and systolic wall stress such that cardiac output increases without an increase in heart rate. The lack of a heart rate response with these agents is believed to be due to an effect on baroreceptor activity as well as inhibition of the normal tonic influence of angiotensin II on the sympathetic nervous system. It is in contrast to the rate-slowing effects of many calcium channel blockers and the direct-acting vasodilators which are associated with a compensatory increase in heart rate.

CLINICAL INDICATIONS FOR ACE INHIBITORS AND ARBS

Congestive Heart Failure

Several large prospective randomized placebo-controlled trials have demonstrated that treatment with ACE inhibitors reduces mortality among patients with ventricular systolic dysfunction, even when asymptomatic (Table 1). Reduced mortality is due primarily to a reduction in the progression toward clinical heart failure. The evidence (Table 1) would suggest that ARB therapy for patients with heart failure and systolic dysfunction should be used in patients who are intolerant of ACE and are a reasonable alternative to ACE I as first-line therapy. There is limited data to support the addition of ARB therapy to an ACE I in persistently symptomatic patients (so called "ACE escape" effect). In patients with heart failure and preserved systolic function (diastolic heart failure) there is little evidence to support a benefit of ACE I or ARB over their blood pressure lowering effects.

Myocardial Infarction

Modulation of the RAS following myocardial infarction favorably affects the early post-infarct ventricular remodeling, thereby limiting the progressive chamber dilatation and increased left ventricular wall stress. ACE inhibition and ARB therapy decrease mortality and the incidence of chronic heart failure when instituted in patients following myocardial infarction (Table 2). These benefits are most apparent in anterior wall infarcts or infarcts complicated by left ventricular systolic dysfunction and/or symptoms or signs of congestive heart failure. The majority of patients enrolled in these trials had ST-segment elevation infarcts.

Hypertension

ACE inhibitors lower mean systolic and diastolic pressures in hypertensive patients as well as in salt-depleted normotensive patients. The decrease in pressure correlates with plasma renin activity and angiotensin levels such that the largest pressure decrease is observed in patients with the highest plasma renin activity. With chronic use of these agents, additional blood pressure lowering occurs independently of plasma renin activity and may involve increased production of vasodilatory prostaglandins by the kallikrein-kinin system. Apart from the specific incidences listed below there is no conclusive evidence that ACE inhibitors should be preferentially used over other antihypertensive therapies. Data has suggested that ACE inhibitors may provide benefit in patients at increased risk for coronary artery disease (such as the HOPE trial). However, the body of evidence (Table 3) suggests that little if any of this benefit is independent of blood pressure reduction. Settings were ACE inhibitors are recommended first-line therapy for hypertension.

- Left ventricular systolic dysfunction.
- Chronic renal failure; diabetic or non-diabetic (exclude renal artery stenosis).
- Following myocardial infarction, particularly if systolic dysfunction.

ACE INHIBITORS IN AFRICAN AMERICANS

There is conflicting literature as to whether African Americans with heart failure have an impaired response to ACE inhibition compared to Caucasians. This does appear to be the case in hypertension where African Americans tend to have less renin-mediated hypertension responding better on average to calcium channel based therapies. There is some evidence to suggest that coadministration of diuretics, which increase plasma renin activity, abolishes racial differences in the response to ACE inhibitors. Too few data exist on clinical outcomes in African Americans to recommend specific guidelines for treatment and it is generally recommended that African Americans be treated the same as Caucasians. Whether higher doses of ACE inhibitors may be more effective is unclear. In contrast to the apparent decreased response to ACE inhibition, African Americans with heart failure appear to have a greater response to hydralazine and nitrate therapy that Caucasians. Whether this combination is more effective than ACE inhibition in a black population is untested.

EMERGING MODULATORS OF THE RENIN-ANGIOTENSIN SYSTEM

Renin itself is the first and rate-limiting enzymatic step in the RAS cascade. Intensive efforts have been committed to the identification and development of potent renin inhibitors. Early clinical trials have demonstrated a clear antihypertensive effect of the renin inhibitor aliskiren in hypertensive patients. Studies to evaluate the role of isolated renin inhibition or the combination of a renin inhibitor with either an ACE inhibitor or an ARB will be necessary to identify the place for renin inhibition in cardiovascular pharmacology (Tables 4 and 5).

Table 1.   Key Clinical Trials of Renin-Angiotensin Modulators in Congestive Heart Failure or LV Dysfunction

Trial	Population	Treatment	Outcome
CONSENSUS	NYHA class IV	Enalapril vs. placebo	Decreased mortality (31% at 1 year) and CHF
SOLVD-T	NYHA classes II and III	Enalapril vs. placebo	Decreased mortality and CHF
V-HeFT II	NYHA classes II and III	Enalapril vs. hydralazine and isosorbide dinitrate	Decreased mortality and sudden death
SOLVD-P	Asymptomatic left ventricular dysfunction	Enalapril vs. placebo	Decreased CHF and hospitalizations
CHARM-Alternative	NYHA classes II and III (intolerant of ACE I) EF<40%	Candesartan vs. placebo	Decreased cardiovascular mortality and CHF
ELITE II	NYHA classes II-IV with EF<40%	Captopril vs. losartan	Losartan as (or slightly less) effective as captopril but better tolerated
Val-HeFT	NYHA classes II-III with EF<40%	Valsartan vs. placebo (93% on ACE I)	No effect on all-cause mortality, but a reduction in combined end point of mortality and morbidity
CHARM-Added	NYHA classes II-III with EF<40%	Candesartan vs. placebo (all on ACE I)	Decreased cardiovascular mortality and CHF
CHARM-Preserved	NYHA classes II-III with EF>40%	Candesartan vs. placebo	Nonsignificant trend towards decreased cardiovascular mortality and CHF

CHARM, Candesartan in Heart Failure: Assessment of Reduction in Mortality and Morbidity; CONSENSUS, Cooperativew North Scandinavian Enalapril Survival Study; ELITE, Evaluation of Losartan in the Elderly Study; NYHA, New York Heart Association; SOLVD, Studies on Left Ventricular Dysfunction (P, prevention and T, treatment); V-HeFT, Veterans Administration Heart Failure Trial; Val-Heft, Valsartan Heart Failure Trial.

Table 2. Key Clinical Trials of Renin-Angiotensin Modulators Following Myocardial Infarction

Trial	Population	Treatment	Time of initial dose	Duration	Outcome
GISSI-3	MI	Lisinopril vs. nitrates	24 hr	6 weeks	Improved survival
ISIS-4	MI	Captopril vs. placebo	24 hr	5 weeks	Improved survival
CONSENSUS II	MI	Enalapril(at) vs. placebo	24 hr	6-26 weeks	No effect on survival. Hypotension with enalaprilat.
CCS-1	MI	Captopril vs. placebo	36 hr	4 weeks	Trend towards improved survival
SAVE	MI with EF<40%	Captopril vs. placebo	3-16 days	24-60 months	Improved survival
AIRE	MI with CHF	Ramipril vs. placebo	3-10 days	>6 months	Improved survival
TRACE	MI with EF<35%	Trandolapril vs. placebo	3-7 days	24-50 months	Improved survival
SMILE	Anterior MI without reperfusion	Zofenopril vs. placebo	24 hr	6 weeks	Improved survival
OPTIMAAL	Anterior MI or MI with CHF	Captopril vs. losartan	<10 days	2.7 years	Trend towards improved survival with captopril
VALIANT	MI with EF<40% or CHF	Captopril vs. valsartan vs. both	12 hr to 10 days	25 months	Valsartan as effective as captopril Combination increased rate of adverse events without improving survival

AIRE, Acute Infarction Ramipril Efficacy; CCS, Chinese Cardiac Study; CONSENSUS, Cooperative North Scandinavian Enalapril Survival Study; GISSI, Gruppo Italino per lo Studio della Streptochinasi nell'Infarto Miocardico; ISIS, International Study for Infarct Survival; OPTIMAAL, Optimal Trial in Myocardial Infarction with Angiotensin II Antagonist Losartan; SAVE, Survival and Ventricular Enlargement; SMILE, Survival of Myocardial Infarction Long-Term Evaluation; TRACE, Trandolapril Cardiac Evaluation; VALIANT, Valsartan in Acute Myocardial Infarction Trial.

Table 3.   Key Clinical Trials of Renin-Angiotensin Modulators in Hypertension and/or Cardiovascular Disease

Trial	Population	Treatment	Outcome
HOPE	CVD or DM + CAD RF	Ramipril vs. placebo	Reduction in CV event rate
EUROPA	CVD	Perindopril vs. placebo	Reduction in CV death or MI
INVEST	HTN and CAD	Verapamil ± trandolapril vs. atenolol ± HCTZ	Equal clinical efficacy between treatment strategies
VALUE	HTN + RF	Valsartan vs. amlodipine	Outcomes similar
ALLHAT	HTN + RF	Chlorthalidone vs. lisinopril	No difference in mortality or MI incidence but higher combined CV outcomes with lisinopril
PEACE	CAD	Trandolapril vs. placebo	No difference in CV event rates
CAMELOT	CAD	Enalapril vs. amlodipine vs. placebo	Amlodipine but not enalapril reduced CV event rates

ALLHAT, Antihypertensive and Lipid-Lowering Treatment to Prevent Heart Attack Trial; CAMELOT, Effect of Antihypertensive Agents on Cardiovascular Events in Patients With Coronary Disease and Normal Blood Pressure; CVD, Cardiovascular disease—i.e. history of coronary artery disease (CAD) or cerebrovascular disease; DM, diabetes mellitus; EUROPA, European Trial on Reduction of Cardiac Events With Perindopril in Stable Coronary Artery Disease; HOPE, Heart Outcomes Prevention Evaluation Study; HTN, hypertension; INVEST, International Verapamil-Trandolapril Study; MI, myocardial infarction; PEACE, Prevention of Events with Angiotensin Converting Enzyme Inhibition; RF, conventional risk factor for CAD; VALUE, Valsartan Antihypertensive Long-Term Use Evaluation.

Table 4.   Adverse Effects of Angiotensin-Converting Enzyme Inhibitors

Effects related to reduced angiotensin II (i.e., also seen with angiotensin receptor blockers, ARBs)

Hypotension   Increased frequency in high renin states and concomitant diuretic use

Hyperkalemia   Frequent and usually minor, stabilizes after 1st week. Risk magnified in renal failure or with concomitant aldosterone antagonist use

Renal failure   Most often due to decreased renal perfusion, e.g., renal artery stenosis or low output state

Teratogenicity   Adverse effects on fetal renal function and development in 2nd and 3rd trimesters. ACE inhibitors or ARBs must be discontinued *immediately* if pregnancy is confirmed or suspected

Effects related to increased kinins (i.e., ACE inhibitor specific)

Dry cough   Common (5-20%). Dose-dependent, often necessitates cessation of therapy

Angioedema   Rare, 1-2/1,000; usually occurs 1st month but may appear later. 90% plus can subsequently safely take an ARB

Sulfhydryl-related effects (i.e., captopril specific)

Neutropenia   Rare (<0.05%), higher incidence in patients with collagen vascular diseases

Rash   1%, usually maculopapular, pruritic; rarely exfoliative dermatitis

Proteinuria   1% of patients receiving captopril, but paradoxically captopril will decrease proteinuria in both diabetic and non-diabetic nephropathy

Table 5. Drug Interactions With Angiotensin-Converting Enzyme (ACE) Inhibitors

Potassium	Potassium supplements, potassium-sparing diuretics, and salt substitutes should be used with caution or discontinued because of the potassium-sparing effect of aldosterone suppression
Diuretics	Increased sensitivity to hypotensive effects of ACE inhibitors because of higher baseline ream levels
NSAIDs	May decrease antihypertensive action of ACE inhibitors, more common in the presence of low renin levels

104

PRINCIPLES OF DIURETIC USAGE

Garvan C. Kane, MD

Joseph G. Murphy, MD

Diuretics decrease sodium chloride reabsorption in the kidney and increase sodium chloride and water excretion in the urine. Their primary uses are in the management of pulmonary and peripheral edema associated with congestive heart failure and the chronic management of hypertension. Aldosterone antagonist diuretics improve survival in advanced heart failure. Diuretics are classified primarily by their site of action.

LOOP DIURETICS

■ Loop diuretics are the most powerful diuretics and act to reduce sodium chloride reabsorption in the thick ascending loop of Henle by blocking the Na^+-K^+-$2Cl^-$ cotransporter. Loop diuretics are highly protein bound and rely on tubular secretion into the proximal kidney tubule to reach their site of action. The accumulation of organic acids as seen in advanced renal insufficiency can block this transportation mechanism and decrease diuretic efficacy necessitating an increased dose of diuretic drug. In patients with normal renal function the maximal diuretic effect is seen with 40 mg of furosemide, 1 mg of bumetanide, 20 mg of torsemide. All loop diuretics are equally efficacious if given in sufficient doses. In renal insufficiency or congestive heart failure higher doses (2-5 fold increase) are required to achieve the maximal diuretic response. There is an increased incidence of side-effects in tandem with increased diuretic dose. All loop diuretics may cause: 1) diuresis-induced hypovolemia and electrolyte abnormalities (hypokalemia, hypomagnesemia, hypocalcemia and metabolic alkalosis) and 2) ototoxicity due to an action on the Na^+-K^+-$2Cl^-$ cotransporter isoform in the inner ear. Sulfonamide mediated allergic reaction including Stevens-Johnson syndrome are occasionally seen with furosemide, bumetanide, and torsemide. Ethacrynic acid is the only nonsulfonamide loop diuretic and may be used in patients with previous sulfonamide allergy, however ethacrynic acid may cause more ototoxicity compared with other diuretic agents. Loop diuretics have a short duration of action (4-6 hours) necessitating at least twice daily dosing typically given in the early morning and early afternoon to avoid nocturia. After oral dosing, furosemide has an onset of action of 60-90 minutes and 15 minutes after intravenous administration. Furosemide also has an acute ill-defined early venodilatory action likely related to release of vasodilatory prostaglandins. Patients with severe cardiac or renal failure loop may require diuretics administered in a high dose intravenous infusion. Loop diuretics cause potent sodium and water excretion.

- Loop diuretics remain efficacious in renal dysfunction, although higher doses needed.
- Loop diuretics can cause hypokalemia, hypomagnesemia, hypocalcemia, and ototoxicity.

THIAZIDE DIURETICS

Thiazide diuretics are moderately powerful diuretics that inhibit sodium chloride reabsorption in the distal convoluted tubule, a site of action distinct from the loop diuretics. Thiazide diuretics are typically administered orally in the chronic management of hypertension. Compared with loop diuretics, they have a longer duration of action and are less efficacious particularly in the setting of renal insufficiency. Metolazone unlike other thiazide diuretics is effective in patients with severe renal dysfunction and is commonly used in combination with high doses of loop diuretics to facilitate a strong diuretic effect. Thiazides are generally well tolerated without serious complications. Adverse effects of thiazides are similar to loop diuretics with diuresis-induced hypovolemia and electrolyte abnormalities (hypokalemia, hypomagnesemia, and metabolic alkalosis). Unlike loop diuretics thiazides tend to cause mild hypercalcemia. In addition thiazides cause a dose-dependent increased incidence of hyperuricemia, hyperglycemia, hyperlipidemia and male impotence, changes that typically reverse on cessation of therapy. Rare idiosyncratic reactions to thiazides include blood dyscrasias and acute pancreatitis. Ototoxicity is not seen with thiazides. Thiazides as sulfonamide derivatives should not be used in sulfonamide allergic patients. Nonsteroidal anti-inflamatory drugs may attenuate the antihypertensive effect of thiazide diuretics.

- Thiazide diuretics cause sodium and water excretion and are commonly used to treat hypertension.
- Thiazide diuretics have impaired efficacy in renal dysfunction, metolazone is an exception.
- Thiazide diuretics can cause hypokalemia, hypomagnesemia and hypercalcemia.
- Thiazide diuretics may exacerbate hyperuricemia, hyperglycemia, hyperlipidemia and impotence.
- Thiazides reduce the renal clearance of lithium and

there is, increased risk of *lithium* toxicity in diuretic-treated patients.

POTASSIUM-SPARING DIURETICS

Potassium-sparing diuretics, such as amiloride and triamterene, are relatively weak diuretics that inhibit sodium reabsorption in the distal convoluted tubule and collecting duct. They indirectly cause relative potassium retention and are mainly used in combination with a loop or thiazide diuretic to offset the associated hypokalemia. Apart from a risk of hyperkalemia and some gastrointestinal upset these agents are relatively free of adverse effects. A subset of potassium-sparing diuretics acts as aldosterone antagonists and has therapeutic benefit in congestive heart failure beyond their diuretic action. Spironolactone significantly lowers blood pressure, decreases the incidence of hypokalemia and reduces hospitalization for heart failure and death in patients with NYHA class III or IV heart failure (RALES study). However spironolactone has nonspecific estrogen-like actions of gynecomastia (10%), decreased libido and impotence in male patients. Much of this occurs in patients who take concomitant digoxin therapy. A newer more specific aldosterone antagonist, eplerenone, lacks the endocrine side effects of spironolactone while maintaining the therapeutic benefits. Eplerenone has demonstrated a mortality benefit when started within 2 weeks in patients with an acute myocardial infarction complicated by heart failure and an LVEF <30% (EPHESUS study). Potassium-sparing diuretics reduce the incidence of serious ventricular arrhythmias in heart failure. The RALES and EPHESUS trials excluded patients with, serum creatinine values of >2.5 mg/dL or baseline serum potassium values of >5.0 mEq/L. The incidence of serious hyperkalemia defined as a potassium of >6.0 mEq/L was 2% and 5% respectively.

- Potassium sparing diuretics are weak agents that inhibit sodium reabsorption in the distal convoluted tubule and collecting duct.
- Aldosterone antagonists decrease morbidity and mortality in patients with symptomatic heart failure.

105

DIGOXIN

Arshad Jahangir, MD

Digitalis compounds have been in use for more than 200 years for the management of congestive heart failure and comprise several active drugs including digoxin and digitoxin. Digoxin is the only positive inotropic agent currently approved for oral use in the U.S.

PHARMACOKINETICS

The bioavailability of digoxin ranges between 60% and 85% (Table 1). Intestinal microflora may metabolize digoxin in about 10% of patients thereby reducing bioavailability and is one of the causes of apparent resistance to standard doses of oral digoxin. This has two main clinical consequences namely higher doses of digoxin are required to achieve therapeutic levels and toxicity may occur with intercurrent use of antibiotics that destroy intestinal microflora. The elimination half-life of digoxin in patients with normal renal function is 36 to 48 hours, with ~70% of the drug eliminated unchanged through the kidneys. Digoxin has a large apparent volume of distribution throughout the body, mostly due to binding to skeletal muscle receptors: thus digoxin is not effectively removed by peritoneal dialysis or hemodialysis. Steady-state blood levels are achieved about 1 week (5 half-lives) after the initiation of oral

maintenance therapy. Digoxin crosses both the blood-brain barrier and the placenta, with similar levels of drug in maternal and umbilical vein blood.

■ Intestinal microflora may metabolize digoxin in about 10% of patients and reduce bioavailability.

MECHANISM OF ACTION

Inotropic Effect

The primary action of digoxin is to inhibit the cell membrane Na^+-K^+- adenosine triphosphatase (ATPase), which normally maintains the transcellular sodium and potassium gradients. Inhibition of the Na^+-K^+ pump increases intracellular sodium, which in turn leads to increased intracellular calcium via the Na^+-Ca^{2+} exchanger (Fig 1). Calcium influx into the myocardial cell is also increased by alteration of the ion selectivity of the membrane voltage-gated sodium channels by "slip-mode conductance." Increased intracellular calcium level enhances calcium in the sarcoplasmic reticulum, which then becomes available for release onto calcium-sensitive proteins of the contractile apparatus during the next cycle of excitation-contraction coupling, thereby

Table 1. Digoxin Pharmacokinetics

Feature	Value
Bioavailability	75%
Serum half-life	36 hr
Steady state blood level	1 wk (5 half-lives)
Therapeutic serum level	1-2 ng/mL
Volume of distribution*	4-7 L/kg
Renal excretion	70%
Microintestinal floral metabolism	~10% of patients
Crosses blood-brain barrier and placenta	

*Bound to muscle receptors and not removed by dialysis.

augmenting the force of myocardial contraction. The inotropic effect of digoxin is present in both normal and failing myocardium and results in increased stroke work for a given ventricular volume.

■ The primary action of digoxin is to inhibit the cell membrane Na^+-K^+-ATPase that leads to increase in intracellular calcium through Na^+-Ca^+ exchanger.
■ The inotropic effect of digoxin is present in both normal and failing myocardium and results in increased stroke work for a given ventricular volume.

Effect on Vascular Smooth Muscle and Neurohumoral System

In normal subjects, digoxin may increase peripheral resistance and venous tone by increasing intracellular calcium in vascular smooth muscle, an effect not present in patients with heart failure because of their increased basal level of autonomic activation.

Digoxin increases parasympathetic activity, resulting in a slowing of sinus impulses and conduction through the atrioventricular (AV) node (Fig. 2). Inhibition of Na^+-K^+-ATPase in vagal afferent fibers sensitizes the cardiac baroreceptors, which in turn reduces sympathetic outflow from the central nervous system. In heart failure, digoxin generally has a sympathoinhibitory effect, believed to be mediated through the central nervous system that results in a decrease in heart rate,

sympathetic nervous activity, and plasma norepinephrine concentration. Renin release is decreased because of inhibition of the renal sodium pump; this leads to a natriuretic effect and vasodilatation that may offset the direct vasoconstrictor effect of digoxin.

■ Digoxin increases parasympathetic activation, resulting in slowing of sinus impulses and conduction through the AV node.

Electrophysiologic Actions

Digoxin alters cardiac electrophysiology by a direct effect on the myocardium and indirectly through parasympathetic activation and sympathetic inhibition. Digoxin at therapeutic plasma concentrations decreases automaticity and conduction velocity in the sinoatrial and AV nodal tissues mainly by an increase in vagal tone and decrease in sympathetic activity. The maximal diastolic resting membrane potential of the nodal tissue is increased and the action potential duration in the atrial tissue shortened. These changes result in sinus bradycardia and/or prolongation or block of AV conduction. At higher (toxic) concentrations, the increased intracellular calcium caused by digoxin enhances automaticity in cardiac tissue and the His-Purkinje system by a shift in resting membrane potential to more depolarized values, increasing phase 4 depolarization and delayed afterdepolarizations that may result in triggered activity and arrhythmias.

The major electrocardiographic (ECG) effects of digoxin are PR prolongation and nonspecific ST-segment changes at rest that may give false-positive ST-T changes during exercise testing.

■ Patients taking digoxin may have false positive EKG changes indicative of myocardial ischemia on treadmill exercise testing.

THERAPEUTIC USES OF DIGOXIN

Arrhythmias

Paroxysmal Supraventricular Tachycardia

Digoxin, through its effects on sinoatrial and AV nodal tissue is effective in terminating or preventing sinus node reentry or AV node-dependent supraventricular

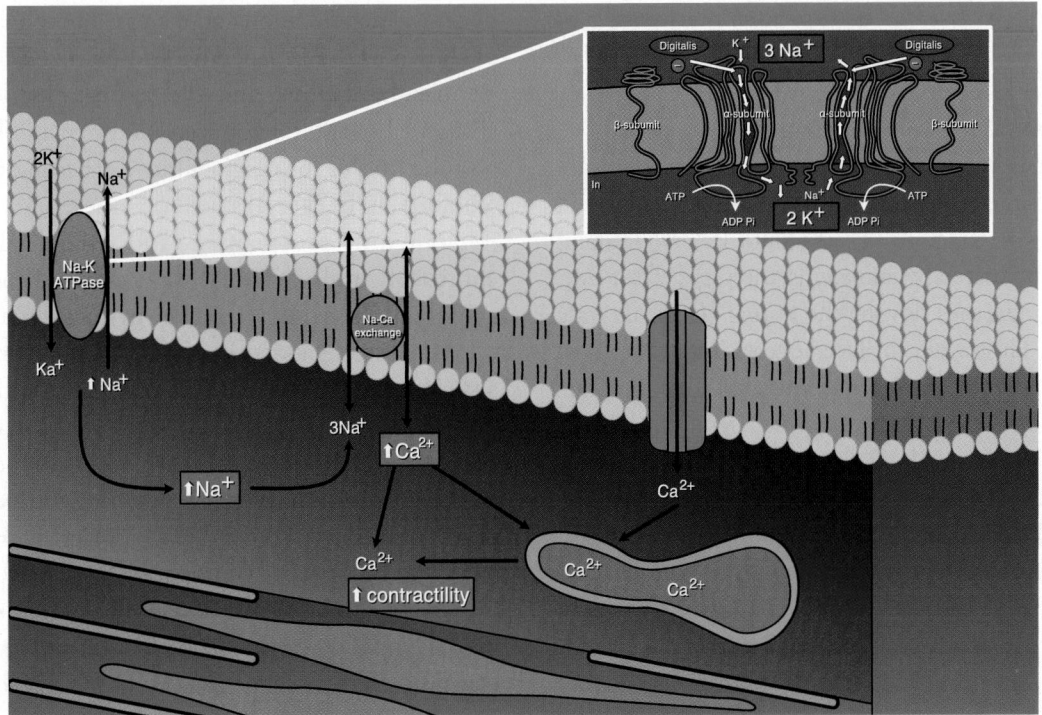

Fig. 1. Inhibition of Na$^+$-K$^+$-ATPase by digoxin. Na$^+$-K$^+$-ATPase (the sodium pump) transports three sodium ions outward and two potassium ions inward. Inhibition of the Na$^+$-K$^+$ pump increases intracellular sodium, which leads to increased intracellular calcium by Na$^+$-Ca^{2+} exchanger. The increased intracellular calcium increases the force of myocardial contraction by increasing both the velocity and extent of sarcomere shortening. Inset shows the proposed structure of the Na$^+$-K$^+$-ATPase consisting of two α-subunits and two surrounding β-subunits. The α-domain contains the ionic channel, the external digitalis binding site, the external potassium binding site, the internal sodium binding site, and the ATP hydrolysis site. (Modified from: Opie LH. The heart: physiology, from cell to circulation. 3rd ed. Philadelphia: Lippincott-Raven Publishers; 1998. p. 108.)

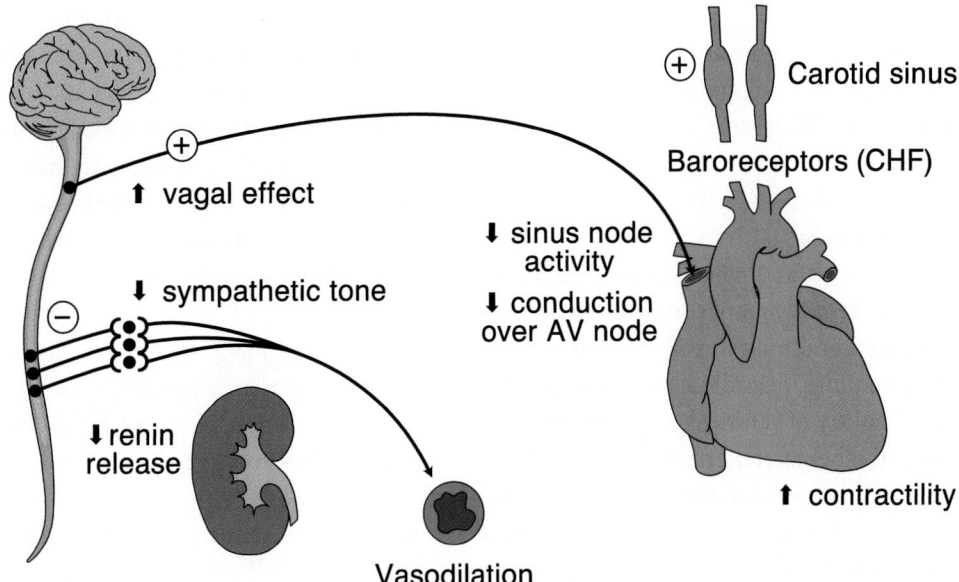

Fig. 2. Digitalis effect on neurocardiovascular system. AV, atrioventricular; CHF, congestive heart failure. (By permission from: Opie LH. Drugs for the heart. 6th ed. Philadelphia: Elsevier Saunders; 2005. p. 152.)

tachycardia, such as AV node reentrant tachycardia or orthodromic AV reentrant tachycardia.

Atrial Fibrillation and Flutter

Digoxin is used to control rapid ventricular rate response in chronic atrial fibrillation particularly in patients with congestive heart failure. Its predominant effect is mediated by enhancing the vagal effect over the AV node, thus slowing the resting ventricular rate response. This vagally mediated effect is easily overcome by sympathetic stimulation. Thus, in high adrenergic states, such as during exercise, post-operatively, thyrotoxicosis or chronic lung disease digoxin alone is only marginally effective and should be used concomitantly with a β-blocker (avoid in chronic lung disease), verapamil or diltiazem for ventricular rate control.

Digoxin is ineffective in terminating or preventing recurrence of paroxysmal atrial fibrillation or atrial flutter and in controlling ventricular rate response during recurrences. Digoxin may make paroxysmal atrial fibrillation worse by prolonging the duration of atrial fibrillation, especially if a strong vagal component is present. Digoxin should not be used in patients with atrial fibrillation and Wolff-Parkinson-White syndrome because anterograde conduction over the accessory pathway could be enhanced precipitating ventricular tachycardia or fibrillation and death.

■ The vagally mediated effect of digoxin is easily overcome by catecholamine and in conditions with high sympathetic tone, digoxin is only marginally effective in slowing ventricular rate response during atrial fibrillation.

Congestive Heart Failure

The positive inotropic and neurohumoral effects of digoxin improve hemodynamics in congestive heart failure. Multiple clinical trials in patients with mild to moderate heart failure, regardless of an ischemic or non-ischemic etiology of ventricular dysfunction have demonstrated the beneficial effect of digoxin with improvement in symptom control, quality of life and exercise capacity with reduction in hospitalizations for heart failure (Table 2). The clinical improvement was seen regardless of the presence of sinus rhythm or atrial fibrillation. The withdrawal of digoxin after chronic use in patients with mild to moderate heart failure results

in clinical deterioration and increased hospitalizations as shown in the Prospective Randomized Study of Ventricular Failure and the Efficacy of Digoxin (PROVED) and Randomized Assessment of Digoxin on Inhibitors of the Angiotensin-Converting Enzyme (RADIANCE) (Fig. 3) studies.

The only prospective randomized, placebo-controlled trial of digoxin that assessed mortality among patients with heart failure in sinus rhythm is the Digitalis Investigation Group (DIG) study. There was a substantial decrease in hospitalizations and deaths due to worsening heart failure but overall mortality was not affected by digoxin usage when added to conventional heart failure therapy including diuretics and angiotensin-converting enzyme (ACE) inhibitor therapy (Fig. 4). Thus, when compared to other positive inotropic agents, which adversely affect overall survival, digoxin appears to be "safe" for long-term use in patients with heart failure. Patients most likely to benefit from digoxin were those at the highest risk for clinical deterioration. Thus, patients with more severe heart failure with functional class III/IV, lower left ventricular ejection fraction (<25%), and a greater cardiothoracic ratio (>0.50) had the greatest benefit from digoxin therapy (Fig. 5). It has been suggested that a balance between a reduction in deaths due to worsening heart failure and an increase in deaths from other causes, such as arrhythmia or myocardial infarction, may occur in these patients. The reduction in risk of worsening heart failure between patients with relatively well preserved left ventricular systolic function and those with markedly impaired left ventricular systolic function was not statistically different, thus alleviating concern about the use of digoxin in patients with relatively well preserved systolic function in whom heart failure was due primarily to diastolic dysfunction.

■ Digoxin therapy in patients with heart failure due to systolic ventricular dysfunction results in reduction in hospitalization and deaths from worsening heart failure; however, overall mortality is not affected.

Digoxin is recommended as a class I indication in the American College of Cardiology/American Heart Association (ACC/AHA) guidelines for the treatment of patients with heart failure due to systolic dysfunction not adequately responsive to ACE inhibitors and

Table 2.   Digoxin in Heart Failure–Randomized, Placebo-Controlled Clinical Trials

	PROVED		RADIANCE		DIG	
	Placebo (n=46)	Digoxin† (n=42)	Placebo (n=93)	Digoxin† (n=85)	Placebo (n=340)	Digoxin (n=3397)
Mean age (yr)	64	64	59	61	63	63
Male (%)	80	90	82	71	77	78
LVEF (%)	29	27	28	26	28	29
NYHA II (%)	83	83	75	71	55	53
NYHA III (%)	15	17	25	29	31	31
NYHA IV (%)	–	–	–	–	2	2
IHD (%)	67	60	56	65	70	71
ACE inhibitor treatment (%)	0	0	100	100	95	94
Mean follow-up (months)	3		3		37	
Progression/worsening of heart failure (%)	39	19	25.0	4.7		
Change in exercise time from baseline (sec)	-96	+4.5 (P=0.003)	-26	+17 (P=0.033)		
Change in body weight (kg)	+0.5	-0.9 (P=0.044)	+1	-1 (P<0.001)		
Change in LVEF (%)	-3	+2 (P=0.016)	-4	-1 (P<0.001)		
Hospital admission for worsening heart failure (%)	13	7	10	2	34.7	26.8

†Withdrawal.
PROVED, Prospective Randomized Study of Ventricular Failure and Efficacy of Digoxin; RADIANCE, Randomized Assessment of Digoxin on Inhibitors of the Angiotensin-Converting Enzyme; DIG, Digitalis Investigation Group.

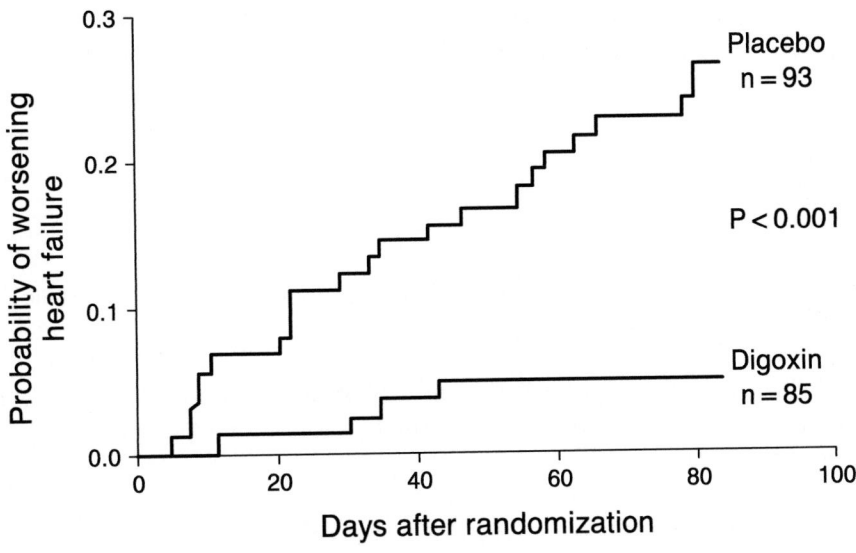

Fig. 3. Kaplan-Meier analysis of the cumulative probability of worsening heart failure in patients continuing to receive digoxin and those switched to placebo. The patients in the placebo group had a higher risk of worsening heart failure throughout the 12-week study (relative risk, 5.9; 95 percent confidence interval, 2.1 to 17.2; P<0.001).

diuretics and in patients with atrial fibrillation and rapid ventricular response not fully controlled with a β-blocker (Table 3). For all other symptomatic patients with heart failure due to left ventricular systolic dysfunction, digoxin has a class IIb indication. The primary benefit of digoxin in heart failure is to improve the clinical status, with attenuation of symptoms and reduction in hospitalizations for heart failure. Because there is no evidence that digoxin decreases mortality, it may not be needed in patients who are asymptomatic after treatment with ACE inhibitors, diuretics, and β-blockers. Patients with heart failure due to amyloid heart disease or restrictive cardiomyopathy respond poorly to treatment with digoxin.

Side Effects and Toxicity

Digoxin has a narrow therapeutic index and toxicity can develop readily if not carefully monitored. The toxic effects increase markedly with digoxin levels greater than 2.0 ng/mL (Fig. 6). The common side effects with chronic digoxin overdose (Table 4) are gastrointestinal (anorexia, nausea, vomiting, diarrhea), visual (colored halos around a light) and cardiac arrhythmias (ectopic rhythm and heart block). Central nervous system effects (malaise, fatigue, confusion, disorientation, insomnia, and vertigo) and gynecomastia may also occur. Adverse effects may occur even with therapeutic serum levels, especially in the presence of hypokalemia or hypomagnesemia, which can independently increase ventricular automaticity and lower threshold for digoxin-induced cardiac arrhythmias.

Because of the direct arterial vasoconstrictive effects of digoxin, intravenous administration can be deleterious in patients with severe atherosclerosis and precipitation of coronary and mesenteric ischemia has been reported. Use of digitalis in the setting of cardiac ischemia, for example, after myocardial infarction, has been suggested to be associated with increased mortality. Recent experimental evidence also suggests that inhibition of Na^+-K^+-ATPase activity with digoxin may prevent the infarct size-limiting effect of ischemic preconditioning.

Digoxin toxicity can result from overdose, decreased excretion, or other factors that may increase the sensitivity of tissue to digoxin even at "therapeutic" serum levels (Table 4). Factors associated with poor prognosis in patients with digitalis toxicity are summarized in Table 5. Disturbances of cardiac conduction, impulse formation or both may occur with digoxin toxicity (Fig. 7). Because of its effect on the shortening of atrial repolarization and dispersion of refractoriness, digoxin may have proarrhythmic effects that prolong the duration of atrial fibrillation. Intracellular calcium overload with digoxin toxicity predispose to delayed afterdepolarization and triggered activity in atrial, junctional or Purkinje tissue giving rise to paroxysmal atrial tachycardia (with AV block due to increased vagal tone), accelerated junctional rhythm, frequent premature ventricular complexes or fascicular or bidirectional ventricular tachycardia. With severe intoxication, hyperkalemia due to Na^+-K^+-ATPase poisoning and profound bradyarrhythmias may occur and may be unresponsive to pacing therapy. If digoxin toxicity is suspected, elective

Table 3.   Recommendations for Therapy with Digoxin

Class I
> Treatment of symptoms of heart failure (stage C) in patients with left ventricular systolic dysfunction in the absence of contraindication to digoxin use

> For control of rapid ventricular rate response with atrial fibrillation that do not respond to electrical cardioversion or recur after a brief period of sinus rhythm, principally in patients with severe left ventricular dysfunction and heart failure.

Class IIb
> To minimize symptoms of heart failure in patients with preserved systolic ventricular function

Class III
> In patients with asymptomatic left ventricular dysfunction (stage B heart failure) who are in sinus rhythm

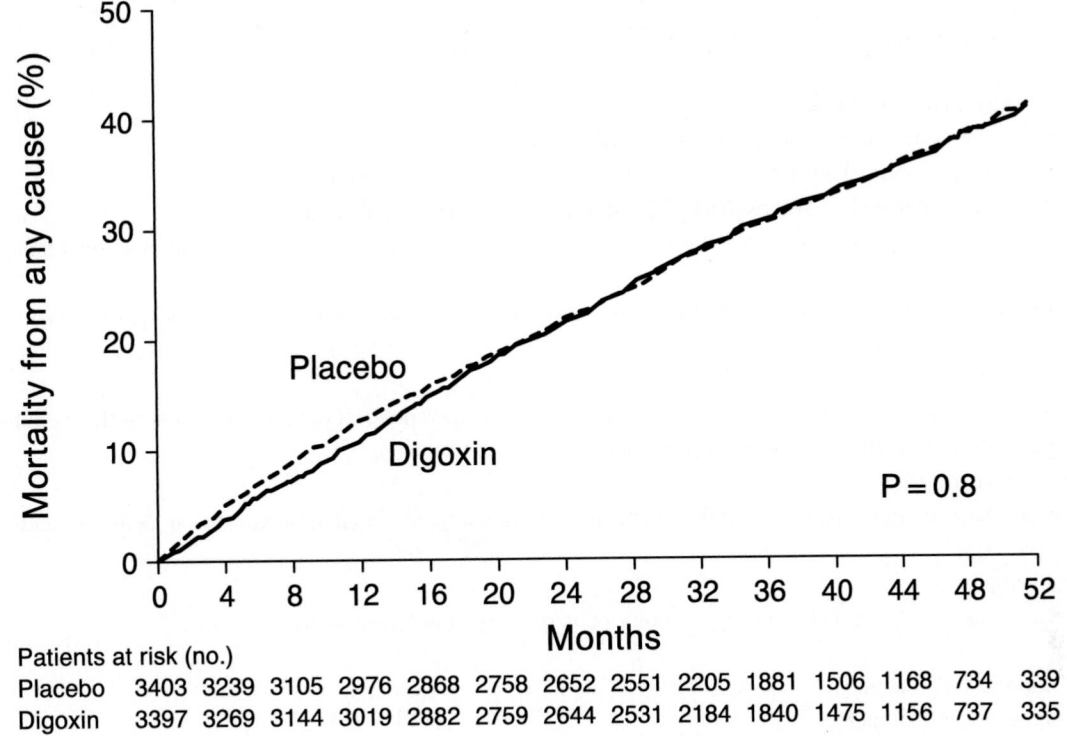

Patients at risk (no.)

Placebo	3403	3239	3105	2976	2868	2758	2652	2551	2205	1881	1506	1168	734	339
Digoxin	3397	3269	3144	3019	2882	2759	2644	2531	2184	1840	1475	1156	737	335

A

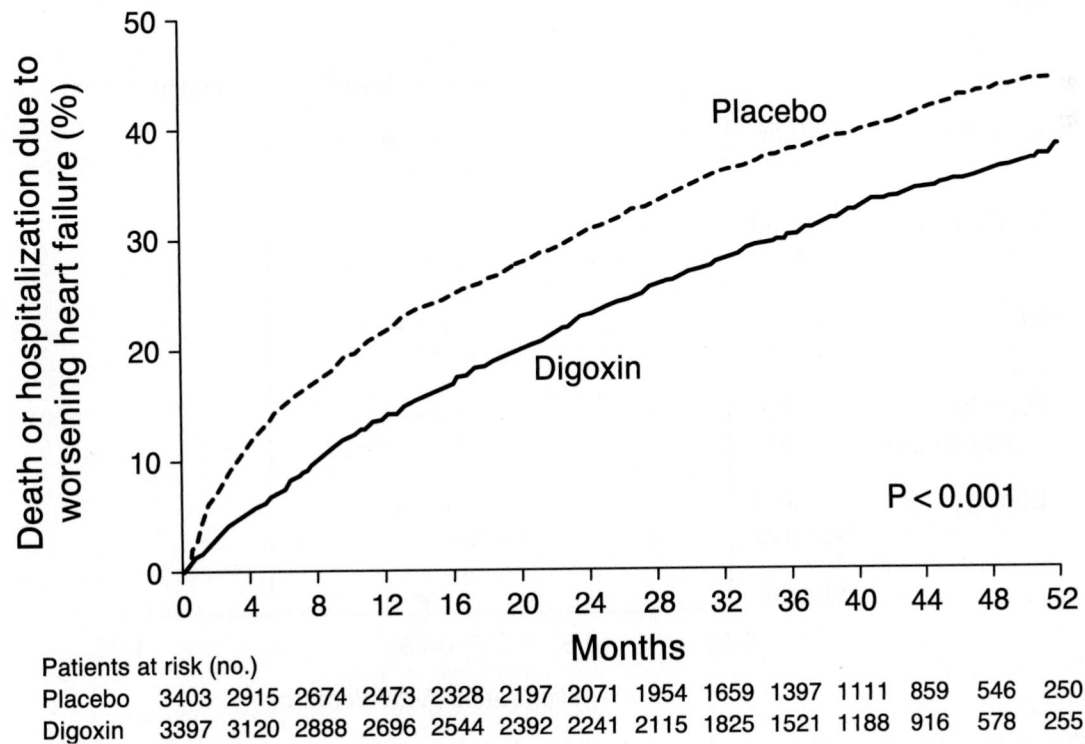

Patients at risk (no.)

Placebo	3403	2915	2674	2473	2328	2197	2071	1954	1659	1397	1111	859	546	250
Digoxin	3397	3120	2888	2696	2544	2392	2241	2115	1825	1521	1188	916	578	255

B

Fig. 4. *A*, Mortality and *B*, incidence of death or hospitalization due to worsening heart failure in the digoxin and placebo groups. The number of patients at risk at each four-month interval is shown below the figure.

Table 4. Major Manifestations of Digitalis Toxicity

Cardiac (vagal and direct effects)
    Sinoatrial node—sinus bradycardia, sinoatrial arrest or exit block
    Atrium—paroxysmal atrial tachycardia, vagally induced atrial fibrillation
    Atrioventricular node—Wenckebach, 2° and 3° AV block, junctional rhythm
    His-Purkinje system—Junctional ectopy, escape or accelerated rhythm, nonparoxysmal junctional tachycardia
    Ventricle—Premature beats (bigeminy or trigeminy, unifocal or multifocal), fascicular or bidirectional ventricular tachycardia
Gastrointestinal
    Anorexia, nausea, vomiting (50%-80% of patients) (chemoreceptors in the area postrema of the medulla)
    Vasoconstrictive effect (mesenteric ischemia)
Central nervous system
    Headeache, fatigue, malaise, neuralgic pain, agitation/anxiety, disorientation, confusion, delirium, and seizures
Visual symptoms
    Scotomas, flickering, halos, change in color perception (yellow/green vision)
Other
    Allergic skin reactions
    Gynecomastia in men
    Sexual dysfunction

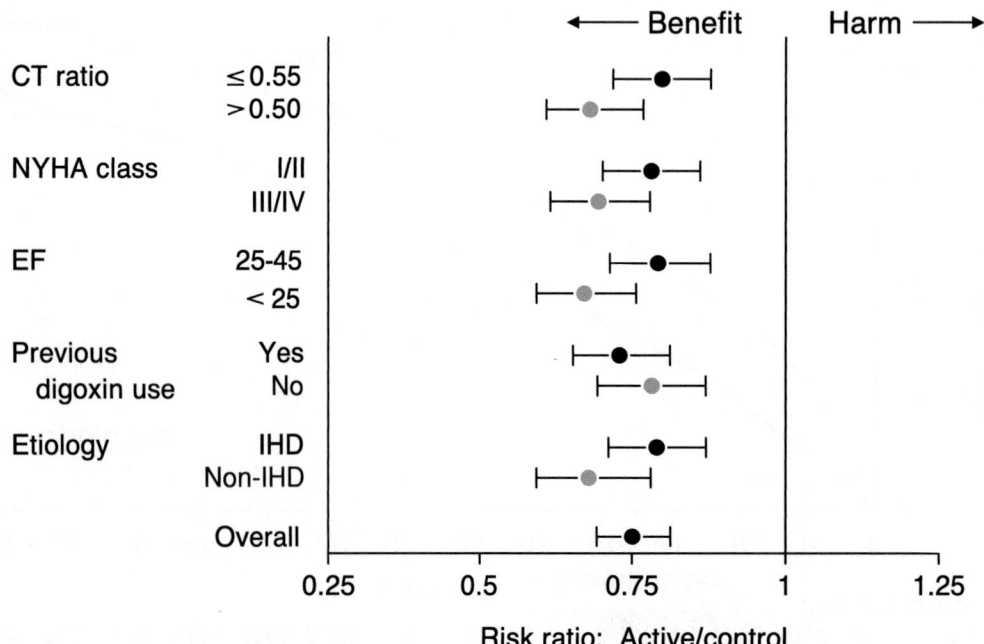

Fig. 5. The effect of digoxin on CHF mortality or related hospitalization: subgroup analysis of the DIG trial. Patients with ejection fraction below 25%, non-ischemic CHF, cardiomegaly on chest X-ray (Cardiothoracic ratio (CT) above 0.55), and NYHA class III/IV symptoms appeared to derive the most benefit from digoxin therapy.

Table 5. Factors Altering Mocardial Sensitivity
to Digoxin Effects

Hypokalemia, hypomagnesemia (diuretic use, gastrointestinal disease, diabetes mellitus, nutritional status, congestive heart failure with prolonged
secondary aldosteronism)

Hypercalcemia (thiazide)

Acid-base imbalance

Acute hypoxemia (enhanced digitalis sensitivity)

Chronic lung disease (hypoxia, hypercapnia,
acidosis, sympathetic activation)

Renal insufficiency

Hypothyroidism or hyperthyroidism

Low lean body mass (decreased binding to skeletal muscle)

Enhanced sympathetic tone (Ca^{2+} loading, afterdepolarization)

Enhanced vagal tone (bradyarrhythmias, pauses,
heart block)

Drugs with negative chronotropic and dromotropic properties (class II, IV, amiodarone)

Type and severity of underlying cardiac disease
(sinus node disease, atrioventricular conduction
disease, amyloidosis [binding], rheumatic or viral
myocarditis, immediately post-myocardial
infarction?)

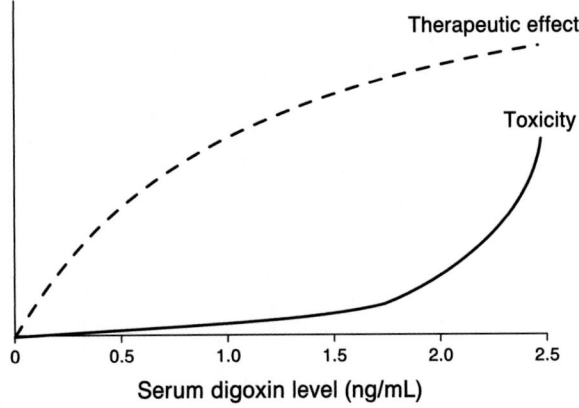

Fig. 6. Relationship between the therapeutic and toxic
effects of digoxin and the serum digoxin level. Above a
level of 1.5 ng/ml, there are minimal additional therapeutic effects and a substantial increase in the frequency
of toxicity.

cardioversion for atrial fibrillation should be delayed. If
urgent cardioversion is required, the energy level should
be minimized.

Management of digoxin toxicity is summarized in
Table 6. The key to successful treatment is early recognition of digoxin intoxication. For mild manifestations,
such as gastrointestinal symptoms or "benign" dysrhythmia (such as occasional ectopy, excessive slowing
of conduction in the AV node with atrial fibrillation),
temporary withdrawal of digoxin and ECG monitoring
is sufficient. In severe bradycardia or heart block associated
with hemodynamic impairment, atropine or temporary
ventricular pacing may be needed. For frequent ectopic
atrial, junctional, or ventricular rhythms, potassium and
magnesium supplementation is often helpful, especially
if hypokalemia is present.

Digoxin-specific antiserum (Digibind) can rapidly
reverse potentially life-threatening digoxin toxicity
manifesting as heart block, hyperkalemia, or ventricular
arrhythmias. The digoxin-specific Fab fragments are
administered intravenously and have a rapid onset of
action, large volume of distribution, and rapid clearance.
Doses of Fab are calculated using a formula based on
either the total body digoxin burden or the estimated
dose of drug ingested and are given intravenously in
saline over 30 to 60 minutes. Serum levels of digoxin
remain abnormal after Fab fragment administration
and are not useful clinically to monitor recovery from
toxicity. Hemodialysis is ineffective in the treatment of

Table 6. Digitalis Toxicity: Poor Prognostic
Factors

Advanced age

Male gender

Initial hyperkalemia (degree of NA$^+$-K$^+$-ATPase
poisoning)

Underlying heart disease (cardiomyopathy,
conduction disease)

Advanced AV block

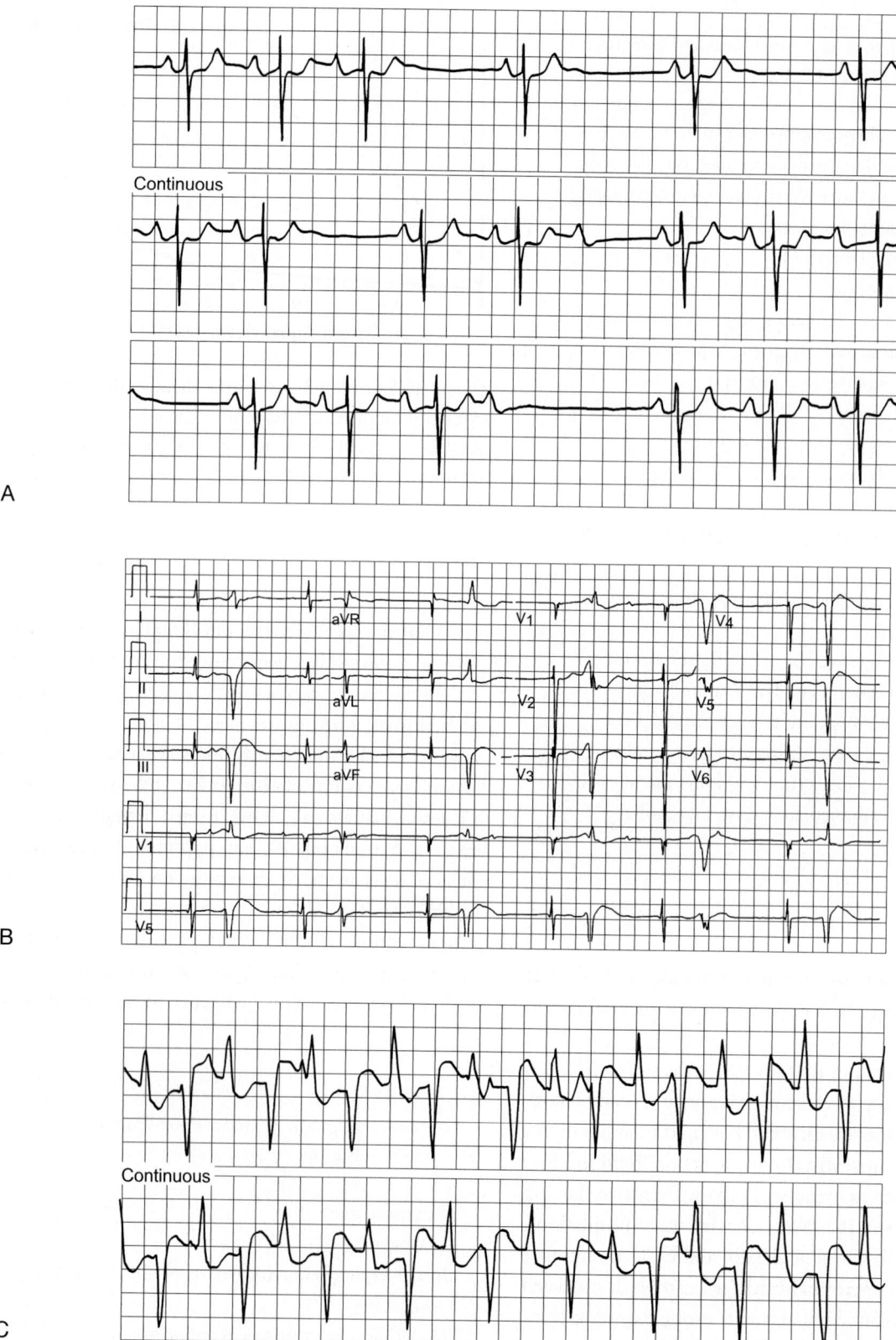

Fig. 7. Cardiac rhythm abnormalities due to digitalis toxicity. *A,* Second degree sinoatrial block and Mobitz I second degree AV block. *B,* Complete AV block, junctional rhythm and premature ventricular complexes *C,* Bidirectional ventricular tachycardia.

digoxin toxicity because of the large volume of distribution of digoxin.

■ Hemodialysis is ineffective in the treatment of digoxin toxicity because of the large volume of distribution of digoxin.

■ Serum digoxin measurement is not an accurate reflection of digoxin toxicity after Digibind administration.

Contraindications to Digoxin Use

1. Digoxin should not be used in patients with Wolff-Parkinson-White syndrome and atrial fibrillation because it may accelerate anterograde conduction over the accessory pathway and precipitate ventricular fibrillation.
2. In patients with hypertrophic obstructive cardiomyopathy, digoxin should not be used because the inotropic effect may worsen the outflow gradient.
3. Digoxin should be used cautiously in all conditions that increase digoxin sensitivity (summarized in Table 4).
4. In patients with preexisting sinus node dysfunction and conduction disease, slowing of the heart rate and symptomatic pauses may occur, causing hemodynamic compromise. Ventricular regularization with atrial fibrillation in a patient taking digoxin suggests toxicity, with AV block and junctional rhythm.

5. In patients with high-output states, such as chronic cor pulmonale or thyrotoxicosis.

Drug Interactions

Antiarrhythmics and other drugs affecting digoxin concentration are summarized in Table 7. Antacids, cholestyramine, metoclopramide, prednisone, and sulfasalazine decrease the serum concentration of digoxin, whereas propafenone, flecainide, amiodarone, quinidine, verapamil, benzodiazepines, spironolactone, and ACE inhibitors may increase the concentration. Several drugs (Table 7) increase plasma digoxin concentration by decreasing its elimination through inhibition of P-glycoprotein, an energy-dependent drug efflux transporter in the intestine and the kidney, thus potentiating toxicity. Patients taking medications that decrease the absorption of digoxin could also develop digoxin toxicity when the concurrent treatment is stopped.

Dosing

Digoxin may be given in daily dose of 0.25 mg or lower (0.125 mg daily or every other day) in those with reduced renal function, lean body mass, elderly or with baseline conduction abnormalities. Steady state levels are reached in approximately 1 week in those with normal renal function and 2 to 3 weeks in those with renal impairment. Dosing is guided by efficacy, tolerance, and serum concentration (goal: 0.6 to 1.0 ng/ml) that should be measured 6 to 8 hours after the last oral dose.

Table 7.   Management of Digitalis Toxicity

Early recognition and withdrawal of digoxin
Correction of underlying abnormalities (electrolytes, hypoxemia)
Electrocardiographic monitoring and treatment of
    Symptomatic bradycardia
        Atropine or temporary pacemaker (with hyperkalemia, failure to capture may occur)
        Digoxin-specific Fab antibody
    Unstable supraventricular tachycardia
        DC shock (low energy; risk of asystole or ventricular arrhythmias is present)
    Ventricular arrhythmias
        Digoxin-specific Fab antibody (watch for K^+, may need to supplement)
        Lidocaine, phenytoin, propranolol
Subsequent adjustment of dosage schedule to prevent recurrences (goal serum level, ~1.0 ng/mL > 6 hours after last dose)

The serum levels are helpful in the evaluation of toxicity and not the efficacy of the drug.

The sensitivity of the patient to digoxin effect may be altered by various factors (Table 4), and clinical judgment should be used to reduce the dose if toxicity is suspected despite apparent "therapeutic serum digoxin levels." The value of regularly determining the serum level of digoxin is uncertain, but it is probably reasonable to check the level once yearly after a steady state has been achieved. Possible interactions with digoxin should be considered whenever treatment is started with a new medication that interacts with digoxin, and the serum level of digoxin should be measured approximately 1 week after the addition of the new drug.

■ Digoxin toxicity may occur despite therapeutic serum levels.

106

Principles of Inotropic Drugs

Garvan C. Kane, MD

Joseph G. Murphy, MD

Arshad Jahangir, MD

Most intravenous inotropic agents work to increase intracellular cyclic adenosine monophosphate (cAMP) which in turn increases intracellular Ca^{2+} which then interacts directly with the myofibril contractile mechanism. Other emerging mechanisms of inotropic action include sensitizing contractile elements to intracellular calcium. An increase in intracellular cAMP is achieved either through the stimulation of adrenergic (isoproterenol, epinephrine, norepinephrine and dobutamine) or dopaminergic receptors (dopamine) or the inhibition of cAMP breakdown by the inhibition of phosphodiesterase III enzyme (PDE III; e.g. milrinone). Blood pressure may be increased through either inotropic- or chronotropic-mediated increases in cardiac output or by α-adrenergic mediated peripheral vasoconstriction. Vasopressors include norepinephrine, phenylephrine and high-dose dopamine. All currently available intravenous inotropic agents exhibit tachyphylaxis (a rapidly decreasing response to a drug following administration of the initial doses).

- β_1 Receptors in atria, ventricles, and AV node are responsible for the positive inotropic and chronotropic effects on the heart.
- β_2 Receptors in arteries, arterioles, veins, and bronchioles are responsible for peripheral vasodilatation.
- α_1 Receptors in arterioles mediate vasoconstriction.
- α_2 Receptors inhibit norepinephrine release from sympathetic nerve endings.
- Dopaminergic DA_1 receptors are present in the renal and mesenteric vascular beds and promote vasodilatation and natriuresis.

Isoproterenol

Isoproterenol is a pure β_1-receptor stimulant ($\beta_1 > \beta_2$). It has strong positive inotropic and chronotropic effects (β_1 effects) with weak vasodilator properties (β_2 effect). It has no effect on α- or dopaminergic receptors. The usual starting dose is 0.5 μg/min, increasing to 5 μg/min, depending on the hemodynamic and heart rate response. Isoproterenol may exacerbate myocardial ischemia. It increase heart rate and is proarrhythmogenic. Isoproterenol is primarily used to stimulate myocardial contraction after heart surgery and to provoke arrhythmias during electrophysiologic study or as treatment for β-blocker overdose (Table 1).

- Isoproterenol is a pure β_1-receptor stimulant.

Table 1.   Summary of the Properties of Common Adrenergic Inotropic Agents

Agent	Contractility	Heart rate	Vascular effect	Arrhythmias
Isoproterenol ($\beta_1 > \beta_2$)	+++	+++	Vasodilatation (+)	+++
Epinephrine ($\beta_1 = \beta_2 > \alpha$)	++	++	Vasoconstriction (+)	+++
Norepinephrine ($\beta_1 > \alpha > \beta_2$)	+	+	Vasoconstriction (++)	+
Phenylephrine (α)	–	–	Vasoconstriction (+++)	–
Dopamine (β_1, α, dopamine)	++	+	Vasoconstriction (++)	++
Dobutamine ($\beta_1 > \beta_2 > \alpha$)	++	+	Vasodilatation (+)	+

EPINEPHRINE

Epinephrine at a high dose stimulates β_1, β_2, and α receptors. It is used primarily in the setting of cardiac arrest or anaphylaxis, because of its powerful inotropic and chronotropic effects in combination with a vasoconstrictor effect to increase blood pressure. The usual dose in the case of cardiac arrest is 1 mg intravenous bolus every 3 to 5 minutes. The intravenous dose in acute shock is 0.1 to 0.4 µg/kg/min. Doses exceeding about 0.2 µg/kg per minute decrease renal blood flow, gastrointestinal motility, and splanchnic vascular bed perfusion. Epinephrine also increases conduction velocity in the myocardium and increases ectopic pacemaker activity.

■ Epinephrine at a high dose stimulates β_1, β_2, and α receptors.

NOREPINEPHRINE

Norepinephrine is an endogenous catecholamine that lacks the vasodilator β_2-receptor effects of epinephrine but has stronger α-receptor stimulating effects. Thus, it is a potent vasoconstrictor with fewer inotropic and chronotropic effects than isoproterenol or epinephrine. It is used primarily to increase arterial blood pressure in severe hypotension especially in the setting of septic shock accompanied by abnormal vasodilatation. The intravenous dose is 2 to 20 µg/min. Norepinephrine produces mesenteric vascular bed vasoconstriction which can induce splanchnic ischemia and facilitate bacterial translocation from the gut resulting in septicemia.

■ Norepinephrine primarily stimulates α receptors.

PHENYLEPHRINE

Phenylephrine is a synthetic catecholamine which, as a pure α-agonist, causes predominantly peripheral vasoconstriction. It is used primarily in septic shock or anesthetic-induced hypotension. It is rarely used in the cardiac intensive care setting apart from situations such as the combination of hypotension and dynamic left ventricular outflow tract obstruction (e.g. hypertrophic cardiomyopathy with ventricular outflow obstruction). A typical dose would be 0.1-0.5 mg bolus with a maintenance rate of 50-100 µg/min. Peripheral vasoconstriction achieved with these vasopressor agents may negatively affect the absorption of drugs, such as insulin or heparin, administered subcutaneously (Table 2).

■ Phenylephrine stimulates α receptors.

VASOPRESSIN

Vasopressin is an analogue of antidiuretic hormone that has vasopressor actions particularly useful in patients with a vasodilatory shock such as sepsis where typically it is administered at an intravenous rate of 0.04 units/min. In the setting of cardiac arrest a 40 IU intravenous or endotracheal dose may be administered in lieu of epinephrine. As with other pressor agents clinically important vasoconstriction of tissue beds including the coronary bed may occur.

Table 2. Relative Receptor Agonist Activity of the Sympathomimetic Agents

	Receptor Type				
	Alpha-1	Alpha-2	Beta-1	Beta-2	Dopamine
Norepinephrine	+++	+++	++	None	None
Epinephrine					None
Low dose			++	+++	
Moderate dose	+		+++	+++	
High dose	+++	+++	+++	+++	None
Dobutamine	+	None	+++	+	None
Dopamine		None		None	
Low dose					+++
Moderate dose			+++		
High dose	+++				
Isoproterenol	None	None	+++	+++	None
Ephedrine (indirect effects via norepinephrine release)	+++	+++	++	None	None
Phenylephrine	+++	None	None	None	None

■ Vasopressin has vasopressor actions and is commonly used in septic shock.

NITRIC OXIDE SYNTHASE INHIBITORS

There is mounting evidence on a pathogenic role for excessive nitric oxide in a variety of shock states and studies with inhibitors of nitric oxide synthase in septic or cardiogenic shock are underway. Preliminary data are mixed with regard to hemodynamic benefit and overall survival.

DOPAMINE

Dopamine is an endogenous catecholamine-like agent that is administered intravenously in the treatment of severe heart failure, hypotension, and cardiogenic shock. The pharmacodynamic actions of dopamine differ with escalating dose. At a low dose (2 μg/kg/min) dopamine has weak tissue-specific vasodilatory actions on DA_1 receptors which may include an increase in renal blood flow aiding diuresis. Dopamine is frequently used when renal blood flow is impaired in severe congestive heart failure although there is no good evidence that "renal-dose" dopamine preserves renal function or promotes significant natriuresis, although it is frequently used for this indication. At intermediate doses (2-8 μg/kg/min) dopamine enhances norepinephrine release from sympathetic neurons, resulting in increased β-adrenergic receptor activation in the heart. A maximal inotropic response is probably observed at 5 μg/kg/min. With increasing doses, particularly at doses greater than 8 μg/kg/min, dopamine acts predominantly on α-receptors to stimulate peripheral vasoconstriction, giving a predominant vasopressor action. Compared with dobutamine (see below), dopamine induces tachycardia and ventricular arrhythmia to a greater degree. Dopamine is the favored inotropic agent in patient with hypotension including shock from any cause who requires both a vasopressor effect (high-dose α-effect) and an increase in cardiac output: tachycardia or propensity to ventricular arrhythmias are relative contraindications to dopamine usage. Dobutamine is the preferred inotropic drug following myocardial infarction when a pure inotropic effect is desired in the absence of a vasoconstrictor response. Dopamine is contraindicated in patients taking monoamine oxidase inhibitors and in those with a significant ventricular arrhythmia, hypertrophic cardiomyopathy, severe aortic stenosis, or pheochromocytoma. Should dopamine or other vasopressors extravasate, they can cause severe tissue necrosis. Hence they are best administered through a central catheter. Should extravasation occur, local treatment with subcutaneous administration of phentolamine is warranted.

- <2 μg/kg/min - vasodilator effect
- 2 to 8 μg/kg/min - adrenergic effect
- > 8 μg/kg/min - vasoconstrictor effect

DOBUTAMINE

Dobutamine is a sympathomimetic that stimulates both β_1 and β_2 adrenergic receptors but has little action on α-adrenergic receptors. The predominant action of dobutamine is a positive inotropic effect (β_1) with some vasodilatation (β_2). Hence, dobutamine increases cardiac output, heart rate and reduces left ventricular end-diastolic filling pressures. Dobutamine does not stimulate dopaminergic receptors and therefore has no selective effects on renal blood flow. Dobutamine does not typically increase myocardial infarct size or cause significant ventricular arrhythmias. Due to the reductions on afterload, dobutamine is preferred to dopamine for most patients in heart failure requiring an inotropic agent. Infusions are initiated at 2 μg/kg/min and titrated up according to the hemodynamic response of the patient (the usual maximal dose is 20 μg/kg/min). If hypotension occurs, a modest dose of dopamine is often co-administered with dobutamine. Dobutamine can be administered as a continuous chronic infusion through a peripheral indwelling central catheter to outpatients with end-stage heart failure. There is no data however that demonstrates a survival benefit from this strategy, in fact there is evidence to suggest an increased long-term mortality. In addition to its therapeutic use as an inotrope, dobutamine is commonly utilized as a pharmacologic stress agent.

- Dobutamine stimulates both β_1 and β_2 receptors.

MILRINONE

- Through the inhibition of the cAMP PDE III enzyme, responsible for the breakdown of cAMP in cardiac and vascular smooth muscle, milrinone increases cardiac contractility and induces peripheral arterial and venous vasodilatation, with little if any effect on heart rate. Milrinone increase ventricular inotropy independent of the action on adrenergic receptors. Like dobutamine, milrinone is indicated for the hemodynamic support of patients with advanced heart failure and provides the inotropic effect irrespective of the use of β-blockers. It may also be used chronically in select outpatients but while having beneficial effects on hemodynamics, may increase long term mortality. Milrinone is started with a typical loading dose of 50 μg/kg over 10 minutes and an infusion rate from 0.25 to 10 μg/kg/min. Two randomized trials of milrinone in chronic heart failure (Milrinone-Digoxin Trial, and OPTIME-CHF Trial) did not show any mortality benefit and there was an increased incidence of arrhythmias in the milrinone treatment arms. The use of milrinone in patients with heart failure protected against arrhythmic death by implantable defibrillators has not been tested.

CALCIUM SENSITIZERS

All currently approved intravenous inotropic agents increase intracellular calcium and are associated with a risk of calcium-induced arrhythmia. Newer "calcium sensitizing" agents have the potential to increase myocardial contractility without the detrimental effects of excess intracellular calcium. Levosimendan is an inotropic agent in clinical use in Europe but not approved as yet in the United States. Levosimendan sensitizes troponin C to intracellular calcium and in addition causes peripheral and coronary vasodilatation through activation of vascular ATP-sensitive K^+ channels with no impairment of myocardial relaxation. Levosimendan has less arrhythmia potential than dobutamine with less mortality in chronically treated patients with severe left ventricular failure (LIDO study).

107

NITRATE THERAPIES

Garvan C. Kane, MD

Peter A. Brady, MD

NITRATE PHARMACOLOGY

Nitrates relax vascular smooth muscle in veins, larger arterioles and arteries through an endothelial dependent pathway. The proposed mechanism involves conversion of administered nitrate to nitric oxide (NO) at or near the plasma membrane (Fig. 1). In turn, NO activates guanylate cyclase to produce cyclic guanosine monophosphate (cGMP). Intracellular accumulation of cGMP causes vasodilation. This mechanism is similar to the vasodilation induced by sodium nitroprusside and endogenous endothelial-derived NO.

The primary effect of nitrates in ischemia is a reduction in the myocardial oxygen demand through their venodilatory effect which reduces preload and end-diastolic volume, thus decreasing myocardial wall tension. In addition, the actions of intracoronary, intravenous, and sublingual nitrates to dilate epicardial coronary arteries and arterioles greater than 100 µm, increases blood flow from the epicardial to the endocardial regions and relieves coronary spasm, leading to better perfusion of ischemic myocardium. These direct effects on the coronary arterial circulation are most beneficial in patients with vasospastic syndromes.

Organic nitrates are prodrugs and, thus, must undergo a biotransformation before they can have a therapeutic effect. Nitrates are rapidly absorbed from the skin, mucous membranes, and gastrointestinal tract.

Both nitroglycerin and isosorbide dinitrate undergo extensive first-pass liver metabolism when taken orally. Liver and intravascular metabolism of nitroglycerin and isosorbide dinitrate yield biologically active dinitrate metabolites with half-lives longer than those of the drug. Isosorbide-5-mononitrate does not undergo first-pass metabolism and is almost 100% bioavailable.

CLINICAL INDICATIONS OF NITRATE THERAPY

Acute Coronary Syndrome

Sublingual nitroglycerin is the recommended initial treatment for patients presenting to the emergency room with a suspected acute coronary syndrome. Sublingual nitroglycerin 0.4 mg should be administered every five minutes as needed. In the absence of relief after a third dose, an intravenous infusion should be administered at an initial dose of 5 to 10 µg/min. The typical blood pressure goal is up to a 30% reduction in systolic pressure, avoiding hypotension. Excessive reduction of blood pressure may lead to detrimental reflexive increases in heart rate and cardiac contractility. Acute tolerance to nitrate therapy will develop within 24 hours: however this can be temporally overcome with escalation of the dose. The use of systemic nitrates are a class I indication in the relief of persistent ischemic

1249

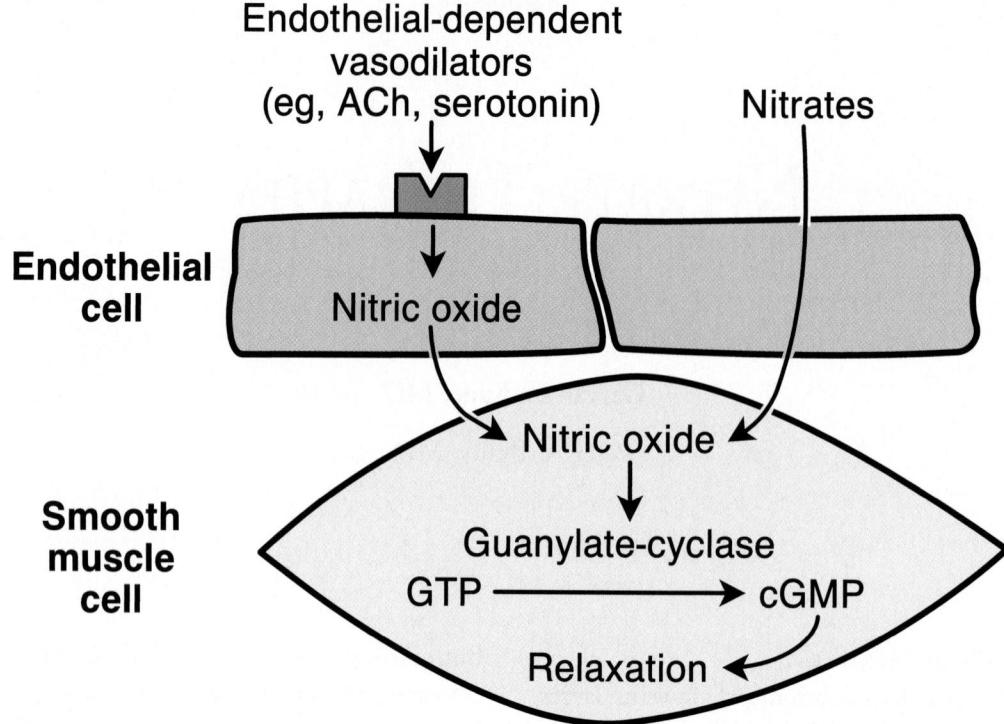

Fig. 1. Mechanism of action of nitrates on vascular smooth muscle cells. ACh, acetylcholine; GTP, guanosine triphosphate.

symptoms, left ventricular failure and in aiding blood pressure control: however have little proven benefit in affecting mortality in patients with an acute coronary syndrome.

In patients with acute infarction and decreased left ventricular function, nitrates appear to limit infarct size and to favorably alter ventricular remodeling. However, these benefits are lost after drug treatment is discontinued. Nitrates do have antiplatelet activity, although the clinical significance of this is unclear. Nitrates appear to have little if any effect on long-term mortality after myocardial infarction. Pooled data from several randomized trials conducted in the prethrombolytic era suggested that intravenous nitroglycerin, given within 24 hours after the onset of symptoms, reduced mortality. However 2 thrombolytic trials, ISIS-4 (with oral mononitrate, Imdur 60 mg) and GISSI-3 (with transdermal nitrates), found no benefit of nitrates over placebo, on either survival or left ventricular function, in patients with an acute infarction (over 70% of whom received thrombolytics). It must be noted that in these trials however, between 50% and 60% of the placebo

groups received non-protocol nitrate therapies.

Left Ventricular Failure
Predominantly by their venodilatory effect, nitrates act acutely to decrease left ventricular filling pressure. They will also lead to potent reduction in afterload in patients who are volume overloaded. Hence they are a first line treatment in normotensive or hypertensive patients in acute left ventricular failure. While the sublingual, oral, and transdermal routes maybe effective acutely the intravenous route allows fast, effective, and easily titratable responses. In patients with chronic congestive heart failure the combination of hydralazine with oral nitrate therapy has proven mortality benefit (although less than that observed with angiotensin converting enzyme inhibitors). These mortality benefits may be even greater in African-American heart failure populations (Table 1).

Nitrate Tolerance
Tolerance or tachyphylaxis, one of the major limitations to nitrate use, can be defined as a loss of the hemodynamic

Table 1. Side Effects, Contraindications and Drug Interactions of Nitrates

Side effects of nitrate use

Headache, nausea	Related to vasodilation
Orthostatic hypotension	More commmon in elderly or with concomitant vasodilator use
Tachycardia	Reflex response to drop in blood pressure
Methemoglobinemia	Nitrate ions oxidize hemoglobin to methemoglobin – seen with prolonged use of sodium nitroprusside
Hypoxia	Patients with severe lung disease may suffer worsening ventilation/perfusion mismatch and hypoxia due to vasodilation

Contraindications to nitrate use

Hypotension	Use with systolic blood pressures <90 mm Hg or >30 mm Hg below baseline will exacerbate ischemia
Hypertrophic cardiomyopathy	May exacerbate or induce a symptomatic outflow tract obstruction
Severe mitral or aortic stenosis	Risk of hypotension and cardiovascular collapse
Right ventricular infarction	Increased risk for hypotension
Potential for drug interactions	See below

Drug interactions with nitrates

Alteplase (tPA)	Decrease efficacy with concurrent i.v. nitroglycerin
Ethanol	Exaggerates hypotensive effects of nitrates
Heparin	Decreased efficacy with concurrent dosese of i.v. nitroglycerin >300 μg/min
Phospodiesterase inhibitors	Profound exaggeration of hypotensive effects of nitrates (avoid concomitant use of nitrates with sildenafil, tadalafil or vardenafil)

nitrate effect with sustained use. This is typically noted as a loss of the antianginal or blood pressure lowering effects or headache. The mechanism of the tolerance phenomenon is unknown but is not related to altered pharmacokinetics. Tolerance is best prevented by allowing a nitrate free window of 12-14 hours. This is typically done at night. Some patients however are highly dependent on nitrates and experience a nitrate rebound on nitrate withdrawal.

Sodium Nitroprusside

Nitroprusside is a potent, fast-acting arterial and venous vasodilator. Given as a continuous intravenous infusion, nitroprusside acts as an NO donor. It remains a first-line agent in the management of hypertensive emergencies, aortic dissection (given with adequate beta-blockade) and left ventricular heart failure with preserved arterial pressure. However, nitroprusside is light-sensitive, requires careful hemodynamic monitoring, and has a short shelf-life. Moreover it carries the risk of both methemoglobinemia and potentially lethal cyanide toxicity when given in high doses or even at low doses for more than a few days. The usual starting dose is 0.5 μg/min. Infusion rates over 2.5 μg/min should be kept short as the risk of cyanide toxicity is high. The maximal dose of 10 μg/min should be limited to no more than 10 minutes of therapy. The hemodynamic and adverse effects of sodium nitroprusside are similar to those seen with intravenous nitroglycerin. In addition vigilance for the signs of cyanide toxicity such as nausea, vomiting, and central nervous system disturbances is essential. If suspected, nitroprusside should be stopped and sodium nitrite 3% solution should be given (Table 2).

Table 2. Commonly Used Nitrate Preparations

Drug	Usual dose	Duration of action	Comments
Short-acting nitrates			
Amyl nitrite (inhilation)	2-5 mg	1-5 min	Diagnostic use for LVOT obstruction
Nitroglycerin tablet (sublingual)	0.3-0.6 mg	10-30 min	Light, heat sensitive, last 3-6 months
Nitroglycerin spray (sublingual)	0.4 mg	10-30 min	More stable, last 2-3 yrs
Isosorbide dinitrate tablet (sublingual)	2.5-5 mg	10-60 min	Provides more sustained prophylaxis
Nitroglycerin, intravenous	5-200 μg/min	mins	Rapid tolerance. Limit use to 48 hr
Long-acting nitrates			
Nitroglycerin, 2% ointment	1-1.5 inch/4 hr	3-6 hr	Care needed to avoid buccal absorption
Nitroglycerin, slow-release patch	0.2-0.8 mg/hr	8-10 hr	Remove for 12-14 hr to avoid tolerance
Isosorbide dinitrate, oral tablet	10-60 mg/4-6 hr	4-6 hr	Careful timing to avoid tolerance
Isosorbide dinitrate, chewable tablet	5-10 mg/2-4 hr	2-3 hr	Provides more sustained prophylasis
Isosorbide mononitrate, oral tablet	20-60 mg/12 hr	6-8 hr	Typically dose at 8 am & 3 pm to avoid tolerance
Isosorbide mononitrate XL, oral tablet	30-120 mg/24 hr	12 hr	Convenient

108

CALCIUM CHANNEL BLOCKERS

Arshad Jahangir, MD

Calcium channel blockers are potent vasodilators with antihypertensive, antianginal, and antiarrhythmic effects. All clinically available calcium channel blockers inhibit the L-type voltage-gated calcium channel, which results in relaxation of vascular smooth muscle and negative inotropic and chronotropic effects in the heart. Mibefradil, a calcium channel blocker that has been withdrawn from the market, blocks both L-type and T-type calcium channels with a greater selectivity for the T-type channels.

PHARMACOLOGY

Calcium channel blockers are a heterogeneous group of drugs that can be chemically classified into dihydropyridine (DHP) and nonDHPs. DHP exhibits greater selectivity for vascular smooth muscle whereas the non-DHPs have additional inhibitory effects on sinoatrial and atrioventricular node. Examples of calcium channel blockers include:

Dihydropyridines
    nifedipine, amlodipine, felodipine, isradipine,
      nicardipine, nisoldipine, nimodipine
Non-dihydropyridines
    Phenylalkylamine
      Verapamil
    Benzothiazepine

    Diltiazem
    Diarylaminopropylamine
      Bepridil

The pharmacokinetic properties of most common calcium channel blockers are summarized in Table 1. Most clinically used calcium channel blockers are absorbed completely after oral administration but have high first-pass liver metabolism that reduces their bioavailability (Table 1). The time to peak concentration and plasma half-life is short, except for newer generation calcium channel blockers, such as amlodipine which has a prolonged effect with a plasma half-life of 35 to 50 hours. Most of these agents are bound extensively to plasma proteins. Metabolites of diltiazem and verapamil are also biologically active and have additional ion channel blocking properties. Plasma drug concentrations are not routinely measured during therapy.

■ All clinically available calcium channel blockers block the L-type voltage-gated calcium channels.

Pharmacodynamics

Mechanisms of Action
Calcium Channel blockers bind in a voltage-dependent manner to specific receptors on the α_1 subunit of the L-type Ca^{2+} channels on cardiac myocytes and vascular smooth muscle cells (Fig. 1). This results in marked

Table 1.　Pharmacokinetics of Oral Calcium Channel Blockers

	Bioavailability (%)	Protein binding (%)	Onset of action after oral intake (hours)	Time to peak concentration (hours)	Plasma half-life (hours)	Route of major elimination
Verapamil	20-35	90	1	1-2	5-12	Renal, hepatic
Diltiazem	40-65	80	1	1-3	5-7	Hepatic
Amlodipine	65-90	97	1-2	6-12	35-50	Hepatic
Felodipine	15-20	99	1-2	2-5	11-16	Hepatic, renal
Isradipine	15-25	95	0.5	1-2	8	Hepatic, renal
Nicardipine	35	95	0.5	1-2	9	Hepatic, renal
Nifedipine (SR)	45-70	95	0.5	2-6	6-11	Hepatic
Nimodipine	13	95		1	8-9	Hepatic
Bepridil	60	99	2-3	8	24-60	Hepatic

reduction in calcium influx into the cells, leading to decreased excitability and contractility. This causes four effects (Fig. 2):

- Vascular smooth muscle relaxation.
- Decreased myocardial contractility.
- Reduced sinoatrial node automaticity.
- Reduced atrioventricular node conductivity.

Under physiologic conditions calcium channel blockers belonging to the DHP group are more selective for vascular smooth muscle cells and are potent vasodilators with less cardiac depressant and electrophysiologic effects than verapamil or diltiazem (Table 2). However, in the presence of myocardial disease and/or β-adrenergic blockers, DHP can also have significant cardiac depressant effects. Short-acting DHPs are potent vasodilators that can abruptly decrease blood pressure causing reflex adrenergic activation and sinus tachycardia. Verapamil and diltiazem, on the other hand have depressant effects on cardiac nodal tissue and myocardium, thus decreasing the sinus rate, AV nodal conduction (prolonging PR and AH interval on electrogram) and myocardial contractility (Table 2).

- Calcium channel blockers bind to specific receptors on the voltage-gated calcium channels in a voltage-dependent manner and results in marked reduction

in calcium influx into the cells, leading to decreased excitability and contractility.

Clinical Use in Cardiovascular Medicine (Table 3)

Ischemic Heart Disease

Effort and Vasospastic Angina
All calcium channel blockers are potent coronary vasodilators and inhibit exercise-induced coronary vasoconstriction. In addition, verapamil and diltiazem decrease myocardial oxygen requirement by reducing myocardial contractility, heart rate, cardiac after-load and ventricular wall stress. Slowing of the heart rate also increases diastolic coronary blood flow thus limiting myocardial ischemia. Heart rate slowing calcium channel blockers are effective in the treatment of exertional or exercise-induced angina decreasing the number of anginal attacks and exercise-induced ST-segment depression.

In Prinzmetal or vasospastic angina, DHP calcium channel blockers are especially effective in relieving and preventing coronary artery spasm and angina symptoms. However, in patients with fixed atherosclerotic narrowing of coronary arteries, these short acting DHPs may aggravate myocardial ischemia due to reflex adrenergic activation that increases heart rate and cardiac workload and therefore, should be avoided unless concomitantly given with a β-blocker. Amlodipine,

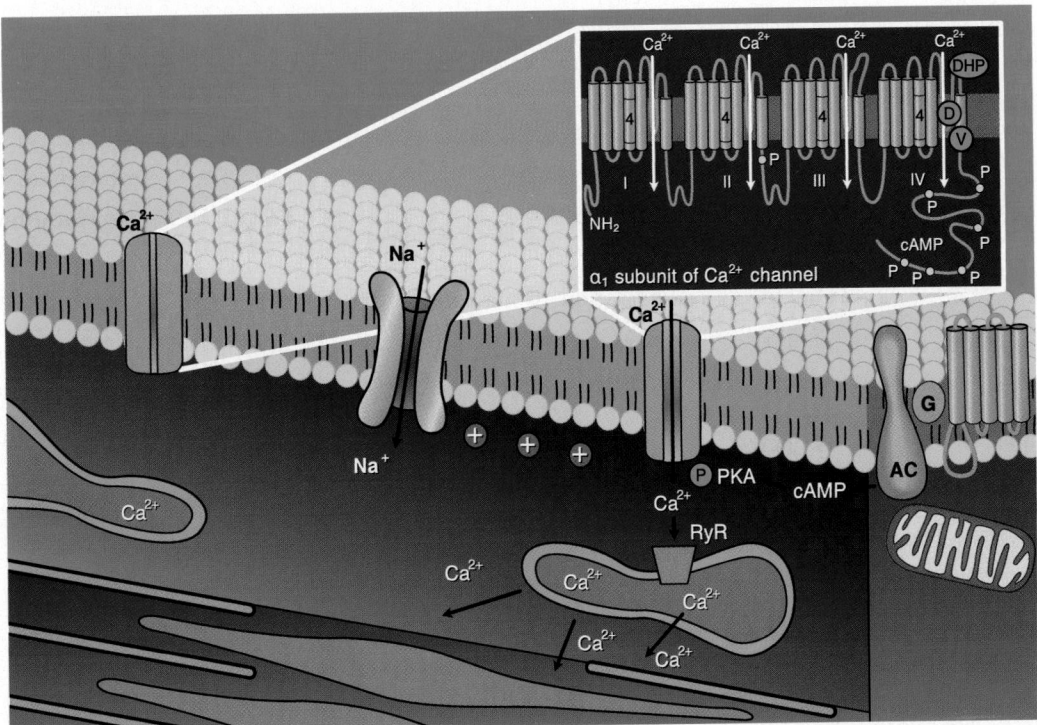

Fig. 1. Proposed molecular model of voltage-gated L-type calcium channel α_1-subunit with binding sites for dihydropyridines (N), diltiazem (D) and verapamil (V). Calcium ions enter through the pore region between segments 5 and 6 of each of the four (I to IV) transmembrane domains of the α_1-subunit. β-Adrenergic stimulation activates adenylate cyclase (AC) through stimulatory G protein (G) resulting in increased production of cyclic adenosine monophosphate (cAMP). This in turn activates protein kinases (PKA) leading to phosphorylation (P) of calcium channel, increased probability of channel opening and calcium (Ca^{2+}) entry into the cell that promotes calcium-induced calcium release from the sarcoplasmic reticulum and increases the rate of development of force and peak contraction. Calcium channel blockers by decreasing channel opening probability decrease intracellular calcium entry and contractility.

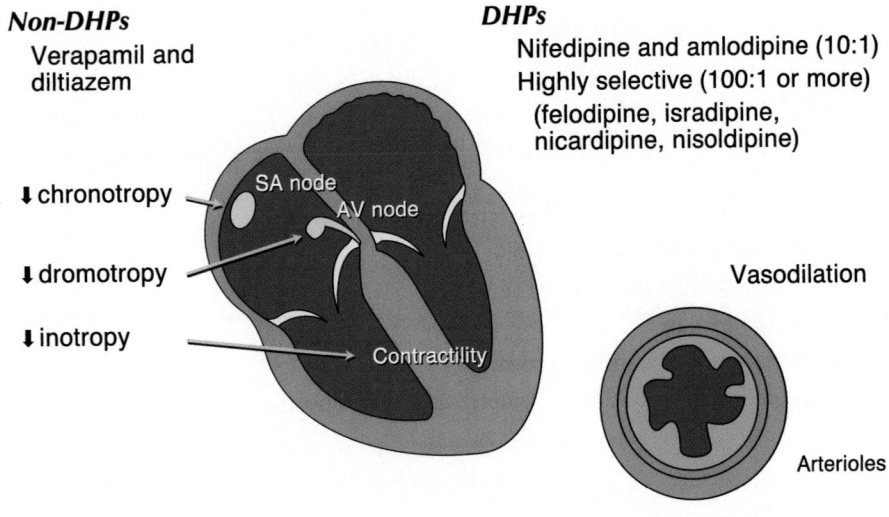

Fig. 2. Cardiovascular effects of nondihydropyridines (Non-DHP) and dihydropyridine (DHP) calcium channel blockers.

Table 2. Summary of Effects of Ca^{2+} Channel Blockers on Ventricular Contractility, Sinus Rate and Surface and Intracardiac Electrograms

	Clinical effects			ECG			Intracardiac electrocardiogram	
	Ventricular contractility	Vasodilatation	Sinus rate	PR	QRS	QT	AH	HV
Dihydropyridines	↔ (↓)	↑↑	↑*	↔	↔	↔	↔	↔
Verapamil	↓↓↓	↑	↓↓	↑↑	↔	↔	↑↑	↔
Diltiazem	↓↓	↑	↓	↑	↔	↔	↑	↔
Bepridil	↔ (↓)	↑	↓	↑		↑	↑	

↔, no effect; ↓, decreased; ↑, increased.
*Due to relfex sympathetic activation secondary to peripheral vasodilation.

Table 3. Therapeutic Uses of Calcium Channel Blockers

Cardiovascular
    Ischemic heart disease
        Stable angina pectoris
        Silent ischemia
        Vasospastic angina
    Systemic hypertension
    Cardiac arrhythmias
        Supraventricular arrhythmias
            Inappropriate sinus tachycardia
            Sinus node reentrant tachycardia
            AV node reentrant tachycardia
            AV reentrant tachycardia
            Atrial tachycardia/flutter/fibrillation with rapid ventricular response
        Ventricular arrhythmias
            Idiopathic right ventricular outflow tract tachycardia
            Idiopathic left ventricular tachycardia
    Primary pulmonary hypertension (second line agent)
    Diastolic ventricular dysfunction
    Hypertrophic obstructive cardiomyopathy (second line agent)
    Cerebral vasospasm following subarachnoid hemorrhage (nimodipine)
Non cardiovascular
    Migraine headache
    Raynaud's phenomenon
    Renal protection in hypertensive diabetics

with a longer plasma half-life produces less reflex tachycardia than other DHPs.

Calcium channel blockers may have a direct antiatherosclerotic action, limiting the progression of coronary atherosclerosis. This is believed to be mediated through a nitric oxide-mediated mechanism, but the extent and clinical importance of this effect have yet to be established.

Myocardial Infarction

Despite well-established anti-ischemic properties, calcium channel blockers do not reduce mortality during or after myocardial infarction. Several clinical trials and meta-analyses of short-acting calcium channel blockers in patients with cardiovascular disease have indicated a detrimental effect on long-term survival. This apparent detrimental effect of short-acting DHPs on survival perfusion pressure, disproportionate dilatation of the coronary arteries adjacent to the ischemic area (steal phenomenon) and reflex tachycardia with consequent increase in myocardial oxygen demand due to activation of the sympathetic nervous system (Table 4).

According to the current guidelines of the American College of Cardiology and American Heart Association (ACC/AHA) (Table 4), calcium channel blockers are not recomended for routine treatment or secondary prevention after acute myocardial infarction; if used, they should be reserved only for patients without heart failure, ventricular dysfunction, or AV block in whom β-blockers are ineffective or contraindicated for relief of ongoing

Table 4. Meta-Analyses of Randomized Trials of Drug Therapy Administered During and After Acute Myocardial Infarction*

Drug class and time administered	No. of trials	No. of patients	Relative risk of death (95% CI)	P value	Strength of evidence†
Beta-adrenergic antagonists					
During MI‡	29	28,970	0.87 (0.77-0.98)	0.02	A
After MI	26	24,298	0.77 (0.70-0.84)	<0.001	A
ACE inhibitors					
During MI	15	100,963	0.94 (0.89-0.98)	0.006	A
After MI, patients with left ventricular dysfunction	3	5,986	0.78 (0.70-0.86)	<0.001	A
Nitrates (during MI)	12	81,908	0.94 (0.90-0.99)	0.03	B
Calcium-channel blockers (during and after MI)	24	20,342	1.04 (0.94-1.14)	0.41	A
Antiarrhythmic drugs					
Lidocaine (during MI)§	14	9,155	1.38 (0.98-1.95)	>0.05	C
Class I drugs (after MI)¶	18	6,300	1.21 (1.01-1.44)	0.04	A
Amiodarone (after MI)	9	1,557	0.71 (0.51-0.97)	0.03	C
Magnesium (during MI)	11	61,860	1.02 (0.96-1.08)	>0.05	A

*CI, denotes confidence interval, and MI myocardial infarction.

†The strength of the evidence in each meta-analysis was graded as follows: a score of A indicates that a randomized trial of adequate size supports the meta-analysis; B, that data from one or more randomized trials of adequate size do not support the meta-analysis; and C, that no large randomized trial was conducted.

‡This study evaluated short-term therapy (mean, 5 weeks).

§This study evaluated prophylaxis administered during and immediately after acute myocardial infarction.

¶This study evaluated long-term oral therapy after acute myocardial infarction.

ischemia or control of a rapid ventricular response with atrial fibrillation. Only the heart rate-slowing calcium antagonists diltiazem or verapamil are acceptable, and short-acting nifedipine is contraindicated (Table 5).

■ Calcium channel blockers are not recommended for routine treatment or secondary prevention after acute myocardial infarction; if used, they should be reserved only for patients without heart failure, ventricular dysfunction, or AV block in whom β-blockers are ineffective or contraindicated for relief of ongoing ischemia or control of a rapid ventricular response with atrial fibrillation.

Hypertension

Calcium channel blockers lower blood pressure mainly by relaxing arteriolar smooth muscle and decreasing peripheral vascular resistance. They are highly effective in all hypertensive patients, including elderly and African-American patients, who have a higher prevalence of low renin status. Despite their efficacy in lowering blood pressure in mild to moderate hypertension, calcium channel blockers are not recommended as first line therapy unless other indications for their use exists, such as supraventricular tachycardia, angina pectoris or Raynaud phenomenon. Short-acting DHPs such as nifedipine have been associated with a dose-related increased risk of myocardial infarction and mortality in

patients with ischemic heart disease, and their use is contraindicated in hypertensive patients with acute ischemic syndrome. Sustained-release or longer-acting calcium channel blockers that provide smoother blood pressure control and cause less adrenergic activation and reflex tachycardia are more appropriate. Recent data from randomized clinical trials do not indicate any difference between long acting calcium channel antagonists and other antihypertensive drug classes with regard to long-term outcomes in those with moderate cardiovascular risk factors. In the Antihypertensive and Lipid-Lowering Treatment to Prevent Heart Attack Trial (ALLHAT) an antihypertensive regimen based on a long-acting calcium channel blocker (amlodipine) or an ACE inhibitor was equal to a thiazide diuretic-based regimen in coronary outcomes. Heart failure and stroke outcomes when compared to diuretics were increased, while new diabetes and deterioration of renal function was slowed by amlodipine.

■ Short-acting dihydropyridines may result in a dose-related increase in the risk of myocardial infarction and mortality in patients with ischemic heart disease and are contraindicated in acute ischemic syndromes.

Antiarrhythmic Effects

Verapamil and diltiazem are Vaughan-Williams class IV antiarrhythmic agents, whereas DHPs have no

---

Table 5.   Recommendations for Therapy with Calcium Channel Blockers in Acute Myocardial Infarction (MI)

Class I
    None
Class IIa
    Verapamil or diltiazem may be given to patients in whom β-adrenoceptor blockers are ineffective or contraindicated (i.e., bronchospastic disease) for relief of ongoing ischemia or control of rapid ventricular response with atrial fibrillation or atrial flutter after acute MI in the absence of congestive heart failure, left ventricular dysfunction, or AV block.
Class III
    Nifedipine (immediate-release form) is contraindicated in the treatment of acute myocardial infarction because of the reflex sympathetic activation, tachycardia and hypotension associated with its use.

    Diltiazem and verapamil are contraindicated in patients with acute MI and associated systolic LV dysfunction and congestive heart failure.

clinically useful antiarrhythmic properties. In the sinoatrial and AV nodes, blockade of the slow inward calcium current results in a decreased rate of automatic discharge, slowed AV node conduction and prolongation of refractoriness, which forms the bases for their antiarrhythmic effects in AV node-dependent reentrant tachycardias and ventricular rate slowing in atrial tachyarrhythmias. Verapamil and to a lesser extent diltiazem possess **use dependence or frequency dependence**, properties that increases the calcium channel blockade as the heart rate increases. In addition to the sinoatrial and AV node, other tissues dependent on the calcium current may be affected by class IV drugs. Class IV agents have no significant effect on intra-atrial, intraventricular, or His-Purkinje conduction or refractoriness.

■ Prolongation of AV node conduction and refractoriness by verapamil and diltiazem are the bases of their antiarrhythmic benefit in AV node-dependent reentrant tachycardias and ventricular rate slowing in atrial tachyarrhythmias.

Paroxysmal Supraventricular Tachycardia (PSVT)

In supraventricular tachycardia circuits requiring conduction through the AV node, such as AV node reentrant or orthodromic AV reentrant tachycardia, verapamil and diltiazem are effective in terminating and suppressing recurrence of tachycardia (efficacy, 65% to 100%). Intravenous verapamil and diltiazem are comparable in safety and efficacy to intravenous adenosine for terminating AV node-dependent arrhythmias. Although the effect of adenosine in this situation is more rapid than that of verapamil, it is short-lived, and in cases in which the arrhythmia recurs after initial termination, verapamil is more effective for controlling the rhythm. Oral calcium channel blockers are less effective when used for the prevention of PSVT recurrence than when used intravenously for acute termination. With increased use of catheter-based ablation of supraventricular tachycardia circuits which effectively cures these arrhythmias, the prophylactic use of drugs, including calcium channel blockers or β-blockers to prevent recurrences has decreased markedly.

■ Recurrence of PSVT after termination with adenosine is best treated with verapamil or diltiazem given intravenously.

Atrial Tachyarrhythmias

In supraventricular tachycardia circuit not dependent on the AV node, calcium channel blockers have a minor role in termination or preventing recurrence of the arrhythmia with the exception of multifocal atrial tachycardia or atrial tachycardia due to digitalis toxicity (probable triggered arrhythmias). Calcium channel blockers have no significant role in converting atrial fibrillation or flutter to sinus rhythm or in maintaining sinus rhythm after it is restored by electrical cardioversion. Both verapamil and diltiazem are however, effective in controlling rapid ventricular rate response with atrial fibrillation at rest and during activity. Because of the negative inotropic effects and concerns regarding increased mortality in patients with ventricular dysfunction after myocardial infarction, use of calcium antagonists is not recommended for long-term rate control in patients after ST-elevation myocardial infarction.

■ Calcium channel blockers have no significant role in converting atrial fibrillation or flutter to sinus rhythm or in maintaining sinus rhythm after it is restored electrically.

Ventricular Arrhythmias

Currently, the role of calcium channel blockers in ventricular arrhythmias is limited to the small subset of patients with idiopathic ventricular tachycardia arising from the right ventricular outflow tract or near the posterior Purkinje fascicle in the left ventricle. This usually occurs in a structurally normal heart, and both β-blockers and verapamil are effective in most cases for terminating and preventing arrhythmia recurrence. No trials comparing the two antiarrhythmic classes have been published.

Although oscillations in cellular calcium level have been suggested to underlie the polymorphic ventricular tachycardia due to early or delayed afterdepolarization-mediated triggered activity, the therapeutic role of calcium channel blockers in suppressing these arrhythmias is not clear.

■ The role of calcium channel blockers in ventricular arrhythmias is limited to a small subset of patients with idiopathic right ventricular outflow tract or left ventricular fascicular tachycardia.

CONGESTIVE HEART FAILURE

Systolic Dysfunction

Calcium channel blockers, with their antianginal and vasodilatory properties appear to have desirable effects for some patients with heart failure; however, their negative inotropic effect and activation of the neurohormonal systems are detrimental and may cause clinical deterioration. Most calcium channel blockers, therefore, should be avoided in patients with congestive heart failure due to systolic dysfunction. Of the available calcium channel blockers, only amlodipine has been shown not to adversely affect survival when used along with angiotensin-converting enzyme (ACE) inhibitors, digoxin, and diuretics.

In the recent ACC/AHA guidelines for the treatment of heart failure, calcium channel blockers are not recommended (class III indication) in patients with left ventricular dysfunction regardless of the presence of symptoms of heart failure (Table 6).

■ Calcium channel blockers should be avoided in patients with congestive heart failure due to systolic dysfunction.

Diastolic Dysfunction

Calcium channel blockers have been proposed to improve diastolic dysfunction by augmenting ventricular relaxation and improving ventricular compliance, but only very limited data are available to support whether these mechanisms are clinically relevant. Verapamil and diltiazem however may have beneficial effects on reducing symptoms of heart failure by heart rate slowing that improves ventricular filling, stroke volume and diastolic coronary perfusion in patients with heart failure with preserved systolic function. Calcium channel blockers are currently recommended as a class IIb indication for patients with heart failure due to diastolic dysfunction (Table 6).

Hypertrophic Cardiomyopathy

β-Blockers are the preferred agent in hypertrophic cardiomyopathy, but in refractory cases, verapamil may improve clinical symptoms, exercise performance, diastolic function and may reduce left ventricular outflow gradient. However, it should be used with great caution because of concerns about hemodynamic collapse with peripheral vasodilatation in patients with significant resting left ventricular outflow obstruction. Negative inotropic agents such as disopyramide or β-blockers without vasodilating properties are preferred in these patients.

■ Verapamil may cause hemodynamic collapse in patients with hypertrophic obstructive cardiomyopathy because of peripheral vasodilatation.

Table 6.   Recommendations for Therapy with Calcium Channel Blockers in Patients with Heart Failure

Asymptomatic LV Systolic Dysfunction (Stage B)
Class III
    Calcium channel blockers with negative inotropic effects may be harmful in asymptomatic patients with low left ventricular ejection fraction and no symptoms of heart failure

Symptomatic LV Systolic Dysfunction (Stage C)
Class III
    Calcium channel blocking drugs are not indicated as routine treatment for HF in patients with current or prior symptoms of heart failure and reduced left ventricular ejection fraction

Heart Failure with Preserved LV Systolic Function
Class IIb
    The use of calcium channel blockers in patients with heart failure and normal left ventricular ejection fraction and hypertension might be effective to minimize symptoms of heart failure

Other Indications

Cerebral Vasospasm

Nimodipine, which has a high affinity for cerebral blood vessels reduces morbidity and improve outcome in patients with cerebral vasospasm following subarachnoid hemorrhage and is recommended for its management.

Aortic Regurgitation

Nifedipine compared with standard management delays the need for valve replacement in patients with severe aortic regurgitation.

Primary Pulmonary Hypertension

High doses of calcium channel blockers (usually amlodipine) appear to be beneficial in a small number of patients with primary pulmonary hypertension. The dose needs to be increased cautiously and the patient needs to be observed for hypotension or heart failure.

Renal Protection

Calcium channel blockers reduce microalbuminuria and preserve kidney function in patients with diabetes. When used in combination with angiotensin-converting enzyme inhibitors they may have an additive beneficial effect on protein excretion in diabetic nephropathy.

Dosage of Calcium Channel Blockers

The usual dosages of commonly used calcium channel blockers are given in Table 7.

Side Effects

Adverse effects due to calcium channel blockers are mainly the result of vasodilatation (dizziness, headache, flushing and ankle swelling) and a decrease in heart rate and blood pressure (fatigue and lassitude). Dizziness and flushing are less common with the sustained-release formulations or DHPs with a long plasma half-life. The ankle edema likely results from increased hydrostatic pressure due to precapillary dilation and reflex postcapillary constriction. Calcium channel blockers can cause or aggravate gastroesophageal reflux due to the inhibition of lower esophageal sphincter contraction. Constipation is also common with verapamil. Occasionally, skin reaction and gingival swelling may occur. These effects are mild and dose-dependent.

Calcium channel blockers should be avoided or used cautiously in conditions summarized in Table 8. In patients with underlying sinus node or conduction system disease, verapamil and diltiazem may cause profound slowing of the heart rate and heart block, which may be exacerbated by the concomitant use of digoxin or β-blockers.

In patients with significant ventricular systolic dysfunction, calcium channel blockers can precipitate heart failure and should be avoided. With intravenous administration, hypotension is common and can be severe. Short-acting nifedipine has been reported to increase the incidence of myocardial infarction and should not be used orally or sublingually for urgent reduction of elevated blood pressure.

In patients with wide complex tachycardia not definitively known to be supraventricular in origin, calcium channel blockers are contraindicated because they may precipitate hemodynamic collapse in patients with ventricular tachycardia or Wolff-Parkinson-White syndrome. Right ventricular outflow tract idiopathic tachycardia is a rare exception to this rule and may be treated with calcium channel blockers. In patients with

Table 7.   Relative Contraindications of Calcium Channel Blocker Use

Overt ventricular failure
Severe sinus node dysfunction
Severe conduction system disease
Wolff-Parkinson-White syndrome
Wide complex tachycardia of unknown cause
History of serious ventricular arrhythmias or prolonged QT interval (Bepridil)
Digitalis toxicity
Severe aortic stenosis
Hypertrophic obstructive cardiomyopathy (dihydropyridines)
Hypotension
Severe constipation (verapamil)
Known hypersensitivity
Pregnancy
Post myocardial infarction or angina at rest (short-acting dihydropyridines in the absence of β-blockade)

Table 8.   Usual Daily Dosage of Calcium Channel Blockers

	Usual Dosage
Verapamil	240-480 mg/day
	For PSVT: IV 5-10 mg over 2 min, repeat in 10 min; then 0.005 mg/kg/min for 30-60 min
Diltiazem	120-360 mg/day
	For PSVT: IV 0.25 mg/kg over 2 min, then 0.35 mg/kg over 2 min; then 5-15 mg/hr infusion
Amlodipine	5-10 mg once/day
Felodipine SR	5-10 mg once/day
Isradipine	2.5-10 mg every 12 hr
Nicardipine SR	30-60 mg twice/day
	IV 5-15 mg/h
Nifedipine SR	30-90 mg/day
Nimodipine	60 mg every 4 hr for 21 days (for subarachnoid hemorrhage)

All doses are for oral preparation, unless indicated.
IV, Intravenously; LD, loading dose; SR, sustained release formulation; PSVT, paroxysmal supraventricular tachycardia.

atrial fibrillation in the setting of Wolff-Parkinson-White syndrome, calcium channel blockers are ineffective for blocking conduction over the accessory pathway and may accelerate conduction, resulting in hypotension or ventricular rate acceleration.

In patients with digitalis toxicity, verapamil is contraindicated because it can increase the blood level of digoxin and lead to complete heart block.

Concerns have been raised in some studies about a possible link between the use of calcium channel blockers and carcinoma. Critical review of these studies and additional studies in which no association was found between therapy with calcium channel blockers and carcinoma suggests that the initial reported association is most likely due to selection bias or chance.

Overdose and Toxicity

In life-threatening situations due to overdose or toxicity of calcium channel blockers, intravenous calcium gluconate (1 to 2 g) or calcium chloride (0.5 to 1 mg) should be used. Managing combined myocardial depression and hypotension with calcium channel blockers is difficult. Positive inotropic agents (dobutamine, dopamine), vasoconstrictive catecholamines (norepinephrine, dopamine), or glucagon (5-10 mg for hypotension) with repeated doses of calcium may be necessary. Intravenous atropine or isoproterenol and a temporary pacemaker might be needed for AV block.

DRUG INTERACTIONS

Drug-drug interactions are common with the use of calcium channel blockers. Verapamil increases the concentration of digoxin when used concomitantly due to inhibition of P-glycoprotein drug transporter in the kidneys and liver. Calcium channel blockers inhibit the hepatic CYP3A isoenzyme, and therefore potentially increases the blood levels of most statins, carbamazepine, cyclosporine, theophylline and sildenafil. Cimetidine increases the bioavailability of calcium channel blockers. Grapefruit juice also inhibits the metabolism of felodipine and DHPs.

Sinus and AV node slowing agents (digoxin and β-blockers) and negative inotropic agents (disopyramide, β-blockers) may increase the negative chronotropic, dromotropic, and inotropic effects of verapamil and diltiazem and may result in symptomatic bradycardia, heart block or congestive heart failure. Concomitant calcium administration may prevent the hypotensive response to intravenous calcium channel blockers.

Unique Calcium Channel Blockers

Bepridil is unrelated structurally to any other calcium channel blocker and has additional sodium and potassium channel blocking properties (class IA and III antiarrhythmic effects). It blocks both voltage- and receptor-operated calcium channels in the myocardium and vascular smooth muscle and inhibits calcium binding to calmodulin. It has direct negative chronotropic, inotropic, and vasodilatory actions that reduce myocardial oxygen consumption and increase coronary blood flow, leading to a significant anti-ischemic and antianginal effect in the absence of reflex tachycardia. In contrast to other calcium channel blockers, bepridil produces only modest peripheral vasodilatation and displays weak antihypertensive activity. It is indicated in patients with stable effort angina who are intolerant of conventional antianginal medications. Bepridil has class I anti-arrhythmic properties and can induce new arrhythmias, including ventricular tachycardia and ventricular fibrillation. Because of its ability to prolong repolarization and the QT interval, bepridil can cause torsades de pointes, especially in the presence of hypokalemia and/or brady-cardia. Agranulocytosis also has been reported.

109

β-Adrenoceptor Blockers

Arshad Jahangir, MD

β-Adrenergic Receptor Antagonists

All β-blockers competitively inhibit catecholamine effects at β-adrenergic receptors.

Pharmacokinetics of β-Blockers

The pharmacokinetics of various β-adrenergic antagonists are summarized in Table 1. More than 30 β-blockers have been developed, but only a few are commonly used in clinical practice. Most are well absorbed after oral administration, with peak concentration occurring 1 to 3 hours after ingestion. β-Blockers exhibit different degrees of lipid solubility (Table 2). Lipid-soluble β-blockers, such as propranolol and metoprolol, are metabolized mainly by the liver and tend to have relatively short plasma half-lives. Hydrophilic β-blockers, such as atenolol and nadolol, are cleared by the kidney and tend to have relatively longer plasma half-lives. The elimination half life of β-blockers varies from 9 minutes for esmolol to 24 hours for nadolol.

■ Lipid-soluble β-blockers are metabolized largely by the liver and have relatively short plasma half-lives, whereas water-soluble β-blockers are cleared by the kidney and have relatively longer plasma half-lives.

Pharmacodynamics of β-Blockers

Classically, β-receptors are divided into:

β_1-receptor (found mainly in the heart),

β_2-receptor (found in vascular and bronchial smooth muscles and myocardium), and

β_3-receptors (found in adipocytes).

At lower concentration, β-blockers exhibit various degrees of cardiac selectivity, i.e., affinity for β_1 versus β_2 receptor (Table 2). The proportion of β_1 and β_2 receptors changes with cardiac disease: in heart failure there is a relative reduction of β_1 receptors but an increase in β_2 receptors. Selectivity for β_1 and β_2 receptors is relative and is overcome by large drug doses. Most β-blocking drugs in clinical use are **pure antagonists**, i.e., they occupy the β-receptor but do not activate the receptor and thus prevent the receptor from being stimulated by β–receptor agonists. In addition to β-blockade, some drugs, such as pindolol and acebutalol also possess **intrinsic** sympathomimetic activity (ISA), which causes weak β-adrenergic activation (**partial agonists**). These drugs decrease resting heart rate and cardiac output less than drugs without intrinsic **sympathomimetic activity**, but prevent the effect of catecholamine stimulation on the heart including the increase in heart rate seen during exercise, emotional reactions, and other stressful events. Third generation β-blockers have additional properties (Table 3), such as vasodilation by β-adrenergic receptor blockade seen with carvedilol, labetalol and bucindolol. Bucindolol

Table 1.   Pharmacokinetics of β-Adrenergic Receptor Antagonists

	Bioavailability (%)	Protein binding (%)	Time to peak action after oral intake (hours)	Elimination half-life (hours)	Route to major elimination
Acebutolol	70	25	3-8	3-10	Hepatic (renal)
Bucindolol	-		0.5-1-6	2-7	Hepatic
Carvedilol	30	95	1.0-1.5	7-10	Hepatic
Labetalol	30	50	2-4 (5 min IV)	3-6	Hepatic (renal)
Metoprolol	50	10	1-2	3-6	Hepatic
Timolol	50	10	1-2	4-5	Hepatic
Propranolol	35	90	1-2	3-5	Hepatic
Esmolol	(100 IV)	55	(2-5 min IV)	9 min	Blood esterase (renal)
Atenolol	50	15	2-4 (10 min IV)	6-9	Renal
Bisoprolol	80	30	2-4	9-12	Renal (hepatic)
Nadolol	30	30	3-4	14-24	Renal
Pindolol	90	55	1-3	3-4	Renal (hepatic)
Sotalol	100	0	2-4	10-15	Renal

IV, Intravenous.

has additional mild direct vasodilating properties that are likely mediated by a cyclic guanosine monophosphate-dependent mechanism. Carvedilol and several of its metabolites are potent antioxidants and may inhibit catecholamine toxicity resulting from the oxidation of norepinephrine and generation of oxygen free radicals. Carvedilol also has antiproliferative effect and blocks the expression of several genes involved in myocardial damage and inhibits free radical-induced activation of transcription factors and programmed cell death (apoptosis). Some of the clinical effects of individual β-blockers may be due to effects independent of β-adrenergic blockade; therefore these drugs should not be considered interchangeable for all clinical applications.

Mode of Action
All β-blockers counteract the effect of catecholamines at the β-adrenergic receptor. This competition decreases catecholamine-receptor interactions, interrupts the production of cyclic AMP, and ultimately inhibits calcium influx across the sarcolemma and calcium release by the sarcoplasmic reticulum (Fig. 1). This results in decreased myocardial contractility (negative inotropic

effect) and reduction in heart rate due to decreased automaticity in the sinus node (negative chronotropic effect) and slowing of conduction in the atrioventricular node (negative dromotropic effect; Fig. 2).

Cardiovascular Effects of β-Blockers and Clinical Use
Various indications for use of β-blockers are summarized in Table 4.

Cardiac Arrhythmias
β-Blockers are effective in treating both supraventricular and ventricular tachyarrhythmias. The beneficial antiarrhythmic effects of β-blockade are especially significant during ischemia and high catecholamine states. Some of the potential antiarrhythmic mechanisms of β-blockers are summarized in Table 5. β-Blockers antagonize catecholamine effects in the sinoatrial node (SAN), atrioventricular (AV) node, His-Purkinje tissue, and atrial and ventricular myocardium. A decrease in the diastolic depolarization rate by a decrease in cyclic AMP results in slowing of sinus and ectopic pacemaker rates and arrhythmias due to enhanced or abnormal automaticity, and a decrease in calcium dependent

Table 2.   β-Blockers: Relative Cardioselectivity, Potency, Lipid Solubility Intrinsic Sympathomimetic Activity, and Membrane-Stabilizing Properties

	Relative β_1 selectivity	β_1 Blockade potency ratio propranolol=1.0	Lipid solubility	ISA	Class I antiarrhythmic effect
Cardioselective					
Acebutolol	+	0.3	+	+β_1	+
Atenolol	++	1.0	−		
Betaxolol	++	1.0	++		
Bisoprolol	+	5-10	+		
Esmolol	++	0.03	+		
Metoprolol	++	1.0	++		±
Noncardioselective					
Bucindolol*‡		3.0	+	+	
Carvedilol*§		2-4	+		++
Labetalol*		0.3	++	+β_2	±
Nadolol		1.0	−		
Pindolol		6.0	++	++	+
Propranolol		1.0	+++		++
Timolol		6.0	+	±	
Sotalol†		0.3	−		

ISA, intrinsic sympathomimetic activity; +, low; ++, moderate; +++, high
*Also alpha-1 adrenergic blockade
†Additional class III antiarrhythmic activity
‡Direct vascular smooth muscle relaxation
§Antioxidant activity

Table 3.   β-blockers

Generation	Properties	Examples
1st	Nonselective No additional properties	Propranolol, timolol
2nd	β_1-Receptor selective No additional properties	Metoprolol, atenolol, bisoprolol
3rd	Nonselective with additional properties (vasodilations, etc.)	Carvedilol, bucindolol, labetalol

afterdepolarization, help suppress arrhythmias due to triggered activity (Fig. 2).

On electrocardiography (ECG), the PR interval is prolonged without any significant effect on the QRS or QT interval. Sotalol with its additional class III antiarrhythmic effect, results in prolongation of the action potential and QT interval.

Supraventricular Arrhythmias
β-Blockers have been used to slow sinus tachycardia when there is a need to control rates (e.g., to reduce ischemia) in patients with hyperthyroidism and in those with inappropriate sinus tachycardia. These drugs are effective in terminating and suppressing AV nodal-dependent tachyarrhythmias, such as AV node reentrant tachycardia and orthodromic AV reentrant tachy-

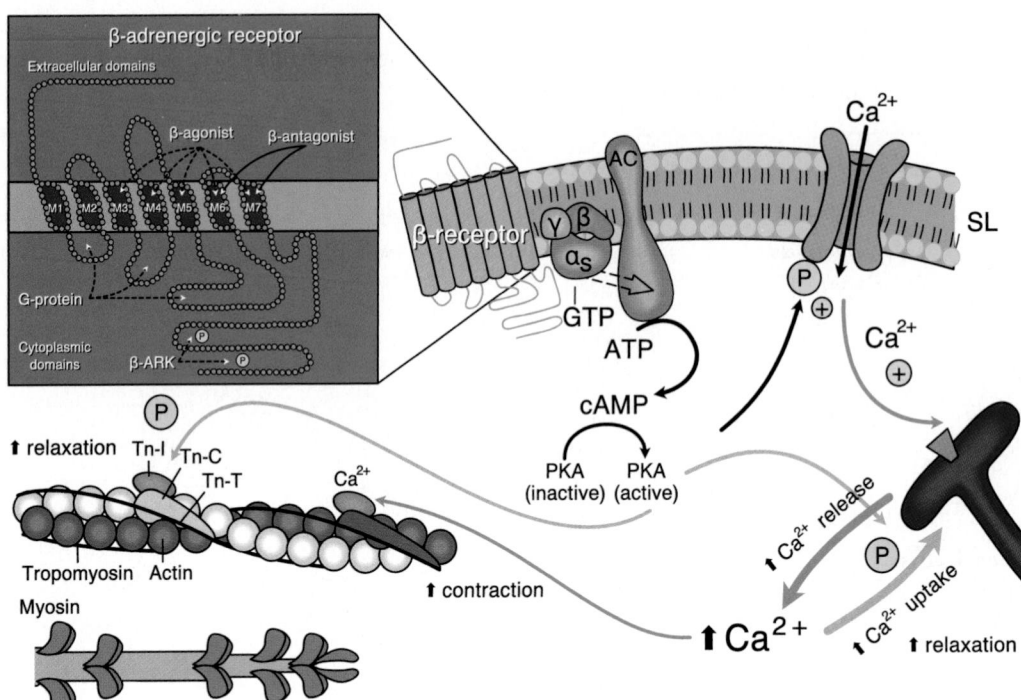

Fig. 1. β-Adrenergic signal systems. β-Adrenergic receptor antagonists block the catecholamine-mediated increase in myocardial rate and peak force of contraction. Catecholamine activates the β-adrenergic receptor, which through a stimulatory G protein (G_{as}) activates adenylate cyclase (AC), resulting in increased production of cyclic adenosine monophosphate (cAMP) from adenosine triphosphate (ATP). This in turn activates protein kinase A (PKA), leading to phosphorylation of sarcolemmal calcium channels, which increase calcium (Ca^{2+}) entry into the cell that leads to calcium-induced calcium release and increased rate of development of force and peak contraction. PKA also phosphorylates troponin I (that decreases the affinity of the myosin head to actin) and phospholamban (that increases Ca^{2+}-uptake into the sarcoplasmic reticulum) thus promoting cardiac relaxation. β-Blockers by antagonizing the effect of catecholamine, thus have negative inotropic and lusitropic effects. *Inset* shows the molecular structure of β-adrenergic receptor. The transmembrane domain (M1-M7) acts as a ligand-binding pocket, with domains M6 and M7 more specific for β-antagonists. β-Agonist binding is more diffuse. β-ARK, β-adrenergic receptor kinase; GTP, guanosine triphosphate; SL, sarcolemma; Tn-C, troponin C; Tn-I, troponin I; Tn-T, troponin T.

cardias. AV node slowing agents, including β-blockers, calcium channel blockers or digoxin do not decrease conduction over accessory pathways and should be avoided during atrial fibrillation with pre-excited ventricular conduction because hemodynamic collapse may occur with rapid ventricular activation over the accessory pathway following blockage of AV node conduction. Patients with Wolff-Parkinson-White syndrome, in whom atrial fibrillation with a rapid ventricular response associated with hemodynamic instability is present, should be immediately cardioverted.

■ Administration of β-blockers, diltiazem, verapamil or digitalis glycosides are contraindicated in patients with

Wolff-Parkinson-White syndrome who have pre-excited ventricular activation during atrial fibrillation.

Atrial Fibrillation and Atrial Flutter

In atrial fibrillation or atrial flutter, β-blockers effectively control the rapid ventricular rate response at rest and during activity by increasing the AV nodal refractory period. They have no significant effect in conversion to or maintenance of sinus rhythm, except in a few patients with high catecholamine states, such as those who develop adrenergically-mediated atrial fibrillation during exercise, with hyperthyroidism or postoperatively. Sotalol in its *dl*-racemic form has both a nonselective β-blocking and class III antiarrhythmic activity and is more effective in preventing recurrences of atrial fibrillation than β-blockers lacking additional antiarrhythmic effects. It is particularly useful in those with atrial fibrillation and ischemic heart disease. When compared with class I antiarrhythmics, such as flecainide, sotalol has an added advantage of controlling the ventricular rate in the event atrial fibrillation recurs during treatment, and thereby reduce associated symptoms.

Perioperative prophylactic β-blockade is recommended as a class I indication to prevent postoperative atrial fibrillation in cardiac patients. β-blockers reduce the incidence of atrial fibrillation from 40% to 20% in patients undergoing coronary artery bypass graft surgery and from 60% to 30% in those undergoing valvular procedures. Withdrawal of beta-blockers in the perioperative period doubles the incidence of postoperative atrial fibrillation after coronary artery bypass surgery. In patients with postoperative atrial fibrillation when hemodynamic instability is a concern, a short-acting beta-blocker, such as esmolol is particularly useful in controlling rapid ventricular rate response. In hemodynamically stable patients, other AV nodal blocking agents, such as calcium channel blockers, can be used as alternative therapy, but digoxin is less effective when adrenergic tone is high. In patients with tachycardia-bradycardia syndrome, associated with episodic tachy-

cardia alternating with periods of bradycardia, β-blockers with intrinsic sympathomimetic activity, such as pindolol and acebutolol may be effective in controlling fast ventricular rate without excessively slowing the resting heart rate.

In the current American College of Cardiology/ American Heart Association guidelines for atrial fibrillation management, the use of oral β-blockers is recommended as a class I indication in patients without contraindications, for the prevention of postoperative atrial fibrillation and for control of rapid ventricular rate in those who develop atrial fibrillation following cardiac surgery. In patients with contraindications to β-blocker use and those at high risk for postoperative atrial fibrillation, preoperative administration of amiodarone is recommended as a class IIa indication and low-dose sotalol as a class IIb indication to reduce the incidence of atrial fibrillation after coronary artery bypass surgery.

Ventricular Arrhythmias

β-Blockers have been used to treat symptomatic premature ventricular complexes in patients with structurally normal heart or with mitral valve prolapse but without convincing evidence that demonstrates any mortality benefit in these conditions. β-Blockers because of their major antiadrenergic actions are likely to be effective in

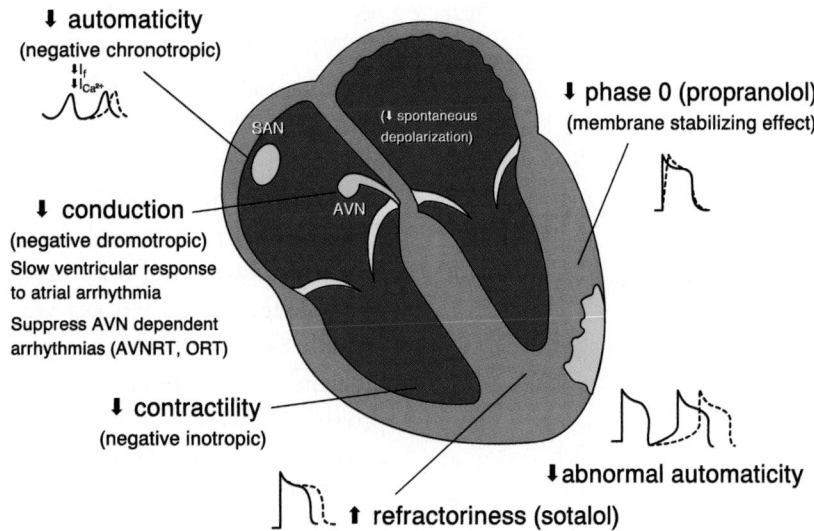

Fig. 2. Cardiac effects of β-adrenergic blocking drugs at the level of the sinoatrial node (SAN), atrioventricular node (AVN) and myocardium. AVNRT. Atrioventricular nodal reentry tachycardia; $I_{Ca^{2+}}$, calcium current; I_f, pacemaker current; ORT, orthodromic reciprocating tachycardia.

arrhythmias in which adrenergic stimulation has a major role, such as those induced by exercise, postoperative state, thyrotoxicosis, pheochromocytoma, anxiety, mitral valve prolapse or "electrical storm" during the early

Table 4.   Therapeutic Uses of β-Blockers

Cardiovascular
   Cardiac arrhythmias
      Supraventricular arrhythmias
         Inappropriate sinus tachycardia
         Sinus node reentry tachycardia
         AV node reentrant tachycardia, AV
            reentrant tachycardia
         Atrial tachycardia, flutter or fibrilla-
            tion with rapid ventricular rate
            response
      Ventricular arrhythmias
         Symptomatic premature ventricular
            complexes
         Idiopathic left ventricular tachycardia
         Digitalis-induced ventricular tachy-
            cardia
         Right ventricular outflow tachycardia
   Ischemic heart disease
      Angina pectoris
      Silent ischemia
      Myocardial infarction
         Acute phase
         Long-term
   Systemic hypertension
   Congestive heart failure
      Systolic ventricular dysfunction
      Diastolic ventricular dysfunction
      Neurocardiogenic syncope
      Hypertrophic obstructive cardiomyopathy
      Aortic dissection
      Aortic aneurysm (Marfan syndrome)
      Mitral valve prolapse
      Congenital long QT syndrome
Noncardiovascular
   Glaucoma
   Hyperthyroidism
   Migraine prophylaxis
   Essential tremor
   Anxiety states (stage fright)
   Alcohol withdrawal
   Esophageal varices due to portal hypertension

phase of acute myocardial infarction. Catecholamine-sensitive ventricular tachycardia, especially in a subset of young patients without structural heart disease, where it originates from the right ventricular outflow tract, is frequently sensitive to β-blockade. This type of ventricular tachycardia is usually exercise-related and can be induced with infusion of isoproterenol but not consistently with electrophysiological programmed stimulation, suggesting a non-reentrant mechanism. In patients with structural heart disease and reentrant ventricular tachycardia, β-blockers have only a limited role and are not effective in preventing inducibility of sustained monomorphic ventricular tachycardia during electrophysiology study, except for patients in whom tachycardia arrhythmia induction is facilitated by isoproterenol infusion. β-Blockers are very effective in reducing the incidence of ventricular fibrillation, sudden death, as well as all-cause mortality in patients who have had myocardial infarction or a history of congestive heart failure, suggesting that these patients are more susceptible to catecholamine-facilitated arrhythmias. Patients with heart failure due to left ventricular systolic dysfunction should be treated with beta-blockers unless they have a contraindication to their use or are unable to tolerate these drugs. In patients with recurrent polymorphic ventricular tachycardia and fibrillation—the so called "electrical storm" that may occur in the setting of acute or recent myocardial infarction and is often unresponsive to standard antiarrhythmic therapy—they may respond to β-blockade.

The actions of several antiarrhythmic drugs, including sodium channel blockers may be attenuated during sympathetic stimulation, thus decreasing their clinical efficacy. β-Blockade might be beneficial in these patients. In the Cardiac Arrhythmia Suppression Trial (CAST), postmyocardial infarction patients with ventricular dysfunction who were receiving a class IC agent along with a β-blocker had lower all-cause and arrhythmia mortality than patients not receiving β-blockers. These findings suggested a possible "antiproarrhythmic effect" of β-blocker therapy that reversed or prevented proarrhythmia associated with class IC antiarrhythmic agents.

In the Electrophysiologic Study versus Electrocardiographic Monitoring (ESVEM) trial, sotalol was more effective in preventing recurrence of ventricular arrhythmia than class I antiarrhythmic agents. In the

Table 5.   Antiarrhythmic and Antiischemic Mechanisms of b-Adrenoceptor Blockade

↓ automaticity (phase 4 depolarization) (sinus/ectopic pacemakers)
↓ membrane excitability
↓ conduction in AV node
↓ electrophysiologic heterogeneity (dispersion of refractoriness in ischemic tissue)
↓ phosphorylation of regulatory proteins of calcium release channel
Raise ventricular fibrillation threshold
Preserves normal serum K^+ levels
Improved myocardial energetics
      ↓ oxygen utilization (↓ heart rate, contractility, afterload, wall-stress)
      ↑ oxygen wastage (myocardial metabolism)
      ↓ oxygen/nutrition supply (↑ diastolic perfusion by slowing heart rate)
      ? O_2-Hgb affinity, ? effect on coronary microvasculature, collateral blood flow)
Antiplatelet (↓ aggregation)
      Limit infarct size and recurrence of infarction
      ↓ catecholamine-induced lipolysis (↓ production of arrhythmogenic fatty acids)
      Prevention of catecholamine toxicity in failing heart (? cellular loss from necrosis and apoptosis)
      Improvement in myocardial force-frequency relationship
      Improvement in baroreflex function (?)

two large multicenter trials of amiodarone therapy, the Canadian Amiodarone Myocardial Infarction Arrhythmia Trial (CAMIAT) and the European Myocardial Infarct Amiodarone Trial (EMIAT) in postmyocardial infarction patients with ventricular dysfunction, β-blockers had a synergistic effect with amiodarone in reducing ventricular arrhythmias and mortality. In the absence of specific contraindications, prophylactic treatment with β-blockers is beneficial, and should be considered in high-risk patients with ischemic or structural heart disease.

In patients with familial long QT syndrome with arrhythmias triggered by physical or emotional stress, β-blockers alone or in combination with permanent pacing decrease the incidence of syncope and sudden death. For asymptomatic persons with a prolonged QT interval and for asymptomatic first-degree relatives of patients with the familial long QT syndrome and a history of syncope or sudden death, prophylactic treatment with β-blockers has been recommended. In the acquired form of long QT syndrome due to electrolyte abnormalities or drugs, β-blockers are not effective in preventing torsades de pointes.

ISCHEMIC HEART DISEASE

Chronic Stable Angina

In patients with chronic stable angina β-blockers reduce the frequency of anginal episodes and improve exercise tolerance. These effects are related to the decrease in cardiac work and oxygen demand with decreased heart rate, blood pressure (ventricular wall tension) and myocardial contractility. Also, the longer diastolic time resulting from slow heart rates lead to better myocardial perfusion, with increased time for diastolic coronary blood flow.

β-Blockers, in combination with nitrates and antiplatelet agents, form the standard treatment for effort angina. In stable exertional angina, these agents decrease the heart rate-blood pressure product, delay ischemic threshold and the onset of angina during exercise, and are superior to long-acting nitrates and calcium channel blockers in reducing angina symptoms and ischemia. β-Blockers are also more effective than calcium channel blockers and nitrates in reducing episodes of silent ischemia. The dose may need to be adjusted to reduce the heart rate at rest to 55 to 60 beats per minute and to limit the increase in heart rate during exercise to less than 75% of the rate response associated with onset of ischemia. The effects of β-blockers in patients with stable angina without prior myocardial infarction or hypertension have been investigated in several randomized, controlled trials. Although effective in reducing angina and silent ischemia, β-blockers are not associated with a reduction in new myocardial infarction or death in patients with chronic stable angina but without a prior myocardial infarction. In pure vasospastic (Prinzmetal) angina, β-blockers may increase coronary spasm from unopposed β-receptor activity and are therefore contraindicated.

β-Blockers reduce the sensitivity of exercise stress testing for the diagnosis of suspected coronary artery disease, by limiting the chronotropic and inotropic response to exercise. β-Blockers should be withheld for four to five hours before a diagnostic exercise study but with the caveat that if abruptly discontinued in patients with ischemic heart disease, because of their increased sensitivity to catecholamine, may cause exacerbation of angina or precipitate myocardial infarction. When discontinuing chronically administered β-blocker, the dosage should be gradually tapered over a period of 1-2 weeks under careful monitoring of patient's status. If angina worsens or acute coronary insufficiency develops, β-blocker should be promptly reinstituted and other measures appropriate for the management of unstable angina undertaken.

- In patients with chronic stable angina without prior myocardial infarction, β-blockers, despite efficacy in reducing angina aggravation and silent ischemia, are not associated with a reduction in new myocardial infarction or death.
- In pure vasospastic angina, β-blockers are contraindicated, because they may increase coronary spasm from unopposed β-receptor activity.

Myocardial Infarction

Early Use of β-Blockers During Acute Myocardial Infarction

The early administration of β-blockers during the acute phase of myocardial infarction decreases the risk of sudden cardiac death, reinfarction, and recurrent ischemia. In patients with suspected myocardial infarction not receiving fibrinolytic therapy, the immediate intravenous administration of a β-blocker (atenolol in ISIS-I, metoprolol in MIAMI trial), followed by the oral administration of a β-blocker significantly reduced short-term mortality compared with placebo. The mortality difference between those who received a β-blocker and those who did not was evident early (within 24 hours) and was sustained in the long-term. The mechanism for this is unclear but may be related to the prevention of cardiac rupture and ventricular arrhythmias.

In patients receiving concomitant fibrinolytic therapy intravenous β-blocker administration in the absence of contraindication to its use, decreases recurrent ischemia, risk of subsequent re-infarction and mortality if given early within 2 hours after onset of symptoms. In the Thrombolysis in Myocardial Infarction (TIMI)-II trial, patients who received metoprolol intravenously at the time of thrombolytic therapy, followed by oral therapy, had fewer subsequent nonfatal reinfarctions and recurrent ischemia than patients who received metoprolol on the sixth day: mortality and ventricular function were not significantly different between the two groups.

The current American College of Cardiology-American Heart Association (ACC/AHA) recommendations for early therapy with β-blocker are summarized in Table 6.

Long-term Use of β-Blockers After Myocardial Infarction

The chronic use of β-blockers in high-risk patients surviving myocardial infarction (i.e., those with recurrent ischemia, a large or anterior infarct, ventricular dysfunction, or cardiac arrhythmias) decreases all-cause mortality, sudden death, and reinfarction (by about 25%). These beneficial effects have been shown in both patients who received and those who did not receive concomitant fibrinolytic therapy (Fig. 3) and are of special benefit in those with ongoing or recurrent ischemia, infarct extension, or tachyarrhythmias. In those with bradycardia or mild-to-moderate heart failure, β-blocker should be initiated after 24 to 48 hours of freedom from such a relative contraindication. Propranolol, atenolol, timolol, metoprolol and carvedilol have been shown to be effective in reducing sudden and non-sudden cardiac death, an effect that is more striking in the setting of reduced left ventricular function. The beneficial effects of β-blockers in postinfarction patients with asymptom-

Table 6. Recommendations for Therapy With β-Blockers in Myocardial Infarction (MI)

Recommendations for early therapy with β-blockers in acute MI

Class I

Oral β-blocker therapy should be administered promptly to all patients without a contraindication, regardless of administration of concomitant fibrinolytic therapy or performance of primary PCI

Class IIa

IV beta-blockers should be administered to STEMI patients without contraindications, especially if a tachyarrhythmia or hypertension is present

Class IIb

Non-Q wave MI

Class III

Patients with moderate or severe ventricular failure or other contraindications to β-blocker therapy

MI precipitated by cocaine use

Recommendations for long-term β-blocker therapy in survivors of MI

Class I

All but low-risk patients without a clear contraindication to β-blocker therapy; treatment should begin within a few days of the event (if not initiated acutely) and continue indefinitely

Class IIa

Low-risk patients without a clear contraindication to β-blocker therapy

Class III

Patients with a contraindication to β-blocker therapy

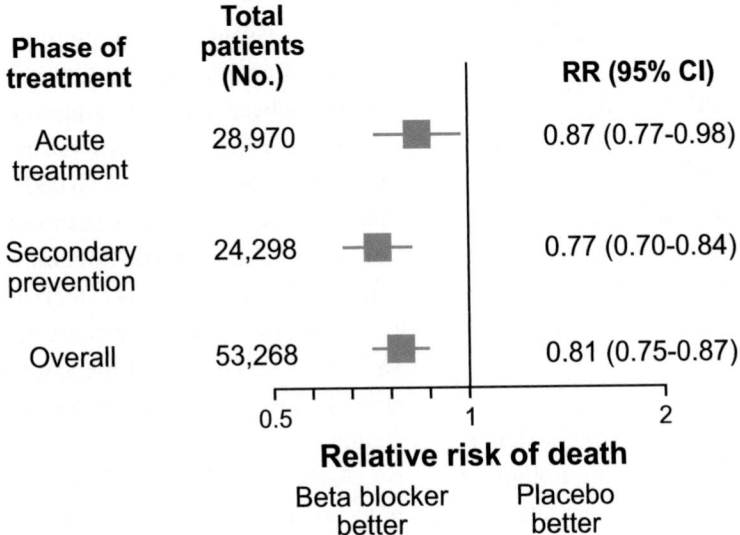

Fig. 3. Summary of data from meta-analysis of trials of β-blocker therapy from the prefibrinolytic era in patients with myocardial infarction. No., number; RR, relative risk; CI, confidence interval.

atic left ventricular dysfunction appear to be additive to those of angiotensin-converting enzyme inhibitors in reducing the risk of cardiovascular mortality (by 30%) and development of heart failure (by 21%). The benefits of β-blockers are greatest in the first year after myocardial infarction compared with the second and third years for angiotensin converting enzyme inhibitors. The beneficial survival effect is maintained in postinfarction patients with coexisting diabetes mellitus and heart failure. The non-selective β-blockers without intrinsic sympathomimetic activity appears to have larger effect on mortality reduction than selective β-blockers. The mechanism of protection by β-blockade in these patients is not clear and may be related to several of the electrophysiologic and antiischemic effects summarized in Table 4.

Low-risk patients (those without previous infarction, anterior infarction, advanced age, ventricular dysrhythmias, or ventricular dysfunction) have a good long-term prognosis, and it is not clear whether adding β-blockers to their therapy improves outcome. Because β-blockers are well tolerated and have several potential beneficial effects, their use in low-risk patient populations is also recommended (Table 6). Therapy with β-blockers should be continued for at least 2 to 3 years following myocardial infarction and longer if well tolerated, although long-term data are lacking. Despite the proven value of β-blocker use in secondary prevention in postinfarction patients, these agents are still underused and should be considered for all patients after infarction, unless clearly contraindicated (Table 7).

- Long-term use of β-blockers in high risk patients surviving myocardial infarction (i.e., those with recurrent ischemia, large or anterior infarct, ventricular dysfunction, or cardiac arrhythmias) may decrease all-cause mortality, sudden death and reinfarction rate.
- Unless contraindicated, β-blockers should be considered for all patients after myocardial infarction.

Congestive Heart Failure

Chronic activation of the adrenergic nervous system is an important component of the pathophysiology of heart failure and is associated with a worse long-term outcome. The adverse cardiovascular effects are mediated by various mechanisms triggered by the interaction of epinephrine and norepinephrine with adrenergic

Table 7.   Contraindications to β-Blocker Therapy

Absolute
    Severe bradycardia
    Severe conduction system disease (sinus node dysfunction or high-grade AV block)
    Overt ventricular failure
    Severe asthma or active bronchospasm
    Severe peripheral vascular disease with rest ischemia
    Severe depression
Relative
    PR interval >0.24 sec
    Systolic arterial pressure <100 mm Hg
    Signs of peripheral hypoperfusion
    Raynaud phenomenon
    Pure vasospastic angina
    Insulin-dependent diabetes mellitus with frequent hypoglycemic reactions
    Mild asthma or severe COPD
    Excessive fatigue
    Hyperlipidemia
    Impotence
    Pregnancy

AV, atrioventricular; COPD, chronic obstructive pulmonary disease

receptors. Antiadrenergic therapy using several β-blockers (metoprolol, carvedilol, nebivolol and bucindolol) has been shown to attenuate the detrimental effects of the sympathetic nervous system and collective experience from more than 10,000 patients with heart failure participating in more than 20 published placebo-controlled clinical trials document their beneficial effects. These beneficial effects include improved hemodynamics, ventricular function, symptoms, overall well-being and quality of life along with reduction in the risk of worsening heart failure, death, and hospitalization (Figs. 4-6).

A reduction in the risk of mortality in patients with heart failure has been demonstrated with non-selective vasodilating (carvedilol) and β_1-selective (immediate-release and slow-release metoprolol and bisoprolol) β-blockers. A number of studies have

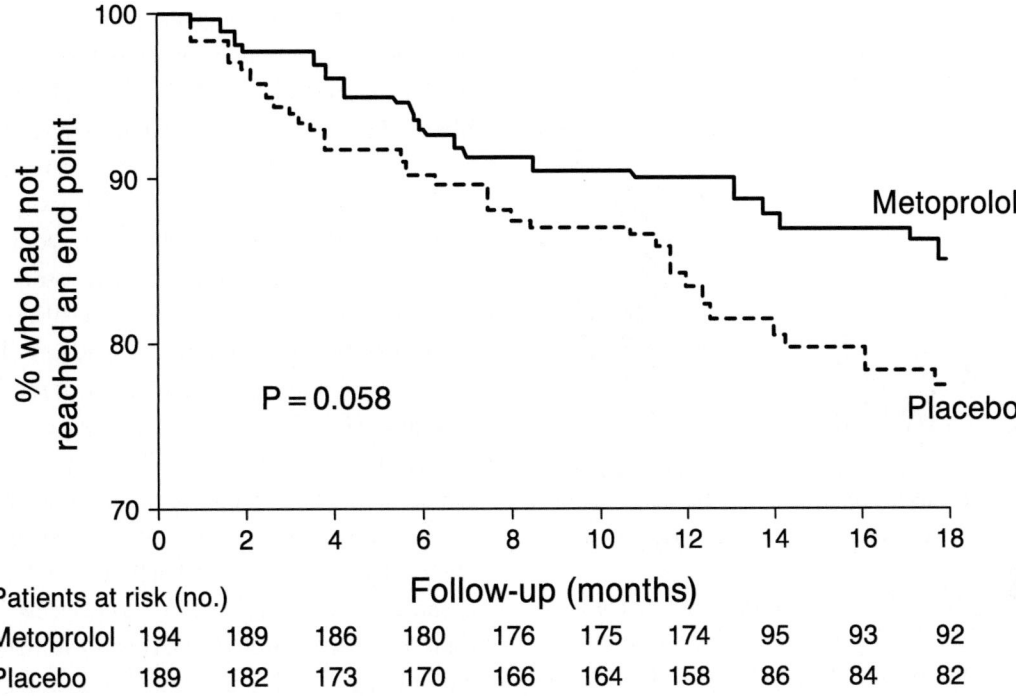

Fig. 4. Metoprolol in Dilated Cardiomyopathy Trial. Percentage of patients who had not reached endpoint of death or need for cardiac transplantation (211 patients were followed for 12 months and 172 for 18 months).

compared clinical effects of metoprolol and carvedilol in patients with heart failure. While some studies revealed no differences between both agents regarding their effects on symptoms and left ventricular ejection fraction others observed more favorable effects of carvedilol compared with metoprolol on ventricular function and pulmonary artery pressure despite similar effects on cardiovascular outcome. Long-term treatment with metoprolol in patients with heart failure results in up-regulation of the ventricular β-adrenoceptor density, restores post-receptor events and increases cardiac norepinephrine release. In contrast, carvedilol does not up-regulate β-adrenoceptors but has additional β-adrenoceptor blocking and antioxidant properties. When switching treatment from one beta-blocker to another, improvement of left ventricular function in patients with heart failure is maintained. The time course of improvement of LV function by β-blockade exceeds 12 months of therapy, irrespective of the β-blocker used. These effects are thought to occur through the prevention of catecholamine toxicity and improved myocardial energetics. β-Blockers are more likely to have an effect on patients with severe heart

failure who have greater sympathetic activation and a higher resting heart rate than on patients with slower heart rates. Carvedilol reduced the risk of all-cause mortality in patients with heart failure by 65% (Fig. 5). The mortality reduction with carvedilol was clearer in patients with a baseline heart rate greater than 82 beats/min and was seen in patients in New York Heart Association (NYHA) functional class II as well as in class III or IV and was seen in patients with either ischemic or nonischemic cardiomyopathy. In the Carvedilol or Metoprolol European Trial (COMET) a larger reduction of mortality was demonstrated with the standard dose of carvedilol (25 mg twice daily) compared to a reduced dose of short-acting formulation of metoprolol (50 mg bid).

In the majority of clinical trials in patients with heart failure both metoprolol and carvedilol treatment improved sub-maximal exercise tolerance, however, maximal exercise tolerance was improved only by metoprolol and not by carvedilol. This may be due to up-regulation of β-adrenergic receptors in metoprolol-treated patients, which is associated with higher maximum heart rate and oxygen consumption. Four clinical

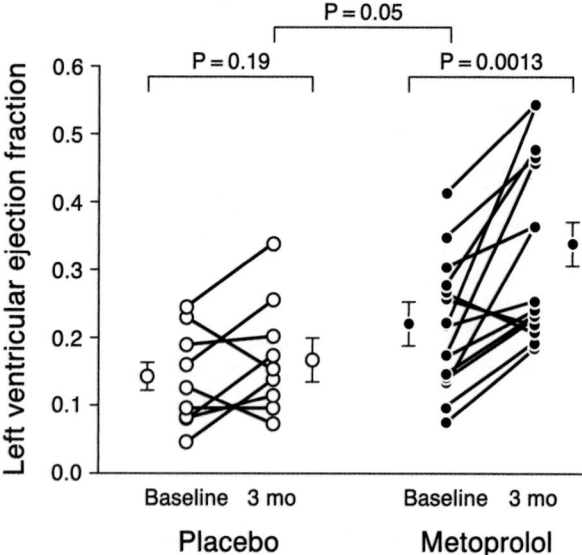

Fig. 5. Changes in left ventricular ejection fraction between baseline and 3 months for placebo and metoprolol groups in patients with dilated cardiomyopathy. A significant increase in ejection fraction was seen only in the metoprolol group.

trials of β-blocker use in patients with heart failure and results on hospitalization and mortality are summarized in Table 8. In a meta-analysis of 18 published double-blind, placebo-controlled, parallel-group trials of β-blockers in heart failure involving more than 3,000 patients, (the majority in NYHA class II or III and only <5% with class IV symptoms), the addition of a β-blocker to conventional therapy was associated with a 32% reduction in the risk of death, a 41% reduction in the risk of being hospitalized for heart failure, and a 37% reduction in the combined risk of morbidity and mortality (Fig. 7). In addition, a 29% increase in left ventricular ejection fraction, a 32% increase in the likelihood of functional improvement, and a 30% decrease in the likelihood of functional deterioration was observed in those treated with a β-blocker. The reduction of mortality risk was greater for nonselective β-blockers than for β1-selective agents. It was estimated that 38 patients will need to be treated to avoid 1 death, 24 patients to avoid 1 hospitalization for heart failure, and

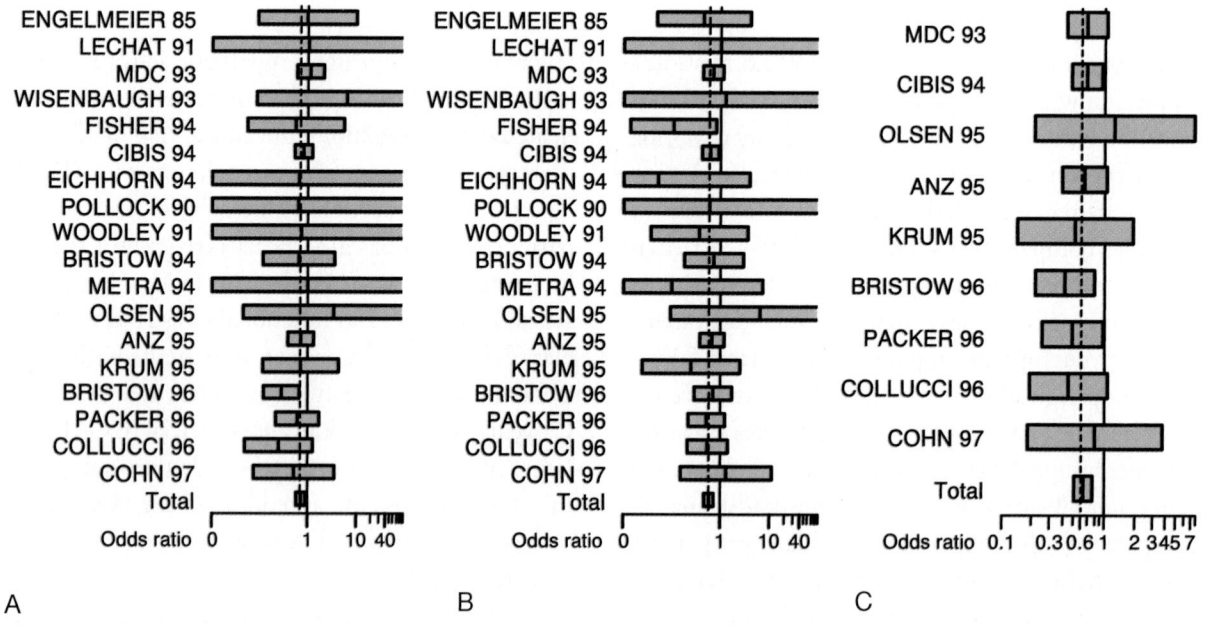

Fig. 6. β-Blockade in heart failure trials (by first author and year of publication) is represented by horizontal bar whose central vertical tick represents point estimate of odds ratio and whose width displays 95% confidence interval of estimate (logarithmic scale). Solid vertical line represents odds ratio of 1 (neutral treatment effect); dotted vertical line represents odds ratio for treatment effect across all trials. Odds ratio <1 indicates lower risk of death with β-blockade, whereas odds ratio >1 indicates higher risk of death with active treatment. Overall, β-blockers reduced risk of death by 31% (P=0.0029) (*A*), hospitalization for heart failure by 41% (P<0.001) (*B*), and death or hospitalization for heart failure by 37% (P<0.001) (*C*).

Table 8.   Major β-Blocker Trials in Heart Failure

	MDC		CIBIS-I		CIBIS-II		US carvedilol trials		COPERNICUS		MERIT HF Metoprolol CR/XL	
	Placebo	Metoprolol	Placebo	Bisoprolol	Placebo	Bisoprolol	Placebo	Carvedilol	Placebo	Carvedilol	Placebo	Metoprolol CR/XL
N	189	194	321	320	1320	1327	398	696	1133	1156	2001	1990
Mean age (yr)	49	49	59	60	61	61	58	58	63	63	64	64
Male (%)	75	70	83	83	80	81	76	77	80	79	78	77
LVEF (%)	22	22	26	25	27	27	22	23	20	20	28	28
NYHA II (%)	47	42	-	-	-	-	52	54	-	-	41	41
NYHA III (%)	47	51	95	95	83	83	44	44	100	100	55	56
NYHA IV (%)	4	4	5	5	17	17	3	3			4	3
IHD (%)	0	0	53	56	50	50	47	47	67	67	66	65
ACE inhibitor (%)	82	78	91	89	96	96	95	95	97	97	90	89
Follow-up (months)	16 (median)		23 (mean)		15 (mean)		6.5 (median)		10.4 (mean)		12 (mean)	
Hospitalization (n) (p-value)	83	51 (=0.04)	90	61 (<0.01)	39%	33% (=0.0006)	19.6%	14.1% (<0.036)			22.5	15.9 (<0.001)
Mortality % (p-value)	11	12	21	17	17	12 (<0.0001)	7.8	3.2 (=0.01)	18.5	11.4 (=0.001)	10.9†	7.5† (<0.001)

MDC, Metoprolol Dilated Cardiomopathy Trial; CIBIS I, First Cardiac Insufficiency Bisoprolol Study.
†Death or heart transplant.

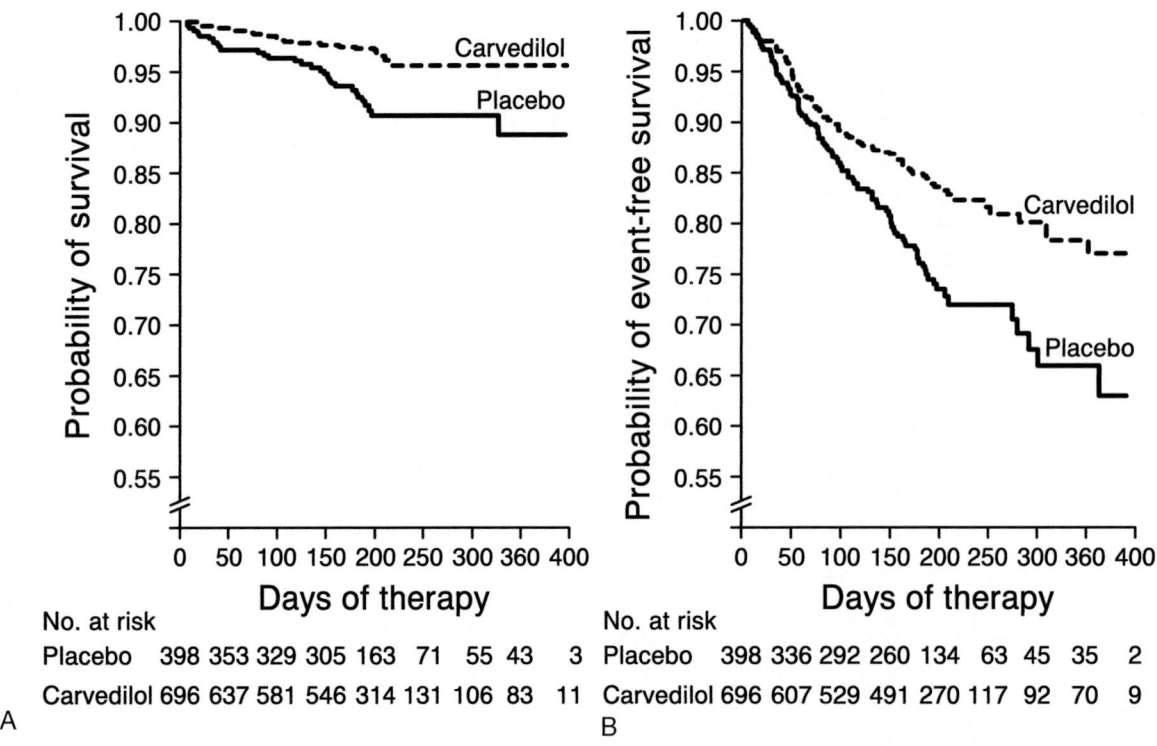

Fig. 7. Carvedilol improves, *A*, survival (65% lower risk of death) and, *B*, event-free survival (38% lower risk of death or hospitalization for cardiovascular disease) in patients with chronic heart failure compared to those on placebo.

15 patients to avoid 1 combined end point for a mean follow-up of 7 months.

The current ACC-AHA guideline for the use of β-blockers in patients with heart failure is summarized in Table 9. Patients with preserved systolic function, low heart rates (<65 beats per min), or low systolic blood pressure (<85 mm Hg) and those with decompensated heart failure or NYHA class IV symptoms were either not recruited or represented only a small proportion of the patients enrolled in clinical trials, therefore, data regarding efficacy and safety in these patients is not available. In those with decompensated heart failure, systolic blood pressure <80 mm Hg or signs of peripheral hypoperfusion or dependence on intravenous inotropic agents, β-blockers should not be used. Otherwise, β-blockers (only carvedilol and long-acting metoprolol are approved in the United States) should be prescribed to all with stable heart failure unless a contraindication to their use is present (Table 7).

When β-blockers are used, treatment should be started at a low dose and the dose titrated up slowly to the maximum tolerated level. The patient should be monitored closely for changes in heart rate, blood pressure and weight gain because severe bradycardia, hypotension or worsening heart failure could be precipitated during initiation of β-blockade. Every effort should be made to achieve the target doses shown to be effective in major clinical trials (Table 10). It may be more than 2 to 3 months before any improvement is noticed, so lack of symptomatic improvement should not lead to discontinuation of therapy because the risk of disease progression, future clinical deterioration and major clinical events, including sudden death are reduced. In case cardiac decompensation occurs but is associated with only mild to moderate symptoms, the dose up-titration should be delayed for 2 to 4 weeks and the schedule of diuretics and angiotensin-converting enzyme inhibitors adjusted. In patients with a history of fluid retention, β-blockers should not be prescribed without diuretics to avoid fluid retention that can accompany the initiation of therapy. General fatigue, weakness or sense of lassitude may develop but usually resolves spontaneously within several weeks. If severe symptoms results, β-blockers should either be

Chapter 109 β-Adrenoceptor Blockers   1279

Table 9. Recommendations for Therapy With β-Blockers in Patients With Heart Failure (HF)

Asymptomatic LV Systolic Dysfunction (Stage B)

Class I

Patients with a recent MI regardless of ejection fraction or presence of heart failure.

Patients with reduced ejection fraction, regardless of history of MI.

Patients with tachyarrhythmias, such as atrial fibrillation with a rapid ventricular rate.

Class III

Absolute contraindications or allergies.

Symptomatic LV Systolic Dysfunction (Stage C)

Class I

All stable patients, unless contraindicated. Patients should have no or minimal fluid retention and have not required recent treatment with an intravenous positive inotropic agent.

Class III

Patients with overt heart failure and pulmonary edema or other contraindications to β-blocker therapy.

Heart Failure With Preserved LV Systolic Function

Class I

Patients with uncontrolled systolic and diastolic hypertension.

Patients with rapid ventricular rate with atrial tachyarrhythmias.

Class IIb

Patients with controlled hypertension to minimize symptoms of heart failure.

decreased by 50% (for pulmonary edema) or held (for cardiogenic shock) and intravenous inotropes whose effects are mediated independently of the β-receptor (such as a phosphodiesterase inhibitor, preferentially milrinone) or vasodilators (nitroprusside or nitroglycerin) used. If β-blocker therapy is discontinued temporarily, it could be started at the previous dose if held for less than 3 days or at one-half the previous dose if held between 3 and 7 days and then resumed and up-titrated as before. If discontinued for more than 7 days, treatment should be resumed at the initial dose and up-titrated as before. An effort should be made to achieve

Table 10. β-Blocker Dosage Scheme Used in Placebo-Controlled Heart Failure Trials

Titration Schedule	Bisoprolol (mg)	Carvedilol (mg)	Metoprolol (mg)	Metoprolol CR/XL (mg)
First dose	1.25	3.125	5	25 (12.5)
Dosing schedule	1.25 x 1 wk	3.125 bid x 2 wk	5 bid x 1 wk	50 x 2 wk
	2.5 x 1 wk	6.25 bid x 2 wk	7.5 bid x 1 wk	100 x 2 wk
	3.75 x 1 wk	12.5 bid x 2 wk	25 bid x 1 wk	
	5.0 x 4 wk	25.0 bid	37.5 bid x 1 wk	
	7.5 x 4 wk	if wt > 75 kg upto	50 bid x 1 wk	
	10.0 qd	50.0 bid	75 bid	200 qd
Target daily dose (mg)	10	50	100-150	200

*12.5 mg was recommended for patients with NYHA class III or IV.
bid, twice daily; qd, once daily; CR/XL, extended release.

the target dose (Table 10); however, if the target dose is not tolerated, a low dose of β-blocker should be maintained even if the symptoms do not improve, because long-term treatment may reduce the risk of major clinical events. Abrupt withdrawal should be avoided (unless clearly indicated), because it could precipitate clinical deterioration.

In patients with diastolic ventricular dysfunction with preserved systolic function, such as those with hypertensive heart disease, hypertrophic cardiomyopathy or elderly, β-blockers are beneficial in reducing symptoms of heart failure by slowing the heart rate and improving ventricular filling and stroke volume. Only limited data is available from clinical trials to guide the management of patients with heart failure due to diastolic dysfunction. β-Blockers are beneficial and recommended for the treatment of comorbid conditions (Table 4), such as hypertension, atrial fibrillation with rapid ventricular rate response or myocardial ischemia to control factors that are known to impair ventricular relaxation.

Hypertension

β-Blockers are recommended as first line treatment for hypertension along with diuretics. β-Blockers may be very valuable in patients with a history of myocardial infarction, coronary artery disease, diabetes, heart failure, and/or tachyarrhythmias. When β-blockers are given chronically, they lower blood pressure by effects on the heart, blood vessels, renin-angiotensin system, central nervous system, and perhaps the autonomic nerve terminals. In the vascular system, β-receptor blockade oppose β_2-mediated vasodilation and, thus, may result in an initial increase in peripheral resistance from unopposed β-receptor-mediated vasoconstriction; however, with chronic use, peripheral resistance decreases.

As a class, β-blockers have proven efficacy in hypertension and are well tolerated when used alone or in combination with diuretics or vasodilator agents. Together with diuretics, β-blockers are recommended as first line therapy for hypertension. Several randomized controlled trials have demonstrated reduction in ventricular hypertrophy, stroke, heart failure, coronary events, and mortality with control of blood pressure with β-blockers in hypertensive patients, but the benefits are less consistent than with diuretics. Successful reduction of blood pressure with β-blockers in diabetic patients produces renal protective effects with reduction in proteinuria and deterioration of glomerular filtration rates. β-Blockers may be less effective in elderly African Americans than elderly white patients or young African Americans.

Labetalol is well tolerated during pregnancy and is recommended for the treatment of acute severe hypertension in preeclampsia. Propanolol and labetalol are preferred if a β-blockers is indicated for the treatment of hypertension during lactation. Intravenous administration of labetalol, which has both β- and α-adrenergic blocking properties and a rapid onset of action, is recommended for the treatment of hypertensive emergencies and severe hypertension.

Aortic Dissection and Aneurysm

By reducing the velocity of left ventricular ejection fraction and the propulsive stress on the aortic wall, β-blockers are useful in the acute and long-term management of aortic dissection. In patients with aortic dilatation, such as with Marfan syndrome, β-blocker may prevent rapid progression of aortic enlargement.

Neurocardiogenic Syncope

In vasovagal syncope, β-blockers are believed to abort the full syncope response by suppressing the neurocardiogenic reflex.

Glaucoma

β-Blockers by suppressing the flow of aqueous humor are effective in lowering intraocular pressure in patients with various forms of glaucoma.

Thyrotoxicosis

β-Blockade is commonly used in thyrotoxicosis to control symptoms due to tachycardia, tremor, and nervousness. β-Blockade also reduces the vascularity of the thyroid gland, thereby facilitating operation.

Side Effects of β-Blockers

The absolute and relative contraindications to β-blocker use are summarized in Table 7. Most of the cardiac side effects of β-blockers are related to their negative chronotropic, dromotropic and inotropic properties. They may cause sinus node slowing and heart block in patients with sinus node dysfunction or AV conduction disease. The use of β-blockers with intrinsic sympathomimetic activity in these patients may be better because these agents may reduce profound slowing of heart rate at rest, while preventing excessive heart rate increases in response to exercise or other stress. Unlike class I and class III antiarrhythmics, β-blockers have a remarkably good safety record in regard to ventricular proarrhythmia.

In patients with ischemic heart disease, abrupt discontinuation of β-blockers after chronic use should be avoided because of possible rebound hypersensitivity to physiologic adrenergic stimulation due to "upregulation" of the number of β-adrenergic receptors that can result in myocardial ischemia or infarction (withdrawal syndrome). In patients with severe ventricular systolic dysfunction, congestive heart failure may be precipitated, especially in those in whom cardiac output is dependent on sympathetic drive. In carefully selected patients with moderate-to-severe heart failure, however, the safety of β-blockade with proper dose titration and monitoring has been demonstrated in several clinical trials.

Other adverse effects, especially with nonselective β-blockers, include bronchospasm in patients with history of asthma, fatigue and central nervous system effects, such as sedation, sleep disturbances, hallucination, depression and rarely psychotic reactions. The lipid soluble β-blockers are more prone to affect the central nervous system; however, adverse nervous system effects may occur with any β-blocker used for a long time. Impotence and worsening of symptoms due to severe peripheral vascular or vasospastic disorders may occur. Because of the overall beneficial effects of β-blockers in diabetic patients, their use should not be avoided due to concerns regarding masking of hypoglycemia symptoms in those requiring insulin therapy or exacerbation of glucose intolerance or insulin resistance. These effects and lipid abnormalities (triglyceride elevation and HDL reduction) are typically greater with noncardioselective agents such as propranolol, nadolol, and timolol than cardioselective ones such as metoprolol and atenolol. In hypertensive patients with type 2 diabetes, initial therapy with atenolol was as effective as the ACE inhibitor captopril in reducing macrovascular end-points. Topical ocular β-blockers (such as timolol) used for treatment of glaucoma may be absorbed from the conjunctival mucosa and have serious adverse effects on the heart (bradycardia and hypotension). Choosing β1-selective drugs with poor lipid solubility, additional intrinsic sympathomimetic

activity, or β-adrenergic blockade may help reduce some of these adverse effects. The safety of β-blockers during pregnancy has not been well established and may decrease placental blood flow, and the potential benefit should be weighed against the risk to the fetus (low birth weight). β-Blockers are excreted in breast milk.

■ In patients with ischemic heart disease, abrupt discontinuation of β-blockers after chronic use can result in withdrawal syndrome, with rebound hypersensitivity to physiologic adrenergic stimulation, and can lead to myocardial ischemia or infarction.

Overdose

In overdose, β-blockers may cause central nervous system depression and potentiate hypotension, hypoglycemia and bronchospasm. In a life-threatening situation with β-blocker overdose or toxicity, the adverse cardiac effects of β-blockers may be counteracted with glucagon (100 mg/kg over 1 min, then 1-5 mg/hr), isoproterenol (up to 0.10 g/kg per minute), or high dose dobutamine (15 μg/kg per minute) infusion. The intravenous administration of atropine should be tried for symptomatic bradycardia, and a temporary pacemaker may be needed in refractory cases.

Drug Interactions

β-Blockers should be used with caution in conjunction with drugs that slow conduction (digitalis and calcium channel blockers), and those that have negative inotropic effects (calcium channel blockers and disopyramide). Hepatically metabolized β-blocker (propranolol, metoprolol, carvedilol, labetalol) levels are increased by cimetidine which reduces hepatic blood flow. β-Blockers by decreasing hepatic flow may effect blood levels of drugs, such as lidocaine that are primarily metabolized in the liver.

Dosing

All β-blockers have about the same antianginal and antiarrhythmic efficacy at comparable doses, and no one agent is superior to other at equipotent doses. Clinical trials have demonstrated that several β-blockers are beneficial in heart failure but currently only carvedilol and extended release metoprolol are approved by the U.S. Food and Drug Administration

Table 11. Usual Daily Doses of β-Adrenergic Agents

	Usual Daily Dosage	Dose Reduction With Renal Impairment
Acebutolol	200-600 mg q 12 hr	Y
Atenolol	50-100 (up to 200 mg) q day	N
Betaxolol	10-20 mg/day	N
Bisoprolol	2.5-10 mg q day	N
Carvedilol	12.5-25 mg q 12 hr	N
Esmolol	IV LD 500 µg/kg over 1 min; then 50-300 µg/kg/min	Y
Labetalol	100 mg q 12 hr (up to 400 mg bid)	N
	IV 20 mg over 2 min, add 40 and 80 mg at 10 min interval. Infusion 2 mg/min	
Metoprolol	50-200 mg q 12 hr, IV 5 mg x 3 at 2 min intervals	N
Nadolol	40-80 mg (up to 240 mg) q day	Y
Pindolol	2.5-7.5 mg 3 times daily	Y
Propranolol	80 160 mg q 12 hr (extended release), IV 1 mg/min (up to 6 mg)	N
Timolol	10-30 mg q 12 hr	N
Sotalol	PO 80-240 mg q 12 hr (for arrhythmias)	Y

All doses are for oral preparation, unless indicated.
IV, intravenously; LD, loading dose; Y, yes; N, no.

for management of chronic heart failure. The usual daily dosage of various β-blockers are summarized in Table 11. The dose should be adjusted to keep resting heart rate of 55 to 60 beats/min and exertional heart rate less than 100 beats/min in patients with angina or atrial fibrillation. In individual patients, ancillary properties, such as β_1-adrenergic receptor selectivity, lipid solubility, vasodilation, intrinsic sympathomimetic activity, longer half-life, and cost may affect selection of one agent over the others.

ANTIPLATELET AGENTS

Garvan C. Kane, MD

Yong-Mei Cha, MD

Joseph G. Murphy, MD

Antiplatelet drugs play a central role in the practice of cardiology and include aspirin, platelet ADP-receptor antagonists and platelet glycoprotein IIb/IIIa inhibitors.

PLATELET BIOLOGY

Platelet arterial wall adhesion, activation and aggregation play a pivotal role in the pathogenesis of arterial thrombosis and acute coronary syndromes. Hence agents with antiplatelet activity are amongst the most commonly prescribed drugs in the prevention and treatment of coronary disease. All antiplatelet agents interrupt one or more of the biological steps that lead from atherosclerotic plaque rupture to arterial thrombosis (Fig. 1). Rupture of an arterial plaque and disruption of the vascular endothelium expose a variety of factors that activate and recruit circulating platelets to aggregate. Some of these factors are released from the subendothelium (collagen, von Willebrand factor) while others are released by activated and degranulated platelets (thromboxane A2, adenosine diphosphate (ADP), serotonin). Intact vascular endothelium functions to prevent platelet activation and aggregation by releasing prostacyclin and nitric oxide. Vascular endothelial damage is an early and prominent feature of vascular disease that facilitates an unfavorable tilt in the balance between antiaggregatory forces and proaggregatory forces. Upon activation, intracellular platelet calcium level rises and platelets undergo a conformational change due to contraction of platelet actin and myosin. Platelets change from smooth discs to spiny spheres with multiple protruding pseudopods thereby increasing the expression of glycoprotein (GP) IIb/IIIa receptors on their cell surface. The activation of these receptors allows crosslinks of fibrinogen to form between platelets initiating a cascade of platelet aggregation with superimposed fibrin thrombus formation.

ASPIRIN

Acetylsalicyclic acid (aspirin) inhibits the synthesis of thromboxane A2 (TX A2) by the irreversible inhibition of the COX-1 isoform of the enzyme cyclooxygenase. It has a potent and long-lasting effect (days) and inhibits a major inducer of platelet activation—TX A2. Mature platelets lack a nucleus and cannot synthesize new enzymatic proteins; thus platelet cyclooxygenase activity is blocked for the lifespan of the platelet and is not restored until new platelets are produced by the bone marrow. Aspirin is a poor inhibitor of the COX-2 isoform of cyclooxygenase which mediates inflammation.

Aspirin also has effects on thromboxane produc-

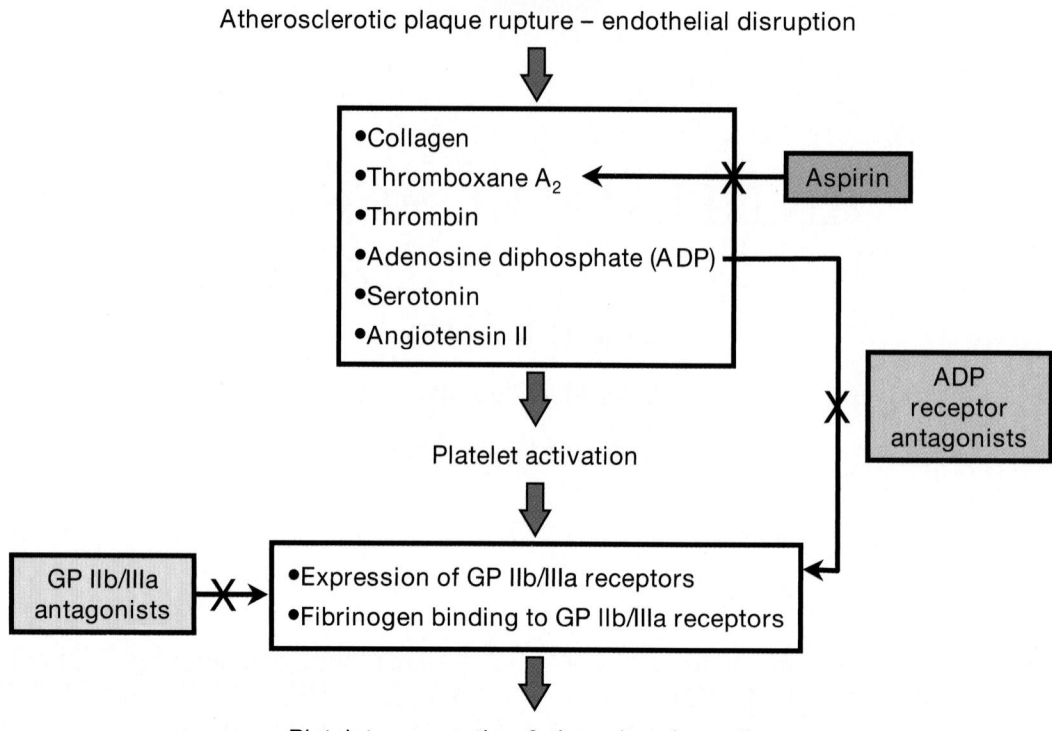

Atherosclerotic plaque rupture – endothelial disruption

• Collagen
• Thromboxane A$_2$ ← ✕ ← Aspirin
• Thrombin
• Adenosine diphosphate (ADP)
• Serotonin
• Angiotensin II

ADP receptor antagonists

Platelet activation

GP IIb/IIIa antagonists ✕

• Expression of GP IIb/IIIa receptors
• Fibrinogen binding to GP IIb/IIIa receptors

Platelet aggregation & thrombus formation

Fig. 1. Steps involved following plaque rupture and targets for antiplatelet activity.

tion in vascular endothelium and during inflammation, although these effects are more transient. The beneficial effect of chronic low dose aspirin administration in the prevention of myocardial infarction is seen particularly in patients with elevated levels of C-reactive protein.

While other nonsteroidal anti-inflammatory agents also inhibit cyclooxygenase they do so reversibly and so their duration of action is limited. Low dose aspirin (75 mg or 81 mg) daily provides maximal chronic antiplatelet inhibition; however in the setting of an acute coronary syndrome 325 mg should be given to achieve rapid and complete cyclooxygenase inhibition as low dose aspirin takes several days to completely inhibit platelet function. This is typically achieved through the administration of four chewable 81 mg aspirin tablets. Aspirin reduces the incidence of death and recurrent myocardial infarction in patients with acute coronary syndromes including ST and non-ST elevation myocardial infarction and unstable angina. Chronic use of aspirin leads to a significant incidence of gastric irritation with a significant gastrointestinal bleeding rate of 0.1-0.2% per annum. Moreover there is a slight increase in the rate of hemorrhagic stroke in

patients taking chronic aspirin therapy. Aspirin may reduce the impact of angiotensin converting enzyme inhibition due to competitive actions on renal hemodynamics. This effect is minimized through the use of only 81 mg daily. There are some data to suggest taking aspirin at night has a beneficial effect on blood pressure control. Some patients are relatively resistant to the antiplatelet effects of aspirin, a condition commonly called "aspirin resistance" in which cardiovascular events recur despite regular aspirin usage. Biochemical aspirin resistance is defined as a failure of suppression of thromboxane generation (measured as high urinary concentrations of thromboxane A$_2$ metabolites) or continued platelet aggregation in vitro with platelet agonists (ADP and arachidonic acid). Aspirin resistance significantly increases the long-term risk of death, myocardial infarct or stroke. Late coronary stent thrombosis (>30 days post procedure) occuring with both bare-metal and drug-eluting stents is strongly linked with cessation of aspirin therapy.

ISIS-2 Trial

The ISIS-2 Trial (Second International Study of

Infarct Survival was the classical randomized trial that demonstrated that aspirin administered within 24 hours of acute ST elevation myocardial infarction reduced cardiovascular mortality (by 23 percent at five weeks' follow-up) comparable to the early mortality benefit of thrombolysis with streptokinase (25 percent mortality benefit). The other key finding of the ISIS-2 trial was that the mortality benefit of streptokinase and aspirin were additive with an absolute mortality reduction of 2.4 cardiovascular deaths per 100 patients treated and a relative cardiovascular mortality benefit of 42%.

INDICATIONS FOR ASPIRIN USE

■ Acute coronary syndromes including ST elevation and non-ST elevation myocardial infarction.
■ Acute thrombotic stroke.
■ Secondary prevention post myocardial infarction.
■ Secondary prevention in stable angina pectoris.
■ Secondary prevention post coronary artery bypass grafting.
■ Secondary prevention in cerebrovascular disease.
■ Pretreatment and lifelong treatment in the setting of percutaneous coronary (or other arterial bed) intervention.
■ Primary prevention in patients at moderate or greater cardiovascular risk (10 year cardiovascular risk >10%) American Heart Association guideline but not FDA approved.
■ Primary prevention in diabetics with one or more additional risk factors.
■ Prevention of stroke in atrial fibrillation when warfarin is contraindicated.
■ In addition to warfarin in patients at high risk for mechanical valve thromboenbolism.
■ Possible benefit in renovascular hypertension by inhibiting formation of prostaglandins involved in renin release.

ADP RECEPTOR ANTAGONISTS

Ticlopidine and clopidogrel are thienopyridine derivatives that act to irreversibly inhibit the ADP-receptor on platelets thereby inhibiting ADP-mediated activation of the GP IIb/IIIa receptors and platelet aggregation. These agents have independent and additive antiplatelet effects to those of aspirin and are key therapies in interventional cardiology and in patients in whom aspirin is contraindicated or ineffective. Either clopidogrel or ticlopidine can be used in addition to aspirin following percutaneous coronary intervention to prevent stent thrombosis. Because of the widespread use of coronary stents in clinical practice there is now a large population of patients who require prolonged treatment with potent antiplatelet agents: this impacts noncardiovascular care as it takes 5-7 days after ADP receptor antagonists cessation for the production of new platelets to occur and a return to normal of platelet function.

The main clinical differences between ticlopidine and clopidogrel are 1) the major side-effect of neutropenia (2.5% incidence with ticlopidine) is much less frequently observed with clopidogrel (0.05%). It is recommended that for the first 3 months on ticlopidine, a complete blood count is measured every two weeks. 2) Meta-analysis comparisons suggest a potential superiority of clopidogrel over ticlopidine with regard to a reduction in cardiovascular risk with a lower risk of gastrointestinal bleeding complications. For this reason, clopidogrel has replaced ticlopidine as the first line ADP receptor antagonist in clinical use.

Clopidogrel when added to aspirin in patients with both ST and non-ST elevation myocardial infarction reduces cardiovascular events even in patients not undergoing percutaneous intervention. The main clinical problem is that clopidogrel increases major bleeding and the need for reoperation for bleeding in patients who need to undergo coronary artery bypass grafting within five days of clopidogrel use. Hence the timing of clopidogrel use in patients with acute coronary syndromes varies with different institutional practice. Current guidelines on non-ST elevation acute coronary syndrome suggest that it may be preferable to delay the loading dose of clopidogrel until the coronary anatomy is defined and it is known that the patient will not require urgent coronary bypass grafting, particularly in the setting of an early invasive strategy when patients go to cardiac catheterization within 24 hours of presentation with an acute coronary syndrome. That said the absolute benefit obtained by the early administration of clopidogrel may be greater than the added overall risk in the subset of patients who require coronary artery surgery.

The antithrombotic effects of clopidogrel and ticlopidine are dose-dependent and both require oral loading to achieve early beneficial effects. After clopidogrel is given at the typical loading dose of 300 mg, within 5 hours approximately 80% of platelet activity is inhibited. Some studies have recommended the higher load of 600 mg load to ensure a more rapid greater inhibition of platelet activity. The maintenance dose of clopidogrel is 75 mg daily, sufficient after loading to achieve maximal platelet inhibition.

Important Clopidogrel Trials

CURE Trial

The CURE trial reported the effects of clopidogrel added to aspirin in acute coronary syndromes without ST-segment elevation. Patients received clopidogrel or placebo in addition to aspirin. The primary outcome was a composite end point of cardiovascular death, nonfatal myocardial infarction, or stroke at one year and occurred in 9.3% of the patients in the clopidogrel group and 11.4% of the patients in the placebo group (relative risk, 80%; $P<0.001$). More major bleeding occurred in the clopidogrel group (3.7% versus 2.7% with a relative risk of 138%; $P=0.001$), but life-threatening bleeding was not significantly more common. Clinical benefit was evident at 24 hours and increased with time. CARE proved that clopidogrel was beneficial in patients with acute coronary syndromes without ST-segment elevation but at an increased risk of major bleeding (Fig. 2 and 3).

CAPRIE Trial

The CAPRIE trial (Clopidogrel versus Aspirin in Patients at Risk of Ischemic Events) evaluated clopidrogel in patients with atherosclerotic vascular disease (recent stroke, MI, or symptomatic peripheral arterial disease). Patients treated with clopidogrel 75 mg daily, showed an 8.7% reduction ($P=0.043$) in the composite end point of ischemic stroke, myocardial infarction, or vascular death compared with patients treated with aspirin 325 mg. Clopidogrel has a lower bleeding risk than aspirin. CAPRIE proved that long-term administration of clopidogrel to patients with atherosclerotic vascular disease was more effective than aspirin in reducing long-term cardiovascular events and at a lower bleeding risk than aspirin.

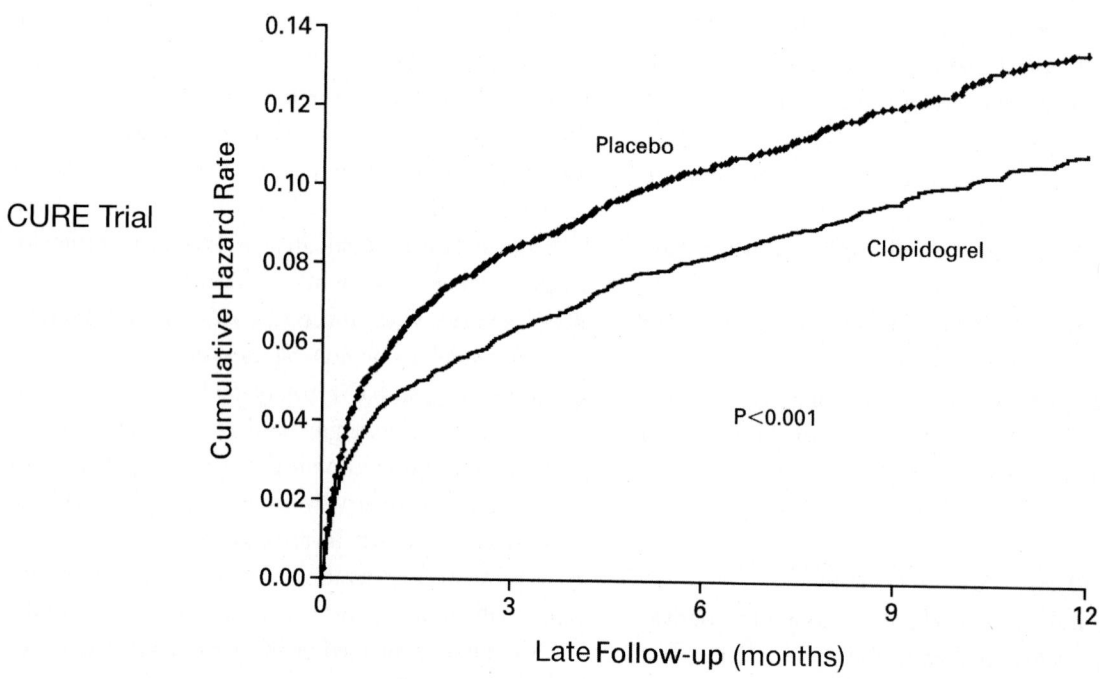

Fig. 2. Cumulative hazard rates for the first primary outcome (death from cardiovascular causes, nonfatal myocardial infarction, or stroke) during the 12 months of the study. The results demonstrate the sustained effect of clopidogrel.

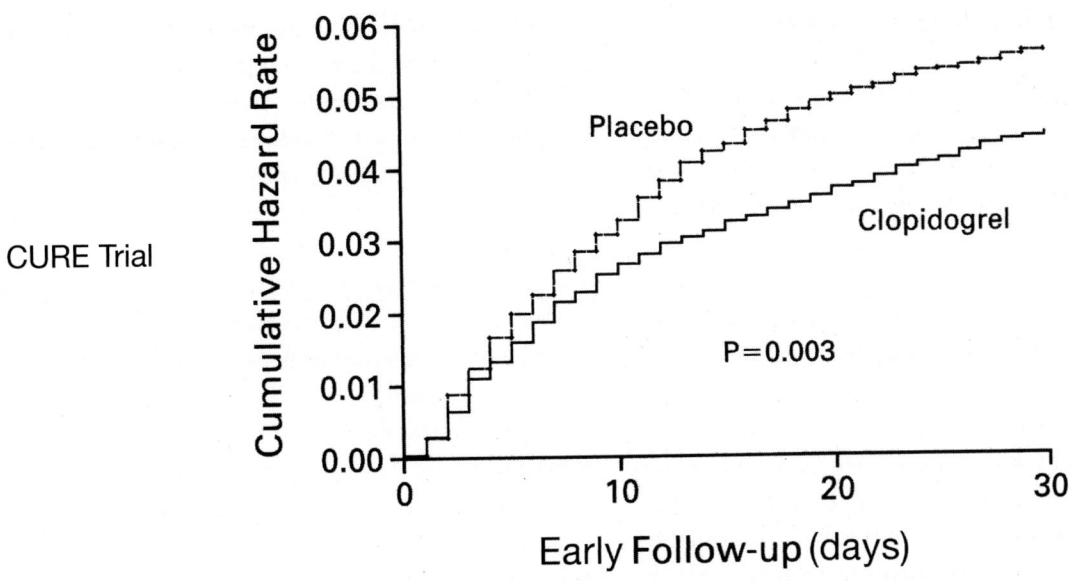

CURE Trial

Fig. 3. Cumulative hazard rates for the first primary outcome (death from cardiovascular causes, nonfatal myocardial infarction, or stroke) during the first 30 days after randomization. The results demonstrate the early effect of clopidogrel.

CREDO Trial

The CREDO trial (Clopidogrel for the Reduction of Events During Observation [CREDO]) investigated pretreatment and long-term clopidogrel combined with aspirin to prevent cardiovascular events in patients undergoing elective PCI. The conclusion of the pretreatment arm was that clopidogrel (300 mg loading dose) needed to be given at least six hours before PCI to achieve a reduction in complications related to stent thrombosis—death, myocardial infarction, urgent target vessel revascularization). The long-term treatment arm concluded that clopidogrel (75 mg daily) added to aspirin achieved at 1 year, a 26.9 percent relative risk reduction (P=0.02) in the composite end point of death, MI, and stroke. This benefit occurred beyond the standard 28-day period of treatment. There was a trend toward an increase in major bleeding in the clopidogrel group.

ACTIVE W Trial

The ACTIVE W Trial (Clopidogrel plus aspirin versus oral anticoagulation for atrial fibrillation trial) proved that oral anticoagulation therapy was superior to clopidogrel plus aspirin for prevention of vascular events in patients with atrial fibrillation at high risk of

stroke, especially in those already taking oral anticoagulation therapy. The primary outcome was first occurrence of stroke, non-CNS systemic embolus, myocardial infarction, or vascular death which occurred with a relative risk of 144%: P=0.0003) in the treatment arm.

CLARITY-TIMI 28 Study

The CLARITY-TIMI 28 Study evaluated the addition of Clopidogrel to Aspirin and Fibrinolytic Therapy for the treatment of patients ≤75 years with ST-Segment Elevation Myocardial Infarction. The trial contained approximately 3,500 patients who presented within 12 hours after the onset of an ST-elevation myocardial infarction and randomly assigned them to receive clopidogrel (300-mg loading dose, followed by 75 mg once daily) or placebo. Patients received a fibrinolytic agent, aspirin, and when appropriate, heparin and were scheduled to undergo angiography 48 to 192 hours after the start of study medication. The primary study end point was a composite of an occluded infarct-related artery (defined by a Thrombolysis in Myocardial Infarction flow grade of 0 or 1) on angiography or death or recurrent myocardial infarction before angiography. The study was not powered to detect a survival benefit, and none was seen.

The rates of the primary end point were 21.7 percent in the placebo group and 15.0 percent in the clopidogrel group, representing an absolute reduction of 6.7 percentage points in the rate and a 36 percent reduction in the odds of the end point with clopidogrel therapy ($P<0.001$). By 30 days, clopidogrel therapy reduced the odds of the composite end point of death from cardiovascular causes, recurrent myocardial infarction, or recurrent ischemia leading to the need for urgent revascularization by 20 percent ($P=0.03$). The rates of major bleeding and intracranial hemorrhage were similar in the two groups.

In patients 75 years of age or younger who have an ST-segment elevation myocardial infarction and receive aspirin and a standard fibrinolytic regimen, the addition of clopidogrel improves the patency rate of the infarct-related artery and reduces ischemic complications without an increase in the risk of major bleeding complications.

COMMIT Trial

The COMMIT Trial (ClOpidogrel and Metoprolol in Myocardial Infarction Trial) also called the Second Chinese Cardiac Study (CCS-2) was a randomized placebo-controlled trial of clopidogrel added to aspirin in the emergency treatment of approximately 46,000 patients with acute myocardial infarction. Most patients (93%) had ST-segment elevation or left bundle branch block while 7% of patients had ST-segment depression. This study took place in a wide range of specialist and nonspecialist hospitals throughout China. Patients who underwent primary PCI for their myocardial infarction were excluded from this study because previous trials had shown that clopidogrel was beneficial in the setting of primary PCI. Addition of clopidogrel produced a highly significant (9%; $P=0.002$) reduction in the combined end point of death, reinfarction, or stroke corresponding to nine fewer events per 1,000 patients treated for about 2 weeks with clopidogrel. There was a significant 7%; ($P=0·03$) reduction in all cause death with clopidogrel. These effects on death, reinfarction, and stroke were consistent across a wide range of patients and independent of other treatments being used. Considering all fatal, transfused, or cerebral bleeds together, no significant excess risk was noted with clopidogrel or in patients aged older than 70 years or in those given fibrinolytic therapy.

The COMMIT trial investigators estimated that if early clopidogrel therapy was given to just 10% of the 10 million patients who have a myocardial infarction worldwide every year then it would save about 5,000 deaths and 5,000 nonfatal reinfarctions and strokes.

INDICATIONS FOR CLOPIDOGREL USE

- Pre and post-percutaneous coronary intervention.
- Acute coronary syndromes particularly non-ST elevation myocardial infarction with or without percutaneous intervention*.
- Secondary prevention in patients with recent stroke, myocardial infarction or documented peripheral vascular disease.
- In place of aspirin in those who are intolerant or clinically resistant to aspirin therapy.

*Typically clopidogrel is withheld until coronary anatomy is defined if there is a reasonable possibility of the need for coronary artery bypass grafting in the immediate future.

Dipyridamole inhibits phosphodiesterase-mediated breakdown of platelet cyclic AMP which in turn prevents platelet activation by multiple mechanisms. It has largely been superseded by other antiplatelet drugs. Dipyridamole may be used in combination with Coumadin in patients with prosthetic mechanical valves. Dipyridamole has a major interaction with adenosine.

GLYCOPROTEIN IIB/IIIA INHIBITORS

Located on the platelet cell surface, the glycoprotein (GP) IIb/IIIa receptor is a member of the integrin family of receptors and plays a central role in platelet aggregation. Platelet activation in turn induces a conformational change that allows the binding of circulating fibrinogen to GP IIb/IIIa receptors on adjoining platelets promoting platelet aggregation. While oral GP IIb/IIIa receptor antagonists have shown no clinical benefit and in fact appear to increase mortality, three intravenous agents with proven therapeutic roles are currently available for clinical use. Abciximab, is a hybrid human/murine monoclonal antibody directed against the GP IIb/IIIa receptor and tirofiban and eptifibatide are high affinity nonantibody inhibitors of the receptor. For this reason both tirofiban and epti-fibatide have a substantially lower cost than abciximab. All three GP IIb/IIIa inhibitors are given by the intra-venous route for a period of hours-days in patients with a medium or high-risk acute coronary syndrome and/or are scheduled to undergo medium-high risk percutaneous coronary intervention. Abciximab com-bined with stenting reduces mortality when compared with stenting alone in high-medium risk PCI patients. In patients with a non-ST elevation acute coronary syndrome GP IIb/IIIa inhibitor use is most beneficial in those patients at high risk (diabetes mellitus, ischemic ECG changes, elevated troponin). Much of the benefit of GP IIb/IIIa inhibitor use in acute coro-nary syndromes is seen in patients who subsequently undergo percutaneous intervention. The GP IIb/IIIa inhibitor infusion should be initiated on admission and continued for 48 to 72 hours or until a fixed time fol-lowing percutaneous intervention. Aspirin and either a reduced dose of unfractionated or low-molecular-weight heparin therapy are always coadministered with GP IIb/IIIa inhibitors. Study data of GP IIb/IIIa inhibitors without supplemental heparin have been dis-appointing.

Given as an initial bolus GP IIb/IIIa receptor antagonists induce a rapid dose-dependent inhibition of platelet function as measured by platelet aggrega-tion in ex vivo studies. Subsequent intravenous infu-sion achieves a sustained inhibition. The half-life of eptifibatide and tirofiban is relatively short with a return of platelet function within a few hours of ter-mination of the infusion. However the effect of abcix-imab on platelets is irreversible and hence the action can persist for a few days until new platelets are pro-duced.

The benefits of the GP IIb/IIIa receptor antago-nists in acute coronary syndromes are at the expense of bleeding risk. Data from multiple randomized trials suggest up to a 2-fold increase in the major bleeding rate and need for blood transfusions. Most of the bleeding complications are either from the arterial puncture and sheath site or mediastinal bleeding in patients requiring urgent coronary artery bypass graft-ing. There appears to be little if any significantly increased risk of intracranial hemorrhage over that seen in the absence of these agents. In rare incidences (<1%) thrombocytopenia, that can be severe, has been seen with GP IIb/IIIa inhibitor use, particularly with abcix-imab. Interestingly the thrombocytopenia occurs very early, typically within the initial 24 hours of use, occa-sionally within a few hours. The incidence of thrombo-cytopenia from GP IIb/IIIa receptor antagonists is associated with both higher rates of severe bleeding and need for blood transfusions and a higher incidence of death, myocardial infarction, or the need for target ves-sel revascularization within 30 days. A proportion of the thrombocytopenia though is not real and is merely due to platelet clumping. Monitoring of platelet counts is recommended before GP IIb/IIIa receptor antago-nist use (particularly abciximab), within a few hours of the initial bolus and then daily as long as drug infusion persists. Pseudothrombocytopenia can be out ruled by checking a blood sample in sodium citrate or a blood smear. If significant bleeding occurrs or the drop in platelet count is sizeable the GP IIb/IIIa receptor inhibitor should be stopped.

The relative efficacy of one intravenous GP IIb/IIIa inhibitor over another is unknown as there is limited direct comparative data. In the TARGET study abciximab had a small short-term but unsustained advantage over tirofiban, likely related to more com-plete initial platelet inhibition. Eptifibatide appears to have similar efficacy to abciximab.

There has been a lot of interest in the combination of GP IIb/IIIa inhibitors with thrombolytics. Trials to date have suggested a trend towards better reperfusion with greater achievement of TIMI III flow rates offset by a tendency for greater bleeding rates resulting in as yet no clear proven overall clinical benefit.

Randomized trial data for glycoprotein IIb/IIIa inhibitors are summarized in the chapter on Interventional Cardiology and Coronary Stents.

Indications for Glycoprotein IIb/IIIa Inhibitors

- Acute coronary syndromes (without ST segment ele-vation) at medium or high risk* particularly if under-going percutaneous intervention.
- High-risk percutaneous intervention**.

*Medium or high risk features include prolonged and/or rest pain; dynamic ischemic ECG changes; ele-vated cardiac biomarkers; diabetes mellitus.
** Acute coronary syndrome, chronically occluded arteries, vein graft lesions, diabetes

Relative Contraindications for Glycoprotein IIb/IIIa Inhibitors

- Bleeding, surgery or recent stroke within previous 30 days.
- Intracranial hemorrhage (ever).
- Uncontrolled systemic hypertension (blood pressure >200/110 mm Hg).
- Aortic dissection.
- Acute pericarditis.
- Platelet count <100,000.

CHARISMA Trial

The CHARISMA trial (Clopidogrel for High Atherothrombotic Risk and Ischemic Stabilization Management and Avoidance) tested the putative benefits of clopidogrel in a broad population of patients at high risk for atherothrombotic events. Approximately 15,500 patients with either a clinical diagnosis of cardiovascular disease or multiple cardiovascular risk factors were randomized to receive clopidogrel plus low-dose aspirin or low-dose aspirin alone for an extended period of time (median of 28 months). The primary end point (composite of myocardial infarction, stroke, or death from cardiovascular causes) was similar in both treatment groups—6.8 percent with clopidogrel plus aspirin versus 7.3 percent with aspirin alone (relative risk, 0.93; P=0.22). There was a suggestion of benefit with clopidogrel in patients with symptomatic atherothrombosis and a suggestion of harm in patients with multiple cardiovascular risk factors. Overall, clopidogrel plus aspirin was not significantly more effective than aspirin alone in reducing the rate of myocardial infarction, stroke, or death from cardiovascular causes in patients with stable cardiovascular disease or strong risk factors for cardiovascular disease.

111

Cardiac Drug Adverse Effects and Interactions

Narith N. Ou, PharmD

Lance J. Oyen, PharmD

Arshad Jahangir, MD

"Primum non nocere": "first, do no harm." Most cardiac drug interactions and side effects can be prevented by a careful review of patient's age, clinical and drug history, and baseline tests including ventricular function (Echo), conduction system function (EKG), liver (AST), and kidney function (creatinine). Adverse drug reactions are often dose-dependent, and correct dosing minimizes patient risk.

PRINCIPLES OF DRUG THERAPY

Drug side effects and interactions can occur for pharmacokinetic or pharmacodynamic reasons.

Basic Concepts

The *half-life* of a drug is the time course necessary for the quantity of the active drug in the body (or plasma concentration) to be reduced to half of its original level through various metabolic and excretory pathways.

Pharmacokinetics is the time course of drug action in the body—what the body does to the drug.

Pharmacodynamics refers to the effect of a drug at its site of action—what a drug does to the body.

Pharmacokinetics includes the totality of drug absorption into the bloodstream, distribution to the site of drug action, metabolism to an inactive form, and final elimination.

Renal or liver failure can markedly decrease the clearance of a drug.

Pharmacodynamics is the effect of the drug at the site of action (cell membrane or receptor). Coadministered drugs, advanced age, and intercurrent disease affect drug dynamics. For example, β-blockers exert a lesser pharmacologic effect in the elderly than in the young, but when doses are titrated, the clinical benefit can be the same regardless of age. More often, cardiac drugs have a heightened effect in the elderly and initiation at half the normal starting doses is prudent in most cases.

- Pharmacokinetics refers to the absorption, distribution, metabolism (bioconversion), and elimination of drugs.
- Pharmacodynamics refers to the effect of the drug at the cellular level.

The *therapeutic index* (Fig. 1) is the ratio of the toxic concentration to the minimally effective concentration. When this ratio is low (i.e., 2 or 3 or less, as with digoxin), small changes in pharmacokinetics can push the drug into the toxic range or pull the drug down and out of the therapeutic window.

- Therapeutic index = $\dfrac{\text{Toxic Effect Concentration}}{\text{Minimal Effective Concentration}}$

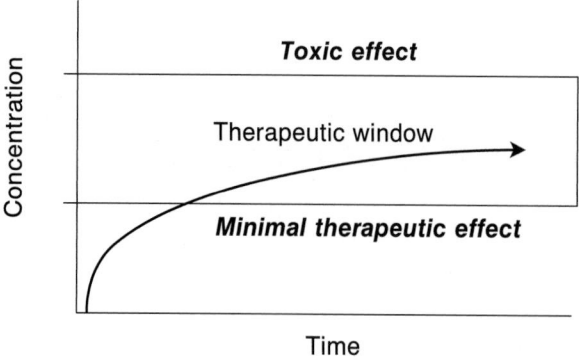

Fig. 1. Therapeutic window.

Liver and Kidney Function and Drug Therapy

Liver or kidney failure can result in decreased metabolism and elimination of specific drugs. For instance, the use of two class Ia antiarrhythmic agents without allowing adequate drug washout (at least 5 half-lives) increases the risk for torsades de pointes (Fig. 2). With renally eliminated drugs, the drug half-life and, consequently, the wash-out period are longer in patients with renal failure.

Renal dose adjustments and patient surveillance minimize the potential for toxic accumulation of drugs and metabolites (Table 1). The initiation of sotalol in a patient with renal dysfunction at routine doses may be well tolerated initially, but drug accumulation may result in torsades de pointes several days later as the concentration increases (Fig. 3).

Renal clearance of drugs eliminated primarily through the kidney is based on correlating drug clearance to the glomerular filtration rate (GFR). Assuming the drug clearance is largely via filtration without active secretion or reabsorption from the renal tubules, an estimated creatinine clearance is as follows:

$$\text{Creatinine Clearance (Cl}_{Cr}) = \frac{140 - \text{Age}}{72} \times \frac{\text{Ideal Body Weight in kg}}{\text{Serum Creatinine in mg/dL}}$$

(For females, answer of above formula multiplied by 0.85.)

$$\text{Ideal Body Weight (IBW)} = [(\text{Height \{in inches\}} - 60) \times (2.3)] + \# \text{ kg}$$
$$\# = 45 \text{ kg for females}$$
$$\# = 50 \text{ kg for males}$$

Drug substitution in renal insufficiency should be by drugs not metabolized by the kidney and therapeutically equivalent. An example would be the use of metoprolol instead of atenolol. Atenolol is eliminated primarily by the kidneys and metoprolol is not, yet both drugs are pharmacologically and clinically equivalent.

Generally, calcium channel blockers, most β-blockers, statins, and anticoagulants have little dependence on renal elimination. Diuretics, angiotensin-converting enzyme (ACE) inhibitors, fibrinic acids, phosphodiesterase inhibitors, and digoxin are all dependent on renal clearance. Cardiac drugs that are potentially nephrotoxic include ACE inhibitors, angiotensin receptor blockers (ARBs), aspirin, hydralazine, methyldopa, diuretics,

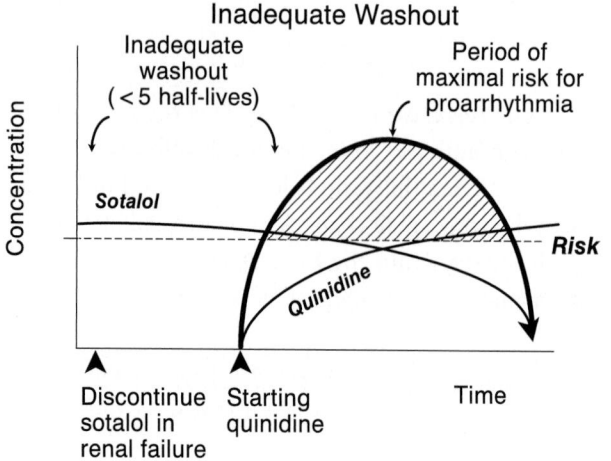

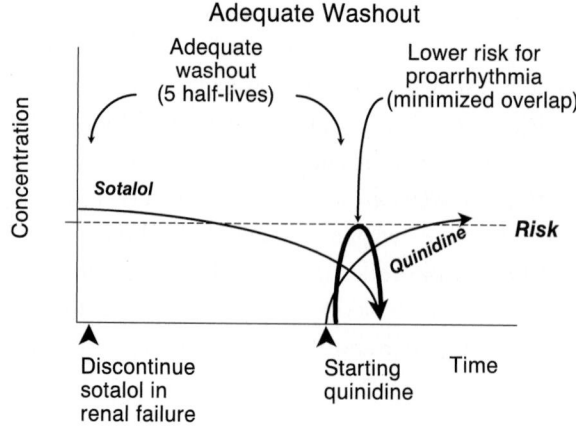

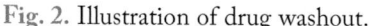

Fig. 2. Illustration of drug washout.

Table 1. Dosage Adjustments of Renally Eliminated Cardiovascular Agents

Drug	Clearance 30-50 ml/min	Clearance 10-30 ml/min	Clearance <10 ml/min	Dialyzed
Acebutolol	↓↓	↓↓↓	↓↓↓	HD
Amiloride	↓↓	↓↓↓	Avoid	
Atenolol	(<35, max 50 mg)	↓↓(<15)	↓↓	HD
Benazepril	↓↓ (max dose 40 mg/day)			
Bisoprolol	↓↓(<40)	max dose 10 mg/day		
Bretylium	↓-↓↓	↓-↓↓	Avoid	
Captopril	↓(35-75)	↓	↓↓	HD
Carteolol	↓↓(20-60)	↓↓(20-60)	↓↓↓(<20)	
Clofibrate	↓	↓↓(10-15)	Avoid	
Digoxin	Consult pahrmacist or package insert for adjustments; follow levels more frequently			
Disopyramide	↓(30-40)	↓↓(15-30)	↓↓↓(<15); follow levels	
Enalapril		↓↓	↓↓	HD, PD
Fenofibrate	Avoid			
Flecainide		Initial dose 100 mg/day	↓-↓↓(<20); follow levels	
Fosinopril			↓	
Hydralazine	↓	↓	↓↓-↓↓↓	
Lisinopril		↓↓	↓↓↓	HD
Low molecular-weight heparins		↓↓	↓↓	
Magnesium	Monitor closely levels and for signs of toxicity			
Milrinone	Consult pharmacist or package insert for adjustments			
Morphine	↓	↓	↓↓(Use caution)	
Nadolol	↓↓	↓↓	↓↓↓	HD
Nitroprusside	Monitor Thiocyanate levels and Cyanide toxicity; Risk: proportional to dosing rate, duration; inversely prortional to Creatininie Clearance			HD,PD
Procainamide	Consult pharmacist or package insert for adjustments: assess drug levels for directing therapy (both procainamide and metabolite, N-acetylprocainamide)			HD
Propranalol	↓↓(10-40)	↓↓	↓↓↓	
Quinapril	↓↓	↓↓↓	Use caution	
Qunidine			↓; Consider following levels	HD
Ramipril	↓-↓↓(max initial dose 5 mg/day)		↓↓-↓↓↓	HD
Sotalol	↓↓(30-60)	↓↓↓	Avoid	HD, PD
Spironolactone	↓↓	↓↓	Avoid	
Thiazide diuretics	Avoid; loop diuretics preferred for diuresis			
Tranexamic acid	↓↓(50-70)	↓↓↓(10-50)	↓↓↓↓	

- *Adult dosing only; HD = Hemodialysis remmoes significant amount—assess additional doses. PD = Peritoneal Dialysis removes significant amount—assess additional does.
- ↓ = 25%, ↓↓ = 50%, ↓↓↓ = 75%, ανδ ↓↓↓↓ = 90% empiric dose reduction required from usual dose or frequency (total daily dose). See table in *Appendix* for more detailed table.
- (ml/min Numbers) = altered Estimated Creatinine Clearance from category.

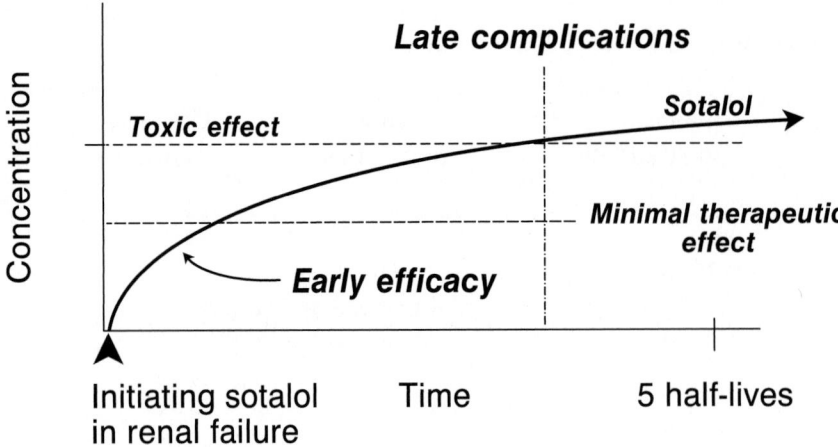

Fig. 3. Drug accumulation.

and thrombolytics as well as the hypotensive potential of many antihypertensives that may exacerbate prerenal renal failure.

Liver function may be important in drug metabolism for two reasons:

1. Drug elimination depends on bioconversion to inactive metabolites (many antiarrhythmics). Conversely, some drugs (enalapril) require conversion by the liver to their active metabolite (enalaprilat).

2. Many cardiac drugs have significant drug-drug interactions by competing for liver enzyme metabolism. Drug bioconversion occurs rapidly with some drugs when administered orally, called the "first-pass effect" (Fig. 4).

With oral intake of a drug, drug absorption occurs via the portal circulation and the drug is immediately subject to liver clearance (Fig. 4). Enzymatic clearance also may occur with cytochrome P-450 (CYP450) enzymes in the small intestine. Both of these degradations yield substantially lower levels of some drugs when given orally instead of intravenously, necessitating much lower doses when given parenterally. Lidocaine cannot be given orally because of the rapid elimination of first-pass clearance. Even when given intravenously, lidocaine clearance diminishes markedly in liver insufficiency. When administering lidocaine in cardiogenic shock after myocardial infarction, presumed liver insufficiency necessitates a 50% dose reduction, with close monitoring of toxicity and drug levels.

Estimation or calculation of liver drug clearance is not as convenient as with estimating renal drug clearance. A method used to modify hepatically cleared drugs is to decrease doses when liver enzymes exceed three times normal. In general, most cardiac drugs have some degree of liver clearance, and drugs to absolutely avoid in liver failure include amiodarone, statins, niacin, methyldopa, ximelagatran, nifedipine, salicylates, bosentan, and verapamil. Dose adjustments may be required in liver failure for many "high first-pass" drugs as well as drugs that are cleared by the kidney and liver, such as flecainide, digoxin, procainamide, and dofetilide. Drug levels are valuable for assessing drug therapy for patients with multiorgan disorders.

- Safe drug therapy depends on appropriate dosing based on patient-specific organ function and individual drug pharmacokinetics.
- Liver metabolism may change the drug from active to inactive (e.g., lidocaine), to another active form (e.g., acebutolol), or from an inactive drug (e.g., enalapril) to an active drug (enalaprilat).

ADVERSE REACTIONS TO CARDIAC DRUGS

Most drug side effects are dose related. Much less frequent are idiosyncratic reactions, which often are immunogenically mediated. Although *all* adverse drug effects may be important, prioritizing surveillance for the most toxic specific side effects simplifies monitoring. The following tables summarize many adverse effects in a manner to simplify your risk-benefit assessment (Tables 2-6).

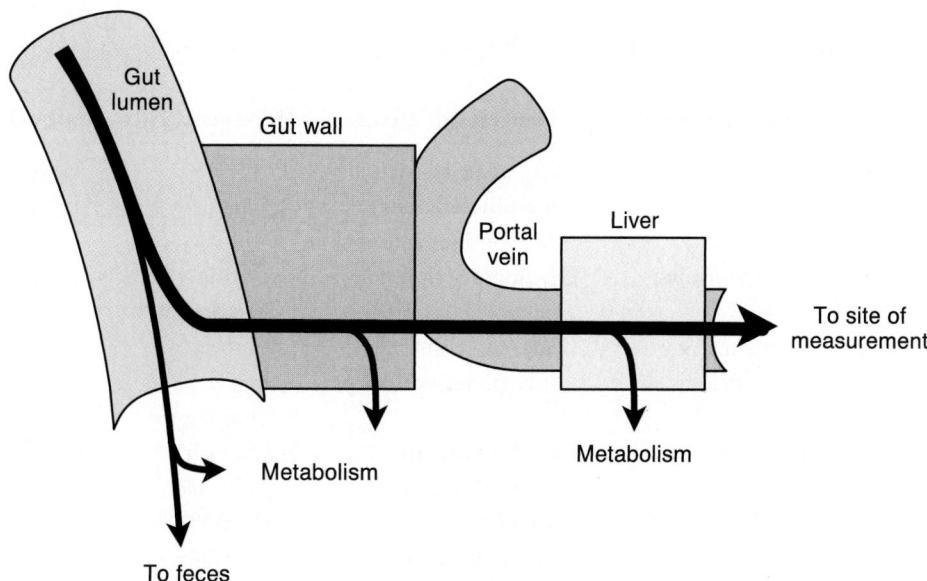

Fig. 4. A drug, given as a solid, encounters several barriers and sites of loss in its sequential movement during gastrointestinal absorption. Dissolution, a prerequisite to movement across the gut wall, is the first step. Incomplete dissolution or metabolism in the gut lumen or by enzymes in the gut wall is a cause of poor absorption. Removal of drug as it first passes through the liver further reduces absorption.

CV Tips: Significant Adverse Effects of Cardiac Medicines and Precautions to Remember Examinations

■ Adenosine	AV node block, risk of VF in atrial fibrillation with WPW
■ ARB/ACE	Hyperkalemia, renal failure, avoid use during pregnancy, cough (ACE inhibitors)
■ β-Blockers	Avoid in acute decompensated heart faillure, advanced AV block or bronchospastic disease
■ Calcium channel blockers	Avoid in LV dysfunction
■ Clonidine and methyldopa	Withdrawal reactions: hypertension, tachycardia, tremors, sweating
■ Fibrates	Cholecystitis, GI symptoms
■ HMG-CoA reductase inhibitors	Myositis, myalgia, liver failure
■ Hydralazine	Rebound tachycardia, lupus-like syndrome
■ Loop diuretics	Ototoxicity (high dose), gout
■ Nitrates	Hypotension, nitrate tolerance—require nitrate-free period
■ Potassium-sparing diuretics	Hyperkalemia in renal insufficiency
■ Thiazide diuretics	Hypercalcemia

Antiarrhythmic agents

■ Disopyramide	Worsening LV dysfunction, anticholinergic (avoid in prostatic hypertrophy, glaucoma, myasthenia gravis)
■ Flecainide	Arrhythmia risk in structural heart disease (avoid in heart failure or post myocardial infarction)
■ Lidocaine/ mexiletine	Seizures, CNS depression
■ Procainamide	Torsades de pointes, hypotension (IV), lupus-like syndrome with long-term therapy
■ Propafenone	Bronchospasm, arrhythmia risk in structural heart disease
■ Quinidine	Anticholinergic effects (prostatic hypertrophy, glaucoma,

Table 2. Adverse Effects of Lipid-Lowering Drugs*

Drug	Toxic side effects	General side effects	Hypersensitivity	Safe use in pregnancy
Binding resins	None	GI, increase triglycerides, **vitamin deficiency (fat-soluble vitamins)**	Possible	May bind fat-soluble vitamins (B)
Fibrates	Rhabdomyolysis (rare) Hepatitis (rare) Renal failure	GI, diuretic (clofibrate), leukopenia, **cholecystitis**, cholelithiasis, rash (photosensitivity)	Arthritis, vasculitis; Stevens-Johnson syndrome (clofibrate)	Safety is unknown (C)
HMG-CoA reductase inhibitors	Rhabdomyolysis (rare) Hepatitis (rare) Pancreatitis **Proteinuria (rosuvastatin)**	GI CNS, **myositis, myalgia, increased serum transaminases (liver)**, conjunctivitis	LLS; rash (lichenoid eruption), arthralgia, thrombocytopenia	Do not use: reports of birth defects (X)
Nicotinic acid derivatives	Hepatitis Rhabdomyolysis (rare) Coronary steal Hypotension Lactic acidosis	Ocular changes, decreased vision, **rash (itching and flushing,** acanthosis nigricans, exfoliation, brown pigmentation), GI, CNS, **hyperglycemia, gout**	Rash (not determined to be allergic-mediated)	(A), Not "toxic" in usual doses for lipid therapy

A, B, C, X, refer to pregnancy class warnings; ANA, antinuclear antibodies; CNS, central nervous system effects; GI, gastro-intestinal effects; LDL, low-density lipoprotein; LLS, lupus-like syndrome.
*Boldface type signifies more prevalence of more severe reactions.

	myasthenia gravis, etc.), Coombs positive
■ Amiodarone	Hypothyroid, hyperthyroid, pulmonary fibrosis, hepatitis, long half-life
■ Bretylium	Hypotension (fast infusion)
■ Sotalol, Dofetilide	Avoid in renal failure

ACE, angiotensin-converting enzyme; AMI, acute myocardial infarction; ARB, angiotensin II receptor blocker; AVB, atrioventricular block; CAD, coronary artery disese; CHF, congestive heart failure; CNS, central nervous system; CV, cardiovascular; IV, intravenous; LV, left ventricular; WPW, Wolff-Parkinson-White syndrome.

Cardiac Drugs in Pregnancy

The U.S. Food and Drug Administration risk factor rating system of drug use in pregnancy is as follows:

Category A—Safe for use during pregnancy. Demonstrated not to pose any risks to human fetuses.

Category B—No evidence of toxicity from animal or human studies but not proven safe in humans.

Category C—Evidence of toxicity in animals but no controlled human studies. Drugs should be given only if the potential benefit justifies the potential risk to the fetus.

Category D—There is evidence of human fetal risk, but the benefits from use in pregnant women may be acceptable despite the risk.

Category X—Contraindicated during pregnancy because of proven teratogenicity and fetal abnormalities

Table 3. Cardiac Drug Side Effects*

Drug	Toxic side effects	General side effects	Hypersensitivity	Safe use in pregnancy
Angiotensin II antagonists	Hypotension, **renal failure, hyper-kalemia**	Headache	Hepatitis, angioedema (rare, cross-reaction with ACE inhibitor)	No (D)
ACE inhibitors	Renal failure, hypotension, hyperkalemia, hepatitis	**Cough**, skin rashes, taste disturbance	**Angioedema**, skin rash, bone marrow suppression, hepatitis, and alveolitis	No (D)
β-Blockers	**Bronchospasm, hypotension,** heart failure	Raynaud phenomenon, impotence, increased serum glucose/lipid levels	None	Yes (B, C)†
Calcium channel antagonists‡	**Hypotension, end-organ ischemia ("steal syndrome")—nifedipine IR**	Dizziness, flushing, peripheral edema, constipation, postural hypotension, taste disturbances	Verapamil, nifedipine, diltiazem: skin eruption, liver and kidney function defects, fever, eosinophilia, lymphadenopathy, maculopapular rash	Unknown (C)
Centrally acting vasodilators (clonidine & methyldopa)	**Withdrawal response, hypotension,** hepatitis (methyldopa)	CNS frequent, sexual dysfunction	Methyldopa: Coombs positive (rarely hemolytic anemia), hepatitis, fever, eosinophilia, rash Clonidine: skin reaction	Unknown (C), methyldopa regarded safe in pregnancy (JNC VII)
Digoxin	Cardiovascular (**heart block,** ectopic proarrhythmias, ventricular extra beats, ventricular tachycardia, **paroxysmal supraventricular tachycardia**)	GI (anorexia, nausea, vomiting, diarrhea) CNS (drowsiness, dizziness, confusion, **vision abnormalities,** photophobia) with toxicity	Rare: thrombocytopenia, rash	May be used therapeutically for fetal arrhythmias (C)
Hydralazine	Hypotension, **hepatitis,** neuropathy	**Flushing**	**Lupus-like syndrome**	Yes (C)
Loop diuretics	Dehydration, pancreatitis, jaundice, **deafness (high dose),** thrombocytopenia, **gout**	Dizziness, postural hypotension, hyponatremia, hypokalemia	Interstitial nephritis, skin reactions (erythema multiforme, Stevens-Johnson syndrome, tissue necrosis)	Use with caution (C)

Table 3   (continued)

Drug	Toxic side effects	General side effects	Hypersensitivity	Safe use in pregnancy
Nitrates	**Hypotension**, transient ischemic attacks, peripheral edema, methemo-globinemia	**Headache**, flushing, palpitation	Contact irritation, allergic contact dermatitis	Unknown (C)
Potassium-sparing diuretics§	**Hyperkalemia**, dehydration	Rashes, **gyneco-mastia in men** (spironolactone) and breast enlarge-ment/soreness (women)§	Skin reactions	Unknown, amiloride (B)
Thiazide diuretics	Dehydration and, rarely, thrombo-cytopenia, chole-static jaundice, pancreatitis, hepatic encepha-lopathy (in patients with cirrhosis)	Dizziness, gout, increased serum glucose/lipid, orthostasis, hypokalemia/ hypomagnesemia, **hypercalcemia**	Skin rashes, allergic vasculitis	No (D)

ACE, angiotensin-converting enzyme; B, C, D, pregnancy class warning; CNS, cenral nervous system effects; GI, gastrointesti-nal effects; IR, immediate release; JNC VII, recommendations of the Seventh Joint National Committee on Hypertension; LLS, lupus-like syndrome.
*Boldface type signifies more prevalence or more severe reactions.
†Metoprolol, atenolol, and labetalol may be used in late pregnancy (JNC VII).
‡Unproven association with internal malignancy.
§Possible association with breast carcinoma and antiandrogenic effect.

in humans. Risk clearly outweighs any possible benefit.

Some of the common drug classes used in cardio-vascular medicine, their potential effects on a fetus, and FDA safety category are summarized in Table 7.

■ Tips for CV Examinations
  ■ ACE inhibitors, ARBs, and statins are con-traindicated in pregnancy.
  ■ For hypertension in pregnancy, methyldopa is the best validated drug or safety.

Drug-Drug Interactions
Drug-drug interactions are summarized in Table 8.

Clinically significant interactions may be difficult to predict because of many variables, including the phar-macology and therapeutic index of each drug, mechanism of drug clearance, gastrointestinal function and metabo-lism, disease states, serum protein status and drug protein binding qualities, and route of administration of the drug (Fig. 5).

■ Patients with certain cardiovascular diseases, including arrhythmias, hypertension, renovascular disease, con-gestive heart failure, and hyperlipidemia, are more susceptible to drug interactions.

Assessing the time course of drug effects depends largely on the half-life of the drugs involved and any

Table 4.   Side Effects of Hematologically Active Agents Used in Cardiology*

Drug	Toxic side effects	General side effects	Hypersensitivity	Safe use in pregnancy
Aspirin	Reye syndrome (children), bleeding, **GI ulceration**, renal toxicity, pulmonary edema, blood	Tinnitus and hearing changes, minor bleeding, hemolytic anemia, **gastritis**	Bronchospasm, urticaria, angioedema, vasomotor rhinitis, anaphylaxis, shock, purpura, hemorrhagic vasculitis, erythema multiforme, Stevens-Johnson syndrome, Lyell syndrome	Yes (C)—no increased risk in large cohort studies
Abciximab	Bleeding (intra-abdominal, retro-peritoneal), **thrombocytopenia**, hypotension, **alveolar hemorrhage**	Pain, sweating	Unknown (none reported with chimeric form); rare with reexposure	Unknown (C)
Clopidogrel	**Hemorrhage**, skin reactions, gastric ulceration	**Gastritis** (similar to aspirin), fatigue, flu-like syndrome, myalgias (all similar to aspirin)	Allergic reactions (necrosis, ischemic)	Unknown (B)
Dipyridamole	Bleeding, myocardial infarction, chest pain, partial seizure	ST-segment abormalities, GI, dizziness, rash, dyspnea, syncope	Allergic reactions reported (skin)	Unknown (C)
Heparin, unfractionated (UFH)	**HIT** type I (mild) and type II (severe), syndrome of thrombohemorrhagic complications (see Hypersensitivity), hypotension; spontaneous arterial emboli	Delayed wound healing, osteoporosis (chronic therapy), minor bleeding, hypoaldosteronism, priapism	Urticaria, conjunctivitis, rhinitis, asthma, cyanosis, tachypnea, feeling of oppression, fever, angioneurotic edema, and anaphylactic shock Rarely—hemorrhagic skin necrosis, vasospastic reactions	Chronic administration: osteopenia for mother (B)
Eptifibatide	Hemorrhage, hypotension, **thrombocytopenia**	Minor bleeding; others rare		Unknown (B)
Low-molecular-weight heparin	Hemorrhage, **thrombocytopenia** (type I [mild] and type II [severe] but lower incidence than UFH; **cross-reactive with UFH-induced events)**	Same as for UFH	Same as for UFH	Yes (B)

Table 4   (continued)

Drug	Toxic side effects	General side effects	Hypersensitivity	Safe use in pregnancy
Protamine	Noncardiogenic pulmonary edema	**Hypotension (with too rapid infusion rates)**	Flushing, urticaria, wheezing, angioedema and hypotension, anaphylaxis, bronchospasm or shock (**IgE or IgG-mediated especially if prior exposure to protamine insulin injections**), pulmonary vasoconstriction, anaphylactoid	Unknown (C)
Ticlopidine	Hemorrhage, hematologic disorders (**leukopenia, agranulocytosis, thrombocytopenia and pancytopenia** [reversible], thrombotic thrombocytopenia (some lethal cases), hepatitis	Skin rashes, severe chronic diarrhea	Rashes (immunogenically mediated unknown)	Unknown (B)
Tirofiban	Hemorrhage, **thrombocytopenia**	Mild bleeding, edema, pain, CNS	Not reported, no repeat exposure information available	(B)
Thrombolytics	Hemorrhage, hemorrhagic stroke, transient hypotensive reactions with streptokinase, embolic phenomena (acute renal failure, cholesterol embolization), reperfusion arrhythmias	Phlebitis at site (streptokinase)	Most associated with streptokinase (history of prior exposure to *Streptococcus* spp), Guillain-Barré, hemolysis, anaphylactic shock, pyrexia, skin rash, angioedema, bronchospasm, ARDS	Yes (urokinase) (B), others unknown (C)
Warfarin	Hemorrhage, hemorrhagic skin necrosis, fetal toxicity Rare—cholestatic hepatitis	Vasodilatation, cholesterol embolization ("purple toe or glove syndrome")	Maculopapular rashes, pruritic purpuritic skin eruptions	No (X) (warfarin, embryopathy) especially in first trimester

ARDS, acute respiratory distress syndrome; B, C, X, pregnancy class warning; CNS, central nervous system effects; DIC, disseminated intravascular coagulation; GI, gastrointestinal effects; HIT, heparin-induced thrombocytopenia; LFT, liver function tests; LLS, lupus-like syndrome.

*Boldface type signifies more prevalence or more severe reactions.

Table 5. Antiarrhythmic Drug Side Effects*

Drug	Toxic side effects	General side effects	Hypersensitivity	Safe use in pregnancy
Adenosine	Chest pain, ische-mia, **bronchocon-striction**, increased ICP, **VF in atrial fibrillation with WPW**	Dyspnea, dizziness, epigastric pain, flushing, GI, headache	Not reported	Unknown (C)
		Type I antiarrhythmic agents		
Disopyramide	Heart failure, **risk of TdP**	Hypoglycemia, **anticholinergic**† **syndromes**	Angioedema (rare)	Uterine contractions (C)‡
Flecainide	Proarrhythmias, Heart failure	CNS, GI, neutro-penia, urinary retention, ankle edema	Not reported	Unknown (C)
Lidocaine	Coma, seizures, respiratory depression, proarrhythmias	**CNS** (nystagmus is early sign of toxicity)	Not reported	Unknown (C)
Mexiletine	Proarrythmias	**CNS**, cholestasis, GI, rash	Thrombocytopenia, ANA	Unknown (C)
Procainamide	**TdP, hypotension (IV)**, worsened myocardial contractility, neutropenia	CNS, rash, cholestasis, Raynaud phenomenon	**Lupus-like syndrome**, ANA, fever, hema-tologic (neutropenia, pancytopenia, pure red cell aplasia, Achilles tendinitis, Coombs-positive hemolytic anemia)	Unknown (C)†
Propafenone	Proarrhythmias, **bronchospasm and dyspnea**, heart failure	SIADH, neutro-penia, GI, CNS (including peripheral neuropathy), impotence, taste disturbance	ANA, LLS	Unknown (C)
Quinidine	**TdP**, heart failure, hypotension	GI (most common), CNS, **cinchonism**, esophagitis, **anti-cholinergic syndrome**†	Fever, rash, thrombo-cytopenia, neutrope-nia, **hemolytic anemia**, hepatitis, Coombs-positive lupus anti-coagulant, asthma, anaphylaxis Rarely, LLS	Unknown (C)‡

Table 5   (continued)

Drug	Toxic side effects	General side effects	Hypersensitivity	Safe use in pregnancy
		Type III antiarrhythmic agents		
Amiodarone	**Hypothyroid, hyperthyroid, hepatitis, pulmonary** (pneumonitis, fibrosis, bronchiolitis obliterans, organizing pneumonia), IV administration—AV block and hypotension, proarrhythmias	Corneal microdeposits, GI, photosensitivity and blue skin, rashes, neuropathy	Interstitial pneumonitis may be hypersensitivity reaction	Neonatal thyroid effects (C)
Bretylium	Hypotension, proarrhythmias	GI, hypertension, hyperthermia	Not reported	Unknown (C)
Sotalol	**TdP**, bronchospasm, hypotension	CNS, GI, reduced peripheral vascular perfusion, impotence, increased serum glucose/lipid, fatigue	Not reported	Unknown (C)

ANA, antinuclear antibodies; AV, atrioventricular; C, pregnancy class C warning; CNS, central nervous system effects; GI, gastrointestinal effects; ICP, intracranial pressure; IV, intravenous; LLS, lupus-like syndrome; SIADH, syndrome of inappropriate antidiuretic hormone; VF, ventricular fibrillation; TdP, torsades de pointes.

*Boldface type signifies more prevalence or more severe reactions.

†Anticholinergic syndrome: dry mouth, dysuria/increased urinary retention, increased intraocular pressure/blurred vision, flushing, agitation/psychosis/dementia, sinus tachycardia.

‡Drugs with anticholinergic effects hae been found to cause neonatal meconium ileus.

active metabolite. Drug interactions may be due to additive or synergistic cellular effects between drugs (pharmacodynamic interactions) or caused by drugs altering the time course of another drug in the body (pharmacokinetic interactions). For example, the half-life of amiodarone averages about 1 month and the drug also has an active metabolite that may further prolong its action. Some pharmacodynamic interactions, such as atrioventricular nodal effects, may occur relatively early in the course of therapy when used with other atrioventricular nodal drugs such as β-blockers, causing exaggerated bradycardia. The metabolic inhibition of amiodarone on warfarin metabolism correlates better with the half-life of the drug and may occur weeks or

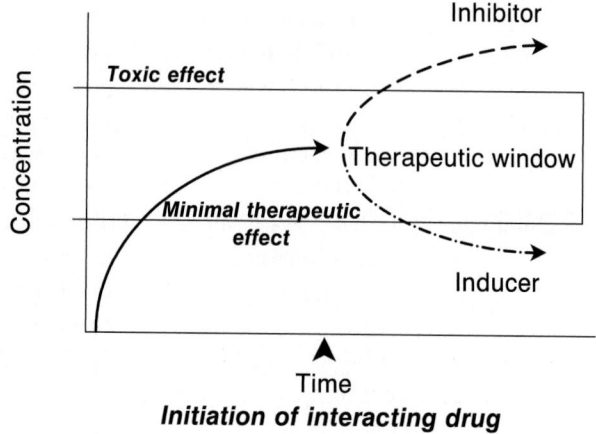

Fig. 5. Clinically significant pharmacokinetic drug interactions.

Table 6.   Metabolic Effects of Cardiac Drugs

Agent	Total cholesterol	LDL	HDL	TG	Insulin sensitivity
High-dose thiazides	↑	↑	↔	↑	↓
Low-dose thiazides	↔	↔	↔	↔	↔
β-Blockers	↔	↔	↓	↑	↓
α-Blockers	↓	↔	↑	↔	↑
ACE inhibitors	↔	↔	↔	↔	↑
Calcium channel blockers	↔	↔	↔	↔	↔

ACE, angiotensin-converting enzyme; HDL, high-density lipoproteins; LDL, low-density lipoproteins; TG, triglycerides.

Table 7.   Common Cardiovascular Drugs and Pregnancy

Drug class	Adverse fetal effects	FDA safety category
ACE inhibitors/ARB	Fetal abnormalities, renal defects, may be lethal	D
β-Blockers*	Bradycardia, neonatal hypoglycemias, growth retardation	C
Ca2+ channel blockers	? Fetal abnormalities	C
Digoxin	...	C
Diuretics		
Furosemide	Electrolyte imbalance, increased fetal urine output	C
Thiazide	? Birth defects, bone marrow depression	D
Nitrates	None (may be useful in delaying premature labor)	B
Anticoagulants		D
Heparin	(Preferable anticoagulant)	
Warfarin	Birth defects, fetal warfarin syndrome, fetal hemorrhage or death	
Antihypertensives†		
Methyldopa	Best validated, preferred antihypertensive	B
Lipid-lowering drugs		
Statins	Toxic	X
Gemfibrozil	? Birth defects	C
Cholestyramine		B

B, C, D, X, refer to pregnancy class warnings.
*Labetolol is the preferred β-blocker in pregancy.
†The preferred medications for treating hypertension in pregnancy are methyldopa, hydralazine labetolol, and nifedipine or amlodipine.

months after the initiation of treatment with the combination of the two drugs.

- Amiodarone–warfarin drug interaction is a good example of a serious delayed interaction.

Torsades de Pointes

Torsades de pointes is a side effect that may occur with high doses of a single drug, including many antiarrhythmic agents, or, more likely, may be the result of drug-drug interactions. Torsades de pointes can be

Table 8. Selected Significant Cardiac Drug Interactions*

Drug	Drug	Net effect and suggested actions
Adenosine	**Dipyridamole**	Increase effect of adenosine. May need to reduce adenosine dose.
	Theophylline	Decrease effect of adenosine. May need to increase adenosine dose.
Amiodarone	**Digoxin**	Increases serum digoxin. Reduce dose of digoxin by 50% and monitor levels.
	Cyclosporine	Increases serum cyclosporine. Monitor cyclosporine levels.
	Dofetilide	Increases dofetilide level resulting in risk of torsades. Must be off amiodarone for at least 3 months or amiodarone level <0.3 mg/mL to start dofetilide.
	Lidocaine/mexiletine	Increase serum lidocaine/mexiletine. Monitor levels.
	Flecainide	Increases flecainide level. Combination is rarely used.
	Fosphenytoin or phenytoin	Phenytoin level can increase 2- to 3-fold. Amiodarone effect may be diminished.
	Procainamide	Increases procainamide level; 20% reduction of procainamide dose is suggested. Combination is rarely used.
	Quinidine	Increases quinidine level; 50% reduction of quinidine dose is suggested. Rarely used together.
	Warfarin	Increases warfarin effect. Decrease warfarin dose by 50% and monitor INR.
Digoxin	**Amiodarone**	Increases serum dogoxin. Reduce dose of digoxin by 50% and monitor levels.
	Propafenone	Increases digoxin levels. Empirically reduce digoxin dose by 50%. Monitor levels and signs of elevated digoxin.
	Quinidine	May increase digoxin levels, monitor ECG and digoxin levels.
	Verapamil	Increases serum digoxin levels. Reduce digoxin dose by 50%. Monitor digoxin levels and signs of elevated digoxin.
	Cholestyramine	Avoid coadministration due to interference of digoxin absorption.
Disopyramide	**Rifampin**, phenytoin, phenobarbital	Initial disopyramide dose increase may be necessary due to enzyme induction. Monitor levels and effects.
	Protease inhibitors	Monitor patients for signs and symptoms of disopyramide toxicity. Reduce dose of disopyramide as required (do not stop protease inhibitors). Protease inhibitors: ritonavir, saquinavir
Dofetilide	**Amiodarone**	Increases level of dofetilide resulting in risk of torsades. Must be off amiodarone for at least 3 months or amiodarone level <0.3 mg/ml to start dofetilide.
	Class I & III anti-arrhythmic agents	Washout out period of at least 3 half-lives before starting dofetilide.
	Cimetidine	Contraindication due to increased serum level of dofetilide.
	Hydrochlorothiazide	Contraindication due to increased serum level of dofetilide and reduction in serum potassium and magnesium.
	Ketoconazole	Contraindication due to increased serum level of dofetilide.
	Megestrol	Contraindication due to increased serum level of dofetilide.
	Prochlorperazine	Contraindication due to increased serum level of dofetilide.

Table 8.   (continued)

Drug	Drug	Net effect and suggested actions
Dofetilide (cont'd)	**SMX/TMP**	Contraindication due to increased serum level of dofetilide.
	Trimethoprim	Contraindication due to increased serum level of dofetilide.
	Verapamil	Contraindication due to increased serum level of dofetilide.
Mexiletine	Phenytoin, Phenobarbital	Initial mexiletine dose increase may be necessary due to enzyme induction. Monitor levels and effects.
	Protease inhibitor: Ritonavir	Monitor patients for signs and symptoms of mexiletine toxicity (nausea, dizziness, cardiac arrhythmias). Reduce dose of mexiletine as required. (Do not stop protease inhibitors.)
	SSRIs	Increase mexiletine levels. Avoid coadministration. SSRIs: fluvoxamine[†]
Lidocaine	**Protease inhibitors:** ritonavir amprenavir	Monitor patients for signs and symptoms of lidocaine toxicity (nausea, dizziness, cardic arrhythmias). Reduce dose of lidocaine as required. (Do not stop protease inhibitors.)
Propafenone	Digoxin	Increases digoxin levels. Empirically reduce digoxin dose by 50%. Monitor levels and signs of elevated digoxin.
	Metoprolol	Increases metoprolol level 1.5- to 5-fold.
	Warfarin	Increases warfarin effect by 25%. Monitor INR when add or withdraw propafenone.
	Phenytoin, phenobarbital	Initial propafenone dose increase may be necessary due to enzyme induction. Monitor effects.
	SSRIs	Increase propafenone levels. Avoid coadministration. SSRIs: fluoxetine, sertraline, paroxetine[†]
Quinidine	**Rifampin,** phenytoin, phenobarbital	Initial quinidine dose increase may be necessary due to enzyme induction. Monitor levels and effects.
	Azole antifungals	Progressive increase in levels of quinidine. Monitor closely.
	Metronidazole	Verapamil: initiate at 50% quinidine dose.
	Verapamil	Azole antifungals: ketoconazole, fluconazole, itraconazole[†]
Simvastatin	**Amiodarone** **Verapamil** **Cyclosporine**	Monitor for toxic side effects of simvastatin (myopathy, rhabdomyolysis). Amiodarone, verapamil: maximum simvastatin dose 20 mg daily. Cyclosporine: maximum simvastatin dose 10 mg daily
Warfarin (this table is not all-inclusive)	**Amiodarone**	Increases warfarin effect. Decrease warfarin dose by 50% and monitor INR.
	Acetaminophen	Increases warfarin effect. Decrease warfarin dose by 25-50% and monitor INR.
	Allopurinol	Increases warfarin effect. Decrease warfarin dose by 25-50% and monitor INR.
	Azole anifungals	Increases warfarin effect. Decrease warfarin dose by 25-50% and monitor INR. Azole antifungals: ketoconazole, fluconazole, itraconazole[†]
	Cholestyramine	Decreases absorption and effectiveness of warfarin. Use colestipol as alternative.
	COX-II inhibitors	Increases INR. Monitor INR closely. COX-II inhibitors: celecoxib, rofecoxib[†]

Table 8. (continued)

Drug	Drug	Net effect and suggested actions
	Propafenone	Increases warfarin effect by 25%. Monitor INR when add or withdraw propafenone.
	GP IIb/IIIa inhibitors (Reopro, Integrilin, Aggrastat)	Should not be used concurrently with warfarin unless the potential benefit outweighs the risk of bleeding.
	Rifampin	Enzyme induction. Increase warfarin dose and monitor INR closely.
	SMX/TMP	Increases warfarin effect. Decrease warfarin dose by 25-50% and monitor INR.
	Thrombolytics	Additive anticoagulation. Monitor INR closely.

*Boldface type signifies more prevalence or more severe reactions.
†SSRIs, selective serotonin reuptake inhibitors; SMX/TMP, sulfamethozaxole/trimethoprim; GP, glycoprotein; INR, international normalized ratio.

idiosyncratic or dose-dependent. The proarrhythmias caused by class Ia antiarrhythmic agents are not directly dose-related, but risk increases with serum concentrations. Most other drug causes of torsades de pointes appear dose-related. Table 9 describes drug and other reported causes of torsades de pointes.

Torsades de pointes drug interactions may be classed as pharmacodynamic or pharmacokinetic. As mentioned above, quinidine plus sotalol share cellular mechanisms for potentially triggering torsades de pointes. Drug antagonism of hepatic cytochrome P-450 isoenzyme metabolism may cause torsades de pointes, whereas antagonism of gut enzymes would prevent absorption. The most common isoenzymes, CYP2D6 and CYP3A4, account for the metabolism of most drugs that cause torsades de pointes. When the isoenzymes are inhibited, the concentrations of torsades de pointes drugs increase, which increases proarrhythmic risks. For example, the combination of erythromycin and astemizole may cause torsades de pointes.

Cardiovascular Adverse Effects of Herbal Remedies

Herbal products are being used increasingly by patients for preventive and therapeutic purposes. These products affect the cardiovascular or hemostatic system directly or indirectly through interactions with cardiovascular drugs. Some of the common herbal remedies, their purported use, and their adverse effects on cardiovascular system are summarized in Table 10.

Table 9. Acquired Forms of Torsades de Pointes*

Drug-induced
   Antiarrhythmic agents
      Type IA (quinidine, procainamide, disopyramide)
      Type III (Sotalol, dofetilide, ibutilide, azimilide, amiodarone)
   Antianginal
      Bepridil,* Ranolazine
   Antibiotics, antimicrobials and antiviral agents
      Erythromycin, clarithromycin, chloroquine, quinine, pentamidine, sparfloxacin,* moxifloxacin,
         TMP-SMX, gatifloxacin
      Foscarnet
   Antidepressant and antipsychotics
      Tricyclic antidepressants, tetracyclic antidepressants, **haloperidol**, paroxetine
      Naratriptan, phenothiazines, pimozide, risperidone
   Antihistamine
      Terfenadine,† astemizole†
   GI motility
      Cisapride†
   Sedative and antinausea
      Dolasetron, **droperidol**, ondansetron, phenothiazines (prochlorperazine, promethazine)
Toxin-induced—organophosphates, arsenic, cocaine
Disease-induced—subarachnoid hemorrhage, cerebrovascular accident, encephalitis, head injury, myocarditis,
   hyperaldosteronism, severe bradycardia
Electrolyte-induced—hypomagnesemia, hypokalemia, hypocalcemia
Nutritional disorders—liquid protein diets, starvation

TMP-SMX, trimethoprim-sulfamethoxazole.
*Boldface indictes hgiher frequency of reports.
†Indicates drugs withdrawn from the market.

Table 10. Herbal Preparations to Avoid in Patients With Cardiovascular Diseases

Herbal preparation	Purported use	Cardiac adverse effect
Alfalfa	Arthritis, asthma, dyspepsia, hyperlipidemia, and diabetes	↑ bleeding risk in patients on warfarin
Angelica (dong quai)	Loss of appetite, peptic discomfort	↑ bleeding risk in patients on warfarin
Capsicum	Shingles, trigeminal and diabetic neuralgia	↑ blood pressure (with MAOI)
Garlic	Cholesterol lowering	↑ bleeding risk in patients on warfarin
Ginger	Cholesterol lowering, motion sickness, digestive aid, and antioxidant	↑ bleeding risk
Ginkgo	Improve circulation and mental function	↑ bleeding risk in patients on warfarin, aspirin, and COX-II inhibitors
Ginseng	Delay aging, boost immunity and resistance to stress improve mental and physyical capacity	↑ blood pressure, ↓ warfarin effectiveness, hypoglycemia
Green tea	Improve cognitive performance, mental alertness, use as diuretic, use in weight loss products	↓ warfarin effectiveness (contains vitamin K)
Hawthorn	Heart faillure and hypertension	Potentiate the action of cardiac glycosides, ↑ blood pressure
Licorice root	Ulcer, cirrhosis, cough	↑ blood pressure, ↓ K⁺, may potentiate digoxin toxicity
Ma-huang (ephedra)	Obesity or cough	↑ heart rate and blood pressure
Saint John's Wort	Depression	↑ in heart rate and blood pressure (with MAOI), ↓ digoxin concentration
Yohimbine	Impotence	↑ in heart rate, ↑ or ↓ blood pressure

112

LIPID-LOWERING MEDICATIONS AND LIPID-LOWERING CLINICAL TRIALS

Joseph G. Murphy, MD

R. Scott Wright, MD

The principal pharmacologic agents used in the treatment of hyperlipidemia are statins, fibric acid derivatives, niacin, ezetimibe, bile acid sequestrants, and sitastanol esters.

STATINS

Statins (HMG CoA reductase enzyme inhibitors) are the most commonly prescribed lipid-lowering medications and are potent agents to reduce LDL cholesterol. These medications act by inhibiting the synthesis of cholesterol in the liver and promoting increased uptake and degradation of LDL cholesterol from the blood. Statins are competitive inhibitors of HMG CoA reductase, the rate-limiting step in cholesterol biosynthesis. Reduced hepatic cholesterol biosynthesis leads to an increase in LDL receptor turnover and increased hepatic LDL receptor cycling.

Most patients with hypercholesterolemia can be managed with monotherapy with a statin agent alone. These drugs are generally very safe and cost-effective and reduce both coronary-related and total mortality in patients with coronary artery disease. The most common side effects in patients treated with statins are muscle cramps, myositis, and an asymptomatic increase of hepatic transaminase enzyme values. These side effects are largely reversible with discontinuation of the medication. Periodic monitoring of hepatic transaminase enzyme levels is important with statins because of the rare occurrence of hepatotoxicity.

Skeletal muscle myopathies associated with statins range from mild muscle aches without muscle enzyme elevation or muscle weakness to muscle weakness and clinical myositis with elevations in serum creatine kinase (CK) enzymes to life-threatening overt rhabdomyolysis with acute renal failure. Myopathies, when they occur, usually begin within weeks of starting statins and usually resolve together with elevated CK concentrations within weeks of drug discontinuation. There is increased susceptibility to statin-associated myopathy and myositis in patients with renal failure, obstructive liver disease, and hypothyroidism, and patients taking cyclosporin, nicotinic acid, or gemfibrozil.

Statins also have multiple secondary beneficial effects, including a reduction in the risk of developing diabetes, a reduced risk of osteoporotic fractures, particularly in older patients, and a mild blood pressure lowering effect in hypertensive patients. Statins appear to have pleiotropic actions on atheromatous plaques and atherogenesis beyond their cholesterol-lowering abilities and may have a beneficial effect when used acutely in patients presenting with acute myocardial infarction.

NICOTINIC ACID

Nicotinic acid (niacin) is a widely used, inexpensive, water-soluble B complex vitamin used in the treatment of hyperlipidemia. Niacin moderately lowers total cholesterol, LDL cholesterol, and triglyceride values and increases HDL cholesterol by a poorly understood biochemical mechanism. It is the most potent currently approved medication for increasing a low HDL value. Torcetrapib, a new investigational CETP inhibitor undergoing clinical trials, may in the future displace nicotinic acid as the agent of choice to raise low HDL cholesterol levels. Nicotinic acid reduces lipoprotein (a) and small, dense LDL. Statins are generally without effect on lipoprotein (a). Nicotinic acid is the least expensive lipid-lowering agent and is a nonprescription medication. The major side effects of nicotinic acid are pruritus, flushing, gastrointestinal distress, glucose intolerance, rash, provocation of gout, and liver toxicity. Aspirin taken 30 to 60 minutes before nicotinic acid can reduce the flushing. There is a rare occurrence of atrial arrhythmia or ocular maculopathy with nicotinic acid. Nicotinic acid increases the risk of myopathy when used concomitantly with a statin. Patient tolerance of medication is increased when using a sustained-release formulation of nicotinic acid.

FIBRIC ACID DERIVATIVES

The fibric acid derivatives include, fenofibrate, gemfibrozil, and benzafibrate (available outside the US) and the discarded medication clofibrate. Fibrates lower serum triglycerides by (30% to 50%) and raise serum high-density lipoprotein (HDL) by (15% to 25%) through a mechanism that includes activation of peroxisome proliferator-activated receptors (PPARs). The fibrates have a variable effect on serum Lp(a). Fenofibrate and benzafibrate lower fibrinogen levels, while gemfibrozil has no effect.

Gemfibrozil is widely used in the treatment of mixed hyperlipidemias that are characterized by an increase in both serum triglyceride and LDL cholesterol, a common occurrence in diabetic patients. The major side effect of fibrate medications are gastrointestinal intolerance and a possible increased risk of cholelithiasis.

Fenofibrate is available commercially in the micronized form (Tricor) and is approved for the treatment of hypertriglyceridemia. Fibric acid derivatives stimulate lipoprotein lipase activity, which results in enhanced triglyceride clearance. They also activate peroxisome proliferator-activated receptors, which are hormone receptors located in the cell nucleus that modify expression of several genes responsible for lipoprotein expression. Fibric acid derivatives also cause a shift from small, dense LDL particles into less dense LDL particles that are less atherogenic. Fenofibrate lowers LDL cholesterol less than pravastatin or simvastatin, but it increases HDL cholesterol level more than either statin agent; it also lowers triglyceride levels (30%-50%), an effect much greater than that seen with statins. Atorvastatin is much more effective than fenofibrate at lowering LDL cholesterol but significantly less effective for increasing HDL cholesterol or lowering triglyceride values. The major side effects of fenofibrate are rash and gastrointestinal upset. Similar to niacin, fibrates potentiate the effects of warfarin by decreasing protein binding.

BILE ACID-BINDING SEQUESTRANTS

The anionic resins, or bile acid-binding sequestrants (cholestyramine, Questran; colestipol, Colestid), are both safe and moderately effective therapy for hyperlipidemia. These agents reduce total cholesterol and low-density lipoprotein (LDL) cholesterol levels by binding positively charged bile acids in the gut to interrupt the enterohepatic circulation of bile acids. This stimulates new bile acid production and a secondary increase in hepatic LDL receptors, which in turn remove LDL cholesterol from the circulation. Resins usually have no significant effect on HDL or triglyceride levels, but, paradoxically, they may increase triglycerides dramatically in rare patients.

As expected from their mode of action, the major side effects associated with the resin agents are gastrointestinal intolerance with gas, bloating, constipation, nausea, and esophageal reflux. This is sufficient to cause about 50% of patients to discontinue therapy at 1 year. These agents help to lower LDL cholesterol, and if the dose is incremented slowly, they can be reasonably tolerated by many patients. They are excellent adjunctive agents in severe hyperlipidemia, when used in combination with statins or nicotinic acid. Bile acid sequestrants are relatively contraindicated in patients with significant hypertriglyceridemia.

A clinical problem with resins is their effect on the absorption of vitamin K, especially in patients receiving warfarin. Resins also inhibit the absorption of digoxin, warfarin, thyroxine, statins, and diuretics if given concomitantly with these agents.

EZETIMIBE

Ezetimibe has a unique mechanism of action different from all other classes of cholesterol-reducing medications. Ezetimibe selectively inhibits absorption of cholesterol at the brush border of the small intestine by about 50%. Intestinal cholesterol is derived primarily from cholesterol secreted in the bile and from dietary cholesterol while hepatic cholesterol is derived from three sources, de novo hepatic synthesis of cholesterol, cholesterol removed from serum lipoproteins and cholesterol absorbed by the small intestine. Ezetimibe does not inhibit cholesterol synthesis in the liver or increase bile acid cholesterol excretion but rather inhibits the intestinal absorption of cholesterol, leading to a decrease in the delivery of intestinal cholesterol to the liver. This in turn causes a reduction of hepatic cholesterol stores and an increase in the clearance of cholesterol from the blood.

Ezetimibe decreases total serum cholesterol, LDL cholesterol (LDL-C), ApoB, and triglycerides (TG) while slightly increasing serum HDL cholesterol (HDL-C). Ezetimibe has a beneficial effect on cholesterol metabolism by blocking both dietary cholesterol absorption and interrupting the enterohepatic recirculation of cholesterol through biliary secretion and intestinal reabsorption.

Ezetimibe (10 mg/day) reduces serum LDL cholesterol by about 18% when used as a sole lipid lowering agent. Ezetimibe, when added to a statin, incrementally lowers LDL cholesterol by a slightly smaller amount (~15%) in addition to the statin-induced lowering of LDL cholesterol.

Statins remain the first drug of choice for pharmacological reduction in LDL-C levels because of their added pleiotropic actions on atheromatous plaques and atherogenesis. Ezetimibe is valuable in patients who do not meet NCEP cholesterol goals on statin therapy alone or in patients who are intolerant of either a high statin dose or any statin dose, because of side effects (generally myopathy or an elevation in liver enzymes) or patients with familial hypercholesterolemia who require a maximum lipid-lowering effect.

Ezetimibe is generally well tolerated when administered alone, the incidence of either myopathy or liver serum transaminase elevations are similar to placebo; when administered in conjunction with a statin, the incidence of serum transaminase elevation is slightly higher than with statin therapy alone.

There have been several postmarketing reports of musculoskeletal side effects including myopathy, CPK elevations, and rhabdomyolysis with etezimibe, while hepatitis, pancreatitis, and thrombocytopenia have been rarely reported. While very rare, of concern is that these side effects have been noted with ezetimibe when used as monotherapy, as well as during combination therapy with HMG-CoA reductase inhibitors. There is a possible drug interaction between ezetimibe and warfarin and gemfibrozil may increase ezetimibe levels.

SITOSTANOL PLANT ESTERS

Sitostanol plant esters are derivatives of naturally occurring plant esters that are present in the Western diet in amounts equal to that of cholesterol. Sitostanol esters reduce the gastrointestinal absorption of cholesterol and are incorporated into some margarine and other food products. Several recent trials have examined the cholesterol-lowering effect of dietary substitution of sitostanol esters for soybean-enriched margarine. A daily consumption of 1.5 to 3.3 grams of sitostanol ester was associated with an 8% to 13% decrease in total cholesterol and LDL cholesterol values and a 1% to 2% increase in the HDL cholesterol value. Additionally, triglyceride levels were reduced 4% to 12% on average. One trial has demonstrated that sitostanol esters can be used in combination with statins to gain additive benefit. No major side effects have been reported.

Tables 1 and 2 provide information on the effects of lipid-lowering medications and their interactions and side effects.

Serum C-Reactive Protein and Cholesterol-Lowering Medications

Epidemiological evidence suggests that inflammation is an important mediator of vascular atherogenesis and plaque rupture. Serum CRP is a marker of inflamma-

Table 1. Drug Treatment of Hyperlipidemia

| Agent | Dosage per day | Typical expected effects | | Triglyceride effect, % |
| | | Cholesterol effect | | |
		↓ LDL, %	↑ HDL, %	
Cholestyramine	12-24 g	15-20	0-2	5-10 ↑
Colestipol	15-30 g	15-20	0-2	5-10 ↑
Sitosterol esters	1.5-3.3 g	10	0-2	4-8 ↓
Niacin	1.5-6 g	20-30	20	30-40 ↓
Gemfibrozil	600-1,200 mg	10	20	50-60 ↓
Fenofibrate	67-200 mg	10-15	5-20	40-50 ↓
Lovastatin	20 mg	25-30	0-10	0-6 ↓
	80 mg	35-40	0-10	25 ↓
Pravastatin	20 mg	25-30	0-10	10 ↓
	40 mg	25-35	0-10	25 ↓
Simvastatin	10 mg	25-30	0-10	0-5 ↓
	80 mg	40-50	0-10	25-40 ↓
Atorvastatin	10 mg	35-40	0-10	20 ↓
	40 mg	40-60	0-10	35 ↓
	80 mg	60	0-10	35-45 ↓
Ezetimibe	10 mg	18	1	8 ↓
Resuvastatin	5 mg	28	3	21 ↓
	10 mg	45	8	37 ↓
	20 mg	31	22	37 ↓
	40 mg	43	17	43 ↓

tion that is statistically linked to an increased risk of future cardiovascular events. CRP is considered a surrogate marker of vascular inflammation and atherosclerotic risk. Measurement of high-sensitivity CRP levels in conjunction with lipid profile analysis improves patient risk stratification. Statins reduces CRP levels independent of their effect on cholesterol levels, suggesting that part of the beneficial effects of statins may lie in their antiinflammatory effects.

■ High-sensitivity CRP is a useful independent marker of vascular inflammation and cardiovascular risk in patients with both stable and unstable cardiovascular disease.
■ Determination of cardiovascular risk by high-sensitivity CRP testing in patients without known cardiovascular disease is based on risk class—low-, average-, and high-risk values for high-sensitivity CRP as defined by <1, 1 to 3, and >3 mg/L.

■ Among patients with known cardiovascular disease, a cutoff value of >3 mg/L is recommended for predicting outcomes in patients with stable cardiovascular disease, while a threshold >10 mg/L is recommended for patients with unstable coronary syndromes.

MAJOR LIPID-LOWERING TRIALS

There is unequivocal clinical evidence from multiple randomized clinical trials that treatment of hypercholesterolemia with statins reduces future cardiovascular events in persons with and without clinically evident ischemic heart disease, although the early studies of cardiovascular prevention with nonstatin agents were disappointing.

Primary Prevention of Cardiac Disease

Primary prevention refers to a reduction in future cardiovascular events in subjects without know cardiovascular disease. The earliest major randomized drug trial of primary prevention of cardiovascular disease was the World

Table 2. Interactions and Side Effects of Lipid-Lowering Agents

Agent	Interactions and side effects
Cholestyramine and colestipol	Other medications should be given 1 hour before or 4-6 hours after resin agent. May impair absorption of vitamins A, D, E, and K and cause vitamin K deficiency. May alter absorption of digoxin, warfarin, thiazide diuretics, propranolol, tetracycline, penicillin G, estrogens and progestins, and thyroid supplements. May produce or worsen constipation, nausea, abdominal pain, flatulence, vomiting, and anorexia
Niacin	Patients may experience flushing, itching, tingling, feelings of warmth, headache, rash, upset stomach, hypotension. May worsen fasting hyperglycemia and cause atrial arrhythmias
Gemfibrozil	Contraindicated in renal failure (creatinine >2.0 mg/dL), hepatic dysfunction (including primary biliary cirrhosis), and preexisting gallbladder disease. Incidence of rhabdomyolysis is increased when agent is used with lovastatin
Fenofibrate	Contraindicated in renal failure (creatinine clearance <50 mL/min), hepatic dysfunction. Doses of warfarin must be reduced and prothrombin time monitored frequently. Dose may need to be adjusted when given with cyclosporine. May increase risk of gallbladder disease
All statins	May increase aspartate aminotransferase. Monitor at initiation of therapy and with any change in dose. Rarely associated with myositis and rhabdomyolysis. Should not be used in pregnant or nursing women. Should not be used with oral or intravenous antifungal agents. May be used with bile acid-binding resins. No effect on β-adrenergic blockers, angiotensin-converting enzyme inhibitors, and diabetic agents
Lovastatin	Should not be used with gemfibrozil. May cause rhabdomyolysis when used with cyclosporine plus itraconazole, or with erythromycin. Widely studied, with good primary and secondary prevention data
Pravastatin	Most widely studied agent, with good primary and secondary prevention data. Little evidence of myopathy when used with cyclosporine, niacin, or gemfibrozil
Simvastatin	Widely studied, with good secondary prevention data. Dose should be decreased when given with cyclosporine. May potentiate effect of digoxin and warfarin
Atorvastatin	Excellent long-term mortality data for primary and secondary prevention effect. A potent agent with a good side-effect profile
Resuvastatin	Very potent statin—trial data pending
Ezetimibe	Blocks cholesterol absorption from the intestine

Health Organization (WHO) Cooperative Trial, which tested clofibrate, a fibric acid derivative, in over 10,500 patients with hyperlipidemia. There were 25% more deaths in the clofibrate-treated group than in the placebo group. Clofibrate is now known to be associated with cholangiocarcinoma and other gastrointestinal cancers, a risk not known to the WHO investigators at the time. Mortality from all causes was higher in the clofibrate-treated group, including deaths from ischemic heart disease and stroke.

The Lipid Research Clinic (LRC) and Helsinki Heart study were also important early trials of non-statin medications in the primary prevention of coronary heart disease in patients with hyperlipidemia. These trials suggested a trend towards benefit with cholesterol lowering, but definitive proof with pharmacologically induced lipid lowering was lacking until the development of powerful statin agents.

LIPID RESEARCH CLINICS (LRC) CORONARY PRIMARY PREVENTION TRIAL (1984)

The Lipid Research Clinics (LRC) Coronary Primary Prevention Trial was an older trial that examined the benefit of lipid-lowering therapy on primary prevention using a combination of cholestyramine and dietary intervention to reduce patient serum cholesterol level. It found a 19% reduction in nonfatal myocardial infarction and a 24% reduction in deaths from cardiovascular disease, but these results were of borderline statistical significance and there was no decrease in overall mortality.

■ In the Lipid Research Clinics Primary Prevention Trial, there was a trend toward a reduction in nonfatal myocardial infarctions and cardiovascular deaths but no statistically significant decrease in overall mortality.

The Helsinki Heart Study (1987)

The Helsinki Heart Study used gemfibrozil for the treatment of hyperlipidemia and resulted in a 34% reduction in the combined end points of death, fatal myocardial infarction, and nonfatal myocardial infarction. Overall mortality was not reduced and there was some statistically significant increase in noncardiovascular mortality in the gemfibrozil-treated group.

■ In the Helsinki Heart Study primary prevention trial, there was a trend toward a reduction in the composite end points of cardiac death and cardiac events but no statistically significant decrease in overall mortality.

The West of Scotland Prevention Study (WOSCOP) (1995)

The West of Scotland Prevention Study tested the hypothesis that primary prevention with pravastatin would reduce mortality and nonfatal infarctions in patients with hyperlipidemia who had not had a prior myocardial infarction. The study randomized, patients

to pravastatin 40 mg/day) versus placebo and included nearly 6,600 middle-aged men with hypercholesterolemia—fasting LDL cholesterol values more than 252 mg/dL—who failed to respond adequately to diet after 4 weeks (LDL >155 mg/dL).

Pravastatin reduced LDL cholesterol by an average of 26% and had the following effects on cardiovascular events. Pravastatin reduced

1. All-cause mortality risk by 22% (P=0.05)
2. All coronary events by 31% (P<0.001)
3. Nonfatal myocardial infarction by 31% (P<0.001)
4. Death from all cardiovascular causes by 33% (P=0.033)
5. Myocardial revascularization (CABG or PTCA) by 37%

In addition there was no increase in noncardiac mortality. There were two major caveats with the WOSCOP study; namely, female patients were excluded and a very high proportion of patients were smokers or exsmokers (78%).

■ The WOSCOP study established that primary prevention with pravastatin in middle-aged men with hyperlipidemia decreased events by about a third and all cause deaths by a fifth in the 5 years following study participation.

(AFCAPS/TexCAPS) Trial (1998)

The Air Force/Texas Coronary Atherosclerosis Prevention Study (AFCAPS/TexCAPS) trial extended the benefit of primary prevention to patient populations with "average" cholesterol values. The investigators randomized just over 6,600 patients, including almost 1,000 women, all without clinical coronary artery disease to lovastatin or placebo for a mean of 5.2 years. The baseline mean triglyceride level was (221 mg/dL), mean LDL-C level was 150 mg/dL), mean HDL-C level was 36 mg/dL for men and 40 mg/dL for women. Treatment with lovastatin decreased LDL cholesterol by 25%, and increased HDL cholesterol by 6%. There was a 37% risk reduction in the occurrence of the composite end point (fatal or nonfatal myocardial infarction, sudden death, or unstable angina) with lovastatin, and coronary revascularization procedures decreased by 32%. The AFCAPS/TexCAPS study demonstrated for the first time a treatment benefit favoring statin therapy in a population without known coronary artery disease and with a previously identified "average" cholesterol value.

■ Taken together, the WOSCOP and AFCAPS/TexCAPS trials established that statin treatment of hyperlipidemia has a beneficial effect in the primary prevention of coronary artery disease.

ASCOT-LLA Trial (2003)

The Anglo-Scandinavian Cardiac Outcomes Trial - Lipid Lowering Arm (ASCOT-LLA) was a European multicenter randomized controlled trial that evaluated atorvastatin in the prevention of coronary and stroke events in high-risk hypertensive patients who have average or lower-than-average cholesterol levels. Just over half of the hypertensive patients had a total serum cholesterol concentration of ≤250 mg/dL (≤6.5 mmol/L) and were randomized to atorvastatin (10 mg/day) or placebo. These 10,300 patients formed the lipid-lowering arm of the study. Follow-up was initially planned for 5 years but the trial was stopped early after a median follow-up of 3.3 years because of a significant benefit in patients receiving atorvastatin. The primary end point of the study was a combination of nonfatal myocardial infarction or coronary heart disease death, which occurred in 1.9% of the atorvastatin patients and 3% of the placebo patients (Hazard ratio 0.64: P=0.0005). Atorvastatin also significantly reduced the stroke risk, total cardiovascular events, and all coronary events but the trial did not show a statistically significant reduction in all-cause mortality or cardiovascular mortality.

■ The ASCOT-LLA Trial established that low-dose atorvastatin reduced cardiovascular events and stroke risk in high risk hypertensive patients with normal or slightly elevated cholesterol levels.

CARDS Trial (2004)

The CARDS Trial (Collaborative Atorvastatin Diabetes Study) was a European study that evaluated the effect of atorvastatin 10 mg per day compared to placebo on primary prevention of cardiovascular events in patients with type 2 diabetes without known cardiovascular disease. The trial enrolled just over 2,800 diabetic patients with a serum LDL concentration ≤160 mg/dL, a fasting triglyceride concentration ≤600 mg, and at least one of the following high-risk features: retinopathy, albuminuria, active smoker, or hypertension.

The trial was terminated two years earlier than planned because of a substantial benefit in the atorvastatin arm. Cardiovascular events were reduced by 37%, and it was estimated that treatment would prevent 37 major cardiovascular events per 1,000 patients treated for a four-year period.

Subgroup analysis also showed a reduced stroke risk by 48%. Atorvastatin reduced the death rate by 27% with marginal statistical significance (P=0.059). An important secondary finding was that the absolute reduction in cardiovascular events with atorvastatin was similar in patients with LDL-cholesterol concentrations above or below 120 mg/dL.

■ The CARDS Trial concluded that atorvastatin 10 mg/daily reduced the risk of first cardiovascular disease event, including stroke, in patients with type 2 diabetes and mild to moderately elevated LDL cholesterol levels.

■ The CARDS study found no scientific justification for a particular threshold level of LDL-cholesterol as the sole arbiter when diabetic patients should receive statins.

SECONDARY PREVENTION OF CARDIOVASCULAR DISEASE

Secondary prevention refers to a reduction in future cardiovascular events in subjects with know cardiovascular disease.

The Scandinavian Simvastatin Survival Study (4S) (1994)

The Scandanavian Simvastatin Survival Study (4S) clearly established the benefit of lipid-lowering therapy for secondary prevention of future coronary events in patients with hyperlipidemia following myocardial infarction.

The 4S study tested the hypothesis that secondary prevention with simvastatin in patients with known coronary artery disease would reduce mortality and nonfatal infarctions in patients with hyperlipidemia. The study randomized patients to simvastatin 20-40 mg/day versus placebo. The study enrolled exactly 4,444 patients (to stay with the 4S theme) with total cholesterol values between 200 and 300 mg/dL. The study excluded high-risk patients—congestive heart failure, recent myocardial infarction or patients requiring revascularization (CABG or PTCA).

Simvastatin decreased total cholesterol by 25% and LDL cholesterol by 35%, with a modest (~8%) increase in HDL.

Simvastatin reduced

1. All-cause mortality by 30%
2. Coronary events by 34%
3. The risk of coronary death by 42%
4. Myocardial revascularization (CABG or PTCA) by 37%

In addition there was no increase in noncardiac mortality. The sickest patients with coronary artery disease were excluded from the study. Female, diabetic, and elderly patients were included in the 4S study.

■ The 4S study established there was a clear benefit for secondary prevention treatment with simvastatin in patients with established coronary artery disease and hypercholesterolemia.

The mortality in the female placebo group in the 4S study was less than 50% of the mortality for men; thus, the study was underpowered to draw statistical conclusions regarding the mortality benefit of lipid lowering in women. Women had a decrease in major coronary events that directly paralleled that seen in men, who in turn showed a mortality benefit with lipid treatment. Patients older than 60 years had both improved all-cause survival and a decreased incidence of major coronary events similar to that which occurred in patients younger than 60 years.

An interesting historical lipid trial was the Program on the Surgical Control of Hyperlipidemia (POSCH), which examined the benefits of partial ileal bypass surgery plus dietary intervention on mortality and cardiac events in 838 patients with hyperlipidemia. There was a 27% reduction in cardiovascular mortality and a 35% reduction in cardiac events in the surgically treated group. The relative risk reductions were similar to those in the 4S trial. There is currently no need to consider ileal bypass in patients with hyperlipidemia because pharmacologic agents can almost always achieve a similar benefit.

The Cholesterol and Recurrent Events (CARE) Study (1996)

The CARE study tested the hypothesis that secondary prevention with pravastatin 40 mg/day compared to placebo would reduce mortality and cardiac events in patients with "average" cholesterol levels. CARE randomized nearly 4,200 patients (21-75 years old) who had history of a myocardial infarction in the previous two years who had a total cholesterol value less than 240 mg/dL, an LDL value between 115 and 174 mg/dL, and a triglyceride value of less than 350 mg/dL. Excluded patients included those with symptomatic congestive heart failure and patients with low ejection fractions (<25%) The follow-up period was a median of 5.0 years.

Pravastatin decreased LDL cholesterol by 32%. In addition, pravastatin reduced

1. All-cause mortality by 9% (not statistically significant)
2. Coronary events by 24%
3. Nonfatal myocardial infarction by 23%
4. The risk of coronary death by 19%
5. Stroke by 31%
6. Myocardial revascularization (CABG or PTCA) by 27%

There was no increase in noncardiac mortality. Women were included in the study and benefited from pravastatin more than men. The CARE study showed a clear nonmortality benefit with secondary prevention treatment with pravastatin in patients with known coronary artery disease and "average" cholesterol levels. It is of interest that women had a more dramatic reduction in fatal and nonfatal myocardial infarction with pravastatin than men (45% versus 19%) in the CARE study. Overall, the CARE study showed no significant decrease in all-cause mortality, and no other significant benefit (mortality or otherwise) occurred in the patient subgroup with a baseline LDL cholesterol of 125 mg/dL or less.

The benefit with pharmacological cholesterol lowering is illustrated in a plot of the degree of LDL cholesterol lowering in the LRC, CARE, WOSCOP, and 4S trials versus the decrease in coronary artery disease relative risk. The greater the degree of LDL cholesterol lowering, the greater the decrease in cardiovascular events (Fig. 1).

Atorvastatin Versus Revascularization Treatment (AVERT) (2000)

The AVERT trial was a randomized trial that directly compared medical therapy with atorvastatin 80 mg/day to interventional therapy with PTCA and usual care in patients with stable coronary artery disease and class I and II angina, all of whom had been recommended to have PTCA, with regard to future cardiac ischemic events.

The study included 341 patients with angiographically proven coronary artery disease with stenosis of 50% or more in at least one vessel recommended for angioplasty with an LDL cholesterol value of at least 115 mg/dL and class I or class II angina. Patients were excluded if there was electrocardiographic evidence of severe ischemia—EKG changes at less than 4 minutes on a Bruce protocol treadmill test. LDL cholesterol was reduced by 46% in the atorvastatin-treated arm and by 18% in the angioplasty/usual-care arm.

At 18 months there was a 36% reduction in ischemic events in the atorvastatin arm compared with PTCA arm. Patients receiving atorvastatin had a 40% or more reduction in LDL cholesterol and had significantly fewer ischemic events than those with less than 40% reduction. Most medically treated patients (87%) who received atorvastatin were able to remain on medical therapy for 18 months without a cardiac ischemic event. This study is important because it highlights the importance of aggressive lipid lowering in all patients who come to coronary intervention. Current cardiology practice would be at variance with the randomization strategy in the AVERT trial and would favor early PCI in patients with a combination of angina, flow limiting coronary stenosis and a coronary anatomy suitable for PCI. Aggressive lipid reduction and PCI should be complementary rather than competitive strategies for the treatment of coronary artery disease.

LIPID Trial (1998)

The Long-Term Intervention With Pravastatin in Ischemic Disease (LIPID) trial examined 9,014 patients with known coronary artery disease who were randomized to treatment with pravastatin or placebo and followed for 6.1 years. Death from coronary artery disease was reduced from 8.3% in the placebo group to 6.4% in the pravastatin group ($P<0.001$). All-cause mortality was reduced from 14.1% to 11.0% ($P<0.001$). In addition, the risk reduction was 19% for stroke, 20% for coronary revascularization, and 29% for myocardial infarction.

TNT Trial (2005)

The Treating to New Targets (TNT) trial randomized 10,000 patients with stable coronary heart disease to low-dose or high-dose statins (atorvastatin low dose, 10

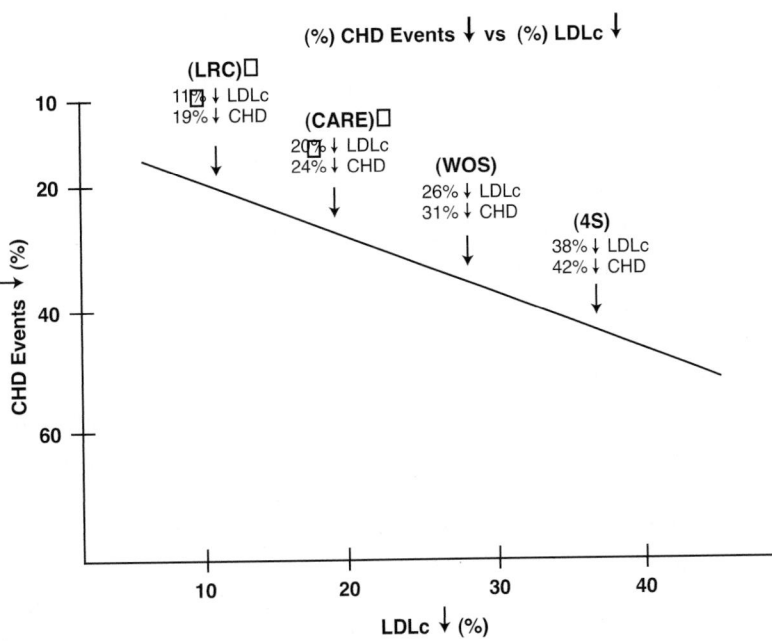

Fig. 1. Management of hyperlipidemia. CARE, Cholesterol and Recurrent Events study; CHD, coronary heart disease; LDLc, LDL cholesterol; LRC, Lipid Research Clinics trial; 4S, Scandinavian Simvastatin Survival Study; WOS, West of Scotland Study. Reduction in LDLc correlated with decrease in cardiovascular events in major lipid lowering trials.

mg/day, or a high dose, 80 mg/day) with goal LDL-cholesterol values of 100 mg/dL or 75 mg/dL respectively. Patients were required to have a baseline LDL-C between 130 mg/dL and 250 mg/dL and achieve an LDL-C below 130 mg/dL on low-dose atorvastatin (10 mg/day) during an initial open label run-in period.

The primary end point of the TNT trial was a major cardiovascular event—coronary death, nonfatal myocardial infarction, cardiac arrest, or stroke during the median follow-up period of 4.9 years.

High-dose atorvastatin had beneficial effects over low-dose statin and significantly lowered the occurrence of the primary end point—any major cardiovascular event—from 10.9% in the low-dose statin arm to 8.7% in the high-dose statin arm This represented an absolute 2.2 % and a relative 22% reduction in cardiovascular risk (hazard ratio, 0.78; *P*<0.001). There was no difference between the two treatment groups in overall mortality. High-dose atorvastatin also reduced the risk of myocardial infarction, fatal or nonfatal stroke, and cardiovascular death. There was a greater occurrence of persistent elevated liver enzymes (1.2% versus 0.2%) in the high-dose statin treatment arm.

IDEAL Study (2005)

The IDEAL study was a Northern European study that compared high-dose atorvastatin 80 mg/day head to head with usual dose simvastatin 20-40 mg/day in 8,888 patients aged 80 years or younger with a history of acute myocardial infarction. The main end point was any major coronary event—defined as coronary death, nonfatal myocardial infarction or cardiac arrest with resuscitation. During treatment, the mean LDL-C levels were 104 mg/dL in the simvastatin group and 81 mg/dL in the atorvastatin group. A major coronary event occurred in 10.4% of the simvastatin patients and in 9.3% of the atorvastatin patients (hazard ratio 0.89; *P*=.07). Aggressive lowering of LDL-C did not result in a significant reduction in the primary outcome of all major coronary events but did reduce the risk of other composite secondary end points and nonfatal acute myocardial infarction. There were no differences in cardiovascular or all-cause mortality between the groups.

Heart Protection Study (2002)

The Heart Protection Study (HPS) was a very large UK trial that randomized over 20,000 subjects aged 40-80 years with coronary disease, arterial vascular disease, treated hypertension, or diabetes to receive simvastatin 40 mg/daily (average compliance: 85%) or a matching placebo (average nonstudy statin use: 17%). Thirty-three percent of patients had a baseline LDL cholesterol <116 mg/dL, 25 percent had a level of 116 to 135 mg/dL, and 42% had levels >135 mg/dL. Patients in all three baseline cholesterol groups benefited equally from simvastatin. The average follow-up was 5.5 years. Simvastatin reduced all-cause mortality by 13% percent, with an 18% reduction in deaths from any cardiovascular cause and a 24% reduction in major cardiovascular events. There was a 25% reduction in the risk of first stroke (ischemic strokes but not hemorrhagic strokes). Diabetics had a larger benefit than nondiabetics, with a 28% reduction in the incidence of myocardial infarction and stroke. The proportional reduction in the event rate was similar (and significant) in each subcategory of participant studied, including those without diagnosed coronary disease; patients with cerebrovascular disease, peripheral artery disease, or diabetes; men, women; subjects aged either under or over 70 years at entry; and most notably even those who presented with an LDL cholesterol below 116 mg/dL or a total cholesterol below 193 mg/dL. The benefits of simvastatin were additional to those of all other cardioprotective treatments.

- Adding simvastatin to existing treatments safely produces substantial additional cardioprotective benefits for a wide range of high-risk patients, irrespective of their initial cholesterol concentrations or specific form of vascular disease.
- For high-risk individuals, as studied in the Heart Protection Study, 5 years of simvastatin would prevent 70-100 people per 1,000 subjects from suffering a major vascular event.
- The size of the 5-year benefit with simvastatin depends chiefly on an individual's overall risk of major vascular events, rather than on their blood lipid concentrations alone.

In summary, clear and compelling evidence now demonstrates that the rate of nonfatal cholesterol events and deaths from cardiovascular disease and total mortality can be reduced with aggressive lipid lowering in patients with known coronary artery disease. This is especially important in patients who have recently had a myocardial infarction in that the CARE study demonstrated benefit in as little as 2 months after initiation of treatment.

■ Early use of statins in unstable coronary syndromes, including myocardial infarction, may be beneficial and is discussed in chapter 69 on adjuvant therapy for myocardial infarction.

Coronary Artery Regression Studies

Several coronary angiographic trials have examined the effect of lipid lowering on the regression of coronary artery disease lesions. These angiographic trials used aggressive lipid management, generally reducing the LDL cholesterol value by 25% to 40%, with a relative decrease in myocardial infarction and coronary mortality by 25% to 45%. Some evidence of coronary disease regression was demonstrated in 14% to 20% of the patients, but the most significant finding was that coronary disease progression was slowed by about 50%. The Multicenter Anti-Atheroma Study (MAAS, simvastatin versus placebo), the Regression Growth Evaluation Statin Study (pravastatin versus placebo), and the Pravastatin Limitation of Atherosclerosis in the Coronary Arteries I Study (PLAC-I, pravastatin versus placebo) all demonstrated significant reductions in the rate of progression of angiographic coronary disease for patients in whom statin treatment significantly lowered serum LDL cholesterol values. The reductions in coronary events and death that were observed in the WOSCOP study, the 4S study, and the CARE study all occurred more quickly than would have been predicted on the basis of coronary atherosclerotic regression. Evidence now suggests that the primary beneficial effect of statin lipid-lowering therapy may be atherosclerotic plaque stabilization.

GAIN Trial (2001)

The GAIN trial was an innovative trial that used intravascular ultrasound to compare the effects of atorvastatin on plaque volume and composition in 130 patients with established coronary artery disease. Following 12 months of atorvastatin therapy there was a reduction in the progression of plaque volume and thickness and increase in plaque echogenicity indicative of change in plaque composition (putatively from a lipid-rich plaque to fibrotic and calcified plaque) that would be consistent with an increase in plaque stability with less risk of precipitation of future unstable coronary syndrome.

ASTEROID Trial 2006

The ASTEROID trial tested the effect of very high-intensity statin therapy (resuvastatin 40 mg daily) on regression of coronary atherosclerosis in 507 patients, as determined by intravascular ultrasound (IVUS) imaging at baseline and after 24 months of treatment. This study was a prospective, open-label, blinded end points trial in which patients were required to have undergone coronary angiography for a standard clinical indication, generally chest pain or an abnormal cardiac stress test. Patients were selected on the basis of an angiographic stenosis greater than 20% narrowing in at least one coronary vessel and a target artery suitable for IVUS with a narrowing of no more than 50%. The primary study end point was change in atheroma volume in the 10-mm subsegment with the greatest disease severity at baseline.

A total of 158 patients (30%) were not included in the final IVUS analysis due to a multiplicity of reasons, including withdrawal of consent (32), adverse events (63), and inadequate IVUS images (33). After 24 months, 349 patients had evaluable serial IVUS examinations.

Mean LDL cholesterol levels decreased by 53% from 130 mg/dL to 61 mg/dL; HDL cholesterol levels increased by 15 percent from 43 to 49 mg/dL. Most patients (78%) had atheroma regression with a mean percent decrease in atheroma volume of 6.1 mm^3 or 8.5 percent in the 10-mm segment with the greatest disease severity.

The study authors concluded that very high-intensity statin therapy for LDL-cholesterol levels below currently accepted guidelines, when accompanied by significant HDL-C increases, can regress atherosclerosis in coronary disease patients. Further studies are needed to determine the clinical effect of these salutary atheroma volume changes.

PROBUCOL

Probucol is a weak LDL cholesterol-lowering agent but a powerful antioxidant that protects LDL and lipoprotein (a) from oxidation. It was withdrawn from the market because of its tendency to prolong the QT interval with resultant ventricular arrhythmias.

FISH OILS
Fish oils contain omega-3 fatty acids, which can significantly reduce elevated triglyceride levels. Their cardiovascular benefit, although much promoted, is scientifically unproved. Fish oils appear to be particularly beneficial in the treatment of retinoid (Accutane)-induced increase of serum triglyceride levels, a drug commonly used in the treatment of severe cystic acne.

COMBINATION THERAPY IN REFRACTORY HYPERLIPIDEMIA OR MIXED HYPERLIPIDEMIA
Combination therapy is frequently necessary to treat refractory hyperlipidemia, often allows lower drug doses, and may reduce the incidence of medication side effects. Combination therapy can often lower LDL cholesterol, increase HDL cholesterol, and lower triglyceride values very effectively.

STATIN + EZETIMIBE
The combination of statin and ezetimibe is an excellent and complementary combination that blocks both hepatic LDL cholesterol production and intestinal cholesterol absorption to give an added decrement in LDL-C beyond that seen with statin therapy alone. There is a minor increase in the risk of statin hepatotoxicity and myositis when ezetimibe is added to a statin.

STATIN + RESIN
The combination of a statin agent and a bile acid-binding resin is very effective when either agent alone fails to reduce the LDL cholesterol to the target goal. The combination of a statin agent and a bile acid-binding agent is particularly effective for lowering LDL cholesterol in type II-A hyperlipidemia. Careful upward titration of the resin dose will often avoid the gastrointestinal side effects frequently observed with resins.

STATIN + FIBRIC ACID DERIVATIVE
The combination of pravastatin and gemfibrozil is excellent for lowering both triglyceride and LDL cholesterol levels, but at an increased risk of myositis. One approach to treatment of mixed hyperlipidemia is to estimate the percentage reduction needed to bring the LDL and triglyceride values into the desired target range.

Monotherapy with high-dose simvastatin or atorvastatin reduces triglyceride values 25% to 40% and LDL cholesterol values by 30% to 60%. Combination therapy with a statin and fenofibrate or gemfibrozil should be considered if the need to lower the triglyceride value exceeds that typically obtained with statin monotherapy. Fenofibrate can be used if a 10% to 20% reduction in LDL cholesterol is desired. If a greater reduction in LDL cholesterol is the goal, then combination therapy of gemfibrozil plus a statin is necessary. The use of fibrates alone is occasionally associated with myopathy, and the combined use of a statin with a fibrate increases the risk of myopathy substantially. Combination therapy must be instituted at low doses of both agents, with careful upward titration until the desired lipid lowering is achieved. Careful monitoring for muscle and liver toxicity is important.

TREATMENT OF AN ISOLATED LOW HDL
An isolated low HDL cholesterol value is a strong risk factor for cardiovascular disease and may be clinically difficult to treat. Niacin, gemfibrozil, and fenofibrate will all increase an isolated low HDL value by 10% to 15%, whereas most statins will increase the HDL level by only 5% to 8%. Niacin, fenofibrate, and gemfibrozil all effectively treat the combination of a low HDL level and an increased triglyceride level. This lipid pattern is often found in patients with diabetes mellitus or obesity with insulin resistance. Combination therapy with a statin plus niacin, gemfibrozil, or fenofibrate effectively treats patients with a lipid profile characterized by a low HDL in combination with high LDL cholesterol with or without increased triglycerides.

SIDE EFFECTS AND DRUG INTERACTIONS OF LIPID-LOWERING DRUGS
The two most common side effects of statins and fibrates are myositis and an increase in hepatic

transaminase enzymes. Both of these side effects are uncommon and usually disappear when drug therapy is discontinued. There is an increased incidence of myositis in patients receiving statins combined with high-dose niacin or fibrates. The use of cyclosporine in combination with statins may increase serum concentrations of the statin and, in turn, increase the incidence of drug-related side effects. It is important to reduce the dose of statin by 50% when a patient is also started on cyclosporin. The dose of statin may be slowly increased with time if the serum cholesterol values necessitate upward titration. Pravastatin is the best statin to use with cyclosporin because of a lower incidence of drug-drug interaction.

COMMON PITFALLS IN LIPID TREATMENT

A major pitfall in the treatment of patients with hyperlipidemia is a failure to achieve the desired LDL cholesterol target goal, despite a maximal dose of the administered drug. This is often the result of patient noncompliance with pharmacologic and, more frequently, nonpharmacologic lipid treatment strategies (diet and exercise). It is important to also consider an exacerbation of a coexisting illness such as diabetes mellitus, hypothyroidism, renal failure, or excess alcohol consumption. Additionally, the lipid-lowering agent should be taken at bedtime, because the liver synthesizes cholesterol predominantly during the sleep cycle.

There are several possible treatment strategies for persistently increased LDL cholesterol despite seemingly adequate lipid-lowering statin medication therapy.

1. Check the lipoprotein (a) value to be certain there is no interaction from this lipoprotein fraction.
2. Switch to a more potent statin, such as atorvastatin, simvastatin, or resuvastatin. Both simvastatin and atorvastatin can be used safely at high doses (80 mg/day) with additional lipid-lowering benefit.
3. Add ezetimibe 10 mg/day to block intestinal cholesterol absorption
4. Add a bile acid-binding resin to the statin.
5. Consider the addition of fenofibrate or gemfibrozil to potentiate the effect of triglyceride lowering plus additional LDL lowering. This strategy increases the risk of side effects
6. Consider referral to a specialized center that per-

forms LDL apheresis for the persistently increased LDL cholesterol value despite maximal pharmacologic therapy. LDL apheresis removes apo-B–containing lipoproteins directly from the blood by extracorporeal circulation through adsorption columns and is indicated in the treatment of refractory hypercholesterolemia despite the use of maximally tolerated lipid-lowering drug therapy and intense dietary modification.

LDL apheresis reduces the following:

- LDL cholesterol by 50% to 75%.
- HDL cholesterol by about 15%.
- Triglycerides by about 50%.
- Lipoprotein (a) by about 60%.

LDL apheresis is approved by the Food and Drug Administration for treatment of medication-refractory hypercholesterolemia defined as:

- LDL >200 mg/dL with coronary disease.
- LDL >300 mg/dL without coronary disease.

LDL apheresis may be beneficially combined with high-dose statin therapy (atorvastatin, 80 mg/day) in some patients with homozygous familial hypercholesterolemia to achieve a further 30% reduction in LDL levels.

SPECIAL POPULATIONS WITH HYPERLIPIDEMIA

Women With Heart Disease

Heart disease is the leading cause of death in women, although in general it develops at an older age in women than in men. The benefit of aggressive lipid-lowering therapy with statin agents in women with hyperlipidemia is now well established. Hormone replacement therapy [HRT] causes a fall in LDL cholesterol by about 15%, an elevation in HDL cholesterol by about 15% and an increase in triglycerides increased by 25% but there is no proven cardiovascular benefit of HRT (Women's Health Initiative [WHI], Heart and Estrogen/Progestin Replacement Study [HERS] Study).

Elderly Patients

Elderly patients derive significant primary and secondary cardiovascular prevention benefit from pharmacological LDL-cholesterol lowering and the decision to start or not start cholesterol-lowering medication should not be based on chronological age. Elderly patients derive a greater benefit in absolute terms than younger patients because the occurrence of cardiovascular events is much higher in the elderly. The following lipid-lowering randomized trials enrolled subjects 65 years and older.

The **Scandinavian Simvastatin Survival Study (4S)**, a secondary prevention study of simvastatin included approximately 1,000 patients greater than 65 years of age with established coronary artery disease and hyperlipidemia. Simvastatin caused a similar reduction in serum lipids in elderly and younger subjects and reduced all-cause mortality and cardiovascular events by about one-third in the elderly.

The **Cholesterol and Recurrent Events (CARE) trial**, a secondary prevention trial of pravastatin also included almost 1,300 patients aged 65 and older and demonstrated a reduction in coronary events by about a third in elderly patients, approximately a twofold greater percentage benefit than that seen in younger patients.

The **LIPID Trial** was a secondary prevention trial with pravastatin that included over 3,500 patients between the ages of 65 and 75 years with established cardiovascular disease and mild-moderate hyperlipidemia. Pravastatin reduced cardiovascular events and all-cause mortality by a similar percentage in older and younger patients, but the absolute benefit to the elderly was greater.

The **PROSPER Trial** was confined to patients aged 70 to 82 years with a history of cardiovascular disease or risk factors for vascular disease. This study randomized over 5,800 patients to pravastatin (40 mg/day) or placebo. Pravastatin lowered serum LDL cholesterol by 34% and significantly reduced the combined cardiovascular end point (coronary death, nonfatal myocardial infarction, stroke) hazard ratio 0.81: P=0.014. Mortality from coronary disease fell by 24% (P=0.043). Overall stroke risk was unaffected by therapy, but pravastatin reduced the hazard ratio for transient ischemic attack by 0.75 (P=0.051). There was no significant reduction in all-cause mortality but the decrease in cardiac deaths was offset by a significant increase in new diagnoses of cancer, a finding considered spurious as a meta-analysis of all major statin trials, including PROSPER, showed no statistical link between statins and cancer.

■ Elderly patients with hyperlipidemia are markedly undertreated with statins, are less compliant with medication, and have more statin-associated side effects (probably more drug interactions) with statins.

Patients With Diabetes

Diabetes mellitus is an important risk factor for the development of cardiovascular disease. Most patients with diabetes die of complications from coronary artery disease, stroke or peripheral vascular disease. Diabetic patients without cardiac symptoms or a diagnosis of known coronary artery disease have a high mortality from cardiovascular causes similar to patients with known cardiovascular disease, suggesting that most diabetes-associated coronary disease is clinically silent or unrecognized. Hypertriglyceridemia is a strong predictor of coronary artery disease in diabetics. Aggressive primary prevention of coronary artery disease is important in diabetic patients with hyperlipidemia with a goal LDL cholesterol value less than 70 mg/dL, HDL cholesterol value more than 40 mg/dL, and triglyceride value less than 200 mg/dL. It can be reasonably argued that all adult diabetics should be on a statin medication for primary prevention of cardiovascular disease unless there is a strong contraindication, such as previous hepatoxicity or myopathy. Pharmacologic therapy with a statin or combination statin and fibrate should be initiated in conjunction with nonpharmacologic measures, including strict diabetes control, diet, exercise and an ACE inhibitor for its cardiorenal protection effect.

Recipients of Organ Transplants

Recipients of heart and other organ transplants often manifest an accelerated form of coronary and peripheral vascular disease (posttransplant vasculopathy) several years after transplantation. The cause of this vasculopathy is probably multifactorial: low-grade transplant rejection, the untoward effects of chronic treatment with immunosuppressive agents (cyclosporine, steroids), hypertension, diabetes, and hypercholesterolemia. Although posttransplantation vasculopathy is not strongly linked to serum LDL cholesterol levels, it is recommended that all transplant patients be treated according to targets established by the National Cholesterol Education Program for patients with known coronary artery disease. This approach will often require pharmacologic therapy with a statin agent. Pravastatin is considered the statin of choice for posttransplant patients when the antirejection drug cyclosporin also is being administered. The use of cyclosporin in conjunction with a statin increases the risk of myopathy significantly, but probably less so with pravastatin than with the other potent statins.

Statins and the Vulnerable Atherosclerotic Plaque

The ultimate target of all lipid-lowering therapy is the vulnerable atherosclerotic plaque. Coronary plaque rupture is the final common pathway for all the unstable coronary syndromes. Experimental data suggest that statin therapy, in addition to its effect on LDL cholesterol metabolism, may stabilize the vulnerable atherosclerotic plaque and convert lipid-rich plaques that are at high risk of rupture into more stable fibrotic plaques. The reduction in cardiovascular events found in all the statin trials occurred earlier than would be expected from coronary plaque regression alone due to pure lipid lowering. This suggests an additional beneficial mechanism by statins on vulnerable plaques. Statin therapy may stabilize the vulnerable plaque through a reduction in macrophages and extracellular lipid accumulation in the plaque region, by an increase in the collagen content of the extracellular plaque matrix, by a reduction in calcification and neovascularization in the intima of the plaque, and through an inhibitory role on the coagulation and inflammatory cascades that accompany plaque rupture.

SECTION XI

Invasive and Interventional Cardiology

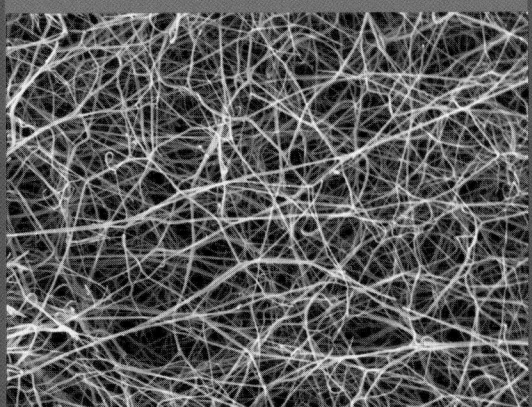

EM of Coronary Thrombus Ultrastructure

113

ENDOTHELIAL DYSFUNCTION AND CARDIOVASCULAR DISEASE

Brian P. Shapiro, MD

Amir Lerman, MD

ENDOTHELIAL CELL PHYSIOLOGY

The endothelium is the largest organ system in the human body and is composed of a monolayer of specialized cells that form the inner surface of blood vessels. Once thought to function as an inert passive vascular barrier, the endothelium is now widely recognized to play a major active role in vascular homeostasis and end organ function blood flow. Endothelium has the ability to sense mechanical and hormonal stimuli and release various vasoactive substances that regulate functions such as the maintenance of vascular tone as well as anti-thrombotic and anti-inflammatory processes (Fig. 1).

The hallmark function of an intact endothelium is its ability to regulate vascular tone by releasing a variety of substances that act as either vascular vasodilators or vasoconstrictors. Vessels are normally in a state of vasodilatation due in large part to endothelial nitric oxide (NO) synthesis and release. In endothelial dysfunction, there is inappropriate vasoconstriction. *Accordingly, endothelial dysfunction has been broadly defined as the reduction of vasodilatation in the presence of increased bioavailability of vascular constricting factors.*

PATHOPHYSIOLOGY OF ENDOTHELIAL DYSFUNCTION AND ATHEROSCLEROSIS

Given the wealth of protective functions of normal endothelium, any damage to these cells can blunt the ability to maintain vascular homeostasis. Endothelial injury often occurs from high shear stress and high oxidative stress (via reactive oxygen and nitrogen intermediates), which lead to the oxidation of low-density lipoproteins (LDLs). These products cause abnormal NO synthesis and the concurrent release of substances that promote vasoconstriction, inflammation and coagulation. A "positive feedback loop" ensues whereby oxidized LDL particles promote the adhesion and infiltration of monocytes and T-cells into the subendothelial space. Inflammatory cells react with the oxidized LDL to form foam cells. This leads to endothelial cell death and/or dysfunction, extracellular matrix digestion and vascular smooth muscle proliferation. Endothelial dysfunction may then progress to subclinical atherosclerosis and finally to acute coronary and vascular syndromes (Fig. 2).

Galley and Webster

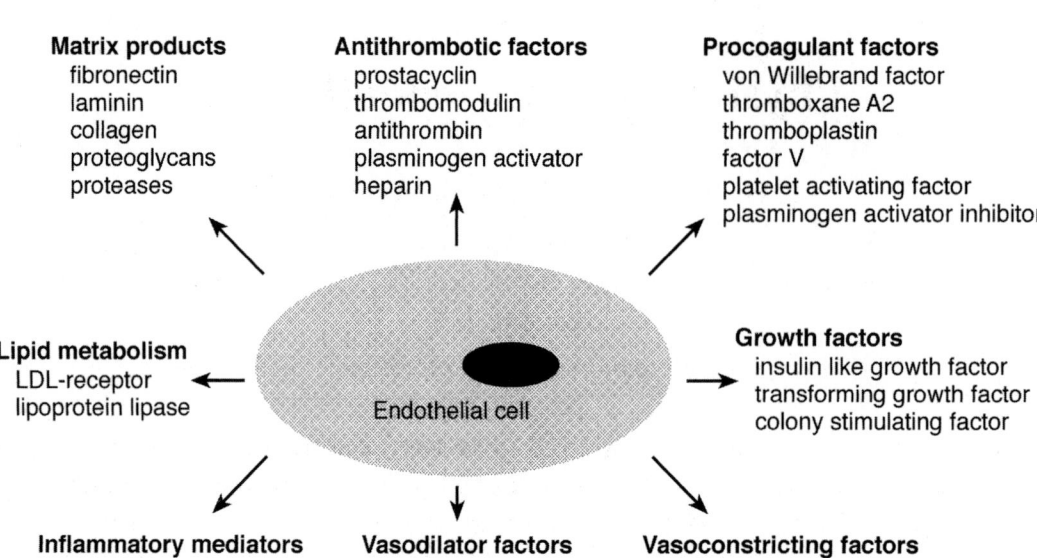

Fig. 1. Normal endothelial cell physiology.

RISK FACTORS ASSOCIATED WITH ENDOTHELIAL DYSFUNCTION

While the exact molecular mechanisms remain unclear, there is a wealth of clinical data that links specific diseases and conditions with endothelial dysfunction. The traditional CV risk factors such as hypertension, hyperlipidemia, diabetes or glucose intolerance, smoking, advanced age and adverse familial cardiovascular history are highly associated with endothelial dysfunction. There is increasing evidence that novel cardiovascular risk factors including the metabolic syndrome, obesity and hyperhomocystinemia among others also play an important role in endothelial dysfunction. There are likely other important environmental and genetic risk factors that remain to be discovered.

CLINICAL CONSEQUENCES AND PROGNOSTIC IMPLICATIONS OF ENDOTHELIAL DYSFUNCTION

Since endothelial dysfunction generally predates atherosclerotic disease, early identification of patient endothelial dysfunction may allow an earlier diagnosis of patients at high risk for atherosclerosis. Endothelial dysfunction predicts the development of classical cardiovascular risk factor such as hypertension and diabetes and also future clinical cardiovascular events. The greater the severity of endothelial dysfunction the greater the risk of CV disease. Thus, endothelial function may serve as a "barometer" for CV health.

Patients with endothelial dysfunction have a greater probability of developing myocardial ischemia or myocardial infarction due to the deleterious effects of vascular vasoconstriction, inflammation and coagulopathy. Patients with endothelial dysfunction may develop myocardial ischemia even with angiographically normal coronary arteries (ie. syndrome X). In the absence of a normal endothelium-dependent coronary vasodilatory response to stress and exercise, patients may experience angina due to a mismatch between myocardial blood supply and demand. In addition endothelial dysfunction may also play a role in acute coronary syndromes via these same processes that may ultimately lead to digestion of the fibrous atherosclerotic cap with subsequent plaque destabilization, plaque rupture and vascular occlusive thrombus formation.

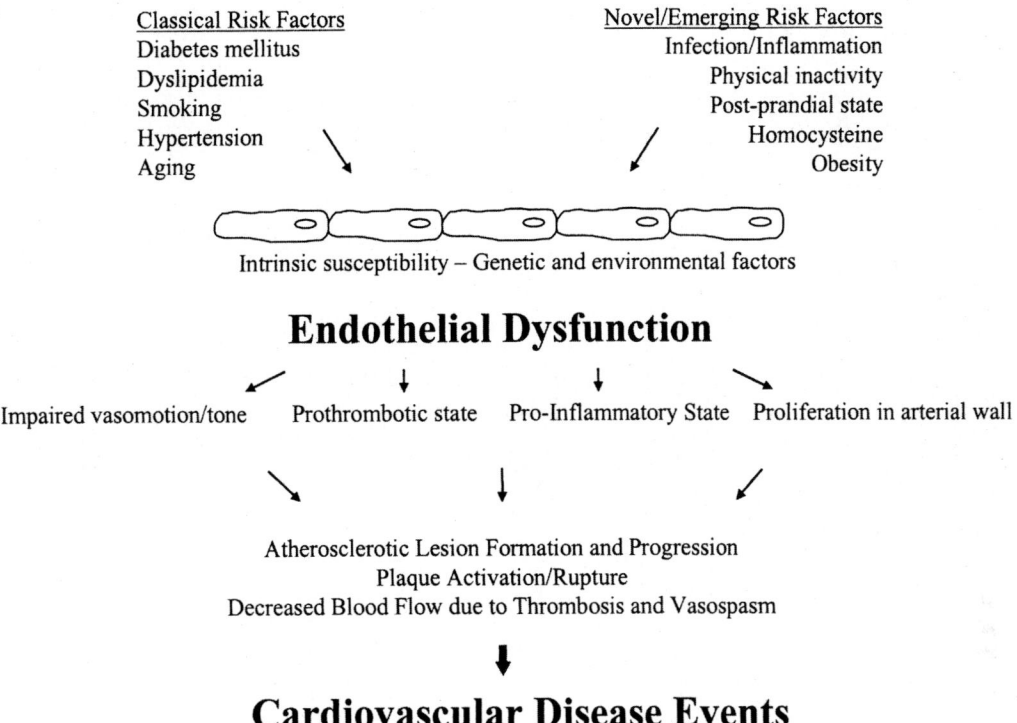

Classical Risk Factors
Diabetes mellitus
Dyslipidemia
Smoking
Hypertension
Aging

Novel/Emerging Risk Factors
Infection/Inflammation
Physical inactivity
Post-prandial state
Homocysteine
Obesity

Intrinsic susceptibility – Genetic and environmental factors

Endothelial Dysfunction

Impaired vasomotion/tone   Prothrombotic state   Pro-Inflammatory State   Proliferation in arterial wall

Atherosclerotic Lesion Formation and Progression
Plaque Activation/Rupture
Decreased Blood Flow due to Thrombosis and Vasospasm

Cardiovascular Disease Events

Fig. 2. Endothelial dysfunction is caused by traditional and novel risk factors, which have deleterious effects on vascular homeostasis. Endothelial dysfunction promotes cardiovascular disease via multiple mechanisms.

Many studies have established the important prognostic role of endothelial dysfunction in cardiovascular disease (Table 1). The existence of endothelial dysfunction predicts worse patient outcome independent of the presence of clinical cardiovascular disease or in the vascular bed where endothelial function was studied. For example, multiple authors have evaluated endothelial dysfunction in the peripheral arteries, which are often without significant atherosclerotic stenotic plaques. The presence of poor vasomotor tone in these conduit vessels correlates well with coronary arterial endothelial dysfunction and is predictive of future cardiovascular events. Thus, endothelial dysfunction is considered a marker of systemic disease that affects the entire vascular tree.

CLINICAL MEASUREMENT AND ASSESSMENT OF ENDOTHELIAL DYSFUNCTION

Normal endothelium responds to shear stress and hormonal stimuli by releasing endothelium-derived relaxing factors, such as NO, which cause vasodilatation. The

change in vessel diameter due to acetycholine (Ach) and other vasoactive substances can be characterized by the calculation of flow-mediated vasodilatation (FMD). Ach works by up-regulating the synthesis of NO from the precursor L-arginine in the presence of endothelial NO synthase (eNOS). Production of NO then activates a cascade of events that ultimately leads to smooth muscle relaxation and vasodilatation (Fig. 3). In endothelial dysfunction, this process is blunted and there is a propensity for paradoxical vasoconstriction due in large part to the release of endothelin.

Although endothelial dysfunction predates atherosclerosis, appropriate patient testing has been limited due its technically challenging nature and the fact that its clinical utility remains undefined. Nevertheless, there are various invasive and noninvasive tests employed to measure vasomotor dysfunction, each with advantages and disadvantages (Table 2).

Functional Coronary Angiography

Considered the gold standard for the assessment of

Table 1.   Studies Evaluating the Predictive Value of Endothelial Dysfunction

Lead author	Design/mean follow-up	Patient population	Vascular bed	Marker of endothelial function	End points examined	Findings
Al Suwaidi	Retrospective/28 months	157 patients with mild CAD	Coronary	Acetylcholine response	Cardiac death, MI, CHF,	6 patients with event. Acetylcholine response independent predictor of events.
Schachinger	Retrospective/7.7 years	147 patients with CAD	Coronary	Acetylcholine, cold pressor test, FMD, NTG	MI, UA, ischemic stroke, CABG, PTCA, peripheral bypass	28 patients with event. Vasomotor function independent predictor of events.
Neunteufl	Retrospective/5 years	73 patients with CAD	Brachial	FMD	Death, MI, PTCA, or CABG	27 patients with event. FMD <10% predictive of events. Effect lost when controlling for extent of CAD.
Heitzer	Prospective/4.5 years	281 patients with CAD	Brachial	Forearm blood flow response to acetylcholine	CVD death, stroke, MI, CABG, PTCA, peripheral bypass	91 patients with event. Acetylcholine response independent predictor of events.
Perticone	Prospective/32 months	225 patients with hypertension	Brachial	Forearm blood flow response to acetylcholine	CVD death, MI, stroke, TIA, UA, CABG, PTCA, PVD	29 subjects with event. Acetylcholine response predictive of events.

Table 1. (continued)

Lead author	Design/mean follow-up	Patient population	Vascular bed	Marker of endo-thelial function	End points examined	Findings
Gokce	Prospective/30 days	187 patients undergoing vascular surgery	Brachial	FMD	CVD death, MI, UA, stroke	45 patients with event. FMD independent predictor of events.
Modena	Prospective/67 months	400 hypertensive post-menopausal women	Brachial	FMD	Hospitalization for CVD event (not otherwise specified)	47 patients with event. Failure to improve FMD with 6 months of anti-hypertensive therapy independent predictor of events.
Halcox	Retrospective/46 months	308 patients referred for cardiac catheterization	Coronary	Acetylcholine response	CVD death, MI, ischemic stroke, UA	35 subjects with event. Acetylcholine response independent predictor of events.
Schindler	Prospective/45 months	130 patients with normal coronary angiograms	Coronary	Cold pressor test	CVD death, UA, MI, PTCA, CABG, stroke, peripheral bypass	26 patients with event. Cold pressor test response independent predictor of events.
Gokce	Prospective/1.2 years	199 patients undergoing vascular surgery	Brachial	FMD	CVD, death, MI, UA, stroke	35 patients with events. FMD independent predictor of long-term events.

CABG, coronary artery bypass graft surgery; CAD, coronary artery disease; CHF, congestive heart failure; CVD, cardiovascular disease; FMD, flow-mediated dilation; MI, myocardial infarction; NTG, nitroglycerin-mediated dilation; PCI, percutaneous coronary intervention (e.g., angioplasty or stent); PTCA, percutaneous transluminal coronary angioplasty; PVD, peripheral vascular disease; TIA, transient ischemic attack; UA, unstable angina.

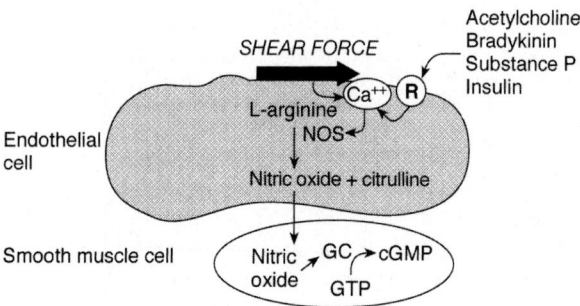

Fig. 3. Endothelial nitric oxide (NO) synthase (eNOS) catalyzes the synthesis of NO from L-arginine. NO activates guanylate cyclase (GC) in the smooth muscle leading to the production of cGMP. This second messenger inhibits calcium influx and, thus, leads to smooth muscle deactivation and vasorelaxation.

endothelial dysfunction, this test evaluates the coronary endothelial response to vasodilators such as Ach (Fig. 4). While normal smooth muscle responds to Ach by vasodilating, patients with endothelial dysfunction often have paradoxical vasoconstriction or blunted vasodilatation. Conversely, the infusion of nitroglycerin or adenosine, drugs that are considered endothelial-independent vasodilators, dilate arterial segments independent of the presence of endothelial dysfunction.

A functional coronary angiogram is performed using a standard protocol (Fig. 5). A Doppler guidewire and coronary infusion catheter are positioned in the mid-left anterior descending artery. Measurements of coronary artery diameter, flow velocity and vascular resistance are taken at baseline and in response to graded intracoronary (IC) infusions of Ach and nitroglycerin. These values are used to calculate flow-mediated vasodilatation (FMD), coronary blood flow (CBF) and coronary flow reserve (CFR) (Fig. 6). FMD is used to assess epicardial vascular tone whereas CBF and CFR evaluate the presence of endothelial dysfunction in the microvasculature. Maximal vasodilatation is achieved with intracoronary (IC) infusion of nitroglycerin or adenosine. N-monomethyl-L-arginine (L-NMMA), an inhibitor of eNOS, can blunt vasodilatation due to acetycholine.

Venous Occlusion Plethysmography

This approach is used to evaluate endothelial dysfunction in the peripheral arteries (Fig. 7). Intra-arterial infusions

Table 2.   Advantages and Disadvantages of Methods to Quantify Endothelial Function in Humans

1. Intracoronary agonist infusion with quantitative coronary angiography
   Advantages
      Direct quantification of endothelial function in the vascular bed of interest
      Allows for mapping dose-response relationships of endothelial agonists and antagonists
      Allows for examination of basal endothelial function (with NOS antagonist infusion)
   Disadvantages
      Invasive
      Expensive
      Carries risks inherent with coronary artery catheterization (stroke, MI, infection, vascular injury)
2. Brachial artery catheterization with venous occlusive plethysmography
   Advantages
      More accessible circulation than coronary arteries
      Allows for mapping dose-response relationships of endothelial agonists and antagonists
      Allows for examination of basal endothelial function (with NOS antagonist infusion)
   Disadvantages
      Invasive
      Risk of median nerve injury, infection, vascular injury
3. Vascular tonometry and measurements of vascular stiffness
   Advantages
      Noninvasive
      Safer and faster than either invasive method
      Lower operator dependence than brachial artery ultrasound
      May reflect basal endothelial function

Table 2.   (continued)

Disadvantages
  Importantly influenced by structural
    aspects of the vasculature beyond the
    endothelium
4. Brachial artery ultrasound with FMD
  Advantages
    Noninvasive
    Safer and faster than either invasive
      method
    Reactivity correlates to endothelial
      dysfunction in coronary circulation
    Flow is a physiological stimulus for
      vasodilation unlike agonists such as
      acetylcholine
  Disadvantages
    Poor resolution relative to arterial size
    Variability in measurements
    Highly operator-dependent

FMD, flow-mediated dilation; MI, myocardial infarction; NOS, nitric oxide synthase.

of vasoactive substances are used to assess vascular hemodynamics (Table 3). FMD can be measured via plethysmography or ultrasound. Unfortunately, this technique is invasive in that it requires an arterial catheter and needs further validation.

Brachial Artery Ultrasound

This is a popular noninvasive technique used to measure endothelial dysfunction and may be the most attractive method for routine clinical assessment. While it correlates well with functional coronary angiography, the need for technical expertise and the existence of many confounding factors (ie. sympathomimetic agents, foods, medications, menstrual cycle and temperature) have limited its use. To control for some of these factors, environmental conditions should be standardized (Table 4).

The principle behind this technique is that there is normally reactive hyperemia (increased FMD) in response to ischemia (Fig. 8). Thus, brachial artery ultrasound imaging is performed at baseline and following the inflation of an occlusive arterial blood pressure cuff. While supine, a cuff is inflated to at least 50 mm Hg above the systolic pressure or to a prespecified value (300 mm Hg and 200 mm Hg in adults and children, respectively) for five minutes. After the cuff is deflated, there should be reactive hyperemia which allows for the calculation of FMD (change in arterial diameter from baseline as a percentage (%). Nitroglycerin can also be given after the hyperemic stage to promote endothelium-independent vasodilatation.

Arterial Stiffness

Vascular stiffness and arterial remodeling are closely tied to the development of endothelial dysfunction. Since measurement of arterial stiffness is highly dependent on structural vascular abnormalities such as fibrosis and calcification, this test should not be used in isolation in the evaluation of endothelial dysfunction.

Biomarkers of Endothelial Dysfunction

Invasive and/or noninvasive assessment of endothelial dysfunction is complemented through the use of circulating biomarkers, which have been found to have prognostic significance. The upregulation of molecules that are involved in vasoconstriction (endothelin), vascular inflammation (soluble adhesion molecules and cytokines) and coagulation (hematologic markers) may help to more accurately predict the presence of endothelial dysfunction (Table 5).

Another potential marker of endothelial dysfunction is the measurement of circulating endothelial progenitor cells (EPCs). Damage to the endothelium needs prompt repair and bone-marrow-derived circulating EPCs are released and migrate to the area of endothelial damage. Unfortunately, the perpetual and continuous process of vascular damage and repair may deplete or cause dysfunction to stores of progenitor cells. Studies have found a strong inverse relationship between the number of EPCs and CV risk factors and CV disease. Further studies using EPCs as a surrogate marker of endothelial dysfunction are under way.

THERAPEUTIC APPROACH TO ENDOTHELIAL DYSFUNCTION

While endothelial dysfunction appears to predate the pathogenesis of atherosclerosis, there is little direct data

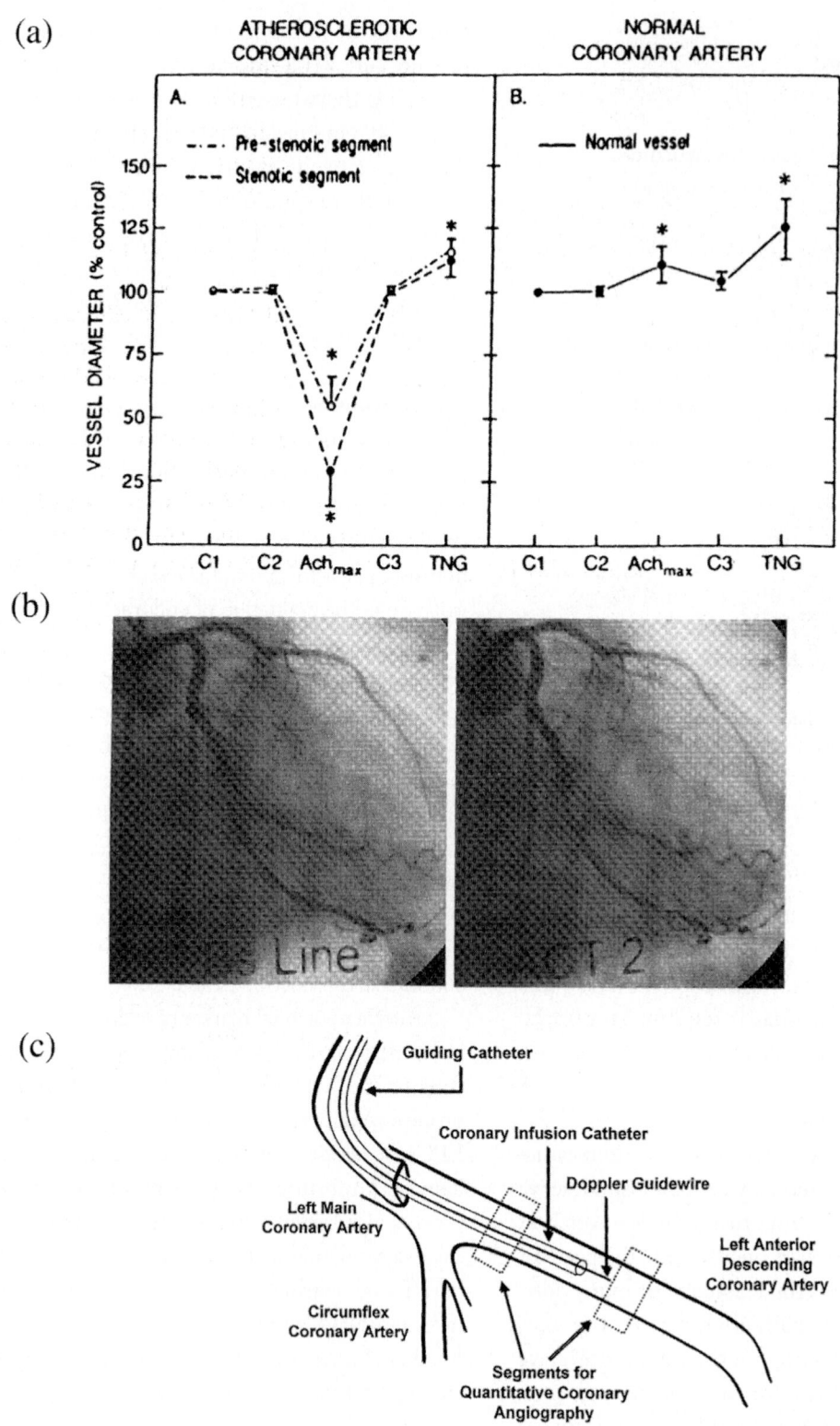

Fig. 4. Functional coronary angiogram. Figure (*a*) depicts flow-mediated dilatation in an atherosclerotic (A) and normal coronary artery (B). C1, control; C2, vehicle control; Ach$_{max}$, response to acetylcholine; C3, repeat control; TNG, nitroglycerin. Corresponding diagnostic angiogram (*b*) shows severe vasoconstriction of the obtuse marginal branch following acetylcholine infusion. Figure (*c*) shows the normal positioning of the infusion catheter and Doppler guidewire.

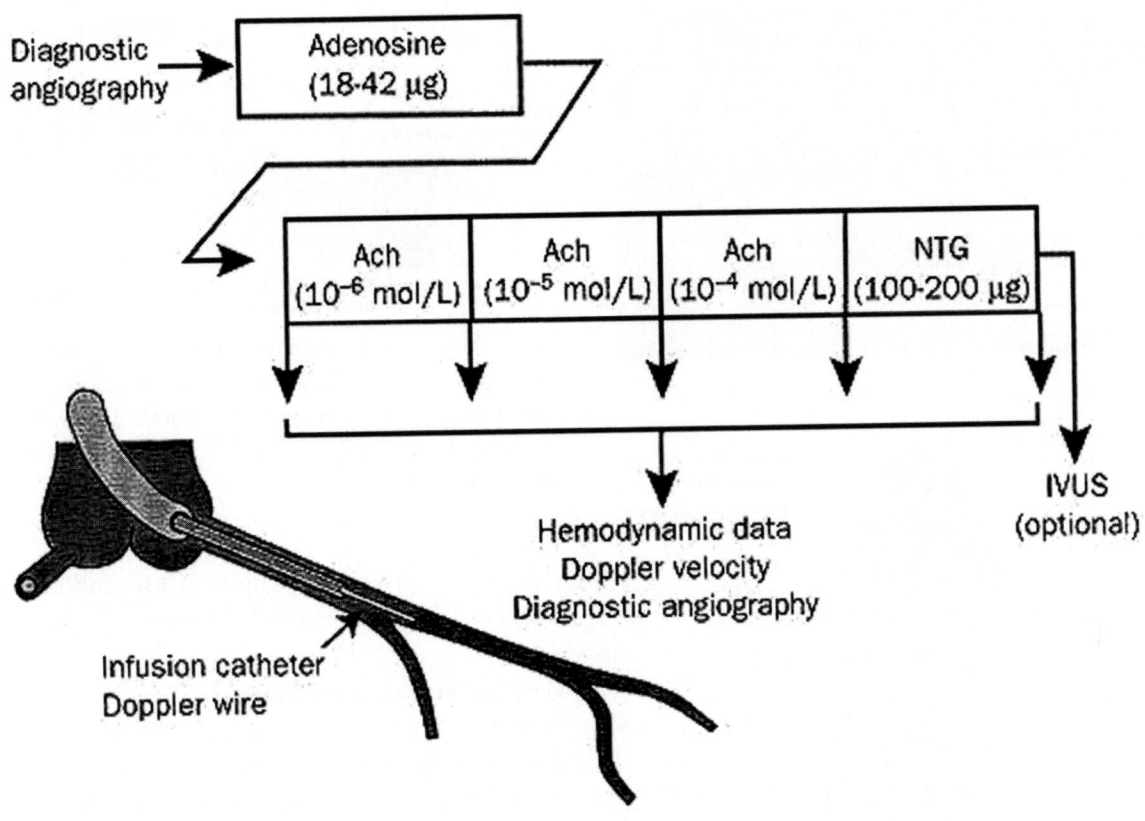

Fig. 5. Clinical protocol for assessing endothelial dysfunction in the coronary arteries. Diagnostic angiography is performed followed by the intracoronary infusion of adenosine to achieve maximal vasodilatation. Then graded doses of acetylcholine (Ach) are given followed by nitroglycerin (NTG) administration.

to conclude that reversal of endothelial dysfunction per se has a direct effect on future CV events. Also, the potential to reverse more significant damage to the endothelium has not been proven. There are a number of therapies to improve endothelial dysfunction that are being currently evaluated and may prove beneficial (Table 6).

Traditional Risk Factor Reduction and Lifestyle Modification

Conventional therapy is aimed at targeting traditional cardiovascular risk factors such as hypertension, hyperlipidemia, diabetes mellitus and tobacco abuse. Guidelines emphasize the importance of weight loss via aerobic exercise and a low fat diet. These measures ameliorate endothelial dysfunction and decrease the risk of future cardiovascular events, and thus, should be regarded as first line therapy for endothelial dysfunction.

Lipid Lowering

Oxidation of LDL particles and the formation of foam cells represent a major mechanism for the development of atherosclerosis. Accordingly, LDL reduction via lifestyle modification and/or pharmacotherapy is critical to the prevention of future cardiovascular events. While LDL reduction itself is highly important, recent data underscore the importance of the pleiotropic effects of HMG CoA reductase inhibitors (statins). These agents restore endothelial function and NO bioavailability while providing antioxidant and anti-inflammatory effects. Recent studies have shown that statins improve endothelial dysfunction independent of changes in LDL levels.

Antioxidants

Free radicals and increased oxidative stress are important triggers of endothelial dysfunction. Therefore, there has

(a)

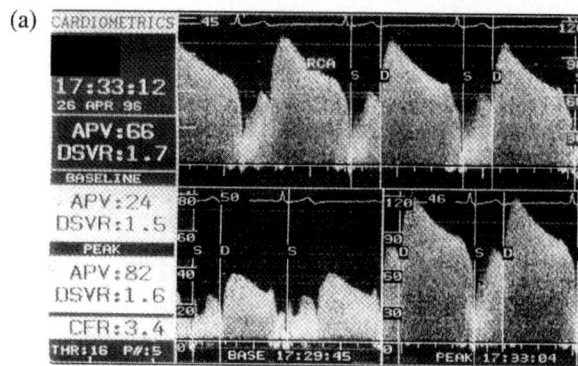

(b)

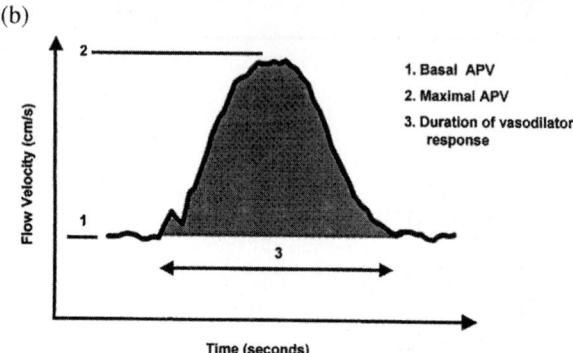

1. Basal APV
2. Maximal APV
3. Duration of vasodilator response

Fig. 6. Functional coronary angiography depicting the normal coronary flow velocity during intracoronary infusion of adenosine (*a*). Average peak velocity (APV) is used (*b*) in the calculation of coronary blood flow (p x 0.125 x APV x diameter^2). Coronary flow reserve (CFR) is the ratio of maximal to basal peak velocity.

been intense interest in using antioxidants such as vitamin E, vitamin C, beta-carotene and *N*-acetylcysteine to treat endothelial dysfunction and atherosclerosis. While many of these agents have positive effects in vitro and in small clinical studies, large randomized clinical trials have failed to show material benefit thus far (Table 7).

Neurohormonal Blockage

Angiotensin converting enzyme inhibitors (ACEIs) and angiotensin II receptor blockers (ARBs) are helpful in restoring vascular homeostasis through their effect on endothelium-derived NO. Large clinical trials have shown benefit when using these medications in high-risk patients or in those with acute coronary syndromes. These agents have a beneficial effect on endothelial function independent of their ability to lower high blood pressure. Thus, blockade of the renin-angiotensin-

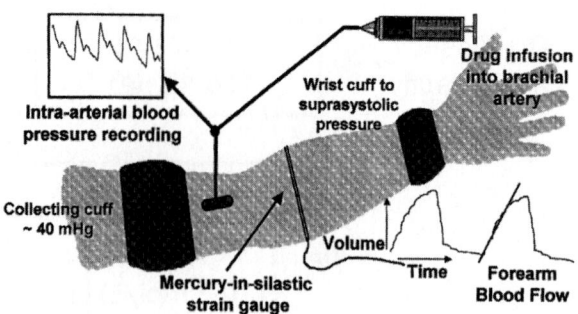

Fig. 7. Venous occlusion plethysmography is a technique that allows the intrabrachial infusion of vasoactive substances to assess conduit vessel endothelial function. Forearm blood flow is calculated from the slope of the volume/time curve.

aldosterone system may help to restore endothelial health and decrease the risk of CV events.

Hormone Replacement Therapy (HRT)

Postmenopausal women have an increased risk of cardiovascular disease compared to premenopausal women. Studies have shown that estrogen only replacement therapy improves markers of endothelial dysfunction via endothelium-dependent vasodilatation and increased NO synthesis. Unfortunately, it appears that progesterone may offset the benefits of estrogen. Large clinical trials have failed to demonstrate any benefit using combined estrogen and progesterone replacement therapy in the prevention of cardiovascular disease in post-menopausal women. Studies to define the effect if any of selective estrogen receptor modulators such as tamoxifen and raloxifene are under way.

SUMMARY

Vascular endothelium plays a pivotal role in vascular homeostasis by promoting vasodilatation while regulating inflammation and coagulation. Injury to the endothelium via traditional and novel risk factors leads to the evolution of atherosclerosis and increases the risk of cardiovascular events. Evaluation of endothelial vasomotor function has strong prognostic importance and may prove valuable as a "barometer" of cardiovascular health. Yet, the clinical utility of routine endothelial function testing remains undefined. Lifestyle modification and risk factor reduction remain the cornerstone of therapy for endothelial dysfunction. Statin drugs, ACE inhibitors, and

Table 3.   Available Substances to Be Used to Assess Endothelial Function in the Forearm Macrocirculation

Agonists to evoke endothelium-dependent vasodilation
 Acetylcholine: the most used; although not physiological it is the only one to have been validated as a prognostic marker of cardiovascular disease.
 Methacholine: stable metabolite of acetylcholine, but not sensitive to L-NMMA.
 Bradykinin: physiological; potent activator of endothelium-derived hyperpolarizing factors.
 Substance P: physiological; mainly used in the coronary circulation
 Isoproterenol: physiological and validated as sensitive to L-NMMA
 Serotonin: physiological and validated as sensitive to L-NMMA
Substances to assess pathways
 NO availability:
  eNOS activation: L-arginine (substrate); sometimes the results are difficult to interpret (L-arginine paradox)
  eNOS inhibition: L-NMMA (competitive specific antagonist); changes basal blood flow, making results difficult to interpret (NO clamp technique highly suggested)
 Hyperpolarization
  Ouabain: inhibitor of Na^+/K^+ ATPase; very nonspecific
  Sulfaphenazole: inhibitor of cytochrome P450; specific
 Oxidative stress
  Vitamin C: nonspecific scavenger of oxygen free radical; effective at very high concentrations (>1 mg/100 mL forearm tissue/min)
  Copper-zinc superoxide dismutase: nonspecific scavenger of oxygen free radical with poor intracellular penetrance
  Oxypurinol: specific inhibitor of xanthine oxidase

Table 3.   (continued)

 Cyclooxygenase activity
  Indomethacin: nonselective COX inhibitor, effective at very high concentration (>15 mg/100 mL forearm tissue/min)

COX, cyclooxygenase; eNOS, endothelial NO synthase; L-NMMA, N^G-monomethyl-L-arginine; NO, nitric oxide.

Table 4.   Practical Setup for Brachial Artery Ultrasound

Quiet, temperature-controlled examination room
Fasting (including caffeine) ≥8 h
No smoking (active and passive)
No exercise, no night work
No mental stress
Stop vasoactive medication ≥4 x drug half-life
In case of long-term follow-up: note changes in BP, cholesterol level, and weight; be aware of stage of menstrual cycle

angiotensin II receptor blockers also appear to be beneficial. Further studies are needed to develop novel therapeutic agents that restore vascular endothelial homeostasis.

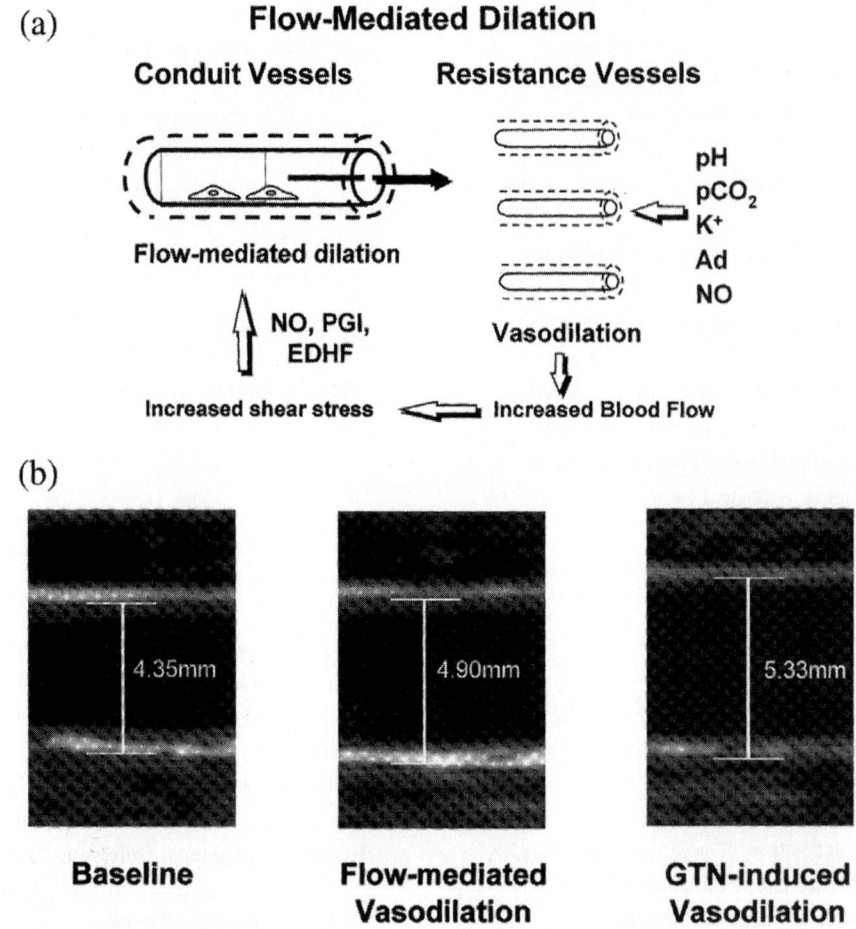

Fig. 8. Mechanical and hormonal stimuli cause flow-mediated dilation (FMD) of conduit vessels (*a*). FMD can be assessed in the brachial artery using high-resolution ultrasound (*b*) at baseline, after occlusion cuff deflation and following the administration of sublingual nitroglycerin.

Table 5. Markers of Endothelial Dysfunction and Vascular Inflammation

Molecule	Main sources	Biological function
Adhesion molecules		
ICAM-1	ECs, circulating leukocytes	Promotes leukocyte adherence and migration
VCAM-1	ECs, VSMC	Promotes leukocyte adherence
E-selectin	Activated ECs	Promotes leukocyte tethering and rolling
P-selectin	ECs, (Weibel Palade bodies), platelets (α granules)	EC/platelet-leukocyte interaction
sCD40L	Activated platelets, T lymphocytes, ECs, VSMCs, macrophages, mast cells	Promotes expression of adhesion molecules, tissue factor and metalloproteinases, release of chemokines, generation of reactive oxygen species, B-cell proliferation, generation of memory B cells and antibody class switching; inhibits B-cell apoptosis.
Cytokines		
Interleukin 6	ECs, macrophages, fibroblast, T cells	Induces acute phase proteins (e.g. CRP), increases antibody production, promotes generation of cytotoxic lymphocytes.
Interleukin 18	Macrophages	Promotes expression of adhesion molecules and metalloproteinases and inflammatory cell recruitment.
TNFα	Macrophages	Promotes expression of adhesion molecules, inflammatory cell recruitment and activation of T and B cells.
hs-CRP	Liver	Promotes upregulation of adhesion molecules, chemoattractants, chemokines and angiotensin type I receptor, generation of reactive oxygen species; reduces endothelial progenitor cell survival and differentiation.
8-iso-PFG$_{2\alpha}$	Nonenzymatic lipid peroxidation	Promotes platelet activation, expression of tissue factor and uptake of oxidized LDL by macrophages.
ET-1	Endothelium, VSMC, others	Vasoconstrictor; upregulates adhesion molecule expression; promotes VSMC proliferation; modulates effect of numerous compounds.
Metalloproteinases	Macrophages, others	Physiologically involved in tissue remodeling; when upregulated favor plaque instability.

ECs, endothelial cells; hs-CRP, high sensitivity C-reactive protein; ICAM-1, intercellular adhesion molecule-1; 8-iso-PgF$_{2\alpha}$, 8-iso-prostaglandin F$_{2\alpha}$; LDL, low-density lipoprotein; sCD40L, soluble CD40 ligand; TNFα, tumor necrosis factor α; VCAM-1, vascular cell adhesion molecule-1; VSMCs, vascular smooth muscle cells.

Table 6.   Effect of Interventions on Endothelial Function and CVD

Intervention	Effect on endothelial function	Effect on CVD events
Lipid-lowering therapy	+	+
Smoking cessation	+	+
Exercise	+	+
ACE inhibitors	+	+
Angiotensin receptor blockers	+	+
N-3 fatty acids	+	+
Glycemic control in diabetes mellitus	+	+
Hormone replacement therapy	±	−
Vitamin E	±	−
Combination antioxidants	−	−
L-arginine	+	?
Dietary flavonoids	+	?
Vitamin C	+	?
Folate	+	?
Tetrahydrobiopterin	+	?
Specific metal ion chelation therapy	+	?
Protein kinase C inhibition	+	?
Cyclooxygenase-2 inhibition	+	?
Thromboxane A_2 inhibition	+	?
Troglitazone treatment in diabetes	+	?
Xanthine oxidase inhibition	+	?
Tumor necrosis factor inhibition	+	?

+, weight of evidence indicates an improvement; −, weight of evidence indicates no effect or worsening; ?, there are insufficient data at the present time.
ACE, angiotensin converting enzyme; CVD, cardiovascular disease.

Table 7.   Potential Strategies for Treating Oxidant Stress

Agent	Mechanisms of action	Summary of clinical trials
Vitamin C	Free radical scavenger	Improves endothelial dysfunction in NIDDM
	↓ Inactivation of NO	Further investigation needed to determine if improves cardiovascular mortality
	↑ eNOS activity	
	↓ Monocyte adhesion	
	↓ LDL oxidation	
Vitamin E	↓ Monocyte adhesion	Conflicting long term trials regarding cardiovascular mortality benefits
	↓ LDL oxidation	
ACE inhibitors	↓ ACE-oxidant production	Improves endothelial dysfunction as well as mortality from cardiovascular death independent of antihypertensive effect
	↓ Inflammatory mediator levels	Tissue-specific may be superior to humorally active ACEIs
	↓ NO bioavailability	
ARBs	↓ NO bioavailability	Conflicting evidence regarding ability to ameliorate endothelial function
Statins	↓ LDL oxidation	Improves endothelial dysfunction as well as mortality from cardiovascular death independent of lipid-lowering effect
	↓ LDL levels	
	↓ eNOS expression	
	↓ $p22^{phax}$ expression	
	↓ Inflammatory mediators	
Metformin	↓ Lipid peroxidation	Improves endothelial dysfunction in NIDDM patients independent of hypoglycemic effect
	↑ SOD and glutathione levels	
TDZ	Promotes less oxidizable LDL conformation	Improves endothelial dysfunction in pre-diabetic and diabetic states while reducing oxidant levels independent of hypoglycemic or antihypertensive effects
	↓ Inflammatory mediator levels	
	↓ $p47^{phax}$ expression	
Folate	↓ eNOS- and XOD-mediated O_2 production	Combination therapy with B_{12} improves endothelial responses
Estrogen	↓ eNOS transcription	Improves endothelial function, yet not effective in secondary prevention of cardiovascular events
	↓ LDL oxidation	

DM II, diabetes type II; TDZ, thiazolidinediones; SOD, superoxide dismutase; eNOS, endothelial nitric oxide synthase; XOD, xanthine oxidase; ↑, increase; ↓, decrease.

CORONARY ARTERY PHYSIOLOGY AND INTRACORONARY ULTRASONOGRAPHY

Abhiram Prasad, MD

NORMAL PHYSIOLOGY

Myocardial Oxygen Consumption

The principal function of the coronary arteries is to provide oxygen and nutrients to the myocardium. Myocardial oxygen consumption ($M\dot{V}O_2$) is equal to the product of coronary blood flow and the arteriovenous oxygen gradient across the coronary vascular bed, that is, arterial oxygen content minus coronary sinus oxygen content. In the resting state, myocardial oxygen extraction is near maximum and coronary sinus oxygen saturations are typically 30% or less (or $PO_2 < 20$ mm Hg). Because myocardial oxygen extraction is already near maximum, $M\dot{V}O_2$ can increase only by increasing coronary blood flow. $M\dot{V}O_2$ is dependent on coronary blood flow, and changes in $M\dot{V}O_2$ closely parallel changes in coronary blood flow. Important determinants of $M\dot{V}O_2$ are heart rate, inotropic state (contractility), and intramyocardial wall stress. $M\dot{V}O_2$ can be approximated clinically by the product of systolic blood pressure and heart rate (called the "rate-pressure product"). The rate-pressure product is an estimate of $M\dot{V}O_2$ (and, thus, coronary blood flow) and is frequently used during exercise testing.

- $M\dot{V}O_2$ can be approximated clinically by the product of systolic blood pressure and heart rate.

- In the resting state, myocardial oxygen extraction is near maximal.
- Important determinants of $M\dot{V}O_2$ are heart rate, inotropic state (contractility), and intramyocardial wall stress.

Coronary Blood Flow Regulation

During rest, normal coronary blood flow is approximately 60 to 90 mL/min per 100 g of myocardium. Its regulation in humans is complex and involves metabolic, autonomic, and mechanical factors. The most important metabolic factors include adenosine, prostaglandins, and endothelial-derived factors (e.g. the vasodilator nitric oxide, and the vasoconstrictor endothelin). Myocardial oxygen and carbon dioxide tensions, ATP-sensitive potassium channels (K-ATP channels) also have a role in regulating coronary blood flow. Of the agents released from myocardial cells, adenosine is probably the most important. Adenosine is produced from the breakdown of high-energy phosphates (adenosine triphosphate [ATP]) which cannot be regenerated during ischemia due to the low oxygen tension. The breakdown product, adenosine monophosphate (AMP) accumulates and is converted to adenosine.

The contribution of the autonomic nervous system to the control of coronary blood flow is likely modest. Changes in coronary blood flow with either sympathetic or parasympathetic stimulation are due predominantly to the accompanying changes in loading conditions and contractility.

Mechanical factors have a major effect on coronary blood flow. During myocardial contraction, intramyocardial pressure increases, causing compression of small vessels and a reduction, or "throttling," of coronary blood flow. The result is a predominant diastolic blood flow pattern (Fig. 1). Approximately 60% of coronary blood flow occurs during diastole in the left coronary artery. The situation is opposite in the proximal right coronary artery, where there is much less vessel compression during low-pressure right ventricular contraction, with the result that there is much less reduction in blood flow during systole. Blood flow in the proximal right coronary artery during systole is nearly equal to that during diastole. However, in the distal right coronary artery (beyond the right ventricular marginal branches), coronary blood flow predominantly perfuses the inferior left ventricle, and diastolic flow again predominates.

The myocardial compressive effects are greater in the subendocardial layer than in the subepicardial layer, thus making the subendocardium at increased risk for ischemia. During maximal vasodilatation, myocardial perfusion is regulated primarily by coronary perfusion pressure and myocardial compressive effects. When coronary blood flow is reduced, as from an epicardial coronary artery stenosis, the subendocardial layer is the first region of the myocardium to become ischemic. Subendocardial ischemia can be detected clinically with ST-segment depression on an electrocardiogram. Although flow may be adequate at rest, subendocardial ischemia may occur with exercise or stress. This effect can be particularly pronounced in hypertrophied left ventricles, even with normal coronary arteries.

Diastolic Pressure-Time Index

Coronary blood flow is closely correlated with the diastolic pressure-time index, which is the product of the average difference between aortic and left ventricular cavity pressure and the duration of diastole (i.e., it is the area between diastolic aortic pressure and left ventricular

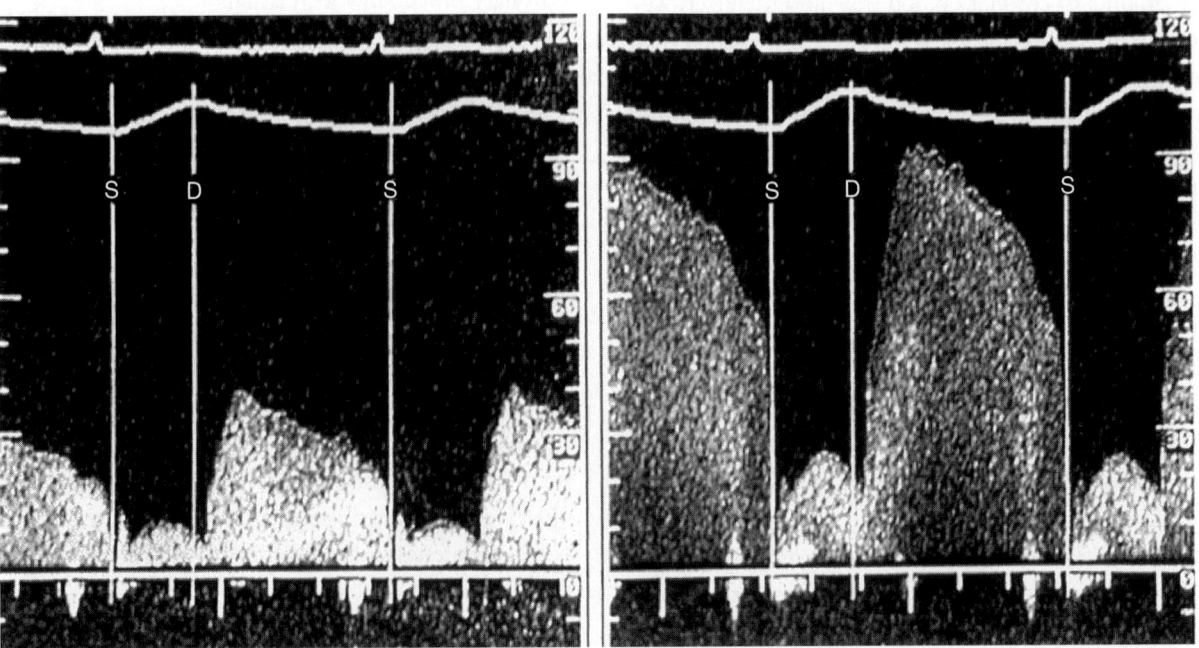

CFR = 2.6 (adenosine 18 μg)

Fig. 1. Intracoronary Doppler velocities from the left anterior descending coronary artery showing predominant diastolic flow. S, onset of systole; D, onset of diastole. Heart rate and aortic pressure are shown. A, Flow during basal conditions and, B, flow after microvessel vasodilatation with adenosine. Coronary flow reserve (CFR) is the ratio of maximal diastolic flow to basal diastolic flow in the coronary vessel.

pressure). The diastolic pressure-time index can be altered by changes in aortic diastolic pressure, left ventricular diastolic pressure, and length of diastole. Coronary blood flow is decreased by systemic hypotension (by decreasing aortic diastolic pressure), increased left ventricular end-diastolic pressure (by increasing left ventricular diastolic pressure), and tachycardia (by shortening diastole). Coronary blood flow can be augmented by increased systemic pressure, decreased left ventricular end-diastolic pressure, and slowing of the heart rate. Intra-aortic balloon pumping can augment coronary blood flow by increasing aortic diastolic pressure.

Myocardial Sinusoids

The coronary circulation drains primarily through the coronary sinus and cardiac veins (Fig. 2). A small portion of the venous return drains into the thebesian veins and myocardial sinusoids, which empty directly into the chambers of the left side of the heart. A small right-to-left shunt occurs at this level, even in normal subjects.

- Approximately 60% of coronary blood flow occurs during diastole in the left coronary artery.
- Blood flow in the proximal right coronary artery during systole is nearly equal to that during diastole.
- Coronary blood flow is decreased by systemic hypotension, increased left ventricular end-diastolic pressure, and tachycardia.

Autoregulation of Coronary Blood Flow

During resting conditions, coronary blood flow is maintained at a fairly constant level over a range of aortic pressures by the process of autoregulation (Fig. 3). As aortic pressure decreases, coronary blood flow is maintained by dilatation of the resistance vessels. The resistance vessels, or arterioles, are small vessels proximal to the capillaries and are below the resolution of coronary angiography. The converse occurs with an increase in aortic pressure. Therefore, during normal resting conditions, coronary blood flow is pressure-independent. At either extreme, however, autoregulation is overcome and coronary blood flow becomes pressure-dependent. At low perfusion pressures, the resistance vessels are dilated maximally and any additional decrease in pressure results in a linear decrease in blood flow. At pressures less than 70 mm Hg, the pressure-flow relationship becomes linear, with blood flow decreasing in direct proportion to the decrease in perfusion pressure. At very high perfusion pressures, vasoconstriction is maximal and an additional increase in pressure results in a linear increase in blood flow. At extremely low perfusion pressures (approximately 20 mm Hg), blood flow ceases altogether. This effect is called the "vascular waterfall phenomenon," which is caused by the compressive effects of extravascular intramyocardial pressure. The pressure at which flow ceases is called the "critical closure pressure," or "the critical flow pressure."

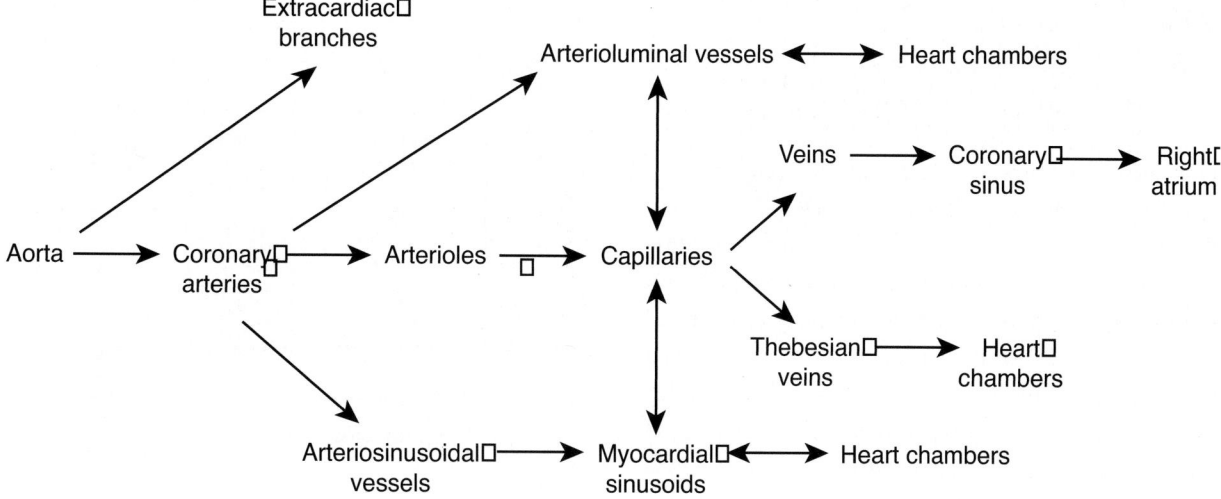

Fig. 2. Diagram of the coronary circulation.

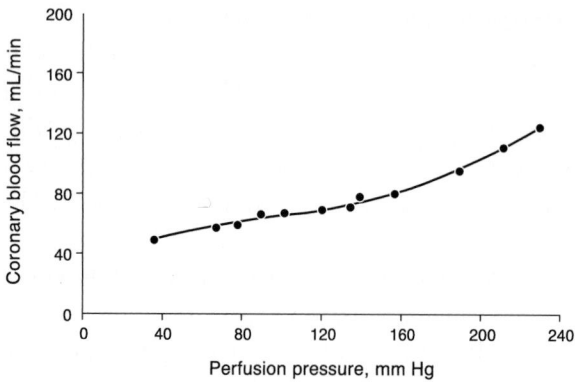

Fig. 3. Autoregulation demonstrated by changes in perfusion pressure.

- During normal resting conditions, coronary blood flow is pressure-independent.
- At pressures less than 70 mm Hg, blood flow decreases in direct proportion to the decrease in perfusion pressure.

Coronary Flow Reserve

With physical or mental stress, the metabolic demands of the myocardium increase and coronary blood flow must increase to increase $M\dot{V}O_2$. Coronary blood flow increases through dilatation of resistance vessels. When the resistance vessels are dilated maximally, coronary blood flow cannot be increased further without an increase in aortic pressure. The vessels proximal to the resistance vessels (i.e., the epicardial and prearteriolar vessels) offer only minimal resistance to coronary blood flow. The ratio of maximal blood flow to resting (or basal) blood flow is termed the "coronary flow reserve" (CFR) (Fig. 4 and Table 1):

$$CFR = \frac{\text{Maximal Coronary Blood Flow}}{\text{Resting Coronary Blood Flow}}$$

Coronary flow reserve, also called the "absolute flow reserve," is a measure of the ability to augment blood flow with stress. It can be measured easily with intracoronary Doppler techniques. Maximal vasodilatation is produced with vasodilators such as adenosine. Adenosine has been the easiest to use because of its short half-life, ability to promote maximal vasodilatation, and safety profile. Bradycardia and complete heart block can occur, particularly with injections into the right coronary artery, but are rare at the recommended doses (intracoronary bolus of 24-60 μg for the left and

12-36 μg for the right coronary arteries, respectively). Papaverine has a longer half-life and can prolong the QT interval, rarely resulting in life-threatening arrhythmias.

- Coronary blood flow increases through dilatation of resistance vessels.
- Maximal vasodilatation is produced with vasodilators such as adenosine.

Endothelial Function

The endothelium comprises the single layer of cells between the vascular smooth muscle and the blood and circulating components. It is the largest "organ" in the body, with approximately one trillion cells, a total surface area equivalent to six tennis courts, and a total weight greater than that of the liver. Although the endothelium functions as a semipermeable membrane, its role in coronary artery physiology is more complex (Table 2). A normally functioning endothelium is essential for maintaining normal coronary blood flow. The increase in coronary blood flow with both physical and mental stress is modulated largely by endothelial-dependent changes in vasomotor tone. Endothelial dysfunction is believed to be one of the earliest stages in pathogenesis of atherosclerosis.

The endothelium continuously produces substances to modulate vascular tone, including nitric oxide, prostacyclin, and endothelial-derived contracting factors such as endothelin. The relaxing factor produced by the endothelium and originally called "endothelium-derived relaxing factor," or "EDRF," was

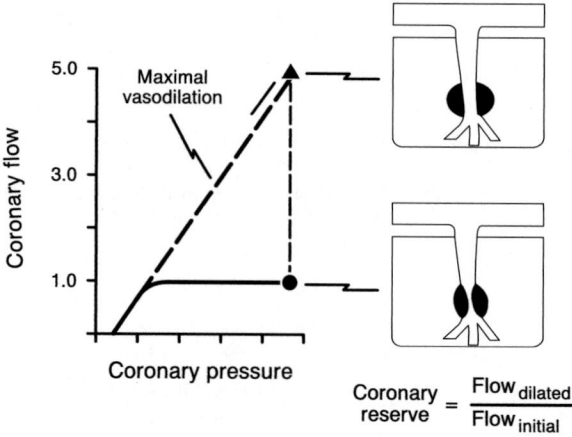

Fig. 4. Coronary flow reserve.

Table 1. Comparison of Three Types of Coronary Flow Reserve

	Absolute flow reserve	Relative flow reserve	Fractional flow reserve
Definition	Ratio of hyperemic to resting flow	Ratio of hyperemic flow in the stenotic region to hyperemic flow in a normal region	Ratio of hyperemic flow in the stenotic region to hyperemic flow in that same region if no lesion is present
Independent of driving pressure	−	+	+
Easily applicable in humans	+	±	+
Applicable to 3-vessel disease	+	−	+
Unequivocal reference value	−	+	+
Abnormal value	<2.0	≤0.65	<0.75

identified subsequently as nitric oxide. The endothelium produces nitric oxide by the action of the enzyme nitric oxide synthase which metabolizes L-arginine to citrulline. Endothelial cells are stimulated to produce nitric oxide by several factors, including acetylcholine, histamine, bradykinin, substance P, and platelet-derived substances. Fluid shear stress also stimulates the release of nitric oxide which contributes to flow-mediated dilation and the arterial remodeling that occurs with changes in coronary blood flow states. Nitric oxide acts by increasing intracellular cyclic guanosine monophosphate (GMP) levels, which mediates smooth muscle relaxation and platelet inhibition. L-Arginine has been used therapeutically to drive nitric oxide synthase and promote nitric oxide production. The endothelial cells also produce endothelin, a vasoactive peptide that directly stimulates receptors on smooth muscle cells. Endothelin, one of the most potent vasoconstrictors known, is produced in response to endothelial cell stimulation by thrombin, transforming growth factor-β, interleukin-1, epinephrine, antidiuretic hormone, and angiotensin II. The endothelium also can convert angiotensin to angiotensin II through tissue-bound angiotensin-converting enzyme, which also causes vasoconstriction.

- A normally functioning endothelium is essential for maintaining normal coronary blood flow.
- Endothelin is one of the most potent vasoconstrictors known.

ALTERED CORONARY PHYSIOLOGY

Obstructive Coronary Disease

Essentially all the clinical manifestations of obstructive coronary artery disease (due to coronary atherosclerosis, and rarely vasculitis or emboli) are caused by altered coronary artery physiology and the resulting myocardial ischemia. Coronary artery stenoses deform the column of blood flowing within the coronary artery. Although minor luminal irregularities have little effect on blood flow, more severe stenoses may cause significant transstenotic pressure gradients. The result is a reduction in the perfusion pressures distal to the stenoses. Resting blood flow is maintained by vasodilatation of the resistance vessels (Fig. 5), also called "autoregulation." Although this mechanism maintains

Table 2. Functions of the Endothelium

Regulate vasomotor tone
Nonthrombogenic surface and regulate thrombosis/fibrinolysis
Regulate vascular cell growth by production of growth factors and inhibitors
Regulate leukocyte and platelet adhesion
Modulate lipid oxidation
Selectively permeable barrier
Modulate thrombogenic response

resting coronary blood flow, the maximal coronary blood flow will be compromised. Furthermore, any attempt to increase flow across the stenosis increases the pressure gradient.

Autoregulation fails when the severity of the stenosis severely decreases the distal pressure beyond the lower limits of autoregulation. At this point, resting coronary blood flow will be decreased, resulting in resting myocardial ischemia and rest angina. Myocardial viability can be maintained with coronary blood flow as low as 10 to 20 mL/min per 100 g if the mechanical activity and metabolic needs of the heart are reduced (as during hypothermic cardioplegia).

■ Myocardial viability can be maintained with coronary blood flow as low as 10 to 20 mL/min per 100 g.

Nonobstructive Coronary Artery Disease

Endothelial Dysfunction
Endothelial dysfunction precedes clinical atherosclerosis and has been detected in patients with normal findings on angiography and intravascular ultrasonography, although microscopic abnormalities likely are present in the endothelial cells. The relationship of endothelial dysfunction to cardiovascular disease is complex. Endothelial dysfunction can be considered the initial pathophysiologic step in the development of atherosclerosis, and its presence is a predictor of adverse cardiovascular events.

Several factors cause endothelial dysfunction:

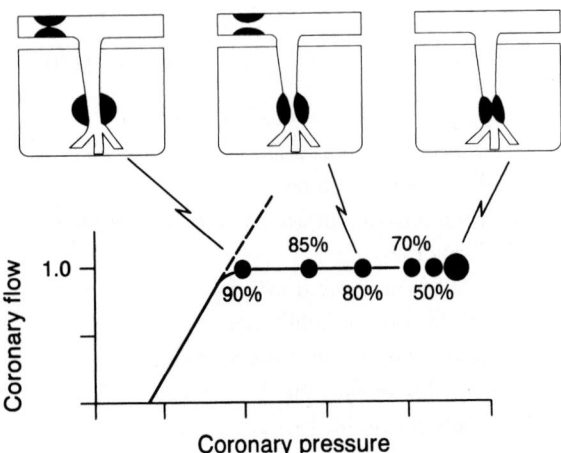

Fig. 5. Effect of stenosis severity on resting flow.

hyperlipidemia, cigarette smoking, uncontrolled hypertension, diabetes mellitus, and loss of estrogen in postmenopausal women. Recent evidence suggests that infectious pathogens and environmental pollution may also lead to endothelial injury. Endothelial dysfunction leads to the expression of adhesion molecules on the cell surface, and increased oxidative stress in the vessels that facilitates leukocyte recruitment, entry and oxidation of low-density lipoprotein into the intima paving the way for the formation of foam cells and atherosclerotic plaques. Endothelial dysfunction also leads to reduced bioavailability of nitric oxide through multiple deleterious mechanisms, and stimulates the formation of endothelin which impairs vasomotion.

Acetylcholine can be selectively infused into the coronary arteries to test for the presence of endothelial dysfunction in humans (see below). In normal individuals, acetylcholine stimulates the production and release of nitric oxide from the endothelium, which results in vasodilatation and increased coronary blood flow. In patients with endothelial dysfunction, acetylcholine is ineffective in releasing nitric oxide uncovering its direct action on smooth muscle cells and causes vasoconstriction; this is called "paradoxical vasoconstriction." Noninvasive methods for testing for endothelial function are being developed for clinical use.

Endothelial cell dysfunction may be treated with lifestyle modification including aerobic exercise, weight loss in obese patients, low fat or Mediterranean diets, and smoking cessation. Aggressive treatment of risk factors such as diabetes mellitus, metabolic syndrome, and hypertension is likely to be effective in improving vascular function. Pharmacological therapy with statins and angiotensin-converting enzyme inhibitors has been shown to reverse endothelial dysfunction. The role of experimental nitric oxide donors, fish oils and antioxidants, has not been established.

■ Endothelial dysfunction can be considered the initial pathophysiologic step in the development of atherosclerosis.
■ Patients with endothelial dysfunction are at increased risk for adverse cardiovascular outcomes.
■ With normally functioning endothelium, acetylcholine stimulates the production and release of nitric oxide, which results in vasodilatation and increased coronary blood flow.

Overload States

Any increase in the workload of the heart increases $M\dot{V}O_2$, and coronary blood flow increases in parallel with $M\dot{V}O_2$. Acute pressure overload increases $M\dot{V}O_2$ more than acute volume overload, although most volume overloads include some element of pressure overload.

Chronic overload results in myocardial hypertrophy, with pressure overload causing concentric hypertrophy and volume overload causing eccentric or dilated hypertrophy. The degree of hypertrophy is related to the workload of the heart or $M\dot{V}O_2$ (and, thus, coronary blood flow). Therefore, coronary blood flow per unit of myocardium (milliliters/minute per 100 g) is frequently normal in hypertrophic states. The increased resting flow often results in a decreased coronary flow reserve. In the pressure-overloaded heart, maldistributions in coronary blood flow occur because of increased compressive forces in the subendocardial layer. Even in patients with normal coronary angiographic findings, decreased subendocardial flow can result in angina pectoris and exercise-induced ST-segment depression, a finding often seen in aortic stenosis, hypertrophic cardiomyopathy, and hypertensive left ventricular hypertrophy.

INTRAVASCULAR ULTRASONOGRAPHY

Although coronary angiography is considered the reference standard for coronary artery imaging, it has several inherent limitations. Angiography is a silhouette technique that detects only arterial disease that indents the luminal column of contrast; it reveals little else about the atherosclerotic plaque. When a normal proximal reference segment does not exist, as in diffuse atherosclerotic disease, it is difficult to detect and to quantitate atherosclerosis with angiography. Angiography also underestimates the amount of atherosclerosis when compensatory arterial enlargement occurs, that is, expansion of the artery at the site of an atherosclerotic plaque (positive remodeling). Positive remodeling is associated with a larger plaque burden, large lipid rich "soft" core, and is believed to occur at sites of active disease with "vulnerable plaques." Negative remodeling can also occur when there is contraction of the vessel. Remodeling index is defined as a ratio of the vessel (external elastic membrane, EEM) area: lesion/proximal reference site. A value of >1.05 is defined as positive and <0.95 as negative remodeling. Intimal lesions frequently

escape detection by angiography, including angioplasty-induced microfractures, intimal dissections, and mural thrombus. Intravascular ultrasonography (IVUS) improves on the angiographic assessment of coronary arteries by allowing better visualization, as well as quantitation of plaque, and assessment of plaque morphology.

- Positive remodeling is associated with a larger plaque burden, large lipid rich "soft" core, and is believed to occur at sites of "vulnerable plaques."
- Remodeling index is defined as a ratio of the vessel (external elastic membrane, EEM) area: lesion/proximal reference site. A value of > 1.05 defines positive and < 0.95 negative remodeling.

Catheter Technology

Small intracoronary ultrasound catheters provide high-resolution cross-sectional images of the coronary arteries. Catheters as small as 2.6 French, or 0.86 mm (0.33 mm/French size) in diameter, can easily reach the distal segments of the coronary arteries in most patients. The two types of intravascular ultrasound catheters are the mechanical and the solid-state. The mechanical catheters are used infrequently. They have a rotating ultrasound crystal in the catheter tip, and most systems have a rotating core driven by a motor outside the body. The solid-state catheters have a phased-array or a dynamic-aperture array, with 64 ultrasound crystals arranged around the circumference of the catheter tip, each activated sequentially to produce a rotating ultrasound beam. By using either a mechanical rotating system or a solid-state phased-array system, the ultrasound beam is rotated around the circumference of the catheter at approximately 1,800 rpm. Excellent arterial images can be obtained with both systems; however, only the mechanical systems are subject to nonuniform rotational defects (NURD).

Image Recognition on Intravascular Ultrasonography

The rotating ultrasound beam produces two-dimensional cross-sectional images of the coronary arteries that are analogous to histologic sections (Fig. 6). High-frequency ultrasound transducers (20 to 40 mHz) are used, and they yield high-resolution images. Often, the three layers of the artery (intima, media, and adventitia) can be imaged. Normal intima may not be visible with intracoronary ultrasonography if it is less than 175-μm thick. Luminal area, wall thickness, and plaque size can be measured accurately. Also, the location of the plaque, concentric or eccentric, can be determined. The atherosclerotic plaque can also be characterized according to its fibrous, lipid, and calcium content. Calcium appears bright and echogenic and results in shadowing of the far field (Fig. 7). Lipid plaques typically are sonolucent or dark-appearing. Fibrous plaques have a heterogeneous appearance. A recent advance in IVUS technology has been the introduction of virtual histology that provides detailed plaque characterization (Fig. 8). Patients with unstable angina more often have soft, lipid-laden plaques. Coronary artery calcification detected with intravascular ultrasonography is predictive of a worse outcome with percutaneous coronary intervention (PCI) (larger and more frequent dissections). An intraluminal thrombus and dissection also can be imaged with intracoronary ultrasonography (Fig. 9).

■ Coronary artery calcification detected with intravascular ultrasonography is predictive of a worse outcome with PCI.

Clinical Utility of Intravascular Ultrasonography

Coronary angiography generates an overview of the coronary arterial tree, whereas intravascular ultrasonography provides an in-depth view of a specific portion of the coronary vasculature. Intravascular ultrasonography is useful for detecting mild coronary atherosclerotic disease, assessing an angiographically indeterminate lesion, and assessing coronary stenoses before and after catheter-based coronary artery interventions. Coronary artery disease in transplanted hearts is studied best with intravascular ultrasonography because of the diffuse nature of the disease, which makes it difficult to detect with angiography.

Indeterminate Coronary Stenoses

Left main coronary artery lesions, which often are difficult to quantitate with angiography because of overlapping branches, diffuse disease, or the ostial location of the disease, are ideally suited for study with intravascular ultrasonography (Fig. 10). A left main cross-sectional area of less than 7 mm^2 is used to identify a significant stenosis. Similarly, a cross-sectional area of less than 4 mm^2 in a major epicardial artery is also considered sufficient to be flow limiting.

Coronary Intervention

Studies have shown that balloon angioplasty is more likely to result in significant dissection if intravascular ultrasonography reveals heavy arterial calcification. If the calcification is superficial, directional atherectomy is less effective however, these lesions are ideally suited for treatment with rotational atherectomy (Rotablator). After balloon angioplasty, lesions with greater plaque volume and smaller lumen area appear to be at high risk for subsequent restenosis.

IVUS guided intervention, compared to routine percutaneous transluminal coronary angioplasty (PTCA) with provisional stenting, has been shown to

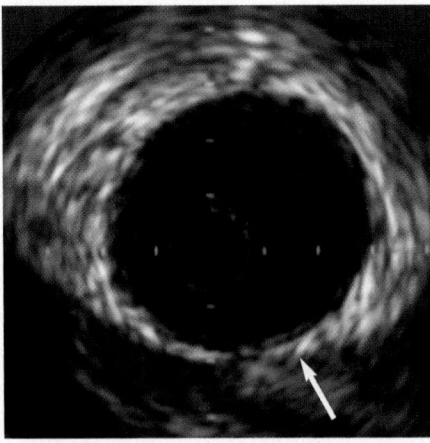

Fig. 6. Intravascular ultrasound image of a normal coronary artery showing the three mural layers: intima, media, and adventitia.

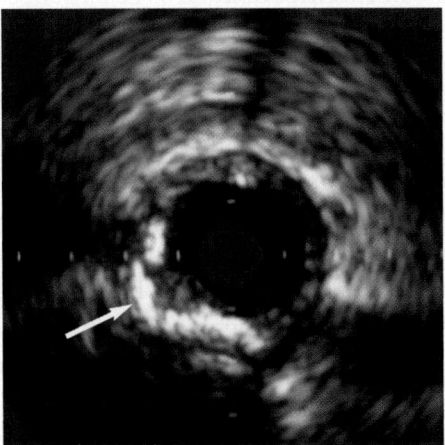

Fig. 7. Intravascular ultrasound image of a calcified atherosclerotic coronary plaque. Calcium is echogenic (bright) and shadows the far field.

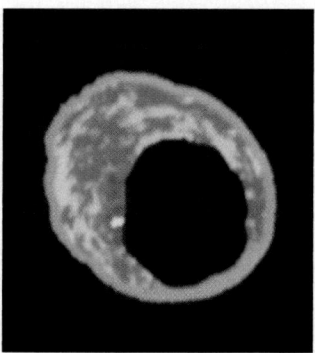

Fig. 8. Virtual histology ᵀᴹ intravascular ultrasound image of a stable plaque. Green-fibrous tissue, yellow-fibrofatty tissue, white-calcium, and red-necrotic core. The plaque is made up of fibrous and fibrofatty material with minimal necrotic tissue.

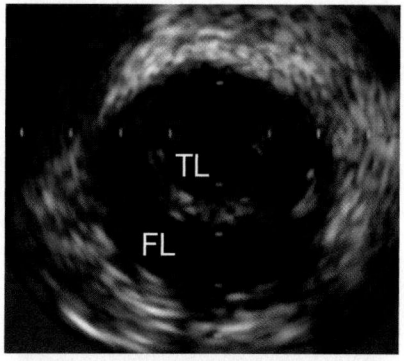

Fig. 9. Intravascular ultrasound image of a coronary dissection (A). The catheter is in the true lumen (TL). FL, false lumen.

result in greater acute gain in luminal diameter by allowing the use of "oversized" (by angiographic criteria) balloons in stenoses with positively remodeled vessels. However, it has not been associated with reduced restenosis, and produces similar clinical outcomes compared with a strategy using angiography alone. Moreover, the use of IVUS is more time consuming, leads to additional expense, and requires expertise in the use of ultrasound. Thus, routine stent implantation is the preferred approach.

IVUS has been instrumental in the development of current high pressure stent deployment techniques which has eliminated the requirement for post procedure anticoagulation and decreased the incidence of subacute thrombosis. Studies with IVUS have established the mechanisms for in-stent restenosis which is largely due to neointimal proliferation with minimal stent recoil. In contrast, restenosis following PTCA is predominantly due to recoil and negative remodeling with a small contribution from neointimal hyperplasia. These observations have been critical to the development of treatments for in-stent restenosis such as brachytherapy and drug-eluting stents (DES).

A strategy of routine IVUS-guided stent deployment has not been shown to be superior to angiographic assessment. However, an IVUS-guided approach may reduce target lesion revascularization in complex lesion subsets such as small vessels and long stenoses when treated with bare metal stents. However, this modest benefit is likely to be offset in clinical practice due to the additional cost, time and expertise

required to use IVUS. Moreover, the use of DES is likely to reduce the impact of IVUS on reducing target lesion revascularization in complex lesions due to the low rates of restenosis. IVUS is occasionally helpful following stent deployment to assess for complete expansion, apposition and presence of edge dissections, if angiographic imaging is inadequate. IVUS studies have demonstrated that the use of DES is associated with an increased frequency of late stent malapposition compared with bare metal stents. This may be a direct effect of the inhibition of neointima formation and postprocedural positive remodeling. The precise prevalence and clinical significance of late stent malapposition remains to be established.

Finally, IVUS is valuable in assessing the mechanism of in-stent restenosis to guide therapy: neointimal formation versus stent under-expansion. The latter may be treated with PTCA alone while the former process needs to be treated with the deployment of a drug-eluting stent.

- Cardiac transplant coronary artery disease is studied best with intravascular ultrasonography because of the diffuse nature of the disease.
- A left main cross sectional area of <7 mm² is significant. A cross sectional area of <4 mm² in a major epicardial artery is also considered to be flow limiting.
- Routine use of IVUS is not recommended to guide PCI.
- Intravascular ultrasonography can detect stent abnormalities that often are not detected with angiography.
- IVUS may be helpful in the evaluation of in-stent restenosis.

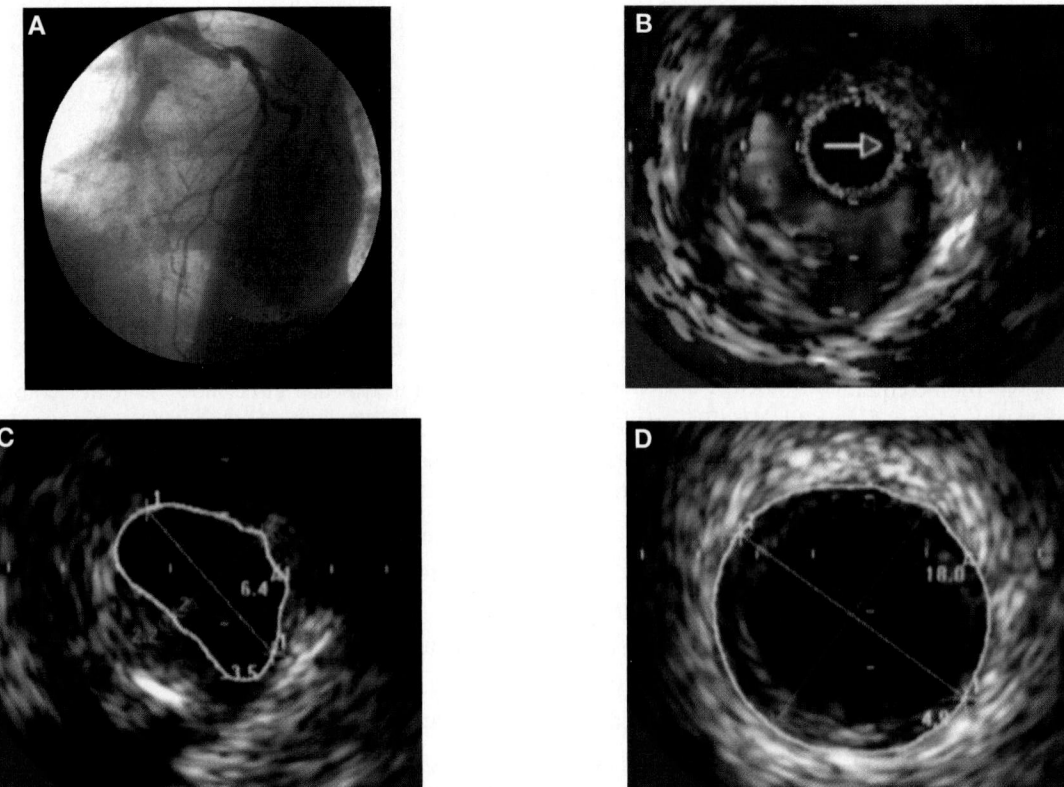

Fig. 10. Coronary angiogram (*A*) and intravascular ultrasound image (*B*) of a moderate ostial stenosis of the left main artery. The cross sectional lumen area is 6.4 mm² at the ostium. The distal reference segment of the left main artery has mild atherosclerosis with a lumen area of 18.0 mm² (*D*).

INTRACORONARY DOPPLER MEASUREMENTS

Doppler Technology

Recent developments in Doppler catheter and guidewire technology have made measurement of coronary blood flow velocity in cardiac catheterization laboratories practical, safe, and reproducible. Doppler guidewires are 0.014 inch (0.36 mm) in diameter and can measure coronary blood flow velocities distal to coronary artery stenoses without impairing blood flow. The Doppler guidewire is an angioplasty guidewire with a Doppler crystal incorporated in its tip. Ultrasound is emitted from the tip of the guidewire in a pulsed-wave fashion. Between pulses, the frequency of the returning, or reflected, ultrasound is recorded at a specific time after the initial pulse. The specific timing of the received ultrasound determines the depth of the sample volume. In the system currently available, the sample volume depth is 5 mm from the guidewire tip. The returning frequency is analyzed relative to the emitted frequency. The frequency will be shifted upward or downward depending on the velocity of its reflector in the sample volume. In the coronary arteries, erythrocytes act as the primary ultrasound reflectors in the moving stream of blood. The ultrasound emitted from the guidewire tip also diverges from the axis of the guidewire by 12.5 degrees, in effect emitting a spray or cone of ultrasound. The effect allows the ultrasound beam to intersect the center of the stream of flow even if it is placed slightly eccentrically in the artery. Although this may add some error in the Doppler equation, the maximal error should be approximately 10%.

Coronary flow velocity is not equivalent to coronary blood flow. Coronary blood flow can be calculated from measurements of coronary flow velocity and coronary cross-sectional area with the hydraulic equation (flow = velocity × area). Several theoretical issues remain a problem. For example, liquids flowing in a tube have characteristic velocity profiles, with zero velocities at the edges and peak velocities near the center of the stream of flow. The Doppler guidewire measures across the entire velocity profile and records the highest velocity flowing in the velocity profile. If this velocity is used in the hydraulic equation, coronary blood flow will be overestimated because the peak velocity is an over-representation of all the velocities flowing in the parabolic velocity profile. A spatial average velocity is required to measure accurately absolute coronary blood flow. If we assume a true parabolic velocity profile, the average velocity is half the peak velocity and flow can be measured with a modified hydraulic equation (flow = 1/2 velocity × area). With this assumption, coronary blood flow can be measured with a high degree of accuracy. Measurement of absolute flow is not required for coronary flow reserve measurements. If we assume that the flow area remains constant and the shape of the velocity profile does not change, coronary flow reserve simplifies to a ratio of the flow velocities.

■ Coronary blood flow can be calculated from measurements of coronary flow velocity and coronary cross-sectional area with the hydraulic equation (flow = velocity × area).

Indications for Intracoronary Doppler Measurements

Indeterminate Coronary Stenoses

Despite a comprehensive angiographic evaluation, coronary stenoses may remain indeterminate. Indeterminate lesions may be angiographically or physiologically indeterminate. Angiographically indeterminate lesions occur when there are overlapping branches, bifurcations, contrast streaming, or ostial lesions. Physiologically indeterminate lesions are ones that are well seen on angiography but are of intermediate severity, in the 50% to 70% range; they also are called "intermediate lesions." Angiographically indeterminate lesions usually require additional anatomical definition, as with intravascular ultrasonography. Indeterminate lesions are evaluated best with additional physiologic testing, as with intracoronary Doppler technique by measuring velocities distal to the stenosis using the Doppler guidewire. Measurement of proximal flow velocities are insufficient because they are affected by flow that is shunted away by any branch vessels proximal to the stenosis. Therefore, in response to maximal vasodilatation, the proximal flow velocity

response represents an integrated response combining both ischemic and nonischemic myocardium. The coronary flow reserve is the single most useful Doppler index of lesion severity.

Coronary Flow Reserve

The hallmark of coronary stenosis is its effect on coronary flow augmentation with stress. Coronary flow reserve is defined as the ratio of the maximally augmented coronary flow velocity to resting flow velocity. Previous studies have shown that the normal coronary flow reserve in animals is 3.5 to 5.0. However, with the Doppler guidewire, it has been suggested that normal coronary flow reserve should be 2.0 or greater. The reason for this discrepancy is unclear. However, if a value greater than 2.0 is used for normal coronary flow reserve, there is an 89% agreement between the results of Doppler-derived coronary flow reserve and adenosine stress sestamibi imaging. Doppler-derived coronary flow reserve is influenced by changes in resting myocardial flow, as might occur with post-PCI reactive hyperemia and changes in heart rate, preload, and contractility. In addition, CFR is frequently abnormal due to microvascular dysfunction which is present in patients with coronary atherosclerosis. Thus, an abnormal CFR does not differentiate between a significant epicardial stenosis and impaired flow response to hyperemia due to an abnormal microcirculation. To address this limitation, relative CFR (rCFR) can be measured but requires additional measurements and instrumentation of a normal vessel. rCFR is the ratio of the CFR in the culprit vessel divided by the CFR in a normal reference vessel. A ratio of ≤0.65 is indicative of a significant epicardial stenosis (Table 1). Due to the complexity of measuring rCFR and limitations of CFR, fractional flow reserve (FFR) has become the preferred physiological index for assessing indeterminate coronary stenoses.

Chest Pain and Normal Coronary Arteries

The incidence of angiographically normal coronary arteries in patients with angina is approximately 10% to 30%. Although angiography provides an excellent *anatomical* road map of the coronary arteries, it gives little information about the physiology of the coronary circulation. Many of these patients have noncardiac causes of their pain (Table 3), but many others have objective evidence of cardiac ischemia, including exercise- or pacing-induced ST-segment depression, scintigraphic perfusion defects, stress-induced left ventricular dysfunction, myocardial lactate production, and decreased coronary sinus O_2 saturation). A reduced coronary flow reserve has been demonstrated in a high percentage of these patients. The mechanism of cardiac ischemia in this syndrome, often called "syndrome X" is unclear but centers on two hypotheses: endothelial dysfunction and prearteriolar defect. Prearterioles function as conduit vessels that carry blood from the epicardial vessels to the arterioles. Unlike arterioles, prearterioles are not under metabolic regulation and, thus, do not respond to myocardial ischemia. Endothelial dysfunction may also limit flow during hyperemia, with excessive vasoconstrictor tone. Both exercise and mental stress require normal endothelial cell function for coronary vasodilatation. Both hypotheses may explain chest pain in some patients.

Patients with typical angina and normal coronary arteriograms may benefit from additional assessment of their endothelial function and microcirculation. Such a "functional angiogram" is performed with an intracoronay Doppler guidewire and an infusion catheter. Graded concentrations of acetylcholine (10^{-6}, 10^{-5}, and 10^{-4} M) are infused selectively into the left anterior descending coronary artery for 2 minutes. Doppler velocities, hemodynamics, and angiographic images are obtained at baseline and with each concentration of acetylcholine as well as with nitroglycerin. A normal response to acetylcholine is vasodilatation. Paradoxical vasoconstriction indicates endothelial dysfunction (Fig. 11). Acetylcholine provocation can be used to test of coronary spasm. Coronary flow reserve is also measured (as described above). Use of vasoactive medications (calcium channel blockers, nitrates, and angiotensin-converting enzyme inhibitors) must be discontinued before the test is performed.

Patients can be stratified into four groups: normal physiology, endothelial cell dysfunction, impaired vasodilatory reserve, and combined defects. Patients with normal results can be reassured. Those with endothelial cell dysfunction can be treated as outlined above, and those with impaired vasodilatory reserve can be treated empirically with conventional antianginal agents, angiotensin-converting enzyme inhibitors, and alpha-blockers. Imipramine has also been used to treat heightened visceral pain sensitivity.

Although the long-term prognosis for patients with normal coronary angiograms is good, there are subsets (e.g., those with left bundle branch block) with a worse prognosis. Patients with endothelial dysfunction are also a group that have worse long-term prognosis, because it is an early stage in the development of atherosclerosis.

Coronary Interventions

The main purpose of coronary interventions is to improve the coronary flow physiology and, thereby, improve symptoms. Physiologic improvement after PTCA has been documented in the Doppler Endpoints Balloon Angioplasty Trial Europe (DEBATE) study. In this study, patients with good angiographic results (quantitative coronary angiography stenosis <35%) and normal Doppler coronary flow reserve (>2.5) had a very low incidence of major adverse cardiac events, equivalent to that seen with the optimal stent results achieved with the stents in the BENESTENT trial. However, only about 20% of the study population had both angiographic and Doppler coronary flow reserve success. The subsequent, larger DEBATE II trial in which optimal results were

Table 3.   Noncardiac Causes of Chest Pain

Psychiatric
    Panic disorders
    Depression
    Anxiety
    Hypochondriasis
Gastrointestinal
    Esophageal spasm
    Peptic ulcer disease
    Gallbladder disease
Musculoskeletal
    Costochondritis
    Herpes zoster
    Arthritis
    Fibromyalgia
Respiratory
    Reactive airways
    Pulmonary embolism
    Pulmonary hypertension
    Pleurisy

achieved in approximately 35% of patients demonstrated that a strategy of Doppler flow velocity and angiography-guided PTCA with provisional stenting was less cost effective than routine stenting.

INTRACORONARY PRESSURE MEASUREMENTS

In assessing coronary stenosis, the important physiologic component, in addition to flow velocity, is the pressure gradient produced by the stenosis. Translesional pressure gradients were used routinely in the early days of coronary intervention. However, a simple resting translesional pressure gradient alone is inadequate for assessing the physiologic significance of a coronary stenosis. The gradient is highly dependent on aortic pressure, and similar resting gradients can have widely differing implications, given different aortic pressures. Furthermore, a pressure gradient alone gives no information about the ability of the artery to augment flow. The distal coronary pressure during hyperemia can be used to derive the FFR, a highly useful measurement of the physiologic effect of a stenosis.

Pressure Guidewires

Pressure guidewires are available, in sizes comparable to those of angioplasty guidewires (0.014 inch), for accurate measurement of distal coronary pressure. Their small size will not cause significant obstruction unless the luminal area is quite small (0.10 mm^2). Pressure gradients can be measured by comparing the aortic pressure (guiding catheter) with the distal coronary pressure (pressure guidewire). The gradient during hyperemia can also be assessed with adenosine (140 µg/kg per minute intravenously for ostial left main or right coronary lesions, or 24 to 60 µg injected into the left coronary artery or 12 to 36 µg injected into the right coronary artery). The gradient equals the difference between the mean pressures in the aorta and the distal coronary segment. Phasic pressures are not used to calculate the gradient, although most of the gradients associated with a mildly stenotic plaque will be seen during diastole.

Myocardial Fractional Flow Reserve

Myocardial fractional flow reserve (FFR$_{myo}$) is defined as the ratio of the hyperemic flow in a diseased target artery and the hyperemic flow in the same target artery if no lesion is present (Table 1). The FFR$_{myo}$ expresses a given hyperemic flow as a fraction of the normal hyperemic flow and can easily be obtained with distal coronary pressure measurements during hyperemia. It is assumed that during hyperemia small resistance vessels are maximally dilated and constant. In normal coronary arteries, the distal pressure equals the aortic pressure during hyperemia and the FFR$_{myo}$ is equal to 1. Values less than 0.75 indicate physiologically significant lesions and are predictive of abnormal findings on noninvasive function tests (Fig. 12).

In contrast to absolute coronary flow reserve measured with Doppler methods, FFR$_{myo}$ is much less dependent on microcirculatory function compared with CFR, and it does not vary appreciably with changing heart rate, blood pressure, or contractility (Table 1). Thus, it is the preferred method for assessing indeterminate lesions.

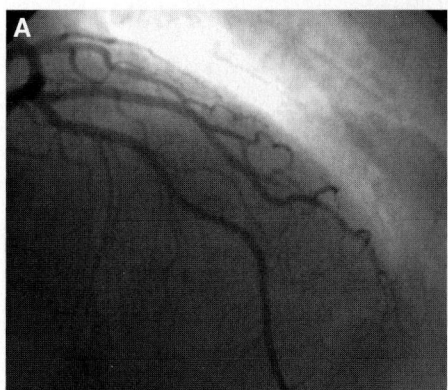
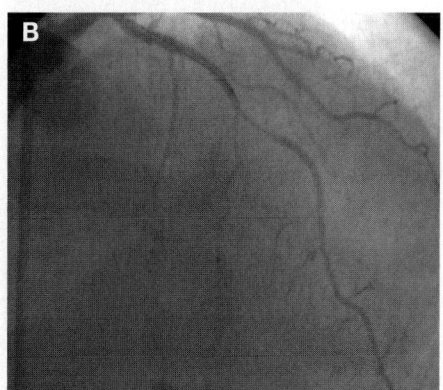

Fig. 11. Coronary angiogram before (*A*) and after (*B*) the infusion of intracoronary acetylcholine into the left anterior descending artery showing diffuse epicardial constriction, indicating the presence of endothelial dysfunction.

Indications for Intracoronary Pressure Measurements

Indeterminate Coronary Stenoses

Intermediate severity stenoses in the 40% to 70% diameter stenosis range are often difficult to assess in a cardiac catheterization laboratory. Frequently, these patients are referred for noninvasive functional testing before considering percutaneous coronary revascularization. The lesions can be assessed physiologically with pressure measurements and the FFR_{myo} in a manner similar to Doppler guidewire and the coronary flow reserve. Several studies have examined the correlation between the FFR_{myo} and noninvasive tests of myocardial ischemia. An FFR_{myo} of 0.75 appears to define lesions that produce ischemia on noninvasive tests. That is, if a vessel cannot produce at least 75% of the expected normal hyperemic flow, ischemia will usually result.

Coronary Interventions

Following PTCA, patients with a low FFR_{myo} value (from 0.75 to 0.90) and adequate angiographic results (<30% residual stenosis by quantitative coronary angiography) have an increased restenosis rate compared with patients with higher FFR_{myo} values (>0.90). A higher FFR_{myo} value reduces the restenosis rate from approximately 30% to 12%, producing stent like results (Table 4). Stents typically produce higher FFR_{myo} values after high-pressure inflation compared with PTCA. In the absence of serial lesions or diffuse disease, optimal stent deployment should result in a

Table 4.　Use of Myocardial Fractional Flow Reserve (FFR_{myo}) for Assessing Results of Percutaneous Transluminal Coronary Angioplasty (PTCA)

FFR_{myo}	Result and anticipated outcome
<0.75	Unsuccessful
0.75-0.90	Moderately successful
	Restenosis rate approximately 30%
	Consider additional PTCA or stent
>0.90	Excellent
	Restenosis rate approximately 12%
	No benefit from stent

FFR_{myo} of >0.90. A lower value predicts higher adverse events during follow-up and may reflect inadequate stent deployment or increased atherosclerotic burden due to diffuse disease.

- Resting pressure gradients are less useful than hyperemic pressure gradients.
- The myocardial fractional flow reserve (FFR_{myo}) is the ratio of the hyperemic flow through an artery with a lesion in question divided by the normal expected hyperemic flow through the same artery if the lesion were not present.
- FFR_{myo} <0.75 is predictive of ischemia on noninvasive testing.

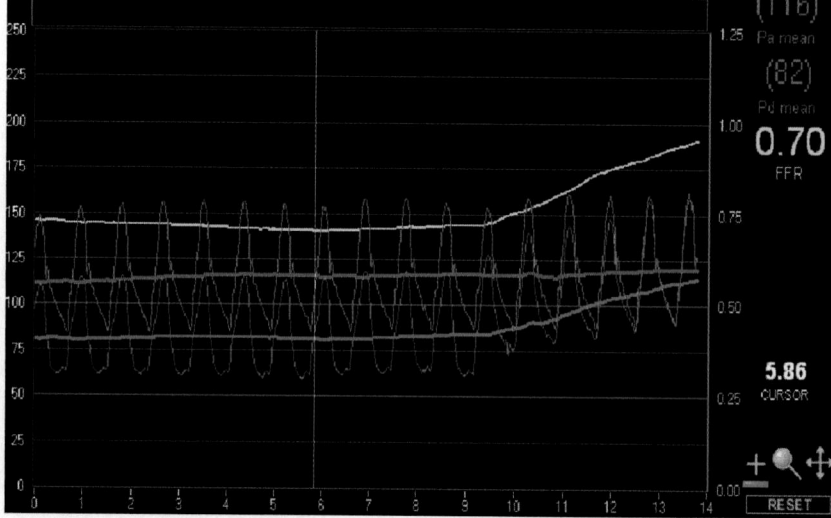

Fig. 12. Intracoronary pressure tracings from the guide (red), and the pressure wire (green) from a patient with a significant stenosis. The fractional flow reserve (FFR) of 0.70 is the ratio between the distal and proximal mean coronary pressures.

Coronary Anatomy and Angiographic Views

André C. Lapeyre III, MD

Basic Concepts

This chapter will focus on the details of coronary angiographic anatomy and the requirements for optimal angiographic visualization of coronary arterial lesions.

The coronary arterial segments need to be visualized in two orthogonal angiographic views, each segment of interest aligned perpendicular to the x-ray beam to avoid the problem of vessel foreshortening. Orthogonal views help to ensure that eccentric or "ribbon-like" coronary lesions are not missed or underestimated by only visualizing the "wide" and not the "edge-on" view of the contrast filled arterial lumen. Overlap with other vessels and the proximal portion of branches from the segment being visualized needs to be avoided to prevent either obscuring true lesions or creating artifacts from edge effect which can simulate lesions. The coronary vessels curve throughout their course. This requires different projections for proper visualization of each portion of the vessel. The heart lies obliquely in the chest with a great degree of variability from individual to individual in its orientation of the reference planes—frontal (or coronal), sagittal, and transverse. Therefore, implicit in the following discussions of the "best view or angle" for each major segment is the understanding that these are the "average or usual" best views and must be individualized based on the individual patient's anatomy and confirmed with a second orthogonal view. These will be summarized in Table 1.

- Since exact angles need to be individualized for the patient, remember the general view needed for specific vessel portions and their origins rather than memorizing specific angles.
- Orthogonal views are needed to avoid missing eccentric and ribbon-like lesions or eccentric results of an intervention.
- Views with the x-ray beam perpendicular to the portion of the artery in question are necessary to avoid missing lesions or problems with an intervention result due to foreshortening.
- Missing vessels should be a reminder to look carefully for collaterals, unsuspected congenital anomalies and coronary grafts.
- Decisions about vessel size should be made by comparison with an object (usually the catheter) of known size at relatively the same level in the chest as the vessel in question.

Left Main Coronary Artery

The origin of the left main coronary artery is usually from the a slightly anterior aspect of the left coronary cusp. The length of the left main is variable and it may be straight or curved in its course and as it divides at its distal end. This often requires different views to best visualize the proximal and distal segments. The ostium of the left main is often best seen straight

Table 1. Angiographic Views for Coronary Arterial Segments

Arterial segment	"Best view"	Orthogonal view
Left main: ostium	Straight AP to LAO 0-5	LAO 60, caudal 30
Left main: distal	RAO 0-20	LAO 60, caudal 30
LAD: proximal	RAO 30, caudal 20	LAO 60, cranial 30
LAD: mid	RAO 30, cranial 30	LAO 60, cranial 20
LAD: distal	RAO 30, cranial 0-15	LAO 60, cranial 0-10
Septal perforators	RAO 15-30, cranial 30-45	Difficult—variable
Diagonals	RAO 30, cranial 30	LAO 60, cranial 20-30
Circumflex	RAO 30, caudal 30-40	LAO 60, caudal 30-40
Obtuse marginals	RAO 30, caudal 30-40	Difficult—variable
Right	LAO 45, cranial 20-30	RAO 30, cranial 20-30

anteroposteriorly (AP) or with minimal left anterior oblique (LAO) projection of 0 to 5 degrees as shown in Figure 1. The distal left main is usually best seen with minimal right anterior oblique (RAO) projection as shown in Figure 2 and possibly slight caudal angulation. The LAO caudal (spider view) is often used as the orthogonal view as shown in Figure 3. This view often suffers from foreshortening, overlap or both due to difficulty achieving sufficient LAO or sufficient caudal angulation.

LEFT ANTERIOR DESCENDING CORONARY ARTERY, SEPTAL PERFORATORS, AND DIAGONAL BRANCHES

The left anterior descending coronary artery takes a curvilinear course from the left main to the apex of the left ventricle and frequently around the apex to supply the distal inferior septum. The course of the left anterior descending follows the plane of the interventricular septum. The plane of the interventricular septum is perpendicular to the x-ray beam when an RAO projection

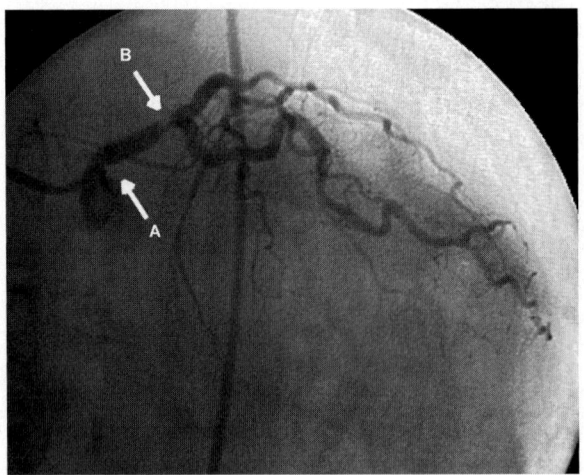

Fig. 1. Shallow LAO view of the left main coronary artery showing its origin (A) perpendicular to the x-ray beam. Notice the slight foreshortening to the lesion (B) in the distal left main.

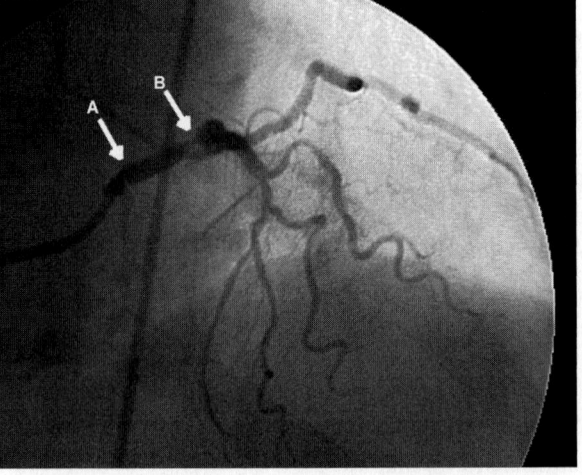

Fig. 2. Shallow RAO view of the left main coronary artery showing the lesion at the origin (A) is not as well seen as in the shallow LAO view (Fig. 1) but that the lesion in the distal portion is better defined. Note the potential problem with overlap from the catheter and the branch vessel.

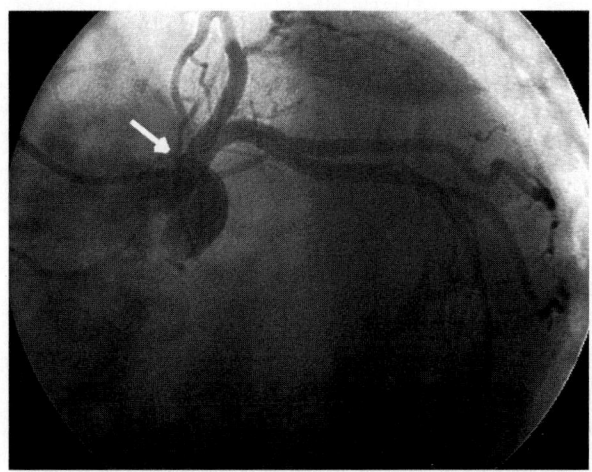

Fig. 3. The LAO caudal (spider) view showing the left main in good profile when adequate angulation can be obtained as in this case. Note however the problem of a branch vessel and of contrast in the aortic cusp overlapping and obscuring the origin of the left main.

of approximately 30 degrees is used. In this projection the only issue is overlap with other vessels. Thus the proximal LAD is best seen with caudal angulation of about 20 degrees which moves the proximal circumflex down and off the proximal LAD (Fig. 4). Because of overlap with the diagonal branches in the caudal projection (Fig. 5), the RAO projection of the middle and

distal left anterior descending coronary segments is usually best with about 30 degrees of cranial angulation (Fig. 6). The orthogonal view of the LAD is more difficult. Depending on the degree of vertical or horizontal orientation of the heart in the chest, the proximal left anterior descending will be better seen either with cranial angulation (Fig. 7) or caudal angulation (Fig. 8). The former is more common. The middle LAD's best orthogonal view is the LAO cranial with the amount of cranial angulation depending on the tilt of the heart in the patient's chest (Fig. 9). As in Figure 9, the left main and proximal LAD are often overlapped or foreshortened in the LAO cranial view that is optimized for the mid-LAD. The distal LAD continues the curve around the narrowing ventricular apex and frequently goes completely around the apex to supply the distal inferior interventricular septum. To maintain this section of the LAD perpendicular to the x-ray beam in the LAO projection very little if any cranial angulation is needed (Fig. 10). Once it wraps around the apex, the very end of the LAD may be foreshortened in this view as it heads back towards the base of the heart on the inferior surface. This "wrap-around" portion of the LAD can usually be adequately visualized in either the LAO 30 degree cranial or the LAO caudal view. Many angiographers take the LAO cranial diagnostic shot of the LAD by "panning." The shot is usually started in LAO with steep cranial angulation and with the patient holding a deep

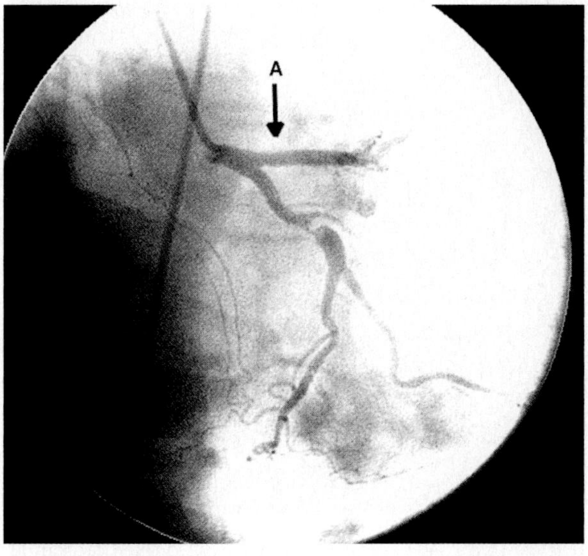

Fig. 4. The RAO caudal view moves the proximal circumflex downward and shows the entire length of the proximal LAD (A) in profile.

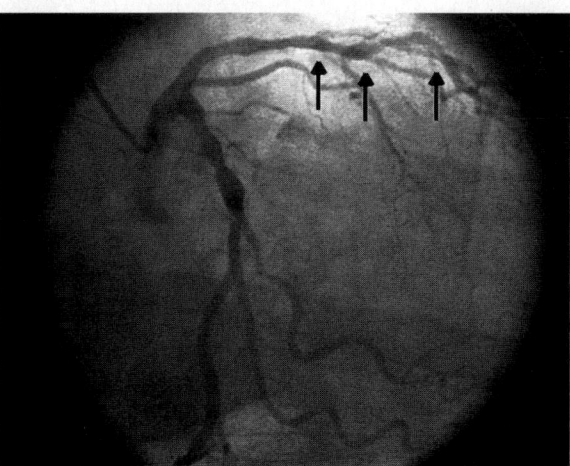

Fig. 5. In the RAO caudal projection the middle and distal LAD are often overlapped with multiple diagonal branches (*arrows*) and sometimes with septal perforators or the ramus intermedius.

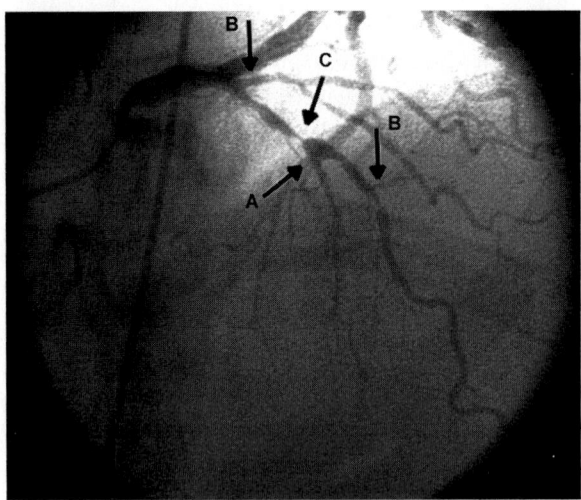

Fig. 6. Notice how cranial angulation on the same LAD seen in Figure 5 moves the septal perforator (A) down off the LAD, the diagonals (B) up off the LAD, and reveals the previously obscured lesion (C).

inspiration. Once the left main and proximal LAD are visualized, the x-ray beam is rotated less cranially in order to visualize the middle and distal LAD. The LAO caudal is usually taken as a separate injection.

Visualization of the septal perforators in the RAO cranial view is usually good throughout the length of the septal perforators (Fig. 11). Obtaining a good orthogonal view to look for eccentric lesions is however

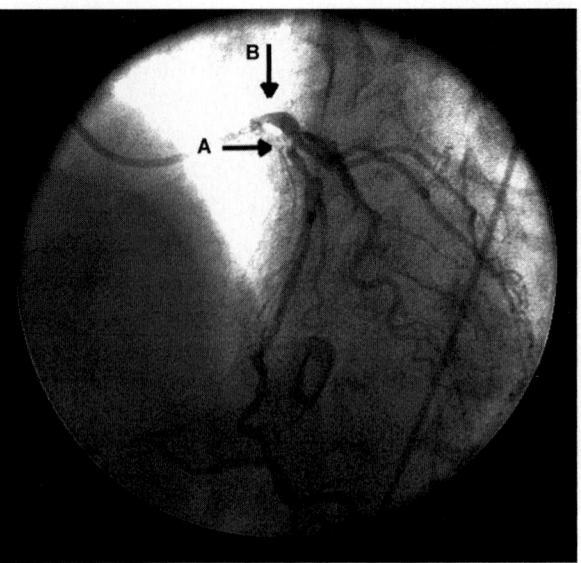

Fig. 7. This LAO cranial injection of the left circulation shows the proximal LAD including the lesion at the origin of the LAD (A) as well as the lesion at the origin of the left main (B). Notice that significant cranial angulation was needed almost to the point of projecting the left main and proximal LAD over the diaphragmatic attenuation. The orientation of this heart in the patient's chest was the more common somewhat vertical orientation with the apex below the base of the heart.

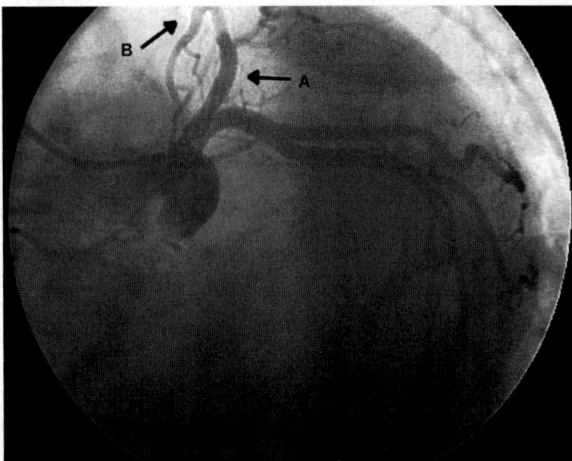

Fig. 8. This LAO caudal shows the proximal LAD (A) very well. This heart was horizontal in the patient's chest with diaphragm pushing the apex upward to the same level as the base of the heart. Notice that the mid-LAD (B) is very foreshortened in this projection.

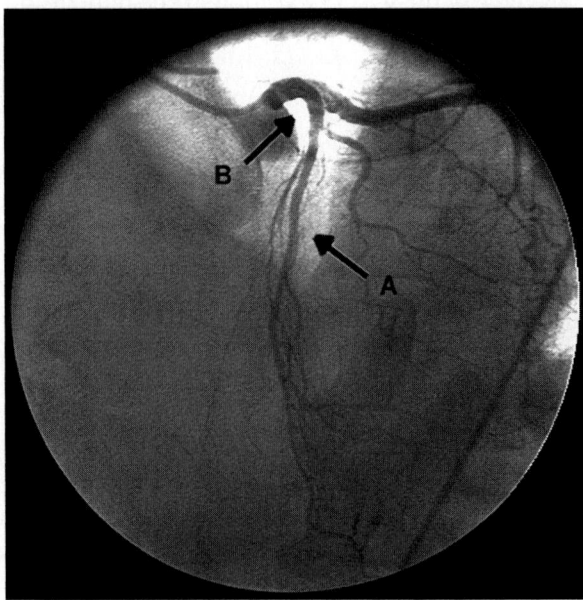

Fig. 9. The LAO cranial view with the degree of cranial angulation optimized to see the mid-LAD (A) often produces foreshortening and overlap with other vessels of the proximal LAD (B).

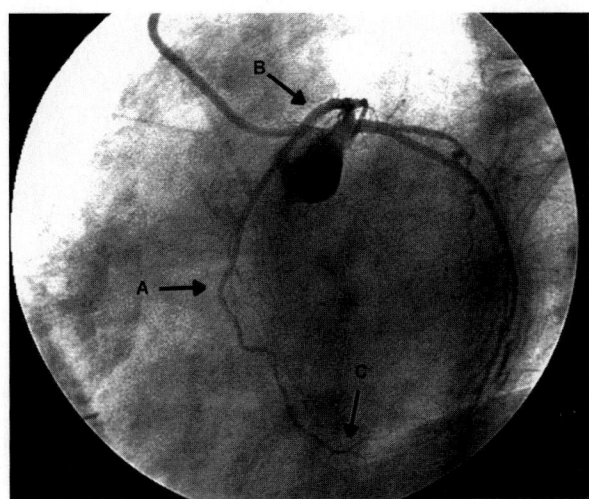

Fig. 10. The LAO with minimal or no (as in this image) cranial angulation is the best orthogonal view of the distal LAD (A). Note the foreshortening of the proximal and middle LAD (B) and of the LAD once it has completely wrapped the apex (C).

very difficult and must be individualized to the patient and artery in question. Despite cranial, straight, or caudal angulation, the LAO view does not reliably produce good visualization of the septal perforators due to overlap (Fig. 12 to 14). They can frequently be seen in a true lateral projection but this is not an orthogonal view

to the RAO as it is closer to 180 degrees away from the RAO than the necessary 90 degrees for an orthogonal view. An RAO caudal angulation will also sometimes visualize the septal perforators but again this is not an orthogonal view for eccentric lesions. A single view is adequate for visualization of proper placement of a catheter for alcohol injections for septal ablation procedures. In most instances, the septal perforators are too small to be considered for angioplasty or coronary bypass grafting and so the need for true orthogonal views is rare.

The diagonal vessels follow the epicardial surface anterolateral left ventricle and do not follow the plane of the interventricular septum. The anterolateral surface of the LV usually describes a curved plane that slopes leftward and toward the diaphragm going from the base of the heart to the apex of the heart. The majority of this surface is perpendicular to an x-ray beam that has between 20 and 45 degrees of cranial angulation (Fig. 14). Orthogonal views can then be obtained by images obtained 90 degrees apart in RAO and LAO both with cranial angulation (Fig. 15). In general the origins of the diagonals are easier to see in the LAO cranial angulation making this the preferred view of many angiographers. However, there can be significant overlap with posterior vessels such as left posterior laterals or the distal circumflex.

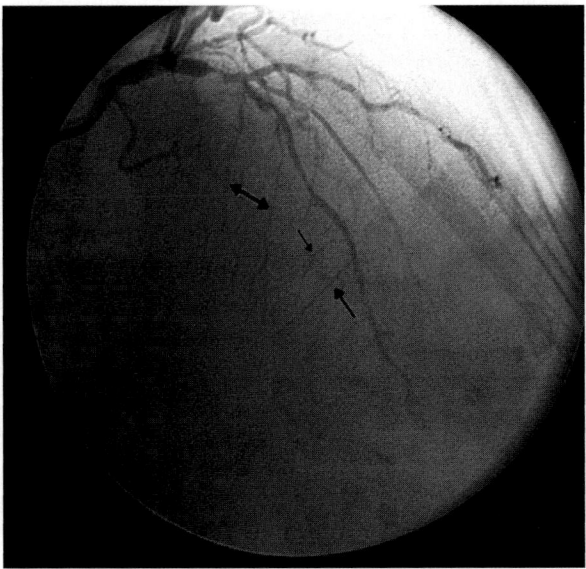

Fig. 11. The RAO cranial view shows the septal perforators in excellent profile from their origin throughout their length (arrows).

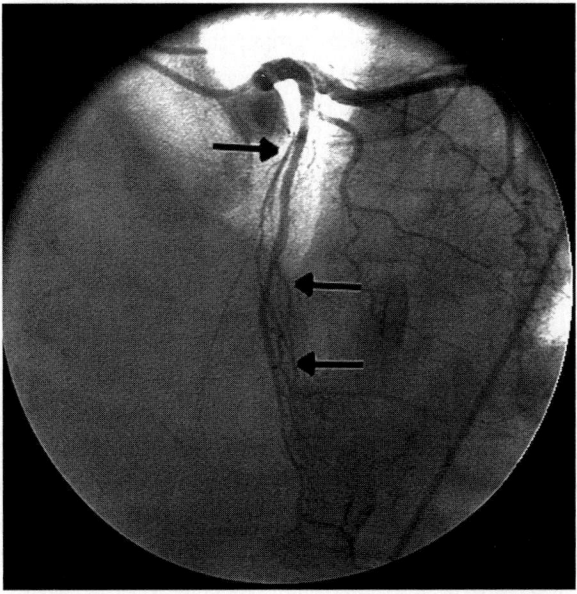

Fig. 12. Note the typical overlap and foreshortening of the septal perforators (arrows) in this LAO cranial view.

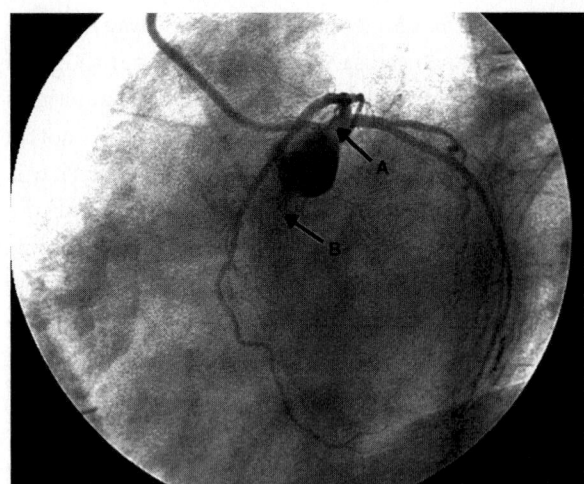

Fig. 13. In this LAO view without cranial or caudal angulation, the large first septal perforator (A) is obscured by the aortic cusp, the proximal LAD and the other septal perforators. The more distal septal perforators (B) are all overlapped on each other and obscured by the "septal blush" of contrast within the "septal muscle" seen "end-on."

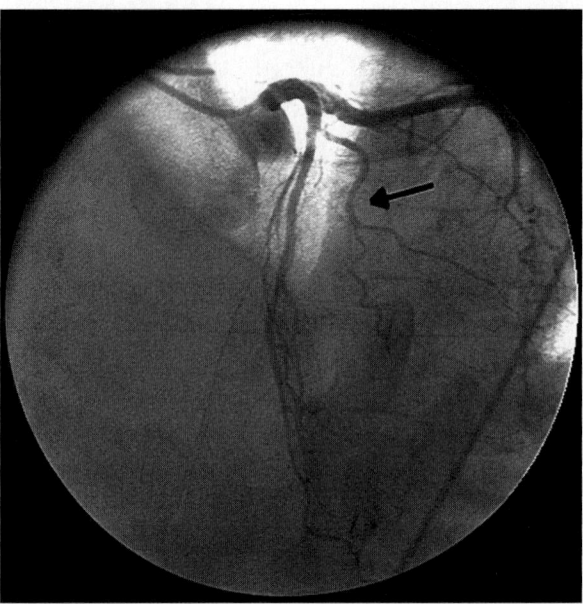

Fig. 14. Notice how the diagonal (*arrow*) is shown in excellent profile throughout its course across the anterolateral wall of the LV in this LAO cranial view.

CIRCUMFLEX, OBTUSE MARGINAL, AND LEFT POSTEROLATERAL CORONARY ARTERIES

The circumflex coronary artery runs in the atrioventricular groove which usually describes a plane that is nearly perpendicular to the LAO caudal projection shot from the apex of the heart. This would make the LAO caudal the optimal projection to view the circumflex were it not for the fact the obtuse marginals come out perpendicular to the circumflex in this view and therefore frequently cause overlap (Fig. 16). The problem of overlap is solved by the RAO caudal projection (Fig. 17) where the proximal circumflex is projected downward off the left main and the proximal LAD. The distal circumflex is seen well with the origins of the obtuse marginals well defined. The problem with this view is foreshortening of the continuing AV groove portion of the circumflex and overlap of the left posterolaterals in a left dominant or balanced circulation (Fig. 18). However, these should be seen well in the LAO cranial angulation taken to visualize the LAD and diagonals if care was taken to avoid overlap (Fig. 19). Since the major proximal vessels are usually seen well in the RAO caudal angulation, this projection is considered the "best view" for the circumflex and obtuse marginals. The LAO caudal angulation is therefore the orthogonal view of the circumflex.

The orthogonal view of the obtuse marginals is much more difficult. As seen in Figure 16, the obtuse marginals are overlapped and foreshortened in LAO projections. Therefore a combination of LAO cranial angulation and LAO caudal angulation are often

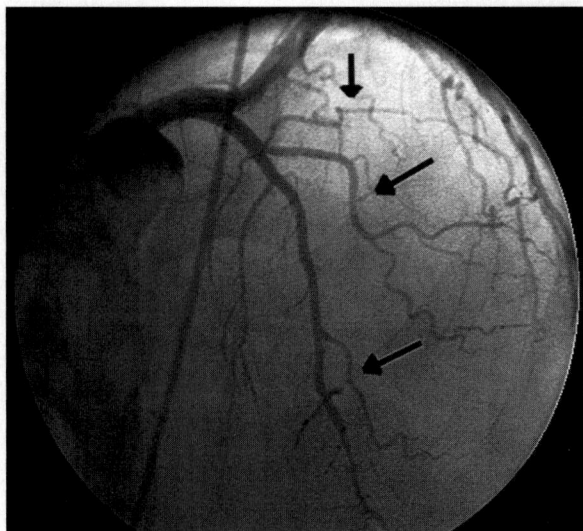

Fig. 15. This RAO cranial view of the diagonals (*arrows*) demonstrates how diagonals supplying the basal, middle and distal anterolateral wall are well seen in this projection.

needed to see lesion in the obtuse marginals which run on the lateral surface of the heart in parallel with the septum both being in the parallel with the x-ray beam in the LAO projection (Fig. 20 and 21).

RIGHT CORONARY, POSTERIOR DESCENDING, AND RIGHT POSTERORLATERAL CORONARY ARTERIES

The right coronary artery is best seen in the LAO view as its entire course runs in the atrioventricular groove, which is perpendicular to an LAO x-ray beam. The major branches are the posterior descending and the posterolateral(s). These are on the inferior surface of the left ventricle and generally have a slightly downward course. Therefore, cranial angulation to the LAO projection usually shows these very well making the LAO cranial the "best" or "preferred" view (Fig. 22). The RAO projection visualizes the mid-right coronary well. In this projection there can be significant foreshortening of the proximal and distal right coronary as

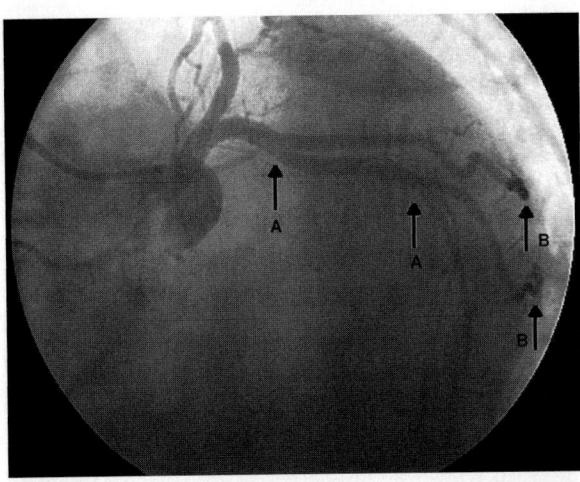

Fig. 16. In this LAO caudal view, the circumflex coronary artery is seen well in profile throughout its course in the atrioventricular groove. However, notice the overlap of the origins of the obtuse marginals with the circumflex (A *arrows*) and the foreshortening of the obtuse marginals as they run parallel with (into) the x-ray beam (B *arrows*).

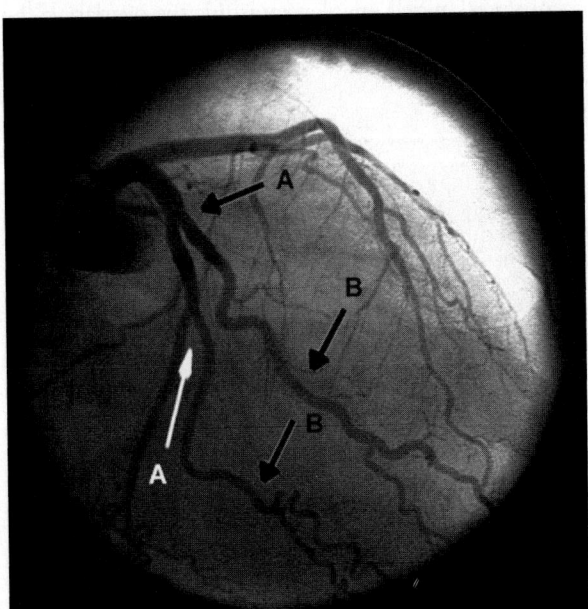

Fig. 17. The RAO caudal view shows the circumflex coronary artery in nice profile from its origin through most of its course to the very distal "continuing AV-groove" or posterolateral segment. The origins of the obtuse marginals (A *arrows*) and the course of the obtuse marginals across the lateral surface of the LV (B *arrows*) also are seen well.

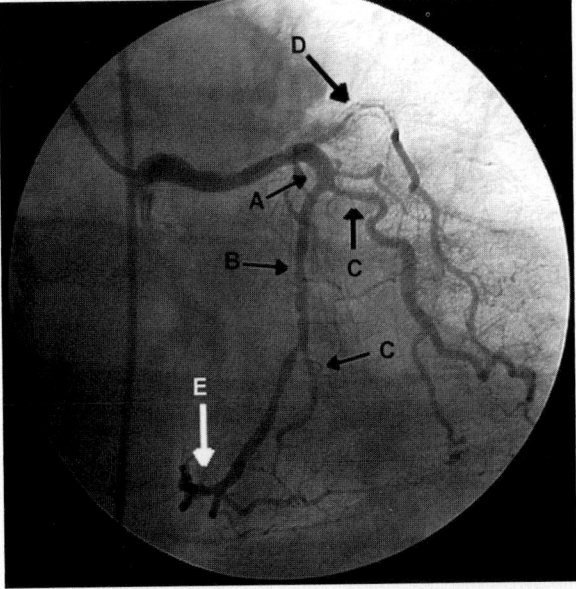

Fig. 18. This RAO caudal angulation demonstrates an excellent view of the proximal circumflex (A *arrow*) the distal circumflex (B *arrow*), the obtuse marginals (C *arrows*), and the diffuse severe in-stent restenosis in the proximal LAD (D *arrow*). It also demonstrates the problem with both foreshortening and overlap in the continuing AV groove portion of the distal vessel as well as overlap of all the left posterolateral vessels (E *arrow*). Note the AV nodal artery just to the left of the "E *arrow*."

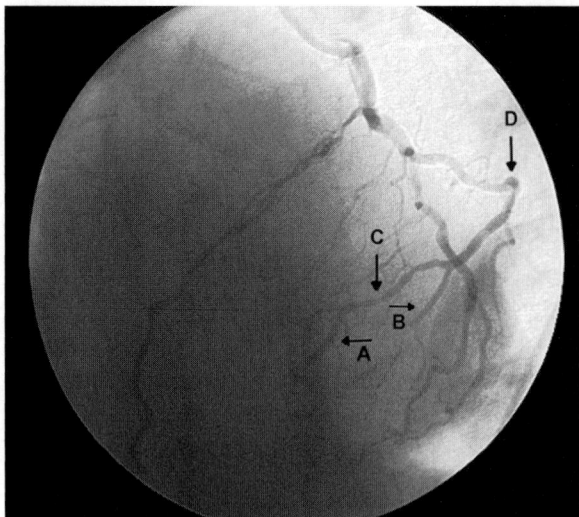

Fig. 19. The LAO cranial view of the same patient's angiogram as Figure 18 shows the left posterior descending (A *arrow*), the left posterolateral (B *arrow*), and the continuing AV groove portion of the circumflex in excellent profile and without overlap or significant foreshortening. However, note the foreshortening and overlap that now occur in the distal circumflex (D *arrow*).

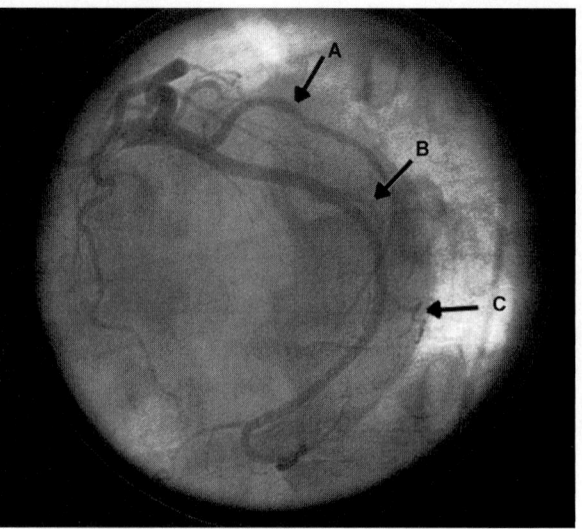

Fig. 20. The LAO caudal view of this circumflex shows the first obtuse marginal to good advantage (A *arrow*) but has considerable overlap and foreshortening of the second (B *arrow*) and third (C *arrow*) obtuse marginals.

well as significant overlap of any or all of the following: the distal right coronary, the right posterior descending, the right posterolateral(s) (Fig. 23). Using slightly less RAO can reduce the foreshortening of the proxi-

mal and distal right coronary. Adding cranial (or less commonly caudal) angulation avoids the overlap of the right posterior descending and right posterolateral(s) (Fig. 24).

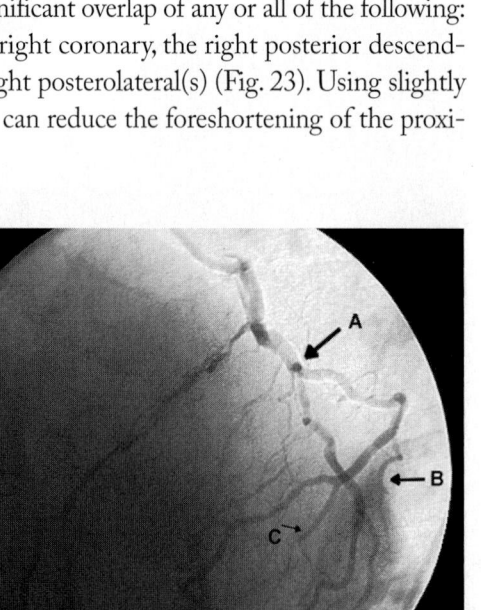

Fig. 21. The LAO cranial view of this circumflex has significant overlap and foreshortening of the origin of the first obtuse marginal (A *arrow*) but shows the second (B *arrow*) and third (C *arrow*) obtuse marginals quite well.

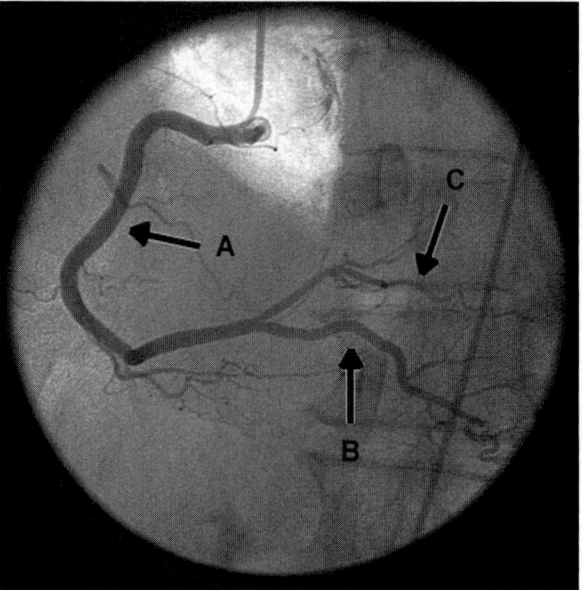

Fig. 22. The LAO cranial view of a dominant right coronary shows a nice profile of the entire right coronary (A *arrow*), the right posterior descending (B *arrow*) and the right posterolateral (C *arrow*).

GRAFTS AND CONGENITAL ANOMALIES

The origin and course of grafts and congenital anomalies are too variable to allow for prediction of the best angles for viewing any particular segment. However a few points are worth mentioning. At least two orthogonal views of each graft or anomaly should be obtained to avoid missing eccentric lesions. Rolling pan shots (cranial to caudal or vice versa) are often helpful to view these vessels throughout their course. If major epicardial vessels are not visualized or are missing on the initial angiographic injections of the native coronary circulations and known bypass grafts, then an additional effort should be made, including cusp injections, review of the ventriculogram or aortic root angiogram if performed, to either visualize or exclude unsuspected collaterals, unsuspected anomalies, or unsuspected grafts.

LESION LOCALIZATION

During interventional procedures, it is frequently important to be able to localize a lesion without being able to directly visualize the lesion with a contrast injection. This occurs because many interventional devices such as directional atherectomy catheters, stents, rotablator burs often totally occlude the lumen of the artery in question. Contrast injections in this situation may not be helpful. An alternative method of device localization relative to the coronary lesion is important.

Reference points that remain relatively fixed in relation to the lesion are used in these situations. Since all points in the chest change relative position on the x-ray image as the projection is changed, this technique requires knowing the exact angles at which the reference picture was obtained and matching those angles exactly when positioning the device. This technique has been variously called "road mapping," "positioning by reference points," "blind positioning," "landmark positioning," etc. Many different reference points can be used including other vessels that will fill with dye, ribs, spine, dense calcifications in some structure, surgical clips, catheter (especially the tip), vessel shape (especially sharp bends), etc. The series of images, Figures 25 *A-C*, demonstrates this technique. You will also note this technique, especially position-relative to the catheter tip, used in the series of images in the discussion of vessel sizing.

VESSEL SIZING

Choosing the correct device size when treating a given arterial segment is a critical interventional issue. Device undersizing and oversizing each carry the potential for significant associated problems.

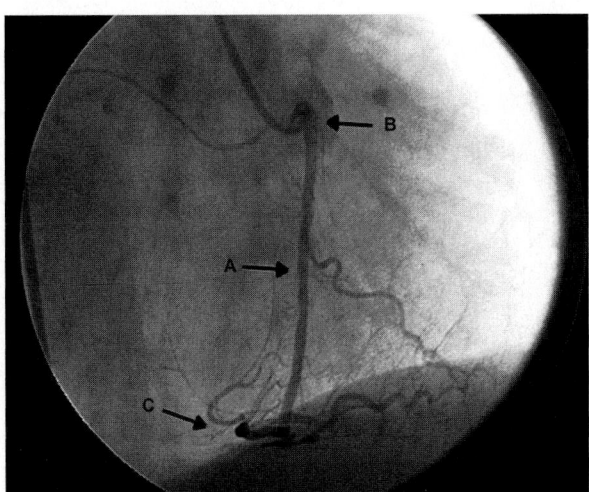

Fig. 23. The RAO straight view of the right coronary shows the middle right (A *arrow*) very well. However, there is foreshortening of the proximal right (B *arrow*) and both foreshortening of the distal right as well as overlap of the distal right, posterior descending, and postero-lateral (C *arrow*).

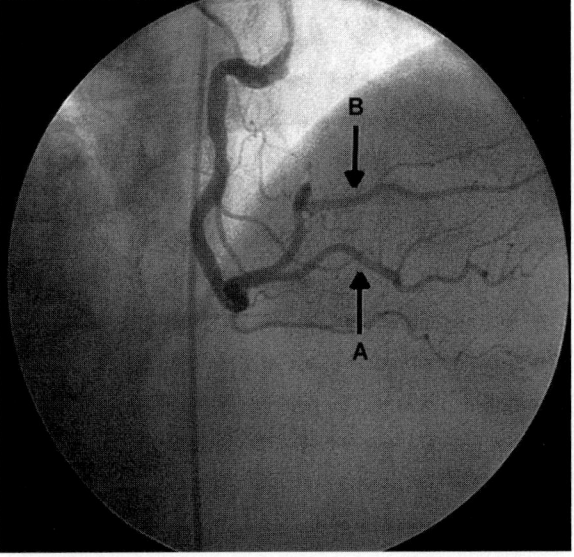

Fig. 24. Addition of cranial angulation with a slight reduction in the degree of RAO gives a nice orthogonal view of the right posterior descending and right postero-lateral that were severely overlapped in Figure 23.

Due to the variability of the size of the coronary arterial segments, there are no "standard" sizes for any of the coronary arteries (except possibly a range for the left main) even after accounting for the patient's gender and body surface area. Thus, empiric tables of coronary artery "standard sizes" are not useful.

The size of the vessel is difficult to judge, as the vessels will be magnified to a different degree on each image depending on the image field size, the distance of the vessel from the x-ray tube, and the distance of the vessel from the image intensifier. If one draws a plane perpendicular to the x-ray beam at the level between the x-ray tube and the image intensifier of the segment being studied, all objects within the field of view in that plane will have similar magnification. Since the diameter of the catheter is known, a segment of the catheter shown in the correct plane and in profile can be measured (either qualitatively or quantitatively) and compared with a measurement of the vessel segment whose size needs to be determined. By calculating the measured ratios and multiplying by the known size of the catheter, the size of the vessel can be determined with sufficient accuracy for the clinical purposes of most interventional procedure. This technique will be demonstrated in the series of images in Figure 26 *A* to *D*. Table 2 provides the values used in our laboratory for

Table 2.* Conversion Table for French Size (Circumference) to Approximate External Catheter Diameter

French size	Catheter external diameter
3	1.0
4	1.3
5	1.7
6	2.0
7	2.3
8	2.7
9	3.0
10	3.3
11	3.7
12	4.0

*Millimeter sizes are approximate and are manufacturer and catheter-line specific. Check the specifics for the catheters in use by your laboratory.

both diagnostic and guide catheters. There is some variability depending on the catheter manufacturer.

The most accurate way to determine vessel size in the catheterization laboratory is with the use of intracoronary ultrasound.

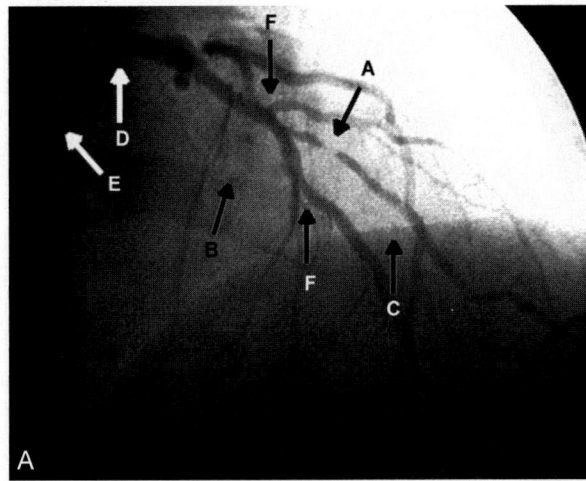

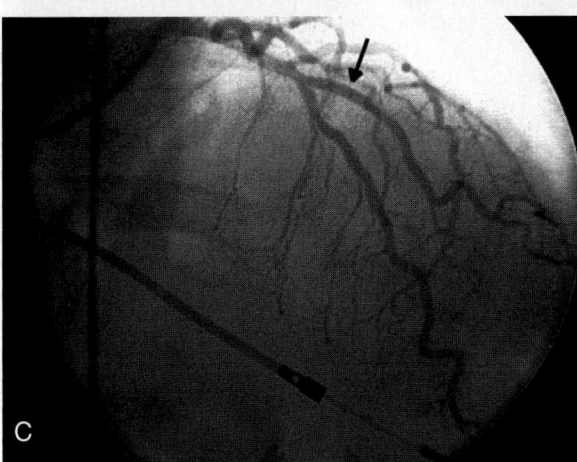

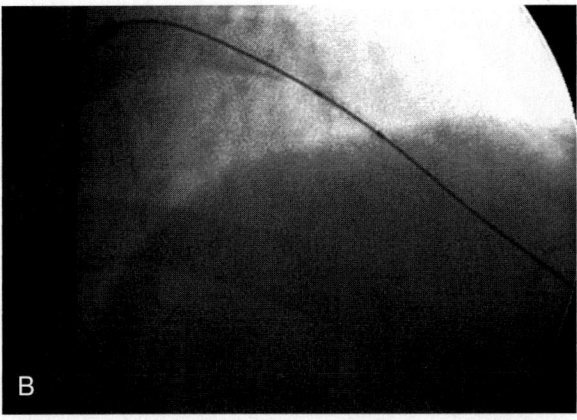

Fig. 25. *A,* This first figure in a series shows a tight lesion in a small caliber second diagonal (A *arrow*). Landmarks or "roadmap" points used by the angiographer to assist in positioning of the balloon include the edge of the rib(s) (B *arrow*), edge of the diaphragm (C *arrow*), distance and relationship from the tip of the guide catheter (D *arrow*), distance and relationship from the intersection catheter in the aortic root and descending thoracic aorta, and the origins of other branches (F *arrows*). *B,* Note how the angiographer is positioning the balloon using all the reference points demonstrated in Figure 25 *A. C,* Although the postprocedure image is taken with slightly more cranial angulation so that the diaphragm is positioned higher in the image, note the excellent result in the second diagonal obtained by using this technique for positioning the balloon.

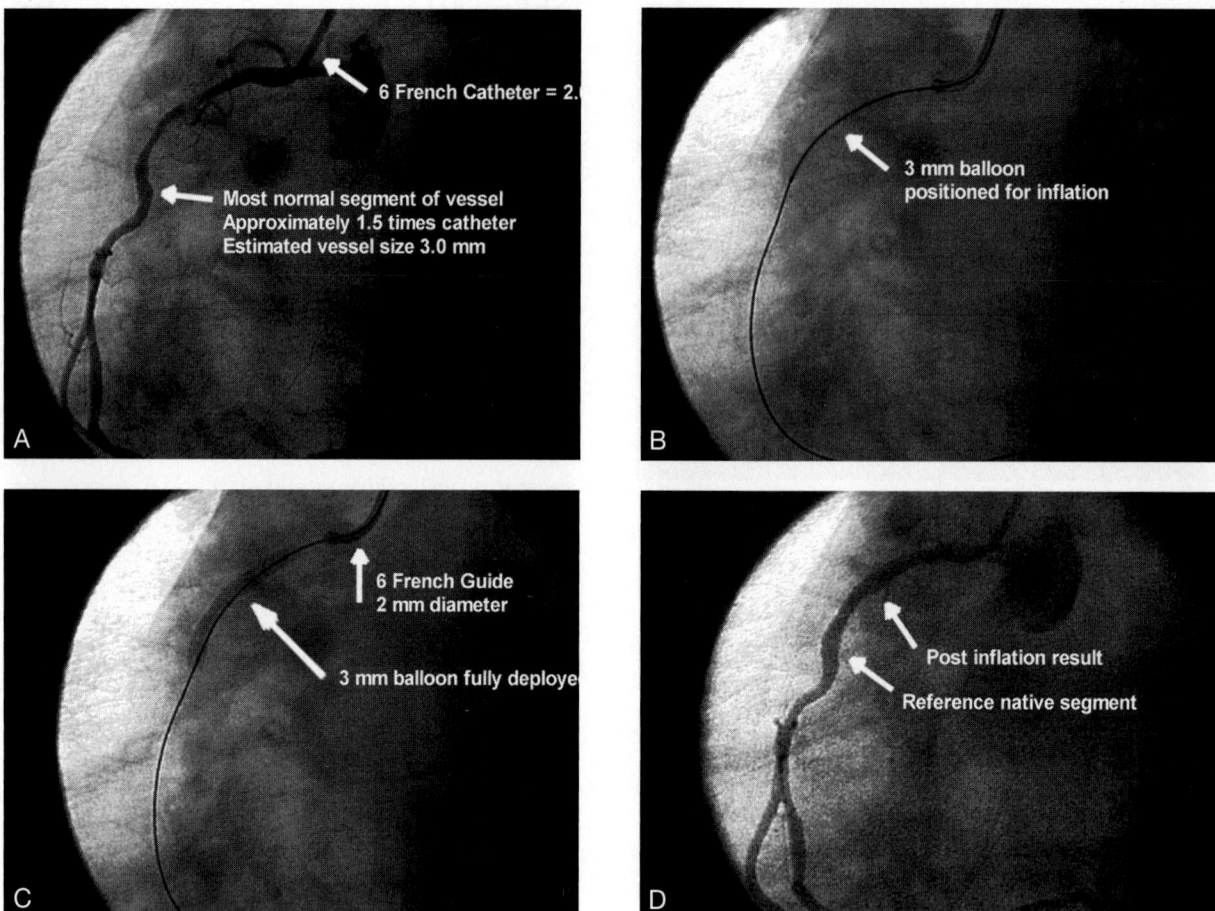

Fig. 26. *A,* The visualized portion of a 6 French diagnostic catheter is in the same angiographic plane as the diseased segment of the proximal right coronary artery and the most normal segment of the proximal right coronary artery. The catheter is 6 French or external diameter of 2 mm. The most normal portion of the proximal right coronary appears to be about 1.5 times as large as the catheter. Calculation of the vessel's size is the ratio of vessel to catheter times catheter conversion in mm. Thus the size of the proximal right coronary is about 1.5 x 2 mm = 3 mm. *B,* Note that the long 3-mm balloon is positioned using the curve in the artery and the distance from the guide tip as landmarks. Comparison of the lesion length to the catheter diameter can also help to estimate the length of vessel requiring treatment. *C,* The inflated 3.0-mm balloon in this image confirms the validity of the method. Note that the inflated balloon appears to be about 1.5 times the external diameter of the 6 French guide catheter. *D,* This postdilatation image shows the good angiographic result obtained by this method of device sizing.

Principles of Interventional Cardiology

Gregory W. Barsness, MD

Joseph G. Murphy, MD

This chapter reviews the principles of interventional cardiology including the indications for percutaneous revascularization (PCI), risk stratification of PCI patients, and complications associated with PCI. Separate chapters are devoted to diagnostic coronary angiography, coronary physiology, coronary stents, endomyocardial biopsy, PCI in acute myocardial infarction, cardiogenic shock, high-risk PCI and PCI in bypass grafts.

Indications for Revascularization in Chronic Coronary Artery Disease

The primary indication for percutaneous coronary revascularization is to improve symptoms of coronary artery disease—angina or an anginal equivalent, or, if the patient is truly asymptomatic, to treat a coronary stenosis associated with objective evidence of myocardial ischemia on myocardial imaging. In addition, there should be a high probability of technical success with PCI, within an acceptable complication range. The coronary lesion(s) dilated should be the culprit lesion(s) generating the anginal symptoms and/or myocardial ischemia either directly, in the stenosed artery itself, or indirectly via collateral vessels to another artery. The short- and long-term risk and benefit associated with PCI should be favorable compared with alternative

management strategies, including coronary bypass surgery or pharmacological therapy.

Survival Benefit With Coronary Revascularization

Coronary surgery data has established that coronary revascularization confers a survival benefit over medical therapy in several situations (Table 1).

Coronary revascularization provides no significant survival benefit compared to medical therapy in patients with one- or two-vessel coronary artery disease (absent

---

Table 1.   Coronary Lesions Proven to Have Survival Benefit With Coronary Revascularization

1. Left main coronary stenosis (>50%),
2. Proximal left anterior descending (LAD) coronary artery stenosis (>75%)
3. Nonproximal LAD multivessel coronary disease (>75% in three or more coronary arteries of significant caliber), particularly when associated with left ventricular dysfunction

left main or proximal LAD stenoses or ischemic left ventricular dysfunction). Paradoxically, coronary revascularization does not significantly reduce the risk of late myocardial infarction in patients with coronary artery disease.

The survival advantage conferred by coronary revascularization diminishes over time due to saphenous vein graft occlusion (50%-60% saphenous graft patency at 10 years) and the development of new stenoses in other coronary vessels. In approximate terms the late cardiac mortality after CABG is about 1 percent per year in patients with mammary grafts and 2.0 percent per year in patients with only saphenous vein grafts—a reflection of the superior patency of internal mammary artery grafts, particularly a LIMA graft to the LAD (>95% patency at 10 years) and RIMA graft patency of about 80% at 10 years. Internal mammary graft failure is generally related to a surgical technical problem (poor distal anastomosis or graft kinking) or intense competitive flow between the native coronary artery and mammary graft rather than late atherosclerosis, as is the case with saphenous vein graft occlusions.

A major extrapolation of early CABG versus PTCA revascularization trials to current PCI practice are the multiple pharmacological and technical PCI innovations, particularly drug-eluting stents that have dramatically lowered the coronary restenosis rate following PCI. In early PTCA versus CABG trials, the principal differentiating advantage of CABG over PTCA was the much lower rate of late target vessel revascularization associated with CABG, due primarily to the high coronary restenosis rate in the PTCA-treated patients. Drug-eluting stents have reduced late restenosis to less than 10%, making PCI the preferred initial approach to coronary revascularization for most patients with obstructive coronary artery disease.

Indications for Percutaneous Coronary Revascularization (PCI)

The leading indication for PCI, independent of whether the patient has anginal symptoms or not, is a large territory of myocardial ischemia due to one or two culprit lesions, deemed technically suitable for PCI in a patient without diabetes mellitus. Patients with and without diabetes mellitus who have one or more coronary lesions that result in a moderate area of

myocardial ischemia should also be considered for PCI. Percutaneous coronary revascularization is indicated for the treatment of moderate to severe anginal symptoms not controlled with medical therapy in patients with anatomic features that place them at increased procedural risk, including vein graft lesions, multivessel disease in patients with diabetes mellitus, and patients with significant left ventricular dysfunction (Tables 2 and 3).

SINGLE-VESSEL CORONARY REVASCULARIZATION

Percutaneous coronary revascularization is a good treatment strategy for most symptomatic patients with

---

Table 2.   Indications for PCI in Patients with Chronic Angina or Asymptomatic Myocardial Ischemia

Class 1
  Nondiabetic patients with one or more hemodynamically significant coronary lesions in one or more coronary arteries suitable for PCI with high likelihood of success and low procedural risk; vessels should subtend a large area of viable myocardium

Class IIa
  Same as class I except the myocardial area at risk is of moderate size or the patient has treated diabetes

Class IIb
  Three or more coronary arteries suitable for PCI with high likelihood of success and low risk; vessels subtend at least moderate area of viable myocardium with evidence of myocardial ischemia

Class III
  Small area of myocardium at risk, absence of ischemia, low likelihood of PCI success, absence of symptoms of ischemia, increased PCI risk, left main stenosis <50%

Table 3.   Indications for PCI in Patients With Unstable Angina

Class I indication for PCI in unstable angina

An early invasive PCI strategy is strongly indicated for patients with unstable angina and coronary lesions amenable to PCI who have no serious comorbidity but who have any of the following high-risk clinical features
    a. Recurrent ischemia despite intensive antiischemic therapy
    b. Elevated troponin level
    c. New ST-segment depression
    d. Heart failure (HF) symptoms or new or worsening mitral regurgitation
    e. Depressed LV systolic function
    f. Hemodynamic instability
    g. Sustained ventricular tachycardia
    h. PCI within 6 months
    i. Prior CABG

Class IIa indication for PCI in unstable angina

PCI should also be considered in patients with unstable angina and single-vessel or multivessel CAD who are undergoing medical therapy with focal saphenous vein graft lesions or multiple stenoses who are poor candidates for repeat CABG. In the absence of high-risk features associated with unstable angina, it is reasonable to perform PCI in patients with amenable lesions and no contraindication for PCI with either an early invasive or early conservative strategy. PCI is considered reasonable in patients with unstable angina and significant left main CAD (greater than 50% diameter stenosis) who are candidates for revascularization but are not eligible for CABG.

Class IIb indication for PCI in unstable angina

In the absence of high-risk features associated with unstable angina, PCI may be considered in patients with single-vessel or multivessel CAD who are undergoing medical therapy and who have 1 or more lesions to be dilated with reduced likelihood of success.

PCI may be indicated in patients with unstable angina who are undergoing medical therapy who have 2- or 3-vessel disease, significant proximal LAD stenosis and treated diabetes or abnormal left ventricular (LV) function.

PCI is not indicated for patients with unstable angina who have only a small area of myocardium at risk or have a culprit lesion with a morphology that conveys a low likelihood of procedural success. PCI is also not indicated in patients with insignificant coronary disease (less than 50% coronary stenosis) or patients with significant left main coronary stenosis who are candidates for CABG or patients otherwise considered to be at high risk of procedure-related morbidity or mortality.

single-vessel coronary disease who have technically suitable coronary anatomy. There is no convincing evidence that patients with single-vessel coronary artery disease (left main or proximal LAD stenosis excepted) have improved survival with coronary revascularization (PCI or CABG) compared with conventional medical therapy, but symptoms and quality of life improve with revascularization.

ACME Trial

The ACME trial compared PTCA with medical therapy in patients with single-vessel coronary disease who had exercise-induced myocardial ischemia. ACME demonstrated an improved quality of life in PTCA patients with reduced angina and improved exercise performance at least out to 3 years. It should be noted that the ACME study was performed prior to the era of coronary stents and by current standards had a relatively high number of acute complications in the PTCA arm (2 percent emergency CABG, 1 percent Q-wave MI) (Fig. 1).

Left Main Coronary Artery (LMCA) Disease

Left main coronary artery stenosis (>50%) is associated with significant patient mortality (~30% two-year mortality with medical management) probably because of the very large area of left ventricular myocardium at risk (~70% of the LV). There is an even higher risk in patients with stenosis ≥75 percent or left ventricular failure. Coronary artery bypass graft surgery is the treatment of choice for patients with left main disease. Surgical revascularization has been demonstrated to improve both symptoms and survival compared to medical therapy alone. Left main PCI is generally limited to patients who decline CABG, are inoperable or at very high risk with CABG, or have "protected" left main disease with a patent CABG graft to either the left anterior descending or circumflex artery from prior CABG surgery.

Indeterminate Left Main Coronary Artery Disease

Patients with indeterminate left main coronary disease at coronary angiography should have intracoronary ultrasonography (ICUS) performed to guide revascularization. In a Mayo study of 121 patients, the lower range of normal left main minimum luminal area (MLA) was 7.5 mm². Surgical revascularization was performed on patients below this cutoff value and medium-term follow-up at a mean 3.3 years showed no significant difference in major adverse cardiac events (target vessel revascularization, acute myocardial infarction, and death) between patients with an MLA <7.5 mm² who underwent revascularization and those with an MLA ≥7.5 mm² deferred from revascularization. Deferring surgical revascularization for patients with a

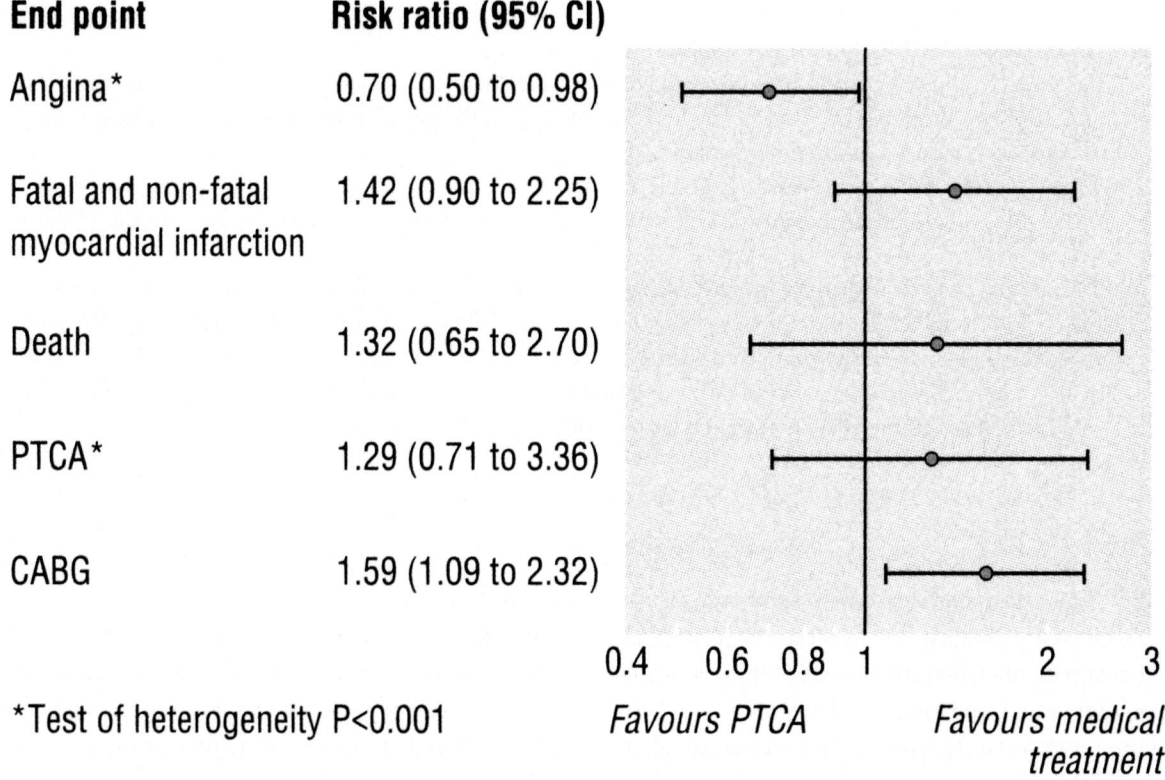

End point	Risk ratio (95% CI)
Angina*	0.70 (0.50 to 0.98)
Fatal and non-fatal myocardial infarction	1.42 (0.90 to 2.25)
Death	1.32 (0.65 to 2.70)
PTCA*	1.29 (0.71 to 3.36)
CABG	1.59 (1.09 to 2.32)

*Test of heterogeneity P<0.001

Favours PTCA   Favours medical treatment

Fig. 1. Adverse event risk ratios with 95% confidence intervals after percutaneous transluminal coronary angioplasty (PTCA) compared with medical therapy in a meta-analysis of 6 trials involving 1,904 patients.

minimum left main lumen area ≥7.5 mm^2 appears to be safe.

Proximal Left Anterior Descending (LAD) Coronary Artery Disease

Critical stenosis of the proximal LAD artery (≥75 percent stenosis) is associated with considerable excess long term mortality, the so-called "widow maker artery" and requires revascularization. Analogous to left main coronary disease, proximal LAD stenosis places a large area of the left ventricular myocardium at risk (~50% of the LV), may precipitate ischemia of the ventricular conduction fibers, and often is associated with left ventricular dysfunction and clinical heart failure. Surgical revascularization of the LAD territory, particularly with a left internal mammary artery graft, improves survival compared to medical therapy alone, particularly if the LAD stenosis is associated with flow-limiting disease in other major coronary vessels or left ventricular dysfunction. Percutaneous coronary intervention of the proximal LAD with stenting appears to offer comparable benefits to CABG at least in the medium term. Technical considerations with PCI include proximity of the lesion to the left main coronary artery and ostia of the left circumflex, or, if anatomically present, a large ramus intermedius vessel, together with the extent of plaque encroachment, if any, on large diagonal and septal branches. Coronary artery bypass grafting with a left internal mammary graft to the LAD is still a good option for patients with complex proximal LAD lesions.

Right Coronary Artery (RCA) Disease

The right coronary artery is dominant in about 85% of patients and typically perfuses about 25% of the left ventricle as well as the right ventricle. In addition, it supplies the artery to the SA node and an AV nodal artery. Compared to the left ventricle, the right ventricle has smaller muscle mass, lower oxygen demand per gram of myocardium, and a lower end-diastolic pressure which facilitates myocardial perfusion (myocardial perfusion pressure = mean coronary perfusion pressure minus ventricular end-diastolic pressure). Right ventricular infarction is generally associated with proximal RCA occlusion or, more rarely, occlusion of a distal "wrap-around" anatomic type LAD or a left dominant circumflex coronary artery. Reperfusion of an occluded RCA may be associated with a profound Bezold-Jarisch reflex with a fall in blood pressure and heart rate slowing that generally responds well to phenylephrine.

Left Circumflex Coronary Artery Disease

The left circumflex coronary artery is dominant in about 15% of patients and can, in selected patients, supply up to 30%-40% of the left ventricular myocardium.

MULTIVESSEL CORONARY REVASCULARIZATION

Extrapolation from the CABG experience suggests that complete myocardial revascularization of all major ischemic territories is important for symptom relief and produces better long-term survival results. The risks of PCI are increased in patients with multivessel disease, which is also a clinical marker for diabetes mellitus, advanced age, renal dysfunction, and poor left ventricular function and heart failure (Tables 4 and 5).

Trials of CABG Versus PCI

RITA Trial

The Randomized Intervention Treatment of Angina (RITA) trial was an early trial of PTCA versus CABG from the United Kingdom in patients with one-, two-, or three-vessel coronary disease with anatomy judged suitable for revascularization by either strategy. Long-term survival and nonfatal infarction rates were similar for PTCA or CABG, while recurrent angina and repeat revascularization were more common in the PTCA arm.

GABI Trial

The German Angioplasty Bypass Surgery Investigation (GABI) compared PTCA and CABG in patients with significant stenoses in at least two coronary vessels with anatomy judged suitable for complete revascularization by either strategy. The GABI investigators concluded that both bypass surgery and angioplasty were equally effective in relieving angina at one year with similar Q wave myocardial infarction rates, but while CABG was associated with higher operative risks than PTCA, CABG patients had a much lower need for repeat intervention. The GABI and RITA trials were performed prior to era of modern PCI with stenting.

Table 4.   Patients with Multivessel Disease in Whom CABG is Generally Preferred Over PCI

- Diffuse multivessel disease with poor targets for stenting
- High-risk patient with poor ventricular function
- Unprotected left main coronary disease
- Patients in whom complete revascularization cannot be accomplished by PCI
- Patients requiring additional heart valve surgery
- Patients with a large amount of myocardium at risk due to triple-vessel disease
- Complex two-vessel disease with significant involvement of the proximal LAD and another major vessel: LAD disease is considered complex if there is ostial LAD disease—generally considered to mean within 3 mm of the left main coronary artery or there is ostial circumflex involvement or the plaque encroaches on a large-caliber diagonal vessel
- Diabetic patients with diffuse multivessel disease

Table 5.   Patients With Multivessel Disease in Whom PCI is Generally Preferred Over CABG

- Focal coronary stenosis in nondiabetic patient with well-preserved left ventricular function (*ideal patient*)
- Focal stenoses in native coronary arteries or in saphenous vein grafts in patients with previous surgical revascularization, particularly in patients with a patent mammary artery graft to the LAD (*increased risk of repeat coronary surgery and risk of LIMA damage with reoperation*)
- Younger patients who will likely need surgical revascularization later in life due to progression of coronary disease (*keep surgical option open*)
- Very elderly and frail patients (*high risk with CABG*)
- Patients with significant comorbidity (e.g., *renal failure on dialysis*)
- Patients with prohibitively high surgical risks (*high risk with CABG*)
- Patients with short life expectancies.(e.g., *metastatic carcinoma*)
- Patients who refuse surgery (*patient choice*)
- Patients who require urgent non cardiac surgery (e.g., *carcinoma of colon*)—Bare metal stenting preferred over drug-eluting stents
- Patients with prior stroke or neurological damage (*risk of further neurological deficit with bypass surgery*)

EAST Trial

The Emory Angioplasty Versus Surgery Trial (EAST) was a single-center study (Emory University) of patients with multivessel coronary disease. Overall, surgery provided more complete revascularization and patients treated with CABG required less revascularization procedures. At the three-year follow-up point both PTCA and CABG groups had a similar rate of the combined end point (mortality, Q-wave MI, or large thallium perfusion defect). While both treatment groups had similar left ventricular function at three years, more patients assigned to PTCA had angina at follow-up. On late follow-up at eight years, two subgroups had a non-statistically significant trend for improved survival—patients with LAD stenosis and diabetics.

CABRI Trial

Coronary Angioplasty Versus Bypass Revascularization Investigation (CABRI) was a large European study that compared CABG to PTCA in over 1,100 patients with multivessel disease and found a similar one-year mortality rate in both groups. PTCA patients required more repeat procedures and had a higher incidence of recurrent angina due both to post PTCA restenosis and a higher likelihood of residual disease after PTCA compared with CABG.

BARI Trial

The Bypass Angioplasty Revascularization Investigation compared CABG versus PTCA in symptomatic patients with two- or three-vessel coronary disease and anatomy suitable for revascularization by either strategy. In nondiabetic patients there was no difference in survival, myocardial infarction or ventricular function at 5-year follow-up between PTCA and CABG patients. This equivalence of PTCA and CABG on cardiac mortality in nondiabetic patients was seen regardless of symptoms, left ventricular function, number of diseased vessels, or stenotic proximal left anterior descending artery. The BARI study was performed prior to the introduction of drug-eluting stents and the CABG patients had more complete revascularization, greater improvement in anginal symptoms, and fewer subsequent revascularization procedures than the PTCA arm almost certainly reflective of restenosis in the PTCA arm.

Diabetic patients overall had better survival with CABG particularly in high-risk insulin-dependent diabetics with diffuse coronary artery disease and left ventricular dysfunction who received internal mammary artery grafts to the LAD at the time of CABG.

New York Registry Study

This very large nonrandomized registry study evaluated approximately 59,000 patients from New York's two cardiac registries, the Cardiac Surgery Reporting System (CSRS) and the Percutaneous Coronary Intervention Reporting System (PCIRS) with multivessel disease who underwent either CABG or bare metal stenting. In patients with two or more diseased coronary arteries, CABG is associated with higher adjusted rates of long-term survival than stenting. A caveat of this study is that it did not include drug-eluting stents and was observational, rather than a randomized, controlled trial.

Bare Metal Stenting Versus CABG for Multivessel Disease

ARTS I Trial

The Arterial Revascularization Therapies Study was a large European study that randomized patients with multivessel disease to bare metal stenting or CABG. At five years there was no overall difference in mortality or the rate of the combined end point of death, myocardial infarction, or stroke between the groups. The incidence of repeat revascularization was significantly higher in the stent group (30.3%) than in the CABG group (8.8%; P<0.001).

An important finding was that diabetics had a five-year mortality of 13.4% in the stent group compared with 8.3% in the CABG group (P=0.27). Repeat revascularizations were also more common in diabetics.

ARTS II Registry

The ARTS II registry was a nonrandomized comparison of drug-eluting stents (sirolimus) in 607 patients with multivessel coronary artery disease matched to the outcomes previously noted in the ARTS I Trial (bare metal stents or CABG). The primary end point was a combination of major adverse cardiac and cerebrovascular events (MACCE).

At one year, the rate of MACCE in ARTS II was similar to the CABG arm in ARTS I and significantly lower than in the PCI with bare metal stent arm in ARTS I—10.4% (DES) and 11.6% (CABG) versus 26.5 percent (bare metal stents) respectively. Repeat revascularization was lowest following CABG (4.1%), greatest with bare metal stenting (21.3%), and intermediate with DES (8.5%) respectively.

Mechanism of Percutaneous Coronary Intervention (PCI)

The mechanism by which PCI improves coronary blood flow is complex and includes two primary pathophysiologic mechanisms, namely fracture of the atheromatous plaque that creates a localized intramural coronary arterial wall dissection and stretching of the nonatheromatous elements of the arterial wall. Other mechanisms of PTCA considered less important include plaque compression and stretching without fracture of the underlying atheromatous plaque.

Complications of Coronary Intervention

Technical improvements have increased the rates of procedural success with PCI over the past 3 decades from approximately 60% to greater than 95%. During the same period, emergency CABG rates following PCI have decreased markedly to about 0.3%, while in-hospital mortality is less than 1%. Asymptomatic small cardiac enzyme elevations occur in about 30% of patients and are of unproven long-term clinical significance. Abrupt vessel closure after PCI may be due to arterial wall dissection, in situ thrombus formation, no reflow (or slow reflow), or distal embolization.

Abrupt Vessel Closure

Abrupt vessel closure is loss of patency of the dilated lesion during or shortly after PCI and is usually due to acute spasm, arterial wall dissection, or thrombosis in situ at the PCI site. Distal embolism, particularly in degenerated saphenous vein grafts, and microembolism after rotational atherectomy are other causes of abrupt vessel closure.

Historically, the incidence of abrupt vessel closure after PTCA was typically about 5% and was a major cause of mortality or myocardial infarction. Coronary stents have dramatically reduced the incidence of abrupt vessel closure due to arterial dissections, but acute or subacute stent thrombosis still occurs in about 1% of patients with equal frequency following bare metal and drug-eluting stent placement, being somewhat more likely in arteries of small caliber and diffusely diseased vessels and strikingly more common in patients not receiving dual antiplatelet therapy (aspirin and clopidogrel).

Predictors of death following abrupt vessel closure after PCI are poor ventricular function, a history of heart failure or unstable angina, advanced age, and a large area of myocardium at risk, including a large amount of myocardium collateralized from the target vessel to another coronary territory.

RISK STRATIFICATION AND PCI

Patient risk models have been developed to identify patients at risk for mortality and major complications after PCI with stenting. The Mayo Clinic predictive point score model is based upon eight clinical and angiographic variables combined to give a total numerical score. Major complications were defined as in-hospital mortality, ST elevation MI, urgent or emergent CABG, and stroke. Other complications such as non-ST elevation MI and vascular access site problems were not included in this model. Most patients had a score between 0 and 25 and the score approximates the risk of complications as shown in Table 6 and Figure 2.

RESTENOSIS FOLLOWING PCI

Restenosis following PTCA develops in about 20% to 40% of patients, most of whom (about 50%-70%) have recurrent angina. Thus the requirement for late target lesion revascularization in most PTCA trials was about 25%. Bare metal stenting reduced the restenosis rate to about 25% with a target lesion revascularization rate of about 15%. Current-generation drug-eluting stents have reduced the overall restenosis rate to less than 10% with a target revascularization rate in single digits.

Several unique features distinguish coronary restenosis from progression of native atherosclerotic coronary disease. These include the time course for clinical restenosis (usually within 6 months of the original procedure), the rare occurrence of myocardial infarction with restenosis lesions, and the lack of a strong association between restenosis and the established risk factors for atherosclerosis.

Histological examination of atherectomy specimens from restenotic lesions has found smooth muscle cell proliferation and neointimal formation in over 95% of samples. In general, the greater the initial luminal gain by PCI, the greater the stimulus to late neointimal proliferation.

Coronary stents are described in detail in Chapter 124 "Coronary Stents."

Adjunctive Interventional Devices

There are a large number of niche interventional devices that were initially designed to debulk atherosclerotic lesions, optimize the results of PTCA and allow an interventional approach to lesions not considered optimal for PTCA (rotational atherectomy, cutting balloon angioplasty, directional atherectomy). Since the advent of modern coronary stenting, these devices are now typically used in <5% of coronary interventions. While most adjunctive interventional devices debulk atheromatous lesions and widen the vessel lumen, they also cause considerable vessel trauma that stimulates aggressive neointimal proliferation.

Table 6.   Risk Stratification and PCI

Very low risk 40% of patients	Score 0 to 5, risk 1% (range 0 to 2 %)
Low risk 39% of patients	Score 6 to 8, risk 3% (range >2% to 5%)
Moderate risk 15% of patients	Score 9 to 11, risk 6.2% (range >5% to 10%)
High risk 4% of patients	Score 12 to 14, risk 19.5% (range >10% to 25%)
Very high risk 2% of patients	Score 15, risk 35% (range >25%)

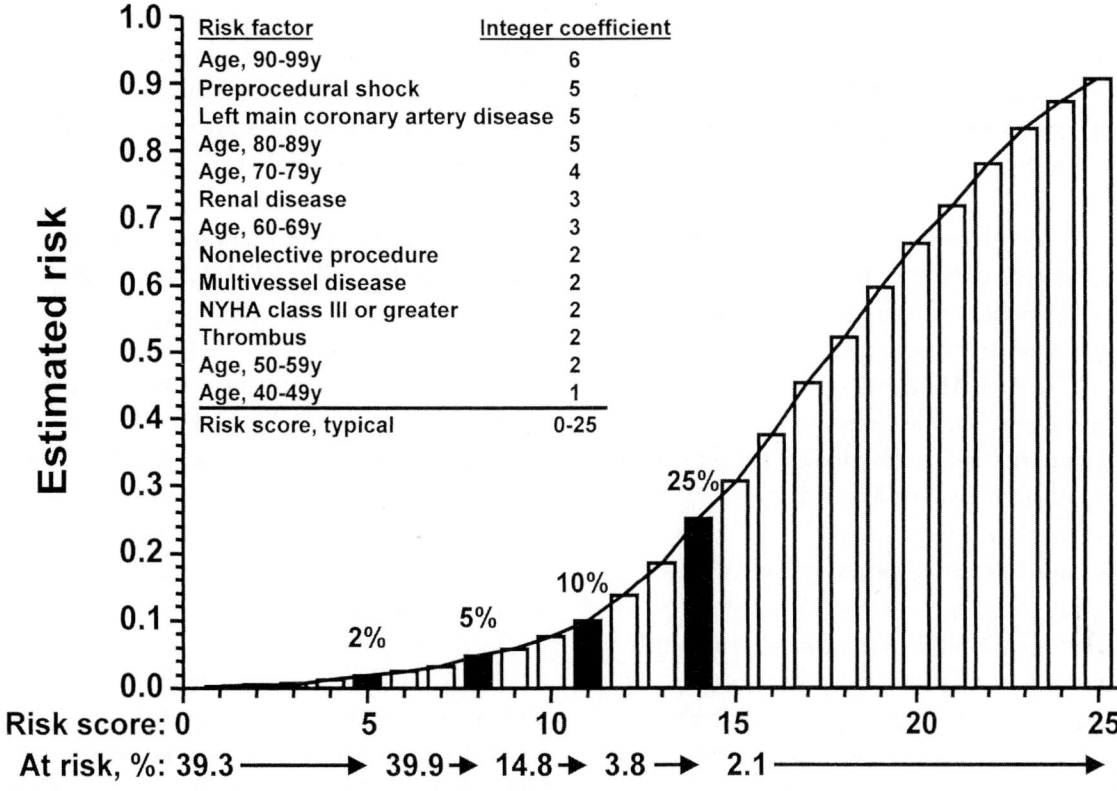

Risk factor	Integer coefficient
Age, 90-99y	6
Preprocedural shock	5
Left main coronary artery disease	5
Age, 80-89y	5
Age, 70-79y	4
Renal disease	3
Age, 60-69y	3
Nonelective procedure	2
Multivessel disease	2
NYHA class III or greater	2
Thrombus	2
Age, 50-59y	2
Age, 40-49y	1
Risk score, typical	0-25

Fig. 2. The Mayo Risk Model for procedural major adverse events.

ATHERECTOMY

Atherectomy is a catheter-based technique in which the atheromatous plaque is removed with interventional cutting devices. Three atherectomy devices are in clinical use.

Directional Coronary Atherectomy

Directional coronary atherectomy (DCA) was the first new interventional device approved by the FDA after PTCA. Directional atherectomy consists of a tiny cylinder atop a catheter which passes over a guidewire down the coronary artery. Conceptually the device is attractive in that it allows atheromatous plaque to prolapse through a window in the cylinder head and to be cut using a contained tiny circular cutting blade, trapping the excised tissue within the cylinder head, which is then removed from the patient completely. The downside is the considerable arterial wall injury and resultant stimulus to neointimal proliferation that result. Atherectomy has been studied in several early large randomized trials (CAVEAT-1, CAVEAT-2,

CCAT, and BOAT) and some more recent trials (DESIRE, AMIGO, ADAPTS, SOLD, ABACAS, OARS).

CAVEAT-1 Trial

The CAVEAT-1 Trial (Coronary Angioplasty Versus Excisional Angioplasty Trial-1) compared DCA with PTCA in de novo native coronary stenoses. DCA was associated with a better initial angiographic result, but an approximate doubling of the procedural complication rate (5% [PTCA] to 11% [DCA] for the combined end point of death, myocardial infarction, or CABG. This excess mortality associated with DCA was still present 1 year postprocedure.

CAVEAT-2 Trial

The CAVEAT-2 Trial (Coronary Angioplasty Versus Excisional Angioplasty Trial-2) and CCAT (Canadian Coronary Atherectomy Trial) found no significant benefit for DCA over PTCA in saphenous vein graft or proximal LAD lesions, respectively.

BOAT Trial

The Balloon Versus Optimal Atherectomy Trial (BOAT) randomized 89 patients to PTCA or DCA. The major complication rate was low with DCA (no death, 2% Q-wave MI, 1% emergency CABG, and 1.4% perforation), with an angiographic restenosis rate of 31% at 7 months compared to 40% in the PTCA arm. At one year, there was no significant difference between PTCA and DCA in major clinical events.

The later atherectomy trials (DESIRE, AMIGO, ADAPTS, SOLD, ABACAS, OARS) showed some improvement in complications in comparison with older atherectomy trails but insufficient benefit to justify routine atherectomy prior to stenting.

- Directional coronary atherectomy showed no statistically significant sustained benefit compared with PTCA in randomized trials performed in either native-vessel or saphenous vein graft disease.
- Directional coronary atherectomy, while generally associated with a better initial angiographic results, does not reduce the restenosis rate compared to PTCA and was associated with more myocardial infarcts at 30 days and major adverse cardiac events at one year.
- DCA currently is occasionally used by some experienced operators in highly selected cases in large coronary vessels (≥3.0 mm) with severely eccentric atheromatous plaques particularly proximal located bifurcation lesions or in-stent restenosis lesions prior to further stenting.
- In the rare cases where DCA is used, it should be used in conjunction with intravascular ultrasound to determine plaque volume and location, which guide DCA use.
- No randomized trials to date have directly compared directional coronary atherectomy with drug eluting stents.

Rotational and Cutting Balloon Atherectomy

Rotational atherectomy utilizes a diamond-studded burr spinning at very high speed (160,000-180,000 revolutions per minute) to selectively abrade the calcified, atheromatous plaque. It is effective in opening many arterial lesions not amenable to conventional PTCA techniques, such as heavily calcified lesions and diffusely diseased vessels, by selectively abrading the relatively more rigid tissues within the arterial wall (calcium and atheromatous plaque), with relative sparing of the normal elastic arterial wall constituents (differential cutting phenomenon). In theory, the abraded arterial wall elements are pulverized to particles less than 10 μm in diameter that should pass through the microcirculation unhindered. In practice, microembolization may lead to no reflow with myocardial infarction or slow reflow (TIMI 2 flow) with regional wall hypokinesis.

- Rotational atherectomy is contraindicated in the presence of intraluminal thrombus or in lesions likely to contain thrombus, such as ulcerated lesions associated with unstable angina or vein graft lesions
- Rotational atherectomy is contraindicated in patients with a preexisting coronary dissection, such as after PTCA with complications.

Rotablator is frequently used is situations where PTCA has failed to open the coronary stenosis due to an inability to either cross or dilate the lesions with the PTCA balloon, although it should not be used if there is any angiographic evidence of dissection. Eccentric lesions can be treated, provided great care is used to ensure the guidewire is coaxial with the vessel lumen (minimize guidewire bias), thus minimizing the risk of vessel perforation.

- The luminal area produced by rotational atherectomy is usually larger greater than the burr size used.
- Rotational atherectomy does not decrease coronary restenosis rates compared to PTCA but the debulking effect on complex calcified lesions makes it a valuable adjunctive tool.
- Rotational atherectomy is generally followed by stent implantation.

COBRA Trial

The COBRA Trial (Comparison of Balloon Angioplasty Versus Rotational Atherectomy) compared PTCA versus rotational atherectomy in just over 500 patients with complex coronary lesions and found no differences in the short- or long-term clinical or angiographic results between these PCI techniques. The trial was performed without stents and the restenosis rate was very high by current standards at approximately 50% in both groups.

■ Rotational atherectomy is associated with unique complications, including slow coronary flow and no coronary reflow phenomenon, arterial wall dissection and perforation, guidewire fracture, burr stall, and, rarely, burr detachment.

Cutting balloon atherectomy is a technique useful in bulky, fibrotic, and ostial or bifurcation lesions. The cutting balloon, handled and delivered in a manner similar to standard balloon catheters, has small cutting microtomes adherent to the surface to "score" lesions as a stand-alone procedure or, more commonly, to facilitate passage of additional devices such as a stent.

■ Rotational atherectomy is valuable for heavily calcified lesions or long, diffusely diseased vessels.
■ Rotational atherectomy provides no restenosis benefit over balloon angioplasty alone.
■ Regional wall hypokinesis after rotational atherectomy use may be due to the slow reflow phenomenon due to microemboli.

HIGH-RISK PERCUTANEOUS CORONARY INTERVENTIONS

Gregory W. Barsness, MD

PERCUTANEOUS CORONARY INTERVENTIONS (PCI) IN SAPHENOUS VEIN GRAFTS

■ Coronary artery saphenous vein bypass grafts have limited long-term longevity. In the first month after coronary revascularization, about 10 percent of vein graft bypass conduits fail due to graft thrombosis secondary to low blood flow often associated with poor distal vessel run-off or competitive blood flow between native coronary artery and graft or due to technical surgical problems such as graft kinking or poor surgical anastomosis. Saphenous vein grafts to the left anterior descending coronary artery have better long-term patency compared to other coronary vessels, as do grafts to native coronary arteries greater than 2.0 mm in diameter.

Sapheous vein graft patency at one week after surgery	90%
1 year after surgery	80%
10 years after surgery	50%

Late saphenous vein occlusion pathologically is characterized by friable, necrotic "gruel" which is a combination of intimal hyperplasia, lipid deposition, cholesterol crystals, foam cells, thrombus and atherosclerotic plaque. Late saphenous vein occlusion increases with years after bypass surgery; poor lipid control including both low HDL concentration, high LDL concentration and high triglyceride levels; left ventricular dysfunction; male sex; and active smoking.

Vein graft failure may lead to recurrent ischemic symptoms or may be asymptomatic in many patients. Repeat bypass surgery is complicated; a periprocedural myocardial infarction rate is 3-5 times that of the first operation, and the operative mortality with second and third bypass procedures may approach 20% in some patients with poor left ventricular function. In addition, repeat coronary bypass grafting is associated with less complete anginal relief and reduced long-term graft patency rates compared to the initial surgery. Advanced age and additional comorbidities contribute to the added-risk nature of repeat bypass surgery. For patients with medically refractory ischemic symptoms related to graft failure, current AHA/ACC guidelines support repeat intervention. Implicit in these guidelines is consideration of a percutaneous intervention as an initial revascularization strategy, particularly in patients with non-LAD territory ischemia or a patent IMA graft (Tables 1 and 2).

Percutaneous vein graft interventions entail greater risk and universally poorer long-term outcome than native vessel interventions (Fig. 1). Much of the frustration regarding vein graft intervention relates to the underlying pathophysiology of the vein graft lesion,

Table 1.   AHA/ACC Guidelines for Coronary Angiography in Patients with Post-CABG Ischemia

Class I (conditions with evidence or general agreement supporting the usefulness and effectiveness of angiography)
  None
Class IIa (conditions with evidence/opinion in favor of the usefulness of angiography)
  Recurrent symptoms and ischemia within 12 months of coronary artery bypass grafting
  High-risk features by noninvasive testing (LVEF <35% at rest or exercise, high-risk treadmill score, extensive area or areas of ischemia by perfusion imaging or stress echocardiography) at any time postoperatively
  Recurrent symptoms after revascularization despite optimal medical management
Class IIb (conditions for which the usefulness of angiography is less well established)
  In patients without high-risk features on noninvasive testing
    1. Recurrent angina occurring more than 1 year postoperatively *or*
    2. No symptoms but deterioration in serial noninvasive tests
Class III (conditions in which angiography is considered, or has been proved to be, useless or possibly harmful)
  Symptoms in a postbypass patient who is not a candidate for repeat revascularization
  Routine angiography after coronary bypass, except in participation in an approved research protocol

which may result in distal embolization, a greater propensity for restenosis, and increased early mortality. While atherosclerotic vein graft plaques are histologically similar to those found in native vessels, at least qualitatively, there is significantly greater plaque mass and a propensity to greater lesion progression with vein graft disease. Experimental evidence suggests that platelet activation is augmented and nitric oxide production is diminished in degenerated vein graft lesions. Risk factors for distal embolization and poor procedural outcome include older graft age, presence of thrombus, and nonfocal lesions. A unique study involving the PercuSurge distal occlusion protection device in 24 degenerated vein graft targets demonstrated that balloon dilatation of degenerated saphenous vein grafts resulted in dislodgement of significant amounts of necrotic core material, foam cells, and cholesterol clefts. To a lesser extent, the aspirate retrieved after balloon dilatation included fibrin, fibrous caps, and a small amount of smooth muscle tissue. These debris elements, when allowed to flow into the distal coronary circulation tree after percutaneous intervention, can contribute to the high incidence of decreased myocardial perfusion, poor TIMI grade flow grade and distal embolization after saphenous vein graft lesion disruption.

Unfortunately, poor initial outcome is not the only problem with saphenous vein graft interventions. Restenosis occurs at rates in excess of that seen in native coronary arteries. Aorto-ostial lesions have the greatest risk of restenosis, with an estimated rate of 50%-80% after balloon angioplasty. Graft bodies have an approximately 50% restenosis rate, while about 40% of distal anastamosis lesions undergo restenosis after balloon angioplasty. Restenosis occurs more commonly in older vein grafts than in vein grafts in situ less than a year which is likely related to the underlying mechanism of the initial stenosis and frequent distal anastamotic lesion location in most early graft failures. The implications of this restenotic process in vein grafts is

Table 2.   ACC/AHA-ASIM Guidelines for Revascularization in Patients With Prior Coronary Bypass Grafting

Class IIa (conditions with evidence/opinion in favor of the effectiveness of revascularization)
  Repeat CABG for surgical candidates with multiple vein graft stenoses, particularly when jeopardizing the LAD distribution
  Percutaneous intervention may be appropriate for patients with focal vein graft lesions or in patients who are poor candidates for repeat CABG with multiple stenoses

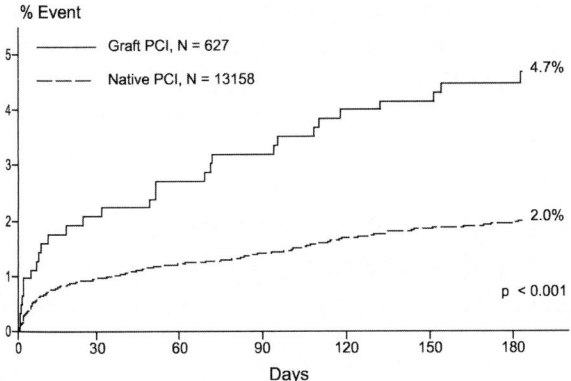

Fig. 1. Kaplan-Meier mortality after PCI in native coronary arteries compared with saphenous vein graft lesions in a pooled analysis from the EPIC, EPILOG, EPISTENT, IMPACTII and PURSUIT trials.

also potentially more significant than that occurring in native vessels, as a large percentage of restenotic vein graft lesions are associated with complete target vessel occlusion at follow-up angiography.

MEDICAL THERAPY VERSUS REPEAT REVASCULARIZATION

Early graft obstruction is generally related to technical problems associated with the surgical procedure and can generally be treated percutaneously with good results. Therefore, patients with signs or symptoms of early postoperative ischemia are generally best evaluated by coronary angiography with an intention of performing percutaneous coronary revascularization, if possible. While balloon dilation across recently placed anastomotic sutures appears safe in most series, care must be exercised to avoid oversizing the balloon. If a graft is thrombosed or if the patient has been incompletely revascularized, it is generally preferable to approach the native vessel percutaneously or consider early coronary reoperation.

For patients with recurrent ischemic symptoms due to saphenous vein graft disease occurring beyond the first postoperative year, there is little information comparing the outcome of patients treated medically with those undergoing repeat revascularization. In some studies, repeat revascularization has been associated with improved long-term outcome, although the

evidence for improved outcome with percutaneous intervention is largely correlative. A retrospective study by Lytle and colleagues of 1,117 patients with vein graft disease found a survival benefit to repeat surgical revascularization. After adjusting for baseline characteristics, there was a significant reduction in mortality associated with repeat surgical revascularization (P=0.0007), particularly among patients with stenotic grafts to the LAD distribution. Patients who are poor surgical candidates should be considered for angiography and percutaneous revascularization (Tables 1 and 2).

PCI VERSUS REPEAT CABG

For patients with older vein grafts affected by atherosclerotic progression, the decision to proceed with percutaneous versus repeat surgical revascularization needs to be individualized based on response to medical therapy, timing after surgery, anatomic suitability for a percutaneous approach, patient preference, and overall surgical risk. Several series have suggested comparable long-term results of percutaneous and surgical revascularization in patients with previous bypass surgery.

In determining the appropriate revascularization strategy for patients with recurrent symptoms after coronary artery bypass grafting, multiple issues must be considered. The patient's age, comorbid conditions, and clinical presentation affect the risks associated with surgical, as well as percutaneous revascularization. In addition, the survival advantage and improved long-term patency rates associated with patent IMA grafts to the LAD necessitate care with reexploration of the chest cavity. Therefore, a patent IMA graft to the LAD may be considered a reason to favor percutaneous intervention rather than repeat surgical revascularization. In addition, associated comorbid conditions may support an initial approach of PCI, as repeat bypass procedures may carry a risk of procedural mortality exceeding 20%. If native vessels are involved and are amenable to PCI, this is often considered a first choice for reintervention.

BALLOON ANGIOPLASTY FOR SAPHENOUS VEIN GRAFT DISEASE

Stand-alone balloon angioplasty is an effective treatment for early anastomotic vein graft stenoses. Balloon angioplasty is plagued by high rates of procedural complications and restenosis when applied to older, degenerated vein graft lesions. Controlled trials have confirmed an angiographic success rates of less than 90%, with major in-hospital cardiac events occurring in about 12% of patients and 6-month restenosis rates of nearly 50 percent (Table 3). Correlates of mortality after balloon angioplasty in patients with prior surgical revascularization include reduced left ventricular ejection fraction, history of heart failure, increased age, vein graft intervention (as opposed to native vessel revascularization in the same territory), older vein grafts, and diabetes mellitus.

ATHEROABLATIVE TECHNOLOGIES IN SAPHENOUS VEIN GRAFT DISEASE

While stand-alone balloon angioplasty of early anastomotic lesions remains a preferred choice, high rates of

Table 3. Contemporary Studies on Percutaneous Interventional Strategies for Saphenous Vein Graft Disease

Study	Year	Device	Patients (n)	Angiographic success (%)	Distal embolization (%)	In-hospital events[1] (%)	6-Month restenosis (%)
Bittl et al.	1994	ELCA	495	92	3.3	6.1	55[2]
Strauss et al.[3]	1995	ELCA	106	91	7.2	5.7	52
Second coronary angioplasty versus excisional atherectomy CAVEAT	1994	Balloon	156	79[5]	5.1[5]	12	51
II) Trial[3]		DCA	149	89[5]	13.4[5]	20	46
NACI registry[3]	1997	DCA	183	91	5.3	7.1[4]	--
William Beaumont Registry[3]	1994	TEC	146	84	11.3	7	69
US TEC Registry	1995	TEC	538	93	3.7	4.3	60[2]
NACI Registry[3]	1997	TEC	243	90	10	6.2	--
Braden et al.	1997	TEC + P-S stent	49	98	2	10	--
US Palmaz-Schatz Stent Registry	1995	P-S Stent	589	98.6	1.9	2.9	29.7[2]
Saphenous Vein De Novo	1997	Balloon	107	86[5]	--	11	46
(SAVED Trial		P-S Stent	108	97[5]	--	6	37
Wallstent CABG Study[3,6]	1997	Wallstent	109	98	--	5.5	--[7]

[1]Death, MI, repeat revascularization; [2]<70% angiographic follow-up; [3]angiographic core laboratory data; [4]includes in-lab abrupt closure; [5]statistically significant difference; [6]interim data only; [7]incomplete follow-up

DCA, directional coronary angioplasty; ELCA, excimer laser coronary angioplasty; NACI, new approaches to coronary intervention; P-S, Palmaz-Schatz; TEC, transluminal extraction-atherectomy catheter.

restenosis and inadequate procedural success rates have led to the evaluation of alternative treatment strategies for advanced vein graft disease. Reducing the total plaque volume through various atheroablative technologies, including Directional Coronary Atherectomy (DCA), transluminal extraction atherectomy (TEC), and excimer laser coronary angioplasty (ELCA) has been the target of considerable investigation. While born of theoretically sound principles, these technologies have not been shown to significantly reduce long-term morbidity or mortality after percutaneous vein graft interventions. The effect on immediate procedural outcomes has varied (Table 3).

STENTING FOR SVG STENOSIS

Elastic recoil after balloon dilation is a greater factor in older, degenerated vein grafts than in native coronary arteries. In addition, the friable cellular debris and thrombus associated with degenerated vein graft lesions is susceptible to distal embolization, a process theoretically modifiable by trapping or immobilizing this material against the conduit wall. These lesions are theoretically well suited for improved outcome after stent placement.

The Saphenous Vein De Novo (SAVED) Trial randomized 220 patients to angioplasty or Palmaz-Schatz stenting (Table 3). These patients all had "ideal" lesions in the body of the vein graft. While angiographic and procedural success were improved with stent use, angiographic restenosis at 6 months, the primary end point of the trial, was not significantly different between groups, occurring in 46% of patients undergoing angioplasty and in 37% of patients undergoing stenting. Stenting had a significantly beneficial effect on the composite end point of death, myocardial infarction, repeat bypass surgery, or repeat PCI of the target lesion (27% versus 42%). At the time of this trial, standard anticoagulation for stenting involved aspirin with dipyridamole and warfarin, which resulted in increased hemorrhagic complications in the stent group. Freedom from adverse outcome six months after the index procedure occurred in 58% of those undergoing angioplasty versus 73% of those in the stent group (P=0.03).

Despite the improved outcome associated with stent placement compared with balloon angioplasty for

lesions in the body of diseased vein grafts, similar data is lacking for other locations. Distal anastomotic lesions occurring early after surgery generally respond well to balloon dilation, with good early and late outcomes. Recent retrospective data suggests that stent placement likely has little impact in decreasing restenosis and target lesion revascularization compared with balloon angioplasty, and stent placement is therefore probably best relegated to a provisional, or bailout, role for distal anastomotic lesions. While the absence of observed benefit may be related to insufficient statistical power in a small, retrospective cohort, it is unlikely that the good results enjoyed after balloon angioplasty at the distal anastomotic site will be readily improved upon with existing technology.

Self-expanding stents, such as the Wallstent, have the potential to improve initial procedural outcome. The cross-hatched wire-mesh design may theoretically improve the restraint of friable graft material and decrease distal embolization. Strauss and colleagues reported an early experience with the first-generation Wallstent, which was limited by imperfect delivery techniques contributing to high rates of early occlusion and restenosis. More recent trials of the second-generation, "less-shortening" Wallstent have produced good initial results, with procedural success rates above 95% and in-hospital event rates of roughly 5 percent. The multicenter Wallstent CABG Study enrolled 109 high-risk patients with symptomatic venous graft disease. All but one patient had successful stent delivery, and postdilation was performed in 87% of cases. In-hospital events occurred in 5.5% of patients, including one death related to graft rupture with postdilation. The preliminary one-year event-free survival rate was 57.8%, including a 9% mortality rate and 22% repeat revascularization. Interim results of the Wallstent Endoprosthesis in Saphenous Vein Graft (WINS) Trial have also been reported and suggest good procedural results and 6-month outcome. While initial clinical results have been favorable, reported restenosis and target lesion revascularization rates have been variable, and the ultimate role of these stents remains to be established.

Drug-eluting stents appear to be superior to bare metal stents in saphenous vein grafts with a significant reduction in the incidence of saphenous vein graft restenosis and target vessel revascularization but no differences in mortality or myocardial infarction. Drug-eluting stents are most commonly used in relatively small caliber saphenous vein grafts.

MANAGING GRAFT THROMBUS AND PREVENTION OF DISTAL EMBOLIZATION

As the acute and long-term results of percutaneous revascularization involving saphenous vein graft conduits have improved and become more predictable with greater utilization of stents, the focus of efforts to improve procedural outcome have turned to the prevention of distal embolization. Distal embolization, the downstream shower of micro- and macroscopic particles, leads to reduced flow and myocardial ischemia. Angiographically apparent in about 10% of vein graft interventions, distal embolization probably occurs more commonly, as evidenced by significantly elevated post-procedural CK-MB levels in 15-17% of cases. Once it occurs, distal embolization cannot be reliably treated and is associated with dramatic increases in in-hospital and long-term morbidity and mortality. Distal embolization in the CAVEAT II trial was associated with a 71% in-hospital adverse event rate compared with 20% for patients without this complication (odds ratio=9.9) as well as a significantly increased 12-month event rate, and an analysis of the NACI TEC Registry demonstrated a significant increase in in-hospital mortality associated with this procedural event (20% versus 3%). Increased postprocedural CK-MB levels, a reflection of distal embolization, is a harbinger of poor long-term outcome even in patients with otherwise successful procedures and no additional in-hospital adverse events.

Preventive efforts have included both pharmacological and mechanical strategies to reduce and control preexisting thrombus and debris. The efficacy of pharmacological therapy is limited in the setting of the complex lesion composition commonly seen in degenerated vein graft disease, which includes not only fresh thrombus, but organized clot and cellular debris as well. Prolonged intra-graft thrombolytic infusions are reasonably effective in reducing large thrombus burdens and improving procedural outcome but have fallen out of favor due to incomplete benefit and a modest rate of associated mortality and hemorrhagic complications. Similarly, platelet glycoprotein IIb/IIIa inhibitors, while having clear benefit in native coronary interventions, have not proven as useful in saphenous vein graft interventions. Initial results from the EPIC trial sparked interest in the use of glycoprotein IIb/IIIa inhibitors in vein graft lesions. Distal embolization was seen in 21 of 29 saphenous vein graft cases when no abciximab was administered. There was a dose-dependent decrease in distal embolization with abciximab therapy. Unfortunately, the exuberance was tempered by later studies demonstrating no long-term benefit to this strategy. In a subsequent pooled analysis of the EPIC and EPILOG trials there was no difference in the combined adverse event rates among 87 patients treated with abciximab (10.4%) and 59 patients treated with placebo (11.9%). The failure of these agents to improve outcome in saphenous vein graft interventions likely relates to the underlying lesion pathology in degenerative vein graft lesions. Antiplatelet agents do not favorably affect the necrotic gruel and cholesterol deposits that are dislodged at the time of percutaneous intervention. In fact, the distal embolization and no reflow phenomena seen in saphenous vein graft lesions appear to be independent of platelet activity and may represent a further manifestation of vein graft pathology, such as the induction of severe distal arteriolar vasospasm.

A variety of mechanical devices to remove or isolate thrombus and debris from the coronary circulation have been under active investigation. A thrombectomy device, the Possis AngioJet, which utilizes the Venturi effect (hydrostatic suction) to remove intravascular debris and thrombus, was evaluated in the randomized VeGAS 2 trial comparing intracoronary urokinase to mechanical thrombectomy. Overall, this trial, which involved vein graft interventions in over 50% of the patients, demonstrated improved safety and efficacy with the use of thrombectomy, as well as decreased costs. While thrombectomy devices successfully remove thrombus and debris during vein graft interventions, improvement in procedural outcome is limited by incomplete prevention of distal embolization.

An alternative strategy to decrease distal embolization and improve procedural outcome involves prophylactic isolation of the treatment segment using a variety of filters or containment systems. The PercuSurge system employs a guidewire with an integrated distal, low-pressure entrapment balloon that is inflated in the vein graft beyond the segment of interest prior to lesion manipulation. This balloon traps debris released during vascular manipulation that is subsequently removed via a proximal aspiration catheter. Studies have confirmed the value of such an approach by demonstrating the large amount of debris recovered in association with each stage of a stenting procedure (predilation, stent placement, and postdilation. Additional devices for distal embolic protection, including braided nitinol "baskets" and a variety of porous "umbrella" filters .

OCCLUDED VEIN GRAFTS

Patients with occluded saphenous vein grafts represent a very high-risk cohort. Despite the axiom that it is impossible to make an occlusion worse, patients with an occluded vein graft but persistent native coronary flow (via collaterals or antegrade via a stenotic native vessel) can experience hemodynamic compromise and even death with no reflow phenomenon occurring after occluded graft procedural manipulation. It is therefore imperative to proceed with caution in such situations, including consideration of repeat surgical revascularization. A study of 77 consecutive patients with occluded vein grafts suggested the futility of such interventions using available percutaneous technologies, even if initially successful. The procedural success rate was only 71%. Thirty-day event rates included death in 5.2% of patients, Q-wave MI in 1.3% of patients, bypass in 7.8% of patients, and angiographically apparent distal embolization in 11.7% of patients, although CK elevation was noted in 43% of patients treated. There was no difference in the 3-year outcome among patients with successful versus unsuccessful initial procedures, with adverse events occurring in about 80% of patients in each group.

Thrombolysis is an alternative strategy in patients with recently occluded saphenous vein grafts. A prolonged urokinase infusion has been studied and modified by multiple investigators. Although recanalization success rates have been modest (70%-80%), complication rates are high, including in-hospital mortality approaching 7%, distal embolization rates of 17%, severe hemorrhage in >10%, and reocclusion rates greater than 50%. In addition, the prolonged hospitalization associated with the 12-30 hour thrombolytic infusion adds significantly to the overall procedural cost.

INTERNAL MAMMARY CONDUIT INTERVENTIONS

Internal mammary conduit interventions require special consideration. Unlike the high attrition rate of saphenous vein grafts, ten- and fifteen-year patency rates of approximately 90% at 7-10 years can be expected for internal mammary artery (IMA) conduits. True atherosclerotic disease of mammary arterial grafts is uncommon, but when it occurs, the histology of atherosclerotic lesions in arterial grafts is similar to native vessel disease. The thromoembolic, no-reflow phenomenon and high restenosis rates often associated with saphenous vein graft procedures are less frequent with IMA interventions, and the short- and long-term procedural results are generally good. However, procedural success varies with lesion location, age of mammary grafts, status of native vessels and procedural technical management issues. Additional considerations include graft caliber and tortuosity and total arterial distance to the lesion, which can often be significant.

Arterial access route and guide catheter selection is critical to procedural success with any of these lesion types, due to the fragile nature of these vessels and susceptibility to disruption. Choice of ipsilateral arm or femoral arterial access and guide catheter selection (most often Judkins right or IMA curves) should be based on a concern to minimizing catheter damping and ostial trauma while attaining adequate guide catheter seating and support. Six- or 7-French guides may allow adequate support and visualization of anatomy without significant damping, although side holes may be necessary. In general, short guides are preferable to provide optimal "reach" to the distal vessel, even for procedures involving the ostium, as distal vascular disruption may occur.

Mammary graft failure may result from a proximal subclavian lesion not appreciated prior to the coronary bypass procedure or a lesion that develops after surgery, atherosclerotic disease of the IMA ostium, or atherosclerotic or mechanical compromise of the IMA graft body. Atherosclerotic lesions can be treated with balloon angioplasty with procedural success rates of about 95% and restenosis rates of about 30%.

Mechanical compromise of the IMA graft is often the result of "kinks" anywhere along the course of the vessel from the point of detachment from the chest wall to the coronary insertion site. These lesions often respond poorly to balloon angioplasty. Stent placement may offer little advantage in highly tortuous segments, as stent delivery is often quite difficult and placement of the stent may simply "move" the lesion to a "hinge-point" on the proximal or distal stent edge.

Most early arterial graft failures are related to anastomotic failures and generally respond well to balloon dilatation with restenosis rates of only about 15%. Stent placement may facilitate optimal expansion of the lesion site and improve antegrade coronary flow.

SUPPORTED INTERVENTIONS

Most patients undergoing percutaneous intervention after coronary bypass surgery require no additional supportive measures. In some patients with severe ventricular dysfunction, however, mechanical support may be required, particularly if the intervention involves the patent's sole patent graft conduit (Table 4). Even in the setting of contemporary interventional techniques, left ventricular dysfunction is associated with increased procedural risk and impaired short- and long-term outcome. Registry data in high-risk patients with combined left ventricular ejection fractions <25%, multivessel coronary disease, and objectively proven myocardial ischemia highlight a high periprocedural event rate and suggest similar early attrition rates with percutaneous coronary interventional procedures or repeat coronary bypass grafting. The risk of hemodynamic collapse due to abrupt closure associated with failed percutaneous coronary angioplasty is related to the presence of multivessel disease, diffuse coronary disease, large areas of myocardial territory at risk, and pre-procedural stenosis severity. Various methods of predicting risk for poor outcome after percutaneous coronary intervention have included the jeopardy score, originally developed by Califf and colleagues, and modified by Ellis. As modified by Ellis, the total jeopardy score is defined as the net ventricular dysfunction anticipated following abrupt closure. This is calculated by allowing one point for each of the 6 myocardial regions (Table 5) in the distribution of a significant (70%) stenosis, and 0.5 points for each area of baseline hypokinesis not supplied through a significant stenosis. A jeopardy score of more than 2.5 is a predictor of patient mortality. The extent of myocardium at risk is of particular concern in the cases where the stenosed vessel supplies collateral circulation to other coronary territories, when the total jeopardized myocardial territory may be quite extensive.

As lesion complexity and the amount of myocardium at risk increases, the anticipated risk of serious adverse results increases. In such high-risk cases, particularly in patients with unstable coronary symptoms recalcitrant to medical therapy, percutaneous support devices, including intraaortic counterpulsation and percutaneous cardiopulmonary support, are essential components of the interventional plan. Assessment of myocardial viability and the extent of ischemic myocardium at risk is essential prior to coronary intervention in such patients. Appropriate assessment of viable and ischemic territories may include PET imaging, sestamibi myocardial perfusion studies, or stress echocardiographic techniques.

Intraaortic Balloon Pump (IABP)

Intraaortic balloon pumping decreases oxygen demand by reducing myocardial workload, providing pulsatile blood flow with an augmentation of cardiac output by 0.5 to 0.8 L/minute, and reducing left ventricular end diastolic pressure by about (10%-20%), with a similar reduction in pulmonary capillary wedge pressure. Although an IABP improves diastolic perfusion pressure and increases oxygen delivery in coronary artery segments without obstructive lesions, aortic counterpulsation has not been demonstrated to improve coronary blood flow past hemodynamically significant stenoses. The benefit of IABP may be more pronounced after coronary intervention, when obstructing lesions have been successfully modified and the resulting improvement in perfusion pressure is translated into an approximate 25% increase in total coronary flow. Prior to coronary intervention or after an unsuccessful intervention, IABP provides benefit primarily through afterload reduction and decreased myocardial oxygen consumption. Reports of elective IABP support in high-risk interventions have described a high procedural success rate and low short-term cardiovascular event rates. However, this success comes at the price of a vascular complication rate of up to 11%, as well as rare instances of gas leak into the arterial circulation, infection, thrombocytopenia, and thromboembolic events. Advantages of IABP use include ready availability; quick, easy insertion; and the availability of routine technical support. The device is contraindicated

Table 4. Support Characteristics

	IABP	pVAD	CPS
Percutaneous insertion	Yes, rapid	Yes	Yes, more difficult
Prophylactic use	Yes	Yes	Usually not
Pulsatile flow	Yes	No	No
Hemodynamic support	Minor (0.5-0.8 L/min)	Complete (≤4.0 L/min)	Complete (3.5-5.0 L-min)
Oxygenation support	No	No	Yes
Support independent of rhythm	No	Yes	Yes
Provides afterload reduction	Yes	No, ↓preload	Some
Augments distal coronary flow			
Past stenosis	No	No	No
Without stenosis	Yes	No	Minimal
Hemolysis	Mild	Intermediate	Significant
Anticoagulation requirements	Low	Intermediate*	High*
Maximal duration of therapy	>48 hours	Weeks	6-8 hours*
Indications	High-risk PCI	High-risk PCI	High-risk PCI*
	Bridge to surgery	Bridge to surgery	
	Refractory angina	Cardiogenic shock	
	Cardiogenic shock	Bridge to transplant or	
	Failure to wean CPS	LVAD	
	Bridge to transplant		
	or LVAD		
Contraindications	Significant AR	Lack of familiarity or	Lack of familiarity or
	Significant AA	technical support	technical support
	Severe PVD	Predominant RV failure	PVD
	Significant arrhythmia	Severe PVD	
Complications	Vascular	Vascular	Vascular
	Nerve injury	Nerve injury	Nerve injury
	Infection	Infection	Infection
	Hemolysis	Hemolysis	DIC, hemolysis
	Bleeding	Bleeding	Bleeding
	Thrombocytopenia	Cannula dislocation	Anemia
	Systemic embolism	May require surgical	Anaerobic metabolism
	Limb ischemia	vascular closure or	Poor CNS perfusion
		prolonged vessel	Fluid third-spacing
		compression	Hypokalemia
		Arterial and/or venous	Hypomagnesemia
		thrombosis	May require surgical
		CNS event	vascular closure or
		Limb ischemia	prolonged vessel
			compression
			Arterial and/or
			venous thrombosis
			Limb ischemia

*See text.

AA, aortic aneurysm; AR, aortic regurgitation; CNS, central nervous system; CPS, cardiopulmonary support system; DIC, disseminated intravascular hemolysis; IABP, intraaortic balloon pump; LVAD, left ventricular assist device; PCI, percutaneous coronary intervention; pVAD, percutaneous ventricular assist device; PVD, peripheral vascular disease.

Table 5. Six Coronary Segments Used to
          Determine the Myocardial Jeopardy
          Score

Coronary segment
    Left anterior descending artery (LAD)
        LAD (body)
        First major septal perforator
        First major diagonal branch
    Left circumflex coronary artery
        Left circumflex (body)
        Major marginal branch
        Left posterior descending (PDA)
    Right coronary artery
        Right PDA

in cases of severe aortoiliac disease or severe aortic
valvular regurgitation.

Percutaneous Cardiopulmonary Support

Percutaneous cardiopulmonary support (CPS) is used
in the extremely high-risk patient when hemodynamic
collapse during a coronary intervention is strongly
anticipated or when the result of such collapse, even if
temporary, would be catastrophic. Successful insertion
and use of CPS depends on team members trained in
the initiation of CPS. The attractiveness of CPS lies in
the fact that, unlike IABP, it provides complete circulatory support, regardless of the underlying rhythm or
left ventricular function. This system can maintain a
cardiac output of up to 5 L/min while unloading the
left ventricle and reducing the pulmonary wedge pressure to less than 5 mm Hg. This may reduce left ventricular workload and oxygen requirements. Additionally,
coronary perfusion may be secondarily improved due
to the reduced left ventricular end-diastolic pressure
and slightly increased diastolic perfusion pressure.
However, CPS offers poor myocardial protection from
prolonged ischemia and is not appropriate for prolonged use. Total bypass times of six to eight hours may
be well tolerated, but hemolysis, disseminated intravascular coagulation, and extracellular fluid shifts prevent
longer support times.

Because CPS initiation is a relatively rare occurrence
for most interventionalists, CPS is probably most helpful
as a planned procedure in very high-risk patients, such as
those undergoing intervention on a lone remaining
patent graft conduit; its standby use may not be reliable
in centers unaccustomed to performing the procedure.
True bailout hemodynamic support with CPS is usually not indicated, as patients who lack an organized cardiac rhythm and those without significant left ventricular function after a coronary intervention typically
have no clearly defined therapeutic end point, unless
imminent cardiac transplantation is a realistic possibility. In this case, CPS may be an appropriate bridge to
early placement of a left ventricular assist device.

MANAGING COMPLICATIONS OF SAPHENOUS VEIN GRAFT INTERVENSIONS

Perforation

Vein graft perforation or rupture, while rare with
stand-alone balloon angioplasty, may occur with
increasing frequency with the use of atheroablative
technologies and oversized balloons and stents.
Perforation may be particularly associated with TEC
and ELCA procedures (up to 2% of cases), and the
combination of perforation or significant dissection
may occur in as many as 35%-45% of these procedures.
In spite of the protective mediastinal scarring common
in postcoronary bypass patients, significant mediastinal
bleeding may still occur with a vein graft perforation,
possibly resulting in vessel occlusion and tamponade.
Initial treatment should be directed at reversing anticoagulation and normalizing coagulation parameters
together with local treatment at the site of perforation.
Prolonged perfusion balloon inflation may effectively
seal the rent, although provision for surgical exploration, and repair must be a consideration.

Abrupt Closure and No Reflow Phenomenon

Abrupt closure is infrequent in saphenous vein graft
interventions. Treatment is directed at the underlying
process, often severe vessel wall dissection or distal
embolization with attendant thrombosis. Perfusion balloon or stent placement may resolve the problem of
severe dissection, which is often associated with an
abrupt point of decreased or absent flow. Aggressive
platelet inhibition may also help alleviate the ongoing
propagation of thrombus. Care must be taken in the
case of severe dissection, as glycoprotein IIb/IIIa recep-

tor blockers may exacerbate mural and extravascular bleeding problems.

No reflow occurs in 10-15% of cases of percutaneous vein graft interventions and may be due to distal embolization of microparticles and vasoactive substances, resulting in mechanical vascular occlusion or microvascular vasoconstriction. While intracoronary calcium channel blockade (verapamil 100-900 mcg) and nitrates have been a standard therapy for no reflow, more recently, the intracoronary or intragraft administration of adenosine has proven promising. The optimal dose and route of administration has yet to be clearly defined, although it may be more effective to deliver 18-36 mcg of adenosine, which is thought to act primarily on the distal microvasculature through an infusion catheter or balloon catheter shaft. In this way, both the mechanical force of injection and medicinal properties of the agent can have an effect. Care must obviously be taken to avoid hydraulic injury to the vessel wall, and heart block and hypotension may accompany the repeated doses of adenosine that are sometimes required. An overall success rate of 80%-90% can be expected with this technique.

Distal Embolization

Distal embolization rates are increased in vein graft intervention due to the underlying complex and unfavorable pathophysiologic milieu. Prevention of this complication is a primary concern in all saphenous vein graft interventions. The incidence of distal embolization in studies from 0%-15% and is greatly dependent on the interventional techniques employed and definition of events (Table 3). Distal embolization is associated with increased rates of periprocedural myocardial infarction and correlated with poorer short- and long-term patient outcome in several series. Studies involving atheroablative techniques have suggested an association between preexisting thrombus and subsequent distal embolization. In an analysis of CAVEAT II and the NACI TEC Registries the presence of vein graft thrombus prior to intervention was a strong, independent predictor of distal embolization. In common with patients who exhibit the no-reflow phenomenon following intervention, patients with severe distal embolization are not be good candidates for emergency bypass surgery as the reduced flow and accumulating thrombus are not easily rectified by surgery.

INVASIVE HEMODYNAMICS

Rick A. Nishimura, MD

CARDIAC OUTPUT

Measurement of volumetric flow rate (i.e., stroke volume or cardiac output) is an important variable for evaluating systolic performance of the heart. Stroke volume is the amount of blood that the heart is able to eject during systole and occurs during the systolic ejection period from aortic valve opening to aortic valve closure. This ejection phase index depends on the loading conditions of the heart (afterload and preload) and on the intrinsic contractility of heart muscle. It provides an overall measurement of the ability of the heart to meet the metabolic demands of the body.

Volumetric flow can be measured by several methods. These include the Fick method, the indicator dilution method, and the Doppler flow velocity method. Cardiac catheterization methods are based on the principle outlined by Fick in 1870: for any circulation, the amount of an indicator substance in the blood leaving the circulation must equal the amount of the substance entering plus any amount added to the circulation during transit. The total amount of substance passing any point in the circulation per unit of time is the product of its concentration (which is measured) and the flow rate (which is the unknown value). The Doppler method is based on the hydrodynamic principle of flow through a rigid tube, in which the velocity of flow times the area through which the flow occurs equals the flow rate.

Each method has inherent advantages and limitations. The Fick measurement of cardiac output is the most accurate measurement for low output states. The indicator dilution method is the most accurate method for high output states. In a properly performed Doppler examination, Doppler-derived cardiac output may be the most accurate and reproducible method overall for determination of volumetric flow rates.

Methods used to measure cardiac output:

- Fick method.
- Indicator dilution method.
- Dopper flow velocity method.
- The Fick measurement of cardiac output is the most accurate measurement for low output states.
- The indicator dilution method is the most accurate method for high output states.

It is important to understand the limitations of cardiac output calculation in both low and high cardiac output states.

Fick Method

The Fick method, a time-honored technique, uses the amount of oxygen extracted by the body, as measured by the arterial-venous oxygen difference, to calculate cardiac output. This difference is divided into the oxygen consumption of the body, which is usually measured through a gas exchange method or, less accurately, by estimation from a patient's body weight. Knowledge of the oxygen-carrying capacity of the blood is required; thus, it is necessary to measure the concentration of hemoglobin in the blood. A properly performed Fick method requires a tight-fitting gas exchange mask at equilibrium (no movement of the patient or movement of catheters inside the patient). Simultaneous measurement of oxygen saturation in the arterial system and in the mixed venous system (main pulmonary artery) is required. The formula for calculating cardiac output is

$$\text{Cardiac Output} = \frac{O_2 \text{ Consumption}}{(A-V)O_2 \times \text{Hemoglobin Concentration} \times (1.36) \times 10}$$

Where $(A-V)O_2$ is the arterial-venous oxygen difference.

The advantage of the Fick method over the other methods is that the variables are measured during steady state. The Fick method of calculating cardiac output is the most accurate method if the heart rate or rhythm is irregular, as in atrial fibrillation. Because lower cardiac output results in a higher arterial-venous oxygen difference, the Fick cardiac output method is most accurate for low output states. The total error in determining cardiac output is 10% to 15%.

The disadvantage of the Fick cardiac output method is that it requires simultaneous measurement of oxygen consumption by the body, and this may be difficult to do because of the logistic problem of obtaining a tight gas exchange coupling. It is not of use in patients undergoing cardiac interventions (e.g., valvuloplasty), because it cannot detect rapid changes in cardiac output.

- The Fick method of calculating cardiac output is the most accurate method if the heart rate or rhythm is irregular, as in atrial fibrillation.
- The pulmonary artery saturation can be used for an overall estimate of cardiac output in the absence of a shunt or arterial desaturation. A saturation >80% indicates a high output and a saturation <65% indicates a low output.

Indicator Dilution Method

The indicator dilution method of calculating cardiac output is the method used most commonly by cardiologists. Originally, the indicator dilution method was performed by injecting indocyanine green into one cardiac chamber and sampling the concentration of dye downstream. A continuous infusion of dye would be the most accurate method, but the use of bolus injections has evolved for logistic reasons. Although the green dye injection method is still used in some laboratories, the thermodilution cardiac output method is more popular. This consists of injecting a bolus of cold liquid in a proximal portion of the heart and sampling the changes in temperature as the solution mixes distally with warm blood.

The measurement of cardiac output is based on a time intensity (or temperature) curve, with concentration on the y-axis and time on the x-axis (Fig. 1). The area underneath the time intensity curve is related inversely to cardiac output if the dye dissipates immediately after measurement. Because of recirculation of dye through the body, extrapolation of the descending limb of the curve is necessary. The disappearance of dye from the human circulation is exponential; thus, the

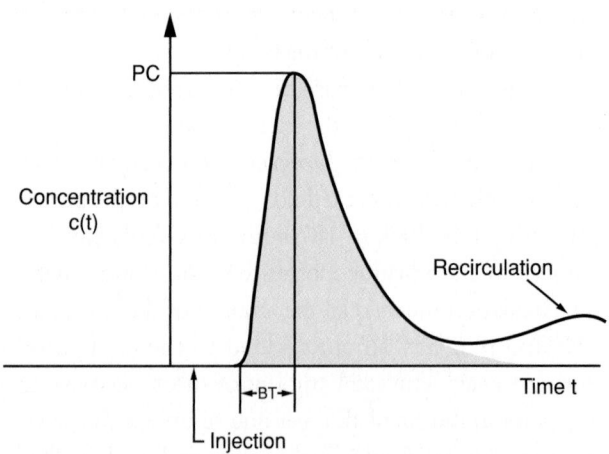

Fig. 1. Catheter pressures of left ventricle (LV) and right atrium (RA). There is elevation of the right atrial pressure. The "A" wave is the right atrial pressure at atrial contraction. The "V" wave is the pressure during atrial filling. The "X" descent is a decrease in pressure during atrial relaxation and anular descent. The "Y" descent is the increase in pressure after atrioventricular valve opening.

area under the curve can be determined by assuming a monoexponential decrease of the curve to baseline:

$$\text{Cardiac Output} = \frac{I}{\int_{0}^{\infty} c(t)dt}$$

where I = amount of indicator injected and c(t) = concentration as a function of time (dt=function of time).

The use of an indicator dye method requires that adequate mixing of the dye (or cold saline) be complete before sampling occurs. Therefore, the optimal method requires that a mixing chamber be interposed between the injection site and the sampling site. The best sampling site is the chamber or great vessel closest to the mixing chamber. The indicator dye solution can be injected into the pulmonary artery or left atrium and the concentration can be sampled in the ascending aorta. For the thermodilution method, the cold solution is injected into the right atrium, and the changes in temperature are sampled in the pulmonary artery.

The indicator dilution method is most accurate in patients with high output states. It is less accurate as cardiac output decreases. This method is inaccurate in the presence of irregular heart rates or rhythms and when coexistent regurgitation of a valve between the ejection site and sampling site is significant. Under the best conditions, the variability in thermodilution cardiac output can be as much as 15% to 20%.

■ The indicator dilution method is inaccurate in the presence of irregular heart rates or rhythms and when coexistent regurgitation of a valve between the ejection site and sampling site is significant.

Doppler Cardiac Output

Volumetric flow rate also can be measured by Doppler echocardiography. This method incorporates the hydraulic principle of flow through a rigid tube. If the area of the tube and the velocity of the flow are known, the product of velocity times area provides a measure of volumetric flow rate. In the pulsatile model, the time velocity integral of the measured Doppler velocity times the area through which the flow occurs provides a measurement of stroke volume, and stroke volume multiplied by heart rate equals cardiac output.

There are limitations to using Doppler echocardiography for measurement of volumetric flow. The orifice through which the flow is measured must be a fixed circular orifice. The velocity profile is assumed to be flat, but in humans, flow profiles are usually parabolic. Changes in the position of the sample volume in relation to the heart with respiration also may cause erroneous measurements. Various sites in the heart and great vessels have been used for measurement of volumetric flow rate by Doppler echocardiography, including the ascending aorta, descending aorta, mitral anulus, mitral valve, tricuspid anulus, tricuspid valve, aortic valve, and right ventricular outflow tract. The sampling site that is most accurate is the left ventricular outflow tract, because the area is relatively constant and the velocity profile is most laminar.

Of all the methods, Doppler measurement of cardiac output potentially is the most accurate on a beat-to-beat basis, but it is also the most operator-dependent method. Care must be taken to obtain an accurate measurement of the diameter of the left ventricular outflow tract, because an error in the diameter measurement is squared when it is converted to area. The velocity profile changes within the left ventricular outflow tract, and different positions of the sample volume may result in different velocity measurements. Also, care must be taken to ensure that the Doppler beam is parallel to the outflow tract velocity.

■ Of the three methods commonly used to calculate cardiac output, Doppler echocardiography is the one most susceptible to operator error.

PRESSURES AND RESISTANCE

Pressures

Direct measurement of intracardiac pressure and pressure in the great vessels can only be done with cardiac catheterization. Indirect noninvasive measurements have been used, including sphygmomanometry and Doppler velocities; however, they rely on several assumptions. Thus, cardiac catheterization is required for accurate measurement of absolute pressures.

Fluid-filled catheter systems are most widely used. The pressure waveforms generated in the cardiac chambers or great vessels are transmitted through the fluid column in the catheter lumen to a pressure transducer. Most pressure transducers are the strain-gauge type, with a diaphragm in direct contact with the fluid column in the catheter. Changes of pressure in the fluid deform this diaphragm and induce a change in electrical potential that is proportional to the pressure change. This potential is calibrated, amplified, and displayed as intracardiac pressure. Zeroing and calibration of the pressure transducers are required before each procedure.

Pressure waves are always distorted with fluid-filled catheters, primarily because of the oscillatory and dampening characteristics of the catheter-fluid column. These distortions may be minimized by 1) minimizing the number and length of stopcocks and connectors between the catheter and the transducer, 2) flushing out all microbubbles in the system, 3) avoiding making measurements after injection of contrast agent or withdrawal of blood, 4) using continuous flushing with heparin, and 5) using catheters of the largest practical size, preferably with a side hole in the ventricles. Artifacts may occur because of incomplete seals between the catheter and the connectors, inadequate initial calibration, and inaccurate zero balance.

The most accurate way of measuring intracardiac pressures is to use high-fidelity manometer-tipped catheters, in which an electronic manometer transducer is placed on the end of the catheter and inserted directly into the cardiac chamber. The electronic pressures need to be balanced and calibrated to the absolute fluid-filled pressures. Normal values for heart pressures are shown in Table 1.

Right and left atrial pressures normally have three distinct positive waves and two negative descents (Fig. 2). The "a" wave is the pressure increase at atrial contraction. The "c" wave is the pressure increase during isovolumic contraction of the ventricle as the atrioventricular valve bulges back into the atrium. The x descent occurs after the "a" and "c" waves and is related to atrial relaxation, descent of the anulus toward the apex, and the compliance of the atrium itself. The "v" wave is the increase in atrial pressure when the atrioventricular valve is closed as blood comes in from either the vena cava or the pulmonary veins. At the peak of the "v" wave, the atrioventricular valve opens and blood rushes from the atria into the ventricles, causing a y descent. On the right side of the heart, the

Table 1.   Normal Values for Heart Pressures

Chamber	Pressure, mm Hg*	
	Average	Range
Right atrium	5	±2
Right ventricle	25/5	±5/±2
Pulmonary artery	25/10	±5/±2
Left atrium	10	±2
Left ventricle	120/15	±20/±5

*The easiest way to remember the normal intracardiac pressures is as multiples of 5.

"a" wave usually is slightly larger than the "v" wave, but on the left side, the "v" wave usually is slightly larger than the "a" wave. The z point on the atrial pressure trace is the pressure of the atria just before the onset of ventricular contraction. The mean right and left atrial pressures are the standard measurements used for clinical assessment.

The left and right ventricular pressures are usually measured at maximal systolic pressure, minimal early diastolic pressure, and ventricular end-diastolic pressure (Fig. 3). End-diastolic pressure is defined as the ventricular pressure just before the onset of ventricular contraction after atrial contraction. The first derivative of the ventricular pressure curves during isovolumic contraction is used as a measurement of systolic contractility, that is, peak positive dp/dt. The peak positive dp/dt may be divided by the absolute pressure at which it occurs to normalize for pressure. The first derivative of the ventricular pressure curve during isovolumic relaxation provides a measurement of the rate of ventricular relaxation, that is, the peak negative dp/dt. The peak positive and negative dp/dt are dependent on the load imposed on the left ventricle.

The time constant of relaxation, or tau, has been used to measure the rate of relaxation and is less dependent on loading conditions. Various methods have been proposed for measuring the time constant of relaxation. In the most commonly used method the ventricular pressure from aortic valve closure to mitral valve opening is fitted to a monoexponential equation

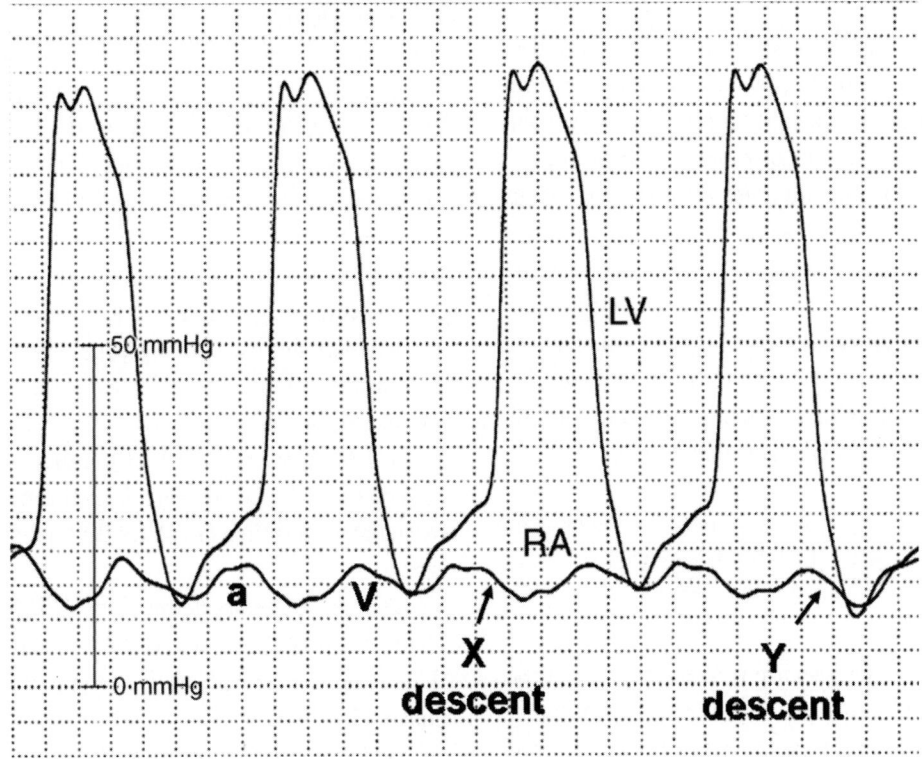

Fig. 2. Normal pressure tracing of LV and RA. a wave, V wave, X and Y descent all labeled.

and allowed to decay to 0 mm Hg. The following equation is used to calculate tau (T) by this method:

$$P(t) = P_0 \times e^{-t/T}$$

Where P(t)=pressure at a point in time (t), T=tau and P_0=pressure at onset of tau.

Other methods of measuring tau include using a nonzero asymptote and a biexponential fit. Other measurements of ventricular pressure during diastole include measurement of the height of the rapid filling wave and the pressure just before the onset of atrial contraction—the "pre-a wave."

Aortic and pulmonary pressures are measured in terms of peak systolic pressure, end-diastolic pressure, and mean pressure. For the aorta, the mean pressure can be assumed to be one-third the difference between the systolic and diastolic aortic pressures. For the pulmonary circulation with normal pulmonary pressures, the mean pressure can be assumed to be one-half the difference between the systolic and diastolic pulmonary pressures.

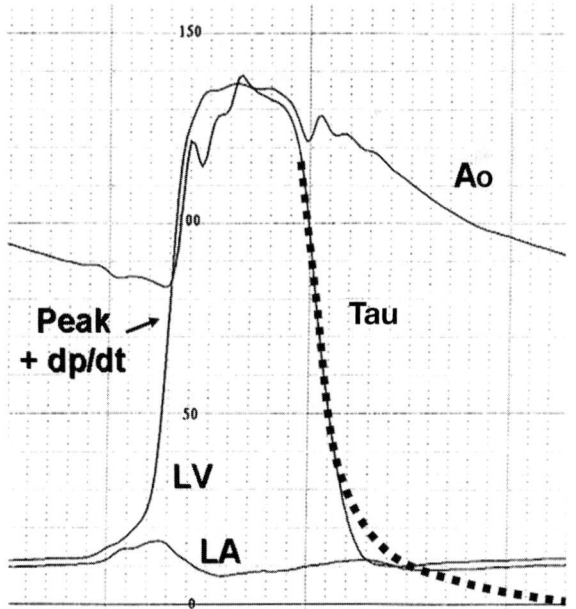

Fig. 3. Catheter pressures of left ventricle (LV), left atrium (LA), and aorta (Ao). The left ventricular pressue is a high fidelity manometer tipped pressure. The time constant of relaxation (Tau) is derived from a mono exponential curve during isovolumic relaxation. The peak (+) (dp/dt) is the first derivative of the left ventricular rise during isovolumic contraction.

Resistance

The great vessels impose an afterload on the ventricles, and this is related to both flow and absolute pressure. Because the cardiovascular system is pulsatile, the ideal measurement of this afterload would be arterial impedance. However, this measurement is difficult to obtain in humans, and its use has been restricted to laboratory investigations. Although arterial resistance is less accurate as a measurement of afterload, it is the clinically used parameter obtained at the time of cardiac catheterization. Resistance is derived from a hydrodynamic model of continuous flow. The resistance of flow through a rigid tube is defined as follows:

$$\text{Resistance} = \frac{\text{Pressure Difference}}{\text{Cardiac Output}}$$

Systemic arterial resistance is mean systemic aortic pressure divided by cardiac output. Pulmonary artery resistance is mean pulmonary artery pressure divided by cardiac output. A measurement of pulmonary arteriolar resistance is mean pulmonary artery pressure minus mean left atrial pressure divided by cardiac output.

Several types of units have been used to describe arterial resistance. A Wood unit is millimeters of mercury times minute divided by liters, with no conversion factor used. Wood units can be indexed to body surface area. Another unit of arterial resistance is "dynes · s · cm^{-5}," which is the same as a Wood unit multiplied by a constant of 80. Normal values for arterial resistance are listed in Table 2.

■ Wood units × 80 = dynes · s · cm^{-5}.

INTRACARDIAC SHUNTS

Intracardiac shunting of blood may be due to either congenital or acquired lesions. Shunting may occur because oxygenated blood from the left heart passes into the systemic venous blood ("left-to-right shunt") or because unoxygenated venous blood passes directly into the arterial circulation ("right-to-left shunt"). In the presence of complex congenital heart disease, it may be confusing to think in terms of left-to-right or right-to-left shunts. The following terms are helpful in describing shunts in complex cases and in calculating shunts (Fig. 4):

1. Effective flow (EF)—Quantity of systemically mixed venous blood that circulates through the lungs, is oxygenated, and then circulates through systemic capillaries.

2. Recirculated systemic flow (RSF)—Amount of relatively desaturated, systemically mixed venous blood that recirculates directly to the aorta without being oxygenated by the lungs.

3. Recirculated pulmonary flow (RPF)—The quantity of fully saturated pulmonary venous blood that recirculates to the pulmonary artery without passing through the systemic capillaries.

4. Total pulmonary flow (PF)—Effective flow plus recirculated pulmonary flow.

5. Systemic flow (SF)—Effective flow plus recirculated systemic flow.

In most cases, the presence of intracardiac shunting has been diagnosed by noninvasive imaging modalities before cardiac catheterization is initiated. However, there may be instances in which a shunt is suspected only at the time of cardiac catheterization, by finding a "step-up" on a routine measurement of right heart oxy-

Table 2. Normal Values for Arterial Resistance

Type	Resistance	
	Wood units	Dynes·s·cm^{-5}
Pulmonary arteriolar resistance	0.84±0.29	67±23
Pulmonary arteriolar resistance index (per m^2)	1.54±0.68	123±54
Total pulmonary resistance	2.56±0.64	205±51
Systemic resistance	14.4±2.2	1,130±178

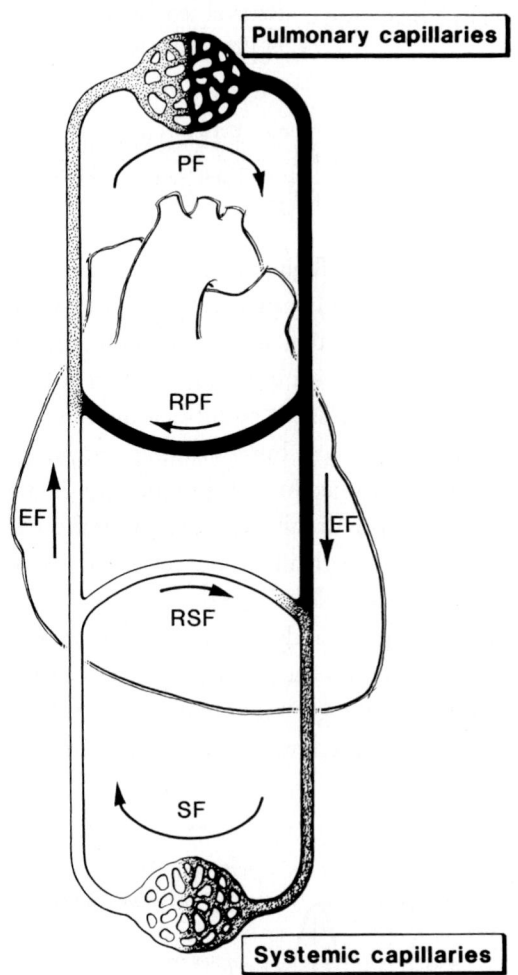

Fig. 4. Schematic depiction of circulation with intracardiac shunting. EF, effective flow; PF, pulmonary flow; RPF, recirculated pulmonary flow; RSF, recirculated systemic flow; SF, systemic flow.

gen saturation or finding desaturation when arterial blood gases are measured. When this is present, it is necessary to perform a complete cardiac catheterization study for shunt determination. This consists of 1) performing a complete measurement of saturation, 2) measuring oxygen consumption, 3) considering administration of 100% oxygen, and 4) obtaining dye curves.

Two Methods of Intracardiac Shunt Detection

Traditionally, the detection and quantitation of intracardiac shunts have been performed in a cardiac catheterization laboratory. With the advent of two-

dimensional and transesophageal echocardiography, the clinical need for invasive evaluation of intracardiac shunts has virtually disappeared. However, it is important to understand the methods used for the detection and measurement of intracardiac shunts at the time of cardiac catheterization. Intracardiac shunts can be detected and quantitated with two separate methods: oximetry and dye curves. The advantage of oximetry is its availability in all laboratories. However, it is a relatively insensitive technique and may miss small shunts. Also, many times, it is difficult to localize the position of the intracardiac shunt by oximetry alone. Dye curves, especially double-sampling dye curves, overcome these limitations of oximetry. However, dye curves are more difficult to perform and their use is limited to a few medical centers in the United States.

Saturations—Left-to-Right

A properly performed saturation measurement should include sampling the saturation at the following sites: the inferior vena cava at the level of the renal arteries, the inferior vena cava below the diaphragm, the inferior vena cava at the diaphragm, the lower right atrium, the mid-right atrium, the high right atrium, the low superior vena cava, the high superior vena cava, the right ventricle, the pulmonary artery, and a systemic arterial location. Hemoglobin and blood gas concentrations should be measured simultaneously at the arterial site. Technical points about catheter position include 1) turning the catheter away from the hepatic vein when sampling from the inferior vena cava, 2) turning the catheter away from the tricuspid valve when sampling from the right atrium, and 3) aspirating all the static blood within the catheter before withdrawing a blood sample in each location for determining oxygen saturation. Normally, the blood in the superior vena cava is less saturated than the blood in the inferior vena cava because of a higher degree of oxygen extraction from the vessels in the head and upper extremity. Therefore, a mixed venous saturation is calculated from the inferior vena cava (IVC) and superior vena cava (SVC):

$$\text{Mixed Venous Saturation} = \frac{3\,\text{SVC} + 1\,\text{IVC}}{4}$$

An oxygen "step-up," which indicates a left-to-right shunt, is significant when there is a step-up of more than 7% at the atrial level, a 5% step-up at the ventricular level, and a 5% step-up at the pulmonary artery level (Table 3).

For measuring shunt flow with oximetry, it is easiest to use the concept of the Fick equation applied to the different circulations. According to this equation (as described above), flow is proportional to oxygen consumption divided by arteriovenous oxygen difference from the most proximal site to the most distal site. Thus, different flows can be determined, as follows:

$$\text{Effective Flow} = \frac{O_2 \text{ Consumption}}{PV\ O_2 - MV\ O_2}$$

$$\text{Total Pulmonary Flow} = \frac{O_2 \text{ Consumption}}{PV\ O_2 - PA\ O_2}$$

$$\text{Total Systemic Flow} = \frac{O_2 \text{ Consumption}}{FA\ O_2 - MV\ O_2}$$

where FA = femoral artery, MV = mixed venous, PA = pulmonary artery, and PV = pulmonary vein.

Recirculated Pulmonary Flow = Total Pulmonary Flow – Effective Flow

Recirculated Systemic Flow = Total Systemic Flow – Effective Flow

The degree of shunt is reported in two ways: Qp/Qs and percentage shunt. A Qp/Qs>1.5 is considered a significant shunt.

$$Qp/Qs = \frac{\text{Total Pulmonary Flow}}{\text{Total Systemic Flow}}$$

Table 3.   Oximetry for Shunts

Location	Step-up, O_2% saturated		Shunt detection, Qp/Qs
	Maximum	Mean	
SVC-IVC/RA	>11	>7	1.5-1.9
RA/RV	>10	>5	1.3-1.5
RV/PA	>5	>5	1.3

IVC, inferior vena cava; PA, pulmonary artery; RA, right atrium; RV, right ventricle, SVC, superior vena cava.

$$\text{\% Left-to-Right Shunt} = \frac{\text{Recirculated Pulmonary Flow}}{\text{Total Pulmonary Flow}}$$

$$\text{\% Right-to-Left Shunt} = \frac{\text{Recirculated Systemic Flow}}{\text{Total Systemic Flow}}$$

Dye Curves—Left-to-Right Shunt

Dye curves are a more sensitive and more accurate method for the detection and quantitation of intracardiac shunts. Single-sampling dye curves consist of injecting dye proximal to an intracardiac shunt and sampling distally to a shunt. Double-sampling dye curves consist of injecting dye proximal to the shunt and sampling both distally to the shunt in the arterial circulation and proximally to the recirculation of the shunt on the venous side (Fig. 5).

A single-sampling dye curve usually is performed by injecting dye into the pulmonary artery and sampling in the ascending aorta or femoral artery. If a left-to-right shunt is present, the descending limb of the

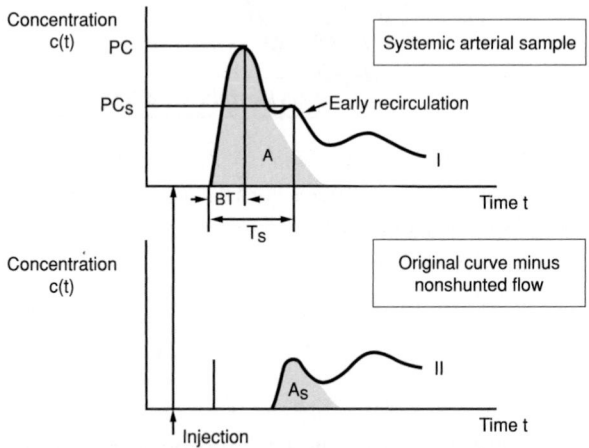

Fig. 5. Pulmonary recirculation, or left-to-right shunt. Curve I, Time-indicator concentration relationship from a typical systemic arterial sample. Total pulmonary flow is proportional to shaded area A. Curve II, Generated by subtracting, point-by-point, from curve I the portion of the curve bounding area A. Shunt flow is then proportional to the shaded area A_s. An approximate formula uses: PC, peak indicator concentration of initial deflection; PC_s, peak indicator concentration of early recirculation from the shunt; BT, buildup time for PC; and T_s, time from initial appearance of dye until PC_s.

dye curve has a secondary bump. Because it may be difficult to determine whether an extra bump is present, double-sampling dye curves have become standard for diagnosing left-to-right shunts. A complete dye curve measurement should consist of injecting dye first into the pulmonary trunk and simultaneously sampling in the ascending aorta and right ventricle. In the absence of a shunt, sampling in the ascending aorta should produce a normal dye curve. Dye should not appear in the right ventricle until after the blood has fully recirculated through the body. In the presence of a left-to-right shunt, dye appears early in the right ventricle, concomitant with the appearance of dye in the ascending aorta. The magnitude of the shunt can be calculated by comparing the area underneath the two curves, using a forward triangle method.

After an intracardiac shunt has been diagnosed, further evaluation by double-sampling dye curves can provide information about shunt localization. This should be done by injecting dye into the right pulmonary artery and sampling the left pulmonary artery and ascending aorta. Next, the dye should be injected into the left pulmonary artery, with sampling in the right pulmonary artery and ascending aorta. In the presence of anomalous pulmonary venous drainage, the dye will appear early after it is injected into one pulmonary artery but not the other. In the presence of an intracardiac shunt, the dye will appear early after it is injected into either pulmonary artery (Fig. 5).

After the question of a partial anomalous pulmonary venous drainage has been answered, injections should be made into the main pulmonary artery, with simultaneous sampling in the ascending aorta and in the right side of the heart. The second sampling site should be made in the right ventricle, then in the right atrium, superior vena cava, and inferior vena cava. The early appearance of dye in the right ventricle alone indicates a shunt at the ventricular level. The appearance of dye in the atrium and ventricle indicates a shunt at the atrial level, and the early appearance of dye in the superior vena cava or inferior vena cava indicates the presence of an anomalous pulmonary venous connection with these venous sites.

Evaluation of Arterial Desaturation

Whenever arterial desaturation (arterial saturation <95%) occurs, an effort must be made to determine whether it is due to a right-to-left shunt, an intrapulmonary shunt, or a pulmonary parenchymal abnormality. The simplest method to determine this is to inject a saline contrast into the right side of the heart under two-dimensional echocardiographic guidance. If no shunt is present, saline contrast will not appear in the left side of the heart. If there is an intracardiac shunt, saline contrast will appear immediately. If there is intrapulmonary shunting, saline contrast will appear after six to seven beats. In orthodeoxia platypnea, intrapulmonary shunting occurs only when the person is standing and not when supine.

If an echocardiographic contrast agent is not available, 100% oxygen can be given over 15 minutes to achieve equilibration, and then saturation can be measured. In the presence of pulmonary abnormalities, arterial saturation increases. If there is an intracardiac shunt, the administration of oxygen does not affect desaturation. If the left atrium can be entered through either an atrial septal defect or a patent foramen ovale, sampling of pulmonary vein saturation also can be used to determine the cause of arterial desaturation.

Single sampling dye curves also can be used to detect right-to-left shunts. In the presence of a right-to-left shunt, the ascending limb of the dye curve has an early rise, reflecting the direct shunting of blood through the cardiac chambers (Fig. 6).

STENOTIC VALVULAR LESIONS

Hemodynamic Assessment of Mitral Stenosis

Mitral stenosis now can be diagnosed readily with two-dimensional and Doppler echocardiography. Many physicians consider Doppler echocardiography to be the standard for determining mitral stenosis hemodynamics.

In mitral stenosis, a gradient occurs between the left atrium and left ventricle during diastole (Fig. 7). This can be measured directly from catheters placed in the left ventricle and left atrium (this requires transseptal cardiac catheterization). In many laboratories, pulmonary artery wedge pressure has been used as an indirect measurement of left atrial pressure in patients with mitral stenosis, but this has inherent problems for determining mean mitral gradient. A properly performed pulmonary artery wedge pressure assessment

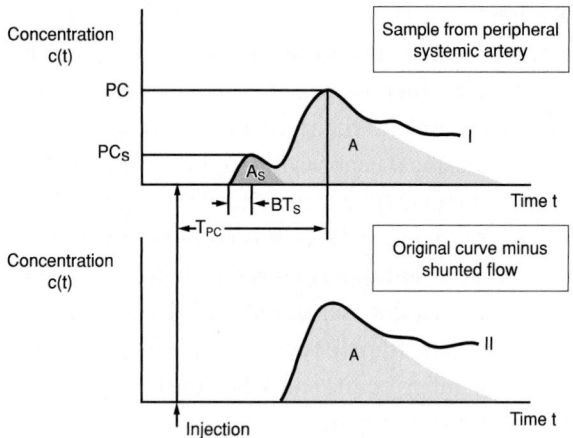

Fig. 6. Time-indicator concentration curves for systemic recirculation, or right-to-left shunt. The magnitude of shunt flow is proportional to the area A_s under curve I. After extrapolation of the downslope of the initial deflection toward zero, the portion of the curve bounding A_s is subtracted from curve I point-by-point to produce curve II. The area A is proportional to systemic flow. An aproximate formula using the forward-triangle technique makes use of: PC_s, peak concentration of initial (shunt flow) deflection; PC, peak concentration of the second (systemic flow) deflection; BT_s, buildup time to PC_s; and T_{pc}, time from injection to PC.

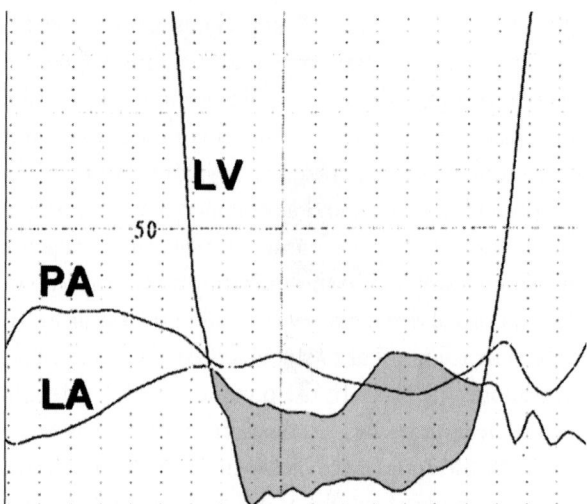

Fig. 7. Catheter pressure traces from a patient with mitral stenosis. The left ventricular (LV), left atrial (LA), and pulmonary artery (PA) pressures are shown. The transmitral gradient between the left atrium and left ventricle (*shaded area*) are a measure of the severity of mitral stenosis. The mean gradient in this patient is 18 mm Hg.

$$\text{Area} = \frac{\text{Flow}}{44.3 \times C \times \sqrt{\Delta P}}$$

where C = 0.85 and ΔP = pressure gradient.

$$\text{Mitral Flow} = \frac{1{,}000 \times \text{Cardiac Output (L/min)}}{\text{Heart Rate (beats/min)} \times \text{DFP (s/beat)}}$$

where DFP = diastolic filling period.

requires an end-hole catheter and confirmation of a saturation more than 97%. Even when a properly obtained pulmonary artery wedge pressure assessment is used, the mean mitral gradient can still be overestimated by up to 50% to 70%. This is due to a delay in the time for transmission of the pulmonary artery wedge pressure and a dampening of the y descent that is normally present in a true left atrial pressure. The pulmonary artery wedge pressure should be "time-shifted" so that the peak of the "v" wave coincides with decreasing left ventricular pressure at the time of mitral valve opening. However, even with this, the gradient may still be overestimated (Fig. 8).

The mean mitral valve gradient depends not only on the degree of obstruction across the mitral valve but also on cardiac output and diastolic filling period. Therefore, the Gorlin equation has been used to derive a calculated mitral valve area, which theoretically takes into consideration flow and duration of flow across the mitral valve:

Measurement of mitral valve area by cardiac catheterization requires accurate measurement of mean mitral valve gradient and cardiac output. The limitations of both of these have been discussed. In addition, the mitral valve area is erroneous at both low and high heart rates. Also, it is not accurate with concomitant significant mitral regurgitation because of a higher flow across the mitral valve than is reflected in the measurement of cardiac output.

Because of problems with the calculated mitral valve area, another indirect measurement of the severity of mitral stenosis is used—diastolic half-time. This is the time it takes for the peak left atrial/left ventricular

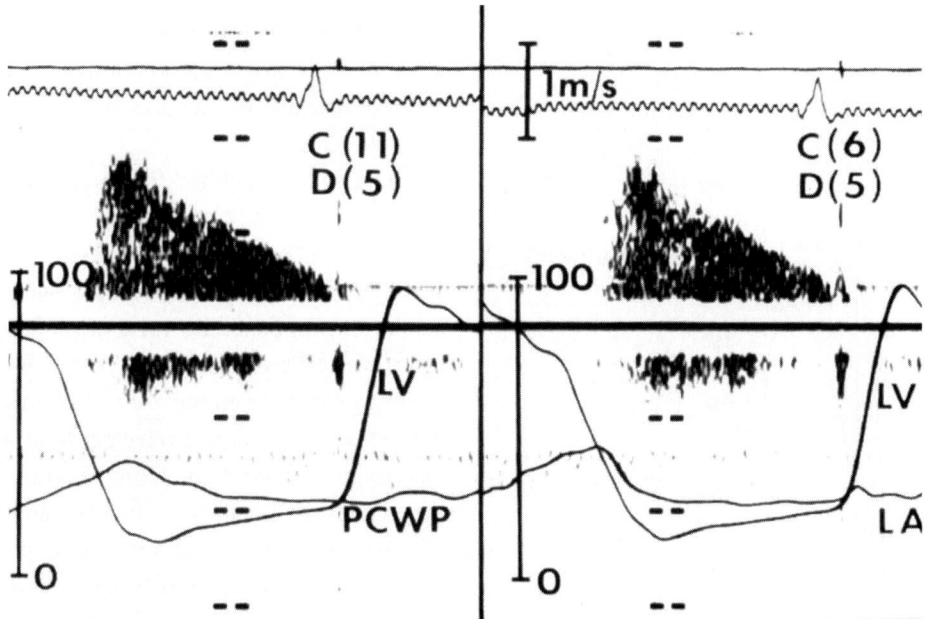

Fig. 8. Simultaneous Doppler (D) and catheterization (C) traces in a patient with mitral stenosis. *Left,* Simultaneous left ventricular (LV) and pulmonary capillary wedge pressures (PCWP) are shown with a simultaneous transmitral Doppler. The gradient derived from catheterization using the pulmonary capillary wedge pressure is 11 mm Hg. This markedly overestimates the true gradient, which is shown by Doppler echocardiography of 5 mm Hg. *Right,* In the same patient, the simultaneous left ventricular and left atrial (LA) pressures are shown. The transmitral gradient measured from left atrial pressure is 6 mm Hg, which corresponds to the Doppler gradient of 5 mm Hg.

pressure gradient to decrease by 50%. It is more accurate than the Gorlin equation for mitral valve area in cases of atrial fibrillation with variable RR intervals and concomitant mitral regurgitation. The original investigations concerning diastolic half-time proposed that a half-time of 100 ms = mild mitral stenosis, of 200 ms = moderate mitral stenosis, and of 300 ms = severe mitral stenosis.

Diastolic half-time for determination of mitral valve severity depends on the relative compliance between the left ventricle and left atrium and will be erroneous when there is a marked abnormality of compliance. This occurs in patients with ventricular compliance abnormalities, such as restriction to filling or severe abnormal relaxation, and in those with acute changes in atrial compliance, for example, immediately after balloon valvuloplasty or after mitral valve surgery.

Hemodynamic Assessment of Aortic Stenosis
In a patient with aortic stenosis, the diagnosis and measurement of the severity of stenosis can be made in most cases by Doppler echocardiography, by obtaining

both the mean aortic valve gradient and the calculated valve area. However, in contrast to mitral stenosis, the Doppler examination in a patient with aortic stenosis is highly operator-dependent, and the severity of stenosis can be grossly underestimated if there is a large theta angle between the Doppler beam and the aortic stenotic jet. Thus, cardiac catheterization may be needed to determine the severity of the stenosis if there is a discrepancy between the clinical impression and the echocardiographic results.

The aortic valve gradient is an important variable to measure in a patient with aortic stenosis (Fig. 9). The peak-to-peak gradient, the one most commonly used in cardiac catheterization laboratories, is the difference between the peak left ventricular and peak aortic pressure. This is a nonphysiologic measurement because it is obtained from nonsimultaneous recordings. Doppler echocardiographic assessment of the aortic valve gradient provides instantaneous gradients between the left ventricle and aorta. The peak aortic velocity is converted to gradient, resulting in a maximal instantaneous gradient. This maximal instantaneous gradient is usual-

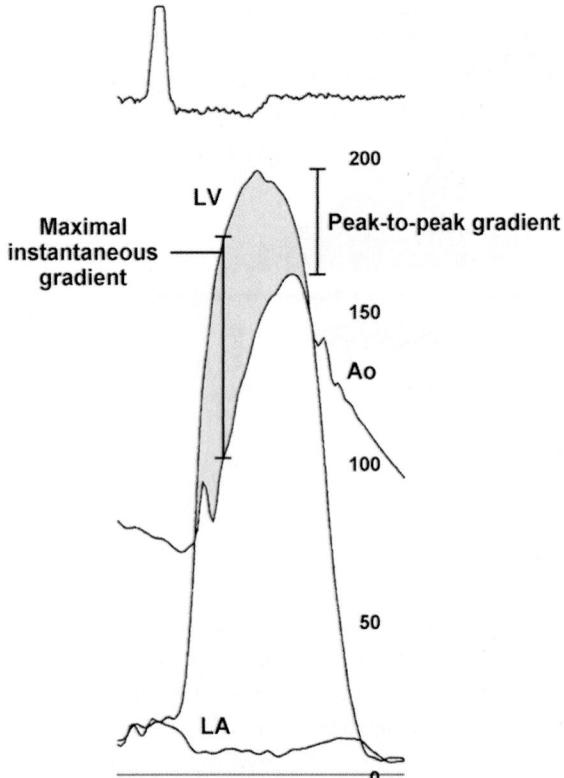

Fig. 9. Catheterization pressures from a patient with aortic stenosis. The left ventricular (LV), left atrial (LA), and aortic (Ao) pressures are shown. The maximum instantaneous gradient is shown. The peak gradient is shown and is the difference between the peak left ventricular and peak aortic pressure, which occur at different times. The mean gradient is the shaded gray area and is the best determinate of the severity of aortic stenosis.

ly 30% to 40% greater than the peak-to-peak gradient. The mean aortic valve gradient provides the most information about the severity of obstruction and should be the gradient used by both Doppler and cardiac catheterization methods. There are several ways the aortic valve gradient can be measured in a cardiac catheterization laboratory. The most common one is the "pull-back" method, in which a catheter is placed in the left ventricle and quickly pulled back into the aorta while the peak pressure is recorded in both places. The difference between the two peak pressures is the gradient across the aortic valve. In most circumstances, this "peak-to-peak" gradient approximates the true mean aortic valve gradient, especially at very high pressure

gradients (>50 mm Hg). However, it will not provide an accurate transaortic gradient in cases of low-output states or irregular rhythms, as with atrial fibrillation or multiple ectopic beats.

The optimal method for obtaining an aortic valve gradient is simultaneously to use two different catheters—one in the left ventricle and one in the aorta—to measure a mean aortic valve gradient. This can be accomplished by a transseptal approach or by using two different arterial accesses. A simultaneous femoral pressure from the sidearm of a sheath has been used to obtain an aortic valve gradient. However, the discrepancy between the femoral artery pressure and the ascending aorta pressure may be significant because of transmission delay and compliance of the peripheral arterial tree, and this may lead to overestimation or underestimation of the mean gradient (Fig. 10).

The aortic valve gradient depends on flow and severity of obstruction. An equation for aortic valve area has been described by Gorlin et al. that incorporates pressure and flow for measurement of the severity of stenosis. For this measurement, mean aortic valve gradient, systolic ejection period, heart rate, and cardiac output are used.

$$\text{Area} = \frac{\text{Flow}}{44.3 \times \text{C} \times \sqrt{\Delta P}}$$

$$\text{Aortic Flow} = \frac{1,000 \times \text{Cardiac Output (L/min)}}{\text{Heart Rate (beats/min)} \times \text{SEP (s/beat)}}$$

$$\text{C} = 10$$

where SEP = systolic ejection period.

A modified Hakke equation can be used for aortic stenosis.

$$\text{Area} = \frac{\text{Cardiac Output}}{\sqrt{\Delta P}}$$

There are limitations to calculation of aortic valve area. Measurement of flow through the aortic valve needs to be accurate. In a patient with severe concomitant aortic regurgitation, neither the Fick method nor the thermodilution method can be used, because they will underestimate aortic flow. Aortic valve areas are inaccurate at low and high heart rates, at low and high cardiac outputs, and in the presence of irregular rhythms.

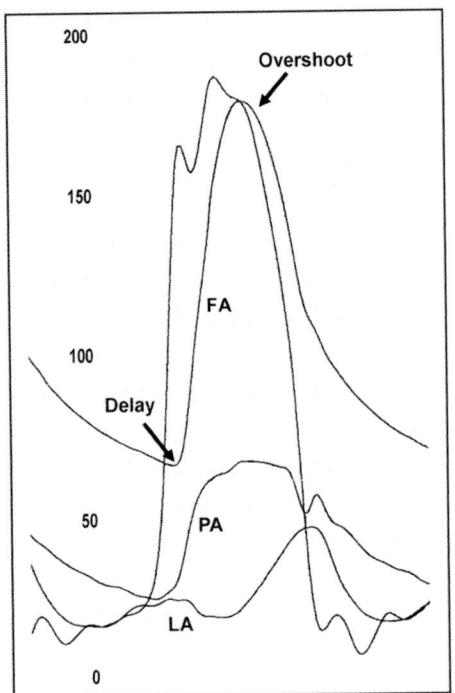
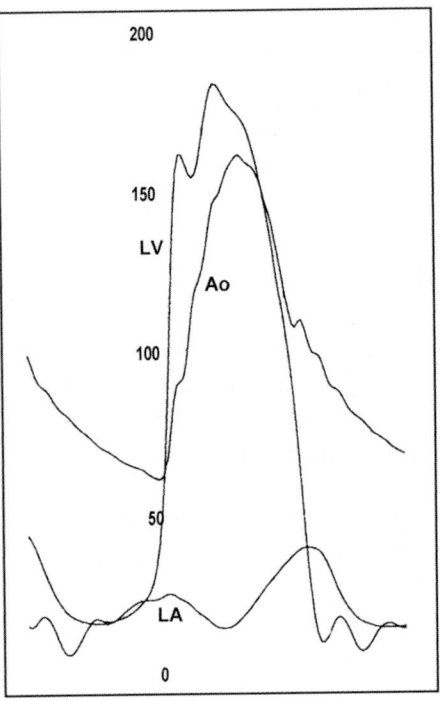

Fig. 10. Catheterization pressures from a patient with aortic stenosis. *Left*, The simultaneous left ventricular (LV) and femoral artery (FA) pressures are shown. This demonstrates that there is a delay in the femoral artery pressure curve and an "overshoot" from peripheral amplification. Therefore, the true aortic valve gradient cannot be determined. *Right*, Simultaneous pressures in left ventricle (LV) and ascending aorta (Ao). This is the methodology to determine the true transaortic gradient. PA, pulmonary artery; LA, left atrium.

REGURGITANT VALVULAR LESIONS

Regurgitant valvular lesions often are assessed in a cardiac catheterization laboratory by injecting contrast into a cardiac chamber or great vessel and visually estimating the amount of contrast that leaks backward into a more proximal chamber. This approach is only semiquantitative, and it has many limitations. Regurgitant fractions have been used in some cardiac catheterization laboratories, but they are cumbersome and have many sources of error. Doppler echocardiographic techniques provide a more quantitative assessment of the severity of a regurgitant lesion (i.e., volumetric regurgitant fractions, proximal isovelocity surface area) but are operator-dependent and should be done only in experienced laboratories.

Injections of Contrast Media

Left ventriculography has been the standard for semi-quantitation of mitral regurgitation. It consists of injecting 45 to 50 mL of contrast medium at a rate of 12 to 14 mL/s into the left ventricle during cineangiography and examining the density, timing, and appearance of the contrast medium in the left atrium. This requires that a large-bore catheter with side holes be well positioned in the left ventricle. Sellars criteria have been established for a semiquantitative estimate of the degree of mitral regurgitation (Table 4).

Left ventriculography has many well-known limitations. The degree to which the contrast medium opacifies the left atrium depends on many factors, including the size and compliance of the left atrium, the size of the left ventricle, the function of the left ventricle, the amount of contrast medium injected, and the rate of injection. Also, catheter entrapment of the mitral apparatus or movement of the catheter into the left atrium can produce erroneous results. Premature beats caused by the catheter or jet of contrast medium also result in erroneous interpretations.

The same concept and grading system are used for determining the severity of aortic regurgitation by aor-

Table 4. Sellars Criteria for Estimating Degree
of Mitral Regurgitation

Grade	Criterion
1+	Contrast medium does not completely fill left atrium
2+	Contrast medium completely opacifies left atrium but does not reach intensity of that in left ventricle
3+	Contrast medium completely opacifies left atrium and reaches intensity of that in left ventricle after 4 or 5 beats
4+	Contrast medium completely opacifies left atrium and reaches intensity of that in left ventricle within first 2 or 3 beats

tic root angiography. At least 50 to 60 mL of contrast medium is injected into the aortic root at a rate of 20 mL/s, and the severity of aortic regurgitation is evaluated by the amount of contrast medium visualized in the left ventricle. As with left ventriculography, the visual estimate of the degree of aortic regurgitation depends on several factors, including the position of the catheter, the amount of contrast medium injected, rate of injection, the size of the aortic root, and the size and function of the left ventricle.

Regurgitant Fractions

Regurgitant fractions and regurgitant volume can be calculated in cardiac catheterization laboratories. Although this method was once considered the standard by early investigators, is prone to error due to the sometimes inaccurate measurement of left ventricular volume; thus, it is not routinely used in many clinical labo-

ratories. However, there may be questions regarding calculation of these parameters on examinations.

For mitral regurgitation, the regurgitant fraction (RF) is the percentage of the total amount of blood ejected by the left ventricle which goes back into the left atrium. The RF is the regurgitant volume (RV) divided by the total amount of blood the ventricle ejects in one beat (total volume [TV]). TV is derived from the left ventriculogram by subtracting the end-systolic volume (ESV) from the end-diastolic volume (EDV). The forward flow volume (FFV) is the amount of blood the ventricle ejects out the aortic valve and is equal to the systemic flow. Thus, this FFV is obtained from the Fick equation. The regurgitant volume is the TV - FFV.

$$TV = EDV - ESV \text{ (from left ventriculography)}$$

$$FFV = \frac{\text{Cardic Output}}{\text{Heart Rate (from the Fick equation)}}$$

$$RV = TV - FFV$$

$$RF = RV/TV$$

■ $\text{Regurgitant Fraction} = \dfrac{\text{Regurgitant Volume}}{\text{Total Ventricular Volume}}$

The major limitation of this technique is the inability to obtain accurate measurements of angiographic stroke volumes. Various methods have been proposed for making such measurements, including monoplane vs. biplane approaches, planimetrically determined area vs. videodensitometry measurements, and various geometric assumptions of left ventricular size. Each of these methods has inherent limitations. A similar approach can be used for patients with aortic regurgitation.

CONTRAST-INDUCED NEPHROPATHY

Patricia J. M. Best, MD

Charanjit S. Rihal, MD

DEFINITION

The most commonly used definition of contrast-induced nephropathy is a rise in the serum creatinine of 0.5 mg/dL. Occasionally, a 1 mg/dL rise in the serum creatinine or a 25% increase in the serum creatinine has been used. More recently, with the improved awareness of the need for estimating glomerular filtration rate (GFR) for its greater accuracy in estimating renal function over the serum creatinine, studies have started to use a 25% decrease in the GFR as the definition of contrast-induced nephropathy.

TIMING

Alterations in renal function usually begin 24-48 hours after contrast exposure. The serum creatinine typically peaks at 3-7 days and usually normalizes by 7-10 days. Because the creatinine often does normalize, the importance of contrast-induced nephropathy has been under appreciated.

EPIDEMIOLOGY

Careful evaluation is needed to determine if contrast-induced nephropathy occurred, otherwise it can easily be undiagnosed. The importance of contrast-induced nephropathy is the potential for progression of renal dysfunction including the need for dialysis, and the association with increased mortality. The significance of contrast-induced nephropathy has been underestimated, yet contrast-induced nephropathy accounts for 12% of in-hospital renal failure. This makes it the third most common cause of in-hospital acute renal failure and it exceeds aminoglycosides in its nephrotoxic potential. Importantly, in the cardiac catheterization laboratory this is one of the most common complications, seen in over 3% of cases. It has been associated with increased in-hospital mortality that is over 11 times higher than those who do not develop contrast-induced nephropathy and it is one of the most powerful predictors for mortality after coronary angiography. In one study, the incidence of contrast-induced nephropathy requiring dialysis after percutaneous coronary revascularization was 7 per 1,000 patients, but these patients had an in-hospital mortality of 27.5%. Contrast-induced nephropathy is also associated with long-term mortality, and the importance of this risk is continued over 4 years after percutaneous coronary intervention (Fig. 1).

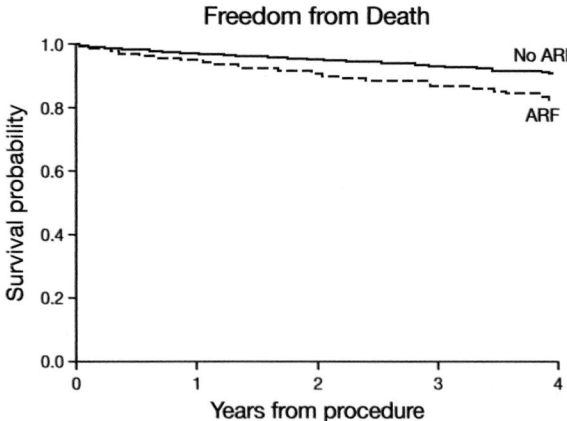

Fig. 1. Kaplan-Meier survival analysis for freedom from death among patients surviving to hospital dismissal. Patients are stratified by presence or absence of contrast-induced nephropathy (ARF), defined as increase in serum Cr ≥0.5 mg/dL from baseline. The survival curve is adjusted for other significant predictors of late survival.

RISK FACTORS FOR CONTRAST-INDUCED NEPHROPATHY

Multiple risk factors for contrast-induced nephropathy have been identified. Consistent strong risk factors are baseline renal function, diabetes mellitus, and age. The incidence of contrast-induced nephropathy based on baseline creatinine and diabetic status from the Mayo Clinic Catheterization Laboratory has been described and is helpful in determining the risk of the procedure (Table 1). Other risk factors which have been identified include female sex, volume depletion, need for an intra-aortic balloon pump, acute coronary syndromes, congestive heart failure, low cardiac output states, and hypotension.

MECHANISMS OF CONTRAST-INDUCED NEPHROPATHY

The specific cause for contrast-induced nephropathy is not known, but it is characterized by acute tubular necrosis. Several potential mechanisms exist. Contrast agents cause vasoconstriction and decrease renal blood flow in the renal medulla. When this occurs it creates a relative hypoxia to the kidney which is undergoing osmotic diuresis from the contrast agent which increases the metabolic demand to the medulla. Pathologically, necrosis may be observed in the thick ascending limb of the loop of Henle. Contrast agents also have a direct toxic effect which is associated with increased renal interstitial inflammation, cellular necrosis, and alterations in cellular enzymes. There are immune mechanisms which have been implicated including activation of the complement system, but these are the least understood mechanisms. Many prevention strategies have tried to target these mechanisms, primarily by preventing renal vasoconstriction and decreasing inflammation and oxidative stress.

RISK SCORES FOR PREDICTING CONTRAST-INDUCED NEPHROPATHY

Two recent risk scores have been formulated to help predict the development of contrast-induced nephropathy and risk-stratify patients. These risk scores may be very useful to determine when patients should undergo staged procedures for percutaneous coronary intervention and to help identify patients which would be at the highest risk for and in greatest need of preventive therapy. Furthermore, these scores are useful in discussions of the risk-benefit ratio, particularly in patients at the highest risk for contrast-induced nephropathy (Fig. 2, Tables 2 and 3).

Table 1.   The Observed Incidence of Contrast-Induced Nephropathy in the Mayo Clinic Catheterization Laboratory Based on Serum Creatinine and Diabetic Status

Creatinine, mg/dL	Risk, all patients, %	Risk, diabetic patients, %	Risk, nondiabetic patients, %
0-1.1	2.4	3.7	2.0
1.2-1.9	2.5	4.5	1.9
2.0-2.9	22.4	22.4	22.3
≥3.0	30.6	33.9	27.4

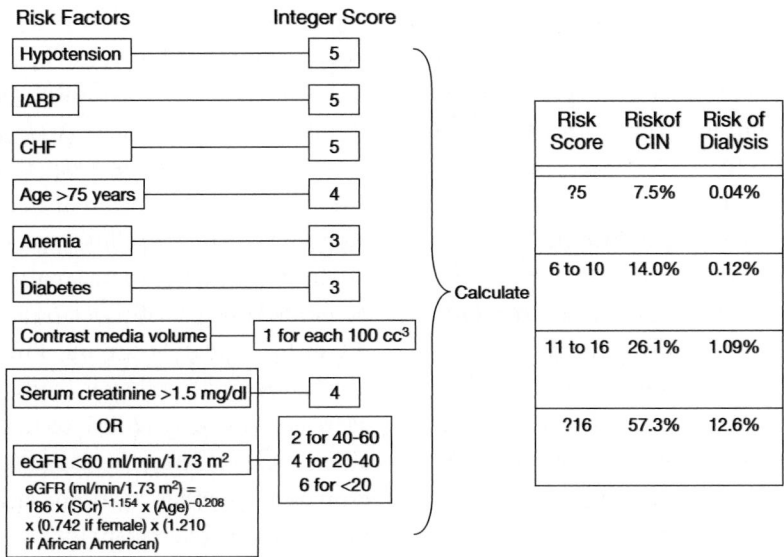

Fig. 2. Scheme to define contrast-induced nephropathy (CIN) risk score. Anemia = baseline hematocrit value <39% for men and <36% for women; CHF = congestive heart failure class III/IV by New York Heart Association classification and/or history of pulmonary edema; eGFR = estimated glomerular filtration rate; hypotension = systolic blood pressure <80 mm Hg for at least 1 h requiring inotropic support with medications or intra-aortic balloon pump (IABP) within 24 h periprocedurally.

PREVENTION OF CONTRAST-INDUCED NEPHROPATHY

Multiple agents have been used to help prevent contrast-induced nephropathy, but the standard of care for the prevention of contrast-induced nephropathy is hydration. Hydration should be performed with normal saline as this has a greater ability to prevent contrast-induced nephropathy compared with one-half normal saline. Agents such as mannitol and furosemide have been utilized to increase urinary output, which were thought to potentially reduce the incidence of contrast-induced nephropathy. However, mannitol and furosemide may increase it. Other agents including L-arginine, atrial natruretic peptide, combined endothelin receptor antagonists, and calcium channel blockers have all been used without success. Furthermore, renal dose dopamine was a potential agent. It increases renal blood flow and could prevent renal vasoconstriction from the

Table 2.   Values for the William Beaumont Hospital Risk Score

Characteristics	Score
Creatinine clearance <60 mL/min	2
Intra-aortic balloon pump usage	2
Urgent/emergency procedure	2
Diabetes mellitus	1
Congestive heart failure	1
Hypertension	1
Peripheral vascular disease	1
Contrast >260 mL	1

Table 3.   Risk of Contrast-Induced Nephropathy and Death Based on the William Beaumont Hospital Risk Score in the Validation Cohort

Risk score group	Contrast-induced nephropathy, %	Death, %
0-4	0.2	0.2
5-6	2.8	2
7-8	10	9
9-11	28	17

contrast agents. However, in multiple studies low-dose dopamine was associated with an increase in serum creatinine and was not beneficial in the prevention of contrast-induced nephropathy. Theories as to why dopamine was not effective include vasoconstriction through the DA_2 receptors. Thus, if not at a low enough dose, dopamine may not have the expected beneficial effect. This observation led to the CONTRAST trial looking at fenoldopam, a selective DA_1 agonist. Fenoldopam acts solely through the DA_1 receptors, and therefore causes only vasodilatation. However, despite multiple prior small studies suggesting that fenoldopam could be beneficial, in the CONTRAST trial of 283 patients undergoing coronary procedures fenoldopam failed to prevent contrast-induced nephropathy.

Another agent which generated great interest for the prevention of contrast-induced nephropathy is N-acetylcysteine. N-acetylcysteine works in-part by reducing local oxidative stress which may be increased by contrast agents. A study evaluated 83 patients undergoing a CT scan who were pretreated with 600 mg twice per day of N-acetylcysteine on the day prior to the procedure and the day of the procedure. They demonstrated a reduction in contrast-induced

nephropathy in their high-risk population from 12% to 2%. This has led to over 23 prospective studies and 11 meta-anaylses. One of these meta-anaylses (Fig. 3) summarized 15 clinical trials and demonstrated marked heterogeneity between the studies. This meta-analysis suggested minimal if any benefit from N-acetylcysteine in the ability to reduce contrast-induced nephropathy. Prior meta-analyses, especially those performed using smaller data-sets, reported a beneficial effect to N-acetylcysteine. The later studies were inconclusive. Recently a study suggested that N-acetylcysteine may reduce serum creatinine without altering GFR. Thus, the use of serum creatinine and estimation of either creatinine clearance or GFR may not be acceptable end-points in studies utilizing N-acetylcysteine. Therefore, the current available literature does not clearly define a role of N-acetylcysteine in the prevention of contrast-induced nephropathy.

The type of contrast agent which is used for the procedure is also an important factor for the risk of contrast-induced nephropathy. In the Iohexonal Cooperative Study evaluating 1,146 patients for the prevention of contrast-induced nephropathy the low-osmolar agent iohexonal was compared with the high-osmolar agent diatrizoate. They found that in high risk

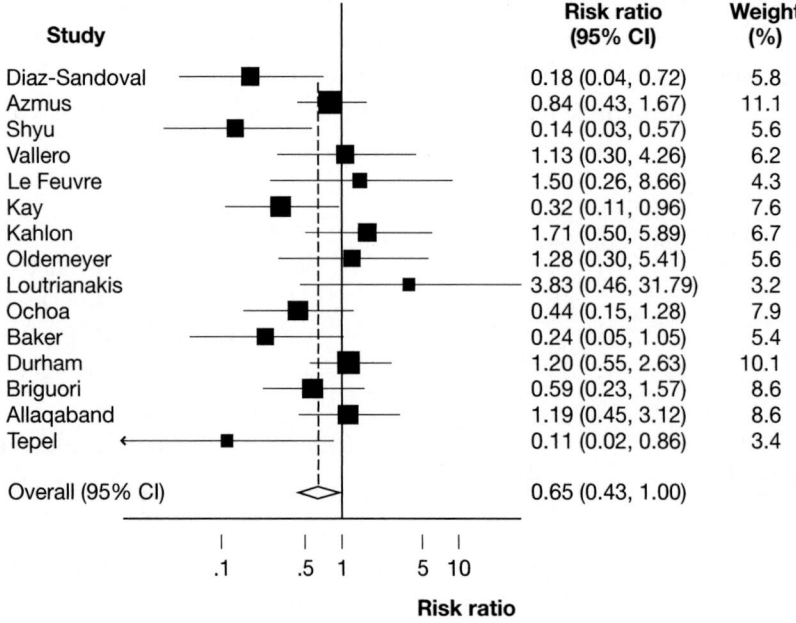

Fig. 3. A meta-analysis of 15 randomized controlled trials of N-acetylcysteine use for the prevention of contrast-induced nephropathy.

patients (those with renal insufficiency or those with renal insufficiency and diabetes mellitus) the low-osmolar contrast agent was associated with a significantly lower incidence of contrast-induced nephropathy. In another study, the patients with neither renal insufficiency nor diabetes mellitus had benefit from the low-osmolar contrast agent. This was in-part because their risk of contrast-induced nephropathy was very low. The NEPHRIC Study subsequently compared the iso-osmolar agent iodixanol with the low-osmolar agent iohexanol in 129 patients. They found that iodixanol was associated with a 10-fold decrease in contrast-induced nephropathy (3% vs. 26%) when defined as a greater than 0.5 mg/dL increase in the serum creatinine and that no patients who received iodixanol had a greater than 1 mg/dL rise in the serum creatinine at 72 hours compared with 15% in those who received iohexanol. This has led to iso-osmolar contrast agents being preferred in patients at significant risk of contrast-induced nephropathy.

Multiple other agents for the prevention of contrast-induced nephropathy have recently been evaluated. In a study of 119 patients who were pretreated with sodium bicarbonate or sodium chloride (154 mEq/liter of sodium chloride compared with sodium bicarbonate given as a bolus of 3 ml/kg/hr for one hour before the procedure and then 1 mg/kg/hr for six hours after the procedure), sodium bicarbonate infusion was associated with a significantly lower incidence of contrast-induced nephropathy (1.7%) compared with sodium chloride (13.6%). Larger studies are needed to confirm that sodium bicarbonate is truly beneficial.

Another potential preventive measure for contrast-induced nephropathy is continuous veno-venous hemofiltration. In a study of 114 patients undergoing coronary procedures hemofiltration was associated with a 5% incidence of contrast-induced nephropathy compared to a 50% incidence in those treated with saline. Further small studies have not shown as significant of a benefit. Due in large part to the challenges and complications of hemofiltration (large vascular catheters) and significant cost (hemofiltration is performed for 4 to 6 hours before and 18 to 24 hours after the procedure), this technique has not gained widespread use.

KEY POINTS ON CONTRAST-INDUCED NEPHROPATHY

- Is associated with increased in-hospital and long term morbidity and mortality.
- Occurs in 3% of catheterization laboratory population.
- Baseline renal function, diabetes, age and age are strong patient risk factors.
- Is associated with contrast volume.
- Is best prevented with normal saline hydration and use of iso-osmolar contrast agents.

DIAGNOSTIC CORONARY ANGIOGRAPHY AND VENTRICULOGRAPHY

Joseph G. Murphy, MD

CORONARY ANGIOGRAPHY

Indications for Coronary Angiography

Coronary angiography is indicated for the diagnosis and treatment of coronary artery disease, usually atherosclerosis, when the procedural risks are outweighed by the likely benefits of accurate diagnosis and the patient is willing to consider a therapeutic procedure (usually PCI or CABG) if hemodynamically significant coronary disease is found. Coronary angiography may also be considered in special situations when coronary artery disease needs to be excluded, although unlikely (airline pilots with mildly abnormal stress tests or preoperatively before heart valve surgery or high-risk noncardiac surgery). Other diseases of the coronary arteries that may be diagnosed with coronary angiography include congenital anomalies of the origin of coronary arteries, coronary fistulas, coronary spasm, coronary emboli, coronary arteritis, and myocardial bridging.

Contraindications to Coronary Angiography

Refusal of a patient to consent to the procedure is an absolute contraindication to coronary angiography.

Relative contraindications that should delay angiography until mitigated include the presence of correctable electrolyte abnormalities or drug toxicity (e.g., hyperkalemia, digitalis toxicity), febrile illness, acute renal failure, decompensated heart failure, severe allergy to radiographic contrast agents, anticoagulated state or a severe bleeding diathesis, severe uncontrolled hypertension, and pregnancy.

■ Virtually the only absolute contraindication to coronary angiography is the refusal of a patient to consent to the procedure.

Complications of Coronary Angiography

Major Complications
The major complications of coronary angiography are death, myocardial infarction, and stroke. The combined frequency of these adverse events is about 0.23% but depends on the case mix. The main risk factors for major adverse events with coronary angiography are left main coronary artery disease and aortic stenosis. Other important risk factors include advanced age,

This chapter has been modified from the previous version by Peter Berger, MD. We would like to acknowledge Peter Berger, MD for his previous contribution.
An atlas of coronary angiograms, ventriculograms, and aortograms is at the end of the chapter.

angina at rest, left ventricular dysfunction, previous stroke, and severe noncardiac disease (including renal insufficiency, cerebrovascular and peripheral vascular disease, and pulmonary insufficiency). Cardiogenic shock increases the risk of coronary angiography by sixfold and acute myocardial infarction by fourfold. Approximately one-half of the complications that occur within 24 hours after coronary angiography are believed to be "pseudocomplications," in that the "complications" may have occurred during the same period had angiography not been performed.

- The two main risk factors for major adverse coronary artery events with coronary angiography are left main coronary artery disease and aortic stenosis.
- One-half of the complications that occur within 24 hours after coronary angiography are believed to be "pseudocomplications," in that the "complications" may have occurred during the same period had angiography not been performed.

Minor Complications (Table 1)

Minor complications include local complications at the vascular access site; the type of complication seen depends on the vascular approach. Complications of percutaneous femoral artery access include hemorrhage, distal embolization, false aneurysm, and local injury to the femoral nerve. Femoral vein thrombosis resulting from compression of the femoral vein during sheath removal has been reported. Complications associated with direct exposure of the brachial artery include thrombosis of the brachial artery. Injury to the brachial nerve, local hemorrhage, and infection may also occur. Percutaneous access of the brachial artery is associated more commonly with hemorrhage than with thrombosis. Significant vascular complications occur in approximately 1% of patients undergoing diagnostic angiography, and are least likely to occur when the radial artery is used. However, a radial artery approach can only be used when there is a patent palmar arterial arch; that is, when the ulnar artery and radial artery communicate via the palmar arch, so that the ulnar artery can supply blood to the hand should the radial artery occlude. Adequacy of the palmar arch can be made clinically by the Allen test.

- Significant vascular complications occur in

approximately 1% of patients undergoing diagnostic angiography.

Arrhythmias During Angiography

Arrhythmias and vasovagal complications occur in approximately 1% of patients. These complications are usually self-limited, but if need be, they generally can be treated readily with electrical cardioversion or defibrillation or the administration of atropine. Pulmonary edema may develop during angiography, most commonly as a result of either increased intravascular volume due to the contrast agent, a cardiac complication (i.e., an acute myocardial infarction), or the recumbent position.

Rare Complications (Less Than 1% of Patients)

Coronary artery dissection is rare. It generally is preventable by meticulous attention to pressure waveforms and avoidance of overly vigorous injection of the contrast agent.

Coronary artery spasm from a reaction to the catheter tip usually responds to removal of the catheter. Nitroglycerin (sublingual or intracoronary) may be required.

Contrast Reactions

Serious reactions to contrast agents can mimic an anaphylactic reaction but are immunologically distinct. These reactions, called "anaphylactoid reactions," are rare. They should be treated with immediate administration intravenously of antihistamines and corticosteroids. Anaphylactoid reactions are more likely to occur in patients with a history of allergy to contrast

Table 1.   Complications of Coronary Angiography

	Percent
Death	0.10
Stroke	0.07
Myocardial infarction	0.05
Significant arrhythmias	0.30
Contrast reaction	0.30
Vascular complication	0.30

agents and can be minimized by prophylactically administering the above drugs and using low ionic agents.

Renal Failure After Angiography

Renal failure from nephrotoxic contrast agents can be reduced by delaying angiography in patients with acute renal failure, avoiding the concomitant administration of other nephrotoxins, and, most importantly, reducing the volume of contrast agent administered. This can be accomplished by minimizing the number of angiographic views taken and using biplane angiography in patients with preexisting renal disease, who are at increased risk for acute renal failure. *N*-acetylcysteine administered before the contrast exposure, can ameliorate contrast nephropathy. Dopamine and fenoldopam cannot. In the presence of normal ventricular function, volume expansion with isotonic saline or isotonic bicarbonate solution may be used to mitigate the nephrotoxic effects of contrast.

Protamine Reactions

Severe protamine reactions may result in shortness of breath, hypotension, flushing, and flank pain. Protamine is given to reverse the effect of intravenous heparin, which is administered in many catheterization laboratories (in doses ranging from 2,500 to 5,000 units) to reduce the risk of thromboembolic complications of the procedure. Such reactions are more likely to occur in patients who have received NPH insulin, because of previous exposure to protamine contained in NPH insulin. Thus, the use of protamine should be avoided in such patients. Patients with an allergy to fish are also at increased risk.

Coronary Artery Anatomy

Dominance

Coronary artery dominance is defined by the artery that gives rise to the posterior descending artery. In approximately 86% of patients, it is the right coronary artery (Fig. 1). In 7% of patients, the circumflex artery is dominant, and 7% of patients have codominant arteries, with both the right coronary artery and the circumflex artery supplying the posterior descending artery. There is no particular clinical significance to whether a patient is right dominant, left dominant, or codominant.

Coronary Arteries

The left main artery is 5 to 10 mm in diameter and generally less than 4 cm long. It bifurcates into the left

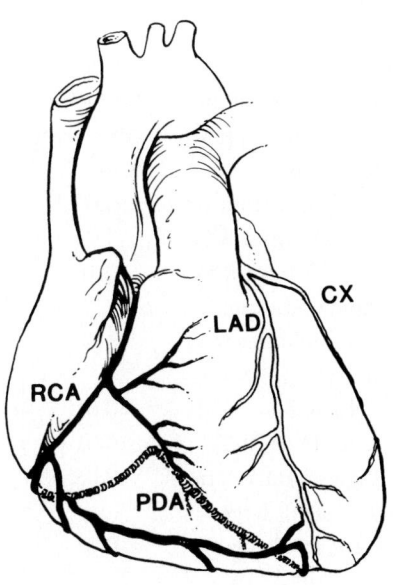

Right dominant

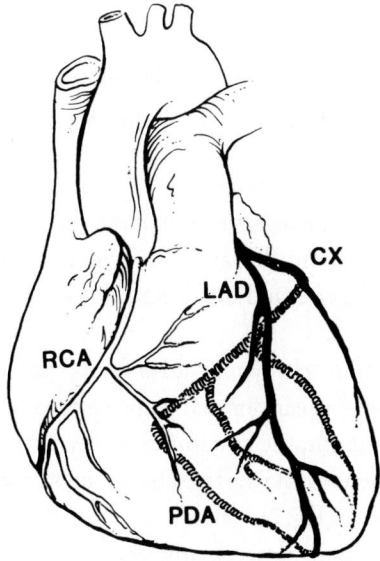

Left dominant

Fig. 1. Coronary artery dominance. In right coronary dominance, the posterior descending branch (PDA) arises from the right coronary artery (RCA). In left dominance, the right coronary artery is a diminutive vessel, and the posterior descending artery arises as a continuation of the left atrioventricular groove artery, a branch of the circumflex (CX) system. LAD, left anterior descending artery.

anterior descending artery and circumflex artery. It may also trifurcate into those branches plus a ramus intermedius artery.

The left anterior descending artery lies in the anterior interventricular groove. It usually wraps around the apex of the left ventricle; its terminal branches reach those of the right posterior descending artery. Diagonal branches supply the lateral wall, and septal branches supply the interventricular septum.

The circumflex artery lies in the left atrioventricular groove. Its terminal branches reach those of the right posterolateral artery. Obtuse marginal branches supply the lateral wall of the left ventricle.

The right coronary artery lies in the right atrioventricular groove. Proximally, it generally gives off the conus artery (50% of patients), the sinoatrial nodal artery (55% of cases), and acute marginal branches to the right ventricle. Frequently, these branches arise from their own coronary ostium in the right coronary sinus. Distally, it most commonly bifurcates into the posterior descending artery and posterolateral artery.

Coronary Artery Anomalies

Coronary artery anomalies are found on 1.0% to 1.5% of coronary angiograms (Table 2). Of these, 90% are abnormalities in the origin or distribution of a coronary artery and 10% are abnormal fistulas. Coronary anomalies are often classified as benign or clinically significant; most of them are benign.

Benign Coronary Artery Anomalies

The most common are separate ostia of the left anterior descending and circumflex arteries. These occur in 0.4% to 1% of patients and may be associated with a bicuspid aortic valve.

The circumflex artery may arise from the right coronary sinus or as an early branch of the right coronary artery. When present, the circumflex artery virtually always travels behind the aorta to lie in the left atrioventricular groove (Fig. 2).

Rarely, there may be no circumflex artery; in this case, a superdominant right coronary artery supplies the entire left atrioventricular groove and left posterolateral wall.

Although these anomalies are benign, they must be recognized by the angiographer.

Clinically Significant Anomalies

The most common is a coronary artery that originates from the contralateral aortic sinus (that is, the left main or left anterior descending coronary artery from the right sinus of Valsalva or the right coronary artery from

Table 2. Coronary Artery Anomalies Among 126,595 Angiograms

Type of anomaly	Incidence, %	Anomalies, %
Benign (80%)		
Separate, adjacent		
LAD and LCx ostia	0.40	30.0
LCx		
LCx origin from		
RSV or RCA	0.40	30.0
Anomalous origin		
from PSV	<0.01	0.3
Anomalous origin		
from aorta		
LMCA	0.01	1.0
RCA	0.15	10.0
Absent LCx	0.003	0.2
Small fistulae	0.10	10.0
Clinically significant (20%)		
Origin of coronary		
artery from opposite		
aortic sinus		
LMCA from RSV	0.02	1.0
LAD from RSV	0.03	2.0
RCA from LSV	0.10	10.0
Anomalous origin		
from pulmonary		
artery		
LMCA	<0.01	<1.0
LAD or RCA	<0.01	<1.0
Single coronary artery	0.05	3.0
Multiple or large		
coronary fistulae	0.05	3.0

LAD, left anterior descending; LCx, left circumflex; LMCA, left main coronary artery; LSV, left sinus of Valsalva; PSV, posterior sinus of Valsalva; RCA, right coronary artery; RSV, right sinus of Valsalva.

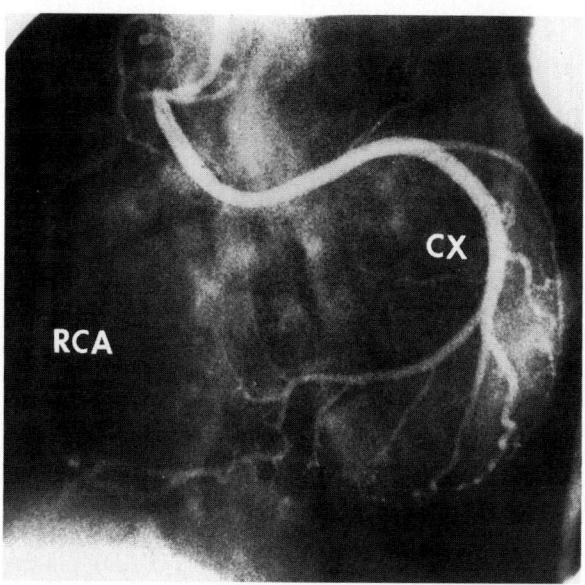

Fig. 2. Anomalous origin of the circumflex coronary artery (CX) from the right coronary artery (RCA). This anomaly occurs in 0.4% of cases. The circumflex branch arises from or near the ostium of the right coronary artery and courses posteriorly to supply the obtuse margin of the heart.

the left sinus of Valsalva). It is important to identify the course as it relates to the great vessels, because if it courses between the aorta and the pulmonary artery, symptoms may occur. In tetralogy of Fallot, the left anterior descending artery arises from the right coronary artery in 4% of patients.

A coronary artery may arise from the pulmonary artery. Most commonly, this is the left main coronary artery, less commonly the left anterior descending artery, and least commonly the right coronary artery. Nearly 90% of patients with these anomalies die during infancy. If the patient survives, the anomalous artery fills retrogradely through collaterals and drains into the pulmonary artery (left-to-right shunt). This condition may cause angina, infarction, and heart failure; it warrants surgical repair (ligation and grafting or reanastomosis to the aorta or subclavian artery).

Coronary Fistula

A coronary artery fistula is an abnormal connection between one of the coronary arteries and another structure, most commonly a venous structure or chamber on the right side of the heart. The right coronary artery is

the site of the fistula in 55% of patients. The majority of coronary artery fistulas empty into the right ventricle, right atrium, or coronary sinus. Less common are fistulas that empty into the pulmonary artery, left atrium, or left ventricle. Generally, the shunt is small, the myocardial blood flow to the terminal branches of the involved coronary artery is not compromised, and the patients are asymptomatic. However, if the shunt is large, pulmonary hypertension, congestive heart failure, bacterial endocarditis, rupture, and myocardial ischemia in the terminal portion of the involved coronary artery can occur.

- Coronary artery dominance is defined by the artery that gives rise to the posterior descending artery.
- In tetralogy of Fallot, the left anterior descending artery arises from the right coronary artery in 4% of patients.

Angiographic Views

Angiography should visualize all segments of the coronary arteries and their branches (and bypass grafts, if present) in at least two orthogonal views. All segments of the coronary arteries must be seen without foreshortening and without being obscured by overlapping branches, so that stenoses can be appropriately evaluated. To do this, multiple projections must be used combining cranial and caudal angulation with right and left angulation.

The four views of the left coronary arteries and two views of the right coronary artery in Figures 3 to 8 are the most commonly encountered views and the views from which one is expected to identify the major coronary arteries and their major branches. Figure 9 shows coronary artery bridging.

Coronary Artery Lesions

The grading of coronary artery stenoses is usually expressed as a percentage of the nearest normal segment of the same artery. For example, the lumen of an artery reduced to 20% of normal is expressed as an 80% stenosis. Because stenoses are often eccentric, orthogonal views must be obtained. When the degree of stenosis appears to differ significantly in orthogonal views, the most severe stenosis is commonly reported. However, some cardiologists report the average stenosis in the two views. Quantitative computer-assisted methods of quantifying coronary artery stenoses have been advocated

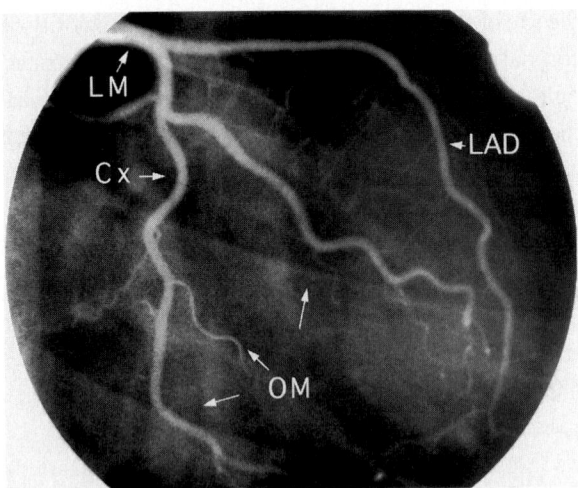

Fig. 3. The circumflex artery (Cx) and its branches are seen clearly on a right anterior oblique caudal projection of the left coronary system. LAD, left anterior descending artery; LM, left main coronary artery; OM, obtuse marginal branches.

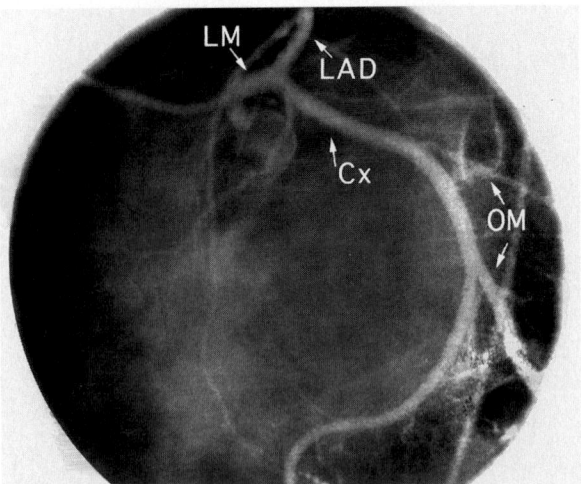

Fig. 4. The distal left main coronary artery (LM), the proximal left anterior descending artery (LAD), and the circumflex artery (Cx) and its branches (especially the proximal portion of its branches) are seen clearly on a left anterior oblique caudal view (termed the "spider view" because it looks somewhat like a spider). OM, obtuse marginal branches.

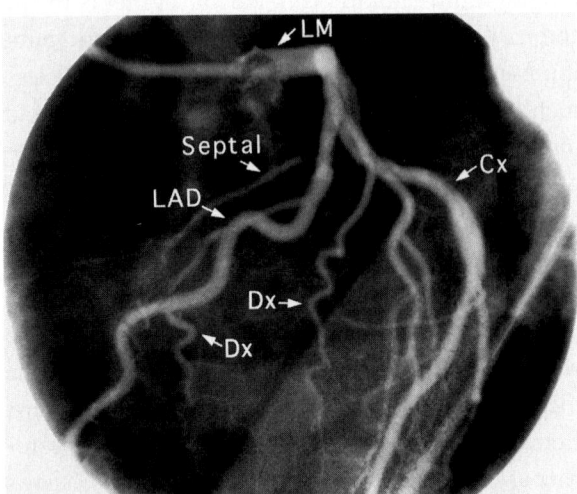

Fig. 5. The left anterior oblique cranial view shows the left anterior descending coronary artery (LAD) and diagonal branches (Dx). (Other abbreviations as in Figure 3.)

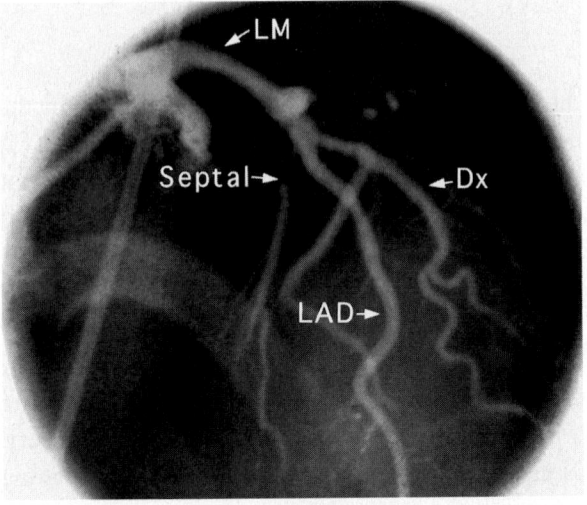

Fig. 6. A right anterior oblique cranial view nicely lays out the LAD and its branches. (Abbreviations as in Figure 5.)

because of their greater accuracy and reproducibility but have not yet become part of routine practice because of the time and expense associated with these methods.

Limitations of Coronary Angiography
It must always be remembered that a coronary angiogram is a "luminogram" and cannot be used to assess changes in wall thickness, a cardinal feature of

atherosclerosis. It relies on the presence of a normal segment of coronary artery, which may not exist, with which to compare a diseased segment. The absence of a normal segment will serve to underestimate the severity and extent of atherosclerosis. Furthermore, measurements of luminal diameter do not take into account any intraluminal obstruction that may be present

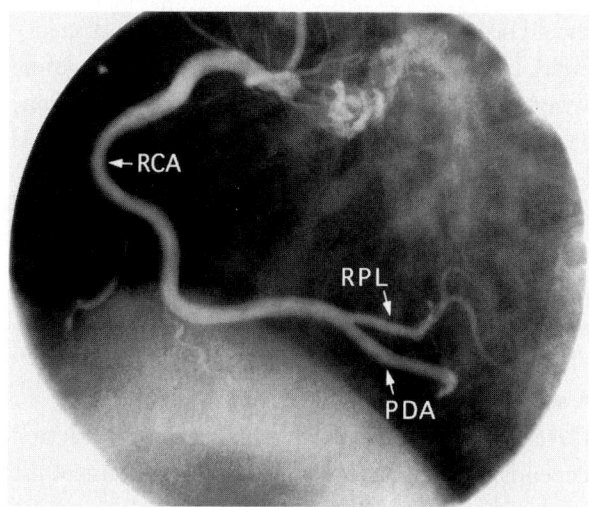

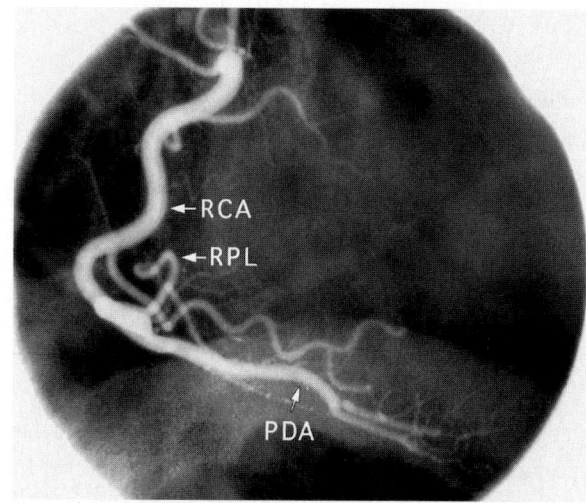

Fig. 7. A left anterior oblique projection of the right coronary artery (RCA) (a dominant right coronary artery) clearly shows the artery and its two main branches, the right posterolateral (RPL) and the posterior descending (PDA) arteries.

Fig. 8. A right anterior oblique projection shows the main portion of the right coronary artery (RCA) and the posterior descending artery (PDA), but individualized views with cranial or caudal angulation are often required to show the right posterolateral (RPL) branch well.

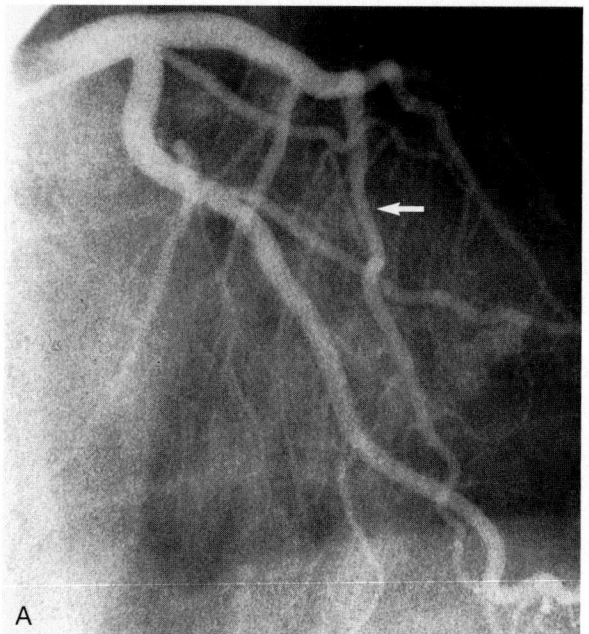

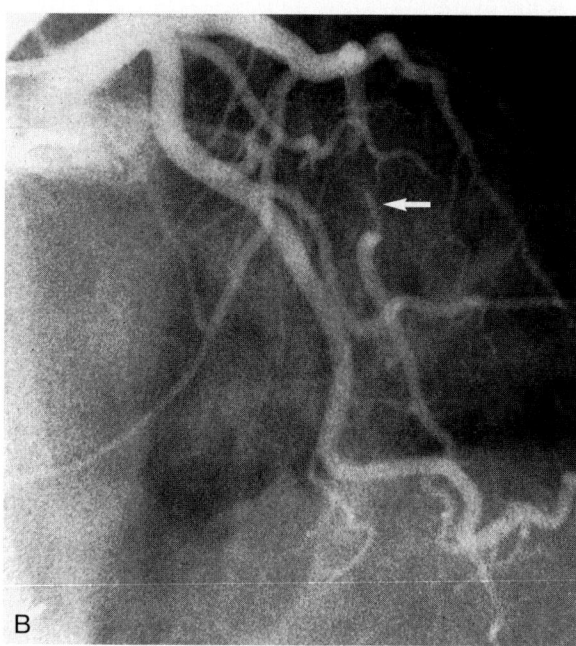

Fig. 9. Coronary artery bridging. *A*, Right anterior oblique view of the left coronary artery in diastole. The left anterior descending coronary artery is only minimally narrowed (*arrow*). *B*, Systolic frame showing obliteration of the middle left anterior descending coronary artery (*arrow*) due to muscular bridging.

because of thrombus or protruding tissue due to a ruptured plaque; these can be suggested only indirectly by the presence of certain characteristic angiographic features such as haziness, a mobile object in the vessel lumen, and the appearance of contrast agent on three sides of an unopacified filling defect. Intravascular ultrasonography and angioscopy are able to provide important information about coronary arteries when the limitations of coronary angiography become relevant in the management of a patient.

Left Ventriculography

Indications for Ventriculography
Indications for left ventriculography include the need to assess left ventricular function or the presence and severity of mitral regurgitation.

Technique
A catheter is advanced to the aortic root, and the aortic valve is crossed retrogradely in a 30° right anterior oblique (RAO) projection. The catheter is placed in a stable position in the left ventricle, and left ventricular pressure is measured. The catheter then is connected to a power injector, and the contrast agent is injected through the catheter into the left ventricle. Biplane images of the ventriculogram are preferred (generally, 30° RAO and 60° LAO), which are more comprehensive and provide a much more accurate assessment of the posterior left ventricle than the RAO view alone.

Contraindications to Ventriculography
Alternative ways of determining left ventricular function should be used for patients at high risk for ventriculography. High-risk patients include those with 1) severe symptomatic aortic stenosis; 2) moderate-severe congestive heart failure or angina at rest from any cause; 3) left ventricular thrombus; 4) endocarditis involving the aortic or mitral valve; and 5) renal failure. Patients with mechanical aortic valve prostheses should not undergo passage of a catheter retrogradely through the prostheses.

Assessment of Ejection Fraction and Wall Motion
Determination of left ventricular ejection fraction depends on defining the endocardial contours of the ventricle at end-systole and end-diastole, accurate calibration, and assumptions about the shape of the left ventricle. The left ventricle is assumed to be an ellipsoid with minor axes that are equal. Wall motion (the motion of each myocardial region) is classified as normal, mildly hypokinetic, moderately hypokinetic, severely hypokinetic, akinetic, or dyskinetic (Fig. 10).

Figures 11 through 16 are examples of uncommon abnormalities demonstrated by ventriculography.

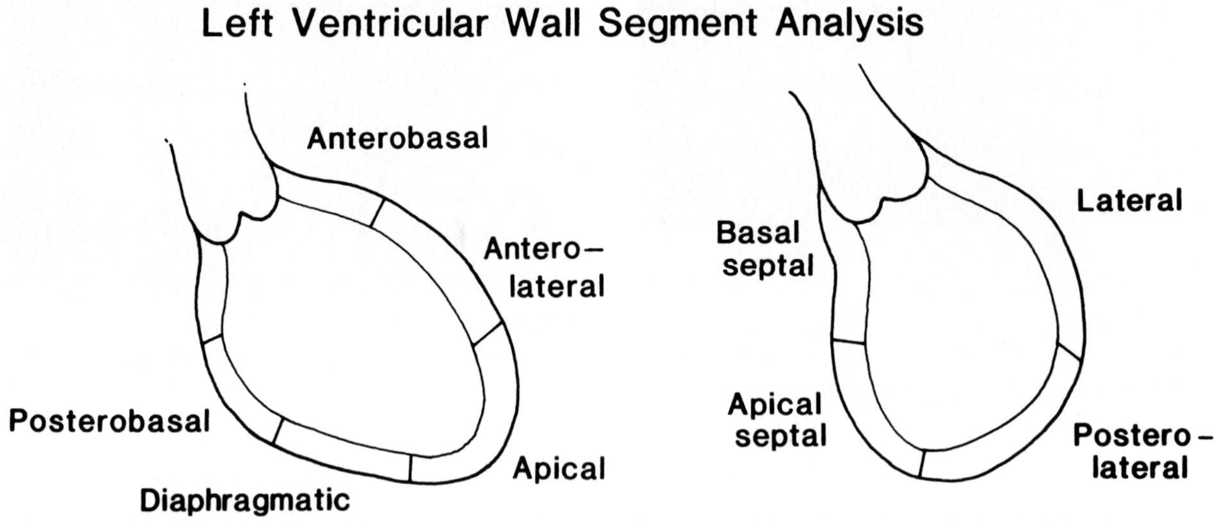

Left Ventricular Wall Segment Analysis

Fig. 10. Analysis of left ventricular wall motion. The outline of the left ventricular cavity in the right anterior oblique (RAO) (*left*) and left anterior oblique (LAO) (*right*) views is demonstrated. The RAO view shows anterobasal, anterolateral, apical, diaphragmatic, and posterobasal segments. The LAO view shows lateral, posterolateral, apical septal, and basal septal segments.

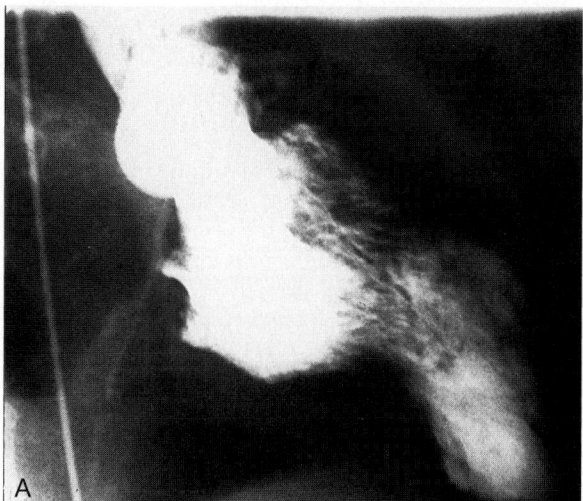
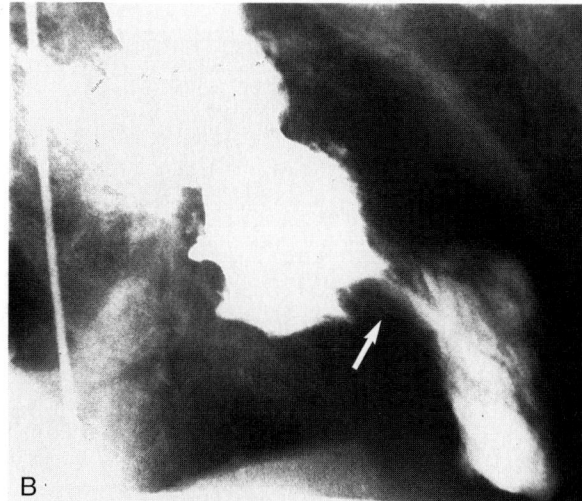

Fig. 11. Right anterior oblique ventriculograms of hypertrophic cardiomyopathy. Diastole (*A*) and systole (*B*) with midcavity obliteration (*arrow*).

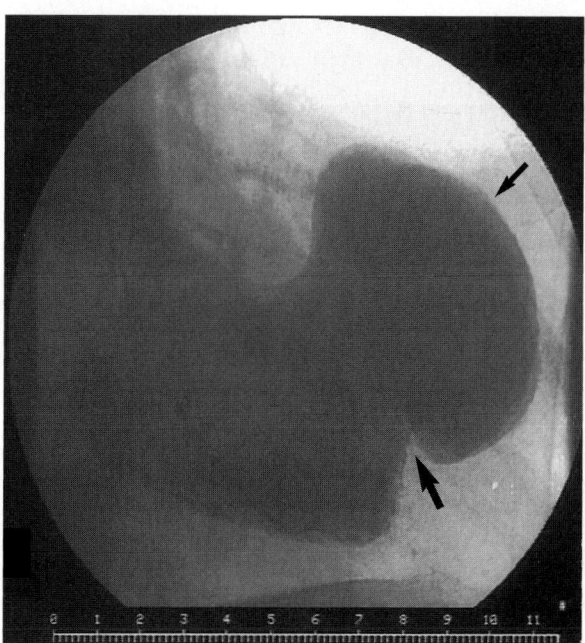

Fig. 12. Pseudoaneurysm of left ventricle (*thin arrow*) with well-defined neck (*thick arrow*).

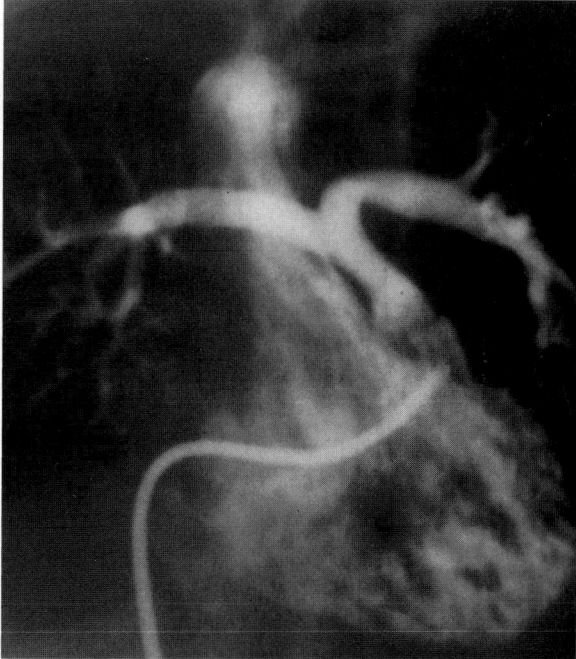

Fig. 13. Right ventriculogram demonstrating anatomy of tetralogy of Fallot. The pulmonary arteries are hypoplastic. The right ventricle is enlarged. The aorta fills with contrast material through the interventricular communication.

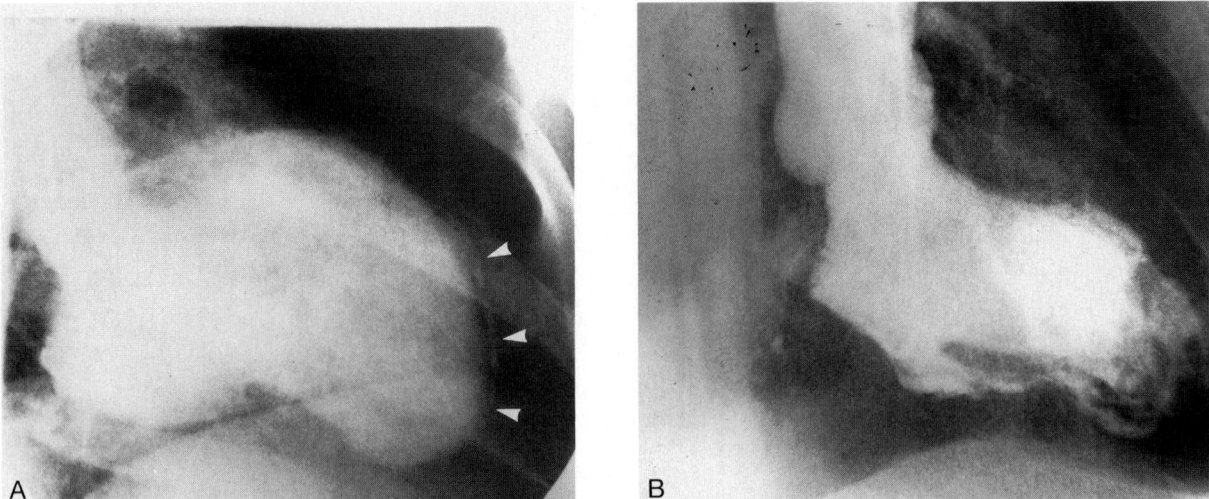

Fig. 14. *A*, Left ventriculogram in the right anterior oblique projection. A large anteroapical left ventricular aneurysm is present. A thin rim of calcification (*arrowheads*) is present along the anterolateral wall. The posterobasal and anterobasal segments showed systolic inward motion, but the remaining segments were dyskinetic. *B*, Anteroapical aneurysm with extensive apical mural thrombus.

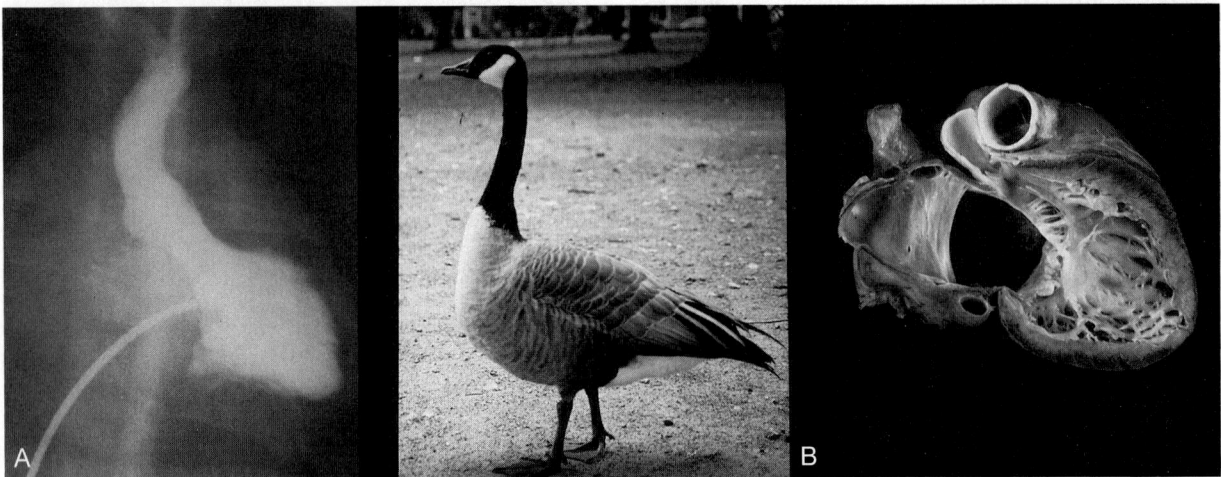

Fig. 15. *A*, Left ventriculogram demonstrating typical appearance in complete atrioventricular canal. *B*, Pathologic specimen. "Gooseneck" appearance of pathologic specimen and angiogram is apparent.

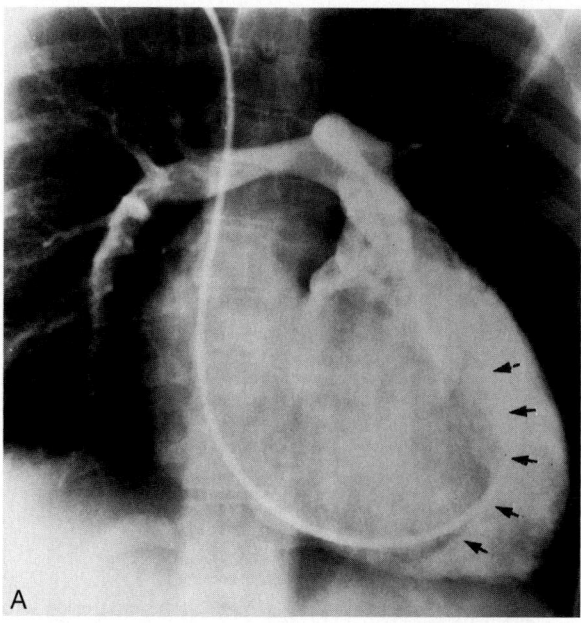

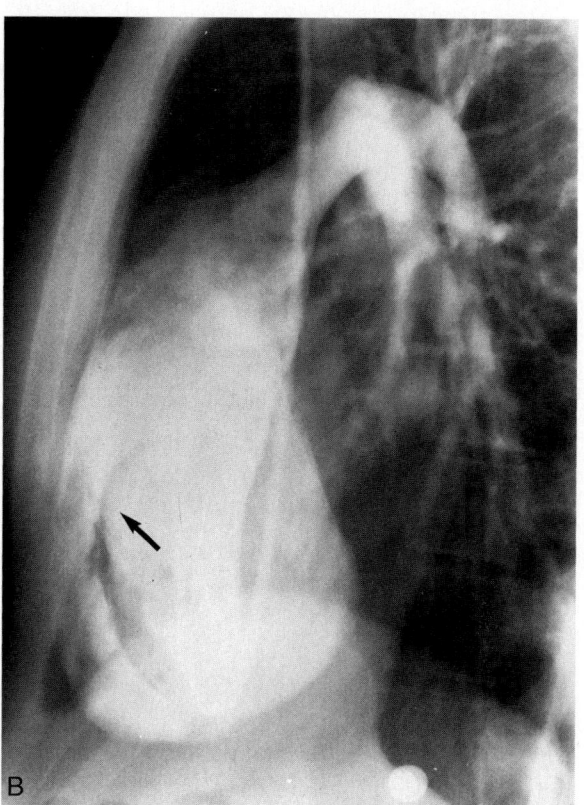

Fig. 16. Anteroposterior (*A*) and lateral (*B*) right ventriculograms from 21-year-old woman with Ebstein anomaly. Anteroposterior view shows large sail-like anterior leaflet (*arrows*) displaced well to left of spine. Severe tricuspid regurgitation is evident. Lateral projection displays pronounced anterior displacement of abnormal anterior tricuspid leaflet.

ATLAS OF CORONARY ANGIOGRAMS, VENTRICULOGRAMS, AND AORTOGRAMS

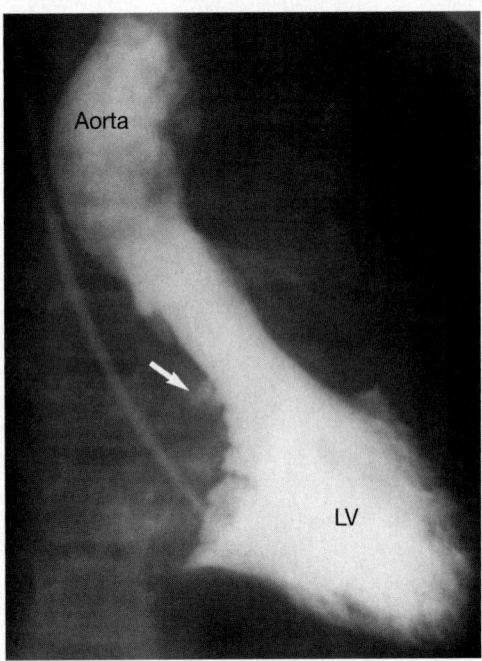

Fig. 17. RAO view. The catheter passed from the right side of the heart through an atrial septal defect and mitral valve into the left ventricle (LV). Left ventriculogram of primum atrial septal defect with typical gooseneck deformity of LV outflow tract (*arrow*).

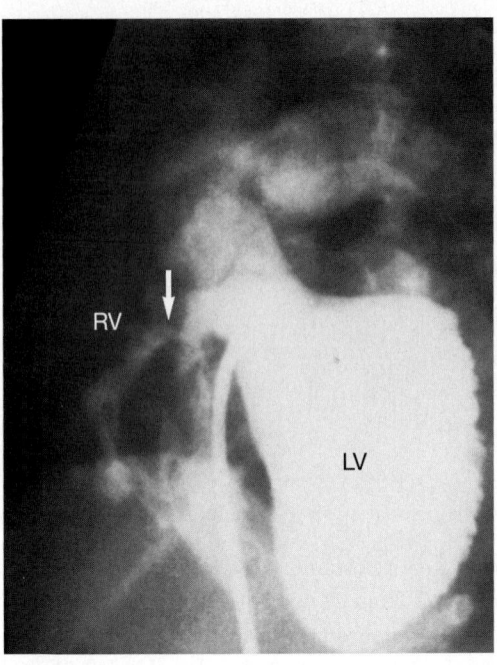

Fig. 18. LAO view. Left ventriculogram in membranous ventricular septal defect (*arrow*). LV, left ventricle; RV, right ventricle.

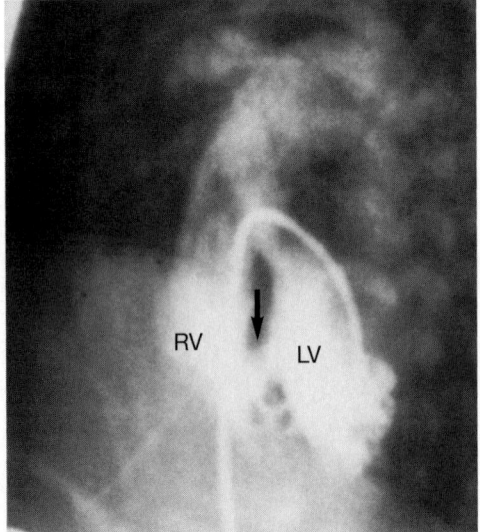

Fig. 19. LAO view. Left ventriculogram showing large muscular ventricular septal defect (*arrow*). RV, right ventricle.

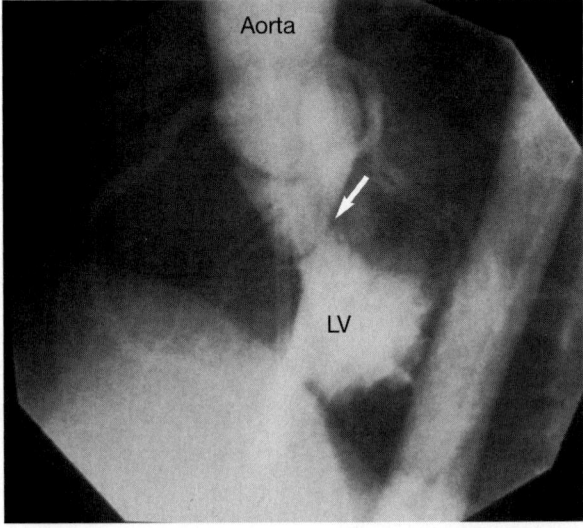

Fig. 20. LAO view. Left ventriculogram showing subvalvular aortic stenosis (*arrow*). LV, left ventricle.

The images in this atlas are typical of ones that may be shown on cardiology examinations. The atlas is not exhaustive for all examination images.

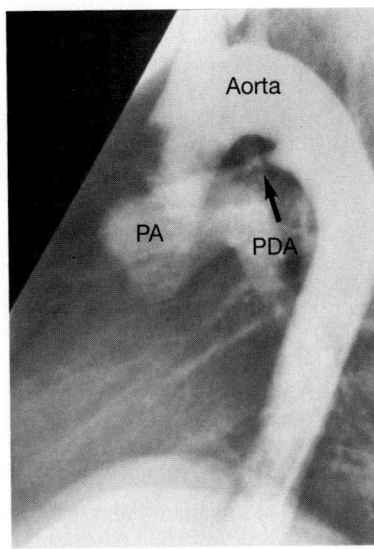

Fig. 21. Aortogram showing a patent ductus arteriosus (PDA) (*arrow*) with a significant left-to-right shunt. PA, pulmonary artery.

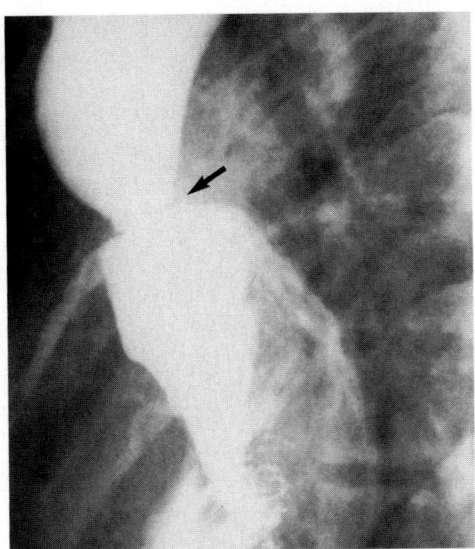

Fig. 22. LAO view. Left ventriculogram showing supravalvular aortic stenosis (*arrow*) (Williams syndrome). Other features (not shown) are pulmonary valve stenosis and infundibular stenosis.

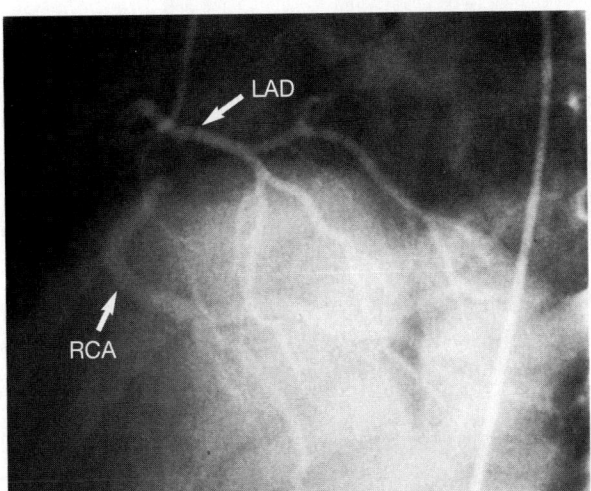

Fig. 23. Abnormal takeoff of the left anterior descending coronary artery (LAD) from the right coronary sinus in a patient with tetralogy of Fallot. RCA, right coronary artery.

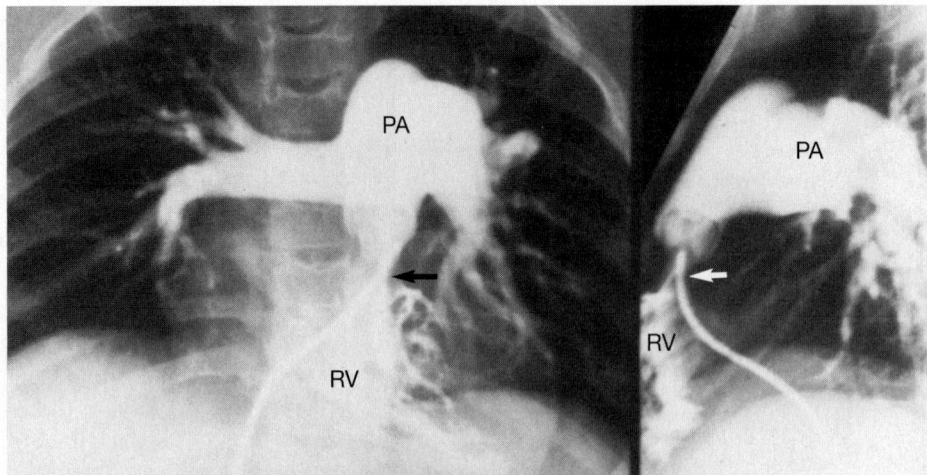

Fig. 24. Pulmonary angiogram showing severe pulmonary valve stenosis (*arrows*). Note unilateral pulmonary artery dilatation. PA, pulmonary artery; RV, right ventricle.

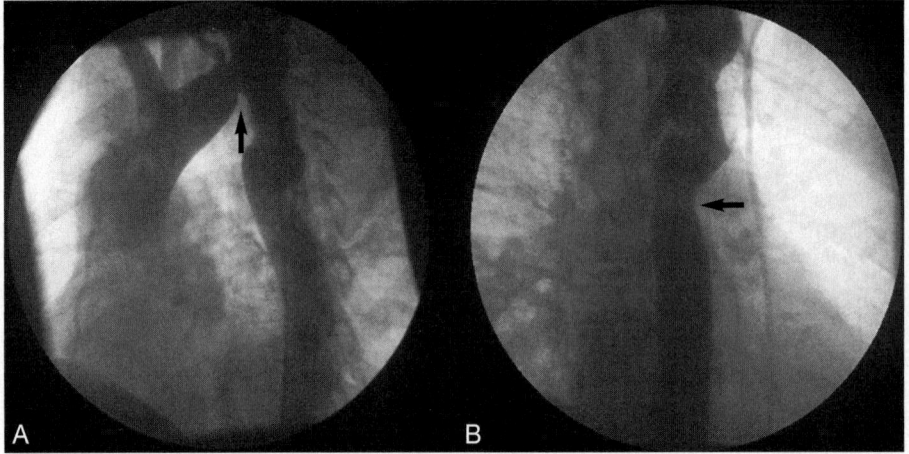

Fig. 25. *A*, LAO and, *B*, AP views of aortic injection. Note mild dilatation of the ascending aorta and moderate aortic coarctation (*arrow*).

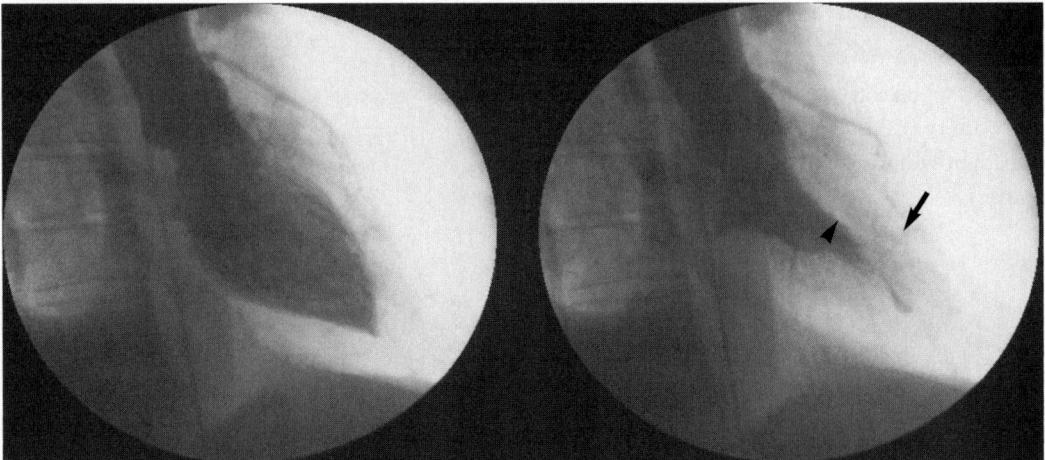

Fig. 26. RAO left ventriculogram showing hypertrophic cardiomyopathy with midcavitary (*arrowhead*) obstruction and apical secondary cavity (*arrow*).

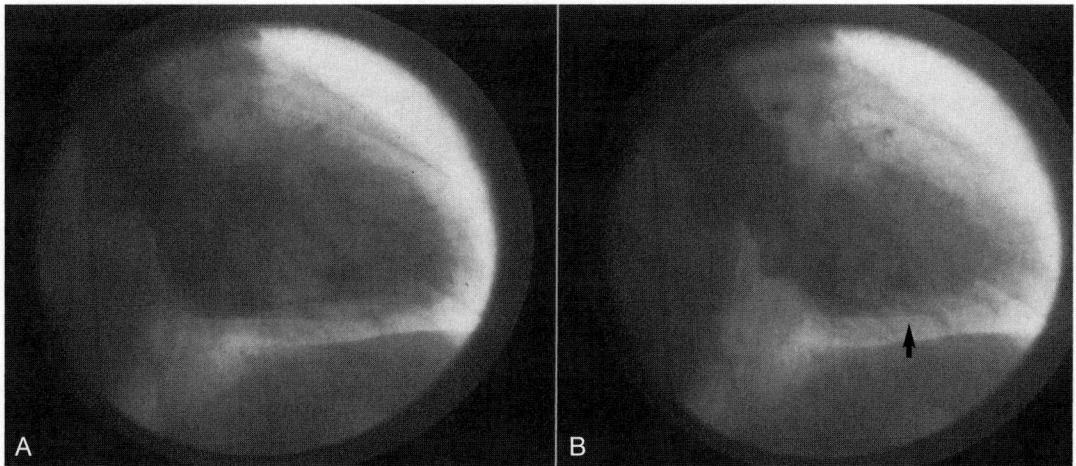

Fig. 27. RAO view of left ventriculogram in, *A*, diastole and, *B*, systole. Moderate left ventricular dilatation and dysfunction. Severe hypokinesis of diaphragmatic, posterobasal, and posterolateral segments (*arrow*).

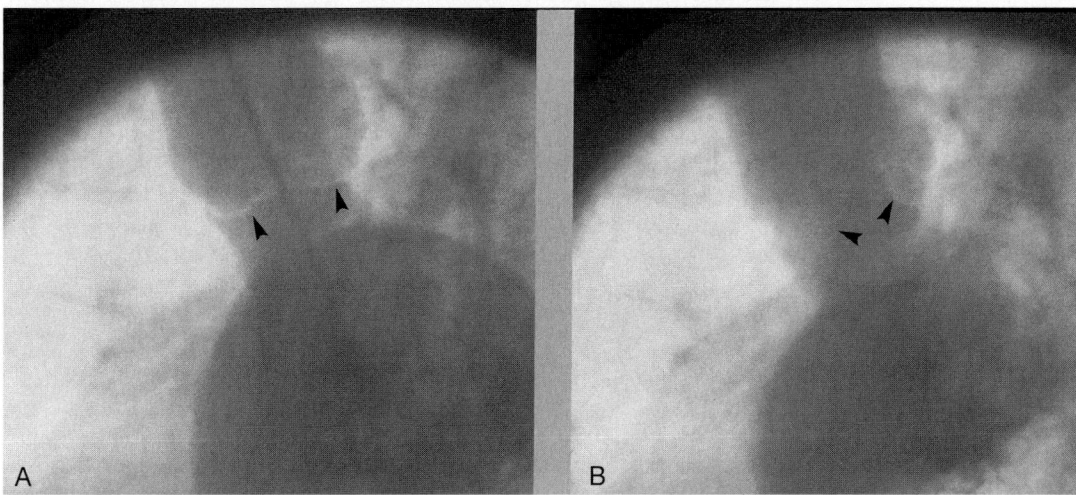

Fig. 28. LAO view of left ventriculogram (magnified) showing normal aortic valve leaflets (*arrowheads*) in, *A*, diastole and, *B*, systole.

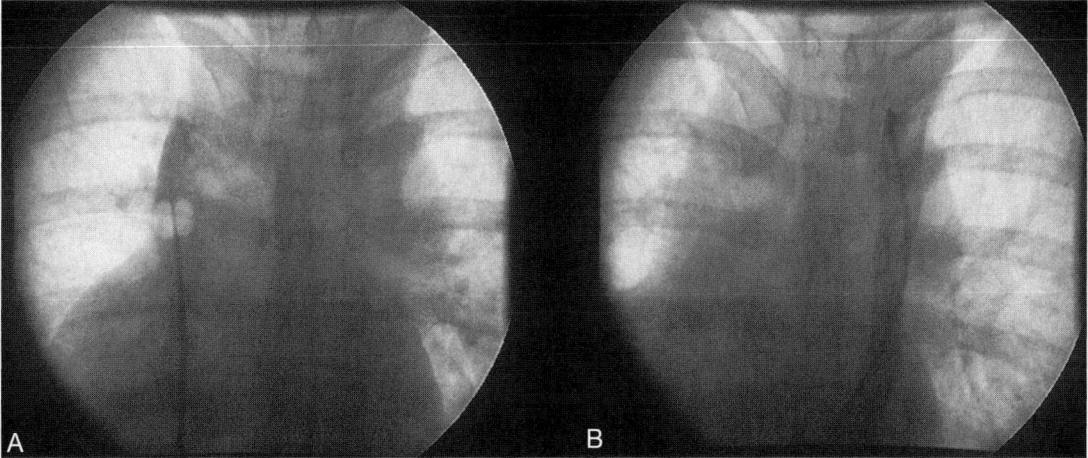

Fig. 29. Dextrocardia (situs solitus). *A*, Catheter progresses from inferior vena cava to right atrium to coronary sinus to left superior vena cava. *B*, Catheter progresses from inferior vena cava to right atrium to right superior vena cava.

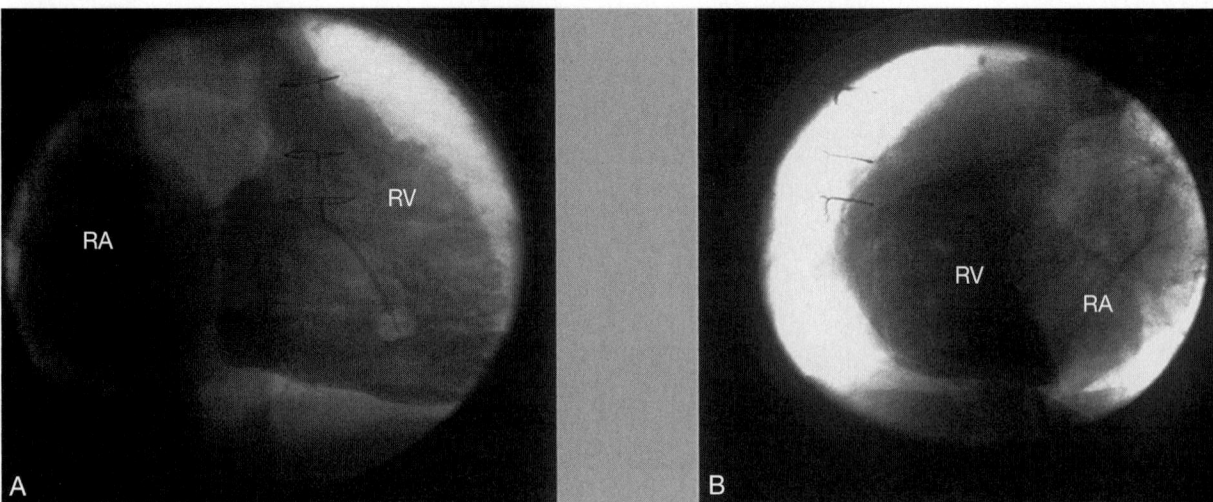

Fig. 30. *A*, RAO and, *B*, LAO images of right ventriculogram with balloon-tipped catheter. Moderate right ventricular (RV) dilatation and hypokinesis. Severe tricuspid regurgitation and moderate right atrial (RA) enlargement. Note sternal wires. LAO view superimposes RA and RV.

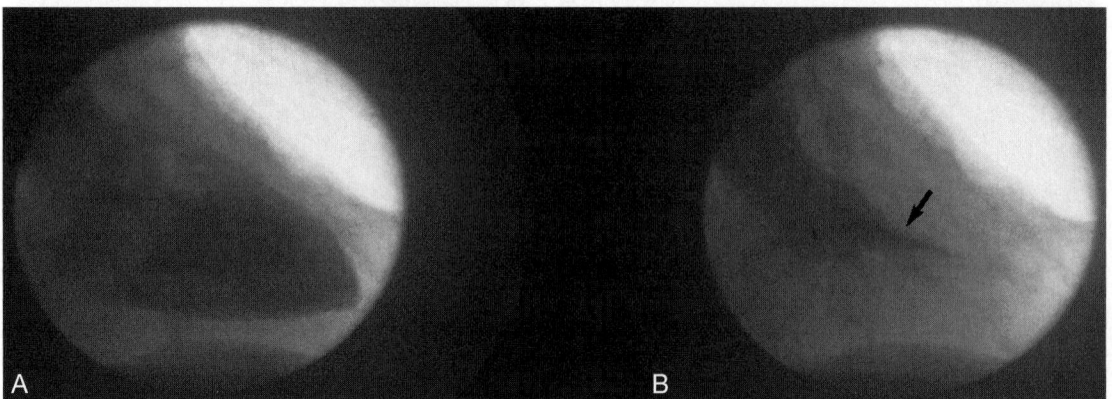

Fig. 31. RAO view of left ventriculogram in, *A*, diastole and, *B*, systole showing apical cavitary obliteration (*arrow*) from apical left ventricular hypertrophy or apical variant hypertrophic cardiomyopathy.

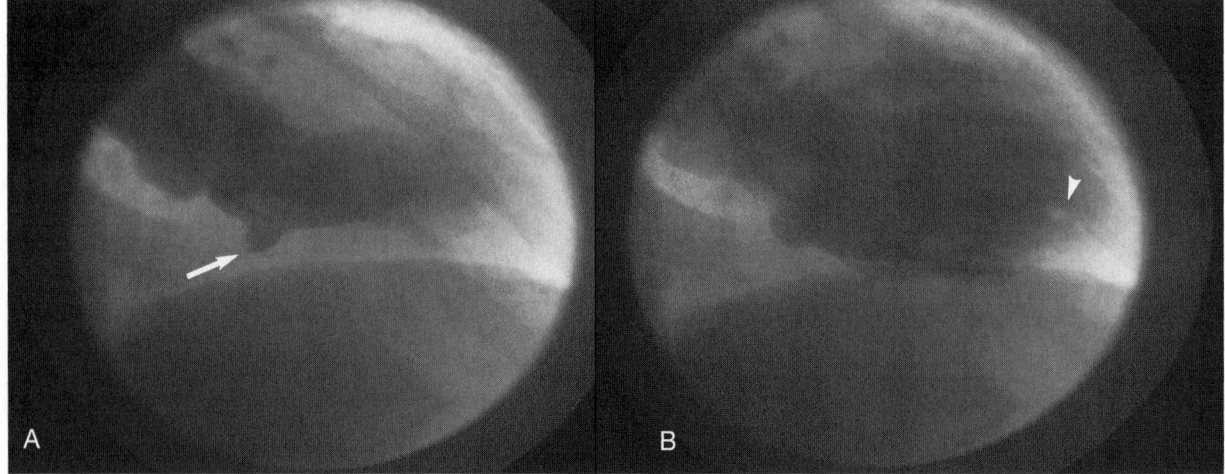

Fig. 32. RAO left ventriculogram. *A*, Mitral valve prolapse (*arrow*) without regurgitation. *B*, Apical filling defect suspicious for mural thrombus (*arrowhead*).

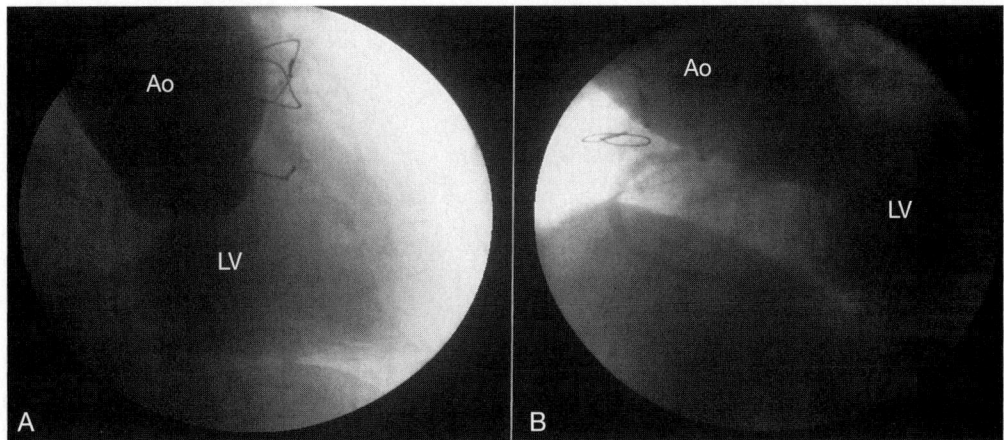

Fig. 33. *A*, RAO and, *B*, LAO views of aortic injection showing moderately severe dilatation of the aortic root (Ao) and probable bicuspid aortic valve with severe aortic regurgitation. Note indirect filling of saphenous vein graft to the right coronary artery. Sternal wires are present. LV, left ventricle.

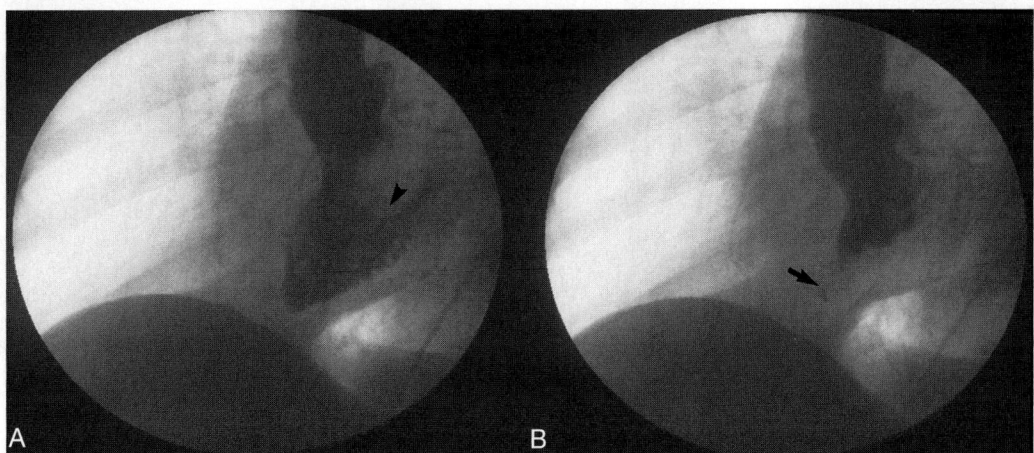

Fig. 34. LAO view of left ventricle in, *A*, diastole and, *B*, systole with hyperdynamic function. Note the prominent washout of contrast from brisk mitral inflow (*arrowhead* in *A*); this likely represents high left atrial pressure (i.e., restrictive filling pattern). Also note hypertrophic cardiomyopathy with mid-cavitary obstruction and apical cavity obliteration (*arrow* in *B*).

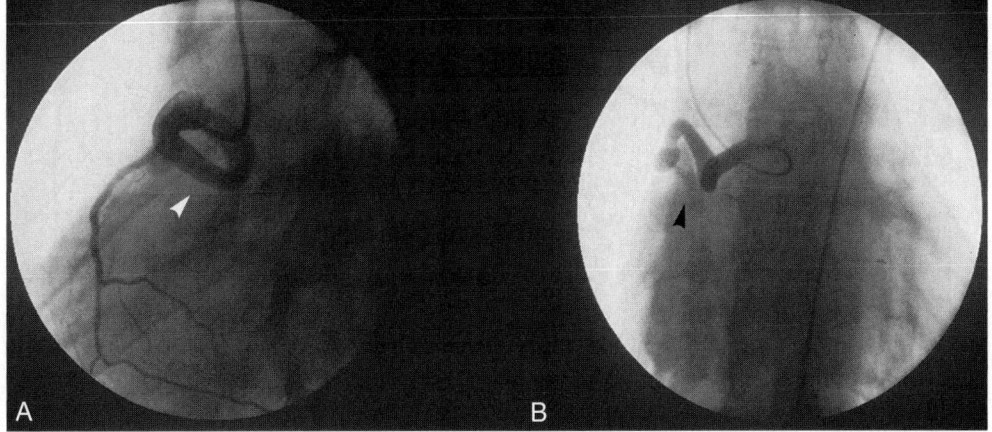

Fig. 35. *A*, LAO and, *B*, AP view of right coronary artery injection showing large fistula from right coronary artery to right atrium. *Arrowheads*, jet of flow.

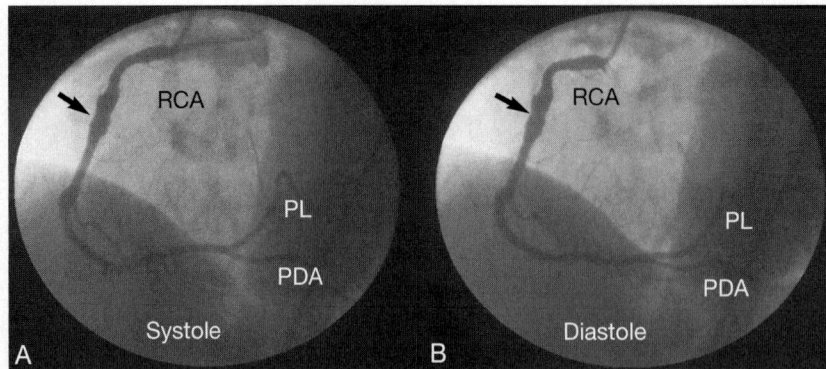

Fig. 36. LAO view in, *A*, systole and, *B*, diastole showing fixation of mid-right coronary (RCA), distal posterolateral (PL), and posterior descending (PDA) arteries from constrictive pericarditis. Note moderate ectasia/aneurysm (*arrows*) of mid-RCA.

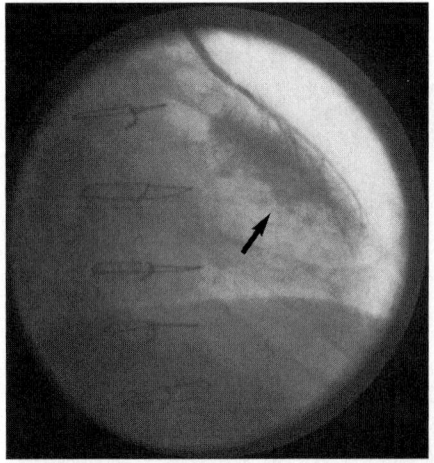

Fig. 37. AP view of saphenous vein graft to first diagonal artery. A large myocardial "blush" (*arrow*) is present after percutaneous transluminal coronary angioplasty of the graft. This likely occurred because of microembolization of the microcirculation.

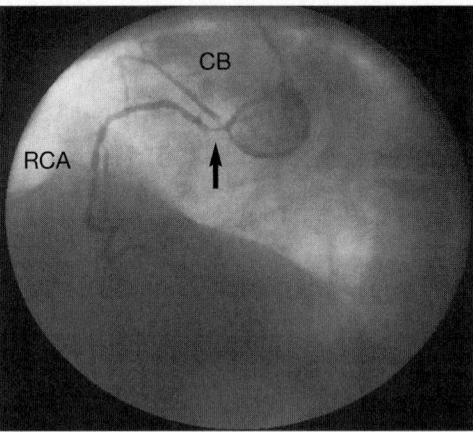

Fig. 38. LAO view of balanced dominant right coronary artery (RCA) with severe stenoses of the ostial and conus branch (CB) (*arrow*). Note contrast agent filling the right sinus of Valsalva.

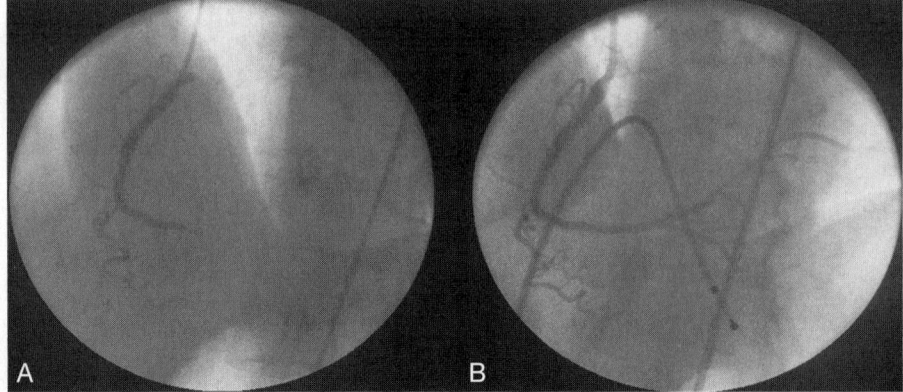

Fig. 39. LAO cranial image of occluded distal right coronary artery. Hazy tapered occlusion suggests thrombus. *B*, During percutaneous transluminal coronary angioplasty (PTCA) there was moderate distal embolization and slow reflow phenomenon. Note placement of temporary pacemaker in right ventricular apex for post-PTCA bradycardia and hypotension (Bezold-Jarisch reflex).

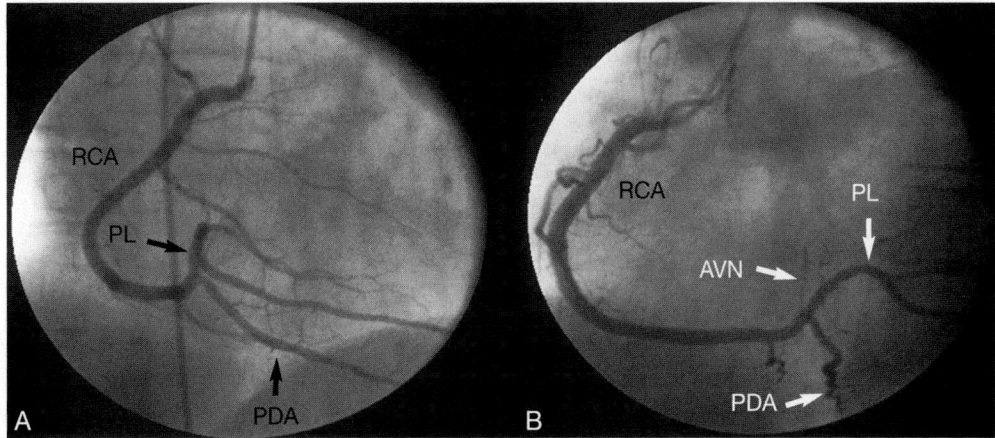

Fig. 40. *A*, RAO and, *B*, LAO views showing normal right coronary artery (RCA) (right dominant), right posterolateral artery (PL), posterior descending artery branch (PDA), and atrioventricular artery (AVN) (determining dominance).

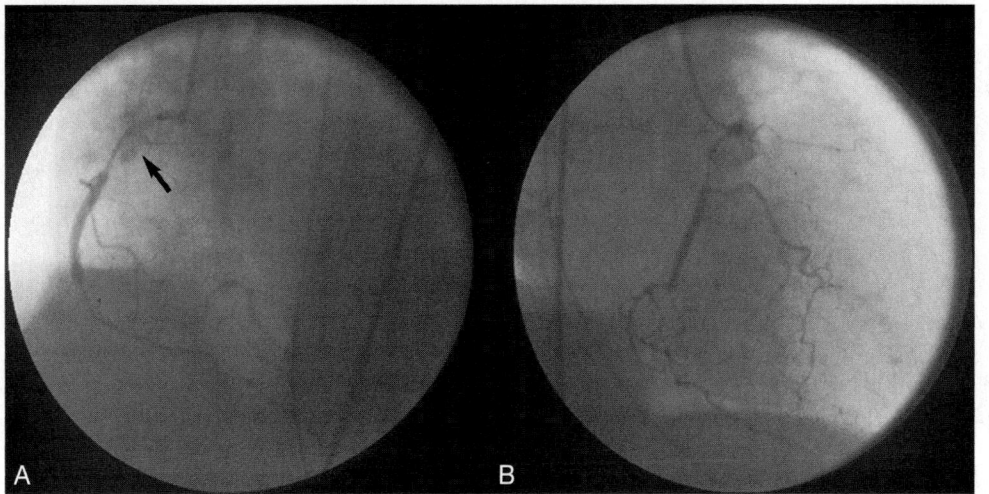

Fig. 41. *A*, LAO and, *B*, RAO views of right coronary artery with diffuse severe spasm (*arrow*) except in stented segment (midsection of the artery).

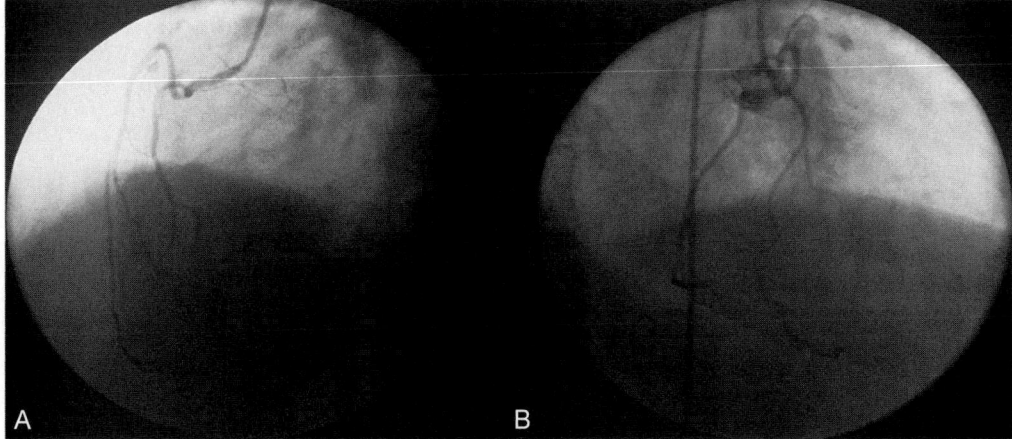

Fig. 42. *A*, LAO and, *B*, RAO views of normal nondominant right coronary artery. Note the diminutive size, predisposing to catheter damping. The artery does not supply the diaphragmatic myocardium. Also note the "shepherd's crook" bend in the proximal right coronary artery.

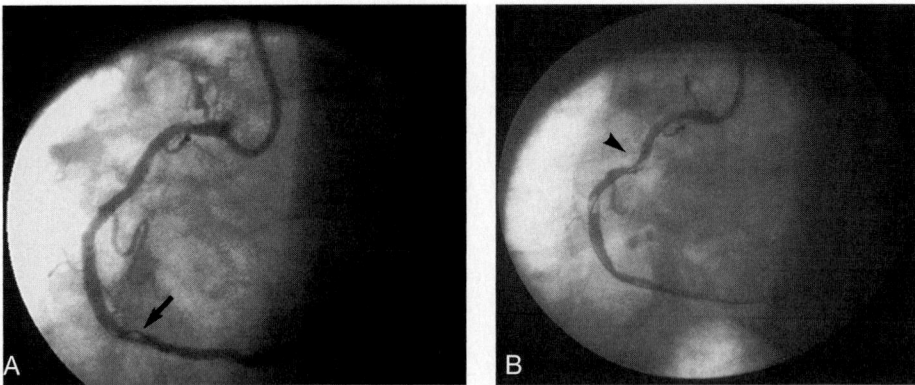

Fig. 43. LAO view of right coronary artery. *A,* A large intracoronary "ball" thrombus (*arrow*) is adherent to the guidewire following percutaneous transluminal coronary angioplasty (PTCA) for acute myocardial infarction. The thrombus was entwined in a second wire and removed successfully without complication. *B,* Note large post-PTCA dissection (*arrowhead*).

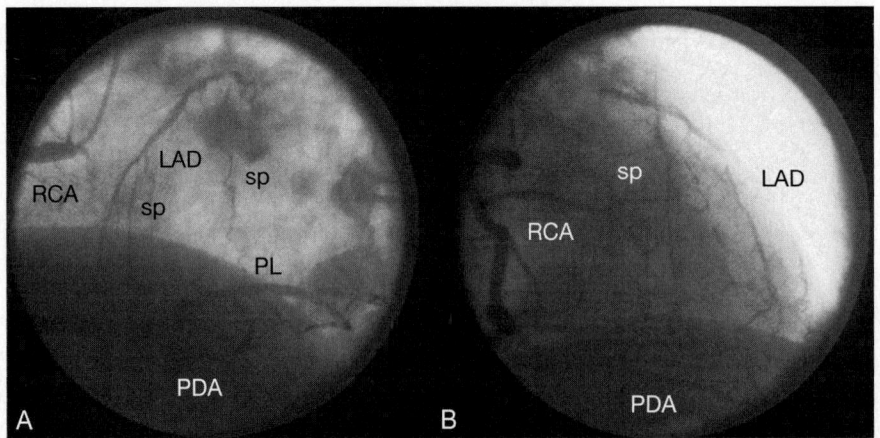

Fig. 44. *A,* LAO and, *B,* RAO views of right coronary artery (RCA) injection. Note mild stenoses of RCA. The left anterior descending artery (LAD) fills retrogradely via collateral vessels to the distal LAD and septal perforators (sp). The LAD is occluded proximally and moderate disease is scattered throughout it. PL, posterolateral artery; PDA, posterior descending artery.

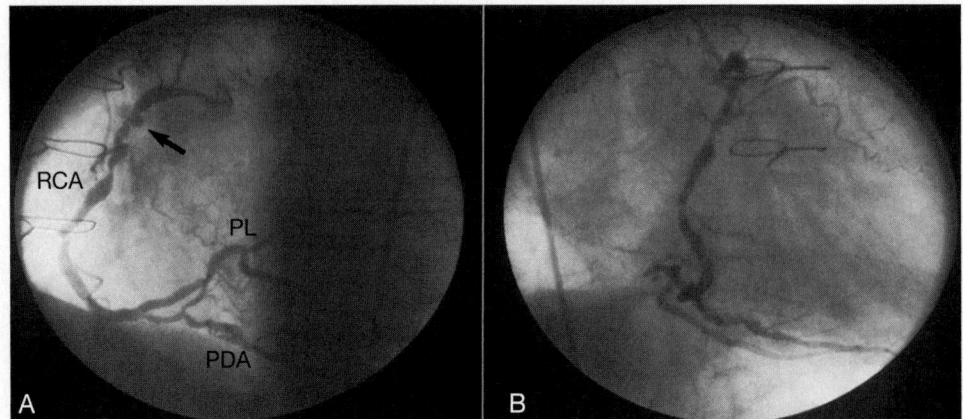

Fig. 45. *A,* LAO and, *B,* RAO views of the right coronary artery (RCA). Note severe stenoses of proximal and mid-RCA and posterolateral branch (PL) and atherosclerotic ulcer of the proximal RCA (*arrow*). Mild vessel ectasia vs. post-stenotic dilatation. PDA, posterior descending artery.

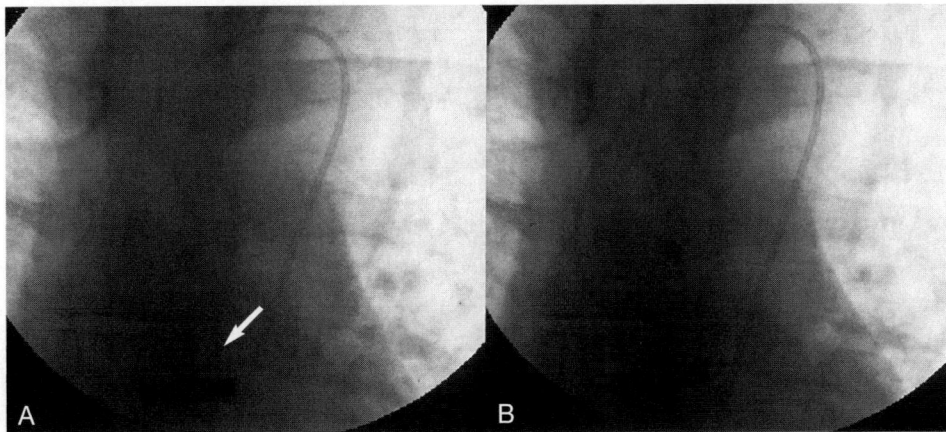

Fig. 46. Tilting disk mechanical prosthetic valve, *A*, open and, *B*, closed. Pigtail catheter is in the ascending aorta. *Arrow*, leaflet.

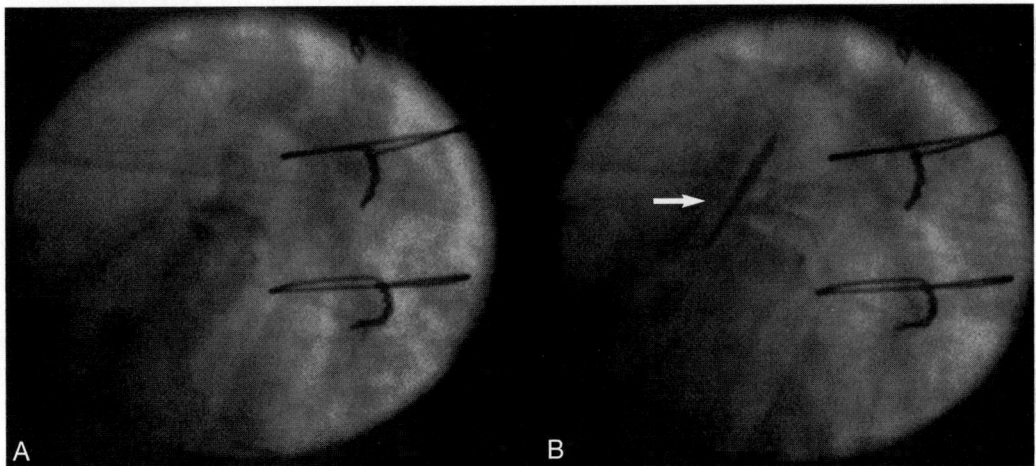

Fig. 47. Normally functioning bileaflet mechanical prosthetic aortic valve in, *A*, systole and, *B*, diastole. *Arrow*, leaflet.

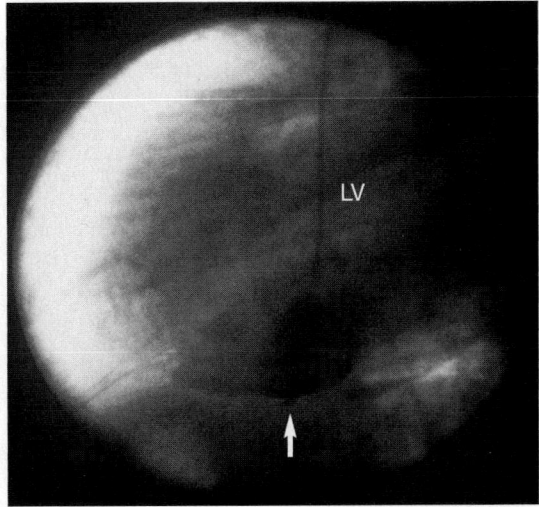

Fig. 48. LAO view of left ventriculogram. Myocardial infarction-associated ventriculoseptal defect. Intraventricular septum is seen as filling defect. Small inferior wall rupture (small jet immediately below catheter) (*arrow*). LV, left ventricle.

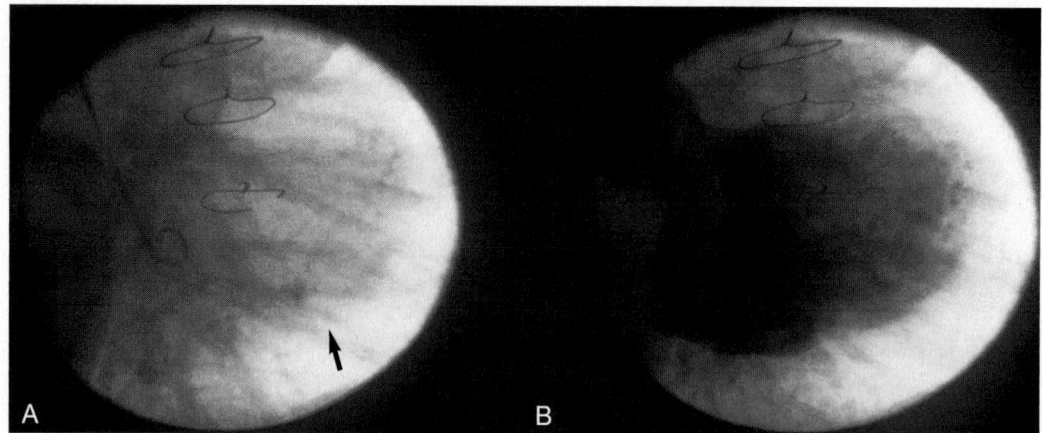

Fig. 49. RAO view of left ventriculogram showing apical mural calcification (*arrow*) compatible with old mural thrombus or calcified myocardial infarction scar or calcified ventricular aneurysm. *A*, Before injection of contrast agent and, *B*, during ventriculogram.

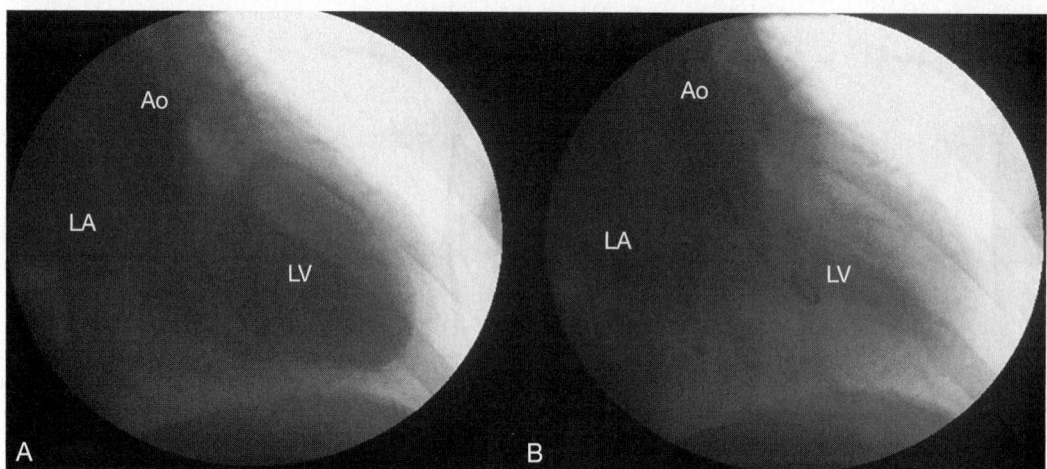

Fig. 50. RAO view of left ventriculogram in, *A*, diastole and, *B*, systole showing moderate left ventricular (LV) dilatation with normal function. Note severe mitral regurgitation. Ao, aorta; LA, left atrium.

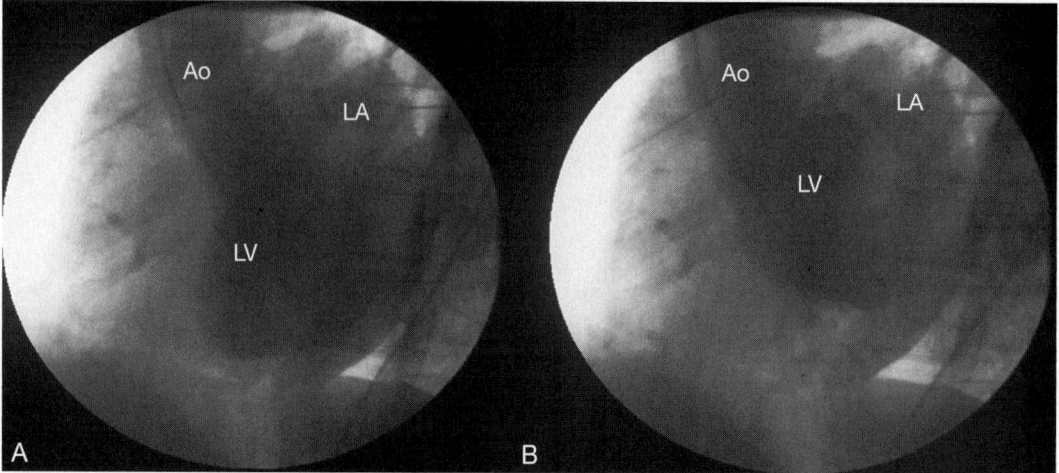

Fig. 51. LAO view of left ventriculogram in, *A*, diastole and, *B*, systole showing moderate left ventricular (LV) dilatation with normal function. Note severe mitral regurgitation. Ao, aorta; LA, left atrium.

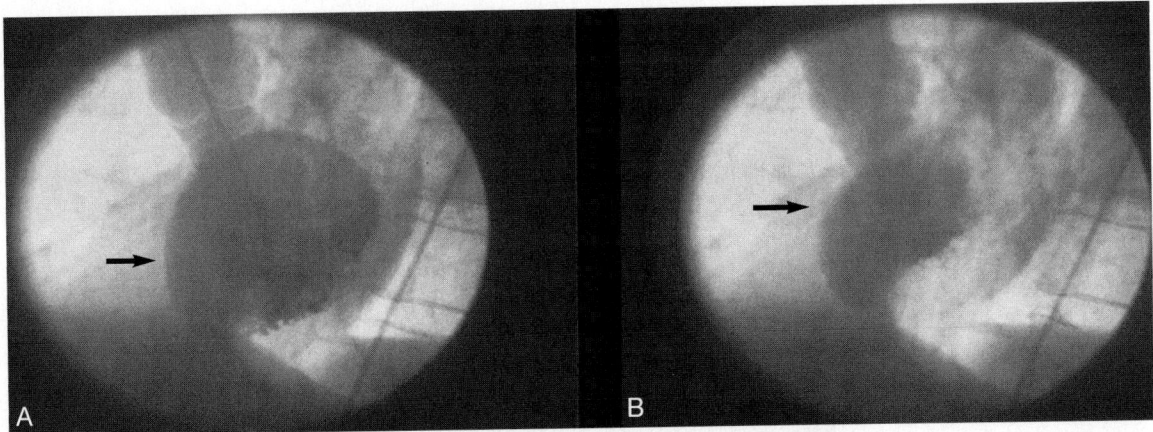

Fig. 52. LAO view of left ventriculogram in, *A*, diastole and, *B*, systole showing akinesis of the anteroapical wall segment (*arrows*).

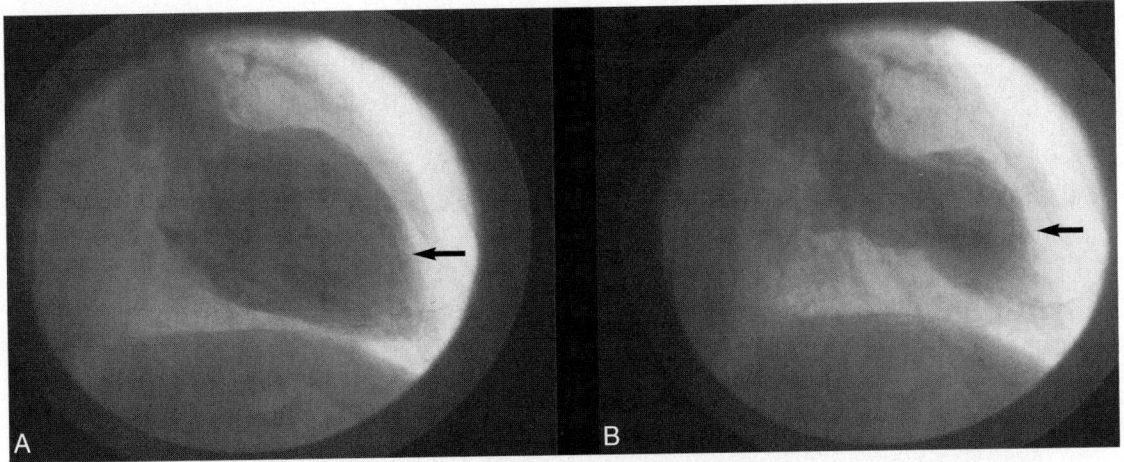

Fig. 53. RAO view of left ventriculogram in, *A*, diastole and, *B*, systole. The left ventricle has normal size but moderately reduced function. Note akinesis of the anterolateral and apical wall segments (*arrows*).

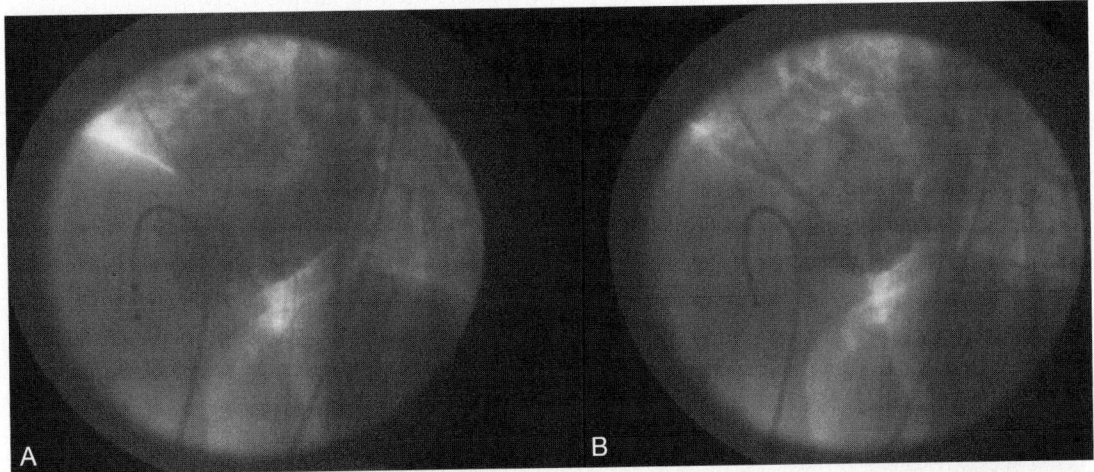

Fig. 54. LAO view of left ventriculogram in, *A*, diastole and, *B*, systole. Note normal size of the left ventricle and akinesis of the posterobasal and posterolateral wall segments. A temporary pacemaker has been placed in the right ventricular apex via the inferior vena cava.

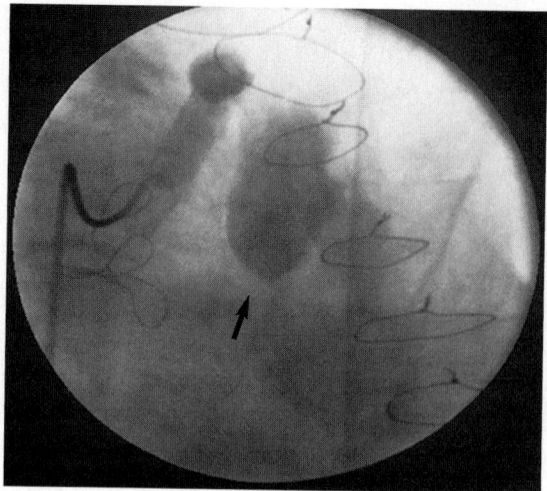

Fig. 55. Large aneurysm (*arrow*) of a saphenous vein graft.

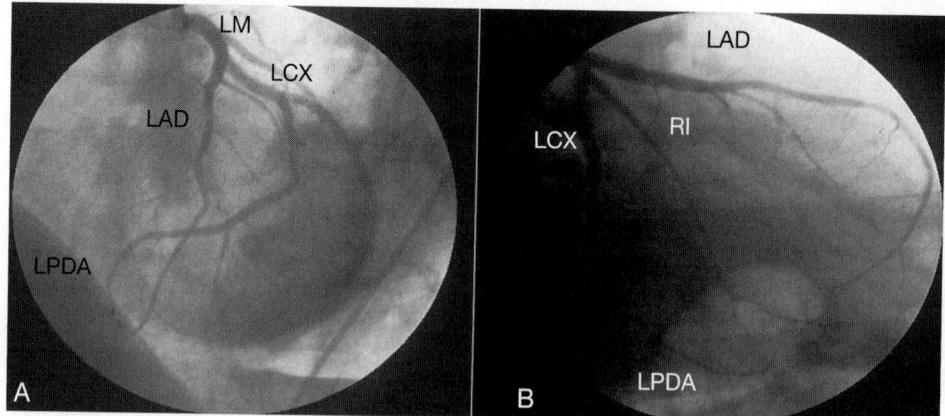

Fig. 56. *A*, LAO cranial and, *B*, RAO caudal views showing (left dominant) normal left main (LM), left anterior descending (LAD), left circumflex (LCX), and ramus intermedius (RI) arteries. Note left posterior descending arery (LPDA) wrapping around from LCX to the inferoseptal wall, meeting the wraparound LAD.

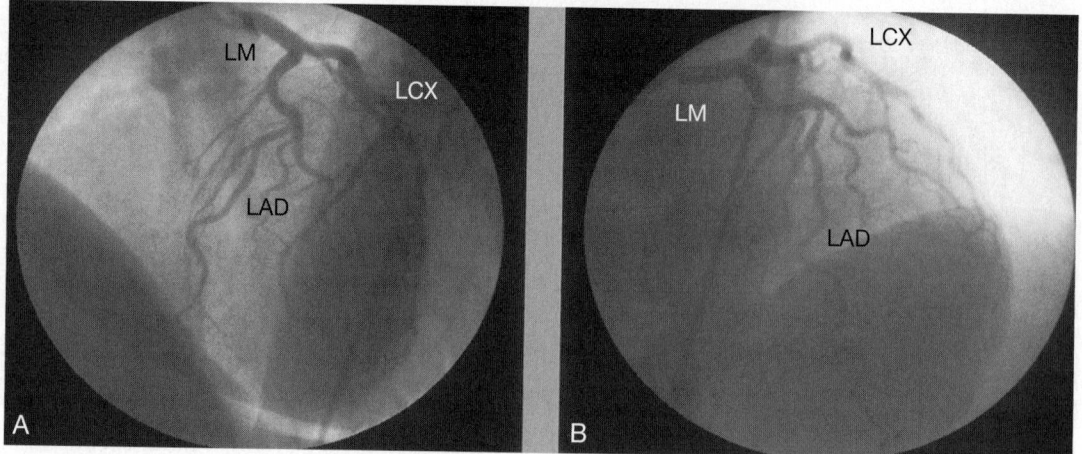

Fig. 57. *A*, LAO and, *B*, RAO cranial views of left main (LM) injection showing normal left anterior descending (LAD) and nondominant left circumflex (LCX) arteries and age-related tortuosity.

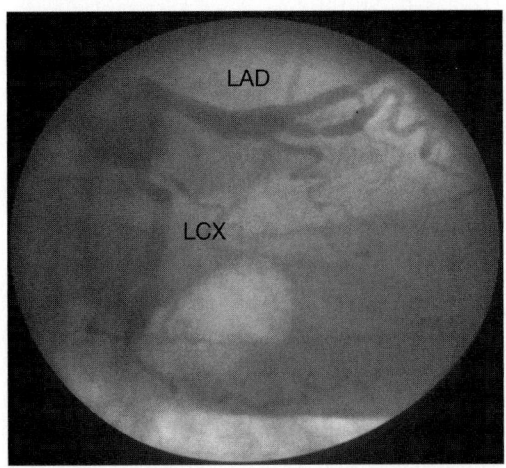

Fig. 58. RAO caudal view of moderate ectasia/aneurysmal disease of the left circumflex (LCX) and left anterior descending (LAD) arteries.

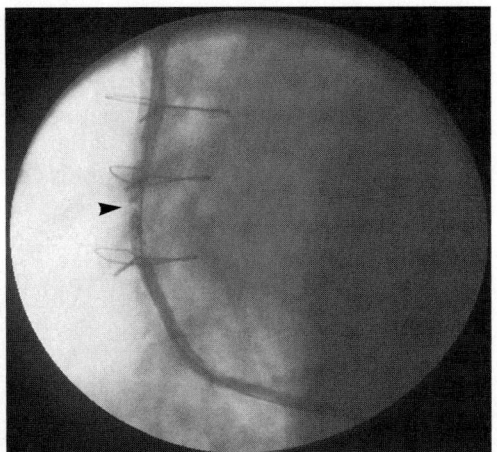

Fig. 59. LAO view of saphenous vein graft to distal right coronary artery. Extensive intraluminal thrombus appears as multiple hazy filling defects (*arrowhead*).

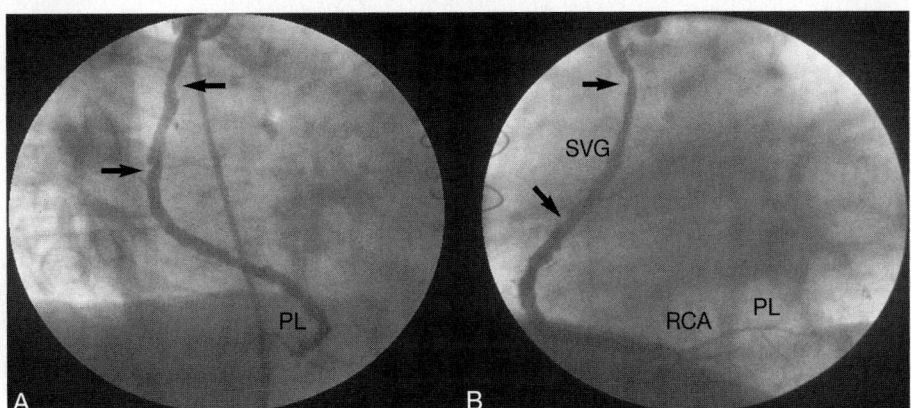

Fig. 60. Saphenous vein graft (SVG) to distal right coronary artery (RCA). Note moderate stenoses in graft body (*arrows*). PL, posterolateral artery.

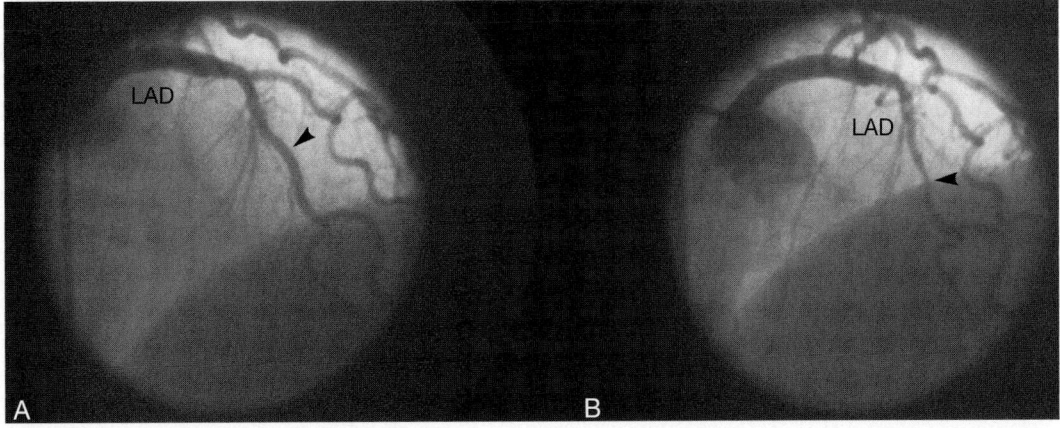

Fig. 61. Moderate bridging (*arrowheads*) of the mid-left anterior descending artery (LAD). RAO, right anterior oblique artery.

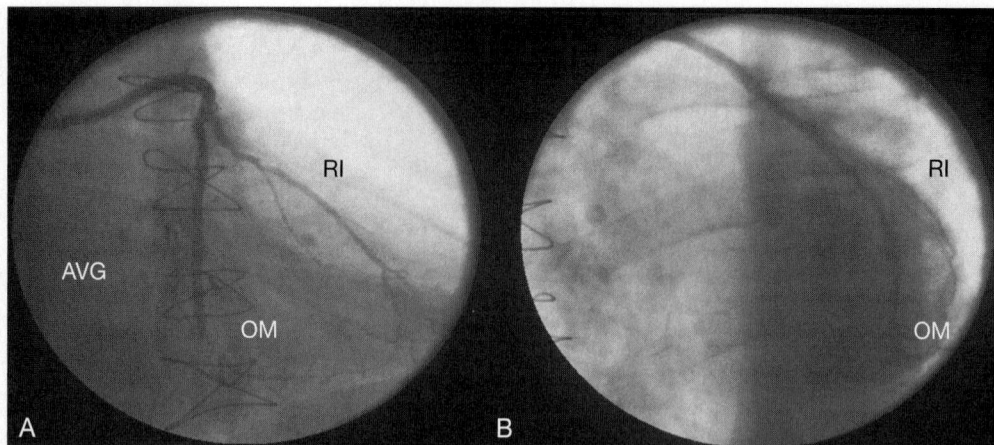

Fig. 62. Normal sequential saphenous vein graft to ramus intermedius artery (RI) and obtuse marginal (OM) artery. Note total occlusion of the distal left circumflex (no retrograde flow beyond the origin of OM and atrioventricular groove branch artery [AVG]).

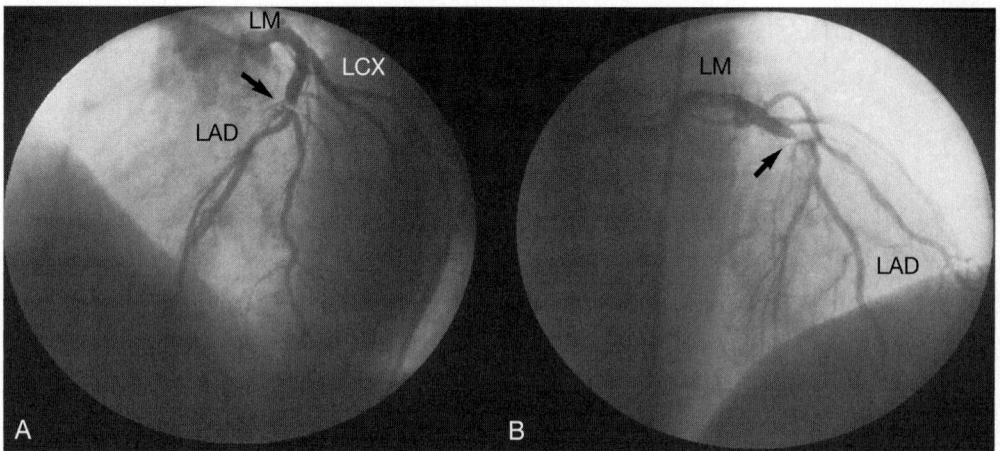

Fig. 63. *A,* LAO and, *B,* RAO cranial views of severe stenosis (*arrow*) of the proximal left anterior descending artery (LAD). LM, left main coronary artery; LCX, left circumflex artery.

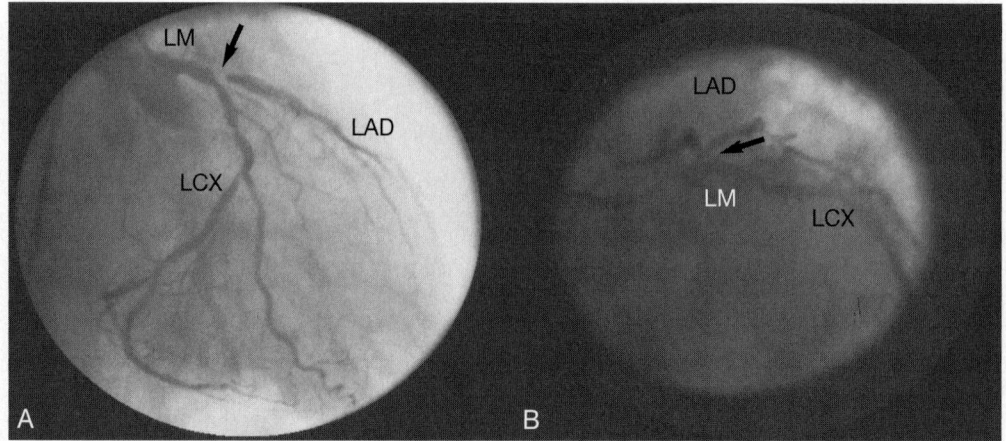

Fig. 64. *A,* RAO and, *B,* LAO caudal views showing severe stenosis (*arrow*) of the origin of the left anterior descending artery (LAD). Note mild stenoses of the left circumflex artery (LCX). LM, left main coronary artery.

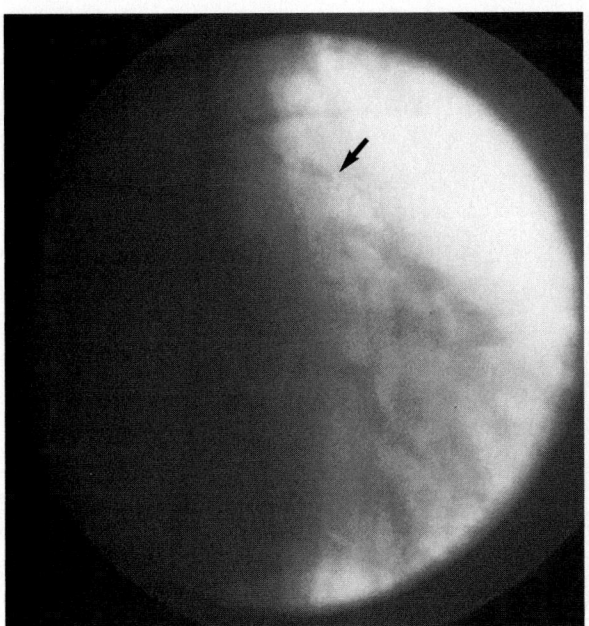

Fig. 65. RAO cranial view showing heavy calcification (*arrow*) of the proximal left anterior descending artery.

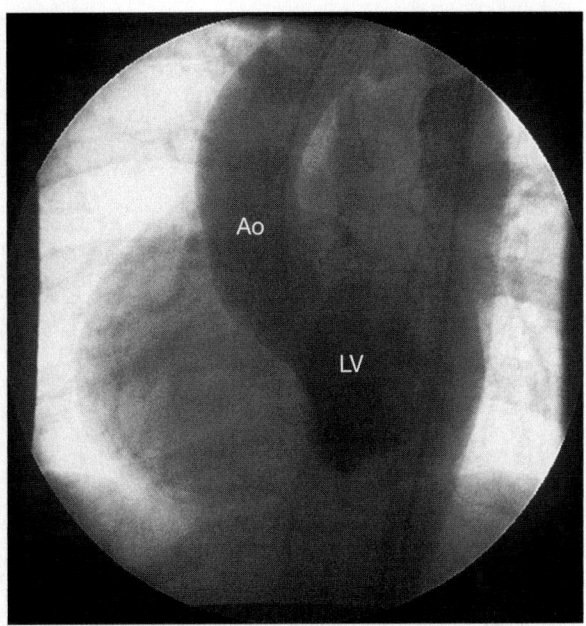

Fig. 66. RAO view of aortic injection showing severe aortic regurgitation. Note the equal density of the aorta (Ao) and left ventricle (LV). Note relatively normal left ventricular size.

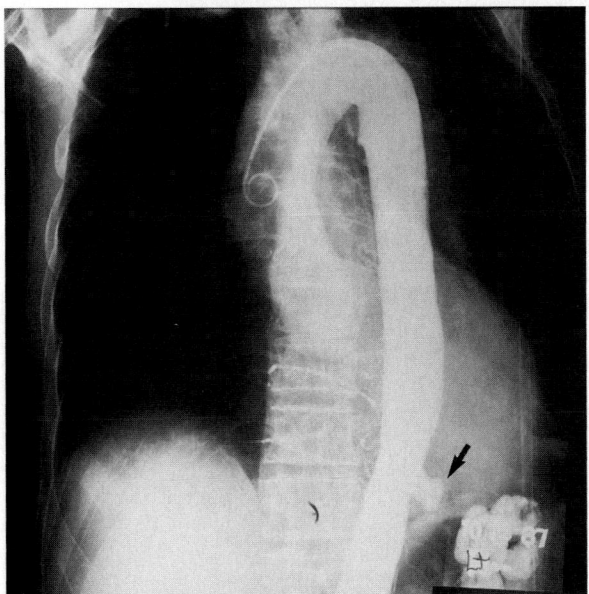

Fig. 67. AP view of aortic injection showing large perforating atherosclerotic ulcer (*arrow*).

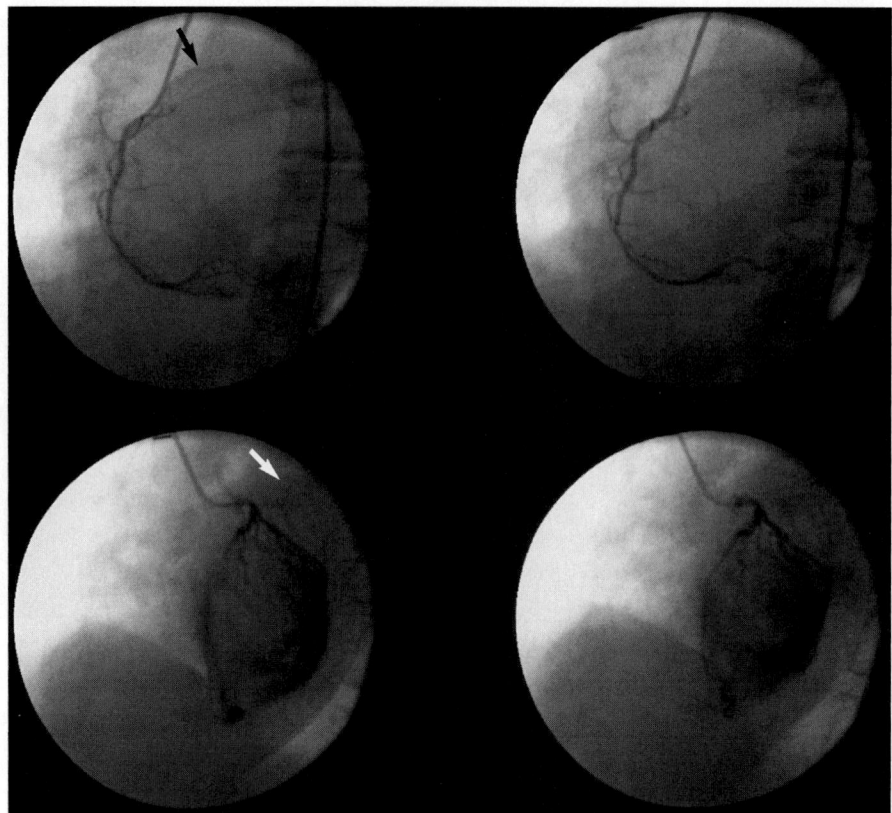

Fig. 68. *Upper,* LAO view of dominant right coronary artery in diastole (*left*) and systole (*right*). *Lower,* LAO cranial view of left main injection in diastole (*left*) and systole (*right*). Fixation of the right coronary artery and branches and the distal left circumflex artery is due to constrictive pericarditis. *Arrows,* Neovascularization of the pericarditis.

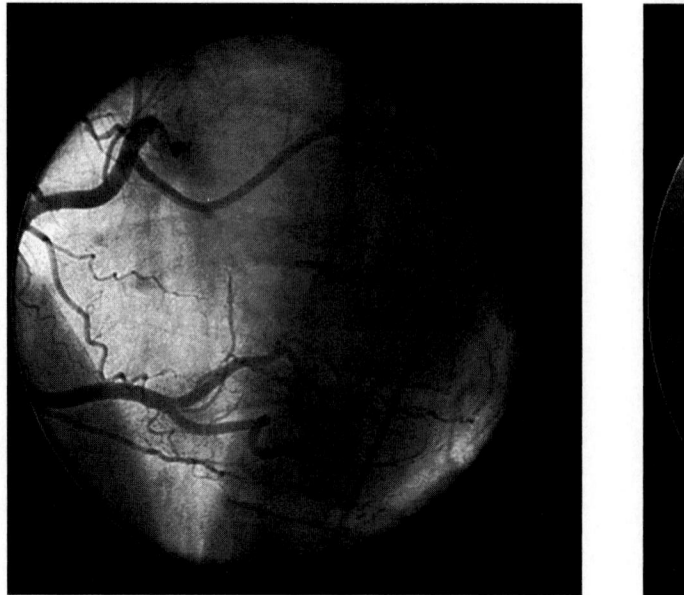
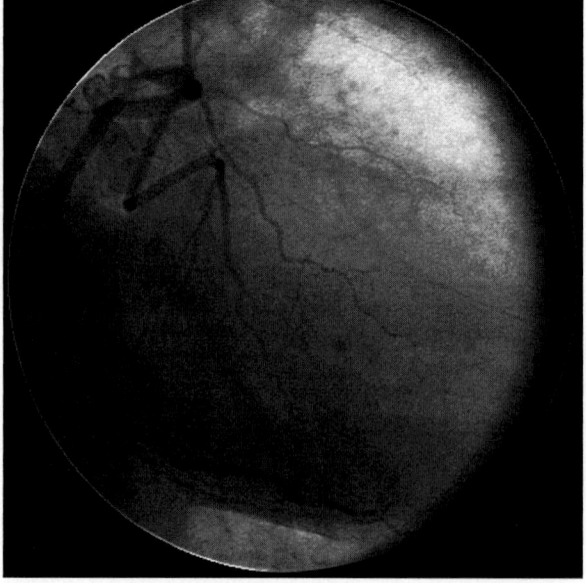

Fig. 69. Anomalous origin of the left circumflex coronary artery from the right coronary artery.

CATHETER CLOSURE
OF INTRACARDIAC SHUNTS

Guy S. Reeder, MD

Percutaneous closure of an atrial septal defect is first-line therapy in carefully selected patients and has been performed in more than 30,000 patients since first described in 1976.

DEVICES FOR ASD/PFO CLOSURE

The features of nine commonly used devices for closure of the atrial septum are shown in Table 1; of these, the largest number of procedures has been performed with the CardioSEAL and Amplatzer systems. The CardioSEAL (and related STARFlex) device employs a double umbrella made of Dacron fabric supported by a metallic framework and in the case of the latter, a self-centering mechanism using nitinol micro-springs. The Amplatzer atrial septal occluder and patent foramen ovale device utilize a nitinol wire-frame mesh with enclosed polyester disks. The differences in device designs are readily apparent in Figure 1. Nonetheless, all devices share in common some type of metallic supporting structure with a fabric portion to occlude interatrial blood flow, and can be collapsed in some fashion to allow catheter deployment.

INDICATIONS AND DEVICE IMPLANTATION

The primary indications for ASD closure is a left-to-right shunt with evidence of right ventricular volume overload. Pre-procedure transesophageal echocardiography is used to determine the extent and borders of the defect. Sinus venosus and primum defects are generally not suitable for percutaneous device closure. Secundum defects with a complete rim of surrounding atrial septum are ideal; many patients with some deficiency in a portion of the rim, usually peri-aortic, can be successfully closed. Defects with major deficient rim and very large defects (>2.5 cm) have a lower success rate and surgical closure may be considered. For PFO, the anatomy is a flap-valve rather than a tissue deficiency; a suitable rim of surrounding tissue is always present. TEE with bubble study (agitated saline injection during Valsalva release) is the most common diagnostic test. In the USA, no percutaneous closure devices have been FDA approved for use in PFO; all patients require either entry into a randomized trial, a device exemption, or off-label use of an ASD device. The latter has been our approach in selected patients with cryptogenic stroke who decline or are not candidates for trial inclusion.

Table 1. Comparative Summary of Percutaneous ASD and PFO Occlusion Devices

Device	Design and construction
Rashkind-PDA-umbrella	Double umbrella made of polyurethane foam, each disc consists of a 4-mm framework. Device sizes: 11 and 17 mm
Sideris buttoned device (3rd and 4th generation)	1) square occluder button; 2) rhomboid counter occluder. Device sizes: 25 to 50 mm
ASDOS	Two self-opening umbrellas (5-arm nitinol wire skeleton) with polyurethane membranes. Device sizes: 25 to 60 mm
Angel wings	Two interconnected square nitinol wire frames covered with Dacron fabric with a central conjoint ring. Device sizes: 18 to 40 mm
CardioSEAL	Non-centering double umbrella device modified from the Clamshell device with a 4-arm metallic framework covered with Dacron. Device sizes: 17 to 40 mm
STARFlex	CardioSEAL modification with a self-centering mechanism achieved by nitinol microsprings. Device sizes: 23 to 40 mm
Amplatzer	Self-centering double disc with a short connecting waist made from nitinol wire frame filled with polyester fabric. Device sizes (ASD): 4 to 40 mm; device sizes (PFO): 25 to 35 mm
Helex	Nitinol wire with ultrathin expanded polytetrafluoroethylene formed into two equal-size opposing discs that bridge the septal defect. Device sizes: 15 to 25 mm
PFO-Star (1st and 2nd generation)	Two Ivalon-square discs, each umbrella is expanded by 4 nitinol arms—1st generation: 2-mm center posts; 2nd generation: 3- and 5-mm center posts. Device sizes: 18 to 30 mm

ASD, atrial septal defect; PFO, patent foramen ovale.

There is controversy regarding indications for PFO closure. Observational studies show an association of PFO with cryptogenic stroke, but prospective data show little or no risk of subsequent stroke in asymptomatic patients with PFO, even with resting or inducible (Valsalva release) right-to-left shunt. The presence of atrial septal aneurysm—usually referring to a redundant atrial septal membrane with mobility during the respiratory cycle—may increase stroke risk—but this also remains controversial. Two ongoing randomized trials—RESPECT—using the Amplatzer PFO device, and Closure-1, using the CardioSEAL—are in progress and hopefully will demonstrate whether PFO device closure is effective in reducing recurrent cryptogenic stroke. Pending results of these trials, we perform PFO closure in some patients with unexplained embolic stroke or definite TIA. Candidates will usually be young individuals with no other documentable embolic source based on normal intra- and extracranial magnetic resonance angiography, carotid ultrasound, TEE examination of the left atrial appendage and aortic arch, and without evidence of hypercoagulable state necessitating warfarin anticoagulation.

The principles of ASD/PFO closure are to establish the size and location of the interatrial defect, usually with prior transesophageal echocardiography, use of transesophageal or intracardiac echocardiography to monitor device deployment, crossing of the defect with a catheter or guidewire, positioning of the delivery system, and deployment first of the left atrial side of the device followed by the right atrial side. In Figure 2, the orientation of the intracardiac imaging catheter is demonstrated; Figure 3 shows the corresponding image

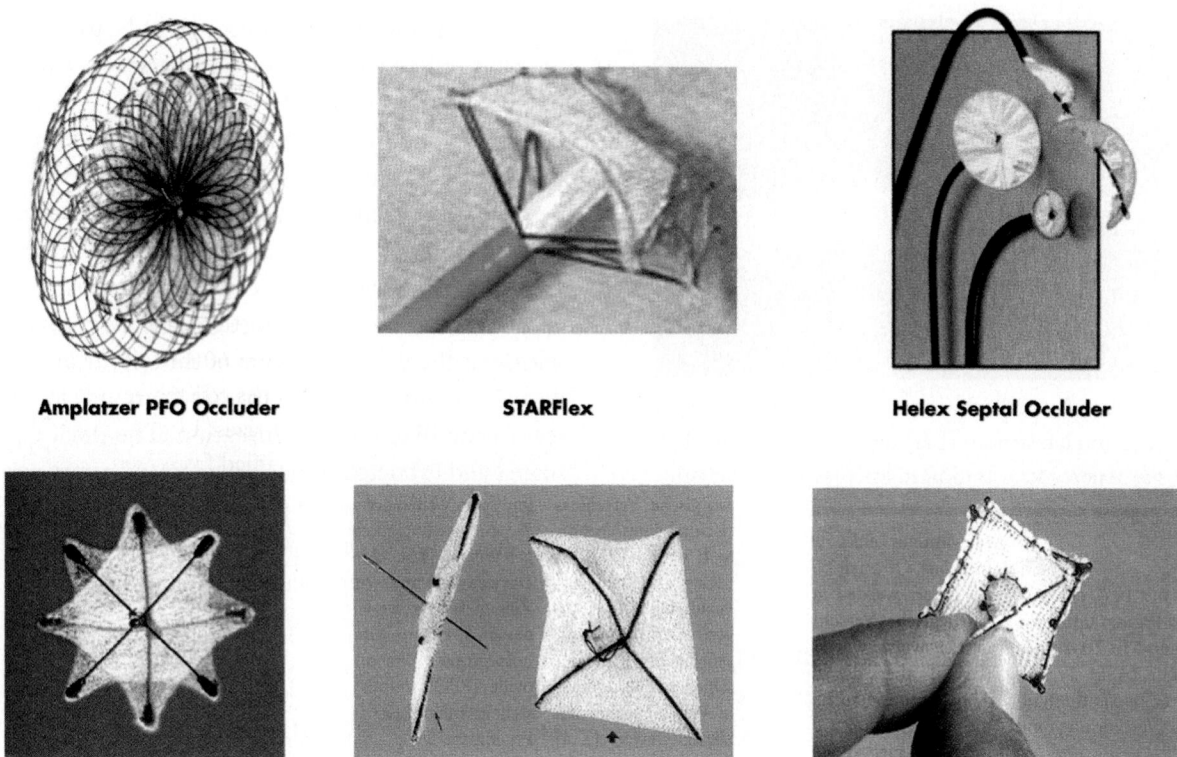

Fig. 1. Various devices used for percutaneous catheter-based patent foramen ovale (PFO) closure.

in a patient with an atrial septal defect. Some patients will have deformation or excessive mobility of the atrial septum characteristic of an atrial septal aneurysm (Fig. 4).

The technique of PFO or ASD closure is usually straightforward (Fig. 5 and 6), but opportunities exist for complications. These include inadvertent trauma or complications related to establishing femoral venous access, cardiac perforation with catheter or guidewire,

thrombus formation with embolism or introduction of air into the right or left heart chambers, and cardiac arrhythmias. Additionally, the device may fail to engage the atrial septum properly, become detached prematurely with embolization, or embolize from its position in the atrial septum following deployment. Fortunately, the occurrence of these complications is very low. A summary of complications is shown in Table 2.

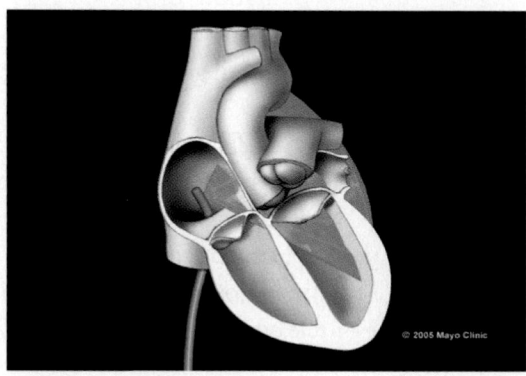

Fig. 2. Artist's rendition of intracardiac echocardiography catheter (ICE) in place in right atrium angled to produce long-axis view of atrial septum.

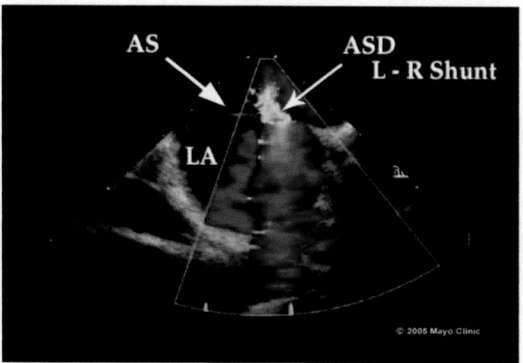

Fig. 3. Resulting imaging from catheter position in Figure 2. Long-axis view of atrial septum (AS) showing color jet of left-to-right shunt through atrial septal defect (ASD). Other abbreviations: LA, left atrium.

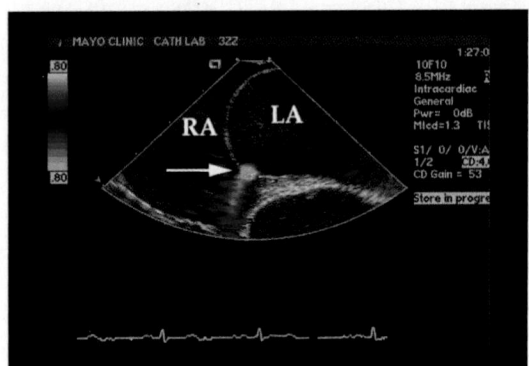

Fig. 4. Atrial septal aneurysm. Atrial septal membrane bulges from left atrium (LA) toward right trium (RA). *Arrow* denotes fenestration in atrial septal aneurysm with left-to-right shunt (blue jet).

MALPOSITION AND DEVICE EMBOLIZATION

Malposition occurs in up to 3.5 percent of cases and is almost exclusively limited to patients with large atrial septal defects (stretched sizes greater than 25 mm) or where there is a markedly deficient rim especially superiorly. The left atrial side of the device may not grasp the atrial septum and can subsequently prolapse into the right atrium during deployment. Echocardiographic monitoring will help the operator appreciate this situation immediately and avoid premature device detachment. Variations in positioning of the delivery system (right versus left superior pulmonary vein) and modest oversizing of the device have been used to reduce this problem. Device embolizations tend to occur early, usually during the procedure, but may rarely occur up to 1 week after implantation. Most devices will embolize within the right heart and can often be retrieved with a gooseneck snare and removed through a venous sheath. In the case of the Amplatzer device, a technique for stabilizing the device with a guidewire and then snaring the right atrial screw pin has been described for removal of embolized devices within the right heart. In our experience with over 500 Amplatzer devices for ASD and PFO closure, we observed 1 embolization. In this patient, premature release of the device occurred in the left atrium. The device embolized through the left heart and came to rest in the iliac artery bifurcation. The device was snared and extracted through the femoral artery and a second, successful device placement was subsequently performed. There were no long-term sequelae. Surgical removal has been reported if percutaneous removal of the embolized device is not possible.

DEVICE MALFUNCTION

Fracture of one of the metallic arms has been reported in 6 to 14 percent of implanted CardioSEAL or STARFlex devices. Arm fractures may or may not be associated with residual leak, and do not require revision unless associated with malposition or large residual shunt.

CARDIAC PERFORATION

Cardiac perforation presents as cardiac tamponade. Twenty-four cases of documented or presumed cardiac perforation involving the Amplatzer device have been described. Most of these events occurred within the

Table 2.   Complications Reported During ASD/PFO Closure

Complication	Frequency, %	Remedy
Malposition/device embolization	0-3.5	Snare and replace, rarely surgery
Device fracture	0-14	Usually observe, replace if large shunt
Cardiac perforation	0.5	Pericardiocentesis; rule out erosion
Air embolism	0-1	None, avoid with careful technique
Arrhythmia	2.6-3.1	Cardioversion, observation, rarely antiarrhythmics
Vascular complications	<1	Usually none needed

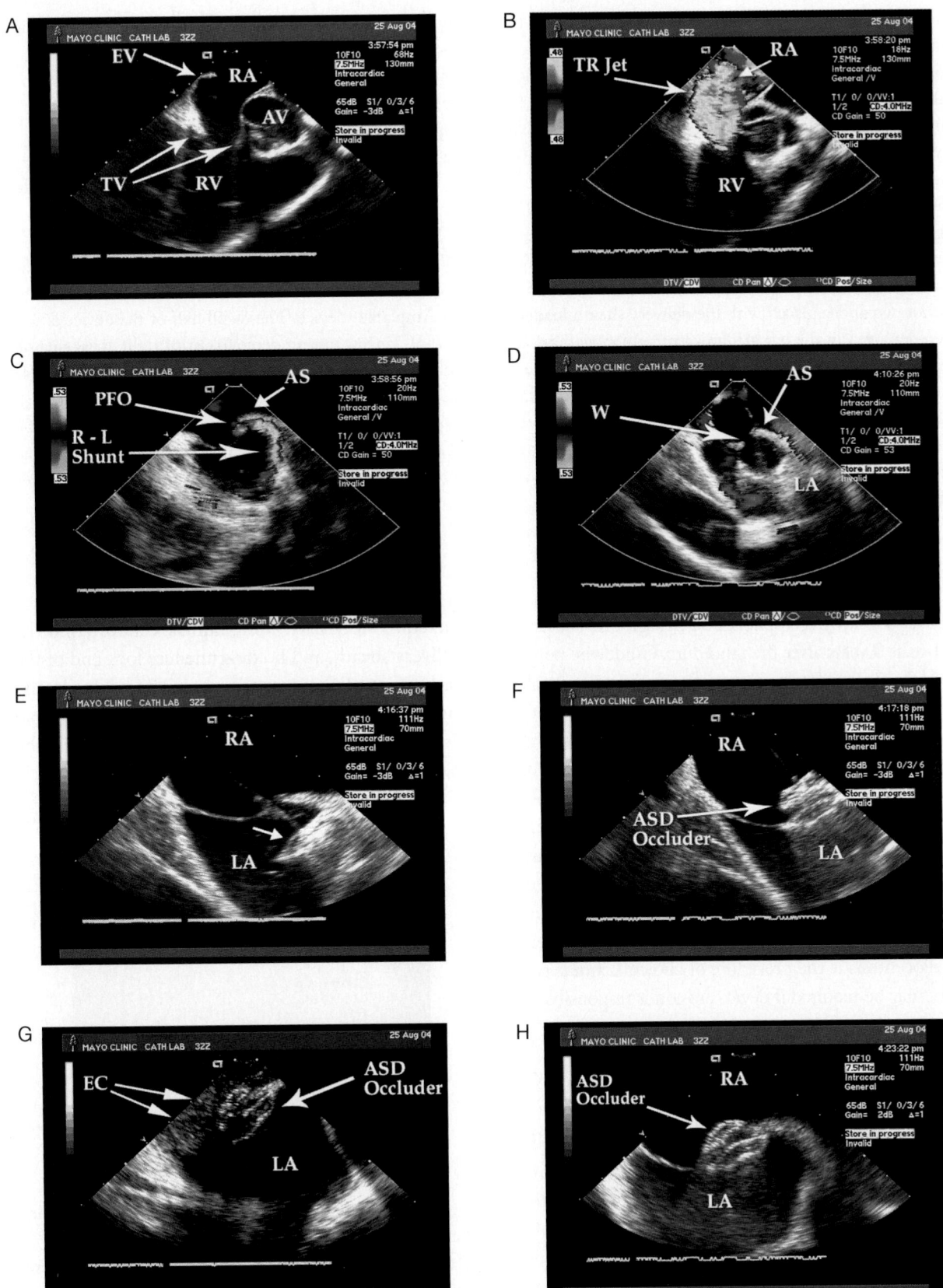

Fig. 5 continued on next page

Fig. 5. Photographs *A* through *H* illustrate sequential findings in closure of PFO using intracardiac echocardiographic guidance. *A*, Intracardiac echocardiography (ICE) image demonstrating tricuspid inflow view in a patient with carcinoid heart disease and progressive desaturation. RA, right atrium; EV, eustachian valve; AV, aortic valve; TV, tricuspid valve leaflets, here thickened and immobile due to carcinoid involvement; RV, right ventricle. The right ventricle is dilated. *B*, Color flow imaging in same view showing large tricuspid regurgitant jet (TR jet). Other abbreviations as before. Significant tricuspid regurgitation caused elevation of the right atrial pressure. *C*, Long-axis view of atrial septum using ICE. The septum bows from the right atrium towards the left atrium and right-to-left shunt is seen continuously during the cardiac cycle (R-L shunt, blue jet). PFO, patent foramen ovale; AS, atrial setpum. This continuous right-to-left shunt was the cause of the patient's desaturation. *D*, In this ICE image, the PFO has been crossed and a low-pressure sizing balloon inflated. The waist of the balloon (W) demonstrates the "stretched" size of the atrial septal communication. AS, atrial septum. *E*, ICE view of atrial septum during PFO closure. The sizing balloon has been withdrawn and replaced with the delivery sheath loaded with the Amplatzer device. The distal half of the device is seen deployed in the left atrium (*arrow*, abbreviations as before). *F*, ICE view during deployment of right atrial side of the ASD occluder device. Abbreviations as before. The ASD occluder covers both sides of the atrial septum. *G*, Bubble study using agitated saline injection in the right femoral vein. EC, echo contrast. Only a few microbubbles cross into the left atrium during Valsalva release after device placement. This step is important to ensure adequate apposition of the device to the margins of the PFO or atrial septal defect. *H*, Device deployment. The ASD occluder (*arrow*) is seated nicely across the PFO. Only minimal residual shunting was present. The patient's desaturation immediately resolved after device placement.

first days following implantation though one occurred as late as 3 years after the procedure. Guidewire perforation as well as late erosion of the device were implicated. Unexplained hypotension during the implantation procedure should suggest cardiac perforation with tamponade and can be confirmed immediately with echocardiography. With intracardiac echocardiography, pericardial effusion may be seen in the pericardial reflection immediately anterior to the aortic root, and should indicate immediate transthoracic echo. Even small pericardial effusions developing acutely can produce tamponade. In our institution, echo-directed pericardiocentesis is the procedure of choice. Cardiac surgery may be required if device erosion is responsible or if pericardial effusion recurs.

AIR EMBOLISM

Air embolism is uncommon and is suggested by ST-segment elevation in the inferior leads during or immediately post-procedure. Entrainment of air into the delivery system may occur during removal of a large central dilating stylet. Embolized air may cross the atrial septum, and obtain access to the most superior coronary sinus and resultantly embolize into the right coronary artery. This complication may be mini-

mized by slowly withdrawing the dilator from the delivery sheath, and holding the lure lock end of the catheter as low as possible on the table during guidewire exchanges and catheter aspiration, to avoid development of an air/fluid meniscus within the catheter.

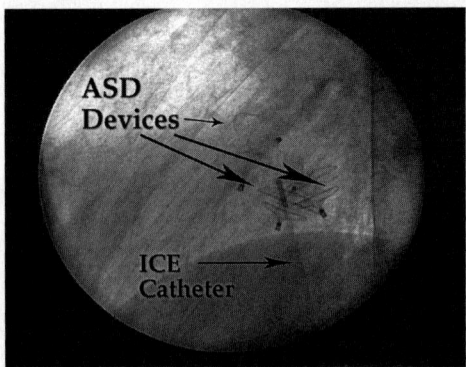

Fig. 6. Patient with atrial septal aneurysm and multiple fenestrations in atrial septum. These were completely closed by placement of 3 Amplatzer devices shown here on fluoroscopic image. Bubble study at 3 months demonstrated no residual intracardiac shunting. Patient has done well over 2-year follow-up.

ARRHYTHMIA

Atrial arrhythmias have been reported in 2-3 percent of patients following device closure of ASD or PFO. This is usually self-terminating within the first few weeks to months after the procedure though can exceptionally require temporary antiarrhythmic therapy. Heart block has occasionally been reported and we have observed 1 case in our practice possibly related to the use of the Amplatzer device.

PATENT FORAMEN OVALE

A large meta-analysis of 10 studies of transcatheter PFO closure involving 1,355 patients documented a 1.5 percent incidence of major complications defined as death, hemorrhage requiring blood transfusion, cardiac tamponade, need for surgical intervention, and massive fatal pulmonary emboli. There was a 7.9 percent incidence of minor complications including bleeding, atrial arrhythmias, transient AV nodal block, device arm fractures, device embolization with successful catheter retrieval, asymptomatic device thrombosis, air embolism, arteriovenous fistula formation, and femoral hematoma.

Late complications occurring after ASD/PFO closure are summarized in Table 3.

COMPLETE CLOSURE

Residual shunt occurs in up to 20 percent of patients with the CardioSEAL/STARFlex device in early series, and as little as 1-4 percent for the Amplatzer device more recently. In our experience with the Amplatzer ASD occluder, complete closure by bubble study is possible in >98 percent of cases.

THROMBUS FORMATION

The prevalence of device-related thrombus was investigated by transesophageal echocardiography at 4 weeks and 6 months in a large prospective follow-up of 1,000 patients undergoing device closure with a variety of devices. Thrombus was found in 1.2 percent of patients who had undergone ASD closure, and in 2.5 percent of patients undergoing PFO closure. Incidence of thrombus was device related; highest in the CardioSEAL/STARFlex/PFO Star devices and lowest in the Amplatzer device group. Risk factors for device thrombus included post-procedure atrial fibrillation and persistent atrial septal aneurysm. A prothrombotic disorder could be identified in only 2 patients with device-related thrombus and pre-existing PFO device placement. In 17 of the 20 patients with device thrombus, anticoagulation was successful in thrombus resolution; in 3 patients surgical thrombus removal was performed. Two patients suffered minor strokes and 1 a TIA in this group of 20 patients with device-related thrombus. Residual atrial septal aneurysm was not a risk factor for development of thromboembolic events. There was no correlation between post-procedure treatment with warfarin versus aspirin versus aspirin plus clopidogrel and subsequent development of thrombus.

Table 3.   Late Complications After ASD/PFO Closure

Complication	Frequency, %	Remedy
Residual shunt	1-20	Observe, 2nd device?
Thrombus	1.2-2.5	Anticoagulation, thrombolysis
TIA or stroke	0.2-4.9	TEE for device thrombus, residual shunt
Device erosion	0.1	Surgical removal
Late device embolization	Rare	Snare or surgery
Infection	Rare	Remove if needed
Atrial arrhythmia	Rare	Observation usually

TIA OR STROKE AFTER ATRIAL SEPTAL CLOSURE

The incidence of TIA or stroke post-procedure is highly related to the characteristics of the patient population, especially past history of stroke or TIA. Thus, in 442 patients undergoing ASD device closure for atrial septal defect, 1 TIA occurred during follow up (0.2%); patients were treated with aspirin alone following device closure. Similarly, in 1,000 patients undergoing ASD and PFO closure reported above, 3 neurologic events occurred (0.3%). On the other hand, in a population of patients with pre-existing cryptogenic stroke undergoing PFO closure for presumed paradoxical thromboemboli, a systematic review of 10 studies showed a wide range of recurrent neurologic events from 0-4.9 percent. The higher incidence of events in some of these studies suggests that non-device (and non-PFO) related causes are the most likely explanation.

DEVICE EROSION

Whereas cardiac perforation has been described during the implantation of a number of different devices, late erosion of the device through a cardiac wall resulting in pericardial tamponade has been described only for the Amplatzer device with an estimated incidence of 0.1 percent. A third of these developed symptoms within 1 day, another third within 3 days, but the remainder presented between 20 days and 3 years from device implantation. Erosions occurred at the superior aspect of either the right or left atrium and sometimes also involved erosion of the aorta with fistula to the left or right atria. Deficiency of the aortic rim of the atrial septal defect was described in 89 percent, and it is likely that deficiency of the superior rim was also present, allowing contact between the left or right atrial flange of the Amplatzer device and the superior left or right atrial wall. It is suspected that repetitive cardiac motion causes tissue erosion by the device. Recommendations for avoidance of this complication include avoidance of device oversizing, an awareness of potential risk in patients with deficient aortic and superior rims, and aggressive evaluation of patients who developed unexplained pericardial effusion at any time following the procedure. Additionally, it seems logical that careful intracardiac echocardiographic inspection of the device flanges and avoidance of contact with the superior

atrial walls prior to device release would be useful. We have not observed device erosion in over 500 Amplatzer device placements.

PERCUTANEOUS CLOSURE OF VENTRICULAR SEPTAL DEFECT

Whereas most atrial septal defects are of the secundum variety and lend themselves to device closure, the opposite is true for ventricular septal defects. At the present time, attempts at closure of VSDs have been mostly limited to defects in the muscular and more recently, perimembranous ventricular septum. The number of cases reported in the literature is somewhat under 500 to date. Impingement on the atrioventricular and semilunar valves, as well as the conduction system, have limited treatment of inflow septal ventricular septal defects.

Devices used for VSD closure have included the Rashkind double umbrella device, the Sideris button device, and more recently the CardioSEAL/STARFlex system and the Amplatzer muscular and perimembranous VSD occluder devices. The technique for implantation of these devices is more complicated than for atrial septal defect or PFO. Most operators have used an arteriovenous loop; using a retrograde approach, the LV is entered and a catheter and guidewire passed across the VSD into the right ventricle, where the wire is snared from a venous catheter and exteriorized to the neck or groin. The delivery system is then placed across the VSD from the right side, and a device subsequently deployed. This sequence of events is shown in Figure 7. Such an approach allows the VSD to be initially crossed from the less trabeculated left ventricular side, and the device implanted from the right ventricular side and provides necessary stabilization of the guidewire and delivery system during deployment.

Complications reported with percutaneous closure of post-infarction muscular ventricular septal defect are shown in Table 4 in a relatively small group of 18 patients. In 2 patients, the device could not be successfully deployed but in patients in whom deployment was possible, there was substantial reduction of shunt. Two of 8 patients presenting for primary closure survived to median follow-up of 332 days. There were no procedure-related deaths; overall mortality was 41 percent. The periprocedural complications were relatively minimal given the high morbidity of this patient popu-

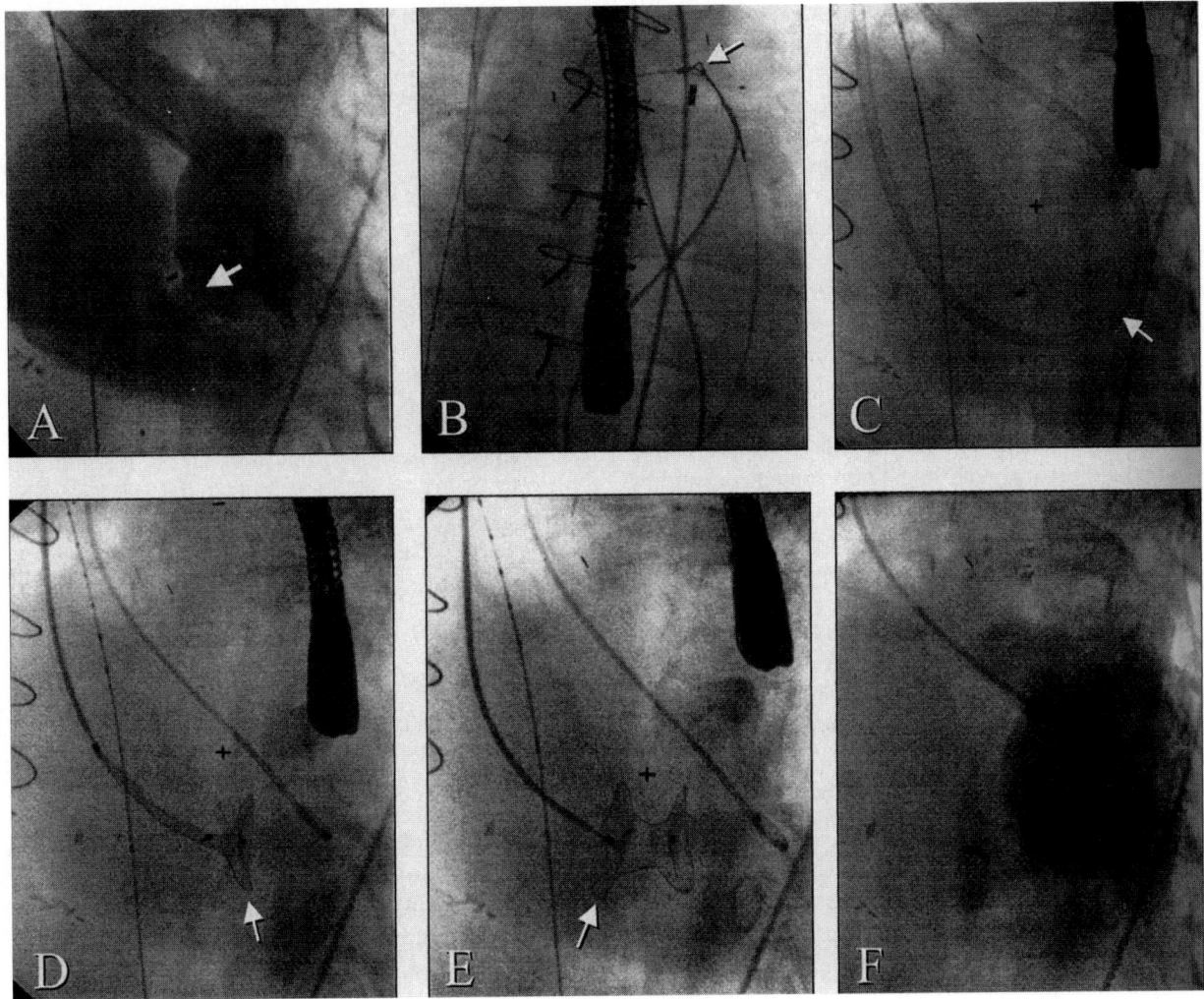

Fig. 7. Technique of percutaneous VSD closure. Cine angiographic images in the four-chamber view (except *B*, straight frontal) in an 81-year-old female patient who sustained myocardial infarction associated with a large mid muscular ventricular septal defect. In all images except *F*, there is a marker wire advanced from the inferior vena cava and positioned in the superior vena cava. *A*, LV angiogram delineating the mid muscular VSD (*arrow*). *B*, Cine image during snaring of the guidewire in the main pulmonary artery (*arrow*) to form the arteriovenous loop. The wire was exteriorized from the right internal jugular vein. *C*, The delivery sheath is advanced over the wire through the VSD (*arrow*) with the tip being positioned in the ascending aorta. *D*, The left ventricular disk (*arrow*) is being deployed and pulled against the interventricular septum. *E*, Connecting waist and right ventricular disk (*arrow*) have been deployed. *F*, Final angiogram in the left ventricle after the device has been released confirming good device position and minimal foaming through central portion of device.

lation. No early or late device embolizations were noted. Given the small number of patients reported in the literature, conclusions regarding efficacy and occurrence of potential complications cannot be conclusively drawn.

Adult cardiologists are unlikely to encounter enough patients with congenital or acquired (post-infarction) VSD to become proficient in device closure. In addition, device closure of VSD is more complex than ASD or PFO, has a higher complication rate, and requires expertise in multiple cardiac imaging modalities including transesophageal and intracardiac echocardiography, and familiarity with right ventricular and atrioventricular valve anatomy.

Table 4. Complications and Residual Shunts After Attempted Percutaneous Device Closure in Postinfarction VSD in 18 Patients

Device released successfully	16 (89%)
Procedure-related complications	4 (22%)
Blood loss-transfusion	2 (11%)
Bradycardia	2 (11%)
LV dysfunction	1 (6%)
Technical complications	0
Death	7 (41%)
Procedure-related	0
Unrelated/unknown	7 (41%)
Residual shunt: immediate result	n=16
Closed	2 (12.5%)
Trivial or small	13 (81.3%)
Moderate or large	1 (6.3%)
Residual shunt: 24-hr results	n=16
Closed	2 (12.5%)
Trivial or small	10 (62.5%)
Moderate or large	4 (25%)
Residual shunt: outpatient follow-up	n=10
Closed	2 (20%)
Trivial or small	6 (60%)
Moderate or large	2 (20%)

122

ATLAS OF HEMODYNAMIC TRACINGS

Deepak R. Talreja, MD

Rick A. Nishimura, MD

Joseph G. Murphy, MD

ARTERIAL PULSES

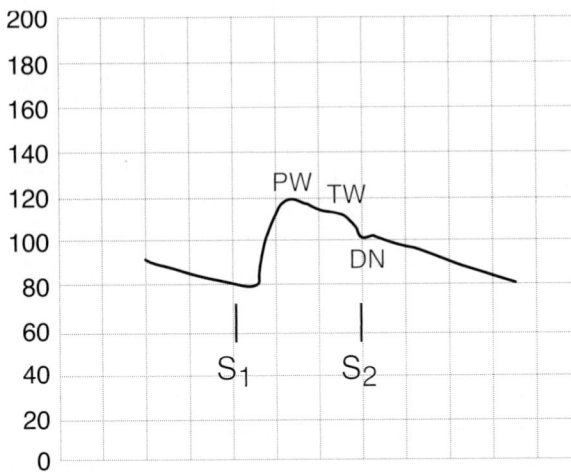

Fig. 1. Normal carotid arterial pulse. It consists of two systolic waves. The initial rise is called the "percussion wave" (PW), and the subsequent wave is called the "tidal wave" (TW), which is due to reflected energy from the aorta. The dicrotic notch (DN) signifies aortic closure. S_1, first heart sound; S_2, second heart sound.

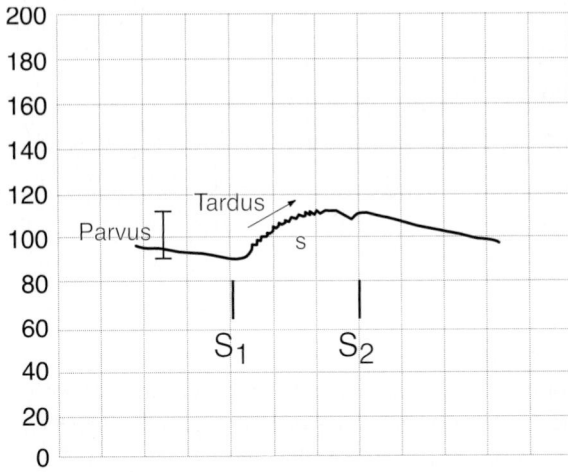

Fig. 2. The parvus (low amplitude) and tardus (slow uprising, *arrow*) pulse of severe calcified aortic stenosis. The irregularity in the slowly uprising pulse is from the turbulence created by the stenotic aortic valve and, on palpation, is often felt as a shudder (s) in the carotid pulse. Note that the degree to which a pulse is parvus and tardus correlates with the severity of aortic stenosis. S_1, first heart sound; S_2, second heart sound.

Special thanks to Naeem K. Tahirkheli, MD, who coauthored the previous version of this text.

Double arterial pulses can be divided into two main categories. In the first category, the double pulses span different cardiac cycles and include pulsus alternans and pulsus bigeminus (not illustrated). Pulsus alternans is frequently associated with heart failure, with one cardiac cycle having a higher pulse pressure while the preceding and following pulses have a lower pulse pressure. Pulsus bigeminus is secondary to a bigeminal rhythm, in which fixed-interval premature ventricular contractions occur after every sinus beat. Therefore, a small-amplitude pulse due to the premature ventricular contraction follows every sinus-mediated larger amplitude pulse.

The second category of double pulses includes bifid, bisferiens, and dicrotic pulses (see below). The split in the pulse in this category is within one cardiac cycle. In the case of a dicrotic pulse, a diastolic component is added to the systolic pulsation. The terms *bifid* and *bisferiens* are sometimes used interchangeably; however, bisferiens (twice-beating pulse) refers to two distinct pulsations and is more appropriate for the pulse character in hypertrophic obstructive cardiomyopathy. A bifid pulse is a double impulse pulse frequently observed in combined aortic stenosis and aortic regurgitation or severe aortic regurgitation alone.

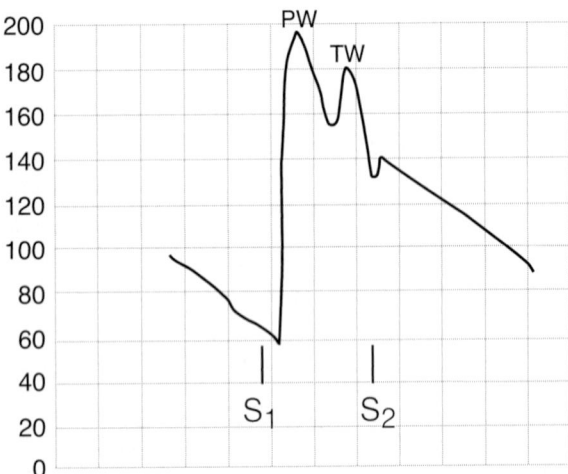

Fig. 3. A bifid pulse in combined aortic regurgitation and stenosis. Note the increased pulse pressure resulting from the lower diastolic blood pressure combined with the increased systolic pressure (blood pressure 200/60 mm Hg). The first peak is the percussion wave (PW) and the second peak is the tidal wave (TW). Note that no specific features of this pulse are related to the severity of the aortic regurgitation. S_1, first heart sound; S_2, second heart sound.

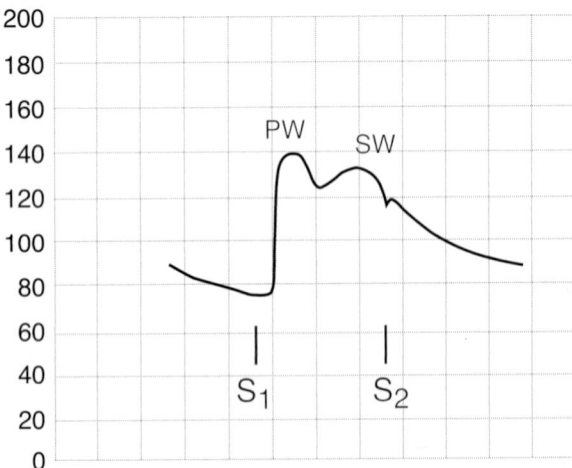

Fig. 4. Spike-and-dome pattern of hypertrophic obstructive cardiomyopathy. After the initial percussion wave (PW), a late systolic secondary wave (SW) can easily be palpated because the two pulsations are frequently distinct. This may also be referred to as a "bisferiens pulse." Note, however, that not all patients with hypertrophic cardiomyopathy have such a pulse, and some may have such a pulse only intermittently (see Figure 37). S_1, first heart sound; S_2, second heart sound.

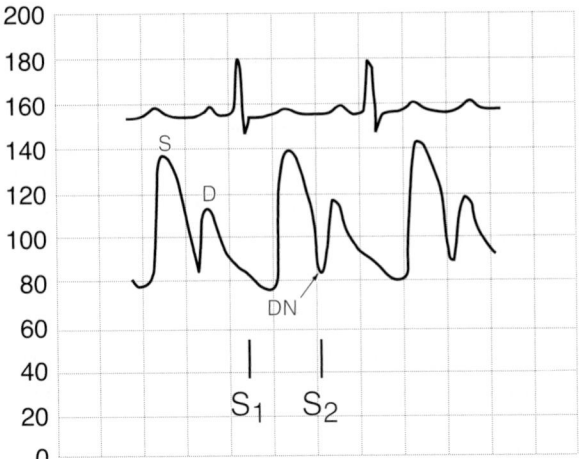

Fig. 5. Dicrotic pulse. This pulse may be seen in significant left ventricular dysfunction and increased peripheral vascular resistance. A systolic wave (S) and a large diastolic wave (D) follow aortic valve closure (dicrotic notch, DN). S_1, first heart sound; S_2, second heart sound.

RIGHT HEART CATHETERIZATION

Considerable controversy surrounds the use of pulmonary artery flotation catheters to monitor critically ill patients. Some authors have reported that after adjustment for treatment selection bias, the use of pulmonary artery flotation catheters was associated with increased mortality and poor use of resources in a group of patients with predominantly multiorgan and respiratory disease rather than cardiac disease.

Technical Considerations When Interpreting Pulmonary Artery Wedge Tracings

Pulmonary artery balloon catheters primarily yield three important hemodynamic measures: pulmonary artery pressure, pulmonary artery wedge pressure, and cardiac output, from which pulmonary arteriolar resistance can be calculated. Pulmonary artery wedge pressure approximates left atrial pressure (in the absence of pulmonary arterial disease), which in turn approximates left ventricular end-diastolic pressure (in the absence of mitral stenosis or other left atrial obstructive lesions).

A fundamental question is, "When in the respiratory cycle should the pulmonary artery wedge pressure be measured?" Measurement at end-expiration is common in intensive care units, whereas most cardiac catheterization laboratories record the mean wedge pressures averaged throughout the respiratory cycle.

Pulmonary artery occlusion pressure accurately reflects pulmonary venous pressure only when pulmonary venous and pulmonary artery pressures exceed pulmonary alveolar pressure (West zone 3 of the lung). In mechanically ventilated patients on positive end-expiratory pressure (PEEP), alveolar pressure may exceed pulmonary artery and venous pressures, thus making measurements of pulmonary capillary wedge pressure (PCWP) inaccurate. Some have suggested subtracting one-half of the wedge pressure from the measured PCWP, but data to support this approach are lacking. While turning off the PEEP can allow accurate measurement of PCWP, the recruitment of alveoli after initiation of PEEP takes up to several hours and this may be deleterious to the care of the patient.

True pulmonary capillary pressure normally exceeds wedge pressure by a few millimeters of mercury, but in septicemia and inflammatory disorders, this discrepancy can be much higher. Left atrial pressure reflects left ventricular mean diastolic pressure only in the absence of significant mitral valve disease (stenosis or regurgitation) or left atrial obstructive lesions. Other discrepancies may occur because of changes in left ventricular compliance which may be present in critically ill patients. Thermodilution cardiac output may be inaccurate in the presence of arrhythmias, significant tricuspid regurgitation, intracardiac shunting, or low cardiac output states. In these cases a Fick cardiac output may be more accurate, particularly if oxygen consumption can be accurately quantified at the time of blood gas measurements.

Indications for the Use of Bedside Right Heart Catheterization

- To differentiate between cardiac (hemodynamic) and noncardiac (abnormal capillary permeability) pulmonary edema.
- In patients with coexisting cardiac and pulmonary disease who have not had a response to conventional heart failure therapy.
- To differentiate cardiogenic from noncardiogenic shock (hypotension); most useful when a trial of intravascular volume expansion has failed to correct hypotension.
- To guide the use of ionotropic or mechanical cardiac support.

- To guide therapy in patients with concomitant forward (hypotension, oliguria, or azotemia) and backward (dyspnea and/or hypoxemia) heart failure.
- To determine whether pericardial tamponade is present when echocardiographic guidance is inadequate.
- To guide perioperative management in selected patients with decompensated heart failure undergoing intermediate- or high-risk noncardiac surgery.
- To detect the presence of pulmonary vasoconstriction and its reversibility in patients being considered for heart transplantation.

Contraindications to Pulmonary Artery Catheter Placement

Absolute Contraindications
- Right-sided endocarditis, mechanical tricuspid or pulmonary valve prosthesis, right-sided thrombus or tumor.
- Patients who are terminally ill, for whom aggressive management would be considered futile, are not candidates for pulmonary artery catheter placement.

Relative Contraindications
- Coagulopathy, including recent thrombolytic therapy, recent implantation of permanent pacemaker, left bundle branch block, or bioprosthetic tricuspid valve.
- In acute myocardial infarction, thrombolytic and/or anticoagulant therapy.

Indications for Pulmonary Artery Catheter Placement

Acute Myocardial Infarction
- To differentiate between cardiogenic and hypovolemic shock when initial therapy with intravascular volume expansion and low-dose ionotropic drugs has failed.
- To guide management of cardiogenic shock with pharmacologic and/or mechanical support in patients with or without coronary reperfusion therapy.
- To guide short-term pharmacologic and/or mechanical management of acute mitral regurgitation before surgical correction.
- To establish severity of left or right shunting and short-term guidance of pharmacologic and/or mechanical management of ventricular septal rupture for surgical correction.
- To guide management of complicated right ventricular infarction.

- To guide management of acute pulmonary edema not responding to the standard treatment.

Perioperative Use in Cardiac Surgery
- To differentiate between causes of low cardiac output when clinical and/or echocardiographic assessment is inconclusive.
- To differentiate between right and left ventricular dysfunction and pericardial tamponade when clinical and/or echocardiographic assessment is inconclusive.
- To guide management of severe low cardiac output syndromes.
- To diagnose and guide management of pulmonary hypertension in patients with systemic hypotension and evidence of inadequate organ perfusion.

Primary Pulmonary Hypertension
- To exclude postcapillary causes of pulmonary hypertension (increased pulmonary artery occlusion pressure).
- To establish the diagnosis and assessment of severity or precapillary pulmonary hypertension.
- To select and establish the safety and efficacy of long-term vasodilator therapy based on acute hemodynamic responses.
- To assess hemodynamic variables before lung transplantation.

Complications of Right Heart Catheterization

Central Venous Access Problems
These include arterial punctures, bleeding at the site of insertion, nerve injury, pneumothorax, and air embolism.

Arrhythmias
Transient arrhythmias frequently occur as the catheter is passed through the pulmonary outflow tract. Sustained ventricular arrhythmias are quite rare and seen primarily in patients with myocardial ischemia or a history of ventricular arrhythmias. Rarely, a right bundle branch block may be precipitated, or in patients with a preexisting left bundle branch block, complete heart block may occur.

Catheter Problems
These complications are related to the catheter residing in the pulmonary artery and include pulmonary artery rupture, thrombophlebitis, venous or intracardiac thrombus formation, pulmonary infarction, and endocarditis.

VENOUS PULSES

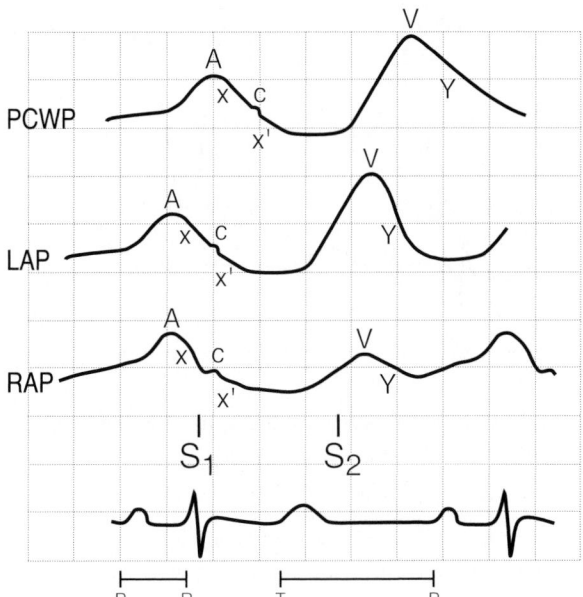

Fig. 6. Top to bottom, tracings of normal pulmonary capillary wedge pressure (PCWP), left atrial pressure (LAP), and right atrial pressure (RAP). The A wave is due to atrial contraction and the downward X descent, to atrial relation. The brief outward C wave is caused by a cephalad motion of the closing atrioventricular valve. The downward X' descent is a continuation of the original X descent after atrioventricular valve closure. The V wave occurs with passive atrial filling against a closed atrioventricular valve. The Y descent denotes atrial emptying into the ventricle after opening of the atrioventricular valve. This figure shows the important differences in the three pressure tracings. The A wave is the first upward deflection on the hemodynamic tracing after the start of the P wave in the ECG and is within the PR segment of the ECG tracing for the right and left atrial pressure tracings. Because of the reflection of the left atrial pressure across the pulmonary vasculature, there is a time delay in the PCWP tracings. Therefore the A wave of the PCWP is toward the end of the PR segment, as shown here. Similarly, the V wave is located in the TP segment of the ECG for the LAP and RAP tracings. In PCWP, the V wave may be in the latter half of the TP segment, occasionally extending into the PR segment. Another difference between the right- and left-sided pressures is that the A wave is the dominant wave of the RAP tracing, whereas the V wave is the larger of the two upward waves in the LAP and PCWP tracings. Finally, the major difference between the LAP and the PCWP is the rapidity of the Y descent. The LAP tracing usually has a distinct sharp Y descent, whereas that of the PCWP tracing is slower. This difference can be important clinically when estimating the pressure gradient across the mitral valve (mitral stenosis), in which the use of PCWP as a surrogate for LAP may tend to overestimate the pressure gradient. S_1, first heart sound; S_2, second heart sound.

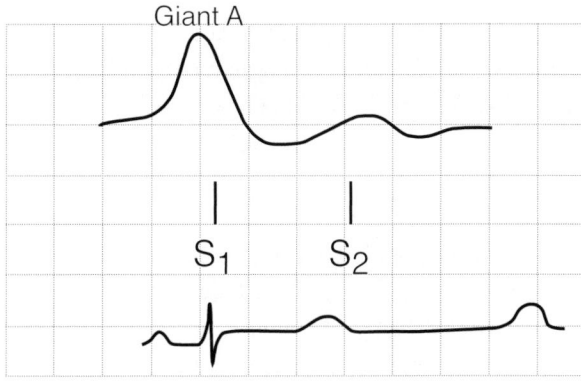

Fig. 7. Right atrial pressure tracing showing a giant A wave. This is usually associated with a poorly compliant ventricle. Note: the *giant* A wave is different from the *cannon* A wave, which refers to the pressure generated when the right atrium contracts against a closed tricuspid valve (not shown here) and is usually seen in patients with complete heart block or the pacemaker syndrome. Cannon A waves are an intermittent phenomenon, whereas giant A waves are seen with every sinus beat. S_1, first heart sound; S_2, second heart sound.

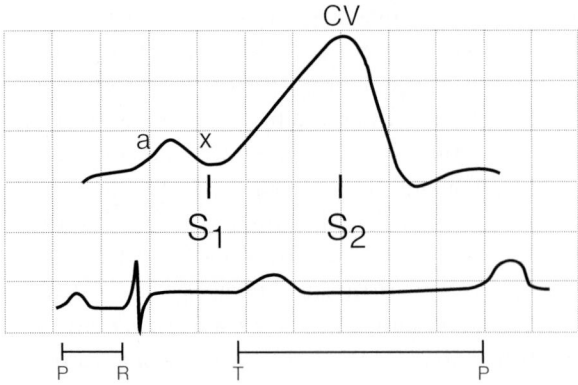

Fig. 8. A CV wave in the pulmonary capillary wedge pressure tracing. This is frequently seen in patients with significant mitral regurgitation. Note that although the A wave is characteristically delayed (end of the PR segment) for a pulmonary capillary wedge pressure tracing, the upward deflection of the CV wave is much earlier (beginning or slightly before the TP segment) than would be expected. Because of the incompetent valve, the CV wave is not only larger, it also starts earlier in systole. S_1, first heart sound; S_2, second heart sound.

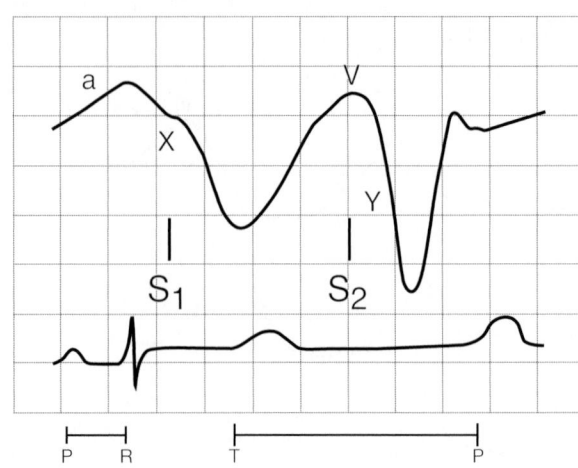

Fig. 9. Right atrial pressure tracing in constrictive pericarditis. Note the sharp X and Y descents. S_1, first heart sound; S_2, second heart sound.

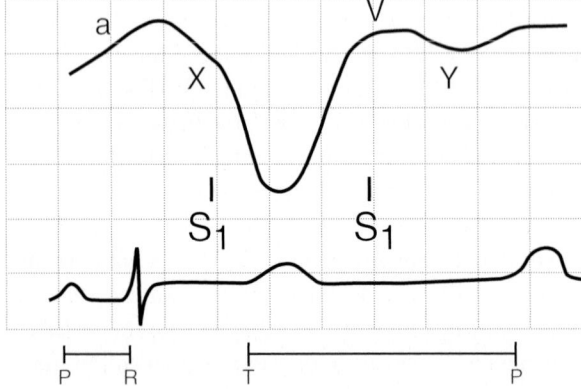

Fig. 10. Right atrial pressure tracing in pericardial tamponade. Note the sharp X descent, but minimal or absent Y descent, consistent with minimal passive atrial emptying. S_1, first heart sound; S_2, second heart sound.

APEX IMPULSES IN DISEASE

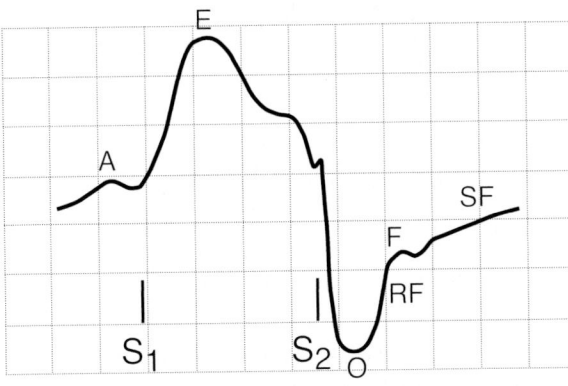

Fig. 11. Normal apex pulse (apex beat cardiogram). The normal apex pulse has several waves. The initial A wave is the outward expansion, "upward deflection on the apex cardiogram," of the apical area due to left atrial contraction. E represents maximal ejection. Note that the upward deflection has occurred entirely in the first half of systole. The notch in the downward slope coincides with the second heart sound (S_2) and the closure of the aortic valve, signifying the end of systole. As systole ends, the left ventricle relaxes, accelerating its retraction from the chest wall (downward slope on the apex cardiogram), which ends at O. The O point marks mitral valve opening. As the left ventricle dilates because of blood flowing through the open mitral valve, an upward deflection is noted, the rapid filling wave (RF). The F point is the peak of this rapid filling and is synchronous with the timing of the third heart sound. The slow filling wave (SF) signifies slow ventricular filling during mid-diastole, before atrial contraction. Note: in a normal heart, only the E point during the early part of systole is palpable. S_1, first heart sound; S_2, second heart sound.

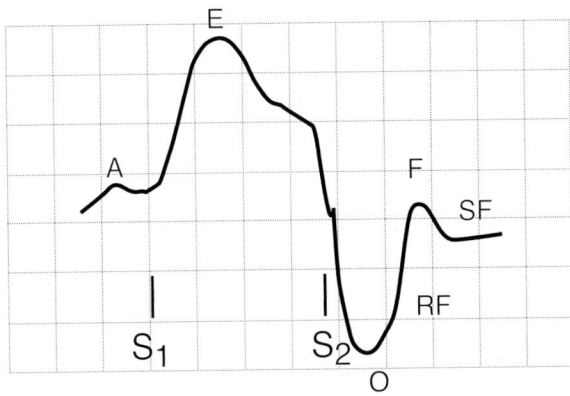

Fig. 12. In conditions in which the the rapid filling wave (RF) is steep and tall (e.g., increased filling due to severe mitral regurgitation or restrictive filling pattern), the F point is more pronounced. This may be appreciated as an audible or palpable third heart sound. S_1, first heart sound; S_2, second heart sound.

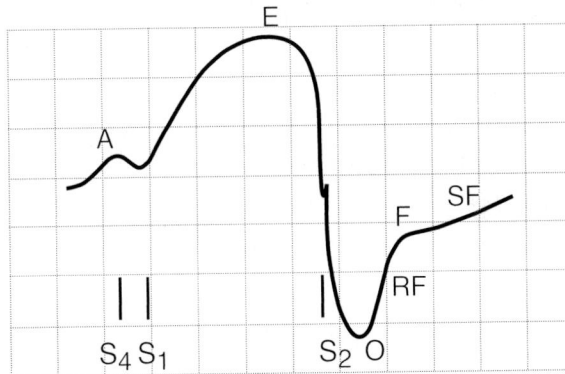

Fig. 13. In aortic stenosis with normal left ventricular function, the apex impulse is strong, prolonged, and reaches a sustained peak, E, in late systole. Contrast this with a normal apex impulse in which peak E is reached in early systole. Also, the amplitude of the A wave may be increased, thereby making it palpable. This would coincide with the fourth heart sound (S_4). S_1, first heart sound; S_2, second heart sound.

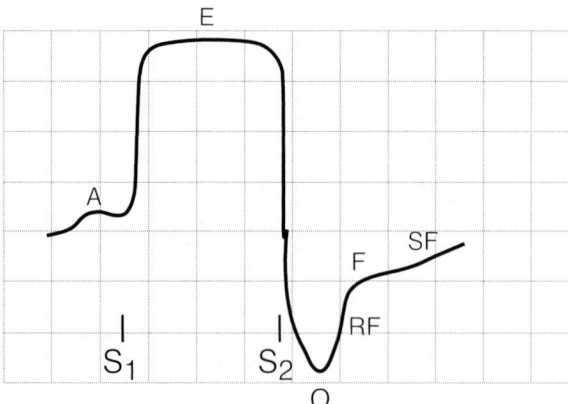

Fig. 14. There is significant dyskinesis of the apical impulse in patients with a left ventricular aneurysm. In contrast to left ventricular hypertrophy, the peak is reached early in systole and, in contrast to the normal impulse, remains sustained throughout systole. Additionally, the apical impulse extends over a wider area corresponding to the ventricular aneurysm. S_1, first heart sound; S_2, second heart sound.

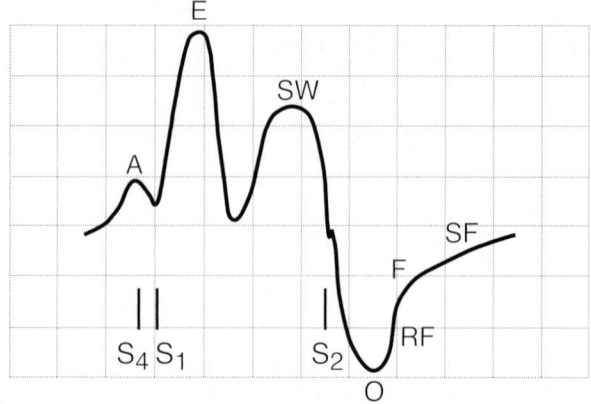

Fig. 15. The classic "triple-ripple" apical impulse of hypertrophic obstructive cardiomyopathy. There is a rapid and early rise to the E point, after which there is sudden cessation and even withdrawal of the apical impulse (corresponds to dynamic outflow obstruction, which peaks in mid-systole) until mid-systole, when a more sustained secondary wave (SW) may be palpable. Additionally, the A wave amplitude may also be increased and, thus, palpable. This corresponds to an audible fourth heart sound (S_4) from the left ventricle. These three peaks are frequently referred to as the "triple-ripple apical impulse of hypertrophic obstructive cardiomyopathy." Note, however, that this classic representation is not universally found in hypertrophic obstructive cardiomyopathy.

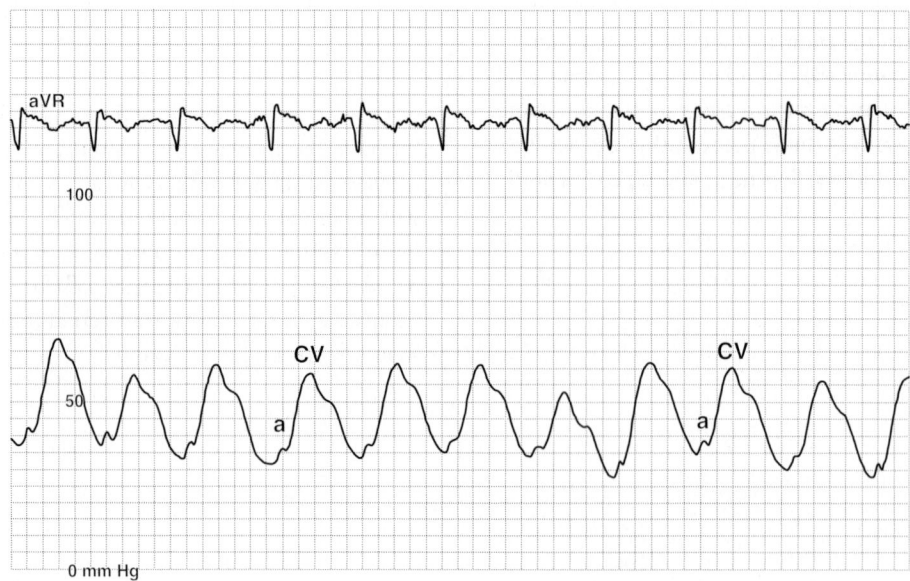

Fig. 16. Pulmonary capillary wedge pressure tracing in a patient with severe mitral regurgitation due to ruptured papillary muscle in association with an acute inferior myocardial infarction. The large CV waves measured on this tracing averaged 60 mm Hg. Note that the start of the CV wave in this tracing (before the TP segment of the ECG) is earlier than would be expected in a normal V wave.

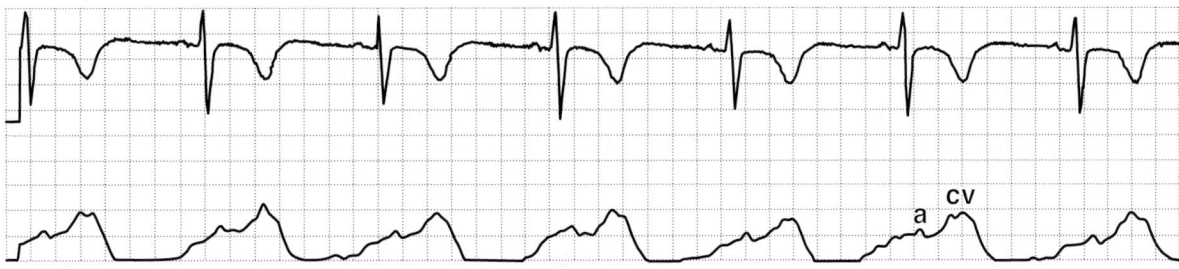

Fig. 17. Pulmonary capillary wedge pressure tracing of a patient with severe mitral regurgitation. Note that the CV waves are not as prominent as in the previous tracing (Fig. 16). Also note the early start of the CV wave in relation to the ECG.

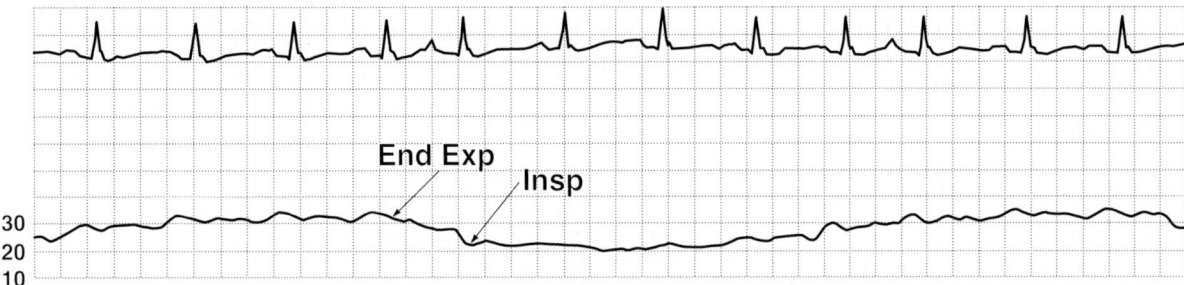

Fig. 18. Variations of the pulmonary capillary wedge pressure (PCWP) during spontaneous breathing. The negative intrathoracic pressure generated during the inspiratory phase (Insp) of spontaneous respiration results in an artificial lowering of the pulmonary capillary wedge pressure. During the end-expiratory phase (End Exp), there is relative apnea and the PCWP here best approximates the left ventricular mean diastolic pressure. As shown in the figure, this point occurs just before the negative dip in the PCWP. During positive pressure ventilation, end expiration remains the optimal time to measure PCWP. However, because of positive pressure ventilation, PCWP is artificially increased during the inspiratory phase and end-expiration occurs just before the upward (positive) shift in the pressure. Therefore, it is important to remember respiratory variations/modes when measuring PCWP. Note that in most catheterization laboratories, multiple cardiac cycles across respiratory phases are averaged to obtain the mean PCWP.

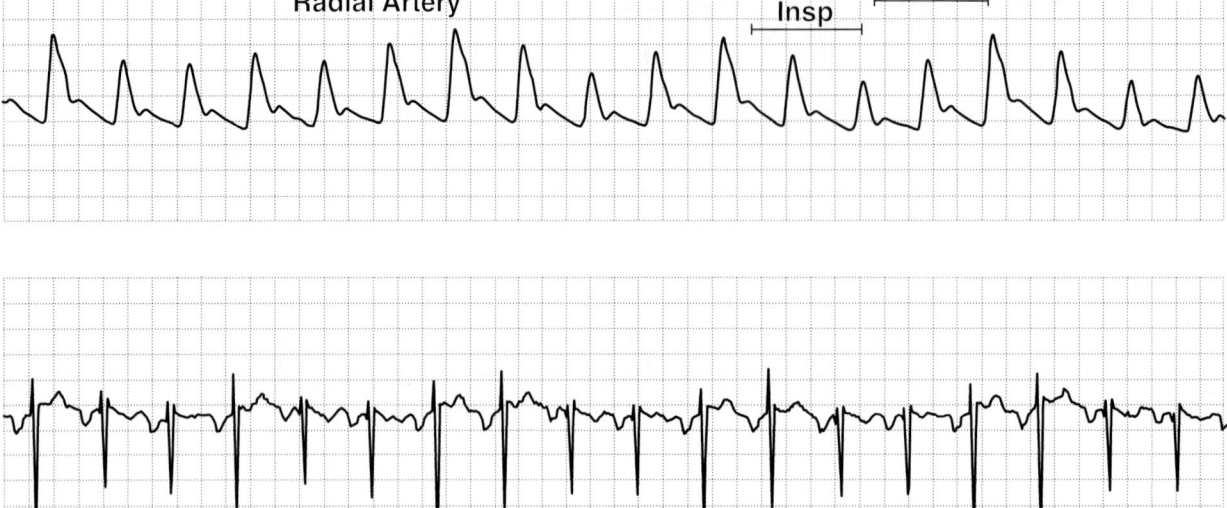

Fig. 19. Pulsus paradoxus and electrical alternans in pericardial tamponade. Radial artery pressure tracing showing a significant decrease in systolic blood pressure and pulse pressure with inspiration consistent with pulsus paradoxus. Electrical alternans is also noted: the changing height of the QRS complexes. Exp, expiration; Insp, inspiration.

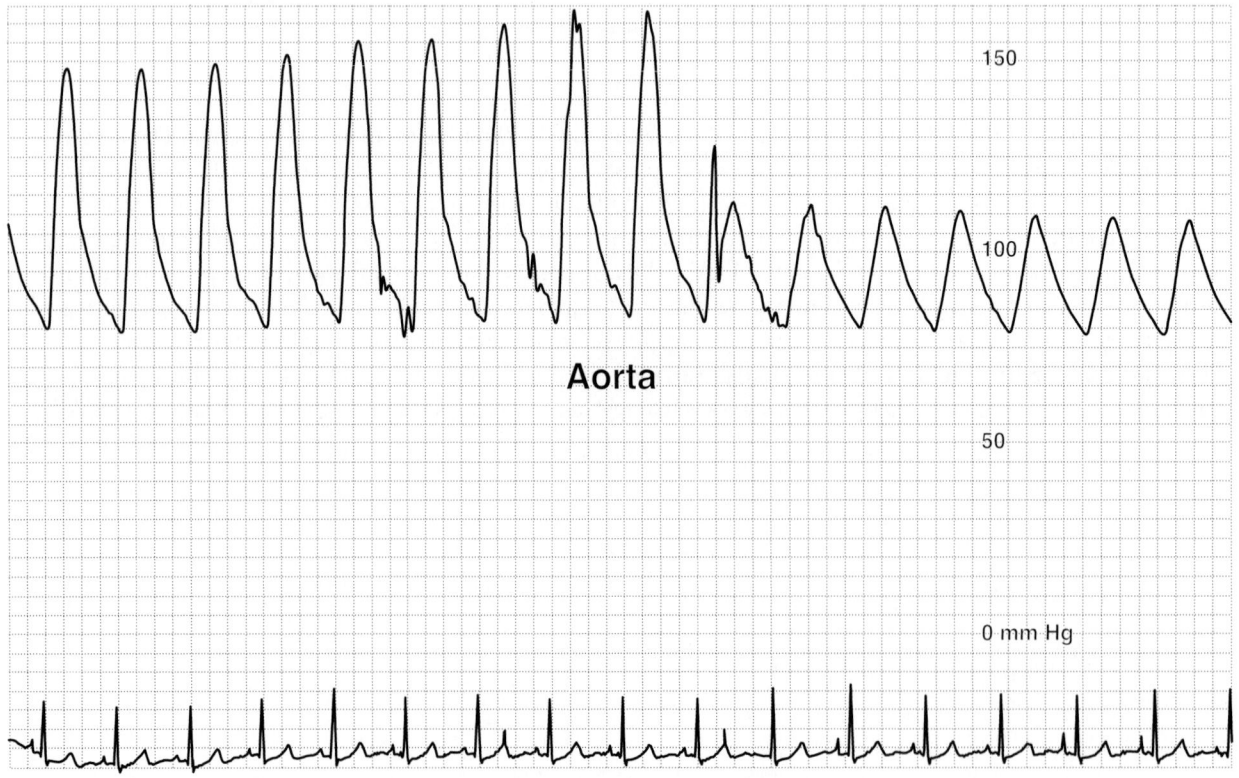

Fig. 20. Coarctation of the aorta. Pullback from the ascending aorta to below the subclavian artery, showing the pressure difference across the coarctation.

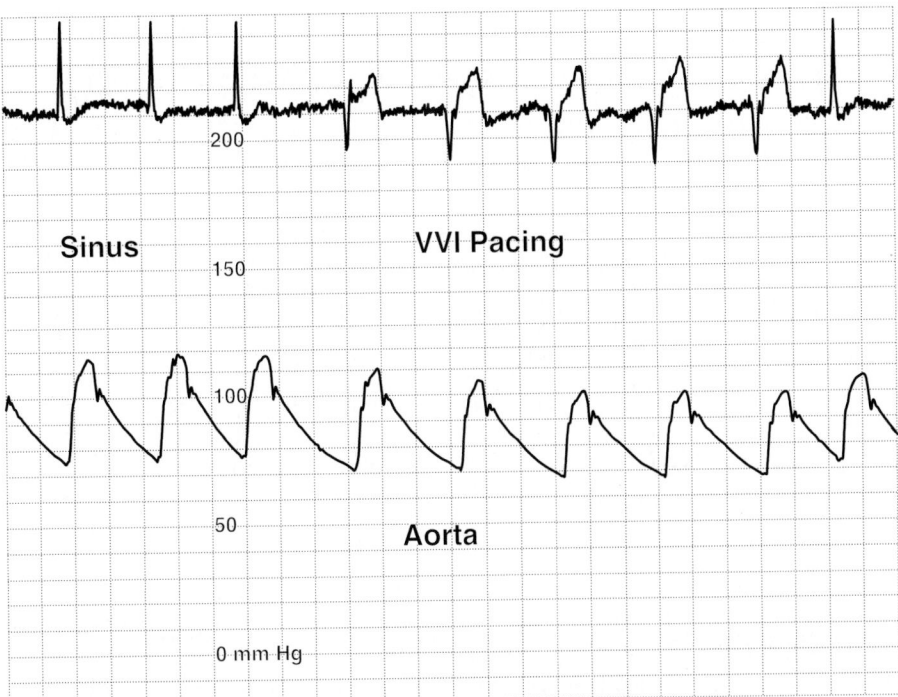

Fig. 21. Pacemaker syndrome. The first 3 beats are sinus-mediated and the next 4 are paced by a VVI permanent pacemaker. Note the decrease in systolic blood pressure while being paced.

VALVULAR HEART DISEASE

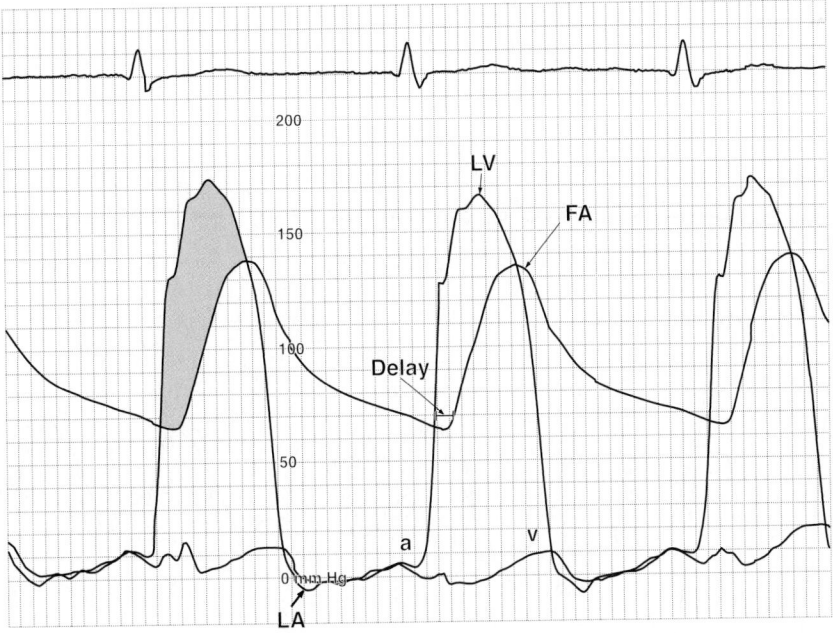

Fig. 22. Aortic stenosis. Aortic valve gradients should not be taken using the femoral artery pressure as a substitute for the ascending aortic pressure. In this patient, pressure tracings from the left ventricle (LV), femoral artery (FA), and left atrium (LA) are displayed. The shaded area represents the gradient between the LV and FA. Because of the transmission of pressure to a peripheral artery, there is a delay (*arrow*) in the upstroke of the FA. Due to the delay in pressure transmission as well as amplification of the pressure, the gradient across the aortic valve can be over- or underestimated when using the femoral artery pressure.

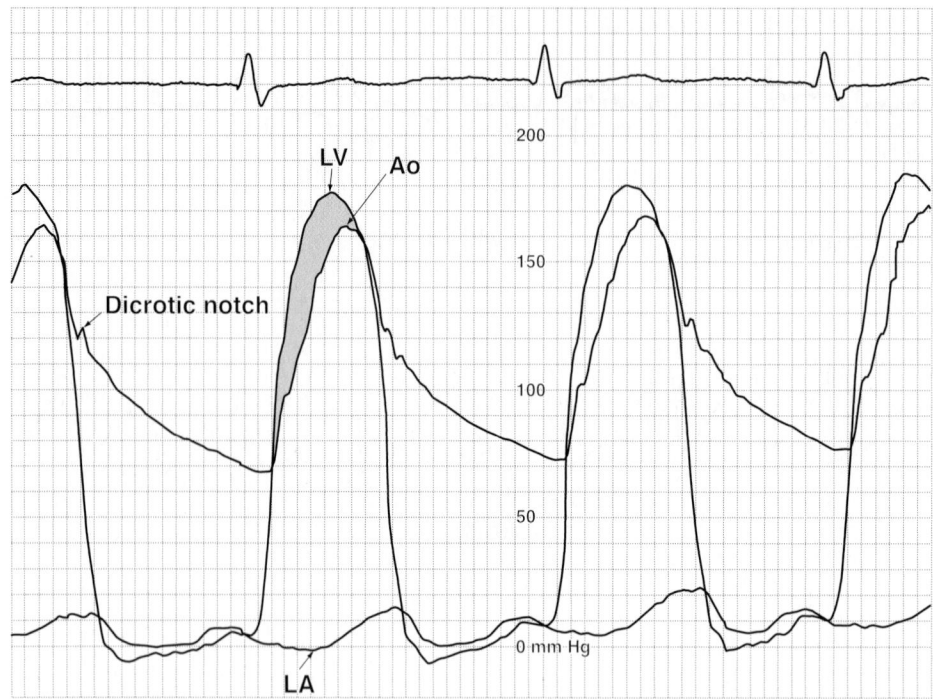

Fig. 23. Aortic stenosis. This is from the same patient as in Figure 22; however, instead of the femoral artery, aortic pressure (Ao) is used to measure the gradient (shaded area) across the aortic valve. Compare this figure with Figure 22, and note the obvious difference in measured gradients.

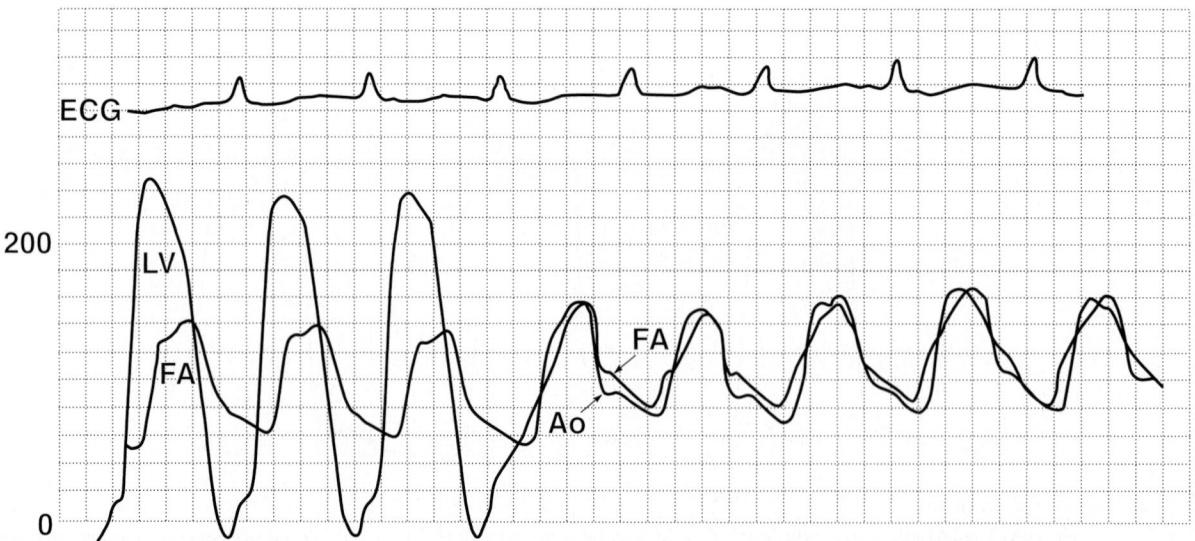

Fig. 24. Carabello sign in aortic stenosis. Pullback of the left ventricular catheter into the femoral artery (FA). The FA pressure increases when the catheter is withdrawn from across the critically stenosed aortic valve (Ao).

LOW-OUTPUT, LOW-GRADIENT AORTIC STENOSIS

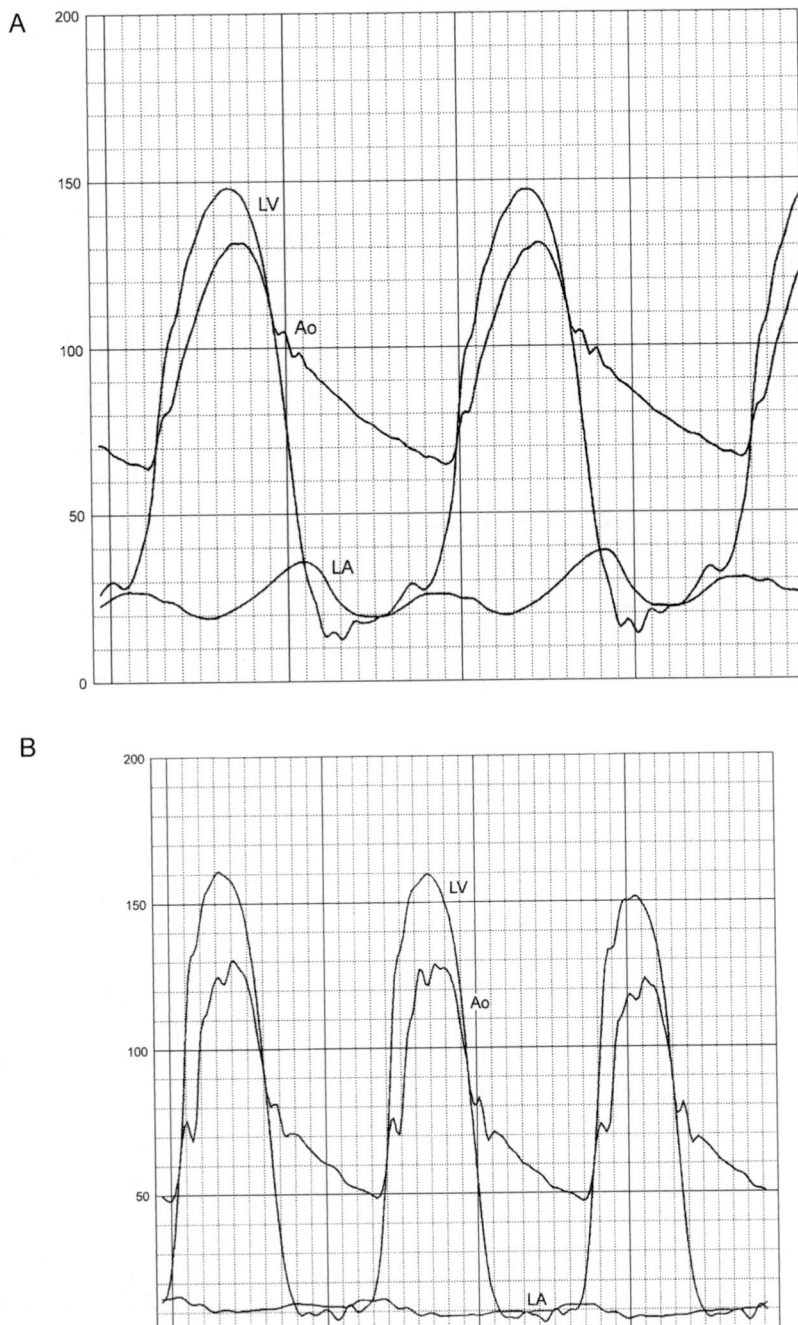

Fig. 25. The question of low-output low-gradient aortic valve stenosis. *A*, Simultaneous left ventricular (LV), left atrial (LA) and aortic (Ao) tracings from a patient referred for evaluation of aortic stenosis. In the resting state there was a low-output, low-gradient aortic stenosis with a mean gradient of 16 mm Hg, a cardiac output of 3.6 L/min and a calculated aortic valve area (AVA) of 0.9 cm2. *B*, During peak dobutamine infusion at 30 µg/kg/min there was normalization of the cardiac output to 6.5 L/min but the gradient increased to 27 mm Hg giving a calculated AVA of 1.1 cm2. Therefore this patient was diagnosed with low cardiac output and moderate aortic stenosis; the low calculated AVA in this patient was due to the low cardiac output rather than severe valvular aortic stenosis.

Aortic Valvuloplasty for Aortic Stenosis

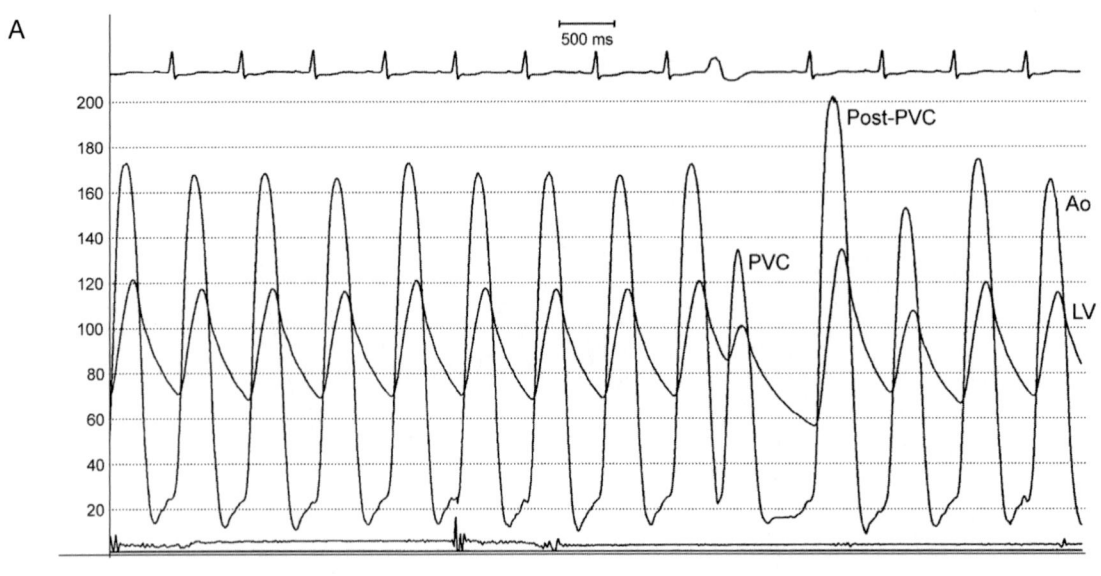

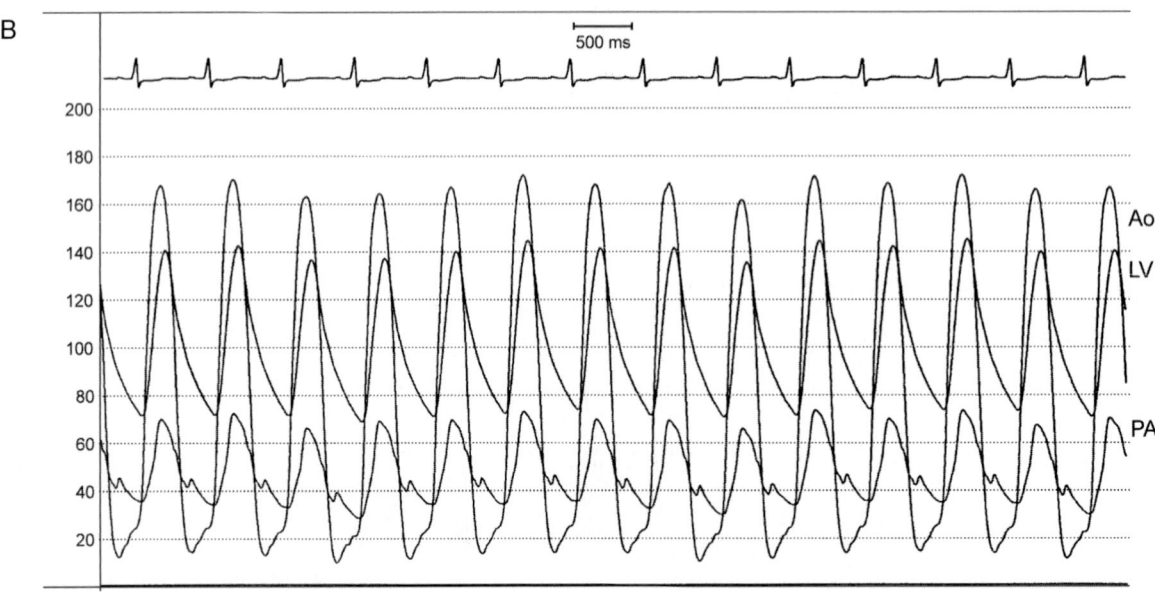

Fig. 26. Aortic valve stenosis. *A*, Simultaneous left ventricular (LV) and aortic (Ao) pressure tracings in a patient with severe symptomatic aortic stenosis. This patient had an ischemic cardiomyopathy with low ejection fraction, a peak-to-peak aortic gradient of 50 mm Hg, and an aortic valve area of 0.4 cm². Note the post-extrasystolic behavior of the gradient across the aortic valve is different in this setting of fixed obstruction compared with that of dynamic obstruction (see the Brockenbrough sign for hypertrophic obstructive cardiomyopathy shown in Figure 37). In the presence of a fixed obstruction, the post-extrasystolic beat may or may not demonstrate an increased gradient, but both the LV and Ao systolic pressures increase significantly. *B*, LV, Ao, and pulmonary artery (PA) pressures are shown after aortic balloon valvuloplasty has been performed. In this patient who was not felt to be a surgical candidate because of multiple comorbidities, a palliative aortic balloon valvuloplasty was performed (class IIa indication). The peak-to-peak gradient has been reduced to approximately 25 mm Hg and the valve area increased to 0.7 cm². The Ao pressure contours and hemodynamic findings are still consistent with moderate aortic stenosis.

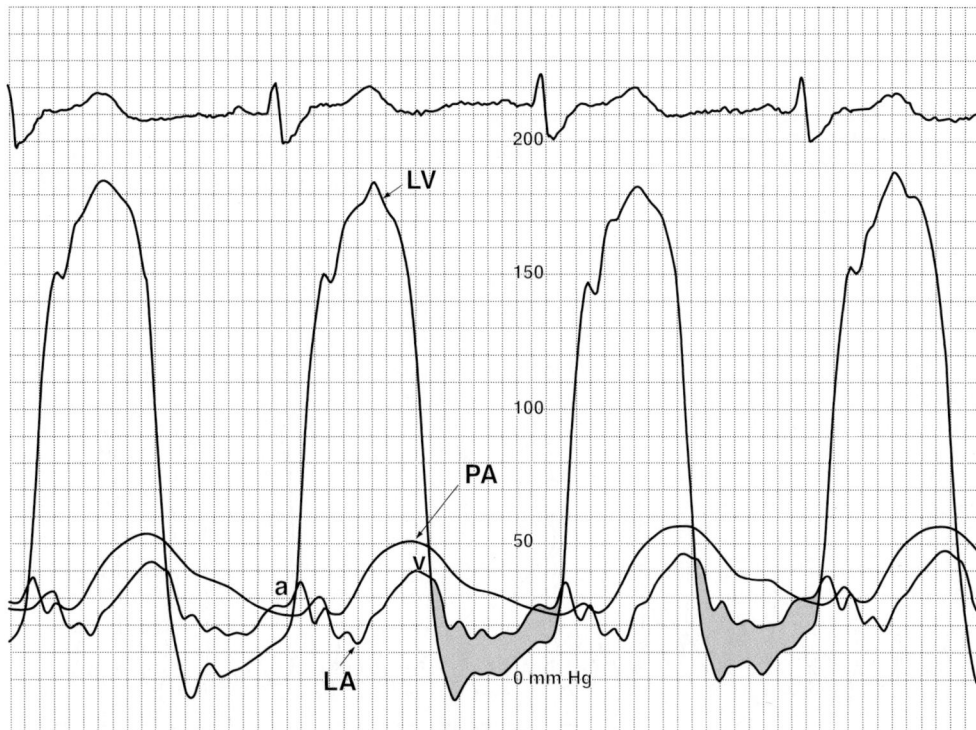

Fig. 27. Mitral stenosis. The shaded area represents the pressure gradient across the mitral valve. LV, left ventricular pressure; PA, pulmonary artery pressure; LA, left atrial pressure; a, left atrial A wave; v, left atrial V wave.

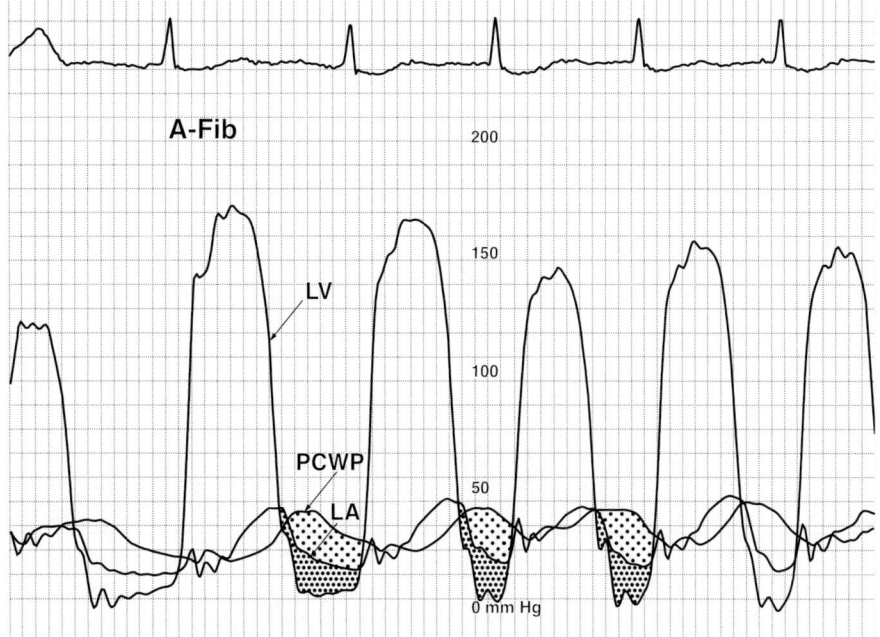

Fig. 28. Severe mitral stenosis. Simultaneous left ventricular (LV), pulmonary capillary wedge pressure (PCWP), and left atrial (LA) pressure tracings. This case illustrates the possibility of overestimating the mitral valve gradient if the PCWP rather than the true LA pressure is measured. Large stipple, gradient between PCWP and LV (false gradient across the mitral valve); small stipple, gradient between LA and LV (true gradient across the mitral valve).

MITRAL BALLOON VALVULOPLASTY FOR MITRAL STENOSIS

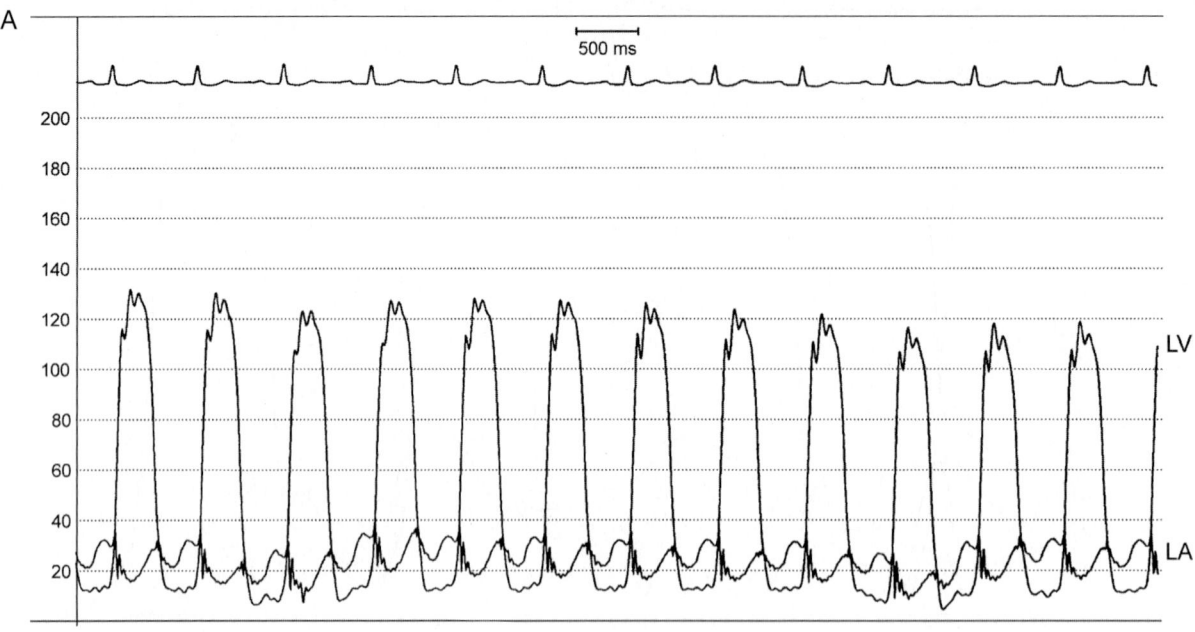

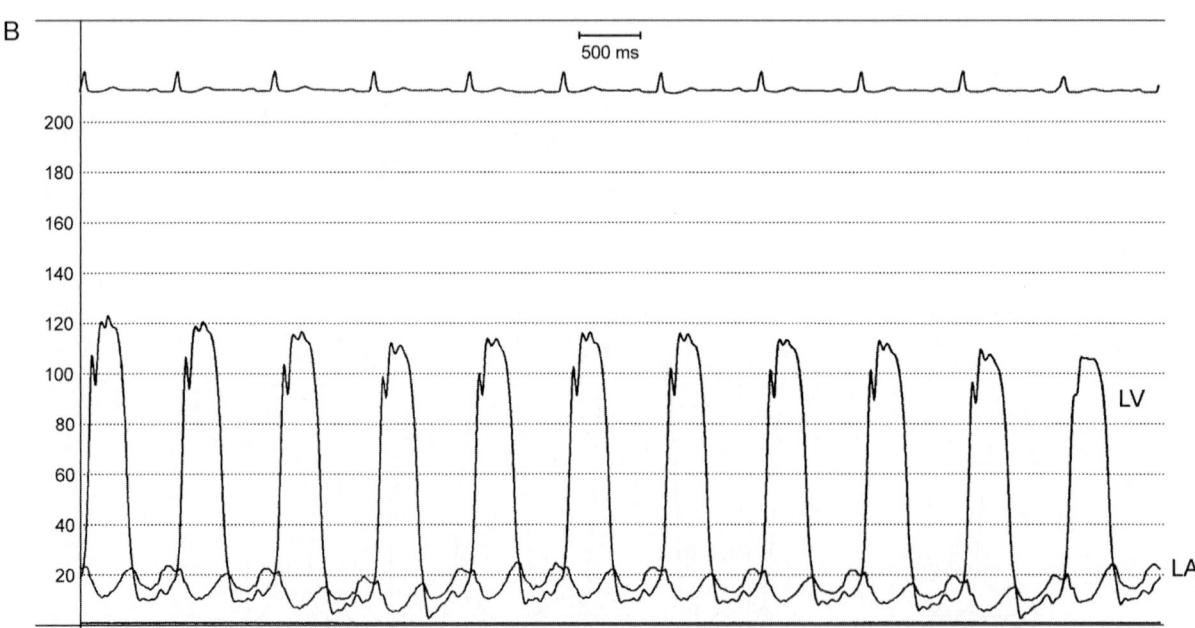

Fig. 29. Mitral valve stenosis. *A*, Simultaneous left ventricular (LV), left atrial (LA) and right atrial (RA) pressure tracings in a patient with severe rheumatic mitral stenosis. This patient had a mean transmitral gradient of 14 mm Hg, and a mitral valve area of 1.4 cm². *B*, LV, LA, and RA pressures are shown after percutaneous mitral balloon valvuloplasty has been performed. The mean transmitral gradient has been reduced to approximately 6 mm Hg and the valve area increased to 2.2 cm². Note that the left atrial V wave is similar in contour before and after the intervention compatible with the absence of severe mitral regurgitation; this finding concurs with an echocardiogram which also documented the absence of significant mitral regurgitation.

PULMONIC BALLOON VALVULOPLASTY OF PULMONIC STENOSIS

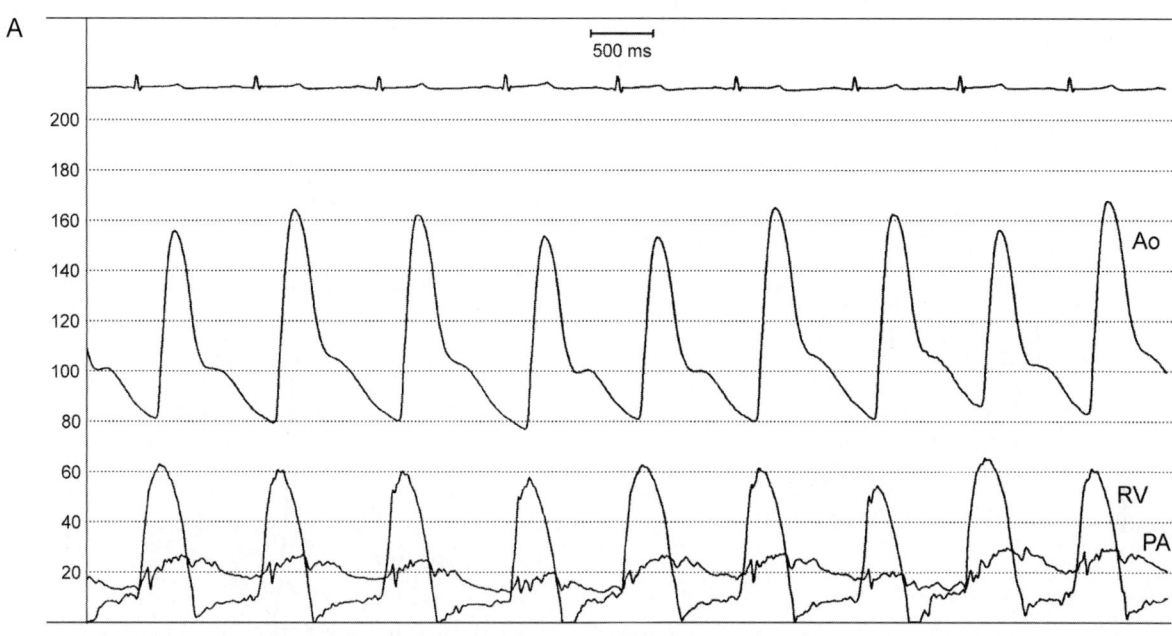

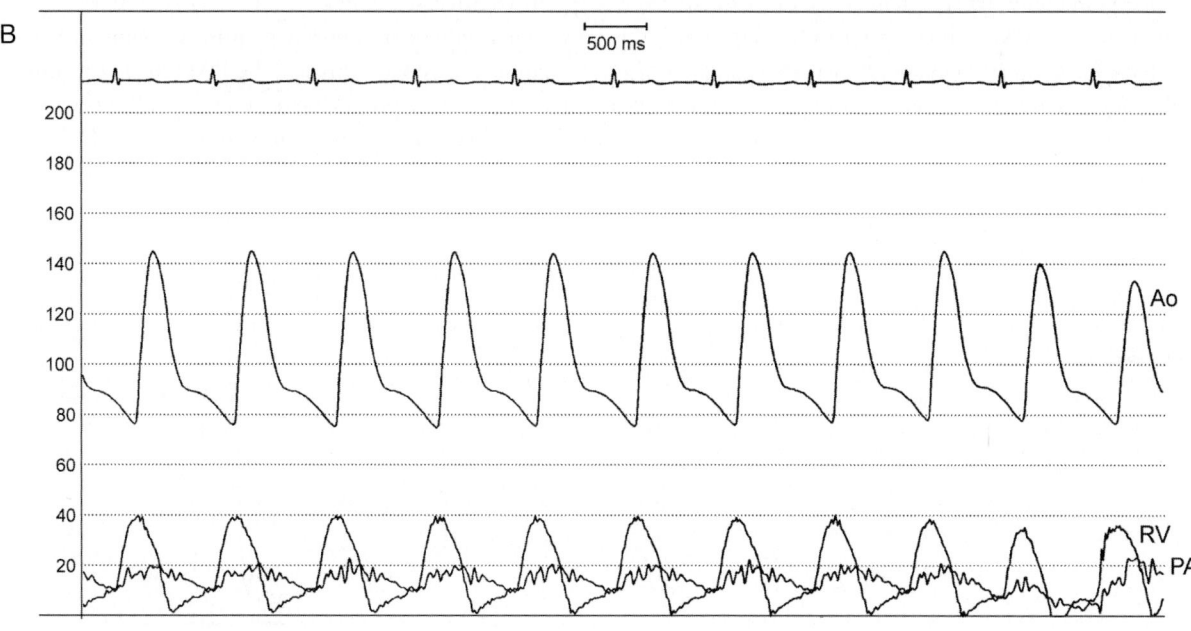

Fig. 30. Pulmonic valve stenosis. *A*, Simultaneous right ventricular (RV), pulmonary artery (PA) and aortic (Ao) pressure tracings in a patient with severe congenital pulmonic stenosis. This patient had a peak-to-peak pulmonary valve gradient of 40 mm Hg, and an pulmonic valve area of 1.1 cm2. *B*, RV, PA, and Ao pressures are shown after pulmonic balloon valvuloplasty has been performed. The peak-to-peak gradient has been reduced to approximately 12 mm Hg and the valve area increased to 1.7 cm2.

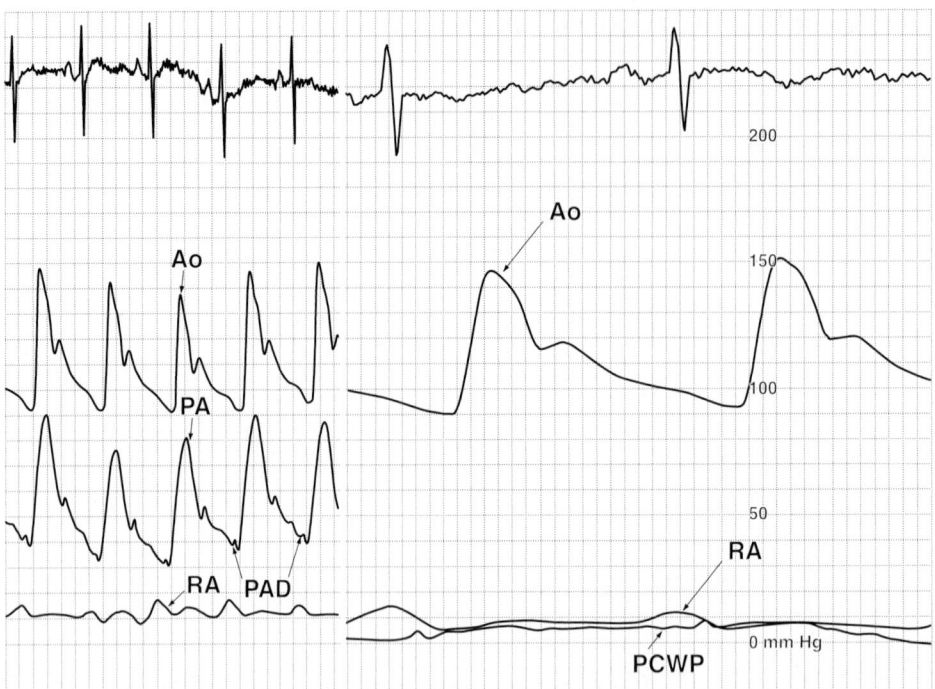

Fig. 31. Pulmonary hypertension. Right heart catheterization is frequently used to identify the cause of pulmonary hypertension, that is, cardiac vs. pulmonary cause. This can be readily appreciated while assessing the relationship of pulmonary artery diastolic pressure (PAD) and pulmonary capillary wedge pressure (PCWP). Normally, and in cases in which pulmonary hypertension is due to a cardiac cause (e.g., left ventricular dysfunction, mitral stenosis), PCWP approximates the PAD. However, when the hypertension has a primary pulmonary cause (e.g., primary pulmonary hypertension, secondary pulmonary hypertension from thromboemboli, pulmonary fibrosis), the PAD may be significantly higher, while the pulmonary artery wedge pressure (PA) remains normal, producing a significant difference between these two pressures. In this figure, the patient had primary pulmonary hypertension with a mean PAD of 35 mm Hg and a PCWP of only 7 mm Hg. Note that the right atrial pressure (RA) is slightly higher than the PCWP. Ao, aorta.

FLOLAN STUDY SHOWING DECREASE IN RIGHT SIDED PRESSURES WITH FLOLAN ADMINISTRATION

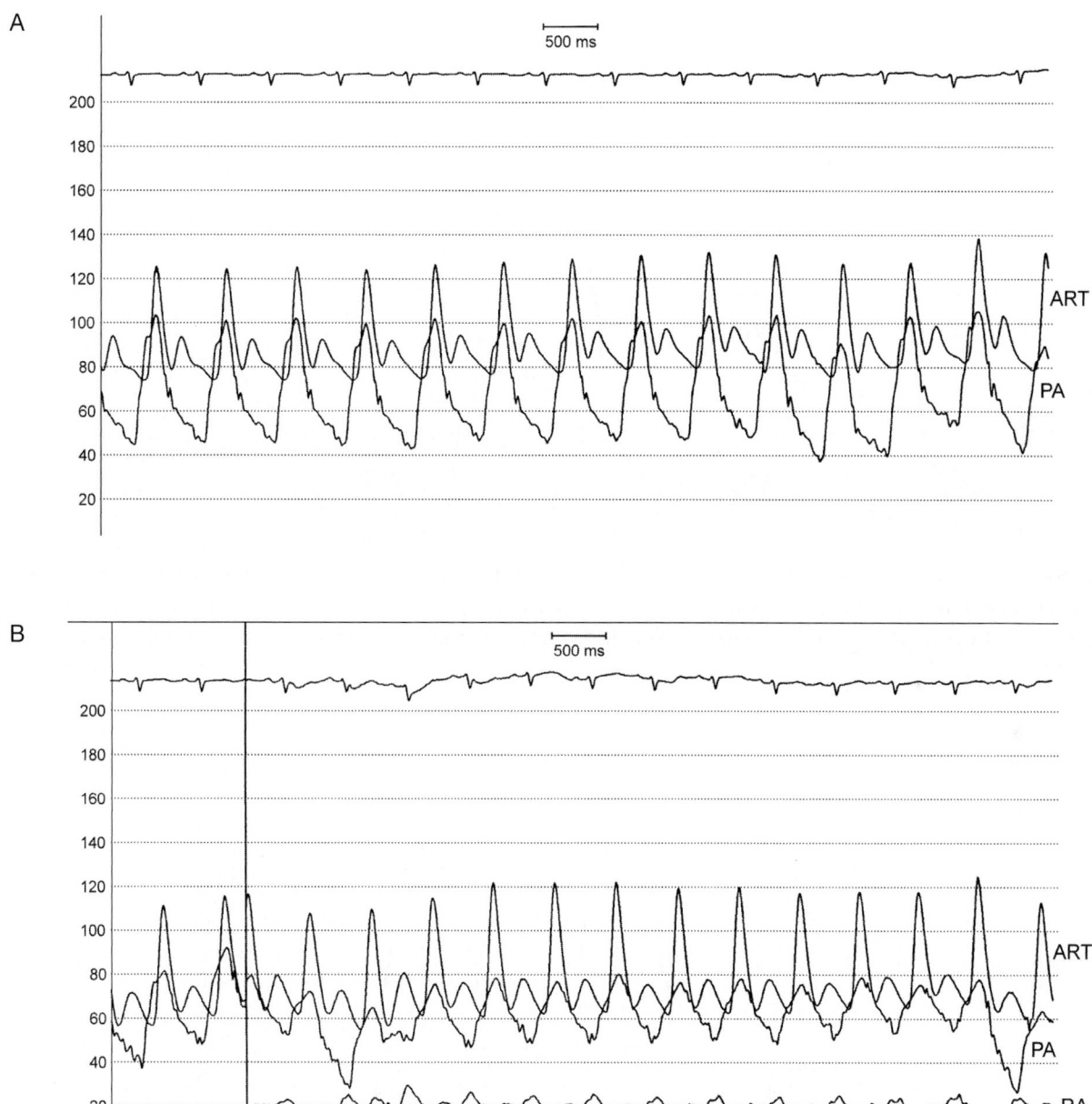

Fig. 32. Pulmonary hypertension. *A*, Simultaneous radial artery (ART), pulmonary atery (PA) and right atrial (RA) tracing from a patient with severe pulmonary hypertension. The mean PA pressure was 64 mm Hg, the mean wedge pressure was 11 mm Hg, and the cardiac output was 5.7 L/min. This allows the calculation of a pulmonary arteriolar resistance of 9.3 Wood units. *B*, Simultaneous ART, PA, and RA tracings during administration of epoprostenol at 12 ng. The mean PA pressure did not change significantly and was 60 mm Hg despite a concurrent decrease in arterial pressure. The mean wedge pressure increased to 20 mm Hg, but the cardiac output increased to 8.8 L/min. This allows the calculation of a pulmonary arteriolar resistance of 4.6 Wood units.

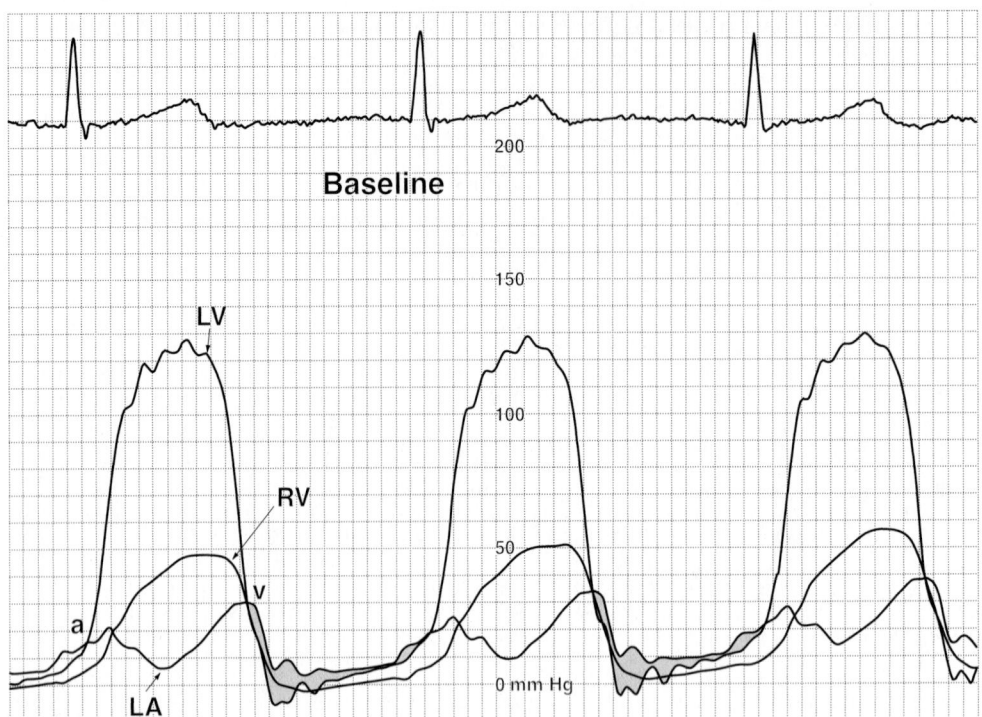

Fig. 33. Mitral stenosis. Pressure tracings in a patient with significant exercise intolerance. The patient was found to have mild mitral stenosis. Rest tracings with a heart rate of approximately 70 beats/min. LV, left ventricular pressure; RV, right ventricular pressure; LA, left atrial pressure. The shaded area represents the pressure gradient across the mitral valve.

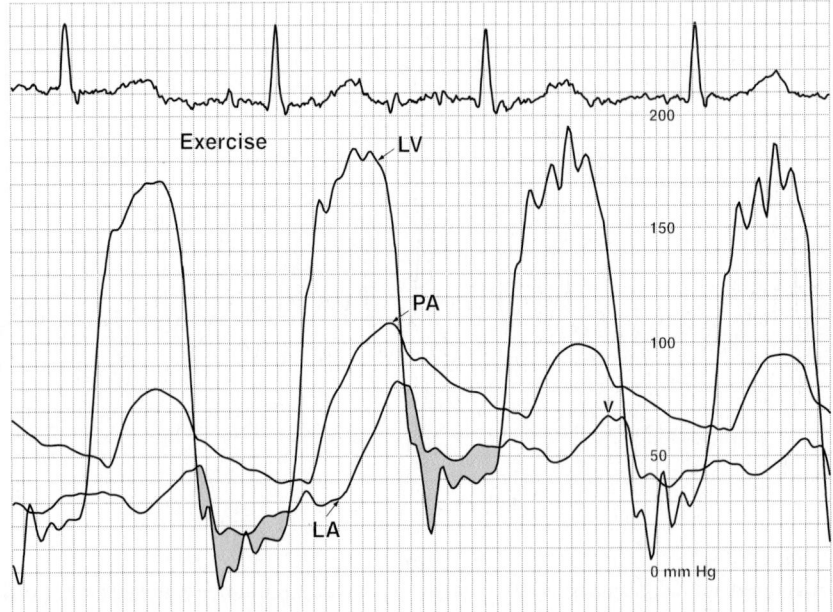

Fig. 34. Effect of exercise. This tracing is from the same patient as in Figure 33. After 4 minutes of exercise, a significant increase in the gradient across the mitral valve was noted. Observe the marked increase in right heart pressures (catheter now in the pulmonary artery [PA]) from 50 mm Hg to about 100 mm Hg and the increase in left atrial pressure (LA) (about 30 mm Hg to about 80 mm Hg at the maximal height of the LA "v" wave). The exercise heart rate was approximately 110 beats/min. The shaded area represents the pressure gradient across the mitral valve.

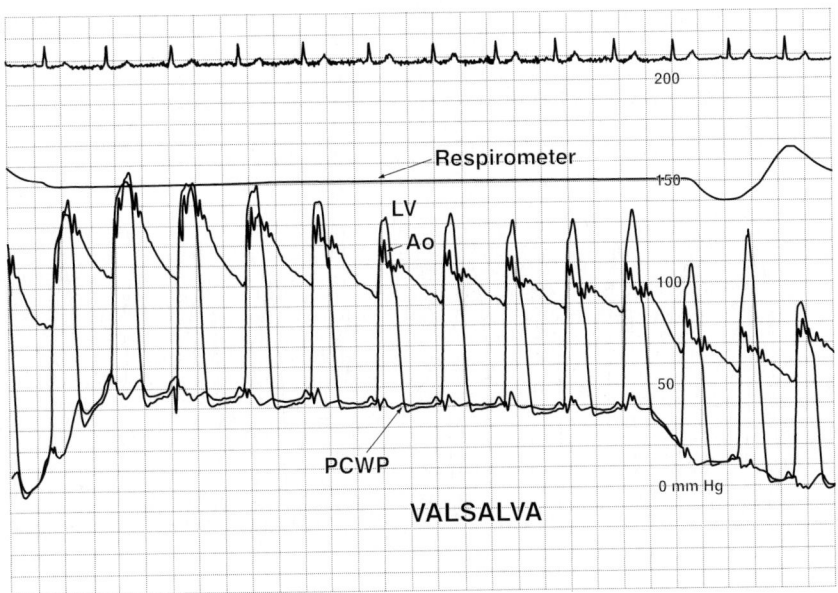

Fig. 35. Hypertrophic obstructive cardiomyopathy. Dynamic left ventricular outflow tract obstruction during phase 2 of the Valsalva maneuver. Note the significant increase in the left ventricular (LV) end-diastolic pressure and steady decrease in LV systolic pressure during phase 2 of the Valsalva maneuver along with an increase in the outflow tract gradient. Ao, aorta; PCWP, pulmonary capillary wedge pressure.

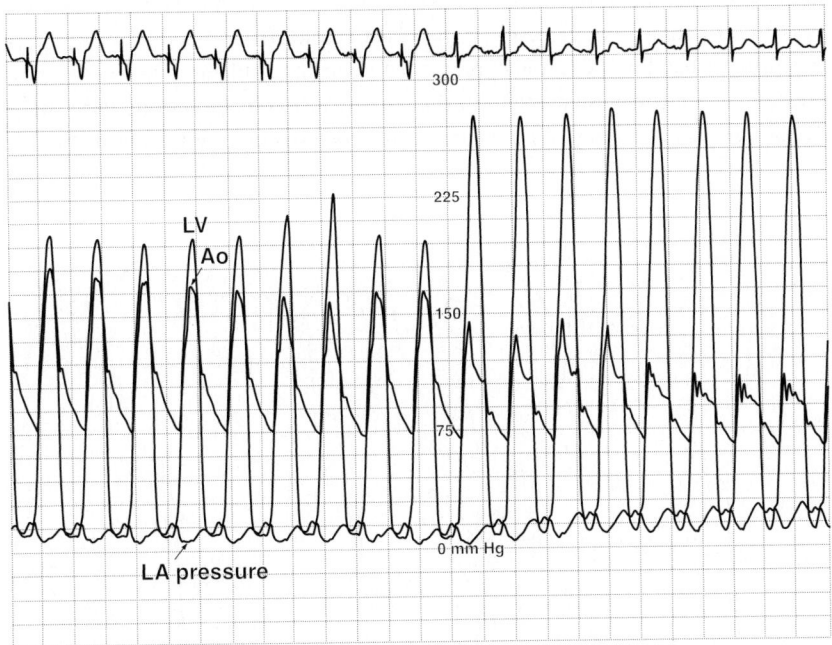

Fig. 36. Effect of pacing on dynamic left ventricular outflow tract gradient. This tracing is from a patient with severe hypertrophic obstructive cardiomyopathy who was evaluated in the cardiac catheterization laboratory to assess whether pacing would be beneficial in decreasing the outflow tract gradient. Both chambers were paced with varying intervals, and the effect of each pacing regimen was assessed. In the first half of the figure, the patient is being paced in a P-synchronized mode with an atrioventricular interval of 100 ms. In the second half of the figure, the pacing is discontinued and the patient is in sinus rhythm. Note the significant worsening of the outflow gradient after the pacing is discontinued. Also note the increase in mean left atrial pressure with discontinuation of pacing secondary to worsening of the outflow gradient. LV, left ventricular pressure; LA, left atrial pressure; Ao, aortic pressure.

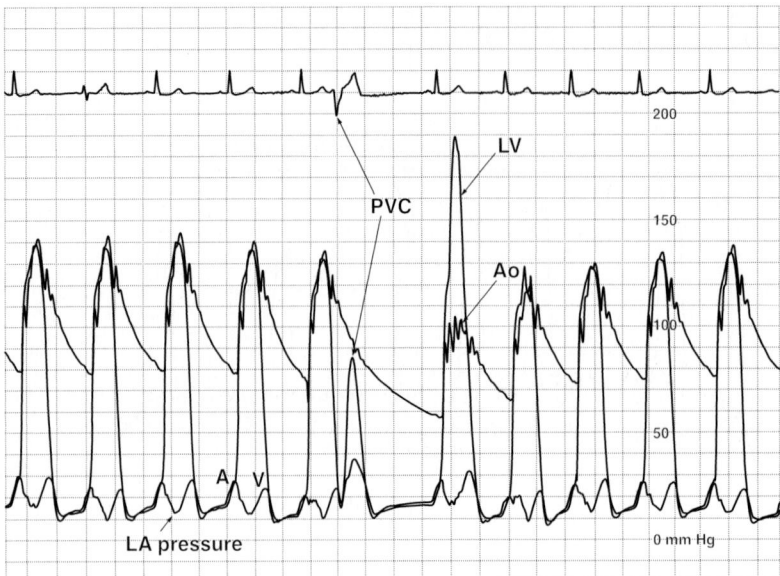

Fig. 37. Brockenbrough sign in hypertrophic obstructive cardiomyopathy. The post-extrasystolic behavior of a gradient across the aortic/outflow tract can differentiate between a fixed and a dynamic obstruction. In a patient with hypertrophic obstructive cardiomyopathy, the post-extrasystolic beat develops more severe obstruction, with a marked increase in gradient and decrease in aortic pressure (Ao). This feature is characteristic of dynamic LV outflow tract obstruction and is called the "Brockenbrough sign." In fixed obstruction like aortic stenosis (in the presence of normal LV function), the gradient increases with the increase in stroke volume but not to the extent that occurs in HCM. Also, the aortic pulse pressure should increase. This patient demonstrates an increased gradient for several beats after a premature ventricular contraction before it returns to baseline. Also, the dynamic nature of the gradient with beat-to-beat variation should be noted. Note the decrease in the aortic pulse pressure in the post-extrasystolic beat along with the increase in the LV systolic pressure. The increase in left atrial (LA) pressure during the post-extrasystolic beat should also be appreciated.

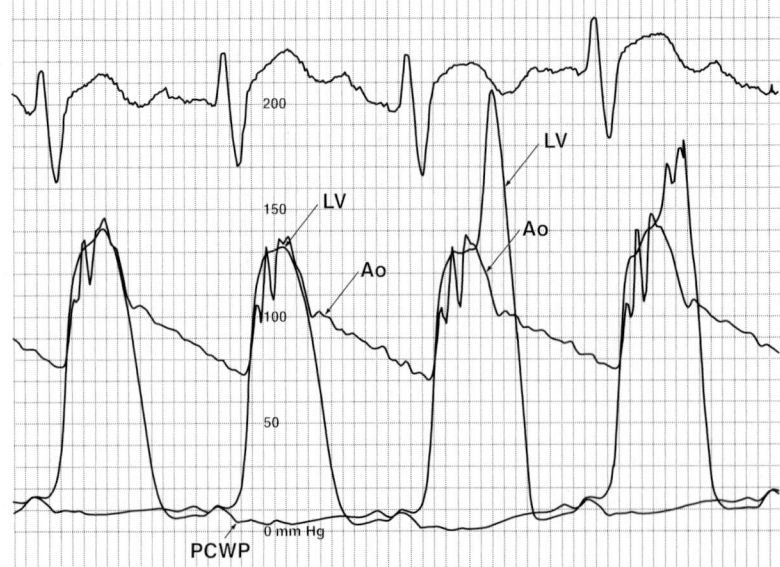

Fig. 38. Artifact. This is a tracing of catheter entrapment. Beat no. 3 is an artifact from left ventricular (LV) catheter entrapment in the small hyperdynamic cavity. The key points that differentiate this from Brockenbrough sign are the absence of a premature ventricular contraction and the fact that the aortic pulse pressure (Ao) did not decrease with the apparent increase in the LV systolic pressure.

ARTIFACTS: DAMPING

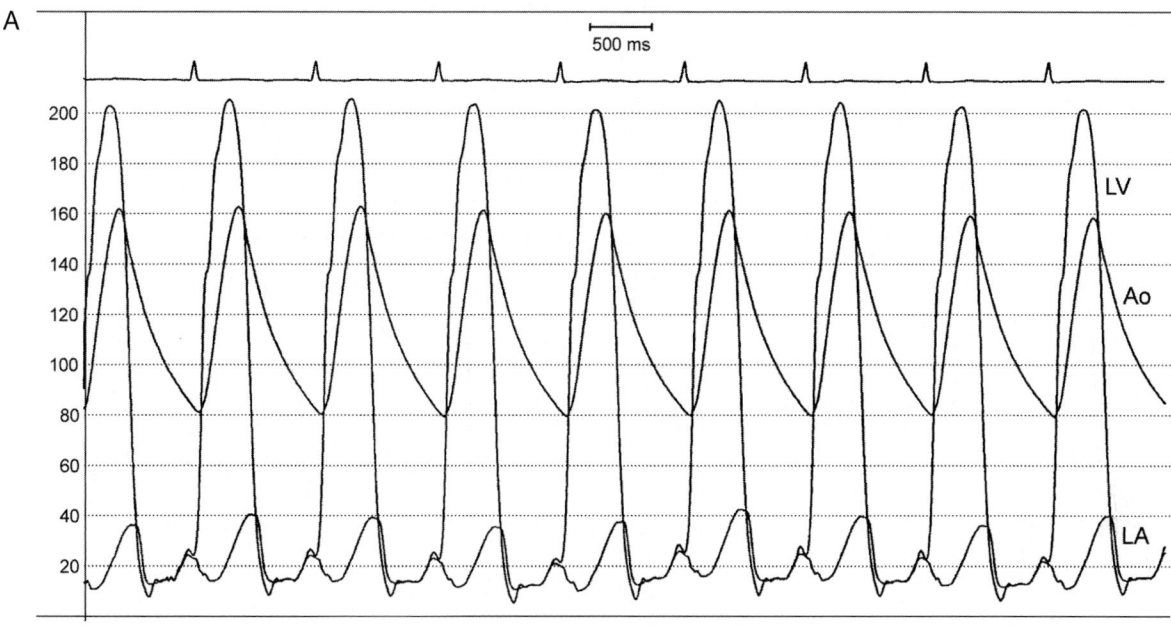

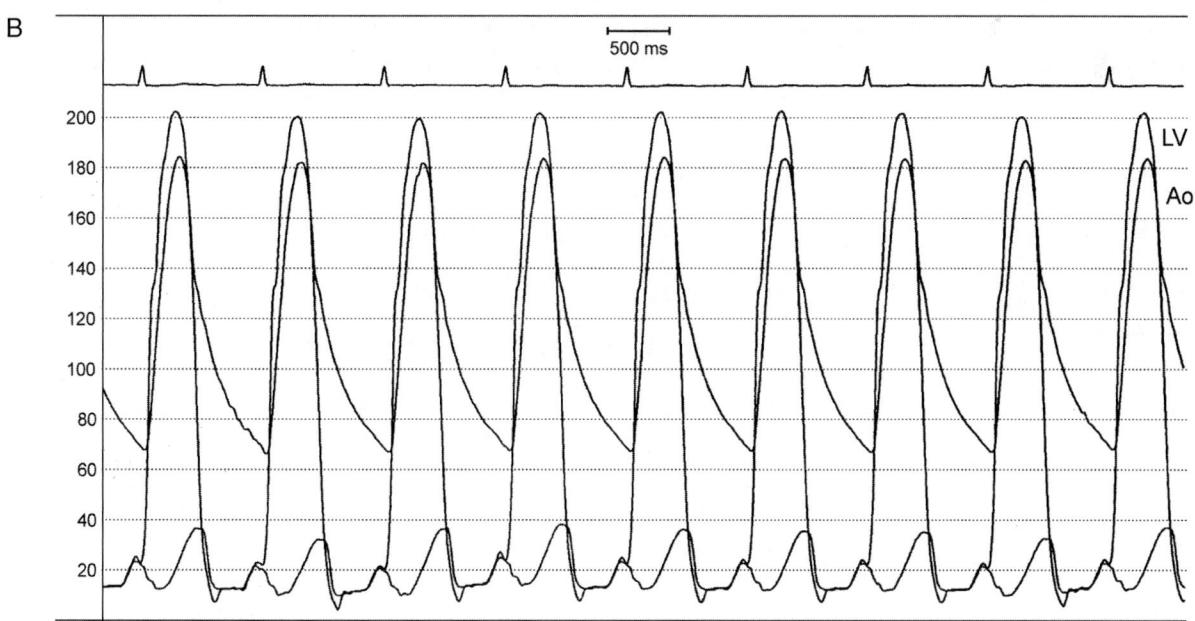

Fig. 39. Artifact. *A,* Simultaneous left ventricular (LV) and aortic (Ao) pressure curves from a patient referred for evaluation of aortic stenosis. At first glance there appears to be a 40-mm Hg peak-to-peak gradient across the aortic valve. However, more careful analysis of the Ao pressure contours reveals the absence of a dicrotic notch consistent with damping of the catheter. *B,* The tracing of the LV and Ao pressures once the catheter has been rotated so that it is no longer damped. Now a dicrotic notch can be seen in the Ao tracing, and the gradient is only 10 mm Hg peak-to-peak.

INTRA-AORTIC BALLOON COUNTERPULSATION

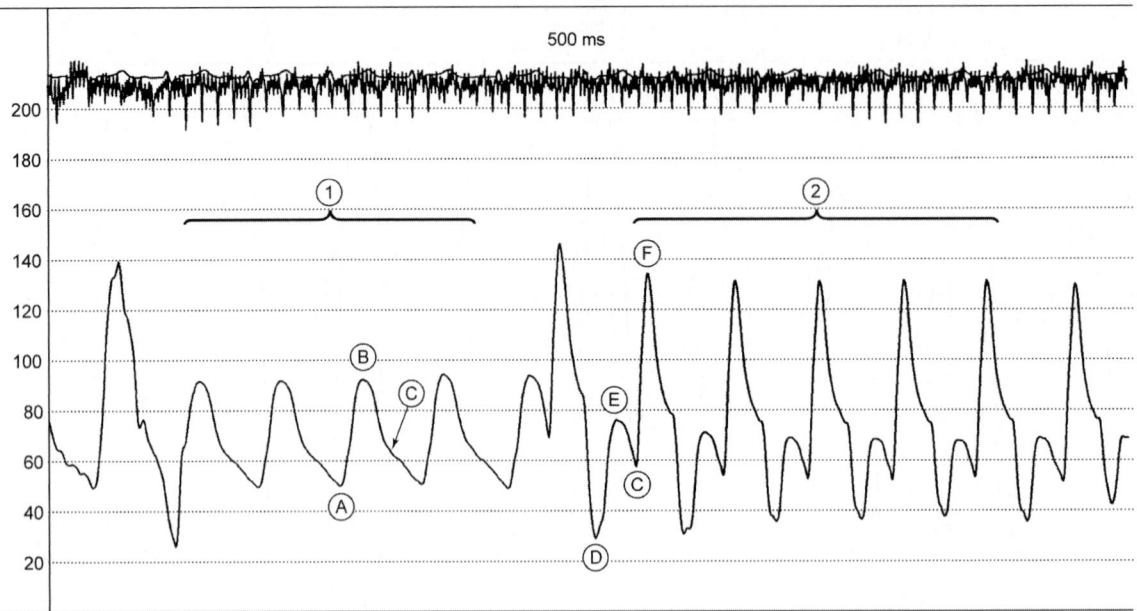

Fig. 40. Intra-aortic balloon counterpulsation. This aortic (Ao) pressure tracing shows the aortic contours before (1) and after (2) application of 1:1 intra-aortic balloon counterpulsation. Before balloon counterpulsation (1), the unassisted aortic end-diastolic pressure (A), unassisted systolic pressure (B) and dicrotic notch (C) can be seen. After initiation of balloon counterpulsation (2), the aortic end-diastolic pressure (D) and systolic pressure (E) are reduced as a result of decreased afterload; this results in decreased myocardial oxygen demand. Simultaneously the aortic diastolic pressure (F) is augmented resulting in increased myocardial perfusion, since most of coronary arterial flow occurs during diastole.

Constrictive Pericarditis and Restrictive Cardiomyopathy

Cases of constrictive pericarditis and restrictive cardiomyopathy are shown below to highlight the traditional hemodynamic criteria and the more recently recognized dynamic respiratory changes noted in these entities. The traditional hemodynamic criteria are sensitive, but lack adequate specificity to distinguish between constrictive pericarditis and restrictive cardiomyopathy. Dynamic respiratory changes have high sensitivity and specificity to allow this distinction. In the following cases, significant overlap of the traditional hemodynamic criteria is found in patients with confirmed constrictive pericarditis and restrictive cardiomyopathy. All the tracings are from high-fidelity pressure micromanometers.

Table 1.   Traditional Hemodynamic Criteria for Differentiating Constrictive Pericarditis and Restrictive Cardiomyopathy in the Catheterization Laboratory

Criterion	Constrictive pericarditis	Restrictive cardiomyopathy
Difference between left ventricular end-diastolic pressure (LVEDP) and right ventricular end-diastolic pressure (RVEDP)	[LVEDP-RVEDP] ≤5 mm Hg	[LVEDP-RVEDP] >5 mm Hg
Pulmonary artery systolic pressure (PASP)	PASP ≤55 mm Hg	PASP >55 mm Hg
Ratio between right ventricular end-diastolic pressure (RVEDP) and right ventricular systolic pressure (RVSP)	RVEDP/RVSP >1/3	RVEDP/RVSP <1/3
Left ventricular rapid filling wave (LVRFW)	LVRFW >7 mm Hg	LVRFW <7 mm Hg
Respiratory variation in mean right atrial pressure (RAP)	RAP variation <3 mm Hg	RAP variation >3 mm Hg

Table 2. Dynamic Respiratory Criteria for Differentiating Constrictive Pericarditis from Restrictive
Cardiomyopathy

Criterion	Constrictive pericarditis	Restrictive cardiomyopathy
Intrathoracic and intracardiac dissociation: Variation in gradient between early left ventricular diastolic pressure and wedge pressure during inspiration when compared with expiration	Variation >5 mm Hg	Variation ≤5 mm Hg
Ventricular discordance due to: Concordant change in right ventricular systolic pressure (RVSP) and left ventricular systolic pressure (LVSP) with respiration	Discordance changes present	Concordant changes present
Concordant change in right ventricular systolic pulse duration and left ventricular systolic pulse duration with respiration	Discordance changes present	Concordant changes present
Relative change in change in area under the right ventricular pulse area to left ventricular pulse area with respiration	Discordance changes present	Concordant changes present

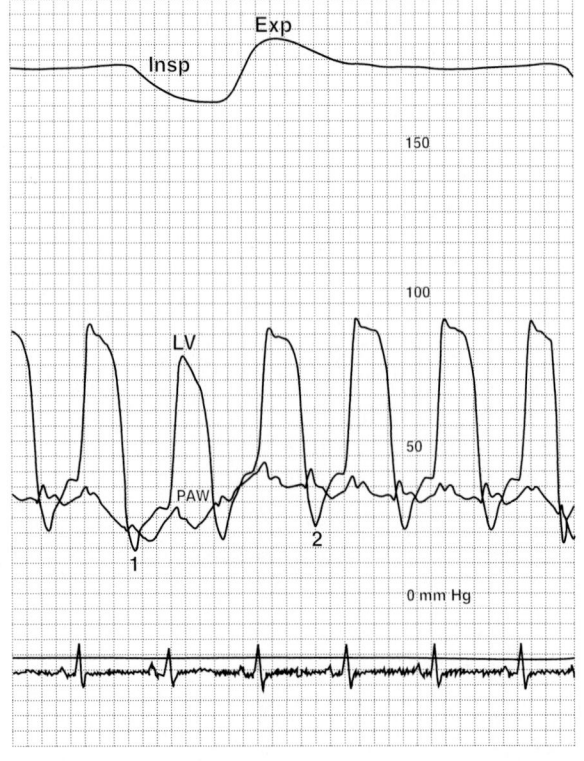

Fig. 41. Dissociation of intrathoracic and intracardiac pressures in constrictive pericarditis. The following 3 tracings are from a patient with surgically proven constrictive pericarditis. Simultaneous recordings of left ventricular and pulmonary capillary wedge pressures demonstrating dissociation of intrathoracic and intracardiac pressures. Note the decrease in early diastolic gradient with inspiration (Insp) (beat marked "1") and the increase with expiration (Exp) (beat marked "2"). Also note the dip-and-plateau morphology of the left ventricular (LV) diastolic pressures. The nasal respirometer tracing is also shown at the top. PAW, pulmonary artery wedge.

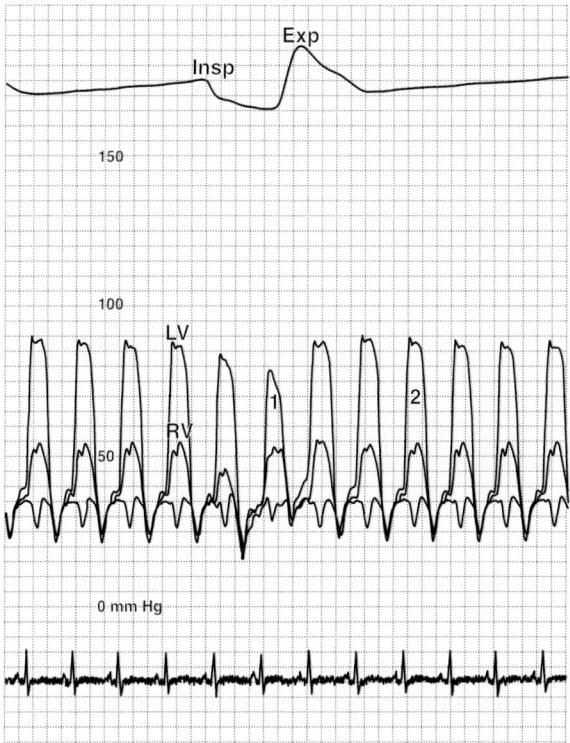

Fig. 42. Ventricular interdependence in constrictive pericarditis. Simultaneous recordings of left ventricular (LV), right ventricular (RV), and right atrial pressures demonstrating ventricular interdependence. Note the discordance in LV and RV systolic pressures with respiration (beats 1 and 2). While the RVSP increases during inspiration, the LVSP pressure decreases; these changes reverse during expiration. As seen in the side panels, the duration of the RV pulse (*arrows*) is also greater relative to the duration of the LV pulse in inspiration than in expiration. The peak pressure and pulse duration are most completely synthesized by comparing the area under the RV curve (shaded area) to the area under the LV impulse (stippled area). The ratio of RV-to-LV area is greater in inspiration than expiration (consistent with a discordant change). Other criteria of constrictive pericarditis are also seen, e.g., a marked "W" or "M" pattern in the right atrial pressure tracing, absence of decrease in right atrial pressure with inspiration (Kussmaul sign), right ventricular end-diastolic pressure (RVEDP) >1/3 of right ventricular systolic pressure (RVSP), and equalization of pressures (<5 mm Hg difference in the left ventricular end-diastolic pressure and RVEDP). However, the RVSP (and, therefore, pulmonary artery systolic pressure, in the absence of RV outflow gradient) is slightly above 55 mm Hg. The nasal respirometer tracing is also shown at the top. Exp, expiration; Insp, inspiration.

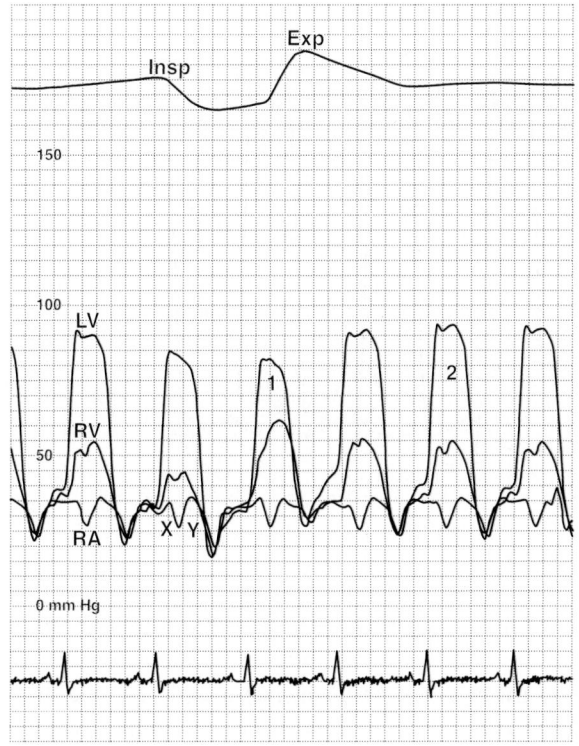

Fig. 43. Hemodynamic tracings in constrictive pericarditis. Higher paper speed (100 mm/s) simultaneous recordings of left ventricular (LV), right ventricular (RV), and right atrial (RA) pressures demonstrating ventricular interdependence. Note the decrease in RV systolic pressure during the first beat and a marked rise in the next ejection at peak inspiration (beat 1) while LV systolic pressure decreases. Note the rapid X and Y descents in the RA tracing. The nasal respirometer tracing is shown at the top. Exp, expiration; Insp, inspiration.

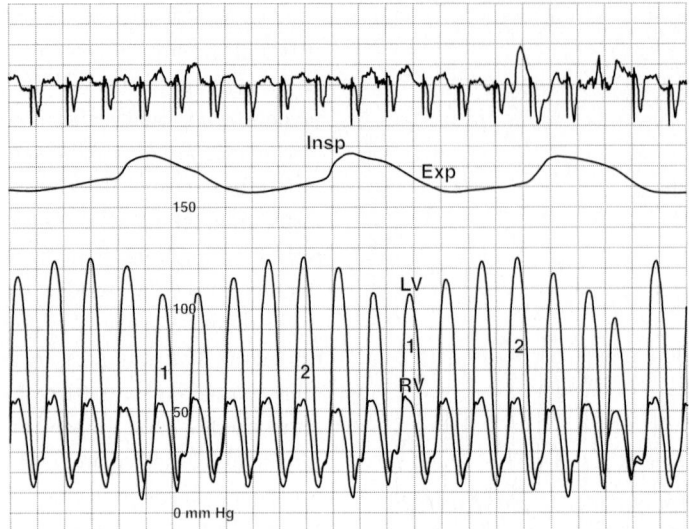

Fig. 44. Simultaneous recordings of left ventricular (LV) and right ventricular (RV) pressure demonstrating subtle ventricular discordance in constrictive pericarditis. This ventricular discordance is more subtle than that seen in Figure 43 and makes the point that ventricular discordance may not be as marked as shown in Figure 43. There are significant changes in LV systolic pressure, whereas those of RV systolic pressure are more subtle but definitely in the *opposite direction*. At peak inspiration (beat 1), LV systolic pressure is significantly lower, but RV systolic pressure is slightly higher than peak expiration (beat 2), although not markedly so. This is absence of concordance, that is, ventricular discordance. The nasal respirometer tracing is shown at the top. Exp, expiration; Insp, inspiration.

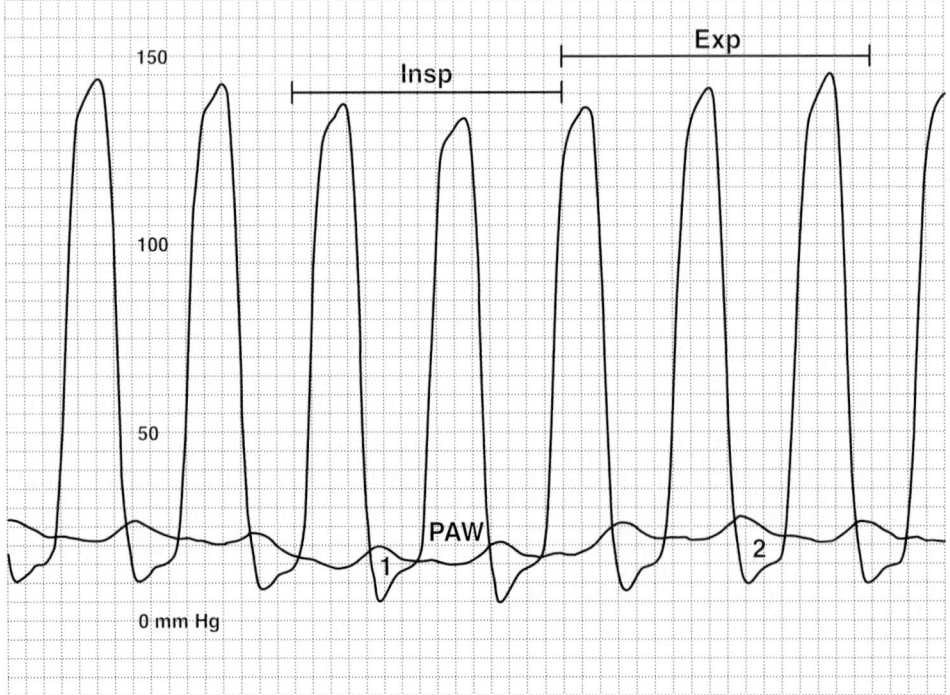

Fig. 45. Restrictive filling in restrictive cardiomyopathy. This tracing is from a patient with idiopathic restrictive cardiomyopathy. Simultaneous recordings of left ventricular and pulmonary capillary wedge pressures demonstrate the lack of dissociation of intrathoracic and intracardiac pressures. Both tracings are from high-fidelity micromanometer catheters. Note the nearly constant early diastolic gradient with respiration (beat 1 vs. 2). Exp, expiration; Insp, inspiration; PAW, pulmonary artery wedge.

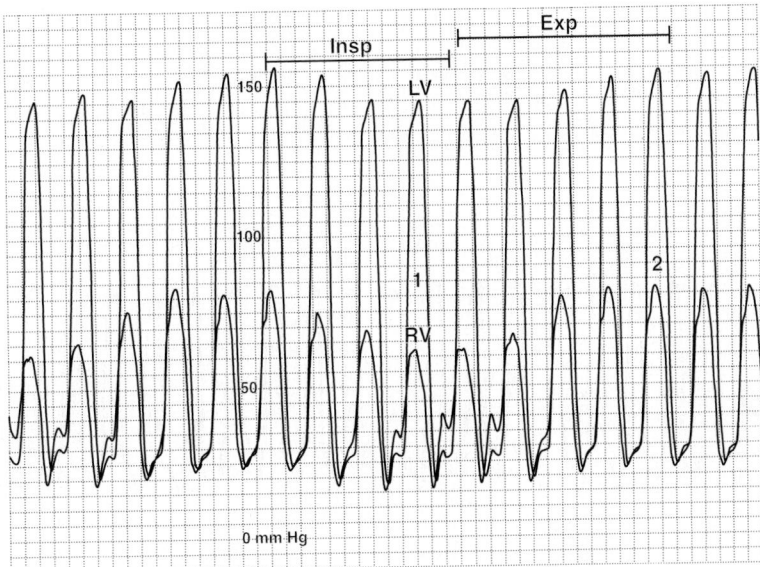

Fig. 46. Simultaneous recordings (from the same patient as in Figure 45) of left ventricular (LV) and right ventricular (RV) pressures demonstrating the absence of ventricular interdependence. Note the concordance in LV and RV systolic pressures with respiration. With inspiration (Insp), the LV and RV systolic pressures decrease and increase in concordance during expiration (Exp) (beat 1 vs. 2). As seen in the side panels, the duration of the RV pulse (*arrows*) does not change relative to the duration of the LV pulse from inspiration to expiration. The peak pressure and pulse duration are most completely synthesized by comparing the area under the RV curve (shaded area) to the area under the LV impulse (stippled area). The ratio of RV-to-LV area similar in inspiration and expiration (consistent with a concordant change). Other features of note are RV systolic pressure (i.e., pulmonary systolic pressure) >55 mm Hg, RV end-diastolic pressure <1/3 of RV systolic pressure, dip-and-plateau morphology of diastolic pressures.

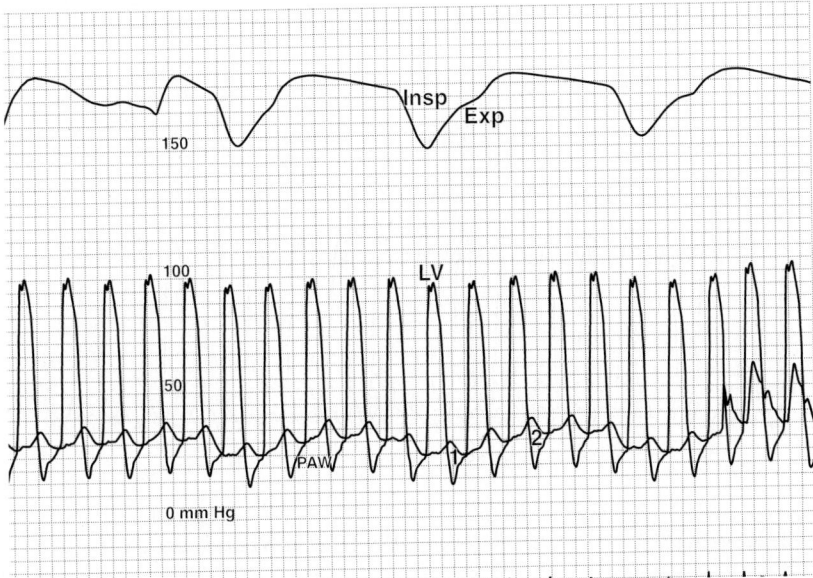

Fig. 47. Tracing from a patient with systemic amyloidosis who had biopsy-proven cardiac involvement resulting in restrictive cardiomyopathy. Simultaneous high-fidelity recordings of left ventricular (LV) and pulmonary capillary wedge pressures demonstrating lack of dissociation of intrathoracic and intracardiac pressures. Note the constant early diastolic gradient (<5 mm Hg change) with respiration (beat 1 vs. 2) and the wedge balloon deflation showing pulmonary artery pressure in the last 3 beats. The nasal respirometer tracing is shown at the top. Exp, expiration; Insp, inspiration; PAW, pulmonary artery wedge.

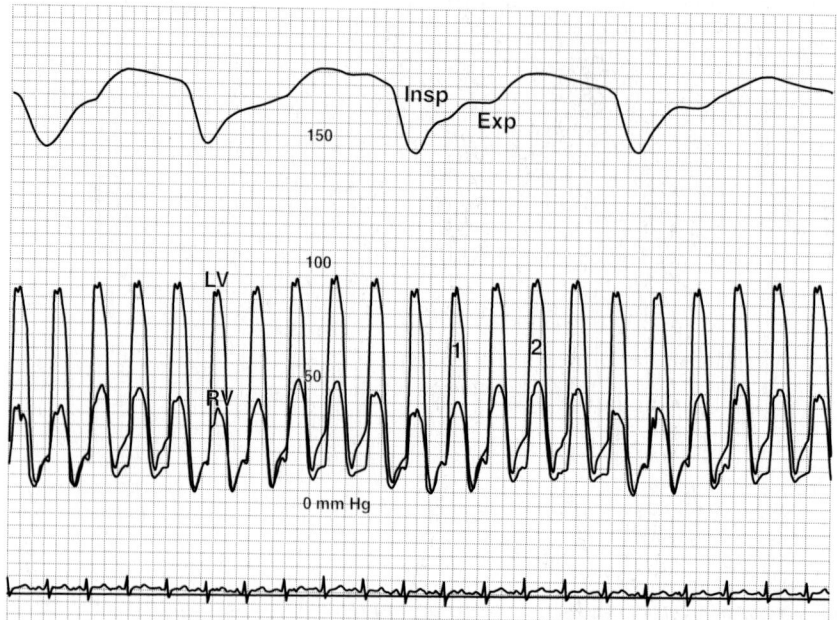

Fig. 48. Simultaneous high-fidelity recordings (from the same patient as in Figure 47) of the left ventricular (LV) and right ventricular (RV) pressures demonstrating the absence of ventricular interdependence. Note the concordance in LV and RV pressures and increase with expiration (beat 2). Also note the dip-and-plateau morphology of diastolic pressures, pulmonary artery pressure of 55 mm Hg, and the RV end-diastolic pressure >1/3 of the RV systolic pressure—all the traditional criteria thought to be consistent with constriction. The nasal respirometer is shown at the top. Exp, expiration; Insp, inspiration.

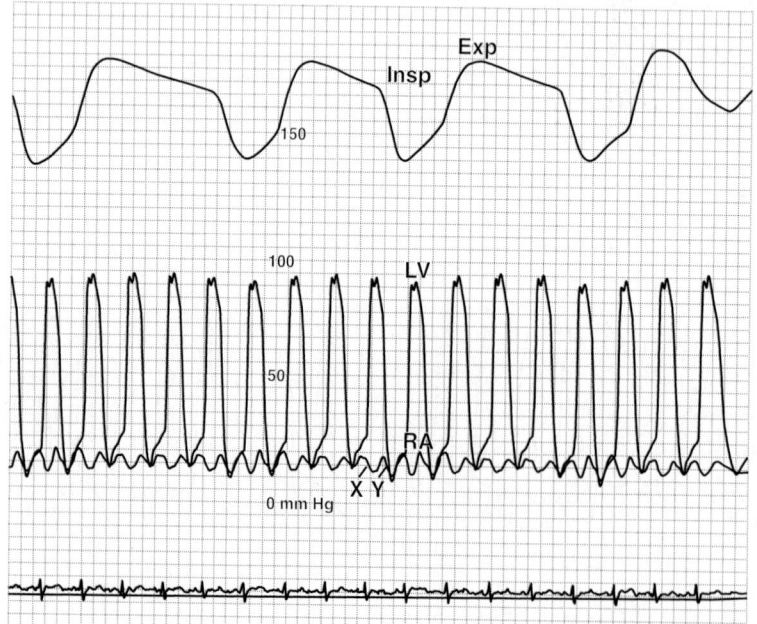

Fig. 49. Simultaneous high-fidelity recordings (from the same patient as in Figures 47 and 48) of the left ventricular (LV) and right ventricular (RV) pressures. Note the marked "W" or "M" pattern in the RA pressure tracing, with prominent X and Y descents and no decrease with inspiration (Insp) (Kussmaul sign). Also note the equalization of the RA and LV diastolic pressures. In summary, this patient has most of the traditional criteria of constrictive pericarditis; however, the dynamic respiratory criteria clearly demonstrate that the patient has restriction and not constrictive pericarditis. The nasal respirometer is shown at the top. Exp, expiration.

123

ENDOMYOCARDIAL BIOPSY

Joseph G. Murphy, MD

Robert P. Frantz, MD

Leslie T. Cooper, Jr., MD

Endomyocardial biopsy (EMB) is a valuable invasive diagnostic modality for selected patients with myocardial disease and remains the proverbial "gold standard" for the diagnosis of cardiac allograft rejection and cardiac involvement in specific rare diseases that may affect the myocardium including sarcoidosis, hemochromatosis, amyloid heart disease and many forms of myocarditis. (Table 1, Fig. 1 and 2). In addition, patients with dilated cardiomyopathy, restrictive cardiomyopathy, and patients with unexplained ventricular arrhythmias may be candidates for endomyocardial biopsy if noninvasive testing does not result in a definitive diagnosis

Patient selection is the key to appropriate use of endomyocardial biopsy and includes three principle considerations: the anticipated diagnostic yield from the procedure given the patient's prebiopsy probability of a specific disease, the physician's judgment regarding the likelihood that the biopsy will lead to a new diagnosis that otherwise would not have be made clinically and the possibility that this in turn will result in a new treatment strategy different from that recommended in the absence of biopsy information. Finally the procedural risk/benefit analysis attendant to the patients from endomyocardial biopsy must be within generally accepted guidelines.

Sampling error is a real problem associated with endomyocardial biopsy that may result in a missed

Table 1. Conditions Which May Be Diagnosed by Endomyocardial Biopsy

Amyloidosis

Sarcoidosis

Hemochromatosis

Myocarditis (e.g., eosinophilic myocarditis, giant cell myocarditis)

Anthracycline cardiomyopathy

Storage diseases such as mucopolysaccharidoses

Carcinoid heart disease

Primary myocardial neoplasms (e.g., rhabdomyosarcoma, lymphoma)

Radiation induced cardiac fibrosis

Cardiac allograft rejection

Chagas disease

Endomyocardial fibroelastosis

diagnosis or an underestimation of the severity of myocarditis or allograft rejection. Absence of pathologic evidence of myocarditis on EMB should not be construed as a definitive negative result in the face of other clinical evidence of allograft rejection or progressive heart failure and repeat EMB may be needed. Gadolinium enhanced MRI has shown some promise in noninvasively detecting areas of myocardial inflammation that may merit targeted biopsy.

Brief descriptions of some clinical scenarios in which endomyocardial biopsy may be clinically valuable are outlined below.

LYMPHOCYTIC MYOCARDITIS

Lymphocytic myocarditis is the most frequent form of myocarditis seen on endomyocardial biopsy (Fig. 3 and 4). Molecular assays show that about 20%-40% of lymphocytic myocarditis cases are associated with the presence of a viral genome in the myocardium. The highest incidence of lymphocytic myocarditis at biopsy is found in patients with acute heart failure with recent symptom onset.

The Myocarditis Treatment Trial was a pivotal trial in which 111 patients with biopsy proven myocarditis and left ventricular dysfunction were randomized to conventional therapy or a 24-week immunosuppressive regimen (prednisone + azathioprine, or prednisone + cyclosporine). There was no significant improvement in ejection fraction or transplant free survival with immunosuppression. Thus endomyocardial biopsy does not usually change treatment in patients with clinically suspected lymphocytic myocarditis.

GIANT CELL MYOCARDITIS (GCM)

Giant cell myocarditis is a rare disorder that can be idiopathic or associated with thymoma or drug hypersensitivity reactions. Endomyocardial biopsy is the only diagnostic method that permits a definitive diagnosis of giant cell myocarditis. While GCM is a rare disorder, prompt identification of patients is critical, since mortality rates are very high due to ventricular arrhythmias and progressive heart failure. Only 11% of patients with GCM were alive without transplant at 4 years' follow-up

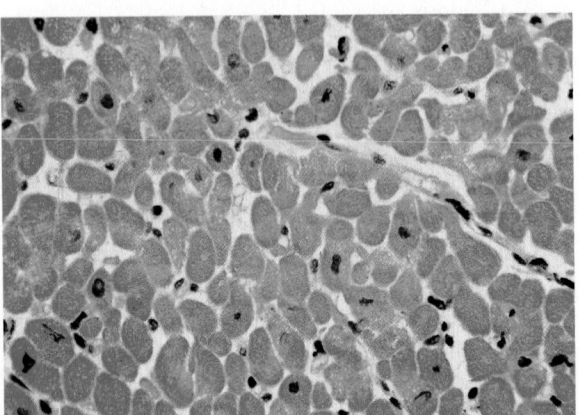
Fig. 1. Normal myocardium.

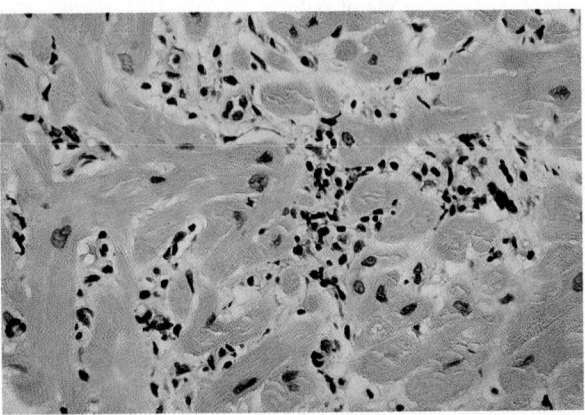
Fig. 2. Borderline myocarditis.

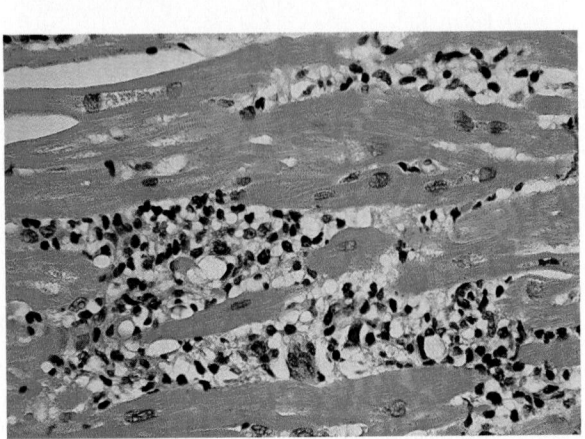
Fig. 3. Moderate focal lymphocytic myocarditis.

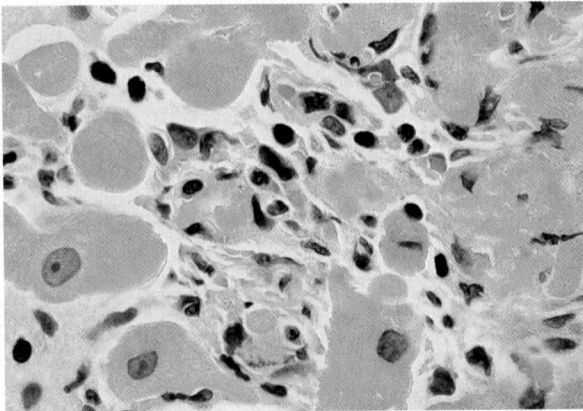
Fig. 4. Lymphocytic myocarditis with myocyte necrosis.

compared to 44% of patients with lymphocytic myocarditis. Anecdotal reports suggest that GCM patients may respond to aggressive immunosuppression and randomized clinical trials to test this hypothesis are under way (Fig. 5).

In a nonrandomized study of patients with GCM treated without immunosuppressive therapy, median transplant-free survival was 3.0 months, compared to a 12.3-month (P=0.003) median transplant-free survival for patients treated with cyclosporine-based immunosuppression. In patients with clinically suspected GCM, endomyocardial biopsy is strongly indicated. Clinical clues to the possibility of giant cell myocarditis include malignant ventricular arrhythmias and an abrupt onset of unexplained cardiac failure. Giant cell myocarditis may recur in the transplanted heart and surveillance for recurrence is required after transplantation.

SARCOID MYOCARDITIS

Histologic evidence of cardiac sarcoidosis is present in approximately 25% of patients with systemic sarcoidosis at autopsy but symptoms referable to cardiac sarcoidosis occur in only 5% of sarcoid patients. Cardiac sarcoidosis should be considered in patients with dilated cardiomyopathy complicated by heart block and/or serious ventricular arrhythmias. Histologically, sarcoidosis can be distinguished from giant cell myocarditis by the presence of noncaseating granulomas with fibrosis and little myocyte necrosis and a few eosinophils (Fig. 6).

While the sensitivity rate of the endomyocardial biopsy in cardiac sarcoidosis is 20% to 30%, a histologic

distinction between cardiac sarcoid and giant cell myocarditis is important for therapeutic decision making and prognosis. Transplant-free survival at 1 year is significantly worse in patients diagnosed with idiopathic GCM versus patients with cardiac sarcoidosis (22% versus 70%).

Case reports suggest that sarcoidosis may respond to treatment with corticosteroids. Survival was better in those who received corticosteroids than in those who received usual care (64% versus 40%, in one retrospective study.

HYPERSENSITIVITY AND EOSINOPHILIC MYOCARDITIS

In addition to acute rash, fever, peripheral eosinophilia, and ECG abnormalities, including, nonspecific ST-segment changes or infarct patterns, hypersensitivity myocarditis may present as sudden death or rapidly progressive heart failure. A temporal relation with recently initiated medications—particularly sulfonamides—and the use of multiple medications are important historical clues.

Early suspicion and recognition of hypersensitivity myocarditis, including findings on EMB, may lead to withdrawal of offending medications and administration of high-dose steroids. The hallmark histologic findings of hypersensitivity myocarditis include an interstitial infiltrate with prominent eosinophils with little myocyte necrosis (Fig. 7). Giant cell myocarditis, granulomatous myocarditis, or necrotizing eosinophilic myocarditis may mimic hypersensitivity myocarditis and EMB may be useful to distinguish these entities. Endomyocardial

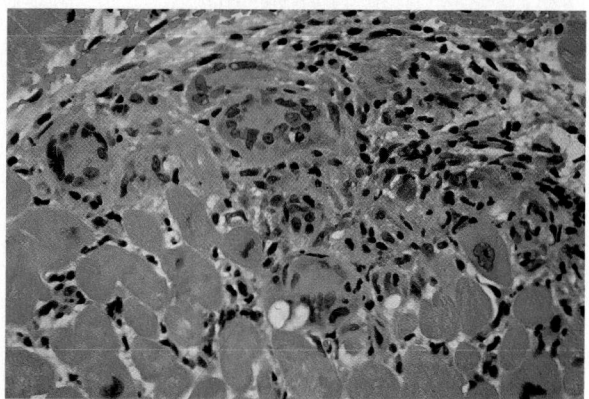

Fig. 5. Giant cell myocarditis.

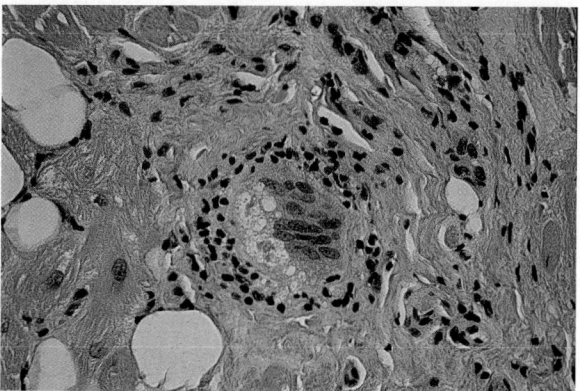

Fig. 6. Cardiac sarcoidosis with solitary granuloma.

biopsy is generally indicated for individuals with new congestive heart failure and peripheral blood eosinophilia. It is important to distinguish hypersensitivity myocarditis from giant cell myocarditis, granulomatous myocarditis, and necrotizing eosinophilic myocarditis both because hypersensitivity myocarditis may respond to corticosteroids and withdrawal of the offending agent while the latter conditions may require more aggressive treatment with immunosuppressive drugs.

HEMOCHROMATOSIS

Hemochromatosis is an inherited disorder of iron metabolism typically manifest clinically as diabetes mellitus, abnormal liver function, skin hyperpigmentation and dilated cardiomyopathy. Serum iron studies will generally show marked elevation of serum iron levels. Patients with alcohol abuse may have similar biochemical abnormalities. An endomyocardial biopsy showing deposits of iron within the sarcoplasm confirms the diagnosis of cardiac involvement in hemochromatosis, if the diagnosis is not apparent on non-invasive testing (Fig. 8).

AMYLOIDOSIS

Amyloidosis is a devastating disease that results from deposits of proteinaceous material in various organs, including the heart. The precise nature of the material depends upon the type of amyloidosis (primary systemic, familial, or senile). Cardiac manifestations include exertional dyspnea, chest pain, atrial arrhythmias, conduction block, and congestive heart failure. Early in the course of cardiac involvement, left ventricular systolic function is preserved, while diastolic function is often abnormal, with a restrictive filling pattern. Increased wall thickness by echo with a low QRS voltage on ECG has an 80% sensitivity for cardiac amyloidosis. Endomyocardial biopsy is the definitive diagnostic procedure to diagnose cardiac amyloidosis (Fig. 9).

CARDIAC ALLOGRAFT REJECTION

Surveillance endomyocardial biopsies are essential for the management of cardiac transplant recipients. Endomyocardial biopsies allow the early diagnosis and treatment of allograft rejection often prior to onset of symptoms. In addition EMB guides immunosuppressive strategies and may also detect cytomegalovirus or toxoplasmosis infection. The International Society for Heart and Lung Transplantation (ISHLT) published a revised grading system for acute cellular rejection in late 2005:

- Grade 0 — no rejection.
- Grade 1 R, mild—interstitial and/or perivascular infiltrate with up to one focus of myocyte damage.
- Grade 2 R, moderate—two or more foci of infiltrate with associated myocyte damage.
- Grade 3 R, severe—diffuse infiltrate with multifocal myocyte damage, with or without edema, hemorrhage, or vasculitis.

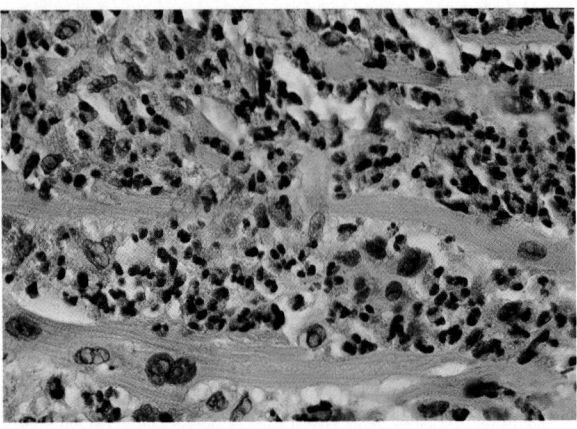

Fig. 7. Eosinophilic myocarditis.

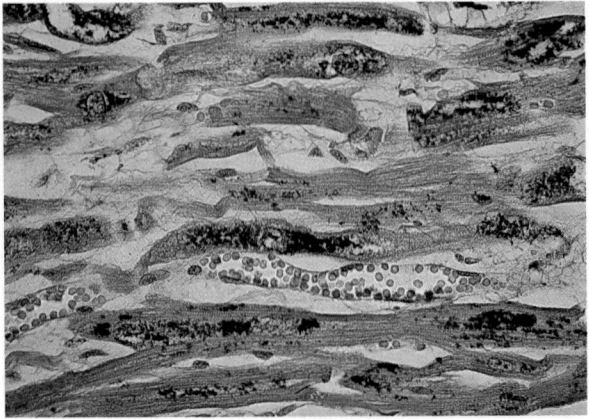

Fig. 8. Hemochromatosis.

Role of the Endomyocardial Biopsy in Immunocompromised Patients

In immunocompromised patients including those undergoing chemotherapy for cancer, steroids for various inflammatory diseases, and AIDS patients—bacteria, fungi, viruses and even parasites may cause myocarditis. In cases where the diagnosis is not apparent, endomyocardial biopsy may allow characterization of the infectious agent and guide optimal antimicrobial treatment (Fig. 10).

Role of the Endomyocardial Biopsy in Individuals Vaccinated for Smallpox

Smallpox vaccination with live *vaccinia* virus has been associated with acute myopericarditis in about 1 in 10,000 vaccinees. While most cases resolve spontaneously a small number of patients develop progressive heart failure associated diffuse ST-segment elevation, heterogeneity of QT intervals, and elevation of cardiac biomarkers.

In cases of progressive severe heart failure, endomyocardial biopsy with viral PCR studies may be helpful in detecting vaccinia genomic sequences in myocardial tissue and allow differentiation between viral myocarditis with active vaccinia replication and myocarditis due to an immune-mediated response, typically an eosinophilic-lymphocytic response without active viral replication that may respond to immunosuppressive therapy with steroids.

Technique of Endomyocardial Biopsy

Endomyocardial biopsies are most frequently performed via vascular access through the right internal jugular or femoral vein with local anesthesia, accompanied by conscious sedation if required. Children may require general anesthesia. Biopsies are usually performed with fluoroscopic guidance in the cardiac catheterization laboratory, but some operators prefer echocardiographic guidance, either alone or combined with use of fluoroscopy.

RIGHT INTERNAL JUGULAR VEIN APPROACH

Anatomic identification of the anatomie triangle containing the internal jugular vein and formed by the clavicle and the medial and lateral heads of the sternocleidomastoid muscle is facilitated by palpating and visualizing the neck while the patient slightly lifts their head tensing the neck muscles. Ultrasound can readily confirm the location of the vein, and demonstrate relative location of the internal jugular vein and carotid artery. An 18 gauge needle with an attached syringe containing saline is advanced along a path toward the ipsilateral nipple, pausing and aspirating while holding slight backward traction on the syringe to confirm venous cannulation. If carotid artery puncture occurs, gentle pressure should be held over the puncture site to reduce the risk of hematoma formation. Rarely carotid dissection and occlusion, or stroke related to emboli from thrombus or atheroma, have been reported in association with inadvertent carotid puncture.

Fluoroscopy should be utilized to confirm appropriate guidewire position, since occasionally the wire

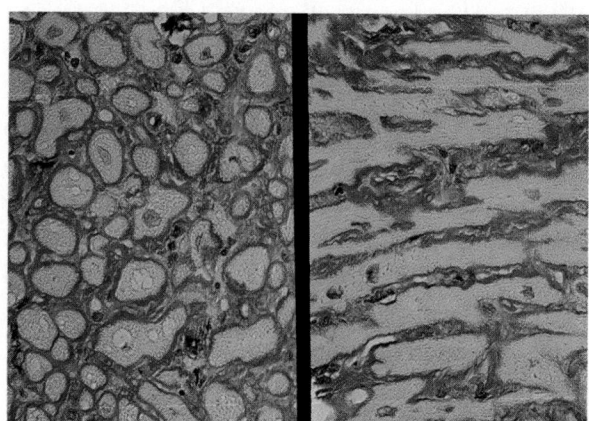

Fig. 9. Amyloid heart disease.

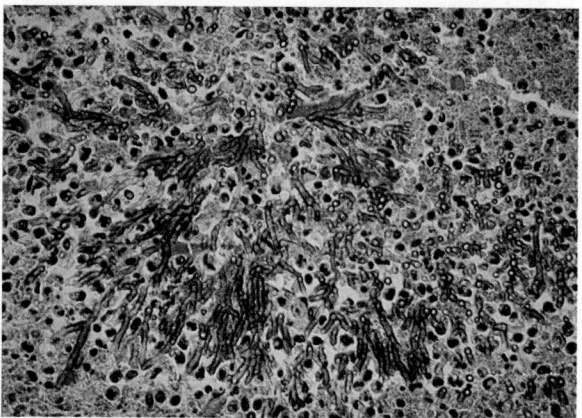

Fig. 10. Aspergillus myocarditis.

will deflect toward the arm instead of advancing toward the right atrium. Following placement of a sheath, the bioptome is advanced under fluoroscopic guidance, with the tip curving medially crossing the tricuspid valve to the apical portion of the ventricular septum. Localization in the right ventricle can be confirmed by the presence of right ventricular ectopic beats (left bundle branch block type morphology). Failure to advance the bioptome sufficiently distally in the right ventricle may result in damage to the tricuspid apparatus, leading to tricuspid insufficiency. This is usually well tolerated, but sometimes results in right sided heart failure that is difficult to manage, particularly if there is an element of pulmonary hypertension. Following gentle advancement to the apical region of the ventricular septum, the bioptome should be withdrawn slightly, the jaws opened, and then advanced gently against the septum (Fig. 11). Gentle pressure is adequate to obtain tissue in patients with dilated cardiomyopathy or myocarditis, who may have a thin-walled or soft inflamed myocardium; patients with multiple prior biopsies may require slightly more pressure because of the presence of endomyocardial scar.

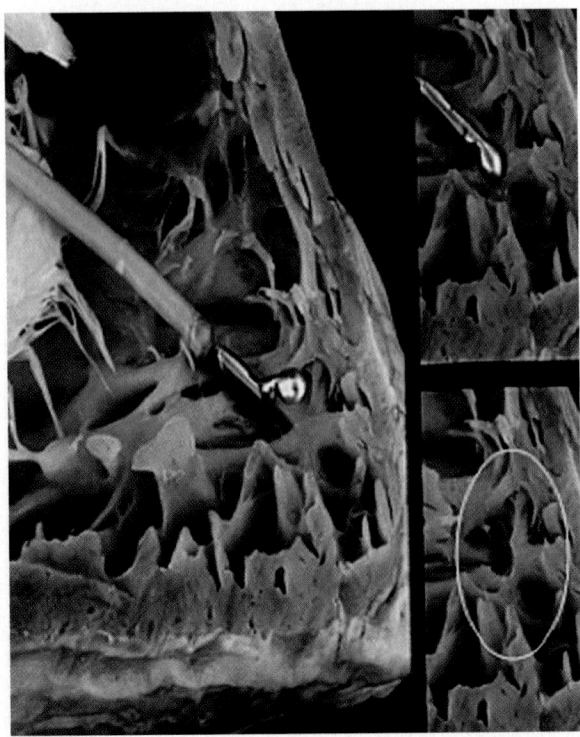

Fig. 11. Endomyocardial biopsy.

Excess force risks perforation of the right ventricle. Sudden onset of sharp pleuritic chest pain is a sign of likely myocardial perforation. Emergency echocardiography should be performed to visualize evidence of pericardial effusion and tamponade. Pericardiocentesis or more rarely thoracotomy may be required.

A hoarse voice, usually transient, but occasionally permanent due to injury of the recurrent laryngeal nerve has rarely been reported following endomyocardial biopsy. Fistulae between the coronary artery and the right ventricle have also been reported. These are usually asymptomatic and are visualized at surveillance coronary angiography; they are generally not associated with clinical sequelae.

FEMORAL VEIN APPROACH

Advantages of the femoral approach include freedom from complications specifically associated with the jugular venous approach such as carotid artery damage and recurrent laryngeal nerve palsy. Disadvantages include the requirement for a long vascular sheath in which thrombus may develop and the risk of deep venous thrombosis in the femoral vein. In addition, directing the bioptome across the tricuspid valve and to the appropriate region of the right ventricle is sometimes difficult from the femoral approach.

Following cannulation of the femoral vein utilizing standard technique, a guidewire is advanced under fluoroscopic guidance. A 7 or 8 French Mullins sheath of the type used for transeptal catheterization is then advanced to the right ventricle. A Mullins sheath with a sidearm to facilitate hemodynamic monitoring, can be used to facilitate bioptome passage. A long reusable Scholten bioptome or a disposable bioptome is passed to the RV apical septum. After the jaws are closed, *both* the bioptome and the Mullins should be gently withdrawn until the bioptome comes free from the endocardium. Failure to hold back pressure on the Mullins will pull the Mullins over the bioptome and into the endocardium, risking RV perforation if the bioptome does not easily come free. It is important to aspirate and flush the sheath carefully after each pass of the bioptome, in order to clear the sheath of possible thrombus.

Left Ventricular Biopsy

Left ventricular biopsy may be performed via a right

femoral approach. A long sheath is advanced over a guidewire into the left ventricle and a long bioptome is then passed through the sheath as far as the endocardial surface. Left ventricular biopsy is associated with a higher complication rate than right ventricular biopsy due to embolism (tissue, air, or thrombus) and ventricular arrhythmias.

■ Right bundle branch block (increased risk of complete heart block from damage to the left bundle) and left ventricular thrombus are contraindications to left ventricular endomyocardial biopsy.

Complications of Right Ventricular Endomyocardial Biopsy

There have been two reported studies of endomyocardial biopsy in large numbers of adult patients. The largest series included 1,300 right ventricular biopsy procedures performed via the right internal jugular venous approach. There were no deaths and the cumulative incidence of complications was less than 1%. Rare extra-cardiac complications included right pneumothorax and air embolism in addition to transient nerve palsies—such as right Horner's syndrome, right recurrent laryngeal nerve paralysis, and right phrenic nerve paresis. Four patients had cardiac perforation with pericardial tamponade; none required surgery and all responded to pericardiocentesis

A small series of 546 endomyocardial biopsies reported a cumulative complication rate of 6%, including inadvertent arterial puncture (2.2%), prolonged bleeding (0.2%), and vasovagal episode (0.4%). Arrhythmias, mostly supraventricular tachycardia, occurred in 1.1% of patients. Transient bradycardia, right bundle branch block, and complete heart block occurred with a cumulative incidence of 1%. Cardiac perforation resulting in death occurred in 2 patients (0.4%).

Techniques such as vascular ultrasound to identify the internal jugular vein, disposable bioptomes, and echocardiographic guidance using 2- or 3- dimensional echocardiography may increase the success and safety of endomyocardial biopsy.

CORONARY STENTS

Joseph G. Murphy, MD

Gregory W. Barsness, MD

Coronary stents were initially introduced as emergency bailout devices to treat obstructive coronary dissections and abrupt vessel closures following PTCA. Stents are now used in more than 95% of all coronary interventions to optimize the angiographic result and reduce the risk of late post PCI coronary restenosis. The early mechanisms by which stents are beneficial in PCI are complex and include a better initial angiographic result compared to PTCA, a scaffolding effect on coronary artery intimal dissections, and endothelial tears with better wound apposition of the endothelial edges, and an improvement in coronary arterial architecture and blood flow characteristics (Fig. 1 and 2). The major late incremental benefit of PCI stent placement over stand-alone PTCA is the marked reduction in coronary restenosis and resultant lower rate of late target lesion revascularization noted in almost all coronary patient subsets and lesions studied. Paradoxically, coronary stents do not have a significant impact on late patient mortality or myocardial infarction rates.

- All current cardiovascular stents are MRI safe and MRI imaging can be done any time following stent implantation

Bare metal stents achieve their late superiority over PTCA by blocking the "nonproliferative modes" of vessel restenosis including acute and chronic vessel wall recoil, arterial spasm, and unfavorable late vascular wall remodeling. The downside of bare metal stents is their increased propensity for in situ thrombosis and stimulation of a more aggressive neointimal proliferative response compared to PTCA.

Bare metal stents improve PCI results by at least four mechanisms (Fig. 3 and 4).

- Emergency rescue of failed PCI, coronary arterial intimal flaps, and medial wall dissections and enhancement of coronary laminar blood flow
- Improve the initial angiographic result and reliability of PCI through optimization of lumen size and stabilization of the vessel wall after PCI injury
- Reduce late restenosis through improved arterial wall architecture and dimensions, facilitating arterial wall wound healing and blocking elastic recoil of the arterial wall on the vessel lumen
- Prevent late unfavorable arterial wall remodeling and arterial spasm

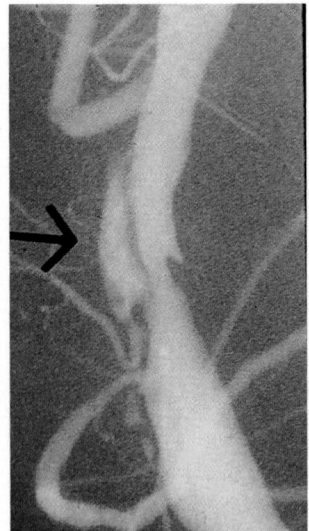
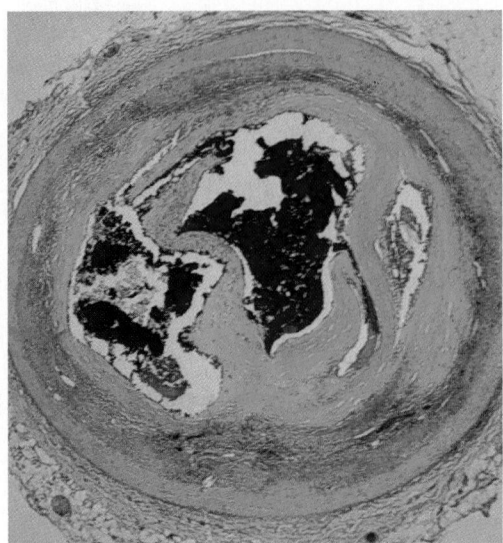

Fig. 1. Atherosclerotic plaque rupture in right coronary artery.

MAJOR EARLY RANDOMIZED COMPARATIVE STUDIES OF BARE METAL STENTS WITH PTCA

STRESS Study

The STRESS Study (STent Restenosis Study) was an early study that randomized 407 patients to a Palmaz-Schatz stent or PTCA for de novo native coronary stenoses. The stent group had a greater primary success rate (96% versus 90%), fewer angiographic dissections (7% versus 34%), less late angiographic restenosis (32% versus 42%, P=0.05) and a trend toward better event-free survival at follow-up (80% versus 74%).

BENESTENT Study

The BENESTENT Study (Belgium and Netherlands Stent Study) was a European study which randomized 516 highly selected patients to a Palmaz-Schatz stent or PTCA for de novo native coronary stenoses. The stent group had a lower restenosis rate (22% versus 32%, P=0.02) and a lower repeat PTCA rate (10% versus 21%, P=0.001) at the time of late follow-up. Vascular and bleeding complications were more common in the stent group.

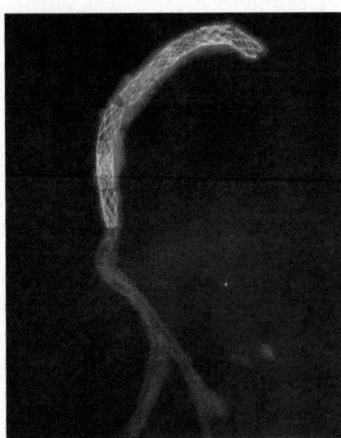

Fig. 2. Radiograph of right coronary artery with five expanded coronary stents.

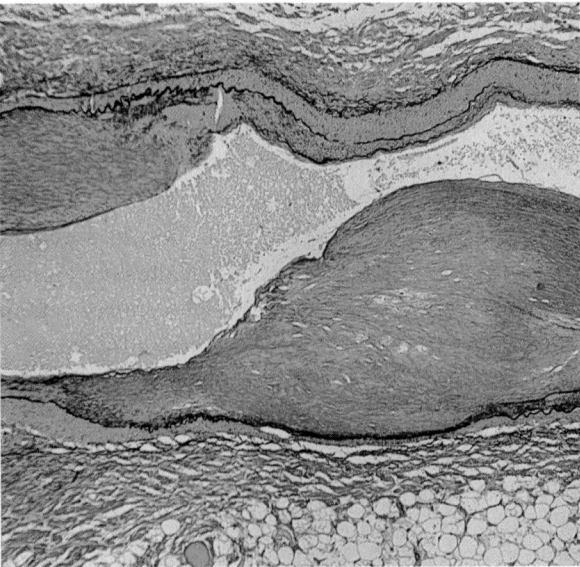

Fig. 3. Coronary artery with stenosis cut in a similar longitudinal section as an angiogram.

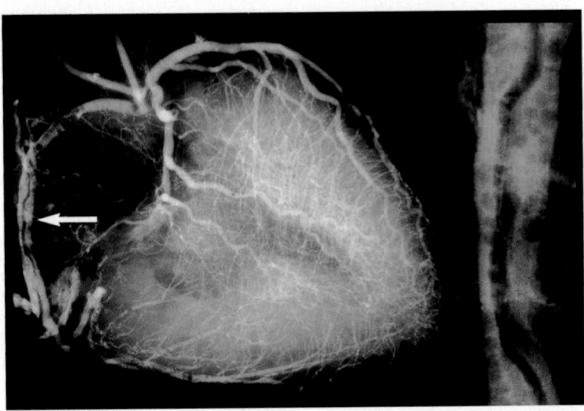

Fig. 4. Postmortem angiogram of right coronary artery with acute dissection (*arrow*). Magnified view on right side.

BENESTENT II

The BENESTENT II trial included a broader patient population and compared the heparin-coated Palmaz-Schatz stent to PTCA. Procedural success was higher in the stent group (97% versus 86%), with 13% of PTCA-assigned patients requiring bail-out stenting. Restenosis was reduced in the stent group (16% versus 30%, P=0.001), as were major adverse coronary events (death, MI, CABG or repeat PCI) at follow-up (13% versus 19%, P=0.03).

■ Stent implantation improves long-term event-free survival compared to PTCA with higher acute procedural success rates and lower rates of restenosis and late repeat revascularization

SAVED Trial

The Saphenous Vein De Novo (SAVED) trial was the first major trial to evaluate stents in saphenous vein grafts and randomly assigned 270 patients to PTCA or Palmaz-Schatz stent implantation for de novo saphenous vein graft lesions. Stent placement was associated with a higher initial procedural success rate and fewer adverse cardiovascular events at 6 months (27% versus 42%, P<0.05), although restenosis was not significantly different at 6-month follow-up (37% versus 46%).

SICCO Trial

The Stenting in Chronic Coronary Occlusion (SICCO) trial evaluated stenting in chronically occluded vessels and demonstrated reduced restenosis 1 year

after stent implantation in chronic total occlusions compared to PTCA in 117 patients (32% versus 74%, P<0.001), with a trend toward reduced reocclusion (12% versus 26%, P=0.058). Several trials have explored the long-term outcome of "optimized" PTCA compared with bare metal stent placement. These trials concluded that intravascular ultrasound (IVUS) guidance improved PTCA results and reduce late PTCA restenosis rates. Final results with optimized PTCA are still inferior to the results obtained with optimally deployed current generation drug-eluting stents in most settings (Fig. 5 and 6).

Drug-Eluting Stents

Drug-eluting stents (DES) possess all the vascular scaffolding benefits of bare metal stents and pharmacologically inhibit the neointimal response during the critical first month after stent implant when re-endothelialization of the injured vascular wall occurs. Current FDA approved DES release either sirolimus (Rapamune), a naturally occurring, lipophilic, macrolide antibiotic with immunosuppressive and antiproliferative properties or paclitaxel, a tubulin inhibitor derived from the Pacific Yew tree, a drug that has previously been used for ovarian cancer treatment. Sirolimus binds to a specific cytosolic receptor protein to upregulate a kinase inhibitor that in turn locks neointimal smooth muscle cells in the G_1 cell cycle phase. Paclitaxel appears to have a selective effect on smooth muscle cells and a much lesser effect on endothelial cells (Fig. 7).

Drug-eluting stents consist of a bare metal stent

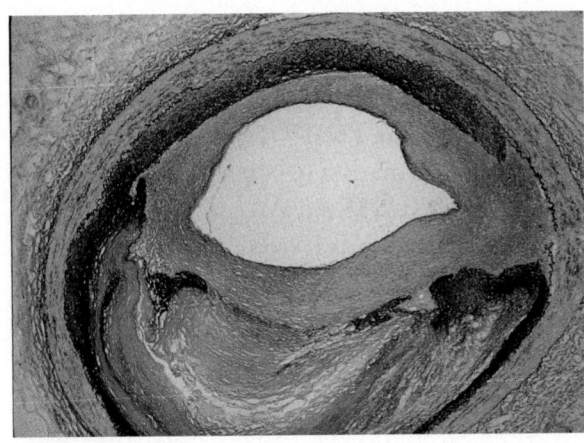

Fig. 5. Post PTCA restenosis.

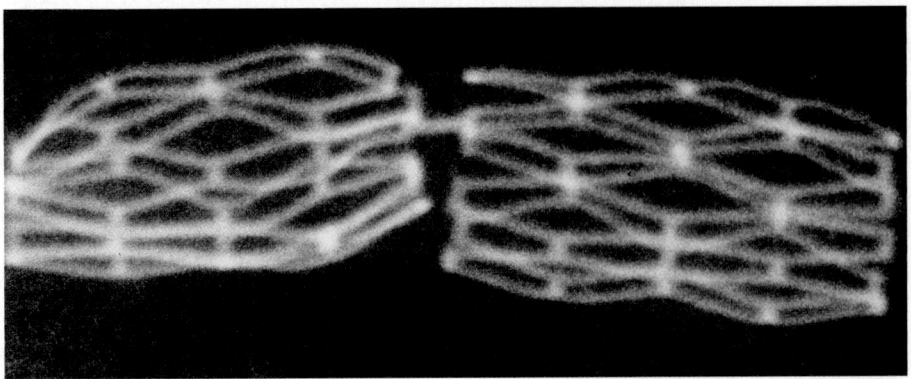

Fig. 6. Radiography of expanded stents in saphenous vein graft.

platform and a slow-release encapsulated drug formulation that inhibits neointimal proliferation delivered from a biostable polymer that coats the bare metal stent and keeps the drug in place. The Taxus stent is coated with a hydrocarbon-based elastomer that binds the drug paclitaxel physically to the stent and allows a controlled release of drug over time, permitting local elution of drug sufficient to inhibit but not completely stop wound healing and re-endothelialization around the stent. Paclitaxel elutes in two distinct phases: an early rapid phase lasting about 48 hours and a slower second phase lasting about 28 days. The Cypher stent elutes sirolimus in a similar but more constant manner also over a period of about 28 days. The goal of DES design is to achieve optimal stent endothelialization but prevent neointimal restenosis (Fig. 7 and 8 *A-C*). Systemic chemotherapy-like side effects are not seen with DES but delayed stent endothelialization may occur, hence the need for prolonged dual anti platelet inhibition (Aspirin and Clopidogrel) after DES implant.

Multiple randomized clinical trials, including four large trials (SIRIUS, RAVEL, TAXUS II and IV trials) compared DES and non-DES (bare metal stents). Intermediate-term data (6-9 months) from trials of paclitaxel (TAXUS II and IV) and sirolimus-eluting stents (SIRIUS, RAVEL) consistently demonstrate reduced rates of restenosis and late target lesion revascularization compared to bare metal stents, but similar intermediate-term rates of cardiovascular death and myocardial infarction.

Drug-eluting stents are an effective treatment strategy against late PCI restenosis in multiple patient groups, including female, elderly, and diabetic patients and multiple lesion subsets including small coronary vessels, diffuse coronary disease, aorto-ostial lesions, saphenous vein graft lesions, chronic total occlusions and patients who present with an unstable coronary syndrome including acute myocardial infarction and unstable angina.

| | Restenosis rates | |
Trials	Bare Metal Stents	DES
TAXUS II (2003)	19.1%	3.5%
TAXUS IV (2004)	27%	8%
SIRIUS (2003)	35%	3%
RAVEL (2002)	27%	0%

$P<0.001$ for all 4 trials.

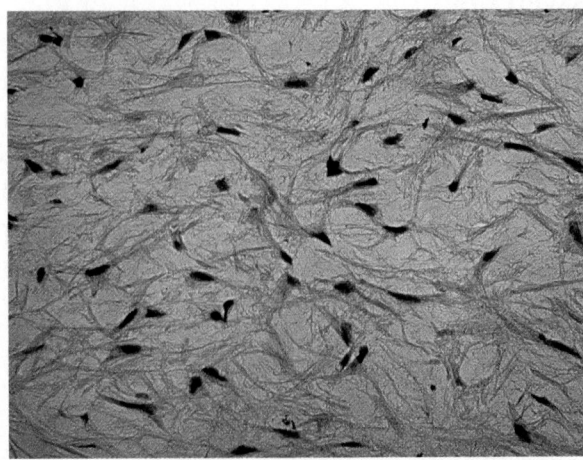

Fig. 7. History of post PTCA restenosis showing neointimal formation.

A

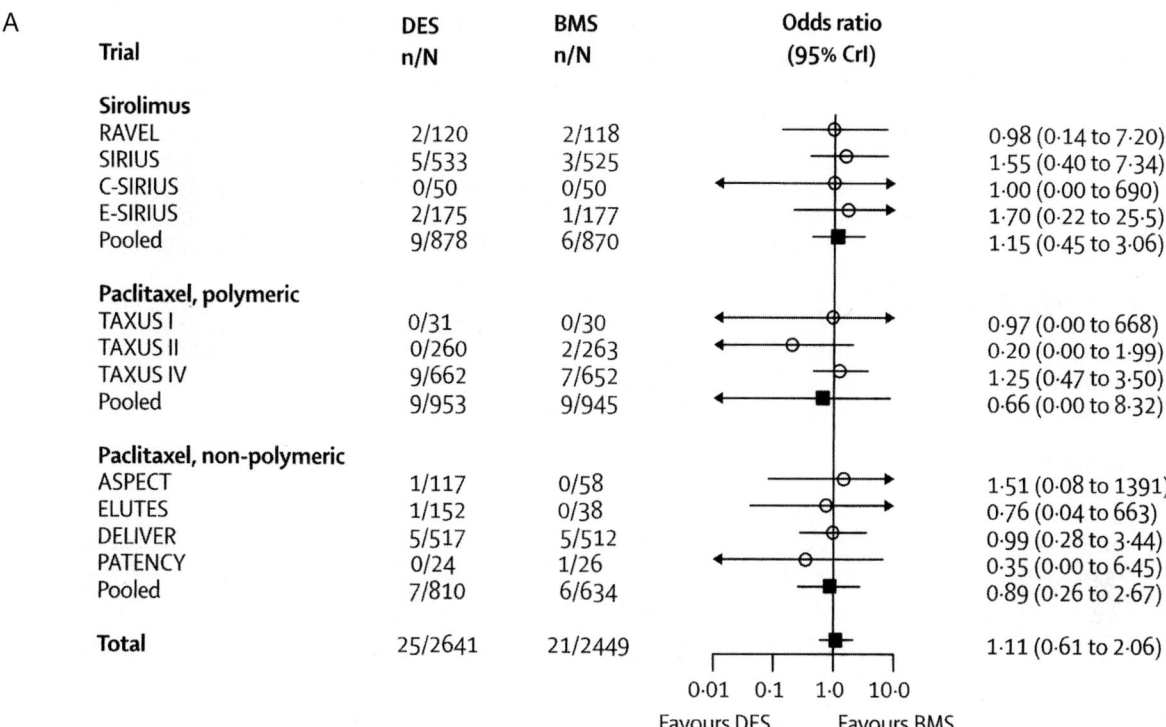

Trial	DES n/N	BMS n/N	Odds ratio (95% CrI)
Sirolimus			
RAVEL	2/120	2/118	0·98 (0·14 to 7·20)
SIRIUS	5/533	3/525	1·55 (0·40 to 7·34)
C-SIRIUS	0/50	0/50	1·00 (0·00 to 690)
E-SIRIUS	2/175	1/177	1·70 (0·22 to 25·5)
Pooled	9/878	6/870	1·15 (0·45 to 3·06)
Paclitaxel, polymeric			
TAXUS I	0/31	0/30	0·97 (0·00 to 668)
TAXUS II	0/260	2/263	0·20 (0·00 to 1·99)
TAXUS IV	9/662	7/652	1·25 (0·47 to 3·50)
Pooled	9/953	9/945	0·66 (0·00 to 8·32)
Paclitaxel, non-polymeric			
ASPECT	1/117	0/58	1·51 (0·08 to 1391)
ELUTES	1/152	0/38	0·76 (0·04 to 663)
DELIVER	5/517	5/512	0·99 (0·28 to 3·44)
PATENCY	0/24	1/26	0·35 (0·00 to 6·45)
Pooled	7/810	6/634	0·89 (0·26 to 2·67)
Total	25/2641	21/2449	1·11 (0·61 to 2·06)

0·01   0·1   1·0   10·0
Favours DES   Favours BMS

B

Trial	DES n/N	BMS n/N	Odds ratio (95% CrI)
Sirolimus			
RAVEL	0/120	27/118	0·01 (0·00 to 0·08)
SIRIUS	22/533	87/525	0·22 (0·13 to 0·35)
C-SIRIUS	2/50	9/50	0·23 (0·03 to 0·80)
E-SIRIUS	7/175	37/177	0·17 (0·06 to 0·35)
Pooled	31/878	160/870	0·15 (0·02 to 0·46)
Paclitaxel, polymeric			
TAXUS I	0/31	3/30	0·12 (0·00 to 1·06)
TAXUS II	11/260	38/263	0·27 (0·13 to 0·51)
TAXUS IV	20/662	74/652	0·25 (0·14 to 0·40)
Pooled	31/953	115/945	0·23 (0·10 to 0·42)
Paclitaxel, non-polymeric			
ASPECT	8/117	2/58	1·75 (0·49 to 11·6)
ELUTES	11/152	6/38	0·41 (0·15 to 1·24)
DELIVER	27/517	35/512	0·75 (0·45 to 1·25)
PATENCY	3/24	5/26	0·64 (0·12 to 2·74)
Pooled	49/810	48/634	0·64 (0·39 to 1·05)
Total	111/2641	323/2449	0·26 (0·14 to 0·45)

0·01   0·1   1·0   10·0
Favours DES   Favours BMS

(Fig. 8 continued on next page)

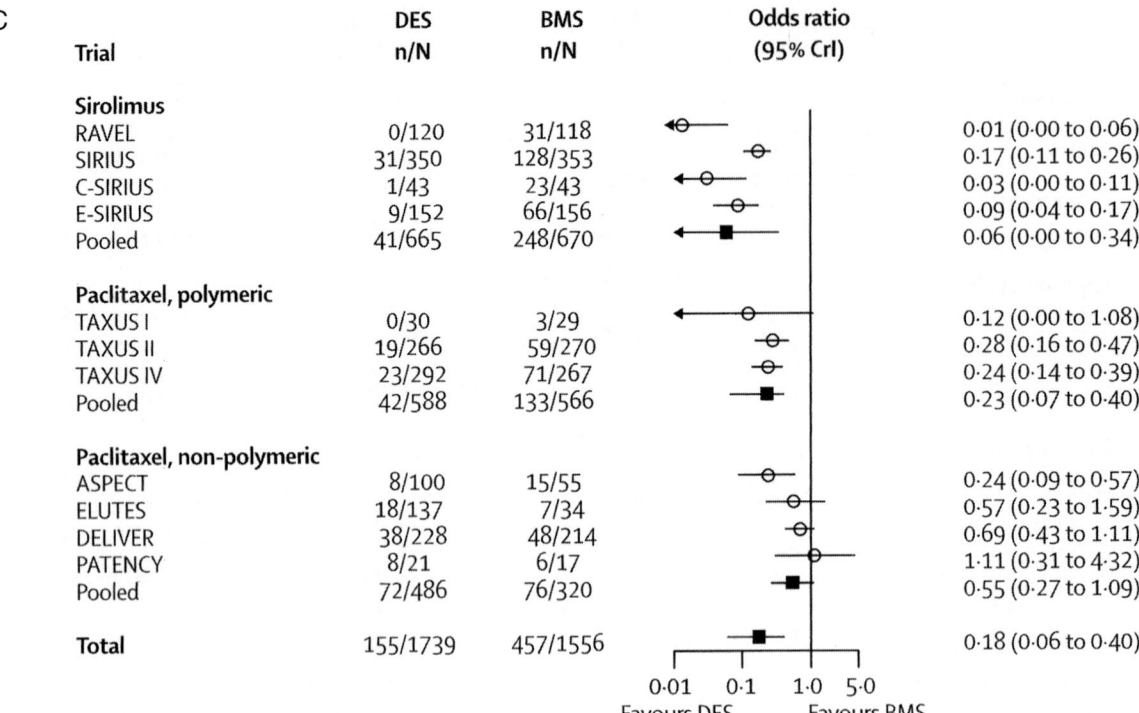

Fig. 8. *A*, Forest plot comparing all-cause mortality rates for DES and for BMS. The TAXUS-II and TAXUS-IV trials reported only cardiac mortality. *B*, Forest plot comparing rates of target-lesion revascularization for DES and for BMS. *C*, Forest plot comparing rates of angiographic restenosis for DES and for BMS. The proportion of patients who underwent repeat angiography in each group was not specified in the RAVEL trial, and was assumed to be 100%. White circles represent the odds ratios for individual trials, and black squares the meta-analytic odds ratios for the indicated subgroups and for the overall (total) results. Horizontal lines represent the 95% credible intervals (CrI) for the data.

COMPLICATIONS OF CORONARY STENTING

The major early complications of coronary stent implantation are failed stent delivery with or without stent embolization, in situ stent thrombosis, asymptomatic cardiac enzyme elevation, clinical myocardial infarction, side branch occlusion, and peripheral vascular and bleeding complications. Other complications of PCI include coronary guide catheter complications (ostial dissection), guide wire complications (coronary perforation) and radiographic contrast complications (allergic reactions and renal failure). Angiographic risk factors associated with an increased risk of cardiovascular events in patients with an initial successful coronary stent deployment include a poor angiographic result (significant residual stenosis, TIMI blood flow grade ≤2, obstructive coronary dissection), failure of close stent apposition to the arterial wall (can be more accu-

rately assessed by IVU) and major side branch occlusion.

Patient-related factors statistically associated with worse outcome with stenting included diabetes mellitus particularly insulin requiring diabetes, renal failure, acute myocardial infarction, poor left ventricular function and poor patient compliance with dual antiplatelet therapy—aspirin and clopidogrel.

■ The current incidence of emergency coronary artery bypass surgery for failed PCI is now about 0.3%.

Failure of Stent Delivery and Stent Loss

Current low-profile stents have a delivery rate of ≥97% with a very low risk of stent loss and peripheral embolization. Failed stent deployment and stent embolization are associated with significant patient morbidity and mortality. Risk factors for failed stent delivery include very tortuous coronary vessels particularly lesions located in the left circumflex and obtuse marginal vessels or saphenous vein graft lesions, long and complex stenoses, and small-caliber vessels.

Side Branch Occlusion

Ideally, stent placement should avoid crossing major side branches, but in many cases adequate atherosclerotic plaque coverage makes stenting across important side branches unavoidable. Most cases of stent-associated side branch occlusion results from plaque shifting, particularly when the atherosclerotic plaque in the vessel to be stented is complex and also involves the ostium of the side branch, or the side branch itself has a baseline plaque stenosis of >50%. The term "stent jail" is used to describe stent coverage of a major side branch. Major side branches considered at high risk of stent occlusion can be protectively prewired with a PCI guidewire before stent placement. Alternatively, a PCI guidewire can often be guided into the jailed branch after stent implant and the branch then dilated through the stent struts. Many jailed side branches do not cause myocardial ischemia and may not need further intervention. Clinical judgment of side branch compromise may be aided by estimation of fractional flow reserve (FFR). An FFR <0.75 indicates physiologic coronary blood flow reserve impairment.

Coronary Artery Perforation

Coronary artery perforation is a rare but potentially serious complication of coronary stenting. Perforation may occur in several situations including overly vigorous manipulation of the PCI guidewire, particularly with stiff guidewires in the setting of chronic total occlusions or due to a PTCA balloon rupture that creates a forceful jet effect that perforates the arterial wall. Perforation is more common with atherectomy devices than with PTCA or stents. Risk factors for coronary perforation with stenting include stent oversizing and high-pressure stent postdilation. Pericardial tamponade, myocardial infarction, emergency CABG and death are all associated with coronary perforation.

Many guidewire perforation can be managed conservatively while emergency treatment of more severe coronary perforations consists of rapid inflation of a PTCA balloon at the site of perforation to limit blood flow into the pericardium. Pericardial tamponade can occur extremely rapidly with coronary perforation and emergency pericardiocentesis may be lifesaving. Small perforations may seal with prolonged PTCA balloon occlusion, while placement of a polytetrafluoroethylene (PTFE)-covered stent is an effective treatment when prolonged PTCA balloon occlusion is unsuccessful. Emergency cardiac surgery may be required for coronary perforation unresponsive to PCI techniques.

Elevated Cardiac Enzymes

Many patients after angiographically successfully stenting have small elevations in cardiac enzymes (CK-MB more than three times the upper limit of normal), popularly called "infarctlets." Distal embolization of friable plaque, coronary thrombus, and platelet embolization and occlusion of minor side branches are considered the most common causes of elevated serum enzymes after PCI. Distal embolic protection devices are particularly useful during PCI in old degenerate saphenous vein grafts and markedly reduce the frequency of distal embolization and periprocedure myocardial infarctions.

Mild asymptomatic elevations in serum CK-MB occur in up to 30 percent of coronary interventions and are linked in some studies to an increased risk of late mortality but not early cardiovascular events. The likely explanation is that an asymptomatic CK-MB enzyme elevation with PCI is an epiphenomenon and a marker for diffuse atherosclerosis which in turn is associated with increased late cardiovascular mortality.

There is considerable debate of the significance of an elevated serum troponin after stenting, and older CK-MB data cannot necessarily be directly extrapolated with troponin data as serum troponins (both troponin I and troponin T) are more sensitive markers of myocardial damage than CK-MB enzyme elevation. Some studies have reported the finding of an elevated serum troponin after stenting as an independent predictor for major in-hospital complications after PCI. A recent Mayo Clinic study of over 2,300 patients reported that baseline troponin elevations before PCI are common in coronary artery disease patients (noted in 31% of Mayo patients) and are associated with worse short- and long-term clinical outcomes. When these baseline cardiac enzyme elevations were taken into account, post-PCI elevations in troponin or CK-MB added no further long-term prognostic information. Postprocedural cardiac enzyme elevations correlated with in-hospital cardiovascular complications, but long-term prognosis was most often related to baseline pre-PCI troponin status and not the biomarker (cardiac enzyme) response to PCI.

The "No-Reflow" or "Slow-Reflow" Phenomenon
The "no-reflow" or "slow-reflow" phenomenon is a marked reduction in forward coronary blood flow (TIMI flow grade 2) without evidence of epicardial coronary obstruction from any cause including residual coronary stenosis, in situ thrombosis, obstructive arterial dissection, coronary spasm, or the loss of a significant distal coronary artery branch due to a large distal embolus. No-reflow and slow-reflow have been linked with distal microembolization and microvascular injury after PCI. Myocardial stunning, reperfusion vascular injury, and α-adrenergic-receptor mediated vasoconstriction may also be important. It may also be more common in diabetics and is usually associated with an elevation in cardiac enzymes. Slow-reflow is estimated to occur in about 5-10 percent of PCI procedures and is associated with primary and rescue PCI for acute myocardial infarction, the presence of intravascular thrombus, saphenous vein interventions, and adjunctive rotablator usage. Paradoxically, a period of pre-infarction angina may attenuate the no-reflow phenomenon, possibly due to ischemic preconditioning.

The "no-reflow" or "slow-reflow" phenomenon may be quantified in the cardiac catheterization laboratory by angiographic visual assessment—Thrombolysis In Myocardial Infarction (TIMI) flow grade 2 or less, TIMI frame count and TIMI myocardial blush score, and coronary Doppler flow wire assessment (systolic retrograde flow with rapid diastolic blood flow deceleration).

Prevention of Distal Microembolism and the "No-Reflow" or "Slow Reflow" Phenomenon
Distal embolic protection devices are effective in reducing distal embolism in saphenous vein grafts but have not been shown to be effective in randomized trials of primary PCI in patients with ST elevation myocardial infarction (STMI). Both the EMERALD trial (PercuSurge) which enrolled 500 patients with acute STMI within six hours of symptom onset and the PROMISE trial (FilterWire) which enrolled 200 patients undergoing primary PCI showed no sustained benefit with distal protection devices. Therapeutic

interventions in which there is evidence of benefit for either the prevention or treatment of the "no-reflow or slow-flow" phenomenon include direct stenting without PTCA predilation and intracoronary infusions of adenosine and verapamil. There is no convincing evidence that GP IIb/IIIa inhibitors are beneficial in this setting.

Endothelial Dysfunction
Most patients who require coronary stenting have some element of baseline endothelial dysfunction prior to PCI and all coronary interventions, by their nature, damage the endothelium to a variable degree, which in turn may not recover for many weeks to months. In general, bare metal stents cause more endothelial dysfunction than PTCA while DES may significantly delay recovery of endothelial function, contributing to the rationale for prolonged dual platelet inhibition in patients with DES.

EMERGENCY CORONARY BYPASS SURGERY FOR FAILED PCI
Emergency CABG for failed PCI is now rare (about 0.3% of patients) compared to the prestent era of PCI when it was 2%-3%. Failed stent deployment, uncontrolled distal or proximal arterial dissections, and inability to revascularize a major territory have replaced abrupt vessel closure and focal coronary artery dissection as the main causes of emergency CABG in patients now undergoing PCI with stenting. The rate of emergency CABG in high-risk patients with high-risk lesions who undergo stenting under cover of clopidogrel and GP IIb/IIIa platelet inhibition is much lower than that observed in the prestent era with PTCA and aspirin alone. Emergency CABG for failed PCI still carries a high operative mortality of about 10%.

Bleeding Complications With Percutaneous Coronary Interventions
The current incidence of vascular access site bleeding complications following stent implant which in the past led to a significant requirement for blood transfusions and surgical vascular repair is currently much improved. This results from the realization that stent thrombosis is primarily a platelet-driven thrombotic process in stents that are poorly apposed to the arterial

wall and that systemic anticoagulation with warfarin is not only unnecessary but harmful.

Glycoprotein IIb/IIIa inhibitors (e.g., abciximab) is useful in complex PCI to reduce the frequency of ischemic complications, especially when intracoronary thrombus is present, but it increases the risk of major and minor bleeding complications. Elderly patients undergoing PCI are at increased risk of bleeding compared to younger patients.

Stroke Risk With PCI

Thromboembolic stroke is a well-recognized complication of PCI with a procedural incidence of between 0.1 to 0.4 percent. Multiple pathogenic mechanisms are likely operative, including incidental catheter and guidewire trauma to the ascending aorta, aortic arch, and ostia of the cerebral vessels and air embolism. More rarely, retrograde thrombus dislodgement for a recently occluded coronary artery may occur during PCI for acute myocardial infarction. Risk factors for cerebral thromboembolism with PCI include a previous history of hypertension, diabetes mellitus, prior stroke, recent thrombolysis and intra-aortic balloon pump usage. Thromboembolism of the cerebral circulation at the time of PCI is statistically associated with concurrent renal and peripheral thromboembolism.

Complications of Drug-Eluting Stent Implantation

Drug-eluting stents carry all the adverse risks associated with bare metal stenting (except high rates of restenosis) and some unique problems. Restenosis, while significantly reduced by DES, is not completely abolished and occurs in about 10% of unselected PCI patients. Randomized drug-eluting stent trials, often highly selected their patients, showed a lower overall rate of restenosis (0-8%) and patients with complex diffuse lesions were generally excluded from the initial DES trials. Restenosis after DES implantation is associated with ostial lesions, diabetes and diffuse coronary disease, small vessel caliber <2.5 mm, prior PTCA or stent restenosis, and previous intracoronary radiation therapy. The preferred treatment for in-stent restenosis or stent edge restenosis associated with significant myocardial ischemia is another DES or, less commonly, CABG.

Stent Thrombosis

Coronary stent thrombosis is a serious complication of stenting that occurs with both bare metal and DES. Stent thrombosis may be asymptomatic if the stented vessel is relatively small and or well collateralized, but most patients with stent thrombosis present emergently with unstable angina, myocardial infarction, or sudden death (Fig. 9).

- More than 50% of patients with stent thrombosis suffer a myocardial infarction.
- The mortality rate with acute stent thrombosis is 10%-15%

Early stent thrombosis (generally defined as stent thrombosis within 30 days of stent placement) develops in approximately 0.5 to 1.0% percent of patients with well deployed stents on dual antiplatelets (aspirin and clopidogrel), with an approximate equal risk of occurrence in bare metal and drug-eluting stents. Most cases of stent thrombosis occur within the first few week after stent placement. Late stent thrombosis (>1 month after implant) is uncommon with bare metal stents (excepting patients with prior intracoronary radiation therapy as a treatment for restenosis) and is strongly associated with patient cessation of aspirin or clopidogrel therapy either by physician design or patient default. The risk of stent thrombosis is similar between drug-eluting and bare metal stents and between sirolimus and paclitaxel stents. Early stent thrombosis typically occurs 7-10 days after cessation of clopidogrel and/or aspirin therapy which correlates well with the

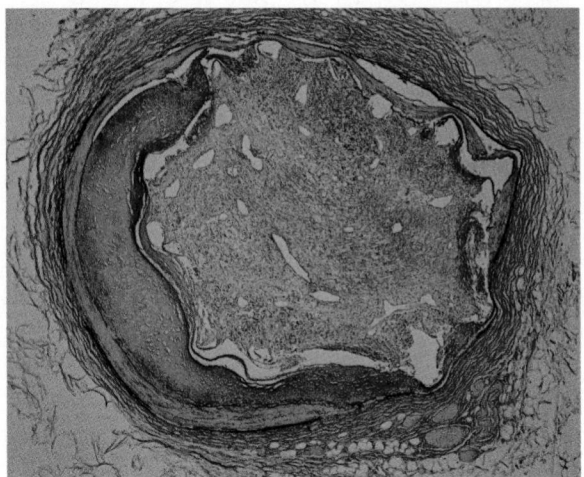

Fig. 9. Chronically thrombosed coronary stent.

time needed for the bone marrow to regenerate functional platelets. Late stent thrombosis which may occur more than a year after stent implant is also associated with cessation of aspirin therapy and typically occurs more than 30 days after stopping antiplatelet therapy, usually in a drug eluting stent possibly related to incomplete stent endothelialization.

Long-term aspirin therapy continues to be important for the long-term prevention of late stent thrombosis in patients who have completed their initial period of dual antiplatelet therapy. Unplanned cessation of aspirin therapy due to bleeding complications or poor patient compliance or planned cessation of aspirin prior to elective surgery remains a strong risk factor for stent thrombosis.

Angiographic risk factors for early stent thrombosis following successful initial stent deployment include residual thrombus or significant stent edge dissection, small-caliber stented artery, a major undilated arterial stenosis proximal or distal to the stented segment, incomplete stent expansion, or poor apposition of the stent to the arterial wall.

- Bifurcation stenting, particularly with the crush technique, increases the risk of early stent thrombosis

Combined antiplatelet therapy (aspirin and a thienopyridine—clopidogrel (Plaid) reduces the risk of stent thrombosis. The STARS trial established that outcomes are better with aspirin plus a thienopyridine (ticlopidine) rather than aspirin alone or aspirin plus warfarin. Further studies established that the combination of aspirin and clopidogrel was as effective as aspirin and ticlopidine and with far fewer side effects. Combined antiplatelet therapy with aspirin and clopidogrel is now standard for all patients receiving coronary stents, aspirin-allergic patients aside. Daily low-dose aspirin (75 mg or 81 mg) should be continued indefinitely while daily clopidogrel (75 mg) should be given for 4-6 weeks with bare metal stents and 3-6 months with DES. Some authorities recommend continuation of clopidogrel therapy for 9 to 12 months or longer in patients who are not considered at high risk for bleeding but who are at increased risk for recurrent cardiovascular events.

- Cessation of antiplatelet therapy is strongly linked to both early and late stent thrombosis.
- High pressure balloon inflation and dual antiplatelet regimens have significantly reduced the incidence of stent thrombosis

Emergency PCI to restore stent patency is the treatment of choice for stent thrombosis The adjunctive use of a glycoprotein IIb/IIIa inhibitor may improve the clinical outcome. Poor prognostic factors following rescue PCI include residual stent stenosis and poor coronary flow ($\leq$TIMI II).

URGENT NONCARDIAC SURGERY IN PATIENTS WITH CORONARY STENTS

The issue of urgent noncardiac surgery in patients with coronary stents generally arises in one of two ways; either a patient is discovered to have a significant flow limiting coronary artery stenosis amenable to PCI at the time of a preoperative evaluation prior to urgent noncardiac surgery or, secondly, a patients who, after coronary stent implant, is found to require urgent noncardiac surgery (e.g., colon carcinoma, fractured femoral head). Surgical procedures promote a prothrombotic milieu. Patients with bare metal stents in whom antiplatelet therapy is stopped within six weeks of coronary stenting have an appreciable risk of perioperative stent thrombosis and consequential myocardial infarction and death. DES require a longer period of dual antiplatelet therapy because of their slower rate of stent endothelialization. If urgent noncardiac surgery is planned, PTCA without stenting is often a reasonable option that is associated with a low incidence of coronary lesion thrombosis or myocardial infarction in the perioperative period provided that PTCA is performed at least a few weeks prior to noncardiac surgery, but at the added price of more target lesion revascularizations at a later date. Stopping aspirin in a coronary stent patient is always a risk and should only be done when continuing aspirin is truly a surgical hazard. In recently stented patients who require emergency surgery, a reasonable strategy is to stop aspirin and clopidogrel and substitute a short-acting intravenous GP IIb/IIIa inhibitor such as eptifibatide which can be stopped several hours before surgery and restarted 12-48 hours following surgery. Many operations (e.g., cataracts) can be safely performed with the patient on aspirin.

IMPORTANT GP IIb/IIIa INHIBITORS TRIALS IN INTERVENTIONAL CARDIOLOGY

Intravenous glycoprotein (GP) IIb/IIIa inhibitors provide substantial benefit when used in high-risk PCI by inhibiting platelet aggregation and attenuating the prothrombotic milieu seen with acute coronary syndromes in which atherosclerotic ulceration and coronary thrombus are common findings.

EPIC (1994) and EPILOGUE (1997) Trials

The EPIC (Evaluation of 7E3 for the Prevention of Ischemic Complications) trial demonstrated that abciximab, a human-murine chimeric monoclonal antibody Fab fragment (abciximab) against the platelet glycoprotein IIb/IIIa fibrinogen receptor reduced the abrupt closure rate, mortality, myocardial infarct rate, and need for emergency CABG by about 35% in high-risk PTCA patients. A subsequent trial aptly named EPILOGUE (Evaluation in PTCA to Improve Long-Term Outcome With Abciximab GP IIb/IIIa Blockade) demonstrated that abciximab, when combined with lower-dose, weight-adjusted heparin (70 units/kg), reduced the risk of acute ischemic complications in patients undergoing PCI without an appreciable increase in bleeding complications.

- The EPIC trial demonstrated that abciximab reduced the risk of abrupt vessel closure in high-risk patients.
- GP IIb/IIIa inhibitors reduce mortality in high-risk PCI patients.
- Major bleeding is increased when excessive heparin is administered or heparin is continued beyond the PCI procedure.

ELECTIVE CORONARY STENTING AND ABCIXIMAB

EPISTENT Trial (1998)

The EPISTENT trial (Randomized Placebo Controlled and Balloon Angioplasty Controlled Trial to Assess Safety of Coronary Stenting with use of Platelet Glycoprotein IIb/IIIa Blockade) tested the efficacy of GP IIb/IIIa inhibitors in elective stenting and randomly assigned almost 2,400 patients undergoing PCI to stenting alone, stenting plus abciximab, or PTCA plus abciximab. Abciximab reduced the 30-day incidence of the primary combined end point (death, myocardial infarction, and urgent revascularization) from 10.8% in the control arm to 5.3% in the stent arm and 6.9% in the PTCA arm. Beneficial effects were seen out to three years. Benefit was seen with abciximab in both younger patients and patients older than 65 years, patients with stable and unstable angina and in diabetics (EPISTENT Diabetic Substudy) and nondiabetics. Paradoxically, women did better with PTCA and abciximab (5.1% combined event rate).

ISAR-REACT Trial (2004)

The ISAR-REACT trial (Intracoronary Stenting and Antithrombotic Regimen–Rapid Early Action for Coronary Treatment) evaluated over 2,000 low-risk patients with stable native vessel coronary disease and no major comorbidities who underwent elective PCI with stenting and were then randomized to either abciximab or placebo plus standard care. This study differed from other PCI studies in that all patients were pretreated with 600 mg of clopidogrel at least 2 hours before PCI. At 30 days, there was no difference in the incidence of the combined end point of death, myocardial infarction, or urgent target vessel revascularization between the abciximab and placebo arms. The overall complication rate was very low, about 4% percent in both groups with major bleeding complications in about 1% percent of both groups. Profound thrombocytopenia occurred in 1 percent of patients in the abciximab group but in none in the placebo group. Patients judged clinically to be at low-to-intermediate PCI procedural risk (not an acute coronary syndrome, age ≤75 years, no diabetes and normal cardiac enzymes) who undergo elective PCI after pretreatment with high-dose clopidogrel (600 mg) derive no benefit with abciximab.

- Low-risk PCI patients do not benefit from a GP IIb/IIIa inhibitor if they are pretreated with a high loading dose (600 mg) of clopidogrel.

ISAR-REACT 2 Trial (2006)

The ISAR-REACT 2 randomized trial evaluated abciximab in patients with acute coronary syndromes undergoing PCI after pretreatment with 600 mg of clopidogrel. Abciximab reduces the risk of adverse events in patients with non-ST-segment elevation acute coronary syndromes in whom troponin levels were elevated.

Acute Coronary Syndromes and Abciximab

GP IIb/IIIa inhibitors are beneficial in patients with non-ST elevation myocardial infarction and unstable angina who undergo PCI, of modest benefit in patients who are not routinely scheduled to undergo PCI (but who may do so if there is evidence of ongoing myocardial ischemia), and of questionable benefit in patients with unstable angina/non-ST elevation myocardial infarction who do not undergo PCI. Patients with elevated troponins benefit substantially more than patients without troponin elevation who in general derive little benefit.

■ GP IIb/IIIa inhibitors are beneficial in patients undergoing primary coronary stenting for acute ST elevation myocardial infarction particularly when there is evidence of residual thrombus, nonobstructive dissection, or ≤TIMI II coronary blood flow.

ADMIRAL Trial (2001)

The ADMIRAL trial (Abciximab before Direct Angioplasty and Stenting in Myocardial Infarction Regarding Acute and Long-term Follow–up) evaluated the incremental benefit of abciximab in addition to primary stenting in patients with acute ST elevation myocardial infarction. Patients were randomized to abciximab or placebo prior to arterial sheath insertion and angiography.

Abciximab improved the occurrence of the primary end point (composite of death, reinfarction, or urgent target vessel revascularization at 30 days) which occurred in 6.0 percent of the abciximab group, compared with 14.6 percent of the placebo group (*P*=0.01); at 6 months, the corresponding figures were 7.4 percent and 15.9 percent (*P*=0.02). The better clinical outcomes in the abciximab group were related to the greater frequency of TIMI grade 3 coronary flow before PCI (16.8 percent vs. 5.4 percent, *P*=0.01), immediately after PCI (95.1 percent vs. 86.7 percent, *P*=0.04), and six months afterward (94.3 percent vs. 82.8 percent, *P*=0.04). Diabetic patients had a very significant benefit with abciximab.

■ Early administration of abciximab in patients with acute myocardial infarction improves coronary patency before stenting, the success rate of the stenting

procedure, late coronary patency at six months, left ventricular function, and clinical outcomes

CADILLAC Trial (2002)

The CADILLAC trial (Controlled Abciximab and Device Investigation to Lower Late Angioplasty Complications) tested the optimal percutaneous revascularization strategy in acute myocardial infarction. CADILLAC randomly assigned over 2,000 patients with acute myocardial infarction to PTCA alone, PTCA and abciximab, stenting alone, or stenting and abciximab. Clopidogrel or ticlopidine was given to all patients at baseline and continued daily in the stented patients. Stenting alone was better than PTCA (with or without abciximab) in reducing the composite end point of death, stroke, reinfarction, or revascularization at 6 months follow-up. There was a modest additional benefit to abciximab in stented patients but not in PTCA patients. Abciximab significantly reduced the rate of subacute stent thrombosis (0.4% versus 1.5 %) and recurrent ischemia leading to repeat revascularization of the target vessel but there was no difference in the rate of reinfarction or in left ventricular function at six months.

■ Stenting is the optimal revascularization strategy in myocardial infarction
■ There was a modest additional benefit to adjunctive abciximab in stented patients

TARGET Trial (2002)

The TARGET trial (Do Tirofiban and Reopro Give Similar efficacy Outcome trial) was a noninferiority randomized trial that directly compared two GP IIb/IIIa inhibitors (abciximab and tirofiban) in just over 4,800 patients who underwent nonemergent coronary stenting. Abciximab was superior to tirofiban in the composite end point of death, infarction, or the need for urgent revascularization at 30 days (6% versus 7.6 percent). The superiority of abciximab was independent of age, gender, or the use of clopidogrel pretreatment. There were no significant differences in the rates of major bleeding complications or transfusions, but tirofiban was associated with a lower rate of minor bleeding and thrombocytopenia. By six months there was no significant difference in any of the end points between the two drugs, and the early advantage of abciximab over tirofiban has fallen to nonsignificant levels.

The early benefit with abciximab was confined to patients undergoing stenting for acute coronary syndromes in whom less periprocedural myocardial infarctions occurred. The superiority of abciximab over tirofiban in acute coronary syndromes has been ascribed to a greater early efficacy of abciximab in blocking platelet glycoprotein IIb/IIIa receptors in the setting of very intense platelet activation. The early benefit seen with abciximab in patients with acute coronary syndrome existed out to six months but had disappeared by one year.

- Abciximab had an early benefit over tirofiban in the TARGET trial due to a reduction in procedure-related myocardial infarction
- Abciximab, but not eptifibatide or tirofiban is associated with an increased risk of thrombocytopenia
- Abciximab has no lasting advantage over tirofiban for nonemergency stenting

Heparin

Unfractionated IV heparin is used at the time of PCI to prevent in situ acute vessel thrombosis. Heparin monitoring is best performed via the activated clotting time (ACT), as the partial thromboplastin time (PTT) is not accurate at high heparin doses. In the absence of GP IIb/IIIa inhibitors, a target ACT of 250 to 350 seconds is the best balance between prevention of stent thrombosis and bleeding risk.

Heparin and GP IIb/IIIa Inhibitors

Heparin dosage should be reduced when used in conjunction with GP IIb/IIIa inhibitors with a target ACT of 200 to 250 seconds. The incidence of major bleeding increased with higher ACT values but without a beneficial effect on patient survival or the occurrence of myocardial infarction. Prolonged heparinization following PCI increases the incidence of major bleeding, prolongs hospitalization and does not reduce the incidence of stent thrombosis.

- Stent deployment may be optimized by using intravascular ultrasound imaging and/or high-pressure PTCA balloon inflation
- Aggressive anticoagulation with warfarin after PCI increases the bleeding risk without reducing the risk of stent thrombosis
- Drug-eluting stents require prolonged administration of dual antiplatelet therapy for several months

DRUG-ELUTING STENTS IN ACUTE MYOCARDIAL INFARCTION

Patients presenting with acute myocardial infarction who underwent primary PCI were excluded from the landmark RAVEL, TAXUS, and SIRIUS drug-eluting stent trials. A period of uncertainty followed regarding the relative risk of acute in-stent thrombosis with DES compared with standard bare metal stents when implanted in the very thrombogenic milieu of acute myocardial infarction, and, secondarily, whether the established late benefits of DES in the prevention of in-stent restenosis seen in noninfarction settings would also acrue when used following primary PCI for acute myocardial infarction.

The STRATEGY trial was a small clinical trial of 175 patients that randomized participants to a sirolimus stent plus tirofiban or a bare metal stent plus abciximab. The study, while underpowered, suggested a benefit with sirolimus and tirofiban on the basis of a reduction in the combined end point of death, reinfarction, stroke, or target vessel revascularization in the tirofiban plus sirolimus-eluting stent group (18%) versus the abciximab plus bare metal stent group (32%) (P=.04), mostly due to a lower rate of target vessel revascularization (7% versus 20%, respectively). Two recent large randomized clinical trials from Europe have compared DES versus bare metal stents in primary PCI and, though shedding further light on the topic, have failed to completely resolve the clinical question.

TYPHOON Trial (2006)

The TYPHOON (Trial to Assess the Use of the Cypher Stent In Acute Myocardial Infarction Treated with Balloon Angioplasty) trial randomized 712 patients to a sirolimus-eluting stent or a bare metal stent. The 1-year rates of death, reinfarction, and in-stent thrombosis were statistically the same for both stents at 2.3% (2.2%), 1.1% (1.4%), and 3.4% (3.6%), respectively, for the sirolimus-eluting and bare metal stents. Target vessel failure—defined as a composite end point of target vessel related death, reinfarction, or target vessel revascularization was reduced by approximately 50% by sirolimus-eluting stents from 14.3% in the bare metal stent arm to 7.3% in the DES arm (P=0.004), while target vessel revascularization was decreased in the respective groups by approximately 60% from 13.4% to 5.6% (P<0.001). An angiographic substudy showed less angiographic in-stent restenosis in the DES patients.

PASSION Trial (2006)

The PASSION (Paclitaxel-Eluting Stent versus Conventional Stent in Myocardial Infarction with ST Segment Elevation Trial) trial randomized 619 patients to the paclitaxel-eluting Taxus Express 2 stent or a bare metal stent. The 1-year rates of death, reinfarction, and in-stent thrombosis were statistically the same for both stents at 4.9% (6.5%), 1.7% (2.0%), and 1.0% (1.0%), respectively, for the paclitaxel-eluting stent and bare metal stent. Target vessel revascularization was also similar in both groups at 5.3% and 7.8% (P=NS), respectively, for the paclitaxel-eluting and bare metal stents.

Comparison of TYPHOON and PASSION

The PASSION and TYPHOON trials had a number of significant design differences that precluded a direct head-to-head comparison of outcome data on paclitaxel- and sirolimus-eluting stents implanted following acute myocardial infarction. These differences included different definitions of in-stent thrombosis, fewer diabetics in the PASSION trial, dissimilar bare metal stents, and distinctively different requirements for follow-up angiography. A marked difference between the trials was the target vessel revascularization rates in the control bare metal stent patients groups, namely 7.8% for PASSION versus 13.4% for TYPHOON.

In summary, the PASSION and TYPHOON trials established that DES placement is safe in the setting of acute myocardial infarction and is not associated with a significantly greater risk of in-stent thrombosis compared to bare metal stent placement. DES may reduce the need for late target vessel revascularization following primary PCI but appear to have no benefit over bare metal stents with regard to mortality at 1 year or recurrent myocardial infarction.

Cardiac Emergencies

Arshad Jahangir, MD

Joseph G. Murphy, MD

This chapter outlines the general principles of managing cardiac emergencies for children 8 years or older and adult patients. It is deliberately not an exhaustive review. Sudden cardiac arrest is a leading cause of death in developed nations and is frequently associated with ventricular fibrillation (VF) at some point in its time course.

Resuscitation for cardiac arrest is most successful if defibrillation is performed within the first 5 minutes after collapse. Cardiopulmonary resuscitation (CPR) markedly increases the victim's chance of survival and should be initiated expeditiously in the unconscious patient and continued until an automated external defibrillator (AED) or manual defibrillator is available. The latest consensus guidelines for CPR stress the importance of high-quality basic life support. Rescuers should "push hard, push fast, allow full chest recoil, minimize interruptions in compressions, and defibrillate promptly when appropriate." In addition, initiation of CPR should not be delayed until after the first defibrillation as CPR before attempted defibrillation has been shown to improve survival rates (Fig. 1).

The stacked sequence of 3 defibrillation shocks previously recommendation for the treatment of ventricular fibrillation/ventricular tachycardia has been superseded by a new one shock recommendation based on the high first-shock efficacy of modern biphasic defibrillators (> 90%). Immediate resumption of CPR is now considered to confer greater value than an immediate second shock (Fig. 2).

There is little scientific evidence that routine administration of any antiarrhythmic drug, epinephrine or vasopressin increases the survival rate of patients post cardiac arrest to hospital discharge and the new guidelines deemphasize drug administration and reemphasizes basic life support for all cardiac arrest victims.

Pulseless Cardiac Arrest

Ventricular Fibrillation (VF) or Pulseless Ventricular Tachycardia

1. **Activate the emergency medical response system** and immediately initiate cardiopulmonary resuscitation (**CPR**) until a defibrillator is available. Initial 2 breaths at 1 second/breath. Check pulse (<10 second).

   Single rescuers: compression-ventilation ratio 30:2.

   Two rescuers: 100 compressions/minute continuously, without pauses with 8 to 10 breaths/minute ventilation by the second rescuer.

   (For every minute without CPR, survival from witnessed VF arrest decreases 7% to 10% vs. 3%

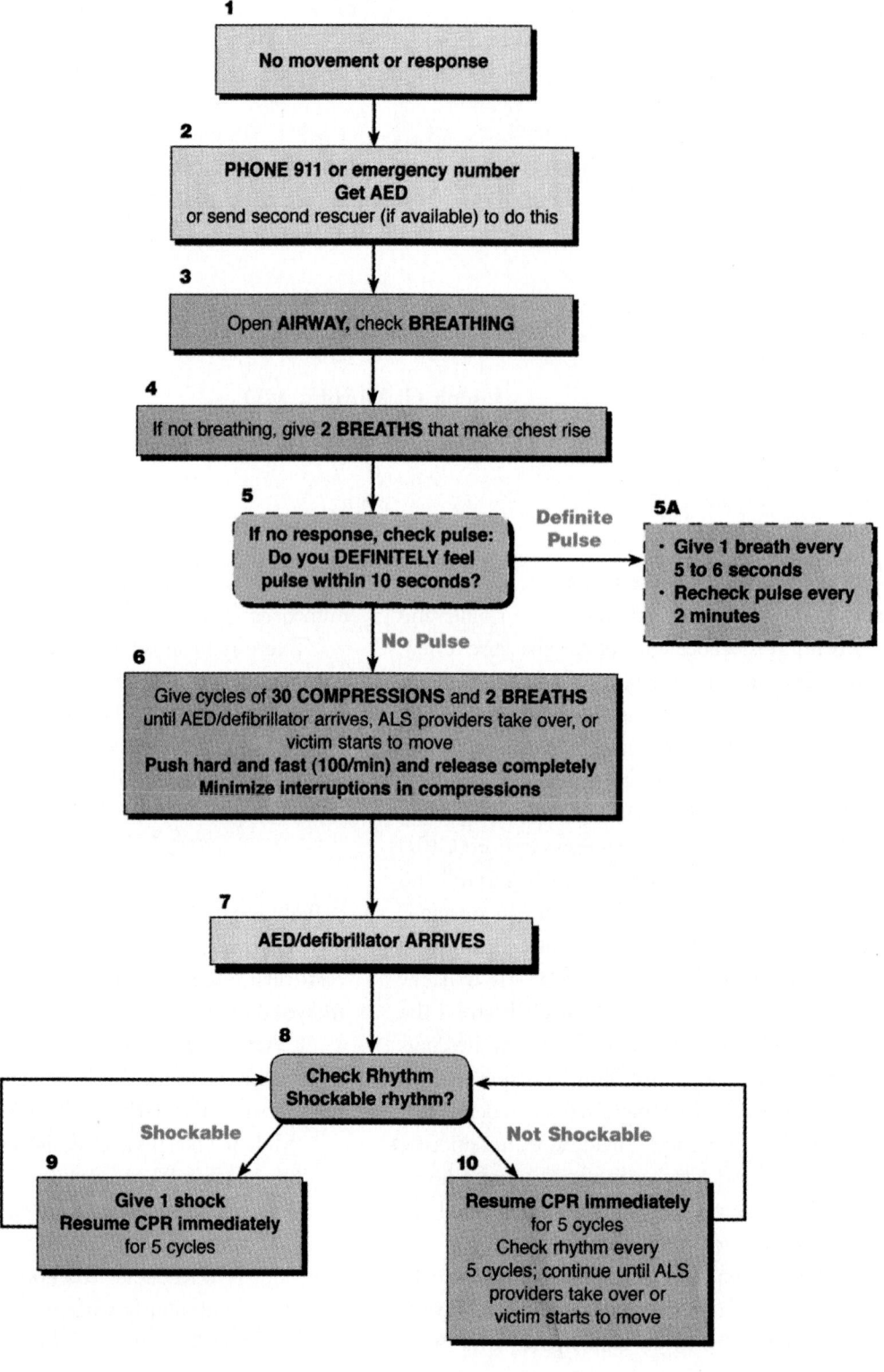

Fig. 1. Adult BLS healthcare provider algorithm. Boxes bordered with dotted lines indicate actions or steps performed by the healthcare provider but not the lay rescuer.

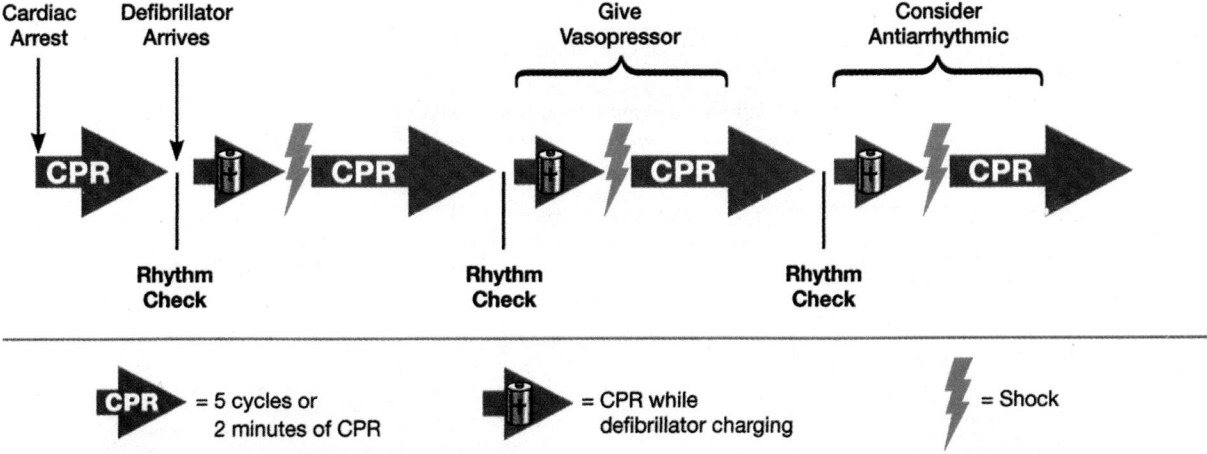

Ventricular Fibrillation/Pulseless Ventricular Tachycardia Sequence: Prepare next drug prior to rhythm check. Administer drug during CPR, as soon as possible after the rhythm check confirms VF/pulseless VT. Do not delay shock. Continue CPR while drugs are prepared and administered and defibrillator is charging. Ideally, chest compressions should be interrupted only for ventilation (until advanced airway placed), rhythm check, and actual shock delivery.

Fig. 2. Treatment sequence for ventricular fibrillation (VF)/pulseless ventricular tachycardia (VT). CPR, cardiopulmonary resuscitation.

to 4% per minute from collapse to defibrillation when bystander CPR is provided).

2. **Defibrillate** once with unsynchronized 200 J biphasic (or 360 J monophasic waveform) shock. Early defibrillation is the key to successful resuscitation (49% to 75% survival rates with CPR plus defibrillation within 3 to 5 minutes of collapse).

3. Immediately resume **CPR** without checking pulse.

4. Check rhythm after 5 cycles of CPR and **defibrillate** 200 J biphasic (360 J monophasic) shock if indicated.

5. Resume **CPR** immediately

6. Give
   a. **Epinephrine** 1 mg intravenously (IV), repeat every 3 to 5 minutes, (2- 2.5 mg endotracheally if IV) , *or*
   b. **Vasopressin** 40 units IV once, epinephrine may then be used 10 minutes after the Vasopressin.

7. **Defibrillate** once (200 J biphasic; 360 J monophasic) and resume **CPR**

8. For recurrent or refractory VF or VT, consider
   ▪ **Amiodarone** (300 mg IV, repeat 150 mg in 3-5 minutes), *or*
   ▪ **Lidocaine** (1-1.5 mg/kg IV, then 0.5-0.75 mg/kg/min max 3 doses)

9. **CPR** 5 cycles

10. Repeat 6-8
    a. Precipitating factors such as myocardial ischemia, electrolyte and acid-base disturbance should be corrected (Fig. 3).

Asystole

1. Activate the emergency medical response system and initiate CPR.

2. Give
   a. **Epinephrine** 1 mg IV, repeat every 3 to 5 minutes, *or*
   b. **Vasopressin** 40 units IV once, epinephrine may then be used 10 minutes after the vasopressin.

3. **Atropine**, 1 mg IV every 3 to 5 minutes up to 3 doses

4. **Check rhythm**

5. Defibrillate if there is any possibility that the rhythm is other than asystole (fine ventricular fibrillation). Randomized controlled trials have failed to show benefit of attempted pacing for cardiac arrest with asystole and pacing is not recommended.

6. Continuously monitor rhythm for ventricular fibrillation and defibrillate if appropriate.

7. Give high dose of epinephrine, 2 to 5 mg

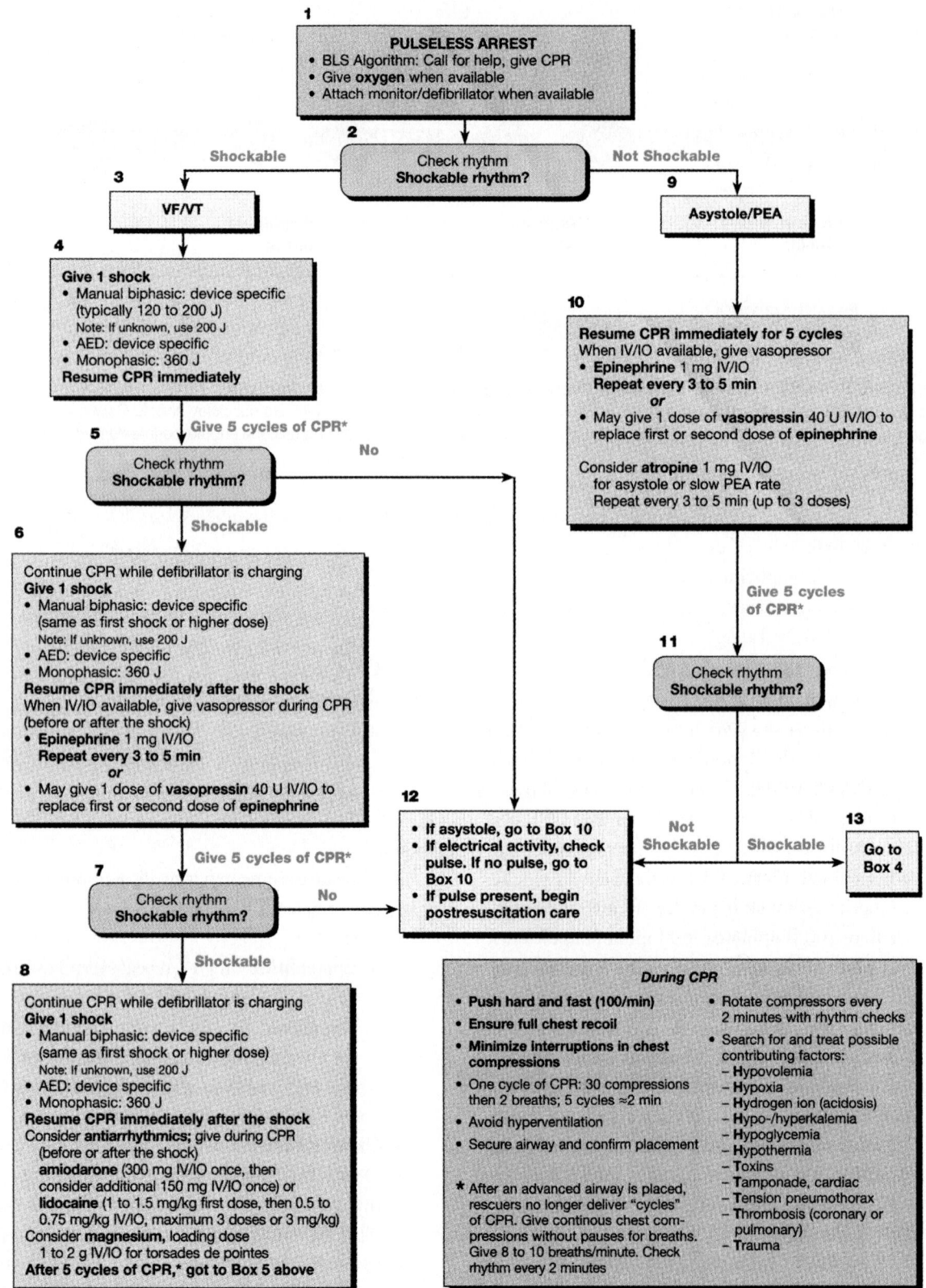

ACLS Pulseless Arrest Algorithm.

Fig. 3. ACLS pulseless arrest algorithm.

intravenously every 3 to 5 minutes.

8. Sodium bicarbonate, 1 mEq/kg intravenously, followed by 0.5 mEq/kg every 10 minutes for documented acidosis not due to hypoventilation.

9. Emergency echocardiography to check for cardiac tamponade and to assess ventricular function. Correct for any reversible cause if possible, such as hypoxia, hypothermia, hyperkalemia, acidosis, drug overdose.

Pulseless Electrical Activity (Electromechanical Dissociation)

Rhythm on monitor without detectable pulse

1. **CPR**
2. Intubate.
3. **Epinephrine**, 1 mg IV every 3 to 5 minutes
4. **Vasopressin** 40 units IV once, epinephrine may then be used 10 minutes after the vasopressin.
5. **Atropine**, 1 mg IV every 3 minutes up to 3 mg.
6. Repeat **epinephrine** every 3 to 5 minutes.
7. Sodium bicarbonate, 1 mEq/kg intravenously, followed by 0.5 mEq/kg 10 minutes for documented acidosis not due to hypoventilation.
8. Look for secondary causes of electromechanical dissociation, and correct if possible.

> Hypovolemia
> Hypoxia
> Hypothermia
> Hypoglycemia
> Hyperkalemia/ hypokalemia
> Hydrogen ion (acidosis)
> Toxins (Drug Overdose)
> Tamponade, Cardiac
> Tension pneumothorax
> Thrombosis (Massive pulmonary embolism or myocardial infarction)
> Trauma

POLYMORPHIC VENTRICULAR TACHYCARDIA (PVT)

A. **PVT in the setting of Prolonged QT Interval (Torsades de Pointes)**

1. **Unsynchronized DC cardioversion** if the patient is hemodynamically unstable, (150-200 J biphasic, 360 J monophasic).

2. Give **magnesium sulfate**, 1 to 2 g dilute in D5W IV over 5 to 60 minutes, even if the serum level of magnesium is within normal limits.

3. Shorten the QT interval and eliminate triggering long-short RR interval by increasing the heart rate to 100 to 120 beats/min with
   a. **Isoproterenol** infusion (start at 1 μg/min up to 20 μg/min)

   or

   b. **Temporary pacemaker**.

4. **Correct underlying electrolyte abnormalities** such as hypokalemia and hypomagnesemia.

5. **Stop treatment with all QT prolonging agents**.
   Antiarrhythmics: quinidine, procainamide, disopyramide, sotalol, ibutilide, amiodarone
   Antipsychotics: haloperidol, thioridazine, droperidol
   Antibiotics: erythromycin
   Antivirals and antiprotozoals: amantidine, pentamidine
   Antifungal agents: ketoconazole, itraconazole
   Antihistamines: terfenadine, astemizole
   Propulsive agents: cisapride
   Hypolipidemic agents: probucol

6. β-Blockers may be effective in preventing torsades de pointes in the setting of congenital long QT syndromes (LQT1).

B. **PVT in the setting of a normal QT interval**

1. Hemodynamically unstable: DC cardioversion (100, 200 J biphasic)

2. Hemodynamically stable:
   - Amiodarone (150 mg intravenously over 10 minutes, then 1 mg/min for 6 hours followed by 0.5 mg/min).
   - Lidocaine (1 to 1.5 mg/kg intravenously, followed by 1 to 4 mg/min, supplemented by boluses of 0.5 to 0.75 mg/kg every 5 to 10 minutes to a maximum of 3 mg/kg), *or*

3. Correct myocardial ischemia or electrolyte disturbances.

C. **Electrical Storm**

Drug-refractory recurrent, hemodynamically destabilizing sustained PVT or VF ("VT Storm") may occur after acute MI related to uncontrolled ischemia and/or increased sympathetic tone and require recurrent cardioversion/defibrillation and may be managed with:

- ■ Sympathetic blockade:
  - **Propranolol** (0.15 mg/kg over 10 minutes and then as a 3- to 5-mg dose every 6 hours to maintain sinus rhythm unless the heart rate dropped below 45 bpm), *or*
  - **Esmolol** (500 μg/kg over 1 min, then 50-250 μg/kg per minute intravenously, titration of maintenance infusion rate at 5- to 10-minute intervals until a maximum dose of 250 μg/kg per minute), *or*
  - **Left stellate ganglionic blockade** (for refractory arrhythmia), *or*
  - **Full sedation with mechanical ventilatory support**
  - **Amiodarone** (150 mg intravenously over 10 minutes, then 1 mg/min for 6 hours followed by 0.5 mg/min)
- ■ Intra-aortic balloon pump
- ■ Emergency revascularization.

VENTRICULAR TACHYCARDIA

1. Maintain **airway**, assist **breathing**, give **oxygen**
2. Assess hemodynamic status
   a. **Unstable: Synchronized DC cardioversion**, stepwise increase 100-200 J (110, 200, 300, 360 J monophasic), sedate first if conscious.
   b. **Stable:** Treat pharmacologically
      - **Amiodarone**, 150 mg IV over 10 minutes, followed by a 1 mg/min infusion for 6 hours and then 0.5 mg/min over 18 hours. Repeat 150 mg every 10 minutes as necessary for recurrent or resistant arrhythmias to a maximum 2.2 g/24 hour, *or*
      - **Lidocaine**, 1 to 1.5 mg/kg IV, followed by 1 to 4 mg/min, supplemented by boluses of 0.5 to 0.75 mg/kg every 5 to 10 minutes to a maximum of 3 mg/kg (lower infusion rates in the elderly and those with congestive heart failure or liver dysfunction, to avoid lidocaine toxicity), or
      - **Procainamide**, 1 g IV over 30 minutes followed by 1 to 4 mg/min (watch for hypotension)
      - **Elective synchronized DC cardioversion** for hemodynamically stable patients (starting at 100 J) who do not have conversion to sinus rhythm pharmacologically (brief

anesthesia is necessary).
3. Correct **precipitating factors**, including myocardial ischemia, electrolyte and acid-base imbalance.

Symptomatic bradycardia with symptoms/signs of poor perfusion

1. Maintain **airway**, assist **breathing**, give **oxygen**
2. **Transcutaneous pacing**
3. While awaiting pacer, give
   a. **Atropine**, 0.5 mg IV every 3 to 5 minutes up to 3 mg, *or*
   b. **Epinephrine**, 2-10 mcg/min IV, *or*
   c. **Dopamine**, 2-10 mcg/kg/min
4. Glucagon, 3 mg IV followed by 3 mg/hour for bradycardia due to β-blocker or calcium channel blocker overdose not responding to atropine
5. Prepare for **transvenous pacing**
6. Treat contributing causes

ATRIAL FLUTTER OR ATRIAL FIBRILLATION WITH RAPID VENTRICULAR RESPONSE

A. **To control rapid ventricular response:**
   1. **Verapamil**, 2.5-5 mg IV over 2-3 minutes, repeat 5-10 mg every 15 to 30 minutes to a total dose of 20 mg, *or*
      Diltiazem, 0.25 mg/kg IV over 2 minutes, repeat 0.35 mg/kg in 15 minutes and then 5-15 mg/hr titrate to heart rate, *or*
      Esmolol, 0.5 mg/kg IV over 1 min, then 50 200 μg/kg/minute, *or*
      Atenolol 5 mg IV over 5 min to a total of 10 mg in 10 to 15 min, *or*
      Metoprolol 5 mg IV every 5 min to a total 15 mg over 15 min, *or*
      Propranolol 0.1 mg/kg by slow IV push divided into 3 equal doses at 2- to 3-minute intervals,
      Magnesium sulfate, 1 to 2 g IV over 5 to 60 minutes.
   2. Elective **synchronized DC cardioversion** (50 to 100 J).

B. **To restore sinus rhythm:**
   1. **Heparin** should be given to patients who were not anticoagulated and if stable a **transesophageal echocardiogram** should be obtained to exclude intracardiac thrombus.
   2. **Ibutilide**, 1 mg over 10 minutes, repeat once after 10 minutes; watch for torsades de pointes, correct hypokalemia or hypomagnesaemia before admin-

istration, *or*

Amiodarone, 150 mg IV over 10 minutes, followed by a 1 mg/min infusion for 6 hours and then 0.5 mg/min over 18 hours

3. Synchronized DC cardioversion (100-120 J biphasic).

4. Rapid atrial or esophageal pacing for type I atrial flutter.

5. Adenosine is not effective therapy for atrial fibrillation or atrial flutter.

6. Anticoagulation should be continued after cardioversion.

7. To prevent recurrence, an antiarrhythmic agent such as Propafenone (structurally normal heart), Sotalol (ischemic heart disease), or amiodarone (LV dysfunction) should be considered.

PAROXYSMAL SUPRAVENTRICULAR TACHYCARDIA

1. Maintain **airway**, assist **breathing**, give **oxygen**
2. Assess hemodynamic status
   a. **Unstable: synchronized DC cardioversion** (50-100 J), sedate first if conscious.
   b. **Stable**:
      i. **Vagal** maneuvers (Valsalva maneuver or carotid sinus massage)
      ii. **Adenosine**, 6 mg rapid IV push followed by saline flush, repeat 12 mg in 1-2 min and then once more.
      iii. **Verapamil**, 2.5-5 mg IV over 2-3 minutes, repeat 5-10 mg every 15 to 30 minutes to a total dose of 20 mg, *or*
      Diltiazem, 0.25 mg/kg IV over 2 minutes, repeat 0.35 mg/kg in 15 minutes and then 5-15 mg/hr titrate to heart rate, or
      iv. **Esmolol**, 500 μg/kg IV over 1 min, then 50-200 μg/kg/minute.
      v. Elective **synchronized DC cardioversion** (50 to 100 J).

RECIPROCATING TACHYCARDIA COMPLICATING WOLFF-PARKINSON-WHITE SYNDROME

1. Maintain **airway**, assist **breathing**, give **oxygen**
2. Assess hemodynamic status

a. **Unstable: Synchronized DC cardioversion** (50-100 J), sedate first if conscious.
b. **Stable**:
   i. With orthodromic conduction (narrow complex QRS), give **Adenosine** IV (may convert from reciprocating tachycardia to atrial fibrillation). Atrial fibrillation with a rapid ventricular response may require emergency synchronized DC cardioversion.
   ii. For conversion to sinus rhythm **Amiodarone**, 150 mg IV over 10 minutes, repeat as needed to max 2.2 g/24 hour, *or* **Procainamide**, 1 g IV over 30 minutes followed by 1 to 4 mg/min (watch for hypotension), *or*
   iii. For atrial fibrillation that complicates WPW syndrome, adenosine is contraindicated, also **avoid AV node blocking agents** (diltiazem, verapamil or digoxin), that can accelerate anterograde conduction over the bypass tract and increase ventricular rate.
   iv. If pharmacologic therapy fails in a hemodynamically stable patient, consider **DC cardioversion**.

MULTIFOCAL ATRIAL TACHYCARDIA

1. Treat the underlying disease (frequently, lung disease and hypoxemia).
2. Stop treatment with provocative agents such as beta-agonists or theophylline.
3. Avoid β-blockers if there is underlying bronchospastic lung disease.
4. Magnesium or potassium given intravenously may be effective even if the serum levels of magnesium and potassium are normal (magnesium sulfate 1 to 2 g intravenously over 10 minutes, then 1 to 2 g/hr over 5 hours).
5. Verapamil given orally or intravenously is usually the drug of choice (5 to 10 mg intravenously, repeat 5 to 10 mg for a total of 20 mg).
6. Digoxin or cardioversion is not effective in treating this arrhythmia due to abnormalities in impulse initiation.
7. In paroxysmal atrial tachycardia with block, always suspect digoxin toxicity and treat accordingly.

PACEMAKER-MEDIATED TACHYCARDIA (PMT)

Pacemaker-mediated tachycardia is a form of reentrant tachycardia that is observed in patients with a dual chamber (DDD) pacemaker and retrograde VA conduction. Ventricular depolarization (paced beat or ventricular premature complex) retrogradely activates the atria via the AV conduction system. Atrial depolarization is sensed by the atrial lead and then triggers the pacemaker to pace the ventricle, which is then again retrogradely conducted to the atria to create a reentrant loop that repeats the sequence resulting in incessant tachycardia at or near the programmed upper rate limit of the pacemaker (commonly set at 120 ppm).

1. **Increase retrograde AV conduction time or induce AV node block**
   - Vagal maneuvers (carotid sinus massage, Valsalva)
   - Adenosine, verapamil or β-blocker
   or
2. **Make atrial lead insensitive to the retrograde P wave**
   - Apply a magnet to disable atrial tracking (especially when pacemaker model is not known or pacemaker programmer is unavailable), *or*
   - Increase the postventricular atrial refractory period (PVARP), *or*
   - Reprogram pacemaker mode to DVI or VVI

New pacemakers have the capability to detect PMT and initiate PMT intervention. This is done by automatically prolonging the PVARP (PVARP extension) for the beat after a ventricular-sensed event that is not preceded by atrial pacing (such as a PVC) or dropping a paced ventricular beat when the pacemaker is pacing at the upper tracking rate for a specified period or shortening the AV interval for a single beat to induce retrograde AV block and terminate the tachycardia.

ACUTE CORONARY SYNDROMES

Unstable Angina or Non-ST-Elevation MI

1. **Oxygen** 4 L/min, maintain O_2 saturation > 90%
2. **Aspirin** orally (160 to 325 mg).
3. **Nitroglycerin** 3 doses sublingual or aerosol at 3-5 minutes, followed by IV (5 to 10 mcg/min,

increase by 10 μg/min every 3 to 5 minutes to a maximal dose of 200 μg/min). Avoid in those with systolic blood pressure <90 mm Hg or in those who have received a phosphodiesterase inhibitor for erectile dysfunction within 24 hours.
4. Sedation and analgesia (**morphine** sulfate, IV 2 to 4 mg every 5 to 10 minutes as tolerated).
5. **β-Blocker** given orally or intravenously unless contraindicated (metoprolol, 5 mg IV, repeat 3 times and then 50 to 100 mg orally twice daily, or esmolol, 0.5 mg/kg per minute initially and then titrate to 50 to 200 mcg/kg per minute).
6. Consider **clopidogrel** orally 300 mg.
7. **Heparin**: Unfractionated, IV bolus 60 U/kg followed by 12 U/kg per hour infusion to keep aPTT around 60 to 70 sec), *or* Low-Molecular Weight Heparin.
7. Consider **glycoprotein IIb/IIIa inhibitor**.
8. Intra-aortic balloon pump for selected patients to stabilize before coronary artery bypass graft or percutaneous coronary intervention (PCI).
9. Emergency coronary angiography and intervention for refractory ischemia (persistent chest pain, recurrent ST deviation, hemodynamic instability, VT, heart failure).
10. ACE inhibitor/angiotensin receptor blocker
11. HMG CoA reductase inhibitor (statin)

ST-Elevation Myocardial Infarction or with New Left Bundle Branch Block

1. **Oxygen** 4 L/min, maintain O_2 saturation > 0%
2. **Aspirin** orally (160 to 325 mg).
3. **Nitroglycerin** sublingual or aerosol followed by IV (5 to 10 mcg/min, increase by 10 μg/min every 3 to 5 minutes to a maximal dose of 200 μg/min). Avoid systolic blood pressure less than 90 mm Hg.
4. Sedation and analgesia (**morphine** sulfate, 2 to 4 mg every 5 to 10 minutes as tolerated).
5. **β-Blocker** given orally or intravenously unless contraindicated (**metoprolol**, 5 mg IV, repeat 3 times and then 50 to 100 mg orally twice daily, or **esmolol**, 0.5 mg/kg per minute initially and then titrate to 50 to 200 mcg/kg per minute). Avoid calcium channel blockers, if possible.
6. Consider **Clopidogrel** orally 300 mg.
7. **Heparin**: Unfractionated, IV bolus 60 U/kg followed by 12 U/kg per hour infusion to keep

aPTT around 60 to 70 sec), *or* low-molecular-weight heparin.

8. Time from chest pain onset ≤12 hours

    Reperfusion Therapy

    Fibrinolysis (Goal: door-to-drug ≤30 minutes),

    or

    Emergency PCI (Goal: door-to-balloon inflation ≤90 minutes).

    Consider fibrinolysis if:
    - Early presentation (<3 hours from symptom onset),
    - Emergency PCI not an option or would be delayed >90 min,
    - No contraindications to fibrinolysis

    Absolute contraindications for **thrombolytic therapy**
    - presence of structural cerebral lesion or intracranial neoplasm
    - any prior intracranial hemorrhage
    - ischemic stroke <3 months except when used to treat an acute stroke within 3 hours of onset
    - suspected aortic dissection
    - significant closed head or facial trauma <3 months
    - major surgery or trauma (including traumatic CPR) <3 weeks
    - known active bleeding or bleeding diathesis

    Streptokinase 1.5 million IU over 1 hour. rtPA, 15-mg bolus, followed by 0.75 mg/kg (up to 50 mg) over 30 minutes, then 0.5 mg/kg (up to 35 mg) infusion over 1 hour. Anistreplase, 30 IU over 2 minutes.

9. Inotropic agents for cardiogenic shock.

    Dobutamine, 2 to 15 µg/kg per minute.

    Dopamine, 0.5 to 10 µg/kg per minute (increases renal blood flow at less than 2 µg/kg per minute only).

    Amrinone, 0.75 mg/kg followed by 5 to 10 µg/kg per minute.

10. Intra-aortic balloon pump for selected patients with hypotension. Or emergency PCI for cardiogenic shock.

11. Fluids given intravenously for right ventricular infarction. (Avoid nitroglycerin or diuretics.)

12. Lidocaine to treat ventricular arrhythmias but not for prophylaxis.

13. Avoid calcium channel blockers.

14. Magnesium sulfate for patients with low serum levels of magnesium.

15. Angiotensin converting enzyme inhibitor unless contraindicated. Captopril orally, start with 6.25 mg and increase to 50 mg twice daily as tolerated.

16. HMG CoA reductase inhibitors.

RIGHT VENTRICULAR ISCHEMIA OR INFARCTION

1. Maintain right ventricular preload with volume loading (intravenous saline). Avoid nitrates and diuretics because they decrease preload. Maintain atrioventricular synchrony, and initiate atrioventricular pacing for symptomatic high-grade atrioventricular block unresponsive to atropine. Prompt cardioversion is important for hemodynamically significant supraventricular tachycardia (atrial fibrillation may occur in up to one-third of patients).

2. Inotropic support—Start intravenous dobutamine if cardiac output fails to improve after infusion of 1 to 2 L of saline solution. Inotropic agents can increase cardiac output in right ventricular infarction by making septal wall motion hyperdynamic even in the presence of severe right ventricular free wall hypokinesia.

PULMONARY EDEMA

1. Identify and treat precipitating factors if possible.

2. Place the patient in a sitting position to improve oxygenation.

3. Give supplemental oxygen by mask or nasal cannula to maintain O_2 saturation > 90%.

4. Intubate and mechanically ventilate the patient if hypoxia and/or hypercapnia cannot be corrected adequately.

5. Give morphine sulfate, 2 to 5 mg intravenously; repeat every 10 to 25 minutes if needed .

6. Give a loop diuretic such as furosemide, 20 to 80 mg intravenously.

7. Start an infusion of nitroglycerin.

    Nitroglycerin is a venodilator that predominantly affects cardiac preload. (Initiate at 5 µg/min and increase 5 to 10 µg/min every 3 to 5 minutes to a maximum of 200 µg/min, as tolerated.)

Nitroprusside is a mixed arterial and venous vasodilator that decreases both cardiac preload and afterload.

Nitroprusside is indicated specifically in pulmonary edema due to systemic hypertension and acute mitral or aortic insufficiency. Start at 0.3 µg/kg per minute, and titrate up to 10 µg/kg per minute as needed.

8. Inotropic agents (dopamine, dobutamine) may be helpful in pulmonary edema due to hypotension and cardiogenic shock. Dopamine, 0.5 to 10 µg/kg per minute; dobutamine, 2 to 15 µg/kg per minute.

9. An intra-aortic balloon pump may be valuable in selected patients.

HYPERTENSIVE EMERGENCIES

1. Nitroprusside, start treatment with 0.3 µg/kg per minute and titrate up to 10 µg/kg per minute.

2. Nitroglycerin, 10 to 400 µg/minute.

3. Esmolol, start treatment with 200 µg/kg for 1 minute and follow with 25 to 300 µg/kg per minute.

4. Labetalol, start treatment with 20 mg given intravenously and repeat with 20 to 40 mg every 10 minutes or 0.5 to 2.0 mg/min continuous infusion up to 300 mg.

5. Captopril, 6.25 to 50 mg orally at hourly intervals or enalapril at 0.625 to 1.25 mg intravenously every 6 hours.

6. Nitroprusside should be administered only in an intensive care setting and with intra-arterial blood pressure monitoring.

7. Nitroprusside is the drug of choice for hypertensive encephalopathy, cerebral hemorrhage, clonidine withdrawal syndrome, and aortic dissection (in combination with a beta-blocker).

8. Captopril or nitroglycerin is the drug of choice after myocardial infarction and in left ventricular failure.

9. Labetalol or phentolamine is the drug of choice for an adrenergic crisis (cocaine overdose, monoamine oxidase inhibitor-induced hypertensive crisis, pheochromocytoma).

AORTIC DISSECTION

1. Dissection of the ascending aorta is an emergency and should be treated surgically/invasively if possible.

2. Dissection of the descending aorta may be treated surgically/invasively or medically in some patients provided there is no organ ischemia.

3. Systemic systolic blood pressure should be lowered to 90 to 100 mm Hg measured by an arterial line or the lowest blood pressure that permits adequate organ perfusion – monitored by urinary output and cerebral function. The blood pressure needs to be controlled without increasing shear forces on the intimal flap of the aorta.

Nitroprusside intravenously (start with 0.3 µg/kg per minute and increase up to 10 µg/kg per minute) can be combined with esmolol intravenously (start with 500 µg/kg for 1 minute and titrate to 250 to 300 µg/kg per minute) to achieve a target heart rate of 60 to 70 beats/min.

4. In dissection of the ascending aortic arch, signs for complications such as acute aortic valve incompetence, inferior myocardial infarction due to extension of the dissection into the right coronary artery, neurologic signs due to dissection into the arch vessels and ischemia of the upper limbs need to be monitored closely.

PERICARDIAL TAMPONADE

1. The treatment of choice for nontraumatic cardiac tamponade is pericardiocentesis under echocardiographic guidance.

2. For traumatic cardiac tamponade and tamponade due to aortic dissection emergency thoracotomy should be performed.

3. Volume expansion with saline, blood, or plasma is valuable pending pericardiocentesis or surgery.

4. Avoid mechanical ventilation and beta-blockade.

5. Diuretics and nitrates are contraindicated.

PULMONARY THROMBOEMBOLISM

1. Supplemental oxygen.

2. Anticoagulation with heparin given intravenously (bolus 7,500 to 10,000 U, maintenance at 20 U/kg per hour to keep aPTT between 60 to 80).

3. Thrombolytic given intravenously for hemody-

namically unstable or profoundly hypoxemic patient with evidence of massive pulmonary embolism even without overt hemodynamic compromise (unless contraindicated, e.g., postoperative state).

Streptokinase, bolus 250,000 U, maintenance 100,000 U/hr for 24 to 72 hours.

Urokinase, bolus 2,000 U/lb, maintenance 2,000 U/lb per hour for 24 to 72 hours.

rtPA, bolus 15 mg, then 50 mg over 30 minutes, then 35 mg over next hour.

Full-dose heparin anticoagulation should be started along with infusion of a lytic agent.

4. Aggressive fluid resuscitation and inotropic or pressor agents if hypotension develops.
5. Surgical thrombectomy (only with severe hemodynamic compromise, when thrombolytic therapy is contraindicated or unsuccessful).

HYPERKALEMIA
1. Continuous ECG monitoring.
2. Calcium gluconate or calcium chloride, (10 mL of 10% solution over 10 minutes).
3. Glucose with insulin (50 mL of 50% dextrose intravenously, with 5 to 10 U regular insulin).
4. Sodium bicarbonate, 50 mEq IV over 5 min.
5. β2-Adrenergic agonists: albuterol nebulized 10-20 mg in 15 min or IV.
6. Diuresis: furosemide 40 to 80 mg IV.
7. Sodium polystyrene sulfonate (Kayexalate) (20 to 30 g orally with equal amount of sorbitol) or retention enema (50-100 g in 200 mL of water and sorbitol).
8. Dialysis may be required for persistent hyperkalemia.
9. Correction of underlying defect (renal failure, potassium-sparing diuretics, or adrenal insufficiency).

DIGOXIN TOXICITY AND OVERDOSE
Specific cardiac arrhythmias include ventricular tachycardia (especially bidirectional ventricular tachycardia), sinus bradycardia, heart block, and paroxysmal atrial tachycardia with block.

Nausea, vomiting, and drowsiness may occur.

1. Induce emesis or perform gastric lavage in digoxin overdose and administer charcoal to decrease further absorption of the drug.
2. Give digoxin-immune Fab: give 10 μg to test for hypersensitivity initially, then give up to 20 vials (dose per calculated digoxin body load if known) through a 0.22-μm membrane filter for

Ventricular tachycardia or fibrillation
High-grade atrioventricular block not responding to atropine or hyperkalemia
Acute ingestion of 10 mg or more
Serum level of 10 ng/mL or greater or severe hyperkalemia

3. Digoxin overdose may cause severe hyperkalemia. Treat in the usual way with insulin, glucose, and bicarbonate but avoid calcium gluconate because it potentiates digoxin toxicity.
4. Treat high-grade atrioventricular block with atropine and temporary pacing if needed.
5. Treat ventricular arrhythmias with lidocaine, phenytoin (100 mg intravenously over 5 minutes and repeat 100 mg over 5 minutes until a full loading dose of 18 mg/kg), esmolol (500 μg/kg intravenously, then 50 to 200 μg/kg per minute intravenously), or magnesium (1 to 2 g intravenously over 10 minutes). If hemodynamically unstable, synchronized DC cardioversion beginning at 10 J, increasing by 10 J to 50 J, then 100 J, 200 J, 300 J, and 360 J if necessary.
6. Correct hypokalemia or hypomagnesemia.

β-BLOCKER OVERDOSE
Emergency care to stabilize the airway, breathing, and circulation is the priority. Patients should have ECG monitoring.

1. Perform gastric lavage and administer charcoal, but avoid emesis because of vagal side effects.
2. Treat hypotension with saline and isoproterenol given intravenously, at 2 to 20 μg/min initially and increase up to 200 μg/min.
3. Glucagon (50 to 150 μg/kg over 1 minute, then 1 to 5 mg/hr in 5% dextrose solution). Calcium chloride or calcium gluconate (10 mL of 10% solution over 10 minutes) given intravenously may be useful for myocardial depression.
4. Treat bronchospasm with β-adrenergic agonists administered systemically or by inhalation or with

theophylline.

5. Treat heart block with atropine (up to 2 mg intravenously) or temporary pacing.

6. Treat hypoglycemia with glucose and glucagon given intravenously if needed.

7. Sotalol overdose may cause torsades de pointes.

CALCIUM CHANNEL BLOCKER OVERDOSE

As with β-blocker overdose, the goal of treatment is to decrease absorption of the drug and increase perfusion to the critical organ system.

1. Perform gastric lavage and administer charcoal, but avoid emesis because of vagal side effects.

2. Treat hypotension and bradycardia with saline infusion and intravenous calcium chloride, 1-g bolus (10 mL of 10% solution over 10 minutes), followed by a continuous infusion (20 to 50 mg/kg per hour). For patients taking digoxin, caution should be used because calcium may have deleterious effects.

3. Treat high-grade heart block with atropine (up to 2 mg) given intravenously or temporary pacing.

4. Glucagon (50 to 150 μg/kg intravenously over 1 minute followed by 1 to 5 mg/hr) may also be helpful for hypotension and heart block.

5. Dobutamine or dopamine should be used for heart failure and norepinephrine for hypotension.

126

CARDIOGENIC SHOCK

Malcolm R. Bell, MD

Cardiogenic shock is a clinical state in which the function of either the left ventricle, right ventricle, or both, is inadequate to maintain adequate perfusion of vital organs. The most common causes of cardiogenic shock are related to acute myocardial infarction, end-stage cardiomyopathy, severe myocarditis from any cause, critical valvular heart disease such as aortic stenosis or mitral stenosis, severe hypertrophic obstructive cardiomyopathy, and as a complication of cardiopulmonary bypass. This chapter addresses cardiogenic shock as a complication of acute myocardial infarction.

Cardiogenic shock is the leading cause of death among hospitalized patients following acute myocardial infarction. It is important to recognize that the majority (70-80%) of patients who develop cardiogenic shock do so in the hospital and that it is uncommon for patients to present to the emergency department in cardiogenic shock. It is important to remain vigilant for the development of cardiogenic shock in all patients following acute myocardial infarction.

INCIDENCE AND MORTALITY

The frequency with which cardiogenic shock complicates acute myocardial infarction has remained essentially unchanged at approximately 8-9% over the last decade as reported by the *National Registry for Myocardial Infarction* database (Fig. 1). Current in-hospital mortality for cardiogenic shock remains extremely high at about 50% - 60% for all age groups: significantly higher among patients over the age of 75 years at 60%-70% compared to younger patients in whom the mortality is about 40%-50%. From the same national registry, mortality rates appear to have declined recently but only very slightly (Fig. 2).

Patients age has a strong impact on mortality in cardiogenic shock. Advanced age in combination with acute myocardial infarction, particularly with shock, is associated with a much worse outcome compared to younger patients. In a German registry of patients undergoing primary percutaneous coronary intervention (PCI) in the setting of cardiogenic shock, the mortality of patients under the age of 55 years of age was 30% compared to 63% in those over the age of 75 years, with a gradation of mortality between these two extremes. Furthermore, in the large SHOCK trial conducting by Judith Hochman and colleagues, the importance of age was very apparent. In this trial patients were randomized to intensive medical therapy versus early revascularization but the benefit of revascularization was only evident in the patients younger than 75 years of age; very high mortality in the older patients was noted.

The other factor that appears to be associated with higher in-hospital mortality is the delay between

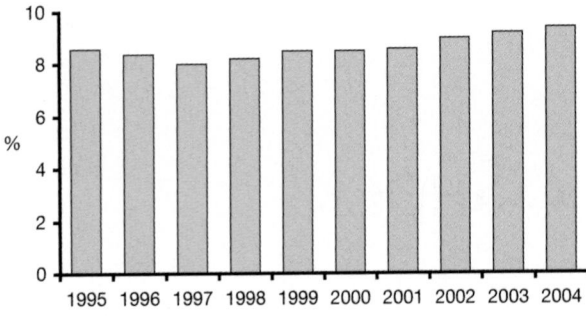

Fig. 1. Frequency of cardiogenic shock over a decade of observations from the National Registry of Myocardial Infarction.

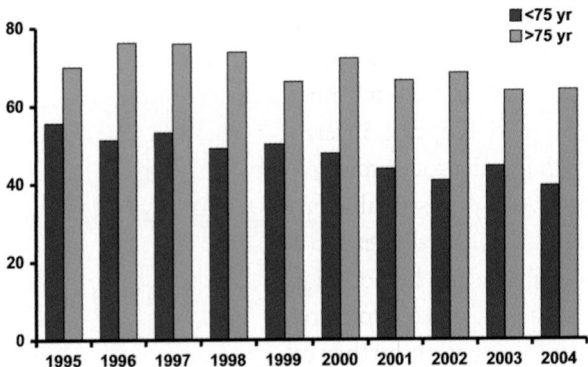

Fig. 2. Mortality from cardiogenic shock according to age (<75 years vs. >75 years).

symptom onset and hospital admission of the patient. It is uncommon for patients to have established cardiogenic shock at the time of presentation. With increasing delay between symptom onset and admission, the risk of development of cardiogenic shock increases, presumably because of progressive and ultimately unsalvageable left ventricular myocardial necrosis. Even when these patients undergo revascularization, as they did in the German PCI registry, patients presenting later than 6-12 hours after symptom onset had a 25% higher in-hospital mortality compared to patients who had presented within 6 hours of symptom onset.

DIAGNOSIS OF CARDIOGENIC SHOCK

It is helpful to define cardiogenic shock both by clinical and invasive hemodynamic criteria. Cardiogenic shock is defined clinically by the finding of a systolic blood pressure <90 mm Hg or a systolic blood pressure ≥90 mm Hg maintained only by pharmacological and/or mechanical support. Hypotension generally needs to be persistent for at least 30 minutes. In addition, these hemodynamic changes are accompanied by evidence of end-organ hypoperfusion, specifically cool extremities and decreased urine output to <30 mL/hour. Significant bradycardia or tachyarrhythmias may also result in serious hemodynamic changes and need to be ruled out and/or treated before a diagnosis of primary cardiogenic shock is made. It is generally accepted that a heart rate ≥60 beats per minute should be present when a diagnosis of shock is made.

The invasive hemodynamic criteria for cardiogenic shock include a cardiac index of <2.2 L/min/m^2 of body surface area and a pulmonary capillary wedge pressure of >15 mm Hg. However, it is important to recognize from a practical standpoint that the clinical criteria are sufficient to make an initial diagnosis of cardiogenic shock and to begin resuscitative measures. Oligemic shock due to hemorrhage or dehydration may simulate cardiogenic shock but will be associated with a low (<15 mm Hg) pulmonary capillary wedge pressure. Septic shock is associated with a low peripheral vascular resistance and a normal or high cardiac index.

Cardiogenic shock usually occurs in the setting of extensive left ventricular damage (Fig. 3) and ventricular dysfunction. It is important to immediately rule out surgically treatable causes of shock in patients following acute myocardial infarction. In particular, mechani-

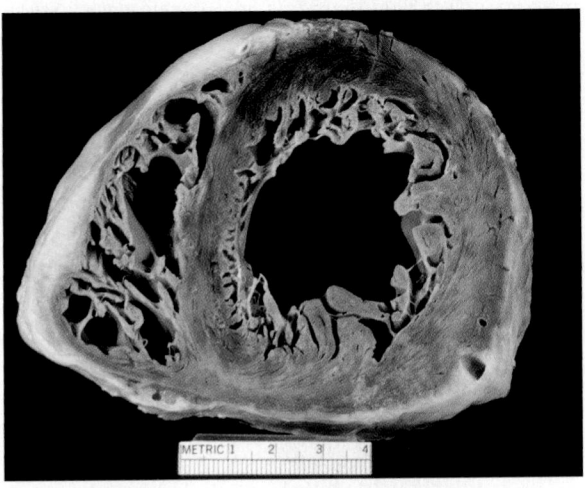

Fig. 3. Cardiogenic shock with large acute myocardial infarction.

cal rupture, such as free wall rupture, ventricular septal rupture (Fig. 4), and papillary muscle rupture (Fig. 5) need to be ruled out immediately with echocardiography and Doppler interrogation, and if necessary, angiography and cardiac catheterization. Aortic dissection can occasionally present as acute myocardial infarction and also lead to a shock-state, either because of rupture and hemorrhage or pericardial tamponade, and this also needs to be ruled out by clinical examination along with further cardiac and aortic imaging.

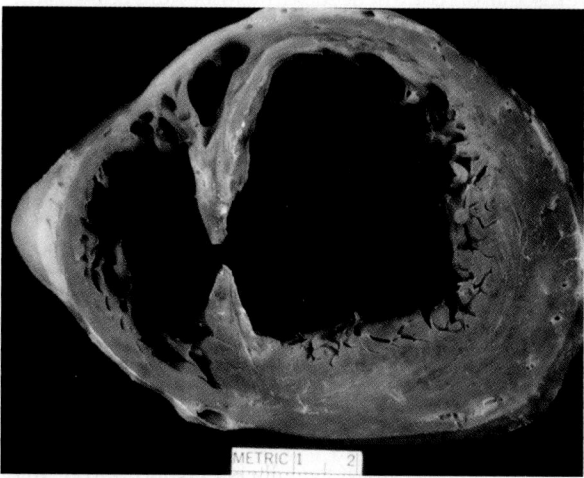

Fig. 4. Ventricular septal rupture after myocardial infarction.

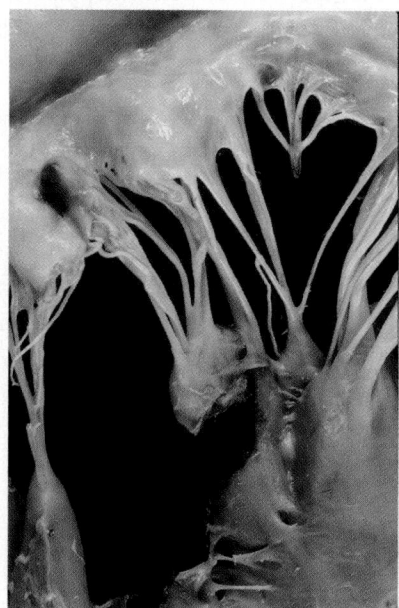

Fig. 5. Partial mitral valve papillary muscle rupture.

Finally, particularly as many of these patients will have received fibrinolytic therapy or undergone primary PCI, hemorrhagic shock needs to be considered and excluded. The differential diagnosis of cardiogenic shock is summarized in Table 1.

Cardiogenic shock can occur in the setting of inferior myocardial infarction complicated by significant right ventricular infarction (Fig. 6), and this needs to be considered when evaluating patients with cardiogenic shock. Right ventricular infarction serious enough to cause hypotension or cardiogenic shock requires a significantly different treatment approach compared to isolated left ventricular infarction. Right ventricular infarction occurs in almost only association with an inferior ST elevation myocardial infarction and can generally be recognized clinically by the triad of hypotension, elevated jugular venous pressure, and clear lung fields. Right-sided electrocardiographic leads, echocardiography, and invasive hemodynamic monitoring will usually establish this diagnosis.

When the physician is faced with a patient who has suffered an acute myocardial infarction and who now has signs of shock or hypoperfusion with or without congestive heart failure, urgent diagnosis and treatment of the underlying problem is required. If a significant bradycardic or tachycardic arrhythmia has been excluded or treated, the physician will be left with three important conditions to distinguish from each other:

- Acute pulmonary edema.
- Hypovolemia.
- Cardiogenic shock (low cardiac output).

Table 1.	Differential Diagnoses of Cardiogenic Shock Secondary to Myocardial Infarction Involving Predominantly the Left Ventricle

Shock secondary to right ventricular infarction (usually with inferior infarction)
Hypovolemia—dehydration, hemorrhagic shock
Myocardial rupture—free wall rupture, ventricular septal rupture, papillary muscle rupture
Acute aortic dissection (DeBakey Type A)
Pulmonary embolism

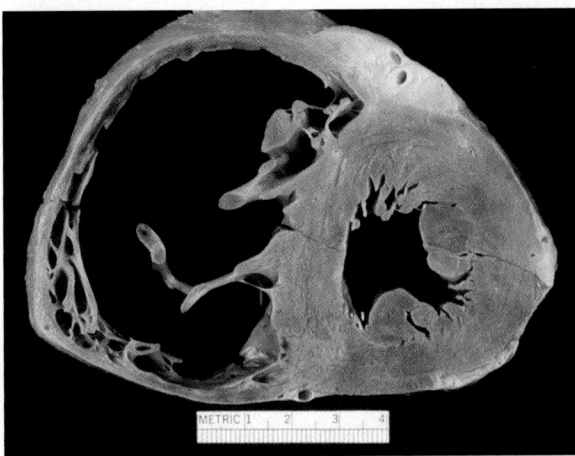

Fig. 6. Acute right ventricle myocardial infarction.

Acute Pulmonary Edema

This should be easily recognized by the clinical findings of rales on chest examination, elevated jugular venous pressure, and radiological evidence of pulmonary congestion. Immediate treatment includes intravenous furosemide, morphine, and oxygen therapy. Obvious respiratory failure will require intubation and ventilation. If the systolic blood pressure is adequate (>100 mm Hg), nitroglycerin, initially sublingual and then by intravenous infusion, should be administered. However, if the systolic blood pressure is <100 mm Hg, intravenous dopamine should be administered (vide infra).

Following these initial resuscitative measures, the systolic blood pressure should be rechecked and if adequate blood pressure is maintained, continued therapy of pulmonary edema, including the addition of an angiotensin-converting enzyme inhibitor is recommended.

Hypovolemia

In a patient who does not have any obvious pulmonary edema, intravenous fluid should be administered and causes for the hypovolemic state evaluated. The most important condition to rule out in these patients is hemorrhagic shock and replacement of blood volume and blood transfusions may be required. The specific cause of the hypovolemic state will necessitate urgent evaluation and treatment.

Cardiogenic Shock

In these patients, a blood pressure of less than 90 mm Hg needs to be confirmed with repeated measurements. Regardless of whether there are early signs of shock, dopamine (5-15 mcg/kg/min) by intravenous infusion should be commenced. If the systolic blood pressure is critically low (<70 mm Hg) with evidence of shock, norepinephrine at a dose of 8-12 mcg/min initially as an intravenous infusion should be immediately commenced and then titrated later to 2-4 mcg/min.

At this point, the patient's diagnosis of shock-state should have been established and immediate bedside resuscitation commenced with either fluid administration, correction of arrhythmias, and initiation of vasopressors. The above measures should be considered to be temporary in nature: the next steps involve immediate diagnosis or exclusion of cardiac rupture and arranging for the patient to undergo urgent coronary angiography with a view to restoring or optimizing coronary blood flow as soon as possible. Unless the patient's general medical condition (for example, terminal malignancy, severe dementia) would make it futile to intervene further or it is against the wishes of the patient, relying on vasopressor support alone is inadequate and is unlikely to impact the survival of the patient.

Clinical examination is always important but may be insufficient to completely diagnose or rule out conditions such as mechanical rupture. Careful examination of the jugular venous pressure, palpation of the peripheral pulses, auscultation of the lungs, and auscultation of the precordium to determine if a new murmur is present are all important. Immediate bedside echocardiography and Doppler examination is required primarily to rule out cardiac tamponade from free wall rupture, ventricular septal defect, and papillary muscle rupture with severe mitral regurgitation. Occasionally, transthoracic echocardiography and Doppler may miss acute severe mitral regurgitation, and further studies with pulmonary capillary wedge pressure measurement, transesophageal echocardiogram, and/or left ventriculography will be required.

ROLE OF INVASIVE MONITORING, INTRA-AORTIC BALLOON PUMPS AND ANGIOGRAPHY

Before discussing the role of invasive monitoring with intra-arterial pressure monitoring and pulmonary artery catheter monitoring (Swan-Ganz catheter) it is important to consider the reperfusion status of the patient. Patients who have already received reperfusion therapy that has been documented to be successful should be distinguished from patients in whom cardiogenic shock is present in the setting of acute myocardial infarction but who have yet to receive reperfusion therapy with either fibrinolysis or PCI. For the latter patients, immediate arrangements should be made for transfer to the cardiac catheterization laboratory for coronary angiography and possible PCI. In a hospital in which no cardiac catheterization or PCI facilities are available, arrangements need to be made for immediate and expeditious transfer of a patient to another suitable facility. If shock has developed in a patient who has recently received a fibrinolytic agent, arrangements should also be made for transfer to the cardiac catheterization laboratory so that patency of the culprit vessel can be assessed and rescue PCI performed if there has been failure of reperfusion. The overall role of early revascularization will be discussed in the next section.

A Swan-Ganz catheter should generally be used in all patients who have cardiogenic shock, particularly in those who have progressive hypotension that appears to be unresponsive to fluid administration or in those patients in whom fluid administration cannot be given, such as those with concomitant pulmonary edema. A Swan-Ganz catheter should certainly be placed if echocardiography is not available or has not been helpful in ruling out myocardial rupture. These are all considered to be class I indications as recommended by the ACC/AHA guideline committee and a Swan-Ganz catheter is considered to be a class IIA recommendation in all other patients who have cardiogenic shock or in any patient who continues to receive vasopressor agents.

Intra-arterial pressure monitoring (for example, radial artery line) should be used in all patients with cardiogenic shock and particularly those who have severe hypotension and/are continuing to receive vasopressor agents. This is currently considered to be a class I indication by the ACC/AHA. In patients who are about to undergo coronary angiography or have recently returned from the cardiac catheterization laboratory, pressure monitoring can be performed via the arterial sheath. Whether these two procedures are performed in the emergency department, the coronary care unit, or the cardiac catheterization laboratory depends entirely on the situation in which the patient is and the local logistics and physician expertise. However, it is critical that transfer to the cardiac catheterization laboratory is not delayed unduly while waiting for these procedures to be performed as they can generally be performed expeditiously at the same time as coronary angiography.

An intra-aortic balloon should be placed as soon as possible in conjunction with the above diagnostic and resuscitative procedures. Intra-aortic balloon counterpulsation has the effects of decreasing afterload, reducing cardiac work and increasing coronary perfusion. It is important to recognize that measured systolic pressure during normal functioning of an intra-aortic balloon counterpulsation is actually lower than when it is not in use. The benefit of intra-aortic balloon counterpulsation is largely due to its augmentation of diastolic blood pressure with a resultant overall increase in mean arterial pressure and coronary artery blood flow. Whether this is placed in the coronary care unit or in the cardiac catheterization laboratory will depend on local practice but again there should be little or no delay in arranging for immediate placement of an intra-aortic balloon. This has received a class I recommendation by the ACC/AHA for all patients being treated for cardiogenic shock.

An intra-aortic balloon pump is required for support of patients with cardiogenic shock with or without mechanical complications of myocardial rupture. In patients with myocardial rupture, it provides a critically important hemodynamic support while angiography is performed and prior to surgery. It is advisable to place the intra-aortic balloon pump prior to coronary angiography and this can be done in the cardiac catheterization laboratory. If coronary angiography and/or PCI are performed before placing an intra-aortic balloon pump in patients with severe hypotension, the patient's clinical condition could deteriorate even further to the point where they may not be able to be resuscitated. In our practice, an intra-aortic balloon pump is placed in the contralateral femoral artery to that used for coronary angiography, although placement of the intra-aortic balloon pump in either femoral artery followed by angiography and PCI via a brachial or radial approach is also acceptable.

A summary of the ACC/AHA recommendations regarding invasive interventions in patients with cardiogenic shock is shown in Table 2.

CORONARY ANGIOGRAPHY AND REVASCULARIZATION

As indicated earlier, patients who have not yet undergone coronary angiography for either primary PCI or to confirm patency of the culprit artery following fibrinolytic therapy, should be transferred for angiography and potential revascularization as soon as possible. Patients who have already undergone successful primary PCI who then later develop shock, should be returned to the cardiac catheterization laboratory without delay to reconfirm the patency, or otherwise, of the culprit vessel. Optimization of coronary blood flow should remain the number one priority in all patients in whom cardiogenic shock has developed. This is true for patients with left ventricular or right ventricular infarction.

Data from various PCI registries and randomized trials, including the SHOCK trial highlighted earlier, have shown that immediate or early revascularization is superior to medical treatment alone. The high mortality rates that continue to be documented for cardiogenic shock, however, include many patients who did undergo revascularization. The use of vasopressor agents and an intra-aortic balloon pump are temporary measures only. At this point, if cardiac catheterization facilities or PCI facilities are not available, the patient should be transferred immediately to an alternative suitable facility.

The importance of restoring normal coronary blood flow has been demonstrated in a registry of the nonrandomized SHOCK population as well as a large German registry. In these two registries, all patients who underwent PCI were evaluated. The success of PCI was a major determinant in in-hospital mortality. In those patients in whom Thrombolysis In Myocardial Infarction (TIMI) coronary blood flow was 0 or 1 at the conclusion of PCI, mortality was in excess of 80%. Among those patients who had residual TIMI-2 blood flow, mortality was approximately 50-60% and among those who had normal (TIMI-3) coronary blood flow, mortality was lowest, at approximately 35%. Thus, the ability to restore normal coronary blood flow had a major impact on patient survival.

Randomized clinical trials, particularly the SHOCK trial, have helped establish that early revascularization therapy is helpful in reducing mortality among patients with cardiogenic shock secondary to left ventricular failure (Fig. 7). These trials have helped shape the current guidelines with respect to the role of revascularization therapy. However, the benefits of revascularization compared to intensive medical therapy (which include the use of intra-aortic balloon pumps in the majority of patients) appear to be confined to younger patients.

Table 2. Summary of American College of Cardiology and American Heart Association Recommendations Regarding Invasive Monitoring and Mechanical Support for Cardiogenic Shock (2004)

Intervention	Recommendation class
Intra-arterial pressure monitoring	Class I
Pulmonary artery catheter monitoring	Class IIa (class I indications include progressive hypotension unresponsive to fluid loading or if myocardial rupture suspected and echocardiography unavailable)
Intra-aortic balloon pump placement	Class I

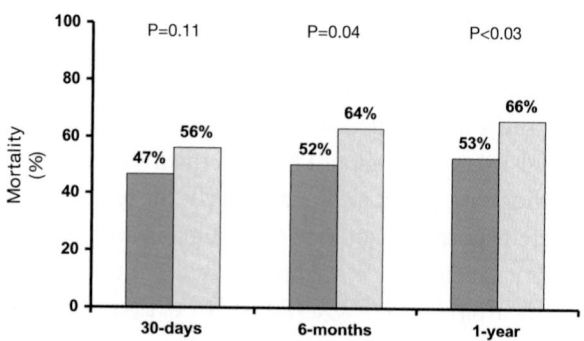

Fig. 7. Mortality at 30 days, 6 months, and 1 year in the SHOCK (Should We Emergently Revascularize Occluded Coronaries for Cardiogenic Shock?) trial, which compared early revascularization (green bars) with intensive medical therapy (yellow bars.)

The current guidelines (Table 3) recommend, as a class I indication, early revascularization with either PCI or coronary artery bypass surgery (CABG) for patients under the age of 75 years with ST elevation myocardial infarction (or left bundle branch block) who have developed shock within 36 hours of the onset of their myocardial infarction. Obviously, such patients need to be suitable for revascularization and the guidelines further recommend that intervention be performed within 18 hours of the development of shock.

With respect to patients over the age of 75 years, the guidelines have recommended early revascularization as a class IIA indication but only in selected patients, using the same time periods as above. Selecting such elderly patients for such therapy can often be a challenge and must be individualized based on the physician's clinical judgment of their overall condition, the patient's prior functional status, and their agreement to proceed with an invasive strategy. As a point of reference, it should be recalled that in the SHOCK trial, the 30-day mortality of patients over the age of 75 years of age was 75% among those who underwent revascularization compared to 53% of those who had been randomized to medical therapy.

In the majority of patients, PCI of the culprit vessel should be performed. Treatment of nonculprit critical coronary artery lesions in a patient with multivessel disease in the setting of cardiogenic shock is controversial. Outside the setting of cardiogenic shock, PCI of nonculprit vessels is strongly discouraged and is current-ly a class III indication according to the ACC/AHA guidelines. The guidelines do not currently state whether CABG is preferable to PCI in cases of shock and there certainly appears to be reluctance among many physicians and surgeons to refer such patients for early CABG. However, it should be noted that in the SHOCK trial, in which early revascularization was shown to be beneficial, more than one-third of patients had undergone coronary artery bypass surgery compared to slightly more than 50% who underwent PCI. In this same population, more than 85% had multivessel disease, including 23% who had left main coronary artery disease.

A recent report from the *National Registry of Myocardial Infarction* that studied practice patterns for patients who had cardiogenic shock showed that only about 3% of patients had undergone CABG while the majority of patients had undergone PCI, although this was only performed in just over 50% of patients. The striking findings from this survey indicated that mortality was significantly reduced in those patients who underwent PCI or CABG surgery. Further interpretation of this study clearly indicates that revascularization, although a class I recommendation, is significantly underutilized in patients with cardiogenic shock and that CABG surgery is very much underutilized. Furthermore, data up to the last few years indicate that less than half of the patients who have cardiogenic shock at hospitals without revascularization facilities are transferred to hospitals with such facilities. Therefore, at least in the United States, the use of

Table 3.   Summary of American College of Cardiology and American Heart Association Recommendations Regarding Early Revascularization (PCI or CABG) for Cardiogenic Shock (2004)

Recommendation	Clinical presentation
Class I	Recommended in patients <75 years with ST elevation or LBBB who present within 36 hours of onset of myocardial infarction and are suitable for revascularization and in whom it can be performed within 18 hours of onset of shock
Class IIa	Reasonable in patients >75 years with ST elevation or LBBB who present within 36 hours of onset of myocardial infarction and are suitable for revascularization and in whom it can be performed within 18 hours of onset of shock. Patients should be selected based on prior functional status and willingness to proceed with intervention

immediate or early revascularization, the only treatment that has ever been shown to decrease mortality from cardiogenic shock, continues to be significantly underutilized.

INOTROPIC AGENTS IN CARDIOGENIC SHOCK

It has previously been emphasized that inotropic or vasopressor agents are important in the initial management of a patient with recently diagnosed cardiogenic shock. They should be used for initial resuscitative purposes and to help maintain improvements in systolic blood pressure during the early hours or days of cardiogenic shock. However, the use of such agents should only be considered to be a temporary measure and they are not a substitute for aggressive invasive management including the use of an intra-aortic balloon pump, coronary angiography, and revascularization. With use of these agents, it is recommended to continuously monitor intra-aortic pressure.

In general, inotropic agents increase myocardial contractility, increase heart rate, and result in varying degrees of vasodilation or vasoconstriction. Intravenous dopamine is generally considered to be the first line agent for patients with hypotension, particularly if there is any evidence of shock. Dobutamine is also often used but should not be used when there are clinical signs of shock. Dobutamine is generally reserved until the systolic blood pressure remains above 90 mm Hg at which time it often provides good support in selected patients due to its additional vasodilator properties (providing afterload reduction). In patients in whom there is severe reduction in systolic blood pressure (generally 70 mm Hg or less) norepinephrine should be used. Other agents such as amrinone or milrinone are considered to be second tier agents and should only be considered if other agents are failing or if there are complications associated with other inotropic agents (for example, severe arrhythmias with dopamine). These second tier agents should be used with extreme caution in patients who have renal failure.

In general, inotropic agents should be used for as short a time as possible and their use is often limited by their toxicity, particularly arrhythmias. As previously emphasized, they should never be considered to be definitive therapeutic agents.

GENERAL MANAGEMENT ISSUES

In addition to revascularization and mechanical and pharmacological support of the patient's blood pressure, there are other general medical issues that will require attention in most patients.

It is important that the workload of the left ventricle is reduced and therefore patients should receive adequate analgesia and sedation to treat pain and any associated anxiety. Cautious and judicious use of morphine is generally excellent in this regard. Any severe anemia should be corrected with cautious red blood cell transfusion.

Oxygen status should be monitored continuously and supplemental oxygen provided; patients who have either demonstrated or incipient respiratory failure should be promptly intubated and ventilated. Pulmonary edema will require use of intravenous furosemide. The risk of sepsis should be minimized by meticulous attention to sterile technique during placement of arterial lines, pulmonary artery catheters, and intra-aortic balloon pumps. Appropriate precautions should also be taken for all patients who are ventilated to decrease the chance of ventilator-associated pneumonia which in itself carries a high mortality.

Early and aggressive treatment of arrhythmias is very important in patients who have cardiogenic shock, particularly with respect to treatment of ventricular tachycardia, atrial fibrillation, severe bradycardia or heart block, and maintaining atrioventricular synchrony.

FAILED TREATMENT

Because of the documented high mortality associated with cardiogenic shock, it will not be uncommon for patients to be unresponsive to aggressive intervention. The overall mortality rate currently is approximately 50%—somewhat lower in younger patients but higher in older patients. In selected younger patients, consideration of alternative therapies may be required or requested by family members. The only additional strategy to consider currently is orthotopic cardiac transplantation. Unfortunately, there is a paucity of suitable donors. However, in selected patients and after discussion with the cardiac transplantation team, patients unresponsive to the above measures might be considered eligible for cardiac transplantation. Placement of a left ventricular assist device will usually be required in such patients, although this should probably only be considered if the patient is free of any significant end-organ damage such as renal failure, liver failure, significant lung injury, or anoxic brain injury.

New Observations of Inflammatory State Accompanying Cardiogenic Shock

Our classic understanding of the pathophysiology of cardiogenic shock revolves around significant damage to the left ventricular myocardium with decreased myocardial contractility. This leads to reduced cardiac output and hypotension which result in further myocardial ischemia caused by decreased coronary blood flow. This additional myocardial ischemia inflicts further myocardial damage with worsening contractility along with further reduction in cardiac output. A vicious cycle ensues. This so-called "pump failure" is compensated, to some extent, by systemic vasoconstriction which can be demonstrated by measurement of high systemic vascular resistance. In patients who succumb to cardiogenic shock following acute myocardial infarction, autopsy studies show that generally at least 40% of the left ventricular myocardium has been infarcted, although this may represent a combination of new and old infarcts in some patients.

Recent observations have perhaps challenged this classical understanding of pathophysiology of cardiogenic shock. Among these observations has been the finding that systemic vascular resistance is not consistently elevated and indeed a wide range of measurements has been found. The left ventricular ejection fraction is generally about 30%, which is interesting when one considers that in daily clinical practice we come across patients with severe cardiomyopathy with ejection fractions as low as 10-20%, and yet these patients may have only minimal symptoms when well compensated and adequately treated. Indeed, the majority of survivors of cardiogenic shock have only class I heart failure or are asymptomatic. Finally, evidence of a systemic inflammatory response has been observed in many patients with cardiogenic shock. The systemic inflammatory response syndrome (SIRS) is a well-recognized state and is most often seen in medical intensive care and trauma units. It is most commonly associated with sepsis, trauma, burns, and pancreatitis.

It is characterized by abnormal temperature >38° centigrade or <36° centigrade, heart rates >90 beats per minute, respiratory rate >20/min, and an elevated white cell count >12,000 × 106/L or low white cell count <4,000 × 106/L. Such a state has been recently recognized and categorized in some patients with cardiogenic shock who also have no objective evidence of systemic vasoconstriction. Indeed, such patients have actually been shown to have low systemic vascular resistance.

The underlying mechanism is uncertain, but an overproduction of nitric oxide (NO), specifically the iNOS isoform, has been postulated. Excessive levels of iNOS have been shown to inhibit myocardial contractility, decrease mitochondrial respiration, be associated with reperfusion injury, have adverse effects on glucose metabolism, and be proinflammatory. Perhaps most relevant is that high levels of iNOS may lead to decreased responsiveness to catecholamines and induce systemic vasodilation. There are ongoing clinical studies, involving large numbers of patients, examining the role of NO synthase inhibitors in preventing excessive release of iNOS in cardiogenic shock patients and determining if there are significant clinical benefits from so doing.

Other markers of inflammation have also been demonstrated in patients who have cardiogenic shock. For example, the cytokine interleukin-6 is generally mildly elevated in patients who have large acute myocardial infarctions. However, in those who develop cardiogenic shock, interleukin-6 levels rise even higher. Furthermore, among patients with shock in whom multiorgan failure occurs, extremely high interleukin-6 levels have been measured and are similar in magnitude to those generally associated with septic shock. Septic shock, of course, is generally characterized by a profound vasodilatory state and thus this challenges our thinking of the underlying pathophysiology of cardiogenic shock.

Remaining questions to be answered include identification of the underlying pathophysiological trigger for the development of an inflammatory state, at what point in the illness the inflammatory state begins, and why this occurs in some patients and not in others. Furthermore, we need to determine whether the mortality is higher among patients who develop an inflammatory state and at what point could preventive interventions interrupt this vicious cycle.

SUMMARY AND CONCLUSIONS

Cardiogenic shock continues to occur with unchanged frequency as a complication of acute myocardial infarction. Although the mortality may recently have decreased slightly, it remains extremely high, particularly in older patients. Aggressive management should include intra-arterial pressure monitoring, Swan-Ganz catheter placement, placement of an intra-aortic balloon pump, and early revascularization with either PCI or CABG. Despite evidence that early revascularization is associated with improved survival, this strategy continues to be significantly underutilized.

Preparing for Cardiology Examinations

Joseph G. Murphy, MD

Margaret A. Lloyd, MD

Important Clinical Clues to the Electrocardiographic Tracing Diagnosis for Cardiology Examinations

Metabolic ECGs

- In the electrocardiographic (ECG) and imaging sections of cardiology examinations, pay special attention to the clinical descriptors that accompany the tracings and images. It is often here that the key to the correct diagnosis is found.
- A history of recent vomiting, pancreatitis, thyroid surgery, or multiple blood transfusions in a patient should suggest a diagnosis of hypocalcemia and prolongation of the QT interval.
- A clinical history of renal failure or dialysis should alert the candidate to the classic ECG findings of both hyperkalemia and hypocalcemia.
- Hyperkalemia—"patient with crush injury" or receiving dialysis.
- Hypokalemia—"patient with diarrhea" or receiving hypertension medications (diuretics).
- Hypercalcemia—"patient with renal cell carcinoma" or parathyroid disease; short QT.
- Hypocalcemia—"patient after blood transfusion" or after thyroidectomy; long QT (narrow T wave).

The Healthy Patient

- Frequently, the examination ECG is of a healthy person who has had an incidental ECG as a requirement for life insurance or employment. This question is geared to test the candidate's knowledge of ECG variants such as juvenile T waves and repolarization changes. The ECG may also show features that suggest previously undiagnosed cardiac disease such as hypertrophic cardiomyopathy, congenital heart disease, atrial septal defect, mitral valve disease, long QT syndrome, or Wolff-Parkinson-White syndrome. Be alert for whether the patient is asymptomatic with a normal cardiac examination or is asymptomatic with a systolic murmur.

The Postoperative Patient

- Immediately after heart surgery, look for hypothermia (Osborne wave), pericarditis (PR-segment depression and concave ST-segment elevation), pericardial effusion (low-voltage ECG), and pericardial tamponade (electrical alternans). If new Q waves are present after surgery, be extremely careful about diagnosing a perioperative myocardial infarction; cardiac manipulation at surgery may simulate infarction. In general, the diagnosis of myocardial infarction following cardiac surgery should not be made solely on the basis of an ECG tracing but should be supported by other clinical, enzyme, and echocardiographic evidence.

- In all postoperative patients who develop dyspnea or pleuritic chest pain or who are hemodynamically unstable, always consider pulmonary embolus ($S_1Q_3T_3$, right ventricular strain pattern, etc.).

Arrhythmias

- A history of aborted sudden death or recurrent syncope in a young patient or a strong family history of sudden death should suggest hypertrophic cardiomyopathy, long QT syndrome, or Brugada syndrome.
- Wide complex tachycardia in the setting of structural heart disease is ventricular tachycardia until proved otherwise.
- In patients with atrial fibrillation, look carefully at the ventricular response to determine whether it is regular—this may signify complete heart block, whereas an excessively fast ventricular response may suggest the possibility of Wolff-Parkinson-White syndrome.
- The presence of sinus bradycardia or the Wenckebach phenomenon may be a normal finding in an athletic patient but should be considered abnormal for examination purposes.
- Digoxin toxicity is an important clinical and ECG diagnosis; be aware of it. The diagnosis of digoxin toxicity appears in some form in most cardiology and internal medicine examinations. Paroxysmal atrial tachycardia with atrioventricular block and bidirectional ventricular tachycardia (originates from both ventricles) are the two cardiac rhythms that strongly suggest the diagnosis. Instead of specifically stating that the patient was taking digoxin, the clinical history may state that the patient was taking cardiac medications. Be alert for patients who develop hypokalemia while taking heart failure medications, because this can precipitate digoxin toxicity.
- Hypertrophic cardiomyopathy—massive left ventricular voltage with T-wave inversion in the anterior leads.
- Amyloid heart disease—low voltage ECG with left ventricular hypertrophy on echocardiography.

Chest Pain

- When coding myocardial infarctions, ST-segment elevation is acute myocardial injury and Q waves are infarction. Watch for posterior infarcts.

- Positional or pleuritic chest pain is pericarditis or pulmonary embolus until proved otherwise.
- The best examination strategy for the ECG section is a conservative approach, with careful coding of significant abnormalities, whereas debatable answers are best left uncoded. In patients with wide complex tachycardia, err on the side of coding ventricular tachycardia rather than supraventricular tachycardia with aberrant conduction, because coding of the latter may lead to inappropriate and dangerous clinical care. When in doubt, for the purposes of the examination, assume that the patient has the more dangerous condition. Look carefully for diagnostic clues that will clinch the diagnosis of ventricular tachycardia such as fusion beats and capture beats. It is quite unlikely that a cardiology examination will show a truly ambiguous ECG.
- The best way to prepare for the ECG section of the examination is to code a large number of patient ECGs using examination-type scoring criteria. The ECG criteria listed in the "Electrocardiographic Diagnoses" chapter in this book are similar to the criteria used on examinations, but minor changes are made from year to year in the examination scoring criteria. These changes are announced in the instructions to candidates several weeks before the examination and may not be completely reflected in the chapter in this book.

IMPORTANT CLINICAL CLUES ON AORTOGRAMS AND VENTRICULOGRAMS

- On the examination, aortograms typically show aortic incompetence, coarctation of the aorta, aortic dissection, patent ductus arteriosus, aberrant subclavian vessels, or an aortic root perivalvular abscess. Clinical clues to the above diagnoses are, respectively, diastolic murmur, differential hypertension between arms and legs, severe back pain, continuous murmur, difficulty swallowing, and recent infective endocarditis or septicemia.
- In left ventriculograms and coronary angiograms in young patients, look for coronary artery anomalies, patent ductus arteriosus, and intraventricular shunt.
- In a right ventricular angiogram, look for interventricular shunt (ventricular septal defect) and pulmonary stenosis.
- In a left ventricular angiogram of a patient with Down syndrome, look for ostium primum or endo-

cardial cushion defect (gooseneck abnormality of left ventricular outflow tract).

- For an unusual catheter path or position shown with an angiogram, look for persistent left superior vena cava, catheter crossing a patent foramen ovale, or patent ductus arteriosis.
- Be familiar with the appearance of mitral valve prolapse on a left ventriculogram.
- Always examine a left ventriculogram for the presence of mitral regurgitation on both right anterior oblique and left anterior oblique projections.
- Examine for a perivalvular leak in an aortic prosthetic valve on an aortogram. Note that a small amount of regurgitation through a prosthetic valve is normal; it "washes" the valve leaflet and inhibits thrombosis.
- Coding of regional wall abnormalities on static ventriculographic images is difficult and should be practiced before the examination.

IMPORTANT ANGIOGRAPHIC IMAGES

- Coronary anomalies, especially an anomalous right coronary artery originating from the left aortic cusp and an anomalous left circumflex coronary artery originating from the right aortic cusp.
- Patent ductus arteriosus.
- Intracoronary dissection after percutaneous transluminal coronary angioplasty (PTCA).
- Intracoronary thrombus.
- Coronary ectasia and aneurysmal disease.
- Specifically look at the left main coronary artery in all coronary angiograms.
- If two identical coronary angiographic projections are shown for comparison, look for coronary vasospasm (before and after nitroglylcerin infusion) or myocardial bridging (systolic vs. diastolic).
- On a coronary angiogram after coronary intervention, look for dissection or thrombus (or both).
- In an angiogram of a patient with acute myocardial infarction or unstable angina, look for intracoronary thrombus.

IMPORTANT ELECTROPHYSIOLOGIC AND PACEMAKER TRACINGS

- His bundle electrograms for *suprahisian* (atrioventricular nodal) and *infrahisian* block.

- His bundle electrograms in atrioventricular dissociation or complete atrioventricular block.
- Sudden AH prolongation before initiation of tachycardia is diagnostic of atrioventricular nodal reentrant tachycardia.
- If the His bundle deflection (H spike) cannot be recognized or the HV spike is negative, the diagnosis is ventricular tachycardia or preexcited tachycardia.
- Atrioventricular nodal blocking agents are *not necessarily contraindicated* for regular (atrioventricular reentrant) or rhythm (narrow or wide complex) tachycardia associated with an accessory bypass tract (Wolff-Parkinson-White syndrome). However, they are *strongly contraindicated* for atrial fibrillation (irregular rhythm) in such a patient.
- If a narrow complex tachycardia becomes a wide complex tachycardia and the cycle length increases (i.e., the rate slows) when the tachycardia becomes wide complex, the diagnosis is atrioventricular reentrant tachycardia via a bypass tract.
- In pacemaker rhythms, even when there is no atrial spike, the patient has a dual chamber pacemaker if the ventricular spike always follows the P wave at a fixed interval.
- Be familiar with pacemaker-mediated tachycardia, safety pacing, pacemaker syndrome, and upper rate limit pacemaker behavior (mode switching, etc.).

IMPORTANT ECHOCARDIOGRAPHIC IMAGES

- Infective endocarditis (vegetations, abscess, and leaflet perforation).
- Atrial thrombus or myxoma.
- Dilated cardiomyopathy.
- Hypertrophic cardiomyopathy with or without dynamic obstruction.
- Restrictive cardiomyopathy, including eosinophilia syndromes and obliterative cardiomyopathy.
- Amyloid heart disease (marked increase in left ventricular thickness with relatively low ECG voltages in contrast to left ventricular hypertrophy or hypertrophic cardiomyopathy (increase in left ventricular thickness with large ECG voltages).
- Tricuspid valve disease, including Ebstein anomaly (large right atrium and apical descent of tricuspid leaflets) and carcinoid syndrome.
- Mitral valve disease, including mitral valve prolapse

(must see prolapse in more than one plane), mitral stenosis, and mitral incompetence (know the basis for proximal isovelocity surface area [PISA] estimation of mitral regurgitation).

- Aortic valve disease, including aortic stenosis, bicuspid nonstenotic aortic valve, and aortic incompetence.
- Simple congenital heart defects, including atrial septal defect, ventricular defect, pulmonary stenosis, tetralogy of Fallot, patent ductus arteriosus, and coarctation of the aorta.
- Pericardial disease, including pericardial effusion and constrictive pericarditis.
- During evaluation of M-mode echocardiographic images, look specifically for mitral valve prolapse, fluttering of the anterior mitral leaflet associated with aortic regurgitation, and systolic anterior motion of the mitral leaflet in hypertrophic cardiomyopathy.

IMPORTANT PHYSICAL SIGNS IN CARDIOLOGY EXAMINATIONS

The following physical signs are particularly important:

1. Jugular venous pulsations
   - Large "V" wave—think of tricuspid regurgitation, especially if it is associated with a pulsating liver.
   - Rapid "Y" descent is usually associated with constrictive pericarditis.
   - Cannon "A" waves with tachycardia suggest ventricular tachycardia.
2. Arterial pulses
   - Bifid arterial pulse of aortic regurgitation and aortic stenosis combined, the characteristic pulse of hypertrophic cardiomyopathy (spike-and-dome pattern), or the dicrotic pulse of advanced heart failure.
   - Pulsus parvus et tardus for severe aortic stenosis.
   - Pulsus alternans for severe heart failure.
   - Pulsus paradoxus of cardiac tamponade or severe lung disease.
3. Apex beat palpation
   - Bifid or trifid apex beat impulse is usually associated with hypertrophic cardiomyopathy.
   - Palpable fourth heart sound (S_4) is frequently associated with left ventricular hypertrophy.

- Palpable third heart sound (S_3) is associated with heart failure and severe mitral regurgitation.
4. Auscultation
   - Loud first heart sound (S_1) of mitral stenosis; however, a soft S_1 does not exclude severe mitral stenosis and may reflect fixed, nonmobile calcified mitral valve leaflets (probably not a good candidate for mitral valve balloon valvuloplasty).
   - If a widely split S_1 occurs, consider Ebstein anomaly.
   - Wide, fixed splitting of the second heart sound (S_2) indicates atrial septal defect.
   - If paradoxical splitting of the S_2 occurs, consider paced rhythms in addition to severe aortic stenosis or left bundle branch block.
   - Absent aortic S_2 indicates severe aortic stenosis.
   - The only right-sided sound (murmur, click, or heart sound) that decreases with inspiration is the pulmonary ejection click.
   - If an opening snap (OS) is present, remember that left atrial pressure, and thus the severity of mitral stenosis, can be gauged by the interval between the S_2 and the OS (similarly for the opening sound associated with some mechanical prosthetic heart valves in the mitral position, e.g., Starr-Edwards valve). The shorter the S_2-OS timing, the higher the left atrial pressure.
   - An S_3 in the absence of overt heart failure may reflect severe mitral regurgitation even if the mitral murmur is soft or absent. A murmur is frequently absent in acute mitral regurgitation. Color Doppler studies may also rarely be negative in the presence of severe mitral regurgitation if no turbulence is present.
   - If on physical examination there are cannon "A" waves or variable splitting or intensity of the S_1 or S_2 in association with a regular wide complex tachycardia on the ECG, think of ventricular tachycardia. Look for flutter waves in the jugular venous waveform (JVP) in cases of suspected atrial flutter.

■ Examination candidates should be conversant with the effects of various maneuvers on heart murmurs: especially amyl nitrite, the Valsalva maneuver, squatting and sudden standing, and the effect following an extrasystolic beat (premature ventricular contraction) (Tables 1 and 2).

SUMMARY OF PHYSICAL SIGNS IN CARDIOVASCULAR DISEASE

Left Ventricular Failure
1. Breathing
   ■ Tachypnea (due to hypoxia and increased intrapulmonary pressures).

Table 1. Interventions Used to Alter the Intensity of Cardiac Murmurs

Respiration
  Right-sided murmurs generally increase with inspiration
  Left-sided murmurs usually are louder during expiration
Valsalva maneuver
  Most murmurs decrease in length and intensity; 2 exceptions are the systolic murmur of HCM, which usually becomes much louder, and that of MVP, which becomes longer and often louder
  Following release of the Valsalva maneuver, right-sided murmurs tend to return to baseline intensity earlier than left-sided murmurs
Exercise
  Murmurs caused by blood flow across normal or obstructed valves (e.g., PS, MS) become louder with both isotonic and submaximal isometric (handgrip) exercise
  Murmurs of MR, VSD, and AR also increase with handgrip exercise; however, the murmur of HCM often decreases with near-maximum handgrip exercise
Positional changes
  With standing, most murmurs diminish; 2 exceptions are the murmur of HCM, which becomes louder, and that of MVP, which lengthens and often is intensified
  With prompt squatting, most murmurs become louder, but those of HCM and MVP usually soften and may disappear; passive leg raising usually produces the same results as prompt squatting
Postventricular premature beat or atrial fibrillation
  Murmurs originating at normal or stenotic semilunar valves increase in intensity during the cardiac cycle following a VPB or in the beat after a long cycle length in AF
  By contrast, systolic murmurs due to atrioventricular valve regurgitation do not change, diminish (papillary muscle dysfunction), or become shorter (MVP)
Pharmacologic interventions
  During the initial relative hypotension following amyl nitrite inhalation, murmurs of MR, VSD, and AR decrease, whereas those of AS increase because of increased stroke volume
  During the later tachycardia phase, murmurs of MS and right-sided lesions also increase
  This intervention may thus distinguish the murmur of the Austin Flint phenomenon from that of MS
  The response in MVP often is biphasic (softer, then louder than control)
Transient arterial occlusion
  Transient external compression of both arms by bilateral cuff inflation to 20 mm Hg greater than peak systolic pressure augments the murmurs of MR, VSD, and AR but not murmurs due to other causes

---

AF, atrial fibrillation; AR, aortic regurgitation; AS, aortic stenosis; HCM, hypertrophic cardiomyopathy; MR, mitral regurgitation; MS, mitral stenosis; MVP, mitral valve prolapse; PS, pulmonic stenosis; VPB, ventricular premature beat; VSD, ventricular septal defect.

Table 2.   Factors That Differentiate the Various Causes of Left Ventricular Outflow Tract Obstruction

Feature	Valvular	Supravalvular	Discrete subvalvular	HOCM
Valve calcification	Common after age 40 y	No	No	No
Dilated ascending aorta	Common	Rare	Rare	Rare
PP after VPB	Increased	Increased	Increased	Decreased
Valsalva effect on SM	Decreased	Decreased	Decreased	Increased
Murmur of AR	Common	Rare	Sometimes	No
Fourth heart sound	If severe	Uncommon	Uncommon	Common
Paradoxic splitting	Sometimes*	No	No	Rather common*
Ejection click	Most (unless valve calcified)	No	No	Uncommon or none
Maximal thrill and murmur	2nd RIS	1st RIS	2nd RIS	4th LIS
Carotid pulse	Normal to anacrotic* (parvus et tardus)	Unequal	Normal to anacrotic	Brisk, jerky, systolic rebound

AR, aortic regurgitation; HOCM, hypertrophic obstructive cardiomyopathy; LIS, left intercostal space; PP, pulse pressure; RIS, right intercostal space; SM, systolic murmur; VPB, ventricular premature beat.
*Depends on severity.

- Cheyne-Stokes breathing, in severe heart failure.
- Central cyanosis due to hypoxia in pulmonary edema.
- Peripheral cyanosis with low cardiac output.
2. Arterial pulse
   - Hypotension in cardiogenic shock and end-stage heart failure.
   - Sinus tachycardia due to increased sympathetic tone.
   - Pulsus alternans (alternate strong and weak beats in end-stage heart failure with regular heart rhythm) differentiated from bigeminal rhythm (alternating regular and ectopic beats that are atrial, junctional, or ventricular).
3. JVP
   - Normal in pure left heart failure, but may be increased in right heart failure due to left heart failure.
4. Apex beat
   - Displaced to the left and inferiorly with left ventricular dilatation from any cause.
   - Dyskinesia of the anterior wall after a large anterior wall myocardial infarction.
   - Palpable S_3 or S_4.

5. Auscultation
   - Left ventricular S_3 or S_4 (or both).
   - Functional mitral incompetence murmur (due to valve ring dilatation and central mitral regurgitation).
6. Lung fields
   - Coarse rales of pulmonary edema (due to pulmonary venous hypertension).

Right Ventricular Failure
1. Breathing
   - Peripheral cyanosis due to low cardiac output.
2. Arterial pulse
   - Low volume due to low cardiac output.
3. JVP
   - Elevated because of increased systemic venous pressure (right heart preload).
   - Positive hepatojugular reflex (increase in JVP with hepatic or abdominal compression).
   - Kussmaul sign (a paradoxical increase in the height of the JVP due to the inability of the dilated right ventricle to stretch farther to accommodate the increased venous return to the right heart during inspiration). This decreased right ventricular compliance typi-

cally occurs with right ventricular myocardial infarction but is also characteristic of tricuspid stenosis and constrictive pericarditis.

- Large "V" waves (functional tricuspid regurgitation due to valve ring dilatation) and central mitral regurgitation.

4. Precordium
   - Right ventricular lift (heave) at the left sternal border.

5. Auscultation
   - Right ventricular S_3 or S_4 (or both), pansystolic murmur of functional tricuspid regurgitation (absence of a murmur does not exclude tricuspid regurgitation).

6. Lung field
   - Pleural effusions (right > left).

7. Abdomen
   - Tender hepatomegaly due to increased venous back pressure transmitted via the hepatic veins; pulsatile liver, if tricuspid regurgitation is present.

8. Peripheral edema
   - Due to a combination of fluid retention and increased venous pressure.
   - Ankle and sacral edema, ascites, or pleural effusions.

Acute Pericarditis

Signs
   - Fever.
   - Three-component pericardial friction rub that may disappear when pericardial fluid accumulates.

Chronic Constrictive Pericarditis

1. General signs
   - Cachexia, jaundice if there is significant liver dysfunction.

2. Pulse and blood pressure
   - Pulsus paradoxus (more than the normal 10–mm Hg decrease in arterial pulse pressure on inspiration, because increased right ventricular filling decreases left ventricle filling and cardiac output).
   - Chronic hypotension.

3. JVP
   - Increased JVP.

- Kussmaul sign (rare).
- Prominent "X" and "Y" descents.

4. Apex beat
   - Frequently impalpable because of thickened pericardium.

5. Auscultation
   - Distant heart sounds
   - Diastolic pericardial knock (rapid ventricular filling abruptly halted by constricted pericardium) occurs later than the S_3.

6. Abdomen
   - Hepatomegaly due to increased venous pressure.
   - Splenomegaly due to increased venous pressure.
   - Ascites.

7. Periphery
   - Peripheral edema.

Cardiac Tamponade

1. General signs
   - Tachypnea.
   - Severe anxiety.
   - Pallor.
   - Syncope or near syncope.

2. Pulse and blood pressure
   - Tachycardia.
   - Pulsus paradoxus.
   - Hypotension.

3. JVP
   - Markedly increased JVP.
   - Kussmaul sign (common).
   - Prominent "X" but absent "Y" descent.

4. Apex beat
   - Usually impalpable because of fluid in pericardial space.

5. Auscultation
   - Soft heart sounds.

6. Lung fields
   - Dullness and bronchial breathing at left base because of compression of the lingula of the lung by the distended pericardial sac (Ewart sign).

Infective Endocarditis

1. General signs
   - Fever.

- Arthropathy (especially metacarpophalangeal joints, wrists, elbows, knees, and ankles).
2. Hands
   - Splinter hemorrhages.
   - Finger clubbing (late sign).
   - Osler nodes (rare), painful skin lesions.
   - Janeway lesions (very rare), painless skin lesions.
3. Arms
   - Evidence of intravenous drug use, especially in right heart endocarditis.
4. Eyes
   - Pale conjunctiva (anemia); retinal or conjunctival hemorrhages.
   - Roth spots (fundal vasculitic lesions with a yellow center surrounded by a red ring).
5. Heart
   - Signs of underlying valvular or congenital heart disease.
6. Abdomen
   - Hepatomegaly.
   - Splenomegaly.
   - Hematuria.
7. Periphery
   - Evidence of embolization to abdominal viscera, limbs, or central nervous system.

Acute Pulmonary Hypertension
- The right ventricle has a limited ability to increase pulmonary artery pressure acutely.
- Acute pulmonary hypertension usually occurs in the setting of an acute pulmonary embolus and is manifested by acute right ventricular failure.
- Acute systemic hypotension, hypoxia, and shock may dominate the clinical picture.

Chronic Pulmonary Hypertension
1. General signs
   - Dyspnea.
   - Tachypnea.
   - Central cyanosis due to arterial desaturation.
   - Peripheral cyanosis and cold extremities due to low cardiac output at end-stage disease.
   - Hoarseness (rare) due to compression of the left recurrent laryngeal nerve by the pulmonary artery.
2. Arterial pulse
   - May be low volume because of the low cardiac output at end-stage disease.
3. JVP
   - Prominent "A" wave as long as sinus rhythm is maintained because of forceful right atrial contraction required to fill hypertrophied right ventricle.
4. Precordium
   - Right ventricular heave.
   - Palpable second pulmonic sound.
   - Palpable dilated pulmonary artery.
5. Auscultation
   - Systolic ejection click due to dilatation of the pulmonary artery.
   - Loud second pulmonic sound because of forceful pulmonary valve closure due to high pulmonary artery pressure.
   - Right ventricular S_3 or S_4 (or both) if right ventricular failure is present.
   - Pulmonary ejection systolic murmur due to turbulent blood flow in dilated pulmonary artery.
   - Diastolic pulmonary incompetence murmur if the pulmonary valve ring is significantly dilated and functional pulmonary valve regurgitation occurs.
6. Other signs
   - Additional signs of right ventricular failure will occur in end-stage pulmonary hypertension (cor pulmonale).

Mitral Stenosis
1. General signs
   - Tachypnea.
   - Mitral facies (combination of vasodilatation and peripheral cyanosis in severe end-stage mitral stenosis).
2. Arterial pulse and blood pressure
   - Normal or decreased pulse volume due to decreased cardiac output at late stages.
   - Atrial fibrillation may be present because of left atrial enlargement.
   - Low blood pressure at late stages of disease.
3. JVP
   - Usually normal.
   - Prominent "A" wave if pulmonary hyperten-

sion is present.

- Loss of the "A" wave if atrial fibrillation supervenes.

4. Precordium
  - Tapping apex beat (due to palpable first heart sound).
  - Right ventricular heave.
  - Palpable second pulmonic sound if pulmonary hypertension is present.
  - Diastolic thrill (rarely present).

5. Auscultation
  - Loud S_1 (indicates that the mitral valve leaflets are widely separated yet mobile at the onset of systole).
  - Loud second pulmonic sound if pulmonary hypertension is present.
  - Opening snap (high left atrial pressure forcefully opens the valve leaflets).
  - Low-pitched, rumbling diastolic murmur.
  - Late diastolic accentuation of the diastolic murmur may occur with atrial contraction if the patient is in sinus rhythm; it is usually absent in atrial fibrillation.

Mitral Regurgitation (Chronic)

1. General signs
  - Tachypnea.

2. Arterial pulse
  - Usually normal.
  - Atrial fibrillation is common.

3. JVP
  - Normal unless right ventricular failure has occurred.
  - Loss of "A" wave in atrial fibrillation.

4. Palpation
  - Apex beat may be displaced laterally, diffuse, greater than 3 cm in diameter, or hyperdynamic, depending on the extent of ventricular dilatation.
  - Pansystolic apical thrill.
  - Parasternal impulse (due to left atrial enlargement behind the right ventricle).

5. Auscultation
  - Soft or absent S_1 (by the end of diastole, atrial and ventricular pressures have equalized and the valve leaflets have drifted back together).

- Left ventricular S_3 even in the absence of heart failure, due to rapid left ventricular filling in early diastole.
- Pansystolic murmur maximal at the apex (usually radiating toward the axilla).

Acute Mitral Regurgitation

- Patients can present with pulmonary edema and cardiovascular collapse.
- A loud apical ejection murmur is usually present (its duration is frequently short because atrial pressure is markedly increased).
- With rupture of the anterior leaflet chordae, the murmur radiates to the axilla and back; with rupture of the posterior leaflet, the murmur radiates to the anterior chest wall.

Mitral Valve Prolapse

1. Auscultation
  - Systolic click (usually mid-systolic) may be the only audible abnormality; note that the click is not always audible in patients with documented mitral valve prolapse.
  - Systolic murmur—high-pitched, late peaking systolic murmur commencing with the click and extending throughout the rest of systole.

2. Dynamic auscultation
  - Murmur and click occur earlier and may be louder with the Valsalva maneuver and with standing, but both occur later and may be softer with squatting and isometric exercise.

Aortic Stenosis

1. General signs
  - Usually no specific signs.

2. Pulse
  - There may be a plateau pulse, or the pulse may be late peaking (tardus).
  - The pulse is frequently of small volume (parvus) and the pulse pressure is decreased.

3. Palpation
  - The apex beat is hyperdynamic (pressure overload) and may be slightly displaced laterally.
  - Systolic thrill at the base of the heart (aortic area).

- Carotid shudder.
4. Auscultation
    - Narrowly split or reversed split S_2 because of prolonged left ventricular ejection.
    - Soft or absent S_2.
    - Rough mid-systolic ejection murmur, maximal over the aortic area and extending into the carotid arteries, is characteristic but may also be heard well at the apex (the murmur is loudest with the patient sitting up and in full expiration).
    - Associated aortic regurgitation is common.
    - In congenital aortic stenosis in which the valve cusps remain mobile and the dome of the valve comes to a sudden halt, an ejection click may precede the murmur (the ejection click is absent if the valve is calcified or if the stenosis is not at the valve level).

Aortic Regurgitation

Named Signs of Aortic Regurgitation
These signs are present only in severe chronic aortic incompetence and are usually not clinically helpful.
1. Quincke sign—marked capillary pulsation in the nailbeds, with blanching during diastole with mild nail pressure
2. Corrigan sign—forceful carotid upstroke with rapid decline
3. De Musset sign—head nodding in time with the heartbeat
4. Hill sign—increased blood pressure in the legs compared with the arms (≥30–mm Hg discrepancy)
5. Müller sign—pulsation of the uvula in time with the heartbeat
6. Duroziez sign—systolic and diastolic bruit over the femoral artery on gradual compression of the vessel by the stethoscope bell
7. Traube sign—a double sound heard over the femoral artery on compressing the vessel distally; this is the "pistol-shot" sound that may be heard with very severe aortic regurgitation

Signs in Aortic Regurgitation
1. General signs
    - Marfan syndrome in a small number of patients.

- Ankylosing spondylitis or other seronegative arthropathy.
2. Pulse and blood pressure
    - The pulse is characteristically collapsing, with a rapid upstroke followed by a rapid decline.
    - Wide pulse pressure.
3. Neck
    - Prominent carotid pulsations (Corrigan sign).
4. Palpation
    - Apex beat is characteristically displaced laterally and hyperkinetic.
    - A diastolic thrill may be felt at the left sternal edge when the patient sits forward in expiration.
5. Auscultation
    - Aortic second sound may be soft.
    - A decrescendo, high-pitched diastolic murmur beginning immediately after the S_2 and extending into diastole (it is loudest at the third and fourth left intercostal spaces).
    - A systolic ejection murmur is usually present (due to associated aortic stenosis or to torrential flow across a nonstenotic aortic valve).
    - Aortic stenosis is distinguished from an aortic flow murmur by the presence of the peripheral signs of significant aortic stenosis, such as a plateau pulse.
    - Listen for an Austin Flint murmur (a low-pitched, rumbling, mid-diastolic murmur audible at the apex—the regurgitant jet from the aortic valve causes the anterior mitral valve leaflet to shudder); the murmur is similar to that of mitral stenosis but can be distinguished from mitral stenosis because the S_1 is not loud and there is no opening snap.

Tricuspid Stenosis
1. JVP
    - Increased giant "A" waves with a slow "Y" descent may be seen.
2. Auscultation
    - Diastolic murmur audible at the left sternal edge and accentuated in inspiration; it is very similar to the murmur of mitral stenosis except for the site of maximal intensity.

- Tricuspid stenosis is rare, usually rheumatic, and frequently accompanied by mitral stenosis.
- There are no signs of pulmonary hypertension.

3. Abdomen
   - Presystolic pulsation of the liver is caused by forceful atrial systole.

Tricuspid Regurgitation

1. JVP
   - Large "V" waves.
   - JVP is increased if right ventricular failure has occurred.
2. Palpation
   - Right ventricular heave.
3. Auscultation
   - A pansystolic murmur that is maximal at the lower end of the sternum and that increases on inspiration is classic, but in its absence, the diagnosis must be made on the basis of peripheral signs alone.
4. Abdomen
   - A pulsatile, large, tender liver is usually present.
   - Ascites, peripheral edema, and pleural effusions may occur.
5. Legs
   - Dilated pulsatile veins.

Pulmonary Stenosis

1. General signs
   - Peripheral cyanosis (due to low cardiac output).
2. Pulse
   - Normal or reduced (because of a low cardiac output).
3. JVP
   - Giant "A" waves because of right atrial hypertrophy; JVP may be increased because of right heart failure.
4. Palpation
   - Right ventricular heave.
   - Thrill over the pulmonary area.
5. Auscultation
   - Murmur may be preceded by an ejection click.
   - Harsh ejection systolic murmur that is heard

best in the pulmonary area and is typically present with inspiration.
   - Right ventricular S_4 may be present (because of right atrial hypertrophy)—augments with inspiration.

6. Abdomen
   - Presystolic pulsation of the liver may be present.

Pulmonary Regurgitation

1. Auscultation
   - A decrescendo diastolic murmur that is high-pitched and audible at the left sternal edge is characteristic; the murmur increases on inspiration.
   - The Graham Steell murmur indicates functional pulmonary incompetence due to severe mitral stenosis.
   - Signs of pulmonary hypertension may also be present.
2. If there is no sign of pulmonary hypertension, a decrescendo diastolic murmur at the left sternal edge is more likely to be due to aortic regurgitation than to pulmonary regurgitation.

Hypertrophic Cardiomyopathy

1. Pulse
   - Sharp-rising and jerky.
   - Rapid ejection by the hypertrophied ventricle early in systole is followed by obstruction caused by the displacement of the mitral valve into the outflow tract. This is very different from the pulse of aortic stenosis.
2. JVP
   - A prominent "A" wave is usually present because of forceful atrial contraction against a noncompliant right ventricle.
3. Palpation
   - Double or triple apical impulse due to presystolic expansion of the ventricle caused by atrial contraction.
4. Auscultation
   - Late systolic murmur at the lower left sternal edge and apex (due to ventricular obstruction) in late systole.
   - Pansystolic murmur at the apex (due to mitral regurgitation).
   - S_4.

5. Dynamic maneuver
  - The outflow murmur is increased by the Valsalva maneuver, by standing, and by isotonic exercise; it is decreased by squatting and isometric exercise.

Ventricular Septal Defect
1. Palpation
   - Hyperkinetic, laterally displaced apex if the defect is large.
   - Thrill at the sternal edge.
2. Auscultation
   - Harsh pansystolic murmur maximal at the lower left sternal edge, with an S_3 or S_4 (the murmur is louder on expiration; sometimes a mitral regurgitation murmur is associated); the murmur is often louder and more harsh when the defect is small.

Atrial Septal Defect
1. Precordium
   - Normal or right ventricular lift.
2. Auscultation
   - Fixed splitting of the S_2.
   - The defect produces no murmur directly, but increased flow through the right side of the heart can produce a low-pitched diastolic flow murmur across the tricuspid valve and a pulmonary systolic ejection murmur (both are louder on inspiration).
   - The signs of an ostium primum defect are the same as for an ostium secundum defect, but associated mitral or tricuspid regurgitation or a ventricular septal defect may be present.
   - The physical signs of a sinus venosus atrial septal defect are the same as those of a secundum atrial septal defect.

Patent Ductus Arteriosus
1. Pulse and blood pressure
   - A collapsing pulse with a sharp upstroke (due to ejection of a large volume of blood into the aorta during systole); there is rapid runoff of blood from the aorta into the pulmonary artery.
   - Low diastolic blood pressure (due to rapid runoff from the aorta).

2. Precordium
   - Hyperkinetic apex beat.
3. Auscultation
   - If the shunt is of moderate size, a single S_2 is heard, but if the shunt is of large size, reversed splitting of the S_2 occurs (a delayed aortic second sound occurs because of the increased left ventricular stroke volume).
   - A continuous, loud machinery murmur that is maximal at the first left intercostal space is usually present.

Eisenmenger Syndrome (Right-to-Left Shunt)
1. Clinical signs
   - Central cyanosis due to the right-to-left shunting.
   - Finger and toe clubbing.
   - Polycythemia.
   - Signs of pulmonary hypertension.
2. It may be possible to decide at what level the right-to-left shunt occurs by listening to the S_2.
   - A wide, fixed splitting of the S_2 suggests an atrial septal defect.
   - The presence of a single S_2 suggests truncus arteriosus or a ventricular septal defect.
   - A normal or reversed S_2 suggests patent ductus arteriosus.

Tetralogy of Fallot
Clinical signs
   - Central cyanosis is common and occurs because of a large right-to-left shunt at the ventricular level, where right and left ventricular pressures are equalized. In addition, the aorta overrides both ventricular outflow tracts and receives a combination of saturated and desaturated blood.
   - Finger and toe clubbing and polycythemia.
   - Signs of right ventricular enlargement, including a parasternal right ventricular lift and a thrill at the left sternal edge.
   - Normal left ventricular impulse.
   - Aortic click.
   - S_2 is single (absent second pulmonic sound).
   - Pulmonary systolic ejection murmur—the louder and longer the pulmonary murmur the better, because this indicates better blood

flow through the pulmonary circulation.

- No significant murmur across the ventricular septal defect (no gradient).
- Continuous murmur from bronchial collaterals or associated patent ductus arteriosus.
- The lungs are protected from pulmonary hypertension by the pulmonary stenosis (valvular and infundibular).

Named Murmurs in Cardiology

- Graham Steell murmur—functional pulmonary regurgitation murmur due to severe pulmonary hypertension usually associated with severe mitral stenosis.
- Austin Flint murmur—functional mitral stenosis murmur due to incomplete mitral valve opening because of severe aortic incompetence.
- Rytand murmur—mid-diastolic mitral flow murmur that occurs in patients with complete heart block.
- Carey Coombs murmur—acute mitral valvulitis due to acute rheumatic fever that causes a short diastolic rumbling-type murmur.
- Dock murmur—very localized, high-pitched diastolic murmur heard in the second and third left intercostal interspaces; it is due to high-grade stenosis of the left anterior descending coronary artery.

TYPICAL CARDIOLOGY EXAMINATION TOPICS

- More than 90% of a cardiology examination is based on clinical cardiology and less than 10% on underlying physiology and biochemistry.
- Most clinical cardiology questions relate to ischemic heart disease, valvular heart disease, or heart failure; approximately 20% of the questions involve related areas of cardiology that are less emphasized, including congenital heart disease, vascular disease, and hypertension.

Arteritis

- Although arteritis is relatively uncommon in clinical cardiology practice, questions about it are commonly asked in cardiology examinations.

- Expect questions on polyarteritis nodosa, Takayasu arteritis, giant cell arteritis, scleroderma, systemic lupus erythematosus, and the phospholipid syndromes.

- Abdominal pain and change in bowel habit in patients with arteritis suggests gut ischemia.
- The question may be asked indirectly by linking abdominal symptoms with photographs of hands (scleroderma) or face (systemic lupus erythematosus) or nails (dermatomyositis).

Coronary Artery Disease

- The topic of coronary artery disease accounts for a large section of cardiology examinations; it is comprehensively covered in multiple areas, including pharmacology of cardiac drugs and imaging studies.
- Several angiograms in the motion studies section may show coronary artery disease.
- In addition to being able to identify the basic coronary anatomy, be able to accurately identify grafts and grafted vessels, including gastroepiploic grafts and free radial artery grafts.
- The left internal mammary artery grafts may be shown from the arm approach.
- Look specifically for ulcerated plaques, spontaneous coronary artery dissections (typically seen in young women without risk factors for atheromatous disease), and intraluminal thrombi.
- Identification (and the mechanism of identification) of the culprit coronary lesion for percutaneous intervention is important:
  1. ST-segment elevation on ECG localizes ischemia; ST-segment depression does not.
  2. Know how to correlate coronary anatomy with ischemia on imaging studies.
  3. An ulcerated plaque or an intraluminal thrombus in association with an unstable coronary syndrome suggests a culprit vessel.
  4. Identification of a culprit vessel in the presence of well-developed collateral circulations or grafts can be extremely difficult.

Mechanical Complications of Myocardial Infarction

- Questions related to the mechanical complications of myocardial infarction (septal rupture, free wall rupture, mitral regurgitation, aneurysm formation, and obstructive cardiomyopathy secondary to myocardial infarction) are asked in some form on all cardiology examinations.

■ Be aware of the timing of complications in relation to infarction and thrombolysis and of the corresponding diagnostic images on both echocardiography and angiography.

Coronary Artery Anomalies

■ Questions about coronary artery anomalies are frequently asked.

■ Be able to distinguish benign abnormalities (separate ostia of the left anterior descending and circumflex coronary arteries) from malignant anomalies (circumflex or left main coronary artery that travels between the aorta and the pulmonary artery). In general, the patient will be asymptomatic and have a normal stress test.

■ Know when a coronary artery bypass graft is indicated from an anatomical abnormality alone.

Magnetic Resonance and Computed Tomographic Imaging

■ Magnetic resonance (MR) and computed tomographic (CT) images are frequently shown in cardiology examinations.

■ Look carefully for apical and right ventricular wall thinning in association with arrhythmias and right ventricular dysplasia.

■ Be aware of the anatomical presentations of CT and MR images.

Stress Testing

■ The topic of stress testing, with or without imaging studies, frequently appears in questions. Be able to distinguish between fixed and stress-induced perfusion defects.

■ Know the optimal imaging study for specific patient situations (e.g., pharmacologic stress testing for patients with left bundle branch block).

■ Know the significance of hypotension, ST elevation, and lung uptake of thallium on stress testing.

Valvular Heart Disease

■ Know the American College of Cardiology/American Heart Association guidelines for management of valvular heart disease. Specifically, know when valve surgery is indicated. Left ventricular dimensions are very important.

■ Be able to diagnose mechanical valve malfunctioning from still-frame echocardiographic images:

1. Mechanical mitral valve Doppler: increased velocity or mean gradient with short deceleration time/pressure half time (DT/PHT) (compatible with significant mitral regurgitation).

2. Mechanical pulmonary valve Doppler with color flow Doppler of pulmonary regurgitation (severe pulmonary regurgitation).

3. Decide whether to replace the valve, increase anticoagulation, or give thrombolytics.

■ Questions about the physical examination findings of mitral valve prolapse are frequently asked, as are questions about the recommendations for endocarditis prophylaxis in mitral valve prolapse.

■ Questions on aortic stenosis are common, especially questions about special situations such as left ventricular dysfunction in the setting of aortic stenosis.

■ Questions about dobutamine assessment of low-output, low-gradient aortic stenosis may be asked. If the patient's cardiac output and aortic area appear to increase with dobutamine, surgery is not necessary. The Gorlin formula is supplied in examinations.

■ Know the indications for aortic valve replacement in patients with moderate aortic stenosis having coronary artery bypass graft surgery for coronary artery disease.

■ Know anticoagulation strategies for patients with prosthetic valves, with specific reference to management of prosthetic valve anticoagulation during pregnancy.

■ Know details of the calculation of aortic and mitral valve areas by different techniques and the possible errors in these techniques.

■ Know calculations for estimation of aortic regurgitation and mitral regurgitation.

■ Know the advantages of mitral valve repair, when possible, over mitral valve replacement.

Hypertrophic Cardiomyopathy

■ Questions on hypertrophic cardiomyopathy are frequently asked in cardiology examinations.

■ Know the effect of pharmacologic interventions in hypertrophic obstructive cardiomyopathy (HOCM), especially the use of phenylephrine therapy for HOCM patients with severe hypotension.

- Know the effects of various maneuvers on the murmurs of aortic stenosis, HOCM, and mitral regurgitation.
- Be able to identify the Brockenbrough sign on a hemodynamic tracing of left ventricular pressure with a premature ventricular contraction.
- Questions on the complications of alcohol septal ablation for HOCM have been asked on cardiology examinations, as have questions on the effect of septal ablation on survival, symptoms, and risk of ventricular tachycardia.
- Remember that late-stage HOCM can change into a condition resembling dilated cardiomyopathy with septal thinning, which should be treated with angiotensin-converting enzyme (ACE) inhibitors.
- Predictors of sudden death in HOCM are important, as are the medicolegal aspects of HOCM care.
- Patients should avoid contact sports and receive endocarditis prophylaxis.

Congestive Heart Failure

- Expect many questions about congestive heart failure.
- Know the indications for cardiac transplantation, specifically the maximum oxygen consumption ($\dot{V}O_{2max}$) that predicts a poor 1-year prognosis.
- Consider transplant vasculopathy in a patient after heart transplantation who has decreased left ventricular function and normal biopsy findings.
- Be aware of eosinophilic heart disease in association with ventricular thrombus.
- Know when to use β-blockers, ACE inhibitors, and spironolactone, and know what the optimal doses are.
- The relationship of brain natriuretic peptide to heart failure is important.
- Know the prognosis of postpartum cardiomyopathy with residual left ventricular dysfunction. If the patient becomes pregnant again, what is the risk of miscarriage and what is the risk of recurrence of the cardiomyopathy?

Pulmonary Hypertension

- Know the causes of pulmonary hypertension and the new drug treatments.
- Be able to calculate pulmonary pressure from a tricuspid regurgitation signal shown.

CREDIT LINES

Permission has been obtained to reuse the following material:

Chapter 1

Figure 1: From Constant J. Bedside cardiology. 5th ed. Philadelphia: Lippincott Williams & Wilkins; 1999. p. 80.

Figure 2: From Sapira JD. The art & science of bedside diagnosis. Baltimore: Urban & Schwarzenberg; 1990. p. 297.

Figures 3 and 5: From Barlow JB. Perspectives on the mitral valve. Philadelphia: F. A. Davis, 1987. p. 23 and p. 138.

Figure 4: From Harvey WP. Innocent vs. significant murmurs. Curr Probl Cardiol. 1976;1(8):1-51.

Table 1: Data from Abrams J. Essentials of cardiac physical diagnosis. Philadelphia: Lea & Febiger; 1987.

Table 12: From Marriott HJL. Bedside cardiac diagnosis. Philadelphia: JB Lippincott Company; 1993. p. 116.

Table 14: From Tavel ME. Clinical phonocardiography and external pulse recordings. 4th ed. Chicago: Year Book Medical Publishers; 1985. p. 198.

Chapter 2

Figure 6: From Edwards WD. Anatomy of the cardiovascular system. In: Spittell JA Jr, editor. Clinical medicine. Vol. 6, Chap 1. Philadelphia: Harper & Row Publishers; 1984. p. 8.

Figures 24, 29, and 30: From Williams PL. Gray's anatomy. The anatomical basis of medicine and surgery. 38th ed. New York: Churchill Livingstone; 1995. p. 1498, p. 1508, p. 1509, p. 1575.

Chapter 3

Figure 1: Modified from Fagan TJ. Nomogram for Bayes's Theorem [letter]. N Engl J Med. 1975;293:257.

Chapter 4

Table 1: From Lee TH, Marcantonio ER, Mangione CM, et al. Derivation and prospective validation of a simple index for prediction of cardiac risk of major noncardiac surgery. Circulation. 1999;100:1043-9.

Table 2: Data from Lee TH, Marcantonio ER, Mangione CM, et al. Derivation and prospective validation of a simple index for prediction of cardiac risk of major noncardiac surgery. Circulation. 1999;100:1043-9.

Tables 3, 4, 5, and 6: From Eagle KA, Brundage BH, Chaitman BR, et al. Guidelines for perioperative cardiovascular evaluation for noncardiac surgery. Report of the American College of Cardiology/American Heart Association Task Force on Practice Guidelines (Committee on Perioperative Cardiovascular Evaluation for Noncardiac Surgery). Circulation. 1996;93:1278-1317; Eagle KA, Brundage BH, Chaitman BR, et al. Guidelines for perioperative cardiovascular evaluation for noncardiac surgery. Report of the American College of Cardiology/American Heart Association Task Force on Practice Guidelines (Committee on Perioperative Cardiovascular Evaluation for Noncardiac Surgery). J Am Coll Cardiol. 1996;27:910-48.

Chapter 5

Figures 2 and 5: From Rosenthal N. DNA and the genetic code. N Engl J Med. 1994;331:39-41.

Figure 3: From Rosenthal N. Regulation of gene expression. N Engl J Med. 1994;331:931-3.

Figure 6 and 9: From Watson JD, Gilman M, Wilkowski J, et al. Recombinant DNA. 2nd ed. New York: Scientific American Books; 1992. p. 164 and 129.

Figures 7 and 10: From Rosenthal N. Tools of the trade—recombinant DNA. N Engl J Med. 1994;331:315-7.

Figure 11: From Rosenthal N. Stalking the gene: DNA libraries. N Engl J Med. 1994;331:599-600.

Figure 14: From Pyeritz RE. Genetics and cardiovascular disease. In: Braunwald E, editor. Heart disease: a textbook of cardiovascular medicine. Vol 2. 5th ed. Philadelphia: WB Saunders Company; 1997. p. 1650-86.

Chapter 8

Figures 1, 2 *A*, 13, 15, and 30: From Oh JK, Seward JB, Tajik AJ. The echo manual. 2nd ed. Philadelphia: Lippincott-Raven Publishers; 1999. p. 9, p. 18, p. 121, p. 126, and p. 217.

Figure 2 *B*: From Tajik AJ, Seward JB, Hagler DJ, et al. Two-dimensional real-time ultrasonic imaging of the heart and great vessels: technique, image orientation, structure identification, and validation. Mayo Clin Proc. 1978;53:271-303.

Figures 3, 7, 12, and 20: From Oh JK, Seward JB, Tajik AJ. The echo manual. Boston: Little, Brown and Company; 1994. p. 18, p. 48, p. 58, and p. 171.

Figure 9: From Sohn DW, Chai IH, Lee DJ, et al. Assessment of mitral annulus velocity by Doppler tissue imaging in the evaluation of left ventricular diastolic function. J Am Coll Cardiol. 1997;30:474-80.

Figures 21 *A*, 22, 23, 24, 26, 27, 28, and 29: From Freeman WK, Seward JB, Khandheria BK, et al. Transesophageal echocardiography. Boston: Little, Brown and Company; 1994. p. 345, p. 374, p. 399, p. 401, p. 440, p. 454, p. 487, and p. 507.

Chapter 13
Figure 2: Courtesy of Dr. Robert Rollings.

Figure 7: From Gerber TC, Kuzo RS, Karstaedt N, et al. Current results and new developments of coronary angiography with use of contrast-enhanced computed tomography of the heart. Mayo Clin Proc. 2002;77:55-71.

Figure 9: From Deibler AR, Kuzo RS, Vöhringer M, et al. Imaging of congenital coronary anomalies with multislice computed tomography. Mayo Clin Proc. 2004;79:1017-23.

Chapter 14
Figure 4: From Schattenberg TT. Chest x-ray films in heart disease. In: Spittell JA Jr, editor. Clinical medicine. Vol 6, Chap 33. Cardiovascular diseases. Philadelphia: Harper & Row, Publishers; 1982. p. 1-13.

Chapter 18
Figures 1, 18, 24, 40, 41, and 42: From Giuliani ER, Gersh BJ, McGoon MD, et al, editors. Mayo Clinic practice of cardiology. 3rd ed. St. Louis: Mosby; 1996. p. 76; p. 83; p. 94; p. 956; p. 958.

Figure 23: From DeGuzman M, Rahimtoola SH. What is the role of pacemakers in patients with coronary artery disease and conduction abnormalities? Cardiovasc Clin. 1983;13 No. 1:191-207.

Figure 31 *D*: Data from Chuang MY, Spodick DH. Electrocardiographic Q-wave inconstancy in inferior wall myocardial infarction. Am J Cardiol. 1990;66:1144-6.

Chapter 20
Tables 1 and 2 and Figures 1, 2, 3, 4, 5, 6, 7, 8, 9, and 10: From Giuliani ER, Gersh BJ, McGoon MD, et al, editors. Mayo Clinic practice of cardiology. 3rd ed. St. Louis: Mosby; 1996. p. 481, p. 483, p. 730, p. 731, p. 734, p. 736, p. 738, p. 772, p. 781, p. 832.

Chapter 21
Figures 1, 2, 3, 6, 10, 11, and 12: From Shen W-K, Gersh BJ. Fainting: approach to management. In: Low PA, editor. Clinical autonomic disorders: evaluation and management. 2nd ed. Philadelphia: Lippincott-Raven; 1997. p. 649-79.

Figures 4 and 5: From Holmes DR Jr. Clinical electrophysiologic assessment. In: Giuliani ER, Fuster V, Gersh BJ, et al, editors. Cardiology: fundamentals and practice. Vol 1. 2nd ed. St. Louis: Mosby Year Book; 1991. p. 601-26.

Figures 7, 8, and 9: From Hammill SC. Ventricular arrhythmias. In: Giuliani ER, Fuster V, Gersh BJ, et al, editors. Cardiology: fundamentals and practice. Vol 1. 2nd ed. St. Louis: Mosby Year Book; 1991. p. 909-38.

Chapter 24
Figure 4: Data from Gurevitz O, Friedman PA. Pulmonary vein exit-block during radio-frequency ablation of paroxysmal atrial fibrillation. Circulation. 2002;105:e124-5.

Figure 5: Modified from Armour JA, Murphy DA, Yuan B-X, et al. Gross and microscopic anatomy of the human intrinsic cardiac nervous system. Anat Rec. 1997;247:289-98.

Chapter 25
Figure 1: From Mazur A, Meisel S, Shotan A, et al. The mechanism of sudden death in the Wolff-Parkinson-White syndrome. J Cardiovasc Electrophysiol. 2005;16:1393.

Figures 2, 3, and 5 (from) and Tables 2 and 3 (modified): From Fuster V, Rydén LE, Asinger RW, et al. ACC/AHA/ESC guidelines for the management of patients with atrial fibrillation: a report of the American College of Cardiology/American Heart Association Task Force on Practice Guidelines and the European Society of Cardiology Committee for Practice Guidelines and Policy Conferences (Committee to Develop Guidelines for the Management of Patients With Atrial Fibrillation). J Am Coll Cardiol. 2001;38:1266i-lxx.

Figure 4: Courtesy of Dr. Samuel Asirvatham.

Table 1: From Gage BF, Waterman AD, Shannon W, et al. Validation of clinical classification schemes for predicting stroke: results from the National Registry of Atrial Fibrillation. JAMA. 2001;2845:2864-70.

Chapter 26
Figure 1: From Wellens HJJ. Contemporary management of atrial flutter. Circulation. 2002;106:649-52.

Chapter 28
Figure 5: Data from The American Heart Association in collaboration with the International Liaison Committee on Resuscitation. Guidelines 2000 for Cardiopulmonary Resuscitation and Emergency Cardiovascular Care. Part 6: advanced cardiovascular life support: section 7: algorithm approach to ACLS emergencies: section 7A: principles and practice of ACLS. Circulation. 2000;102 (suppl):I-136-I-139.

Chapter 31
Table 4: From McKenna WJ, Thiene G, Nava A, et al. Diagnosis of arrhythmogenic right ventricular dysplasia/cardiomyopathy. Br Heart J. 1994;71:215-218.

Chapter 32
Tables 1, 2, 7, 8, 9, and 10: Modified from Task Force on Syncope, European Society of Cardiology. Guidelines on management (diagnosis and treatment) of syncope. Eur Heart J. 2001;22:1256-1306.
Table 4: From Task Force on Syncope, European Society of Cardiology. Guidelines on management (diagnosis and treatement) of syncope update 2004. Europace. 2004;6:467-537.

Chapter 33
Table 1: From Bernstein AD, Daubert J-C, Fletcher RD, et al. The revised NASPE/BPEG generic code for antibradycardia, adaptive-rate, and multisite pacing. PACE. 2002;25:260-4.

Chapter 34
Table 1: From Yu C-M, Hayes DL, Auricchio A. Cardiac resynchronization therapy. Malden (MA): Blackwell Futura; 2006. p. 243-4.
Figures 1 *A* and 1 *B*: From Asirvatham SJ. Biventricular device implantation. In: Hayes DL, Wang PJ, Sackner-Bernstein J, et al, editors. Resynchronization and defibrillation for heart failure. A practical approach. Oxford: Blackwell Futura; 2004. p. 99-137.

Chapter 36
Figure 1: From Bardy GH, Lee KL, Mark DB, et al. Amiodarone or an implantable cardioverter-defibrillator for congestive heart failure. N Engl J Med. 2005;352:225-37.
Figure 2: From Bigger JT Jr, The Coronary Artery Bypass Graft (CABG) Patch Trial Investigators. Prophylactic use of implanted cardiac defibrillators in patients at high risk for ventricular arrhythmias after coronary artery bypass graft surgery. N Engl J Med. 1997;337:1569-75.
Table 4: Courtesy of Stephen C. Hammill, MD

Chapter 37
Figure 1: From Antezano ES, Hong M. Sudden cardiac death. J Intensive Care Med. 2003;18:313-29.
Figure 2: From Belhassen B, Viskin S, Antzelevitch C. The Brugada syndrome: Is an implantable cardioverter defibrillator the only therapeutic option? PACE. 2002;25:1034-40.
Figure 3: From Antzelevitch C, Brugada P, Borggrefe M, et al. Brugada syndrome: report of the Second Consensus Conference. Heart Rhythm. 2005;2:429-40.
Table 1: From John RM. Sudden cardiac death. Curr Treat Options Cardiovasc Med. 2004;6:347-55.
Table 3: From Calkins H. Arrhythmogenic right-ventricular dysplasia/cardiomyopathy. Curr Opin Cardiol. 2006;21:55-63.
Table 4: From Maron BJ, Chaitman BR, Ackerman MJ, et al. Recommendations for physical activity and recreational sports participation for young patients with genetic cardiovascular diseases. Circulation. 2004;109:2807-16.
Table 5: From Huikuri HV, Castellanos A, Myerburg RJ. Sudden death due to cardiac arrhythmias. N Engl J Med. 2001;345:1473-82.

Chapter 38
Figures 1 and 2: Hammill SC. Syncope, palpitations, family history should cause closer look in athletes' physicals. Cardiovasc Update. 2003;1 no. 4:1-2.

Chapter 43
Figures 4, 5, and 6: Courtesy of William D. Edwards, MD.

Chapter 44

Figures 4, 5, and 6: From Freeman WK, Seward JB, Khandheria BK, et al. Transesophageal echocardiography. Boston: Little, Brown and Company; 1994. p. 279; p. 280; p. 281.

Table 3: Modified from Rahimtoola SH, Chandraratna PAN. Valvular heart disease. In: Spittell JA Jr (editor). Clinical Medicine. Vol 6. Cardiovascular Diseases. Philadelphia: Harper & Row, Publishers; 1982; chap 15. p. 1-51.

Table 4: Modified from Bonow RO, Carabello B, de Leon AC Jr. ACC/AHA guidelines for the management of patients with valvular heart disease: a report of the American College of Cardiology/American Heart Association Task Force on Practice Guidelines (Committee on Management of Patients With Valvular Heart Disease). J Am Coll Cardiol. 1998;32:1486-588.

Table 5: Data from Bonow RO, Carabello B, de Leon AC Jr. ACC/AHA guidelines for the management of patients with valvular heart disease. A report of the American College of Cardiology/American Heart Association Task Force on Practice Guidelines (Committee on Management of Patients With Valvular Heart Disease). J Am Coll Cardiol. 1998;32:1486-588.

Chapter 55

Figures 7 and 8: From McGovern PG, Jacobs DR Jr, Shahar E, Arnett DK, Folsom AR, Blackburn H, Luepker RV. Trends in acute coronary heart disease mortality, morbidity, and medical care from 1985 through 1997: the Minnesota heart survey. Circulation. 2001;104:19-24.

Chapter 57

Figures 1, 9, and 15: From Giuliani ER, Gersh BJ, McGoon MD, et al, editors. Mayo Clinic practice of cardiology. 3rd ed. St. Louis: Mosby; 1996. p. 478; p. 1060; p. 1069.

Chapter 58

Table 3: From Lavie CJ, Gau GT, Squires RW, et al. Management of lipids in primary and secondary prevention of cardiovascular diseases. Mayo Clin Proc. 1988;63:605-21.

Table 5: From Giuliani ER, Gersh BJ, McGoon MD, et al, editors. Mayo Clinic practice of cardiology. 3rd ed. St. Louis: Mosby; 1996. p. 492.

Chapter 59

Figure 1: Modified from Kullo IJ, Ballantyne CM. Conditional risk factors for atherosclerosis. Mayo Clin Proc. 2005;80:219-30.

Figure 2: Modified from Danesh J, Wheeler JG, Hirschfield GM, et al. C-Reactive protein and other circulating markers of inflammation in the prediction of coronary heart disese. N Engl J Med. 2004;350:1387-97.

Figure 3: Modified from Danesh J, Lewington S, Thompson SG, et al, Fibrinogen Studies Collaboration. Plasma fibrinogen level and the risk of major cardiovascular diseases and nonvascular mortality: an individual participant meta-analysis. JAMA. 2005;294:1799-809.

Figure 4: Modified from Clarke R, Collins R, Lewington S, et al, The Homocysteine Studies Collaboration. Homocysteine and risk of ischemic heart disease and stroke: a meta-analysis. JAMA. 2002;288:2015-22.

Figure 5: Modified from Danesh J, Collins R, Peto R. Lipoprotein(a) and coronary heart disease: meta-analysis of prospective studies. Circulation. 2000;102:1082-5.

Chapter 60

Figure 1: From CDC/NCHS and National Heart, Lung, and Blood Institute.

Figure 2: From Health, United States, 2004. CDC/NCHS.

Chapter 62

Figure 1: From American Heart Association. Heart disease and stroke statistics—2006 Update. Dallas, Texas: American Heart Association; 2006, p. 9.

Figure 2: From American Heart Association. Women and cardiovascular diseases – statistics (revised). c2004 [cited 2006, June 8]. Available from: http://www.americanheart.org/presenter.jhtml?identifier=3000941.

Chapter 64

Table 1: From Kostis JB, Jackson G, Rosen R, et al. Sexual dysfunction and cardiac risk (the Second Princeton Consensus Conference). Am J Cardiol. 2005;96:313-21.

Chapter 65

Figure 1: From Jaffe AS, Babuin L, Apple FS. Biomarkers in acute cardiac disease. The present and the future. J Am Coll Cardiol. 2006;48:1-11.

Figure 3: From Apple FS, Murakami AM, Pearce LA, et al. Predictive value of cardiac troponin I and T for subsequent death in end-stage renal disease. Circulation. 2002-106:2941-5.

Table 3: From Jeremias A, Gibson M. Narrative review: alternative causes for elevated cardiac troponin levels when acute coronary syndromes are excluded. Ann Intern Med. 2005;142:786-91.

Table 4: From Casey PE. Markers of myocardial injury and dysfunction. AACN Clin Issues. 2004;15:547-57.

Chapter 66

Tables 2 and 3: Modified from Braunwald E, Mark DB, Jones RH, et al. Unstable angina: diagnosis and management. Public Health Service, Agency for Health Care Policy and Research, National Heart, Lung, and Blood Institute. Rockville (MD): US Department of Health and Human Services; 1994. AHCPR Publication no. 94-0602.

Figure 3: Modified from Antman EM, Cohen M, Bernink PJLM, et al. The TIMI risk score for unstable angina/non-ST elevation MI: a method for prognostication and therapeutic decision making. JAMA. 2000;284:835-42.

Figure 4: Modified from Khot UN, Jia G, Moliterno DJ, et al. Prognostic importance of physical examination for heart failure in non-ST-elevation acute coronary syndromes: the enduring value of Killip classification. JAMA. 2003;290:2174-81.

Chapter 67

Figure 2: From Hubbard BL, Gibbons RJ, Lapeyre AC III, et al. Identification of severe coronary artery disease using simple clinical parameters. Arch Intern Med. 1992;152:309-12.

Table 1: From Goldman L, Hashimoto B, Cook EF, et al. Comparative reproducibility and validity of systems for assessing cardiovascular functional class: advantages of a new specific activity scale. Circulation. 1981;64:1227-34.

Table 2: From Gibbons RJ, Abrams J, Catterjee K, et al. ACC/AHA 2002 guideline update for the management of patients with chronic stable angina: a report of the American College of Cardiology/American Heart Association Task Force on Practice Guidelines (Committee to Update the 1999 Guidelines for the Management of Patients with Chronic Stable angina). 2002. Availabale at www.acc.org/clinical/guidelines/stable/stable.pdf.

Table 3: Modified from Yusuf S, Zucker D, Peduzzi P, et al. Effect of coronary artery bypass surgery on survival: overview of 10-year results from randomised trials by the Coronary Artery Bypass Graft Surgery Trialists Collaboration. Lancet. 1994;344:563-70.

Chapter 69

Figure 2: From Williams BA, Wright RS, Murphy JG, et al. A new simplified immediate prognostic risk score for patients with acute myocardial infarction. Emerg Med J. 2006;23:186-92.

Figure 7: From Pitt B, Remme W, Zannad F, et al. Eplerenone, a selective aldosterone blocker, in patients with left ventricular dysfunction after myocardial infarction. N Engl J Med. 2003;348:1309-21.

Figure 8: From Ferrières J, Cambou J-P, Guéret P, et al. Effect of early initiation of statins on survival in patients with acute myocardial infarction (the USIC 2000 registry). Am J. Cardiol. 2005;95:486-9.

Figure 9: From Ridker PM, Canon CP, Morrow D, et al, for the Pravastatin or Atorvastatin evaluation and infection therapy—thrombolysis in myocardial infarction 22 (PROVE IT-TIMI 22) investigators. C-reactive protein levels and outcomes after statin therapy. N Engl J Med. 2005;352:20-8.

Table 1: Modified from Williams BA, Wright RS, Murphy JG, et al. A new simplified immediate prognostic risk score for patients with acute myocardial infarction. Emerg Med J. 2006;23:186-92.

Chapter 70

Figure 1: From Freeman WK, Seward JB, Khandheria BK, et al. Transesophageal echocardiography. Boston: Little, Brown and Company; 1994. p. 554.

Chapter 71

Appendix graph: From Antman EM, Cohen M, Bernink PJLM, et al. The TIMI risk score for unstable angina/non-ST elevation MI: a method for prognostication and therapeutic decision making. JAMA. 2000;284:835-42.

Chapter 72

Tables 1, 2, and 3: Modified from Antman EM, Anbe DT, Armstrong PW, et al, American College of Cardiology, American Heart Association Task Force on Practice Guidelines, Canadian Cardiovascular Society. ACC/AHA guidelines for the management of patients with ST-elevation myocardial infarction: a report of the American College of Cardiology/American Heart Association Task Force on Practice Guidelines (Committee to revise the 1999 guidelines for the management of patients with acute myocardial infarction). Circulation. 2004;110:e82-292.

Table 5: Modified from Antman EM. ST-Elevation myocardial infarction: management. In: Zipes DP, Libby P, Bonow RO, Braunwald E, editors. Braunwald's heart disease: a textbook of cardiovascular medicine. Vol 2. 7th ed. Philadelphia: Elsevier Saunders; 2005. p. 1167-1226.

Figure 1: From Boersma E, Maas ACP, Deckers JW, et al. Early thrombolytic treatment in acute myocardial infarction: reappraisal of the golden hour. Lancet. 1996;348:771-5.

Figure 2: From Morrison LJ, Verbeek PR, McDonald AC, et al. Mortality and prehospital thrombolysis for acute myocardial infarction: a meta-analysis. JAMA. 2000;283:2686-92.

Chapter 73
Table 2: From Singh M, Reeder GS, Jacobsen SJ, et al. Scores for post-myocardial infarction risk stratification in the community. Circulation. 2002;106:2309-2314.

Figures 1 and 2: From Antman EM, Anbe DT, Armstrong PW, et al. ACC/AHA guidelines for the management of patients with ST-elevation myocardial infarction: executive summary: a report of the ACC/AHA Task Force on Practice Guidelines (Committee to Revise the 1999 Guidelines on the Management of Patients With Acute Myocardial Infarction). Circulation. 2004;110:588-636.

Chapter 74
Table 2: Data from AHCPR supported clinical practice guidelines: cardiac rehabilitation. Clinical Guideline No. 17. (AHCPR Publication No. 96-0672, October 1995.) Available from: http://www.ncbi.nlm.nih.gov/books/bv.fcgi?rid=hstat2.chapter.6677.

Figure 2: From Hämäläinen H, Luurila OJ, Kallio V, et al. Long-term reduction in sudden deaths after a multifactorial intervention programme in patients with myocardial infarction: 10-year results of a controlled investigation. Europ Heart J. 1989;10:55-62.

Chapter 75
Table 1: Modified from Eagle KA, Guyton RA, Davidoff R, et al, American College of Cardiology; American Heart Association. ACC/AHA 2004 guideline update for coronary artery bypass graft surgery: a report of the American College of Cardiology/American Heart Association Task Force on Practice Guidelines (Committee to Update the 1999 Guidelines for Coronary Artery Bypass Graft Surgery). Circulation. 2004;110:e340-437.

Figure 2: Modified from Maniar HS, Sundt TM, Barner HB, et al. Effect of target stenosis and location on radial artery graft patency. J Thorac Cardiovasc Surg. 2002;123:45-52.

Chapter 76
Figures 2 *B*, 2 *C*, 11, 21, and 22: From Oh JK, Seward JB, Tajik AJ. The echo manual. 2nd ed. Philadelphia: Lippincott-Raven Publishers; 1999. p. 182, p. 184, p. 187, p. 188.

Figure 12: From Burstow DJ, Oh JK, Bailey KR, et al. Cardiac tamponade: characteristic Doppler observations. Mayo Clin Proc. 1989;64:312-24.

Figure 14: Courtesy of William D. Edwards, MD.

Figure 16: From Tavel ME. Clinical phonocardiography and external pulse recording. 4th ed. Chicago: Year Book Medical Publishers; 1985. p. 378.

Figure 25 *B*: From Vaitkus PT, Kussmaul WG. Constrictive pericarditis versus restrictive cardiomyopathy: a reappraisal and update of diagnostic criteria. Am Heart J. 1991;122:1431-41.

Chapter 77
Table 1: Modified from Nachman RL, Silverstein R. Hypercoagulable states. Ann Intern Med. 1993;119:819-27.

Table 2: From Morehead RS, Tzouanakis AE, Berger R. Preventing VTE: a guide to nonpharmacologic therapies. J Crit Illness. 1998;13:486-95.

Table 3: From Fedullo PF, Tapson VF. The evaluation of suspected pulmonary embolism. N Engl J Med. 2003;349:1247-56.

Table 4: From Colavita A, Wirth JA. Three decdes of thrombolysis for acute PE: where do we stand? J Respir Dis. 1997;18:474-86.

Figure 6: From Wells PS, Ginsberg JS, Anderson DR, et al. Use of a clinical model for safe management of patients with suspected pulmonary embolism. Ann Intern Med. 1998;129:997-1005.

Figure 7: From Blann AD, Lip GYH. Venous thromboembolism. BMJ. 2006;332:215-9.

Figure 8: From Goldhaber SZ, Elliott CG. Acute pulmonary embolism: Part I: Epidemiology, pathophysiology, and diagnosis. Circulation. 2003;108:2726-9.

Chapter 78
Table 8: Modified from Giuliani ER, Gersh BJ, McGoon MD, et al, editors. Mayo Clinic practice of cardiology. 3rd ed. St. Louis: Mosby; 1996. p. 1827.

Figure 3: From Humberg M, Sitbon O, Simonneau G. Treatment of pulmonary arterial hypertension. N Engl J Med. 2004;351:1425-36.

Figure 14: From McLaughlin VV, Shillington A, Rich S. Survival in primary pulmonary hypertension. The impact of epoprostenol therapy. Circulation. 2002;106:1477-82.

Chapter 79
Figure 1: From Longo LD. Maternal blood volume and cardiac output during pregnancy: a hypothesis of endocrinologic control. Am J Physiol. 1983;245:R720-9.

Figures 2 and 4: From Alexander RW, Schlant RC, Fuster V, editors. Hurst's the heart, arteries and veins. Vol 2. 9th ed. New York: McGraw-Hill; 1998. p. 2392, 2401.

Figure 6: Modified from Elkayam U, Singh H, Irani A, et al. Anticoagulation in pregnant women with prosthetic heart valves. J Cardiovasc Pharmacol Ther. 2004;9:107-15.

Chapter 80

Figure 2: From Fuster V, Brandenburg RO, McGoon DC, et al. Clinical approach and management of congenital heart disease in the adolescent and adult. Cardiovasc Clin. 1980;10(3):161-97.

Figure 3: From Bonchek LI, Brooks HL, editors. Office management of medical and surgical heart disease: a concise guide for physicians. Boston: Little, Brown & Company; 1981. p. 183-217.

Figures 5 and 6: Giuliani ER, Gersh BJ, McGoon MD, et al, editors. Mayo Clinic practice of cardiology. 3rd ed. St. Louis: Mosby; 1996. p. 1575; p. 1576.

Chapter 82

Figure 16: From Peters W, Gilles H. A colour atlas of tropical medicine and parasitology. 2nd edition. London: Wolfe Medical Publications; 1981, p. 77.

Table 2: Modified from Mandell GL, Bennett JE, Dolin R, editors. Principles and practice of infectious diseases. 4th edition. New York: Churchill Livingstone; 1995, p. 748.

Table 4 *A*: From Li JS, Sexton DJ, Mick N, et al. Proposed modifications to the Duke Criteria for the diagnosis of infective endocarditis. Clin Infect Dis. 2000;30:633-8.

Table 4 *B*: Modified from Li JS, Sexton DJ, Mick N, et al. Proposed modifications to the Duke Criteria for the diagnosis of infective endocarditis. Clin Infect Dis. 2000;30:633-8.

Table 5: Non-injection drug abusers from Scheld WM, Sande MA. Endocarditis and intravascular infections. In: Mandell GL, Bennett JE, Dolin R, editors. Principles and practice of infectious diseases. 4th edition. New York: Churchill Livingstone; 1995, p. 753. Injection drug addicts modified from Mathew J, Addai T, Anand A, et al. Clinical features, site of involvement, bacteriologic findings, and outcome of infective endocarditis in intravenous drug users. Arch Intern Med. 1995;155:1641-8.

Table 7: Modified from Wilson WR, Karchmer AW, Dajani AS, et al. Antibiotic treatment of adults with infective endocarditis due to streptococci, enterococci, staphylococci, and HACEK microorganisms. JAMA. 1995;274:1706-13

Table 8: From Berbari EF, Cockerill FR III, Steckelberg JM. Infective endocarditis due to unusual or fastidious microorganisms. Mayo Clin Proc. 1997;72:532-42.

Tables 9 and 10: Modified from Task Force on Practice Gidelines (Committee on Management of Patients with Valvular Heart Disease). ACC/AHA guidelines for the management of patients with valvular heart disease. A report of the American College of Cardiology/American Heart Association. J Am Col Cardiol 1998;32:1486-188.

Tables 11, 12, 13, 14, and Figure 17: From Dajani AS, Taubert KA, Wilson W, et al. Prevention of bacterial endocarditis. Recommendations by the American Heart Association. JAMA. 1997;277:1794-1801.

Table 15: From Baddour LM, Bettmann MA, Bolger AF, et al. Nonvalvular cardiovascular device-related infections. Circulation 2003;108;2015-31.

Chapter 84

Tables 1 and 2 and Figure 1: From Giuliani ER, Gersh BJ, McGoon MD, et al, editors. Mayo Clinic practice of cardiology. 3rd ed. St. Louis: Mosby; 1996. p. 1675, p. 1679, p. 1681.

Figures 2, 5, and 8: From Freeman WK, Seward JB, Khandheria BK, et al. Transesophageal echocardiography. Boston: Little, Brown and Company; 1994. p. 342, p. 349, p. 350.

Chapter 85

Figure 2: From Somers VK, Dyken ME, Clary MP, et al. Sympathetic neural mechanisms in obstructive sleep apnea. J Clin Invest. 1995;96:1897-1904.

Figure 3: From Shamsuzzaman AS, Gersh BJ, Somers VK. Obstructive sleep apnea: implications for cardiac and vascular disease. JAMA. 2003;290:1906-14.

Figure 4: From Shamsuzzaman AS, Winnicki M, Lanfranchi P, et al. Elevated C-reactive protein in patients with obstructive sleep apnea. Circulation. 2002;105:2462-4.

Figure 5: From Wolk R, Shamsuzzaman AS, Somers VK. Obesity, sleep apnea, and hypertension. Hypertension. 2003;42:1067-74.

Figure 6: From Kanagala R, Murali NS, Friedman PA, et al. Obstructive sleep apnea and the recurrence of atrial fibrillation. Circulation. 2003;107:2589-94.

Figure 7: From Becker HF, Jerrentrup A, Ploch T, et al. Effect of nasal continuous positive airway pressure treatment on blood pressure in patients with obstructive sleep apnea. Circulation; 2003;107:68-73.

Chapter 86
Table 1: From Giuliani ER, Gersh BJ, McGoon MD, et al, editors. Mayo Clinic practice of cardiology. 3rd ed. St. Louis: Mosby; 1996. p. 1699.
Figures 1 and 2: From Freeman WK, Seward JB, Khandheria BK, et al. Transesophageal echocardiography. Boston: Little, Brown and Company; 1994. p. 458, p. 566.

Chapter 87
Figure 1: From Gray H. Anatomy of the human body. 20th ed. Philadelphia: Lea & Febiger; 1918. Available from http://www.bartleb.com/107/illus839.html. .

Chapter 88
Figure 1: From Eagle KA, Berger PB, Calkins H, et al. ACC/AHA guideline update for perioperative cardiovascular evaluation for noncardiac surgery: executive summary; a report of the American College of Cardiology/American Heart Association Task Force on Practice Guidelines (Committee to Update the 1996 Guidelines on Perioperative Cardiovascular Evaluation for Noncardiac Surgery). Circulation. 2002;105:1257-67.
Figure 2: From Williams PL. Gray's anatomy. The anatomical basis of medicine and surgery. 38th ed. New York: Churchill Livingstone; 1995. p. 1293.
Table 1: Modified from American Society of Anesthesiologists. ASA physical status classification system. [cited 2006 July 24]. Available from: http://www.asahq.org/clinical/physicalstatus.htm.
Tables 2 and 4: From Fleisher LA, Beckman JA, Brown KA, et al. ACC/AHA 2006 guideline update on perioperative cardiovascular evaluation for noncardiac surgery: focused update on perioperative beta-blocker therapy. A report of the American College of Cardiology/American Heart Association Task Force on Practice Guidelines (Writing Committee to update the 2002 guidelines on perioperative cardiovascular evaluation for noncardiac surgery). J Am Coll Cardiol. 2006;47:2343-55.
Table 3: From Eagle KA, Berger PB, Calkins H, et al, Committee to Update the 1996 Guidelines on Perioperative Cardiovascular Evaluation for Noncardiac Surgery. ACC/AHA guideline update for perioperative cardiovascular evaluation for noncardiac surgery: a report of the American College of Cardiology/American Heart Association Task Force on Practice Guidelines. c2002. Available from: http://www.acc.org/clinical/guidelines/perio/dirIndex.htm.

Chapter 89
Table 1: Modified from Giuliani ER, Gersh BJ, McGoon MD, et al, editors. Mayo Clinic practice of cardiology. 3rd ed. St. Louis: Mosby; 1996. p. 560.
Table 3: From Giuliani ER, Gersh BJ, McGoon MD, et al, editors. Mayo Clinic practice of cardiology. 3rd ed. St. Louis: Mosby; 1996. p. 562.

Chapter 90
Figure 1 and 2: From Giuliani ER, Gersh BJ, McGoon MD, et al, editors. Mayo Clinic practice of cardiology. 3rd ed. St. Louis: Mosby; 1996. p. 552, p. 554.

Chapter 91
Figure 1: From Senni M, Tribouilloy CM, Rodeheffer RJ, et al. Congestive heart failure in the community: a study of all incident cases in Olmsted County, Minnesota, in 1991. Circulation. 1998;98:2282-9.
Figure 2: Modified from Senni M, Tribouilloy CM, Rodeheffer RJ, et al. Congestive heart failure in the community: a study of all incident cases in Olmsted County, Minnesota, in 1991. Circulation. 1998;98:2282-9.
Figure 3: From Little WC, Downes TR. Clinical evaluation of left ventricular diastolic performance. Prog Cardiovasc Dis. 1990;32:273-90.
Figure 4: From Perreault CL, Williams CP, Morgan JP. Cytoplasmic calcium modulation and systolic versus diastolic dysfunction in myocardial hypertrophy and failure. Circulation 1993;87 Suppl 7:VII-31-VII-37.
Figure 5: From Nishimura RA, Housmans PR, Hatle LK, et al. Assessment of diastolic function of the heart: background and current applications of Doppler echocardiography. Part I. Physiologic and pathophysiolgic features. Mayo Clin Proc. 1989;64:71-81.
Figure 8: Modified from Appleton CP, Hatle LK. The natural history of left ventriclar filling abnormalities: assessment by two-dimensional and Doppler echocardiography. Echocardiography. 1992;9:437-57.
Figure 10: From Ommen SR, Nishimura RA, Appleton CP, et al. Clinical utility of Doppler echocardiography and tissue Doppler imaging in the estimation of left ventricular filling pressures: a comparative simultaneous Doppler-catheterization study. Circulation. 2000;102:1788-94.
Figure 11: From Pinamonti B, DiLenarda A, Sinagra G, et al, Heart Muscle Disease Study Group. Restrictive left ventricular filling pattern in dilated cardiomyopathy assessed by Doppler echocardiography: clinical, echocardiographic and hemodynamic correlations and prognostic implications. J Am Coll Cardiol. 1993;22:808-15.

Chapter 92
Figure 2: Data from Pfeffer MA, Braunwald E, Moye LA, et al, the SAVE Investigators. Effect of captopril on mortality and morbidity in patients with left ventricular dysfunction after myocardial infarction: results of the survival and ventricular enlargement trial. N Engl J Med. 1992;327:669-77 and The SOLVD Investigators. Effect of enalapril on mortality and the development of heart failure in asymptomatic patients with reduced left ventricular ejection fractions. N Engl J Med. 1992;327:685-91.

Chapter 94
Figure 1 *A*: Courtesy of William D. Edwards, MD.
Figure 1 *B*: Courtesy of Henry D. Tazelaar, MD.
Figure 2: From Nippoldt TB, Edwards WD, Holmes DR Jr, et al. Right ventricular endomyocardial biopsy: clinicopathologic correlates in 100 consecutive patients. Mayo Clin Proc. 1982;57:407-18.
Figure 3: From Cooper LT Jr, Berry GJ, Shabetai R, Multicenter Giant Cell Myocarditis Study Group Investigators. Idiopathic giant-cell myocarditis: natural history and treatment. N Engl J Med. 1997;336:1860-6.
Table 2: Modified from From Giuliani ER, Gersh BJ, McGoon MD, et al, editors. Mayo Clinic practice of cardiology. 3rd ed. St. Louis: Mosby; 1996. p. 643-4.
Tables 4, 5, and 6: From Giuliani ER, Gersh BJ, McGoon MD, et al, editors. Mayo Clinic practice of cardiology. 3rd ed. St. Louis: Mosby; 1996. p. 661; p. 678.
Table 7: Modified from Hagar JM, Rahimtoola SH. Chagas' heart disease in the United States. N Engl J Med. 1991;325:763-8.

Chapter 95
Figure 1 and Table 1: From Maron BJ, Towbin JA, Thiene G, et al. Contemporary definitions and classification of the cardiomyopathies: an American Heart Association Scientific Statement From the Council on Clinical Cardiology, Heart Failure and Transplantation Committee; Quality of Care and Outcomes Research and Functional Genomics and Translational Biology Interdisciplinary Working Groups; and Council on Epidemiology and Prevention. Circulation. 2006;113:1807-16.

Chapter 96
Table 2: From: Kushwaha SS, Fallon JT, Fuster V. Restrictive cardiomyopathy. N Engl J Med. 1997;336:267-76.
Figure 7: From Hatle LK, Appleton CP. Popp RL. Differentiation of constrictive pericarditis and restrictive cardiomyopathy by Doppler echocardiography. Circulation. 1989;79:357-70.

Chapter 100
Figure 1: From McGregor CGA. Current state of heart transplantation. Br J Hosp Med. 1987;37:310-8.
Figure 3: Courtesy of William D. Edwards, MD.

Chapter 101
Figure 1: Modified from Atkinson AJ Jr. Drug absorption and bioavailability. In: Atkinson AJ Jr, Daniels CE, Dedrick RL, et al, editors. Principles of clinical pharmacology. 1st ed. San Diego (CA): Academic Press; 2001. p. 31-41.
Figure 10: From Lilja JJ, Kivisto KT, Neuvonen PJ. Duration of effect of grapefruit juice on the pharmacokinetics of the CYPA4 substrate simvastatin. Clin Pharmacol Ther. 2000;68:384-90.

Chapter 102
Figure 10 *A*: From The Cardiac Arrhythmia Suppression Trial (CAST) Investigators. Preliminary report: effect of encainide and flecainide on mortality in a randomized trial of arrhythmia suppression after myocardial infarction. N Engl J Med. 1989;321:406-12.
Figure 10 *B*: The Cardiac Arrhythmia Suppression Trial II Investigators. Effect of the antiarrhythmic agent moricizine on survival after myocardial infarction. N Engl J Med. 1992;327:227-33.
Figure 11: Torp-Pedersen C, Moller M, Bloch-Thomsen PE, et al, Danish Investigations of Arrhythmia and Mortality on Dofetilide Study Group. Dofetilide in patients with congestive heart failure and left ventricular dysfunction. N Engl J Med. 1999;341:857-65.

Chapter 105
Figure 1: Modified from: Opie LH. The heart: physiology, from cell to circulation. 3rd ed. Philadelphia: Lippincott-Raven Publishers; 1998, p. 108.
Figure 2: Modified from: Opie LH. Drugs for the heart. 4th ed. Philadelphia: WB Saunders Company; 1995, p. 146.
Figure 3: From Packer M, Gheorghiade M, Young JB, et al. Withdrawal of digoxin from patients with chronic heart failure treated with angiotensin-converting-enzyme inhibitors. N Engl J Med. 1993;329:1-7.
Figure 4: From The Digitalis Investigation Group. The effect of digoxin on mortality and morbidity in patients with heart failure. N Engl J Med. 1997;336:525-33.
Figure 5: From Dangas G, Gorlin R. The role of digitalis in the management of heart failure: old molecule new respectability. In: Coats

A, editor. Controversies in the management of heart failure. Edinburgh: Churchill Livingstone; 1997. p. 83-96.

Figure 6: From Lewis RP. Digitalis. In: Leier CV, editor. Cardiotonic drugs: a clinical survey. New York: Marcel Dekker; 1987. p. 85.

Figure 7: A and C from Chou T-C, Knilans TK. Electrocardiography in clinical practice: adult and pediatrics. 4th ed. Philadelphia: WB Saunders Company; 1996. p. 508, p. 512.

Chapter 108

Table 4: From Hennekens CH, Albert CM, Godfried SL, et al. Adjunctive drug therapy of acute myocardial infarction—evidence from clinical trials N Engl J Med. 1996;335:1660-7.

Chapter 109

Figure 1: Modified from Opie LH: The heart: physiology, from cell to circulation. 3rd ed. Philadelphia: Lippincott-Raven Publishers; 1998. p. 173-231.

Figure 3: From Antman EM, Braunwald E. Acute myocardial infarction. In: Braunwald E, Zipes DP, Libby P, editors. Heart disease: a textbook of cardiovascular medicine. Vol 2. 6th ed. Philadelphia, PA: WB Saunders; 2001. p. 1114-231.

Figure 4: From Waagstein F, Bristow MR, Swedberg K, et al. Beneficial effects of metoprolol in idiopathic dilated cardiomyopathy. Lancet. 1993;342:1441-6.

Figure 5: From Eichhorn EJ, Heesch CM, Barnett JH, et al. Effect of metoprolol on myocardial function and energetics in patients with nonischemic dilated cardiomyopathy: a randomized, double-blind, placebo-controlled study. J Am Coll Cardiol. 1994;24:1310-20.

Figure 6: Packer M, Brostow MR, Cohn IN et al. The effect of carvedilol on morbidity and mortality in patients with chronic heart failure. N Engl J Med. 1996;334:1349-55.

Figure 7: Lechat P, Backer M, Chalon S, et al. Clinical effects of β-adrenergic blockade in chronic heart failure: a meta-analysis of double-blind, placebo-controlled, randomized trials. Circulation. 1998;98:1184-91.

Chapter 110

Figures 2 and 3: From The Clopidogrel in Unstable Angina to Prevent Recurrent Events Trial Investigators. Effects of clopidogrel in addition to aspirin in patients with acute coronary syndromes without ST-segment elevation. N Engl J Med. 2001;345:494-502.

Chapter 111

Figure 4: From Rowland M, Tozer TN. Clinical pharmacokinetics: concepts and applications. 2nd ed. Philadelphia: Lea & Febiger; 1989, p. 114.

Chapter 113

Tables 1, 2, 6 and Figure 2: From Widlansky ME, Gokce N, Keaney JF Jr, et al. The clinical implications of endothelial dysfunction. J Am Coll Cardiol. 2003;42:1149-60.

Tables 3 and 5: From Deanfield J, Donald A, Ferri C, et al. Endothelial function and dysfunction. Part I: Methodological issues for assessment in the different vascular beds: a statement by the Working Group on Endothelin and Endothelial Factors of the European Society of Hypertension. J Hypertens. 2005;23:7-17.

Table 4: From Moens AL, Goovaerts I, Claeys MJ, et al. Flow-mediated vasodilation: a diagnostic instrument, or an experimental tool? Chest. 2005;127:2254-63.

Table 7: From Fenster BE, Tsao PS, Rockson SG. Endothelial dysfunction: clinical strategies for treating oxidant stress. Am Heart J. 2003;146:218-26.

Figures 1 and 3: From Galley HF, Webster NR. Physiology of the endothelium. Br J Anaesth. 2004;93:105-13.

Figures 4, 6, 7, and 8: From Farouque HMO, Meredith IT. The assessment of endothelial function in humans. Coron Artery Dis. 2001;12:445-54.

Figure 5: From Al Suwaidi J, Higano ST, Holmes DR Jr, et al. Pathophysiology, diagnosis, and current management strategies for chest pain in patients with normal findings on angiography. Mayo Clin Proc. 2001;76:813-22.

Chapter 114

Figure 1: From Higano ST, Nishimura RA. Coronary circulation. B. Intravascular ultrasonography. In: Giuliani ER, Gersh BJ, et al, editors. Mayo Clinic practice of cardiology. 3rd ed. St. Louis: Mosby; 1996. p. 1054.

Figure 2: From Milnor WR. Regional circulations. In: Mountcastle VB, editor. Medical physiology. 14th ed. St Louis: CV Mosby Company; 1980. p. 1098.

Figure 3: Modified from Berne RM. Cardiodynamics and the coronary circulation in hypothermia. Ann N Y Acad Sci. 1959;80:365-83.

Figures 4 and 5: From Klocke FJ. Cognition in the era of technology: "seeing the shades of gray." J Am Coll Cardiol. 1990;16:763-9.

Figure 6: From Nishimura RA, Edwards WD, Warnes CA, et al. Intravascular ultrasound imaging: in vitro validation and pathologic correlation. J Am Coll Cardiol. 1990;16:145-54.

Figures 7 and 9: From Giuliani ER, Gersh BJ, McGoon MD, et al, editors. Mayo Clinic practice of cardiology. 3rd ed. St. Louis: Mosby; 1996. p. 1051, p. 1053.

Figure 8: From Nishimura RA, Higano ST, Holmes DR Jr. Use of intracoronary ultrasound imaging for assessing left main coronary artery disease. Mayo Clin Proc. 1993;68:134-40.

Table 1: From De Bruyne B, Paulus WJ, Pijls NHJ. Rationale and application of coronary transstenotic pressure gradient measurements. Cathet Cardiovasc Diagn. 1994;33:250-61.

Chapter 116

Tables 2 and 3: Modified from Smith SC Jr, Feldman TE, Hirshfeld JW Jr, et al. ACC/AHA/SCAI 2005 guideline update for percutaneous coronary intervention—summary article: a report of the American College of Cardiology/American Heart Association Task Force on Practice Guidelines (ACC/AHA/SCAI) Writing Committee to Update the 2001 Guidelines for Percutaneous Coronary Intervention. Circulation. 2006;113:156-75.

Figure 1: From Bucher HC, Hengstler P, Schindler C, et al. Percutaneous transluminal coronary angioplasty versus medical treatment for non-acute coronary heart disease: meta-analysis of randomised controlled trials. BMJ. 2000;321:73-7.

Figure 2: From Singh M, Lennon RJ, Holmes DR Jr, et al. Correlates of procedural complications and a simple integer risk score for percutaneous coronary intervention. J Am Coll Cardiol. 2002;40:387-93.

Chapter 117

Figure 1: From Roffi M, Mukherjee D, Chew DP, et al. Lack of benefit from intravenous platelet glycoprotein IIb/IIIa receptor inhibition as adjunctive treatment for percutaneous interventions of aortocoronary bypass grafts: a pooled analysis of five randomized clinical trials. Circulation. 2002;106:3063-7.

Chapter 118

Figures 1, 4, 5, and 6: From Brandenburg RO, Fuster V, Giuliani ER, et al. Cardiology: fundamentals and practice. Vol 1. Chicago: Year Book Medical Publishers; 1987. p. 423; p. 425; p. 426.

Figure 8: From Nishimura RA, Rihal CS, Tajik AJ, et al. Accurate measurement of the transmitral gradient in patients with mitral stenosis: a simultaneous catheterization and Doppler echocardiographic study. J Am Coll Cardiol. 1994;24:152-8.

Chapter 119

Figure 1: From Rihal CS, Textor SC, Grill DE, et al. Incidence and prognostic importance of acute renal failure after percutaneous coronary intervention. Circulation. 2002;105:2259-64.

Figure 2: From Mehran R, Aymong ED, Nikolsky E, et al. A simple risk score for prediction of contrast-induced nephropathy after percutaneous coronary intervention. Development and initial validation. J Am Coll Cardiol. 2004;44:1393-9.

Figure 3: From Pannu N, Manns B, Lee H, et al. Systematic review of the impact of N-acetylsteine on contrast nephropathy. Kidney Int. 2004;65:1366-74.

Table 1: Modified from Rihal CS, Textor SC, Grill DE, et al. Incidence and prognostic importance of acute renal failure after percutaneous coronary intervention. Circulation. 2002;105:2259-64.

Tables 2 and 3: From Bartholomew BA, Harjai KJ, Dukkipati S, et al. Impact of nephropathy after percutaneous coronary intervention and a method for risk stratification. Am J Cardiol. 2004;93:1515-9.

Chapter 120

Figures 1, 2, 9, 10, 13, 14, and 15: From Giuliani ER, Gersh BJ, McGoon MD, et al, editors. Mayo Clinic practice of cardiology. 3rd ed. St. Louis: Mosby; 1996. p. 341; p. 342; p. 345; p. 357; p. 359; p. 1570; p. 1606.

Figure 12: Courtesy of Dr. Andre Lapeyre.

Figure 16: From Giuliani ER, Fuster V, Brandenburg RO, et al. Ebstein's anomaly: the clinical features and natural history of Ebstein's anomaly of the tricuspid valve. Mayo Clin Proc. 1979;54:163-73.

Table 2: Modified from Giuliani ER, Gersh BJ, McGoon MD, et al, editors. Mayo Clinic practice of cardiology. 3rd ed. St. Louis: Mosby; 1996. p 342.

Chapter 121

Table 1: Modified from Krumsdorf U, Ostermayer S, Billinger K, et al. Incidence and clinical course of thrombus formation on atrial septal defect and patient foramen ovale closure devices in 1,000 consecutive patients. J Am Coll Cardiol. 2004;43:302-9.

Table 4 and Figure 7: From Holzer R, Balzer D, Amin Z, et al. Tanscatheter closure of postinfarction ventricular septal defects using the new Amplatzer muscular VSD occluder: results of a U. S. Registry. Cathet Cardiovasc Interven. 2004;61:196-201.

Figure 1: From Meier B. Closure of patent foramen ovale: technique, pitfalls, complications, and follow up. Heart. 2005;91:444-8.

Chapter 124

Figure 8 *A-C*: From Babapulle MN, Joseph L, Bélisle P, Brophy JM, Eisenberg MJ. A hierarchical Bayesian meta-analysis of randomised clinical trials of drug-eluting stents. Lancet. 2004;364:583-91.

Chapter 125

Figure 1: From 2005 American Heart Association Guidelines for Cardiopulmonary Resuscitation and Emergency Cardiovascular Care, Part 4: Adult basic life support. Circulation. 2005;112 Suppl IV:IV-19-IV-34.

Figure 2: From Handbook of emergency cardiovascular care. Dallas: American Heart Association; 2006.

Figure 3: From 2005 American Heart Association Guidelines for Cardiopulmonary Resuscitation and Emergency Cardiovascular Care, Part 7.2: Management of cardiac arrest. Circulation. 2005;112 Suppl IV:IV-58-IV-66.

Chapter 126

Figure 1: From Babaev A, Frederick PD, Pasta DJ, et al, NRMI Investigators. Trends in management and outcomes of patients with acute myocardial infarction complicated by cardiogenic shock. JAMA. 2005;294:448-54.

Figure 2: Data from the National Registry of Myocardial Infarction.

Appendix

Table 1: From Bonow RO, Carabello B, de Leon AC Jr, et al. ACC/AHA guidelines for the management of patients with valvular heart disease: a report of the American College of Cardiology/American Heart Association Task Force on practice guidelines (Committee on management of patients with valvular heart disease). J Am Coll Cardiol. 1998;32:1486-588.

Table 2: Modified from Marriott HJL. Bedside cardiac diagnosis. Philadelphia: JB Lippincott Company; 1993. p. 116.

Section Images

   I: Courtesy of William D. Edwards, MD.
  II: Courtesy of Peter C. Spittell, MD.
 III: Courtesy of Stephen C. Hammill, MD.
  IV: Courtesy of William D. Edwards, MD.
   V: Courtesy of William D. Edwards, MD.
  VI: Courtesy of William D. Edwards, MD.
 VII: Courtesy of Thomas C. Gerber, MD, PhD.
VIII: Courtesy of William D. Edwards, MD.
  IX: Courtesy of William D. Edwards, MD.
   X: Courtesy of William D. Edwards, MD.
  XI: Courtesy of Bernard B. C. Lim, MB, ChB, PhD.

INDEX

ABBREVIATED TABLE OF CONTENTS